Nutrition and Diagnosis-Related Care

SEVENTH EDITION

Sylvia Escott-Stump, MA, RD, LDN

Dietetic Internship Director
East Carolina University
Greenville, North Carolina

Consulting Dietitian
Nutritional Balance
Winterville, North Carolina

2011-2012 President
American Dietetic Association

Wolters Kluwer | Lippincott Williams & Wilkins
Health

Philadelphia • Baltimore • New York • London
Buenos Aires • Hong Kong • Sydney • Tokyo

Acquisitions Editor: David B. Troy
Product Manager: John Larkin
Marketing Manager: Allison Powell
Creative Director: Doug Smock
Compositor: Aptara, Inc.

Seventh Edition

351 West Camden Street
Baltimore, MD 21201

Two Commerce Square
2001 Market Street
Philadelphia, PA 19103

Printed in China

First Edition, 1985
Second Edition, 1988
Third Edition, 1992
Fourth Edition, 1997
Fifth Edition, 2002
Sixth Edition, 2008

9 8 7 6 5 4 3 2 1

Library of Congress Cataloging-in-Publication Data

Escott-Stump, Sylvia.
Nutrition and diagnosis-related care / Sylvia Escott-Stump. – 7th ed.
p. ; cm.
Includes bibliographical references and index.
ISBN 978-1-60831-017-3 (alk. paper)
1. Diet therapy–Handbooks, manuals, etc. 2. Nutrition–Handbooks, manuals, etc. I. Title.
[DNLM: 1. Nutrition Therapy–Handbooks. 2. Nutritional Physiological Phenomena–Handbooks. WB 39]
RM217.2.E83 2012
615.8′54–dc22 2010041550

DISCLAIMER

Care has been taken to confirm the accuracy of the information present and to describe generally accepted practices. However, the authors, editors, and publisher are not responsible for errors or omissions or for any consequences from application of the information in this book and make no warranty, expressed or implied, with respect to the currency, completeness, or accuracy of the contents of the publication. Application of this information in a particular situation remains the professional responsibility of the practitioner; the clinical treatments described and recommended may not be considered absolute and universal recommendations.

The authors, editors, and publisher have exerted every effort to ensure that drug selection and dosage set forth in this text are in accordance with the current recommendations and practice at the time of publication. However, in view of ongoing research, changes in government regulations, and the constant flow of information relating to drug therapy and drug reactions, the reader is urged to check the package insert for each drug for any change in indications and dosage and for added warnings and precautions. This is particularly important when the recommended agent is a new or infrequently employed drug.

Some drugs and medical devices presented in this publication have Food and Drug Administration (FDA) clearance for limited use in restricted research settings. It is the responsibility of the health care providers to ascertain the FDA status of each drug or device planned for use in their clinical practice.

To purchase additional copies of this book, call our customer service department at **(800) 638-3030** or fax orders to **(301) 223-2320**. International customers should call **(301) 223-2300**.

Visit Lippincott Williams & Wilkins on the Internet: **http://www.lww.com.** Lippincott Williams & Wilkins customer service representatives are available from 8:30 am to 6:00 pm, EST.

FOREWORD

This book is a valuable resource for registered dietitians, dietetic interns and students, and other health care professionals involved or interested in medical nutrition therapy. Given the increasing time demands confronting health care professionals, efficient time management is essential for delivering high-quality patient care. The ever-changing health care environment necessitates that registered dietitians efficiently and effectively maintain their high level of practice skills. Thus, this book remains a key resource for prioritizing patient care and appropriately planning nutrition therapy. The guidance provided by *Nutrition and Diagnosis-Related Care* is of immense value in charting the clinical course for each patient, especially for clinical conditions that the practitioner does not routinely treat. This book continues to present an extensive, succinct compilation of nutrition information. The most impressive attribute is that the germane information required by dietitians is presented in a single resource. This greatly simplifies the development of nutrition care plans. Thus, this book provides dietetic practitioners with superb guidance they can use to maintain outstanding practice skills. This book is a resource that can help achieve excellence in dietetic practice.

Penny Kris-Etherton, PhD, RD
Pennsylvania State University

Karen Kubena, PhD, RD
Texas A & M University

PREFACE

Health care professionals must identify all elements of patient care capable of affecting nutritional status and outcomes. The registered dietitian must provide nutritional care in a practical, efficient, timely, and effective manner regardless of setting. Various environments provide unique and special considerations. The astute dietitian is sensitive to the patient/client's current status in the continuum of care, meticulously adapting the nutritional care plan. Communication between staff of different facilities will save time for screenings and assessments and will promote the implementation of strategic interventions. With electronic health records, data and summary reports can be shared from one practitioner to the next while maintaining confidentiality.

Nutrition and Diagnosis-Related Care has evolved since 1985 to supplement other texts and references and to quickly assimilate and implement medical nutrition therapy (MNT.) This guide can be used to help write protocols, to establish priorities in nutrition care, to demonstrate cost-effective therapies, and to categorize disorders in which nutrition interventions can decrease complications, further morbidity, mortality, or lengthy hospital stays. Adequate nutritional intervention often results in financial savings for the patient, the family, and the health care system. Indeed, current knowledge solidifies the role of nutrition as therapy, and not just adjunctive support.

The seventh edition updates guidance in MNT, adding commentary about nutritional genetics and nutrition care process concepts for each condition. The format of the book continues to promote easy navigation for quick retrieval of information. Appendix A summarizes the nutrients and their major food sources and functions. Appendix B promotes use of the Nutrition Care Process approved for the profession of dietetics. Sample forms are included, including language related to the critical thinking involved with A-D-I (assessment, nutrition diagnosis, interventions) and M-E (monitoring and evaluation) as follow-up documentation. The Nutritional Acuity Level Ranking for dietitian services is found in Appendix C. Content previously in appendices D and E has been moved into the text.

Using evidence-based practice guides from the American Dietetic Association, and use of this manual can improve nutrition therapy in any setting. The profession of dietetics continues to evolve and develop a deeper understanding of the prominence of nutrition in health promotion and disease management.

ASSUMPTIONS ABOUT THE READER

For this text, the following assumptions have been made:

1. The reader has an adequate background in nutrition sciences, physiology, pathophysiology, medical terminology, biochemistry, basic pharmacotherapy, and interpretation of biochemical data to understand the abbreviations, objectives, and interventions in this book.
2. An individualized drug history review is essential, as only a few medications are listed in this manual.
3. Herbs, botanicals, and dietary supplements are included because they are often used without prior consultation with a dietitian or a physician; they have side effects as well as perceived or real benefits.
4. For patient education, the reader must provide appropriate handouts, printed materials and teaching tools to prepare the patient for independent functioning. The nutrition counselor must share relevant information, as deemed appropriate, with the patient and significant other(s). The educator must identify teachable moments and share what is needed at the time. Follow-up interventions are highly recommended to assess successful behavioral changes by the patient/client.
5. Providers must prioritize key nutritional diagnoses that can be managed within the given time frame. With roles in ambulatory centers, extended care facilities, subacute or rehabilitative centers, private practices, grocery stores, Web-based practices, rehabilitation facilities, and home care, the "seamless" continuum affords registered dietitians the possibility of lifelong patient relationships, a reality that promotes more effective monitoring, follow-up, and evaluation.
6. The Clinical Indicators section for each condition lists tests, disease markers, and common biochemical evaluations reviewed by physicians or dietitians for that condition. Because few laboratory tests are available in nonhospital settings for monitoring nutritional status, appetite and weight changes are the most viable screening factors. Physical changes and signs of malnutrition are important for assessment and should be identified.
7. A current diet manual and MNT text should be used to acquire diet modification lists; comprehensive lists are not included with this book.
8. Use of evidence-based guides from American Dietetic Association must be used to provide predictable types of interventions over multiple visits, especially for reimbursement. Use the www.eatright.org Web site to select current guidelines for practice.
9. Except where specifically noted for children, nutrition therapy plans are for individuals over the age of 18.
10. Vitamin and mineral supplements are needed in cases of a documented or likely deficiency. However, in large doses, they may cause food–drug interactions. Plan meals and nourishments carefully to avoid the need for individual supplements.
11. Use of a general multivitamin–mineral supplement may be beneficial for many adults; monitor intakes judiciously from all food and supplemental sources. Athletes, women, elderly individuals, and vegetarians tend to take vitamin and mineral supplements more often than other individuals and may be at risk for overdoses if not carefully monitored.

12. Most evidence points to the benefits of whole foods to acquire phytochemicals and yet unknown substances. Healthy persons should obtain nutrients from a balanced diet as much as possible. The use of functional food ingredients, such as antioxidant foods, is highly recommended. A well-balanced, varied diet uses the US Department of Agriculture (USDA) MyPyramid Food Guidance System and various ethnic, vegetarian, pediatric, geriatric, or diabetes food guides for menu planning and design.
13. Ethics, cultural sensitivity, and a concern for patient rights should be considered and practiced at all times. When available, the wishes and advanced directives of the patient are to be followed. This may preclude aggressive use of artificial nutrition.
14. Interesting and varied Web sites have been included for the reader for additional insights into various diseases, conditions, and nutritional interventions.

ACKNOWLEDGMENTS

Thanks to all reviewers who made valuable suggestions for changes.

I wish to thank John Larkin, Samir Roy and Shelley Opremcak, RD, LDN and other colleagues for their valuable suggestions, insights, and edits. This book is dedicated to my family and to my students, interns and colleagues.

Sylvia Escott-Stump, MA, RD, LDN

COMMON ABBREVIATIONS

AA	amino acid
abd	abdomen, abdominal
ABW	average body weight
ACE	angiotensin-converting enzyme
ACTH	adrenocorticotropic hormone
ADA	American Dietetic Association
Alb	albumin
Alk phos	alkaline phosphatase
ALT	alanine aminotransferase
amts	amounts
ARF	acute renal failure
ASHD	atherosclerotic heart disease
AST	aspartate aminotransferase
ATP	adenosine triphosphate
BCAAs	branched-chain amino acids
BEE	basal energy expenditure
BF	breastfeeding
BMR	basal metabolic rate
BP	blood pressure
BS	blood sugar
BSA	body surface area
BUN	blood urea nitrogen
BW	body weight
bx	biopsy
C	cup(s)
C	coffee
CA	cancer
Ca^{++}	calcium
CABG	coronary artery bypass grafting
CBC	complete blood count
CF	cystic fibrosis
CHD	cardiac heart disease
CHF	congestive heart failure
CHI	creatinine-height index
CHO	carbohydrate
Chol	cholesterol
Cl^-	chloride
CNS	central nervous system
CO_2	carbon dioxide
CPK	creatine phosphokinase
CPR	cardiopulmonary resuscitation
CrCl	creatine clearance
CRP	C-reactive protein
CT	computed tomography
Cu	copper
CVA	cerebrovascular accident
DAT	diet as tolerated
dec	decreased
decaf	decaffeinated
def	deficiency
DJD	degenerative joint disease
dL	deciliter
DM	diabetes mellitus
DNA	deoxyribonucleic acid
DOB	date of birth
DRI	dietary reference intakes
DV	daily value
Dx	diagnosis
D5W	5% dextrose solution in water
EAA	essential amino acid
ECG, EKG	electrocardiogram
EEG	electroencephalogram
EFAs	essential fatty acids
Elec	electrolytes
EN	enteral nutrition
ESRD	end-stage renal disease
ETOH	ethanol/ethyl alcohol
Fe^{++}	iron
F & V	fruits and vegetables
FSH	follicle-stimulating hormone
FTT	failure to thrive
FUO	fever of unknown origin
G, g	gram(s)
GA	gestational age
GBD	gallbladder disease
GE	gastroenteritis
gest	gestational
GFR	glomerular filtration rate
GI	gastrointestinal
Gluc	glucose
GN	glomerular nephritis
GTT	glucose tolerance test
H & H	hemoglobin and hematocrit
HbA_{1c}	hemoglobin A_{1c} test (glucose)
HBV	high biological value
HBW	healthy body weight
HCl	hydrochloric acid
Hct	hematocrit
HDL	high-density lipoprotein
HLP	hyperlipoproteinemia or hyperlipidemia
HPN, HTN	hypertension
ht	height
Hx	history
I	infant
I & O	intake and output
IBD	inflammatory bowel disease
IBS	irritable bowel syndrome
IBW	ideal body weight
IEM	inborn error of metabolism
INR	international normalized ratio
IU	international units
IUD	intrauterine device
IV	intravenous
K^+	potassium
kcal	food kilocalories
kg	kilogram(s)
L	liter(s)
lb	pound(s)
LBM	lean body mass
LBV	low biological value
LBW	low birth weight
LCT	long-chain triglycerides

LDH	lactate dehydrogenase
LDL	low-density lipoproteins
LE	lupus erythematosus
LGA	large for gestational age
LH	luteinizing hormone
lytes	electrolytes
M	milk
MAC	midarm circumference
MAMC	midarm muscle circumference
MAO	monoamine oxidase
MBF	meat-base formula
MCH	mean cell hemoglobin
MCT	medium-chain triglycerides
MCV	mean cell volume
Mg^{++}	magnesium
mg	milligram(s)
μg	micrograms
MI	myocardial infarction
mm	millimeter(s)
MODS	multiple organ dysfunction syndrome
MSG	monosodium glutamate
MUFA	monounsaturated fatty acids
N&V	nausea and vomiting
N	nitrogen
Na	sodium
NCEP	National Cholesterol Education Program
NCP	Nutrition Care Process
NEC	necrotizing enterocolitis
NG	nasogastric
NPO	nil per os (nothing by mouth)
NSI	Nutrition Screening Initiative
O_2	oxygen
OP	outpatient
OT	occupational therapist
oz	ounce(s)
P	phosphorus
PCM	protein—calorie malnutrition
pCO_2	partial pressure of carbon dioxide
PG	pregnant, pregnancy
PKU	phenylketonuria
PN	parenteral nutrition
pO_2	partial pressure of oxygen
prn	pro re nata (as needed)
Prot	protein
PT	prothrombin time or physical therapy
PTH	parathormone
PUFA(s)	polyunsaturated fatty acid(s)
PVD	peripheral vascular disease
RAST	radioallergosorbent test
RBC	red blood cell count
RDA	recommended dietary allowance (specific)
RDS	respiratory distress syndrome
REE	resting energy expenditure
RQ	respiratory quotient
Rx	treatment
SFA	saturated fatty acids
SGA	small for gestational age
SI	small intestine
SIADH	syndrome of inappropriate antidiuretic hormone
SIDS	sudden infant death syndrome
SOB	shortness of breath
Sub	substitute
Sx	symptoms
t	teaspoon(s)
T	tablespoon
TB	tuberculosis
TF	tube feeding; tube fed
TG	triglycerides
TIBC	total iron-binding capacity
TLC	total lymphocyte count
TPN	total parenteral nutrition
TSF	triceps skinfold
UA	uric acid
UTI	urinary tract infection
UUN	urinary urea nitrogen
VMA	vanillylmandelic acid
VO_{2max}	maximum oxygen intake
WBC	white blood cell count
WNL	within normal limits
Zn	zinc

LIST OF TABLES

SECTION 1

SECTION 2

SECTION 3

SECTION 8

SECTION 9

SECTION 10

SECTION 11

SECTION 12

SECTION 13

SECTION 14

SECTION 15

SECTION 16

SECTION 17

APPENDIX A

APPENDIX B

APPENDIX C

APPENDIX D

CONTENTS

SECTION 8

HEPATIC, PANCREATIC, AND BILIARY DISORDERS 471

SECTION 9

ENDOCRINE DISORDERS 519

SECTION 10

MALNUTRITION—OBESITY AND UNDERNUTRITION 601

SECTION 11

MUSCULO-SKELETAL AND COLLAGEN DISORDERS 637

SECTION 12

HEMATOLOGY: ANEMIAS AND BLOOD DISORDERS 687

ALPHABETICAL LIST OF TOPICS

SECTION 1

Normal Life Stages

CHIEF NUTRITION SCREENING AND ASSESSMENT FACTORS

Public health measures are established to promote wellness and reduce disease for all ages; Table 1-1.

- Priority Factors: Unintentional Weight Loss with Appetite Changes in Adults, Protein-Energy Deficiency, or Growth Retardation in Children
- Body Fat and Muscle Mass: Weight, Height, Body Mass Index (BMI), Percentage of Healthy Body Weight (HBW) for Height, Loss of Lean Body Mass (LBM), Previous Weight Percentile or Curve, Weight Changes, Waist Circumference, Skinfold Measurements, Visceral Proteins, Estimated Basal Energy Expenditure, Nitrogen Balance
- Illiteracy or Low Educational Level: Low Socioeconomic Status, Food Insecurity
- Hair or Nails: Changes, Rashes, Itching, Lesions, Turgor, Petechiae, Pallor
- Eyes: Glasses, Blurred Vision, Glaucoma, Cataracts, or Macular Degeneration
- Ears, Nose: Hearing Loss, Chronic Otitis Media, Altered Sense of Smell, Nasal Obstruction, Sinusitis
- Dental and Mouth: Ill-fitting Dentures, Loose or Missing Teeth, Caries, Bleeding Gums, Severe Gum Disease, Poor Oral Hygiene, Taste Alterations, Dysphagia
- Neurological: Headache, Seizures, Convulsions, Altered Speech, Paralysis, Altered Gait, Anxiety, Memory Loss, Altered Sleep Patterns, Depression, Substance Abuse, Low Motivation, Fatigue, Weakness, Fever or Chills, Excessive Sweating, Tremors
- Heart: Chest Pain, Dyspnea, Wheezing, Cough, Hemoptysis, Ventilator Support, Altered Blood Gas Levels, Abnormal Blood Pressure, Electrolyte Imbalance, Cyanosis, Edema, Ascites, Low Cardiac Output
- Blood: Anemias, Altered Heart Rate, Arrhythmias, Blood Loss
- Gastrointestinal (GI): Cachexia, Anorexia, Nausea, Diarrhea, Vomiting, Jaundice, Constipation, Indigestion, Ulcers, Hemorrhoids, Melena, Altered Stool Characteristics, Gluten Intolerance, Lactase Insufficiency
- Therapies: Radiation, Chemotherapy, Physical Therapy, Dialysis, Recent Surgery or Hospitalizations
- Urinary and Renal: Hematuria, Fluid Requirements, Specific Gravity, Urinary Tract Infections, Renal Disease or Stones
- Hormonal Balance: Altered Blood Glucose, Hyper or Hypothyroidism, Goiter, Glucose Intolerance or Metabolic Syndrome

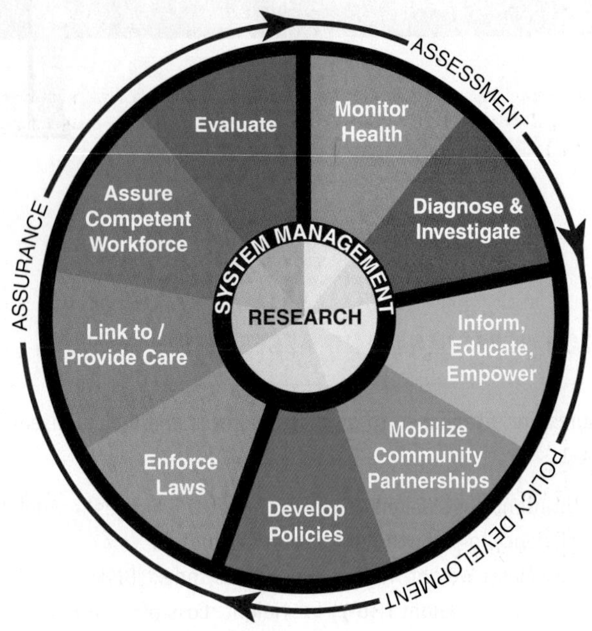

- Immunity: Food Allergy or Intolerances, Sensitivities, Cellular Immunity, HIV or Other Chronic Infections, Inflammation
- Musculoskeletal System: Pain, Arthritis, Numbness, Amputations, Limited Range of Motion or Muscular Strength
- Phenotype or Genotype (see the adult nutrition content in this section)
- Nutrition: Any Special Diets or Nutrition Support, Dietary Pattern, Typical Intake of Food and Alcohol, Use of Vitamin/Minerals/Herbs/Botanicals/Supplements, Over-the-Counter and Prescribed Medications, Knowledge of Food and Nutrition

TABLE 1-1 Public Health: Ten Achievements and Ten Essential Services

10 Public Health Achievements in the 20th Century

- Development of vaccines
- Increased motor vehicle safety
- Safer workplaces
- Control of infectious diseases
- Decline in deaths from coronary artery disease and stroke
- Safer and healthier foods
- Healthier mothers and babies
- Better family planning
- Fluoridation of drinking water
- Recognition of tobacco as a health hazard

10 Essential Public Health Services

- Monitor health status to identify community health problems.
- Diagnose and investigate health problems and hazards in the community.
- Inform, educate, and empower people about health issues.
- Mobilize community partnerships to identify and solve health problems.
- Develop policies and plans that support individual and community health efforts.
- Enforce laws and regulations that protect health and ensure safety.
- Link people to needed personal health services and assure the provision of health care when otherwise unavailable.
- Assure competent public health and personal health care workforce.
- Evaluate effectiveness, accessibility, and quality of personal and population-based health services.
- Research for new insights and innovative solutions to health problems.

Adapted from: Centers for Disease Control and Prevention, http://www.cdc.gov/mmwr/preview/mmwrhtml/00056796.htm and American Public Health Association, http://www.health.gov/phfunctions/public.htm; accessed January 11, 2009.

Life Stage–Specific Assessments

- Pregnancy: Vegan or disordered eating pattern; presence of diabetes, hepatitis B, hypothyroidism, obesity, AIDS or HIV infection, phenylketonuria (PKU), sexually transmitted disorders; use of accutane, alcohol, anticoagulant, or antiepileptic medications; poor foliate intake; lack of rubella immunity; and smoking habits (March of Dimes, 2009)
- Lactating Women: Mother's Intake and Breastfeeding Practices; Extent to Which Infant Is Breastfeeding; Composition of Milk Variable with Use of Medications
- Infants: Breast Milk; Formula Intake; Mixed Feedings with Other Foods; Disordered Eating Patterns Including Supplemented with Nutrients or Foods
- Preschool Children: Variable Intakes; Food Jags; Anemia
- School Children: Limited Ability to Recall Foods Eaten; Limited Attention Span; Use of Any Medications or Special Therapies; Anemia; Exposure to Lead
- Adolescents: Intakes Altered by Growth Spurts; Meal Skipping; Dieting; Fasting; Disordered Eating; Abuse of Drugs, Alcohol, Diuretics, Prescription Drugs, Laxatives
- Adults: Illiteracy; Biased or False Reporting; Failure to Report Use of Herbs, Alcohol, Supplements; Unusual Work Patterns such as Shift Work; Vegan or Disordered Eating Pattern
- Older Adults: Limited Dietary Recall; Limitations in Hearing or Sight; Chronic Illness that Affects Intake; Polypharmacy; Monotonous or Limited Intake

For More Information on MyPyramid and Food Guidance Systems, See the Dietary Guidelines in Table 1-2

- American Dietetic Association Fact Sheets
  http://www.eatright.org/cps/rde/xchg/ada/hs.xsl/nutrition_350_ENU_HTML.htm
- Food and Nutrition Information Center (FNIC)
  http://www.nal.usda.gov/fnic/about.shtml
- FNIC—Dietary guidance
  http://grande.nal.usda.gov/nal_display/index.php?tax_level=1&info_center=4&tax_subject=256
- MyPyramid Food Guidance System Tools
  http://www.mypyramid.gov/

TABLE 1-2 Dietary Guideline Systems

The Food and Agriculture Organization (FAO) and the World Health Organization (WHO) have frequently brought together scientists and experts in agriculture to address nutrition and malnutrition. Dietary guidelines offer dietary advice for the population to promote overall nutritional wellbeing. As a result, many countries have established food-based dietary guidelines. Several principles and guidelines are included here.

Source: http://www.fao.org/docrep/v7700t/v7700t02.htm

Energy

- Nutritional guidelines should aim to prevent the consequences of either energy deficit or excess.
- Food-based dietary guidelines should promote appropriate energy intakes by encouraging adequate food choices from a balance of foods containing carbohydrates, fats, proteins, vitamins, and minerals.
- The role of physical activity in the energy balance equation should be addressed.

Protein

- For high-quality proteins, requirements for most people are met by providing 8–10% of total energy as protein.
- For predominantly vegetable-based, mixed diets, which are common in developing country settings, 10–12% is suggested to account for lower digestibility and increased incidence of diarrheal disease.
- In the case of the elderly, where energy intake is low, protein should represent 12–14% of total energy.

Fat

- In general, adults should obtain at least 15% of their energy intake from dietary fats and oils.
- Women of childbearing age should obtain at least 20% to better ensure an adequate intake of essential fatty acids needed for fetal and infant brain development.
- Active individuals who are not obese may consume up to 35% fat energy as long as saturated fatty acids do not exceed 10% of energy intake.
- Sedentary individuals should limit fat to not more than 30% of energy intake.
- Saturated fatty acids should be limited to less than 10% of intake.

Carbohydrate

- Carbohydrates are the main source of energy in the diet (>50%) for most people.
- Grain products, tubers, roots, and some fruits are rich in complex carbohydrates. Generally, they need to be cooked before they are fully digestible.
- Sugars usually increase the acceptability and energy density of the diet. Total sugar intake is often inversely related to total fat intake. Moderate intakes of sugar are compatible with a varied and nutritious diet, and no specific limit for sugar consumption is proposed in the report.

Micronutrients

- Vitamins and minerals include compounds with widely divergent metabolic activities and are essential for normal growth and development and optimal health.
- Micronutrients may help to prevent infectious and chronic diseases. Epidemiological, clinical, and experimental studies define the role of specific foods and nutrients in disease development and prevention.

American Dietary Guidelines

An evidence-based, scientific approach is used for updates to the Dietary Guidelines for Americans (Nicklas et al, 2005). The guidelines are updated every 5 years. In 2010, the guidelines were enhanced to describe the need for a Total Diet approach. There is no single "American" or "Western" diet. According to the National Health and Nutrition Examination Survey (NHANES), Americans eat too many calories and too much solid fats, added sugars, refined grains, and sodium. Americans also eat too little dietary fiber, vitamin D, calcium, potassium, and unsaturated fatty acids (specifically omega-3s), and other important nutrients that are mostly found in vegetables, fruits, whole grains, low-fat milk and milk products, and seafood. See the website at http://www.cnpp.usda.gov/DGAs2010-DGACReport.htm for the evidence-based recommendations.

Balance Nutrients With Calories

Eat a variety of nutrient-dense foods and beverages within and among the basic food groups.

Choose foods that limit the intake of saturated and trans fats, cholesterol, added sugars, salt, and alcohol.

Meet recommended intakes within energy needs by adopting a balanced eating pattern, such as the U.S. Department of Agriculture (USDA) Food Guide or the Dietary Approaches to Stop Hypertension (DASH) Eating Plan.

Manage Weight

To maintain body weight in a healthy range, balance calories from foods and beverages with calories expended.

To prevent gradual weight gain over time, make small decreases in food and beverage calories and increase physical activity.

Maintain Physical Activity

Engage in regular physical activity and reduce sedentary activities to promote health, psychological well-being, and a healthy body weight.

To reduce the risk of chronic disease in adulthood, engage in at least 30 minutes of moderate-intensity physical activity, above usual activity, at work or home on most days of the week. For most people, greater health benefits can be obtained by engaging in physical activity of more vigorous intensity or longer duration.

To help manage body weight and prevent gradual, unhealthy body weight gain in adulthood, engage in approximately 60 minutes of moderate- to vigorous-intensity activity on most days of the week, while not exceeding caloric intake requirements.

(continued)

TABLE 1-2 Dietary Guideline Systems *(continued)*

To sustain weight loss in adulthood, participate in at least 60–90 minutes of daily physical activity.
Achieve physical fitness by including cardiovascular conditioning, stretching exercises for flexibility, and resistance exercises or calisthenics for muscle strength and endurance.

Food Groups to Emphasize

Consume nine 1/2-cup servings of fruits and vegetables daily (2 cups of fruit and 2½ cups of vegetables for reference 2000-calorie intake).
Choose a variety of fruits and vegetables each day. In particular, select from all five vegetable subgroups (dark green, orange, legumes, starchy vegetables, and other vegetables) several times a week.
Consume ≥3-oz equivalents of whole-grain products per day, with the rest of the recommended grains coming from enriched or whole-grain products; half the grains should come from whole grains.
Consume 3 cups per day of fat-free or low-fat milk or equivalent milk products.

Eat the Right Fats

Aim for 20–35% of total calories from fats, mostly from polyunsaturated and monounsaturated sources, such as fish, nuts, and vegetable oils.
Consume less than 10% of calories from saturated fatty acids and less than 300 mg/d of cholesterol, and keep trans fatty acid consumption as low as possible.
When selecting and preparing meat, poultry, dry beans, and milk or milk products, make choices that are lean, low fat, or fat free.

Carbohydrates Do Matter

Choose fiber-rich fruits, vegetables, and whole grains.
Choose and prepare foods and beverages with little added sugars or caloric sweeteners, such as amounts suggested by the USDA Food Guide and the DASH Eating Plan.
Consuming sugar- and starch-containing foods and beverages less frequently for good oral hygiene.

Less Sodium and More Potassium

Consume less than 2300 mg (approximately 1 teaspoon of salt) of sodium per day. Choose and prepare foods with little salt. Eat more potassium-rich foods, such as fruits and vegetables.

Take It Easy on Alcoholic Beverages

Those who choose to drink alcoholic beverages should limit to one drink per day for women and up to two drinks per day for men.
Alcoholic beverages should not be consumed by individuals who cannot restrict their alcohol intake, women of childbearing age who could become pregnant, pregnant and lactating women, children and adolescents, individuals taking medications that can interact with alcohol, and those with specific medical conditions.
Alcoholic beverages should be avoided by individuals engaging in activities that require attention, skill, or coordination, such as driving or operating machinery.

Keep Food Safe

Wash hands, food contact surfaces, and fruits and vegetables. Meat and poultry should not be washed or rinsed.
Separate raw, cooked, and ready-to-eat foods while shopping, preparing, or storing foods.
Cook foods to a safe temperature to kill micro-organisms.
Chill (refrigerate) perishable food promptly and defrost foods properly.
Avoid raw (unpasteurized) milk or any products made from unpasteurized milk, raw or partially cooked eggs or foods containing raw eggs, raw or undercooked meat and poultry, unpasteurized juices, and raw sprouts.

Sources: Dietary guidelines http://www.health.gov/DietaryGuidelines/; Kris-Etherton PM, Weber JA. Dietary Guidelines 2005: contributions of registered dietitians to the evolution and dissemination of the guidelines. *J Am Diet Assoc.* 105:1362, 2005; and Nicklas TA, et al. The 2005 Dietary Guidelines Advisory Committee: developing a key message. *J Am Diet Assoc.* 105:1418, 2005. Dietary Guidelines 2010: http://www.cnpp.usda.gov/DGAs2010-DGACReport.htm.

Canada's Food Guide to Healthy Eating

- Provide energy consistent with the maintenance of body weight within the recommended range.
- Include essential nutrients in amounts specified in the Recommended Nutrient Intakes.
- Include no more than 30% of energy as fat (33 g/1000 kcal or 39 g/5000 kJ) and no more than 10% as saturated fat (11 g/1000 kcal or 13 g/5000 kJ).
- Provide 55% of energy as carbohydrate (138 g/1000 kcal or 165 g/5000 kJ) from a variety of sources.
- Reduce sodium content.
- Include no more than 5% of total energy as alcohol, or 2 drinks daily, whichever is less.
- Contain no more caffeine than the equivalent of 4 cups of regular coffee per day.
- Use community water supplies that are fluoridated.

Source: Health Canada, http://www.hc-sc.gc.ca/fn-an/food-guide-aliment/index-eng.php

Chinese Nutrition Society—Balance Dietary Pagoda

- Eat a variety of foods, with grains as the staple food.
- Eat more vegetables, fruits, and tubers.
- Eat milk and legumes, and their products, every day.
- Increase appropriately the consumption of fish, poultry, egg, and/or lean, meat, and decrease the consumption of fat meat and/or animal fat.
- Balance the amount of food consumed with physical activity to maintain a healthy body weight.
- Eat a diet with less fat/oil and salt.

(continued)

TABLE 1-2 Dietary Guideline Systems *(continued)*

- For those who consume alcohol, be moderate.
- Do not eat putrid and deteriorated foods.

Source: Chinese Nutrition Society, http://www.cnsoc.org/asp-bin/EN/?page=8&class=92&id=144

South African Dietary Guidelines

- Enjoy a variety of foods; this is difficult but necessary in developing countries.
- Be active.
- Make starchy foods the basis of most meals.
- Eat plenty of vegetables and fruits every day.
- Eat more legumes for better overall health.
- Foods from animals can be eaten every day.
- Eat fats sparingly—implications for health and disease.
- Eat salt sparingly—sprinkle, do not shake!
- Drink water—the neglected nutrient.
- If you drink alcohol, drink sensibly.

Source: http://www.sahealthinfo.org/nutrition/safoodbased.htm

PREGNANCY AND LACTATION

PREGNANCY

NUTRITIONAL ACUITY RANKING: LEVEL 1 (UNCOMPLICATED); LEVEL 3 (HIGH RISK)

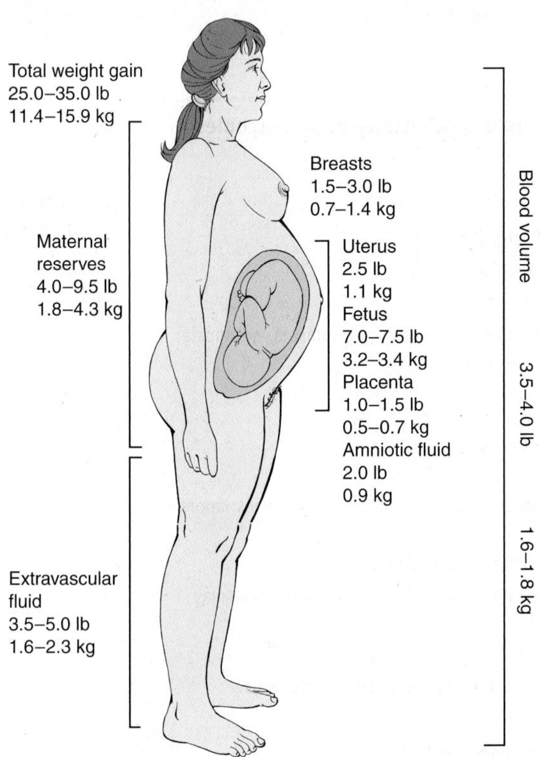

Reprinted with permission from: Weber J RN, EdD and Kelley J RN, PhD. *Health Assessment in Nursing,* 2nd ed. Philadelphia: Lippincott Williams & Wilkins, 2003.

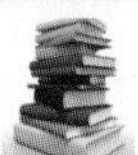

DEFINITIONS AND BACKGROUND

Women who are interested in becoming pregnant need a "preconception risk assessment" (March of Dimes, 2009). They should be aware of their personal genetic biomarkers that could cause problems with infertility, pregnancy, childbirth, or chronic diseases.

Pregnancy is an anabolic state that affects maternal tissues using hormones synthesized to support successful pregnancy. Progesterone induces fat deposition to insulate the baby, supports energy reserves, and relaxes smooth muscle, which will cause a decrease in intestinal motility for greater nutrient absorption. Estrogen increases tremendously during pregnancy for growth promotion, uterine function, and water retention. Progesterone and estrogen secreted during pregnancy in combination also help prepare for successful lactation.

Adequate weight gain is needed to ensure optimal fetal outcome. Underweight is associated with small for gestational age (SGA) or preterm deliveries. Energy costs of pregnancy vary by the BMI of the mother (Butte et al, 2004). Tissue growth in pregnancy is approximately: breast, 0.5 kg; placenta, 0.6 kg; fetus, 3–3.5 kg; amniotic fluid, 1 kg; uterus, 1 kg; increase in blood volume, 1.5 kg; and extracellular fluid, 1.5 kg. Rapid weight losses or gains are not desirable during pregnancy.

Higher maternal weight before pregnancy increases the risk of late fetal death, although it protects against the delivery of an SGA infant. Obesity increases risk of first trimester or recurrent miscarriages and the need for caesarean delivery; obesity should be corrected before pregnancy whenever possible (Rasmussen and Yaktine, 2009). Some obese women will seek bariatric surgery to enhance fertility. Women who have had bariatric surgery usually have a positive outcome (Maggard et al, 2008).

A short span between pregnancies or an early pregnancy within 2 years of menarche increases the risk for preterm or growth-retarded infants. Maternal nutrient depletion of energy and protein leads to poor nutritional status at conception and may alter pregnancy outcomes. Poor maternal iron and folate intakes have been associated with preterm births and intrauterine growth retardation, two outcomes for which women with early or closely spaced pregnancies are at high risk.

Brain development starts during pregnancy and continues into adulthood. Deficiency of various micronutrients has long-term implication for cognitive development (Benton, 2008). Major diseases including heart disease, hypertension, and type 2 diabetes may originate from impaired intrauterine growth and development as consequences of an insult at a critical, sensitive time. People who are small or disproportionate (thin or short) at birth may later have CHD, high BP, high cholesterol concentrations, and abnormal glucose–insulin metabolism, independent of length of gestation (Godfrey and Barker, 2000).

Nutritional deficits are serious during pregnancy. Living with marginal food security has been found to correlate with greater weight gain, more complications, and gestational diabetes (Laraia et al, 2010). Planned pregnancies usually have the most favorable outcomes. Continuous dietary monitoring of pregnant women and pregnant teens is essential, especially for calcium, iron, folate, vitamins A, C, B_6, and B_{12} (ACOG, 2009). Other nutrients of importance include magnesium, fiber, zinc, vitamin D, and biotin (Zempleni et al, 2008). Table 1-3 lists risk assessments and indicators of potentially poor maternal or fetal outcomes.

Many cardiac defects may be prevented by maternal use of multivitamins during the periconceptual period. To prevent SGA births, a mother is encouraged not to smoke, to manage any cardiac disease or conditions such as elevated blood pressure (BP), and to gain sufficient weight. Women who are HIV positive may experience undesirable weight loss (Villamore, 2004). Bulimia nervosa during pregnancy can lead to miscarriage, inappropriate weight gain (excessive or inadequate), complicated delivery, low birth weight (LBW), prematurity, infant malformation, low Apgar scores, and other problems. Women with unmanaged PKU may also have poor reproductive outcomes. Prevention requires initiation of the low Phe diet before conception or early in pregnancy, with metabolic control and sufficient intake of energy and proteins.

For twin and multiple pregnancies, twice-monthly visits, sufficient energy intake, multimineral supplementation, and patient education may reduce complications such as LBW and neonatal morbidity (Luke et al, 2003). The American Dietetic Association suggests at least three visits for medical nutrition therapy in high-risk pregnancies. The individual may require more visits if there are complex or multiple risk factors, such as diabetes and celiac disease.

TABLE 1-3 Prenatal Risk Assessments and Indicators of Potentially Poor Outcomes

Prepregnancy

- Adolescence (poor eating habits, greater needs for growth of teen and fetus).
- History of three or more pregnancies in past 2 years, especially miscarriages.
- History of poor obstetrical/fetal performance.
- Overweight and obesity, which can cause a higher risk for gestational diabetes, preeclampsia, eclampsia, C-section, and/or delivery of infant with macrosomia.

Prepregnancy or During Pregnancy

- Economic deprivation.
- Food faddist; smoker; user of drugs/alcohol; practice of pica with related iron or zinc deficiencies; anorexia nervosa or bulimia.
- Modified diet for chronic systemic diseases, such as diabetes, celiac disease, PKU.
- Prepartum weight of less than 85% or more than 120% of desirable BMI for height and age; these may reflect inability to attain proper weight or poor dietary habits.
- Deficient Hgb (<11 g) or hematocrit (Hct) (<33%) with medical diagnosis of anemia.
- Weight loss during PG or gain <2 lb/month in the last two trimesters; dehydration; hyperemesis.
- Risk of toxemia (2-lb weight gain per week or more).
- Poorly managed vegetarian diet, especially vegan diet without supplementation.
- Poor nutrient or energy intakes over the duration of the pregnancy.
- Poor intake of magnesium, zinc, calcium, iron, folate, vitamins A and C, and other key nutrients.

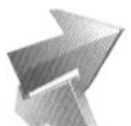

ASSESSMENT, MONITORING, AND EVALUATION

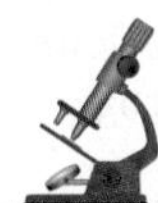

CLINICAL INDICATORS

Genetic Markers: Each individual has a unique genetic profile and phenotype. Because both parents contribute genes and chromosomes to the fetus, a genetic history may be beneficial. Epigenetics involves inherited changes in chromatin and DNA that affect human pathologies, including inflammatory disorders and cancers, and nutritional factors can have a profound effect on gene expression (Wilson, 2008).

Clinical/History
- Gravida (number of pregnancies)
- Para (number of births)
- Abortus (number of abortions)
- Height
- Prepregnancy weight (% standard)
- Weight grid or prenatal BMI (19.8–20.0)
- Present weight for gestational age
- Desired weight at term
- BP
- Multiple gestation?
- Diabetes or other chronic disease?
- Hx of births with neural tube defects, preterm delivery, multiple births
- Uterine or cervical abnormalities
- Diet history, including use of alcohol
- Smoking habits, herbs, botanicals, and drug use
- Exposure to accutane, diethylstilbestrol (DES), anticoagulants, antiepilepsy drugs
- Nausea or vomiting (frequency, duration, impact on intake)
- Pica, harmful beliefs, or disordered eating patterns

Lab Work
- Hemoglobin and hematocrit (H & H)
- Serum Fe
- Urea N
- Glucose (by 24–28 weeks)
- Ca^{++}, Mg^{++}
- Albumin (Alb)
- Transferrin
- Ceruloplasmin
- T3, T4, TSH
- Blood urea nitrogen (BUN)
- Creatinine
- Homocysteine
- Cholesterol (may be increased)
- Alkaline phosphatase (alk phos) (may be increased)
- Total iron-binding capacity (TIBC) (often increased in late pregnancy)

INTERVENTION

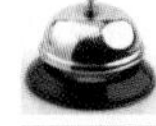

OBJECTIVES

- Maintain adequate gestational duration; avoid preterm delivery.
- Provide adequate amount of weight gain during the pregnancy; prevent delivery of LBW infants. Underweight women (BMI <18.5) should gain 28–40 lb. Normal weight women (BMI = 19–24.9) should gain 25–35 lb total. Overweight women (BMI = 25–29.9) should gain 15–25 lb. Obese women (BMI >30) should gain 11–20 lb, as obesity is a risk for undesirable consequences, including neural tube defects (Rasmussen and Yaktine, 2009; Scialli, 2006).
- Encourage proper rate of weight gain: 2–4 lb first trimester, 10–11 lb second trimester, and 12–13 lb third trimester. More weight should be gained if patient is below ideal weight range before pregnancy, especially in younger women. Adolescents are at high risk of gaining an excessive amount of weight during pregnancy and should be closely monitored.
- Provide additional nutrients and energy (net cost of pregnancy varies from 20,000–80,000 kcal total). Women carrying more than one fetus must add extra kilocalories to support multiple births.
- Prevent or correct hypoglycemia and ketosis.
- Provide adequate amino acids to meet fetal and placental growth. Approximately 950 g of protein are synthesized for the fetus and placenta. Low protein intake may lead to a smaller infant head circumference.
- Promote development of an adequate fetal immune system.
- Prevent or correct deficiencies of iron, which are common in 50–75% of pregnancies. Iron deficiency may cause low infant birth weight and premature birth (Luke, 2005).

SAMPLE NUTRITION CARE PROCESS STEPS

Inadequate Protein Intake for Multiple Gestation

Assessment Data: Dietary recall indicating low use of protein-rich foods; labs such as albumin, BUN, and H & H; insufficient rate of weight gain on prenatal grid.

Nutrition Diagnosis (PES): Inadequate protein intake related to needs for twin pregnancy as evidenced by dietary intake records (60% of goal) and slow growth on prenatal growth grid.

Intervention: Education on protein and protein-sparing kilocalories during pregnancy for twins. Counseling for individual needs, snack habits, recipes, tips for reducing nausea, physical activity.

Monitoring and Evaluation: Changes in dietary intake, improved lab values, improved weight gain on prenatal growth grid, successful pregnancy outcomes.

Rapid Weight Gain in Pregnancy

Assessment Data: Dietary history reflects high-caloric food intake; patient statements reflect misinformation; weights and rate of weight gain exceed recommended rate.

Nutrition Diagnosis (PES): Excessive energy intake related to misinformation about nutrition needs during pregnancy as evidenced by dietary recall showing daily intake of high-calorie foods, 3-lb body weight gain per week during the second trimester, and 20-lb weight gain by the middle of the second trimester.

Intervention: Education on food and nutrient needs during pregnancy. Referral to Women-Infants-Children Program (WIC) if eligible financially and medically.

Monitoring and Evaluation: Monthly appointment; include diet history and rate/amount of weight gain.

- Folate deficiency and elevated homocysteine levels may lead to miscarriage, club foot, structural heart disease, anencephaly and neural tube defects (Wilson et al, 2008). A woman with a history of spontaneous abortion in her immediate prior pregnancy and short interpregnancy interval is especially vulnerable. L-methylfolate is the natural, active form of folate used for DNA reproduction and regulation of homocysteine levels. Women with altered genetic alleles may not have sufficient methyl-tetrahydrofolate (MTHFR) enzymes to use folic acid properly; these women may benefit from using special prenatal supplements, such as Neevo®. Vitamins B_6 and B_{12} will also be needed if homocysteine levels are elevated.
- Vitamin A deficiency is strongly associated with depressed immune system and higher morbidity and mortality due to infectious diseases such as measles, diarrhea, respiratory infections. On the other hand, doses of 10,000–30,000 IU vitamin A/d may cause birth defects.
- Avoid zinc, vitamin D, or calcium deficiencies.
- Supply sufficient iodine (250 μg) to prevent cretinism with mental and physical retardation (Angermayr and Clar, 2004). Systematic provision of iodine supplementation is recommended, especially if women are cutting back on intake of iodized salt (Glinoer, 2007).
- Limit caffeinated beverage intake to two cups daily.
- Avoid alcohol. Mothers who drink relatively high levels of alcohol around the time of conception increase the risk for orofacial clefts and spina bifida.
- Support the individual patient; pregnant women who are fatigued, stressed, and anxious tend to consume more macronutrients and decreased amounts of micronutrients (Hurley et al, 2005).
- Develop or improve good eating habits to prevent or delay onset of chronic health problems postnatally. The interaction between genes, nutrition, and environmental stimuli has been found to cause permanent changes in metabolism; these Developmental Origins of Health And Disease (DHOaD) are just beginning to be understood (Waterland and Michaels, 2007).
- Discuss the importance of a high-quality prenatal diet. Fetal under-nutrition can predispose to hypercholesterolemia and program food preferences that are more atherogenic (Lussana et al, 2007).
- Women should drink plenty of fluids to remain adequately hydrated (Klein, 2005).
- Multiple gestation creates new challenges and magnified nutritional requirements (Luke, 2005). There are more risks for adverse outcomes, including diabetes, hypertension, eclampsia, delivery of a premature or LBW infant (Klein, 2005; Luke, 2005). For twins, weight gain should reflect the period of gestation and prepartum BMI; 35–45 lb is often recommended with twins, and 50 lb overall is recommended for triplets.
- Monitor BP and blood glucose regularly to prevent or to identify complications such as preeclampsia or gestational diabetes.
- Monitor or treat other complications, such as nausea and vomiting of pregnancy (NVP) and hyperemesis gravidarum. See appropriate disorder entries.

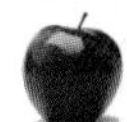

FOOD AND NUTRITION

- Include in diet: 1 g protein/kg body weight daily (or 10–15 g above recommended dietary allowances for age). Young teens: 11–14 years (1.7 g/kg); 15–18 years (1.5 g/kg); over 19 years of age (1.7 g/kg); high risk (2 g/kg).
- Energy: In women of normal weight, energy requirements increase minimally in the first trimester, by 350 kcal/d in the second trimester, and by 500 kcal/d in the third trimester (Butte et al, 2004). Add more or less, depending on level of physical activity. Evaluate teens individually according to age and prepregnancy weight. With twins, dietary prescription of 3000 to 4000 kcal/d may be needed (Luke et al, 2003). See nutrient chart.

Recommendations for Pregnant Women

Nutrient	Age 18 Years or Under	Ages 19–30 Years	Ages 31–50 Years
Energy	1st tri = +0 kcal/d; 2nd tri = +340 kcal/d; 3rd tri = +452 kcal/d	1st tri = +0 kcal/d; 2nd tri = +340 kcal/d; 3rd tri = +452 kcal/d	1st tri = +0 kcal/d; 2nd tri = +340 kcal/d; 3rd tri = +452 kcal/d
Protein	71 g/d	71 g/d	71 g/d
Calcium	1300 mg/d	1000 mg/d	1000 mg/d
Iron	27 mg/d	27 mg/d	27 mg/d
Folate	600 μg/d	600 μg/d	600 μg/d
Phosphorus	1250 mg/d	700 mg/d	700 mg/d
Vitamin A	750 μg	770 μg	770 μg
Vitamin C	80 mg/d	85 mg/d	85 mg/d
Thiamin	1.4 mg/d	1.4 mg/d	1.4 mg/d
Riboflavin	1.4 mg/d	1.4 mg/d	1.4 mg/d
Niacin	18 mg/d	18 mg/d	18 mg/d

Data from: Food and Nutrition Board, Institute of Medicine. *Dietary reference intakes for energy, carbohydrate, fiber, fat, fatty acids, cholesterol, protein, and amino acids (macronutrients)*. Washington, DC: National Academy Press, 2002.

- The diet and supplement should include 27 mg of ferrous iron and a 5-mg increase in intake of zinc, easily obtained from meat or milk.
- Encourage use of vitamin C foods with iron-rich foods or an iron sulfate supplement.
- Use adequate vitamins A and D to match DRIs for age; avoid hypervitaminosis, which may lead to fetal damage. Monitor use of dietary supplements and fortified foods carefully.
- Be sure to use iodized salt, but avoid salt intake greater than that recommended for healthy adults.
- Desired pattern of food intake: Two to three servings of milk–yogurt–cheese group (for calcium, protein); 6 oz of meat or protein substitute (protein, iron, zinc); 3 fruits and 4 vegetables, including citrus (vitamin C) and rich sources of vitamin A and folacin; 9 servings of grains and breads, 3 of which are whole-grain or enriched breads/substitutes (iron, energy); 3 servings of fat.
- Omit alcohol. Reduce caffeine intake to the equivalent of two cups of coffee or less per day; this includes intake from colas, chocolate, and tea.
- Use cereal grains, nuts, black beans, green vegetables, and seafood for magnesium. Magnesium plays a role in preventing or correcting high BP; follow the Dietary Approaches to Stop Hypertension (DASH) diet whenever possible.
- Essential fatty acids (EFAs) from fats, such as corn oil or safflower oil and walnuts, should equal 1–2% of daily calories. Arachidonic acid and docosahexaenoic acid (DHA) are essential for brain growth and cognitive development; supplementation supports higher IQ in young children (Helland et al, 2008). Fish and seafood (e.g., tuna, mackerel, salmon) can be encouraged for their omega-3 fatty acids twice weekly, if allergies and cautions about mercury intake have been considered.
- Extra vitamin B_6 and copper are readily obtained from a planned diet and a prenatal supplement.
- See Table 1-4 for a description of special problems in pregnancy.

Common Drugs Used and Potential Side Effects

- After the fourth month, encourage use of a basic vitamin-mineral supplement between meals (with liquids other than milk, coffee, or tea) for better utilization. Supplements vary greatly; read labels carefully. Discuss the relevance of tolerable upper intake levels (ULs) from the latest dietary reference intakes of the National Academy of Sciences. These levels were set to protect individuals from receiving too much of any nutrient from diet and dietary supplements.
- Iron is the only nutrient that cannot be met from diet alone (30 mg needed after the first trimester). Avoid taking iron supplements with antacids; bedtime is often the best time.
- Avoid taking isotretinoin (Accutane,) 13-*cis*-retinoic acid (CRA) or vitamin A as 10,000 IU or more, especially in the first trimester, as birth defects may result.
- Insulin may be needed with consistently high blood glucose levels over 120 mg/dL; monitor and avoid overfeeding.
- Antiemetic agents may be used to control NVP and include ondansetron (Zofran), cyclizine (Marezine), buclizine (Bucladin-S), metoclopramide (Reglan), meclizine (Antivert), prochlorperazine (Compazine), promethazine (Phenergan), or antihistamines such as Benadryl. Side effects vary but may include sedation, dizziness, changes in BP, and/or tachycardia.
- Women who have chronic diseases such as epilepsy, thyroid disorders, diabetes and cardiac disorders will need to manage all medications with careful medical supervision.
- Women who develop preterm labor are often treated with one of several drugs (tocolytics) to stop premature labor. Drugs include calcium channel blockers, terbutaline, ritodrine, magnesium sulfate, indomethacin, ketorolac, and sulindac. Use is short term, and side effects are not significant.
- Neevo® contains 1.13 mg L-methylfolate Calcium (as Metafolin®). It may be used for women who have MTHFR alleles.

Herbs, Botanicals, and Supplements

- Pregnant women should not use herbs, botanical supplements, and herbals teas. There are no rigorous scientific studies of the safety of dietary supplements during pregnancy. The Teratology Society has stated that it should not be assumed that they are safe for the embryo or fetus (Marcus and Snodgrass, 2005). Women who are using such supplements should stop immediately when they discover they are pregnant.
- Pregnant women should avoid supplements containing aloe, apricot kernel, black cohosh, borage, calendula, chaparral, chasteberry, comfrey, dong quai, ephedra, euphorbia, feverfew, foxglove, gentian, ginseng, golden seal, hawthorne, horehound, horseradish, juniper, licorice root, nettle, plantain, pokeroot, prickly ash, red clover, rhubarb, sassafras, saw palmetto, senna, skullcap, St. John's wort, tansy, wild carrot, willow, wormwood, yarrow, or yohimbe (American Dietetic Association, 2008). Willow bark, which contains salicilin, may cause stillbirth, prolonged gestation, and LBW.
- Ginger may be an effective treatment for nausea and vomiting in pregnancy (Borrelli et al, 2005). Sips of ginger ale or use of small amounts of ginger in cooking may be useful. However, when taking blood thinners or preparing for surgery, discontinue use.

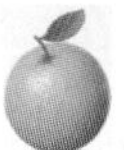

NUTRITION EDUCATION, COUNSELING, CARE MANAGEMENT

- Describe adequate patterns and rates of weight gain in pregnancy; explain the rationale. Individualize according to goals (e.g., shorter women at lower range of gain). Excess equals more than 6.5 lb gained monthly after 20 weeks. Inadequate intake is 2 lb or less gained monthly after the first trimester.
- Encourage adequate calcium intake. If needed, discuss what to do for milk allergy/intolerance and lactose intolerance.
- Discourage trendy diets, pica, fads, and the habit of skipping breakfast. Discuss ketosis related to low glucose levels and its undesirable effect on fetal brain development.

TABLE 1-4 Special Issues in Pregnancy

Issue	Considerations
Allergies, personal or family history	Avoidance of common food allergens during pregnancy does not prevent allergies in offspring (Kramer and Kakuma, 2003). Women may wish to take probiotics to stimulate health-producing microbes in their fetuses and to delay onset of eczema and allergies (Kukkonen et al, 2007; Wickens et al, 2008).
Hyperemesis (intractable, dehydrating vomiting)	This affects 20% of pregnancies in the first trimester. Half of these patients have some liver dysfunction (Hay, 2008). Early hospitalization with tube feeding may be needed (Paauw et al, 2005; Quinla and Hill, 2003). Metoclopramide (Reglan) may help. When eating orally, liquids taken between meals, extra B-complex vitamins and vitamin C, and limited fat may be beneficial. Low birth weight and greater length of hospital stay are common (Paauw et al, 2005). Avoid electrolyte imbalances.
Liver dysfunction such as viral hepatitis, gallstones or intrahepatic cholestasis in pregnancy	With pruritus, elevated bile acids in the second half of pregnancy, high levels of aminotransferases and mild jaundice, immediate delivery may be needed (Hay, 2008).
Multiple gestation	Energy regimen of 20% protein, 40% carbohydrate, and 40% fat may be particularly useful (Luke, 2005). Supplement with calcium, magnesium, and zinc, as well as multivitamins and essential fatty acids (Luke, 2005).
Nausea and vomiting of pregnancy (NVP)	Initial treatment of nausea and vomiting should be conservative with dietary changes, emotional support, and perhaps use of ginger (Quinla and Hill, 2003). NVP affects 80% of pregnancies. It is reasonable to suspect *H. pylori* (Goldberg et al, 2007). Frequent, small meals should be consumed separately from fluids. Offer high-protein snacks, such as cheese or lean meat. Avoid lying down immediately after meals and suggest not skipping meals. Do not force eating; suck on ice chips or other frozen items and make up lost calories later. Eat meals and snacks in a well-ventilated area, free of odors; avoid strong spices and aromas. Eat and drink slowly and rest after meals. Try lemonade and potato chips or saltines. Avoid large meals, very sweet, spicy or high-fat foods if not tolerated. Eat dry crackers before rising in the morning. If necessary, drink fluids between meals rather than with meals. Multivitamin-mineral supplements may also trigger NVP; it may be helpful to try a different brand. Minimize offensive odors. Rehydration may be essential. NVP often abates by 17 weeks of pregnancy.
Pica (intake of nonnutritive substances)	Intake of ice, freezer frost, baking soda, baking powder, cornstarch, laundry starch, baby powder, clay, or dirt. As pica practices are associated with significantly lower hemoglobin levels at delivery, WIC and prenatal counselors must be aware. Discussion of practices should be nonjudgmental because pica may have strong cultural implications. Food cravings and aversions usually subside after pregnancy.
Severe gastrointestinal problems	Consider total parenteral nutrition with adequate lipids (10–20% of energy) for the fetus, as well as protein and carbohydrate. Check blood sugar regularly. Use adequate fluid according to estimated needs. Complications may include bacteremia, decreased renal function with preexisting disease, neonatal hypoglycemia, or subclavian vein thrombosis.
Vegan vegetarians	Vitamin B_{12}, zinc, calcium, and vitamin D supplements may be needed.
Women with high levels of inflammatory cytokines	Reduced placental perfusion and a tendency toward preeclampsia (LaMarca et al, 2007). New tests and treatments are being identified.
Women who have previously given birth to an infant with neural tube defect or anencephaly	Test for folic acid alleles; consider use of Neevo® or 600 μg folate daily throughout PG.
Women with preeclampsia	Test for folic acid alleles; consider use of Neevo® or 600 μg folate daily throughout pregnancy (Klein, 2005).

- Encourage intake of high-density nutrients, especially among women with pregravid obesity, as their diets tend to be poorer quality (Laraia et al, 2007).
- Encourage pleasant meal times and a healthy appetite. Stress has negative effects on nitrogen and calcium.
- Encourage breastfeeding. Explain the reasons for doing so (e.g., immunological benefits, bonding, and weight stabilization). Mothers who are HIV-positive should consider HAART, which can drastically reduce the risk of transmission of HIV; infant prophylaxis can also reduce the transmission rate (Slater et al, 2010).
- For excessive weight gain, the goal should be to restore eating patterns to match a normal growth curve. Severe calorie restriction should be avoided. At least 175 g of CHO will be needed.
- A balanced intake of fluoride and iodine from water, table salt, and seafood is needed. Avoid excesses.
- Discuss effects of tobacco and drug use (cocaine, alcohol, and marijuana), such as decreased birth weight and congenital malformations.
- Eligible women should be referred to the WIC Program, especially to prevent LBW. Many barriers hinder participation in nutrition education programs, including lack of transportation or child care. Facilitated discussions, support groups, cooking classes, and websites may be useful.

TABLE 1-5 March of Dimes Campaign to Reduce Preterm Births

- Consume a multivitamin containing 400 μg of the B vitamin folic acid before and in the early months of pregnancy. Women who need L-methylfolate should receive that special formulation.
- Stop smoking, drinking and/or using illicit drugs; avoid prescription or over-the-counter drugs (including herbal preparations) unless prescribed by a doctor who is aware of the pregnancy.
- Once pregnant, get early regular prenatal care, eat a balanced diet with enough calories (about 300 more than a woman normally eats), and gain enough weight (usually 25–35 lb).
- Talk to a doctor about signs of premature labor and what to do if warning signs are evident.

Source: http://www.marchofdimes.com/pnhec/240_48590.asp; accessed January 2, 2009.

- For constipation, suggest extra fiber, activity, and fluid (35–40 cc/kg); avoid laxatives.
- For swelling of ankles, hands, and legs, become more physically active. Avoid excessive salt at the table but do not restrict salt severely.
- For heartburn, eat smaller meals more frequently, eat slowly, and cut down on spicy or high-fat foods. Avoid antacids unless approved by the physician.
- All infections are cause for concern among pregnant women because they pose a risk to the health of the baby. Prostaglandins may stimulate early labor and cause delivery of an LBW infant. Women should have a periodontal evaluation to rule out gum disease and to eliminate infection.
- Discuss postpartum issues, including physical activity, breastfeeding, anemia, and control of hyperglycemia. Adherence to dietary guidelines may be limited in low-income women because of neglect of self-care, weight-related distress, negative body image, stress, and depressive symptoms (George et al, 2005). Attention to psychosocial needs may help to improve dietary intakes.
- The March of Dimes has launched a campaign to reduce rates of preterm birth; see Table 1-5.

Patient Education—Food Safety

- *Helicobacter pylori* should be suspected as one possible cause of nausea and vomiting (Goldberg et al, 2007). Hepatitis A, *Salmonella*, *Shigella*, *Escherichia coli*, and *Cryptosporidium* are common causes of diarrhea during pregnancy (American Dietetic Association, 2008). Careful hand washing is recommended.
- Avoid soft cheeses such as feta, brie, camembert, Roquefort, and Mexican soft cheese; they may have been contaminated with *Listeria*, which can cause fetal death or premature labor.
- Avoid raw or undercooked eggs, fish or shellfish, and meats because of potential foodborne illnesses.
- Do not eat or drink raw (unpasteurized) milk or products made from it.
- Avoid eating unpasteurized juices and raw sprouts.
- Pregnant women should not eat shark, swordfish, king mackerel, and tilefish. These long-lived larger fish contain the highest levels of methyl mercury, which may harm an unborn baby's developing nervous system. Pregnant women should select a variety of other kinds of fish, such as shellfish, canned fish, smaller ocean fish, and farm-raised fish. They can safely eat 12 oz of cooked fish per week, with a typical serving size being 3–6 oz. Keep fish and shellfish refrigerated or frozen until ready to use.

For More Information

- American Association of Birth Centers
  http://www.birthcenters.org/
- American College of Nurse-Midwives (ACNM)
  http://www.midwife.org
- American Academy of Periodontology in pregnancy
  http://www.perio.org/consumer/mbc.baby.htm
- Centers for Disease Control and Prevention—Geriatrics
  http://www.cdc.gov/ncbddd/pregnancy_gateway/default.htm
- Farmers' Markets, Agricultural Marketing Service of USDA
  http://www.ams.usda.gov/farmersmarkets/
- Institute of Medicine, Weight Gain During Pregnancy
  http://www.nap.edu/catalog/12584.html
- My Pyramid for Pregnant Moms
  http://www.mypyramid.gov/mypyramidmoms/
- National Healthy Mothers, Healthy Babies Coalition
  http://www.hmhb.org/
- National Center for Education in Maternal-Child Health
  http://www.ncemch.org/
- National Foundation—March of Dimes
  http://www.modimes.org/
- National Women's Health Information Center
  www.4woman.gov
- WIC Program—Supplemental Food Programs Division
  http://www.fns.usda.gov/wic/

PREGNANCY—CITED REFERENCES

American College of Obstetrics and Gynecology. Accessed October 1, 2009, at http://www.acog.org/publications/patient_education/bp001.cfm.

American Dietetic Association. Position of the American Dietetic Association: nutrition and lifestyle for a healthy pregnancy outcome. *J Am Diet Assoc.* 108:553, 2008.

Angermayr L, Clar C. Iodine supplementation for preventing iodine deficiency disorders in children. *Cochrane Database Syst Rev.* 2:CD003819, 2004.

Benton D; ILSI Europe. Micronutrient status, cognition and behavioral problems in childhood. *Eur J Nutr.* 47:38S, 2008.

Borrelli F, et al. Effectiveness and safety of ginger in the treatment of pregnancy-induced nausea and vomiting. *Obstet Gynecol.* 105:849, 2005.

Butte NF, et al. Energy requirements during pregnancy based on total energy expenditure and energy deposition. *Am J Clin Nutr.* 79:1078, 2004.

George GC, et al. Compliance with dietary guidelines and relationship to psychosocial factors in low-income women in late postpartum. *J Am Diet Assoc.* 105:916, 2005.

Glinoer D. The importance of iodine nutrition during pregnancy. *Public Health Nutr.* 10:1542, 2007.

Godfrey KM, Barker DJ. Fetal nutrition and adult disease. *Am J Clin Nutr.* 71S:1344, 2000.

Goldberg D, et al. Hyperemesis gravidarum and Helicobacter pylori infection: a systematic review. *Obstet Gynecol.* 110:695, 2007.

Hay J. Liver disease in pregnancy. *Hepatology.* 47:1067, 2008.

Helland IB, et al. Effect of supplementing pregnant and lactating mothers with n-3 very-long-chain fatty acids on children's IQ and body mass index at 7 years of age. *Pediatrics.* 122:e472, 2008.

Hurley KM, et al. Psychosocial influences in dietary patterns during pregnancy. *J Am Diet Assoc.* 105:963, 2005.

Klein L. Nutritional recommendations for multiple pregnancy. *J Am Diet Assoc.* 105:1050, 2005.

Kukkonen K, et al. Probiotics and prebiotic galacto-oligosaccharides in the prevention of allergic diseases: a randomized, double-blind, placebo-controlled trial. *J Allergy Clin Immunol.* 119:192, 2007.
LaMarca BD, et al. Inflammatory cytokines in the pathophysiology of hypertension during preclampsia. *Curr Hypertens Rep.* 9:480, 2007.
Laraia BA, et al. Pregravid body mass index is negatively associated with diet quality during pregnancy. *Public Health Nutr Rep.* 10:920, 2007.
Laraia BA, et al. Household food insecurity is associated with self-reported pregravid weight status, gestational weight gain, and pregnancy complications. *J Am Diet Assoc.* 110:692, 2010.
Luke B. Nutrition and multiple gestation. *Semin Perinatol.* 29:349, 2005.
Luke B, et al. Specialized prenatal care and maternal and infant outcomes in twin pregnancy. *Am J Obstet Gynecol.* 189:934, 2003.
Lussana F, et al. Prenatal exposure to the Dutch famine is associated with a preference for fatty foods and a more atherogenic lipid profile. *Am J Clin Nutr.* 88:1648, 2007.
Maggard MA, et al. Pregnancy and fertility following bariatric surgery: a systematic review. *JAMA.* 300:2286, 2008.
March of Dimes. Preconception risks. Accessed January 11, 2009, at http://www.marchofdimes.com/professionals/19695.asp.
Marcus DM, Snodgrass WR. Do no harm: avoidance of herbal medicines during pregnancy. *Obstet Gynecol.* 105:1119, 2005.
Paauw JD, et al. Hyperemesis gravidarum and fetal outcome. *JPEN J Parenter Enteral Nutr.* 29:93, 2005.
Rasmussen KM, Yaktine AL. Weight gain during pregnancy: reexamining the guidelines. Institute of Medicine, National Research Council. Accessed May 29, 2009, at http://www.nap.edu/catalog/12584.html.
Scialli AR. 2005 Josef Warkany lecture: clinicians. *Birth Defects Res A Clin Mol Teratol.* 76:1, 2006.
Slater M, et al. Breastfeeding in HIV-positive women: what can be recommended? *Paediatr Drugs.* 12:1, 2010.
Waterland RA, Michels KB. Epigenetic epidemiology of the developmental origins hypothesis. *Annu Rev Nutr.* 27:363, 2007.
Wickens K, et al. A differential effect of 2 probiotics in the prevention of eczema and atopy: a double-blind, randomized, placebo-controlled trial. *J Allergy Clin Immunol.* 122:788, 2008.
Wilson AG. Epigenetic regulation of gene expression in the inflammatory response and relevance to common diseases. *J Periodontol.* 79:1514, 2008.
Wilson RD, et al. Pre-conceptional vitamin/folic acid supplementation 2007: the use of folic acid in combination with a multivitamin supplement for the prevention of neural tube defects and other congenital anomalies. *J Obstet Gynaecol Can.* 30:193, 2008.
Zempleni J, et al. Epigenetic regulation of chromatin structure and gene function by biotin: are biotin requirements being met? *Nutr Rev.* 66:S46, 2008.

LACTATION

NUTRITIONAL ACUITY RANKING: LEVEL 1

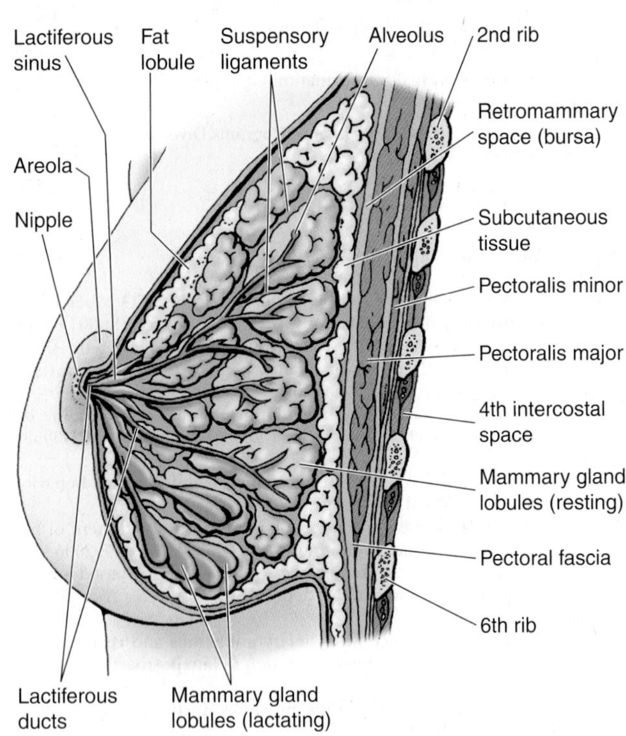

Reprinted with permission from: Moore KL, PhD, FRSM, FIAC & Dalley AF II, PhD. *Clinical Oriented Anatomy,* 4th ed. Baltimore: Lippincott Williams & Wilkins 1999.

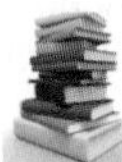

DEFINITIONS AND BACKGROUND

Breastfeeding should be supported and encouraged because of its immunological, physiological, economic, social, and hygienic effects on mother and infant. Exclusive breastfeeding for the first 6 months of life provides the best form of nutrition (James et al, 2005). Because maternal intake and breastfeeding practices vary over the duration of lactation, assess regularly and determine whether or not the infant needs supplemental foods or nutrients. Only rarely is supplementation needed. In fact, adding formula or solids to the diet of the exclusively breastfed infant almost guarantees lactation failure. Unless mom is severely malnourished, she can keep making good milk.

Breastfeeding is an anabolic state, requiring extra energy. The composition of breast milk varies over time. Colostrum contains mainly immunological factors (days 1–4); a short transition occurs (days 5–9); breast milk secreted between days 9 and 28 is primarily nutritional; and breast milk content is equally valuable for immunity and nutrition thereafter.

Human milk is better digested and absorbed by infants than other forms of milk; it has more DHA and arachidonic acid for normal cognitive and visual development, and carnitine for mitochondrial oxidation of these long-chain fatty acids. It also has less sodium and a proper protein ratio. Levels of DHA and arachidonic acid are lower in women who have diabetes; insulin resistance is higher among their infants (Min et al, 2005).

Breast milk has 1.5 times as much lactose as cow's milk; consequently, protein is absorbed better. The whey to casein ratio of 80:20 is more desirable than that of many formulas. In comparison, cow's milk has twice as much protein and mineral content. The composition of breast milk changes to meet the developing baby's needs (i.e., the fat content decreases over time). In many cases where a mother cannot breastfeed, the use of banked human milk may be a better option than cow's milk formulas (Wojcik et al, 2009). See Table 1-6 for the nutrient content of human milk.

TABLE 1-6 Nutrient Content of Mature Human Milk

Nutrients	Units	1 Cup/ 240 g
Proximates		
Water	g	215.25
Energy	kcal	171.125
Protein (casein, IgA, IgG, lactalbumin, lactoferrin, albumin, B-lactoglobulin)	g	2.53
Total lipid (fat)	g	10.775
Carbohydrate (lactose, oligosaccharides)	g	16.95
Fiber, total dietary	g	0.00
Amino acids		
Tryptophan	g	0.042
Threonine	g	0.113
Isoleucine	g	0.138
Leucine	g	0.234
Lysine	g	0.167
Methionine	g	0.052
Cystine	g	0.047
Phenylalanine	g	0.113
Tyrosine	g	0.130
Valine	g	0.155
Arginine	g	0.106
Histidine	g	0.057
Alanine	g	0.089
Aspartic acid	g	0.202
Glutamic acid	g	0.413
Glycine	g	0.064
Proline	g	0.202
Serine	g	0.106

Nutrients	Units	1 Cup/ 240 g
Vitamins		
Vitamin C	mg	12.300
Thiamin	mg	0.034
Riboflavin	mg	0.089
Niacin	mg	0.435
Pantothenic acid	mg	0.549
Vitamin B_6	mg	0.027
Folate	μg	12.792
Vitamin B_{12}	μg	0.111
Vitamin A, IU	IU	592.860
Vitamin A, RE	μg	157.440
Vitamin D	IU	9.840
Vitamin E	mg	2.214
Lipids		
Fatty acids, saturated	g	4.942
Fatty acids, monounsaturated	g	4.079
Fatty acids, polyunsaturated	g	1.223
Cholesterol	mg	34.194
Minerals		
Calcium, Ca	mg	79.212
Iron, Fe	mg	0.074
Magnesium, Mg	mg	8.364
Phosphorus, P	mg	33.702
Potassium, K	mg	125.952
Sodium, Na	mg	41.574
Zinc, Zn	mg	0.418
Copper, Cu	mg	0.128
Manganese, Mn	mg	0.064
Selenium, Se	μg	4.428

Other

Antimicrobial Factors
- Secretory IgA, IgM, IgG
- Lactoferrin
- Lysozyme
- Complement C3
- Leucocytes
- Bifidus factor
- Lipids and fatty acids
- Antiviral mucins, GAGs
- Oligosaccharides

Cytokines and Anti-inflammatory Factors
- Tumor necrosis factor; interleukins; interferon-γ; prostaglandins; acetyl hydrolase; α_1-antichymotrypsin; platelet-activating factor

Growth Factors
- Epidermal (EGF)
- Nerve (NGF)
- Insulin-like (IGF)
- Transforming (TGF)
- Taurine
- Polyamines

Digestive Enzymes
- Amylase
- Bile acid-stimulating esterase
- Bile acid-stimulating lipases
- Lipoprotein lipase

Potentially Harmful Substances
- Viruses (e.g., HIV)
- Aflatoxins
- *Trans*-fatty acids
- Nicotine, caffeine
- Food allergens
- PCBs, DDT, dioxins
- Radioisotopes
- Drugs

Hormones
- Feedback inhibitor of lactation (FIL)
- Insulin
- Prolactin
- Thyroid hormones
- Corticosteroids, ACTH
- Oxytocin
- Calcitonin
- Parathyroid hormone
- Erythropoietin

Sources: U.S. Department of Agriculture, November 1999; Jensen RG, ed. *Handbook of milk composition.* New York: Academic Press, 1995; Scrimshaw NS. *Food Nutr Bull.* 17(4), 1996.

Food allergies are less frequent in infants who are exclusively breastfed, even more so if maternal diets are higher in omega-3 fatty acids. Compared with cow's milk formulas, breast milk has more antibodies and over 45 bioactive factors such as digestive enzymes, hormones, immune factors, and growth factors. The promotion of breastfeeding has played an important role in improving child health by providing optimum nutrition and protection against common childhood infections and by promoting child spacing.

Breast milk is a living fluid. Infants receive beneficial nucleotides, macrophages, leukocytes, lymphocytes, and neutrophils from human milk, which protect against diarrhea, allergies, ear infections, necrotizing enterocolitis, urinary tract infection, and pneumonia. Bacterial flora of breastfed infants are generally *Lactobacillus*, not *Escherichia coli* like those of formula-fed infants. Formula-fed infants may be more prone to wheezing, Gastroesophageal (GE) reflux, urinary tract infection, influenza, sepsis, and *Giardia;* therefore, exclusive breastfeeding for 6 months or longer is highly recommended.

If the mother uses alcohol or illicit drugs, is receiving chemotherapy or has HIV infection, or if the infant has galactosemia, breastfeeding is not recommended unless HAART therapy is given (Slater et al, 2010). Women must be fully informed about the risks of breastfeeding transmission of HIV versus the expense and availability of obtaining formula.

Women should be encouraged to breastfeed until the child is 1 year of age or as long as mutually desirable. In developing countries, mothers may be encouraged to increase the breastfeeding time to 2 years, but mothers should not deprive themselves. The volume of milk decreases in a poorly nourished mother (American Dietetic Association, 2009).

New mothers who are breastfeeding should try not to lose weight rapidly. Women who are obese before pregnancy need extra encouragement to breastfeed. Prolonged breastfeeding helps to lower postpartum weight, although this benefit may slow in older mothers.

The long-term effects of breastfeeding an infant include lower incidences of type 2 diabetes, Crohn's disease, some types of cancer, allergies, and neurological disabilities. The relation of vitamin D insufficiency in the fetus or neonate to long-term outcomes such as type 1 diabetes and other chronic diseases needs to be investigated (Kovacs, 2008). Several minerals and peptides found in milk have a BP lowering effect, which may be protective later in life. Exclusive and prolonged breastfeeding is also associated with higher cognitive development than formula feeding, likely from long-chain fatty acids Docosahexaenoic acid (DHA) and Eicosapentaenoic acid (EPA) (Kramer et al, 2008).

Breastfeeding reduces the risk of breast and ovarian cancers, protects bone density in the mother, improves glucose profiles in gestational diabetes, and saves money not spent on formula (James et al, 2005). While it has been proposed that breastfeeding helps adults maintain a desirable BMI, this needs further evaluation (Owen et al, 2005). A recent study found that breastfeeding did not reduce adiposity at age of 6.5 years (Kramer et al, 2009).

There is an essential role for dietetics professionals in promoting and supporting breastfeeding by providing up-to-date, practical information to pregnant and postpartum women, involving family and friends in breastfeeding education and counseling, removing institutional barriers to breastfeeding, collaborating with community organizations that promote and support breastfeeding, and advocating for policies that position breastfeeding as the norm (James et al, 2005). Because prenatal WIC participation is associated with a greater likelihood of providing babies infant formula rather than breastmilk after birth, it is critical to educate these women about the health risks of introducing cow's milk complementary foods too early (Ziol-Guest and Hernandez, 2010).

The nutrition counselor should encourage mothers to continue breastfeeding for 6–12 months, and somewhat longer in developing countries. The Ten Steps to Successful Breastfeeding (WHO/UNICEF) provide an evidence-based standard used to assess individual hospitals and their support for mothers to breastfeed (Grizzard et al, 2006). Billions of dollars would be saved if breastfeeding were increased to 6 months or longer to reduce otitis media, gastroenteritis, and necrotizing enterocolitis.

In a survey of physicians about their breastfeeding promotion practices, over half indicated that they had had little or no education about breastfeeding; more education for solving common problems is desired (Krogstrand and Parr, 2005). See Table 1-7 for common problems that occur during breastfeeding and guidance to support the mother.

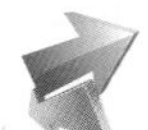

ASSESSMENT, MONITORING, AND EVALUATION

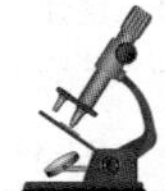

CLINICAL INDICATORS

Genetic Markers: Each individual has a unique genetic profile and phenotype. Mothers with galactosemia should not breastfeed.

Clinical/History

- BP
- Smoking
- Height
- Current weight
- Weight history
- Prepregnancy weight
- Healthy body weight (HBW) range for height
- Date of birth (DOB) for infant
- Goal for return to usual body weight
- Diet history

Lab Work

- Glucose
- Albumin (Alb) or transthyretin (if needed)
- H & H, serum Fe
- Alk phos
- Protime or INR
- Chol
- Triglycerides (Trig)
- Homocysteine
- Ca^{++}
- Serum phosphorus
- Serum 25-hydroxyvitamin D [25(OH)D]

INTERVENTION

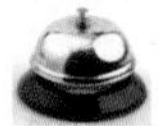

OBJECTIVES

- Support adequate lactation (usual secretion, 750–800 mL/d). Human milk provides 67 kcal/dL. Good energy intake improves milk production, especially in undernourished women.

TABLE 1-7 Common Problems in Breastfeeding and Reasons Why Women Discontinue Breastfeeding

Birth Control Pills: High estrogen-types are not recommended as they can decrease milk supply. A progestin-only pill is usually recommended by a physician.

Colic and Fussiness: A randomized, controlled trial of a low-allergen maternal diet was conducted among exclusively breastfed infants presenting with colic; when mothers excluded cow's milk, eggs, peanuts, tree nuts, wheat, soy, and fish from their diet, crying/fuss duration was reduced by a substantially greater amount in the low-allergen group (Hill et al, 2005).

Engorgement: The best way to prevent engorgement is to begin breastfeeding as soon as possible after birth followed by nursing regularly throughout the day. Rapid filling of the breasts and blocked mammary ducts may cause a painful engorgement. Frequent nursing, breast massage or warm shower before feedings, use of cold packs shortly after nursing, wearing a firm bra that is not too tight, and avoiding the use of nipple shields can help alleviate this condition.

Inadequate Milk Supply: Poor milk supply can be a cause of failure to thrive in breastfeeding infants. Maternal causes of poor milk supply are hypothyroidism, excessive antihistamine use, smoking, oral contraceptive use, illness, inadequate intake after gastric bypass surgery, poor diet, decreased fluid intake, infrequent nursing, or fatigue. Correction of any of these causes may improve milk supply. Increasing frequency of nursing is the best way to increase milk supply.

Jaundice: Breast milk jaundice occurs in about 1% of the population of breastfeeding newborns, is caused by the presence of a substance that alters liver function, and may cause red cell hemolysis. Mothers should breastfeed 10–12 times per day to correct elevated serum bilirubin levels.

Latching On: For problems with baby latching on, the trick is to have the baby open his or her mouth wide. Brush baby's lips with the nipple to encourage him or her to open wide, as if yawning. Once baby's mouth is open wide, quickly pull the baby onto the breast by pulling the baby toward mom with the arm that is holding him or her (not moving mom towards the baby). Baby's gums should cover an inch of the aerola behind the nipple. Be sure the baby's lips are everted and not inverted (turned in). Almost the entire areola should be in the baby's mouth.

Mastitis: Breast infection causes fever, chills, redness, flu-like symptoms, and breast sensitivity. A clogged mammary duct, maternal anemia, stress, or an infection carried from the baby may cause mastitis. The primary goal is emptying the infected breast; frequent nursing (every 1–3 hours during the day and 2–3 hours at night) is encouraged. The physician should be notified so that antibiotics or pain relievers can be prescribed. Application of heat to the breast, drinking plenty of fluids, and adequate rest are useful measures for treatment.

Nipple Confusion: Infants who are breastfeed may refuse to take a bottle as the weaning of breastfeeding occurs. Mothers should be encouraged to continue attempts at breastfeeding.

Sore Nipples: Frequent, short nursing, repositioning the infant at the breast, applying cold packs or heat to breasts, avoiding irritating soaps or lotions on nipples, air-drying nipples after nursing, exposing nipples to direct sunlight or 60-watt bulb for 15 minutes several times per day, applying vitamin E squeezed from capsules or ointment such as vitamin A and D or pure lanolin cream to nipples, and avoiding the use of nipple shields may help ease the pain. Occasionally, sore nipples are caused by *Candida albicans*; the breasts may not appear to have a fungal infection, but cultures of nipple surfaces will be positive for Candida albicans.

Reasons Why Women Discontinue Lactation

Acute infections in the mother

Employer attitudes toward breastfeeding mothers; lack of private space with a locking door, adequate time to express milk, inadequate refrigeration (Stewart-Glenn, 2008)

Hospital practices that do not support breastfeeding (Grizzard et al, 2006) including physician and nurse apathy or misinformation

Infant's inability to nurse due to weakness or oral anomalies

Lack of information and support and/or inadequate preparation

Lack of part-time jobs, flexible scheduling, and convenient day care for mothers who must work

Maternal depression

Mother's chronic illness (e.g., tuberculosis, severe anemia, chronic fevers, cardiovascular or renal disease) and/or use of medications

Mother's inability to provide 50% of the infant's needs

Mother's return to work by 12 weeks postpartum (Taveras et al, 2003)

Obesity: poor infant feeding behavior and reduced hormonal responses in the early postpartum period result in delayed lactogenesis and early cessation of breastfeeding (Lovelady, 2005)

- Breast milk can meet nutrient needs during the first 6 months, with possible exception of vitamin D and iron in certain populations.
- Exclusive breastfeeding for 6 months has many nutritional benefits. Have the mother continue breastfeeding for up to 1 year when possible. Exclusive breastfeeding should be encouraged for at least 4–6 months in infants at risk of atopy (Friedman and Zeigler, 2005).
- Decrease nutritional risks from use of alcohol, stimulants, and medications while mother is breastfeeding. Alcohol intake inhibits the letdown reflex from oxytocin. Discourage excessive use of stimulants, including caffeine from coffee (limit to 2 cups daily) and from tea, colas, and chocolate.
- Omit known food allergens while breastfeeding if infant shows signs of colic (Hill et al, 2005). Eliminate cow's milk, eggs, peanuts, tree nuts, wheat, soy, and fish, especially if members of the immediate family have allergies.
- Promote adequate infant growth and development, including bone mineralization. Lactation increases the normal daily loss of calcium for the mother, yet is generally beneficial for protecting bone health.
- Normalize body composition gradually so that the mother returns to ideal weight. Promote gradual weight

SAMPLE NUTRITION CARE PROCESS STEPS

Harmful Beliefs about Food and Nutrition

Assessment Data: Food records; signs of infant GI distress or excessive sleep.

Nutrition Diagnosis (PES): Harmful beliefs/attitudes about food or nutrition-related topics related to consumption of 4 beers daily while breastfeeding as evidenced by food diary, discussion with mom about "beer making more breastmilk," and reports that the infant is lethargic during daytime.

Intervention: Education about appropriate dietary and substance intake for pregnancy. Counseling about dangers of consuming alcohol.

Monitoring and Evaluation: Omission of alcohol intake while breastfeeding. Infant weight and infant growth charts; reports about infant sleep and GI patterns.

loss even in obese women. Weight loss by the mother of 0.5 kg per week after delivery does not affect the growth of breastfed infants (Lovelady, 2005).

- Support brain health and visual acuity by including fatty acids in the mother's diet (Anderson et al, 2005; Lauritezen et al, 2005). Both EPA and DHA should be included.

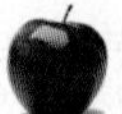

FOOD AND NUTRITION

- In the first 6 months, increase the mother's energy by 330 kcal over RDA for age. In the next 6 months, increase energy by 400 kcal over RDA for age. Recommendations may vary because individuals vary in prepregnancy weights, activity levels, and rates of weight gain.
- Consider the special needs of adolescents or women older than 35 years of age. Energy and nutrient requirements will change accordingly.
- Increase the mother's intake of protein (approximately 65 g daily), especially sources of high-quality protein.

Recommendations for Lactation

Nutrient	Age 18 Years or Under	Ages 19–30 Years	Ages 31–50 Years
Energy, 1st 6 months	+330 kcal/d	+330 kcal/d	+330 kcal/d
Energy, 2nd 6 months	400 kcal/d	400 kcal/d	400 kcal/d
Protein	61 g/d or 1.1 g/kg/d	61 g/d or 1.1 g/kg/d	61 g/d or 1.1 g/kg/d
Calcium	1200 mg/d	1300 mg/d	1300 mg/d
Iron	10 mg/d	9 mg/d	9 mg/d
Folate	500 μg/d	500 μg/d	500 μg/d
Phosphorus	1250 mg/d	700 mg/d	700 mg/d
Vitamin A	1200 μg	1300 μg	1300 μg
Vitamin C	115 mg/d	120 mg/d	120 mg/d
Thiamin	1.4 mg/d	1.4 mg/d	1.4 mg/d
Riboflavin	1.6 mg/d	1.6 mg/d	1.6 mg/d
Niacin	17 mg/d	17 mg/d	17 mg/d

Data from: Food and Nutrition Board, Institute of Medicine. *Dietary reference intakes for energy, carbohydrate, fiber, fat, fatty acids, cholesterol, protein, and amino acids (macronutrients).* Washington, DC: National Academy Press, 2002.

- Encourage intake of usual sources of vitamins and minerals. Intake of calcium should be 1200–1300 mg/d. Increases of B-complex vitamins, vitamins A and C should be included. Supplementation may be needed for women with poor dietary intakes or chronic illnesses.
- Adequate vitamin D is needed for the infant if maternal intake is poor, if infant receives little sunshine exposure or has high levels of skin pigmentation. Daily vitamin D supplements of 400 IU/L will keep serum 25(OH)D concentrations higher than 50 nmol/L and prevent rickets in infants and young children (Greer, 2008).
- Levels of both iron and copper decrease with progression of lactation; there is no evident need for supplementation in the first 6 months.
- Increase intake of fluids. Omit alcohol unless permitted by a physician.
- After 3 months of lactation, mothers should increase energy intake if weight loss has been excessive.
- Women who follow vegan diets may need zinc, calcium, vitamin D, or vitamin B_{12} supplementation. These diets also may be low in carnitine.
- If tube feeding is needed using breast milk, some fat losses can occur. Formula enhancers may be added if long-term use is required.
- Breastfeeding by adolescent mothers is associated with greater bone mineral density (BMD) during young adulthood; lactation may be protective to their bone health.

Common Drugs Used and Potential Side Effects

- Discuss the relevance of tolerable ULs from the latest dietary reference intakes of the National Academy of Sciences. These levels were set to protect individuals from receiving too much of any nutrient from diet and dietary supplements. Lactating mothers should be especially aware of what they are consuming between diet and supplements to avoid hypervitaminosis A and D. Read food and supplement labels carefully.
- Alcohol and nicotine are transmitted through breast milk to infants; discourage use. Cigarette smoking reduces the amount of milk produced.
- Moderate amounts of caffeine are acceptable in the equivalent of 2 cups of coffee.
- Cimetidine, Prozac, lithium, cyclosporine, cold medicines, and some other drugs may be contraindicated. Otherwise, prescribed medications are used only under supervision of the doctor.
- Drugs that may be used during breastfeeding include acetaminophen, some antibiotics and antihistamines, codeine, decongestants, insulin, quinine, ibuprofen, and thyroid medications.
- Parlodel (bromocriptine mesylate) inhibits secretion of prolactin and decreases lactation; it is used for women who do not wish to breastfeed. Constipation or anorexia may result.

Herbs, Botanicals, and Supplements

- Herbs and botanical supplements should not be used without first discussing with the physician. In general, these supplements have not been proven to be safe for breastfeeding mothers and their infants. Fenugreek, anise, fennel, garlic, and echinacea have been suggested for breastfeeding but have not been studied in this population for side effects. Lactating women should not take kava, chasteberry, dong quai, Asian ginseng, licorice root, or saw palmetto.
- IgM-, IgA-, and IgG-secreting cells are higher in infants who are breastfed exclusively for at least for 3 months and supplemented with probiotics compared with breastfed infants receiving placebo; use of probiotics during breastfeeding may positively influence gut immunity (Rinne et al, 2005).

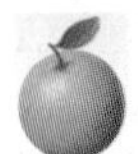

NUTRITION EDUCATION, COUNSELING, CARE MANAGEMENT

- "Best practice" counseling includes one prenatal and one postpartum home contact and telephone consultation by a lactation consultant (Bonuck et al, 2005). Explain the composition of breast milk, the benefits of breastfeeding, nipple care, and what to do during illness or infection.
- Self-esteem is crucial. Help mom believe that she can do it; give positive feedback and help her handle negative comments from others. Promotion of self-efficacy is useful. To prevent early discontinuation, lay support (peer counseling) is effective (Chung et al, 2008). Primary care physicians should support breastfeeding efforts during early, routine visits (Labarere et al, 2005).
- Help mom address barriers, such as short maternity leave, lack of private places to pump, coworker comments, minor health barriers, lack of support from doctor or nurses, and old wives' tales (e.g., breastfeeding spoils the baby, restrictive diet).
- Women with delayed onset of lactation need additional support during the first week postpartum; recommend frequent nursing.
- To ensure baby receives enough milk, mom should nurse at least eight times in each 24-hour period, no longer than one hour at a time. Baby should be able to rest for about 2 hours between feedings.
- Breastfed infants should have at least five wet diapers in each 24 hours. Stools of breastfed babies differ from formula-fed infants by being more loose. By day 4, there should be three stools a day, yellowish in hue.
- Explain the meaning of a balanced diet. Stress food sources of nutrients often limited in their diets: calcium, zinc, folate, and vitamins E, D, and B_6.
- Breastfed infants may be deficient in vitamin B_{12}, especially after 6 months (Hay et al, 2008). Vegetarian women may need supplemental vitamin B_{12} and vitamin D.
- Amounts of food antigens in breast milk may be controlled by modifying the maternal diet (Hill et al, 2005). Infants fed formulas of intact cow's milk or soy protein compared with breast milk have a higher incidence of type 1 diabetes autoantibodies, atopic dermatitis and wheezing in early childhood; exclusive breastfeeding should be encouraged (Friedman and Zeigler, 2005; Kull et al, 2005).
- Encourage the mother to normalize weight after delivery, but not start a weight loss program while she is nursing. Other than postpartum diuresis, average loss is 0.67 kg/month. Total weight gained during pregnancy affects weight loss afterwards. Mothers should try to maintain their postpartum weight during lactation. Weight loss should not be initiated until breastfeeding is discontinued, with no more than 1 lb/wk.
- Moderate exercise has no adverse effects on breastfeeding among healthy mothers. However, extra energy intake is needed with vigorous exercise (Lovelady, 2004).
- Exercise alone is not always sufficient to promote the desired level of weight reduction. Once lactation is established, overweight women can reduce energy intake by 500 kcal per day to allow gradual weight loss of 0.5 kg/wk (Lovelady, 2004).
- Lactating women are at high risk for energy and nutrient inadequacies, especially in low-income communities. Strategies must ensure adequate intakes. For example, in 2009, the WIC food package changed to use lower fat milk, whole grains, canned beans, salmon and tuna, a fruit/vegetable cash voucher. The program now offers the formula/BF option to encourage breastfeeding.
- Depressive symptoms in postpartum mothers should be identified and addressed (Hatton et al, 2005).
- Exposure to pesticides and polychlorinated biphenyls (PCBs) is undesirable. Some exposure occurs from breastmilk, with similar content in both colostrum and mature milk (Yu et al, 2007).
- Discuss issues related to safe handling of breast milk (see the following Food Safety recommendations).

Patient Education—Food Safety

- Avoid soft cheeses such as feta, brie, camembert, Roquefort, and Mexican soft cheese; they may have been contaminated with *Listeria*, which can cause fetal death or premature labor. If they are used, cook until boiling first.
- Avoid raw eggs, raw fish, and raw and undercooked meats because of potential viral and bacterial foodborne illnesses. *Helicobacter pylori* should be suspected as one possible cause of nausea or vomiting; careful hand washing is recommended.
- Nursing mothers should not eat shark, swordfish, king mackerel, and tilefish. These long-lived larger fish contain the highest levels of methyl mercury, which may harm a baby's developing nervous system. Nursing women should select a variety of other kinds of fish, such as shellfish, canned fish, smaller ocean fish, or farm-raised fish. They can safely eat 12 oz of cooked fish per week, with a typical serving size being 3–6 oz.
- After expressing milk, it should be stored in a clean, tightly enclosed container. An opaque container may help to protect riboflavin more than a clear container if there is any exposure to light.
- Human milk can be stored safely if refrigerated but not at room temperature because bacterial growth and lipolysis are rapid. Milk to be used within 48 hours can be refrigerated; if milk is to be used after 48 hours, try freezing (up to 6 months) immediately.

For More Information

- Academy of Breastfeeding Medicine
  http://www.bfmed.org/Default.aspx
- American Academy of Pediatrics
  http://www.aap.org/
- American Academy of Pediatrics Nutrition Resources
  http://www.medicalhomeinfo.org/Publications/Nutrition.html
- Benefits of breastfeeding
  http://www.4woman.gov/Breastfeeding/index.cfm?page=227
- Breastfeeding a Cleft-Lip/Palate Baby
  http://www.cleft.org/breastfeeding.htm
- Breastfeeding Basics Course
  http://www.breastfeedingbasics.org/
- Breastfeeding Promotion Committee
  Healthy Mothers, Healthy Babies National Coalition
  http://www.hmhb.org/
- CDC Breastfeeding topics
  http://www.cdc.gov/breastfeeding/
- Center for Breastfeeding Information
- La Leche International
  http://www.lalecheleague.org/
- Consumer Tips
  http://www.breastfeeding.com/helpme/consumer_friendly%20_bftips.html
- Got Mom: Breastfeeding Resources
  http://www.gotmom.org/
- Human Milk Banking Association of North America
  http://www.hmbana.org/
- International Lactation Consultant Association Directory
  http://www.breastfeeding.com/directory/lcdirectory.html
- Keep Kids Healthy
  http://www.keepkidshealthy.com/breastfeeding/
- Medline Plus
  http://www.nlm.nih.gov/medlineplus/ency/article/002452.htm
- Mother's Best
  http://www.breastfeeding.com/
- My Pyramid: Tips for Breastfeeding Moms
  http://www.nal.usda.gov/wicworks/Topics/BreastfeedingFactSheet.pdf
- National Women's Health Information Center
  http://www.4woman.gov/Breastfeeding/
- Storage Guidelines for Human Milk
  http://www.guideline.gov/summary/summary.aspx?ss=15&doc_id=11225&nbr=5872

LACTATION—CITED REFERENCES

American Dietetic Association. Position of the American Dietetic Association: Promoting and Supporting Breastfeeding. *J Am Diet Assoc.* 109:1926, 2009.

Anderson JG, et al. Can prenatal N-3 fatty acid deficiency be completely reversed after birth? Effects on retinal and brain biochemistry and visual function in rhesus monkeys. *Pediatr Res.* 58:865, 2005.

Bonuck KA, et al. Randomized, controlled trial of a prenatal and postnatal lactation consultant intervention on duration and intensity of breastfeeding up to 12 months. *Pediatrics.* 116:1413, 2005.

Chung M, et al. Interventions in primary care to promote breastfeeding: an evidence review for the U.S. Preventive Services Task Force. *Ann Intern Med.* 149:565, 2008.

Friedman NJ, Zeigler RS. The role of breast-feeding in the development of allergies and asthma. *J Allergy Clin Immunol.* 115:1238, 2005.

Greer FR. 25-Hydroxyvitamin D: functional outcomes in infants and young children. *Am J Clin Nutr.* 88:592S, 2008.

Grizzard TA, et al. Policies and practices related to breastfeeding in Massachusetts: hospital implementation of the ten steps to successful breastfeeding. *Matern Child Health J.* 10:247, 2006.

Hatton DC, et al. Symptoms of postpartum depression and breastfeeding. *J Hum Lact.* 21:444, 2005.

Hay G, et al. Folate and cobalamin status in relation to breastfeeding and weaning in healthy infants. *Am J Clin Nutr.* 88:105, 2008.

Hill DJ, et al. Effect of a low-allergen maternal diet on colic among breastfed infants: a randomized, controlled trial. *Pediatrics.* 116:709, 2005.

James DC, Dobson B, American Dietetic Association. Position of the American Dietetic Association: promoting and supporting breast feeding. *J Am Diet Assoc.* 105:810, 2005.

Kovacs CS. Vitamin D in pregnancy and lactation: maternal, fetal, and neonatal outcomes from human and animal studies. *Am J Clin Nutr.* 88:520S, 2008.

Kramer MS, et al. Breastfeeding and child cognitive development. *Arch Gen Psychiatry.* 65:578, 2008.

Kramer MS, et al. A Randomized Breast-feeding Promotion Intervention did not reduce child obesity in Belarus. *J Nutr.* 139:417S, 2009.

Krogstrand KS, Parr K. Physicians ask for more problem-solving information to promote and support breastfeeding. *J Am Diet Assoc.* 105:1943, 2005.

Kull I, et al. Breast-feeding reduces the risk for childhood eczema. *J Allergy Clin Immunol.* 116:657, 2005.

Labarere J, et al. Efficacy of breastfeeding support provided by trained clinicians during an early, routine, preventive visit: a prospective, randomized, open trial of 226 mother-infant pairs. *Pediatrics.* 115:e139, 2005.

Lauritezen L, et al. Maternal fish oil supplementation in lactation: effect on developmental outcome in breast-fed infants. *Reprod Nutr Dev.* 45:535, 2005.

Lovelady CA. The impact of energy restriction and exercise in lactating women. *Adv Exp Med Biol.* 554:115, 2004.

Lovelady CA. Is maternal obesity a cause of poor lactation performance? *Nutr Rev.* 63:352, 2005.

Min Y, et al. Unfavorable effect of type 1 and type 2 diabetes on maternal and fetal essential fatty acid status: a potential marker of fetal insulin resistance. *Am J Clin Nutr.* 82:1162, 2005.

Owen CG, et al. The effect of breastfeeding on mean body mass index throughout life: a quantitative review of published and unpublished observational evidence. *Am J Clin Nutr.* 82:1298, 2005.

Rinne M, et al. Effect of probiotics and breastfeeding on the bifidobacterium and *Lactobacillus/Enterococcus* microbiota and humoral immune responses. *J Pediatr.* 147:186, 2005.

Slater M, et al. Breastfeeding in HIV-positive women: what can be recommended? *Paediatr Drugs.* 12:1, 2010.

Stewart-Glenn J. Knowledge, perceptions, and attitudes of managers, coworkers, and employed breastfeeding mothers. *AAOHN J.* 56:423, 2008.

Wojcik KY, et al. Macronutrient analysis of a nationwide sample of donor breast milk. *J Am Diet Assoc.* 109:137, 2009.

Yu Z, et al. Comparison of organochlorine compound concentrations in colostrum and mature milk. *Chemosphere.* 66:1012, 2007.

Ziol-Guest K, Hernandez DC. First- and second-trimester WIC participation is associated with lower rates of breastfeeding and early introduction of cow's milk during infancy. *J Am Diet Assoc.* 110:702, 2010.

INFANCY, CHILDHOOD, AND ADOLESCENCE

INFANT, NORMAL (0–6 MONTHS)

NUTRITIONAL ACUITY RANKING: LEVEL 1

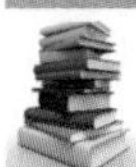

DEFINITIONS AND BACKGROUND

Normal gestation is 40 weeks. The average birth weight of an infant ranges between 5.5 and 10 lb; the average is approximately 7–7.5 lb. Healthy, full-term infants lose some weight in the first days after birth but tend to regain it within the first week. Infants often double their birth weight by 4–6 months and triple it within 1 year. For assessment of an infant, monitoring growth is the best way to evaluate intake. Head circumference increases about 40% during the first year, and brain weight should almost double.

Breastfeeding takes longer than cup or bottle feeding but has more benefits and is the preferred method. (American Dietetic Association, 2009). When breastfeeding is not possible or not desired, formula feeding is used. For formula feedings in infants with oral or developmental problems, administration times, amounts ingested, and physiological stability of infants are similar when newborn infants are fed using a bottle or a cup. Section 3 describes conditions where alternative feeding methods may be needed.

Infants are composed of approximately 75–80% water, whereas adults are composed of 60–65% water. Infants may become dehydrated easily, especially in hot weather or after bouts of diarrhea.

When infants are ill, special techniques (doubly labeled water studies or test weighing) may be used to determine intakes of breast milk.

Mineral status should be carefully assessed. Infants are born with a 4- to 6-month supply of iron if maternal stores were adequate during gestation. Anemia from severe iron deficiency (ID) is the most prevalent and widespread nutrition-related health problem in infants and young children in low-income countries (Lutter, 2008). Correcting ID anemia may prevent developmental and behavioral delays.

Calcium is another important mineral during infancy to set the stage for healthy bones. Zinc and copper may also be nutrients that are insufficient, especially in low-income populations (Schneider et al, 2007). Infants of vegan mothers may require calcium, zinc, and vitamin B_{12} supplementation (American Dietetic Association and Dietitians of Canada, 2003; Weiss et al, 2004). Another common problem in infancy is low vitamin D intake in breast milk, leading to growth failure, lethargy, irritability and rickets (Hollis and Wagner, 2004). Excesses of vitamin D should also be avoided.

The American Academy of Pediatrics supports the following practices during infancy (American Academy of Pediatrics, 2009):

- Breastfeed exclusively for the first 6 months. Supplement with vitamin D from birth and use iron supplementation as ferrous sulfate drops or iron-fortified cereal after 4 months of age. Fluoride supplementation may be required after 6 months of age, depending on the fluoride content of the city water. Feeding of iron-fortified commercial infant formula may be done for the first year as an alternative to breastfeeding.
- Delay the use of whole cow milk until after 1 year of age. Early introduction of whole cow milk protein during infancy may contribute to ID anemia by increasing gastrointestinal (GI) blood loss. Whole cow milk has an increased renal solute load compared to infant formulas.
- Reduced-fat milks should be delayed until after the second year of life. Adequate fat intake is important for the developing brain, and milk is usually the primary source of fat for infants and toddlers.
- Delay the introduction of semisolid foods until 4–6 months of age or until the infant demonstrates signs of developmental readiness, such as head control and ability to sit with support.

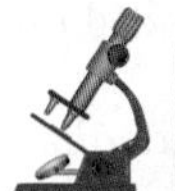

CLINICAL INDICATORS

Clinical/History		Lab Work
Birth weight	Appetite changes	H & H, serum ferritin
Birth length	No. of wet diapers in 24 hours	Glucose
Present weight for gestational age	No. of dirty diapers in 24 hours	Cholesterol
Height-weight percentile	BP	Other labs as indicated by medical exam or family history
Head circumference	Pink, firm gums	
Feeding pattern	Use of vitamins, herbs, supplements	

INTERVENTION

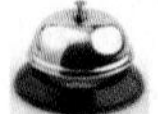

OBJECTIVES

- Promote normal growth and development: assess sleeping, eating, and attentiveness habits. Compare infant's growth to the chart of normal growth patterns. Weight for length (height) is the most meaningful measurement. Use updated Centers for Disease Control and Prevention

SAMPLE NUTRITION CARE PROCESS STEPS

Inadequate Iron Intake

Assessment Data: Food records; lab reports for H & H, serum ferritin.

Nutrition Diagnoses (PES): Inadequate mineral intake related to intake of insufficient amounts of iron-fortified formula as evidenced by mother's report of diluting formula with cow's milk for infant at 3 months of age to save money.

Intervention: Education about appropriate preparation and use of formula for infants. Referral to WIC program if eligible.

Monitoring and Evaluation: Lab reports for H & H, serum ferritin; dietary history indicating proper use of iron-fortified formula.

(CDC) growth charts and monitor growth trends, not a singular value. Chronic malnutrition results in decreased weight, then height, and then head circumference.

- Overcome any nutritional risk factors or complications, such as otitis media or dehydration.
- Evaluate use and discourage early introduction of cow's milk and solids, including gluten-containing cereals. Follow recommended guidelines for timing of introduction of new foods.
- Encourage the mother to use breast milk as the infant's main source of nutrition for the first 6 months, introducing solids and juices slowly beginning at approximately 4 months of age.
- If the infant is breastfed, assess the mother's prepregnancy nutritional status and risk factors, weight gain pattern, food allergies, and medical history (such as preeclampsia, chronic illnesses, or anemia). Discuss any current conditions that may affect lactation (e.g., smoking, use of alcohol, family history of allergies).
- If the infant is formula fed, the mother should learn about early childhood caries (ECC) prevention and about potential overfeeding problems.
- Promote growth and development through adequate fatty acid intake, especially for visual acuity.
- Effects of soy formulas on the thyroid must be monitored in infants with hypothyroidism. Iodine has been added to most infant formulas; check labels. Iodized salt has been found to be beneficial for maintaining desirable infants, especially in developing countries (Zimmerman, 2007).

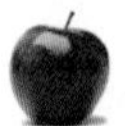

FOOD AND NUTRITION

- Fluid requirements may include the following: 60–80 mL/kg water in newborns; 80–100 mL/kg by 3 days of age; 125–150 mL/kg up to 6 months of age. Assess individual needs according to status.
- Energy needs are estimated to decrease between birth and 6 months; this can be met in about 28–32 oz of human milk or infant formula.
- Protein requirement is generally 1.52 g/kg, or about 9.1 g/d. Sick infants may need a higher ratio. Use the nutrient recommendation chart (see below).

Nutrient	Recommendation for Infants Ages 0–6 Months
Energy	570 kcal/d males; 520 kcal/d females
Protein	9.1 g/d or 1.52 g/kg/d
Calcium	210 mg/d
Iron	0.27 mg/d
Folate	65 mg/d
Phosphorus	100 mg/d
Vitamin A	400 μg
Vitamin C	40 mg
Thiamin	0.2 mg/d
Riboflavin	0.3 mg/d
Niacin	2 mg/d

Data from: Food and Nutrition Board, Institute of Medicine. *Dietary reference intakes for energy, carbohydrate, fiber, fat, fatty acids, cholesterol, protein, and amino acids (macronutrients)*. Washington, DC: National Academy Press, 2002.

- *Breastfed infants:* discourage the mother from using drugs and alcohol; limit caffeine intake to the equivalent of 2 cups of coffee per day. Breast milk yields an 80:20 whey to casein ratio and approximately 20 kcal/oz. These infants will need information on vitamin D (Casey et al, 2010), fluoride, and sometimes iron supplements (at about 3 months of age). Mothers of infants predisposed to allergies should avoid fish, cow's milk, and nuts. Teach parents about use of diluted fruit juice (perhaps apple) at 4 months of age. Introduce cow's milk only after 12 months of age.
- *Formula-fed infants*: Review type of formula, such as milk-based, soy; significant ingredients; and volume for 24 hours. No sweetened beverage or calorie-containing formula should be given in between meals or at bedtime. Warm bottles carefully because folic acid and vitamin C may be destroyed by heat. Iron-fortified formula can be used after 2–3 months (American Academy of Pediatrics, 2009). Discourage use of evaporated milk formula, which is low in vitamin C and high in protein, sodium, and potassium. Standard formulas have a 60:40 whey to casein ratio, which is desirable; they provide 20 kcal/oz. Standard formulas include Enfamil, Similac, Gerber Formula, Good Start, and other products. Fluoride supplements are needed only if the water supply provides less than 0.3 ppm, or if unfluoridated bottled water is used to prepare formula.
- Soy formulas are available for cow's milk allergies; they are fortified with zinc, iron, and carnitine. Nutramigen, Alimentum, or Pregestimil are used for complex GI problems. Nutramigen may also be used for allergies to both soy and cow's milk protein. Alimentum and Pregestimil are for malabsorption with inclusion of medium-chain triglycerides (MCT).
- Ensure that the daily requirements are being met for all nutrients for each stage of growth. When in doubt, a liquid multivitamin–mineral supplement is advisable.
- For tube-feeding, several products are available. Formula should contain 10–20% protein, 30–40% fat, and 40–60% carbohydrates.
- An elemental diet may be needed for severe protein intolerance or cow's milk allergy. Monitor carefully for hydration; do not modify nutrients because of altered osmolality. Breast milk has an osmolality of 285 mOsm/kg; formulas vary from 150 to 380 mOsm/kg. Formulas with over 400 mOsm/kg can cause diarrhea or vomiting.
- Minimal enteral feeding (MEF) protects against necrotizing entercolitis and other infection and should be started early.
- TPN may be used when the infant cannot tolerate oral or tube feedings. Include 1–2% EFAs (linoleic and linolenic acids) to prevent outcomes of deficiency, such as inadequate wound healing, growth, immunocompetence, and platelet formation.
- *Introduction of solids:* At 4–6 months, introduce plain (not mixed, sweetened, or spiced) strained or pureed baby cereals, then nonallergenic vegetables (such as carrots or green beans), and then fruits. Start with 1–2 teaspoons, and progress as appetite indicates. Try a single new item for 7–10 days to detect any signs of food allergy. The intake of solids should not decrease breast milk or formula intake to less than 32 oz daily. Avoid giving too much juice; 4–6 oz daily is sufficient.

Herbs, Botanicals, and Supplements

- Infants and children may be highly susceptible to some of the adverse effects and toxicity of herbs and botanical products because of their physiology, immature metabolic enzyme systems, and different doses for body weights.
- Most topical preparations are benign; however, garlic poultices can cause burns. Internal use of herbs containing saturated pyrrolizidine alkaloids (comfrey) should be avoided.
- Discuss the relevance of tolerable ULs from the latest dietary reference intakes of the National Academy of Sciences. These levels were set to protect adults from receiving too much of any nutrient from diet and dietary supplements; infants are especially at risk for toxicities.

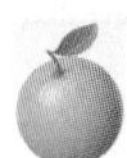

NUTRITION EDUCATION, COUNSELING, CARE MANAGEMENT

- Explain the proper timing and sequence of feeding. Discuss successful feeding as trusting and responding to cues from the infant about timing, pace, and eating capacity.
- Explain growth patterns (e.g., an infant who is 4–6 months of age should double his or her birth weight). Discuss problems related to inadequate growth.
- Emphasize the importance of adequate bonding between mother and child.
- Explain the proper care of infant's teeth, including risks of early childhood caries. Ad lib nocturnal feeding should be discontinued after the first teeth erupt. Bottle-fed infants should not be put to sleep with the bottle.
- Explain the proper timing and sequence of solid food introduction. Avoid use of stringy foods or foods such as peanut butter that are hard to swallow. Hard candies, grapes, and similar foods may increase the risk of aspiration.
- Discuss the rationale for delaying introduction of cow's milk (risks for allergy, GI bleeding).
- Discuss why fluid intake is essential; explain that infant needs are much greater (as a percentage of total body weight) than for adults. Breastfed infants usually have 4–6 soft stools each day. After the first month, they will tend to have fewer bowel movements than before; by 2 months, they have even fewer. However, a doctor should be consulted if the baby has not had a bowel movement in 3 days, or whenever diarrhea occurs.
- For resolution of special feeding problems, see Table 1-8.

Patient Education—Food Safety

- Hand washing with soap and hot water is recommended before breastfeeding or before formula preparation. Use clean utensils and containers for mixing formula. Wash the top of cans before opening.
- Before using tap water for formula preparation or to give as a beverage, let cold tap water run for 2 minutes to remove any lead that may be in the pipes.
- Well water should not be used since it may contain bacteria.
- Follow the 2-hour rule: discard any formula that has been left at room temperature for 2 hours or longer. Do not reuse.
- Avoid honey to decrease potential exposure to botulism in infancy.
- Avoid using raw or partially cooked eggs, raw or undercooked fish or shellfish, and raw or undercooked meats because of potential foodborne illnesses.
- Avoid using raw (unpasteurized) milk or products made from it.
- Avoid using unpasteurized juices and raw sprouts.

TABLE 1-8 Special Problems in Infant Feeding[a]

Allergy. Dietary exposures in pregnancy and the early postnatal period can modify gene expression and disease susceptibility. Avoidance of food allergens in infancy has provided no clear evidence in allergy prevention and is no longer recommended; focus is on their role in tolerance induction (West et al, 2010.)

Colic. Check for hunger, food allergy, incorrect formula temperature, stress, or other underlying problems. Give small, frequent feedings and parental encouragement. Colic is equally common in breastfed or formula-fed infants. If breastfed, continue to breastfeed. Rarely, removal of cow's milk products from the mother's diet is useful. If formula fed, discontinue expensive elemental formulas if symptoms do not improve. Curved bottles allow infants to be fed while they are held upright. Collapsable bags decrease swallowing of air. Infants should be burped regularly during feedings.

Constipation. The doctor will make a careful assessment and may suggest adding 1 teaspoon of a carbohydrate source to 4 oz of water or formula, one to two times daily. Avoid use of honey and corn syrup to prevent infant botulism.

Diarrhea. Replace fluids and electrolytes (e.g., Pedialyte) as directed by the doctor. After an extended period of time, have the doctor rule out allergy. Monitor weight loss and fluid intake carefully. FDA approved a vaccine (RotaTeq) to prevent rotavirus, which causes severe diarrhea and fever and dehydration in infants and results in many hospitalizations each year (Glass and Parashar, 2006).

Regurgitation. Position the infant in an upright, 40–60° position after feeding for approximately 30 minutes; have the doctor rule out other problems. Use smaller, more frequent feedings to avoid overfeeding. Use prethickened formulas if the doctor thinks it is necessary.

Pale, oily stools. Check for fat malabsorption. Use a formula containing medium-chain triglycerides if necessary.

Spitting Up or Reflux. If there is no weight loss concern, just offer encouragement that the problem will resolve in a few months. Positioning is an important consideration during feeding. Feed more slowly and burp often. Use feeding volumes and a schedule that is set. Avoid exposure to second-hand smoke. Offer parental reassurance.

[a]See also: American Dietetic Association *Pediatric manual of clinical dietetics* and *Children with special health care needs: NutritionCare handbook.*

For More Information

- Abbott Laboratories (products for infants)
  http://abbottnutrition.com/
- American Academy of Pediatrics
  http://www.aap.org/
- Bright Futures–Babies
  http://www.nal.usda.gov/wicworks/Learning_Center/BF_babies.pdf
- Centers for Disease Control and Prevention—Infants and Toddlers
  http://www.cdc.gov/LifeStages/infants_toddlers.html
- Complementary Foods
  http://www.nal.usda.gov/wicworks/Topics/infant_nut_solids.html
- Feeding Kids Newsletter
  http://www.nutritionforkids.com/Feeding_Kids.htm
- Gerber—Start Healthy, Stay Healthy
  http://www.gerber.com/Nutrition_Feeding/SHSH_Nutriton_101.aspx
- Growth Charts
  http://www.cdc.gov/nchs/about/major/nhanes/growthcharts/clinical_charts.htm
- Heinz Baby Foods
  http://www.heinzbaby.com/
- Infant Nutrition
  http://www.nal.usda.gov/fnic/etext/000106.html
- Kids Health
  http://www.kidshealth.org/
- National Perinatal Association
  http://www.nationalperinatal.org/
- National Center for Maternal and Child Health
  http://www.healthystartassoc.org/
- Nestle Very Best Kids
  http://www.verybestkids.com/
- Pediatric Nutrition Practice Group
  http://www.pediatricnutrition.org/
- Sudden Infant Death Syndrome
  http://www.sidscenter.org/
- USDA/ARS Children's Nutrition Research Center
  http://www.bcm.tmc.edu/cnrc/
- WIC Topics A-Z
  http://www.nal.usda.gov/wicworks/Topics/Infant_Nutrition.html
- World Health Organization
  http://www.who.int/child-adolescent-health/NUTRITION/infant.htm

INFANT, NORMAL (0–6 MONTHS)—CITED REFERENCES

American Academy of Pediatrics. *Pediatric nutrition handbook.* 6th ed. Chicago, IL: AAP Committee on Nutrition, 2009.

American Dietetic Association and Dietitians of Canada. Position of the American Dietetic Association: Vegetarian Diets. *J Am Diet Assoc.* 109:1266, 2009.

American Dietetic Association. Position of the American Dietetic Association: Promoting and Supporting Breastfeeding. *J Am Diet Assoc.* 109:1926, 2009.

Butte N, et al. The start healthy feeding guidelines for infants and toddlers. *J Am Diet Assoc.* 104:455, 2004.

Casey CF, et al. Vitamin D supplementation in infants, children, and adolescents. *Am Fam Phys.* 81:745, 2010.

Glass RI, Parashar UD. The promise of new rotavirus vaccines. *N Engl J Med.* 354:75, 2006.

Hollis BW, Wagner CL. Assessment of dietary vitamin D requirements during pregnancy and lactation. *Am J Clin Nutr.* 79:717, 2004.

Lutter CK. Iron deficiency in young children in low-income countries and new approaches for its prevention. *J Nutr.* 138:2523, 2008.

Schneider JM, et al. The prevalence of low serum zinc and copper levels and dietary habits associated with serum zinc and copper in 12- to 36-month-old children from low-income families at risk for iron deficiency. *J Am Diet Assoc.* 107:1924, 2007.

Weiss R, et al. Severe vitamin B_{12} deficiency in an infant associated with a maternal deficiency and a strict vegetarian diet. *J Pediatr Hematol Oncol.* 26:270, 2004.

West CE, et al. Role of diet in the development of immune tolerance in the context of allergic disease. *Curr Opin Pediatr.* 22:2010.

INFANT, NORMAL (6–12 MONTHS)

NUTRITIONAL ACUITY RANKING: LEVEL 1–2

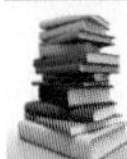

DEFINITIONS AND BACKGROUND

Infants older than 6 months of age are beginning the developmental stages that will lead to walking and talking. Many of the same principles associated with infant feeding during the first 6 months will continue with the greater use of solids. The growth pattern of breastfed and formula-fed infants differs in the first 12 months of life. The new CDC growth charts were developed with a larger proportion of breastfed infants.

Timing of the introduction of complementary foods (solids) is an important consideration. The Feeding Infants and Toddlers Study (FITS) evaluated the introduction of complementary foods into the diets of young children, and the findings show that healthcare professionals play an important role in improving feeding practices (Stang, 2006). Early introduction is considered to be at 3–4 months of age, and late introduction is considered to be at 6 months of age. Many foods that are introduced are of low nutritional value, including sweetened beverages, cookies, processed meats, cakes, and pies (Stang, 2006).

Introduction of cow's milk at 12 months of age brings new problems and risks related to EFA deficiency if low-fat or skim milks are used. Long-chain fatty acids are useful in normal growth and development of infants and young children. It is not necessary to alter the diets of infants to prevent heart disease or to lower cholesterol. Breastfed and formula-fed infants maintain a characteristic serum cholesterol ester fatty acid pattern after age 7 months even after they begin to receive solid food; breastfed infants have higher levels of arachidonic acid and DHA with better cognitive development (Daniels et al, 2004).

Growth and development at this stage are affected by underlying or acute illnesses, nutritional intake, and related factors. Breast-fed infants have a strong prevalence of bifidobacteria and lactobacilli, which stimulate formation of oligosaccharides with a protective prebiotic effect (Coppa et al, 2004). Infants who are breastfed for four months or longer also have stronger lung function (Ogbuanu et al, 2009).

Sodium and chloride intakes may be higher than desirable in infants and toddlers; delaying the introduction of cows' milk, limiting the amount of salt used in food processing and preparation, and increasing intake of fruits and vegetables are reasonable measures that can be applied (Heird et al, 2006). Overall, interventions for improving the diets of young children should focus on breastfeeding and the whole continuum of diet in order to promote healthy guidelines (Couch and Falciglia, 2006).

Lead poisoning should be monitored in growing children, especially children who live in older homes or spend time in older buildings or day care centers. Toddlers may eat lead-based paint that is chipping away from walls. Lead depletes iron and replaces calcium in the bone; deposition may be seen in x-rays of the knee, ankle, or wrist.

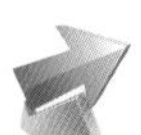

ASSESSMENT, MONITORING, AND EVALUATION

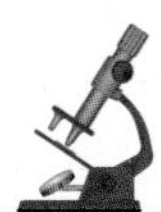

CLINICAL INDICATORS

Genetic Markers: Each individual has a unique genetic profile and phenotype. Because both parents contribute genes and chromosomes to the fetus, a genetic history may be beneficial.

Clinical/History

- Length
- Current weight
- Birth length/weight
- Percentile weight/length
- Diet/intake history
- Age in months
- Head circumference
- Developmental stage
- Tooth development
- Physical handicaps
- Appetite
- Hydration status
- Intake and output (I & O)
- Persistent vomiting
- Diarrhea

Lab Work

- Glucose
- Cholesterol
- H & H, serum ferritin

SAMPLE NUTRITION CARE PROCESS STEPS

Inadequate Energy Intake

Assessment Data: Food records; weight loss or failure to thrive on growth charts.

Nutrition Diagnoses (PES): Inadequate energy intake related to mother's withholding of formula and infant cereal when infant cries "excessively" as evidenced by intake diary and perceptions of colic.

Intervention: Education about appropriate dietary intake for age of infant. Counseling about desired foods for a healthy growth; tips for introducing new foods to the diet and for handling an infant with colic.

Monitoring and Evaluation: Weight and growth charts; successful growth for child; lab reports for H & H, serum ferritin; dietary history indicating improved variety of food choices.

INTERVENTION

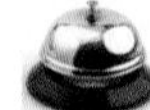

OBJECTIVES

- Continue to promote normal growth and development during this second stage of very rapid growth. Use updated CDC growth charts. Monitor trends in growth, not a singular value.
- Prevent significant weight losses from illness or inadequate feeding. Malnutrition results in decreased weight, then height, and then head circumference.
- Avoid dehydration.
- Prevent or correct such complications as diarrhea, constipation, and otitis media.
- Begin to encourage greater physical activity; prepare for walking by ensuring adequate energy intake.
- Continue to emphasize the role of good nutrition in the development of healthy teeth.
- Delay food allergens until 12 months of age (e.g., citrus, egg white, cow's milk, corn, peanut and nut butters.)
- Use of follow-up formulas with higher percentage of kilocalories from protein and carbohydrates (CHO) and less from fat have questionable benefits at this time.
- Prevent nutrient deficiencies upon weaning (e.g., zinc, iron). Iron supplementation, even during breastfeeding, may be beneficial.
- Support feeding skills and introduce solids, at appropriate periods of time, singly.

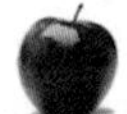

FOOD AND NUTRITION

Start Healthy Feeding Guidelines for Infants and Toddlers (Butte et al, 2004; http://www.bcm.edu/cnrc/consumer/nyc/vol_2004_3/guidelines_ADA.pdf)

- Repeated exposure to a particular food is usually necessary before it is accepted by the infant or toddler; up to 10–15 exposures may be necessary. Introduction of a variety of flavors in the first 2 years of life may lead to acceptance of a wider variety of flavors in later childhood.
- After 6 months, most breastfed infants need complementary foods to meet current recommendations (DRI) for energy, manganese, iron, fluoride, vitamin D, vitamin B_6, niacin, zinc, vitamin E, magnesium, phosphorus, biotin, and thiamin; amounts needed from complementary foods will vary depending upon the intake of human milk or formula.
- Although iron-fortified infant formula provides the recommended intakes of energy and nutrients until about 1 year of age depending on intake, all infants need complementary foods for exposure to flavors and textures as well as to master eating skills. Complementary foods such as meats and fortified cereals contribute significant amounts of iron; this is helpful in preventing deficiency, which is common in toddlers under the age of 2 years; see Table 1-9 for additional tips on feeding infants.
- Because rickets due to vitamin D deficiency has been observed recently in dark-skinned, breastfed infants and other infants without adequate sun exposure, 200 IU of vitamin D_3 is recommended as a supplement for breastfed infants and infants receiving less than 500 mL of formula

TABLE 1-9 Feeding Babies in the First Year of Life

Foods	Birth	1	2	3	4	5	6	7	8	9	10	11	12 Months
Breast milk or iron-fortified formula	Breast milk or formula				Continue breast milk or iron fortified formula								Start whole cow's milk from cup
Cereals and grain products					Iron-fortified plain infant cereal (no fruit flavor or mixed grains). Start with rice, then oatmeal or barley			Teething biscuits		Mixed grain cereals. Noodles, rice. Bread and toast strips			
Vegetables					Strained, single vegetables					Cooked vegetables, mashed or chopped		Sliced cooked vegetables for finger-feeding	
Fruit and fruit juices					Strained, single fruits			Unsweetened fruit juices		Cooked, canned, or soft fresh fruits, mashed or chopped		Sliced soft fruit for finger feeding	
Meat and other protein foods					Strained single meats. Pureed dried beans, peas. Plain yogurt					Same foods, chopped or mashed. Cottage cheese, mashed egg yolk		Same foods, bite-sized pieces for finger feeding. Creamy peanut butter	
Egg white and fish												Egg white. Tender, flaked boneless fish	

The infant's developmental readiness, age, appetite, and growth rate are factors that help determine when to feed solid foods.

Before feeding solid foods, the baby should be able to swallow and digest solid foods, sit with support and have neck and head control, and close their lips over a spoon. Semisolid foods and juices are a significant change and should not be started until 4–6 months.

Introduce single-ingredient foods one at a time; wait 5–7 days before introducing a new food. This process helps identify any food sensitivities the child might have. Offer new food when baby is in a good mood, not too tired and not too hungry. Serve solids after the baby has had a little breast milk or formula. Hold the baby on the lap or use an infant seat or feeding chair if the baby can sit. Use a baby spoon and place a small amount (about 1/2 teaspoon) of food on the baby's tongue. Give the baby time to learn to swallow these foods and get used to the new tastes.

The sequence of new foods is not critical, but rice cereal mixed with breast-milk or formula is a good first choice. Add vegetables, fruits, and meats to the infant's diet one at a time. Serving mixed foods is not recommended in the beginning.

Introduce juices when the baby can drink from a cup, around 6–9 months. Dilute adult juices half and half with water or strain them before giving to a baby. Avoid sweet drinks; they can promote tooth decay. In addition, avoid sweetened foods because they also can promote tooth decay and may cause a preference for sweets. Do not offer fruit desserts that contain unnecessary sugar.

Food can be homemade or commercially prepared Choose plain, strained fruit such as applesauce, peaches or mashed ripe bananas. Boil fruits until tender; cool; blend until there are no lumps. If it is too thick, add breast milk, baby formula or a little water. Use the same process for vegetables.

Feed the baby when he or she is hungry, but do not overfeed. Make meal time a happy time. Never force a child to finish bottles or food; watch for cues that he or she is full.

Delay introduction of the major food allergens, such as eggs, milk, wheat, soy, peanuts, tree nuts, fish, and shellfish, until well after the first year of life. Foods that are associated with lifelong sensitization (e.g., peanuts, tree nuts, and shellfish) should not be introduced until even later years.

Combination foods (instead of single-ingredient foods) may be given to older infants after tolerance for the individual components has been established.

Hungry toddlers may point at foods or beverages, ask for foods or beverages, or reach for foods. Full toddlers may slow the pace of eating, become distracted or notice surroundings more, play with food, throw food, want to leave the table or chair, and/or not eat everything on the plate. To help avoid underfeeding or overfeeding, parents and caregivers must be sensitive to the hunger and satiety cues of the healthy infant and young child.

Avoid raw carrots, nuts, seeds, raisins, grapes, popcorn, and pieces of hot dogs during baby's first year as they may cause choking.

Age-appropriate, daily physical activity in a safe, nurturing environment may help promote physical development and movement skills and teach the healthy habit of activity. Encourage parents and caregivers to promote enjoyment of movement and motor skill confidence at an early age. Fundamental motor skills (e.g., walking, running, jumping, etc.) begin to develop. When activity is encouraged, these skills can further develop into advanced patterns of motor coordination.

Television viewing should be discouraged for children under 2 years of age.

[a]Start Healthy Feeding Guidelines for Infants and Toddlers (Butte et al, 2004).

per day. Intakes of EFAs may require emphasis once breast milk or formula is replaced with cow's milk.

- Children often eat small frequent meals and snacks throughout the day, generally three regular meals and two to three appropriate, healthy snacks. Portions should provide essential nutrients but not exceed energy requirements for the child.
- Occasional picky eating, a normal stage of development, is not associated with changes in nutrient intake or height and weight. Consuming a single food or foods for extended periods of time (food jag) may require monitoring of growth more frequently if it persists for a long time.

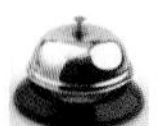

OTHER GUIDELINES

- For energy needs, the current DRI recommends about 743 kcal/d for males and 676 kcal/d for females. Monitor according to the CDC growth charts, and identify problems early.
- Continue to provide breast milk or iron-fortified formula during this stage. The presence of DHA and arachidonic acid (ARA) in human milk, along with reports of higher IQ in individuals who were breastfed versus formula fed as infants, suggest that exogenous DHA and ARA are essential for optimal development (Heird and Lapillone, 2005).
- Special milk substitutes are not necessary unless there is an allergy to soy protein or cow's milk.
- Fluid requirements may include approximately 125–150 mL/kg up to 1 year of age. Fluid needs may begin to decline slightly during this stage.
- Protein requirement for a 6-month-old infant is generally 1.5 g/kg and changes as the infant grows; this equals about 13.5 g/d. By 12 months, the need is only 1.1 g/kg. See nutrient recommendations chart:

Nutrient	Recommendation for Infants Ages 6 Months to 1 Year
Energy	743 kcal/d males; 676 kcal/d females
Protein	13.5 g/d
Calcium	270 mg/d
Iron	11 mg/d
Folate	80 mg/d
Phosphorus	275 mg/d
Vitamin A	500 μg
Vitamin C	50 mg/d
Thiamin	0.3 mg/d
Riboflavin	0.4 mg/d
Niacin	4 mg/d

Data from: Food and Nutrition Board, Institute of Medicine. *Dietary reference intakes for energy, carbohydrate, fiber, fat, fatty acids, cholesterol, protein, and amino acids (macronutrients)*. Washington, DC: National Academy Press, 2002.

- Avoid raw vegetables and fruits (other than ripe banana or soft, peeled apple). Beware of foods that may cause choking (e.g., hot dogs, popcorn, nuts, grapes, seeds) because toddlers do not have molars for proper chewing (Morley et al, 2004).
- As tolerated, introduce coarsely ground table foods by 10–12 months of age.
- Introduce cow's milk at 12 months of age, ensuring that intake does not go above 1 quart daily to prevent anemia. Use whole milk to include sufficient access to fatty acids.
- Begin to offer fluids by cup at approximately 9–12 months of age; weaning often occurs by about 1 year of age. Avoid sweetened beverages at this age whenever possible.
- Spicy foods often are not liked or not tolerated. Taste buds are very acute at this stage. This is also affected by culture and the seasoning of foods that are introduced.
- Continue use of iron-fortified baby cereal after 12 months of age to ensure adequate intake. Approximately 10 mg of iron is required. WIC-approved cereals are iron fortified. Adult cereals often are inappropriate for infants and children younger than 4 years of age.
- Discourage use of low-density, high-energy foods such as carbonated beverages, French fries, candy, and other sweets.
- Generally, healthy infants and toddlers can achieve recommended levels of intake from food alone; use foods rather than supplements as the primary source of nutrients for children (Briefel et al, 2006). When indicated, vitamin-mineral supplements can help infants and toddlers with special nutrient needs or marginal intakes. However, avoid excessive intakes of vitamin A, zinc, and folate, which are commonly fortified in the food supply (Briefel et al, 2006).
- Children who require tube feeding require specialty care. If the infant needs a tube feeding (e.g., for poor weight gain, low volitional intake, 5th percentile or lower for weight for height and age, slow and prolonged feeding times over 4–6 hours because of oral/motor problems), a standard isotonic tube feeding formula that provides 30 kcal/oz of intact proteins may be used. If necessary, lactose-free and gluten-free formulas are available. Added fiber and a mix of long- and medium-chain fatty acids may be useful. Osmolality of 260–650 mOsm/kg is common; monitor tolerances regularly. Be sure to use sufficient water. The infant may tolerate bolus feedings in the day and continuous feedings at night.

Common Drugs Used and Potential Side Effects

- Drugs and medications used for infants should be prescribed only by a physician.

Herbs, Botanicals, and Supplements

- Infants and children may be even more susceptible to some of the adverse effects and toxicity of these products because of differences in physiology, immature metabolic enzyme systems, and dose per body weight.
- Herbs and botanical supplements should not be used without discussing with the physician. In general, these types of supplements have not been proven to be safe for infants.
- Discuss the relevance of tolerable ULs from the latest dietary reference intakes of the National Academy of Sciences. These levels were set to protect adults from receiving

too much of any nutrient from diet and dietary supplements; infants are even more at risk for toxicities.

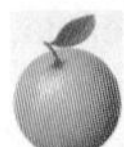

NUTRITION EDUCATION, COUNSELING, CARE MANAGEMENT

- Early childhood is a critical time for development of appropriate food choices and eating habits, which are complex processes for parents to understand (Stang, 2006).
- Discuss adequate weight pattern: infants generally double or triple birth weight by 12 months of age; body length increases by about 55%; head circumference increases by about 40%; and brain weight doubles.
- Discuss the healthy guidelines that are available.
- For lunches at home, parents will need suggestions about appropriate and easy to serve foods, homemade or commercial, for toddler lunches and snacks (Ziegler et al, 2006).
- Special attention should be given to counsel mothers who are single, whose child is in day care, whose education or literacy is limited, or who are enrolled in the Special Supplemental Nutrition Program for Women, Infants, and Children (Hendricks et al, 2006).
- Assure parents and caregivers that, while infants and toddlers have an innate ability to regulate energy intake, there is potential for environmental cues to diminish natural hunger-driven eating behaviors, even among young toddlers (Fox et al, 2006). Overfeeding may result if children are not taught to recognize their natural cues about hunger and satiety.
- Encourage consumption of milk at home and other locations, such as restaurants and friends' homes, in place of fruit-flavored drinks or other sweetened beverages (Ziegler et al, 2006).
- All day care providers should be encouraged to use menu planning aids, such as those available from the U.S. Department of Agriculture (Ziegler et al, 2006).
- Discuss iron intake, fluid intake, and other nutritional factors related to normal growth and development, including calcium for bone health.
- Plan toddler snacks to complement meals by including additional fruits, vegetables, and whole grains that are culturally appropriate rather than fruit drinks, cookies, and crackers; this will increase fiber intake and limit fat and sugar intakes (Ziegler et al, 2006).
- To develop healthful eating patterns, introduce toddlers to foods 8 to 10 times to increase food acceptance and the likelihood of establishing healthful eating patterns (Ziegler et al, 2006).
- Discuss the role of fat-soluble vitamins, their presence in whole milk, and the role of EFAs in normal growth and development of the nervous system.
- Bottled waters are not a substitute for formula. Hyponatremia may result.
- Fluoridated water is recommended; check the community status. Fluoride supplements are not needed when the water supply is fluoridated and the infant receives adequate water from this source. Note that well water and most bottled waters are not fluoridated; supplementation should be discussed with the physician.
- When brushing teeth, be carefully not to use a large amount of fluoridated toothpaste. A very small amount suffices.
- For planning vegan diets in infancy, breast milk should be the sole food, with soy-based formula as an alternative. Breastfed vegan infants may need supplements of vitamin B_{12}, zinc, and vitamin D. Protein sources for older vegan infants may include tofu and dried beans.
- Intensive nutrition education can help mothers provide more effective feeding practices. This is especially important in developing countries where inappropriate feeding, poor hygiene, and poor health often lead infants to a malnourished state (Roy et al, 2007).

Patient Education—Food Safety

- Hand washing with soap and hot water is recommended before breastfeeding or before formula preparation. Use clean utensils and containers for mixing formula. Wash the top of the can before opening.
- Before using tap water for formula preparation or to give as a beverage, let cold tap water run for 2 minutes to remove any lead that may be in the pipes.
- Well water should not be used since it may contain bacteria.
- Follow the 2-hour rule: discard any formula, beverage, or food that has been left at room temperature for 2 hours or longer. Do not reuse.
- Do not use honey in the diets of infants to decrease potential exposure to botulism.
- Avoid using raw or partially cooked eggs, raw or undercooked fish or shellfish, and raw or undercooked meats because of potential foodborne illnesses.
- Do not use raw (unpasteurized) milk or products made from it.
- Avoid using unpasteurized juices and raw sprouts.
- For hospital preparation of infant formula, use available guidelines.

For More Information

- Abbott Laboratories (products for infants)
  http://abbottnutrition.com/
- American Academy of Pediatrics
  http://www.aap.org/
- Bright Futures–Babies
  http://www.nal.usda.gov/wicworks/Learning_Center/BF_babies.pdf
- Centers for Disease Control and Prevention—Infants and Toddlers
  http://www.cdc.gov/LifeStages/infants_toddlers.html
- Complementary Foods
  http://www.nal.usda.gov/wicworks/Topics/infant_nut_solids.html
- Feeding Kids Newsletter
  http://www.nutritionforkids.com/Feeding_Kids.htm
- Gerber—Start Healthy, Stay Healthy
  http://www.gerber.com/Nutrition_Feeding/SHSH_Nutriton_101.aspx
- Growth Charts
  http://www.cdc.gov/nchs/about/major/nhanes/growthcharts/clinical_charts.htm
- Heinz Baby Foods
  http://www.heinzbaby.com/
- Infant Nutrition
  http://www.nal.usda.gov/fnic/etext/000106.html
- Kids Health
  http://www.kidshealth.org/
- Medline Plus
  http://www.nlm.nih.gov/medlineplus/infantandtoddlernutrition.html

- National Center for Maternal and Child Health
  http://www.healthystartassoc.org/
- Nestle Very Best Kids
  http://www.verybestkids.com/
- Pediatric Nutrition Practice Group
  http://www.pediatricnutrition.org/
- USDA/ARS Children's Nutrition Research Center
  http://www.bcm.tmc.edu/cnrc/
- WIC Topics A-Z
  http://www.nal.usda.gov/wicworks/Topics/Infant_Nutrition.html
- World Health Organization
  http://www.who.int/child-adolescent-health/NUTRITION/infant.htm

INFANT, NORMAL (6–12 MONTHS)—CITED REFERENCES

Briefel R, et al. Feeding infants and toddlers study: do vitamin and mineral supplements contribute to nutrient adequacy or excess among US infants and toddlers? *J Am Diet Assoc.* 106:52S, 2006.

Butte NF, et al. The start healthy feeding guidelines for infants and toddlers. *J Am Diet Assoc.* 104:442, 2004.

Coppa GV, et al. The first prebiotics in humans: human milk oligosaccharides. *J Clin Gastroenterol.* 38:S80, 2004.

Couch SC, Falciglia GA. Improving the diets of the young: considerations for intervention design. *J Am Diet Assoc.* 106:10S, 2006.

Daniels JL, et al. Fish intake during pregnancy and early cognitive development of offspring. *Epidemiology.* 15:394, 2004.

Fox MK, et al. Relationship between portion size and energy intake among infants and toddlers: evidence of self-regulation. *J Am Diet Assoc.* 106:77S, 2006.

Heird WC, et al. Current electrolyte intakes of infants and toddlers. *J Am Diet Assoc.* 106:43S, 2006.

Heird WC, Lapillone A. The role of essential fatty acids in development. *Annu Rev Nutr.* 25:549, 2005.

Hendricks K, et al. Maternal and child characteristics associated with infant and toddler feeding practices. *J Am Diet Assoc.* 106:135S, 2006.

Morley RE, et al. Foreign body aspiration in infants and toddlers: recent trends in British Columbia. *J Otolaryngol.* 33:37, 2004.

Ogbuanu IU, et al. Effect of breastfeeding duration on lung function at age 10 years: a prospective birth cohort study. *Thorax.* 64:62, 2009.

Pac S, et al. Development of the start healthy feeding guidelines for infants and toddlers. *J Am Diet Assoc.* 104:455, 2004.

Roy SK, et al. Prevention of malnutrition among young children in rural Bangladesh by a food-health-care educational intervention: a randomized, controlled trial. *Food Nutr Bull.* 28:375, 2007.

Stang J. Improving the eating patterns of infants and toddlers. *J Am Diet Assoc.* 106:7S, 2006.

Ziegler P, et al. Nutrient intakes and food patterns of toddlers' lunches and snacks: influence of location. *J Am Diet Assoc.* 106:124S, 2006a.

Ziegler P, et al. Feeding infants and toddlers study: meal and snack intakes of Hispanic and non-Hispanic infants and toddlers. *J Am Diet Assoc.* 106: 107S, 2006b.

Zimmerman MB. The impact of iodized salt or iodine supplements on iodine status during pregnancy, lactation and infancy. *Public Health Nutr.* 10;1584, 2007.

CHILDHOOD

NUTRITIONAL ACUITY RANKING: LEVEL 1–2

DEFINITIONS AND BACKGROUND

The American Dietetic Association (2008) has taken the position that children between the ages of 2 and 11 years should have appropriate eating habits so they can achieve optimal physical and cognitive development, a healthy weight, enjoyment of their meals, and reduction of the risk for chronic disease.

While children are not "little adults" and should be treated individually, conversation with an adult is usually required to discuss actual food intake by a child. The ability to recall by children is often limited because of vocabulary and attention span. Children benefit from training, such as with pictures, food models and cups.

Growth during this stage involves changes in appetite, physical activity, and frequency of illnesses. The CDC growth charts provide a guideline for monitoring successful growth related to weight, height, and age. Body mass index (BMI) calculations are now available for use with children, and calculations may be used to identify underweight, potential stunting, or obesity. Prevalence of low height for age (stunting) low weight for age (wasting) and health issues can be higher than desirable.

During the early years of life, eating occurs primarily as a result of hunger and satiety cues. Evidence suggests that, by the time children are 3 or 4 years of age, eating is no longer driven by real hunger but is influenced by a variety of environmental factors, including presentation of larger portions (Rolls et al, 2000) and parenting behaviors. Girls with mothers who are dieting have more ideas about dieting than girls with moms who do not diet (Abramovitz and Birch, 2000).

Children from underserved population groups may have increased risk for obesity, increased serum lipids, and poor dietary consumption patterns of dairy products, fruits, and vegetables. In the past few decades, children's dietary intakes have changed dramatically, and children are eating more meals away from home (Nicklas et al, 2004). Children are becoming more overweight and less active, often from physical inactivity and intake of energy-rich, nutrient-poor foods (American Dietetic Association, 2008). Intake of foods that are less healthful than desired (such as sugar-sweetened beverages, high-fat foods, and refined carbohydrates) plays a role in displacing nutrient-dense foods and can contribute to the risk of childhood obesity, type 2 diabetes, and adult chronic diseases (Stroehla et al, 2005). See Section 3 for childhood obesity and Section 9 for type 2 diabetes in children.

Many children live in poverty; some may be exposed to lead poisoning, others risk ID anemia. The preschool period (1–5 years of age) is a time of rapid and dramatic postnatal brain development, neural plasticity, and of fundamental acquisition of cognitive development such as working memory, attention and inhibitory control (Rosales et al, 2009). Because even mild undernutrition affects brain growth and function, food assistance programs should be used whenever possible. Children need nutritious snacks to eliminate transient hunger. Attention is easily diverted at this age; total intake may vary from day to day. Scheduling of lunch after physical activity encourages greater intake of all foods and energy.

Misconceptions must be corrected, such as "good foods/bad foods" or "foods that are good for you taste bad." Dietary fat restriction may compromise growth and should not be implemented. There is no proof of long-term safety and efficacy for restricting fat in children's diets; lowered calcium, zinc, magnesium, phosphorus, vitamins E and B_{12}, thiamin, niacin, and riboflavin intakes can be a problem.

The National Academy of Sciences recommends adequate dietary intake of calcium for the development of peak bone mass and prevention of fractures and osteoporosis later in life (Food and Nutrition Board, 2002). The current recommended adequate intake for children 9–18 years of age is 1300 mg/d, based on calcium-balance studies that show that, in healthy children of this age, maximal net calcium balance is achieved with this intake (Food and Nutrition Board, 2002).

Adequate calcium and vitamin D are essential during growth and into puberty, especially during rapid bone growth and mineralization. Current mean dietary intakes are below desired levels; families may need information (Greer and Krebs, 2006). Dietary calcium needs of children who take medications that alter bone metabolism are likely higher than usual.

Infectious diseases of childhood may be related to poor nutrition, especially lack of vitamin C, zinc, and vitamin A (Long et al, 2007). Children who are prone to repetitive illness may benefit from a basic multivitamin–mineral supplement in addition to a carefully planned diet. ID is another major concern in young children (Skalicky et al, 2006). Participation in WIC programs may be helpful (Altucher et al, 2005). Children should have access to an adequate supply of healthful and safe foods that promote optimal physical, cognitive, and social growth and development; nutrition assistance programs play a vital role (American Dietetic Association, 2010).

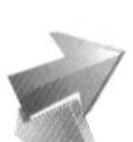

ASSESSMENT, MONITORING, AND EVALUATION

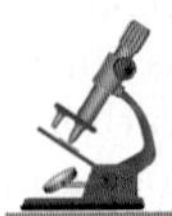

CLINICAL INDICATORS

Genetic Markers: Each individual has a unique genetic profile and phenotype. Because both parents contribute genes and chromosomes to the fetus, a genetic history may be beneficial.

Clinical/History

- Age
- Weight
- Height
- Growth percentile for age
- Diet/intake history
- Dental status
- Physical handicaps
- Appetite
- Hydration (I & O)
- Triceps skinfold (TSF)
- Midarm muscle circumference (MAMC), midarm circumference (MAC)

Lab Work

- Glucose
- H & H, serum Fe
- Chol, Trig (check family history for risks)
- Homocysteine
- Alk phos
- Ca^{++}
- Alb (if needed)

INTERVENTION

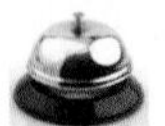

OBJECTIVES

- Assess growth patterns, feeding skills, dietary intake, activity patterns, inherited factors, and cognitive development. Promote adequate growth and development patterns such as increased independence at 12–18 months (stop bottle, begin eating with a spoon) and growth slowdown from 18 months to 2 years (less interest in food, begin eating with utensils); energy intake varies from 2 to 3 years (control exerted), and brain growth triples by age 6.

SAMPLE NUTRITION CARE PROCESS STEPS

Lead Poisoning in Childhood

Assessment Data: Dietary recall; labs such as H & H, serum ferritin, and serum lead levels; growth charts.

Nutrition Diagnosis (PES): Excessive bioactive substance intake related to lead consumption from lead-based paint exposure in environment as evidenced by high serum lead levels, documented ID anemia, and deposition seen on x-rays.

Intervention: Education and counseling tips on avoiding accidental lead intake; increasing sources of iron and calcium in the diet; tips on reducing environmental lead sources; running water awhile before drinking.

Monitoring and Evaluation: Reduced intake of sources of lead; improved lab values, improved weight gain on growth grid; successful growth and development.

Limited Fruit-Vegetable Consumption

Assessment Data: Dietary recall; growth charts; physical signs of malnutrition.

Nutrition Diagnosis (PES): Inadequate vitamin intake (vitamin C) related to minimal consumption of fruits and vegetables as evidenced by diet history, no use of children's vitamins or fortified foods, and signs of bleeding gums, petechiae, irritability, and easy bruising.

Intervention: Education and counseling tips on improving intake of fruits and vegetables; recipes and tips for increasing citrus fruits and good sources of vitamin C in foods well accepted by children. Referral to WIC program if eligible.

Monitoring and Evaluation: Improved signs of nutrition and resolution of bleeding gums, etc; diet history and mother's description of improved vitamin C intake and financial assistance from WIC.

- Avoid food deprivation, which may decrease ability to concentrate, cause growth failure or anemia, aggravate stunting, and lead to easy fatigue.
- Monitor long-term drug therapies and related side effects, such as use of anticonvulsants and the effects on folate, vitamin D and growth.
- Assess nutritional deficiencies, especially iron. If possible, detect and correct pica (eating nonfood items or any one food to the exclusion of others—even ice chips). Prevent "milk anemia" from drinking too much milk with meals and not consuming enough iron-rich meats, grains, and vegetables.
- Evaluate status of the child's dental health. Prevent dental decay.
- Support adequate nutritional immunity through a balanced diet; encourage vaccinations to prevent infectious diseases such as measles, mumps, and tetanus.
- Promote adequate intake of calcium, vitamin D, fiber, and zinc, which are nutrients that are often poorly consumed by young children.
- Help reduce onset of chronic diseases later in life by prudent menu planning and meal intakes. Early lesions of atherosclerosis begin in childhood; diet, obesity, exercise, and certain inherited dyslipidemias influence progression of such lesions (American Heart Association, 2006; Holmes and Kwiterovich, 2005). Good nutrition, a physically active lifestyle, and absence of tobacco use can delay or prevent the onset of cardiovascular disease (American Heart Association, 2006).
- Avoid mislabeling overweight children as "fat," which may trigger eating disorders (EDs) later. All providers should be aware of the problems of childhood obesity and refer accordingly. See entry in the text about childhood obesity.
- To promote proper growth, especially for stature, parents and caretakers should limit sweetened beverage intake to 12 fl oz/d; fruit juice should be only 4–6 oz daily for proper dental health and to prevent diarrhea. Encourage sufficient calcium intake from dairy beverages.
- Emphasize food variety to reduce fear of new foods (neophobia), which may reduce nutritional status. Introduction of many new foods and flavors before age 4 may be an important way to enhance children's acceptance of new food items (Nicklas et al, 2005).

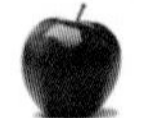

FOOD AND NUTRITION

- Energy and nutrient requirements vary by age and sex; see charts below.

	Recommendation		
Nutrient	**Ages 1–3 Years**	**Ages 4–8 Years**	**Ages 9–13 Years**
Energy	1046 kcal/d	1742 kcal/d	2279 kcal/d males; 2071 females
Protein	13 g/d or 1.1 g/kg	19 g/d or 0.95 g/kg	34 g/d or 0.95 g/kg
Calcium	500 mg/d	800 mg/d	1300 mg/d
Iron	7 mg/d	10 mg/d	8 mg/d
Folate	150 μg/d	200 μg/d	300 μg/d
Phosphorus	460 mg/d	500 mg/d	1250 mg/d
Vitamin A	300 μg	400 μg	600 μg
Vitamin C	15 mg/d	25 mg/d	45 mg/d
Thiamin	0.5 mg/d	0.6 mg/d	0.9 mg/d
Riboflavin	0.5 mg/d	0.6 mg/d	0.9 mg/d
Niacin	6 mg/d	8 mg/d	12 mg/d
Fiber	19 g	25 g	26 g females; 31 g males
Sodium	<1500 mg	<1900 mg	<2200 mg
Potassium	3000 mg	3800 mg	4500 mg

Data adapted from: A Report of the Panel on Macronutrients, Subcommittees on Upper Reference Levels of Nutrients and Interpretation and Uses of Dietary Reference Intakes, and the Standing Committee on the Scientific Evaluation of Dietary Reference Intakes; Food and Nutrition Board; and Institute or Medicine. *Dietary reference intakes for energy, carbohydrate, fiber, fat, fatty acids, cholesterol, protein, and amino acids.* Washington, DC: The National Academies Press, 2005:1357.

- The American Dietetic Association (2008) supports the following macronutrient distribution:

Carbohydrates—45–65% of total calories. Added sugars should not exceed 25% of total calories (to ensure sufficient intake of essential micronutrients).

Fat—30–40% of energy for 1–3 years and 25–35% of energy for 4–18 years.

Protein—5–20% for young children and 10–30% for older children. Include protein foods with 50% high biological value when possible.

- The American Heart Association and the American Academy of Pediatrics support portion control and energy intake as shown in Table 1-10. Where there is evidence or high risk for cardiovascular disease, start with a diet low

TABLE 1-10 Daily Estimated Calories and Recommended Servings in Children and Teens

	1 Year	2–3 Years	4–8 Years	9–13 Years	14–18 Years
Kilocalories[a]					
Female	900	1000	1200	1600	1800
Male	900	1000	1400	1800	2200
Fat,% of total kcal	30–40	30–35	25–35	25–35	25–35
Milk/dairy, cups[b]	2[c]	2	2	3	3
Lean meat/beans, oz	1.5	2		5	
Female			3		5
Male			4		6
Fruits, cups[d]	1	1	1.5	1.5	
Female					1.5
Male					2
Vegetables, cups[d]	3/4	1			
Female			1	2	2.5
Male			1.5	2.5	3
Grains, oz[e]	2	3			
Female			4	5	6
Male			5	6	7

Calorie estimates are based on a sedentary lifestyle. Increased physical activity will require additional calories: increase of 0–200 kcal/d if moderately physically active and increase of 200–400 kcal/d if very physically active.

[a]For child 2 years and older; adapted from Tables 2 and 3 and Appendix A-2 in U.S. Department of Health and Human Services, U.S. Department of Agriculture. *Dietary guidelines for Americans*. 6th ed. Washington, DC: U.S. Government Printing Office, 2005; www.healthierus.gov/dietaryguidelines. Nutrient and energy contributions from each group are calculated according to the nutrient-dense forms of food in each group (e.g., lean meats and fat-free milk).

[b]Milk listed is fat free (except for children under the age of 2 years). If 1%, 2%, or whole-fat milk is substituted, this will use, for each cup, 19, 39, or 63 kcal of discretionary calories and add 2.6, 5.1, or 9.0 g of total fat, of which 1.3, 2.6, or 4.6 g are saturated fat, respectively.

[c]For 1-year-old children, calculations are based on 2% fat milk. If 2 cups of whole milk are substituted, 48 kcal of discretionary calories will be utilized. The American Academy of Pediatrics recommends that low-fat/reduced-fat milk not be started before 2 years of age.

[d]Serving sizes are 1/4 cup for 1 year of age, 1/3 cup for 2–3 years of age, and 1/2 cup for ≥4 years of age. A variety of vegetables should be selected from each subgroup over the week.

[e]Half of all grains should be whole grains.

Sources: American Heart Association, 2006, and Pediatrics Web site, http://pediatrics.aappublications.org/cgi/content/full/117/2/544/T3; accessed February 2, 2009.

in total and saturated fat, trans fats, and cholesterol; use water-soluble fiber and plant sterols; promote weight control and exercise (Holmes and Kwiterovich, 2005). For example, select lower fat foods, use low-fat cooking techniques, spread jelly on bread instead of butter.

- Offer calcium to increase mineral density. Yogurt, plain or flavored milks, calcium-fortified juices or soy milk, soft-serve ice cream, and cheeses are generally well accepted by children. If dairy foods are not used, include foods such as 1 oz of cooked dried beans (161 mg), 10 figs (169 mg), spinach (120 mg), 1 packet of oatmeal (100 mg), 1 medium orange (50 mg), 1/2 cup of mashed sweet potato (44 mg), or 1/2 cup of cooked broccoli (35 mg).
- Phosphorus intake should be relatively similar to calcium intake.
- Give 50–60 mL/kg of fluids daily. Milk, fruit juice, vegetable juices, and water should be the basic fluids offered. Cut out carbonated beverages as much as possible.
- Encourage exposure to sunlight and monitor dietary intake of vitamin D. Adequate folate, magnesium, selenium, and vitamin E are important to obtain from dietary sources.
- Day care meals given for a 4- to 8-hour stay should provide for one third to one half of daily needs. School lunch programs generally provide one third of daily needs. Meals at home should be planned carefully to make up the difference.
- Fiber from fruits, vegetables, grains, and legumes may help to prevent or alleviate constipation. Ensure that adequate fluid is consumed each day.

Common Drugs Used and Potential Side Effects

- Anticonvulsants may cause problems with the child's growth and normal body functions. Diet should be adjusted carefully, such as increasing intake of folate.
- Corticosteroids may cause growth stunting if given over an extended time in large doses.
- Drug therapy with inhibitors of hydroxymethylglutaryl CoA reductase, bile acid sequestrants, and cholesterol absorption inhibitors may be considered in those with a positive family history of premature coronary artery disease and a low-density lipoprotein (LDL) cholesterol level above 160 mg/dL after dietary and lifestyle changes (Holmes and Kwiterovich, 2005).
- Nutritional supplements should be taken only when prescribed by a physician, although over-the-counter use is

common. Avoid serving cereals to children that fulfill the adult RDAs for vitamins and minerals. Poly-Vi-Fluor contains fluoride; use caution in areas where water is fluoridated. Too much can cause fluorosis.
- Stimulants such as methylphenidate (Ritalin) or dextroamphetamine (Dexedrine) work on dopamine levels and may cause anorexia, growth stunting, nausea, stomach pain, or weight loss; use frequent snacks. Strattera (atomoxetine) works on norepinephrine; it may also decrease appetite.
- Tofranil (imipramine,) used for bedwetting, can cause dry mouth. Include adequate liquids.

Herbs, Botanicals, and Supplements

- Herbs and botanical supplements have not been proven to be safe for children. While not needed or desirable, use of nutrient supplements is common in the first 2 years of life (Eichenberger Gilmore et al, 2005).
- Discuss the relevance of tolerable ULs from the dietary reference intakes of the National Academy of Sciences. These levels were set to protect individuals from receiving too much of any nutrient from diet and dietary supplements.
- Children are more prone to toxicity than adults. For example, jinbuhuan causes bradycardia and CNS and respiratory depression and is to be avoided in children; fenugreek may trigger asthma in susceptible individuals.

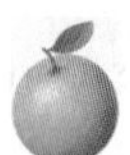

NUTRITION EDUCATION, COUNSELING, CARE MANAGEMENT

- Children should be treated respectfully. Converse with the child and not only with parents or caregivers. A personalized conversation elicits the most effective response. Review Erikson's developmental phases of childhood (1963): toddlers 1–3 years of age want autonomy; preschoolers 4–6 years of age seek initiative; and school-age children (6–12 years of age) are industrious. Age-appropriate games, projects, or tasks help in learning nutrition concepts.
- Explain the age-appropriate diet for children. Encourage parents to use finger foods for toddlers. Young children have food jags, and they often prefer single foods. Older children need nutritious snacks such as cheese cubes and iron-rich desserts. Avoid use of high-energy foods with low nutrient value.
- Encourage a relaxed atmosphere at mealtime, without pressure to eat, hurry, or finish meals. Bribery or rewards for eating should not be used; rewards can actually decrease acceptance. Parents must not "control" meals or foods; disordered eating may result.
- Education is needed to support optimal nutrition and physical activity; see Table 1-11 (American Heart Association, 2006).
- With toddlers, continue use of iron-fortified cereal and juices that are naturally high in vitamin C.
- Children should be allowed to vary in their food acceptance, choices, and intake. An authoritative feeding style is generally more effective than an authoritarian style (Patrick et al, 2005).
- Proper atmosphere is important to children since their eating patterns are strongly influenced by both the physical and social environment. Children are more likely to eat foods that are available and easily accessible; they tend to eat greater quantities when larger portions are provided; and structured family mealtimes are important (Patrick and Nicklas, 2005).
- Many children skip breakfast each day. Discuss the importance of eating breakfast for enhancing the abilities to concentrate, learn, and retain new information. Breakfasts should contain a variety of foods, with high-fiber and nutrient-rich whole grains, fruits, and dairy products (Rampersaud et al, 2005).
- Promote healthy meals at school. School-aged children need adequate meals and snacks to eliminate transient hunger. Recess before lunch is a good way to increase intake.
- Both school and the community have a shared responsibility to provide students with high-quality foods and school-based nutrition services (American Dietetic Association, 2006). Establish at least one "champion" for nutrition issues at school (e.g., a parent, the principal, the foodservice manager), and promote teamwork (Making It Happen, 2009). Standards should allow children to have access to nutritious choices.
- Knowledge and training are needed to improve food consumption patterns as children consume foods away from home and as they take on greater responsibility for meal preparation and food selection.
- Zinc absorption is improved when consumed with dairy products (Baylor, 2009).
- Vegan children should be encouraged to consume adequate sources of vitamin B_{12}, riboflavin, zinc, and calcium, and vitamin D if sun exposure is not adequate.
- Children who have chronic illnesses fare better if parents give them responsibilities, such as meal planning and taking their own medications. Tasks should be age appropriate. Section 3 addresses pediatric illnesses in greater detail.
- Nutrition education targeting low-income African–American parents should address planning and preparing convenient and economical meals and snacks that include fruits and vegetables using social support strategies (Hildebrand and Shriver, 2010).
- Specific considerations about lead poisoning and measles are found in Table 1-12.
- Adult diseases often have a fetal or childhood onset. Childhood height, growth, diet and BMI have been associated with breast cancer later in life (Ruder et al, 2008). Size at birth, rapid weight gain, and childhood growth patterns affect the onset of type 2 diabetes (Dunger et al, 2007). Elevations in homocysteine levels begin in childhood and have implications for stroke and heart disease (Kerr et al, 2009).
- A dramatic increase in childhood obesity is related to many things, including decreased physical activity and fitness. Too much time in front of the television or computer results in low energy expenditure. Promote healthy forms of activity; the USDA Kids' Activity MyPyramid Food Guidance System is a useful guide. Table 1-13 provides suggestions for increasing physical activity.

TABLE 1-11 General Dietary Recommendations for Children Aged 2 years and Older

Balance dietary calories with physical activity to maintain normal growth.

Get 60 minutes of moderate to vigorous play or physical activity daily.

Use fresh, frozen, and canned vegetables and fruits and serve at every meal.

Limit high-calorie sauces such as Alfredo sauce, cream sauces, cheese sauces, and hollandaise.

Use canola, soybean, corn, safflower, or olive oils in place of solid fats during food preparation.

Reduce the intake of sugar-sweetened beverages and foods. Limit juice intake to 1–2 servings.

Use nonfat (skim) or low-fat milk and dairy products daily.

Remove the skin from poultry before eating.

Use only lean cuts of meat and reduced-fat meat products.

Introduce and regularly serve fish as an entree, especially oily fish, broiled, or baked.

Use recommended portion sizes on food labels when preparing and serving food.

Eat whole-grain breads and cereals rather than refined products; read labels and ensure "whole grain" as the first ingredient on the food label (Thane et al, 2005).

Eat more legumes (beans) and tofu in place of meat several times a week.

Reduce salt intake, including salt from processed foods (breads, breakfast cereals, soups).

Read food labels and choose high-fiber, low-salt/low-sugar alternatives.

Patient Education—Food Safety

- Children should be taught to wash their hands before eating and after use of the toilet, sneezing, etc., to prevent foodborne illness and the spread of various infections.
- Children can be taught to avoid food and beverages that have an unusual flavor or odor.
- Avoid raw or partially cooked eggs, raw or undercooked fish or shellfish, and raw or undercooked meats because of potential foodborne illnesses.
- Five of the most commonly eaten varieties of fish are low in mercury (shrimp, canned light tuna, salmon, pollack, and catfish); AHA continues to recommend two servings of fish weekly (American Heart Association, 2006).

TABLE 1-13 Tips for Encouraging Children to Enjoy Nutrition and Physical Activity

Children should be empowered to make food choices that reflect the Dietary Guidelines for Americans.

Good nutrition and physical activity are essential to children's health and educational success.

School meals that meet the Dietary Guidelines for Americans should appeal to children and taste good.

Programs must build upon the best science, education, communication, and technical resources available.

School, parent, and community teamwork is essential to encouraging children to make food and physical activity choices for a healthy lifestyle.

Messages to children should be age appropriate and delivered in a language they speak, through media they use, and in ways that are entertaining and actively involve them in learning.

Focus on positive messages regarding the food choices children can make.

Support education and action at national, state, and local levels to improve children's eating behaviors.

Source: USDA Team Nutrition, http://www.fns.usda.gov/tn; accessed January 31, 2009.

- Do not use raw (unpasteurized) milk or products made from it.
- Avoid serving unpasteurized juices and raw sprouts.
- Only serve certain deli meats and frankfurters that have been reheated to steaming hot temperature.
- Child care centers should follow guidelines for safe food handling and for inclusion of nutritious meals and snacks (American Dietetic Association, 2010). A safe and sanitary setting is needed.

For More Information

- Activity Pyramid for Children http://extension.missouri.edu/explorepdf/hesguide/foodnut/n00386.pdf
- American Academy of Pediatrics http://www.aap.org/
- American Dietetic Association http://www.eatright.org
- American Dietetic Association—Fact sheets http://www.eatright.org/cps/rde/xchg/ada/hs.xsl/nutrition_350_ENU_HTML.htm
- American School Foodservice Association http://www.asfsa.org/

TABLE 1-12 Special Considerations in Children: Lead Poisoning and Measles

Lead Poisoning: Lead poisoning is the most common environmental health problem affecting American children. Exposure occurs through ingestion of lead-contaminated household dust and soil in older housing containing lead-based paint. Lead replaces calcium in the bone; deposition may be seen in x-rays of the knee, ankle, or wrist. Anemia may also occur. Lead is also a confirmed neurotoxicant; lower arithmetic scores, reading scores, nonverbal reasoning, and short-term memory deficits occur. Nutritional interventions suggest regular meals with adequate amounts of calcium, and iron supplementation. Parents need education about lead exposure, hygiene, and housekeeping measures to prevent ingestion of dust and soil. Use drinking water from the cold tap, not hot water tap. Bottled water is not guaranteed as a safe alternative. Blood lead screening may be recommended universally at ages 1 and 2 years. For more information, visit the CDC website: http://www.cdc.gov/nceh/lead/lead.htm and the Environmental Protection Agency website at: http://www.epa.gov/lead/pubs/nlic.htm.

Measles and Blindness in Children: Childhood blindness and visual impairment in developing countries remains a significant public health issue (Maida et al, 2008). Control of blindness in children is a priority within the World Health Organization's VISION 2020 program. Vitamin A supplementation and measles immunizations and have caused a decrease in xerophthtalmia; cataract is more treatable (Maida et al, 2008).

- Bright Futures
  http://www.brightfutures.org
- Centers for Disease Control and Prevention—Children
  http://www.cdc.gov/LifeStages/children.html
- Children's Nutrition Research Center—Baylor University
  http://www.bcm.tmc.edu/cnrc/
- Growth Charts
  http://www.cdc.gov/growthcharts
- Healthy School Meals
  http://schoolmeals.nal.usda.gov/
- Kids Activity Pyramids
  http://www.uwex.edu/ces/cty/waupaca/documents/KidsActivityPyramid.pdf
- Kids Nutrition
  http://www.kidsnutrition.org/consumer/archives/
- My Pyramid for Preschoolers
  http://www.mypyramid.gov/preschoolers/index.html
- Pediatric Nutrition Practice Group
  http://www.pediatricnutrition.org/
- Team Nutrition
  http://www.fns.usda.gov/tn/Healthy/execsummary_makingithappen.html
- USDA Kids MyPyramid Food Guidance System
  http://www.cnpp.usda.gov/FGP4Children.htm

CHILDHOOD—CITED REFERENCES

Abramovitz BA, Birch LL. Five-year-old girls' ideas about dieting are predicted by their mothers' dieting. *JAMA.* 100:1157, 2000.

Altucher K, et al. Predictors of improvement in hemoglobin concentration among toddlers enrolled in the Massachusetts WIC program. *J Am Diet Assoc.* 105:709, 2005.

American Dietetic Association. Position of the American Dietetic Association: local support for nutrition integrity in schools. *J Am Diet Assoc.* 106:122, 2006.

American Dietetic Association. Position of the American Dietetic Association: dietary guidance for healthy children ages 2 to 11 years. *J Am Diet Assoc.* 108:1038, 2008.

American Dietetic Association. Position of the American Dietetic Association: child and adolescent nutrition assistance programs. 110:791, 2010.

American Heart Association. Dietary recommendations for children and adolescents: a guide for practitioners. *Pediatrics.* 117:544, 2006.

Baylor. Children's Nutrition Research Center. Accessed January 31, 2009, at http://www.bcm.edu/cnrc/consumer/nyc/vol_2005_1/page4.htm.

Dunger DB, et al. Session 7: Early nutrition and later health early developmental pathways of obesity and diabetes risk. *Proc Nutr Soc.* 66:451, 2007.

Eichenberger Gilmore JM, et al. Longitudinal patterns of vitamin and mineral supplement use in young white children. *J Am Diet Assoc.* 105:763, 2005.

Food and Nutrition Board, Institute of Medicine. *Dietary reference intakes for energy, carbohydrate, fiber, fat, fatty acids, cholesterol, protein, and amino acids (macronutrients).* Washington, DC: National Academy Press, 2002.

Greer FR, Krebs N. Optimizing bone health and calcium intakes of infants, children, and adolescents. *Pediatrics.* 117:578, 2006.

Hildebrand DA, Shriver LH. A quantitative and qualitative approach to understanding fruit and vegetable availability in low-income African-American families with children enrolled in an urban head start program. *J Am Diet Assoc.* 110:710, 2010.

Holmes KW, Kwiterovich PO Jr. Treatment of dyslipidemia in children and adolescents. *Curr Cardiol Rep.* 7:445, 2005.

Kerr MA, et al. Folate, related B vitamins, and homocysteine in childhood and adolescence: potential implications for disease risk in later life. *Pediatrics.* 123:627, 2009.

Long KZ, et al. The comparative impact of iron, the B-complex vitamins, vitamins C and E, and selenium on diarrheal pathogen outcomes relative to the impact produced by vitamin A and zinc. *Nutr Rev.* 65:218, 2007.

Making It Happen. School nutrition success stories. Accessed February 1, 2009, at http://www.fns.usda.gov/tn/Healthy/execsummary_makingithappen.html.

Maida JM, et al. Pediatric ophthalmology in the developing world. *Curr Opin Ophthalmol.* 19:403, 2008.

Nicklas TA, et al. Children's meal patterns have changed over a 21-year period: the Bogalusa Heart Study. *J Am Diet Assoc.* 104:753, 2004.

Nicklas TA, et al. A prospective study of food variety seeking in childhood, adolescence and early adult life. *Appetite.* 44:289, 2005.

Patrick H, et al. The benefits of authoritative feeding style: caregiver feeding styles and children's food consumption patterns. *Appetite.* 44:243, 2005.

Patrick H, Nicklas TA. A review of family and social determinants of children's eating patterns and diet quality. *J Am Coll Nutr.* 24:83, 2005.

Rampersaud GC, et al. Breakfast habits, nutritional status, body weight and academic performance in children and adolescents. *J Am Diet Assoc.* 105:743, 2005.

Rolls B, et al. Serving portion size influences 5-year-old but not 3-year old children's food intakes. *J Am Diet Assoc.* 100:232, 2000.

Rosales FJ, et al. Understanding the role of nutrition in the brain and behavioral development of toddlers and preschool children: identifying and addressing methodological barriers. *Nutr Neurosci.* 12:190, 2009.

Ruder EH, et al. Examining breast cancer growth and lifestyle risk factors: early life, childhood, and adolescence. *Clin Breast Cancer.* 8:334, 2008.

Skalicky A, et al. Child food insecurity and iron deficiency anemia in low-income infants and toddlers in the United States. *Matern Child Health J.* 10:177, 2006.

Stroehla BC, et al. dietary sources of nutrients among rural Native American and white children. *J Am Diet Assoc.* 105:1908, 2005.

Thane CW, et al. Whole-grain intake of British young people aged 4–18 years. *Br J Nutr.* 94:825, 2005.

ADOLESCENCE

NUTRITIONAL ACUITY RANKING: LEVEL 2

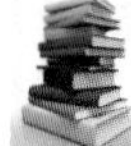

DEFINITIONS AND BACKGROUND

Adolescents need to consume food and beverages that provide adequate energy and nutrients to reduce risk for poor outcomes including growth retardation, ID anemia, poor academic performance, development of psychosocial difficulties, and an increased likelihood of developing diseases such as heart disease and osteoporosis (American Dietetic Association, 2010). Breakfast consumption is important to enhance cognitive function related to memory, test grades, and school attendance (Rampersaud et al, 2005).

Physiological growth is more accurately assessed by using Tanner Stages than by chronological age alone. Girls often start their growth spurt by age 10–11 and generally stop by age 15, whereas boys begin at 12–13 and generally stop by age 19. Teens require increased nutrients for accelerated growth; deficiencies can lead to loss of height, osteoporosis, and delayed sexual maturation.

Skeletal growth is unpredictable, and girls may gain 3.5 inches in 1 year, and boys may gain 4 inches in 1 year. When the teen years begin, the adolescent has achieved 80–85% of final height, 53% of final weight, and 52% of final skeletal mass. Teens may almost double their weight and can add 15–20% in height. Maintaining adequate calcium intake during childhood and adolescence is necessary for the development of peak bone mass, which may be important in reducing the risk of fractures and osteoporosis later in life (Greer and Krebs, 2006).

Some teens develop more rapidly than others (early maturers), while others may develop more slowly (late maturers). The Tanner stages of development are more useful than just use of chronological age. Girls who mature early may be prone to depression, EDs, and anxiety. Obesity is an increasing trend. Parental pressure and weight status concerns are evident among girls who are "picky eaters" (Galloway et al, 2005).

Intakes change often during teen years, especially during growth spurts and stages of physical maturation. Sociocultural influences affect adolescent eating patterns and behaviors. Some teens reject a meat-based diet to become vegetarians; others take up dieting to lose weight or develop an ED. Meal skipping, snacks at odd hours, laxative or diuretic use, fasting, bulimia, self-induced vomiting, and sports requirements are issues that should be addressed in a nutritional assessment. Food choices established during childhood and adolescence tend to persist into adulthood (Fitzgerald et al, 2010). Adolescents need improved diets. Fast food is one factor that impacts adolescents' intake of nutrient-dense foods (Sebastian et al, 2009).

Daily requirement tables separate preteens as ages 9–13 years and teen years as ages 15–18 years. The growth spurt of girls occurs at 9½ to 13½ years of age; menarche generally occurs at 12½ years. For boys, the growth spurt occurs between 11 and 14½ years. Sexual maturation occurs at ages 10–12 years for girls and at ages 12–14 years for boys. The increase in percentage of total body fat in girls is 1.5–2 times that in boys at this time. Boys have greater increases in lean body mass (LBM, muscle) and greater increases in height before epiphyseal closure of long bones occurs. Most skeletal growth is completed by 19 years of age. Girls have more total body fat and less total body water than boys.

According to Erickson's psychological stages of development (1968), teens (12–18 years of age) are working on "identity." In cognitive development, the concrete, "here and now" stage lasts from ages 11 to 14 years in girls and from ages 13 to 15 years in males. Early abstract thinking and daydreams are common among 15- to 17-year-old females and 16- to 19-year-old males. True abstract thinking and idealism (faith, trust, and spirituality) occur for young women at ages 18–25 years and for males at 20–26 years of age.

The brain continues developing through late adolescence, especially with the nerve fiber system that transmits messages from one hemisphere to the other. There is an increase in gray matter at the onset of adolescence, followed by a substantial loss in the frontal lobes from the mid-teens through the mid-twenties, where inhibiting impulses and regulating emotions may be altered. Teens should make the most of their brains during this time, when they can "hard wire" their ability to process skills in academics, sports, and music. Among adolescents, parental control begins to diminish; teens exercise more autonomy over their food choices as compared with children (Fitzgerald et al, 2010).

Dietary intake and body size influence age at menarche and growth patterns in teen girls. Puberty comes early for some girls because of a gene (*CYP1B1*) that speeds up the body's breakdown of androgensas well as percentage of energy intake from dietary protein. These factors have implications for later development of diseases, including breast cancer and heart disease. Another concern is polycystic ovarian syndrome (PCOS). The genetic polymorphisms are not yet clearly identified, but the risks for metabolic syndrome, diabetes, infertility and heart disease must be managed. Diet, physical activity, insulin-sensitizers or anti-androgen medications may be useful. Weight loss of 5–10% may help improve blood functions and ovarian function.

Teens should have access to an adequate supply of healthful and safe foods that promote optimal physical, cognitive, and social growth and development; nutrition assistance programs play a vital role (American Dietetic Association, 2010).

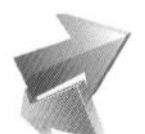

ASSESSMENT, MONITORING, AND EVALUATION

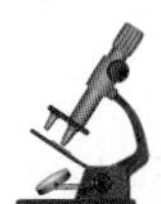

CLINICAL INDICATORS

Genetic Markers: Each individual has a unique genetic profile and phenotype. Because both parents contribute genes and chromosomes to the fetus, a genetic history may be beneficial.

Clinical/History
- Age
- Height
- Weight
- Weight/height percentile
- BMI or HBW
- Waist to hip ratio
- Recent changes (height, weight)
- Diet history
- Tanner stage of sexual maturation
- Hydration status (I & O)
- Physical activity level or athletics
- Physical handicaps
- Disordered eating patterns
- GI complaints
- Signs of PCOS in girls
- Sleep disorder screening

Lab Work
- H & H, serum Fe
- Glucose
- Chol
- Trig
- Albumin (if needed)
- Na^+, K^+
- Ca^{++}, Mg^{++}, phosphorus
- Homocysteine

SAMPLE NUTRITION CARE PROCESS STEPS

Disordered Eating Pattern

Assessment Data: Dietary recall; labs such as H & H, serum ferritin; growth charts; recent growth spurt; age at menarche.

Nutrition Diagnosis (PES): Disordered eating pattern related to dieting behavior as evidenced by restricted eating, skipping breakfast, frequent infections, BMI of 19, low H & H, irregular intake of nutrient-dense foods and daily consumption of fast foods.

Intervention: Education and counseling tips on desirable nutritional intake in adolescence; consequences on energy, appearance and health from poor dietary habits.

Monitoring and Evaluation: Improved intake of nutrient-dense foods; improved lab values, improved quality of life (energy for school, recreation, and physical activity) and fewer illnesses.

INTERVENTION

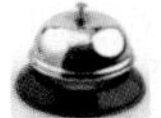

OBJECTIVES

- Provide adequate energy for growth and development, especially for current and future growth spurts.
- Evaluate the patient's weight status. Offer appropriate guidance.
- Prevent or correct nutritional anemias. Determine a girl's sexual maturity, onset of menstruation, and growth spurts, which are often associated with iron depletion. Alter diet accordingly to provide sufficient vitamins and minerals.
- Evaluate use of fad diets, skipping meals, unusual eating patterns, or tendency toward EDs. If problems are noted, seek immediate assistance. Family therapy may be beneficial.
- To prevent obesity in a teen whose parents are obese, a family approach focused on regular breakfast consumption is most beneficial (Fiore et al, 2006).
- Prevent future tendency toward osteoporosis. Because of the influence of the family's diet on the diet of children and adolescents, adequate calcium intake by all members of the family is important; low-fat dairy products, fruits and vegetables, and appropriate physical activity are important for achieving good bone health (Greer and Krebs, 2006).
- Encourage healthy food choices according to the factors of greatest interest to teens (taste and appearance). Health, energy, and price are often not viewed as essential at this stage. Introduce food changes one at a time.
- Vegetarians should be encouraged to consume adequate sources of vitamin B_{12}, riboflavin, zinc, iron, calcium, protein, and energy for growth. Cobalamin deficiency, in the absence of hematologic signs, may lead to impaired cognitive performance. Vegan children tend to have higher intakes of fiber and lower intakes of saturated fatty acids and cholesterol than omnivore children; they may need to increase intake of omega-3 fatty acids.
- Girls may have higher total serum cholesterol concentration than boys, somewhat related to differences in male and female hormones.

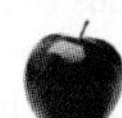

FOOD AND NUTRITION

- The MyPyramid Food Guidance System: 4 cups of milk or equivalent source of calcium; 2–3 servings of meat or equivalent; 6–12 servings from the bread group; 2–4 servings of fruit or juices; 3–5 servings from vegetable group.
- Protein intake should be sufficient to support growth. For energy needs, see nutrient recommendation charts.

	Recommendation	
Nutrient	**Males 14–18 Years**	**Females 14–18 Years**
Energy	3152 kcal/d	2368 kcal/d
Protein	52 g/d or 0.85 g/kg/d	46 g/d or 0.85 g/kg/d
Calcium	1300 mg/d	1300 mg/d
Iron	12 mg/d	15 mg/d
Folate	400 μg/d	400 μg/d
Phosphorus	1250 mg/d	1250 mg/d
Vitamin A	900 mg	700 mg
Vitamin C	75 mg/d	75 mg/d
Thiamin	1.2 mg/d	1.0 mg/d
Riboflavin	1.3 mg/d	1.0 mg/d
Niacin	16 mg/d	14 mg/d

Data from: Food and Nutrition Board, Institute of Medicine. *Dietary reference intakes for energy, carbohydrate, fiber, fat, fatty acids, cholesterol, protein, and amino acids (macronutrients)*. Washington, DC: National Academy Press, 2002.

- Snacks should be planned as healthy options. Snacking frequency affects intake of macronutrients and a few micronutrients and promotes consumption of fruits; an excess of discretionary calories as added sugars and fats (Sebastian et al, 2009).
- Adequate zinc and iodine are needed for growth and sexual maturation; use iodized salt and foods such as meat and dairy products.
- Calcium is needed for bone growth; vitamins D and A are also essential in this age group. Iron is needed for menstrual losses in girls.
- Debut age of drinking alcohol is important to note. If drinking begins before age 15, there is twice the risk of substance abuse and four times the risk of dependence.
- Diet for athletes: an acceptable diet for the athlete would be a normal diet for age, sex, and level of activity plus adequate intake of carbohydrates and fluids. Avoid excess of protein and inadequate replacement of electrolytes (see Sports Nutrition entry).
- For pregnant teens, follow guidelines listed in Table 1-14.

TABLE 1-14 **Special Considerations for Adolescent Pregnancy**

Issue	Comments
Mother is still growing	Check gynecological age (chronological age less age of menarche) to determine future potential growth of the mother.
Low birth weight (LBW) and prematurity	Fetuses grow more slowly in 10- to 16-year-olds. Increased weight in the last trimester is helpful in lessening the incidence of LBW.
Fetal growth and optimal nutritional status during and after gestation	By the end of the pregnancy, the mother's desired weight gain should be between 25 and 35 lb. Add desired increments for energy for requirements of same-age nonpregnant teens, or monitor the weight gain pattern to assess the adequacy of the present diet. Adolescents are at high risk of gaining an excessive amount of weight during pregnancy and should be monitored during pregnancy by dietetics professionals.
Protein requirements	Protein requirement is 1.1 g/kg body weight for most adolescents.
Prenatal supplements	The physician will prescribe prenatal vitamins.
Meal patterns	Mom will need 5 cups of milk, 3 servings of protein or meat, 4 servings of fruits/vegetables, 4 servings of breads/cereals. Three snacks daily will be needed.
Nutrients needed	Frequently missing nutrients include calcium, zinc, iron, folate, vitamins A and B_6 and C. Nutrient-dense choices include: Vitamin A: Chicken liver, cantaloupe, mango, spinach, apricots. Vitamin C: Citrus fruits and juices, broccoli, spinach, melon, strawberries. Calcium: Low-fat milk, yogurt, broccoli, cheddar cheese, low-fat shakes, skim-milk cheeses. Iron: Liver, rice, whole milk, raisins, baked potatoes, enriched cereal. Vitamin B_6: White meats, bananas, potatoes, egg yolks. Folacin: Wheat germ, spinach, asparagus, strawberries. Zinc: Apples, chicken, peanut butter, tuna, rice, whole milk.
Bad habits, cravings, and aversions	Discourage skipping of meals. Cravings are common, especially for chocolate, fruit, fast foods, pickles, and ice cream. Watch for aversions to meat, eggs, and pizza during this time.
Iron deficiency anemia (IDA) during pregnancy	Women who conceive during or shortly after adolescence are likely to enter pregnancy with low or absent iron stores. IDA during pregnancy is associated with significant morbidity for mothers and infants; supplementation is a strategy to improve iron balance in pregnant teens.
Smoking	Pregnant teens are more likely to smoke, to deliver preterm infants, and to have their infants die in the first year than other mothers (Markovitz et al, 2005).
Resistance to authority figures	Encourage the teen to see herself as having a key role in providing good nutrition for her new family. Allow her to express her feelings and concerns.
WIC Program	Encourage enrollment in programs such as WIC where an individualized nutrition risk profile is developed for each pregnant teen. Positive outcomes are noted in birth weight, rates of low or very low birth weight, preterm delivery, maternal morbidity, and perinatal morbidity/mortality (Dubois et al, 1997).

Common Drugs Used and Potential Side Effects

- Vitamin-mineral supplements are not needed, except for pregnant teens or teens whose diets are generally inadequate (such as those following an unplanned vegetarian pattern or restricted energy plans). The majority of American teens do not use supplements; those who do use them tend to eat a more nutrient-dense diet than those who do not. Vitamins A and E, calcium, and zinc tend to be low regardless of use of supplements. In addition, excesses of these nutrients are not recommended and may lead to toxic levels of vitamins A and D if taken indiscriminately.
- Discuss the relevance of tolerable ULs from the dietary reference intakes of the National Academy of Sciences. These levels were set to protect individuals from receiving too much of any nutrient from diet and dietary supplements.
- Monitor use of nonprescription medications (such as aspirin and cold remedies) and use of illegal drugs, including marijuana and alcohol. Side effects may include poor oral dietary intakes of several nutrients. Smoking cigarettes tends to decrease serum levels of vitamin C.

Herbs, Botanicals, and Supplements

- Herbs and botanical supplements should not be used without discussing with the physician. In general, these supplements have not been proven to be safe for adolescents. There may be subgroups that are at risk for inappropriate use of these products (e.g., individuals with EDs and athletes).
- The use of multivitamin–mineral preparations is most common. More males than females use creatine and diuretics. Females consume herbal weight control products significantly more than males.
- Athletes reported supplementing with creatine and protein. There may be misguided beliefs in performance enhancement by these products.

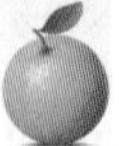

NUTRITION EDUCATION, COUNSELING, CARE MANAGEMENT

- Explain the MyPyramid Food Guidance System and the rationale behind the concepts. School-based interventions to promote healthy choices are beneficial.

- Diets of teens are often low in vitamins A and C, folate, and iron. Discuss the concept of nutrient density; food comparison charts are useful. Encourage a minimum of five servings of fruits and vegetables daily. Having easy access to ready-to-eat, appealing fruits and vegetables is important (Befort et al, 2006). Educate about desirable snacks; link discussions to dental and oral health.
- Limit intake of sweetened beverages (soda, sweetened tea, fruit drinks) to improve nutrient density (Nelson et al, 2009) and to prevent or correct obesity (Dubois et al, 2007).
- Explain the relation of diet to the needs of the adolescent athlete, as well as its influence on skin, weight control, and general appearance.
- Discuss body image, heroes, and peer pressure. Boys generally want larger biceps, shoulders, chests, and forearms. Girls often want smaller hips, waistlines, and thighs, and larger bustlines.
- The 5-year period between adolescence and adulthood is a time of potential weight gain. Emphasize the importance of not skipping meals, especially breakfast. Discourage obsessions with dieting and weight and promote safe dieting practices when needed.
- Discuss calcium and vitamin D; many adolescent girls consume inadequate amounts. Assess current intake by asking questions such as: How many times a day do you drink milk or eat cheese and yogurt? Have you had any bone fractures? Low-fat dairy products may be helpful for maintaining or achieving a HBW; use 3–4 servings daily. Teens who live in northern climates may need extra vitamin D intake (Sullivan et al, 2005).
- Teens respond well to discussions that respect their independence, sense of justice, and idealism. One of their roles is to establish a clear identity of how they fit into the world. Teens spend increased amounts of time with their friends but still tend to conform to parental ideals when it comes to values, education, and long-term life plans. Help the family recognize the adolescent's need for independence in choosing meals and snack items.
- Teens often feel that "it can't happen to me," prompting them to take unnecessary risks like drinking and driving ("I won't crash this car"), having unprotected sex ("I can't possibly get pregnant"), or smoking ("I can't possibly get cancer"). Effects of various nutrients on appearance or energy levels may be helpful.
- Encourage family meals and discuss options for nourishing meals eaten away from home ("portable foods"). Parents play a large role in modeling eating behavior; today's access to low density, high-energy foods must be carefully managed to prevent obesity (Savage et al, 2007). Parents need to limit soft drink consumption and encourage intake of calcium-rich beverages (Cluskey et al, 2008).
- Parents need to work closely with physicians when there are childhood-onset disorders, especially when it is time to change from a pediatrician to a doctor treating young adults (Peter et al, 2009).
- Consumption of fast food is common and may contribute to weight gain if not carefully monitored. A focus on eating or physical activity behaviors without discussing weight specifically is preferred over direct approaches about weight (Shrewsbury et al, 2010).

Patient Education—Food Safety Tips

- Since teens may not think about the consequences of their actions, gentle reminders about hand washing and safe food handling may be important. Use of hand sanitizers may be popular among teen girls.
- Avoid raw or partially cooked eggs, raw or undercooked fish or shellfish, and raw or undercooked meats because of potential foodborne illnesses.
- Do not use raw (unpasteurized) milk or products made from it.
- Avoid serving unpasteurized juices and raw sprouts.
- Only serve processed deli meats and frankfurters that have been reheated to steaming hot temperature.
- Safe food handling is an important part of school food service (American Dietetic Association, 2006).

For More Information

- American Academy of Child and Adolescent Psychology http://www.aacap.org/
- Attention Deficit Hyperactivity Disorder http://www.nimh.nih.gov/publicat/adhd.cfm#adhd14
- Body and Mind (BAM) http://www.bam.gov/index.html
- Body Image http://www.focusas.com/BodyImage.html
- Bright Futures—Adolescence http://brightfutures.aap.org/web/
- Calorie King http://www.calorieking.com/
- Centers for Disease Control and Prevention—Adolescents http://www.cdc.gov/HealthyYouth/az/index.htm
- Food Safety for Teens http://www.fsis.usda.gov/food_safety_education/for_kids_&_teens/index.asp
- National Institute of Health and Human Development http://www.nichd.nih.gov/health/
- Polycystic Ovarian Syndrome http://women.webmd.com/tc/polycystic-ovary-syndrome-pcos-topic-overview
- President's Challenge for Physical Activity http://www.presidentschallenge.org/
- Teens Health http://kidshealth.org/teen/
- Vegetarian Nutrition for Teens http://www.vrg.org/nutrition/teennutrition.htm

ADOLESCENCE—CITED REFERENCES

American Dietetic Association. Position of the American Dietetic Association: child and adolescent nutrition assistance programs. *J Am Diet Assoc.* 110:791, 2010.

Befort C, et al. Fruit, vegetable, and fat intake among non-Hispanic black and non-Hispanic white adolescents: associations with home availability and food consumption settings. *J Am Diet Assoc.* 106:367, 2006.

Cluskey M, et al. At-home and away-from-home eating patterns influencing preadolescents' intake of calcium-rich food as perceived by Asian, Hispanic and non-Hispanic white parents. *J Nutr Educ Behav.* 40:72, 2008.

Dubois L, et al. Regular sugar-sweetened beverage consumption between meals increases risk of overweight among preschool-aged children. *J Am Diet Assoc.* 107:924, 2007.

Fiore H, et al. Potentially protective factors associated with healthful body mass index in adolescents with obese and nonobese parents: a secondary data analysis of the third national health and nutrition examination survey, 1988–1994. *J Am Diet Assoc.* 106:55, 2006.

Fitzgerald A, et al. Factors influencing the food choices of Irish children and adolescents: a qualitative investigation. *Health Promot Int.* 2010 Apr 10. [Epub ahead of print]

Galloway AT, et al. Parental pressure, dietary patterns and weight status among girls who are "picky eaters." *J Am Diet Assoc.* 105:541, 2005.

Greer FR, Krebs N. Optimizing bone health and calcium intakes of infants, children, and adolescents. *Pediatrics.* 117:578, 2006.
Markovitz BP, et al. Socioeconomic factors and adolescent pregnancy outcomes: distinctions between neonatal and post-neonatal deaths? *BMC Public Health.* 5:79, 2005.
Nelson MC, et al. Five-year longitudinal and secular shifts in adolescent beverage intake: findings from project EAT (Eating Among Teens)-II. *J Am Diet Assoc.* 109:308, 2009.
Peter NG, et al. Transition from pediatric to adult care: internists' perspectives. *Pediatrics.* 123:417, 2009.
Rampersaud GC, et al. Breakfast habits, nutritional status, body weight and academic performance in children and adolescents. *J Am Diet Assoc.* 105:743, 2005.
Savage JS, et al. Parental influence on eating behavior: conception to adolescence. *J Law Med Ethics.* 35:22, 2007.
Sebastian RS, et al. US adolescents and mypyramid: associations between fast-food consumption and lower likelihood of meeting recommendations. *J Am Diet Assoc.* 109:225, 2009.
Shrewsbury VA, et al. Adolescent-parent interactions and communication preferences regarding body weight and weight management: a qualitative study. *Int J Behav Nutr Phys Act.* 7:16, 2010.
Sullivan SS, et al. Adolescent girls in Maine are at risk for vitamin D insufficiency. *J Am Diet Assoc.* 105:971, 2005.

PHYSICAL FITNESS AND STAGES OF ADULTHOOD

SPORTS NUTRITION

NUTRITIONAL ACUITY RANKING: LEVEL 2

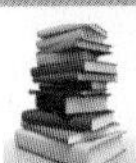

DEFINITIONS AND BACKGROUND

Many athletes are involved in active sports (running, jogging, weight-lifting, or wrestling) when they seek nutritional guidance. Questions about weight control, disordered eating patterns, and wellness are common; fewer athletes have questions about conditions such as diabetes. During high physical activity, energy and protein intakes must be met to maintain body weight, replenish glycogen stores, and provide adequate protein for building and repairing tissues (American Dietetic Association, 2009). Use of carbohydrate drinks can maintain energy intake and prevent dehydration.

Female children and adolescent athletes may develop nonanemic ID (Unnithan and Goulopoulu, 2004), disordered eating, menstrual dysfunction, or decreased BMD. Pediatricians need to carefully monitor their health. All athletes should be screened for ID using serum ferritin, serum transferrin receptor, and hemoglobin (Sinclair and Hinton, 2005).

Female athletes who are under intense pressure to have a low percentage of body fat for performance, may have disordered eating with subsequent amenorrhea and osteoporosis, the "female athlete triad." This triad is serious and requires a multidisciplinary approach. Perfectionism enhances the risk for disordered eating, especially in varsity athletes. Prevention requires de-emphasis on percentage of body fat and adequate emphasis on good nutrition. The consequences of lost BMD can be devastating; premature osteoporotic fractures can occur, and lost BMD might never be regained. Winter sports may protect bone density because of the vigor required.

The primary fuel for athletic events using less than 50% VO_{2max} (or aerobic capacity) is fat. Muscle glycogen and blood glucose supply half of the energy for aerobic exercise during a moderate workout (at or below 60% of VO_{2max} or aerobic capacity) and nearly all the energy during a hard workout (above 80% of aerobic capacity). In short-duration events of more than 70% VO_{2max} (as in events like swimming or sprint running), glycogen is the key fuel. In long-duration events or activities of more than 70% VO_{2max} (such as long-distance running, cycling, or swimming), muscle glycogen can be depleted in 100–120 minutes; maintaining a high-carbohydrate daily diet while training for adequate glycogen replenishment is necessary.

Carbohydrate (CHO) ingestion during prolonged exercise and CHO loading before exercise can have different effects on fuel substrate kinetics. The glycemic index of the carbohydrates consumed during the immediate postexercise period might not be important as long as sufficient carbohydrate is consumed; high insulin concentrations following a high–glycemic index meal later in the recovery period could facilitate further muscle glycogen resynthesis (Stevenson et al, 2005). Elite athletes may metabolize CHO more effectively than nonathletes, but nutritional factors still affect glycemic control (Chou et al, 2005).

Performance in endurance events depends upon maximal aerobic power, sustained by the availability of substrates (carbohydrates and fats). Fatigue is associated with reduced muscle glycogen; increasing muscle glycogen or blood glucose prolongs performance, while increasing fat and decreasing CHO decreases performance.

A sports diet aligns 20% protein, 30% CHO, and 30% fat, with the remaining 20% of the energy distributed between CHO and fat based on the intensity and duration of the sport. Table 1-15 lists the position statements of the International Society of Sports Nutrition.

Trained individuals have higher levels of fat oxidative capacity, which spares glycogen during endurance sports. Endurance runners who eat a low-fat diet may not consume enough energy, EFAs, and some minerals, especially zinc; these inadequate intakes may compromise their performance. Gymnasts often have a lower weekly calorie intake but a higher dietary protein intake than nonathletes; this places them at risk of malnutrition and immunosuppression.

A qualified sports dietitian who is Board-Certified Specialist in Sports Dietetics can provide individualized nutrition direction and advice following a comprehensive nutrition assessment (American Dietetic Association, 2009). Athletes should be well hydrated before the start of exercise and should drink enough fluid during and after exercise to balance fluid losses. Consumption of sports drinks containing

TABLE 1-15 International Society of Sports Nutrition Position Statements

Individuals engaged in regular exercise training require more dietary protein than sedentary individuals. Protein intakes of 1.4–2.0 g/kg/d for physically active individuals are not only safe, but may improve the training adaptations to exercise training. When part of a balanced, nutrient-dense diet, protein intakes at this level are not detrimental to kidney function or bone metabolism in healthy, active persons.
While it is possible for physically active individuals to obtain their daily protein requirements through a varied, regular diet, supplemental protein in various forms are a practical way of ensuring adequate and quality protein intake for athletes. Different types and quality of protein can affect amino acid bioavailability; superiority of one protein type over another in terms of optimizing recovery and/or training adaptations remains to be demonstrated.
Appropriately timed protein intake is an important component of an overall exercise training program, essential for proper recovery, immune function, and the growth and maintenance of lean body mass. Under certain circumstances, specific amino acid supplements, such as branched-chain amino acids (BCAAs), may improve exercise performance and recovery from exercise.
Maximal endogenous glycogen stores are best promoted by following a high-glycemic, high-carbohydrate diet (600–1000 g CHO or 8–10 g CHO/kg/d). Ingestion of free amino acids and protein (PRO) alone or in combination with CHO before resistance exercise can maximally stimulate protein synthesis.
Ingesting CHO alone or in combination with PRO during resistance exercise increases muscle glycogen, offsets muscle damage, and facilitates greater training adaptations after either acute or prolonged periods of supplementation with resistance training.
Nutrient timing incorporates methodical planning and eating of whole foods, nutrients extracted from food, and other sources. The timing of the energy intake and the ratio of ingested macronutrients allow for enhanced recovery and tissue repair following high-volume exercise, augmented muscle protein synthesis, and improved mood states when compared with unplanned or traditional strategies of nutrient intake.

Sources: Kerksick et al, 2008; Campbell et al, 2007.

carbohydrates and electrolytes during exercise will provide fuel for the muscles, help maintain blood glucose and the thirst mechanism, and decrease the risk of dehydration or hyponatremia (American Dietetic Association, 2009).

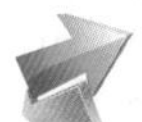

ASSESSMENT, MONITORING, AND EVALUATION

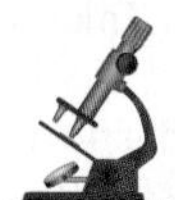

CLINICAL INDICATORS

Genetic Markers: Each individual has a unique genetic profile and phenotype. Because both parents contribute genes and chromosomes to the fetus, a genetic history may be beneficial.

Clinical/History	Lab Work	
Height	H & H, serum Fe	Total Chol
Weight	Transferrin	High-density lipoprotein (HDL)
Goal weight	Na^+, K^+, chloride	LDL
BMI	Serum glucose	Trig
HBW range for height	BP	Serum insulin
Diet/intake history	Alb, transthyretin (if needed)	Ca^{++}, Mg^{++}
Hydration (I & O)		Alk phos
		Homocysteine

INTERVENTION

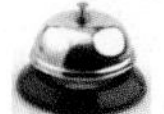

OBJECTIVES

- Promote healthy, safe eating habits and activities that can be continued throughout life. Aerobic activity and resistance training are especially beneficial. Participation in sports activity can be an important component of obesity prevention.
- Because physical activity, athletic performance, and recovery from exercise are enhanced by optimal nutrition, adequate energy intake is needed to support peak performance (American Dietetic Association, 2009).
- Correct faddist beliefs, dangerous dieting trends, meal skipping, and other unhealthy eating behaviors.
- Prevent or correct amenorrhea, which may result from poor energy and fat intake. Runners may be especially vulnerable (Barrack et al, 2008). Monitor or correct EDs, including bulimia and anorexia nervosa.
- Help prevent injuries, dehydration, overhydration, and hyponatremia.
- Enhance overall health and fitness. A certain amount of fat is essential to bodily functions. Fat regulates body temperature, cushions and insulates organs and tissues. Fat intake provides EFAs and fat-soluble vitamins, as well as energy for weight maintenance (American Dietetic Association, 2009).

SAMPLE NUTRITION CARE PROCESS STEPS

Inadequate Fluid Intake in Athlete

Assessment Data: Dietary recall; labs (BUN, sodium); I & O descriptions.

Nutrition Diagnosis (PES): Inadequate fluid intake related to marathon preparation as evidenced by altered labs, poor skin turgor, frequent headaches, reports of dehydration and limited intake of fluids on workout days.

Intervention: Education on fluid intake for body size, extent of training, and types of physical activities. Counseling on use of any supplements or sports drinks.

Monitoring and Evaluation: Improved hydration status; improved lab values (BUN, sodium); fewer headaches and signs of dehydration; I & O levels that are balanced.

TABLE 1-16 **Percent Body Fat Standards**[a]

Stages	Men	Women
Essential for life	4–5%	10–12%
Athletes	6–13%	14–20%
Very lean/Underweight	≤8%	≤21%
Recommended	8–20%	21–32%
Overweight	20–25%	32–38%
Obese	>25%	>38%
Children[b]	14% newborn	14% newborn
	13% 10-year-old boy	19% 10-year-old girl

[a]These standards are for 20–40 years of age. Add approximately 1% body fat for each additional decade above 40 years of age.
[b]Shils M, et al. *Modern nutrition in health and disease*. 9th ed. Philadelphia: Lippincott Williams & Wilkins, 1999, p. 799.

Ranges of body fat standards are listed below to evaluate and counsel accordingly (see Table 1-16).

- Body weight and composition should not be a criterion for sports performance and daily weigh-ins are discouraged (American Dietetic Association, 2009).

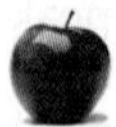

FOOD AND NUTRITION

- For active individuals, use a normal diet for age and sex with special attention to energy needs for the specific activity and frequency. Most athletes should consume 6–10 g of CHO per kg of body weight on a daily basis. Female athletes may not consume sufficient levels of protein and energy, often because they want to lose weight.
- Maintain total fat intake at a level determined by age, medical status, type of performance and endurance required. Focus on heart healthy fats such as olive oil and canola oil.
- Protein eaten in excess of recommendations is used by the body as a fuel; the body will store the excess as fat tissue. Athletes who eat many high-protein foods and take protein supplements in addition may be at risk for dehydration or kidney problems. Protein requirements should be calculated by age and sex, with a slightly higher requirement in endurance sports activity (Gleeson, 2005). Table 1-17 provides a chart for calculating protein needs.
- Vitamin and mineral supplements are not needed if adequate energy to maintain body weight is consumed from a variety of foods, but may be needed if the individual's diet is imbalanced (American Dietetic Association, 2009). Extra riboflavin may be needed to meet muscle demands; this is easily met by dairy products (Manore, 2000).
- Fluid replacement may be essential with a calculation of 1 mL/kcal used for an average. With too much, there is a risk for hyponatremia in slow runners and marathon walkers; drink too little, risk dehydration as in marathon runners.
- Electrolytes must be carefully monitored and replaced. Sports drinks are formulated to have between 6 and 8% CHO along with an appropriate amount of electrolytes; they should not be diluted. Newer sports drinks on the market contain glucose polymers with lower osmolality than sugared drinks or fruit juice. Gatorade and other recently formulated sports drink products are acceptable.
- When athletes omit meat from their diets, other sources of zinc and heme iron must be obtained. Dried beans, nuts, seeds, peanut butter, soy products, tofu, and enriched cereals provide protein and some iron. A good rule of thumb is to consume twice the iron in nonheme foods as would have been available from heme sources.
- Adequate calcium intake may prevent osteoporosis, reduce muscle cramping and protect against stress fractures. For maximum bone density, include 4 servings of dairy or calcium-fortified foods (or 3 servings plus a 500 mg calcium supplement) until age 24.
- Avoid skipping meals. Breakfast is especially important; small meals or frequent snacks are useful for some individuals.
- Glucose loading is not recommended for athletes who train daily for endurance sports. Complex CHO in the form of starch promotes glycogen storage. Table 1-18 lists tips on planning meals for athletes.

Common Drugs Used and Potential Side Effects

- If an athlete is in a sport that requires drug testing, check first with the U.S. Olympic Committee or the National Collegiate Athletic Association (NCAA) before using any drug. Androstenedione and anabolic steroids do promote muscle mass enhancement but are not allowed. Steroids affect numerous nutritional parameters. Take a careful drug history and discuss all side effects.
- Salt tablets should be discouraged. A balanced sports drink is more desirable.
- Discuss the relevance of tolerable ULs from the latest dietary reference intakes of the National Academy of

TABLE 1-17 **Protein for Athletes**

Protein Needs: Group	Protein Intake Per Day
Sedentary men and women	0.8–1.0 g/kg or 0.4 g /lb body weight
Moderate-intensity endurance athletes, 45–60 minutes 4–5 times per week	1.2 g/kg or 0.6 g/lb body weight
Elite male endurance athletes	1.6 g/kg or 0.8 g/lb body weight
Competitive sports which emphasize building muscle mass	1.4 g/kg or 0.7 g/lb body weight
Recreational endurance athletes, 30 minutes at <55% VO_2 peak 4–5 times per week	0.8–1.0 g/kg or 0.5 to 0.6 g/lb body weight
Football, power sports	1.4–1.7 g/kg
Resistance athletes (early training)	1.5–1.7 g/kg
Resistance athletes (steady state)	1.0–1.2 g/kg

Adapted from: Burke L, Deakin V. *Clinical sports nutrition*. 3rd ed. McGraw-Hill, 2006, pp. 73–112; Clark N, *Nancy Clark's sports nutrition guidebook*. 4th ed. Champagne, IL: Human Kinetics Publishers, 2008, pp. 127–146.

TABLE 1-18 Guidelines for Planning Meals for Athletes

	Number of Servings Per Day		
	Female Nonathletes	**Female Athletes, Male Nonathletes**	**Male Athletes**
Bread/Grains Group	6–11	9–15	11–18
Vegetable Group	3+	3+	3+
Fruit Group	2–4	3–5	4–8+
Dairy Group	4	4+	4–5+
Protein/Meat Group	2 (= 5 oz)	2 (= 6 oz)	3 (= 7–11 oz)
Fats/Lipids	20–35% calories	20–35% calories	20–35% calories

Source: *U.S. Department of Agriculture* and *the U.S. Department of Health and Human Services.*

Preexercise

- Consumption of a CHO + PRO supplement may result in peak levels of protein synthesis.
- Eat lightly before an athletic competition; chew foods well. Remember, it takes 4–5 hours to fully digest a meal. Focus on complex carbohydrates (about 65% of the meal).
- Avoid bulky foods (raw fruits and vegetables, dry beans and peas, and popcorn), which may stimulate bowel movements; avoid gas-forming foods (cabbage family and cooked dry beans).
- Drink water to be adequately hydrated: drink 2 cups of cool water 1–2 hours before the event and 1–2 cups of fluid 15 minutes before the event.
- Avoid drastic changes in normal diet routine immediately prior to competition; focus on well-tolerated or favorite foods.

During Exercise

- CHO should be consumed at a rate of 30–60 g of CHO/hour in a 6–8% CHO solution (8–16 fluid ounces) every 10–15 minutes. CHO:PRO ratio of 3–4:1 may increase endurance performance and maximally promotes glycogen resynthesis during acute and subsequent bouts of endurance exercise.

Postexercise (within 30 minutes)

- Consumption of CHO at high dosages (8–10 g CHO/kg/d) stimulates muscle glycogen resynthesis Adding 0.2–0.5 g protein/kg/d to CHO at a ratio of 3–4:1 (CHO: PRO) further enhances glycogen resynthesis. Fruits, juices, and high-carbohydrate drinks are examples (Kerksick et al, 2008).
- Replace fluids that have been lost; drink 2 cups of fluids for every lost pound. Replace any potassium or sodium that has been lost during competition or training; fruits and vegetables are excellent sources of potassium. Replace sodium by eating salty foods; if activity was vigorous and exceeded 2 hours, a sports beverage may be useful (Kerksick et al, 2008).

Postexercise Ingestion (immediately to 3 hours post)

- Protein (essential amino acids) has been shown to stimulate robust increases in muscle protein synthesis, while the addition of CHO may stimulate even greater levels of protein synthesis (Kerksick et al, 2008).
- Meat and soy substitutes have 7 g protein/serving; dairy products have 8 g protein/serving; and breads/cereals/grains have 3 g protein/serving.

During Consistent, Prolonged Resistance Training

- Postexercise consumption of CHO plus PRO supplements in varying dosages have been shown to stimulate improvements in strength and body composition when compared to control or placebo conditions. The addition of creatine (0.1 g Cr/kg/day) to a CHO + PRO supplement may facilitate even greater adaptations to resistance training (Kerksick et al, 2008).
- The following list estimates for carbohydrates (CHO):

5 g CHO
1 serving of nonstarchy vegetables
12 g CHO
1 serving of milk and dairy products
15 g CHO
1 serving each of breads, cereals, grains, "starchy" vegetables corn, peas, lima beans; fruits
40–45 g CHO
4 graham crackers
4 fig newtons
1 Power Bar
12 oz can soda
1 cup cranberry juice cocktail
1 baked potato with skin
3 oz pretzels
20 saltine crackers
6 cups popcorn (any kind)
1 cup rice (any kind)
1 large flour tortilla
2 hamburger buns
16 oz PowerAde
22 oz Gatorade
8 graham crackers, 2-1/2" squares
3 slices of bread (any kind)

Resource: Brown University, 2009.

Sciences. These levels were set to protect individuals from receiving too much of any nutrient from diet and dietary supplements. Discuss the fact that excessive use of vitamin-mineral supplements can lead to toxicity, especially for vitamins A and D.

Herbs, Botanicals, and Supplements

- Herbs and botanical supplements should not be used without discussing with the physician, especially for underlying medical conditions. Use of supplements is common in athletes, and there may be undesirable side effects (Burns et al, 2004). FDA has taken steps to implement the Dietary Supplementation Health and Education Act (DSHEA) with a stronger stance than in the past.
- Some supplements may be contaminated with banned substances. If an athlete is found to have taken a banned substance, actions are taken by the regulatory agency (such as the International Olympic Committee, NCAA, or other sports sanctioned agencies). Athletes must be advised accordingly.
- Because regulations specific to nutritional ergogenic aids are poorly enforced, they should be used with caution, and only after careful product evaluation for safety, efficacy, potency, and legality (American Dietetic Association, 2009). Athletes often use supplements such as those found in Table 1-19 (Brown University, 2009).

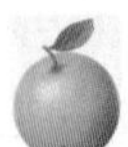

NUTRITION EDUCATION, COUNSELING, CARE MANAGEMENT

- A well-balanced diet will suffice for most events (American Dietetic Association, 2009). Dispel myths, such as "milk is for children only," "meat is bad for you," "carbohydrates are fattening," or "dieting is the key to fluid control."
- Athletes with traits such as perfectionism, compulsive or controlling behaviors, and a need for attention may need referral to counseling from an appropriate health provider. Restrictive eating behaviors practiced for physical activities that emphasize leanness are a concern. Educate athletes, parents, coaches, trainers, judges, and administrators about the dangers of restrictive eating (Nattiv et al, 2007). Where there are weight problems, address body weight, family genetics, body type, parenting styles, socioeconomic issues, and environmental cues.
- Pre-event diets should be eaten up to an hour before the activity. Complex carbohydrates should be consumed, using less fat and protein because of their effect on digestive processes. After an event, recovery carbohydrate intake is suggested.
- There is no such thing as "quick energy." The habit of eating candy before a game can cause an insulin overshoot, leading to hypoglycemia. A balanced diet is more practical. Discuss how to obtain a high-calorie, high-complex carbohydrate diet with attention to individual preferences. In vigorous training programs such as ultramarathons, 3000–6000 kcal may be needed.
- Prevent dehydration. Drink fluids before, during, and after exercising. Weigh before and after events and replace lost weight (such as 2 cups of fluid per pound lost). Avoid use of alcoholic beverages as they do nothing to promote performance and may negatively affect neurologic and cardiac systems.
- Some populations have lower resting metabolic rates and physical activity energy expenditures than others. If confirmed, target interventions to decrease energy intake and to increase physical activity (Gannon et al, 2000).

TABLE 1-19 Supplements Commonly Used by Athletes

Androstenedione "andro" (hormone)	Banned by the NCAA, the IOC, the U.S. Olympic Committee, the National Football League, and the Association of Tennis Professionals.
Caffeine	Ergogenic aid for endurance athletes when taken before and/or during exercise in moderate quantities, such as 3–6 mg/kg body mass (Ganio et al, 2009). However, caffeine use is limited in competitive sports.
Chromium Picolinate (CrPl)	Widely available in many foods; supplements are not necessary.
Creatine	Increases the capacity of skeletal muscle to perform work during periods of alternating intensity exercises, possibly because of increased aerobic phosphorylation (Rico-Sanz and Mendez Marco, 2000). Creatine is useful for strength training (Becque et al, 2000), but not for endurance sports. If used, use 20–25 g daily for 5–7 days, followed by maintenance at 5 g/d. It requires a month to completely leave the bloodstream after stopping.
Ephedra/Ephedrine (Ma Huang)	Raises heart rate. Does not increase energy. Removed from the market by FDA.
Ginseng	Often used for performance enhancement. Avoid use with warfarin, insulin, oral hypoglycemics, CNS stimulants, caffeine, steroids, hormones, antipsychotics, aspirin, or antiplatelet drugs.
Tryptophan	Precursor to serotonin. Sometimes used for performance enhancement. May cause psychosis if used with antidepressants, MAO inhibitors
Yohimbe, smilax, tribulus, and wild yams	Cannot be converted by the body to anabolic steroids or enhance muscle mass.
Zinc	Sometimes taken to enhance performance. Zinc should not be taken with immunosuppressants, fluoroquinolones, and tetracycline.

- Women who are breastfeeding can exercise reasonably without adverse effects and may find that return to normal weight is easier than while being sedentary (Lovelady et al, 2004).
- Female athletes with subclinical EDs tend to have dietary intakes of energy, protein, and CHO below desired levels. Micronutrient status is generally unaffected, probably due to use of supplements (Hinton et al, 2004). The aim here is to increase energy intake or reduce excessive energy expenditure (Nattiv et al, 2007). Signs that someone is exercising excessively include rigid rules about exercising, anxiousness, or restlessness when off schedule, working out more than a coach or athletic trainer recommends, rigid or calculated eating patterns to exactly match calories expended on exercise (Brown University, 2009).

Patient Education—Food Safety Tips

- Reminders about hand washing and safe food handling may be important, especially for athletes with busy lifestyles. Use of hand sanitizers can be encouraged.
- Athletes who are on the road may find that they are vulnerable to foodborne illnesses. They should be advised to choose foods carefully when traveling.
- Athletes who compete in other countries should become aware of potential risks where they will be traveling. For example, food and water sources are not always reliably safe.

For More Information

- American Academy of Family Physicians: Nutrition Prescription
  http://familydoctor.org/298.xml
- American College of Sports Medicine
  http://www.acsm.org/
- American College of Sports Medicine Position Stand: Female Athlete Triad
  http://www.acsm-msse.org
- American Council on Exercise
  http://www.acefitness.org
  ACE Recipes: http://www.acefitness.org/getfit/recipes.aspx
- American Alliance for Health, Physical Education, Recreation and Dance
  http://www.aahperd.org
- American Dietetic Association: Sports and Cardiovascular Nutritionists
  http://www.scandpg.org/
- Brown University Guidelines for Athletes
  http://www.brown.edu/Student_Services/Health_Services/Health_Education/nutrition/sportsnut.htm):
- Centers for Disease Control and Prevention—Nutrition and Physical Activity
  http://www.cdc.gov/nccdphp/dnpa/
- Food and Nutrition Information Center
  http://www.nal.usda.gov/fnic/etext/000054.html
- Health and Human Services: Physical Activity Guidelines for Americans
  http://www.health.gov/paguidelines/
- Hydration
  http://www.aces.edu/pubs/docs/H/HE-0749/
- Gatorade Sports Science Institute
  http://www.gssiweb.com/
- Intelihealth—Fitness
  http://www.intelihealth.com/IH/ihtIH/WSIHW000/7165/7165.html
- National Institutes of Health
  http://www.nlm.nih.gov/medlineplus/exerciseandphysicalfitness.html
- Penn State University Fitness and Sports Nutrition
  http://nirc.cas.psu.edu/fitness.cfm
- President's Council on Physical Fitness and Sports
  http://www.fitness.gov/
- Sports Science Peer Reviewed Information
  http://www.sportsci.org/index.html?jour/03/03.htm&1
- Women's Sports Foundation
  http://www.womenssportsfoundation.org/
- Young Men's Health Site
  http://www.youngmenshealthsite.org/nutrition-sports.html
- Young Women's Health Site
  http://www.youngwomenshealth.org/nutrition-sports.html

SPORTS NUTRITION—CITED REFERENCES

American Dietetic Association. Position of the American Dietetic Association and the Canadian Dietetic Association: nutrition and athletic performance. *J Am Diet Assoc.* 109:509, 2009.

Barrack MT, et al. Prevalence of and traits associated with low BMD among female adolescent runners. *Med Sci Sports Exerc.* 40:2015, 2008.

Burns RD, et al. Intercolleagiate student athlete use of nutritional supplements and the role of athletic trainers and dietitians in nutrition counseling. *J Am Diet Assoc.* 104:246, 2004.

Campbell B, et al. International society of sports nutrition position stand: protein and exercise. *J Int Soc Sports Nutr.* 4:8, 2007.

Chou SW, et al. Characteristics of glycemic control in elite power and endurance athletes. *Prev Med.* 40:564, 2005.

Ganio MS, et al. Effect of caffeine on sport-specific endurance performance: a systematic review. *J Strength Cond Res.* 23:315, 2009.

Gannon B, et al. Do African Americans have lower energy expenditure than Caucasians? *Int J Obes Relat Metab Disord.* 24:4, 2000.

Gleeson M. Interrelationship between physical activity and branched-chain amino acids. *J Nutr.* 135:1591S, 2005.

Hinton PS, et al. Nutrient intakes and dietary behaviors of male and female collegiate athletes. *Int J Sport Nutr Exerc Metab.* 14:389, 2004.

Kerksick C, et al. International society of sports nutrition position stand: nutrient timing. *J Int Soc Sports Nutr.* 5:17, 2008.

Lovelady C, et al. Immune status of physically active women during lactation. *Med Sci Sports Exerc.* 36:1001, 2004.

Manore MM. Effect of physical activity on thiamine, riboflavin, and vitamin B-6 requirements. *Am J Clin Nutr.* 72:598S, 2000.

Nattiv A, et al. American College of Sports Medicine position stand. The female athlete triad. *Med Sci Sports Exerc.* 39:1867, 2007.

Rico-Sanz J, Mendez Marco MT. Creatine enhances oxygen uptake and performance during alternating intensity exercise. *Med Sci Sports Exerc.* 32: 379, 2000.

Sinclair LM, Hinton PS. Prevalence of iron deficiency with and without anemia in recreationally active men and women. *J Am Diet Assoc.* 105:975, 2005.

Stevenson E, et al. The metabolic responses to high carbohydrate meals with different glycemic indices consumed during recovery from prolonged strenuous exercise. *Int J Sport Nutr Exerc Metab.* 15:291, 2005.

Unnithan VB, Goulopoulou S. Nutrition for the pediatric athlete. *Curr Sports Med Rep.* 3:206, 2004.

ADULTHOOD

NUTRITIONAL ACUITY RANKING: LEVEL 2

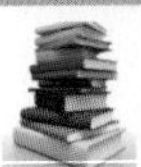

DEFINITIONS AND BACKGROUND

Nutrition is involved in the 10 leading causes of death in women. Heart disease is the number one disabler and killer of women in the United States, whereas cancer is the leading cause of premature death. Table 1-20 lists special considerations for men.

From the Human Genome project, scientists know that variations occur in all humans, even though they are 99.5% identical for DNA sequencing. At a particular chromosome, slight variations can occur; these are recognized as single nucleotide polymorphisms (SNPs). Some of these changes (alleles) lead to chronic diseases such as heart disease, cancer, diabetes, and others. There are 2400 known phenotypes affecting disease onset; 3700 more are suspected to have a genetic origin (McKusick, 2007) or have gene–environmental interactions (see http://www.ncbi.nlm.nih.gov/Omim/mimstats.html. Many diseases are caused by different mutations in genes, with variable age of onset, severity and outcome. Polymorphisms can lead to differences in susceptibility of individuals to adverse environments or to reproductive success. For example, methylenetetrahydrofolate reductase (MTHFR) and folate metabolism affects early pregnancy loss and infertility. Table 1-21 lists some of the disorders that have a genetic link for which mutations have been identified.

"Healthy life expectancy" measures the distribution of health status within a population. People living in poor countries face low life expectancy and a life of poor health. Changes in health and nutritional behaviors can improve quality of life and promote longevity; peer support may be needed. In young adulthood between 18 and 40 years, careers are a priority. In middle adulthood (40–65 years,) family is the primary focus. Peer pressure and family persuasion can promote long-term changes in behavior.

Weight control is another major concern. Over the past 40 years, height, BMI, and weights have increased in both sexes, all ethnic groups, and all ages. There are health implications with this weight increase. Both men and women should attempt to maintain a HBW.

Up to 60% of adults may have prehypertension, especially African Americans, older people, individuals with low socioeconomic status, and overweight individuals. Lifestyle modification and appropriate medications may be needed.

Both genetics and conditioning influence taste preferences and intake. Taste seems to be innate, whereas responses to odors are more conditioned. The influence of genetic variation in taste on food intake depends on how perceptible sweet, fat, or bitter components are in foods and beverages (Duffy and Bartoshuk, 2000). Bitterness "supertasters" may avoid high-fat or sweet foods because the oral sensations are too intense and less pleasant. Supertasters may taste more bitterness in vegetables but still enjoy eating them if condiments are added (Duffy and Bartoshuk, 2000).

It is important to work with individuals to identify foods and taste preferences that will help to achieve healthy eating patterns. When adults are hospitalized, nutritional declines occur and lead to higher hospital charges and more complications. Longstanding dietary habits from childhood, confusion about oral instructions, coexisting depression, inadequate referral or information, literacy deficits, social influences or barriers, and even the right to refuse treatment make it difficult for patients to follow a modified diet (Stein, 2005).

Understanding why patients refuse to follow a diet prescription is a priority. The use of the Standardized Language and Nutrition Care Process from the American Dietetic Association promotes thorough assessment, selection of nutrition diagnoses, targeted goals and interventions, and careful monitoring for evaluation of outcomes.

TABLE 1-20 Leading Causes of Death and Nutritional Implications for Men in the United States

1. **Heart disease:** hyperlipidemia and hypertension are commonly related (see appropriate entries).
2. **Cancer:** prostate, testicular, esophageal, and stomach cancers have special nutritional implications (see appropriate entries). Increasing intake of soy products, fruits, and vegetables and reducing red meat intake may be beneficial.
3. **Stroke:** high intake of sodium and alcohol are problematic, as is chronic hypertension that is untreated (see appropriate entry).
4. **Accidents:** excessive alcohol intake may be related (see appropriate entry).
5. **Chronic lower respiratory diseases:** weight loss or gain may aggravate breathing problems.
6. **Diabetes:** carbohydrate intake should be consistent and consumed at regular intervals.
7. **Influenza and pneumonia:** infectious diseases burn more energy; weight loss can occur if energy intake is poor.
8. **Suicide:** depression and excessive alcohol intake may play a role (see appropriate entries).
9. **Kidney disease:** many renal diseases have implications for control of protein, sodium, electrolytes, and fluid. Kidney stones are more common in men than in women and drinking plenty of fluids and consuming adequate calcium may prevent onset or recurrence (see appropriate entries).
10. **Chronic liver disease and cirrhosis:** excessive alcohol intake is often related (see appropriate entry).

TABLE 1-21 Disorders and Their Related Genes

Neurological Disorders	Related Genes
Premature family Alzheimer's disease	*APP* gene *PSEN1* gene *PSEN2* gene
Late-onset Alzheimer's disease	*APOE* gene
Huntington's disease	CAG triplet-repeat expansion in the IT15 region of the *HD* gene
Frontotemporal dementia	*MAPT* gene
Tay-Sachs disease	*HEXA* gene
Pantothenate kinase neurodegeneration	*PANK2* gene
Hereditary neuropathy with pressure palsies (HNPP)	17p11.2 deletion in the *PMP22* gene *PMP22* gene
Familial Parkinson disease (PARK1)	*SNCA* gene
Early-onset Parkinson disease (PARK2)	*PARK2* gene
Autosomal dominant Lewy body parkinsonism (PARK4)	*SNCA* gene
Rett syndrome	*MECP2* gene
Fragile X syndrome (FRAX)	CGG triplet-repeat expansion analysis of the *FMR-1* gene
Hematological and Cardiovascular Disorders	
Thrombophilia	Mutation of G1691 A (Arg506Gln) in the *Factor V (Leiden)* gene Mutation of G20210 A in the *Prothrombin* (Factor II) gene Mutation C677 T (Ala222Val) and A1298 C (Glu429Ala) in the *MTHFR* gene *PAI1* gene, pasminogene activator inhibitor Angiotensine enzime converter gene
Fanconi anemia (complementation group A)	*FANCA* gene
Fanconi anemia (complementation group C)	Mutation of IVS4+4 A-T in the *FANCC* gene *FANCC* gene
Hemophilia	Intron 22 inversion mutation of *F8* gene *F8* gene Type A; F9 gene in Type B
Glucocorticoid-remediable aldosteronism type 1	*CYP11B1/CYP11 B2* chimeric gene
Marfan syndrome	*FBN1* gene
Congenital thrombocytopenia	*MPL* gene
Metabolic Disorders	
Pituitary hormone deficiency	*POU1F1* and *PROP1* genes
Alpha-1-antitrypsin deficiency	Mutation of E264 V (Allele S) and E342 K (Allele Z) in the *PI* gene
Fructose-1,6-diphosphatase deficiency	*FBP1* gene
Growth hormone deficiency	*GH1* gene
Hereditary hemochromatosis	Mutation of C282Y, H63D and S65 C in the *HFE* gene
Familial hypercholesterolemia	*LDLR* gene Mutation of Arg3500Gln, Arg 3531Cys and Arg3480Trp in the *APOB* gene Mutations of the *CYP11B1* gene and *CYP21A2* gene
Homocystinuria	Mutation of Gly307Ser and Ile278Thr in the *CBS* gene Mutation of C677 T and A1298 C in the *MTHFR* gene
Muscular and Skeletal Disorders	
Achondroplasia	Mutation of G1138 A, G1138 C and G375 C in the *FGFR3* gene
Myoclonus-dystonia (DYT11)	*SGCE* gene
Rapid-onset dystonia-parkinsonism (DYT12)	*ATP1A3* gene
Duchenne/Becker muscular dystrophy	*DMD* gene
Amyotrophic lateral sclerosis (ALS1)	*SOD1* gene
Osteoporosis	BsmI, ApaI, TaqI and FokI polymorphism in the *VDR* gene Pro463Leu polymorphism detection in the *CTR* gene PCOL2 (-1997 G/T) and Sp1 (1546 G/T) polymorphisms in *COL1A1* gene PvuII (397 T>C) and XbaI (351 C>G) polymorphism in *ESR1* gene Polymorphisms in the *IL-6* gene

(continued)

TABLE 1-21 Disorders and Their Related Genes *(continued)*

Reproductive Disorders	Related Genes
Preeclampsia, eclampsia, Hellp syndrome or recurrent spontaneous pregnancy loss	Mutation of G1691 A (Arg506Gln) in the *Factor V* gene Mutation of G20210 A in the *Factor II* gene Mutation of C677 T (Ala222Val) and A1298 C (Glu429Ala) in the *MTHFR* gene
Neoplastic Disorders	
Breast/ovarian cancer	Mutation in exons 2, 3, 5, 8, 11, 18, 20, and 23 of the *BRCA1* gene *BRCA1* gene Mutation in exons 2, 10, 11, and 23 of the *BRCA2* gene *BRCA2* gene
Hereditary nonpolyposis colon cancer—Lynch syndrome	Microsatelites instability *MLH1* gene or *MSH2* gene
Medullary thyroid carcinoma	Mutation in exons 10, 11, 13, 14, and 16 of the *RET* gene *RET* gene
Cutaneous malignant melanoma 2	*CDKN2 A* gene
Familial adenomatous polyposis (FAP)	*APC* gene
Colorectal polyposis	*MUTYH* (MYH) gene
Retinoblastoma	*RB1* gene
Wilms' tumor	*WT1* gene
Multisystemic Disorders	
Cystic fibrosis	30 prevalent European mutations of the CFTR gene IVS8-Tn (poli-T) polymorphism detection in the CFTR gene
Polycystic kidney disease	*PKD1* gene *PKD2* gene
Pharmacogenetics	
Breast cancer	*HER2* (NEU) overexpression detection and Herceptin (trastuzumab) treatment
Nonsmall cell lung cancer (NSCLC)	Mutation screening in exons 18–21 of the *EGFR* gene and Gefinitib treatment
CYP2D6 for psychiatric and cardiovascular disorders treatment	Polymorphism of the *CYP2D6* gene. This gene is involved in metabolizing different drugs such as, Prozac, Zoloft, Haldol, Metoprolol, Tagamet, Tamoxifen, Paxil, Effexor, Hydrocodone, Amitryptiline, Claritin, Cyclobenzaprine, Allegra, Dytuss, Tusstat, Rythmol
CYP2C9 linked to thrombosis, diabetes and other disorders treatment	Polymorphism of the *CYP2C9* gene. This gene is involved in metabolizing Coumadin (Warfarin), Viagra, Amaryl, Isoniazid, Sulfa, Ibuprofen, Amitriptiline, Dilantin, Hyzaar, Tetrahidrocannabinol, Naproxen
CYP2C19 linked to psychiatric diseases, epilepsies, malaria and anesthesia	Polymorphism of the *CYP2C19* gene. This gene is involved in metabolizing different drugs: Carisoprodol, Diazepam, Dilantin, Premarin and Prevacid
Chronic myeloide leukemia	Mutation screening in exons 4–10 of the *ABL* gene, for the treatment with Gleevec (Imatinib)
Acute myeloide leukemia	Mutation in the *KIT* (CD117) gene, for the treatment with Gleevec (Imatinib) Mutation of the *FLT3* gene
5-Fluorouracil toxicity	Allele 2 A (IVS14+1G-A) determination in the *DPD* gene
Thiopurines toxicity	For the treatment of thrombosis, diabetes, and a variety of diseases. The TPMT gene is associated to the different tiopurines metabolism: azatioprine (Imuran,) 6-mercaptopurina (Purinetol,) and 6-tioguanina (Lanvis)
Mitochondrial Disorders	
Neuropathy, ataxia and retinitis pigmentosa (NARP)	Mutation of T8993G and T8993 C in the *MTATP6* gene
Maternal hereditary deafness	Mutation of A1555G, A827G, T961 C, T961insC, T961delT+C(n)ins, T1005 C, A1116G and C1494 T in the *MTRNR1* gene Mutation screening of T7445 C and A7443G in the *MTCO1* gene

Source: LabGenetics, www.labgenetics.com.es; accessed March 1, 2009.

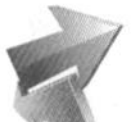

ASSESSMENT, MONITORING, AND EVALUATION

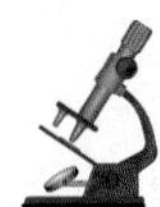

CLINICAL INDICATORS

Genetic Markers: Each individual has a unique genetic profile and phenotype. Because both parents contribute genes and chromosomes to the fetus, a genetic history may be beneficial.

Clinical/History	Lab Work	
BP	Glucose	C-reactive protein (CRP)
Height	Chol—HDL, LDL, total	Alb, transthyretin (if needed)
Weight, current	Trig	BUN, Creat
Weight, usual	Na^+, K^+	Sleep disorder screening
BMI and waist to hip ratio	Mg^{++}, Ca^{++}	
Recent weight changes	H & H, serum Fe	
HBW range	Homocysteine	
Diet history	Serum folic acid and vitamin B_{12}	
Body fat analysis		
Smoking		
Alcohol use		

SAMPLE NUTRITION CARE PROCESSES

Imbalance of Nutrients

Assessment Data: Dietary recall, nutrient analysis for vitamins and minerals, results of genetic testing.

Nutrition Diagnosis (PES): Imbalance of nutrients related to low micronutrient intake (vitamins A and C, magnesium, and potassium) and C>T genetic allele of methyltetrahydrofolate reductase (MTHFR) as evidenced by consistent omission of fruits and vegetables in dietary intake records, genetic inability to metabolize folic acid, and history of three miscarriages in past 5 years.

Intervention: Education about a healthy diet for promoting optimal reproductive health. Counseling about use of L-methylfolate and multivitamin–mineral supplement in preparation for a healthy pregnancy.

Monitoring and evaluation: Dietary intake records, increased intake of fruits and vegetables; successful pregnancy where possible.

Menopause

Assessment Data: Dietary recall, side effects of taking multiple herbs, weight history, labs.

Nutrition Diagnosis (PES:) Harmful beliefs about food/nutrition related to regular intake of dietary supplements as evidenced by dietary recall indicating use of large doses of Chinese herbal remedies that are unsubstantiated by medical efficacy.

Intervention: Education about safe use of herbs and supplements for menopausal symptoms (soy, black cohosh, multivitamin-mineral supplements). Counseling about acceptable choices.

Monitoring and Evaluation: Dietary recall, dietary supplement usage pattern, side effect reports, improvement of symptoms of menopause.

INTERVENTION

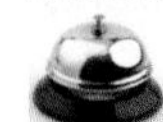

OBJECTIVES

- Maintain quality of nutrition while compensating for energy needs that are lower than those during periods of growth.
- Maintain a healthy lifestyle, which offers greater longevity than genetics alone. Losing excess weight, exercising, and eating a nearly meat-free diet are tips shared by many centenarians.
- Prevent obesity resulting from a sedentary lifestyle where relevant. Highly sedentary people lose 20–24% of overall muscle mass and strength. Every adult should accumulate 30 minutes or more of moderate-intensity physical activity on most days of the week. Also useful are strength training (resistance or weight training with 8–12 repetitions), isotonics, and aerobics (20 minutes of walking, jogging, swimming, or bicycling).
- Prevent or delay the onset of conditions such as, hypertension, osteoporosis, cardiovascular disease, diabetes, renal disorders, Alzheimer's disease, and cancers. Focus on a plant-based diet, rich in colorful fruits and vegetables plus nuts, seeds, and whole grains. Include fish and sources of omega-3 fatty acids, including walnuts, flaxseed, and dark-green leafy vegetables. The Mediterranean diet is a good pattern to follow.
- Improve nutrient density of meals, especially those eaten away from home. The average American eats 3–4 meals away from home each week. Making "each calorie count more" is a message that encourages selecting foods that offer more quality per "bite." The Naturally Nutrient Rich (NNR) approach is also helpful; encourage "super foods" such as salmon, blueberries, bananas, whole-wheat grains, fat-free yogurt, broccoli, and top round steak (Drewnoski, 2004).
- Use of a multivitamin–mineral supplement can assure that the basics are met, but a balanced diet provides other beneficial phytochemicals. Lutein and zeaxanthin from food protect against age-related eye diseases such as macular degeneration.
- Promote adequate bone mass density, which peaks at 25–30 years of age. Osteopenia is common in women over age 40, and testing of bone density is recommended. Men are also at risk as they age.
- Identify food insecurity and its relationship to availability of varied foods and intake patterns. For example, food insecurity is common among migrant workers and farm worker households. The impact of hunger varies by factors such as participation in food banks, dependence on family members or friends outside the household for food, inadequate transportation, and not having a garden (Holben et al, 2010).

TABLE 1-22 Special Nutrition-Related Concerns of Adult Women[a]

Fibrocystic breast changes	50–60% of all women present with breast nodularity, swelling, and pain with monthly hormonal changes. A low-fat (15–20% kcal), adequate fiber diet (30 g/d) and soy isoflavones seems to be useful. Fruit and vegetable intake should be high. Studies fail to support nutrition interventions with decreased sodium or fluid and caffeine; increased use of primrose oil, herbal teas, vitamins A, C, E, B_6, iodine, selenium.
Infertility	Women desiring to become pregnant should stop smoking and drinking alcohol, and increase intakes of folate and vitamin B_{12} (American Dietetic Association, 2004).
Premenstrual syndrome (PMS) and premenstrual dysphoric disorder (PMDD)	Up to 40% of women experience symptoms including edema, migraines, depression, and mastalgia. PMDD is generally more severe, although women experience anxiety and irritability in both conditions. A basic multivitamin-mineral supplement can help assure adequacy of all micronutrients, especially calcium, vitamin B_6 and magnesium (American Dietetic Association, 2004). Herbal supplements have limited supporting evidence (Johnson, 2007).
Perimenopause	In the 2- to 10-year stage before menopause, women may experience hot flashes, night sweats, fatigue, insomnia, weight gain, loss of libido, irregular periods, fibroids or heavy bleeding, breast pain, mood swings and irritability, cravings for sweets or alcohol, digestive problems, hair loss, stiffness or joint pain, anxiety, and depression. Women should exercise regularly and consume a balanced, healthy diet. Herbal remedies are not very effective.
Menopause	Declining levels of estrogens and other hormones, cessation of menstrual periods, and a decreased need for iron. Hormone replacement therapy is no longer the mainstay for preventing osteoporosis and fractures because of the risk for cancer. Exercise, calcium, vitamin D and physical examinations are needed. A diet that is moderate in carbohydrate slows insulin shifts; lean proteins and moderate fat help to prevent weight gain. Food sources of selenium, vitamins C and E contribute antioxidant benefits. Whole grains, flax seed, and other omega-3 fatty acids may reduce the inflammation that aggravates hot flashes. Phytoestrogens from isoflavones, lignans, and coumestans (soy foods, flaxseed, and red clover) are useful for some women. Avoid large amounts of soy if breast cancer is a known risk. Black cohosh has some merit but may also have undesirable side effects (see herbal guidelines).
Postmenopause	Older women may be at risk for poor nutritional intake because their diets tend to be more limited; they may have difficulty chewing; and they may no longer enjoy cooking (American Dietetic Association, 2004). Nutrient supplementation may be beneficial, especially for calcium, zinc, and the vitamins.

[a]See related disorder sections for specific disease advice.

- ID affects approximately one half of all women. Correct through diet as far as possible. Avoid iron excesses in men and in post menopausal women. Table 1-22 provides a summary of conditions that affect women specifically.

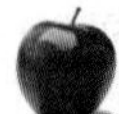

FOOD AND NUTRITION

- Ensure intake from the MyPyramid Food Guidance System: 2–3 servings of milk, 2–3 servings of meat or substitute, 3–5 servings of vegetables, 2–4 servings of fruits, and 6–12 bread group servings. Control fats, oils, sugars, alcohol, and sweets as needed to increase or decrease energy intake; foods from this group often replace nutrient-dense foods in the American diet. Limit or eliminate foods that contain trans-fatty acids.
- Follow the dietary guidelines. Modify diet as needed for special medical conditions, such as hypertension, heart disease, and osteoporosis.
- Energy needs will vary by sedentary or active status; 30 kcal/kg/d is average. Use 20–25 kcal/kg/d when weight loss is desired and 35–40 kcal/kg/d when weight gain is needed. Adults are encouraged to maintain weight rather than gaining weight after reaching adulthood. See nutritional recommendation charts.

Nutrient Recommendations for Adults

Nutrient	Males 19–50 Years	Males 51–70 Years
Energy	3067 kcal/d	3067 kcal/d
Protein	56 g/d or 0.8 g/kg/d	56 g/d or 0.8 g/kg/d
Calcium	1000 mg/d	1200 mg/d
Iron	8 mg/d	8 mg/d
Folate	400 mg/d	400 mg/d
Phosphorus	700 mg/d	700 mg/d
Vitamin A	900 μg/d	900 μg/d
Vitamin C	90 mg/d	90 mg/d
Thiamin	1.2 mg/d	1.2 mg/d
Riboflavin	1.3 mg/d	1.3 mg/d
Niacin	16 mg/d	16 mg/d

- For most healthy adults, 0.8 g of protein/kg will suffice. Use fish, poultry, and nonmeat entrees (e.g., dry beans, peas, nuts as tolerated) regularly instead of just meat-centered meals. Soy products such as tofu, textured soy protein, soynut butter, or tempeh can be useful. The Continuing Survey of Food Intakes by Individuals (CSFII) has found that households with higher income tend to use more chicken and less beef and pork (Guenther et al, 2005).

- For carbohydrate, the Institute of Medicine has set the minimum intake at 130 g daily. In general, use of whole grains, fresh fruits or vegetables, and low-fat dairy products will provide high-quality carbohydrate. Refined carbohydrates in sweetened beverages, desserts, and candy should be limited.
- Mineral and phytochemical balance is important, including sodium, potassium, calcium, and magnesium. The DASH diet may be useful for designing meal patterns to lower BP and lipids, when needed.
- Eat a balanced diet. The most recent national study of What We Eat in America (United States Department of Agriculture, 2006) identified that vitamins A, C, and E and magnesium tend to be low in most diets; teen girls and older men and women tend to be low in zinc intakes; and potassium, calcium, vitamin D, vitamin K, and fiber are low as well.
- Hyperhomocysteinemia is an independent risk factor for cardiovascular disease in men and women as well as for Alzheimer's disease, and stroke. B-complex vitamins (folic acid, vitamins B_6 and B_{12}) are needed. If an individual has an MTHFR allele, L-methylfolate may be needed.
- Women of childbearing age should include foods rich in folic acid, now available through fortification of grains, to prevent neural tube defects. Men may need to eat more folic acid–rich foods to lower risk for colorectal cancer. Cold cereals, cooked pinto or navy beans, asparagus, spinach, orange juice, lentils, and avocado should be planned into the diet regularly.
- Fiber-rich foods may help protect against heart disease, stroke, diabetes, high BP, some types of cancer, constipation, and diverticulosis. They are also helpful with management of weight by increasing satiety with meals. Soluble fiber is found in pectins, gums, plums, apples, berries, figs, broccoli, potatoes, and okra. Insoluble fibers are found in bran cereal, whole-wheat bread, brown rice, legumes, vegetables, and many fruits. Nuts and seeds are also good sources of fiber.
- Favorable dietary habits promote health, whereas unfavorable habits are linked to various chronic diseases; an individual's "sense of coherence" (SOC) correlates with prevalence of some diseases to which dietary habits are linked (Lindmark et al, 2005).
- Family meals are associated with positive dietary intakes and healthy behaviors. Family interaction can lower risks for obesity, enhance language skills and academic performance, and improve social skills. A positive atmosphere is beneficial; see http://www.cfs.purdue.edu/CFF/promotingfamilymeals/index.html.
- Use spices and herbs liberally in cooking. Oregano, cinnamon, dill, savory, coriander, cumin, and other herbs have potent antioxidant properties.
- A Mediterranean-style diet can enhance cholesterol-lowering plans; design menus accordingly.
- Adequate vitamins A, C, and E and selenium foods should be consumed for their antioxidant properties. Foods rather than supplements are recommended because of the phytochemical and biological properties that may prevent or delay some chronic diseases.
- Functional food ingredients, including fortified, enriched, or enhanced foods, have a potentially beneficial effect on health when consumed as part of a varied diet on a regular basis (American Dietetic Association, 2005). Functional foods may reduce the risk of coronary heart disease, cancers, hypertension, and osteoporosis. Each food or ingredient should be assessed individually for its relative merit. Soybeans, fruits, and vegetables seem to yield the greatest risk reductions. Soy protein, as in tofu and meat extenders, may reduce serum cholesterol and possibly reduce risks of some forms of cancer. Quercetin (found in apples, broccoli, oranges, tomatoes, kale, and onions) may help protect against cataracts. Phytosterols in sunflower seeds, pistachio nuts, sesame seeds, and wheat germ are good for the heart. Plant sterols and stanols help to lower serum cholesterol levels and are less expensive than statin drugs. Polyphenols (flavonoids from tea, cocoa, red wine, Concord grape juice, blueberries, and chocolate) also support heart health. See Table 1-23 for a list of functional food ingredients and their beneficial effects.

Common Drugs Used and Potential Side Effects

- In general, discuss the relevance of tolerable ULs from the latest dietary reference intakes of the National Academy of Sciences. These levels were set to protect individuals from receiving too much of any nutrient from diet and dietary supplements. Table 1-24 provides a useful chart.

Herbs, Botanicals, and Supplements

- Herbs, botanical products, and supplements should not be used without discussing with a physician, especially with underlying medical conditions (Boullata, 2005). The Food and Drug Administration implement guidelines for DSHEA.
- Supplement use is common among middle-aged men and women in the United States, it should be recognized that micronutrient intakes of vitamins A, C, and E, niacin, folate, and iron are often higher than from foods alone (Archer et al, 2005). Section 2 provides an extensive list of herbs and botanicals; see Table 2-1.
- Use of multivitamins/minerals (MVMs) has grown rapidly; dietary supplements are now used by more than half of the adult population in the United States (NIH, 2006). The NIH consensus report (2006) reported that fortification of foods has reduced vitamin and mineral deficits. Now there are safety concerns about exceeding upper levels and there is limited evidence for beneficial health-related effects of supplements taken singly, in pairs, or in combinations of three or more (NIH, 2006).

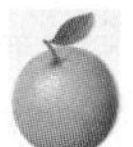

NUTRITION EDUCATION, COUNSELING, CARE MANAGEMENT

- Help plan a diet in accordance with individual lifestyle. Explain nutrient density, food cost, and portion sizes. Meal and snack patterns are markers for nutrient intakes and diet quality (Kerver et al, 2006).

TABLE 1-23 Functional Foods and Ingredients

Food	Function
Almonds	Lower LDL and total cholesterol to reduce heart disease. Source of potassium, vitamin E, riboflavin, magnesium, and zinc.
Apples	Good source of fiber, quercetin in the skin. May protect against cancer, asthma, and Alzheimer's disease.
Apricots	Good source of vitamins A and C, as well as lycopene. Cancer prevention.
Avocado	Reduces risk of heart disease, high blood pressure, and osteoporosis. Contains vitamins B_6 and E, folate, potassium, and fiber.
Bananas	Good source of potassium and magnesium, which are helpful to prevent heart disease, bone loss, and hypertension.
Barley	Good whole grain source.
Blueberries and other berries	Reduce risk of cancer; may improve cognitive function. Contain vitamin C as well as anthocyanins, fiber, and ellagic acid.
Brazil nuts	Supply of selenium, which is a cancer preventive. Use no more than 2 per day.
Broccoli	Reduces risk of cancer and maintains healthy immune system. Sulforaphane detoxifies carcinogens. Source of quercetin.
Brown rice	Rich whole grain with phosphorus and potassium in greater amounts than white rice.
Brussels sprouts	Source of sulforaphane to prevent cancer; also good source of vitamin K.
Cabbage	Contains sulforaphane; consume often as a cancer prevention measure.
Canola oil	Good source of fatty acids, which reduce heart disease and cancer.
Cantaloupe	Great source of beta-carotene and vitamin C.
Carrots	Rich source of beta-carotene.
Cauliflower	Rich in sulforaphane and vitamin C; may protect against cancer.
Cheese	May decrease risk of colon cancer because of calcium content.
Chicken or turkey breast	Skinless poultry is a great source of protein and zinc; turkey is also high in B vitamins and selenium.
Chocolate	May decrease risk for cardiovascular disease; flavonoid content is a powerful antioxidant.
Cinnamon	May lower LDL cholesterol and blood glucose levels. Anti-clotting effect. Anti-inflammatory effect in arthritis.
Citrus fruits	Limonoids reduce risk of certain cancers. Oranges are a source of quercetin.
Cloves	Ground cloves are the richest source of polyphenols among the spices.
Cocoa	Rich source of flavonols; reduces risk of cancer and heart disease.
Collard greens and kale	Great source of carotenoids, vitamin C, lutein, sulforaphane, and calcium.
Cranberries	Improves urinary tract health and prevents infection; reduces risk of heart disease; may reduce periodontitis/gingivitis.
Cruciferous vegetables	Sulforaphane content helps to prevent cancer. Brussels sprouts, cauliflower, broccoli, and bok choy are in this family.
Edamame	Green soybeans, a staple in Asia. They can lower LDL cholesterol and may protect against colon cancer.
Fatty fish	Source of omega-3 fatty acids; helpful for brain, eye, and neurological health.
Flaxseed	Reduces risk of heart disease, high blood pressure, and osteoporosis. Provides lignans and alpha linolenic acid, an omega-3 fatty acid.
Garlic	Reduces risk of cancer; lowers cholesterol levels and blood pressure.
Kale	High in antioxidants lutein and zeaxanthin; protects eye health. Source of quercetin.
Kiwifruit	High in potassium, vitamin C, fiber, folate, magnesium, vitamin E, copper, and lutein. Great antioxidant fruit.
Legumes and beans	Lentils, dried beans, and peas provide folate, which reduces DNA damage and helps with cancer prevention. Rich in fiber, magnesium, potassium, protein, iron.
Lycopene	Lycopene is especially rich in tomatoes, pink grapefruit. A substance called Fru-his in rehydrated tomato products protects against prostate cancer.
Marjoram	Good source of polyphenols.
Milk, nonfat	Reduces risk of osteoporosis, high blood pressure, and colon cancer. Good source of vitamin D, calcium, and potassium.
Nuts, Seeds	Good source of arginine, magnesium, fiber.
Oatmeal	Reduces total and LDL cholesterol levels.
Olive oil	Good source of monounsaturated fatty acids (MUFA), which reduce heart disease risk by improving cholesterol levels.
Onions	Sulfur-rich and full of quercetin (red or yellow are richer). Blood thinning to help lower blood pressure and LDL cholesterol levels.
Oranges	Great source of potassium and vitamin C. Source of quercetin.
Oregano	Good source of polyphenols.
Peaches	Good source of vitamin C, carotenoids, niacin, and potassium.
Peanut butter	Good source of protein, MUFA, and niacin.

(continued)

TABLE 1-23 Functional Foods and Ingredients *(continued)*

Food	Function
Pistachio nuts	Good source of phytosterols for heart health.
Pomegranate	Antioxidant that protects against hormonal and lung cancers, Alzheimer's disease and heart disease.
Pork loin	Leanest cut of "red meat" sources. Protein, zinc, and iron source.
Prunes	Great source of antioxidants, fiber, potassium, and vitamins A and B_6.
Pumpkin seeds	Good source of phytosterols; B vitamins, along with C, D, E, and K; calcium, potassium, niacin, and phosphorous. May protect against depression and learning disabilities. Excellent source of magnesium.
Pycogenol	Antioxidant plant extract from the bark of a French pine tree; reduces blood sugar in type 2 diabetes patients, allows people to lower their antihypertensive medication, and improves cardiovascular disease risk factors.
Quinoa	Seed containing high amounts of protein, fiber, magnesium, potassium, vitamin E, riboflavin, zinc, copper, and iron.
Sage, tarragon, thyme	Moderately good sources of polyphenols.
Salmon, sardines, mackerel	Improve mental and visual function; reduce risk of heart disease and may prevent cancers. Rich omega-3 fatty acid source.
Shredded wheat	Great source of whole-grain fiber, as well as magnesium; helpful in maintaining normal blood glucose levels.
Soy	Reduces risk of heart disease by lowering LDL cholesterol; eases menopausal symptoms. Isoflavones have weak estrogenic effects.
Spinach and romaine lettuce	Great source of lutein, carotenoids, and vitamin C; maintain healthy vision.
Squash, acorn	Rich in carotenoids, folate, vitamin C, and potassium; all helpful in reducing heart disease and cancer risk.
Strawberries	May lower blood pressure, reduce the risk of heart disease and some cancers, and improve memory.
Sunflower and sesame seeds	Good source of phytosterols for heart health.
Tea, black, green or white	Reduces risk for stomach, esophageal, and skin cancers, and heart disease. Flavonoids neutralize free radicals.
Tofu	Great meat substitute; rich in protein and isoflavones and may be high in calcium.
Tomatoes	Reduce risk of prostate cancer and heart attack; rich in lutein, lycopene, and vitamin C. Lycopene protects cell membranes. Source of quercetin.
Tuna	Reduces risk of heart disease; high in vitamins B_6 and B_{12}, omega-3 fatty acids, and protein.
Turmeric	Natural anti-inflammatory that reduces cancer risk. Thought to slow Alzheimer's disease.
Walnuts	Lower total and LDL cholesterol and reduces risk of heart disease. Good source of vitamin E, alpha linolenic acid, minerals, and folate.
Whey protein	Immune-enhancing properties including lactoferrin, beta-lactoglobulin, alpha-lactalbumin, and immunoglobulins. Useful for intracellular conversion of cysteine to glutatione, a powerful antioxidant. Whey protein is found naturally in milk.
Whole grains	Reduce risk of certain cancers and heart disease. Contain saponins, flavonoids, and lignans.
Wine, red, grapes and grape juice	Reduce risk of cardiovascular disease and cancer because of resveratrol, a flavonoid (polyphenol).
Winter squash	Butternut squash is one example. Good source of beta-carotene, calcium, potassium, and folate.
Yogurt	Improves intestinal health because of bacterial (probiotic) content; reduces risk of cancer; lowers cholesterol. Rich source of calcium, vitamin B_{12}, magnesium, and protein. May also use cultured dairy products.

Derived from: Functional Foods List, http://www.mealsmatter.org/EatingForHealth/FunctionalFoods/func_list.aspx; accessed February 9, 2009; Fruits and Veggies More Matters, http://www.fruitsandveggiesmorematters.org/; accessed February 9, 2009.

- Explain the benefits of weight management for adults to prevent or delay the onset of chronic diseases. Start with BMI; select a healthy weight goal as needed. Successful weight losers tend to follow a low-fat, high-carbohydrate food plan with high levels of physical activity; they eat breakfast regularly.
- Popular low-carbohydrate, high-protein diet plans may contribute to problems such as kidney stones and are not advised for most adults. The South Beach diet, by recommending olive oil and fatty fish, mimics the Mediterranean diet plan more than the Atkins plan.
- Encourage planned meals. Skipping breakfast may lead to overeating later at night.
- Describe the effects of alcohol at the "business lunch;" alcohol intake may equal 300 calories or more. Discourage intake of more than two alcoholic drinks per day for men or one drink for women.
- Being physically fit can improve the odds against chronic diseases. Goal setting may be an effective strategy. The Surgeon General recommends 1 hour daily of physical activity. Using a pedometer to count steps is very motivating; "10,000 steps a day" is the goal; one mile is approximately 2000 steps. Other forms of exercise should be encouraged as well; yoga, pilates, and Tai chi can help increase flexibility.
- Fluid intake may be lower than desirable. Dehydration can contribute to kidney stones, strain on the heart and cardiovascular system, or even drug toxicity. Encourage daily intake of 30 mL/kg of water and other liquids.

TABLE 1-24 **Medications Commonly Used by Adult Women and Men**

Infertility	Smoking can reduce the ability of sperm to bind to an egg and can also reduce fertility in women (Bordel et al, 2006). Oxidative stress is detrimental to sperm function and a significant factor in male infertility. Dietary and supplementary intake of the antioxidants vitamin C, vitamin E, and beta-carotene on sperm chromatin integrity (Silver et al, 2005).
Women: Childbearing Age	
Infertility and miscarriages	Genetic defects in the MTHFR (methyltetrahydrofolate reductase) enzyme can cause spontaneous abortions and infertility; forms of L-methylfolate (such as Deplin® or Neevo®) may be needed.
Intrauterine devices	May increase menstrual losses of iron and vitamin C.
Interstitial cystitis (IC)	Acidic foods and beverages such as coffee, alcoholic beverages, fruit juices, carbonated beverages, tomato products, hot peppers, and other spicy foods or beverages may cause irritation. Use buffering products or pain relievers.
Women: Menopause	Low doses of Megace (megestrol acetate) may be used to decrease hot flashes in postmenopausal women who cannot take estrogen. Megace can cause increased appetite, edema, and sodium retention.
Bone density loss	Alendronate (Fosamax) may be used to maintain bone density without breast cancer risk.
Men: Baldness	Androgenic alopecia (baldness) may suggest higher risk for prostate cancer or for early, severe coronary heart disease.
	Rogaine (minoxidil) can cause diarrhea, low blood pressure, nausea, vomiting, and weight gain; it is a vasodilator. A low-sodium, low-calorie diet may be beneficial.
	5-Alpha reductase catalyzes the conversion of testosterone to dihydrotestosterone. Disturbances in 5-alpha reductase activity in skin cells might contribute to male pattern baldness, acne, or hirsutism. Plant homologs are being tested.
Men: Prostate Problems	Proscar (finasteride) and other medications are used with some relief. Monitor blood pressure; no nutritional side effects are noted. Saw palmetto may be useful (see following herb section).
	Antioxidant foods may help protect against prostate cancer (Kranse et al, 2005). Brazil nuts, seafood, and whole grains are natural sources of selenium. Lycopene from dietary sources (tomato sauce, pink grapefruit) are preferable over supplements. Broccoli and cauliflower also be protective.

- Coffee and tea contain antioxidants that can be preventive against cancers, diabetes, heart disease, and Parkinson's disease; moderate daily inclusion may be promoted.
- Annual doctor visits are reasonable. Cholesterol, dental check-ups, BP screening should start at age 20; women need Pap smears and vaccinations against Human papilloma virus (HPV) and cervical cancer (Gardisil®). Women more than 35 years of age should be tested for thyroid status (as with the thyroid stimulating hormone (TSH) test) and should schedule mammograms at least every 3 years. Periodic electrocardiograms (EKGs) and fasting blood glucose are useful after age 40. After age 50, a fecal occult blood test, bone density scan, and (for men), a prostate-specific antigen test should be added. Vaccines for tetanus, flu, shingles, and pneumonia are useful after age 60.
- Help clarify conflicting information about a "serving" and a "portion" on food labels.
- The American Council on Science and Health (ACSH) ranks consumer magazines as sources of reliable nutrition information; *Parents, Cooking Light,* and *Good Housekeeping* rank highly.
- Discuss food choices when eating away from home. For travelers who experience jet lag, adjust meal times to match new time zone, which may help the liver adjust more readily.
- Discuss calcium alternatives for people who exclude milk products. There are calcium-fortified foods and beverages, such as fortified orange juice, cereals, mineral waters, and margarine.
- For people living in northern climates, taking vitamin D_3 may be important.
- Discuss the role of managing BP and how diet can help. Ignoring high BP can set the stage for stroke, dementia, and heart disease later in life. Intensive diet and physical activity modifications can greatly reduce disease risk (Aldana et al, 2005).
- Determine psychological readiness for dietary and lifestyle change and the individual's current stage. The Transtheoretical Model for Stages of Change (precontemplation, contemplation, preparation, action, maintenance, or termination) is a useful tool that defines motivation as a dynamic process (Prochaska and DiClemente, 1982). People in the action stages tend to display healthier eating; demographic and psychosocial factors help to mediate readiness to change dietary factors; and precontemplators need individually tailored interventions.
- Many primary care patients are ready to lose weight, improve diet, and increase exercise (Wee et al, 2005). Concentrate on small changes with the client.
- The "Slow Food" movement is trying to counter the fast-food culture by returning to traditional foods, having pleasurable mealtimes, and enjoying the aroma and flavors of foods more fully.

TABLE 1-25 Tips for Eating More Fruits and Vegetables

- Eat at least one vitamin A–rich fruit or vegetable, such as apricots, cantaloupe, carrots, sweet potatoes, spinach, collards, or broccoli each day.
- Eat at least one vitamin C–rich fruit or vegetable such as oranges, strawberries, green peppers, or tomatoes each day.
- Eat several high-fiber fruits or vegetables daily, such as apples, grapefruit, broccoli, baked potato with skin, or cauliflower.
- Eat berries often; blueberries have been highly rated for their antioxidant properties (anthocyanins). Other berries are equally nutritious and contain fiber, quercetin, and other flavonoids.
- Eat cabbage family vegetables, such as cauliflower, broccoli, Brussels sprouts, and cabbage, several times every week.
- Add fruit to cereal or plain yogurt.
- Use fruit juice instead of water when preparing cakes and muffins.
- Drink 100% fruit juice instead of soda.
- Eat a piece of fruit for a morning snack; choose a grapefruit or an orange for an afternoon snack.
- Choose the darkest green or red leaf lettuce greens for salads; add carrots, red cabbage, and spinach.
- Add more vegetables or add tomato juice to soups and stews for vitamins A and C.
- Choose pizza with extra mushrooms, green pepper, onion, broccoli, and tomatoes.
- Munch on raw vegetables with a low-fat dip for an afternoon snack.
- When dining out, choose a side dish of vegetables.
- Fill up most of the plate with vegetables at lunch and dinner.
- Choose fortified foods and beverages, such as juice with added calcium.
- Snack on dried fruits, such as dried apricots, peaches, raisins, or "craisins."
- Use dried plums (prunes) for a natural laxative.
- Use dried plum puree as a butter or margarine substitute in recipes to reduce fat; use half the measure required.

Refer clients to: (1) *Centers for Disease Control and Prevention. Resources for Fruits and Vegetables*. http://www.fruitsandveggiesmorematters.org/?page_id=71

- If needed, provide resources to alleviate food insecurity (American Dietetic Association, 2006).
- Discuss fiber, nonmeat vegetarian meals, cooking methods for nutrient preservation, and phytochemicals. Nutrition messages that lead to increased consumption of dietary fiber need to be strengthened.
- The "Total Diet" message is important to share with consumers (American Dietetic Association, 2007). Peer support is effective for increasing fruit and vegetable intake; Table 1-25 lists ways to include more fruits and vegetables and Table 1-26 describes their key nutrients.
- Nutrition information on packaged food labels is useful to teach point-of-purchase tips, and adults can be encouraged to use them (Satia et al, 2005). However, many adults do not know how to use the food label as well as they might. Consumers are confronted with food and dietary supplement products that claim to improve health, manage conditions, and reduce disease risks (Turner et al, 2005). Label reading may be a marker for other dietary behaviors that predict healthful food choices. Table 1-27 describes food labeling terms. Table 1-28 briefly describes Health Claims that are approved and under review by the Food and Drug Administration.

Patient Education—Food Safety Tips

- Reminders about hand washing and safe food handling may be important, especially for those adults who prepare and serve meals for others.
- Avoid food preparation when sick with viral or bacterial infections. Use latex gloves if there are any cuts on the hands. Thoroughly cook meat, poultry, and fish entrees. Keep cold foods cold and hot foods hot.
- Bacteria are commonly found on foods such as green onions (scallions), cantaloupe, cilantro, and many types of imported produce. Wash all fresh fruits and vegetables. Scrub the outside of produce such as melons and cucumbers before cutting.
- Avoid tap water and ice made from tap water, uncooked produce such as lettuce, and raw or undercooked seafood when traveling. Moderate use of alcoholic beverages may prevent foodborne illness; studies are under way to determine why.
- Airline water may not be free from contamination. Use of bottled water is recommended. Coffee and tea may not be hot enough to kill all bacteria.
- Throw out cooked foods that have been at room temperature for longer than 2 hours.
- Consumption of sulforaphane in foods such as broccoli, cauliflower, cabbage and Brussels sprouts may reduce the presence of *Helicobacter pylori.*
- Avoid raw or partially cooked eggs, raw or undercooked fish or shellfish, and raw or undercooked meats because of potential foodborne illnesses.
- Do not use raw (unpasteurized) milk or products made from it.
- Avoid serving unpasteurized juices and raw sprouts.
- Only serve processed deli meats and frankfurters that have been reheated to steaming hot temperature.

TABLE 1-26 **Key Nutrients in Fruits and Vegetables**[a]

Food	Vitamin A, >500 IU	Vitamin C, >6 mg	Folate, >0.04 mg	Potassium, >350 mg	Dietary Fiber, >2 g
Fruits					
Apple, with skin (1 medium)		X			X
Apricot, dried (3)	X	X		X	X
Banana (1 medium)		X		X	X
Blackberries (1/2 cup)					X
Blueberries (1 cup)		X			X
Cantaloupe (1 cup)	X	X		X	
Grapefruit (1/2 medium)		X			
Grapefruit juice (3/4 cup)		X		X	
Grapes (1/2 cup)		X			
Honeydew melon (1 cup)		X		X	X
Kiwifruit (2 medium)		X	X	X	X
Mango (1 medium)	X	X			X
Nectarine (1 medium)	X	X			X
Orange (1 medium)		X	X		X
Orange juice (3/4 cup)		X	X	X	
Papaya (1 medium)	X	X	X	X	X
Peach, with skin (1 medium)	X	X			X
Pear, with skin (1 medium)		X			X
Pineapple (two 3/4″ slices)		X			X
Plum, with skin (2 medium)		X			X
Prunes (4) (dried plums)	X				X
Raspberries (1 cup)		X			X
Strawberries (1/2 cup)		X			X
Watermelon (1 cup)	X	X			
Vegetables					
Artichokes (1 medium)					X
Asparagus (5 spears)		X	X		X
Beans, kidney (1/2 cup)			X	X	X
Beans, lima (1/2 cup)			X	X	X
Black-eyed peas (1/2 cup)			X		X
Bok choy (1 cup cooked)		X			
Broccoli (1/2 cup)	X	X	X		X
Brussels sprouts (1/2 cup)		X			
Carrots (1 medium)	X	X			X
Cauliflower (1 cup)		X	X		X
Collards (1/2 cup)	X	X	X		X
Corn (1 cup)		X	X	X	X
Green beans (1/2 cup)		X			X
Green pepper (1 medium)	X	X			X
Kale (1/2 cup)	X	X			X
Lentils (1/2 cup)			X	X	X
Peas, green (1/2 cup)		X	X		X
Peas, split (1/2 cup)			X	X	X
Potato (1 medium)		X		X	
Potato, with skin (1 medium)		X		X	X
Romaine lettuce (6 leaves)	X	X	X		
Spinach, cooked (1/2 cup)	X	X	X	X	X
Squash, winter (1/2 cup)	X	X		X	X
Sweet potato (1 medium)	X	X		X	X
Tomato (1 medium)	X	X		X	
Turnip greens (1/2 cup)	X	X	X		

Adapted from: *Supermarket Savvy* newsletter, Linda McDonald Associates Inc., www.supermarketsavvy.com. Used with permission.

[a]X indicates that the item provides 10% or more of the daily value in the serving size specified or at least 2 g of dietary fiber.

TABLE 1-27 Food Labeling Terms

Labeling Terms	
% Fat free	Food must be a low-fat or fat-free food to include this value
Free	Food contains 0% of the indicated nutrient
Good source	Contains 10–19% of the daily value (DV) for a nutrient
High	Contains 20% or more DV for a nutrient
Lean	Contains 10 g fat or less and 95 mg cholesterol or less (extra lean 5% fat by weight)
Less	Food contains 25% less than original food
Light/lite	Food contains fewer calories or 50% less fat than original food OR description of color (if indicated on the label)
Low	Low fat as 3 g or less; low sodium as 140 mg or less; very low sodium as 35 mg or less; low cholesterol as 20 mg or less; low calorie as 40 calories or less
More	Food contains 110% or more DV than original food
Reduced	Product has 25% or less of a nutrient or the usual calories of that food
Reduced cholesterol	The food contains 75% or less of the cholesterol found in the original product

Source: U.S. Food and Drug Administration.

TABLE 1-28 Health Claims

(1) Authorized Health Claims		**Health claims must be supported by significant scientific agreement among experts that the proclaimed benefit of a food or food component on a disease or health-related condition is true (Turner et al, 2005).**
Diet	**Disease**	**Model Claim**
Calcium	Osteoporosis	Regular exercise and a healthful diet with enough calcium help teens and young adult white and Asian American women maintain good bone health and may reduce their risk of osteoporosis.
Sodium	Hypertension	Diets low in sodium may reduce the risk of high blood pressure, a disease associated with many factors.
Dietary fat	Cancer	Development of cancer depends on many factors. A diet low in total fat may reduce the risk of some cancers.
Dietary saturated fat and cholesterol	Coronary heart disease	While many factors affect heart disease, diets low in saturated fat and cholesterol may reduce the risk of this disease.
Fiber-containing grain products, fruits, and vegetables	Cancers	Low-fat diets rich in fiber-containing grain products, fruits and vegetables may reduce the risk of some types of cancer, a disease associated with many factors.
Fruits, vegetables, and grain products that contain fiber, particularly soluble fiber	Coronary heart disease	Diets low in saturated fat and cholesterol and rich in fruits, vegetables, and grain products that contain some types of dietary fiber, particularly soluble fiber, may reduce the risk of heart disease, a disease associated with many factors.
Fruits and vegetables	Cancer	Low-fat diets rich in fruits and vegetables may reduce the risk of some types of cancer, a disease associated with many factors.
Folate	Neural tube birth defects	Healthful diets with adequate daily folate may reduce a woman's risk of having a child with a brain or spinal cord birth defect.

(continued)

TABLE 1-28 Health Claims *(continued)*

(2) Authorized Health Claims after Petition		**When significant scientific agreement is lacking, qualifying statements may be required on the label to describe the strength of the evidence that supports the claim (Turner et al, 2005).**
Diet	**Disease**	**Approved Health Claim**
Sugar alcohols	Dental caries	"Frequent eating of foods high in sugars and starches as between-meal snacks can promote tooth decay. The sugar alcohol [name of product] used to sweeten this food may reduce the skin of dental caries."
Foods that contain fiber from whole-oat products	Coronary heart disease	"Diets low in saturated fat and cholesterol that include soluble fiber from whole oats may reduce the risk of heart disease."
Foods that contain fiber from psyllium	Coronary heart disease	"Diets low in saturated fat and cholesterol that include soluble fiber from psyllium seed husk may reduce the risk of heart disease."
Soy protein	Coronary heart disease	"Diets low in saturated fat and cholesterol that include 25 g of soy protein a day may reduce the risk of heart disease. One serving of [name of food] provides 6.25 g of soy protein."
Plant sterol/stanol esters	Coronary heart disease	Plant sterols: "Foods containing at least 0.65 g per serving of plant sterols, eaten twice a day with meals for a daily total intake of at least 1.3 g, as part of a diet low in saturated fat and cholesterol, may reduce the risk of heart disease. A serving of [name of the food] supplies ___ g of vegetable oil sterol esters." Plant stanol esters: "Foods containing at least 1.7 g per serving of plant stanol esters, eaten twice a day with meals for a total daily intake of at least 3.4 g, as part of a diet low in saturated fat and cholesterol, may reduce the risk of heart disease. A serving of [name of the food] supplies ___ g of plant stanol esters."
(3) Qualified Health Claims NOT Approved by FDA		**Qualified health claims, where FDA has found some support but not enough clear evidence to allow an approved health claim.**
Diet–Disease Relationship	**Disease**	**Qualified Health Claim**
Omega-3 fatty acids	Coronary heart disease	Consumption of omega-3 fatty acids may reduce the risk of coronary heart disease. FDA evaluated the data and determined that, although there is scientific evidence supporting the claim, the evidence is not conclusive.
Folic acid, B_6, B_{12}	Vascular disease	As part of a well-balanced diet that is low in saturated fat and cholesterol, Folic Acid, Vitamin B_6 and Vitamin B_{12} may reduce the risk of vascular disease. FDA evaluated the above claim and found that, while it is known that diets low in saturated fat and cholesterol reduce the risk of heart disease and other vascular diseases, the evidence in support of the above claim is inconclusive.
Selenium	Cancer	Selenium may reduce the risk of certain cancers. Some scientific evidence suggests that consumption of selenium may reduce the risk of certain forms of cancer. However, FDA has determined that this evidence is limited and not conclusive.
Phosphatidylserine	Dementia	Very limited and preliminary scientific research suggests that phosphatidylserine may reduce the risk of dementia [cognitive dysfunction] in the elderly. FDA concludes that there is little scientific evidence supporting this claim.

From: Hasler CM. Functional foods: benefits, concerns and challenges—a position paper from the American Council on Science and Health. *J Nutr.* 132:3772–3781, 2002. Reprinted with permission.

For More Information

- American Association of Family and Consumer Sciences
  http://www.aafcs.org/
- American Pregnancy Association: Preconceptual Nutrition
  http://www.americanpregnancy.org/gettingpregnant/preconceptionnutrition.html
- American Public Health Association
  http://www.apha.org/
- Centers for Disease Control and Prevention—Young Adults
  http://www.cdc.gov/lifestages/youngAdults.html
- Centers for Disease Control and Prevention—Men
  http://www.cdc.gov/men/
- Centers for Disease Control and Prevention—Women
  http://www.cdc.gov/women/
- Chronic Disease Prevention and Health Promotion
  http://www.cdc.gov/nccdphp/index.htm
- Dietary Supplements
  http://www.foodsafety.gov/~dms/supplmnt.html
- Eating Well
  http://www.eatingwell.com
- Family Mealtime
  http://www.cfs.purdue.edu/CFF/promotingfamilymeals
- Food and Drug Administration
  http://www.fda.gov/
- Gardisil® and Human Papilloma Virus Vaccines
  http://www.gardasil.com/
- Healthfinder—Information
  http://www.healthfinder.gov/
- Health Statistics
  http://www.cdc.gov/nchs/fastats/Default.htm
- Human Genome Project
  http://www.genome.gov/
- Human Variome Project
  http://www.humanvariomeproject.org/
- International Food Information Council
  http://ific.org/
- Interstitial Cystitis Association
  http://www.ichelp.org/
- Menopause—Women's Healthcare Forum
  http://www.womenshealthcareforum.com/menopause.cfm
- Men's Health
  http://www.nlm.nih.gov/medlineplus/menshealth.html
- Men's Health Network
  http://www.menshealthnetwork.org/
- MyPyramid Food Guidance System
  http://www.mypyramid.gov/
- National Center for Complementary and Alternative Medicine
  http://nccam.nih.gov/
- National Institutes of Health
  http://www.nih.gov/
- National Women's Health Resource Center
  http://www.4woman.org/
- Recipes:
  http://www.deliciousdecisions.org
  http://www.cookinglight.com
  http://www.mealsforyou.com
  http://www.allrecipes.com
- Shape Up America
  http://www.shapeup.org/
- Slow Food Movement
  http://slowfood.com
- Sustainable Food Systems
  http://www.localharvest.org
- Web MD—Men's Health
  http://men.webmd.com/
- Women's Health Initiative
  http://www.nhlbi.nih.gov/whi/index.html

ADULTHOOD—CITED REFERENCES

Aldana SG, et al. Effects of an intensive diet and physical activity modification program on the health risks of adults. *J Am Diet Assoc.* 105:371, 2005.

American Dietetic Association. Position of the American Dietetic Association: fortification and dietary supplements. *J Am Diet Assoc.* 105:1300, 2005.

American Dietetic Association. Position of the American Dietetic Association: food insecurity and hunger in the United States. *J Am Diet Assoc.* 106:446, 2006.

American Dietetic Association. Position of the American Dietetic Association: total diet approach to communicating food and nutrition information. 107:1224, 2007.

Archer SL, et al. Association of dietary supplement use with specific micronutrient intakes among middle-aged American men and women: the INTERMAP study. *J Am Diet Assoc.* 105:1106, 2005.

Bordel R, et al. Nicotine does not affect vascularization but inhibits growth of freely transplanted ovarian follicles by inducing granulose cell apoptosis. *Hum Reprod.* 21:610, 2006.

Boullata J. Natural health product interactions with medication. *Nutr Clin Pract.* 20:33, 2005.

Drewnoski A. *Indices of nutrient density: making each calorie count.* Anaheim, CA: Lecture, American Dietetic Association Symposium, 2004.

Duffy VB, Bartoshuk LM. Food acceptance and genetic variation in taste. *J Am Diet Assoc.* 100:647, 2000.

Guenther PM, et al. Sociodemographic, knowledge, and attitudinal factors related to meat consumption in the United States. *J Am Diet Assoc.* 105:1266, 2005.

Holben DH, et al. Position of the American Dietetic Association: food insecurity in the United States. *Am Diet Assoc.* 110:1368, 2010.

Kerver JM, et al. Meal and snack patterns are associated with dietary intake of energy and nutrients in US adults. *J Am Diet Assoc.* 106:46, 2006.

Kranse R, et al. Dietary intervention in prostate cancer patients: PSA response in a randomized double-blind placebo-controlled study. *Int J Cancer.* 113:835, 2005.

Lindmark U, et al. Food selection associated with sense of coherence in adults. *Nutr J.* 4:9, 2005.

MuKusick VA. Mendelian Inheritance in Man and its online version, OMIM. *Am J Hum Genet.* 80:588, 2007.

NIH. State-of-the-Science Conference Statement on Multivitamin/Mineral Supplements and Chronic Disease Prevention. *NIH Consens State Sci Statements.* 23(2):1, 2006.

Prochaska JO, DiClemente CC. Transtheoretical therapy: toward a more integrative model of change. *Psychother Theory Res Pract.* 19:276, 1982.

Satia JA, et al. Food nutrition label use is associated with demographic, behavioral, and psychosocial factors and dietary intake among African Americans in North Carolina. *J Am Diet Assoc.* 105:392, 2005.

Silver EW, et al. Effect of antioxidant intake on sperm chromatin stability in healthy nonsmoking men. *J Androl.* 26:550, 2005.

Stein K. Refusal to follow dietary prescriptions. *J Am Diet Assoc.* 105:1188, 2005.

Turner RE, et al. Label claims for foods and supplements: a review of the regulations. Label claims for foods and supplements: a review of the regulations. *Nutr Clin Pract.* 20:21, 2005.

United States Department of Agriculture. What we eat in America, 2001–2002. Accessed January 2, 2006, at http://www.ars.usda.gov/Services/docs.htm?docid=7674.

Wee CC, et al. Stage of readiness to control weight and adopt weight control behaviors in primary care. *J Gen Intern Med.* 20:410, 2005.

NUTRITION IN AGING

NUTRITIONAL ACUITY RANKING: LEVEL 2

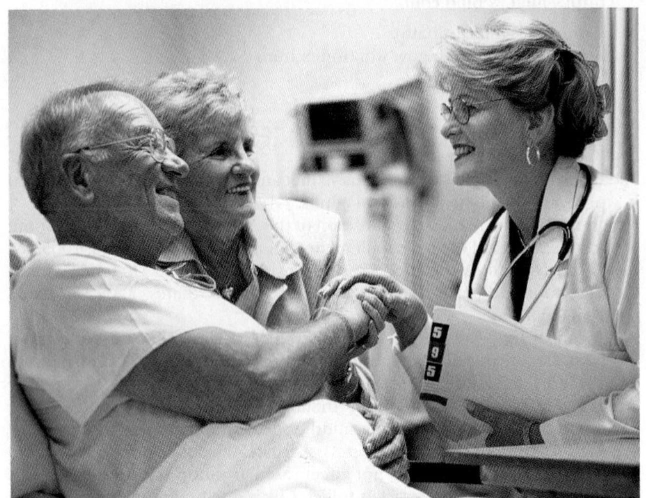

DEFINITIONS AND BACKGROUND

Aging involves a progression of physiological changes with cell loss and organ decline. Decreased glomerular filtration rate (GFR) and creatine-height index (CHI), constipation, decreased glucose tolerance, and lowered cell-mediated immunity can occur. Energy needs for basal metabolism decrease as much as 10% for ages 50–70 years and by 20–25% thereafter.

Life span is the length of time an organism could live; for humans, this is between 120 and 140 years. But life expectancy (average life span) is seldom beyond 114 years. Many gerontologists prefer to have patients start out a little overweight to support immunity. Nutrition density is an integral part of successful aging; culturally appropriate food and nutrition services should be customized to the individual's needs (American Dietetic Association, 2005).

It is estimated that most of the older population have one or more chronic conditions that would benefit from nutrition interventions. Challenges of nutritional assessment in older adults include limited recall, hearing and vision losses, changes in attention span, and variations in dietary intake from day to day. The inability to perform activities of daily living can be a major concern. Older adults may need assistance with shopping, meal preparation, and in ensuring adequate intake. Food insecurity exists among senior citizens and should be addressed (American Dietetic Association, 2006).

According to the U.S. Census Bureau, people older than 65 years of age comprise 13% of the United States population. Only about 5% of senior citizens are in nursing homes, the others live in the community, often alone. Approximately 20–50% of patients admitted to hospital are malnourished, especially older adults. Although the stress response to surgery (decrease in albumin and transferrin) is not affected by age, serum protein levels return to normal more slowly in older individuals, a factor to consider in older surgical patients. In addition, it is important to consider the wishes of the individual about nutrition and hydration (American Dietetic Association, 2008).

Loss of teeth, decreased salivation, lower nutrient absorption, as well as declining taste and smell, are common problems in the aged. More importantly, BMR declines 2% with each decade of life. LBM declines with each decade, generally replaced by fat. Being too thin is risky to the immune system; weight loss is not desirable in older adults because it is usually difficult for them to recover lost muscle mass. Essentially, older persons consume less food, about one third few calories, than younger people. Over 30% of seniors consume less energy than recommended levels, and 50% have low mineral and vitamin intakes. Lower food intake by this population appears to be a result of smaller meals eaten at a slower rate. In addition, protein intake is below the desired levels in many older adults.

Inflammatory chronic conditions such as obesity, cardiovascular disease, insulin resistance, and arthritis are associated with aging (Jensen, 2008). Seniors exhibit loss of muscle strength, easy fatigue, physical inactivity, slow or unsteady gait, poor appetite, unintentional weight loss, impaired cognition, depression and mortality. Muscle loss with aging (sarcopenia) comes from changes in anabolic hormones, decreased intake of dietary protein, a decline in physical activity, and inflammation driven by cytokines and oxidative stress with elevated levels of interleukin-6 and CRP (Jensen, 2008).

Protein-energy undernutrition contributes to pressure ulcers, immune dysfunction, infections, hip fractures, anemia, muscle weakness, fatigue, edema, cognitive changes, and mortality. While weight loss, depression, dehydration, and feeding problems are the easy to detect, elevated CRP levels should also be noted. Interventions for sarcopenia include enhanced physical activity, resistance exercise, calorie restriction, use of anabolic hormones, anti-inflammatory agents, nutritional supplements, and antioxidants (Jensen, 2008). Nutrition alone is not sufficient.

Growth hormone (GH) supports appetite and intake. Because GH secretion declines after puberty, researchers have developed oral ghrelin mimetics to improve intake, prevent declines in fat-free muscle mass, and reduce abdominal visceral fat in older adults (Hanauer, 2009). Multivitamin–mineral supplementation should be recommended; extra vitamins E, B_{12}, $B_{6,}$ folate, calcium, and zinc are needed to counteract gastric atrophy, decreased levels of hydrochloric acid, and poor nutrient intakes. Folate and vitamin D_3 seems to play a role in depression and dementia.

Use of medications including digoxin, furosemide, warfarin, paroxetine, nifedipine, ranitidine, theophylline, amlodipine, ciprofloxacin, and sertraline may cause anorexia or nausea. Scrutiny of the rationale of all medications should be undertaken.

Always follow abnormal lab work with evaluation of nutritional intake. Request labs that are truly warranted or cost effective. Low albumin may indicate infection or a draining wound, and not dietary inadequacy. Precipitously declining cholesterol (<150 mg/dL) appears to be a marker for depression, poor nutrition, or mortality. At the opposite end of the spectrum, lowering high cholesterol and homocysteine levels, obesity management, smoking cessation are beneficial for heart and brain health. The Mediterranean diet has been found to be especially useful. This diet improves cholesterol levels, blood sugar levels and blood vessel health, and reduces inflammation (Scarmeas et al, 2009).

When done properly, medical nutritional therapy can save thousands of dollars *per patient, per hospital stay*. Studies by the American Dietetic Association demonstrate that for every dollar spent on nutrition screening and intervention, at least $3.25 is saved in healthcare costs.

Common factors used for nutritional risk assessments are found in Table 1-29. The CNAQ, MNA and DETERMINE assessments are short, simple appetite assessment tools that predict anorexia-related weight loss in community-dwelling adults and long-term care residents (Wilson et al, 2005).

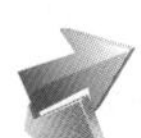

ASSESSMENT, MONITORING, AND EVALUATION

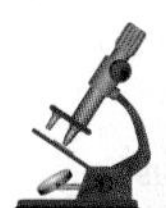

CLINICAL INDICATORS

Genetic Markers: Each individual has a unique genetic profile and phenotype. Because both parents contribute genes and chromosomes to the fetus, a genetic history may be beneficial.

Clinical/History

- Age
- Height (actual)
- Weight, current
- Weight, usual
- Recent weight changes
- BMI
- Waist circumference
- Diet history
- Temperature (hypothermia?)
- BP
- Dentition
- Eyesight
- Hearing
- Difficulty in chewing
- Dysphagia
- Constipation, diarrhea
- Fecal impaction
- Changes in bowel habits or incontinence
- Urinary incontinence or indwelling catheter
- Skin condition and pressure ulcers
- Hx of surgery, radiation, chemotherapy
- Mini-Mental State Examination
- Hydration status, I & O
- Clinical signs of malnutrition
- DXA for sarcopenia or osteopenia
- Changes in appetite
- Nausea, vomiting, indigestion
- Pain
- Infection
- Abnormal gait or motor coordination
- Sleep disorder screening

Lab Work

- Glucose
- CRP
- Ca^{++}, Mg^{++}
- Urinary N
- Na^{+}, K^{+}
- H & H, serum Fe
- Serum vitamin B_{12}, methylmalonic acid
- Serum folate
- Serum homocysteine
- Chol, Trig
- Alb or transthyretin (can be high in dehydration)
- TSF, MAC, MAMC
- BUN, Creat
- Transferrin
- TLC
- Protime (PT) or international normalized ratio (INR)

SAMPLE NUTRITION CARE PROCESS STEPS

Unintentional Weight Loss In Long-Term Care

Assessment: Intake reports and food preferences, I & O records, weight changes, lab values, psychological issues.

Nutrition Diagnosis (PES): Involuntary weight loss related to inadequate food and beverage intake as evidenced by 24-lb weight loss and dining room records indicating intake less than 50% at meals.

Intervention: Offer more favorite foods; promote consumption of between-meal nourishments, collaboration with social worker.

Monitoring and Evaluation: Changes in weight, verbalized improvement in appetite, dining room food intake records.

Palliative Care Nutrition

Assessment: Individual not eating or drinking; physician-ordered palliative care; resident wishes to have "no heroic measures" including tube feeding as per Advanced Directives.

Nutrition Diagnosis (PES): Inadequate food and beverage intake related to patient's choice to withdraw nutritional support as evidenced by minimal oral intake and palliative care status.

Intervention: Make food and fluids available upon patient or family request.

Monitoring and Evaluation: Check measures taken for meeting patient or family requests.

INTERVENTION

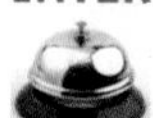

OBJECTIVES

- Provide proper nutrition for weight control, healthy appetite, prevention of acute illness, and complications of chronic diseases such as osteoporosis, fractures, anemia, obesity, diabetes, heart disease, and cancer.
- Avoid rapid unintentional weight loss, which often indicates underlying disease and accelerated muscle loss (Miller and Wolfe, 2008). Determine baseline functional level and evaluate changes over time.
- Monitor signs of malnutrition. Prevalence increases with age, is more common in institutionalized individuals, and is associated with susceptibility to infection, longer hospital stay, and increased mortality (Hudgens and Langkamp-Henken, 2005). Malnutrition may be caused by poverty, ignorance, chronic disease, poor dietary intake, chewing or swallowing problems, polypharmacy, mental or physical disability, even depression. MIA syndrome reflects the triad of malnutrition, inflammation, and atherosclerosis that often includes oxidative stress and elevated cytokines.
- Correct existing nutritional deficiencies. Avoid restrictive diets as much as possible (Niedert, 2005).
- Recognize cachexia syndromes that are not reversible by hypercaloric feeding. Sometimes failure of nonpharmacologic therapies warrant consideration of orexigenic drug therapy. Malnourished older adults benefit from receiving oral supplemental beverages.
- Vitamin B_{12} deficiency in older people is most often from malabsorption of food-bound vitamin B_{12} (Johnson, 2007). High serum folate levels along with vitamin B_{12} deficiency

TABLE 1-29 Nutrition Assessment Tools for the Elderly

DETERMINE Checklist	*Warning signs for malnutrition* (from the Nutrition Screening Initiative, a project of the American Academy of Family Physicians, The American Dietetic Association and the National Council on the Aging, Inc., and Abbott Laboratorie, 1994. No longer published.)
D	Disease (illness affects nutritional intake)
E	Eating poorly, especially fewer than two meals daily
T	Tooth loss, mouth pain, chewing difficulty
E	Economic hardship (too few dollars to buy food)
R	Reduced social contact; eating meals alone
M	Multiple medicines (three or more prescribed or over-the-counter medications)
I	Involuntary weight loss or gain (10 lb in 6 months)
N	Needs assistance with self-care (shopping, cooking, eating)
E	Elderly years (older than 80 years of age), with increasing frailty
MNA: Mini Nutrition Assessment	MNA is a reliable and easy-to-use nutritional assessment tool for physicians, dietitians, medical students, or nurses to quickly evaluate the nutritional status of an individual (Nestle.) http://www.mna-elderly.com/clinical-practice.htm
18 questions, 4 categories: anthropometric assessment, general assessment, dietary assessment, subjective assessment	Asks questions relating to the last 3 months, such as: • Weight loss; BMI • Mobility problems; psychological stress; acute disease • Food intake, digestive problems, chewing or swallowing difficulties • Depression or dementia
SGA: Subjective Global Assessment	SGA classification technique can aid in the recognition of undernutrition by assessing a patient's nutritional status based on features of the medical history and physical examination. See Section 13 for examples of the SGA.
SNAP: Malnutrition Screening in Senior Citizens	Common factors to assess (adapted from the Australian College of Royal General Practitioners. SNAP: a population guide to be behavioral risk factors in general practice. *Austr Fam Phys*. 33:1, 2004.)
Protein and muscle mass	Impaired synthesis of new tissue Decline of the protein reserve of the body Diminished capacity to meet the extra demand of protein synthesis associated with disease or injury Increased frailty Sarcopenia
Nutrient deficits	Decreased energy intake; anorexia of aging
Changes in mobility	Falls Illness Hospitalization Immobilization

Nonphysiological Causes of Undernutrition	
Social factors	Poverty Inability to shop Inability to prepare and cook meals Inability to feed oneself Living alone, social isolation, or lack of social support network Failure to cater to ethnic food preferences
Psychological factors	Dementia Alcoholism Bereavement Depression Phobia about cholesterol, fat, calories
Medical factors	Anorexia, early satiety, malabsorption, increased metabolism, cytokine-mediated and impaired functional status Cancer Alcoholism Cardiac failure Chronic obstructive pulmonary disease Infection Dysphagia Rheumatoid arthritis Parkinson disease Hyperthyroidism, HIV or AIDS
Gastrointestinal issues	Malabsorption syndromes Dyspepsia, atrophic gastritis, vomiting Diarrhea or constipation Poor dentition
CNAQ: Council on Nutrition Appetite Questionnaire	Eight questions from the Council on Nutrition http://medschool.slu.edu/agingsuccessfully/pdfsurveys/appetitequestionnaire.pdf.
A. My appetite is	1. Very poor 2. Poor 3. Average 4. Good 5. Excellent
B. When I eat, I feel full after	1. Eating only a few mouthfuls 2. Eating about 1/3 of a plate or meal 3. Eating over 1/2 of a plate or meal 4. Eating most of the food 5. Hardly ever
C. I feel hungry	1. Never 2. Occasionally 3. Sometimes 4. Most of the time 5. All of the time
D. Food tastes	1. Very bad 2. Bad 3. Average 4. Good 5. Very good
E. Compared to when I was 50, food tastes	1. Much worse 2. Worse 3. Just as good 4. Better 5. Much better
F. Normally, I eat	1. Less than one regular meal a day 2. One meal daily 3. Two meals daily 4. Three meals daily 5. Over three meals daily including snacks
G. I feel sick or nauseated when I eat	1. Most times 2. Often 3. Sometimes 4. Rarely 5. Never
H. Most of the time my mood is	1. Very sad 2. Sad 3. Neither happy nor sad 4. Happy 5. Very happy
Total Score	Add the numbers associated with the patient's response. 8–16 at risk for anorexia and needs nutrition counseling 17–28 patient needs frequent reassessment >28 patient is not at risk at this time.

exacerbate anemia and can worsen cognitive symptoms, therefore careful monitoring is important (Clarke et al, 2007; Johnson, 2007; Tangney et al, 2009).

- Provide foods of proper consistency by dental status. Dentures alter the taste of foods by increasing bitter and sour taste sensations (Duffy et al, 1999). Chop foods as needed; puree only if necessary.
- Provide a diet of correct texture; exclude hard, sticky foods that are difficult to chew and swallow.
- Older individuals have fewer taste buds. More sweet flavors and stronger seasonings may be required to satisfy the appetite.
- Evaluate for laxative and enema use or abuse; recommend suitable alternatives and interventions, such as oat fiber, prunes or other dried fruits, extra liquid.
- Evaluate for alcohol abuse; make appropriate referrals as needed.
- "If the gut works, use it." Maintain oral diet as much as possible. For individuals who are unable to regain unintentional weight losses, artificial nutrition may be needed. Review advance directives and proceed accordingly.
- Investigate hydration status and any major weight shifts. Diminishing thirst mechanisms and incontinence contribute to dehydration. Generally, older adults should ingest 25–30 mL/kg of fluids per day. Alterations would be needed for heart, liver, or renal failure.
- Indices of overweight and obesity such as BMI do not correlate as strongly with adverse health outcomes in older as compared to younger individuals (Miller and Wolfe, 2008).
- Assess the behavioral and environmental situations (i.e., Who shops? Who cooks? How are finances handled? How often are meals eaten away from home? Is this person dependent or independent?). Evaluate family and social support. If there is a need for assistance, make appropriate referrals.
- Correct frailty where possible by addressing depression, use of multiple medications, underlying medical illnesses. Low levels of serum cholesterol (<189 mg/dL) may indicate signs of occult disease or rapidly declining health.
- Encourage physical activity, especially resistance training. This can help to maintain metabolically active tissue, stimulate appetite, improve sleep, correct mild constipation, improve cognitive function, enhance nitrogen balance, and promote positive outcomes in memory, self-esteem, and independence.

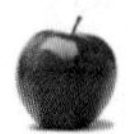

FOOD AND NUTRITION

- Ensure intake of the MyPyramid Food Guidance System: 3–4 servings of milk, dairy products, or calcium substitutes; 2–3 servings of protein foods (meat or substitute); 3–5 servings of vegetables; 2–4 servings of fruits; and 6–12 bread group servings. Recommend fats, oils, alcohol, sugars, and sweets to increase or decrease energy intake, as appropriate for the individual.
- Diet should provide adequate intake of protein: 0.8–1 g/kg body weight. This may mean 63 g for men and 50 g for women. Considering liver and renal impairments, decrease protein intake if needed. Increase protein intake in case of pressure ulcers, cancers, infections and other conditions requiring tissue repair.
- Energy: 25–35 kcal/kg. The Institute of Medicine suggests that the average 75-year-old female and male need 2403 and 3067 kcal, respectively, if ambulatory. Fewer kilocalories are needed if nonambulatory (e.g., living in an institution). Nutritional supplements may provide needed energy and protein for nursing home residents (Avenell and Handoll, 2010). See Table 1-30.
- Consume 1200 mg of calcium from milk, yogurt, and related dairy products when possible. Include sources of the B vitamins and zinc. Iron needs are lower in women after menopause, but include at least the RDA. Ensure sufficiency of other nutrients according to the patient's age and sex, using Table 1-29.
- If patient has heart disease or hypertension, encourage the Mediterranean diet or the DASH diets. Liberalize where possible to keep intake at a sufficient level. Extra natural vitamin E may be used from nuts, olive and canola oils, and some fruits and vegetables.
- The consistency of the food should be altered (i.e., ground, pureed, or chopped) only as required. Try to maintain whole textures as often as possible to enhance the food's appeal and to increase chewing with saliva. Mechanically altered diets are often not necessary, may have been started inappropriately, and may compromise taste, acceptability, and micronutrient intake.
- Adequate fiber and fluid intakes are necessary. Prudent increases in fiber (e.g., from prunes and bran) can reduce laxative abuse. Dehydration is a common cause of confusion and should be identified or avoided.
- A low-fat, vegan diet is associated with significant weight loss in overweight postmenopausal women, even without prescribed limits on portion size or energy intake (Barnard et al, 2005). If obesity is present, this change may improve health status.
- Adequate amounts of vitamins C and D, folic acid, and iron are often deficient in the diets of older individuals. Vitamin C levels must be increased for those individuals who smoke. Consider a multivitamin–mineral supplement.
- When taste and olfactory sensations are weak, the diet should provide adequate intake of zinc, folate, and vitamins A and B_{12}. Season with herbs and spices; add butter-flavored seasonings, garlic, maple or vanilla extract, and cheese or bacon-flavored seasonings. Consider all possible taste enhancers.
- Increased thiamin may be needed because of decreased metabolic efficiency. Men are especially susceptible.
- Reduce intake of excessive sweets; poor glucose tolerance and insulin resistance are common after 65 years of age.
- If early satiety is a problem, serving the main meal at noon may help with overall intake.
- Encourage socialization at mealtimes. Healthy individuals have food intakes that are greater when eating with other people, especially family or friends.
- Offer substitutes for major foods not consumed. If the individual resides in an institution, it is recommended to try other menu alternatives before offering a nutritional supplement as a meal replacement. Consult a dietitian if intake is chronically poor. If necessary, liquid supplements can provide needed energy, protein, and micronutrients.
- Offer tips for those who must eat alone. Menus and shopping tips may be needed, such as cooking in batches and freezing extra portions.
- For hospice patients, provide comfort foods and liquids as requested.

TABLE 1-30 Dietary Reference Intakes for Older Adults

	Vitamins and Elements									
	Vitamin A (μg)[a,b]	Vitamin C (mg)	Vitamin D (μg)[c,d]	Vitamin E (mg)[e,f,g]	Vitamin K (μg)	Thiamin (mg)	Riboflavin (mg)	Niacin (mg)[g,h]	Vitamin B_6 (mg)	Folate (μg)[g,i]
RDA or AI[j]										
Age 51–70 Male	**900**	**90**	10*	**15**	120*	**1.2**	**1.3**	**16**	**1.7**	**400**
Female	**700**	**75**	10*	**15**	90*	**1.1**	**1.1**	**14**	**1.5**	**400**
Age 70+ Male	**900**	**90**	15*	**15**	120*	**1.2**	**1.3**	**16**	**1.7**	**400**
Female	**700**	**75**	15*	**15**	90*	**1.1**	**1.1**	**14**	**1.5**	**400**
Tolerable upper intake levels[k]										
Age 51–70 Male	3000	2000	50	1000	ND	ND	ND	35	100	1000
Female	3000	2000	50	1000	ND	ND	ND	35	100	1000
Age 70+ Male	3000	2000	50	1000	ND	ND	ND	35	100	1000
Female	3000	2000	50	1000	ND	ND	ND	35	100	1000

	Vitamin B_{12} (μg)[l]	Pantothenic Acid (mg)	Biotin (μg)	Choline (mg)[m]	Boron (mg)	Calcium (mg)	Chromium (μg)	Copper (μg)	Fluoride (mg)	Iodine (μg)
RDA or AI[j]										
Age 51–70 Male	**2.4**	5*	30*	550*	ND	1200*	30*	**900**	4*	**150**
Female	**2.4**	5*	30*	425*	ND	1200*	20*	**900**	3*	**150**
Age 70+ Male	**2.4**	5*	30*	550*	ND	1200*	30*	**900**	4*	**150**
Female	**2.4**	5*	30*	425*	ND	1200*	20*	**900**	3*	**150**
Tolerable upper intake levels[k]										
Age 51–70 Male	ND	ND	ND	3500	20	2500	ND	10,000	10	1100
Female	ND	ND	ND	3500	20	2500	ND	10,000	10	1100
Age 70+ Male	ND	ND	ND	3500	20	2500	ND	10,000	10	1100
Female	ND	ND	ND	3500	20	2500	ND	10,000	10	1100

	Elements and Macronutrients								
	Iron (mg)	Magnesium (mg)[n]	Manganese (mg)	Molybdenum (mg)	Nickel (mg)	Phosphorus (mg)	Selenium (ug)	Vanadium (mg)[o]	Zinc (mg)
RDA or AI[j]									
Age 51–70 Male	**8**	**420**	2.3*	**45**	ND	**700**	**55**	ND	**11**
Female	**8**	**320**	1.8*	**45**	ND	**700**	**55**	ND	**8**
Age 70+ Male	**8**	**420**	2.3*	**45**	ND	**700**	**55**	ND	**11**
Female	**8**	**320**	1.8*	**45**	ND	**700**	**55**	ND	**8**
Tolerable upper intake levels[k]									
Age 51–70 Male	45	350	11	2000	1	4000	400	1.8	40
Female	45	350	11	2000	1	4000	400	1.8	40
Age 70+ Male	45	350	11	2000	1	3000	400	1.8	40
Female	45	350	11	2000	1	3000	400	1.8	40

(continued)

TABLE 1-30 Dietary Reference Intakes for Older Adults *(continued)*

		Elements and Macronutrients							
		Energy (kcal)[b]	Protein (g)[c]	Carbohydrates (g)[d]	Total Fat (% kcal)[e,f]	*n* -6 PUFA (g)	*n* -3 PUFA (g)	Total Fiber (g)	Drinking Water, Beverages, Water in Food (L)
RDA or AI[a]									
Age 51–70	Male	2204	**56**	**130**		14*	1.6*	30*	3.7*
	Female	1978	**46**	**130**		11*	1.1*	21*	2.7*
Age 70+	Male	2054	**56**	**130**		14*	1.6*	30*	2.6*
	Female	1873	**46**	**130**		11*	1.1*	21*	2.1*
AMDR[a]			10–35%	45–65%	20–35%	5–10%	0.6–1.2%		

[a]Recommended dietary allowances (RDAs) are in **bold type** and adequate intakes (AIs) are in ordinary type followed by an asterisk (*).
[b]Values are based on Table 5-22 estimated energy requirements (EER) for men and women 30 years of age. Used height of 5′7″, "low active" physical activity level (PAL), and calculated the median BMI and calorie level for men and women. Caloric values based on age were calculated by substracting 10 kcal/d for males (from 2,504 kcal) and 7 kcal/d for females (from 2,188 kcal) for each year of age above 30. For ages 51–70, calculated for 60 years old, for 70+, calculated for 75 years old. 80 year old male calculated to require 2,004 kcal, female, 1,838 kcal.
[c]The RDA for protein equilibrium in adults is a minimum of 0.8 g/kg body weight for reference body weight.
[d]The RDA for carbohydrate is the minimum adeqaute to maintain brain function in adults.
[e]Because percentage of energy consumed as fat can vary greatly and still meet energy needs, an AMDR is provided in absence of AI, EAR, or RDA for adults.
[f]Values for mono- and saturated fats and cholesterol not established as "they have no role in preventing chronic disease, thus not required in the diet."
[g]Acceptable macronutrient distribution ranges (AMDRs) for intakes of carbohydrates, proteins, and fats expressed as percentage of total calories.
The values for this table were excerpted from the Institute of Medicine, *Dietary reference intakes: Applications in dietary assessment,* 2000, and *Dietary reference intakes for energy, carbohydrates, fiber, fat, protein and amino acids (macronutrients),* 2002.
[j]Recommended dietary allowances (RDAs) are in bold type and adequate intakes (AIs) are in ordinary type followed by an asterisk (*).
ND—Indicates values not determined.
The values for this table were excerpted from the Institute of Medicine, *Dietary reference intakes: Applications in dietary assessment,* 2000, and *Dietary reference intakes for energy, carbohydrates, fiber, fat, protein and amino acids (macronutrients),* 2002.

		Electrolytes		
		Potassium (g)	Sodium (g)	Chloride (g)
RDA or AI[a]				
Age 51–70	Male	4.7	1.3*	2.0*
	Female	4.7	1.3*	2.0*
Age 70+	Male	4.7	1.2*	1.8*
	Female	4.7	1.2*	1.8*
Tolerable upper intake levels[a]				
Age 51–70	Male		2.3	3.6
	Female		2.3	3.6
Age 70+	Male		2.3	3.6
	Female		2.3	3.6

[a]Recommended dietary allowances (RDAs) are in bold type and adequate Intakes (AIs) are in ordinary type followed by an asterisk (*).
ND—Indicates values not determined.
The values for this table were excerpted from the Institute of Medicine, *Dietary reference intakes: Water, potassium, sodium, chloride, and sulfate,* 2004.

Common Drugs Used and Potential Side Effects

- Discuss the relevance of tolerable ULs from the latest dietary reference intakes of the National Academy of Sciences. These levels were set to protect individuals from receiving too much of any nutrient from diet and dietary supplements.
- Many drugs affect the nutritional status of the patient. A thorough drug history is needed.
- Drug metabolism and detoxification require an adequate diet containing methionine and other sulfur amino acids; vitamins A, B_{12}, C, and E; choline; folate and selenium.
- Polypharmacy is common in older adults, especially those living in institutionalized settings.
- Long-term use of high-carbohydrate, low-protein diets is undesirable when protein-bound drugs are prescribed. Drug metabolism is slowed, a potentially dangerous occurrence. See Table 1-31.

Herbs, Botanicals, and Supplements

- Herbs and botanical supplements should not be used without discussing with the physician, especially for underlying medical conditions.
- Older people should be encouraged to report the use of herbs and nutritional supplements to their doctors. Doctors should provide comprehensive and current information about potential herb–drug interactions. Among older

TABLE 1-31 Drugs with Potentially Undesirable Side Effects in Seniors

Effect	Medications
Addiction	Amphetamines, anorexic agents, and barbituates
Anorexia	Antibiotics, digoxin
Calcium and fat-soluble vitamin depletion	Mineral oil as a laxative
Confusion	Cimetidine (Tagamet) can decrease vitamin B_{12} levels
Constipation	Opiates, iron supplements, diuretics
Decreased sense of taste	Metronidazole, calcium channel blockers, angiotensin-converting enzyme (ACE) inhibitors, metformin
Diarrhea	Laxatives, antibiotics
Dysphagia	Potassium supplements, NSAIDs, bisphosphonates, prednisolone
Early satiety	Anticholinergic drugs, sympathomimetic agents
Hypotension	Cardiac drugs (amiodarone, guanethidine, guanadrel, doxazosin, nifedipine, and clonidine)
Hypermetabolism	Thyroxine, ephedrine
Nausea/vomiting	Antibiotics, opiates, digoxin, theophylline, nonsteroidal anti-inflammatory drugs (NSAIDs)
Neurological effects	Indomethacin
Reduced feeding ability	Sedatives, opiates, psychotropic agents
Renal clearance, decreased	Digoxin
Urinary excretion of electrolytes and water-soluble vitamins	Diuretics: thiamin deficiency; a low-dose thiamin supplement may be useful to prevent subclinical beri-beri (McCabe-Sellers et al, 2005). Diuretics can also decrease serum levels of potassium, magnesium, calcium, and zinc.
Vitamin C, iron and folic acid depletion	Large amounts of aspirin
Vitamin K and B-complex depletion	Sulfonamides

adults, herbal supplement users are more likely to perceive their supplements as safe and to consider conventional medicine to be less effective than nonusers (Shahrokh et al, 2005).

- Increases in prostaglandin E2 production contribute to the decline in T-cell–mediated function with age. Black currant seed oil is rich in both gamma and alpha linoleic acids.
- Creatine supplements have been used to increase strength in older individuals; results are mixed.
- Echinacea may be used as an immune system stimulant. It should not be taken with steroids, cyclosporine, or immunosuppressants. It may aggravate allergies in susceptible individuals.
- Gingko biloba is proposed for memory support; studies show no effectiveness.
- Ginseng may be used for stress adaptation, impotence, or as a digestive aid. It should not be taken with warfarin, insulin, oral hypoglycemics, CNS stimulants, caffeine, steroids, hormones, antipsychotics, aspirin, or antiplatelet drugs.
- Kava is sometimes used as a sleep aid. Discourage use with sedatives, alcohol, antipsychotics, or other CNS depressants.
- Vitamin E supplements may ward off colds or flu in older people (Meydani et al, 2004).

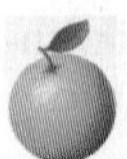

NUTRITION EDUCATION, COUNSELING, CARE MANAGEMENT

- Efforts to correct malnutrition in seniors are beneficial. Numerous tools are available and can be used in a variety of settings.
- Dietitians should handle nutritional discharge planning (Baker and Wellman, 2005). Senior citizens often improve protein intake after appropriate counseling (Rousset et al, 2006).
- Emphasize the need to consume adequate amounts of calcium, folic acid, vitamins A, E, and D. Review the desired nutrient intakes with the client; supplemental iron is not often needed unless there is anemia. Vitamin B_{12} and thiamin may be needed, depending on medications used and concurrent chronic disease.
- Be aware of income limitations when planning a menu—less-expensive protein sources may be necessary. Discuss shopping and meal preparation tips.
- Prevent excessive use of caffeine from coffee, colas, and tea if it prevents intake of other desirable juices and beverages. Three 6- to 9-oz cups of coffee per day pose no specific health risk and caffeine may also promote improved cognition.
- Make every effort to determine whether the patient is using alcohol because multiple deficiencies may result, especially for thiamin, vitamin B_{12}, folate, and zinc. Make appropriate referrals. Older adults may not admit the true amount of alcohol being consumed because of embarrassment.
- Encourage participation in Meals on Wheels, SNAP (food stamps,) congregate feeding programs, and Senior Farmers' Market programs.
- Ensure adequate fluid intake for age and medical condition. Ensure that the diet provides adequate fluid and fiber to alleviate constipation.
- Encourage physical activity such as strength conditioning and walking. Yoga may help to prevent weight gain with aging.

TABLE 1-32 Weight Table for Men Aged 70 and Over

Height (inches)	Ages 70–74	Ages 75–79	Ages 80–84	Ages 85–89	Ages 90–94	Ages Over 94
61	128–156	125–153	123–151	120–145	118–142	113–139
62	130–158	127–155	125–153	122–148	119–143	114–140
63	131-161	129–157	127–155	122–150	120–146	115–141
64	134–164	131-161	129–157	124–152	122–148	116–142
65	136–166	134–164	130–160	127–155	125–153	117–143
66	139–169	137–167	133–163	130–158	128–156	120–146
67	140–172	140–170	136–166	132–162	130–160	122–150
68	143–175	142–174	139–169	135–165	133–163	126–154
69	147–179	146–178	142–174	139–169	137–167	130–158
70	150–184	148–182	146–178	143–175	140–172	134–164
71	155–189	152–186	149–183	148–180	144–176	139–169
72	159–195	156–190	154–188	153–187	148–182	143–173
73	164–200	160–196	158–192	157–189	156–187	155–177
74	169–205	165–201	163–197	162–190	160–188	158–181

Adapted from: *J Am Med Assoc.* 177:658, with permission of American Medical Association, Copyright 1960.

- Olfactory decline is common. Flavorful foods release endorphins, which boosts the immune system (Duffy et al, 1999). Discuss adding herbs, spices, and other flavor enhancers to foods.
- Hypothermia (body temperature of 95°F or lower) can occur, with fatigue, weakness, poor coordination, lethargy, slurred speech, and drowsiness. Give hot beverages and keep patient in a warm bed. If body temperature reaches 90°F, death is likely.
- Support intake of antioxidants to protect the aging brain. Top choices include: grape juice, blueberries, pomegranate, papaya, kiwifruit, cantaloupe, mango, apricot, broccoli, spinach, tomato, sweet potato, and collards.
- Encourage physical activity. Peer and leader encouragement for strength training is especially beneficial in this age group (Layne et al, 2008).
- Restorative dining may require attention. The American Dietetic Association has suggested three visits for medical nutrition therapy for restorative dining procedures.
- For patients with a history of, current status of, or risk for dehydration, the American Dietetic Association recommends two or more medical nutrition therapy visits.
- For end of life, advanced directives document a patient's wishes, regardless of the setting. If advance directives

TABLE 1-33 Weight Table for Women Aged 70 and Over

Height (inches)	Ages 70–74	Ages 75–79	Ages 80–84	Ages 85–89	Ages 90–94	Ages Over 94
55	117–143	106–132	107–132	94–113	86–108	85–107
56	118–144	108–134	108–133	95–114	88–110	87–109
57	119–145	110–136	109–134	96–115	90–112	89–110
58	120–146	112–138	111–135	97–118	94–115	93–114
59	121–147	114–140	112–136	100–122	99–121	98–120
60	122–148	116–142	113–139	106–130	102–124	101–123
61	123–151	118–144	115–141	109–133	104–128	103–129
62	125–153	121–147	118–144	112–136	108–132	107–131
63	127–155	123–151	121–147	115–141	112–136	107–131
64	130–158	126–154	123–151	119–145	115–141	108–132
65	132–162	130–158	126–154	122–150	120–146	112–136
66	136–166	132–162	128–157	126–154	124–152	116–142
67	140–170	136–166	131–161	130–158	128–156	120–146
68	143–175	140–170	137–164	134–162	131–160	124–150
69	148–180	144–176	Not available	Not available	Not available	Not available

Adapted from: *J Am Med Assoc.* 177:658, with permission of American Medical Association, Copyright 1960.

TABLE 1-34 Formula for Calculating Stature Using Knee Height

Knee height can be used to estimate standing height in a bedridden or handicapped person. Knee height is not affected by aging. Different populations may require the use of different equations; equations derived from taller statured populations (e.g., Caucasians) may be less accurate when applied to shorter statured populations. Sample formulas are as follows:
Stature for Caucasian men = 64.19 − (0.04 × age in years) + (2.02 × knee height in cm)
Stature for Japanese men = 71.16 − (0.56 × age in years) + (2.61 × knee height in cm)
Stature for Caucasian women = 84.88 − (0.24 × age in years) + (1.83 × knee height in cm)
Stature for Japanese women = 63.06 − (0.34 × age in years) + (2.38 × knee height in cm)

Sources: Chumlea, 1984; Chumlea et al, 1994; Knous and Arisawa, 2002; and Mendoza-Nunez et al, 2002.

indicate "no heroic measures," be sure to identify if that includes tube feeding and hydration. Both terminally ill patients and their caregivers need education, information, advocacy, and emotional support. Effective end of life discussions lead to earlier hospice referral and less-aggressive treatments (Wright et al, 2008).

- Depression affects 20–40% of older Americans but is not a normal part of aging. It causes a lot of weight loss in nursing homes and in the community and must be treated. Tables 1-32, 1-33, and 1-34 can be used to follow weight changes in older adults.

Patient Education—Food Safety Tips

- Reminders about hand washing and safe food handling may be important, especially for adults who prepare and serve meals for older adults. Check out the home food safety website at http://www.homefoodsafety.org/pages/tips/tips/adults.jsp
- Avoid food preparation when sick with viral or bacterial infections; use gloves if needed.
- Thoroughly cook meat, poultry, and fish entrees. Keep cold foods cold and hot foods hot.
- Because bacteria are commonly found on foods such as green onions (scallions), cantaloupe, cilantro, and imported produce, wash all fresh fruits and vegetables. Scrub the outside of produce such as melons and cucumbers before cutting.
- When traveling, avoid tap water and ice made from tap water, uncooked produce such as lettuce, and raw or undercooked seafood.
- Airline water may not be free from contamination. Use of bottled water is recommended. Coffee and tea may not be hot enough to kill all bacteria.
- Throw out cooked foods that have been at room temperature for longer than 2 hours.
- Consumption of sulforaphane in foods such as broccoli, cauliflower, cabbage, and Brussels sprouts may reduce the presence of *Helicobacter pylori*, which is beneficial.
- Avoid raw or partially cooked eggs, raw or undercooked fish or shellfish, and raw or undercooked meats because of potential foodborne illnesses.
- Do not use raw (unpasteurized) milk or products made from it.
- Avoid serving unpasteurized cider, juices, and raw sprouts because they may contain *Escherichia coli.*
- Only serve processed deli meats and frankfurters that have been reheated to steaming hot temperature. If the patient is immunocompromised, it may be best to avoid deli meats and ready-to-eat meat and poultry products; smoked fish; and soft cheese such as brie and blue-veined varieties because of the risk for *Listeria.* Homemade egg nog, cookie and cake batter, and other foods prepared with raw eggs should be avoided because of the risks of *Salmonella.*
- Raw seafood such as oysters, clams, and mussels may contain *Vibrio* bacteria. Caution or avoidance is recommended.

For More Information

- American Association of Retired Persons (AARP)
  http://www.aarp.org/
- Administration on Aging
  http://www.aoa.gov/
- Aging Well
  http://agingwell.state. ny.us/
- Aging with Dignity
  http://www.agingwithdignity.org/
- American Federation for Aging Research
  http://www.afar.org/
- American Geriatrics Society
  http://www.americangeriatrics.org/
- American Society on Aging
  http://www.asaging.org/
- Centers for Medicare & Medicaid Services (CMS)
  http://www. cms.hhs.gov/home/medicare.asp
- Colorado State Extension
  http://www.ext.colostate.edu/pubs/foodnut/09322.html
- Diabetes and Aging
  http://diabetes.niddk.nih.gov/about/dateline/spri02/8.htm
- Food and Drug Administration—Aging
  http://www.fda.gov/opacom/lowlit/eatage.html
- Food Safety for Seniors
  http://www.cfsan.fda.gov/~dms/seniors.html
- Gerontological Society of America
  http://www.geron.org/
- Government Page for Seniors
  http://www.firstgov.gov/Topics/Seniors.shtml
- Health and Age
  http://www.eldercare.com/
- Hearing Loss
  http://www.nia.nih.gov/HealthInformation/Publications/hearing.htm
- Homecare and Hospice
  http://www.nahc.org/consumer/home.html
- Hospice Foundation
  http://www.hospicefoundation.org/

- Human Nutrition Resource Center on Aging (Tufts University)
  http://hnrc.tufts.edu/1191590448205/
  HNRCA-Page-hnrca2 w_1191937436491.html
- Meals on Wheels
  http://www.mowaa.org/
- Medicare Information
  http://www.medicare.gov/
- National Association Directors of Nursing Administration in Long Term Care
  http://www.nadona.org/
- National Association of Nutrition and Aging Services Programs
  http://www.nanasp.org/
- National Council on Aging (NCOA)
  http://www.ncoa.org/
- National Eye Institute
  http://www.nei.nih.gov/about/
- National Institute on Aging (NIA)
  http://www.nih.gov/nia/
- National Institutes of Health—Senior Health
  http://nihseniorhealth.gov/
- National Policy and Resource Center on Nutrition and Aging
  http://nutritionandaging.fiu.edu/
- Okinawa Centenarians Study
  http://www.okicent.org/
- Older Americans Resource Toolkit
  http://nutritionandaging.fiu.edu/OANP_Toolkit/
- U.S. Department of Disability, Aging and Long-Term Care
  http://aspe.hhs.gov/_/office_specific/daltcp.cfm
- U.S. Senate Committee on Aging
  http://aging.senate.gov/
- Young at Heart—Tips for Seniors
  http://win.niddk.nih.gov/publications/
  young_heart.htm

NUTRITION IN AGING—CITED REFERENCES

American Dietetic Association. Position of the American Dietetic Association: nutrition across the spectrum of aging. *J Am Diet Assoc.* 105:616, 2005.

American Dietetic Association. Position of the American Dietetic Association: food Insecurity and Hunger in the United States. *J Am Diet Assoc.* 106:446, 2006.

American Dietetic Association. Position of the American Dietetic Association: ethical and legal issues in nutrition, hydration and feeding. *J Am Diet Assoc.* 108:873, 2008.

Avenell A, Handoll HH. Nutritional supplementation for hip fracture aftercare in older people. *Cochrane Database Syst Rev. 2010 Jan* 20;(1): CD001880, 2005.

Baker EB, Wellman NS. Nutrition concerns in discharge planning for older adults: a need for multidisciplinary collaboration. *J Am Diet Assoc.* 105:603, 2005.

Barnard ND, et al. The effects of a low-fat, plant-based dietary intervention on body weight, metabolism, and insulin sensitivity. *Am J Med.* 118:991, 2005.

Chumlea WD et al. Prediction of stature from knee height for black and white adults and children with application to mobility-impaired or handicapped persons. *J Am Diet Assoc.* 94:1385, 1994.

Clarke R, et al. Low vitamin B-12 status and risk of cognitive decline in older adults. *Am J Clin Nutr.* 86:1384, 2007.

Duffy V, et al. Measurement of sensitivity to olfactory flavor: application in a study of aging and dentures. *Chem Senses.* 24:671, 1999.

Hanauer SB. Sarcopenia and the elusive fountain of youth. *Nat Clin Pract Gastroenterol Hepatol.* 6:1, 2009.

Hudgens J, Langkamp-Henken B. The mini nutritional assessment as an assessment tool in elders in long-term care. *Nutr Clin Pract.* 19:463, 2005.

Jensen GL. Inflammation: roles in aging and sarcopenia. *JPEN J Parenter Enteral Nutr.* 32:656, 2008.

Johnson MA. If high folic acid aggravates vitamin B_{12} deficiency what should be done about it? *Nutr Rev.* 65:451, 2007.

Knous BL, Arisawa Estimation of height in elderly Japanese using region-specific knee height equations. *J Am J Hum Biol.* 14:300, 2002.

Layne JE, et al. Successful dissemination of a community-based strength training program for older adults by peer and professional leaders: the people exercising program. *J Am Geriatr Soc.* 56:2323, 2008.

McCabe-Sellers B, et al. Diuretic medication therapy use and low thiamin intake in homebound older adults. *J Nutr Elder.* 24:57, 2005.

Meydani SN, et al. Vitamin E and respiratory tract infections in elderly nursing home residents: a randomized controlled trial. *JAMA.* 292:828, 2004.

Miller SL, Wolfe RR. The danger of weight loss in the elderly. *J Nutr Health Aging.* 12:487, 2008.

Niedert K. Position of the American Dietetic Association: liberalized diets for older adults in long-term care. *J Am Diet Assoc.* 105:1955, 2005.

Rousset S, et al. Change in protein intake in elderly French people living at home after a nutritional information program targeting protein consumption. *J Am Diet Assoc.* 106:253, 2006.

Scarmeas N, et al. Mediterranean diet and mild cognitive impairment. *Arch Neurol.* 66:216, 2009.

Shahrokh LE, et al. Elderly herbal supplement users less satisfied with medical care than nonusers. *J Am Diet Assoc.* 105:1138, 2005.

Tangney CC, et al. Biochemical indicators of vitamin B_{12} and folate insufficiency and cognitive decline. Biochemical indicators of vitamin B_{12} and folate insufficiency and cognitive decline. *Neurology.* 72:361, 2009.

Wilson MM, et al. Appetite assessment: simple appetite questionnaire predicts weight loss in community-dwelling adults and nursing home residents. *Am J Clin Nutr.* 82:1074, 2005.

Wright AA, et al. Associations between end-of-life discussions, patient mental health, medical care near death, and caregiver bereavement adjustment. *JAMA.* 300:1665, 2008.

SECTION 2

Nutrition Practices, Food Safety, Allergies, Skin and Miscellaneous Conditions

CHIEF ASSESSMENT FACTORS

- Complementary and Integrative Medicine, Including Use of Herbs, Spices, and Botanical Products
- Cultural or Religious Preferences with Special Diets or Practices
- Vegetarian Diets (see also Table 2-4)
- Mouth: Dental Problems, Periodontal Diseases, Dentures (Ill-Fitting), Missing or Loose Teeth, Caries, Oral Hygiene and Dental Care, Increased or Decreased Salivation, Dryness, Lesions (see also Tables 2-5 and 2-6)
- Problems with Self-Feeding
- Vision: Cataracts, Visual Field Changes, Diplopia, Glaucoma, Macular Degeneration, Blindness (see also Table 2-7)
- Skin: Texture or Color Changes, Dryness, Ecchymoses, Lesions, Masses, Petechiae, Pressure Ulcers (see also Table 2-8)
- Physical Signs of Nutrient Deficiencies
- Head/Face: Pain, Past Trauma, Syncope, Unusual or Frequent Headaches
- Ears: Hearing Problems, Discharge, Infections, Tinnitus, or Vertigo
- Food Allergies or Intolerances
- Food-Borne Illnesses

Possible Nutrition Diagnoses

- Inadequate intake of bioactive substances?
- Excessive intake of bioactive substances?
- Harmful beliefs about food and nutrition?
- Inadequate oral food and beverage intake (if foods served are unfamiliar or forbidden)?
- Harmful beliefs about food and nutrition (such as pica)?
- Inadequate protein intake?
- Inadequate mineral (iron, calcium, zinc) or vitamin intakes (B_{12}, D)?
  - Disordered eating pattern (unusual diet excluding multiple food groups)?
  - Underweight or involuntary weight loss?
  - Excessive fiber intake (phytates)?
  - Inadequate intake of fat (omega 3 fatty acids)?
  - Difficulty chewing?
    - Inadequate oral food and beverage intake?
    - Difficulty swallowing?
    - Involuntary weight loss?
    - Excessive carbohydrate intake (sugars, sweets, beverages)?

- Inadequate vitamin or mineral intakes?
- Self-feeding difficulty (functional, physical, psychological)?
- Malnutrition?
- Inadequate oral food and beverage intake?
- Involuntary weight loss?
- Altered nutrition-related lab values?
- Inadequate protein intake?
- Inadequate fluid intake?
- Underweight?
- Inadequate protein intake or increased nutrient needs (protein)?
- Inadequate vitamin intake (list specifics)?
- Increased nutrient needs (vitamins)?
- Excessive sodium intake?
- Inadequate oral food and beverage intake (from nausea, anorexia)?
- Intake of unsafe food (allergens)?
- Altered GI function (diarrhea)?
- Intake of unsafe food (pathogens)?

For More Information

- American Dietetic Association—Nutrition Education for the Public
http://www.nepdpg.org/
- Centers for Disease Control and Prevention—Index for Consumer Questions
http://www.cdc.gov/health/diseases.htm
- Evidence-Based Practice Centers
http://www.ahrq.gov/clinic/epcquick.htm
- Federal Trade Commission
http://www.ftc.gov/
- Health Finder
http://www.healthfinder.gov/
- Health Fraud and Quackery
http://www.quackwatch.com/
- Health Statistics
http://www.cdc.gov/nchswww/
- Healthy People (2010, 2020)
http://www.healthypeople.gov/
- Human Anatomy Online
http://www.innerbody.com/
- International Food Information Council—Functional Foods
http://www.ific.org/nutrition/functional/index.cfm
- PubMed
http://www.ncbi.nlm.nih.gov/PubMed/
- USDA: Food Composition Tables
http://www.nal.usda.gov/fnic/foodcomp/Data/HG72/hg72.html

COMPLEMENTARY OR INTEGRATIVE NUTRITION

COMPLEMENTARY OR INTEGRATIVE NUTRITION

NUTRITIONAL ACUITY RANKING: LEVEL 2 (NUTRITIONAL ADVISING)

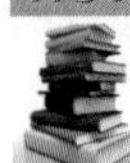

DEFINITIONS AND BACKGROUND

The philosophy that food can be health promoting beyond its nutritional value has gained acceptance within the public arena. Functional foods are so named because whole foods and fortified, enriched, or enhanced foods have a potentially beneficial effect on health when consumed as part of a varied diet on a regular basis, at effective levels (American Dietetic Association, 2009). Fish provides fish oils; fermented dairy products have probiotics; and beef has conjugated linoleic acid. Oats provide beta-glucan, soy provides isoflavones, flaxseed provides lignins and alpha-linolenic acid, garlic provides organosulfur compounds, broccoli and cruciferous vegetables provide isothiocyanates and indoles, citrus fruits provide liminoids, cranberry provides polymeric compounds, tea provides cachectin, and wine provides phenolics (American Dietetic Association, 2009).

Many plants and herbs contain biologically active phytochemicals with potential for disease prevention. Patients may use herbal medicines but not tell their healthcare providers (van der Voet et al, 2008). About one third of Americans take a vitamin–mineral supplement daily (Thomson et al, 2005). Nutrition is an integral part of many complementary therapies for cancer, arthritis, chronic pain, human immunodeficiency (HIV) virus, and gastrointestinal (GI) problems. Dried culinary herbs (e.g., oregano, sage, peppermint, garden thyme, lemon balm, clove, allspice, and cinnamon) contain very high concentrations of antioxidants (i.e., >75 mmol/100 g) and contribute significantly to the total intake of plant antioxidants by many people (Dragland et al, 2003).

Dietitians are uniquely qualified to translate sound scientific evidence into practical applications, yet many are not confident about the roles of herbs in prevention and treatment of illnesses. Education and training are important for the dietetic practitioner in preparing to answer questions about complementary nutrition. Dietitians should be able to describe implications of FDA structure/function claims, explain how to read labels, identify sound resources, associate common dietary supplements and their appropriate uses, and assess the science behind the supplement claims (Thomson et al, 2005).

Dietetics professionals are trained to assess dietary adequacy and the need for nutrient modifications (American Dietetic Association, 2005). Therefore, this text focuses on herbs, spices, and botanical products and does not cover the additional concepts and practices of homeopathy, acupuncture, traditional Chinese or Indian medicine. While some individuals need dietary supplements because of disease states, certain life stages, or chronic conditions, it is important to respect those cultural patterns and habits in which herbs and botanicals are used as medical or dietary enhancements. Clinicians should be aware of all the dietary supplements that their patients consume, and help their patients make informed decisions (Sadovsky et al, 2008). Table 2-1 lists questions to ask and Table 2-2 lists products that are used. Consider any adverse effects and discuss as needed.

TABLE 2-1 Herbal, Botanical, and Dietary Supplement Intake

1. **Identify types of supplements that you use:** ___None ___Multivitamin/mineral supplement ____Vitamin C ____Calcium/Vitamin D ___Protein supplement ___Fiber supplement ___Fish oil ___Herbal supplement (such as aloe, black cohosh, calcium, ginseng, gingko biloba, valerian) specify:___________
2. **For how long?** ___1 month or less ___3–6 months ___6–12 months ___>1 year
3. **How long will you use these supplements?** ___Indefinitely ___1–6 months ___6–12 months
4. **Why do you take this supplement(s)?** ___Prevention against disease ___General wellness ___Energy ___Weight loss ___Other reason (specify) ____________________To help treat a disease. If so, what are your medical symptoms? __________________and how long have you had this medical condition? ___<week ___1–3 months ___3–12 months ___>1 year
5. **How have symptoms improved since you started taking this supplement?** ___Feel better ___More energy ___Fewer symptoms ___Other (explain):____________________
6. **List any allergies to medications, foods, plants, or flowers** ____________
7. **List any additional illnesses or medical conditions** ____________________**Women: pregnant or breastfeeding?** _____No ___Yes
8. **List other over-the-counter and prescription medications (such as aspirin, diuretics, heart medicines, fish oil, oral contraceptives) that you take** ________________
9. **How much alcohol do you drink in a day?** ___None ___1 glass ___2 glasses ___More than 2 glasses
10. **How much do you smoke in a day?** ___None ___Less than one pack ____One pack or more
11. **Name any diet or eating plan you follow**________________How long?___________Was this prescribed for you? ___No ___Yes

Adapted from: American Dietetic Association. *Sports nutrition: a guide for the professional working with active people.* Chicago: American Dietetic Association, 2000; and American Dietetic Association. *Special report from the Joint Working Group on Dietary Supplements.* Chicago: American Dietetic Association, 2000. Used with permission.

TABLE 2-2 Herbs, Botanicals, Spices, Commentary and Adverse Effects

Herb, Botanical, Spice	Common Uses	Adverse Effects
Alfalfa (*Medicago sativa*)	Used for diuretic properties in asthma, diabetes, thyroid gland malfunction, arthritis, high cholesterol, and peptic ulcers. Said to promote menstruation and lactation.	Rats fed with this are prone to colon cancer. Fatalities reported due to ingestion of contaminated Alfalfa.
Alpha Lipoic Acid	Used to prevent cancer, HIV, AIDS, and liver disease. Used to lower triglycerides by reducing endothelial dysfunction. Most studies have been done with rats; more human studies are needed. Contained in broccoli, spinach, and tomato.	Its antioxidant activity may antagonize the effects of chemotherapy.
Aloe Vera (*Aloe barbadensis*)	Topical administration of Aloe vera gel for burns is generally safe. It may help reduce radiation-induced skin changes, but clinical trials are inconsistent.	FDA rules that it is not safe as a stimulant laxative; causes strong GI cramping. Chronic use can lead to loss of potassium. Do not use with diuretics, corticosteroids, or antihyperglycemic or cardiovascular agents.
Arnica (*Arnica montana*)	Used as a topical ointment for bruises, osteoarthritis in homeopathy preparations.	If taken orally, causes hypotension and shortness of breath; can be fatal.
Artemesia (*Wormwood*)	Used as an antimalarial; also used in cancer, fever, infections.	GI upset is a common side effect; causes hyperacidity.
Avlimil	Used to alleviate symptoms of female sexual dysfunction. Contains cloves, capsicum, black cohosh, ginger, and licorice.	Contraindicated in women having hormone-sensitive cancers. Stomach upset is an adverse reaction.
Ayurveda	Used in diabetes, rheumatoid arthritis (RA), Parkinson's disease, obesity, cancer, anemia, edema, and postpartum complications of pregnancy. Meditation helps in reducing anxiety, lowering blood pressure, and enhancing general well-being. The herbs show antioxidant, antitumor, antimicrobial, hypoglycemic, and anti-inflammatory properties.	Lead poisoning is a potential complication.
Barberry	Used as a coagulant herb.	May inhibit effects of anticoagulant medications such as warfarin.

(continued)

TABLE 2-2 Herbs, Botanicals, Spices, Commentary and Adverse Effects *(continued)*

Herb, Botanical, Spice	Common Uses	Adverse Effects
Bilberry (*Vaccinium myrtillus*)	Used in Europe as an antioxidant to prevent diabetic retinopathy; improves visual acuity and retinal function. Used for cataracts, cancer, circulatory disorders, diabetic retinopathy, glaucoma, macular degeneration, hemorrhoids, and varicose veins. Relative of blueberry. Do not use with anticoagulants or antiplatelet medications. No adverse reactions reported.	Exhibits antiplatelet activity. May enhance effects of anticoagulant medications such as warfarin and potentiate bleeding.
Bitter Melon (*Momordica charantia*)	Used in cancer prevention, diabetes, fever, HIV, infections, menstrual disorders.	Contraindicated in children and pregnant women because it causes bleeding, contraction of the uterus, and abortion. Adverse reactions include hypoglycemia and hepatotoxicity, headache, fever, abdominal pain, and coma.
Black Cohosh (*Cimicifuga racemosa*)	Used with hot flashes, headaches, vaginal dryness, mood swings, cough, dysmenorrhea, RA, and sedation. It functions as an antispasmodic, sedative, or relaxant. Controversial whether black cohosh possesses estrogenic activity.	May cause hypotension, vomiting, headache, dizziness, GI distress, and limb pain. May increase the toxicity of doxorubicin and docetaxel or interact with drugs that are metabolized by CYP3A4 enzyme. **Warning: should not be confused with blue cohosh** (*Caulophyllum thalictroides*), **which is toxic** and may be used in attempts to induce abortion.
Borage Oil (*Borago officinalis*)	Used for RA, infantile seborrheic dermatitis, cough, chest congestion, and menopausal symptoms.	Contains pyrrolizidine alkaloid and amabiline, which are hepatotoxic. Unsafe during pregnancy due to teratogenic effects and premature labor. Adverse effects include constipation and hepatotoxicity after chronic administration.
Boswellia (*Boswellia serrata*)	Used for arthritis, asthma, colitis, inflammation, and menstrual cramps.	Long-term affects on humans are unknown, but it has cytotoxic activity.
Brewer's Yeast	Used as a natural source of chromium.	Avoid supplement use with MAO inhibitors such as Nardil, Parnate.
Bromelain, from pineapple stem (*sulfhydryl proteolytic enzyme*)	Used for arthritis, bruises, burns, cancer prevention and treatment, edema, indigestion, and circulatory disorders. Exhibits antiplatelet activity.	Diarrhea, GI disturbances, allergic reactions. May enhance effects of anticoagulant medications such as warfarin and potentiate bleeding.
Buckthorn Bark	Used as laxative herb to speed digestion, which reduces absorption time of drugs.	Chronic use results in a loss of potassium, thereby strengthening effects of cardiac glycosides and antiarrhythmic agents. Use with thiazide diuretics, corticosteroids, or licorice root increases potassium loss.
Bupleurum (*Bupleurum chinense, B. scoizone—raefolium*)	Used for colds, fever, infections, cirrhosis, hepatitis, liver disease, malaria, and cancer treatment.	**Warning: may be associated with interstitial pneumonitis** as an ingredient of shosaiko. Adverse reactions include nausea, vomiting, edema, GI disturbance.
Burdock (*Arctium majus*)	Used for arthritis, HIV, AIDS, psoriasis, diabetes, eczema, and anorexia; no human studies on these proposed claims. Promotes urination.	Contraindicated in pregnancy, lactation or allergy to chrysanthemum. **Warning: burdock tea sometimes is contaminated** with belladonna alkaloids.
Butcher's Broom (*Ruscus aculeatus*)	Used for hemorrhoids, varicose veins, circulatory diseases, lymphedema, leg cramps, constipation, and inflammation.	Diarrhea.
Calendula (*Calendula officinalis*)	Used for conjunctivitis, eczema, GI disturbance, inflammation, menstrual cramps, and radiation therapy.	Contraindicated in pregnancy and lactation. Possible allergic reactions.
Capsicum, Capsaicin (*Capsicum frutescens* and *C. annuum*)	Used as a circulatory stimulant to aid in digestion. Used externally to relieve pain, as from arthritis, circulatory disorders, and diabetic and herpes zoster neuropathy. Suggested to lower high cholesterol or to lessen motion sickness, muscle pain, or toothache.	Avoid contact with eyes and irritated or broken skin. Burning skin, urticaria, and contact dermatitis. Drug interactions: increases the incidence of cough associated with ACE inhibitors.
Cascara (*Rhamnus purshiana*)	Used for cancer treatment and constipation. Often found in over-the-counter laxatives. **FDA has ruled that cascara is not safe as a stimulant laxative.**	Contraindications: should not be used in intestinal obstruction, undiagnosed abdominal symptoms, and inflammatory bowel disease. Adverse reactions include vomiting, intestinal cramps; excessive use can cause diarrhea, weakness, or cholestatic hepatitis. Drug interactions: excess loss of K^+ with digoxin that potentiates cardiac effects; avoid use with cardiovascular agents.

(continued)

TABLE 2-2 Herbs, Botanicals, Spices, Commentary and Adverse Effects *(continued)*

Herb, Botanical, Spice	Common Uses	Adverse Effects
Cayenne	Used for muscle spasms and relief of pain in arthritis. Large doses may lead to chronic gastritis and kidney or liver damage. Exhibits anticoagulant activity.	May enhance effects of anticoagulant medications such as warfarin and potentiate bleeding; avoid with anticoagulants or antiplatelet medications.
Chamomile (*Matricaria recutita*)	Used for colic, GI disturbance, hemorrhoids, infections, skin ulcers, mucositis. Chamomile soothes indigestion, flatulence. Topical and oral administration is safe except in patients with allergies to ragweed or chrysanthemum.	Contact dermatitis or anaphylaxis in those allergic to ragweed or chrysanthemum. Drug interactions: increases anticoagulant effects due to its natural coumarin content; avoid with warfarin.
Chasteberry (*Vitex agnus castus*)	Used for premenopausal symptoms, dysmenorrhea, or menopause.	GI upset, nausea, rash, urticaria, and headache. Should not be taken with hormone replacement therapy or oral contraceptives; an itchy rash can occur. It may interact with dopamine antagonists.
Chinese Asparagus (*Asparaguscochinchinensis*)	Used for cancer treatment, constipation, cough, and hepatitis.	No adverse reactions or drug interactions reported.
Chitosan	Used as an ingredient in many weight loss supplements, with claims to bind and trap dietary fat.	It is clinically insignificant (Gades and Stern, 2005).
Cholesterol Spinach (*Gynura crepioides*)	Used for control of high cholesterol; no scientific evidence.	Contraindications: immunocompromised patients due to the possibility of contamination.
Chondroitin	Used to support healthy connective tissue and synovial fluid that lubricates joints. Improves functional status of people with hip or knee osteoarthritis, relieves pain, and reduces joint swelling and stiffness. Used with glucosamine in many products. Third most widely used supplement by elderly (Wold et al, 2005).	
Chromium Picolinate	Often used by athletes. May have some merit in diabetes management. Naturally found in mushrooms, nuts, bread, yeast.	Chronic use may lead to impaired iron and zinc metabolism, GI intolerance, nephritis, or chromosomal damage.
Cinnamon	Increases sensitivity of insulin to help manage diabetes (Anderson et al, 2004).	
Chrysanthemum (*Chrysanthemum morifolium*)	Used for angina, hypertension, fever, common cold. No human studies.	Contraindications: those with allergy to ragweed. Adverse reactions include contact dermatitis, photosensitivity.
Coenzyme Q10	Used for patients with heart failure or early signs of Parkinson's disease.	Coenzyme Q10, superoxide dismutase (SOD), S-adenosyl-L-methionine methionine (SAM-e), and other products have not been proven to reduce the effects of aging.
Coleus or Forskolin	Exhibits antiplatelet activity.	May enhance effects of anticoagulant medications such as warfarin and potentiate bleeding.
Cone Flower (*Echinacea purpurea, E. pallida, E. augustifolia*)	Used for common cold, immunostimulation, infections, viral infections, wound healing.	Contraindications: patients with autoimmune disorders (systemic lupus erythematosus, RA, multiple sclerosis, tuberculosis, HIV). Adverse reactions include headache, dizziness, nausea, rash, dermatitis, anaphylaxis.
Cranberry	Used to prevent urinary tract infection caused by *Escherichia coli* bacteria, especially after menopause.	
Creatine	Used to increase strength in some older individuals and in athletes. More studies are needed.	Heavy use may lead to cardiomyopathy, hypertension, renal impairment.
Curcumin and Curry	Used for antioxidant effects in cystic fibrosis, cognitive function in Alzheimer's disease, cancer prevention, and other conditions.	
Dandelion (*Taraxacum mongolicum*)	Used for diabetes, lactation stimulation, promote urination, rheumatoid arthritis, liver disease. Used as salad greens and in teas. Only a few clinical studies.	Allergic reactions, contact dermatitis, dyspepsia. Contraindication in patients with obstruction of the bile duct or gallbladder. Drug interactions: additive effect on hypoglycemic activity.
Da Qing Ye (*Isatis tinctoria*)	Used for cancer treatment, diarrhea, GI disorders, hepatitis, HIV and AIDS, respiratory infections.	Adverse reactions include nausea, vomiting, hematuria following injection.
Devil's Claw (*Harpagophytum procumbens*)	Used for analgesic, anti-inflammatory, osteoarthritis, muscle pain, GI disturbances.	Contraindication in pregnancy. Adverse reactions include dyspepsia, diarrhea, bradycardia.

(continued)

TABLE 2-2 Herbs, Botanicals, Spices, Commentary and Adverse Effects *(continued)*

Herb, Botanical, Spice	Common Uses	Adverse Effects
Dong Quai (*Angelica sinensis*)	Used as Chinese tonic for menstrual cramps, peripheral vasodilator, and pain reliever. It has not shown effectiveness for reducing hot flashes.	Exhibits anticoagulant activity. May enhance effects of anticoagulant medications such as warfarin and potentiate bleeding. It should not be used in pregnancy. Increased doses are carcinogenic. Adverse effects include bloating, loss of appetite, diarrhea, photosensitivity, gynecomastia.
Echinacea (see *Cone Flower*)	Used as an immune system stimulant. Echinacea is no more effective for upper respiratory tract infections than placebo. Avoid taking for longer than 2 months at a time.	Avoid with corticosteroids, cyclosporine, or immunosuppressants. It may trigger allergies since it is related to the ragweed family (as are butterbur, chamomile, goldenrod, and yarrow).
Eucalyptus	Used for asthma, coughs, arthritis in small doses.	Overdoses can be fatal.
Evening Primrose Oil (*Oenothera biennis*)	Used for RA, mastalgia, eczema, fatigue, diabetic neuropathy, premenstrual syndrome, menopausal symptoms, cancer treatment. Contains essential fatty acid known as gamma linolenic acid (GLA), which may be useful in cardiac or arthritic conditions.	Contraindication: pregnant women. Adverse reactions are headache, nausea, GI upset. Drug interactions: may lower the seizure threshold in patients taking phenothiazines. Avoid use also with chlorpromazine, fluphenazine, mesoridazine, anticoagulants or antiplatelet medications.
Fenugreek (*Trigonella foenum-graecum*)	Used for laxatives, lactation stimulation, diabetes, high cholesterol, wounds, alopecia, arthritis, GI disturbance, induce child birth.	Contraindication: infants and pregnant women. Adverse reactions: flatulence, diarrhea, bleeding, bruising, hypoglycemia.
Feverfew (*Tanacetum parthenium*)	Used for migraine, psoriasis, arthritis, dysmenorrhea. DISCONTINUE 2 WEEKS BEFORE SURGERY	Avoid use with nonsteroidal anti-inflammatory drugs (NSAIDs) because they negate its usefulness (Miller, 1998). Avoid use with warfarin, antiplatelet, or migraine headache medicines. Contraindicated in those who are allergic to ragweed or marigold. Adverse reactions are mouth ulcers. Withdrawal causes anxiety, muscle stiffness, and pain.
Flaxseed (*Linum usitatissimum*)	Used for cancer prevention, constipation, high cholesterol, menopausal symptoms, periodontal diseases.	Exhibits antiplatelet activity. May enhance effects of anticoagulant medications such as warfarin and potentiate bleeding. Avoid with radiation therapy.
Folk Remedy Oils	Used for childhood ailments in Mexican culture.	May cause pneumonia in infants and children.
Forskolin (*Coleus forskohlii*)	See Coleus.	
Gamma Linolenic Acid (GLA)	Used for reducing signs of PMS or menopause. Black currant oil contains GLA.	Avoid with anticonvulsants or anabolic steroids. Liver toxicity may occur.
Garcinia cambogia (hydroxycitric acid)	Used as ingredient of many weight loss products.	
Garlic	Used to help lower cholesterol. Antibacterial, antifungal, antiviral, and hypotensive benefits have also been noted. Fourth most widely used supplement by elderly (Wold et al, 2005). DISCONTINUE 2 WEEKS BEFORE SURGERY	Garlic appears to induce cytochrome P450 3A4 and may enhance metabolism of many medications such as cyclosporine and saquinavir. Avoid using capsules with warfarin and with diabetes medications (may cause drop in blood glucose).
Ginger (*Zingiber officinale*)	Used as a treatment for nausea, motion sickness, vomiting, anorexia, drug withdrawal, RA.	Adverse reactions include heartburn, dermatitis, CNS effects, depression, arrhythmias. Drug interactions: increases risk of bleeding if used with anticoagulant or antiplatelet medications. Additive effects with hypoglycemic drugs and histamine antagonists.
Gingko Biloba	Used to improve blood flow to the brain; to help with memory, hearing loss, dementias, circulatory disturbance, Raynaud's disease, sexual dysfunction, stress, tinnitus, asthma. Second most widely used supplement by elderly (Wold et al, 2005). DISCONTINUE 2 WEEKS BEFORE SURGERY	Gingko biloba may cause allergic skin reactions or bleeding. Avoid use with warfarin, antihyperglycemic agents, vitamin E, or aspirin. Warning: discontinue before surgery. Adverse reactions include headache, dizziness, GI upset, diarrhea, and seizures in patients predisposed to seizures or on medications that lower seizure threshold.

(continued)

TABLE 2-2 Herbs, Botanicals, Spices, Commentary and Adverse Effects *(continued)*

Herb, Botanical, Spice	Common Uses	Adverse Effects
Ginseng (*panax*)	American ginseng (*panax quinquefolius*) is often used for stress adaptation, cognitive or performance enhancement, impotence, a digestive aid, protection against cancer. Siberian ginseng (*Acanthopanax senticosus*) is used for lessening chemotherapy side effects; for health maintenance, strength, stamina, and immunostimulation. DISCONTINUE 2 WEEKS BEFORE SURGERY	It should not be taken with warfarin, insulin, oral hypoglycemics, CNS stimulants, caffeine, steroids, hormones, antipsychotics, aspirin, cardiovascular agents, warfarin, or other antiplatelet drugs. May interfere with digoxin action (Miller, 1998). Ginseng may add to the effects of estrogens or corticosteroids and can elevate BP. Contraindicated in hypertension and in perimenopausal, pregnant or lactating women.
Glehnia (*Glehnia littoralis*)	Used for bronchitis, chest congestion, whooping cough.	Photosensitivity may occur due to psoralens component. Contraindicated in radiation therapy.
Glucosamine Sulfate	Used to build new cartilage, rebuild old cartilage, lubricate joints, mount a healthy inflammatory response, and ease symptoms of osteoarthritis. It is often taken with chondroitin. Most widely used supplement by elderly (Wold et al, 2005).	Side effects are mild.
Gotu Kola (*Centella asiatica, Hydrocotyle asiatica*)	There are wide variations in terpenoid concentrations depending on the location in which gotu kola is grown. Used for burns, cancer treatment, circulatory disorders, GI disorders, hypertension, memory loss, psoriasis, scars, sedation, varicose veins. Gotu kola should not be confused with kolanut; gotu kola does not contain any caffeine and has not been shown to have stimulant properties. Products should be standardized as to asiaticoside, asiatic acid, madecassic acid, and madecassoside content.	Adverse effects: contact dermatitis, pruritus, photosensitization, and headache; reduced fertility may occur in women wishing to become pregnant. With toxic levels, hyperglycemia, hyperlipidemia, and sedation have occurred.
Green Tea	Used for activation of thermogenesis, fat oxidation, or both (Dulloo et al, 1999). Green tea is popular in several cultures. Both black and green tea may be preventive for cancers and strokes; they are also a good source of fluoride. Green tea contains a class of polyphenols called catechins, which consist mainly of epigallocatechin gallate (EGCG), epicatechin gallate, and gallocatechin gallate with various physiological and pharmacological properties. Green tea extract (GTE) may improve endurance capacity and may support weight loss (Nagao et al, 2005). GTE boosts exercise endurance by using fat as energy source, accompanied by higher rates of fat oxidation. Results come from the equivalent of about 4 cups of tea a day.	Avoid use with MAO inhibitors and warfarin since green tea contains vitamin K. Avoid use in pregnancy and infants.
Guggul	Used to treat osteoarthritis and bone fractures; suppresses the nuclear factor-κB activation induced by various carcinogens (Ichikawa and Aggarwal, 2006). Guggul may induce CYP3A4 activity.	Not enough scientific evidence to support the use of guggul for any medical condition. Guggul may cause stomach discomfort or allergic rash. It should be avoided in pregnancy and lactation and in children.
Hawthorn (*Crataegus monogyna*)	Used for angina, atherosclerosis, heart failure, HTN, indigestion. It seems to be safe for long-term use.	Contraindications: pregnancy, lactation. Adverse reactions: nausea, sweating, fatigue, hypotension, arrhythmia. Because hawthorn lowers blood pressure and cholesterol levels, never take with digoxin. In high doses, it can cause hypotension and sedation and should be monitored carefully. Avoid use with cardiovascular agents.
Horseradish	Used as a natural decongestant.	
Horse Chestnut	Exhibits anticoagulant activity.	May enhance effects of anticoagulant medications such as warfarin and potentiate bleeding.
Huang Lian (*Coptis chinensis*)	Used for diarrhea, hypertension, bacterial and viral infections, ear infections, and cancer treatment.	Contraindications in jaundiced neonates. Adverse reactions: nausea, vomiting, dyspnea. Toxicity: seizures, hepatotoxicity, cardiac toxicity.

(continued)

TABLE 2-2 Herbs, Botanicals, Spices, Commentary and Adverse Effects *(continued)*

Herb, Botanical, Spice	Common Uses	Adverse Effects
Indirubin (*Indigofera tinctoria*)	Used for cancer treatment, inflammation. There are limited clinical data	Adverse reactions: nausea, vomiting, abdominal pain. Long-term treatment has caused pulmonary arterial hypertension and cardiac insufficiency
Juniper	Used as a diuretic or for indigestion in some cultures.	Avoid in pregnancy and kidney disease.
Karela	Used to lower blood glucose.	Because it effect blood glucose levels, it should not be used by patients with diabetes mellitus.
Kava	May cause drowsiness, dizziness, and intoxication.	Avoid with sedatives or hypnotics.
Kudzu (*Pueraria mirifica, P. thunbergiana, P. montana* var. *lobata, P. montana* var. *thomsonii*)	Used for estrogenic effects. Promoted for alcoholism, common cold, diabetes, eye pain, fever, menopausal symptoms, neck pain.	Avoid in hormone-sensitive cancers, tamoxifen use, hypersensitivity to kudzu, and estrogen receptor-positive (ER+) breast cancer.
Kyushin	Used as a cardiotonic medicine in China.	Kyushin may interfere with digoxin.
Licorice (*Glycyrrhiza glabra, G. uralensis*)	Used for bronchitis, chest congestion, constipation, GI disorders, hepatitis, inflammation, menopausal symptoms, microbial infection, peptic ulcers, primary adrenocortical insufficiency, prostate cancer. Active ingredient (glycyrrhizin) has an anti-inflammatory role.	Avoid in renal or liver dysfunction, pregnancy and breast-feeding. Licorice can offset the pharmacological effect of spironolactone or digoxin. Large doses can produce headache, lethargy, or high blood pressure. May increase sodium retention and potassium losses when used with thiazide diuretics. Avoid use in cirrhosis, hypertension, cholestatic liver disease, hypokalemia, kidney failure.
Lycium (*Lycium barbarum; L. chinense; L. europeaum*)	Used for anemia, burns, cancer treatment, cough, inflammation, pain, sedation, skin infections, visual acuity.	May prolong bleeding time in some individuals.
Mayapple	Common in Native American medicine. Used for venereal warts (condyloma acuminata); it contains podophyllotoxins.	
Meadowsweet	Exhibits antiplatelet activity.	May enhance effects of anticoagulant medications such as warfarin and potentiate bleeding.
Melatonin	Used as a sleep aid or a jet lag adjuster	Avoid use with CNS depressants such as alcohol, barbiturates, corticosteroids, or immunosuppressants.
Milk Thistle (*silymarin*)	Used for alcoholic liver disease, cirrhosis, infectious hepatitis, drug-induced hepatitis. Best administered by injection. Serves as a natural antidote for death-cap mushroom poisoning.	It may have a mild laxative effect or can cause uterine or menstrual stimulation.
Mint	Used in oil form for colds, bronchitis, fever, indigestion.	Mild GI distress may result. Worsens gastroesophageal reflux disease (GERD) or hiatal hernia symptoms.
Motherwort	Exhibits antiplatelet activity.	May enhance effects of anticoagulant medications such as warfarin and potentiate bleeding.
Mushrooms, Edible	Used to prevent hormone-related cancers (breast, prostate). AHCC is obtained from mycelia of several species of basidiomycetes mushrooms. *Agaricus blazei*, native to Brazil and Japan, is used to treat arteriosclerosis, hepatitis, hyperlipidemia, diabetes, dermatitis, and cancer. Oral administration of *Agaricus* extract may improve natural killer cell activity and quality of life in cancer patients undergoing chemotherapy.	May enhance resistance to *Klebsiella pneumoniae* due to its antioxidant effects.
N-Acetyl-L-Cysteine (NAC)	Used to fight aging, alleviate allergies, and fight viruses. It may work as an antioxidant to protect against sun damage and skin lesions. May be useful in managing addictions.	
Oregano	Used for antioxidant effect. Destroys *Helicobacter pylori* and *Giardia*.	
Oregon Grape Root	Coagulant herb.	May inhibit effects of anticoagulant medications such as warfarin and potentiate bleeding.
Parsley	Used for flatulence, indigestion, topical antibiotic. Breath freshener after a meal.	Avoid use in pregnancy as it may stimulate uterine contractions. May work as a diuretic in large doses.

(continued)

TABLE 2-2 Herbs, Botanicals, Spices, Commentary and Adverse Effects *(continued)*

Herb, Botanical, Spice	Common Uses	Adverse Effects
Peppermint	Used to relieve excess gas as a digestive aid (Koretz and Rotblatt, 2004). It has antispasmodic action which can be useful for irritable bowel syndrome and GI cramping.	
Policosanols	Used to protect against cancers, cardiovascular disease, and obesity (Awika and Rooney, 2004) by reducing platelet aggregation and hepatic synthesis of cholesterol (Varady et al, 2003). Policosanols are phytochemicals extracted from sugar cane.	
Poplar	Exhibits antiplatelet activity.	May enhance effects of anticoagulant medications such as warfarin and potentiate bleeding.
Probiotics (Good bacteria such as *Lactobacillus* and *Lactobacillus acidophilus*)	Used in inflammatory bowel disease and other GI disorders or to replenish gut flora after antibiotic use. May reduce presence of harmful bacteria in the gut and may decrease vaginal infections. Select yogurt and products made with live cultures.	
Psyllium	Use as a laxative to alleviate chronic constipation.	Avoid use with cardiovascular agents.
Red Clover	Used for hot flashes because it contains isoflavones. It may also be used for coughs, eczema, and psoriasis.	Evidence suggests that it has limited effectiveness (Krebs et al, 2004).
Rhodiola (*Rhodiola rosea*), arctic root	Used for depression, fatigue.	Side effects are insomnia and irritability.
Rhubarb or Da-Huang (*Rheum palmatum, R. officinale*)	Used for cancer treatment, constipation, fever, hypertension, immunosuppression, inflammation, microbial infection, peptic ulcers.	Avoid prolonged stimulant laxative use over 7 days without medical supervision. Patients with arthritis, kidney or hepatic dysfunction, history of kidney stones, inflammatory bowel disease, or intestinal obstruction should not take this herb. Rhubarb may cause uterine stimulation; avoid in pregnancy. Reported effects include abdominal cramps, nausea, vomiting, diarrhea with possible hypokalemia, anaphylaxis, and renal and hepatic damage.
Rice Bran Oil	It contains tocotrienols, powerful antioxidants in the vitamin E family that protect against coronary heart disease and some forms of cancer.	
Rosemary	Used for antioxidant and anticarcinogenic potential. Often used for lowering blood pressure.	Do not use in pregnancy in large doses.
Royal Jelly	It is a milky substance secreted by young worker honey bees. Apalbumin 1 (Apa1) is the major royal jelly and honey glycoprotein and has various biological properties, such as cancer prevention. It seems to stimulate macrophages to release TNF-α.	Avoid use with asthma; may cause allergic reactions.
Saw Palmetto	Used with benign prostatic hyperplasia to increase urine flow. Tannic acids are present.	Saw palmetto should not be taken with oral contraceptives, estrogens, or anabolic steroids. Can cause GI upset in rare cases.
Schisandra (*Schisandra chinensis*)	Used for asthma, cough, influenza, diarrhea, indigestion, liver disease, premenstrual syndrome, strength, and stamina.	Adverse reactions include depression and heartburn.
Senna	Used as a laxative herb; it contains anthraquinone, which stimulates bowel contractions. Safe for constipation, but dependence or obstruction can occur with long use. Psyllium and other naturally high-fiber foods (such as prunes), extra fluids, and exercise are better choices.	Laxative herbs speed digestion, which reduces absorption time of drugs. Chronic use results in a loss of potassium, thereby strengthening effects of cardiac glycosides and antiarrhythmic agents. Simultaneous use of thiazide diuretics, corticosteroids, or licorice root increases potassium loss. Because fluid and electrolyte losses may be severe, avoid during pregnancy and lactation.
Sheep Sorrel (*Rumex acetosella*)	Used for cancer treatment, diarrhea, scurvy, fever, inflammation.	Contraindications: patients with kidney stones should not use this herb. Adverse reactions: abdominal cramps, gastroenteritis, diarrhea leading to hypokalemia, adrenal and liver damage.

(continued)

TABLE 2-2 Herbs, Botanicals, Spices, Commentary and Adverse Effects *(continued)*

Herb, Botanical, Spice	Common Uses	Adverse Effects
Shepherd's Purse	Coagulant herb.	May inhibit effects of anticoagulant medications such as warfarin and potentiate bleeding.
Slippery Elm (*Ulmus rubra*)	Used for bronchitis, cancer treatment, cough, diarrhea, fever, inflammation, peptic ulcer, skin abscess, skin ulcers, sore throat.	Adverse reactions: none known, but no human studies have been done to evaluate its actions.
Spirulina (Blue-green algae)	Used to treat cancers, viral infections, weight loss, oral leucoplakia, increased cholesterol, attention-deficit hyperactivity disorder (ADHD). Sold as an immune enhancer or to lower cholesterol levels.	Expensive as a protein source. Adverse effects are uncommon unless contaminated; if contaminated, it is hepato-, nephro-, and neurotoxic. Adulterated form can cause allergies or gastroenteritis.
Stillingia (*Stillingia sylvatica*)	No clinical data to support its uses in bronchitis, chest congestion, cancer treatment, hemorrhoids, constipation, skin abscess, laryngitis, spasm, syphilis.	Warning: the diaterpene esters in this herb are irritants to the skin and mucous membranes. Adverse reactions: vertigo, burning sensation over the mucous membrane, diarrhea, nausea, vomiting, pruritus, skin eruptions, cough, fatigue, and sweating.
St. John's Wort (*Hypericum perforatum*)	Laboratory reports have suggested but not confirmed that the mechanism of action for St. John's wort may involve monoamine oxidase (MAO) inhibition, SSRI reuptake inhibition, increased melatonin production, and others. Used to alleviate anxiety and nervousness; does not alleviate depression. This herb has been shown to induce the drug-metabolizing enzyme cytochrome p4503A4 and has the potential to interact with many medications. DISCONTINUE 2 WEEKS BEFORE SURGERY	It can inhibit iron absorption. May enhance effects of narcotics and selective serotonin reuptake inhibitors (SSRIs). Increases side effects of photosensitizing drugs, alcohol, and melatonin. Avoid use with statins, blood pressure medications, donepezil, antidepressants and other CNS medications, and chemotherapy.
Tannins and Saponins (*Acacia pennata, Hibiscus spp., Lasianthicaafricana Gouanialupiloides*)	Used for dental hygiene and to treat gingivitis.	
Tea Tree Oil	Used for acne treatment, wound healing, or as an antiseptic for thrush (as in HIV infection). Natural fungicide.	Topical use only; toxic if consumed. Allergy is possible in sensitive individuals.
Tribulus terrestris	Used by athletes. Contains steroidal glycosides and saponins that cause secretion of luteinizing hormone, testosterone.	It is phototoxic, cytotoxic, and neurotoxic.
Tryptophan	Used to promote sleep or to correct depression.	L-tryptophan is the precursor to serotonin. It should not be used with MAO inhibitors, antidepressants, or serotonin receptor antagonists; it can exaggerate psychosis.
Turmeric (*Curcuma longa*)	Used for immune system enhancement, correcting anorexia, carcinoma prevention, reducing infections (such as reducing *H. pylori*) and inflammation, kidney stones.	Warning: breast cancer patients on cyclophosphamide should restrict intake because it inhibits the antitumor action of chemotherapeutic agents. Contraindications: patients with bile duct obstruction, gallstones, GI disorders.
Ukrain (*Chelidonium majus* alkaloid-theophosphoric acid derivative)	Used for cancer prevention and treatment, hepatitis, HIV and AIDS, immunostimulation.	Warning: it is not regulated by FDA. Adverse reactions: soreness at the injection site, nausea, diarrhea, dizziness, fatigue, drowsiness, polyuria, hematological side effects, and tumor bleeding have been reported.
Valerian (*Valeriana officinalis, Valerianae radix*, garden heliotrope)	Used for insomnia, anxiety, colic, menstrual cramps, migraine treatment, sedation, spasms, stomach and intestinal gas. Effective as a sleep aid and is not habit forming. DISCONTINUE 2 WEEKS BEFORE SURGERY	Headache, uneasiness, cardiac disturbances, morning drowsiness, and impaired alertness can occur. Benzodiazepines, sedatives, alcohol, antipsychotics, and antidepressants should not be used at the same time because of the risk of additional sedation. Long-term use can cause headaches, sleeplessness, cardiac dysfunction, hepatotoxicity. Patients should be warned not to drive or operate dangerous machinery when taking valerian. Valerian should be stopped about 1 week before surgery because it may interact with anesthesia.

(continued)

TABLE 2-2 Herbs, Botanicals, Spices, Commentary and Adverse Effects *(continued)*

Herb, Botanical, Spice	Common Uses	Adverse Effects
Vanadium (*vanadyl sulfate*)	Used to mimic insulin; it may restore plasma DHEA and seems to improve insulin action. There may be a role for its use in the metabolic syndrome. Found in mushrooms and shellfish.	May cause GI bleeding.
Vitex (chaste tree)	Used for relief of menstrual disorders. Fruits are used; approved for use in Germany.	
White Willow	Used for fever, headache, pain, and rheumatic complaints. Aspirin is derived from white willow.	GI irritation or stomach ulcers can occur with long-term use; similar reactions as aspirin. Avoid use with alcohol, methotrexate, phenytoin, and valproate. Do not use in pregnancy or lactation.
Wild Yam (*Dioscorea villosa*)	Used for amenorrhea, dysmenorrhea, colic, cough, GI symptoms, rheumatoid arthritis, menopausal symptoms, urinary tract disorders, sexual dysfunction, spasms.	Efficacy of hormonal actions is not proven. Topical creams that say that they contain yam extracts as a source of natural progesterone are not accurate.
Willow Bark (*Salix alba*)	Used for fever, headache, inflammation, influenza, muscle pain.	Adverse reactions: nausea, vomiting, GI bleed, tinnitus, renal damage. Drug interactions: increases risk of bleeding with anticoagulants and GI bleed with NSAIDs.
Witch Hazel	Used as astringent with bruises or varicose veins. Approved for use with hemorrhoid products.	Not for oral use.
Yew (*Taxus baccata, T. wallachiana, T. media*)	Used in treatment of some breast tumors. Cultivated varieties are being used to prepare triterpenoid precursors which are used to create paclitaxel and docetaxel, which in turn, have an antiestrogenic effect.	
Zinc	Used to prevent viral illness, enhance performance, and correct male infertility.	It should not be taken with immunosuppressants, fluoroquinolones, or tetracycline. Large doses may also conflict with copper metabolism.
Hazardous Products	These products should never be consumed.	
Aristolochic acid (*Aristolochia*, birthwort, snakeroot, snakeweed, snagree root, sangrel, serpentary, wild ginger)	**Definitely Hazardous**	Documented human cancers. Also linked to kidney failure.
Belladonna	**Definitely Hazardous**	Causes GI pain and spasms; contains toxic alkaloids, which can cause coma and death.
Very Likely Hazardous	***These are banned in other countries, have an FDA warning, or show adverse effects in studies.***	
Androstenedione (4-androstene-3, 17-dione, andro, androstene)	**Very Likely Hazardous**	Increased cancer risk and decrease in "good" HDL cholesterol have been reported.
Chaparral (*Larrea divaricata*, creosote bush, greasewood, hediondilla, jarilla, larreastat)	**Very Likely Hazardous** Often used for anti-inflammatory and anticancer effects, arthritis, carcinoma treatment, inflammation, spasm.	Abnormal liver function and hepatitis or even cirrhosis have been linked to use.
Comfrey (*Symphytum officinale*, ass ear, black root, blackwort, bruisewort, *Consolidae radix*, consound, gum plant, healing herb, knitback, knitbone, salsify, slippery root, *Symphytum radix*, wallwort)	**Very Likely Hazardous** Used for bronchitis, cancer treatment, rheumatoid arthritis, wound healing.	Abnormal liver function or damage, often irreversible. It contains pyrrolizidine alkaloids and causes hepatic veno-occlusive disease or death. Avoid in infants, pregnancy, lactation. FDA has asked all manufacturers to remove products containing comfrey because it is hepatotoxic.
DHEA	**Very Likely Hazardous** Used as an immune enhancer or to prevent heart disease. No evidence that it works.	Can actually aggravate heart disease and have effects like steroids; may promote cancers in breast, prostate, or ovaries.

(continued)

TABLE 2-2 Herbs, Botanicals, Spices, Commentary and Adverse Effects *(continued)*

Herb, Botanical, Spice	Common Uses	Adverse Effects
Ephedra (ma huang)	**Very Likely Hazardous** Often used in weight loss products. Banned by FDA. DISCONTINUE 2 WEEKS BEFORE SURGERY	Contains cardiac toxins linked to dozens of deaths. Ephedra can cause stroke, insomnia, hypertension, or heart attack. Avoid taking with caffeine, sedatives, antipsychotics, antidepressants, antihyperglycemic agents, decongestants, and cardiovascular agents.
Germander (*Teucrium chamaedrys*, wall germander, wild germander)	**Very Likely Hazardous** Germander contains flavanoids.	Abnormal heart and liver function have been linked to use.
Goldenseal (*Hydrastis canadensis*)	**Very Likely Hazardous** Used for anorexia, heart disease, coughs, upset stomach, menstrual problems, and arthritis. It has long been used by Native Americans for antiseptic and wound-healing properties. DISCONTINUE 2 WEEKS BEFORE SURGERY	GI complaints are common side effects. With toxicity: stomach ulcerations, constipation, convulsions, hallucinations, nausea, vomiting, depression, nervousness, bradycardia, respiratory depression, seizures. It can raise blood pressure, complicating treatment for those taking beta-blockers. For patients taking medication to control diabetes or kidney disease, this herb can cause dangerous electrolyte imbalance. Patients with hypertension or cardiovascular disease and women who are pregnant should not take this herb.
Kava (*Piper methysticum*, ava, awa, gea, gi, intoxicating pepper, kao, kavain, kawapfeffer, kew, long pepper, malohu, maluk, meruk, milik, rauschpfeffer, sakau, tonga, wurzelstock, yagona, yangona)	**Very Likely Hazardous** Used as a stimulant.	Abnormal liver function has been linked to use.
Kelp	**Very Likely Hazardous**	If ingested as a source of iodine, it may interfere with thyroid replacement therapies. May worsen hyperthyroidism.
Red yeast rice	**Very Likely Hazardous** The fermented product of rice on which red yeast has been grown. A dietary staple in Asian countries to lower total cholesterol levels (Heber et al, 1999).	It has been removed from the market in the United States. Avoid use with grapefruit juice or niacin.
Likely Hazardous	***These have adverse event reports or theoretical risks.***	
Astragalus	**Likely Hazardous** Used in Chinese and Indian medicine for its immune enhancement.	Do not take with antihyperglycemic agents. Not recommended for use, especially in immunosuppressed patients.
Bitter orange (*Citrus aurantium*, green orange, kijitsu, neroli oil, Seville orange, shangzhou zhiqiao, sour orange, zhi oiao, zhi xhi)	**Likely Hazardous**	High blood pressure and increased risk of heart arrhythmias, heart attack, and stroke are risks associated with use.
Borage	**Likely Hazardous**	May cause liver toxicity or even cancers.
Horse chestnut (*Aesculus hippocastanum*; aescin 50 mg)	**Likely Hazardous** Studies have shown clinical efficacy in chronic venous insufficiency, but no data support the reversal of varicose veins.	Patients with compromised renal or hepatic functions should not consume horse chestnut. It may also interact with anticoagulants and increase the risk of bleeding.
Kombucha tea	**Likely Hazardous** It is sometimes suggested for acne or insomnia or in AIDS.	Can cause liver damage or intestinal problems or death.

(continued)

TABLE 2-2 Herbs, Botanicals, Spices, Commentary and Adverse Effects *(continued)*

Herb, Botanical, Spice	Common Uses	Adverse Effects
Lobelia (*Lobelia inflata*, asthma weed, bladderpod, emetic herb, gagroot, lobelie, Indian tobacco, pukeweed, vomit wort, wild tobacco)	**Likely Hazardous**	Difficulty breathing and rapid heart rates are associated with lobelia. Large doses can lead to rapid heartbeat, paralysis, coma, or death. Avoid in children, infants, pregnant women, smokers, and people with cardiac diseases.
Mistletoe/Eurixor (*Viscum album*)	**Likely Hazardous** Used for arthritis, cancer treatment, hepatitis, HTN, spasm, immunostimulation.	Warning: berries and leaves are highly poisonous. Contraindication in pregnancy. Adverse reactions include fever, headache, chest pain, bradycardia, hypotension, coma.
Organ/glandular extracts (brain/adrenal/pituitary/placenta/other gland "substance" or "concentrate")	**Likely Hazardous**	Theoretical risk of mad cow disease, particularly from brain extracts.
Passion flower	**Likely Hazardous** Sometimes recommended for sedative use.	It can cause seizures, hypotension, hallucinations.
Pennyroyal oil (*Hedeoma pulegioides*, lurk-in-the-ditch, mosquito plant, piliolerial, pudding grass, pulegium, run-by-the-ground, squaw balm, squawmint, stinking balm, tickweed)	**Likely Hazardous**	Liver and kidney failure, nerve damage, convulsions, abdominal tenderness, and burning of the throat are risks; deaths have been reported.
Poke root	**Likely Hazardous**	May cause low blood pressure and respiratory depression. Extremely toxic.
Sassafras (*Sassafras albidum*)	**Likely Hazardous** Used for detoxification, inflammation, health maintenance, rheumatoid arthritis, mucositis, sprain, syphilis, urinary tract disorders.	Produces sweat and contains safrole, which is banned as a carcinogen. Warning: risk of liver cancer with prolonged use, so it is not safe to use. Adverse reactions: hot flashes, diaphoresis, hallucinations, hypertension, tachycardia, liver cancer, and death.
Skullcap (*Scutellaria lateriflora*, *S. baicalensis*, baikal, blue pimpernel, helmet flower, hoodwort, mad weed, mad-dog herb, mad-dog weed, quaker bonnet, scutelluria, scullcap)	**Likely Hazardous** Used for epilepsy, hepatitis, infections, cancer.	Toxicity causes stupor, confusion, seizures. Adverse reactions include hepatotoxicity and pneumonitis.
Wheat grass (*Triticum aestivum*)	**Likely Hazardous** Used for carcinoma treatment, chronic fatigue syndrome, immunostimulation, ulcerative colitis. An antioxidant.	Adverse reactions: nausea because of contamination. No safety guidelines available.
Yohimbe (*Pausinystalia yohimbe*, johimbi, yohimbehe, yohimbine, yohimbe bark)	**Likely Hazardous** May be used for male impotence. It causes CNS stimulation and vasodilation. In high doses, it is an MAO inhibitor. It is to be avoided in individuals with hypotension, CHF, diabetes, and kidney and liver diseases.	Blood pressure changes, heartbeat irregularities, heart attacks, and paralysis have been reported. Yohimbe is not effective for male impotence and can cause side effects such as hypertension and kidney failure; it can also aggravate bipolar disorder or decrease antidepressant effectiveness.

Sources:

1. National Institutes of Health. Accessed March 21, 2009, at http://www.nlm.nih.gov/medlineplus/herbalmedicine.html.
2. Office of Dietary Supplements. Accessed March 21, 2009, at http://ods.od.nih.gov/Health_Information/Information_About_Individual_Dietary_Supplements.aspx.
3. Kumar NB, et al. Perioperative herbal supplement use in cancer patients: potential implications and recommendations for presurgical screening. *Cancer Control.* 12:149, 2005.

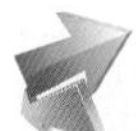

ASSESSMENT, MONITORING, AND EVALUATION

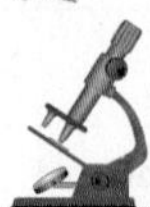

CLINICAL INDICATORS

Clinical/History
- Use of vitamin/mineral supplements
- Herbs and botanical products—amount, frequency
- Special diets or nutrition support
- Dietary pattern for food and alcohol
- Over-the-counter and prescribed medications
- Knowledge of food and nutrition
- Family or genetic history

Lab Work
- Hemoglobin and hematocrit (H & H)
- Serum Fe
- Glucose
- Na^+, K^+, Cl^-
- Ca^{++}, Mg^{++}
- Albumin (Alb)
- T3, T4, TSH
- Blood urea nitrogen (BUN)
- Creatinine (Creat)
- Homocysteine (tHcy)
- Cholesterol (Chol), triglycerides (TG)
- Other values as determined by products consumed

INTERVENTION

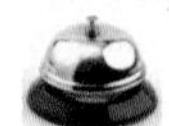

OBJECTIVES

The White House Commission on Complementary and Alternative Medicine Policy Executive Summary (2002) supported the following guiding principles for counseling individuals:

- Apply a "wholeness orientation" in health care delivery. Health involves all aspects of life—mind, body, spirit, and environment.
- Evaluate for evidence of safety and efficacy. Promote the use of science and appropriate scientific methods to help identify safe and effective CAM services and products.
- Identify the healing capacity of the individual person. People have a remarkable capacity for recovery and self-healing; support and promote this capacity.
- Respect individuality, recognizing that each person is unique and has the right to health care that is appropriately responsive to him or her, respecting preferences and preserving dignity.
- Recognize patient rights. Each has the right to choose treatment; to choose freely among safe and effective care or approaches; and to choose among qualified practitioners who are accountable for their claims and actions and responsive to the person's needs.
- Support health promotion, self-care, and early intervention for maintaining and promoting health.
- Develop partnerships. Good health care requires teamwork among patients, health care practitioners (conventional and CAM), and researchers committed to creating optimal healing environments and to respecting the diversity of all health care traditions.
- Educate about prevention, healthy lifestyles, and the power of self-healing.
- Disseminate comprehensive and timely information. The quality of health care can be enhanced by promoting efforts that thoroughly and thoughtfully examine the evidence on which CAM systems, practices, and products are based and make this evidence widely, rapidly, and easily available.
- Integrate public involvement. The input of informed consumers and other members of the public must be incorporated in setting priorities for health care and health care research and in reaching policy decisions.

SAMPLE NUTRITION CARE PROCESS STEPS

Harmful Beliefs about Food or Nutrition-Related Topics

Assessment Data: Food records; adverse side effects with specific products and amounts taken; blood pressure (BP), lab reports for serum electrolytes.

Nutrition Diagnoses (PES): Harmful beliefs/attitudes about food or nutrition-related topics related to intake of unsafe substances as evidenced by intake of ephedra in products otherwise removed from the market by FDA and complaints of rapid heartbeat and undesirable changes in BP.

Intervention: Education about appropriate use of herbs and botanical products; dangers of consuming substances with unknown side effects. Counseling about desired foods and use of evidence-based complementary products.

Monitoring and Evaluation: Improved quality of life and reduced symptoms; improvements in heart rate and BP.

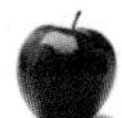

FOOD AND NUTRITION

- Promote the appropriate use of herbal and botanical products that have shown efficacy and safety. The best strategy for promoting optimal health and for reducing chronic disease is to choose a wide variety of foods (American Dietetic Association, 2005).
- Functional foods are available that have health benefits beyond basic nutrition (e.g., omega-3–enriched eggs, stanol- and sterol-fortified soft chews and related margarines, or high-flavanol chocolate snacks). Use relevant products and recipes.
- Special attention may be needed for intake of iron and folic acid for females in teen and childbearing years; vitamin B_{12} for adults over age 50; and vitamin D for older adults, those with dark skin, and those exposed to ultraviolet radiation (American Dietetic Association, 2005).

Common Drugs Used and Potential Side Effects

- Plants have been used throughout history to improve health. Modern medicines often come from plants (e.g., aspirin from willow bark). Therefore, herbs used for health purposes are drugs and chemicals that affect the human body (O'Hara et al, 1998).

- About 15 million Americans are at risk for drug–supplement interactions (Boullata, 2005). Natural health products often interfere with medications, and caution is necessary.

Herbs, Botanicals, and Supplements

- Many cultures use herbs and botanicals as part of their meal patterns, rituals, and celebrations. Remember that plant products are not necessarily safe, even if they are "natural" or "organic."
- Individual reports of safety for any herbal product are not reliable; some people who use a herb will feel better even if there is no evidence of its efficacy (the placebo effect).
- The use of dietary supplements may be associated with adverse events (Sadovsky et al, 2008). Although there are new regulatory requirements for dietary supplements, these products do not require FDA approval, submission of efficacy and safety data prior to marketing, or prospective, randomized clinical trials (Sadovsky et al, 2008). Check www.consumerlab.com to identify brand names that are reliable before making recommendations.
- Herbs commonly used by children enrolled in the Women-Infants-Children (WIC) program children include aloe vera, chamomile, garlic, peppermint, lavender, cranberry, ginger, echinacea, and lemon, as recommended by family or friends (Lohse et al, 2006). Identify those that are used and monitor for potential side effects. Because herbs with safety issues, such as St. John's wort, dong quai, and kava, may also be used, herbal education is highly recommended for WIC clinics, especially for Latinos (Lohse et al, 2006).

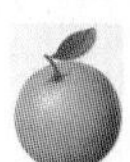

NUTRITION EDUCATION, COUNSELING, CARE MANAGEMENT

- Demonstrate respect for the beliefs, values, and practices of the patient and family members. Discuss CAM in a nonjudgmental way; encourage sharing the information with their primary physician.
- Discuss evidence that is known about different types of herbs and botanical products. Counsel that herbs are considered dietary supplements and not medicines, that FDA has no oversight on ingredients or safety and efficacy, and that there is no guarantee that the herb will work.
- Many physicians are not aware of the frequency of use and adverse events related to dietary supplements (Ashar et al, 2007).
- Alcohol interacts with many medications and possibly with herbs. Mix with caution.

Patient Education—Food Safety

- Discuss food handling, preparation, and storage of herbs and botanical products.
- Because bacteria are commonly found on foods such as green onions (scallions), cilantro, and imported produce, wash all fresh fruits and vegetables.
- Store spices as directed and discard after shelf-life expiration. Spices such as paprika are easily contaminated.

For More Information

- American Botanical Council
  http://www.herbalgram.org/
- American Council on Science and Health
  http://www.acsh.org/
- American Dietetic Association
  http://www.eatright.org/
- American Herbal Products Association
  http://www.ahpa.org/
- Alternative Medicine Foundation
  http://www.amfoundation.org/
- Botanical Dietary Supplements
  http://ods.od.nih.gov/factsheets/BotanicalBackground.asp
- CAM on PubMed—Searchable database
  http://www.nlm.nih.gov/nccam/camonpubmed.html
- Cochrane Collaboration—Complementary Medicine
  http://www.compmed.umm.edu/cochrane/index.html
- Complementary and Integrative Medicine
  http://www.mdanderson.org/departments/cimer/
- Consumer Lab.com
  http://www.consumerlab.com/
- Dietary Supplements
  http://www.cfsan.fda.gov/~dms/supplmnt.html
- Drug Digest
  http://www.drugdigest.org/wps/portal/ddigest
- Facts about Dietary Supplements
  http://www.cc.nih.gov/ccc/supplements/intro.html
- Federal Trade Commission (FTC)
  http://www.ftc.gov/
- Food and Nutrition Information Center—Dietary Supplements
  http://fnic.nal.usda.gov/nal_display/index.php?tax_level=1&info_center=4&tax_subject=274
- Herbal Monographs and Frequently Asked Questions on Herbs from RxList.com
  http://www.rxlist.com/alternative.htm#herbal_mon
- HerbMed—Interactive, electronic herbal database
  http://www.herbmed.org/
- Herb Research Foundation
  http://www.herbs.org/
- Herbs and Cultural Uses
  http://asiarecipe.com/herb.html
- Herbs Database
  http://nccam.nih.gov/health/herbsataglance.htm
- Intelihealth, Vitamin and Nutrition Resource Center
  http://www.intelihealth.com/IH/ihtIH/WSIHW000/325/325.html
- Institute of Food Technologists
  http://www.ift.org/
- International Food Information Council—Functional Foods
  http://www.ific.org/nutrition/functional/index.cfm
- Labels Database
  http://dietarysupplements.nlm.nih.gov/dietary/
- Mayo Clinic
  http://www.mayoclinic.com/health/alternative-medicine/CM99999
- MEDLINE, Vitamin and Mineral Supplements
  http://www.nlm.nih.gov/medlineplus/vitaminandmineralsupplements.html
- National Center for Complementary and Alternative Medicine (NCCAM)
  http://altmed.od.nih.gov/
- NIH Herbal Listing:
  http://www.nlm.nih.gov/medlineplus/druginfo/herb_All.html
- National Institutes of Health, Office of Dietary Supplements
  http://ods.od.nih.gov/
- Rosenthal Center for Complementary and Alternative Medicine
  http://www.rosenthal.hs.columbia.edu/index.html
- Sloan-Kettering Herbs and Cancer
  http://www.mskcc.org/mskcc/html/58481.cfm
- Special Nutritionals Adverse Event Monitoring System—Searchable database from the FDA
  http://www.fda.gov/medwatch/how.htm

- Tufts University Nutrition
  http://www.tufts.edu/med/ebcam/nutrition/
- University of Illinois Botanical Supplement Research
  http://www.uic.edu/pharmacy/centers/uic_nih_botanical_dietary_supplement_research/index.php
- U.S. Pharmacopeia
  http://www.usp.org/
- USP Verified Program
  http://www.uspverified.org/

COMPLEMENTARY NUTRITION—CITED REFERENCES

American Dietetic Association. Position of the American Dietetic Association: fortification and nutritional supplements. *J Am Diet Assoc.* 105:1300, 2005.

American Dietetic Association. Position of the American Dietetic Association: functional foods. *J Am Diet Assoc.* 109:735, 2009.

Anderson RA, et al. Isolation and characterization of polyphenol type-A polymers from cinnamon with insulin-like biological activity. *J Agric Food Chem.* 52:65, 2004.

Ashar BH, et al. Physicians' understanding of the regulation of dietary supplements. *Arch Int Med.* 167:966, 2007.

Boullata J. Natural health product interactions with medication. *Nutr Clin Pract.* 20:33, 2005.

Dragland S, et al. Several culinary and medicinal herbs are important sources of dietary antioxidants. *J Nutr.* 133:1286, 2003.

Gades MD, Stern JS. Chitosan supplementation and fat absorption in men and women. *J Am Diet Assoc.* 105:72, 2005.

Ichikawa H, Aggarwal BB. Guggulsterone inhibits osteoclastogenesis induced by receptor activator of nuclear factor-kappaB ligand and by tumor cells by suppressing nuclear factor-kappaB activation. *Clin Cancer Res.* 12:662, 2006.

Lohse B, et al. Survey of herbal use by Kansas and Wisconsin WIC participants reveals moderate, appropriate use and identifies herbal education needs. *J Am Diet Assoc.* 106:227, 2006.

Nagao T, et al. Ingestion of a tea rich in catechins leads to a reduction in body fat and malondialdehyde-modified LDL in men. *Am J Clin Nutr.* 81:122, 2005.

Sadovsky R, et al. Patient use of dietary supplements: a clinician's perspective. *Curr Med Res Opinion.* 24:1209, 2008.

Thomson CA, et al. Practice paper of the American Dietetic Association: dietary supplements. *J Am Diet Assoc.* 105:460, 2005.

van der Voet GB, et al. Clinical and analytical toxicology of dietary supplements: a case study and a review of the literature. *Biol Trace Elem Res* 125(1):1, 2008.

White House Commission on Complementary and Alternative Medicine Policy. Final report. Accessed November 1, 2000, at http://www.whccamp.hhs.gov.

Wold RS, et al. Increasing trends in elderly persons' use of nonvitamin, nonmineral dietary supplements and concurrent use of medications. *J Am Diet Assoc.* 105:54, 2005.

CULTURAL FOOD PATTERNS, VEGETARIANISM, RELIGIOUS PRACTICES

CULTURAL FOOD PATTERNS

NUTRITIONAL ACUITY RANKING: LEVEL 2 (DIETARY ADAPTATIONS, ADVISEMENT)

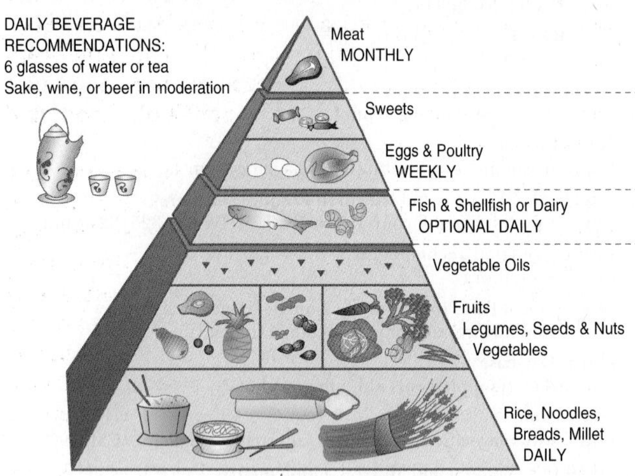

Reprinted with permission from: Weber J RN, EdD and Kelley J RN, PhD. *Health Assessment in Nursing,* 2nd ed. Philadelphia: Lippincott Williams & Wilkins, 2003.

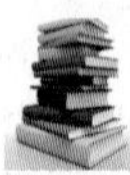

DEFINITIONS AND BACKGROUND

Varied dietary intakes by age, culture, gender, and years in the United States are common. Assessment of a patient's cultural food preferences is essential to determine adequacy of nutritional intake. Nutrition planning will be more effective if tailored to the individual (Sucher and Kittler, 2007). Disease prevention strategies must use available knowledge about individual cultures.

Soon, over half of the U.S. population will consist of people from different cultural backgrounds (Goody and Drago, 2010). The process by which immigrants adopt the dietary practices is multidimensional, dynamic, complex, varying by personal, cultural, and environmental factors (Unger et al, 2004). Adoption of U.S. dietary patterns that are high in fat and low in fruits and vegetables is not positive. Neighborhood grocery stores may have limited availability of fresh produce, making healthy choices a struggle (Larson et al, 2009).

Dietetics practitioners can use the information to study nutrition education efforts directed toward ethnic-specific groups. It is important to become aware of diverse traditions and preferred food resources. Clinicians should be able to offer a wide variety of self-management support systems to meet the needs of diverse patient populations that vary by race/ethnicity, language proficiency, and health literacy (Sarkar et al, 2008).

The Joint Commission has set the standard for meeting individual needs for cultural and religious preferences. Whereas most hospitals attend to the religious (97%), dietary (85%), and psychosocial (78%) cultural needs of patients, fewer institutions respond to patients' cultural needs related to health literacy (57%); complementary/alternative medicine (43%); cultural brokers, folk remedies, traditions, rituals and traditional healers (Stein, 2009). It is important to reinforce positive traditional habits while encouraging inclusion of new, healthy ones.

SAMPLE NUTRITION CARE PROCESS STEPS

Unintentional Weight Loss

Assessment Data: Food records indicating lack of appetite for new foods; weight records; low blood glucose and Chol levels.

Nutrition Diagnoses (PES): Unintentional weight loss related to limited access to preferred foods as evidenced by 15# weight loss since moving to this country 6 months ago with a current BMI of 17.

Intervention: Education about where to find ethnic food choices for protein choices, whole grains, fruits and vegetables. Counseling about culturally appropriate choices that are accessible in neighborhood or area stores.

Monitoring and Evaluation: Improved BMI and weight for height; lab reports showing improvement in glucose and Chol.

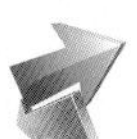

ASSESSMENT, MONITORING, AND EVALUATION

Race/ethnicity
Language proficiency
Health literacy
Cultural food preferences
Traditional dietary habits

INTERVENTION

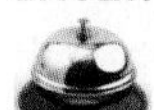

OBJECTIVES

- Be aware of personal cultural values but avoid imposing them on others. For example, the desire to be thin is more common among Caucasians than people from many other ethnic backgrounds.
- Assess values, attitudes, beliefs, practices, and rituals of the client before attempting to discuss any lifestyle changes. Observe and interact appropriately.
- Provide individualized patterns when they differ from the local standard. Be prepared to understand the differences from a "typical American" diet.
- Determine which habits, if any, are detrimental for a healthy lifestyle. Review patterns or foods that aggravate existing or predisposed conditions for each person. Build on healthy practices.
- Correct dietary intake patterns for nutrient deficits, such as calcium and riboflavin where dairy products or milk are excluded or not tolerated. Identify other nutrients that are at risk for insufficiency.
- Offer suggestions for changes in food preparation (e.g., ways for reducing fat or salt) rather than changing the foods themselves, whenever possible.
- Each culture has functional foods and ingredients that have special attributes. Identify and acknowledge these foods or ingredients.
- Understand customs, festive occasions, fasting, ceremonial activities, and celebrations. Promote the traditions and welcome special events or activities, as appropriate for the setting.

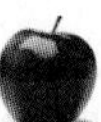

FOOD AND NUTRITION

- Review and identify specific ethnic and religious food patterns. Table 2-3 lists a brief overview of religious dietary patterns and common practices. More extensive information can be found on the internet and in many cookbooks.
- The WIC food package was updated to include foods to help families from diverse backgrounds. Most participants prefer whole versus low-fat milk; whole grain products and peanut butter are preferred over beans or soy foods (Black et al, 2009).
- *African/African American patterns.* Foods such as peanuts, peppers, and corn are traditional, as are fruits, vegetables, meats, and milk. Starch is a main consideration in the diet. Access to healthy foods such as fruits, vegetables, and whole grains should be noted as some community resources may be limited (Franco et al, 2009). In the South, dietary habits may include healthy foods prepared with unhealthy ingredients (such as fried chicken, greens prepared with lard). Spices and seasonings may vary. Alterations in recipes may be needed for taste and acceptance if healthier choices are offered.
- *Asian patterns.* Asian diets vary from one country to another. Diets may be low in calcium and riboflavin because milk often is not tolerated or consumed. Encourage use of tofu, green vegetables, and fish containing small bones. Diet may be high in sodium if monosodium glutamate (MSG) and soy sauces are used. The traditional Chinese diet contains 80% grains, legumes, and vegetables. Stir-frying, deep fat frying, and steaming are common cooking methods. Pork is the preferred meat. Hot peppers may be used daily. "Hot" and "cold" foods may be used during pregnancy or illness but these terms do not refer to food temperatures. Korean Americans tend to have a greater intake of carbohydrates, vitamins A and C than of saturated and total fat or Chol (Goody and Drago, 2010).
- *Hmong (Southeast Asian) patterns.* Milk is seldom used, related to lactose intolerance; calcium intake may be low. Fish, chicken, and pork are common entrees. Rice may be eaten at nearly every meal. A highly salted fish sauce is used. Snacking is rare in the family diet. Anemia may result from parasite infestation in those individuals who have been refugees. Like Chinese patterns, hot–cold patterns are often observed. A website for Vietnamese food is available at http://www.ivietbusiness.com/vietnamese-food-recipe.htm
- *Hispanic/Latino patterns.* Whole milk is used rarely, but cheese is a common additive to meals. Chili peppers, mangos, and avocados are the primary fruits and vegetables consumed. The main starch is corn or flour tortilla. Rice is the major contributor of energy among the elderly. The diet may be high in sugar and saturated fat (lard). A common main dish is beans with rice. Hot and cold foods are concepts commonly found. Salsa or sofrito seasonings are used frequently. Obesity, type 2 diabetes, hypertension, cardiovascular disease, dental caries, snacking, and undernutrition may be problems. Most Hispanic countries use folk remedies, such as garlic to treat hypertension and cough; chamomile to treat nausea, gas, colic, and anxiety; and peppermint to treat dyspepsia.

TABLE 2-3 Common Religious Food Practices

	Seventh-Day Adventist	Buddhist	Eastern Orthodox	Hindu	Jewish	Mormon	Moslem	Roman Catholic
Beef	A	A		X				
Pork	X	A		A	X		X	
All meat	A	A	R	A	R		R	R
Eggs/dairy	O	O	R	O	R			
Fish	A	A	R	R	R			
Shellfish	X	A	O	R	X			
Alcohol	X			A		X	X	
Coffee/tea	X					X	A	
Meat and dairy at same meal					X			
Leavened foods					R			
Ritual slaughter of meats					+		+	
Moderation	+	+					+	
Fasting[a]		+	+	+	+	+	+	+

[a]Fasting varies from partial (abstention from certain foods or meals) to complete (no food or drink).
X, prohibited or strongly discouraged; A, avoided by the most devout; R, some restrictions regarding types of foods or when a food may be eaten; O, permitted, but may be avoided at some observances; +, practiced.

REFERENCES

http://asiarecipe.com/religion.html.
http://www.betterhealth.vic.gov.au/bhcv2/bhcarticles.nsf/pages/Food_culture_and_religion?open.

- *Indian/Pakistani patterns.* India has some of the most diverse populations and diets in the world. In India, rates for oral and esophageal cancers are high. Indian immigrants in the United States are largely Hindus; Pakistani immigrants are mostly Muslims. Vegetarianism is a primary practice among Indians, deriving from religious beliefs in which the cow is sacred. Lentils and legumes are a primary source of protein; sometimes milk, eggs, fish, shrimp are consumed. Sattvic foods are believed to create a healthy life; these include milk products (except cheese made from rennet), rice, wheat, and legumes. Rajasic foods are believed to contribute to aggression; these include meats, eggs, and rich or very salty foods. Tamasic foods are believed to contribute to slothfulness or dullness; these include garlic, pickled foods, stale or rotten foods, and alcohol used for pleasure or to excess. Lack of portion control may be a factor in diabetes, which is common (Goody and Drago, 2010). Combination foods include biryani (grain, meat), samosas (grain, vegetable, meat, fat), kheer "rice pudding" (grain, milk), and curry (meat, vegetable). Turmeric (curcumin) is an ingredient in Indian curry spice that has strong antioxidant properties.
- *Mediterranean diet pattern (MDP).* The MDP reflect the habits of populations of Italy, Crete, and Greece. Olive oil; fish, poultry, and eggs rather than beef; breads, fruits, and vegetables in abundance; and lots of beans/legumes, yogurt, and cheeses make up this pattern. Exercise and wine are also mainstays. MDP is more often found among older people and people in rural areas, among males more than females, and among people who are more physically active (Tur et al, 2004). A Mediterranean-style diet rich in whole grains, fruits, vegetables, legumes, walnuts, and olive oil is effective in reducing both the prevalence of the metabolic syndrome and cardiovascular risks. Urban young people should be encouraged to return to this pattern.
- *Middle Eastern patterns.* Countries usually include Egypt, Iran, Jordan, Lebanon, Saudi Arabia, and Turkey. Lamb and beef are consumed; pork is eaten only by Christians. Yogurt and cheese provide calcium sources as lactose intolerance is prevalent. Because olive oil is commonly used, lower BP is often found (Goody and Drago, 2010).
- *Native American patterns (American Indian and Alaskan Native).* Food has great religious and social significance and is commonly part of many celebrations. Fried foods, fried bread, corn, mutton, and goat are frequently used by American Indians, whereas seafood and game are more common among Alaskan natives. Obesity and type 2 diabetes are very common (Goody and Drago, 2010). For recipes, see website http://www.kstrom.net/isk/food/recipes.html. More information is available at http://www.usda.gov/news/pubs/indians/open.htm

Common Drugs Used and Potential Side Effects

- Drugs may interact with various herbs botanicals and supplements. Individualize care and counseling.
- In the Multi-Ethnic Study of Atherosclerosis, white, African-American, Hispanic, and Chinese-American participants aged 45–84 years were studied; some met DRI guidelines for calcium, vitamin C, and magnesium but

effects of supplementation varied according to ethnicity and sex (Burnett-Hartman et al, 2009). Counselors should always ask about use of vitamin–mineral supplements.

Herbs, Botanicals, and Supplements

- Knowledge of integrative medicine incorporates herbal and botanical products that are used for preventive or medicinal purposes. Different cultures apply different herbs and practices in folk medicine.
- Many cultures use herbs and botanicals as part of their meal patterns, rituals, and celebrations. Identify those that are used and monitor for potential side effects. See the first part of this chapter, which describes complementary medicine products.

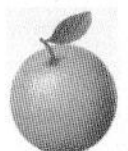

NUTRITION EDUCATION, COUNSELING, CARE MANAGEMENT

- Culturally appropriate counseling and awareness of religious practices are important for improving health issues, such as obesity and intake of fruits and vegetables (Goody and Drago, 2010). Different methods may be needed for dietary modification for obesity, diabetes, and hypertension, taking into account differences in cultural understanding and food practices. First, demonstrate respect for the beliefs, values, and practices of the patient and family members.
- Interpreters may be needed. Bilingual staff or community volunteers are helpful. Speak directly to the individual and not to the interpreter during sessions to show respect.
- Alternative solutions to dietary patterns must be gently offered. There is no "one right way" for dietary patterns. Understanding background, health problems, statistics, social issues, and disease patterns is useful when providing multicultural education.
- Build relationships through sensitivity and communication. Remove assumptions and stereotypes; cultures are changing, growing, and dynamic.
- Family beliefs and behaviors may sabotage a client's efforts; be aware and be helpful. Develop an intuitive counseling style, reading body language, eye contact, and other behaviors.
- Offer tips on food selection, preparation, and storage; identify available resources, ethnic stores, and agencies.
- Interpreting food labels and preparing unfamiliar foods can be part of the educational session.
- Body language differs between cultures. For example, Hispanic/Latino cultures prefer being close to others in space; sitting within 2 feet demonstrates interest. Oriental cultures may prefer a greater distance to demonstrate respect.

Patient Education—Food Safety

- Discuss food handling, preparation, and storage within a cultural context.
- When traveling, avoid tap water and ice made from tap water, uncooked produce such as lettuce, and raw or undercooked seafood.
- Avoid raw or partially cooked eggs, raw or undercooked fish or shellfish, and raw or undercooked meats because of potential foodborne illnesses.
- Do not use raw (unpasteurized) milk or products made from it. Avoid serving unpasteurized juices and raw sprouts.

For More Information

- Association for the Study of Food and Society http://www.food-culture.org/
- Center for Cross-Cultural Health http://www.crosshealth.com/links.htm
- Cultural and Ethnic Resources http://www.nal.usda.gov/fnic/pubs/bibs/gen/ethnic.pdf
- Cultural and Ethnic Food Pyramids http://www.semda.org/info/
- Eating Healthy with ethnic Foods http://www.nhlbi.nih.gov/health/public/heart/obesity/lose_wt/eth_dine.htm
- Ethnic Grocer http://www.ethnicgrocer.com/
- Food History Timeline http://www.foodtimeline.org/
- Food Habits and Anthropology http://www.foodhabits.info/
- Food and Nutrition Information Center, National Agricultural Library http://www.nal.usda.gov/fnic/
- Georgia State Nutrition Handouts http://monarch.gsu.edu/multiculturalhealth
- Joint Commission—Culture http://www.jointcommission.org/PatientSafety/HLC/about_hlc.htm
- Journal of Food and Culture http://www.gastronomica.org/
- National Center for Cultural Competence http://gucchd.georgetown.edu/nccc/index.html
- Ohio State University Extension Fact Sheets http://ohioline.osu.edu/hyg-fact/5000/index.html
- Oldways Cultural Food Pyramids http://www.oldwayspt.org/
- Religious Food Practices http://asiarecipe.com/religion.html#help
- Seventh Day Adventist Foodways http://www.sdada.org/position.htm
- USDA Food Pyramid—Ethnic and Cultural Versions http://www.nal.usda.gov/fnic/Fpyr/pyramid.html

CULTURAL FOOD PATTERNS—CITED REFERENCES

Black MM, et al. Participants' comments on changes in the revised special supplemental nutrition program for women, infants, and children food packages: the Maryland food preference study. *J Am Diet Assoc.* 109:116, 2009.

Burnett-Hartman AN, et al. Supplement use contributes to meeting recommended dietary intakes for calcium, magnesium, and vitamin C in four ethnicities of middle-aged and older Americans: the Multi-Ethnic Study of Atherosclerosis. *J Am Diet Assoc.* 109:422, 2009.

Franco M, et al. Availability of healthy foods and dietary patterns: the Multi-Ethnic Study of Atherosclerosis. *Am J Clin Nutr.* 89:897, 2009.

Goody CM, Drago L. *Cultural food practices.* Chicago, IL: American Dietetic Association, 2010.

Kittler PG, Sucher KP. *Food and culture.* 5th ed. Belmont, CA: Wadsworth, 2008.

Larson NI, et al. Neighborhood environments: disparities in access to healthy foods in the U.S. *Am J Prev Med.* 36:74, 2009.

Sarkar U, et al. Preferences for self-management support: findings from a survey of diabetes patients in safety-net health systems. *Patient Educ Couns.* 70:102, 2008.

Stein K. Navigating cultural competency: in preparation for an expected standard in 2010. *J Am Diet Assoc.* 109:1676, 2009.

Unger JB, et al. Acculturation, physical activity, and fast-food consumption among Asian-American and Hispanic adolescents. *J Community Health.* 29:467, 2004.

VEGETARIANISM

NUTRITIONAL ACUITY RANKING: LEVEL 2 FOR MEAL PLANNING

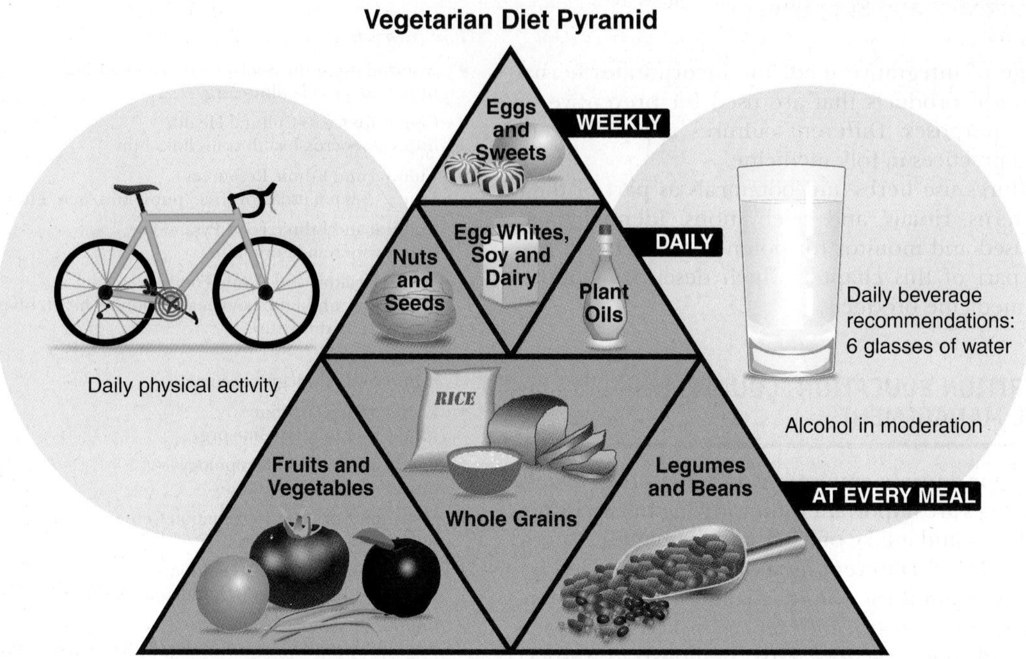

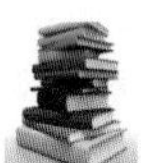

DEFINITIONS AND BACKGROUND

Vegetarian diets are plant-based with large amounts of cereals, fruits, vegetables, legumes, seeds, and nuts (Key et al, 2006). These diets generally omit meat, poultry, and fish. The vegan plan is a very strict vegetarian food pattern ("pure" vegetarianism); lacto is a vegetarian food pattern using milk; and lacto–ovo, a vegetarian food pattern using milk and eggs. While a Macrobiotic diet consists mainly of beans and whole grains, some individuals also consume fish. Conscious combining of complementary protein sources does not appear to be necessary on a regular basis (American Dietetic Association, 2003).

Vegetarian diets can be healthful when carefully planned. The Institute of Medicine recommends 25–35 g of fiber per day; vegetarian diets can easily provide this level. Individuals following vegetarian diets tend to have less obesity, constipation, diabetes, hypertension, diverticular disease, appendicitis, hiatal hernia, hemorrhoids, and varicose veins. Vegetarians usually consume less-saturated fats and Chol and often have more favorable lipid levels. Long-term vegetarians have a better antioxidant status and coronary heart disease risk profile than do apparently healthy omnivores; plasma ascorbic acid is a useful marker of overall health status (Szeto et al, 2004). Finally, there may be fewer kidney stones among vegetarians. A balanced diet with a moderate animal protein and purine content, an adequate fluid intake, and a high-alkali load with fruits and vegetables results in low risk of uric acid crystallization (Siener and Hesse, 2003).

Hindus, Seventh Day Adventists, Buddhists, and some other religious groups may suggest following a vegetarian lifestyle. Vegetarian diets are usually rich in carbohydrates, n-6 fatty acids, dietary fiber, carotenoids, folic acid, vitamin C, vitamin E and Mg, and relatively low in protein, saturated fat, long-chain n–3 fatty acids, retinol, vitamin B_{12} and Zn (Key et al, 2006). See Table 2-4 for guidance on nutrients that are at risk.

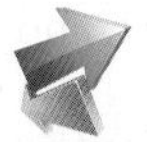

ASSESSMENT, MONITORING, AND EVALUATION

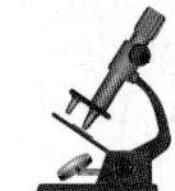

CLINICAL INDICATORS

Clinical/History

Height
Weight
BMI
Diet history

Lab Work

Mean cell volume (MCV)
Serum Fe and ferritin
Transferrin
Albumin (alb), transthyretin
chol, Trig
Glucose (gluc)
Serum folate
Serum B_{12}
tHcy
Ca^{++}, Mg^{++}
Na^{+}, K^{+}
Serum zinc
Alkaline phosphatase (alk phos)
Serum vitamin D

TABLE 2-4 Potential Complications of a Vegetarian Diet

Calcium absorption may be inhibited as a consequence of the presence of phytates in plant foods; vegetarian diets are a risk for pregnant women, children, and adolescents if calcium intake is not carefully planned.

Iron Deficiency Anemia. Females should be sure to obtain an adequate amount of absorbable iron (Sharma et al, 2003). The iron in dairy, eggs, and plant foods is largely nonheme, of which only about 2–20% is absorbed.

Excess Fiber or Inadequate Energy Intake. In some circumstances, this regimen can restrict energy intake in the first few years of life (Murphy and Allen, 2003). This is also true for adults who consume large amounts of fiber to the extent that other nutrients are not able to be absorbed in the small intestine.

Omega-3 Fatty Acids and essential amino acids **methionine** and **lysine** are found in significantly lower amounts in vegetarian diets (Mezzano et al, 2000). It may be necessary to use a supplemental form.

Protein may be limited. Suggest complementary food combinations to acquire all amino acids.

Vitamin B_{12} Deficiency. An individual following a vegan diet should use supplements to obtain this vitamin (Stabler and Allen, 2004).

Vitamin D Deficiency or Rickets. The human body can synthesize vitamin D from sunlight, but this is only possible when the sun reaches a certain intensity level. For people who live in northern latitudes, for a few months of the year, they will have to seek other sources of vitamin D. Milk is generally fortified with vitamin D; for vegans who do not consume dairy products, supplements are necessary (Outila et al, 2000). A very low-fat vegan diet can be nutritionally adequate with the exception of vitamin D; supplementation is needed (Dunn-Emke et al, 2005).

Zinc intake may be lower in vegetarian diets (Hunt, 2003).

INTERVENTION

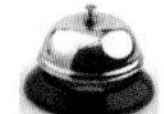

OBJECTIVES

- Encourage use of a wide variety of foods in adequate quantity with a mix of nutrients and amino acids throughout the day.

SAMPLE NUTRITION CARE PROCESS STEPS

Excessive Fiber Intake

Assessment Data: Food records; adverse side effects from high fiber intake; low BP; altered nutritional labs for calcium and iron.

Nutrition Diagnoses (PES): Excessive fiber intake related to vegan lifestyle as evidenced by complaints of excessive gas at night and intake of 45+ g of fiber daily, especially with large amounts at dinner.

Interventions: Food and Nutrition Delivery: ND 3.2.1 and ND 3.2.3 provide supplementation of a multivitamin and vitamin B_{12}; ND-1.4 educate and counsel patient on following a healthy vegan diet and teach patient how to plan and monitor diet carefully.

Nutrition Education: E-2.2 Registered dietitian (RD) to provide recommend modifications to patient's diet through instruction and training to lead to a better understanding of the importance of monitoring vegan diet and supplementing to get required nutrients not supplied through diet.

Counseling: C-2.4 Problem Solving: RD will teach and counsel patient on how to get nutrients she needs while continuing to follow a vegan diet. They will discuss solutions to patient's vitamin B_{12} deficiency by discussing vegan foods that are fortified with vitamin B_{12} and foods such as nutritional yeast that will provide her with a source of vitamin B_{12} in her diet.

Coordination of Care: RC-1.2 Refer patient to RD specializing in vegetarianism.

Monitoring and Evaluation: Improved quality of life with reduced symptoms of gas; lab reports for calcium, iron, ferritin; diet history revealing intake of fiber within desired range of 25–35 g/d.

- Provide nutritionally adequate menus with sufficient energy for weight goals. Discourage excessive use of sweets.
- Monitor the vegetarian diet carefully if the client is a pregnant woman, lactating mother, or elderly person. Infants, children, and teens on vegan diets should be monitored even more closely to ensure adequate energy intake and mineral and vitamin intakes (Perry, 2002). High-fiber diets may replace calories and cause some stunting or other growth deficits.
- Monitor fiber intake in general; excesses may interfere with absorption of calcium, zinc, and iron.
- Prevent or correct anemias, which could be either microcytic or macrocytic.
- The limiting amino acids in typical protein foods include wheat (lysine), rice (lysine and threonine), corn (lysine and tryptophan), beans (methionine), and chickpeas (methionine). Vary food mixtures such as using bread with milk, rice with cheese, or pasta with cheese; rice with beans, bread with beans, or corn and beans; garbanzo beans with sesame seeds (as in dips or in roasted snacks). Serve vegetables with nuts, dairy products, rice, sunflower seeds, or wheat germ. Different food combinations provide essential amino acids that produce higher quality proteins (American Dietetic Association, 2003).
- Plant sources of protein can provide adequate amounts of essential amino acids. Using a variety of plant foods is key, and energy needs should readily be met. Although vegetarian diets are lower in total protein, protein intake in both lacto–ovo–vegetarians and vegans appears to be adequate (Messina and Messina, 1996).
- Soy foods can be useful in reducing elevated Chol as part of a healthy vegetarian diet (Rosell et al, 2004).

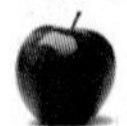

FOOD AND NUTRITION

The American Dietetic Association recommends that vegetarians consult with a registered dietitian or other qualified nutrition professional, especially during periods of growth, breastfeeding, pregnancy, or recovery from illness.

- For a balanced diet, minimize intake of less nutritious foods such as sweets and fatty foods. Choose whole or

unrefined grain products instead of refined products. Choose a variety of nuts, seeds, legumes, fruits, and vegetables, including good sources of vitamin C to improve iron absorption. Choose low-fat or nonfat varieties of dairy products, if they are included in the diet.
- Vegetarian foods rich in iron include many breakfast cereals, oatmeal, raisins, black beans, cashews, lentils, kidney beans, black-eyed peas, soybeans, hempseed, sunflower seeds, chickpeas, molasses, whole-wheat bread. Follow the food guide for North American vegetarians by including: 6–12 servings from the bread group, 2–3 servings of protein-rich foods such as legumes, nuts and seeds, or eggs (if used), 2–3 servings from the dairy group as tofu, yogurt, or fortified soy milk, 4 or more servings of vegetables, 3 or more servings of fruits, 2–3 servings of fats and oils, including olives and avocado.

Common Drugs Used and Potential Side Effects

- Monitor use of medications that deplete vitamins and minerals, especially iron and B-complex vitamins.

Herbs, Botanicals, and Supplements

- Many cultures use herbs and botanicals as part of their meal patterns, rituals, and celebrations. Identify those that are used and monitor side effects. Counsel about use of herbal teas, especially regarding toxic substances.

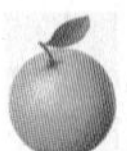

NUTRITION EDUCATION, COUNSELING, CARE MANAGEMENT

- Beneficial changes to diet may occur on changing to a self-selected vegetarian diet; for example, it is one way of achieving a better blood lipid profile (Robinson et al, 2002).
- Explain patterns of food intake that provide complementary amino acids. Whole grains, legumes, seeds, nuts, and vegetables contain sufficient essential and nonessential amino acids if taken in the right combinations.
- Emphasize the importance of a balanced diet.
- Describe the role vegetarian diets play in lowering serum Chol, TG, and glucose. These are beneficial changes that can result after starting a vegetarian diet (Phillips et al, 2004).
- Counsel about appropriate products for infants and children, as protein may be the biggest problem. Soy milk should be fortified with calcium and vitamin B_{12}.
- Unless otherwise advised by a doctor, those taking dietary supplements should limit the dose to 100% of the Daily Reference Intakes.

Patient Education—Food Safety

- Discuss food handling, preparation, and storage, especially careful washing of fruits and vegetables. Spinach and sprouts have been contaminated in recent years; wash produce thoroughly. Discuss hand washing.
- Starches such as hot cereals and rice should not be prepared and held in large batches because of the risks of *Bacillus cereus.*

For More Information

- Food and Nutrition Information Center
http://www.nal.usda.gov/fnic/pubs/bibs/gen/vegetarian.pdf
- Hindu Food Practices
http://monarch.gsu.edu/WebRoot$/multiculturalhealth/handouts/Hindi/Hindi_food_pyramid.pdf.
- Lacto-Ovo Vegetarian Cuisine
http://www.nhlbi.nih.gov/health/public/heart/obesity/lose_wt/lacto_ov.htm
- North American Vegetarian Society
http://www.navs-online.org/
- Oldways Preservation and Trust
http://www.oldwayspt.org/
- Soy Connection
http://www.soyconnection.com/newsletters/soy-connection/health-nutrition/index.php
- Seventh-Day Adventist Diet
http://www.sdada.org/aboutsda.htm
http://www.andrews.edu/NUFS/veggiediet.html
- UCLA Vegetarian Nutrition
http://apps.medsch.ucla.edu/nutrition/vegetarianism.htm
- Vegetarian Cuisine and Recipes
http://vegweb.com/
- Vegetarian Diets for pregnancy
http://my.clevelandclinic.org/healthy_living/pregnancy/hic_nutrition_during_pregnancy_for_vegetarians.asp
- Vegetarian Network (Victoria, Australia)
http://www.vnv.org.au/
- Vegetarian Recipes
http://allrecipes.com/HowTo/Vegetarian-Cuisine/Detail.aspx
- Vegetarian Resource Group
http://www.vrg.org/
- Vegetarian Recipes for Teens
http://kidshealth.org/teen/recipes/
- Vegetarian Society of the United Kingdom
http://www.vegsoc.org/
- World Guide to Vegetarianism
http://www.veg.org/veg/

VEGETARIANISM—CITED REFERENCES

American Dietetic Association. Position of the American Dietetic Association: vegetarian diets. *J Am Diet Assoc.* 103:748, 2003.

Dunn-Emke SR, et al. Nutrient adequacy of a very-low-fat vegan diet. *J Am Diet Assoc.* 105:1442, 2005.

Hunt JR. Bioavailability of iron, zinc, and other trace minerals from vegetarian diets. *Am J Clin Nutr.* 78:633S, 2003.

Key TJ, et al. Health effects of vegetarian and vegan diets. *Proc Nutr Soc.* 65:35, 2006.

Messina M, Messina V. *The dietitian's guide to vegetarian diets: issues and applications.* Gaithersburg, MD: Aspen Publishers, 1996.

Mezzano D, et al. Cardiovascular risk factors in vegetarians. Normalization of hyperhomocysteinemia with vitamin B_{12} and reduction of platelet aggregation with omega-3 fatty acids. *Thromb Res.* 100:153, 2000.

Murphy SP, Allen LH. Nutritional importance of animal source foods. *J Nutr.* 133:3932S, 2003.

Outila TA, et al. Dietary intake of vitamin D in premenopausal, healthy vegans was insufficient to maintain concentrations of serum 25-hydroxyvitamin D and intact parathyroid hormone within normal ranges during the winter in Finland. *J Am Diet Assoc.* 100:434, 2000.

Perry CL, et al. Adolescent vegetarians: how well do their dietary patterns meet the Healthy People 2010 objectives? *Arch Pediatr Adolesc Med.* 156: 431, 2002.

Phillips F, et al. Effect of changing to a self-selected vegetarian diet on anthropometric measurements in UK adults. *J Hum Nutr Diet.* 17:249, 2004.

Robinson F, et al. Changing from a mixed to self-selected vegetarian diet—influence on blood lipids. *J Hum Nutr Diet.* 15:323, 2002.

Rosell MS, et al. Soy intake and blood cholesterol concentrations: a cross-sectional study of 1033 pre- and postmenopausal women in the Oxford arm of the European Prospective Investigation into Cancer and Nutrition. *Am J Clin Nutr.* 80:1391, 2004.

Sharma JB, et al. Effect of dietary habits on prevalence of anemia in pregnant women of Delhi. *J Obstet Gynaecol Res.* 29:73, 2003.

Siener R, Hesse A. The effect of a vegetarian and different omnivorous diets on urinary risk factors for uric acid stone formation. *Eur J Nutr.* 42:332, 2003.

Stabler SP, Allen RH. Vitamin B_{12} deficiency as a worldwide problem. *Annu Rev Nutr.* 24:299, 2004.

Szeto YT, et al. Effects of a long-term vegetarian diet on biomarkers of antioxidant status and cardiovascular disease risk. *Nutrition.* 20:863, 2004.

EASTERN RELIGIOUS DIETARY PRACTICES

NUTRITIONAL ACUITY RANKING: LEVEL 2 (ADVISEMENT/PLANNING)

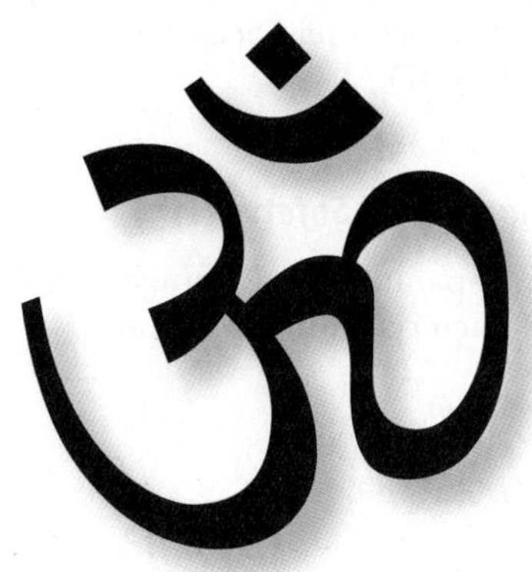

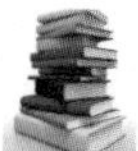

DEFINITIONS AND BACKGROUND

Hinduism, Jainism, and Sikhism

Hindus may be vegetarian while adhering to *ahimsa*, related to nonviolence as applied to the infliction of pain on animals. Beef is never eaten (the cow is considered sacred), and pork is usually avoided. Foods prohibited may include snails, crab, poultry, cranes, ducks, camels, boars, and some types of fish. The Brahmins, "high caste" folk, have stricter rules and practices, and there are differences between the North Indian Brahmins and the South Indian Brahmins. Some foods promote purity of the body, mind, and spirit. Devout Hindus avoid alcoholic beverages and foods that stimulate the senses, such as garlic and onions. Feast days include Holi, Dusshera, Pongal, and Divali (varying each year according to the lunar calendar). In addition, personal feast days include the anniversaries of birthdays, marriages, and deaths. Fasting depends on a person's social standing (caste), family, age, gender, and degree of orthodoxy. Fasting can be complete, adopting a completely vegetarian diet, or it can be abstaining from favorite foods.

Jainism is a branch of Hinduism that also promotes the nonviolence of ahimsa. Jains are expected to practice nonviolence, including against animals. Devout Jains are complete vegans. They avoid blood-colored foods (tomatoes) and avoid root vegetables, which may result in the death of insects clinging to the vegetable when it is harvested. Jains drink only boiled water. Fasting is a tool for connecting with the inner being during festivals. Fasting is based on three levels of austerity: Uttam, Madhyam, and Jaghanya. When one has finished with the roles of life, he or she willingly gives up food and drink; this can take up to 12 years with a gradual decline in eating.

Sikhs participate in many Hindu practices but differ by their belief in a single God. Sikhs abstain from beef and alcohol, but pork is permitted. Everyone is equal, no matter what color, sex, race, wealth, height, weight or religion; there is only one true race, the human race. Everyone sits on the floor when eating, as equals.

Buddhism

Buddhist dietary customs vary considerably depending on sect (Theravada or Hinayana, Mahayana, Zen) and on country of origin. Most Buddhists also subscribe to the concept of ahimsa, and many are lacto–ovo–vegetarians. Some eat fish, whereas some only abstain from beef. Some believe that unless they personally slaughter an animal, they may eat its meat.

Buddhist monks fast completely on the days of the new moon and full moon each lunar month; they also avoid eating any solid food after the noon hour. Buddhist feasts vary from one region to another. Celebrations include the birth, enlightenment, and death of Buddha in Mahayana Buddhism; the 3 days are unified into the single holiday of Vesak for Theravada Buddhism.

Buddhist vegetarian diets tend to allow more natural insulin sensitivity, so diabetes is less common (Kuo et al, 2004). However, serum tHcy should be monitored because of possibly lower intakes of vitamin B_{12} (Hung et al, 2002).

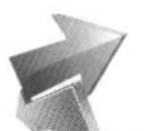

ASSESSMENT, MONITORING, AND EVALUATION

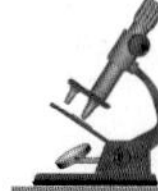

CLINICAL INDICATORS

Clinical/History	Diet history	Serum Na^+, K^+
Height	BP	Ca^{++}, Mg^{++}
Weight		Alk phos
BMI	**Lab Work**	H & H, serum Fe
Recent weight changes	Gluc	
	Chol, Trig	

SAMPLE NUTRITION CARE PROCESS STEPS

Inadequate Mineral (Iron) Intake

Assessment Data: Food records showing low intake of heme iron; altered nutritional labs for iron and ferritin; normal folate and B_{12} levels; complaints of easy fatigue and irritability.

Nutrition Diagnoses (PES): Inadequate iron intake related to Hindu (vegan) lifestyle as evidenced by intake of 4–5 g nonheme iron daily and low-serum Fe and ferritin levels.

Intervention: Education about increasing intake of iron-rich foods while decreasing excess of wheat bran. Counseling about using iron-fortified cereals or a supplement that provides 100% DRI for iron.

Monitoring and Evaluation: Improved energy and less fatigue; improved lab reports for iron and ferritin; diet history revealing improved intake of nonheme iron with supplements as needed.

INTERVENTION

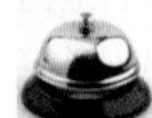

OBJECTIVES

- Serve appropriate menu choices, and omit foods or beverages that are not permitted.
- Respect traditions and preferences of the individual and family members.

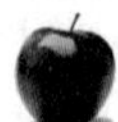

FOOD AND NUTRITION

- Support dietary practices as followed by the individual and family members.
- Counsel about specific nutritional changes according to the medical diagnosis and current condition.

Common Drugs Used and Potential Side Effects

- During periods of fasting, identify potential interactions from drugs that are dependent on energy sources for their metabolism.

Herbs, Botanicals, and Supplements

- Many cultures use herbs and botanicals as part of their meal patterns, rituals, and celebrations. Identify those that are used and monitor side effects.
- Counsel about use of herbal teas, especially regarding toxic substances.

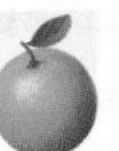

NUTRITION EDUCATION, COUNSELING, CARE MANAGEMENT

- Show the patient how to prepare foods to reduce Chol, fat, or sodium if heart disease or hypertension is present.
- Various types of cancer may prevail in different parts of the world and in different cultures. Discuss diet in relationship to what is common.
- While medical students and physicians with healthful personal practices (such as vegetarianism) are more likely to encourage such behaviors in their patients, these beliefs do not affect their actual nutrition counseling (Spencer et al, 2007).

Patient Education—Food Safety

- Discuss safe preparation and storage of foods to reduce likelihood of bacterial contamination.

For More Information

- Asian Foods
  http://www.asiafood.org/
- Asian Society
  http://www.asiasociety.org/
- Buddhism
  http://www.buddhanet.net/
- Ethnic Recipes
  http://asiarecipe.com/religion.html
- Hinduism
  http://www.hindunet.org/vegetarian/
- International Studies
  http://www.internationaled.org/
- Jainism
  http://www.diversiton.com/religion/main/jainism/holydays-festivals-rituals.asp
- Sikhism
  http://jainguru.com/diets.html

EASTERN RELIGIOUS DIETARY PRACTICES—CITED REFERENCES

Hung CJ, et al. Plasma homocysteine levels in Taiwanese vegetarians are higher than those of omnivores. *J Nutr.* 132:152, 2002.

Kuo CS, et al. Insulin sensitivity in Chinese ovo-lactovegetarians compared with omnivores. *Eur J Clin Nutr.* 58:312, 2004.

Spencer EH, et al. Personal and professional correlates of US medical students' vegetarianism. *J Am Diet Assoc.* 107:72, 2007.

WESTERN RELIGIOUS DIETARY PRACTICES

NUTRITIONAL ACUITY RANKING: LEVEL 2 (ADVISEMENT/PLANNING)

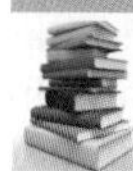

DEFINITIONS AND BACKGROUND

Judaism (Edited by Rabbi Allan Bernstein)

Jewish congregations in the United States are either identified as Orthodox, Conservative, or Reform. Orthodox Jews believe the laws are the direct commandments of God, to be explicitly followed by the faithful. Reform Jews follow the moral law but believe that the laws are still being interpreted (some are considered dated or currently irrelevant) and may be observed selectively. Conservative Jews fall in between the other congregations in their beliefs and adherence to the laws. About 25–30% of Jews in America keep kosher to one extent or another (http://www.jewfaq.org/kashrut.htm).

Jewish dietary laws are known as *Kashrut* and are among the most complex of all religious food practices. The term *kosher*, or *kasher*, means "fit" and describes all foods that are permitted for consumption. Kosher is loosely used to identify Jewish dietary laws, and to "keep kosher" means that the laws are followed. The dietary laws are complex. Briefly, they include what foods are fit to eat, what foods are prohibited (a lengthy list that includes pork, shellfish, and other foods), how animals must be slaughtered, how they must be prepared, and when they may be consumed (specifically, rules regarding when milk products can be consumed with meat products).

Jewish feast days include Rosh Hashanah, Sukkot, Hanukkah, Purim, Passover, and Shavout (dates vary because Judaism uses a lunar calendar). Specific foods are associated with the feasts but may differ nationally. Complete fast days (no food or water from sunset to sunset) include Yom Kippur and Tisha b'Av. Partial fast days (no food or water from sunrise to sunset) include Tzom Gedaliah, Tenth of Tevet and Seventeenth of Tamuz, Ta'anit Ester, and Ta'anit Bechorim. Special kosher laws are observed during Passover, including the elimination of any products that can be leavened.

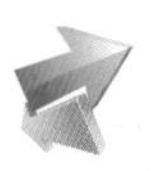

ASSESSMENT, MONITORING, AND EVALUATION

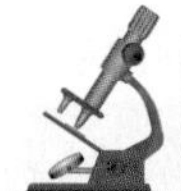

CLINICAL INDICATORS

Clinical/History
- Height
- Weight
- BMI
- Recent weight changes
- Diet history
- BP

Lab Work
- Gluc
- Chol, Trig
- Serum Na^+, K^+
- Ca^{++}, Mg^{++}
- Alk phos
- H & H, serum Fe

INTERVENTION

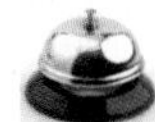

OBJECTIVES

- Observe dietary practices as followed by the laws of Judaism: meats are limited to cud-chewing animals with cloven hooves (cows and sheep) that are properly slaughtered. Pork (including ham and all pork products), shellfish, and scavenger fish are forbidden.
- Separate utensils are used for preparation and eating and especially for separating meat and milk foods.
- Monitor the kosher diet, which tends to be high in Chol, saturated fats, and sodium. Encourage application of the DASH diet principles where possible, but reduce lactose and sodium if necessary.

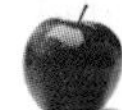

FOOD AND NUTRITION

The Jewish dinner table follows these guidelines (http://www.jewfaq.org/kashrut.htm):

- Certain animals may not be eaten at all. This restriction includes the flesh, organs, eggs, and milk of the forbidden animals. No pork, ham, bacon, pork products, rabbit, shellfish, or eel may be eaten.
- Of the animals that may be eaten, the birds and mammals must be killed in accordance with Jewish law. All blood must be drained from the meat or broiled out of it before it is eaten. Certain parts of permitted animals may not be eaten. Sheep, cattle, goats, and deer are kosher.
- Meat (the flesh of birds and mammals) cannot be eaten with dairy. Fish, eggs, fruits, vegetables, and grains can be eaten with either meat or dairy. According to some views, fish may not be eaten with meat.
- Dairy: Milk may be consumed before a meal, but once meat is eaten, 3–6 hours (depending on individual traditions) must pass before dairy products can be consumed. Omit lactose if not tolerated; provide other sources of calcium and riboflavin.
- Utensils that have come into contact with meat may not be used with dairy and vice versa. Utensils that have come into contact with nonkosher food may not be used with kosher food.
- Fruits, vegetables, and grains can be used, except that breads made with milk products are forbidden with meat meals. Grape products made by non-Jews may not be eaten.
- Leavened (raised) bread is forbidden during Passover. Matzoh bread or crackers may be used. Haroset and fried matzoh are traditional Passover foods. Seder plates and other items appropriate for the Seder dinner are important additions to the menu at this time.
- Common food choices include matzoh ball soup, chicken soup with kreplach, gefilte fish with beet horseradish,

cheese blintz with sour cream, flanken tzimmes, chopped liver, noodle Kugel, and kishka. Frozen kosher meals may be available in some areas.
- Fasting is common during Yom Kippur.
- Traditional Hanukkah foods include latkes and sour cream or applesauce.

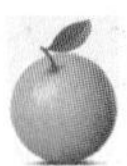

NUTRITION EDUCATION, COUNSELING, CARE MANAGEMENT

- Show the patient how to limit foods high in Chol/fat if weight and elevated lipid levels are a problem.
- Discuss sodium and obesity in relationship to hypertension, as appropriate. Recommend other herbs, spices, and cooking methods.
- Low-fat cheeses should be substituted for high-fat cheeses such as cream cheese.
- Note that food labels with a "U" with an "O" encircling it are considered kosher. Many other foods are considered kosher, but an inquiry should be made.
- Discuss holiday preferences and alternatives when needed.

Patient Education—Food Safety

- Discuss safe preparation and storage of foods to reduce likelihood of bacterial contamination.

For More Information

- Determining Kosher
  http://www.ou.org/kosher/primer.html
- Hebrew Food Pyramid
  http://monarch.gsu.edu/WebRoot$/multiculturalhealth/handouts/hebrew//Hebrew_food_pyramid.pdf
- Judaism 101
  http://www.jewfaq.org/kashrut.htm
- Kashrut–Dietary Laws
  http://www.myjewishlearning.com/daily_life/Kashrut.htm
- Kosher certification
  http://www.okkosher.com/
- Kosher recipes
  http://www.okkosher.com/Content.asp?ID=79
- Kosherfest
  http://www.kosherfest.com/
- Union for Traditional Judaism
  http://www.utj.org/

Christianity

There are three major branches of the Christian faith: Roman Catholicism, Eastern Orthodox Christianity, and Protestantism. Dietary practices vary; some are minimal.

(1) Roman Catholicism: Devout Catholics observe several feast and fast days during the year. Feast days include Christmas, Easter, the Annunciation (March 25th), Palm Sunday (the Sunday before Easter), the Ascension (40 days after Easter), and Pentecost Sunday (50 days after Easter). Catholics in each country observe many food traditions. Fasting (one full meal per day permitted; snacking according to local custom) and/or abstinence (meat is prohibited, but eggs, dairy products, and condiments with animal fat are permitted) may be practiced during Lent, on the Fridays of Advent, and Ember Days (at the beginning of the seasons) by some Catholics; some fast or abstain only on Ash Wednesday and Good Friday. Today, Catholics may avoid meat only on the Fridays of Lent (40 days before Easter). Food and beverages (except water) are to be avoided for 1 hour before communion is taken.

(2) Eastern Orthodox Christianity: The 14 self-governing churches that form the Orthodox Church differ from Catholicism in their interpretation of the Biblical theology, including the use of leavened bread instead of unleavened wafers in communion. Numerous feast and fast days are observed (dates vary according to whether the Julian or Gregorian calendar is used). Feast days include Christmas, Theophany, Presentation of the Lord into the Temple, Annunciation, Easter, Ascension, Pentecost Sunday, the Transfiguration, Dormition of the Holy Theotokos, Nativity of the Holy Theotokos, and Presentation of the Holy Theotokos. In addition, Meat Fare Sunday is observed the third Sunday before Easter (all meat in the house is consumed, and none is eaten again until Easter). Cheese Fare Sunday is observed on the Sunday before Easter (all cheese, eggs, and butter are consumed). On the next day, Clean Monday, the Lenten fast begins. Food and drink are avoided before communion.

Meat and all animal products (milk, eggs, butter, and cheese) are prohibited on fast days; fish is avoided, but shellfish is permitted. Some devout followers may avoid olive oil on fast days, too. Fast days include every Wednesday and Friday (except for three fast-free weeks each year), the Eve of Theophany, the Beheading of John the Baptist, and Elevation of the Holy Cross. Fast periods include Advent, Lent, the Fast of the Apostles, and Fast of the Dormition of the Holy Theotokos.

(3) Protestantism: The only feast days common in most Protestant religions are Christmas and Easter. Few practice fasting.

(4) Mormons (Church of Jesus Christ of Latter Day Saints): Mormons avoid alcoholic beverages, hot drinks (coffee and tea), and caffeine-containing drinks. Followers are encouraged to eat mostly grains and to limit meats. Some Mormons fast 1 day a month and donate that food money to the poor.

(5) Seventh-Day Adventists avoid overeating. Most are lacto–ovo–vegetarians, but when meat is consumed, most avoid pork. Tea, coffee, and alcoholic beverages are prohibited. Water is consumed before and after meals. Eating between meals is discouraged. Strong seasonings and condiments, such as pepper and mustard, are avoided.

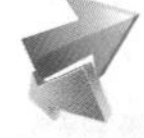

ASSESSMENT, MONITORING, AND EVALUATION

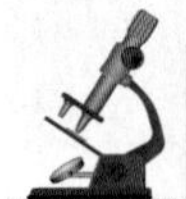

CLINICAL INDICATORS

Clinical/History	Lab Work	
Height	Gluc	H & H, serum Fe
Weight	Chol, Trig	C-reactive protein (CRP)
BMI	Serum Na^+, K^+	
Recent weight changes	Ca^{++}, Mg^{++}	
Diet history	Alk phos	
BP		

INTERVENTION

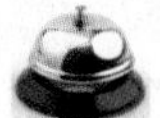

OBJECTIVES

- Observe dietary practices as followed by the individual. Discuss the role of special meals, fasting, or events and plan menus accordingly.
- Assist guests and immigrants in maintaining their healthy dietary practices and religious traditions, as appropriate (Kaplan et al, 2004).

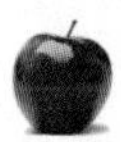

FOOD AND NUTRITION

- Promote a healthy diet. For example, principles of a Mediterranean diet may be suitable for many individuals (Bilenko et al, 2005).
- Fasting may be common during special holidays. Discuss concerns related to pregnancy, children, the elderly or those in a malnourished state.
- Some individuals avoid caffeine and alcohol as part of their religious preferences; honor those wishes.
- Determine if any foods are avoided on special days of the week and plan alternatives accordingly.

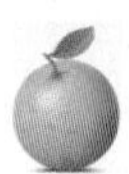

NUTRITION EDUCATION, COUNSELING, CARE MANAGEMENT

- Show the patient how to limit foods high in Chol/fat if weight and elevated lipid levels are a problem.
- Discuss sodium and obesity in relationship to hypertension, as appropriate. Recommend other herbs, spices, and cooking methods.
- Discuss holiday preferences and alternatives where needed.
- There tend to be few specific relationships between religion, fat intake, and physical activity in contemporary U.S. society; religion may play only a small role in the context of how diet and exercise are developed and maintained (Kim and Sobal, 2004).

Patient Education—Food Safety

- Discuss safe preparation and storage of foods to reduce likelihood of bacterial contamination.

For More Information

- Andrews University–Seventh Day Adventist diet http://www.sdada.org/position.html

WESTERN RELIGIOUS DIETARY PRACTICES—CITED REFERENCES

Bilenko N, et al. Mediterranean diet and cardiovascular diseases in an Israeli population. *Prev Med.* 40:299, 2005.

Kaplan MS, et al. The association between length of residence and obesity among Hispanic immigrants. *Am J Prev Med.* 27:323, 2004.

Kim KH, Sobal J. Religion, social support, fat intake and physical activity. *Pub Health Nutr.* 7:773, 2004.

MIDDLE EASTERN RELIGIOUS DIETARY PRACTICES

NUTRITIONAL ACUITY RANKING: LEVEL 2 (ADVISEMENT/PLANNING)

DEFINITIONS AND BACKGROUND

Islam is an Arabic word that means submission, surrender, and obedience; it also means peace, as it is derived from the word "Salam," which means peace. As a religion, Islam stands for complete submission and obedience to God. Followers of the Islamic faith are known as Muslims. Muslims promote the concept of eating to live, not living to eat. They advise sharing food.

Prohibited foods as described in the Koran are called *haram*; those in question are *mashbooh.* Pork and birds of prey are haram; meats must be slaughtered properly. Alcohol is prohibited, and stimulants, such as coffee and tea, are allowed. *Halal* is the term for all permitted foods. The flesh of animals must be slaughtered according to Islamic law or *halal*; kosher items may be used for this reason. Feast days (dates vary according to the lunar calendar) include Eid al-Fitr, Eid al-Azha, Nau-Roz (a Persian holiday), Al-Ghadeer, and Maulud n'Nabi. Fasting is considered an opportunity to earn the approval of Allah, to wipe out sins, and to understand the suffering of the poor. Fasting includes abstention from all food and drink from dawn to sunset. Voluntary fasting is common on Mondays and Thursdays; it is undesirable to fast on certain days of the month and on Fridays. Muslims are required to fast during the entire month of Ramadan and are encouraged to fast 6 days during the month of Shawwal, on the Al-Ghadeer day, and on the 9th day of Zul Hijjah.

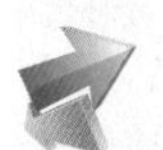

ASSESSMENT, MONITORING, AND EVALUATION

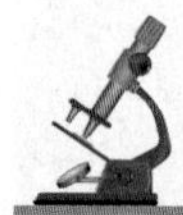

CLINICAL INDICATORS

Clinical/History	Diet history	Serum Na^{+}, K^{+}
Height	BP	Ca^{++}, Mg^{++}
Weight		Alk phos
BMI	**Lab Work**	H & H, serum Fe
Recent weight changes	Gluc	
	Chol, Trig	

INTERVENTION

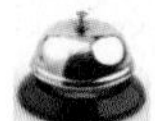

OBJECTIVES

- During fasting, eating occurs only before dawn and after sunset. Plan accordingly.
- Monitor dietary patterns, which include fasting 3 days a month. Pregnant and breastfeeding mothers need not fast.
- Monitor need for vitamin D in women if sun exposure is minimal.

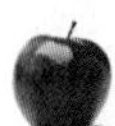

FOOD AND NUTRITION

- Pork and pork products are forbidden, including gelatin.
- Alcohol is not used, even in vanilla extract and other preparations.
- Foods such as dates, seafood, honey, sweets, yogurt, milk (goat's milk also), meat, and olive or vegetable oils are encouraged. Beef, chicken, and lamb are commonly used. Couscous, pita bread, rice, millet, and bulgur are frequently included. Eggplant, cucumbers, green peppers, pomegranates, and tomatoes are readily available.
- Typical combination foods include: falafel (grain, fat), hummus (grain, fat), kibbeh (meat, grain, fat), tabouli (vegetable, grain, fat), baba ghanouj (vegetable, fat), pilaf (grain, fat), stuffed grape leaves (meat, grain, fat), and shawarma (meat, grain, fat). Khoresh is a stew with meats (lamb, beef, or veal), poultry, or fish with vegetables; fresh or dried fruits; beans, grains, and even nuts.

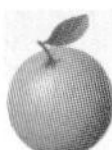

NUTRITION EDUCATION, COUNSELING, CARE MANAGEMENT

- If diet is low in heme iron, anemia may occur. Discuss options if necessary.
- Fasting is not recommended for persons who have diabetes, cancer, or HIV/AIDS. Discuss menu planning for religious occasions.
- Discuss useful dietary changes for managing obesity and diabetes.

Patient Education

- Discuss periods of fasting if there are undesirable side effects, such as hypotension or fainting.

For More Information

- Catering for Muslim Patients
  http://www.med.umich.edu/multicultural/ccp/culture/muslim.htm
- Iranian Cooking
  http://www.asiafood.org/persiancooking/index.cfm
- Islamic Food and Nutrition Council of America
  http://www.ifanca.org/
- Jordanian Food
  http://www.gondol.com/English/food.htm
- Muslim Consumer group
  http://www.muslimconsumergroup.com/hfs.htm

OROFACIAL CONDITIONS

DENTAL DIFFICULTIES AND ORAL DISORDERS

NUTRITIONAL ACUITY RANKING: LEVEL 2–3

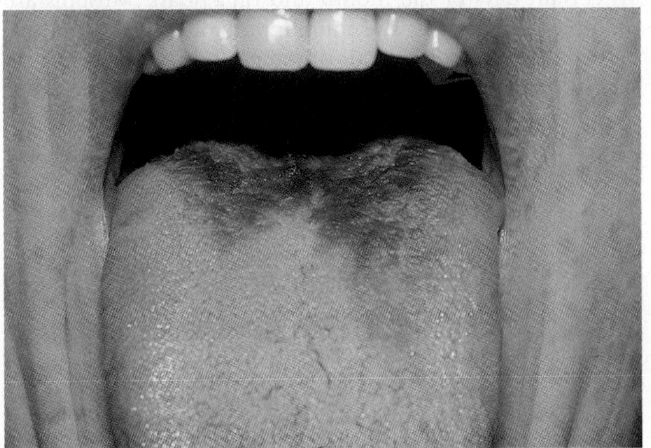

Reprinted with permission from: Goodheart HP, MD. *Goodheart's Photoguide of Common Skin Disorders,* 2nd ed. Philadelphia: Lippincott Williams & Wilkins, 2003.

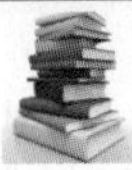

DEFINITIONS AND BACKGROUND

Diet and nutrition affect many oral diseases. Cell turnover is rapid in the tongue and oral mucosa; therefore, the oral cavity is one of the first areas where signs of systemic disease appear. Two oral infectious diseases are diet related: dental caries (tooth decay related to diet composition and frequency), and periodontal disease, associated with malnutrition (Touger-Decker et al, 2003). In dental caries, chronic infectious disease leads to progressive destruction of tooth substances from interactions between bacteria and organic tooth compounds. *Streptococcus mutans* and *Lactobacillus* form acids within 20 seconds to 30 minutes after contact. Erosion of tooth enamel may occur in patients who chronically consume acidic beverages and/or keep such beverages or foods in the mouth for a period of time (e.g., sucking lemons, chewing vitamin C tablets, chewing lemon hard candies). Tooth loss can prevent proper bite and may lessen the ability

to chew foods properly. Dietary advice given when dentures are placed results in increased consumption of fruits and vegetables during stages of change (Moynihan, 2005a).

Health professionals should check the oral and dental health of their patients. Many Americans lack fluoridated water, an effective safeguard against dental cavities. Those who are poor or have no dental insurance are also at risk for caries. Water fluoridation can reduce caries by 20–40% (American Dental Association, 2009).

Some dental problems are age specific. Infants should be monitored for early childhood caries (ECC); dental decay often occurs during the growth spurts of adolescents; and older patients should be monitored for changes in eating habits, inadequate diet, and caries. Elderly persons who wear dentures are more prone to malnutrition (de Oliveria and Frigerio, 2004) and problems with chewing, swallowing, and mouth pain often precede hospitalizations (Bailey et al, 2004).

Poor oral hygiene can increase the likelihood of gingival abnormalities when vitamin C and D intakes have been poor. Some conditions, such as diabetes, can also make individuals prone to dry mouth and dental decay. An increase in water intake, extra care with oral hygiene, chewing sugarless gum, and prevention of periodontal disease are important steps.

With tongue disorders, mastication of food may be affected. The ability to push mashed food with the tongue and anterior hard palate will be affected. Other oral problems may cause pain, problems with chewing, dysphagia, mouth dryness, or infection including aphthous stomatitis, cheilosis, oral cancer, lichen planus, oral herpes, candidiasis, thrush, or xerostomia. Many of these conditions occur because of altered immunity and debility, as in cancer or HIV infection.

Fracture of the lower jaw (mandible) is an injury that requires intermaxillary fixation (wiring). Patients with wired jaws face a whole new lifestyle for up to 6 weeks following surgery. Patients have to eat liquefied meals; proper presurgical patient education is essential.

Proper nutrition is essential for good dental and oral health. Table 2-5 provides a list of the key nutrients needed for healthy oral mucosa and teeth. Vitamins A and C are significant for prevention and treatments of leukoplakias (Scully, 2000; Sheiham et al, 2001). Treatment with beta-carotene or retinoids is often recommended (Lodi et al, 2004). Table 2-6 lists dental problems, treatment, and prevention.

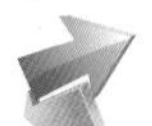

ASSESSMENT, MONITORING, AND EVALUATION

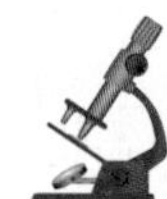

CLINICAL INDICATORS

Clinical/History

Height
Weight
BMI
Recent weight changes
Diet history
Mouth, gum or tongue lacerations
Dental caries
Missing or loose teeth
Dentures, missing, loose or ill-fitting
Taste alterations
Sore or bleeding gums
High intake of sugars and sticky starches?

Lab Work

Alb, transthyretin
Serum Na^+, K^+
Ca^{++}, Mg^{++}
Alk phos
H & H, serum Fe
X-rays (mandible)
Serum folate
Serum ascorbate and retinol

TABLE 2-5 Nutrients Needed for Proper Oral Tissue Synthesis and Dental Care

Nutrient	Role
Protein	Needed for healthy tissue growth and maintenance.
Vitamin A	Necessary for epithelial tissue and enamel. Beta-carotene may play a role in oral cancer prevention (Lodi et al, 2004).
Vitamin B-complex	Deficiencies show a bright scarlet tongue and stomatitis in niacin deficiency; magenta tongue, glossitis, and angular cheilitis in riboflavin deficiency; smooth tongue in vitamin B_{12} deficiency.
Folate	Needed for a healthy blood supply.
Vitamin C	Enables connective tissue cells to elaborate intercellular substances. Deficiency can lead to easy bleeding or swelling of gums and gingivitis. Forms collagen; helps to heal wounds and bleeding gums.
Vitamin K	Aids with calcium absorption in bone; adequate blood clotting; helps in healing.
Vitamin D	Protects against chronic inflammation of the gums, which can lead to gingivitis or periodontal disease (Dietrich et al, 2004). Necessary for dentin, bony tissue synthesis; mineralization; and jawbone sufficiency.
Calcium and phosphorus	Necessary for dentin and bony tissue synthesis. Poor mineralization occurs with deficiency. Maintains jawbone sufficiency.
Chromium	Needed for proper glucose metabolism. Controlled intake of carbohydrates helps to maintain healthier gums and overall health status (Moynihan, 2005b).
Copper	Needed for production of blood and nerve fibers.
Fluoride	Consumption of fluoridated water coupled with a reduction in nonmilk sugar intake is an effective means of caries prevention (American Dietetic Association, 2000; Moynihan, 2005a). Keeps bones healthy. Drinking water should contain 1 ppm; toothpaste, mouth rinses, and topical treatments also help.
Iron	Helps produce red blood cells; promotes resistance to disease; improves health of the teeth, skin, and bones. Maintains energy.
Magnesium	Helps in bone development. Enhances use of vitamin C. Deficiency may lead to calcium resorption.
Potassium	Needed for muscle contraction and proper nerve function.
Zinc	Regulates the inflammatory process; aids in wound healing. Deficiencies can lead to poor healing, susceptibility to infection, loss of taste, and altered metabolism.

TABLE 2-6 Dental Problems, Treatment, and Prevention

Symptoms	Likely Cause	Treatment	Prevention
Bad Breath			
Odor from mouth; bad, metallic taste; coated tongue	Food caught around and between teeth; infection in gums; improper brushing; sinusitis; digestive problems, such as preulcerative conditions; diabetes	Practice good oral hygiene, including rinsing with mouthwash; brush tongue often; see dentist to evaluate throat, sinuses, tongue, and possible gum infection, and professionally clean teeth and gums; review diet	Regular dental visits; flossing, brushing, and rinsing; good nutrition
Broken Tooth or Filling			
Tooth feels sharp; tooth sensitivity to temperature and pressure	Accidental trauma; decay; weak tooth from grinding or improper bite	Do not irritate; place piece of soft dental wax from drugstore over cracked or fractured tooth; see a dentist immediately	Regular dental checkups to discover possible weak teeth, decay, or large, unstable fillings
Canker Sores			
Painful red circular area that develops on the tongue, gums, lips, or cheeks; in certain phases, sores have a yellow or white center area; sore to touch; sensitivity to spicy, salty foods	Bacterial or viral infection; trauma from denture in mouth; stress	Use over-the-counter remedies recommended by the dentist; coat lesions after meals; see dentist to make sure there is no infection or for additional medication if pain persists; the dentist will evaluate dentures for weight-bearing points to be certain the problem does not exist there	Avoid irritating the area; avoid spicy, acidic foods while mouth is sore
Dental Abscess (swelling around tooth or cheek)			
Pain, throbbing in gum or tooth; swelling; sensitive bite; loose teeth; sensitivity to heat	Tooth decay; initial eruption of tooth through the gums or fractured tooth; tooth nerve damage	Rinse with salt water solution; use mouthwash; avoid eating on or near tooth; see dentist immediately; may require antibiotics or root canal treatment to prevent spread of infection	Regular dental checkups; good oral hygiene; brushing, flossing, and rinsing
Discolored Teeth			
Teeth have unsightly and discolored appearance; single tooth begins to turn yellow or gray	Surface stain from certain foods, such as tea and coffee; internal staining from tooth nerve damage or from rheumatic fever; stains from tetracycline	Improve oral hygiene; brush frequently; diminish coffee or tea intake; rinse with peroxide; consult dentist to check nerve in darkened tooth; consider supervised tooth bleaching/whitening	Good oral hygiene; avoid foods and liquids that can stain teeth, such as tea and coffee
Gum Disease			
Gum pain; nonthrobbing ache; swelling; gum bleeding; blood in saliva when brushing; metallic taste	Food debris between teeth; tartar beneath gums; infection; poor bite may worsen this condition	Improve oral hygiene by brushing often and flossing; rinse with mouthwash; consult dentist to evaluate extent of condition; treatment by removing plaque and tartar may require surgery and/or bite adjustment	Good oral hygiene; regular dental checkups and cleanings
Red Inflamed Gums			
Color of gums around teeth progresses from pink to red with swelling or puffiness; dry mouth; snoring	Mouth breathing; some medications, such as antihistamines, blood pressure medications, and antidepressants, decrease salivary flow	Use oral salivary rinses and toothpastes for dry mouth; improve oral hygiene; consult dentist because this condition can lead to tooth decay, advanced gum disease, or other mouth infections	Ask physician if medications can be changed; consult dentist about obtaining oral rinses and a snoreguard

(continued)

TABLE 2-6 Dental Problems, Treatment, and Prevention *(continued)*

Symptoms	Likely Cause	Treatment	Prevention
Loose Teeth			
Teeth move; spongy feel to bite; teeth sensitive or even painful when chewing	Gum disease; tooth grinding; orthodontic appliances too tight; cyst, tumor, abscess, or trauma to teeth	See dentist as soon as possible to determine cause; practice good oral hygiene; be aware of tooth grinding or clenching and use appliance to prevent grinding	Regular dental visits; good oral hygiene; have your dentist evaluate your bite; use a bite appliance if your dentist advises
Lumps Under Jaw or Neck Muscle			
Neck sore to touch or movement; swelling in neck; sore throat; difficulty swallowing	Cold/flu; tooth abscess or infection; tumor	Treat cold/flu symptoms; limit neck movement; check temperature; take pain relievers such as aspirin; see a dentist if symptoms persist to evaluate the extent of swelling and infection	Regular dental checkups; patients should pay special attention to any growth or changes in the head or neck
Toothache (tooth pain on biting or chewing)			
Tooth pain related to temperature change or touch or from chewing or biting; dark brown spots on teeth may indicate new decay	Bacterial acids; large filling broken out of tooth; tooth grinding	Rinse mouth often with vanilla extract to soothe discomfort; avoid chewing on tooth; see a dentist as soon as possible to determine cause and further treatment	Regular dental visits for prevention; the sooner examined, the better the chance of success
Tooth Sensitivity to Temperature Change			
Breathing outside in cold air causes pain; waking up with toothache; pain when eating/drinking cold things	Inflamed gums; gum recession that exposes root surfaces; tooth decay; teeth clenching or grinding that has worn away tooth enamel	Use desensitizing toothpaste on a daily basis; use a soft bristle brush; avoid temperature differences; consult dentist for appropriate treatment	Good oral hygiene; apply fluoride gel; use desensitizing toothpaste; avoid food temperature differences; avoid hard bristle toothbrushes; become aware of and avoid tooth grinding or squeezing teeth together; have fillings bonded to seal areas of sensitivity; dentist may recommend a biteguard for grinding

Adapted from Rhode Island Dental Association, 200 Centerville Road, Warwick, RI 02886; Phone: (401) 732-6833. Web site accessed March 28, 2009, at http://www.ridental.com/dentalproblems.cfm. Used with permission.

INTERVENTION

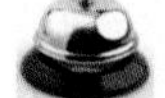

OBJECTIVES

Broken or Wired Jaw

- Provide adequate nourishment to allow healing while reducing jaw movement.
- Decrease complications such as fever, nausea, and vomiting.
- Prevent excessive weight loss; up to 10% is common.
- Maintain a patent airway.

Dental Caries

- Alter dietary habits; deprive bacteria of substrate; reduce acid by keeping pH at 7.0.
- Maintain frequent fluoride contact with tooth surfaces as directed by a dental professional.

Early Childhood Caries (ECC)

- ECC is a preventable dental disease in which enamel erodes, and tooth surfaces are permanently damaged from long exposure to liquid carbohydrate sources.
- Education is the biggest factor. Children with significant risk factors for caries (e.g., inadequate home dental care, poor oral hygiene, a mother with a high number of cavities, a high sugar intake, enamel defects, premature birth, special health care needs, low socioeconomic status) should be referred to a dentist (Douglass et al, 2004).

Edentulism

- Provide proper consistency to allow the patient to eat.
- Monitor for deficiencies in fiber, vitamins A and C if whole grains, fruits, and vegetables are not consumed (Touger-Decker, 2004).

Mouth Ulcers or Pain

- Lessen mouth soreness to increase dietary intake; mouth sprays may be available to lessen pain while eating.
- Promote healing for a return to normal eating patterns.
- Prevent weight loss or other consequences.

Tongue Disorders

- Provide adequate nourishment despite acute or chronic disability.

SAMPLE NUTRITION CARE PROCESS STEPS

Chewing Difficulty

Assessment Data (sources of info): Food records and intake calculations; dental evaluation for loose dentures; weight changes.

Nutrition Diagnosis: Chewing difficulty related to inability to chew foods from poor dentition as evidenced by weight loss of 2 lb in 14 days and ill-fitting dentures.

Interventions: Food and Nutrient Delivery

ND 1.2 Modify current diet to puree diet until otherwise noted from Dentist/MD.

ND 3.1.1 Continue with shakes BID to enhance energy intake.

Recommend dental referral for dentures.

Monitoring and Evaluation: Intake records, reduction in chewing problems, improved weight after fitting of new dentures.

Inadequate Energy Intake—Early Childhood Caries

Assessment Data (sources of info): Food records (high intake of juice, sweetened beverages throughout the day from the bottle); intake calculations; dental evaluation for ECC; weight loss from inability to chew solids and refusal to drink from a cup.

Nutrition Diagnosis: Inadequate energy intake (NI-1.4) related to inability to chew foods as evidenced by early childhood dental caries with poor weight gain.

Interventions

Goals: Wean from bottle completely. Increase solid food intake and decrease fluids, especially sweetened fluids. Follow a weight gain of at least 0.6 oz/wk, 2.7 oz/mo, or 1 lb/6 mo. Educate parents on importance of healthy oral hygiene and not allowing child to carry liquids around during day or fall asleep with liquids.

Food and Nutrient Delivery: ND-1.1 Provide general/healthful diet, provide information on weaning from the bottle, educate on importance of oral hygiene, increase intake of water, decrease intake of juice to a maximum of 4 oz/d diluted with water, eliminate other sweet drinks, alter diet to reduce need to chew (puree, mash, or chop foods).

Nutrition Education: E-1.2 Provide information on weaning, calorie boosters, importance of oral hygiene, limiting sweetened beverages. DDS to perform oral surgery for removal of dental caries to decrease pain and increase intake of solid foods for weight gain. RD to continue to monitor weight gain and food intake.

Counseling: C-2.5 Counsel patient's mother and father on supporting each other through weaning and the importance of good oral hygiene.

Coordination of Care: RC-1.3 Collaborate with MD and DDS on patient's care through oral surgery and monitoring weight status.

Monitoring and Evaluation: Intake records, reduction in chewing problems, improved weight, and health status.

Tube Feeding

- Children on tube feedings often have dental problems; attend to oral hygiene more carefully than for those fed orally.
- Adults will require special attention to oral hygiene and mouth care while on tube feedings.

Xerostomia

- Dry mouth may be more severe after radiation therapy than with other causes, such as diabetes.
- Artificial saliva agents may be useful for some. Reduced saliva affects patient perception of swallowing ability and changes dietary choices (Logemann et al, 2003).
- Good oral hygiene may prevent dental decay.

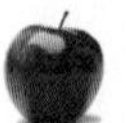

FOOD AND NUTRITION

Broken or Wired Jaw

- A diet of pureed or strained foods and liquids of high protein/calorie content are necessary. Use high-energy supplemental beverages (perhaps 2 kcal/mL). Double-strength milk may also be used to keep protein intake at a high level.
- Take adequate amounts of vitamin C for healing.
- Monitor food temperatures carefully, as extremes may not be tolerated.
- Six to eight meals are needed.
- Follow meals with salt water rinse.

Dental Caries

- Decrease sucrose and cooked or sticky starches, as well as the frequency of snacking and duration of exposure time. *Streptococcus mutans* is a common bacterial culprit; others include *Lactobacillus casein* and *Streptococcus sanguis* (Touger-Decker, 2004).
- Use a balanced diet, avoid eating sweets or starches with meals.
- Fluoride exposure should be adequate, including from water supplies.
- The sequence of eating foods, the combination of foods, the form of foods and beverages consumed, and nutrient composition of foods/beverages must be evaluated and altered accordingly (Touger-Decker, 2004).

Early Childhood Caries (ECC)

The following are guidelines for prevention (American Academy of Pediatric Dentistry, 2005–2006; Clarke et al, 2006; Wagner, 2006):

- Do not allow a child to fall asleep with a bottle containing milk, formula, fruit juices, or other sweet liquids. Never let a child walk around with a bottle in his/her mouth. Never put an infant or child to bed with a bottle that is filled with sugar-containing beverages, including fruit juice or Kool-Aid.
- Comfort a child who wants a bottle between regular feedings or during naps with a bottle filled with cool water.
- Always make sure a child's pacifier is clean, and never dip a pacifier in a sweet liquid.
- Introduce children to a cup as they approach 1 year of age. Children should stop drinking from a bottle soon after their first birthday.
- Notify the parent of any unusual red or swollen areas in a child's mouth or any dark spot on a child's tooth so that the parent can consult the child's dentist.
- Maintain good oral hygiene.
- Monitor for iron deficiency anemia, which is common (Clarke et al, 2006).

Edentulism

- A chopped, ground, strained, or pureed diet should be followed as required. Use the least restricted diet and progress as tolerated.
- Identify potential solutions such as obtaining new dentures or repairing current dentures.

Mouth Ulcers or Pain

- Foods low in acid and spices should be consumed; avoid citrus juices, vinegar and other similar foods.
- Supplement the diet with vitamin C, protein, and calories to speed healing.
- Small, frequent meals and oral supplements may be beneficial to prevent weight loss.
- Moist or blenderized foods with additional liquid are helpful.
- Soft, cold foods such as canned fruits, ice cream, popsicles, yogurt, cottage cheese, or cold pasta dishes may be used.
- Use of a straw may be helpful.
- Cut or grind meats or vegetables.
- Extra butter, mild sauces, and gravies may be needed.
- Follow meals by brushing teeth to reduce possibility of dental caries.

Tongue Disorders

- If the patient is unable to chew, tube feeding should be considered (Fig. 2-3).
- Liquids may be added to the diet as tolerated. Many foods are tolerated if liquefied and blenderized.

Tube Feeding

- Good oral hygiene and mouth care will be needed, even if a patient is not fed by mouth. Tube feeding should include all key nutrients to meet patient needs; see Section 17.

Xerostomia

- Moisten foods, adding water or milk when possible. Use sauces or gravies if needed.
- Avoid excessive spices.
- Avoid excessively chewy foods such as steak, crumbly foods such as crackers or cake, dry foods such as chips, or sticky foods such as peanut butter (Touger-Decker, 2004).

Common Drugs Used and Potential Side Effects

- Luride is a fluoride supplement for children to strengthen teeth against tooth decay. Avoid use with calcium or dairy products because it may form a nonabsorbable product.
- For patients with cancer, various therapies affect the mouth and gums. Monitor closely.
- Oral side effects of drugs interfere with functioning and increase risks for infection, pain, and possible tooth loss (Spolarich, 2000).

Herbs, Botanicals, and Supplements

- Herbs and botanicals may be used; identify and monitor side effects.
- Counsel about use of herbal teas, especially unsuitable products such as comfrey tea.

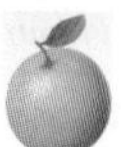

NUTRITION EDUCATION, COUNSELING, CARE MANAGEMENT

- If needed for oral or dental problems, blended foods and/or tube feedings should be prepared. Sometimes, using a bulb syringe to feed may be useful.
- Provide creative ideas for the seasoning and flavoring of foods. Discuss acceptable restaurant options for persons who are at home.
- Ensure that fluoride is provided in some way by the diet, water supply, or dental office.
- Read milk labels to ensure vitamin D fortification.
- Dental status is an especially important part of assessment and care for the elderly (Sahyoun et al, 2003; Sheiham et al, 2001).
- Integrating dietary counseling into the dental setting warrants further investigation (Moynihan, 2005a).

To Prevent Caries

- Encourage good habits in oral hygiene and diet: detergent foods (raw fruits and vegetables) should be recommended rather than sticky or impactant foods (soft cookies, bread, sticky sweets, dried fruits). Cariostatic foods should be encouraged, such as cheese, raw fruits and vegetables, peanuts, and cocoa.
- Avoid cariogenic foods such as dried fruits, candy, cookies, pies, cakes, ice cream, canned fruit, soft drinks, fruit drinks, lemonade, gelatin desserts, snack crackers, pretzels or chips, and muffins. Brush teeth or eat cheese after meals and sugary snacks to normalize pH.
- Regular use of fluoride daily can help reduce the incidence of root caries (Richards, 2009).

Patient Education—Food Safety

- When traveling, avoid ice made from tap water. Airline water may not be free from contamination.
- Use of bottled water is recommended for brushing teeth in countries where water is not safe.

For More Information

- American Academy of Pediatric Dentistry
  http://www.aapd.org/
- American Academy of General Dentistry
  http://www.agd.org/
- American Academy of Periodontology
  http://www.perio.org/
- American Dental Association
  http://www.ada.org/
- Colgate
  http://www.colgate.com/app/Colgate/US/OralCare/HomePage.cvsp
- International Association for Disability and Oral Health
  http://www.iadh.org/
- Medline—dental health
  http://www.nlm.nih.gov/medlineplus/dentalhealth.html
- National Institute of Dental and Craniofacial Research (NIDCR)
  http://www.nidcr.nih.gov/
- Oral Health America
  http://www.oralhealthamerica.org/

DENTAL DIFFICULTIES AND ORAL DISORDERS—CITED REFERENCES

American Academy of Pediatric Dentistry. Policy on early childhood caries (ECC): classifications, consequences, and preventive strategies. *Pediatr Dent.* 27:31, 2005–2006.

American Dietetic Association. Position of the American Dietetic Association: the impact of fluoride on health. *J Am Diet Assoc.* 100:1208, 2000.

American Dental Association. Accessed March 29, 2009, at http://www.ada.org/prof/resources/positions/statements/fluoride_community_safety.asp.

Bailey RL, et al. Persistent oral health problems associated with comorbidity and impaired diet quality in older adults. *J Am Diet Assoc.* 104:1273, 2004.

Clarke M, et al. Malnourishment in a population of young children with severe early childhood caries. *Pediatr Dent.* 28:254, 2006.

de Oliveria TR, Frigerio ML. Association between nutrition and the prosthetic condition in edentulous elderly. *Gerodontology.* 21:205, 2004.

Dietrich T, et al. Association between serum concentrations of 25-hydroxyvitamin D_3 and periodontal disease in the US population. *Am J Clin Nutr.* 80:108, 2004.

Douglass JM, et al. A practical guide to infant oral health. *Am Fam Phys.* 70: 2113, 2004.

Lodi G, et al. Interventions for treating oral leukoplakia. *Cochrane Database Syst Rev.* 3:CD001829, 2004.

Logemann JA, et al. Xerostomia: 12-month changes in saliva production and its relationship to perception and performance of swallow function, oral intake, and diet after chemoradiation. *Head Neck.* 25:432, 2003.

Moynihan P. The interrelationship between diet and oral health. *Proc Nutr Soc.* 64:571, 2005a.

Moynihan P. The role of diet and nutrition in the etiology and prevention of oral diseases. *Bull World Health Org.* 83:694, 2005b.

Richards D. Fluoride has a beneficial effect on root caries. *Evid Based Dent.* 10:12, 2009.

Sahyoun NR, et al. Nutritional status of the older adult is associated with dentition status. *J Am Diet Assoc.* 103:61, 2003.

Scully C. Advances in oral medicine. *Prim Dent Care.* 7:55, 2000.

Sheiham A, et al. The relationship among dental status, nutrient intake, and nutritional status in older people. *J Dent Res.* 80:408, 2001.

Spolarich A. Managing the side effects of medications. *J Dent Hyg.* 74:57, 2000.

Touger-Decker R. Oral and dental health. In: Mahan K, Escott-Stump S, eds. *Krause's food, nutrition, and diet therapy.* 11th ed. Philadelphia: WB Saunders, 2004.

Touger-Decker R, Mobley C, American Dietetic Association. Position of the American Dietetic Association: oral health and nutrition. *J Am Diet Assoc.* 103:615, 2003.

Wagner R. Early childhood caries. *J Am Dent Assoc.* 137:150, 2006.

PERIODONTAL DISEASE AND GINGIVITIS

NUTRITIONAL ACUITY RANKING: LEVEL 1–2

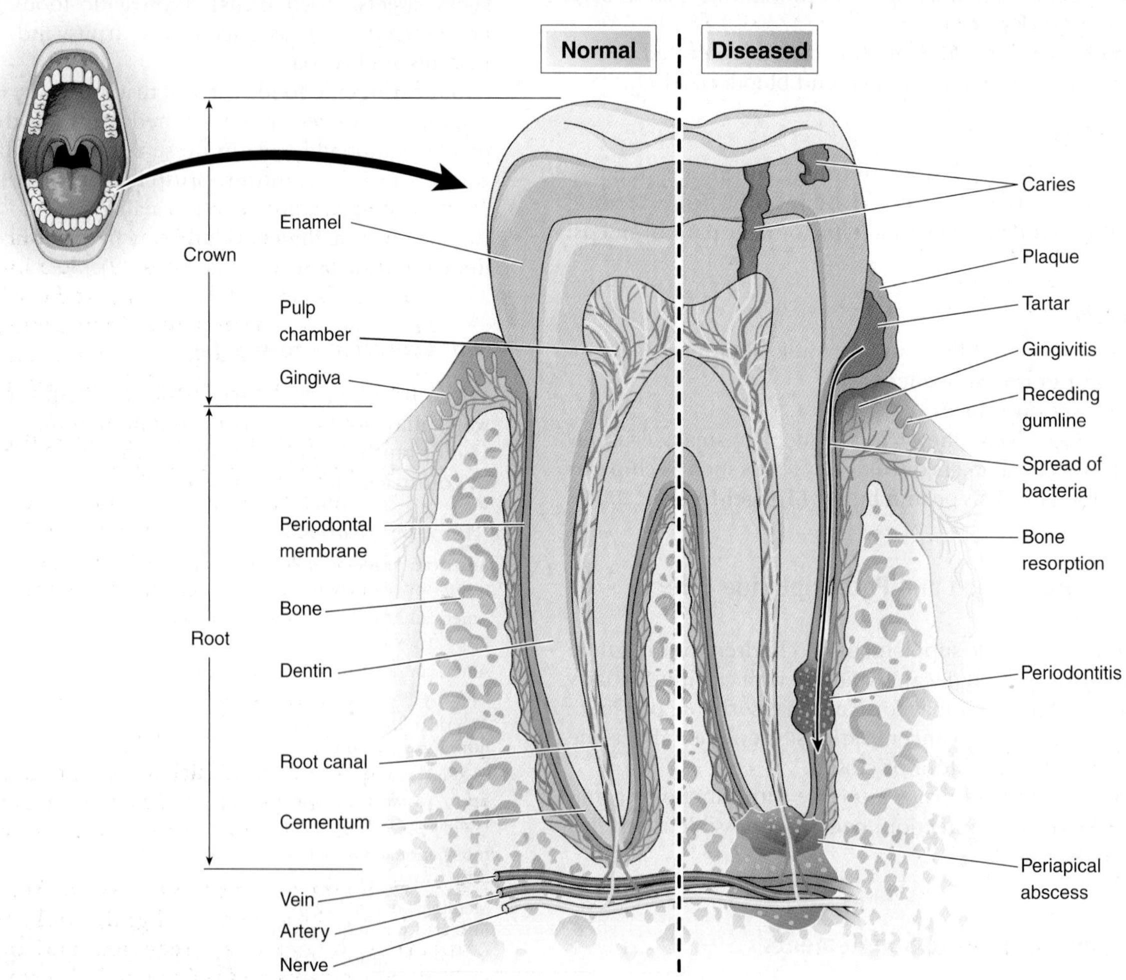

Reprinted with permission from: Thomas H. McConnell, *The Nature Of Disease Pathology for the Health Professions,* Philadelphia: Lippincott Williams & Wilkins, 2007.

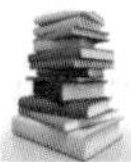

DEFINITIONS AND BACKGROUND

Gingivitis involves minor inflammatory changes in the gums; it may be acute or chronic, local or generalized. Vitamins C and D may reduce gingivitis (Dietrich et al, 2005). *Acute necrotizing ulcerative gingivitis* (Vincent's disease or trench mouth) is an acute ulceration affecting marginal gingiva with inflamed or necrotic interdental papillae. The onset is abrupt and painful with slight fever, malaise, excess salivation, and bad breath. It can be caused by systemic disease.

Tissues that support teeth in the jaws are collectively known as the periodontium (gums, alveolar bone, periodontal membrane). Any abnormality that leads to a visible change or loss of integrity of any component of the supporting tissue is a periodontal disease. Periodontal disease is a painless, chronic inflammatory disease that most commonly manifests as *pyorrhea alveolaris.* It involves a gross breakdown of supporting tissues with progressive loosening and loss of teeth inflammatory disease initiated by oral microbial biofilm (Van Dyke, 2008). It is a major cause of tooth loss in adults.

Periodontoclasia involves destruction of tissues around the teeth. A poor diet and inadequate dental hygiene can cause destruction of the jawbone. Osteoporosis and inflammation-associated bone degradation in periodontitis have a common pathogenesis (Serhan, 2004). Periodontal disease is evident approximately 10 years before osteoporosis.

Periodontal disease can start in the second decade; wisdom teeth are a breeding ground for bacteria that cause problems. Children and teens are also at risk if their oral and dental health needs are not addressed (Cummins, 2006). Nutrient deficiencies are prevalent and smokers are especially vulnerable to vitamin C deficiency (Nishida et al, 2000). Immune-enhancing nutrients for good oral health include protein, zinc, vitamins C and E, calcium, and the B-complex vitamins.

In the United States, periodontal disease affects a large portion of the population. At risk in particular are pregnant women, women after menopause, obese individuals, diabetics, alcoholics, smokers, persons with AIDS or rheumatoid arthritis, persons with respiratory ailments, and persons on medications including heart medicines, antidepressants, and antihistamines. Periodontal disease may precede bacterial pneumonia, so treatment is important. Evidence-based periodontology includes antimicrobial therapy, regenerative periodontal surgery, periodontal plastic surgery, bone regeneration surgery and implant treatment, and advanced soft tissue management at implant sites (Tonetti, 2000).

SAMPLE NUTRITION CARE PROCESS STEPS

Inadequate Oral Food and Beverage Intake—Periodontal Disease

Assessment Data (sources of info): Food records and intake calculations; dental evaluation.

Nutrition Diagnosis: Inadequate oral food and beverage intake related to sore and inflamed gums as evidenced by diet history revealing low use of antioxidant foods and vitamin C from fruits and vegetables; weight loss of 5# in past month; and diagnosis of periodontal disease.

Intervention: Education about the role of diet and oral hygiene in periodontal disease. Recommend nutrient and dietary changes to improve quality of food intake, reduce inflammation, and promote healing.

Monitoring and Evaluation: Intake records, rate of healing of gum disease.

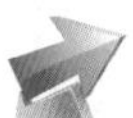

ASSESSMENT, MONITORING, AND EVALUATION

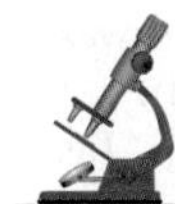

CLINICAL INDICATORS

Clinical/History

- Height
- Weight
- BMI
- Diet history
- Gums—color, friability, receding
- Oral examination for tooth mobility, calculus
- Sore mouth
- Overall nutritional status
- History of smoking, diabetes, other chronic diseases

Lab Work

- Serum glucose
- Serum Na^+, K^+
- Ca^{++}, Mg^{++}
- Serum ascorbic acid
- H & H, serum Fe
- Alb, transthyretin
- CRP

INTERVENTION

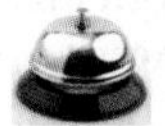

OBJECTIVES

- Reduce inflammation and promote healing.
- Correct poor nutritional habits that can lead to chronic subclinical deficiencies in levels of vitamins A, C, D, amino acids, riboflavin, folacin, zinc, and calcium.
- Prevent further decline in status of bones and gums. Protect the jawbone with adequate calcium and vitamin D (Hildebolt et al, 2004), especially in postmenopausal women.
- Review medications and consider alternatives to those causing dry mouth or other problems.
- Pregnant women with this condition are at risk for preterm birth and other adverse obstetric outcomes, such as preeclampsia and low birth weight; they should be closely monitored with prenatal medical and dental care.

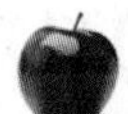

FOOD AND NUTRITION

- Ensure adequate intake of calcium, protein, zinc, phosphorus, vitamin C, fluoride, and vitamin A. A multivitamin–mineral supplement and vitamin-D fortified milk should be used.
- Use high-detergent foods (firm, fresh fruits and raw vegetables or those that are lightly cooked). Include cranberries, blueberries, green tea, and other foods rich in antioxidants and polyphenols (Kushiyama et al, 2009).

- Control timing and frequency of meals and snacks to reduce exposure of susceptible gum tissue and teeth to the acids that form plaque. Control blood glucose in diabetes.
- Promote a diet containing foods naturally rich in antioxidants and omega-3 polyunsaturated fatty acids (DHA, EPA), and low in refined carbohydrates (Chapple, 2009).

Common Drugs Used and Potential Side Effects

- Sodium bicarbonate may be used as a mouthwash. Patients with high BP should not swallow this wash.
- Peridex is an oral rinse to control bleeding gums. Taste changes may occur with its use.
- Triclosan-containing dentifrices may slow periodontal disease progression (Niederman, 2004).
- Antibiotic treatment of periodontitis includes amoxicillin/clavulanic acid, metronidazole, and clindamycin.
- Nonsteroidal anti-inflammatory agents may be used, such as Ibuprofen.

Herbs, Botanicals, and Supplements

- Herbs and botanicals may be used; identify and monitor side effects. Counsel about use of herbal teas, especially those containing toxic substances.
- For gingivitis, bloodroot, Echinacea, purslane, chamomile, licorice, and sage have been recommended but not confirmed for efficacy.
- A "Connective Tissue Nutrient Formula" that contains vitamins A, C, and D, glucosamine sulfate, magnesium, oligoproanthocyanidins, copper, zinc, manganese, boron, silicon, and calcium may be prescribed to enhance the integrity of key connective tissue elements.
- Naturopathic physicians may prescribe *Panax ginseng, Withania somnifera*, and *Eleutherococcus senticosus* to reverse the impact of bacterial and psychosocial stressors.

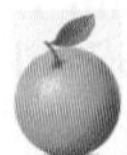

NUTRITION EDUCATION, COUNSELING, CARE MANAGEMENT

- Encourage a proper diet, especially sources of omega-3 fatty acids, calcium and vitamins C and D.
- Recommend meticulous oral hygiene and regular dental examinations to maintain dental hygiene. Brush often and floss after eating sticky foods such as candy, sticky buns, and fruit rolls. Drink lots of water.
- Encourage pregnant women and persons with dentures, diabetes, cancer, HIV/AIDS, rheumatoid arthritis, or leukemia to pay special attention to oral hygiene.
- Encourage intake of polyphenols and antioxidant-rich foods, including green tea (Kushiyama et al, 2009).

Patient Education—Food Safety

- Periodontitis involves host-mediated inflammation, with modulation of inflammation at a cellular and molecular level. Avoidance of infection with added inflammatory response will be needed, especially related to food handling and sanitation.

For More Information

- American Academy of Periodontology
  http://www.perio.org/index.html
- Dental Societies
  http://www.perio.org/links/links.html#dental
- Periodontal Societies
  http://www.perio.org/links/links.html#perio

PERIODONTAL DISEASE AND GINGIVITIS—CITED REFERENCES

Chapple IL. Potential mechanisms underpinning the nutritional modulation of periodontal inflammation. *J Am Dent Assoc.* 140:178, 2009.

Cummins D. The impact of research and development on the prevention of oral diseases in children and adolescents: an industry perspective. *Pediatr Dent.* 28:118, 2006.

Dietrich T, et al. Association between serum concentrations of 25-hydroxyvitamin D and gingival inflammation. *Am J Clin Nutr.* 82:575, 2005.

Hildebolt CF, et al. Estrogen and/or calcium plus vitamin D increase mandibular bone mass. *J Periodontol.* 5:811, 2004.

Kushiyama M, et al. Relationship between intake of green tea and periodontal disease. *J Periodontol.* 80:372, 2009.

Niederman R. Triclosan-containing dentifrice may slow periodontal disease progression. *Evid Based Dent.* 5:107, 2004.

Nishida M, et al. Dietary vitamin C and the risk for periodontal disease. *J Periodontol.* 71:1215, 2000.

Serhan CN. Clues for new therapeutics in osteoporosis and periodontal disease: new roles for lipoxygenases? *Expert Opin Ther Targets.* 8:643, 2004.

Tonetti M. Advances in periodontology. *Prim Dent Care.* 7:149, 2000.

Van Dyke TE. The management of inflammation in periodontal disease. *J Periodont.* 79(8S):1601, 2008.

TEMPOROMANDIBULAR JOINT DYSFUNCTION

NUTRITIONAL ACUITY RANKING: LEVEL 1

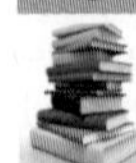

DEFINITIONS AND BACKGROUND

Temporomandibular joint (TMJ) disorders result from local or systemic causes, such as rheumatoid or osteoarthritis and connective tissue disorders. The TMJ is a diarthrodial joint with moving elements (mandible) and fixed elements (temporal bone). With this dysfunction, overuse or abuse of any part of normal action affects the mastication process. Patients with TMJ disorder pain dysfunction have toothaches, facial pains, and food-intake problems. The National Institute of Dental and Craniofacial Research (2009) indicates that over 10 million people in the United States suffer from TMJ problems at any given time. Osteoarthrosis and internal derangement may coexist in the same joint in about 33% of cases; pathological tissue changes should be examined in patients with TMJ (Dimitroulos, 2005).

Women between the ages of 30 and 60 years account for 75% of all cases. Mandibular deviation may occur from repetitive overloading (stress or habit such as gum chewing, grinding), from functional masseter muscle coordination problems, or from incorrect occlusion (as with missing teeth). Structural problems are treated by surgery (e.g., fusion can be treated by removing the area of fused bone and replacing it with silicon rubber). Sometimes an artificial joint is the answer; but surgery is recommended for only a few patients. Undue muscle tension causes most TMJ, with some other problems stemming from inadequate bite (as from a high filling or a malocclusion). People with TMJ benefit from a visit to their dentist or ear, nose, and throat specialist.

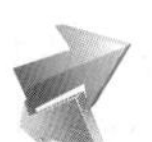

ASSESSMENT, MONITORING, AND EVALUATION

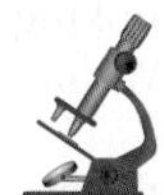

CLINICAL INDICATORS

Clinical/History		
Height	Mouth/jaw pain or clicking noise	Ca^{++}, Mg^{++}
Weight	Headaches	H & H, serum Fe
BMI	Shoulder or neck pain	Chol, Trig
Diet history	**Lab Work**	Alb
Stiff neck, face, or shoulders	Gluc	CRP
Locking of affected joint	Serum Na^+, K^+	
Trismus		
Gum status		

INTERVENTION

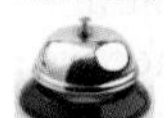

OBJECTIVES

- Reduce repetitive overloading by use of a splint or by breaking bad habits such as grinding (bruxism).
- Reduce stress with relaxation techniques. Relieve pain and muscle spasms.
- Prevent or correct malnutrition or weight loss.
- Ensure adequate intake of soft, nonchewy sources of fiber.
- Reduce any existing inflammation and prevent complications such as mitral valve prolapse.

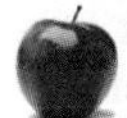

FOOD AND NUTRITION

- Use a normal diet with soft foods to prevent pain while chewing.
- Cut food into small, bite-sized pieces. Avoid chewy foods such as caramel, nuts, toffee, chewy candies, and gummy bread and rolls.

> **SAMPLE NUTRITION CARE PROCESS STEPS**
>
> **Chewing Problems**
>
> ***Assessment Data:*** Food records and intake calculations; dental evaluation; pain when chewing.
>
> ***Nutrition Diagnosis:*** Chewing problems related to TMJ and pain when eating as evidenced by diet history
>
> ***Intervention:*** Education about soft foods and liquids of high nutrient density. Recommend individualized dietary changes to improve intake and prevent weight loss.
>
> ***Monitoring and Evaluation:*** Intake records, reduction in TMJ pain, improved intake from nutrient-dense foods.

- Avoid opening mouth widely, as for large and thick sandwiches. Grate vegetables (e.g., carrots) to reduce need for chewing.
- Use adequate sources of vitamin C for adequate gingival health.
- Suggest foods rich in antioxidants, such as green tea, to promote health.

Common Drugs Used and Potential Side Effects

- Pain medicines may be needed when the condition is active. Monitor side effects for the specific drugs used.

Herbs, Botanicals, and Supplements

- Herbs and botanicals may be used; identify and monitor side effects. Counsel about use of herbal teas, especially avoiding toxic ingredients.

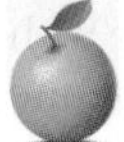

NUTRITION EDUCATION, COUNSELING, CARE MANAGEMENT

- Discuss the role of dental care in maintaining adequate health.
- Monitor for any tooth or gum soreness; advise the dentist as necessary. Regular oral hygiene must be continued despite mouth pain.
- Physical therapy may be needed to correct functioning of muscles and joints.
- Nail biting, gum chewing, use of teeth to cut thread, or similar habits should be stopped.
- Smoking is often a cause of bruxism, and programs to stop smoking should be considered if needed.

Patient Education—Food Safety

- Use general safe food handling measures.

For More Information

- Jaw Joints and Allied Musculoskeletal Disorders Foundation
  http://www.tmjoints.org/
- TMJ Disorder
  http://www.tmj.org/

TEMPOROMANDIBULAR JOINT DYSFUNCTION—CITED REFERENCES

Dimitroulos G. The prevalence of osteoarthrosis in cases of advanced internal derangement of the temporomandibular joint: a clinical, surgical and histological study. *Int J Oral Maxillofac Surg.* 34:345, 2005.

National Institute of Dental and Craniofacial Research. TMJ diseases and disorders. Accessed March 28, 2009, at http://www.tmj.org/basics.asp.

SELF-FEEDING PROBLEMS: VISION, COORDINATION, CHEWING, HEARING LOSS

NUTRITIONAL ACUITY RANKING: LEVEL 1–2 (VARIES BY SEVERITY)

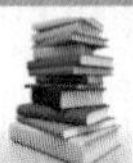

DEFINITIONS AND BACKGROUND

Self-feeding ability, one of the activities of daily living (ADLs), can be limited by low vision or blindness, lack of coordination, and chewing problems. Where appropriate, these factors are mentioned in other sections. Dysphagia is a fourth problem, described in Section 7. Assessment for vision changes, self-feeding difficulty, hearing, continence, gait and balance, and cognition can reveal a great deal about an individual's ability to function independently (Rao et al, 2004).

Low vision or blindness can affect any age; children with developmental disabilities and older persons may have cataracts or macular degeneration. The World Health Organization defines "low vision" as visual acuity between 20/70 and 20/400 with the best possible correction, or a visual field of 20 degrees or less. "Blindness" is defined as a visual acuity worse than 20/400 with the best possible correction. Someone with a visual acuity of 20/70 can see at 20 feet what someone with normal sight can see at 70 feet. Someone with a visual acuity of 20/400 can see at 20 feet what someone with normal sight can see at 400 feet. Normal visual field is about 160–170 degrees horizontally. Age-related macular degeneration and cataract are the leading causes of visual impairment and blindness in the United States; both diseases increase dramatically after age 60.

Age-related macular degeneration (AMD) is a vascular condition that damages the retina and affects 25–30 million people worldwide. The Age-Related Eye Disease Study (AREDS), sponsored by the National Eye Institute, found that taking high levels of antioxidants and zinc can reduce the risk of developing advanced AMD by about 25%. The specific daily amounts are 500 mg vitamin C; 400 IU vitamin E; 15 mg beta-carotene; 80 mg zinc oxide; and 2 mg copper as cupric oxide to prevent copper deficiency anemia. Protective foods include nuts, fish (Miljanovic et al, 2005; Seddon et al, 2003) lycopene, lutein and zeanthin. Lutein and zeaxanthin are carotenoids that have a role in filtering destructive blue light as photosensitive antioxidants. Smokers should not take beta-carotene supplements (Age-Related Eye Disease Research Group, 2001). In addition to the AREDS supplement, a lower dietary glycemic index (dGI) with higher intakes of DHA and EPA reduces progression to advanced AMD (Chiu et al, 2009). Diets high in saturated fat, animal fat, linoleic acid, and trans-fatty acids promote higher risk of AMD (Seddon et al, 2003). Abdominal obesity, smoking, and diets high in glycemic index should be avoided. Women tend to have a higher risk than men.

Cataract causes clouding in the crystalline lens of the eye, causing opacity and less passage of light. Blindness occurs if not treated. Regular intake of antioxidant foods, including rich sources of vitamins A, C, E and selenium, can be protective.

Diabetic retinopathy is a major cause of vision loss. All individuals who have diabetes should have a dilated eye exam annually. Diabetic retinopathy affects as many as 80% of individuals who have had diabetes for 10 years or longer. Careful control of blood glucose and hypertension are important measures to protect the small vessels of the eye. Treatment often involves laser surgery.

Glaucoma also has nutritional implications. Risk factors for chronic glaucoma include age over 40; a family history of glaucoma, diabetes, myopia; or being African American. Acute glaucoma may occur in persons with a family history of acute glaucoma, older age, presbyopia, or use of systemic anticholinergic medications. Prostagladins regulate inner eye pressure; glaucoma may be related to a higher intake ratio of omega-3 fatty acids to omega-6 fatty acids (Kang et al, 2004). Soybean, safflower, and sunflower oils may be protective.

Hemianopia yields loss in half of the field of vision; quadrantanopia affects a quarter of the visual field. Vision loss may range from slight to severe. Patients may need guidance about their meals, as they may not see the full plate or tray of food. Vision restoration therapy and the brain's ability to repair itself have made advances for these patients.

Coordination problems may occur at any age. Conditions that can cause coordination problems include Alzheimer's disease, alcohol abuse, attention deficit disorder, brain cancer, chorea, Down syndrome, encephalitis, fetal alcohol syndrome, advanced HIV infection, hydrocephaly, multiple sclerosis, Parkinson's disease, Rett syndrome, stroke, and Wilson's disease. Hand–eye coordination is needed for self-feeding, and when this is not working properly, assistance is needed. Other problems affecting meal intake may include falling forward, feet not touching the floor, leaning to one side, poor balance while sitting, and poor neck control. Sometimes, it is possible to adjust table height, offer pillows or other positioning equipment, offer a footstool, or adjust pedals on a wheelchair. It is recommended to work with an occupational therapist for the proper types of adjustments to allow for better mealtime food intake.

Chewing problems may cause inability to consume enough food or foods of varying texture. Total edentulism without dentures may contribute to deterioration in health. Without chewing, there is less production of saliva and food is not properly mixed before swallowing. **Dry mouth (xerostomia)**, from a variety of causes, may interfere with chewing and swallowing; it should be corrected where possible.

Hearing loss, while not always affecting food intake, may be related to underlying cardiovascular disease, hypertension, or diabetes. Cochlear vulnerability from microvascular changes may occur (Agrawal et al, 2009). Hearing loss is more common than previously believed and preventive measures, such as lifestyle changes, may be needed as early as adolescence (Helzner et al, 2005).

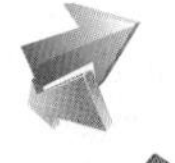

ASSESSMENT, MONITORING, AND EVALUATION

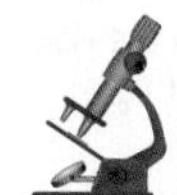

CLINICAL INDICATORS

Genetic Markers

Clinical/History
- Height
- Weight
- BMI
- Recent weight changes
- Diet history
- Mouth or tongue lacerations
- Sore or bleeding gums
- Missing or loose teeth, edentulism
- Dentures, especially poorly fitting
- Blindness, cataracts, AMD
- Hemianopia, low vision
- Chewing problems
- Dysphagia (see Section 7)
- Signs of dehydration or edema
- Coordination problems
- Dry mouth (xerostomia)
- Needs feeding assistance
- Needs adaptive feeding equipment

Lab Work
- Gluc
- Alb, transthyretin
- Serum Na^+, K^+
- Ca^{++}, Mg^{++}
- I & O
- H & H, serum Fe
- X-rays (such as mandible)

INTERVENTION

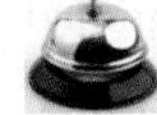

OBJECTIVES

- Promote independence in self-feeding, when possible.
- Address all nutritional deficiencies and complications individually. Select nutrient-dense foods.
- Promote overall wellness and health.
- Increase interest in eating. Increase pleasure associated with mealtimes.
- Prevent malnutrition and weight loss.

SAMPLE NUTRITION CARE PROCESS STEPS

Self-Feeding Problems—Low Vision

Assessment Data: Food records and intake calculations; vision and self-feeding problems.

Nutrition Diagnosis: Self-feeding difficulty related to blindness and no adaptive equipment as evidenced by limited intake at meals and long period required for eating.

Intervention: Education about adaptive equipment with careful orientation to items served at meals. Reading menu choices aloud.

Refer to Occupational Therapy for proper equipment, techniques for cueing, positioning at mealtime, and encouragement tips.

Counsel about dietary changes to improve intake and prevent weight loss, such as finger foods and easy to handle foods.

Monitoring and Evaluation: Intake records showing better intake when using adaptive equipment; weight records; improved quality of life with greater independent functioning at mealtimes.

- Decrease instances in which constipation, anorexia, or other problems affect nutritional status.
- Educate the caregiver about adaptive equipment, utensils, and special food modifications. Patients with hemianopia may require special training to be able to see and eat all of the meals served to them.

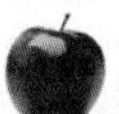

FOOD AND NUTRITION

Low Vision, Blindness, AMD, Cataracts

- Provide special plate guards, utensils, double handles, and compartmentalized plates with foods placed in similar locations at each meal. Place all foods within 18″ reach at mealtime. Explain placement of foods. Open packets if needed.
- Work with occupational therapist (OT) or family to practice kitchen safety and to determine ability to be independent at mealtimes. Allow sufficient time to complete meals; refrigerate or reheat items as needed.
- Create a feeling of usefulness by delegating appropriate tasks related to mealtime, such as drying dishes and assisting with simple meal tasks that are safe for the individual.
- Support companionship during meals, especially if problems occur or if anything else is needed.
- Use straws for beverages unless there is dysphagia.
- Include a balance of fatty acids (omega 3 and omega 6). Use rich sources of DGA and EPA, such as salmon, sardines, herring, tuna, or a fish oil supplement as needed. Use more oils such as olive and canola. Linoleic acid from vegetable oils reduces the positive effects and should be used less often.
- For a diet lower in dGI, include whole grains, soybeans and lentils more often and exclude desserts, candy, sweetened beverages, potatoes and white bread.
- Include more lycopene from pink grapefruit, tomato sauce, tomato juice, and watermelon. Lutein and zeaxanthin are found in broccoli, spinach, other leafy greens, egg yolk. Antioxidant-rich foods that include good sources of

TABLE 2-7 Nutrients for Healthy Vision[a]

Protein and Amino Acids	Protein undernutrition is associated with increased risk of cataract. Low protein intake may induce deficiencies of specific amino acids that are needed to maintain the health of the lens, or other nutritional deficiencies, particularly niacin, thiamin, and riboflavin (Delcourt et al, 2005).
Vitamin A, Lutein and Zeaxanthin	Vitamin A is needed for healthy cornea and conjunctiva. Many studies have shown that lutein and zeaxanthin reduce the risk of chronic eye diseases, including age-related macular degeneration and cataracts. Cataract and AMD patients tend to be deficient in vitamin A and the carotenes, lutein, and zeaxanthin (Head, 2001; Krinsky et al, 2003; Seddon et al, 2003). Lutein and zeaxanthin are found in green leafy vegetables (kale, collards, spinach, turnip greens, broccoli) as well as eggs, yellow corn, peas, tangerine, and orange bell peppers. Eggland's Best eggs contain 185 mg of lutein. Lutein is facilitated with ascorbic acid supplementation (Tanumihardjo et al, 2005).
Thiamin	For normal retinal and optic nerve functioning. Protective against cataracts (Jacques et al, 2005).
Riboflavin	For corneal vascularization. Protective against cataracts (Jacques et al, 2005). Riboflavin appears to play an essential role as a precursor to flavin adenine dinucleotide (FAD), a cofactor for glutathione reductase activity (Head, 2001).
Niacin	For healthy vision. Avoid excesses, which can cause nicotinic acid maculopathy (Spirn et al, 2003).
Folate	A strong protective influence on cortical cataract from use of folate or vitamin B_{12} supplements is a recent finding (Kuzniarz et al, 2001).
Vitamin B_6	For healthy conjuntiva. Untreated homocystinuria is known to cause ocular changes; vitamin B_6 can help to lower homocysteine levels.
Vitamin B_{12}	For retinal and nerve fibers. Protective against cataract (Kuzniarz et al, 2001). Found only in animal foods such as meat and milk.
Vitamin C	For healthy conjuntiva and vitreous humor. Long-term use of adequate vitamin C may delay or prevent early age-related lens opacity (Ferrigno et al, 2005; Valero et al, 2002). Orange and grapefruit juices, cantaloupe, oranges, green peppers, tomato juice, broccoli, kiwifruit, and strawberries are good sources. Vitamin C (ascorbic acid) is an antioxidant that lowers the risk of developing cataracts, and when taken in combination with other essential nutrients, can slow the progression of age-related macular degeneration and visual acuity loss (American Optometric Association, 2009).
Vitamin D	Helps prevent cancer, heart disease, diabetes, and age-related macular degeneration; it is the most potent steroid hormone in the human body, and is the only vitamin formed with the help of sunlight (American Optometric Association, 2009).
Vitamin E	Important for antioxidant properties. Protects the eyes from free radical damage and may slow the onset of cataracts. Long-term use of supplements may be beneficial (Jacques et al, 2005). Vitamin E is found in almonds, peanuts, peanut butter, sunflower seeds, safflower oil, margarines, fortified cereals, sweet potatoes, and creamy salad dressings.
Omega-3 Fatty Acids	Omega-3 fatty acids and fish are protective against AMD (Cho et al, 2001). Eating fish (sardines, salmon, herring, tuna, fortified eggs) weekly and cutting back on saturated fatty acids are important (Smith et al, 2000). Infants need a supply of DHA for up to a year for healthy visual development (Hoffman et al, 2004). Avoid use of large doses of alpha linolenic acid.
Omega-6 Fatty Acids	Omega-6 fatty acids in soybean, safflower, and sunflower oils may be protective against glaucoma (Kang et al, 2004) but not against cataracts. High doses of canola, flaxseed, and soybean oils may actually increase the risk of cataracts (Jacques et al, 2005).
Selenium	Pathophysiological mechanisms of cataract formation include deficient glutathione levels contributing to a faulty antioxidant defense system within the lens of the eye; nutrients that increase glutathione levels and activity include selenium (Head, 2001; Flohe, 2005).
Sodium	Sodium-restricted diets may protect against cataracts (Cumming et al, 2000).
Zinc	For healthy retina, choroid, and optic nerve. Found in beef, chicken, oysters, mixed nuts, and milk. Zinc is an essential trace mineral, bringing vitamin A from the liver to the retina in order to produce melanin for a protective pigment in the eyes (American Optometric Association, 2009). Zinc is highly concentrated in the eye.

American Optometric Association. Web site accessed March 29, 2009, at http://www.aoa.org/x11813.xml.

[a]Long-term use of multivitamin, B group, and vitamin A supplements is associated with reduced prevalence of either nuclear or cortical cataract (Kuzniarz et al, 2001).

vitamins C and E and zinc should also be consumed daily. Snacking on nuts is an excellent choice.

Coordination Problems

- Self-feeding requires the ability to suck, to sit with head and neck balanced, to bring hand to mouth, to grasp cup and utensil, to drink from a cup, to take food from a spoon, to bite, to chew, and to swallow. Each person should be assessed individually to determine which, if any, aspects of coordination have been affected by his or her condition. Adjust self-feeding accordingly.
- Use clothing protectors at mealtime to maintain dignity.
- Assist with feeding if needed; use adaptive feeding equipment as needed (such as weighted utensils, large-handled cups, larger or smaller silverware than standard). Adjust table or chair height.
- Place all foods within 18″ reach at mealtime.

Chewing Problems

- Dentures should fit well and be adjusted or replaced as needed, such as after weight loss.
- Decrease texture as necessary; use a mechanical soft, pureed, or liquid diet. Season as desired for individual taste. Try to progress in textures if possible because chewing

is important for saliva production and for proper digestion of foods.

- Liquid or blenderized foods may be beneficial. If needed, use a tube feeding.
- For some persons, a straw may be helpful; for others, it is not. Speech therapists can assess this ability.
- Protein foods such as tofu, cottage cheese, peanut butter, eggs, cheese, and milk products can be used when meats or nuts cannot be chewed.
- If fresh fruits and vegetables cannot be consumed, use cooked or canned sources and juices. Use pureed foods when needed. If whole grain breads and cereals are not tolerated, use cooked cereals. Avoid rice or foods with small particles in dysphagia (see Section 7).

Hearing Loss

- Researchers and international scientists have found a gene that causes deafness in humans: *LRTOMT*.
- Alter diets as needed if diabetes, cardiovascular disease, or hypertension are present. A controlled carbohydrate diet, therapeutic lifestyle diet (low saturated fat), or the DASH diet may be appropriate.

Common Drugs Used and Potential Side Effects

- For glaucoma, a combination of medications is used to reduce elevated intraocular pressure and prevent damage to the optic nerve. Some may cause dry mouth or fatigue; monitor individually.
- For AMD, Chol-lowering medications (statins) may be protective. Clinical trials are in order.

Herbs, Botanicals, and Supplements

- Nutrients and botanicals that may prevent cataracts include folic acid, melatonin, and bilberry (Head, 2001). Flavonoids, particularly quercetin, and ginkgo biloba may increase circulation to the optic nerve (Head, 2001). Curcumin is also under study.
- Lutein and zeaxanthin, in whole food or supplemental form, have an impact on retinal function with the potential to preserve vision and prevent degeneration in AMD; further research is needed to determine an effective dose (Carpentier et al, 2009).
- Herbs and botanicals may be used; identify and monitor side effects. For glaucoma, oregano, jaborandi, kaffir potato, and pansy have been recommended but not confirmed as effective. For cataract, rosemary, catnip, and capers have not been found to be effective.

Counsel about use of herbal teas to avoid intake of toxic substances.

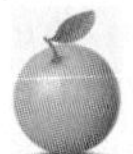

NUTRITION EDUCATION, COUNSELING, CARE MANAGEMENT

- Discuss the importance of using the various therapies and medications.
- Discuss the role of nutrition in health, weight control, recovery and repair processes.
- For healthy eyes, nutrition plays an essential role; see Table 2-7. Consume 10 mg of lutein weekly, the equivalent of one cup of cooked spinach four times a week. Orange juice is a good choice for vitamin C. The DASH diet is a good plan.
- Provide instruction regarding simplified meal planning and preparation. Refer to agencies such as Meals-on-Wheels if needed.
- Discuss the tips appropriate for the individual (texture, finger foods, ease of placement at meals).

Patient Education—Food Safety

- Discuss simple hand washing or use of hand sanitizers before meals.

For More Information

- Age-Related Macular Degeneration Alliance
  http://www.amdalliance.org/
- American Association of Ophthalmology
  http://www.eyenet.org/
- American Academy of Ophthalmology
  http://www.aao.org/
- American Council for the Blind
  http://www.acb.org/siteindex.html
- American Occupational Therapy Association
  http://www.aota.org/
- American Optometric Association
  http://www.aoanet.org/conditions/eye_coordination.asp
- Coordination Problems: National Center for Education in Maternal and Child Health
  http://www.brightfutures.org/physicalactivity/issues_concerns/10.html
- Hearing Loss Association
  http://www.hearingloss.org/
- Hearing Disorders and Deafness
  http://www.nlm.nih.gov/medlineplus/hearingdisordersanddeafness.html
- Help for Vision Loss
  http://www.visionaware.org/getstarted_professionals
- Low Vision
  http://www.lowvision.org/
- National Library Service for the Blind and Physically Handicapped (NLS)
  http://www.loc.gov/nls
- National Eye Institute, NIH
  http://www.nei.nih.gov/health/
- Prevent Blindness America
  http://www.preventblindness.org/
- Save your vision
  http://www.aoa.org/documents/nutrition/Save-Your-Vision-Month-Release.pdf
- Vision Loss for Seniors
  http://www.afb.org/seniorsitehome.asp

SELF-FEEDING PROBLEMS—CITED REFERENCES

Age-Related Eye Disease Research Group. A randomized, placebo-controlled, clinical trial of high-dose supplementation with vitamins C and E, beta-carotene, and zinc for age-related cataract and vision loss. AREDS Report No. 9. *Arch Ophthalmol.* 119:1439, 2001.

Agrawal Y, et al. Risk factors for hearing loss in US adults: data from the National Health and Nutrition Examination Survey, 1999 to 2002. *Otol Neurotol.* 30:139, 2009.

Bainbridge KE, et al. Diabetes and hearing impairment in the United States: audiometric evidence from the National Health and Nutrition Examination Survey, 1999 to 2004. *Ann Int Med.* 149:1, 2008.

Carpentier S, et al. Associations between lutein, zeaxanthin, and age-related macular degeneration: an overview. *Crit Rev Food Sci Nutr.* 49:313, 2009.

Chiu CJ, et al. Does eating particular diets alter the risk of age-related macular degeneration in users of the Age-Related Eye Disease Study supplements? *Br J Ophthalmol.* 93:1241, 2009.

Cho E, et al. Prospective study of dietary fat and the risk of age-related macular degeneration. *Am J Clin Nutr.* 73:209, 2001.

Cumming R, et al. Dietary sodium intake and cataract: the Blue Mountains Eye Study. *Am J Epidemiol.* 151:624, 2000.

Delcourt C, et al. Albumin and transthyretin as risk factors for cataract: the POLA study. *Arch Ophthalmol.* 123:225, 2005.

Ferrigno L, et al. Associations between plasma levels of vitamins and cataract in the Italian-American Clinical Trial of Nutritional Supplements and Age-Related Cataract (CTNS): CTNS Report #2. *Ophthalmic Epidemiol.* 12:71, 2005.

Flohe L. Selenium, selenoproteins and vision. *Dev Ophthalmol.* 38:89, 2005.

Head KA. Natural therapies for ocular disorders, part two: cataracts and glaucoma. *Altern Med Rev.* 6:141, 2001.

Helzner EP, et al. Race and sex differences in age-related hearing loss: the Health, Aging and Body Composition Study. *J Am Geriatr Soc.* 53:2119, 2005.

Hoffman DR, et al. Maturation of visual acuity is accelerated in breast-fed term infants fed baby food containing DHA-enriched egg yolk. *J Nutr.* 134:2307, 2004.

Jacques PF, et al. Long-term nutrient intake and 5-year change in nuclear lens opacities. *Arch Ophthalmol.* 123:517, 2005.

Kang JH, et al. Dietary fat consumption and primary open-angle glaucoma. *Am J Clin Nutr.* 79:755, 2004.

Krinsky NI, et al. Biologic mechanisms of the protective role of lutein and zeaxanthin in the eye. *Annu Rev Nutr.* 23:171, 2003.

Kuzniarz M, et al. Use of vitamin supplements and cataract: the Blue Mountains Eye Study. *Am J Ophthalmol.* 132:19, 2001.

Miljanovic B, et al. Relation between dietary n-3 and n-6 fatty acids and clinically diagnosed dry eye syndrome in women. *Am J Clin Nutr.* 82:887, 2005.

Rao AV, et al. Geriatric assessment and comorbidity. *Semin Oncol.* 31:149, 2004.

Seddon JM, et al. Progression of age-related macular degeneration: association with dietary fat, transunsaturated fat, nuts, and fish intake. *Arch Ophthalmol.* 121:1728, 2003.

Smith W, et al. Dietary fat and fish intake and age-related maculopathy. *Arch Ophthalmol.* 118:401, 2000.

Spirn MJ, et al. Optical coherence tomography findings in nicotinic acid maculopathy. *Am J Ophthalmol.* 135:913, 2003.

Tanumihardjo SA, et al. Lutein absorption is facilitated with cosupplementation of ascorbic acid in young adults. *J Am Diet Assoc.* 105:114, 2005.

Valero MP, et al. Vitamin C is associated with reduced risk of cataract in a Mediterranean population. *J Nutr.* 132:1299, 2002.

SKIN CONDITIONS, PRESSURE ULCERS, AND VITAMIN DEFICIENCIES

SKIN DISORDERS

NUTRITIONAL ACUITY RANKING: LEVEL 1

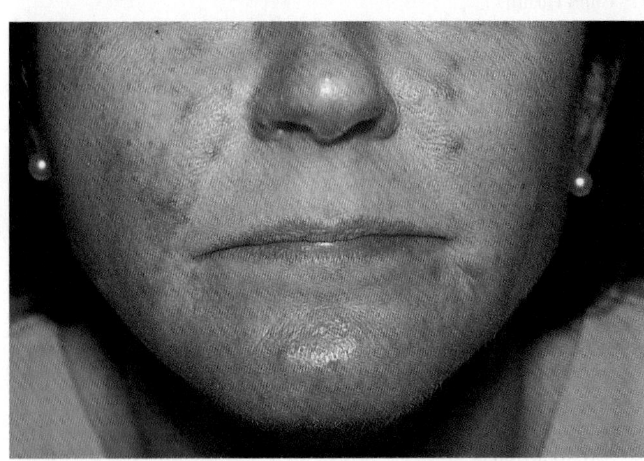

Adapted from: *Goodheart HP. Goodheart's Photguide of Common Skin Disorders.* 2nd ed. Philadelphia: Lippincott Williams & Wilkins, 2003.

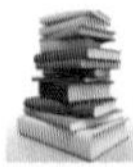

DEFINITIONS AND BACKGROUND

Human skin is the largest, independent peripheral endocrine organ of the body (Zouboulis, 2000). Skin is affected by both internal and external influences, which may lead to photo aging, inflammation, immune dysfunction, imbalanced epidermal homeostasis, and other disorders (Boelsma et al, 2001). The skin often reflects internal problems such as GI disturbances, alcoholism, or general malnutrition.

Nutritional factors impact hydration status, sebum production, elasticity, and skin cancer (Greenwald, 2001). A low-fat diet and foods rich in vitamin D and carotenoids may protect against some forms of skin cancer and actinic keratoses (Millen et al, 2004).

Many carotenoids found in nature are also found in the human body. Lutein and zeaxanthin are present in the skin and have shown significant efficacy against ultraviolet light-induced skin damage (Roberts et al, 2009). Retinoids have vitamin A biological activity; they have benefits for skin diseases and reversal of photo aging. Supplementation with vitamins, carotenoids, and polyunsaturated fatty acids has been shown to provide protection against ultraviolet light; however, sunscreen is still important (Boelsma et al, 2001).

Enzymes of the cytochrome P450 (P450 or CYP) family are drug-metabolizing enzymes that are induced in skin in response to xenobiotic exposure; they also play important roles in metabolism of fatty acids, eicosanoids, sterols, steroids, vitamins A and D (Ahmad and Mukhtar, 2004). In psoriasis, for example, many CYP enzymes are elevated; some relationship with celiac disease has been noted.

Acne affects many young people and may cause psychological distress. Iodine can aggravate acne; milk and dairy products contain a high level of iodine, but more studies are needed (Arbesman, 2005). Changes in diet are not the primary solution. Benzoyl peroxide is efficacious in mild-to-moderate acne, whereas adapalene and tretinoin are better for greater severity. Green tea polyphenols have anti-inflammatory effects, both taken internally and in topical creams.

Atopic dermatitis (AD), or eczema, causes itchy, inflamed skin. It usually affects the insides of the elbows, backs of the knees, and the face, but can cover much of the body.

AD often affects people who either suffer from asthma and/or hay fever or have family members who do (the "atopic triad"). AD flares when the person is exposed to trigger factors, such as dry skin, irritants, allergens, emotional stress, heat and sweating, and infections; avoiding triggers is the key. Because essential fatty acids (EFAs) form an important component of cell membranes, are eicosanoid precursors, and are required for both the structure and function of every cell, EFAs may benefit persons who have AD or psoriasis (Das, 1999).

Dermatitis herpetiformis (DH or Durhing's disease) is related to celiac disease (Karpati, 2004). There is the presence of villous atrophy and endomysial antibodies (EMAs) as markers (Kumar et al, 2001). A gluten-restricted diet is needed.

Epidermolysis bullosa is a hereditary condition in which blistering of the skin occurs with even slight trauma. It affects two of every 100,000 live births, occurring in both sexes and all ethnic groups. Nail dystrophy can occur, with rough, thickened, or absent fingernails or toenails. There may be blisters and problems with the soft tissue inside the mouth; protein–energy malnutrition, stunting, anemia, vitamin and mineral deficiencies are common. Treatment involves careful skin and wound care, and prevention of infections.

Nickel dermatitis affects 8–15% of women and 1% of men. Sensitization to nickel is often associated with ear piercing (Garner, 2004). In severe cases, reduce exposure to nickel from foods (Antico and Soana, 1999), and other sources.

Nummular eczematous dermatitis occurs with a rash; etiology is unknown. The rash is coin shaped and worsens in very hot or cold weather. Wool, soaps, frequent bathing (more than once a day), detergents, and rough clothing may be irritants. No special diet is needed unless food allergies are identified.

Psoriasis has patches of scaly red skin that burn, itch, or bleed. Calcitriol and vitamin D analogs are useful, along with controlled exposure to sunlight (Lehmann et al, 2004; May et al, 2004). Omega-3 fatty acids (specifically EPA) with a drug regimen of etretinate and topical corticosteroids may improve symptoms. Enbrel (etanercept), a tumor necrosis factor alpha (TNFα) inhibitor, relieves the clinical symptoms and may also clear up related depression and fatigue. There may be a relationship with celiac disease; if tests are positive, a gluten-free lifestyle will be needed.

Rosacea is a disorder of the central portion of the facial skin with onset in the third decade and peak in the fourth or fifth decade. A chronic and progressive condition of flare-ups and remissions, rosacea can be disfiguring if left untreated. Rosacea resembles other dermatological conditions, especially acne vulgaris. It affects one in 20 people, or 13 million people in the United States. Members of the same family tend to be affected; fair-skinned individuals of Northern and Eastern European descent (English, Scottish, Welsh, or Scandinavian) are most commonly affected (Litt, 1997). Green tea extract in creams may have benefits.

SAMPLE NUTRITION CARE PROCESS STEPS

Psoriasis

Assessment Data: Food records and intake calculations; many skin rashes, with psoriasis diagnosed 15 years ago.

Nutrition Diagnosis: Inadequate vitamin and fatty acid intake related to chronic history of psoriasis and poor diet as evidenced by diet history revealing high intake of beer, low intake of vitamin D and omega 3 fatty acids, and low serum vitamin D.

Intervention: Education about careful exposure to sunshine and use of vitamin D-fortified foods, fatty fish such as salmon and mackerel. Counsel about dietary changes to improve intake of omega-3 fatty acids and vitamin D_3. Advise cutting beer intake down or out. Coordinate care with physician to evaluate for celiac disease.

Monitoring and Evaluation: If positive for celiac, discuss gluten-free lifestyle. Intake records showing better food intake and lower intake of beer; improved quality of life with fewer outbreaks of psoriasis.

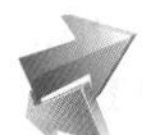

ASSESSMENT, MONITORING, AND EVALUATION

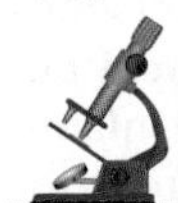

CLINICAL INDICATORS

Genetic Markers: Single genes control mediators such as enzymes, neuroendocrine transmitters, and cytokines that promote rosacea and probably other skin disorders.

Clinical/History	Lab Work	
Height	Alb (decreased in exfoliative dermatitis)	Thyroid-stimulating hormone (TSH), T4 level
Weight	Transthyretin	H & H, serum Fe
BMI	Serum zinc	Gluc
Growth pattern in children	Serum histamine (may be elevated)	Chol, Trig
Diet history	Skin tests for allergies	Serum Na^+, K^+
Family history of skin disorders, allergies	Anti-tTG, AGA, and/or EMA tests (for celiac)	Ca^{++}, Mg^{++}
Psoriasis?		Serum carotene
Rashes, blisters, pustules?		Retinol-binding protein (RBP)
Dermatitis?		CRP

INTERVENTION

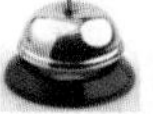

OBJECTIVES

- Reduce inflammation, redness, or edema where present. Prevent further exacerbations of the condition.
- Apply nutritional principles according to the particular condition (such as vitamin D, omega-3 fatty acids, carotenoids, zinc).
- Identify any offending foods; omit from the diet any food allergens or intolerances, such as gluten.

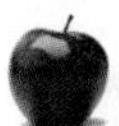

FOOD AND NUTRITION

- **Acne.** Encourage intake of adequate zinc, carotenoids, and vitamin A foods. This condition is hormone dependent. It is less common in non-Western societies, so a high-fat diet that is low in fruit and vegetable intake should be avoided (Cordain et al, 2002). Drinking green tea can be highly recommended.
- **Acrodermatitis enteropathica.** Supplement with zinc because absorption is often impaired. Use protein of high biological value. Decrease excess fiber, if necessary, to normalize bowel function.
- **Atopic dermatitis.** Eczema is a general term for any type of dermatitis; AD is the most severe and chronic form. AD is a disease that causes itchy, inflamed skin. It typically affects the insides of the elbows, backs of the knees, and the face, but can cover most of the body. Diet therapies do not work well; do not automatically eliminate important foods such as milk and wheat. A trial without salicylates (berries and dried fruits), aspirin, penicillin, food molds, some herbs and spices, and FD&C yellow 5 may be useful. Infants may have hypersensitivity to milk, egg albumin, wheat, or linoleic acid but tend to outgrow it. Control energy excess in obese infants. Avoid herbal products, such as chamomile tea, for which allergy is possible. Green tea is safe and may be recommended.
- **Dermatitis herpetiformis.** A gluten-free diet is quite successful in treating this condition; see Section 7.
- **Epidermolysis bullosa (EB).** A balanced diet that includes extra protein, calories, and a multivitamin–mineral supplement will be useful. Highlight the nutrients that are beneficial, including omega-3 fatty acids, vitamin A, and zinc. Dysphagia is common, and may even lead to esophageal strictures. Anemia, contractures, gastroesophageal reflux (GERD), or scarring of the tongue may occur. Gastrostomy feeding may be needed.
- **Nickel dermatitis.** Avoid canned foods, such as tuna fish, tomatoes, corn, spinach, and other canned vegetables. Do not cook with stainless steel utensils. Chocolate, nuts, and beans may have slightly higher naturally occurring nickel than other foods; avoid large quantities (Christensen et al, 1999).
- **Psoriasis.** Psoriasis may precede arthritis by months or years; both are inflammatory processes. Because of their antiproliferative effects, calcitriol and other vitamin D analogs are highly efficient in the treatment of psoriasis (Lehmann et al, 2004; May et al, 2004). The therapeutic effect of UVB light therapy may be related to its skin synthesis of calcitriol. If celiac sensitive, omit gluten from diet, beverages such as beer, and medications.
- **Rosacea.** Alcoholic beverages (especially red wine), spicy foods, hot beverages, some fruits and vegetables, marinated meats, and dairy products may trigger flare-ups; avoid as needed. Limit use of all forms of pepper, paprika, chili powder, and curry. Substitute with cumin, oregano, sage, thyme, marjoram, turmeric, cinnamon, basil, and milder spices. Recommend drinking green tea.

Common Drugs Used and Potential Side Effects

When using cortisone ointments, use just a little and massage in well. Application once daily does as much good as using it more often. The potential for long-term use to suppress the adrenal gland exists (Matsuda et al, 2000; Woo and McKenna, 2003).

Acne

- Isotretinoin (Accutane) may be used for acne. Watch for a decrease in high-density lipoprotein (HDL) and an increase in TG. An increase in depression or suicide attempts seem to be related. Avoid taking with vitamin A supplements. Dry mouth can occur. Do not use during pregnancy.
- Retin A (retinoic acid) is useful for moderate cases of acne; side effects are mild.
- Tetracycline should not be taken within 2 hours of use of milk products or calcium supplements. Excesses of vitamin A can cause headaches or hypertension. Use more riboflavin, vitamin C, and calcium in the diet. Protein and iron malabsorption may result from prolonged use. Diarrhea is the major GI effect. Minocycline causes less GI distress and does not affect calcium metabolism as dramatically. Antibiotics are used their anti-inflammatory effect.

Atopic Dermatitis

- Topical cortisone (steroid) creams, such as Aclovate, usually have a mild effect on the nutritional status of the patient. Stronger brands or dosages may act like oral steroids and can suppress the adrenal system if taken for prolonged periods.

Epidermolysis bullosa

- Wound care products are used for tissue regeneration. Fluid replacement and protein loss may be associated with blistering.

Psoriasis

- Calcitriol and other vitamin D analogs are often highly effective. Topical products such as tazarotene (Tazorac) and calcipotriene, a form of vitamin D, have been available for years.
- Enbrel (enteracept), Humira (adalimumab), or Remicade (infliximab) are used for severe chronic plaque psoriasis. TNF inhibitors such as efalizumab (Raptiva) yield less-frequent itching and better quality of life (Ricardo et al, 2004).

Rosacea

- Antibiotic creams such as metronidazole (MetroCream) and azelaic acid (Finacea) are commonly prescribed. Tetracycline may also be prescribed; avoid taking within an hour of dairy or calcium-related supplements.
- Taking an antihistamine about 2 hours before a meal may counter the effects of histamine.
- Aspirin may reduce the effects of niacin-containing foods in sufferers affected by the flushing effect of these foods. Monitor multivitamin supplements and intakes carefully.

Herbs, Botanicals, and Supplements

- Counsel about use of herbal teas, especially related to potentially toxic ingredients. Herbs and botanicals may be used; identify and monitor side effects.
- For **acne**, salicylic acid helps break down blackheads and whiteheads and helps cut down the shedding of cells lining the hair follicles. Tea tree oil topical solutions may be beneficial for **acne** because of anti-inflammatory effects (Koh et al, 2002; Liao, 2001). Ointment containing tea leaf extract is effective for in impetigo, acne, and methicillin-resistant *Staphylococcus aureus*; results equal conventional treatments (Martin and Ernst, 2003).
- For prevention of **AD**, Chinese herbs, dietary restrictions, homeopathy, house dust mite reduction, massage therapy, hypnotherapy, evening primrose oil, emollients, topical coal tar, and topical doxepin are not proven effective (Hoare et al, 2000). Extracts of arnica (*Arnica montana*), chamomile (*Chamomilla recutita*), tansy (*Tanacetum vulgare*), and feverfew (*Tanacetum parthenium*) may cause allergic reactions. Calendula is often recommended but not proven effective.
- For **psoriasis**: bishop's weed, avocado, licorice, red pepper, Brazil nut, and purslane are not confirmed. Red clover is sometimes used for dermatitis or psoriasis; avoid use with warfarin or hormone replacement therapy.
- For **scabies**: evening primrose, onion, neem, and mountain mint have been proposed. No confirming studies are available.
- For **sunburn**: eggplant, plantain, and calendula have been proposed. Topical aloe is used for sunburn and mild burns; it causes GI cramping and hypokalemia if ingested.

NUTRITION EDUCATION, COUNSELING, CARE MANAGEMENT

- Encourage the patient to read food, medication, and supplement labels. A symptom and food diary may be quite useful to identify any relationship between diet, allergies, and skin flare-ups.
- Encourage adequate fluid intake. Hydration of the skin is important. Drinking green tea can be highly recommended.
- Help the patient modify his or her diet as specifically indicated by the condition.
- Discuss the roles of nutrients in skin care. Sunscreens may prevent vitamin D from penetrating the skin, especially formulas with higher protective factors. Therefore, if dietary intakes are low in vitamin D, a supplement may be needed. Protein, vitamin A, and zinc are also important nutrients for healthy skin; describe good sources.
- Discuss the effect of EFAs on membrane function and how to include them in the diet. Omega-3 fatty acids reduce inflammation for some skin conditions. Eskimo skin care products, containing natural stable fish oil, is quite beneficial for improving skin elasticity (Segger et al, 2008). Otherwise, avoid topical products, except as recommended by the doctor.
- Flavones in medicinal plants, some vegetables and spices, have natural anti-oxidant with cytoprotective properties. Carrots, peppers, celery, olive oil, peppermint, rosemary and thyme contain natural levels of luteolin; more research is needed to identify its usefulness in medicine.

Patient Education—Food Safety

- The usual food safety habits are needed for good skin health. With open sores or exudative lesions on hands, a bandaid might be needed when preparing or serving food.

For More Information

- Acne Hotline
  http://www.niams.nih.gov/hi/topics/acne/acne.htm
- Acne Resources
  http://www.acne-resource.org/
- American Academy of Dermatology
  http://www.aad.org/
- Dystrophic Epidermolysis Bullosa Research Association of America
  http://www.debra.org/
- National Eczema Association
  http://www.nationaleczema.org/home.html
- National Psoriasis Foundation
  http://www.psoriasis.org/
- National Quality Measures Clearinghouse
  http://www.qualitymeasures.ahrq.gov/
- National Rosacea Society
  http://www.rosacea.org/
- NIH—Dermatitis
  http://www.niams.nih.gov/hi/topics/dermatitis/
- NIH—Eczema
  http://www.nlm.nih.gov/medlineplus/eczema.html

SKIN DISORDERS—CITED REFERENCES

Ahmad N, Mukhtar H. Cytochrome p450: a target for drug development for skin diseases. *J Invest Dermatol.* 123:417, 2004.

Antico A, Soana R. Chronic allergic-like dermatopathies in nickel-sensitive patients. Results of dietary restrictions and challenge with nickel salts. *Allergy Asthma Proc.* 20:235, 1999.

Arbesman H. Dairy and acne—the iodine connection. *J Am Acad Dermatol.* 53:1102, 2005.

Boelsma E, et al. Nutritional skin care: health effects of micronutrients and fatty acids (review). *Am J Clin Nutr.* 73:853, 2001.

Christensen JM, et al. Nickel concentrations in serum and urine of patients with nickel eczema. *Toxicol Lett.* 108:185, 1999.

Cordain L, et al. Acne vulgaris: a disease of Western civilization. *Arch Dermatol.* 138:1584, 2002.

Das U. Essential fatty acids in health and disease. *J Assoc Physicians India.* 47:906, 1999.

Garner LA. Contact dermatitis to metals. *Dermatol Ther.* 17:321, 2004.

Greenwald P. From carcinogenesis to clinical interventions for cancer prevention. *Toxicology* 166:37, 2001.

Hoare C, et al. Systematic review of treatments for atopic eczema. *Health Technol Assess.* 4:1, 2000.

Karpati S. Dermatitis herpetiformis: close to unravelling a disease. *J Dermatol Sci.* 34:83, 2004.

Koh KJ, et al. Tea tree oil reduces histamine-induced skin inflammation. *Br J Dermatol.* 147:1212, 2002.

Kumar V, et al. Tissue transglutaminase and endomysial antibodies-diagnostic markers of gluten-sensitive enteropathy in dermatitis herpetiformis. *Clin Immunol.* 98:378, 2001.

Lehmann B, et al. Vitamin D and skin: new aspects for dermatology. *Exp Dermatol.* 13:11S, 2004.

Liao S. The medicinal action of androgens and green tea epigallocatechin gallate. *Hong Kong Med J.* 7:369, 2001.

Litt J. Rosacea: how to recognize and treat an age-related skin disease. *Geriatrics* 52:39, 1997.

Martin KW, Ernst E. Herbal medicines for treatment of bacterial infections: a review of controlled clinical trials. *J Antimicrob Chemother.* 51:241, 2003.

Matsuda K, et al. Adrenocortical function in patients with severe atopic dermatitis. *Ann Allergy Asthma Immunol.* 85:35, 2000.

May E, et al. Immunoregulation through 1,25-dihydroxyvitamin D_3 and its analogs. *Curr Drug Targets Inflamm Allergy.* 3:377, 2004.

Millen AE, et al. Diet and melanoma in a case-control study. *Cancer Epidemiol Biomarkers Prev.* 13:1042, 2004.

Ricardo RR, et al. Clinical benefits in patients with psoriasis after efalizumab therapy: clinical trials versus practice. *Cutis.* 74:193, 2004.

Roberts RL, et al. Lutein and zeaxanthin in eye and skin health. *Clin Dermatol.* 27:195, 2009.

Segger D, et al. Supplementation with Eskimo Skin Care improves skin elasticity in women. A pilot study. *J Dermatolog Treat.* 19:279, 2008.

Woo WK, McKenna KE. Iatrogenic adrenal gland suppression from use of a potent topical steroid. *Clin Exp Dermatol.* 28:672, 2003.

Zouboulis C. Human skin: an independent peripheral endocrine organ. *Horm Res.* 54:230, 2000.

PRESSURE ULCERS

NUTRITIONAL ACUITY RANKING: LEVEL 2–3 (STAGES 1–2), LEVEL 4 (STAGES 3–4)

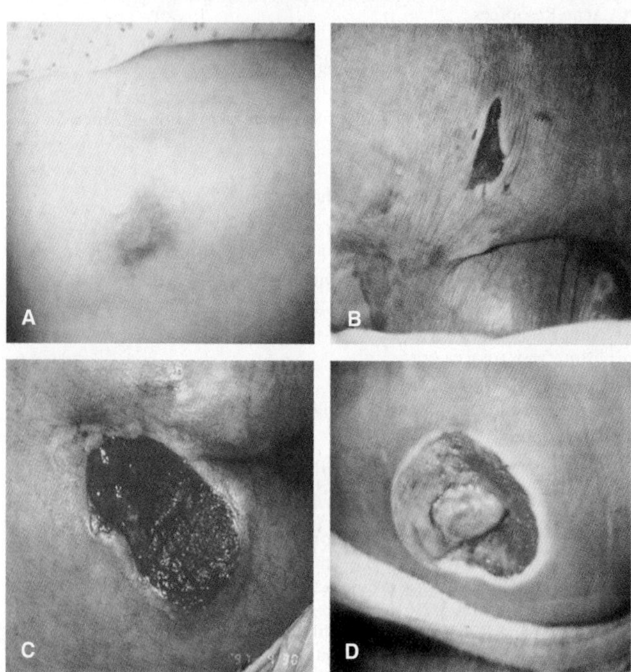

A = stage 1 B = stage 2 C = stage 3 D = stage 4
Adapted from: Nettina, Sandra M., MSN, RN, CS, ANP, *The Lippincott Manual of Nursing Practice,* 7th ed. Lippincott, Williams & Wilkins, 2001.

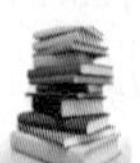

DEFINITIONS AND BACKGROUND

Pressure, friction, or shear and a lack of oxygen and nutrition to an affected area are associated with the development of pressure ulcers over bony or cartilaginous prominences (hip, sacrum, elbow, heels, back of the head). Pressure ulcers are common among patients with protein-energy malnutrition in HIV infection, pulmonary and cardiac cachexia, rheumatological cachexia, cancers, renal diseases, and among bedridden or paralyzed patients. With immobility, loss of lean body mass in muscle and skin, and lowered immunity, the risk of pressure ulcers increases by 74% (Harris and Fraser, 2004).

Many patients with pressure ulcers are below their usual body weight, have a low transthyretin level, and are not taking in enough nutrition to meet their needs (Guenter et al, 2000). Poor nutritional status and decreased oxygen perfusion are predictors of pressure ulcers; nutritional status and length of stay are predictors of ulcer severity in institutions (Williams et al, 2000). Patients with malnutrition are at risk for many complications, including incidence, progression, and severity of pressure ulcers. Risk factors should be assessed frequently: unintentional weight loss, incontinence, immobility, poor circulation (as in diabetes, peripheral vascular disease, or anemia), infection, prolonged pressure, multiple medications, serum albumin <3.4 g/dL, reduced functional ability, poor oral intake (<50% of meals over 3 days or longer), chewing or swallowing problems, and Chol levels below 160 mg/dL.

The mini-nutritional assessment (MNA) is a useful tool, with better results than using albumin levels or visceral proteins alone (Langkamp-Henken et al, 2005). Causes of malnutrition that should be carefully monitored include (Harris and Fraser, 2004): decreased appetite, requirement of assistance with meal intake, impaired cognition and/or communication, poor positioning, frequent acute illnesses with GI losses, medications that decrease appetite or increase nutrient losses, polypharmacy, decreased thirst response, decreased ability to concentrate urine, intentional fluid restriction because of fear of incontinence, fear of choking with dysphagia, isolation or depression, monotony of diet, and higher nutrient requirements. Reversible protein-energy malnutrition should be treated. A "MEALS ON WHEELS" mnemonic helps in identifying individuals at risk (Morley and Thomas, 2004): **M**edications—**E**motional problems—**A**norexia/alcoholism—**L**ate-life paranoia—**S**wallowing disorders—**O**ral problems—**N**osocomial infections—**W**andering/other dementia behaviors—**H**yperthyroidism or hypercalcemia—**E**nteric problems—**E**ating problems—**L**ow-salt, low-Chol diets—**S**tones (cholelithiasis).

Wound healing is complex and has three distinct phases. In each phase of wound healing, energy and macronutrients are required. Studies have established specific roles for nutrients including arginine; vitamins A, B, and C; selenium, manganese, zinc, and copper (Mathus-Vliegen, 2004). Administration of nutrition is an important part of wound healing.

Medicare costs attributable to pressure ulcer treatment are over $2 billion annually. The cost of caring for these preventable pressure ulcers is over $60,000 per patient (Edlich et al, 2004) and affects 10% of hospital admissions (Harris and Fraser, 2004). Pain, amputations, and osteomyelitis may result; mortality is often secondary to sepsis (Brem et al, 2003). In most cases, it is difficult to determine whether a pressure ulcer led to the terminal event, or whether the process of dying (decreased cardiac output, severe catabolic state) led to an unpreventable pressure ulcer (Braden, 1996).

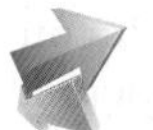

ASSESSMENT, MONITORING, AND EVALUATION

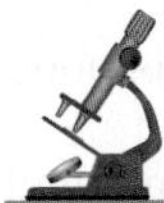

CLINICAL INDICATORS

Clinical/History

Height
Weight
Weight changes
BMI
BP
Diet history
Number, size and stage of ulcer(s)—see Table 2-8
Exudate, infection or sepsis, fever
Pain
Abnormal motor coordination
Changes in appetite, anorexia, indigestion
Nausea/vomiting
Diarrhea, bowel incontinence
Urinary tract infections or incontinence
Recent or frequent surgeries
Prognostic Inflammatory and Nutritional Index (PINI)
Braden scale: intense or prolonged pressure (activity, mobility, sensory perception) and tissue tolerance for pressure (nutrition, moisture, friction, and shear); scores range from 6 to 23, lower scores suggest higher risk
Norton scale: physical condition, mental status, activity, mobility, and incontinence; rating >16 suggests high risk

Lab Work

Gluc
C-reactive protein
Serum Chol
BUN, Creat
Serum Na^+, K^+
Ca^{++}, Mg^{++}
H & H, serum Fe, serum ferritin
Alb, transthyretin, RBP (usually decreased)
N balance, transferrin
Total lymphocyte count (TLC)
Protime or INR
Serum zinc
Serum B_{12}

TABLE 2-8 **Skin Changes with Aging and Pressure Ulcer Stages**

Skin Change	Consequences
Thinning of epidermis	Increased vulnerability to trauma and skin tears
Decreased epidermal proliferation	Slower production of new skin cells
Atrophy of dermis	Underlying tissue more vulnerable to injury; decreased wound contraction
Decreased vascularity of dermis	Easy bruising and injury; decreased wound capillary growth
Compromised vascular response	Impaired immune and inflammatory responses
Fragility	Easy bruising and tearing
Suspected deep tissue injury	Purple or maroon localized area of discolored intact skin or blood-filled blister due to damage of underlying soft tissue from pressure and/or shear. The area may be preceded by tissue that is painful, firm, mushy, boggy, warmer or cooler as compared to adjacent tissue

*Staging**

Stage I	Intact skin with nonblanchable redness of a localized area usually over a bony prominence. Darkly pigmented skin may not have visible blanching; its color may differ from the surrounding area. The area may be painful, firm, soft, warmer or cooler as compared to adjacent tissue. Stage I may be difficult to detect in individuals with dark skin tones. May indicate "at risk" persons (a heralding sign of risk)
Stage II	Partial thickness loss of dermis presenting as a shallow open ulcer with a red pink wound bed, without slough. May also present as an intact or open/ruptured serum-filled blister. Presents as a shiny or dry shallow ulcer without slough or bruising. This stage should not be used to describe skin tears, tape burns, perineal dermatitis, maceration or excoriation. Bruising indicates suspected deep tissue injury
Stage III	Full thickness tissue loss. Subcutaneous fat may be visible but bone, tendon or muscle are not exposed. Slough may be present but does not obscure the depth of tissue loss. May include undermining and tunneling The depth of a stage III pressure ulcer varies by anatomical location. The bridge of the nose, ear, occiput and malleolus do not have subcutaneous tissue and stage III ulcers can be shallow. In contrast, areas of significant adiposity can develop extremely deep stage III pressure ulcers. Bone/tendon is not visible or directly palpable
Stage IV	Full thickness tissue loss with exposed bone, tendon or muscle. Slough or eschar may be present on some parts of the wound bed. Often include undermining and tunneling. The depth of a stage IV pressure ulcer varies by anatomical location. The bridge of the nose, ear, occiput and malleolus do not have subcutaneous tissue and these ulcers can be shallow. Stage IV ulcers can extend into muscle and/or supporting structures (e.g., fascia, tendon or joint capsule) making osteomyelitis possible. Exposed bone/tendon is visible or directly palpable
Unstageable	Full thickness tissue loss in which the base of the ulcer is covered by slough (yellow, tan, gray, green or brown) and/or eschar (tan, brown or black) in the wound bed. Until enough slough and/or eschar is removed to expose the base of the wound, the true depth, and therefore stage, cannot be determined. Stable (dry, adherent, intact without erythema or fluctuance) eschar on the heels serves as "the body's natural (biological) cover" and should not be removed

*Adapted from: National Pressure Ulcer Advisory Panel, 2007 staging. Web site accessed April 1, 2009, at http://www.npuap.org/.

SAMPLE NUTRITION CARE PROCESS STEPS

Pressure Ulcer

Assessment Data: Food intake records, weight records, need for enteral nutrition or feeding assistance, pressure ulcer team reports, other nutritional evaluations and risk measures. Check that Nursing is turning and repositioning every 2 hours and offering fluids.

Nutrition Diagnosis: Inadequate protein intake related to poor appetite and intake as evidenced by new stage 2 and stage 4 sacral pressure ulcers this past month with intake records showing limited protein consumption from milk, eggs, cheese and entrees; poor nutritional lab values (H & H, transthyretin) and elevated CRP.

Intervention: Education of patient, staff, or family members about the role of nutrition in wound healing. Counseling about acceptable sources of protein and enhancing menu items with protein powders or liquid supplements. Encourage use of oral supplements with medication passes; adequate fluid intake calculated as 30 mL/kg. Careful calculation of fluid, protein, and energy requirements according to stage of ulcers; recalculate as needed if healing does not occur. Micronutrient provision with vitamin–mineral supplement meeting 100% DRIs and RDA levels for zinc, copper, vitamins A and C.

Monitoring and Evaluation: Healing of pressure ulcers by 14 days after initiation of treatment; improved intake of protein foods to meet higher needs. Greater understanding by patient, family, or staff about the importance of nutrient-dense foods or formulas. Intake and output records indicating sufficient protein and energy intake. Labs improving for H & H, albumin, CRP.

INTERVENTION

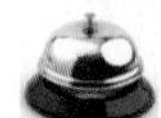

OBJECTIVES

- Restore to a healthy nutritional status. Correct protein-energy malnutrition; this is of paramount importance.
- Monitor risk assessments. Nutrition risks evaluate the person's usual food intake pattern; intake of 3–5 days can be useful.
- Improve low-grade infections, fever, diarrhea, and vomiting. Support the patient's immune system to prevent sepsis.
- Heal the pressure ulcer(s) and prevent further tissue breakdown. Assess healing using an appropriate scale, such as the PUSH scale from the National Pressure Ulcer Advisory Panel at http://www.npuap.org/PDF/push3.pdf.

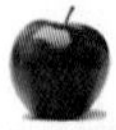

FOOD AND NUTRITION

- Provide a high-quality protein diet (Mathus-Vliegen, 2004). The guidelines for the treatment of pressure ulcers (2006) recommend 1.0–1.5 g protein/kg body weight. A deep ulcer or multiple sites may require 1.5–2 g/kg. It may be necessary to add protein powders to beverages, casseroles, tube feedings, and liquid supplements to get the adequate amount. Intake of protein greater than 2 g/kg of body weight may not be metabolized to increase protein synthesis.
- Recommended calorie levels for wound healing vary from 25 to 35 kcal/kg body weight; use lower levels for obese patients and higher levels for underweight patients. Whether or not pressure ulcers are preventable is controversial, but removing nutritional deficits is essential (Thomas, 2006).
- Provide small, frequent feedings if oral intake is poor, four to six times daily.
- Supplement diet with a general multivitamin–mineral supplement to supply adequate B vitamins, vitamin A, vitamin C, zinc, and copper; excesses are wasteful, do not necessarily speed the healing process, and may harm the immune system.
- A concentrated, fortified, collagen protein hydrolysate supplement may be of benefit to residents of long-term care facilities who have pressure ulcers (Lee et al, 2006).
- Feed by tube if necessary. With a large sacral pressure ulcer, central parenteral nutrition (CPN) may be the only way to feed if bowel incontinence is present; avoid. EFA deficiencies by including at least 2% of calories from lipid.
- Follow the algorithm given on page 117.

Common Drugs Used and Potential Side Effects

- Monitor the drug profile for potential side effects, especially for depletion of serum proteins or blood-forming nutrients. Drugs that can affect skin include antibacterials, antihypertensives, analgesics, tricyclic antidepressants, antihistamines, antineoplastic agents, antipsychotic agents, corticosteroids, diuretics, and hypoglycemic agents. Antibiotics may be needed in bacterial sepsis.
- Recommend, if needed, an appetite stimulant. Unintentional weight loss may be corrected by using dronabinol or cannabinoids (Marinol); megestrol acetate (Megace); oxymetholone.

Herbs, Botanicals, and Supplements

- Herbs and botanicals may be used; identify and monitor side effects and potential drug interactions.
- Counsel about use of herbal teas, especially regarding ingredients that may be toxic or ineffective.

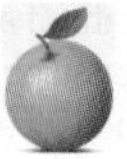

NUTRITION EDUCATION, COUNSELING, CARE MANAGEMENT

- Instruct nursing personnel and patient's family about the importance of adequate nutrition for healing of tissues.
- Discuss importance of maintaining healthy, intact skin. Skin should be kept clean and dry; avoid massage over bony prominences.
- Provide information about high-protein diets, and appropriate calorie and fluid levels.
- Where possible, improve ambulation and circulation to all tissues. Physical activity can help improve appetite.
- Discuss the role of nutrition in wound healing: collagen and fibroblasts require protein, zinc, and vitamin C for proper formation; adequate vitamins A and K, B-complex vitamins for healthy nerves and muscles.
- Discuss degree of assistance needed at mealtimes and provide ideas for self-help devices to increase overall intake (wet cloth under plate, curved flatware, two-handled cup, other adaptive equipment if needed.

INTERDISCIPLINARY NUTRITION CARE PLAN

Pressure Ulcer

Client Name: ______________________ **#:** __________ **Initiated by:** __________ **Date:** __________

SCREEN
Nutrition Screen diagnosis: Pressure Ulcer
Signed: ______________ Date: ________

GOALS (Check any/all):

❑ Maintain or improve nutritional status in ____ (goal time).

❑ Correct causes of involuntary weight loss where possible in ____ (goal time).

❑ Maintain or improve hydration status to prevent dehydration in ____ (goal time).

Weight ❑ maintained, or ❑ loss / ❑ gain of ______lb in ____ (goal time).

❑ Support pressure ulcer healing in ____ (goal time).

ASSESS *(Check any/all)*
- ❑ **Multiple pressure ulcers**
- ❑ **Stage III or IV pressure ulcer**
- ❑ **Receiving enteral or parenteral nutrition support**

Weight/BMI
- ❑ Weight change >3 lb/wk, >5%/mo, or >10%/6 mo
- ❑ BMI <20
- ❑ BMI >27

❑ **Infection (UTI, URI)**

Poor Oral Intake Symptoms
- ❑ Complex diet order
- ❑ Nausea/vomiting
- ❑ Poor appetite/early satiety
- ❑ Problems chewing/swallowing
- ❑ Depression/anxiety
- ❑ GI distress

Signed: ______________ Date: ________

None →

MODERATE RISK INTERVENTIONS
(Check any/all)
- ❑ **Power packing your diet** provided and explained
- ❑ **Food record** provided and explained
- ❑ **Fluid intake encouraged**
- ❑ **Wound care explained**

Obtain Dr. orders as needed:
- ❑ RD chart consult
- ❑ Monitor weight q:_____
- ❑ Multiple vitamin/mineral supplement
- ❑ BID/TID supplements

❑ **Other:**______________
(See notes for documention.)

Signed: ______________ Date: ________

Next visit ↓

ASSESS RESPONSE *(Check any/all)*
- ❑ Weight change not appropriate per goal
- ❑ Dehydration
- ❑ Development of Stage III or IV pressure ulcer
- ❑ Development of multiple pressure ulcers
- ❑ Onset of new infection
- ❑ Exhibiting poor oral intake symptoms
- ❑ **Other:**______________
(See notes for documention.)

Signed: ______________ Date: ________

None →

OUTCOMES ACHIEVED
- ❑ Pressure ulcers improved
- ❑ Weight Maintained or improved
- ❑ Hydration status maintained or improved
- ❑ Development of multiple pressure ulcers
- ❑ **Other:**______________
(See notes for documentation.)
- ❑ Repeat Nutrition Risk Screen in ____ days

Signed: ______________ Date: ________

← 1 or more

1 or more ↓

HIGH-RISK INTERVENTIONS *(Check any/all)*
- ❑ **Power packing your diet** provided and explained
- ❑ **Food record** provided and explained
- ❑ **Fluid intake stressed**

Obtain Dr. orders as needed:
- ❑ RD referral for home visit(s)
- ❑ Monitor weight q:_____
- ❑ Monitor I & O q: _____
- ❑ Multiple vitamin/mineral supplement
- ❑ BID/TID supplements
- ❑ Tube feeding

❑ **Other:**______________
(See notes for documentation.)

Signed: ______________ Date: ________

Next visit ↓

ASSESS RESPONSE *(Check any/all)*
- ❑ Stage III or IV pressure ulcer
- ❑ Multiple pressure ulcers
- ❑ Weight change not appropriate per goal
- ❑ Infection worsened
- ❑ Continued dehydration
- ❑ Continued Poor Oral Intake Symptoms
- ❑ **Other:**______________
(See notes for documention.)

Signed: ______________ Date: ________

None →

OUTCOMES ACHIEVED
- ❑ Pressure ulcers improved
- ❑ Weight Maintained or improved
- ❑ Hydration status maintained or improved
- ❑ Development of multiple pressure ulcers
- ❑ **Other:**______________
(See notes for documention.)
- ❑ Repeat Nutrition Risk Screen in ____ days

Signed: ______________ Date: ________

1 or more ↓

OUTCOMES NOT ACHIEVED
Reassess/evaluate need for EN/PN (refer to Tube Feeding Nutrition Care Plan). Document on Nutrition Variance Tracking form.

Adapted with permission from www.RD411.com, Inc.

Patient Education—Food Safety

- Hand washing will be important for patients, caretakers, and nurses before and after meals.

For More Information

- Agency for Healthcare Research and Quality
  http://www.ahrq.gov/consumer/bodysys/edbody6.htm
- Centers for Medicare and Medicaid Services
  http://www.cms.hhs.gov/
- European Pressure Ulcer Advisory PanelNutrition Guidelines
  http://www.epuap.org/guidelines/english1.html
- National Pressure Ulcer Advisory Panel
  http://www.npuap.org/
- Wound Care Network
  http://www.woundcarenet.com/index.html

PRESSURE ULCERS—CITED REFERENCES

Braden B. Using the Braden scale for predicting pressure sore risk. *Support Line.* XVIII:14, 1996.

Edlich RF, et al. Pressure ulcer prevention. *J Long Term Eff Med Implants.* 14:285, 2004.

Guenter P, et al. Survey of nutritional status in newly hospitalized patients with stage III or stage IV pressure ulcers. *Adv Skin Wound Care.* 13:164, 2000.

Harris CL, Fraser C. Malnutrition in the institutionalized elderly: the effects on wound healing. *Ostomy Wound Manage.* 50:54, 2004.

Langkamp-Henken B, et al. Mini nutritional assessment and screening scores are associated with nutritional indicators in elderly people with pressure ulcers. *J Am Diet Assoc.* 105:1590, 2005.

Lee SK, et al. Pressure ulcer healing with a concentrated, fortified, collagen protein hydrolysate supplement: a randomized controlled trial. *Adv Skin Wound Care.* 19:92, 2006.

Mathus-Vliegen EM. Old age, malnutrition, and pressure sores: an ill-fated alliance. *J Gerontol A Biol Sci Med Sci.* 59:355, 2004.

Morley JE, Thomas DR. Update: guidelines for the use of oregigenic drugs in long-term care. *Supplement to the Annals of Long-Term Care.* St. Louis: St. Louis University, 2004.

Thomas DR. Prevention and treatment of pressure ulcers. *J Am Med Dir Assoc.* 7:46, 2006.

Williams D, et al. Patients with existing pressure ulcers admitted to acute care. *J Wound Ostomy Continence Nurs.* 27:216, 2000.

VITAMIN DEFICIENCIES

NUTRITIONAL ACUITY RANKING: LEVEL 3

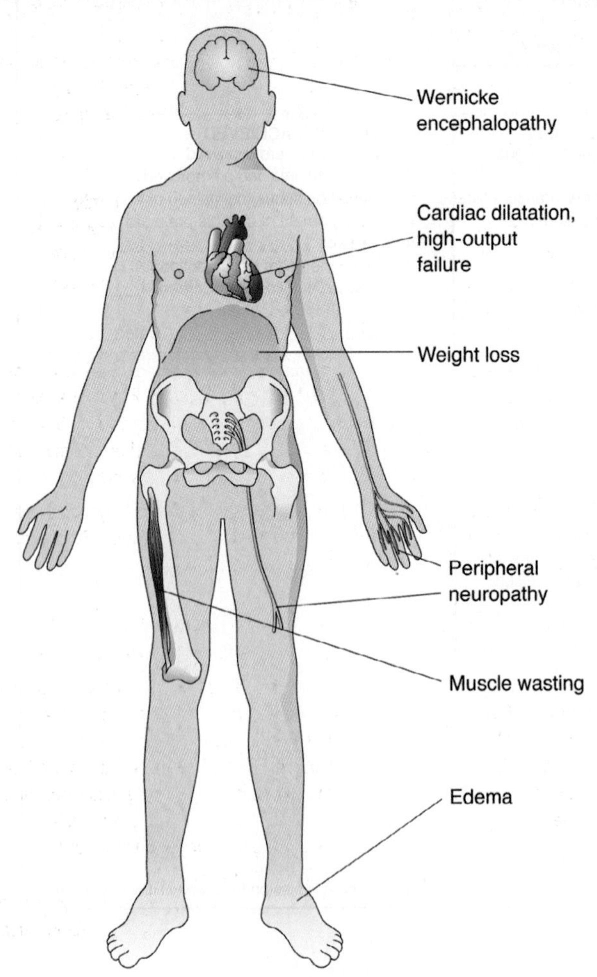

Adapted from: Rubin E MD and Farber JL MD. *Pathology,* 3rd ed. Philadelphia: Lippincott Williams & Wilkins, 1999.

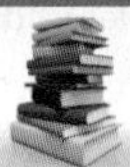

DEFINITIONS AND BACKGROUND

Vitamins are a part of a healthy diet. If a person eats a variety of foods, deficiency is less likely. However, people who follow restricted diets may not get enough of one or more particular nutrients. Deficiencies may be primary (self-induced by inadequate diet) or secondary to disease process. They are especially common in alcoholics, people who live alone and eat poorly, and among those who follow restrictive food fads. Vegetarians are also susceptible, especially for vitamin B_{12} deficiency. Appendix A provides greater detail about the vitamins, their sources, toxicities, and deficiencies. Table 2-9 summarizes concerns and physical signs of deficiency.

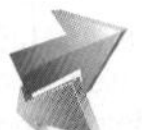

ASSESSMENT, MONITORING, AND EVALUATION

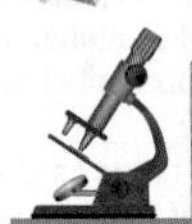

CLINICAL INDICATORS

Clinical/History

Height
Weight
BMI
Diet history
Neurological, hepatic or renal changes
Physical signs of malnutrition (see Table 2-9 and Appendix A)

Lab Work

Vitamin A—serum retinol <0.35 mmol/L
Vitamin C—plasma concentrations <0.2 mg/dL
Vitamin D—25-OHD values <25 nmol/L
Vitamin E—plasma alpha-tocopherol <18 μmol/g

TABLE 2-9 Vitamin Deficiency Summary

Vitamin	Issues	Physical Signs
Vitamin A	Common in children. Night blindness and eye changes are often early signs. Many infections (such as measles) may cause deficiency. Vitamin A helps form and maintain healthy teeth, mucous membranes, skeletal and soft tissues, and skin. Retinol generates the pigments in the retina. Vitamin A promotes good vision (especially in dim light) and is required for healthy reproduction and lactation. Because beta-carotene is a precursor for vitamin A and because so many carotenoids play a role in maintaining good health, deficiencies of these phytochemicals may play an even larger role in maintaining vitamin A adequacy in the body.	Night blindness, Bitot's spots, xerophthalmia, follicular hyperkeratosis Reduced growth, changes in epithelial tissue, failure of tooth enamel and/or degeneration, loss of taste and smell.
Thiamin	Common in alcoholics, patients with heart failure, and persons with poor-quality diets. Thiamin helps convert carbohydrate (CHO) into energy; a high-CHO diet can deplete thiamin. It is also important for proper functioning of the heart, nervous system, and muscles.	Impairment of cardiovascular, nervous, and gastrointestinal systems.
Niacin and riboflavin	Often in conjunction with other B-complex vitamin deficiencies. Riboflavin (B_2) is important for growth, red cell production, and releasing energy from carbohydrates. Niacin assists in the functioning of the digestive system, skin, and nerves; it is important in the conversion of food to energy. A deficient diet or failure of the body to absorb niacin or tryptophan can cause signs of deficiency or pellagra. It is common in certain parts of the world where people consume large quantities of corn and is characterized by dermatitis, diarrhea, and schizophrenia-like dementia. It sometimes develops after gastrointestinal diseases or among alcoholics.	Niacin: Symmetrical, pigmented rash on areas exposed to sunlight, bright red tongue, Dermatitis, diarrhea, depression, and (sometimes) death (the 4 Ds). Riboflavin: Sore throat, hyperemia, edema of pharyngeal and oral mucous membranes, cheilosis, angular stomatitis, glossitis, seborrheic dermatitis, and normochromic, normocytic anemia. Magenta tongue.
Vitamin B_6	Can occur after surgery or as a result of poor diet. Vitamin B_6 deficiency has role in cardiac disorders (atrial fibrillation, hyperhomocysteinemia) and inflammation (Friso et al, 2004) and in dopamine release in the brain. Because vitamin B_6 plays a role in the synthesis of antibodies and red blood cells, a healthy immune system and circulatory system depend on it. The higher the protein intake, the more need there is for vitamin B_6; a high protein–low CHO diet may deplete vitamin B_6.	Seborrheic dermatitis, stomatitis, cheilosis, glossitis, confusion, depression. Convulsions or intractable seizures in infants and young children (Gospe, 2006); anemias; nerve and skin disorders.
Folic acid	May result in a megaloblastic anemia; supplementation is needed (see Section 12). Folic acid acts as a coenzyme with vitamins C and B_{12} in the metabolism and synthesis of proteins. It is needed to make red blood cells, to synthesize DNA, and to support tissue growth and cell function. There are roles for folic acid in disease prevention (e.g., neural tube defects, cancers, heart disease).	Depapillation of the tongue, rarely. Pregnancy-induced anemias; neural tube defects (Tamura and Picciano, 2006). Cardiovascular disease with elevated homocysteine levels.
Vitamin B_{12}	May also result in megaloblastic anemia (see Section 12 on anemias). Peripheral neuropathy and a positive Schilling test are needed to indicate B_{12} deficiency. Folic acid supplementation may mask a B_{12} deficiency; both should be given.	Tingling and numbness in extremities, diminished vibratory and position sense, motor disturbances including gait disturbances. Pernicious anemia and other anemias; poor vision; some psychiatric symptoms.
Pantothenic acid and biotin	Not common. Pantothenic acid is essential for metabolism and in the synthesis of hormones and cholesterol. Biotin is essential for metabolism of proteins and carbohydrate and the synthesis of hormones and cholesterol.	*Pantothenic acid:* No visible physical signs of note *Biotin*. Inflammation of the lips and skin.
Choline	May occur in long-term TPN use without lipid replacement. Plays a role in preventing neural tube defects along with folic acid.	No visible physical signs of note. Liver damage and altered DNA function.
Vitamin C	Occurs overtly with scurvy after 3 months without intake from inadequate consumption of fresh fruits and vegetables. Hypovitaminosis C can occur in the elderly and the homeless, among those who live alone or have psychiatric diseases, and in those who follow food fads. It is more common than realized in the general population. Long-term deficiency can be a concern for people with cancer or cataracts.	Follicular hyperkeratosis, petechiae, ecchymosis, coiled hairs, inflamed and bleeding gums, perifollicular hemorrhages, joint effusions, arthralgia, delayed wound healing. Weakness, myalgia, vascular purpura, loss of teeth. Biological signs include anemia, hypocholesterolemia, and hypoalbuminemia.

(continued)

TABLE 2-9 **Vitamin Deficiency Summary *(continued)***

Vitamin	Issues	Physical Signs
Vitamin D	Insufficiency is a low threshold value for plasma 25-OHD (50 nmol/L). Secondary hyperparathyroidism, increased bone turnover, bone mineral loss, and seasonal variations in plasma PTH can occur with insufficiency. Deficiency is defined as 25-OHD values below 25 nmol/L; common among community-dwelling elderly who live in higher latitudes and among institutionalized elderly and patients with hip fractures. Vitamin D is produced in the skin by exposure to the sun and is found in fortified milk and other foods. For individuals who are not getting enough vitamin D in the diet, supplements may be helpful. The average adult under 50 needs 200 IU of vitamin D a day; 1 cup of vitamin D-fortified milk provides 50 IU of vitamin D (Surgeon General's Report, 2004). Recent studies suggest a role for vitamin D in autoimmune disorders, including multiple sclerosis (Mark and Carson, 2006); ovarian cancer (Zhang et al, 2006); type 1 diabetes or hypertension (Holick, 2006).	Widening at ends of long bones, rachitic rosary in children, rickets. Abnormal bone growth and repair; osteomalacia in adults; muscle spasms. Decreased immunity (Villamor, 2006).
Vitamin E	It is an antioxidant, protects body tissue from the damage of oxidation, helps form red blood cells, and supports the use of vitamin K. Abetalipoproteinemia is the most severe deficiency and occurs mainly in premature and sick children. Fat malabsorption occurs in deficiency, especially in children.	Rupture of red blood cells; nerve damage.
Vitamin K	Rare except in intestinal problems and short gut syndromes because intestinal bacteria in the healthy gut can make vitamin K. Healthy bones require sufficient vitamin K.	Poor wound healing or blood clotting. Osteopenia (Duggan et al, 2004).

Vitamin K—elevated prothrombin time, altered INR
Thiamin—erythrocyte transketolase activity >1.20 µg/mL/h; AST is often decreased
Riboflavin—erythrocyte glutathione reductase >1.2 IU/mg hemoglobin
Niacin—*N*-methyl-nicotinamide excretion <5.8 µmol/d
Vitamin B_6—plasma pyridoxal 5′phosphate <20 nmol/L
Vitamin B_{12}—serum concentration <180 pmol/L; elevated tHcy
Folic acid—serum concentration <7 nmol/L; red cell folate <315 nmol/L
Choline—plasma choline and phosphatidylcholine concentrations fall when humans are fed a choline-deficient diet, but otherwise there are no definitive tests; abnormal liver function tests may occur

INTERVENTION

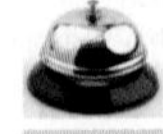

OBJECTIVES

- Replenish the deficient nutrient and restore normal serum levels.
- Prevent or correct signs, symptoms, and effects of nutrient deficiency. For example, reduced immunity and high maternal and child mortality occur in populations with poor intakes of vitamin A (Cox et al, 2006). Vitamin D deficiency can lead to increased incidence of hip fracture (Cauley et al, 2008).

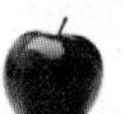

FOOD AND NUTRITION

- **Vitamin A deficiency.** Use a diet including foods high in vitamin A and carotene: carrots, sweet potatoes, squash, apricots, collards, broccoli, cabbage, dark leafy greens, liver, kidney, cream, butter, and egg yolk.
- **B-Complex vitamins:**
- **Thiamin deficiency** (beri-beri). Use a diet including foods high in thiamin: pork, whole grains, enriched

SAMPLE NUTRITION CARE PROCESS STEPS

Vitamin A Deficiency

Assessment Data: Food intake records, physical signs of deficiency, frequent bouts of infectious illnesses.

Nutrition Diagnosis: Inadequate vitamin A intake related to poor appetite and intake as evidenced by prolonged recovery after measles, recent onset of night blindness, serum retinol <0.35 mmol/L, complaints of lethargy and frequent illnesses.

Intervention: Education of patient, staff, or family members about the role of vitamin A for healthy immunity and vision. Counseling about good sources of vitamin A and carotenoids. Micronutrient provision meeting 100% DRI for vitamin A.

Monitoring and Evaluation: Total recovery after measles. Improvement in vision. Labs improving for retinol. Fewer infectious illnesses, colds, flu, etc. Improved quality of life.

cereal grains, nuts, potatoes, legumes, green vegetables, fish, meat, fruit, and milk in quantity. A high-protein/high-carbohydrate intake should be included.

- **Riboflavin deficiency.** Use a diet including foods high in riboflavin: milk, eggs, liver, kidney, and heart. Caution against losses resulting from cooking and exposure to sunlight.
- **Niacin deficiency or pellagra.** Use a diet including foods high in niacin and other B vitamins: yeast, milk, meat, peanuts, cereal bran, and wheat germ.
- **Folic acid deficiency.** Use fresh, leafy green vegetables, oranges and orange juice, liver, other organ meats, and dried yeast.
- **Vitamin B_6 deficiency.** Use dried yeast, liver, organ meats, whole-grain cereals, fish, and legumes.
- **Vitamin B_{12} deficiency.** Use liver, beef, pork, organ meats, eggs, milk, and dairy products.
- **Biotin deficiency.** Use liver, kidney, egg yolks, yeast, cauliflower, nuts, and legumes.
- **Pantothenic acid deficiency.** Use live yeast and vegetables.
- **Choline.** Include eggs, liver, beef, milk, oatmeal, soybeans, peanuts, and iceberg lettuce.
- **Vitamin C deficiency or scurvy.** Use a diet high in citrus fruits, tomatoes, strawberries, green peppers, cantaloupe, and baked potatoes.
- **Vitamin D deficiency.** Use fortified milk, fish liver oils, and egg yolks. Expose skin to sunlight if possible.
- **Vitamin E deficiency.** Use vegetable oil, wheat germ, leafy vegetables, egg yolks, margarine, and legumes.
- **Vitamin K deficiency.** Use a diet high in leafy vegetables, pork, liver, and vegetable oils.

Common Drugs Used and Potential Side Effects or Toxicity

Note: The DRI "tolerable upper intake levels" (UL) address the toxic side.

- **Vitamin A.** Absorption of vitamin A depends on bile salts in the intestinal tract. Controlled high doses may be prescribed for a short period of time. Beware of doses greater than the recommended upper limit per day for a long time, especially for children.
- **Thiamin.** A common dose is 5–10 mg/d of thiamin; anorexia and nausea may be common at the beginning of treatment. Intravenous therapy may be better tolerated.
- **Riboflavin.** Achlorhydria may precipitate a deficiency and may preclude successful correction. Alkaline substances destroy riboflavin.
- **Niacin.** Treatment with niacin may cause flushing. Niacinamide is a better choice; 200–400 mg of niacin or niacin equivalents may be used for a short time. Nicotinic acid can cause nausea, vomiting, and diarrhea.
- **Vitamin B_6.** Pyridoxine hydrochloride is the common content.
- **Pantothenic acid.** Pantholin is a drug that is prescribed as needed.
- **Choline.** Choline hydrochloride salt may be degraded by intestinal bacteria and cause a fishy body odor. This does not occur when lecithin is eaten in the diet.
- **Vitamin C.** Excesses can cause false-positive glucosuria tests. Cevalin or Cevita are drug sources; 50–300 mg/d may be given to correct scurvy. Excesses may have an antihistamine effect or cause diarrhea.
- **Vitamin D.** Calderol, Rocaltrol, Hytakerol, and Calciferol are common drug sources. Be sure to use vitamin D_3 [25-hydroxyvitamin D (25-OHD)] for greater effectiveness.
- **Vitamin E.** Aquasol E has no adverse side effects if used within measured dosage for age and daily requirements.
- **Vitamin K.** Vitamin K is usually injected to correct deficiency rather than using diet alone. Synkayvite, Mephyton, and Konakion are trade names.

Herbs, Botanicals, and Supplements

- Herbs and botanicals may be used by many individuals; identify and monitor side effects.
- Counsel about use of herbal teas, especially regarding ingredients that may be toxic.

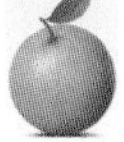

NUTRITION EDUCATION, COUNSELING, CARE MANAGEMENT

- Explain where sources of the specific nutrient may be found.
- Demonstrate methods of cooking, storage, etc., that prevent losses.
- Help the patient plan a menu incorporating his or her preferences.
- Discuss the use of vitamin and mineral supplements. Although they may be appropriate to correct a deficiency state, they may not be warranted for continuous or long-term use.

For More Information

- American Cancer Society—Vitamins http://www.cancer.org/docroot/eto/eto_5_2_5.asp
- Food and Nutrition Information Center http://www.nal.usda.gov/fnic/
- Medline Plus http://www.nlm.nih.gov/medlineplus/vitamins.html
- Merck Manual http://www.merck.com/mmpe/sec01/ch004/ch004a.html
- NIH Office of Dietary Supplements http://www.cc.nih.gov/ccc/supplements/intro.html
- Nutrient Data Laboratory http://www.ars.usda.gov/main/site_main.htm?modecode=12354500
- Nutrition Information http://www.nutrition.org/
- U.S. Department of Health and Human Services http://www.dhhs.gov/
- Vitamin Information Service http://www.vitamins-nutrition.org/

VITAMIN DEFICIENCIES—CITED REFERENCES

Cauley JA, et al. Serum 25-hydroxyvitamin D concentrations and risk for hip fractures. *Ann Intern Med.* 149:242, 2008.

Cox SE, et al. Vitamin A supplementation increases ratios of proinflammatory to anti-inflammatory cytokine responses in pregnancy and lactation. *Clin Exp Immunol.* 144:392 2006.

Duggan P, et al. Vitamin K status in patients with Crohn's disease and relationship to bone turnover. *Am J Gastroenterol.* 99:2178, 2004.

Friso S, et al. Low plasma vitamin B-6 concentrations and modulation of coronary artery disease risk. *Am J Clin Nutr.* 79:992, 2004.
Gospe SM. Pyridoxine-dependent seizures: new genetic and biochemical clues to help with diagnosis and treatment. *Curr Opin Neurol.* 19:148, 2006.
Holick MF. High prevalence of vitamin D inadequacy and implications for health. *Mayo Clin Proc.* 81:353, 2006.
Mark BL, Carson JA. Vitamin D and autoimmune disease—implications for practice from the multiple sclerosis literature. *J Am Diet Assoc.* 106:418, 2006.
Surgeon General's Report on Bone Health. By 2020, one in two Americans over age 50 will be at risk for fractures from osteoporosis or low bone mass. Available at http://www.hhs.gov/news/press/2004pres/20041014.html; 2004.
Tamura T, Picciano MF. Folate and human reproduction. *Am J Clin Nutr.* 83:993, 2006.
Villamor E. A potential role for vitamin D on HIV infection? *Nutr Rev.* 64:226, 2006.
Zhang X, et al. Vitamin D receptor is a novel drug target for ovarian cancer treatment. *Curr Cancer Drug Targets.* 6:229, 2006.

FOOD ALLERGY AND MÉNIÈRE'S SYNDROME

FOOD ALLERGY AND INTOLERANCES

NUTRITIONAL ACUITY RANKING: LEVEL 2–3 (SIMPLE); LEVEL 3–4 (COMPLEX)

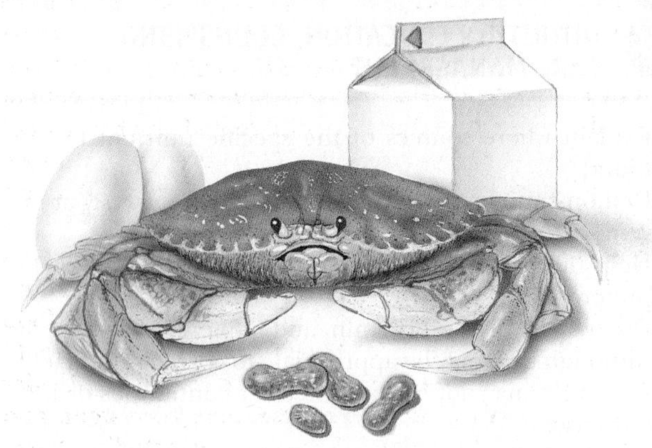

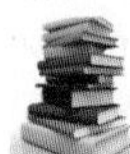

DEFINITIONS AND BACKGROUND

It is important to distinguish food allergies from intolerances caused by toxins or drugs and metabolic disorders such as lactase deficiency or celiac disease. People who have a tendency toward allergy may develop sensitivity to new foods at any time. The manifestations of allergy are caused by the release of histamine and serotonin.

Prevalence of food allergies in the United States is about 6 million people; worldwide, they affect 3.5–4% of all individuals (Taylor, 2008). Allergic tendencies are inherited but not necessarily to a specific antigen (i.e., a parent with a genetic predisposition to severe bee sting reactions could have a child with a bee sting allergy, food allergy, or other allergy). Immune deviation and disturbed gut motility occurs in children with multiple food allergies, along with a maternal history of autoimmunity (Latcham et al, 2003). It is now recognized that children who have a fever before age 1 are less likely to develop allergies by age 6–7 years, and exposure to pets such as dogs at an early age builds immunity.

The most common symptoms of food allergies affect the GI tract (GIT): diarrhea, nausea, vomiting, cramping, abdominal distention, and pain. GI allergic manifestations can be classified as immunoglobulin E-mediated; "mixed" GI allergy syndromes, involving some IgE components and some non-IgE or T cell–mediated components; or eosinophilic gastroenteritis (Garcia-Careaga and Kerner, 2005; Lee and Burks, 2009). **GI food allergies** include a spectrum of disorders that result from adverse immunologic responses to dietary antigens, as defined by the National Institute of Allergy and Infectious Diseases (NIAID) in 2010:

- **Immediate GI hypersensitivity** refers to an IgE-mediated FA in which upper GI symptoms may occur within minutes and lower GI symptoms may occur either immediately or with a delay of up to several hours. This is commonly seen as a manifestation of anaphylaxis. Among the GI conditions, acute immediate vomiting is the most common reaction and perhaps the one best documented as immunologic and IgE mediated.
  - **Eosinophilic esophagitis** (EoE) involves localized eosinophilic inflammation of the esophagus. While EoE is commonly associated with the presence of food-specific IgE, the precise causal role of FA in its etiology is not well defined. Both IgE- and non-IgE-mediated mechanisms seem to be involved.
  - **Eosinophilic gastroenteritis (EG)** also is both IgE- and non-IgE-mediated, and commonly linked to food allergies. EG symptoms vary depending on the portion of the GIT involved and a pathologic infiltration of the GIT by eosinophils that may be quite localized or very widespread.
  - **Dietary protein-induced proctitis/proctocolitis** typically presents in infants who seem generally healthy but have visible specks or streaks of blood mixed with mucus in the stool. [5]IgE to specific foods is generally absent.
  - **Food protein-induced enterocolitis syndrome** (FPIES) is another non-IgE-mediated disorder presenting in infancy with vomiting and diarrhea severe enough to cause dehydration and shock. Cow's milk and soy protein are the most common causes. It typically manifests in the first few months of life, with severe projectile vomiting, diarrhea, and failure to thrive. A similar

condition has also been reported in adults, most often related to crustacean shellfish ingestion. Children will often outgrow an allergy to milk and soy by age 5 or 6. Recent research suggests that many children tolerate products containing egg or milk if extensively heated (Sicherer and Leung, 2009).

- **Oral allergy syndrome** (OAS), or pollen-associated FA syndrome, is a form of localized IgE-mediated allergy. Reaction is usually from direct contact with fresh fruits or vegetables, confined to the lips, mouth, and throat. OAS most commonly affects patients who are allergic to pollens. Symptoms include itching of the lips, tongue, roof of the mouth, and throat, with or without swelling, and/or tingling of the lips, tongue, roof of the mouth, and throat. There is a rapid onset of symptoms, but it is rarely progressive. Cross-reactivity occurs between certain pollen and food allergens, such as ragweed allergy with ingestion of bananas or melons; birch pollen allergy with ingestion of raw carrots, celery, potato, apple, hazelnut, or kiwi; or latex-fruit allergy with apples, avocado, banana, bell pepper, cherries, chestnut, kiwi, nectarines, peach, plums, potato and tomato.

Over 170 different foods have been known to produce an allergy or intolerance. Yet, over 90% of food allergies are caused by eight foods: eggs, milk, wheat, soy, fish, shellfish, peanuts, and tree nuts (TNs). Peanut and TN allergies are the leading cause of fatal or near-fatal food allergic reactions, including respiratory arrestand shock (Sicherer, 2003). The greatest danger comes from anaphylaxis, a violent allergic reaction that involves many parts of the body. Signs include itchy lips, tongue, or palate; metallic taste; flushing and itching or urticaria of skin; angioedema and edema of lips and tongue; nausea, vomiting, or diarrhea; tightness in chest or throat; dysphagia; hoarseness; dry cough; shortness of breath or wheezing; rhinorrhea or congestion; bronchospasm; syncope; chest pain; and hypotension.

Food allergy reactions usually occur within 2 hours. Immediate (1 minute–2 hours) or delayed reactions (2–48 hours) may also occur. **Food-induced anaphylaxis** is an IgE-mediated, rapid-onset, potentially life-threatening systemic reaction in which the affected individual may experience cardiovascular shock and/or serious respiratory compromise due to airway obstruction or bronchoconstriction (NIAID, 2010). Anaphylaxis occurs when a person is exposed to an allergen after being sensitized by at least one previous exposure. Peanuts, TNs, shellfish, milk, eggs, and fish are the most problematic. Tropomyosin is the protein that causes allergic reactions in shellfish (Taylor, 2008). Peanut allergy is quite serious, where even miniscule amounts have caused deaths (Lee and Burks, 2009; Scurlock and Burks, 2004).

Histamine mediates anaphylaxis by triggering a cascade of inflammatory mediators (Winbery and Lieberman, 2002). Histamine occurs naturally in foods such as cheese, red wines, spinach, eggplant, and yeast extract; it may elicit a response, including hives, urticaria, GI irritability, nausea, and flushing (Maher, 2002). A nonallergic reaction may occur from eating spoiled (scombroid) fish, which tends to be high in histamine; it may cause a reaction similar to anaphylaxis.

The GIT is highly involved in nutritional, physiological and immunological health. Gut-associated lymphoid tissue (GALT) is developed after birth with bacterial colonization, supporting development of protective IgA. An imbalance in T cells (type th2 greater than type th1) promotes autoimmune disease, Crohn's disease, or gut disease such as NEC (Walker, 2008). Persons with chronic urticaria may have impaired small bowel enterocyte function, with higher sensitivity to histamine-producing foods (Guida et al, 2000). Probiotics are being widely promoted for a role in reducing undesirable GIT responses to pathogens and allergens. In addition, retinoids regulate immunosuppressive factors within the mucosa; this role is just becoming understood (Strober, 2008).

Exercise and aspirin may facilitate allergen absorption from the GI tract (Matsuo et al, 2005). Food-dependent exercise-induced anaphylaxis (FDEIA) is an allergic reaction induced by intense exercise with the ingestion of a causative food (Matsuo et al, 2005). FDEIA is often associated with celery, chicken, shrimp, oyster, peaches, and wheat.

Alcoholic beverages may also contribute to hypersensitivity reactions: flushing syndrome, anaphylactoid reactions of urticaria/angioedema, asthma, food allergy, or exercise-induced anaphylaxis in susceptible subjects (Gonzalez-Quintela et al, 2004). Alcohol may promote development of IgE-mediated hypersensitivity to different allergens; alcohol abuse and even moderate alcohol consumption are associated with increased total serum IgE levels (Gonzalez-Quintela et al, 2004).

The Food Allergen Labeling and Consumer Protection Act (FALCPA) became effective January 1, 2006. Food ingredient labeling is the first line of defense for those with food allergies and their caregivers. Food ingredient labels should be read every time a food is purchased and used. Under FALCPA, food labels are to provide clear, consistent, and reliable ingredient labeling information by including "common English" names of the top eight major food allergens in food labeling. Legislation requires one of two options for food labeling with these common terms. The first is to list the food allergen in parentheses following the required ingredient term; for example, "whey (milk)" or "semolina (wheat)." The second option is to follow the ingredient declaration with a statement such as "contains flounder, pecan, wheat, and soy." In addition, all spices, flavors, and incidental additives that contain or are derived from a major food allergen will be labeled with the name of an allergen under either ingredient labeling option. For example, a flavor that contains an ingredient derived from milk might say "natural butter flavor (milk)."

Genetically modified (GM) foods are the product of biotechnology. Genetic bioengineering may, eventually, be able to reduce the level of allergens in the food supply (Lehrer, 2004), a common concern among members of the public (Celec et al, 2005). For GM foods, possible allergenicity of proteins is evaluated by comparison of their amino acid sequence with that of known allergens and determination of their stability during processing. GM crops that have been grown commercially are regularly evaluated for allergenic properties (Goodman et al, 2005). Overall, biotechnology can enhance the safety, nutritional value, and variety of foods without promoting allergies (American Dietetic Association, 2006).

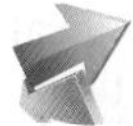

ASSESSMENT, MONITORING, AND EVALUATION

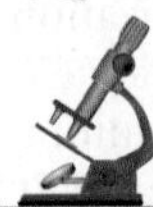

CLINICAL INDICATORS

Genetic Markers: Both genetics and environment play a role in promoting food-specific IgE responses (Tsai et al, 2009). Major food allergens are water-soluble glycoproteins. In normal individuals, allergens cause an IgA response along with suppressor CD8+ lymphocyte production. Antigen uptake is altered in children with cow's milk allergy; this affects about 3% of children in the U.S. Soy allergy affects about 1% of children. Peanuts have an Ara h 1 component that promotes IgE-mediated mast cell degranulation; tree nuts have similar effects (Khodoun et al, 2009). Gliadin is often found to be a factor in wheat allergy. Latex contains Hev b protein, to which some people are hypersensitive.

Clinical/History	Lab Work	
Height	H & H, serum Fe	Double-blind food challenge
Weight	Serum tryptase (elevated)	Patch tests for delayed hypersensitivity reactions
BMI	Serum histamine	CRP
Recent weight changes	Allergen microarray test for IgE profiling	Alb, transthyretin
Food diaries and symptoms history	Radioallergosorbent test (RAST)	BUN, Creat
BP	Allergen-specific IgE levels: skin prick tests (SPT) give 50% false-positives but are very reliable if negative	
Temperature		
Chronic GI distress, diarrhea		
Asthma or rhinitis		
Angioedema, urticaria		
Double-blind food challenge test		

SAMPLE NUTRITION CARE PROCESS STEPS

Intake of Unsafe Foods—Food Allergies

Assessment: Food diaries, food history, history of previous anaphylaxis and known food allergens.

Nutrition Diagnosis: Intake of unsafe food related to knowledge deficit as evidenced by anaphylaxis reaction after consuming peanuts.

Intervention: Education and counseling about identified food allergies (peanuts,) food labeling, recipes, and ingredients; evaluation of nutritional adequacy. Teach how to keep a food diary, keeping a chronological record of all foods eaten and any associated adverse symptoms. If needed, implement an elimination diet.

Monitoring and Evaluation: Review of food diaries; reports of no further problems with anaphylactic reactions to foods.

INTERVENTION

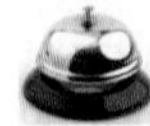

OBJECTIVES

- Careful clinical history, diagnostic studies, endoscopy, or double-blind food challenge may be needed. Children with AD could have a food allergy that can be diagnosed using a skin prick test and double-blind food challenge. Assist as needed in obtaining information; teach how to keep a food diary to track reactions to food.
- The therapy is avoidance of incriminating foods, plus education to avoid inadvertent exposures. Exclude or avoid the offending allergen. If it is not known, use an elimination diet to discover the cause. Note that "rotation diets" are not effective and are potentially dangerous.
- Monitor speed of onset of reactions, delayed versus immediate. The onset of delayed reaction may take from several hours to as long as 5 days. An immediate response is more common with raw foods; patient history may include diarrhea, urticaria, dermatitis, rhinitis, and asthma (see Asthma, Section 5). Allergic diarrhea is almost entirely IgE and mast-cell dependent, mediated by platelet-activating factor (PAF) and serotonin (Finkelman, 2007).
- Treatment of GI allergic disorders includes strict dietary elimination of offending food (Garcia-Careaga and Kerner, 2005). Use of protein hydrolysates has not been proven to be necessary (Osborn and Sinn, 2006).
- Breastfeeding should be promoted for primary prevention of allergic infants who are not lactose-intolerant (Garcia-Careaga and Kerner, 2005).
- Treat nutritional deficiencies or ensure adequate supplementation. Children who have multiple food allergies tend to have growth problems. The nutritional consequences of food allergy by various allergens are listed in Table 2-9.

Follow the new guidelines at http://www.niaid.nih.gov/topics/foodAllergy/clinical/Documents/guidelines.pdf.

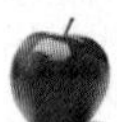

FOOD AND NUTRITION

- The most common allergens in infants are eggs, wheat, milk, and fish. For children, cow's milk, eggs, soy, peanuts, wheat, TNs, and fish are often a problem. For adults, common allergens include shellfish, peanuts, and TNs. Peanuts are implicated in approximately one third of all cases of anaphylaxis.
- After skin testing, a double-blind, placebo-controlled food challenge (DBPCFC) can be useful (Perry et al, 2004). This should only be used under the guidance

of a physician in case there are immediate or severe reactions.

- For an elimination diet, use an unflavored elemental diet as a hypoallergenic base to which other foods are added as test challenges. Foods that seldom cause an allergic reaction include apples, apricots, artichokes, carrots, gelatin, lamb, lettuce, peaches, pears, rice, squash, and turkey; they may be used in this protocol.
- Read labels of foods prepared for the patient. Check all menu items served to patients. See Table 2-10.
- Monitor food preparation methods to exclude possible cross contact with the allergen.
- Monitor nutrient needs specific for the patient's age; evaluate for possible "hidden" ingredients.
- For infants, exclusive breastfeeding is best as it is nonallergenic.
- Lactating mothers may want to omit cow's milk, eggs, fish, and nuts from their own diets. See Table 2-11. Do not give cow's milk to infants until after they are 1-year old.
- Children should not eat peanuts, nuts, or fish until they are 3-year old. Toddlers should not eat eggs until after 2 years of age.
- Persons with rhinitis may be sensitive to monosodium benzoate in fruit juice, pie filling, pickles, olives, salad dressings, and fruit drinks.

Common Drugs Used and Potential Side Effects

- Aspirin may trigger skin reactions, which are associated with the inhibition of cyclooxygenase-1 (COX-1) and characterized by overproduction of cysteinyl leukotrienes; these reactions are due to the interference of aspirin-like drugs with arachidonic acid metabolism (Mastalerz, 2005).

TABLE 2-10 Major Food Allergens and Nutritional Consequences

Most Common	Nutrients of concern
Milk	Check for deficiencies in protein, riboflavin, calcium, and vitamins A and D.
Eggs	Check for iron from other sources.
Fish and shellfish	Other protein sources will be needed. Niacin, vitamin B_6, vitamin B_{12}, omega-3 fatty acids, phosphorus, and selenium should be available from other foods.
Nuts, tree	Protein, fatty acids, and other nutrients will be needed from other sources in the diet. Often, children outgrow a tree nut allergy.
Peanuts	Protein, fatty acids, and other nutrients will be needed from other sources in the diet.
Soy	Protein and other nutrients may be needed from other sources.
Wheat	Check for sufficiency of B vitamins and iron from other sources.
Less Common	Most frequently tied to adverse reactions that can be confused with food allergy are yellow dye number 5, monosodium glutamate (MSG), and sulfites.
Food additives: Tartrazine (not a true food allergen)	Yellow dye number 5 can cause hives, although rarely. FD&C Yellow No. 5, or tartrazine, is used to color beverages, dessert powders, candy, ice cream, custards, and other foods. The color additive may cause hives in fewer than one out of every 10,000 people. By law, whenever the color is added to foods or taken internally, it must be listed on the label so those who may be sensitive to FD&C Yellow No. 5 can avoid it (http://www.cfsan.fda.gov/~dms/qa-top.html).
MSG (not a true food allergen)	Dietary glutamate is a major energy source for the intestines and placenta. The brain is well protected against a flux of glutamate, and it is not toxic. Glutamate is found naturally in foods such as tomatoes and cheeses and is released in protein hydrolysis during stock or soup preparation. It is added to foods in crystalline form as MSG. MSG, which is 14% sodium, is used as a flavor enhancer, known as "umami." Glutamate helps to stimulate the vagus nerve and helps to facilitate digestion and nutrient absorption (Fernstrom and Garattini, 2000). MSG enhances flavor, but when consumed in large amounts, it can cause flushing, sensations of warmth, lightheadedness, headache, facial pressure, and chest tightness; these effects are temporary. These adverse reactions, "Chinese restaurant syndrome," have not been confirmed in double-blind studies (Geha et al, 2000).
Mustard	Mustard allergy is not as uncommon as previously believed (Figueroa et al, 2005). There is a relationship with mugwort pollinosis and plant-derived food allergies. A relationship between this syndrome and food-dependent exercise-induced anaphylaxis has also been reported (Figueroa et al, 2005).
Rice	Certain ethnic groups may have sensitivities to foods that may not be as allergenic for other populations. An example is an Asian person who develops an allergy to rice. Some of this may be dose-related exposure.
Spices	Spices may cause delayed-typed contact allergic or immediate allergic reaction. Sesame seed is a fairly common allergen. Carmine/cochineal is another minor allergen.
Sulfites (not a true food allergen)	Although not an IgE-mediated allergic response, sulfites can produce life-threatening reactions similar to the major food allergens. To help sulfite-sensitive people avoid problems, FDA requires the presence of sulfites in processed foods to be declared on the label and prohibits the use of sulfites on fresh produce intended to be sold or served raw to consumers (FDA Consumer: http://vm.cfsan.fda.gov/~dms/wh-alrg1.html). Foods such as wine, beer, dried fruits and vegetables, maraschino cherries, and dried or frozen potatoes may contain sulfites. No specific nutrient deficits are likely if omitted from the diet.

TABLE 2-11 Food Processing Concerns

Manufacturing processes	The food industry has taken steps to address the needs of consumers with food allergies, including changes to manufacturing processes to reduce the potential for cross-contact with major food allergens. Under existing good manufacturing practice (GMP) regulations, reasonable precautions must be taken to prevent cross-contact with major allergenic proteins. In instances when cross-contact cannot be avoided, even when complying, food and ingredient manufacturers use labeling that informs the food allergic consumer of the possible presence of allergens in the food. Food manufacturers label the ingredients in their products in accordance with existing regulatory requirements. The rule is, "no protein, no problem."
Oils in processing	Most oils used in food processing and for sale to the public contain no protein and are extracted from the oilseed or nut using solvents and then are degummed, refined, bleached, and deodorized. Some oils are mechanically extracted (cold pressed) and left unrefined to purposely maintain the flavor; these oils may contain protein and be allergenic.
Product recalls	Undeclared food allergens have been responsible for many food product recalls during the past decade, and the food industry has made significant investment, effort, and improvements in allergen control during this time (Hefle and Taylor, 2004). More research will be important.

- Cyclosporine, when used, can be steroid sparing; monitor BUN, Creat, and BP (Kaplan, 2004).
- Epinephrine is the synthetic version of naturally occurring adrenaline. It is the first line of defense for anaphylaxis and often requires an emergency room visit. Injectable epinephrine should be carried by those who are prone to allergic reactions to food and other allergens. An Epi-Pen provides a single dose; the Ana-Kit provides two doses.
- Oral antihistamines, such as Benadryl or Atarax or Vistaril, should be taken with food. Dry mouth, constipation, and GI distress are potential side effects.
- H_1-antihistamines (such as ranitidine, cimetidine) are adjunctive treatment therapy for acute anaphylactoid reactions, but they have a slow onset of action when compared with epinephrine, the medication of choice (Winbery and Lieberman, 2002). They are a mainstay of therapy for urticaria; nonsedating products include fexofenadine, loratadine, and desloratadine (Monroe, 2005).
- Treatment with topical or systemic steroids is used if all dietary measures are unsuccessful (Garcia-Careaga and Kerner, 2005).
- Consumption of omega-3 fatty acids can reduce the severity of asthma symptoms. With fish allergy, use nonfish oil sources.
- Probiotics have possible use for treatment of AD (Vanderhoof, 2008). Other new treatments for AD, urticaria and angioedema include biologics, vitamin D, and skin creams (Sicherer and Leung, 2009).
- Scientists at NIH fed mice a mixture of whole peanut extract (WPE) and a toxin called staphylococcal enterotoxin B (SEB) to simulate the human anaphylactic reaction to peanuts in mice. They are trying to develop a method for desensitizing people who are allergic to peanuts over time.

Herbs, Botanicals, and Supplements

- The pathway that activates transcription factors can be interrupted by phytochemicals derived from turmeric (curcumin); red pepper (capsaicin); cloves (eugenol); ginger (gingerol); cumin, anise, and fennel (anethol); basil and rosemary (ursolic acid); garlic (diallyl sulfide, S-allylmercaptocysteine, ajoene); and pomegranate (ellagic acid) (Aggarwal and Shishodia, 2004).
  - Bee pollen does not prevent allergies. It may, in fact, cause asthma, urticaria, rhinitis, or anaphylaxis after eating plants that cross-react with ragweed, such as sunflowers or dandelion greens.
  - Food/plant sensitivities are common (e.g., melon/ragweed, apple/birch, wheat/grasses). Be wary of herbal teas.
  - Jewelweed, parsley, stinging nettle, amaranth, gingko, chamomile, and feverfew have been proposed for use in allergies or with hives; no long-term studies are needed.
  - Sweeteners are not usually allergenic. After reviewing scientific studies, the FDA determined in 1981 that aspartame is safe for use in foods. Persons who have phenylketonuria (PKU) should not use it because it is made from phenylalanine.
  - For conditions such as allergic asthma, clinical trials are underway to determine effectiveness of Traditional Chinese Medicines (TCM).

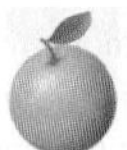

NUTRITION EDUCATION, COUNSELING, CARE MANAGEMENT

- Education on reading ingredient labeling is essential. Ensure extensive nutrition counseling and health education for those who have food allergies to avoid nutrient deficiencies, to limit unnecessary restrictions, and to prevent reactions. Nutrient deficiencies will depend on the food groups involved and omitted.
- Signs of anaphylaxis (hoarseness, throat tightening, difficulty breathing, tingling in hands or feet or scalp, wheezing) should be taken seriously; call 911 immediately.
- Teach about possible cross-reactivity, such as cow's milk with goat's milk, or various types of fin fish.
- Tips to share with individuals who have allergies are found in Table 2-12.

Patient Education—Food Safety

- Intake of food allergens is actually "intake of unsafe food" in susceptible individuals. With GI disturbances and reactive symptoms, individuals with food allergies may be more sensitive to foodborne illness. Teach good hand washing, food preparation and storage tips.
- Children who have allergies should wear a Medic Alert tag or bracelet.

TABLE 2-12 Specifics of Food Allergies

Egg	Reactions are usually mild. Flu shots may contain egg albumin. Yolks are often tolerated. ALWAYS CONTAINS IT: Eggs, egg whites, dried eggs, egg solids, egg nog, albumin, cake, some candies or creamed foods, cookies, custard, doughnuts, egg rolls, some frostings, hollandaise sauce, some ice creams, lecithin, mayonnaise, meringue, some puddings, pretzels, Simplesse sweetener, souffle, waffles. MAY CONTAIN IT: Egg may appear as "albumin" in marshmallows, frozen dinners, and dry food mixes. Egg washes are often used on bakery goods to make them look shiny. Eggs are often used in glazes and icings.
Fish and shellfish	Avoid seafood restaurants. Abalone, clams, crab, crawfish, lobster, oysters, scallops, shrimp, cockle (sea urchin), and mussels are the shellfish that should be avoided. ALWAYS CONTAINS IT: Fish, shellfish, agar, alginic acid, ammonium alginate, anchovies, calcium alginate, caviar, disodium ionsinate, potassium alginate, propylene glycol alginate sodium alginate, imitation crab or "surimi," roe. MAY CONTAIN IT: Asian sauces, Caesar salad dressing, omega-3 fatty acid capsules or oils; Chinese, Vietnamese, Japanese, Indian, Indonesian, and Thai foods; fried foods, i.e., French fries, chicken nuggets (often cooked in the same oil as fish/shellfish); steak or Worcestershire sauces.
Latex	Natural rubber latex contains more than 35 proteins that may be related to type IgE–mediated allergy (Perkin, 2000). Latex-specific IgF may be responsible. Cross-reactivity has been documented with banana, avocado, kiwi, and European chestnuts; less commonly with potatoes; tomatoes; and peaches, plums, cherries, and other pitted fruits. Individuals with latex allergy also tend to report food allergies, including fish and shellfish (Kim and Hussain, 1999). Children with spina bifida and atopic dermatitis are a high-risk group for latex sensitization. Increasing age, additional sensitization to ubiquitous inhaled allergens, and enhanced total serum IgE values seem to be important variables for latex sensitization and further sensitization to the latex-associated foods (Tucke et al, 1999).
Milk	ALWAYS CONTAINS IT: Casein, caseinates, lactalbumins, lactoglobulins, lactose, nougat, rennet, milk, milk solids, nonfat or powdered milks, buttermilk, evaporated milk, condensed milk, yogurt, cream, cream cheese, sour cream, cheese, cheese sauces, cottage cheese, butter, butter fat, curds, whey, white sauces. MAY CONTAIN IT: Artificial butter flavor. Caramel color or flavoring, flavorings or seasonings, puddings, custards, sauces, sherbet. It may be necessary to acquire sufficient calcium from greens and broccoli or clams, oysters, shrimp, and salmon if not allergic to fish Calcium supplementation may also be warranted. Persons with a milk allergy can add vanilla or other flavorings to soy milk. Goat's milk has less lactalbumin, vitamin D, and folacin than cow's milk and supplements may be required. Some people may also be allergic to goat's milk, so caution must be used. Avoid early introduction of cow's milk in infancy.
Nuts, tree	Tree nuts include almonds, Brazil nuts, cashews, chestnuts, filberts, hazelnuts, hickory nuts, macadamia nuts, pecans, pine nuts, pistachios, and walnuts. Monitor food labels for nut paste, nut oil, and nut extracts. Avoid nut butters also. Read labels for ground or mixed nuts.
Peanut	Peanuts are a type of legume, but a person is more likely to be allergic to tree nuts than to beans, peas, and lentils. Avoid nut butters also; aflatoxins can cause an allergic-like reaction. For the food industry, new inexpensive kits are available to test for presence of peanut proteins in cookies, cereal, ice cream, and milk chocolate. Despite severity and reaction frequency to peanut and tree nut allergy, only 74% of children and 44% of adults in a large study sought evaluation for the allergy, and fewer than half who did were prescribed self-injectable epinephrine (Sicherer et al, 2003). It may be recommended that those children who outgrow their peanut allergy be encouraged to eat peanut frequently and carry epinephrine until they demonstrate true peanut tolerance (Fleischer et al, 2004). ALWAYS CONTAINS IT: Peanuts, mixed nuts, peanut butter, peanut oil, peanut flour, ground or mixed nuts, artificial nuts, nougat, many types of candy or cookies, ethnic dishes made with peanut oil, some egg rolls, marzipan. MAY CONTAIN IT: Peanut butter may be used to keep egg rolls from falling apart or in chili as a thickener.
Soybean	Some people are also allergic to legumes such as chickpeas, navy beans, kidney beans, black beans, pinto beans, lentils, and peanuts. ALWAYS CONTAINS IT: Soybeans, soybean oil, margarines made from soybean oil, soy sauce, soy nuts, soy milk. Reading food labels will be very important. COMMON SOURCES: Soy protein, textured vegetable protein, hydrolyzed plant protein, lecithin, miso, soy sauce, Worcestershire sauce, tofu, tempeh, some vegetable broths.
Wheat	Wheat-dependent, exercise-induced anaphylaxis (WDEIA) and baker's asthma are different clinical forms of wheat allergy (Mittag et al, 2004). ALWAYS CONTAINS IT: Whole-wheat or enriched flour, high-gluten flour, high-protein flour, bran, farina, bulgur, durum, wheat malt, wheat starch, modified starch, wheat germ, graham flour, wheat gluten, matzoh/matzoh meal, semolina, bread crumbs, cereal extract, dextrin, malt flavoring, modified starch. COMMON SOURCES: Baby food, baked goods, baking mixes, breaded foods, processed meats, pastas, snack foods, soups, breads, cookies, cakes and other baked goods made with wheat flour; crackers, many cereals, some couscous, cracker meal, pasta, gelatinized starch, hydrolyzed vegetable protein, wheat gluten, vegetable gum, vegetable starch.

- Always work with an RD to identify foods and ingredients to avoid, and develop an eating plan to ensure that each child gets all the nutrients needed to grow and develop properly.

For More Information

- American Academy of Allergy, Asthma, and Immunology
http://www.aaaai.org/
- American College of Allergy, Asthma, and Immunology
http://www.acaai.org/
- Asthma and Allergy Foundation of America
http://www.aafa.org/
- Cherrybrook Kitchens: Allergy free
https://www.cherrybrookkitchen.com/index.html
- Food Allergy and Anaphylaxis Network
http://www.foodallergy.org/

- Food Allergies Database
  http://allergyadvisor.com/
- Food Allergy Initiative
  http://www.foodallergyinitiative.org/
- Food and Nutrition Information Center
  http://www.nal.usda.gov/fnic/pubs/bibs/gen/allergy.htm
- Food Labeling
  http://www.fda.gov/fdac/special/foodlabel/food_toc.html
- Grocery Manufacturers Association
  http://www.gmaonline.org/
- Hidden Allergens
  http://allergyadvisor.com/hidden.htm
- International Food Information Council Foundation
  http://ific.org
- Kids with Allergies
  http://www.kidswithfoodallergies.org
- Mayo Clinic
  http://www.mayoclinic.com/health/food-allergy/DS00082
- Medline: Food Allergy
  http://www.nlm.nih.gov/medlineplus/foodallergy.html
- National Institute on Allergy and Infectious Diseases
  http://www3.niaid.nih.gov/
- Nutrition MD—allergies
  http://www.nutritionmd.org/nutrition_tips/nutrition_tips_managing_diseases/allergies.html
- Nutrition MD—Diet Makeover
  http://www.nutritionmd.org/makeover/basics/not.html
- RAST Testing
  http://www.labtestsonline.org/understanding/analytes/allergy/test.html
- Teen Allergies
  http://kidshealth.org/teen/food_fitness/nutrition/food_allergies.html

FOOD ALLERGY AND INTOLERANCES—CITED REFERENCES

Aggarwal BB, Shishodia S. Suppression of the nuclear factor-kappaB activation pathway by spice-derived phytochemicals: reasoning for seasoning. *Ann N Y Acad Sci.* 1030:434, 2004.

American Dietetic Association. Position of the American Dietetic Association: agricultural and food biotechnology. *J Am Diet Assoc.* 106:285, 2006.

Celec P, et al. Biological and biomedical aspects of genetically modified food. *Biomed Pharmacother.* 59:531, 2005.

Figueroa J, et al. Mustard allergy confirmed by double-blind placebo-controlled food challenges: clinical features and cross-reactivity with mugwort pollen and plant-derived foods. *Allergy.* 60:48, 2005.

Finkelman FD. Anaphylaxis: lessons from mouse models. *J Allergy Clin Immunol.* 120:506, 2007.

Fleischer DM, et al. Peanut allergy: recurrence and its management. *J Allergy Clin Immunol.* 114:1195, 2004.

Garcia-Careaga M Jr, Kerner JA Jr.. Gastrointestinal manifestations of food allergies in pediatric patients. *Nutr Clin Pract.* 20:526, 2005.

Gonzalez-Quintela A, et al. Alcohol, IgE and allergy. *Addict Biol.* 9:195, 2004.

Goodman RE, et al. Assessing genetically modified crops to minimize the risk of increased food allergy: a review. *Int Arch Allergy Immunol.* 137:153, 2005.

Guida B, et al. Histamine plasma levels and elimination diet in chronic idiopathic urticaria. *Euro J Clin Nutri.* 54:155, 2000.

Hefle SL, Taylor SL. Food allergy and the food industry. *Curr Allergy Asthma Rep.* 4:55, 2004

Kaplan AP. Chronic urticaria: pathogenesis and treatment. *J Allergy Clin Immunol.* 114:465, 2004.

Khodoun M, et al. Peanuts can contribute to anaphylactic shock by activating complement. *J Allergy Clin Immunol.* 123:342, 2009.

Latcham F, et al. A consistent pattern of minor immunodeficiency and subtle enteropathy in children with multiple food allergy. *J Pediatr.* 143:39, 2003.

Lee LA, Burks AW. New insights into diagnosis and treatment of peanut allergy. *Front Biosci.* 14:3361, 2009.

Lehrer SB. Genetic modification of food allergens. *Ann Allergy Asthma Immunol.* 93:S19, 2004.

Maher TJ. Pharmacological actions of food and drink. In: Brostoff J, Challacombe S, eds. *Food allergy and intolerance.* 2nd ed. London: Saunders, 2002.

Mastalerz L, et al. Mechanism of chronic urticaria exacerbation by aspirin. Mechanism of chronic urticaria exacerbation by aspirin. *Curr Allergy Asthma Rep.* 5:277, 2005.

Matsuo H, et al. Exercise and aspirin increase levels of circulating gliadin peptides in patients with wheat-dependent exercise-induced anaphylaxis. *Clin Exp Allergy.* 35:461, 2005.

Mittag D, et al. Immunoglobulin E-reactivity of wheat-allergic subjects (baker's asthma, food allergy, wheat-dependent, exercise-induced anaphylaxis) to wheat protein fractions with different solubility and digestibility. *Mol Nutr Food Res.* 48:380, 2004.

Monroe E. Review of H1 antihistamines in the treatment of chronic idiopathic urticaria. *Cutis.* 76:118, 2005.

Munoz-Furlong A. Food allergy in schools: concerns for allergists, pediatricians, parents, and school staff. *Ann Allergy Asthma Immunol.* 93:S47, 2004.

National Institute of Allergy and Infectious Diseases. Guidelines for the diagnosis and management of food allergies. Accessed April 24, 2010, at http://www.niaid.nih.gov/topics/foodAllergy/clinical/Documents/guidelines.pdf.

Osborn DA, Sinn J. Soy formula for prevention of allergy and food intolerance in infants. *Cochrane Database Syst Rev.* (4):CD003741, 2006.

Perry TT, et al. Risk of oral food challenges. *J Allergy Clin Immunol.* 114:1164, 2004.

Scurlock AM, Burks AW. Peanut allergenicity. *Ann Allergy Asthma Immunol.* 93:S12, 2004.

Sicherer SH, et al. Prevalence of peanut and tree nut allergy in the United States determined by means of a random digit dial telephone survey: a 5-year follow-up study. *J Allergy Clin Immunol.* 112:1203, 2003.

Sicherer SH, Leung DY. Advances in allergic skin disease, anaphylaxis, and hypersensitivity to foods, drugs and insects in 2008. *J Allergy Clin Immunol.* 123:319, 2009.

Stone KD. Advances in pediatric allergy. *Curr Opin Pediatr.* 16:571, 2004.

Strober W. Vitamin A rewrites the ABCs of oral tolerance. *Mucosal Immunol.* 1:92, 2008.

Taylor SE. Molluscan seafood allergy. *Adv Food Nutr Res* 54:139, 2008.

Tsai HJ, et al. Familial aggregation of food allergy and sensitization to food allergens: a family based study. *Clin Exp Allergy* 39:101, 2009.

Vanderhoof JA. Probiotics in allergy management. *J Pediatr Gastroenterol Nutr* 47:S38, 2008.

Walker WA. Mechanisms of action of probiotics. *Clin Infect Dis.* 46:S87, 2008.

Winbery SL, Lieberman PL. Histamine and antihistamines in anaphylaxis. Histamine and antihistamines in anaphylaxis. *Clin Allergy Immunol.* 17:287, 2002.

MÉNIÈRE'S SYNDROME (AUTOIMMUNE INNER-EAR DISEASE)

NUTRITIONAL ACUITY RANKING: LEVEL 1

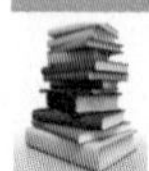

DEFINITIONS AND BACKGROUND

Ménière's syndrome is also known as autoimmune inner-ear disease (AIED;) it affects the inner ear, causing disturbed fluid flow. Patient may have a history of otitis media, smoking, or allergies. Attacks last from a few hours to several days, but the vertigo causes disability in many patients. Ménière's disease affects about 1% of the population and presents with episodic vertigo, fluctuating hearing loss, tinnitus and aural fullness (Hamid, 2009).

Sodium restriction and diuretic treatment are early management measures (Devaiah and Ator, 2000; Minor et al, 2004).

Aggressive medical therapy can prevent disease progression and hearing loss. Treatment options are limited and usually targeted toward reducing endolymphatic hydrops (Hamid, 2009).

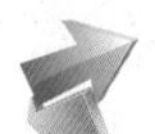

ASSESSMENT, MONITORING, AND EVALUATION

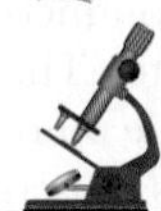

CLINICAL INDICATORS

Clinical/History
Height
Weight
BMI
Diet history
Fluctuating hearing loss
Tinnitus with roaring sensation
Vertigo, blurred vision
Nausea and vomiting
Known allergies?
BP

Lab Work
IgE levels
H & H, serum Fe
Alb
Electrocochleography (ECOG)
Electronystagmography, or balance test (ENG)
Auditory brainstem response
CT scan or MRI
Serum Na^{++}, K^{+}
I & O

INTERVENTION

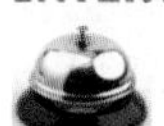

OBJECTIVES

- Correct nausea and vomiting; replace any electrolyte losses.
- Avoid or decrease edema and fluid retention, which can aggravate an attack.
- Omit any known food allergens from the diet.

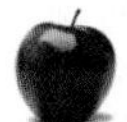

FOOD AND NUTRITION

- Low-sodium (1000–2000 mg) diet may be useful.
- Use a multivitamin–mineral supplement and foods that are nutrient dense. Calcium and vitamin D strengthen the bones of the inner ear. Folate, vitamins B_6 and B_{12} reduce high levels of tHcy, which can reduce blood flow to the cochlea. Vitamin B_{12} also protects the nerves of the ear.
- Provide a diet that is free of known allergens, specific for the individual.
- Some people report feeling better after eliminating caffeine, aspartame, or alcohol.

SAMPLE NUTRITION CARE PROCESS STEPS

Knowledge Deficit

Assessment: Food diaries and frequency of intake of high sodium foods, history of previous anaphylaxis or food allergens.

Nutrition Diagnosis: Knowledge deficit related to high sodium foods as evidenced by chronic fluid retention in the ear.

Intervention: Education and counseling about high sodium foods, food labeling, recipes, and ingredients. Teach how to keep a food diary, keeping records of foods eaten and any adverse symptoms related to Ménière's.

Monitoring and Evaluation: Review of food diaries; reports of fewer problems related to Ménière's syndrome.

Common Drugs Used and Potential Side Effects

- Diuretics are used to reduce edema in the ear. If thiazides are used (such as furosemide, Lasix), monitor for the need for a potassium replacement. Other treatments to lower the pressure within the inner ear include antihistamines, anticholinergics, or steroids.
- Diazepam (Valium) may cause nausea, drowsiness, fatigue, and other effects. Limit caffeine.

Herbs, Botanicals, and Supplements

- Herbs and botanicals may be used; identify and monitor side effects. Counsel about use of herbal teas, especially regarding toxic substances.
- For *earache*: ephedra, goldenseal, forsythia, gentian, garlic, honeysuckle, and Echinacea are sometimes recommended but have not been proven as effective.
- For *tinnitus*: black cohosh, sesame, goldenseal, and spinach have been suggested; no long-term studies are on record that prove effectiveness. Gingko biloba has been approved for tinnitus in Europe but research has proven little effect (Karkos et al, 2007).

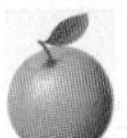

NUTRITION EDUCATION, COUNSELING, CARE MANAGEMENT

- Discuss how a balanced diet can affect general health status.
- Discuss sources of sodium and hidden ingredients that could aggravate the condition.
- Relaxation and biofeedback techniques may be useful for enhancing pain tolerance.

For More Information

- Ear Surgery Center
  http://www.earsurgery.org/meniere.html
- Ménière's Disease Information Center
  http://www.menieresinfo.com/
- National Institute on Deafness
  http://www.nidcd.nih.gov/
- NIH—Ménière's
  http://www.nidcd.nih.gov/health/balance/meniere.asp

MÉNIÈRE'S SYNDROME—CITED REFERENCES

Devaiah A, Ator G. Clinical indicators useful in predicting response to the medical management of Ménière's disease. *Laryngoscope*. 110:1861, 2000.
Hamid M. Ménière's disease. *Pract Neurol*. 9:157, 2009.
Karkos PD, et al. 'Complementary ENT': a systematic review of commonly used supplements. *J Laryngol Otol*. 121:779, 2007.
Minor LB, et al. Ménière's disease. *Curr Opin Neurol*. 17:9, 2004.

FOODBORNE ILLNESS

FOODBORNE ILLNESS

NUTRITIONAL ACUITY RANKING: LEVEL 1 (PREVENTIVE COUNSELING); LEVEL 2 (CORRECTIVE THERAPY)

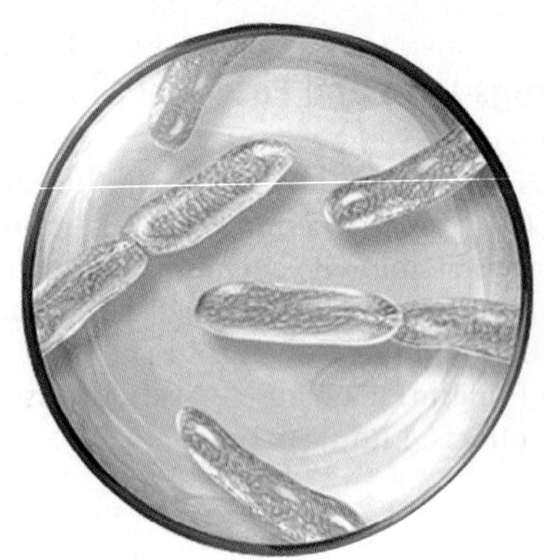

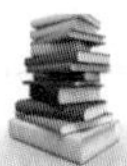

DEFINITIONS AND BACKGROUND

True foodborne illness involves GIT insults, infections, or intoxications resulting from contaminated beverages or food. Millions of cases occur annually, but only a few hundred are reported. The Centers for Disease Control and Prevention report that there are millions of cases each year in the United States alone. The most vulnerable are elderly people, pregnant women, immune-compromised people, and children. Bacterial pathogens cause the largest percentage of outbreaks; chemical agents, viruses, and parasites are often implicated. In addition, multistate outbreaks caused by contaminated produce and outbreaks caused by *Escherichia coli* O157:H7 remain a concern. See Table 2-13.

Pathogens often transmitted via food contaminated by infected food handlers are *Salmonella typhi* and other species, *Shigella, Staphylococcus aureus, Streptococcus pyogenes,* hepatitis A virus, norovirus, *Listeria,* and *E. coli* O157:H7. Personal hygiene is one of the most important steps in food safety. The Centers for Disease Control and Prevention and most health departments require that food handlers and preparers with gastroenteritis ***not*** work until 2 or 3 days after they feel better. Strict hand washing after using the bathroom and before handling food items is important in preventing contamination. Food handlers who were recently sick can be given different duties in the foodservice operation so that they do not have to handle food.

An outbreak occurs when two or more individuals develop the same symptoms over the same time period. Infants and children younger than age 6, people with chronic illnesses (such as HIV infection or cancer), pregnant women, and elderly individuals are most at risk. For most infections, reported incidence is highest among children aged <4 years (CDC, 2010). Table 2-14 lists the most common foodborne illnesses, their onset and duration.

Nausea, vomiting, diarrhea, abdominal cramping, vision problems, fever, chills, dizziness, and headaches may occur. Some people attribute their symptoms mistakenly to "stomach flu." The Foodborne Diseases Active Surveillance Network (FoodNet) of CDC's Emerging Infections Program conducts active, population-based surveillance in the United States. The incidence of Vibrio infection continues to increase while there have been declines in reported incidence of infections caused by Campylobacter, Listeria, Salmonella, Shiga toxin-producing Escherichia coli (STEC) O157, Shigella, and Yersinia have been observed (CDC, 2010).

A recent legislative provision requires school food authorities participating in the National School Lunch Program (NSLP) or the School Breakfast Program (SBP) to develop a school food safety program for the preparation and service of school meals served to children, based on the hazard analysis and critical control point (HACCP) system (Food and Nutrition Services, 2009). Figure 2-11 shows the Food Safety Pyramid of how issues are handled by health departments and the Centers for Disease Control and Prevention (CDC).

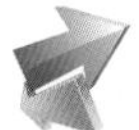

ASSESSMENT, MONITORING, AND EVALUATION

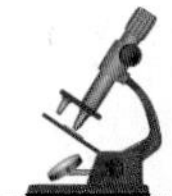

CLINICAL INDICATORS

Clinical/History

Height
Weight
BMI
Usual weight
Weight loss/changes during illness
Diet history
Vomiting
Diarrhea
Nausea
Abdominal cramps
Blood or parasites in stools?
Fever?
Timing of symptoms after suspected meal
Signs of dehydration; I & O

Lab Work

Na^+, K^+
Chloride (Cl^-)
H & H, serum Fe

SAMPLE NUTRITION CARE PROCESS STEPS

Foodborne Illness

Assessment: Food diary reveals intake of unsafe food or beverage, altered GI function (diarrhea, nausea, vomiting).

Nutrition Diagnosis: Intake of unsafe food related to salmonella as evidenced by onset of multiple episodes of vomiting and foodborne gastroenteritis, diarrhea, and lethargy in past several days.

Intervention: Education about rehydration with foods containing sodium, potassium, fluids (such as Gatorade). Counseling about food safety measures, including hand washing, avoidance of cross-contamination, safe food storage.

Monitoring and Evaluation: Review of food diaries; fewer problems related to foodborne illness from intake of unsafe food.

TABLE 2-13 Tips for Educating Individuals about Food Allergies

Shopping in Food Stores

DELI: Ask to have the deli slicer cleaned before preparing the order. Avoid prepared foods because they often share bins and serving utensils. Request that clean gloves to be worn.

ICE CREAM SHOPS: Make sure they do not share scoops for different flavors.

PACKAGED FOODS: Read labels to detect hidden allergens. Choose foods made in facilities that do not make other problematic products. Re-read labels often as ingredients may change; if unsure, call the manufacturer.

SALAD BARS: Be careful with severe allergies because food can drop from one container into another.

Dining Out

AVOID FRIED FOODS, which often share oil with other problem foods.

INQUIRE AHEAD if possible and consult the chef on best menu picks for safe dining.

USE A PLEASANT BUT ASSERTIVE MANNER in explaining the situation to wait staff. Let them know that eating even a small amount of a certain food(s) will make you severely ill.

BE CAREFUL of sauces and soups. Make sure you know exactly what is in them before eating.

REGULAR PATRONAGE. Choose a favorite eatery that accommodates well and visit often.

At School

EDUCATE. Schools need to educate their entire staff, improve prevention and avoidance measures, make sure epinephrine is readily available and that the staff knows how to administer it, and use consumer agency resources (Munoz-Furlong, 2004). The Food Allergy Network has educational kits targeted at schools to assist in the training of the staff on food allergies.

MEDIC ALERT. Students should be encouraged to wear a Medic-Alert bracelet.

CAFETERIA MEALS. Food allergy continues to rise in childhood, and careful meal planning is needed.

At Home

KEEP A FOOD DIARY. Identify all symptoms, timing, and foods eaten.

READ FOOD LABELS every time a food is purchased and used.

FIND RECIPE BOOKS THAT PROVIDE ALTERNATIVES. Recipe books are available from formula companies, food manufacturers, the Food Allergy and Anaphylaxis Network, and registered dietitians.

PATIENT OR PARENT EDUCATION. Patients and parents must stay informed about how to handle allergic reactions (Stone, 2004).

At the Doctor's Office

TESTING. Cytotoxic testing, sublingual provocative tests, pulse tests, kinesiologic testing, yeast hypersensitivity, and brain allergy theories should be dismissed entirely.

After Anaphylaxis

To work with anaphylaxis, remember the "3 Rs": RECOGNIZE symptoms; REACT quickly; REVIEW what happened to prevent it from happening again.

INTERVENTION

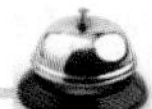

OBJECTIVES

- Allow the GIT to rest after rehydration; progress diet as tolerated.
- Prepare and store all foods using safe food-handling practices and good personal hygiene. Temperatures should be maintained below 40°F or above 140°F for safe food handling, storage, and holding.
- Teach the importance of hand washing, care of food contact surfaces, and insect or rodent extermination. This is especially important in foodservice operations where members of the public are fed.
- Any person operating a foodservice operation should know and use Hazard Analysis and Critical Control Point (HACCP) procedures to evaluate critical control points where foodborne illness risk is high and use precautions and safeguards (McCluskey, 2004). Careful monitoring is recommended. For the aging population in particular, barriers against the use of HACCP should be minimized (Strohbehn et al, 2004).
- Sanitize all surfaces before food preparation; sanitize after each food item is prepared when using the same surface (e.g., cutting boards and slicers). See Table 2-15 for more safe food practices.

TABLE 2-14 **Symptoms, Sources, and Pathogens That Cause Foodborne Illness**

General Source of Illness	Symptoms	Bacteria	
Raw and undercooked meat and poultry	Abdominal pain and cramping, diarrhea, nausea, and vomiting	*Campylobacter jejuni, Escherichia coli* 0157:H7, *Listeria monocytogenes, Salmonella*	
Raw (unpasteurized) milk and dairy products, such as soft cheeses	Nausea and vomiting, fever, abdominal cramps, and diarrhea	*L. monocytogenes, Salmonella, Shigella, Staphylococcus aureus, C. jejuni*	
Fresh or minimally processed produce	Diarrhea, nausea, and vomiting	*E. coli* 0157:H7, *L. monocytogenes, Salmonella, Shigella, Yersinia enterocolitica*, viruses, and parasites	
Specific Illness	**Symptoms**	**Bacteria**	**Onset and Duration**
Meats, milk, vegetables, and fish (diarrhea). Rice products; potato, pasta, and cheese products (vomiting) Consider also: sauces, puddings, soups, salads, casseroles, pastries	Watery diarrhea, abdominal cramping, vomiting	*Bacillus cereus* Gram-positive, aerobic spore former	6–15 hours after consumption. Duration = 24 hours
Raw and undercooked meat and poultry; raw milk and soft cheeses	Abdominal pain and cramping, diarrhea (often bloody), nausea, and vomiting. Note: 40% of Guillain–Barré syndrome (GBS) cases in the United States are caused by campylobacteriosis	*Campylobacter jejuni*	2–5 days after exposure. Duration = 2–10 days
Improperly canned goods especially with low acid content—asparagus, green beans, beets, and corn; chopped garlic in oil; chile peppers; improperly handled baked potatoes wrapped in aluminum foil; home-canned or fermented fish. Honey contains spores	Muscle paralysis caused by the bacterial toxin; double vision, inability to swallow, slurred speech and difficulty speaking, and inability to breathe Infants appear lethargic with poor muscle tone, feed poorly, are constipated, and have a weak cry	*Clostridium botulinum*	18–36 hours after eating contaminated food; can occur as early as 6 hours or as late as 10 days. Duration may be weeks or months
Canned meats, contaminated dried mixes, gravy, stews, refried beans, meat products, and unwashed vegetables	Nausea with vomiting, diarrhea, acute gastroenteritis	*Clostridium perfringens*	Within 6–24 hours from ingestion; lasting 1 day
Contaminated food from poor handling	Watery stools, diarrhea, nausea, vomiting, slight fever, and stomach cramps; especially in immunocompromised patients	*Cryptosporidium parvum* (protozoa)	2–10 days after infection
Contaminated water with human sewage may lead to contamination of foods; infected food handlers. More common with travel to other countries	Watery diarrhea, abdominal cramps, low-grade fever, nausea, and malaise. In infants or debilitated elderly persons, electrolyte replacement therapy may be necessary	*Escherichia coli*; Enterotoxigenic *E. coli* (ETEC)	With high infective dose, diarrhea can be induced within 24 hours
Undercooked ground beef and meats; unpasteurized fruit juices such as apple cider; unwashed fruits and vegetables (lettuce, alfalfa sprouts); dry-cured salami, game meat; cheese curds. *E. coli* 0157:H7 can survive in refrigerated acid foods for weeks	Hemorrhagic colitis (painful, bloody diarrhea) The condition may progress to hemolytic anemia, thrombocytopenia, and acute renal failure requiring dialysis and transfusions	*E. coli* 0157:H7; Enterohemorrhagic *E. coli* (EHEC)	Onset is slow, 3–8 days after ingestion Antibiotics are not used as they can spread the infection Hemolytic uremic syndrome can be fatal, especially in young children

(continued)

TABLE 2-14 **Symptoms, Sources, and Pathogens That Cause Foodborne Illness *(continued)***

Specific Illness	Symptoms	Bacteria	Onset and Duration
Processed, ready-to-eat products (undercooked hot dogs, deli or lunchmeat, unpasteurized dairy products). Postpasteurization contamination of soft cheeses, milk, or commercial coleslaw. Cross-contamination between food surfaces	Mild fever, headache, vomiting, and severe illness in pregnancy; sepsis in immunocompromised patients; febrile gastroenteritis in adults; meningoencephalitis in infants. May lead to meningitis or septicemia if untreated	*Listeria monocytogenes* (LM)	Onset is 2–30 days. Can be fatal
Direct contact or droplets from contaminated hands or work surfaces (stool or vomit). Most common on cruise ships	Gastroenteritis with nausea, vomiting, diarrhea; fever with chills; abdominal cramps; headache; muscle aches. Vomiting may be frequent and quite violent, but subsides within a few days. Drink liquids to prevent dehydration	*Norovirus* Virus cannot multiply outside human body. Once on food, it can be transmitted easily to humans	24–48 hours after ingestion of the virus but may appear as early as 12 hours. Lasts only 1 or 2 days
Raw or undercooked meat, poultry, fish, unpasteurized dairy products; unwashed fruits and raw vegetables (melons and sprouts). Need thorough cooking, hygiene, and sanitation	Diarrhea, fever, and abdominal cramps. Most people recover without treatment. However, elderly, infants, and those with impaired immune systems are more likely to have a severe illness requiring hospitalization and antibiotics	*Salmonella typhimurium*	12–72 hours after infection. Duration = 4–7 days
Raw or undercooked eggs; eggs in foods such as homemade hollandaise sauce, caesar and other salad dressings, tiramisu, homemade ice cream, homemade mayonnaise, cookie dough, frostings	Nausea and vomiting, fever, abdominal cramps, and diarrhea	*Salmonella enteriditis*	12–72 hours after infection. Duration = 4–7 days
Milk and dairy products; cold mixed egg, tuna, chicken, potato, and meat salads	Bloody diarrhea, fever, and stomach cramps	*Shigella* (causes Shigellosis)	24–48 hours after exposure
Meat, pork, eggs, poultry, tuna salad, prepared salads, gravy, stuffing, cream-filled pastries	Nausea, vomiting, retching, abdominal cramping, and prostration	*Staphylococcus aureus* Cooking does not destroy the toxin. Refrigerate foods immediately after preparation and meal service	Within 1–6 hours; rarely fatal. Duration = 1–2 days
Milk, ice cream, eggs, steamed lobster, ground ham, potato salad, egg salad, custard, rice pudding, shrimp salad Foodstuffs at room temperature for several hours between preparation and consumption	Sore and red throat, pain on swallowing, tonsillitis, high fever, headache, nausea, vomiting, malaise, rash, rhinorrhea Complications are rare and are treated with antibiotics	*Streptococcus pyogenes* Entrance into the food is the result of poor hygiene, ill food handlers, or the use of unpasteurized milk	Onset = 1–3 days
Raw or undercooked shellfish, especially raw clams and oysters, contaminated with human pathogen	Vomiting, diarrhea; chills, fever, and collapse Can be fatal in immunocompromised individuals	*Vibrio vulnificus, V. parahaemolyticus* This bacterium is in the same family as cholera. It yields a norovirus	16 hours after eating contaminated food. Duration = 48 hours
Raw or undercooked pork products. Postpasteurization contamination of chocolate milk, reconstituted dry milk, pasteurized milk, and tofu	Fever, abdominal pain, and diarrhea (often bloody) in children In older children and adults, right-sided abdominal pain and fever may be predominant, mimicking appendicitis. Rarely, skin rash, joint pains, and sepsis may occur	*Yersinia enterocolitica* Occurs most often in young children. Cold storage does not kill the bacteria	1–2 days after exposure. Duration = 1–3 weeks or longer

Adapted from the following Web sites (accessed April 7, 2009):
CDC: http://www.cdc.gov/az.do.
FDA: http://www.cfsan.fda.gov/~MOW/intro.html.
NIDDK: http://digestive.niddk.nih.gov/ddiseases/pubs/bacteria/#10.

TABLE 2-15 Safe Food Handling and Food Safety Guidelines

Food Preparation

- Clean hands, food contact surfaces, and fruits and vegetables.
- Meat and poultry should not be washed.
- Because bacteria are commonly found on foods such as cantaloupe, cilantro, and imported produce, wash all fresh fruits and vegetables. Scrub the outside of produce such as melons and cucumbers before cutting. Scallions have been linked to hepatitis A outbreak; cook them thoroughly.
- Discard cracked eggs; avoid using products from dented cans.
- Avoid food preparation when sick with viral or bacterial infections; use gloves if needed.
- Sanitize work surfaces and sponges daily with a mild bleach solution (2 teaspoons per quart of water is sufficient). However, if a work surface comes into contact with raw food, it should be sanitized after contact with each food.
- Separate raw, cooked, and ready-to-eat foods while shopping, preparing, and storing foods.
- Sanitize work surfaces after each food. Ideally, keep one board for poultry, another for meats, and another for produce to prevent cross-contamination. Discard cutting boards that are badly damaged.
- Chill (refrigerate) perishable food promptly and defrost foods properly. Thaw meats and poultry in the refrigerator, not at room temperature. If necessary, thaw in a sink with cold running water that allows continuous drainage or thaw quickly in the microwave and use immediately.
- Do not partially cook meat or poultry in advance of final preparation. Bacteria may still grow rampantly.
- Cook foods to a safe temperature to kill micro-organisms. Cook beef to proper internal temperature of 160°F, pork to 165°F, and poultry to 175°F. Cook hamburger to the proper temperature of 165°F; "pink in the middle, cooked too little." Monitor internal temperatures with an accurate food thermometer placed correctly into the meat or poultry.
- Boil water used for drinking when necessary; hold at boiling temperature for 1 minute.
- Avoid raw or partially cooked eggs, raw or undercooked fish or shellfish, and raw or undercooked meats because of potential foodborne illnesses.
- Avoid raw (unpasteurized) milk or products made from it.
- Avoid serving unpasteurized juices and raw sprouts.

Holding and Serving Foods

- Hold and serve foods at 140–165°F during meal service.
- Reheat foods to at least 165°F. Discard leftovers after the first reheating process.
- Keep hot foods above 140°F and cold foods below 40°F.
- Discard cooked foods that are left at room temperature for more than 2 hours.
- Reheat home-canned foods appropriately. In institutional settings, do not allow home-cooked foods at all.
- Only serve certain deli meats and frankfurters that have been heated to steaming hot temperature.
- Keep pet foods and utensils separate from those for human use.
- Use clean plates and separate utensils between raw and cooked foods.
- Cool foods quickly in shallow pans (2–4 inches deep). Temperature should reach 70°F within 2 hours. If food has not cooled to that level, place in the freezer for a short time. Then, wrap lightly and return to refrigerator.

Other Tips

- When traveling, avoid tap water and ice made from tap water, uncooked produce such as lettuce, and raw or undercooked seafood.
- Airline water may not be free from contamination. Use of bottled water is recommended. Coffee and tea may not be hot enough to kill all bacteria.
- See Fight BAC guidelines at http://www.fightbac.org.

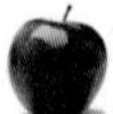

FOOD AND NUTRITION

- For patients with extreme diarrhea or vomiting, feed with intravenous glucose (NPO) until progress has been made.
- Oral rehydration therapy may be a useful adjunct treatment in the recovery process.
- Start with bland or soft foods and then progress to a normal diet.
- Prolonged inability to eat orally may require tube feeding.

Common Drugs Used and Potential Side Effects

- Hydrochloric acid in the stomach protects against pathogens ingested with food or water. A gastric fluid pH of 1–2 is deleterious to many microbial pathogens. Neutralization of gastric acid by antacids or the inhibition of acid secretion by various drugs can alter stomach pH and may increase the risk of acquiring food- or waterborne illnesses (Smith, 2003).
- Octreotide (Sandostatin) may be used parenterally only. It may alter fat absorption and fat-soluble vitamin absorption.

- Antibiotics such as Puromycin, erythromycin, or a fluoroquinolone may be prescribed.
- For *Salmonella*, ampicillin, gentamicin, trimethoprim/sulfamethoxazole, or ciprofloxacin may be used. New strains of this bacteria have evolved so that they are more resistant to antimicrobial treatment (Foley and Lynne, 2008).
- *V. vulnificus* infection is treated with doxycycline or ceftazidime.

Herbs, Botanicals, and Supplements

- Note that herbs and botanicals themselves could be a source of foodborne bacteria and thus exacerbate an existing foodborne infection. If herbs and botanicals are used, identify and monitor for potential contamination and side effects.
- Counsel about use of herbal teas, especially regarding toxic substances.

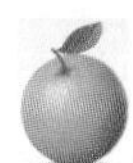

NUTRITION EDUCATION, COUNSELING, CARE MANAGEMENT

- Encourage safe methods of food handling. More males, African Americans, and adults aged between 30 and 54 years consume raw/undercooked ground beef than any other group; males, Caucasians, Hispanics, and young adults aged between 18 and 29 years often engage in poor hygienic practices (Patil et al, 2004).
- Monitor water supply for unexpected odors or color changes; report to authorities.
- Discuss ways to prevent further episodes of foodborne illness. See Table 2-15.
- Hand washing is important. Wash hands with soap before handling raw foods of animal origin, after handling raw foods of animal origin, and before touching anything else. Prevent cross-contamination in the kitchen. Proper refrigeration and sanitation are also essential.
- Avoid raw milk and cook all meats and poultry thoroughly. Drink only pasteurized milk.
- Bacteria may be found in raw vegetables and fruits. Wash before eating.
- Throw out bulging, leaking, or dented cans and jars that are leaking. Safe home canning tips can be obtained from county extension services or from the U.S. Department of Agriculture.
- Commercial mayonnaise, salad dressings, and sauces appear to be safe due to their content of acetic acid and lesser amounts of citric or lactic acids (Smittle, 2000). Thus, if items are prepared using cold dressings, they stay at proper temperatures longer.
- To prevent parasite infestation (such as *Giardia*), sewage treatment, proper hand washing, and use of bottled water is recommended (Kucik et al, 2004).
- Food handlers need more education to understand their role in food safety, especially non-English speaking staff members (DeBess et al, 2009). Correct hand washing procedures, involvement of both managers and food handlers, and support from health departments are all important (Pragle et al, 2007). Errors in methods of washing hands, utensils, and preparation surfaces between food preparation tasks are common (Kendall et al, 2004).
- Three key practices are needed for safe food handling: careful hand washing, using thermometers, and proper handling of food surfaces (Pilling et al, 2008). Barriers in the workplace often include time constraints, inconvenience, inadequate training, and insufficient resources (Howells et al, 2008).
- Cancer and imunocompromised patients are especially vulnerable to foodborne illness. Risk-reducing behaviors, better food handling of routine foods, and hand washing should be encouraged (Medeiros et al, 2008).
- Young adults also need education about food safety for themselves and for their future families (Byrd-Bredbenner et al, 2007).
- Low socioeconomic status has been shown to be linked with poorer quality produce and an increased reliance on small retail stores (Koro et al, 2010).
- Biotechnology has developed food crops that are more resistant to pests and have better nutritional value as well as having longer shelf-life for food safety. Some consumers are concerned about the safety of food irradiation, genetically modified foods (GMOs), and potential allergens. Nutrition professionals should reassure the public that GM items are safe to eat.

TABLE 2-16 Recommended Refrigerator Food Storage

Food	Time Period
Butter	1–3 months
Cheese, hard	6 months unopened; 3–4 weeks opened
Cheese, soft	1 week
Chicken, turkey	1–2 days
Eggs in shell	3–5 weeks
Eggs, raw	2–4 days
Fish, cooked	3–4 days
Fish, raw	1–2 days
Gravy	1–2 days
Hamburger, raw	1–2 days
Juices, chilled	3 weeks unopened, 7–10 days opened
Luncheon meat	3–5 days opened, 2 weeks in sealed package
Margarine	4–5 months
Milk	1 week
Pizza	3–4 days
Roast or steak	3–5 days (uncooked)
Sausage, raw	1–2 days
Sausage, smoked	1 week
Shellfish, fresh	1–2 days
Soups, stews	3–4 days
Yogurt	1–2 weeks

For More Information

- American Dietetic Association Home Food Safety Program
  http://www.homefoodsafety.org/index.jsp
- Biotechnology and Food Safety
  http://www.foodsafety.gov/~lrd/biotechm.html
- Bioterrorism and Food Safety
  http://www.fda.gov/oc/opacom/hottopics/bioterrorism.html
  http://www.foodsafety.gov/~fsg/bioterr.html
- Botulism
  http://www.cdc.gov/nczved/dfbmd/disease_listing/botulism_gi.html
- CDC Foodborne, Bacterial and Mycotic Diseases
  http://www.cdc.gov/nczved/dfbmd/disease_listing.html
- CDC Wonder—single access site
  http://wonder.cdc.gov/
- Codex Alimentarius—International Food Regulations
  http://www.fsis.usda.gov/Codex_Alimentarius/index.asp
  http://www.fsis.usda.gov/codex_alimentarius/Codex_Publications/index.asp
- Division of Emerging Infections and Surveillance Services (DEISS)
  http://www.cdc.gov/ncpdcid/deiss/index.html
- Drinking Water Safety
  http://www.epa.gov/safewater/dwh/index.html
- Frequently Asked Questions—Drinking Water
  http://www.epa.gov/safewater/faq/faq.html
- Federal Consumer Information Center
  http://www.pueblo.gsa.gov/food.htm
- Fight BAC
  http://www.fightbac.org/
- Food and Drug Administration Center for Food Safety and Applied Nutrition (CFSAN)
  http://www.cfsan.fda.gov/
- Food Defense and Emergency Response
  http://www.fsis.usda.gov/food_defense_&_emergency_response/index.asp
- FoodNet Incidence Figures
  http://www.cdc.gov/foodnet/factsandfigures.htm
- Food Safety Education
  http://www.fsis.usda.gov/Food_Safety_Education/index.asp
- Food Safety and Inspection Service (FSIS)
  http://www.fsis.usda.gov/
- Food Safety and Inspection—Risk Assessment
  http://www.fsis.usda.gov/Science/Risk_Assessments/index.asp
- Food Safety for Kids, Teenagers and Educators
  http://www.foodsafety.gov/~fsg/Fsgkids.html
- Food Safety for Seniors
  http://www.pueblo.gsa.gov/cic_text/food/foodsafetyfs/seniors.htm
- Government Food Safety Website
  http://www.foodsafety.gov/
- HACCP
  http://www.fsis.usda.gov/Science/Hazard_Analysis_&_Pathogen_Reduction/index.asp
  http://www.who.int/foodsafety/fs_management/haccp/en/index.html
  http://foodsafety.nal.usda.gov/nal_display/index.php?info_center=16&tax_level=1&tax_subject=178
- HACCP—International Alliance
  http://www.haccpalliance.org/sub/index.html
- Image Library
  http://www.fsis.usda.gov/News_&_Events/FSIS_Images/index.asp?src_location=IWT&src_page=FSE
- International Food Safety Sites
  http://www.foodsafety.gov/?7Efsg/fsgintl.html
- North Carolina State University
  http://www.ces.ncsu.edu/depts/foodsci/agentinfo/
- USDA Home Canning Guide
  http://www.uga.edu/nchfp/publications/publications_usda.html
- USDA Food Safety Index
  http://www.fsis.usda.gov/help/site_map/index.asp
- Water Quality Association
  http://www.wqa.org/
- World Health Organization—Biotechnology and GM Foods
  http://www.who.int/foodsafety/biotech/en/
- World Health Organization—Foodborne Illnesses
  http://www.who.int/topics/foodborne_diseases/en/index.html
- World Health Organization—Food Safety
  http://www.who.int/topics/food_safety/en/
- World Health Organization—International Travel and Health
  http://www.who.int/ith/en/index.html

  http://www.who.int/foodsafety/publications/consumer/travellers/en/index.html
- World Health Organization—Water Sanitation
  http://www.who.int/water_sanitation_health/mdg1/en/index.html

FOODBORNE ILLNESS—CITED REFERENCES

Byrd-Bredbenner C, et al. Food safety self-reported behaviors and cognitions of young adults: results of national study. *J Food Prot.* 70:1917, 2007.

Centers for Disease Control and Prevention. Preliminary FoodNet data on the incidence of infection with pathogens transmitted commonly through food—10 states, 2009. *MMWR Morb Mortal Wkly Rep.* 16;59:418, 2010.

DeBess EE, et al. Food handler assessment in Oregon. *Foodborne Pathog Dis.* 6:329, 2009.

Foley SL, Lynne AM. Food-animal associated Salmonella challenges: pathogenicity and microbial resistance. *J Anim Sci.* 86:E173, 2008.

Food and Nutrition Service (FNS), USDA. School food safety program based on hazard analysis and critical control point principles. Final rule. *Fed Regist.* 74:66213, 2009.

Howells AD, et al. Restaurant employees' perceptions of barriers to three food safety practices. *J Am Diet Assoc.* 108:1345, 2008.

Kendall PA, et al. Observation versus self-report: validation of a consumer food behavior questionnaire. *J Food Prot.* 67:2578, 2004.

Koro ME, et al. Microbial quality of food available to populations of differing socioeconomic status. *Am J Prev Med.* 38:478, 2010.

Kucik CJ, et al. Common intestinal parasites. *Am Fam Physician.* 69:1161, 2004.

Mayerhauser C. Survival of enterohemorrhagic *Escherichia coli* O157:H7 in retail mustard. *J Food Prot.* 64:783, 2001.

McCluskey KM. Implementing hazard analysis critical control points. *J Am Diet Assoc.* 104:1699, 2004.

Medeiros LC, et al. Discovery and development of educational strategies to encourage safe food handling behaviors in cancer patients. *J Food Prot.* 71:1666, 2008.

Patil SR, et al. An application of meta-analysis in food safety consumer research to evaluate consumer behaviors and practices. *J Food Prot.* 67:2587, 2004.

Pilling VK, et al. Identifying specific beliefs to targetto improve restaurant employees' intentions for performing three important food safety behaviors. *J Am Diet Assoc.* 108:991, 2008.

Pragle AS, et al. Food workers' perspectives on handwashing behaviors and barriers in the restaurant environment. *J Environ Health.* 69:27, 2007.

Smith JL. The role of gastric acid in preventing foodborne disease and how bacteria overcome acid conditions. *J Food Prot.* 66:1292, 2003.

Smittle R. Microbiological safety of mayonnaise, salad dressings, and sauces produced in the United States. *J Food Prot.* 63:1144, 2000.

Strohbehn CH, et al. Food safety practice and HACCP implementation: perceptions of registered dietitians and dietary managers. *J Am Diet Assoc.* 101:1692, 2004.

Woteki C. Dietitians can prevent listeriosis. *J Am Diet Assoc.* 101:285, 2001.

SECTION 3

Pediatrics: Birth Defects and Genetic and Acquired Disorders

BACKGROUND AND CONSIDERATIONS

Because good nutrition is essential for achieving growth and development, screening and assessment should be an integral part of health care. Efforts should be made to enhance appetite and intake in children who are not with their families; familiarity is important. Simple nutritional screening tools can help identify children at risk for malnutrition, affecting one fourth to one third of children admitted to a hospital. When there are problems with growth, proper interventions and referrals are important. A checklist of "ABCDE" factors can be used to assure completion of all assessments. Poor health habits, limited access to services, and long-term use of multiple medications are common health risk factors (American Dietetic Association, 2010). See Table 3-1 for assessments and calculations and see Table 3-2 for common pediatric problems. Nationally credentialed dietetics professionals are best able to provide appropriate nutrition information as it pertains to wellness, good health, and quality of life (American Dietetic Association, 2010). In particular, children with developmental disabilities and special health care needs frequently have growth alterations (failure to thrive (FTT), obesity, or growth retardation), metabolic disorders, poor feeding skills, medication–nutrient interactions, or dependence on enteral or parenteral nutrition (PN; American Dietetic Association, 2010). Nutrition services should be provided throughout life in a manner that is interdisciplinary, family-centered, community-based, and culturally competent (American Dietetic Association, 2010).

TABLE 3-1 Useful Assessments in Pediatrics

Anthropometric

Use age-, gender-, and disease-specific growth charts from the Centers for Disease Control and Prevention (CDC) with trained personnel and appropriate equipment. *Figure 1 shows how to measure the length of an infant properly.*

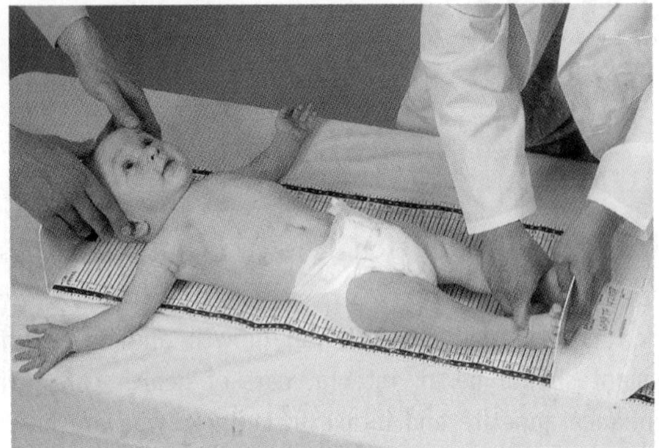

Figure 1. Measuring an infant. (From Bickley LS, Szilagyi P. *Bates' guide to physical examination and history taking,* 8th ed. Philadelphia: Lippincott Williams & Wilkins, 2003).

- Birth data (Weight, length, head circumference, size, gestational age)
  - Low birthweight ≤2500 g or 5.5 lb
  - Very low birth weight ≤1500 g or 3.5 lb
- Growth parameters: *Figure 2 provides the pediatric BMI tables*
  - Current height (ht) and weight (wt)
  - Wt/age <10th percentile or >85th percentile (overweight) or >95% (obese)
  - Ht/age <5th percentile
  - Wt/ht <5th percentile (underweight or FTT) or >85th percentile (overweight)
  - Head circumference <5th percentile (under 3 years of age)
- Pubertal staging (Tanner Stages), skeletal maturity staging
- Small for gestational age—need catch up growth to normalize length and weight; may later have CKD or metabolic syndrome as adults
- Unintentional weight loss

Behavioral—Psychosocial

- Developmental disorders: mental retardation, learning disorders, motor skills disorder, communication disorders, or PDDs
- Growth and development milestones

CALCULATED BODY MASS INDEX (BMI) FOR CHILDREN AND ADOLESCENTS

WEIGHT (in pounds)

HEIGHT (in inches)	50	55	60	65	70	75	80	85	90	95	100	105	110	115	120	125	130	135	140	145	150	155	160	165
3'9"	17.4	19.1	20.8	22.6	24.3	26	27.8	29.5	31.2	33	34.716	36.452	38.2	39.9	41.66	43.395	45.131	46.87	48.6	50.34	52.07	53.81	55.546	57.28
	17	18.7	19	20	23.8	25.5	27.2	28.9	30.6	32.3	33.957	35.655	37.4	39.1	40.75	42.447	44.144	45.84	47.54	49.24	50.94	52.63	54.332	56.03
3'10"	16.6	18.3	18	20	23.3	24.9	26.6	28.2	29.9	31.6	33.223	34.884	36.5	38.2	39.87	41.529	43.19	44.85	46.51	48.17	49.83	51.5	53.157	54.82
	16.3	17.9	18	19.5	22.8	24.4	26	27.6	29.3	30.9	32.512	34.138	35.8	37.4	39.01	40.641	42.266	43.89	45.52	47.14	48.77	50.39	52.02	53.65
3'11"	15.9	17.5	19.1	20.7	22.3	23.9	25.5	27.1	28.6	30.2	31.824	33.416	35	36.6	38.19	39.78	41.372	42.96	44.55	46.15	47.74	49.33	50.919	52.51
	15.6	17.1	18.7	20.3	21.8	23.4	24.9	26.5	28	29.6	31.158	32.716	34.3	35.8	37.39	38.947	40.505	42.06	43.62	45.18	46.74	48.29	49.853	51.41
4'0"	15.3	16.8	18.3	19.8	21.4	22.9	24.4	25.9	27.5	29	30.512	32.038	33.6	35.1	36.61	38.14	39.666	41.19	42.72	44.24	45.77	47.29	48.819	50.35
4'1"	14.6	16.1	17.6	19	20.5	22	23.4	24.9	26.4	27.8	29.279	30.743	32.2	33.7	35.14	36.599	38.063	39.53	40.99	42.46	43.92	45.38	46.847	48.31
4'2"	14.1	15.5	16.9	18.3	19.7	21.1	22.5	23.9	25.3	26.7	28.12	29.526	30.9	32.3	33.74	35.15	36.556	37.96	39.37	40.77	42.18	43.59	44.992	46.4
4'3"	13.5	14.9	16.2	17.6	18.9	20.3	21.6	23	24.3	25.7	27.028	28.379	29.7	31.1	32.43	33.785	35.136	36.49	37.84	39.19	40.54	41.89	43.245	44.6
4'4"	13	14.3	15.6	16.9	18.2	19.5	20.8	22.1	23.4	24.7	25.999	27.298	28.6	29.9	31.2	32.498	33.798	35.1	36.4	37.7	39	40.3	41.598	42.9
4'5"	12.5	13.8	15	16.3	17.5	18.8	20	21.3	22.5	23.8	25.027	26.278	27.5	28.8	30.03	31.283	32.535	33.79	35.04	36.29	37.54	38.79	40.043	41.29
4'6"	12.1	13.3	14.5	15.7	16.9	18.1	19.3	20.5	21.7	22.9	24.108	25.314	26.5	27.7	28.93	30.135	31.341	32.55	33.75	34.96	36.16	37.37	38.573	39.78
4'7"	11.6	12.8	13.9	15.1	16.3	17.4	18.6	19.8	20.9	22.1	23.24	24.402	25.6	26.7	27.89	29.05	30.212	31.37	32.54	33.7	34.86	36.02	37.183	38.35
4'8"	11.2	12.3	13.5	14.6	15.7	16.8	17.9	19.1	20.2	21.3	22.417	23.538	24.7	25.8	26.9	28.021	29.142	30.26	31.38	32.5	33.63	34.75	35.867	36.99
4'9"	10.8	11.9	13	14.1	15.1	16.2	17.3	18.4	19.5	20.6	21.637	22.719	23.8	24.9	25.96	27.047	28.129	29.21	30.29	31.37	32.46	33.54	34.62	35.7
4'10"	10.4	11.5	12.5	13.6	14.6	15.7	16.7	17.8	18.8	19.9	20.898	21.943	23	24	25.08	26.122	27.167	28.21	29.26	30.3	31.35	32.39	33.436	34.48
4'11"	10.1	11.1	12.1	13.1	14.1	15.1	16.2	17.2	18.2	19.2	20.195	21.205	22.2	23.2	24.23	25.244	26.254	27.26	28.27	29.28	30.29	31.3	32.313	33.32
5'0"	9.76	10.7	11.7	12.7	13.7	14.6	15.6	16.6	17.6	18.6	19.528	20.504	21.5	22.5	23.43	24.41	25.386	26.36	27.34	28.32	29.29	30.27	31.244	32.22
5'1"	9.45	10.4	11.3	12.3	13.2	14.2	15.1	16.1	17	17.9	18.893	19.837	20.8	21.7	22.67	23.616	24.561	25.51	26.45	27.39	28.34	29.28	30.228	31.17
5'2"	9.14	10.1	11	11.9	12.8	13.7	14.6	15.5	16.5	17.4	18.288	19.203	20.1	21	21.95	22.86	23.775	24.69	25.6	26.52	27.43	28.35	29.261	30.18
5'3"	8.86	9.74	10.6	11.5	12.4	13.3	14.2	15.1	15.9	16.8	17.712	18.598	19.5	20.4	21.25	22.14	23.026	23.91	24.8	25.68	26.57	27.45	28.34	29.23
5'4"	8.58	9.44	10.3	11.2	12	12.9	13.7	14.6	15.4	16.3	17.163	18.021	18.9	19.7	20.6	21.454	22.312	23.17	24.03	24.89	25.74	26.6	27.461	28.32
5'5"	8.32	9.15	9.98	10.8	11.6	12.5	13.3	14.1	15	15.8	16.639	17.471	18.3	19.1	19.97	20.799	21.631	22.46	23.29	24.13	24.96	25.79	26.622	27.45
5'6"	8.07	8.88	9.68	10.5	11.3	12.1	12.9	13.7	14.5	15.3	16.139	16.946	17.8	18.6	19.37	20.173	20.98	21.79	22.59	23.4	24.21	25.01	25.822	26.63
5'7"	7.83	8.61	9.4	10.2	11	11.7	12.5	13.3	14.1	14.9	15.661	16.444	17.2	18	18.79	19.576	20.359	21.14	21.92	22.71	23.49	24.27	25.057	25.84
5'8"	7.6	8.36	9.12	9.88	10.6	11.4	12.2	12.9	13.7	14.4	15.203	15.963	16.7	17.5	18.24	19.004	19.764	20.52	21.28	22.04	22.8	23.57	24.325	25.09
5'9"	7.38	8.12	8.86	9.6	10.3	11.1	11.8	12.6	13.3	14	14.766	15.504	16.2	17	17.72	18.457	19.196	19.93	20.67	21.41	22.15	22.89	23.625	24.36
5'10"	7.17	7.89	8.61	9.33	10	10.8	11.5	12.2	12.9	13.6	14.347	15.064	15.8	16.5	17.22	17.934	18.651	19.37	20.09	20.8	21.52	22.24	22.955	23.67
5'11"	6.97	7.67	8.37	9.06	9.76	10.5	11.2	11.9	12.6	13.2	13.946	14.643	15.3	16	16.73	17.432	18.129	18.83	19.52	20.22	20.92	21.62	22.313	23.01
6'0"	6.78	7.46	8.14	8.81	9.49	10.2	10.8	11.5	12.2	12.9	13.561	14.239	14.9	15.6	16.27	16.951	17.629	18.31	18.99	19.66	20.34	21.02	21.698	22.38
6'1"	6.6	7.26	7.92	8.57	9.23	9.89	10.6	11.2	11.9	12.5	13.192	13.852	14.5	15.2	15.83	16.49	17.15	17.81	18.47	19.13	19.79	20.45	21.107	21.77
6'2"	6.42	7.06	7.7	8.34	8.99	9.63	10.3	10.9	11.6	12.2	12.838	13.48	14.1	14.8	15.41	16.047	16.689	17.33	17.97	18.61	19.26	19.9	20.541	21.18
6'3"	6.25	6.87	7.5	8.12	8.75	9.37	10	10.6	11.2	11.9	12.498	13.123	13.7	14.4	15	15.622	16.247	16.87	17.5	18.12	18.75	19.37	19.996	20.62
6'4"	6.09	6.69	7.3	7.91	8.52	9.13	9.74	10.3	11	11.6	12.171	12.78	13.4	14	14.61	15.214	15.822	16.43	17.04	17.65	18.26	18.87	19.474	20.08
6'5"	5.93	6.52	7.11	7.71	8.3	8.89	9.49	10.1	10.7	11.3	11.857	12.45	13	13.6	14.23	14.821	15.414	16.01	16.6	17.19	17.79	18.38	18.971	19.56
6'6"	5.78	6.36	6.93	7.51	8.09	8.67	9.24	9.82	10.4	11	11.555	12.133	12.7	13.3	13.87	14.444	15.021	15.6	16.18	16.75	17.33	17.91	18.488	19.07
6'7"	5.63	6.2	6.76	7.32	7.88	8.45	9.01	9.57	10.1	10.7	11.264	11.827	12.4	13	13.52	14.08	14.643	15.21	15.77	16.33	16.9	17.46	18.023	18.59

Figure 2. Pediatric BMI tables (*continued*)

(continued)

TABLE 3-1 Useful Assessments in Pediatrics *(continued)*

- Hunger and satiety; use of food for reward or as pacifier
- Home environment and family economics (access to food)
- Access to interdisciplinary, family-centered, community-based and culturally relevant services (American Dietetic Association, 2004)

Clinical

- Altered gastrointestinal function: nausea, vomiting, acute diarrhea, constipation, GERD
- Altered nutrition-related biochemical values—such as serum cholesterol. Total serum cholesterol should be <170 mg/dL in children and teens. If >170–199 mg/dL, take a second total serum cholesterol, and average the two together. If >200 mg/dL, a fasting lipid profile is needed
- Birth defects: some can be diagnosed before birth, using prenatal ultrasound, amniocentesis, and chorionic villus sampling (CVS). Ultrasound can help diagnose structural birth defects, such as spina bifida and heart or urinary tract defects. Amniocentesis and CVS are used to diagnose chromosomal abnormalities, such as DS
- Chewing and swallowing difficulties (such as from cleft lip or palate, oral lesions)
- Chronic illnesses (cancer, cardiac disease or heart failure, diabetes, elevated lipids, FTT, hypertension, kidney disease, malabsorption, HIV/AIDS, trauma)
- Congenital or chromosomal abnormalities, inborn metabolic disorders
- Digestive and malabsorptive problems from celiac disease, lactose deficiency, or inflammatory bowel disease; sugar intolerance; foul-smelling, bulky stools indicate fat malabsorption
- Food allergies
- Inadequate intake because of depression, pain or dyspnea, poor appetite >3 days
- Increased nutrient demands, as from protein–energy malnutrition, pressure ulcers

WEIGHT (in pounds)																			
170	175	180	185	190	195	200	205	210	215	220	225	230	235	240	245	250	255	260	265
59.017	60.753	62.489	64.225	65.96	67.7	69.432	71.1679	72.9037	74.64	76.375	78.111	79.84691	81.583	83.31852	85.054321	86.7901	88.5259	90.2617	91.998
57.727	59.425	61.123	62.821	64.52	66.22	67.915	69.6124	71.3102	73.01	74.706	76.404	78.10168	79.8	81.4974	83.195266	84.8931	86.591	88.2889	89.987
56.479	58.14	59.802	61.463	63.12	64.78	66.446	68.1073	69.7684	71.43	73.091	74.752	76.41304	78.074	79.73535	81.396503	83.0577	84.7188	86.38	88.041
55.271	56.897	58.522	60.148	61.77	63.4	65.025	66.6505	68.2761	69.9	71.527	73.153	74.77859	76.404	78.02983	79.655451	81.2811	82.9067	84.5323	86.158
54.101	55.693	57.284	58.875	60.47	62.06	63.649	65.2399	66.8311	68.42	70.014	71.605	73.19602	74.787	76.37845	77.96967	79.5609	81.1521	82.7433	84.335
52.968	54.526	56.084	57.642	59.2	60.76	62.316	63.8737	65.4316	66.99	68.547	70.105	71.66316	73.221	74.77895	76.336842	77.8947	79.4526	81.0105	82.568
51.871	53.396	54.922	56.447	57.97	59.5	61.024	62.5499	64.0755	65.6	67.127	68.652	70.17795	71.704	73.22917	74.754774	76.2804	77.806	79.3316	80.857
49.775	51.239	52.703	54.167	55.63	57.09	58.559	60.0229	61.4869	62.95	64.415	65.879	67.34277	68.807	70.27072	71.734694	73.1987	74.6626	76.1266	77.591
47.804	49.21	50.616	52.022	53.43	54.83	56.24	57.646	59.052	60.46	61.864	63.27	64.676	66.082	67.488	68.894	70.3	71.706	73.112	74.518
45.948	47.299	48.651	50.002	51.35	52.7	54.056	55.4075	56.7589	58.11	59.462	60.813	62.16455	63.516	64.86736	66.218762	67.5702	68.9216	70.273	71.624
44.197	45.497	46.797	48.097	49.4	50.7	51.997	53.297	54.5969	55.9	57.197	58.497	59.7966	61.097	62.39645	63.696376	64.9963	66.2962	67.5962	68.896
42.545	43.797	45.048	46.299	47.55	48.8	50.053	51.3047	52.5561	53.81	55.059	56.31	57.56141	58.813	60.06408	61.315415	62.5667	63.8181	65.0694	66.321
40.984	42.19	43.395	44.6	45.81	47.01	48.217	49.4222	50.6276	51.83	53.038	54.244	55.44925	56.655	57.86008	59.065501	60.2709	61.4763	62.6818	63.887
39.507	40.669	41.831	42.993	44.16	45.32	46.479	47.6413	48.8033	49.97	51.127	52.289	53.45124	54.613	55.77521	56.93719	58.0992	59.2612	60.4231	61.585
38.109	39.23	40.351	41.472	42.59	43.71	44.834	45.955	47.0759	48.2	49.318	50.438	51.55931	52.68	53.80102	54.921875	56.0427	57.1636	58.2844	59.405
36.784	37.865	38.947	40.029	41.11	42.19	43.275	44.3567	45.4386	46.52	47.602	48.684	49.76608	50.848	51.92982	53.011696	54.0936	55.1754	56.2573	57.339
35.526	36.571	37.616	38.661	39.71	40.75	41.795	42.8404	43.8853	44.93	45.975	47.02	48.0648	49.11	50.15458	51.199465	52.2444	53.2892	54.3341	55.379
34.332	35.342	36.352	37.361	38.37	39.38	40.391	41.4005	42.4102	43.42	44.43	45.44	46.4493	47.459	48.46883	49.478598	50.4884	51.4981	52.5079	53.518
33.197	34.174	35.15	36.126	37.1	38.08	39.056	40.0319	41.0083	41.98	42.961	43.938	44.91389	45.89	46.86667	47.843056	48.8194	49.7958	50.7722	51.749
32.118	33.062	34.007	34.952	35.9	36.84	37.786	38.7302	39.6748	40.62	41.564	42.509	43.45337	44.398	45.34265	46.287288	47.2319	48.1766	49.1212	50.066
31.09	32.004	32.919	33.833	34.75	35.66	36.576	37.4909	38.4053	39.32	40.234	41.149	42.06296	42.977	43.89178	44.806191	45.7206	46.635	47.5494	48.464
30.111	30.996	31.882	32.768	33.65	34.54	35.425	36.3102	37.1958	38.08	38.967	39.853	40.73822	41.624	42.50945	43.395062	44.2807	45.1663	46.0519	46.938
29.177	30.035	30.894	31.752	32.61	33.47	34.326	35.1843	36.0425	36.9	37.759	38.617	39.4751	40.333	41.19141	42.049561	42.9077	43.7659	44.624	45.482
28.286	29.118	29.95	30.782	31.61	32.45	33.278	34.1101	34.942	35.77	36.606	37.438	38.26982	39.102	39.93373	40.76568	41.5976	42.4296	43.2615	44.093
27.436	28.243	29.05	29.857	30.66	31.47	32.277	33.0843	33.8912	34.7	35.505	36.312	37.11892	37.926	38.73278	39.539715	40.3466	41.1536	41.9605	42.767
26.623	27.406	28.189	28.972	29.75	30.54	31.321	32.104	32.8871	33.67	34.453	35.236	36.01916	36.802	37.58521	38.368233	39.1513	39.9343	40.7173	41.5
25.846	26.606	27.366	28.126	28.89	29.65	30.407	31.1667	31.9269	32.69	33.447	34.207	34.96756	35.728	36.48789	37.248054	38.0082	38.7684	39.5285	40.289
25.102	25.84	26.578	27.317	28.06	28.79	29.532	30.2699	31.0082	31.75	32.485	33.223	33.96135	34.7	35.43793	36.176223	36.9145	37.6528	38.3911	39.129
24.39	25.107	25.824	26.542	27.26	27.98	28.694	29.4112	30.1286	30.85	31.563	32.281	32.99796	33.715	34.43265	35.15	35.8673	36.5847	37.302	38.019
23.708	24.405	25.102	25.799	26.5	27.19	27.891	28.5886	29.2859	29.98	30.68	31.378	32.07499	32.772	33.46955	34.166832	34.8641	35.5614	36.2587	36.956
23.054	23.732	24.41	25.088	25.77	26.44	27.122	27.8	28.478	29.16	29.834	30.512	31.1902	31.868	32.5463	33.224344	33.9024	34.5804	35.2585	35.937
22.426	23.086	23.746	24.405	25.06	25.72	26.384	27.0435	27.7031	28.36	29.022	29.682	30.34153	31.001	31.66072	32.320323	32.9799	33.6395	34.2991	34.959
21.824	22.466	23.108	23.75	24.39	25.03	25.676	26.3176	26.9595	27.6	28.243	28.885	29.52703	30.169	30.81081	31.452703	32.0946	32.7365	33.3784	34.02
21.246	21.871	22.496	23.121	23.75	24.37	24.996	25.6204	26.2453	26.87	27.495	28.12	28.74489	29.37	29.99467	30.619556	31.2444	31.8693	32.4942	33.119
20.691	21.299	21.908	22.516	23.13	23.73	24.342	24.9507	25.5592	26.17	26.776	27.385	27.99342	28.602	29.21053	29.819079	30.4276	31.0362	31.6447	32.253
20.157	20.75	21.343	21.935	22.53	23.12	23.714	24.3068	24.8996	25.49	26.085	26.678	27.27104	27.864	28.45674	29.049587	29.6424	30.2353	30.8281	31.421
19.643	20.221	20.799	21.377	21.95	22.53	23.11	23.6875	24.2653	24.84	25.421	25.999	26.57627	27.154	27.73176	28.3095	28.8872	29.465	30.0427	30.62
19.149	19.712	20.276	20.839	21.4	21.97	22.528	23.0917	23.6549	24.22	24.781	25.344	25.90771	26.471	27.03413	27.59734	28.1606	28.7238	29.287	29.85

(continued)

TABLE 3-1 Useful Assessments in Pediatrics *(continued)*

- Marked weight loss (malabsorption, IBD, hyperthyroidism, or malignancy)
- Medications with nutritional side effects:
  - Antibiotics (energy, protein, minerals; GI problems)
  - Anticonvulsants (vitamins C, K, D, and B-complex, and calcium)
  - Corticosteroids (calcium, phosphorus, glucose levels; weight gain or stunting)
  - Diuretics (potassium, magnesium, calcium, energy; GI problems)
  - Stimulants such as ritalin (energy and protein intake, growth, appetite)
  - Sulfonamides (vitamin C, protein, folate, and iron)
  - Tranquilizers (energy intake; weight gain)
- Inability to consume oral diet:
  - Pediatric tube feeding: prematurity, developmental delays, orofacial defects, CP, anorexia nervosa, cystic fibrosis, metabolic disorders, renal failure, HIV infection, or inflammatory bowel disorders
  - Pediatric TPN: biliary atresia, Hirschsprung's disease with enterocolitis, Crohn's disease, ulcerative colitis, congenital short-bowel, GI ischemia or fistulas, severe burns or trauma, and bowel transplantation. It may be possible to wean from TPN to tube or oral feeding in some conditions; for others, PN may be permanent. Children cannot tolerate fasting as long as adults
- Increased nutrient needs for trauma, surgery, recent hospitalizations, acute illnesses, chemotherapy or radiation

Developmental Disabilities

- Altered nutritional status, feeding skills, feeding behaviors including positioning
- Use specific screening tools for each physical, motor, sensory, or developmental delays. Use arm span where height is difficult to measure
- In children whose weight is hard to maintain, catch-up growth is important with a focus on protein and kilocals
- Individualize care: design the desired outcomes, determine necessary resources, and seek regular feedback on progress or obstacles. Personal control, independence, and choice must be considered

Eating and Feeding Skills

- Avoidance of easily aspirated foods
- Biting, chewing or swallowing difficulty requiring texture modifications
- Coordination for safe and proper chewing, sucking, swallowing
- Feeding: length of time, feeding method, skill level, persons involved
- Food allergies, multiple or severe
- Food Intake: ability to eat and retain food
- Food preferences, dislikes, and intolerances
- Special formula or supplements, tube feeding or PN

Genetic and Metabolic Disorders

- Growth failure, skin rashes, developmental delays, vomiting or diarrhea and other concerns affect nutrition and health status in:
  - Amino acid metabolism: *phenylketonuria (PKU); maple syrup urine disease (MSUD); glutaric acidemia type 1(GA1); argininosuccinic academia (ASA); tyrosinemia (TYR); propionic academia (PA); isovaleric academia (IVA); citrullinemia type 1 (CIT)*
  - Carbohydrate metabolism: *galactosemia; glycogen storage disease (GSD); galactose-phosphate uridyltransferase (GALT)*
  - Fatty acid metabolism: *medium chain acyl dehydrogenase deficiency (MCAD); carnitine uptake deficiency (CUD); very long-chain acyl-CoA dehydrogenase (VLCAD); abetalipoproteinemia (ABL)*
- Presently, screening for 29 disorders is recommended for newborns in the United States; many states are doubling or tripling the number of tests offered (Isaacs and Zand, 2007). Newborn screening consists of testing; follow-up of abnormal screening; diagnostic testing; disease management; continuous evaluation and improvement of the system. Clues that suggest a genetic condition or an inherited susceptibility to a common disease include the following:
  - Two or more seemingly unrelated medical conditions (e.g., hearing loss and renal disease, diabetes and muscle disease)
  - A medical condition and dysmorphic features
  - Developmental delay with dysmorphic features and/or physical birth anomalies
  - Developmental delay associated with other medical conditions
  - Progressive mental retardation, loss of developmental milestones
  - Progressive behavioral problems
  - Unexplained hypotonia
  - A movement disorder
  - Unexplained seizures
  - Unexplained ataxia
  - Two or more major birth anomalies
  - Three or more minor birth anomalies
  - One major birth defect with two minor anomalies
  - A cleft palate, or cleft lip with or without cleft palate
  - Unusual birthmarks (particularly if associated with seizures, learning disabilities, or dysmorphic features)
  - Hair anomalies (hirsute, brittle, coarse, kinky, sparse or absent)
  - Congenital or juvenile deafness
  - Congenital or juvenile blindness
  - Cataracts at a young age
  - Primary amenorrhea
  - Ambiguous genitalia

(continued)

TABLE 3-1 Useful Assessments in Pediatrics *(continued)*

	A Fetus With
Proportionate short stature with dysmorphic features and/or delayed or arrested puberty	A major structural anomaly
Disproportionate short stature	Significant growth retardation
Premature ovarian failure	Multiple minor anomalies
Proportionate short stature and primary amenorrhea	(Gilchrist, 2002; March of Dimes, 2009)
Males with hypogonadism and/or significant gynecomastia	
Congenital absence of the vas deferens	
Oligozoospermia/azoospermia	

TABLE 1A: Examples of Single Gene Disorders in Adults[a]

Neurology

Muscular dystrophy
Spinocerebellar ataxia
Hereditary neuropathy
Dystonia
Early onset Alzheimer's disease
Familial multiple sclerosis
Familial amyotrophic lateral sclerosis
Neurofibromatosis

Nephrology

Autosomal dominant polycystic kidney disease
Hereditary nephritis
Disorders of renal physiology

Hematology

Hemoglobinopathies
Hereditary disorders of hemostasis
Hereditary hypercoagulability

Pulmonary disorders

Adult-onset cystic fibrosis
Alpha-1-antitrypsin deficiency

Cardiac disorders

Conduction abnormalities
Cardiomyopathy

Infectious disease

Immune deficiencies

Metabolic disorders

Hemochromatosis
Lipid disorders
Homocysteine

Gastroenterology

Osler-Weber-Rendu disease
Polyposis

Oncology

BRCA1/2
Familial adenomatous polyposis and hereditary nonpolyposis colon cancer
Familial prostate cancer
Multiple endocrine neoplasia
Hippel-Lindau disease
Li-Fraumeni syndrome

Musculoskeletal disorders

Inherited disorders of connective tissue—
Marfan's, Ehlers-Danlos, osteogenesis imperfecta

Dermatology

Icthyosis
Bullous disorders

Notes: Inborn metabolic disorders are usually due to defects of single genes that code for enzymes, intended to convert substrates into products.
[a]This is a far from complete list.

REFERENCES

American Dietetic Association. Position paper: providing nutrition services for infants, children and adults with developmental disabilities and special health care needs. *J Am Diet Assoc*. 104:97, 2004.

Gilchrist DM. Medical genetics: 3. An approach to the adult with a genetic disorder. *CMAJ*. 167:1021, 2002.

Harris AB. Evidence of increasing dietary supplement use in children with special health care needs: strategies for improving parent and professional communication. *J Am Diet Assoc*. 105:34, 2005.

Institute of Medicine. *Dietary reference intakes for energy, carbohydrate, fiber, fat, fatty acids, cholesterol, protein, and amino acids*. Washington, DC: National Academy of Sciences, 2002.

Isaacs JS, Zand DJ. Single-gene autosomal recessive disorders and Prader-Willi syndrome: an update for food and nutrition professionals. *J Am Diet Assoc*. 107:466, 2007.

Lucas B, ed. *Children with special care needs: nutrition care handbook*. Chicago: The American Dietetic Association, 2004.

March of Dimes. Accessed May 9, 2009, at http://www.marchofdimes.com/.

(continued)

TABLE 3-1 Useful Assessments in Pediatrics *(continued)*

Estimating Daily Energy Requirements (EER) and Total Energy Expenditure (TEE) for Infants and Children (Derived from Institute of Medicine, 2002; Lucas, 2004)

Age (months)	Equation
0–3	(89 × Wt − 100) + 175
4–6	(89 × Wt − 100) + 56
7–12	(89 × Wt − 100) + 22
13–35	(89 × Wt − 100) + 20

Boys: Age (years)	Equation
3–8	EER = 88.5 − 61.9 × age (y) + PA × (26.7 × Wt + 903 × Ht) + 20
9–19	EER = 88.5 − 61.9 × age (y) + PA × (26.7 × Wt + 903 × Ht) + 25
3–19, overweight	TEE = 114 −50.9 × age (y) + PA × (19.5 × Wt + 116.4 × Ht)

Girls: Age (years)	Equation
3–8	EER = 135.3 −30.8 × age (y) + PA × (10.0 × Wt + 934 × Ht) + 20
9–19	EER = 135.3 − 30.8 × age (y) + PA × (10.0 × Wt + 934 × Ht) + 25
3–19, overweight	TEE = 389 − 41.2 × age (y) + PA × (15.0 × Wt + 701 × Ht)

Physical Activity (PA) Coefficients for Children Aged 3–19 Years

	Coefficient for Boys Aged 3–19 years	Boys	Coefficient for Girls Aged 3–19 years	Girls
Activity Level	Normal Wt	Overweight	Normal Wt	Overweight
Sedentary	1.0	1.0	1.0	1.00
Low active	1.13	1.12	1.16	1.18
Active	1.26	1.24	1.31	1.35
Very Active	1.42	1.45	1.56	1.60

Acceptable Macronutrient Ranges

	Range (% of energy)		
Age	CHO	Fat	Protein
Full-term infant	35–65	30–55	7–16
1–3 years	45–65	30–40	5–20
4–18 years	45–65	25–35	10–30

TABLE 3-2 **Nutritional Risks Associated with Selected Pediatric Disorders**

	Low weight	Over-weight	Short Stature	Low Energy Needs	High Energy Needs	Feeding Problems	Constipation	Chronic Meds
Autism spectrum disorders	X				X	X		X
Bronchopulmonary dysplasia	X	X			X	X		X
Cerebral palsy	X	X	X	X	X	X	X	X
Cystic fibrosis	X		X		X	X		
Down syndrome		X		X		X		
Fetal alcohol syndrome	X		X					
Heart disease, congenital	X				X	X		X
HIV infection, AIDS	X				X			X
Phenylketonuria	X					X		
Prader-Willi syndrome		X	X	X				
Prematurity or low birth weight	X		X		X	X		
Seizure disorder								X
Spina bifida; neural tube defects	X	X	X	X			X	X

Adapted from: Baer M, Harris A. Pediatric nutrition assessment: identifying children at risk. *J Am Diet Assoc.* 97:107A, 1997.

For More Information About Birth Defects and Genetic Disorders

- Centers for Disease Control and Prevention (CDC) Birth Defects Research
  http://www.cdc.gov/ncbddd/bd/research.htm
- Coalition of State Genetics Coordinators
  http://www.stategeneticscoordinators.org
- Family Voices
  http://www.familyvoices.org/
- Genetic Alliance Disease InfoSearch
  http://www.geneticalliance.org
- Human Genome Project
  http://www.ornl.gov/sci/techresources/Human_Genome/home.shtml
- March of Dimes
  http://www.modimes.org/
- National Center for Education in Maternal and Child Health
  http://www.ncemch.org/
- National Dissemination Center for Children with Disabilities
  http://www.nichcy.org/
- National Folic Acid Campaign
  http://www.cdc.gov/ncbddd/folicacid/council.htm
- National Coalition for Health Professional Education in Genetics
  http://www.nchpeg.org
- National Institutes of Health Office of Rare Diseases
  http://rarediseases.info.nih.gov
- National Newborn Screening and Genetics Resource Center
  http://genes-r-us.uthscsa.edu
- National Urea Cycles Disorders Foundation
  http://www.nucdf.org/
- Online Mendelian Inheritance in Man (OMIM)
  http://www.ncbi.nlm.nih.gov/entrez/dispomim
- Organic Acidemia Association
  http://www.oaanews.org

For More Information About Feeding Problems and Assistance

- American Occupational Therapy Association, Inc.
  http://www.aota.org/
- The Oley Foundation for Home Enteral/Parenteral Therapy
  http://www.oley.org/

For More Information About Specialty Foods and Formulas

- Abbott Pediatric Products
  http:// www.ross.com/productHandbook/default.asp
- Applied Nutrition
  http://www.medicalfood.com
- Cambrooke Foods
  http://www.cambrookefoods.com/
- Dietary Specialties
  http://www.dietspec.com/
- Ener-G Foods
  http://www.ener-g.com/
- Glutino
  http://www.glutino.com/
- Kingsmill Foods
  http://www.kingsmillfoods.com/
- Loprofin (SHS)
  http://www.shsna.com/pages/loprofin.htm
- MedDiet
  http://www.med-diet.com/
- Mead Johnson
  http://www.meadjohnson.com/professional/prodinfo.html
- Milupa North American
  http://www.milupana.com
- Novartis
  http://www.novartis.com
- Scientific Hospital Supply
  http://www.shsna.com

For More Information About Rare Disorders and Health Laws

- Alliance of Genetic Support Groups
  http://geneticalliance.org/
- Genetics Home Reference
  http://ghr.nlm.nih.gov/
- Metabolic Disorders
  http://themedicalbiochemistrypage.org/inborn.html
- National Health Law Program
  http://www.healthlaw.org

- National Organization for Rare Disorders
  http://www.rarediseases.org/
- Newborn Screening
  http://www.savebabies.org/
- Office of Rare Diseases—NIH
  http://rarediseases.info.nih.gov/

REFERENCE

American Dietetic Association. Position of the American Dietetic Association: providing nutrition services for people with developmental disabilities and special health care Needs. *J Am Diet Assoc.* 110:296, 2010.

ABETALIPOPROTEINEMIA

NUTRITIONAL ACUITY RANKING: LEVEL 2–3

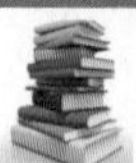

DEFINITIONS AND BACKGROUND

Abetalipoproteinemia (ABL) is a rare, inherited disease characterized by the inability to make low-density lipoproteins (LDL), very low–density lipoproteins (VLDL), and chylomicrons or to fully absorb dietary fats through the gut. Other names for this condition are Bassen-Kornzweig syndrome, acanthocytosis, or apolipoprotein B deficiency.

Acanthocytosis refers to the altered shape of the normal erythrocyte into one with a few irregularly shaped external projections that are thorny in appearance (Rampoldi et al., 2002; Wong, 2004). Infants present with FTT and fatty and pale stools that are frothy and foul smelling. They may also have a protruding abdomen, developmental delays, slurred speech, and problems with balance and muscle coordination after age 10. Mental deterioration and scoliosis also occur.

Prognosis is related to the progression of neurological and visual problems. Severe forms lead to irreversible neurological disease before age 30 and often to blindness. Progressive ataxic neuropathy and retinopathy are related to oxidative damage resulting from deficiencies of vitamins E and A (Granot and Kohen, 2004). Therefore, vigorous nutritional supplementation is essential (Chardon et al, 2008). Other treatments such as stem-cell therapy and gene product replacement are under evaluation.

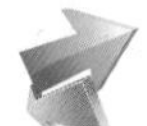

ASSESSMENT, MONITORING, AND EVALUATION

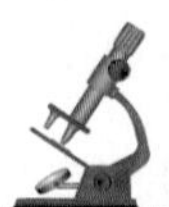

CLINICAL INDICATORS

Genetic Markers: Microsomal triglyceride transfer protein (MTTP or MTP) deficiency

Clinical/History

Height
Weight
Growth chart
Diet/intake history
Scoliosis
Retinal degeneration, retinitis pigmentosa
Low vision or blindness
Developmental delay?
Neurological changes

Lab Work

CBC with abnormal, thorny-shaped cells

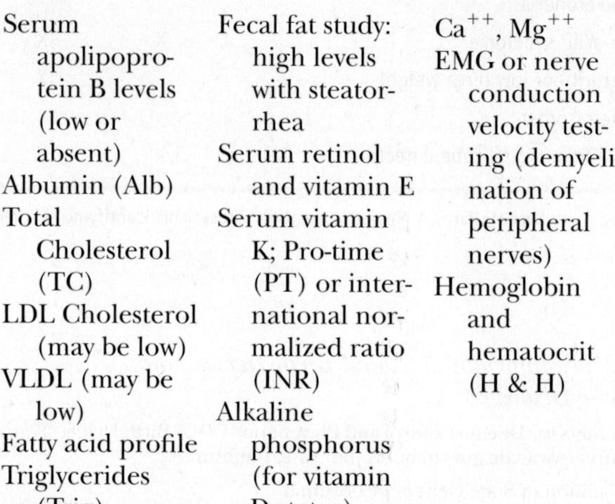

Serum apolipoprotein B levels (low or absent)
Albumin (Alb)
Total Cholesterol (TC)
LDL Cholesterol (may be low)
VLDL (may be low)
Fatty acid profile
Triglycerides (Trig)
Fecal fat study: high levels with steatorrhea
Serum retinol and vitamin E
Serum vitamin K; Pro-time (PT) or international normalized ratio (INR)
Alkaline phosphorus (for vitamin D status)
Ca^{++}, Mg^{++}
EMG or nerve conduction velocity testing (demyelination of peripheral nerves)
Hemoglobin and hematocrit (H & H)

INTERVENTION

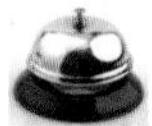

OBJECTIVES

- Decrease rapid progression of disorder by giving large doses of fat-soluble vitamin supplements. This may help prevent deterioration of vision and degeneration of the retina (retinitis pigmentosa).

SAMPLE NUTRITION CARE PROCESS STEPS

Steatorrhea

Assessment Data: Food records indicating poor intake; changes in weight; cholesterol levels.

Nutrition Diagnoses (PES): Inadequate fat soluble vitamin intake (especially E) related to fat malaborption in ABL as evidenced by frothy stools four to five times daily, low serum cholesterol level, low serum levels of vitamin E, and abdominal distention.

Intervention: Education of parents about the need for fat-soluble vitamin supplementation and for linoleic acid supplementation for condition.

Monitoring and Evaluation: Improved lab reports for vitamin E and cholesterol; weight improvement; fewer frothy stools and less abdominal distention.

- Avoid use of long-chain triglycerides; use medium-chain triglycerides (MCT) instead.
- Prevent nutrient deficiency symptoms and conditions, such as FTT; impaired balance; difficulty walking, and other complications. Provide linoleic acid supplementation for essential fatty acids (EFAs).

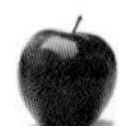

FOOD AND NUTRITION

- The diet should contain no more than 5 oz of lean meat, fish, or poultry per day.
- Use skim milk instead of whole milk; reduce fats from other types of dairy products.
- Use MCT oil in food preparation and with gravies, sauces, and other cooked foods. Avoid excesses to prevent liver problems.
- The diet should be supplemented with fat-soluble vitamins A, D, E, and K plus linoleic acid to prevent deficiency. Water-miscible forms will be needed.

Common Drugs Used and Potential Side Effects

- Large doses of supplemental vitamins A and E may be needed and prescribed by the physician (Chowers et al, 2001).

Herbs, Botanicals, and Supplements

- Herbs and botanicals are not recommended for this condition because there are no clinical trials proving efficacy.

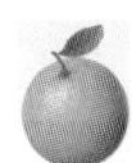

NUTRITION EDUCATION, COUNSELING, CARE MANAGEMENT

- Advise that MCT products should be consumed slowly to avoid side effects such as diarrhea.
- Discuss the need for intake of linoleic acid.
- A multivitamin–mineral supplement will be recommended. Identify food sources of the fat-soluble vitamins and discuss how the disorder prevents use of these vitamins accordingly.
- For persons with low vision, teaching with food models or large pictures may be more beneficial than use of text. Audiotapes may also be developed.

Patient Education—Food Safety

- Hand washing with soap and hot water is recommended before preparing formula or meals. Use clean utensils and containers for mixing formula.
- Before using tap water for formula preparation or to give as a beverage, let cold tap water run for 2 minutes to remove any lead that may be in the pipes.
- Follow the 2-hour rule: discard any beverage or food that has been left at room temperature for 2 hours or longer.
- Do not use honey in the diets of infants to decrease potential risk of botulism.

For More Information

- Prevent Blindness
  http://www.preventblindness.org/
- Prevent Blindness Foundation
  http://www.pbf.org.au/

ABETALIPOPROTEINEMIA—CITED REFERENCES

Chardon L, et al. Identification of two novel mutations and long-term follow-up in abetalipoproteinemia: a report of four cases. [published online ahead of print December 09, 2008] *Eur J Pediatr.* 168:983, 2009.

Chowers I, et al. Long-term assessment of combined vitamin A and E treatment for the prevention of retinal degeneration in abetalipoproteinaemia and hypobetalipoproteinaemia patients. *Eye.* 15:525, 2001.

Granot E, Kohen R. Oxidative stress in abetalipoproteinemia patients receiving long-term vitamin E and vitamin A supplementation. *Am J Clin Nutr.* 79:226, 2004.

Rampoldi D, et al. Clinical features and molecular bases of neuroacanthocytosis. *J Mol Med.* 80:475, 2002.

Wong P. A basis of the acanthocytosis in inherited and acquired disorders. *Med Hypotheses.* 62:966, 2004.

ATTENTION-DEFICIT DISORDERS

NUTRITIONAL ACUITY RANKING: LEVEL 1

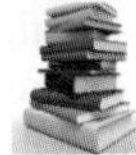

DEFINITIONS AND BACKGROUND

Attention-deficit disorder (ADD) and attention-deficit hyperactivity disorder (ADHD) were formerly called "hyperkinesis." Adults can have symptoms as well and may find relief from certain medications and therapies. ADD is a neurobiological condition characterized by developmentally inappropriate level of attention, concentration, activity, distractibility, and impulsivity; it is more common in males.

ADHD is the most commonly diagnosed behavioral disorder of childhood, affecting an estimated 7% of school-aged children (Schonwald, 2005). Three types are designated: predominantly hyperactive-impulsive, predominantly inattentive, and combined hyperactive-impulsive and inattentive; most children have the combined form. The Preschool ADHD Treatment Study (PATS) provides guidance for diagnostic considerations and intervention strategies for children between the ages of 3 and 5. Most ADHD is identified by age 6. Children with ADHD with a particular version of a certain gene have thinner brain tissue in the areas of the brain associated with attention, which is usually outgrown.

Glucose is the brain's energy source. In ADD, brain regions that inhibit impulses and control attention actually use less glucose; this decreased activity in the brain leads to inattention. PET scan comparisons between the brain of a normal child and the brain of an ADHD child show a significant difference. Children should be assessed for brain injury or seizure disorders, which may cause inattention and sleep disturbances (Schubert, 2005).

Exposure to lead is neurotoxic. Lead is found in trace amounts in everything from children's costume jewelry to imported candies to soil and drinking water (Nigg et al, 2010). It attaches to sites in the brain's striatum and frontal cortex, causing genes there to turn on or remain inactive, disrupting brain activity, decreasing cognitive control and contributing to hyperactivity and lack of vigilance (Nigg et al, 2010).

Children with ADHD may have low levels of other nutrients. Iron deficiency causes abnormal dopaminergic neurotransmission and may also contribute to ADD (Konofal et al, 2004). Zinc and EFAs (EPA and DHA) may be needed along with pharmacotherapy (DiGirolamo and Ramirez-Zea, 2009).

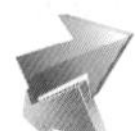

ASSESSMENT, MONITORING, AND EVALUATION

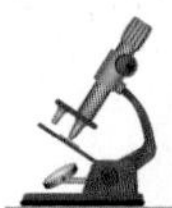

CLINICAL INDICATORS

Genetic Markers: ADHD often runs in families. Several genes make people more susceptible: SLC6A1, SLC9A9, HES1, ADRB2, HTR1E, DDC, ADRA1 A, DBH, DRD2, BDNF, TPH2, HTR2 A, SLC6A2, PER1, CHRNA4, SNAP25, and COMT but SLC9A9 has the strongest relationship (Lasky-Su et al, 2008). While genes account for 70% of hyperactivity and inattention in children, 30% is environmental (Nigg et al, 2010).

Clinical/History	EEG	Lab Work
Height	Sleep disturbances	Glucose (Gluc)
Weight	Middle ear infections with hearing loss	H & H, serum Fe
Growth chart	Learning disabilities	Ferritin levels
Diet/intake history	Anxiety or depression	Serum lead (elevated?)
Mental retardation, other developmental delay?	Nocturnal enuresis	Serum zinc (low?)
Head injury?		Alb
Seizures or hx of epilepsy?		Chol
		Liver function tests (LFTs)

INTERVENTION

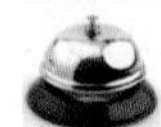

OBJECTIVES

- Prevent nutrient deficiencies if diet is inadequate or with extensive documented food allergies.

> **SAMPLE NUTRITION CARE PROCESS STEPS**
>
> **Poor Food Choices**
>
> ***Assessment Data:*** Food records indicating poor intake; weight loss and food jags. Low H & H levels.
>
> ***Nutrition Diagnoses (PES):***
>
> NI 1.4. Inadequate energy intake related to insufficient energy intake from a diet compared to estimated needs as evidenced by weight loss and dietary intake records.
>
> NI 55.1. Inadequate iron intake related to a disordered eating pattern as evidenced by a low Hgb of 10 g/L and low iron food choices.
>
> ***Interventions:*** Food-nutrient delivery to include iron-rich foods. Educate parents about introducing new iron-rich food items, reducing distractions at mealtime, scheduling of activities to give structure, and the use of small snacks throughout the day to improve overall intake of nutrients and energy. Counseling about the importance of nutrient density in children's diets. Coordinate care with medical team to test and identify other risks, such as high serum lead or low zinc levels.
>
> ***Monitoring and Evaluation:*** Improved nutrient density in food intake records. Better attention in school, fewer complaints about hyperactivity.

- Address poor intake and appetite, where present. Offer foods that are liked along with one to two new tastes to encourage expanding preferences.
- Correct zinc deficiency and iron deficiency anemia, where indicated.
- Rule out lead poisoning.
- Provide sufficient intake of omega-3 fatty acids and other micronutrients.

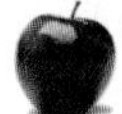

FOOD AND NUTRITION

- The diet should be balanced and sufficient in energy and protein for age and sex. The MyPyramid food guidance system should be the basis for planning; see Section 2.
- Omit any food allergens that have been medically diagnosed and verified (McCann et al, 2007).
- Elimination of sugar is not required; moderation is reasonable. Small, frequent healthy snacks may be beneficial.
- EFA supplementation may be useful (Murphy et al, 2005; Schnoll et al, 2003). Include DHA and EPA in the diet from tuna, mackerel, herring, sardines, and salmon (Ramakrishnan et al, 2009). The use of fortified foods requires some long-term studies (Riediger et al, 2009).
- Offer plenty of whole grains, low-fat dairy, fruits, and vegetables in greater proportion than sugary foods to provide more micronutrients and phytochemicals.
- Discuss good food sources of zinc and iron, especially for children with a limited diet or food jags. They may not eat meats, poultry, fish, eggs, and fortified cereals in sufficient amounts.

Common Drugs Used and Potential Side Effects

- Stimulants such as Ritalin (methylphenidate) have been used for many years. They may cause weight loss, appetite change, sleep problems or irritability. Newer, long-acting medications will alleviate some of the burden of ADD (Connor and Steingard, 2004). See Table 3-3.
- Nonstimulant Strattera (atomoxetine) is used to increase attention and the ability to focus; long-term use may cause liver damage or suicidal thoughts, so monitor carefully.
- Antiepileptic drugs phenobarbital, gabapentin, and topiramate may alter attention whereas lamotrigine and carbamazepine may have beneficial effects on attention span.
- Mood stabilizers, beta-blockers, or serotonin reuptake inhibitors be used in managing aggression or self-injury. There are many side effects, such as weight gain or loss, elevation of glucose with possible diabetes, gastrointestinal distress; monitor closely.

Herbs, Botanicals, and Supplements

- Many parents try complementary medicine (CAM) as an alternative to stimulant medicines as the marketing for herbal remedies, elimination diets, and food supplements for ADHD has increased. There are key questions regarding safety and efficacy of these treatments in children (Sawni, 2008). Herbs and botanicals are not recommended for this condition because there are no clinical trials proving efficacy.

TABLE 3-3 **ADHD Medications Approved by U.S. Food and Drug Administration (FDA)**[a]

Trade Name	Generic Name	Approved Age
Adderall	Amphetamine	3 and older
Adderall XR	Amphetamine (extended release)	6 and older
Concerta	Methylphenidate (long acting)	6 and older
Daytrana	Methylphenidate patch	6 and older
Desoxyn	Methamphetamine hydrochloride	6 and older
Dexedrine	Dextroamphetamine	3 and older
Dextrostat	Dextroamphetamine	3 and older
Focalin	Dexmethylphenidate	6 and older
Focalin XR	Dexmethylphenidate (extended release)	6 and older
Metadate ER	Methylphenidate (extended release)	6 and older
Metadate CD	Methylphenidate (extended release)	6 and older
Methylin	Methylphenidate (oral solution and chewable tablets)	6 and older
Ritalin	Methylphenidate	6 and older
Ritalin SR	Methylphenidate (extended release)	6 and older
Ritalin LA	Methylphenidate (long acting)	6 and older
Strattera	Atomoxetine	6 and older
Vyvanse	Lisdexamfetamine dimesylate	6 and older

[a]Not all ADHD medications are approved for use in adults.

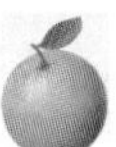

NUTRITION EDUCATION, COUNSELING, CARE MANAGEMENT

- Different causes of the symptoms of ADD may include allergies, food intolerances, anxiety, depression, family problems, poor discipline, or acute illnesses. A healthy, balanced diet is important (Marcason, 2005).
- Since glucose is the brain's source of energy, a sufficient intake of carbohydrate is needed. Assure that healthy choices are made from dairy, fruit and vegetable, and bread and cereal items. Reduce intake of sugary sweets, beverages, and snacks as a commonsense approach.
- Identify and remove sources of lead in the environment, especially if serum levels are found to be high.
- EFAs are important; include adequate amounts of fats in the daily diet (Ross et al, 2007).
- Zinc intake also plays an important role (Arnold and DiSilvestro, 2005; DiGirolamo and Ramirez-Zea, 2009).
- Identify and treat nocturnal enuresis, which may be present.
- Children need clear, consistent rules and praise when rules are followed.
- Individual psychotherapy may be quite beneficial. Encourage full participation.
- Children need help to stay organized and follow directions. Use of a schedule is important; organize everyday items; use notebook organizers.

Patient Education—Food Safety

- Hand washing with soap and hot water is recommended before preparing meals and snacks. Use clean utensils and containers.
- Before using tap water for formula preparation or to give as a beverage, let cold tap water run for 2 minutes to remove any lead that may be in the pipes.
- Follow the 2-hour rule: discard any beverage or food that has been left at room temperature for 2 hours or longer.
- Do not use honey in the diets of infants to decrease potential risk of botulism.

For More Information

- Attention Deficit Disorder Association
  http://www.add.org/
- National Institute for Mental Health
  http://www.nimh.nih.gov/publicat/adhd.cfm

ATTENTION-DEFICIT DISORDERS—CITED REFERENCES

Arnold LE, DiSilvestro RA. Zinc in attention-deficit/hyperactivity disorder. *J Child Adolesc Psychopharmacol.* 15:619, 2005.

Connor DF, Steingard RJ. New formulations of stimulants for attention-deficit hyperactivity disorder: therapeutic potential. *CNS Drugs.* 8:1011, 2004.

DiGirolamo AM, Ramirez-Zea M. Role of zinc in maternal and child mental health. *Am J Clin Nutr.* 88:940S, 2009.

Konofal E, et al. Iron deficiency in children with attention-deficit/hyperactivity disorder. *Ach Pediatr Adolesc Med.* 158:1113, 2004.

Lasky-Su J, et al. Genome-wide association scan of quantitative traits for attention deficit hyperactivity disorder identifies novel associations and confirms candidate gene associations. *Am J Med Genet B Neuropsychiatr Genet.* 147:1345, 2008.

Marcason W. Can dietary intervention play a part in the treatment of attention deficit and hyperactivity disorder? *J Am Diet Assoc.* 105:1161, 2005.

McCann D, et al. Food additives and hyperactive behaviour in 3-year-old and 8/9-year-old children in the community: a randomised, double-blinded, placebo-controlled trial. *Lancet.* 370:1560, 2007.

Murphy P, et al. Effect of the ketogenic diet on the activity level of Wistar rats. *Pediatr Res.* 57:353, 2005.

Nigg JT, et al. Confirmation and extension of association of blood lead with attention-deficit hyperactivity disorder (ADHD) and ADHD symptom domains at population-typical exposure levels. *J Child Psychol Psychiatry.* 51:58, 2010.

Ramakrishnan U, et al. Role of docosahexaenoic acid in maternal and child mental health. *Am J Clin Nutr.* 89:958S, 2009.

Riediger ND, et al. A systemic review of the roles of n-3 fatty acids in health and disease. *J Am Diet Assoc.* 109:668, 2009.

Ross BM, et al. Omega-3 fatty acids as treatments for mental illness: which disorder and which fatty acid? *Lipids Health Dis.* 6:21, 2007.

Sawni A. Attention-deficit/hyperactivity disorder and complementary/alternative medicine. *Adolesc Med State Art Rev.* 19:313, 2008.

Schnoll R, et al. Nutrition in the treatment of attention-deficit hyperactivity disorder: a neglected but important aspect. *Appl Psychophysiol Biofeedback.* 28:63, 2003.

Schonwald A. Update: attention deficit/hyperactivity disorder in the primary care office. *Curr Opin Pediatr.* 17:265, 2005.

Schubert R. Attention deficit disorder and epilepsy. *Pediatr Neurol.* 32:1, 2005.

AUTISM SPECTRUM DISORDER

NUTRITIONAL ACUITY RANKING: LEVEL 1–2

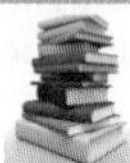

DEFINITIONS AND BACKGROUND

Autism spectrum disorder (ASD) begins in childhood as developmental disabilities caused by abnormalities in the brain. Generalized enlargement of gray and white matter cerebral volumes is present at 2 years of age. Increased rate of brain growth occurs in the latter part of the first year of life (Hazlett et al, 2005). The ASDs are part of a broader category of pervasive developmental disorders (PDDs), affecting over 500,000 individuals in the United States.

Autism is a neurodevelopmental condition affecting 1 in 160 children in the United States (West et al, 2009). Children with ASDs have unusual ways of learning, paying attention, or reacting to different sensations. They like to repeat certain behaviors and do not want change in their daily activities. They are hypersensitive to sensory stimuli (tastes, smells, sounds, sights) and withdraw from what is perceived as distressing or painful. People with ASDs have problems with social and communication skills. Up to 40% of persons with an ASD do not speak. Rather than conversing in a dialogue fashion, they may repeat back what has been said (echolalia).

Autism is considered to be genetic. Environmental factors with exposure to toxins, infections such as measles, mumps, or rubella, and diet play a role (White, 2003). Mental retardation and seizures of mild-to-moderate intensity can be present, especially in **fragile X syndrome** (found mostly in males). **Rett syndrome** occurs primarily in girls and is evident by repetitive hand movements. In **Asperger's disorder**, speech occurs at the usual time, intelligence is normal or above average, but social skills are stunted and interests are limited or obsessive.

Pica with anemia is common, such as eating paper, string, or dirt. Ritualistic eating behaviors, food limitations, messy eating habits and food jags are common; variety in texture or colors may not be accepted. Foods that could cause choking should be avoided. A quiet environment for eating is best tolerated.

High use of oral antibiotics or higher mercury exposure can aggravate oxidative stress and decrease detoxification capacity, leading to decreased plasma methionine, glutathione, cysteine, SAM, and sulfate (Adams et al, 2007; James et al, 2004). A methylation problem is likely (Deth et al, 2007). Allergies or sensitivities are also relevant. Autistic children often have IgA deficiency, decreased natural killer (NK) cell numbers, antibodies against serotonin receptors, and a tumor necrosis factor (TNF) response to casein, gluten, and soy (Schneider, 2007; Vojdani et al, 2008). Mega doses of nutrients are not helpful.

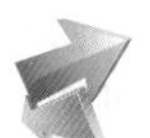

ASSESSMENT, MONITORING, AND EVALUATION

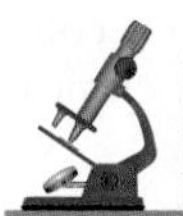

CLINICAL INDICATORS

Genetic Markers: At least 10 genes and enzymes have been implicated (Campbell, 2006; Muhle et al, 2004; Schneider, 2007): Adenosine Deaminase; Cystathionine-B-Synthase; Catecholamine-O-Methyltransferase (COMT 472G > A); FOXP2, RAY1/ST7, IMMP2 L; GABA(A) receptor; Glutathione-S-transferase (GST M1); MET Receptor Tyrosine Kinase (MET); Methionine Synthase (MS); Methionine Synthase Reductase (MSR); MTHFR C677 T and A1298 C; Paraoxonase (PON1); Reduced folate carrier (RFC 80G > A); Reelin and RELN genes at 7q22-q33; Serotonin transporter gene (5-HTT); Transcobalamin II (TCN2 776G > C); UBE3 A genes.

Clinical/History

Height
Weight
Head circumference
Growth chart
Diet/intake history
Childhood Asperger Syndrome Test (CAST), a parental questionnaire
MRI or CT scan of the brain
Pica
Endoscopy
Sleep patterns

Lab Work

CBC with differential
Gluc
H & H, Serum Fe, Ferritin
Celiac screening panel
Lactose breath test
Thyroid studies
LFTs Lipid profile
RAST or allergy testing
Alb
Chol, Trig
Serum lead (with pica)
C-reactive protein (CRP)

SAMPLE NUTRITION CARE PROCESS STEPS

Intake of Unsafe Foods

Assessment Data: Food records indicating intake of gluten; loss of weight; chronic rashes, infections and diarrhea; small bowel biopsy indicating celiac disease.

Nutrition Diagnoses (PES):

NI 5.3. Inadequate protein-energy intake related to highly restricted eating behaviors and pickiness as evidenced by parental report of insufficient intake, below 50% for age for weight, growth failure, and frequent lack of interest in food.

NB 3.1. Intake of unsafe foods related to sensitivity to gluten in autistic child as evidenced by biopsy positive for celiac disease, rashes, chronic diarrhea.

Intervention: Educate parents about gluten-free diet, food labeling, simple meal preparation. Counseling about use of food diaries and routines; how to include frequent nutrient-dense snacks of desired food items.

Monitoring and Evaluation: Improved weight records; fewer loose stools, infections and rashes.

INTERVENTION

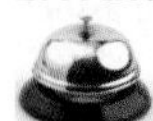

OBJECTIVES

- Prevent or lessen complications of the disorder, such as feeding problems. Offer consistency in food textures and tastes to prevent sensory overload.
- Evaluate carefully and analyze which nutrients should be replaced in the diet. If the diet has been severely limited, nutritional status may be at risk.
- Correct constipation if fiber intake is low and if symptoms are present.
- Work with other therapies, such as speech therapy or occupational therapy, to determine how to best offer foods of greater texture and variety that can be consumed by the child or offered by the caregiver.
- Monitor food jags, pica, history of choking on foods, and intolerances for varied textures, and adapt meals and menu items accordingly. Goal is to eat foods from all parts of the food pyramid regardless of texture.
- Autism seems to be related to altered immunity (Ashwood et al, 2004). Frequent infections, gastro-intestinal (GI) concerns (including chronic constipation or diarrhea) thyroid problems, and allergies are common and require nutritional management. A high prevalence of non-IgE-mediated food allergies exist in young children with ASDs, with GI symptoms (Jyonouchi, 2008).
- Monitor use of the popular gluten casein–free diet, as more clinical trials are needed to confirm efficacy (Millward et al, 2008).

FOOD AND NUTRITION

- Offer foods of texture and variety that are desired by the child. Follow a usual pattern and enhance with nutrient-dense additives in food preparation that will not alter flavor and texture.
- If a multivitamin–mineral supplement is needed, use one that has acceptable taste to the individual.
- Gluten-casein-soy elimination diets have some success, but can also lead to nutrient deficiencies. Use under supervision of a dietitian.
- Offer extra energy if weight is low, a common finding. Assess needs according to activity levels, weight and nutritional status, and medications that are prescribed.
- Since the brain requires omega-3 fatty acids for membrane integrity and to reduce inflammation, it is beneficial to include them in the diet or to use them in supplemental form.
- Some autistic children have disaccharide deficiencies; alter diet accordingly.

Common Drugs Used and Potential Side Effects

- Only risperidone has Food and Drug Administration approval for the pharmacologic management of autism in children (West et al, 2009).
- Atypical antipsychotic agents, selective-serotonin reuptake inhibitors, stimulants, and *N*-methyl-D-aspirate receptor antagonists may be used off-label to decrease core behaviors and associated symptoms (West et al, 2009). If clonidine, clomipramine, haloperidol, naltrexone, or desipramine is prescribed for behavioral or learning problems, monitor for GI side effects, nausea, and diarrhea. Olanzapine (Zyprexa) may cause weight gain, dry mouth, and constipation. Fluoxetine (Prozac) may cause anorexia or weight loss, GI distress, and diarrhea.
- Medications to control seizures may be needed (Tuchman, 2004).
- D-cycloserine treatment may improve social withdrawal without side effects (Posey et al, 2004).
- Folinic acid, betaine, and methylcobalamin may be needed normalize metabolic imbalances or to treat cerebral folate deficiency (James et al, 2004; Moretti et al, 2005).

Herbs, Botanicals, and Supplements

- Over half of children with autism are using CAM (Golnick and Ireland, 2009). Melatonin, sulfation glutathione, amino acids, chelation, probiotics, thyroid supplements, antifungals are common. In one report (Golnick and Ireland, 2009) physicians encouraged multivitamins (49%), EFAs (25%), melatonin (25%), and probiotics (19%) and discouraged withholding immunizations (76%), chelation (61%), anti-infectives (57%), delaying immunizations (55%), and secretin (43%). Evidence-based studies are needed.
- Herbs and botanicals are not recommended for these conditions because clinical trials have not proven efficacy.
- "Improved diet" techniques may include organic foods, which adds expense to the cost of meals.
- Vitamin–mineral mega doses such as vitamin B_6 and magnesium may have been used; discuss the implications and potential risks.

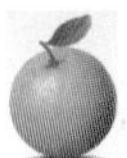

NUTRITION EDUCATION, COUNSELING, CARE MANAGEMENT

- Evaluate for behaviors such as pica; discuss how this may lead to anemia.
- Assist with tips on how to handle picky eating, rigid food behaviors, and nutrient insufficiency. Discuss various ways to include nutrient-dense foods in the diet.
- Discuss the importance of maintaining a quiet environment with few interruptions or distractions.
- Keep language simple and concrete; do not offer abstract text. Pictures and simple words are more effective when working with an older child or teen.
- Artificial colors and preservatives may have a detrimental effect on behavior, especially red and yellow food dyes. Limit their use in the diet.
- Avoid allergens, where documented.
- Support various therapies, such as speech therapy, occupational therapy, use assistive technology and biomedical applications that are evidence-based.

Patient Education—Food Safety

- Hand washing with soap and hot water is recommended before preparing formula or meals. Use clean utensils and containers. Sanitize work surfaces before food preparation.
- Before using tap water for formula preparation or to give as a beverage, let cold tap water run for 2 minutes to remove any lead that may be in the pipes.
- Follow the 2-hour rule: discard any beverage or food that has been left at room temperature for 2 hours or longer. To avoid wasting foods, serve small portions more frequently.

For More Information

- Asperger's Syndrome
  http://www.aspergers.com/
- Asperger Syndrome Coalition of the United States
  http://www.irsc.org/
- Autism Research Institute
  http://www.autism.com/
- Autism Society of America
  http://www.autism-society.org/
- CDC—About Autism
  http://www.cdc.gov/ncbddd/autism/
- Center for Collaborative Genetic Studies on Mental Disorders
  http://www.nimhgenetics.org
- Defeat Autism Now (DAN)
  http://www.defeatautismnow.com/
- National Fragile X Foundation
  http://www.nfxf.org/
- Report to Congress on Autism
  http://www.nimh.nih.gov/autismiacc/autismreport2004.pdf
- Rett Syndrome
  http://www.rettsyndrome.org/
- Vaccines
  http://www.cdc.gov/ncbddd/autism/documents/vaccine_studies.pdf

AUTISM SPECTRUM DISORDER—CITED REFERENCES

Adams JB, et al. Mercury, lead, and zinc in baby teeth of children with autism versus controls. *J Toxicol Environ Health.* 70:1046, 2007.

Ashwood P, et al. Spontaneous mucosal lymphocyte cytokine profiles in children with autism and gastrointestinal symptoms: mucosal immune activation and reduced counter regulatory interleukin-10. *J Clin Immunol.* 24:664, 2004.

Campbell DB, et al. A genetic variant that disrupts MET transcription is associated with autism. *Proc Natl Acad Sci USA.* 103(45):16834, 2006.

Deth R, et al. How environmental and genetic factors combine to cause autism: A redox/methylation hypothesis. *Neurotoxicol.* 29:190, 2007.

Golnick AE, Ireland M. Complementary alternative medicine for children with autism: a physician survey. *J Autism Dev Disord.* 39:996, 2009.

Hazlett HC, et al. Magnetic resonance imaging and head circumference study of brain size in autism: birth through age 2 years. *Arch Gen Psychiatry.* 62:1366, 2005.

James SJ, et al. Metabolic endophenotype and related genotypes are associated with oxidative stress in children with autism. *Am J Med Genet B Neuropsychiatr Genet.* 141:947, 2006.

Jyonouchi H. Non-IgE mediated food allergy. *Inflamm Allergy Drug Targets.* 7:173, 2008.

Millward C, et al. Gluten- and casein-free diets for autistic spectrum disorder. *Cochrane Database Syst Rev.* 16(2):CD003498, 2008.

Moretti P, et al. Cerebral folate deficiency with developmental delay, autism, and response to folinic acid. *Neurology.* 64:1088, 2005.

Muhle R, et al. The genetics of autism. *Pediatrics.* 113:472, 2004.

Posey DJ, et al. A pilot study of D-cycloserine in subjects with autistic disorder. *Am J Psychiatry.* 161:2115, 2004.

Schneider C. Center for Autism Research and Education. Genetic vulnerability to environmental toxins: the gene/environment interface. Accessed October 7, 2008, at http://www.autism.com/danwebcast/presentations/alexandria/Saturday/Schneider.pdf.

Tuchman R. AEDs and psychotropic drugs in children with autism and epilepsy. *Ment Retard Dev Disabil Res Rev.* 10:135, 2004.

Vojdani A, et al. Low natural killer cell cytotoxic activity in autism: the role of glutathione, IL-2 and IL-15. *J Neuroimmunol.* 205:148, 2008.

West L, et al. Pharmacological treatments for the core deficits and associated symptoms of autism in children. *J Pediatr Health Care.* 23:75, 2009.

White JF. Intestinal pathophysiology in autism. *Exp Biol Med (Maywood).* 228:639, 2003.

BILIARY ATRESIA

NUTRITIONAL ACUITY RANKING: LEVEL 2–3

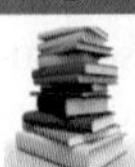

DEFINITIONS AND BACKGROUND

Biliary atresia (neonatal hepatitis) is a serious condition, affecting one in 15,000 births. Incidence is highest in the Asian population. Unconjugated hyperbilirubinemia occurs in approximately 60% of normal-term infants and in 80% of preterm infants; persistence beyond 2 weeks of age demands evaluation (Gubernick et al, 2000).

Complete degeneration or incomplete development of one or more of the bile duct components occurs due to arrested fetal development. CD4(1) lymphocytes and CD56(1) NK cells predominate in the liver of infants with extrahepatic biliary atresia (Davenport et al, 2001). Lymphocyte-mediated inflammatory damage of the bile ducts plays a role (Shinkai et al, 2006), as does altered *HLA-DR* gene expression in bile ductules (Feng et al, 2004).

Biliary atresia results in persistent jaundice, enlarged spleen, liver damage, portal hypertension, clay-colored stools, dark urine, irritability, and swollen abdomen. The condition becomes evident between 2 and 6 weeks after birth. Treatment involves having a surgical procedure done, the Kasai procedure, which bypasses the ducts to connect the liver to the small intestine. It is more successful if performed early. Complications of the surgery can include liver failure, infections, and sepsis.

If a donor is available, the patient may be a candidate for a liver transplantation. This is the most common disease in childhood that requires liver transplantation. Malnutrition is a critical predictor of mortality and morbidity in children with biliary atresia. Immunosuppressive drugs are then necessary to overcome organ rejection.

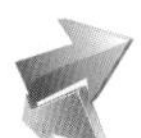

ASSESSMENT, MONITORING, AND EVALUATION

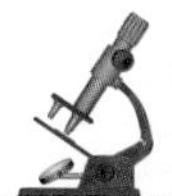

CLINICAL INDICATORS

Genetic Markers: *HLA-DR* gene in bile ductules has been noted, but otherwise not likely inherited.

Clinical/History

- Birth weight
- Height
- Growth (%)
- Diet/intake history
- Dark urine
- Steatorrhea
- Swollen abdomen; edema
- Jaundice >1 month
- Clay-colored stools
- Nuclear hepato imino diacetic acid (HIDA) test
- Liver scan or biopsy

Lab Work

- Alb
- Transthyretin
- H & H
- Alk phos
- Chol
- Trig
- Transferrin
- Blood urea nitrogen (BUN)
- Aspartate aminotransferase (AST)
- Alanine aminotransferase (ALT)
- Alpha-1 antitrypsin deficiency
- PT or INR
- Serum zinc
- Serum copper

INTERVENTION

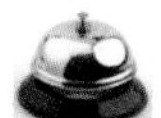

OBJECTIVES

Preoperatively

- Correct malabsorption and alleviate steatorrhea from decreased bile.
- Correct malnutrition of fat-soluble vitamins and zinc. Prevent rickets, visual disturbances, peripheral neuropathy, and coagulopathies.
- Prevent hemorrhage from high blood pressure (BP) if there is portal hypertension.
- Prepare for surgery or transplantation.

SAMPLE NUTRITION CARE PROCESS STEPS

Altered GI Function

Assessment Data: Stool and urine tests; abdominal girth; weight changes; poor intake.

Nutrition Diagnoses (PES): Altered GI function related to degenerating bile ducts and biliary atresia as evidenced by clay-colored stools, abdominal distention, jaundice, and dark urine.

Intervention: Educate parents about the needed surgery and need for protein, fat-soluble vitamins.

Monitoring and Evaluation: Improved weight and intake after surgery; reduced abdominal distention and normalized stools and urine color.

Postoperatively

- Support proper wound healing by providing all necessary nutrients (e.g., vitamin C, zinc) using appropriate and tolerated feeding method.
- Promote normal growth and development.
- Provide regular nutritional assessments to evaluate progress and improvement or decline.
- Reduce inflammation, which may continue even after surgery (Asakawa et al, 2009).

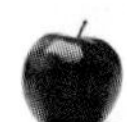

FOOD AND NUTRITION

Preoperative

- Infants need 1.5–3.0 g protein/kg dry weight to avoid protein catabolism, dependent on enteral versus parenteral source. This translates to 2–2.5 g/kg for PN and 2.5–3 g/kg for enteral nutrition, 1–1.5 g/kg if encephalopathic.
- Identify products enriched with branched-chain amino acids (BCAAs).
- Small, frequent feedings may be useful.
- Use low total fat from the diet. Supplement with oil high in MCTs; add EFAs for age and body size. Pregestimil or Alimentum or other elemental formulas may be needed to decrease fiber and prevent hemorrhage anywhere along the GI tract.
- With edema, limit intake of sodium to 1–2 g/d.
- Supplement with vitamins A, D, E, and K. Intravenous or water-miscible forms can be used.
- Provide antioxidants as serum levels of minerals, such as selenium, zinc, and iron, tend to be low. Avoid use of copper in total parenteral nutrition (TPN) or supplements to prevent toxic build-up.
- Tube feed especially if recurrent or prolonged bleeding from the GI tract occurs. If nasogastric (NG) feeding is not tolerated, a percutaneous gastrostomy (PEG) tube may be used. Failing nutrition should prompt aggressive support (Utterson et al, 2005).

Postoperative

- Control sodium, protein, and other nutrients only if necessary based on symptoms such as edema and renal failure. Carefully monitor vitamin and mineral requirements.
- Use of antioxidants will be needed to reduce inflammatory processes (Asakawa et al, 2009).

- For needed catch-up growth, tube feeding may be beneficial. Assure that all key nutrients are included over a long-term basis.

Common Drugs Used and Potential Side Effects

- Ursodiol (Actigall, Urso) promotes bile flow and may be used after surgery. Side effects are minimal.
- Phenobarbital and cholestyramine are often used to control hyperlipidemia and pruritus. Increase vitamin D, calcium, vitamin B_{12} and folate intake. Constipation can result.
- Corticosteroids may be needed to stimulate independent bile flow. Long-term use can deplete stores of calcium and phosphorus; may elevate glucose, cause stunting, or cause weight gain.
- Diuretics may be used; monitor for depletion of potassium, magnesium, calcium, and folate. Anorexia can occur.
- Antibiotics such as Bactrim or Septra may be needed to manage cholangitis, common following the Kasai procedure. Anorexia, nausea, or vomiting may result. Use of acidophilus and probiotic products may alleviate loss of intestinal bacteria.
- Growth hormone (GH) may be useful to promote catch-up growth.

Herbs, Botanicals, and Supplements

- Herbs and botanicals are not recommended with this condition because the liver is not able to perform its usual role of detoxification.
- Probiotics may be helpful; more studies are needed.

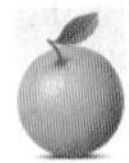

NUTRITION EDUCATION, COUNSELING, CARE MANAGEMENT

- Teach parents about proper feedings or supplements. Indicate which foods provide antixodants, including vitamins C and E, selenium.
- If bile flow improves after surgery or transplantation, a regular diet may be used, although continuing use of MCT oil may be better tolerated for awhile.
- Teach that the fat-soluble vitamins A, D, E, and K can be used only when they are bound to fat. It may be important to take supplemental forms.

Patient Education—Food Safety

- Hand washing with soap and hot water is recommended before preparing formula or meals. Use clean utensils and containers for mixing formula.
- Before using tap water for formula preparation or to give as a beverage, let cold tap water run for 2 minutes to remove any lead that may be in the pipes.
- Follow the 2-hour rule: discard any beverage or food that has been left at room temperature for 2 hours or longer.
- Do not use honey in the diets of infants to decrease potential risk of botulism.

For More Information

- American Liver Foundation http://www.liverfoundation.org/
- Canadian Liver Foundation http://www.liver.ca/Home.aspx
- Children's Liver Association for Support Services http://www.classkids.org/library/biliaryatresia.htm

BILIARY ATRESIA—CITED REFERENCES

Asakawa T, et al. Oxidative stress profile in the post-operative patients with biliary atresia. *Pediatr Surg Int.* 25:93, 2009.

Davenport M, et al. Immunohistochemistry of the liver and biliary tree in extrahepatic biliary atresia. *J Pediatr Surg.* 36:1017, 2001.

Feng J, et al. The aberrant expression of HLA-DR in intrahepatic bile ducts in patients with biliary atresia: an immunohistochemistry and immune electron microscopy study. *J Pediatr Surg.* 39:1658, 2004.

Gubernick J, et al. U.S. approach to jaundice in infants and children. *Radiographics.* 20:173, 2000.

Shinkai M, et al. Increased CXCR3 expression associated with CD3-positive lymphocytes in the liver and biliary remnant in biliary atresia. *J Pediatr Surg.* 41:950, 2006.

Utterson EC, et al. Biliary atresia: clinical profiles, risk factors, and outcomes of 755 patients listed for liver transplantation. *J Pediatr.* 147:180, 2005.

BRONCHOPULMONARY DYSPLASIA

NUTRITIONAL ACUITY RANKING: LEVEL 3–4

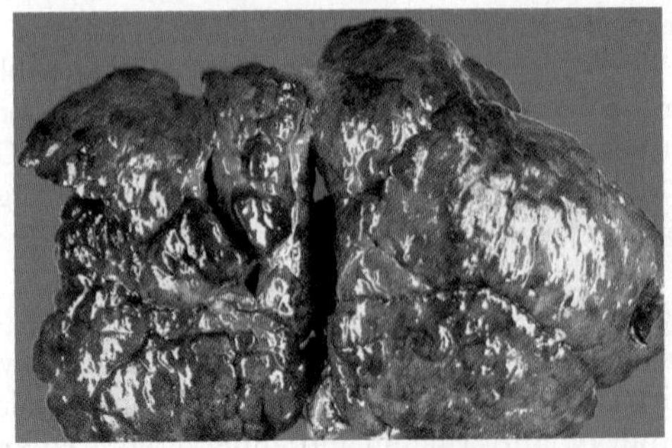

Adapted from: Cagle PT, MD. *Color Atlas and Text of Pulmonary Pathology.* Philadelphia: Lippincott Williams & Wilkins, 2005.

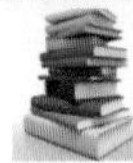

DEFINITIONS AND BACKGROUND

Bronchopulmonary dysplasia (BPD) is a chronic lung disease with abnormal growth of the lungs, often following the respiratory distress syndrome of prematurity. One third to one half of all infants born before the 28th week of gestation develop BPD and inflammatory regulators appear to be involved in the pathogenesis in the fetus (Cohen et al, 2007). Chronic aspiration of GI contents is common; measurement of pepsin is one marker (Farhath et al, 2008). The use of supplemental oxygen, while necessary, may also aggravate the condition (Bancalari and Claure, 2006).

Very low-birth-weight (VLBW) infants with severe respiratory disease need extra nutrients for epithelial cell repair and to support catch-up growth. VLBW infants should be given adequate nutritional attention (e.g., parenteral or enteral nutrition, fluid restriction) from the first day of life to enhance growth and minimize respiratory morbidity (Biniwale and Ehrenkranz, 2006). Respiratory failure, supplemental oxygen use, mechanical ventilation, endotracheal intubation, and congenital heart disease all affect nutritional status (D'Angio and Maniscalco, 2004). Slow growth occurs and feeding problems are common. Long-term chronic care is required.

Infants with BPD benefit from comprehensive nutrition and feeding therapy with adequate energy, parental support and education, and feeding evaluation (Biniwale and Ehrenkranz, 2006). Between 10% and 25% of preterm infants with BPD have malnutrition after 2 years of age, and 30–60% of them will continue to suffer from persistent airway obstruction or asthma (Bott et al, 2004).

Glutamine is the main source for lung energy; inositol is necessary for surfactant synthesis; vitamin E and selenium have antioxidant effects (Bott et al, 2004). Vitamin A provides benefit in these patients (Biniwale and Ehrenkranz, 2006; Spears et al, 2004). Long-chain polyunsaturated fatty acids and surfactant replacement therapy are sometimes used to prevent BPD in susceptible infants (D'Angio and Maniscalco, 2004), but controlled trials are needed to verify efficacy (Biniwale and Ehrenkranz, 2006).

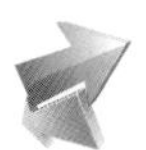

ASSESSMENT, MONITORING, AND EVALUATION

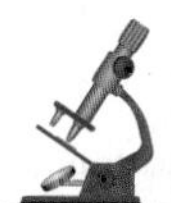

CLINICAL INDICATORS

Genetic Markers: Gene expression of the newborn umbilical cord implicates chromatin remodeling pathways in premature infants with BPD (Cohen et al, 2007).

Clinical/History
- Gestational age
- Length
- Body mass index (BMI)
- LBW or VLBW growth charts for height and weight
- Size for gestational age (use intrauterine growth chart if available)
- Head circumference
- Diet/intake history
- Emesis
- Stool pattern
- Urinary output
- BP
- Pulmonary hypertension

Lab Work
- H & H
- Pepsin levels
- pH
- Chol, Trig
- K^+ and Cl^- (tend to be low)
- Na^+
- Alb
- Alkaline phosphatase (alk phos)
- White blood cell (WBC) count
- Gluc
- Oxygen saturation levels
- Partial pressure of carbon dioxide (pCO_2)
- Partial pressure of oxygen (pO_2)
- Ca^{++}, Mg^{++}
- Urine-specific gravity

SAMPLE NUTRITION CARE PROCESS STEPS

Overfeeding

Assessment Data: Weight and growth charts, presence of Gastroesophageal reflux disease (GERD) or vomiting, low serum potassium and chloride.

Nutrition Diagnoses (PES): Excessive oral intake of formula in VLBW infant related to respiratory distress and BPD as evidenced by vomiting after most feedings and GERD.

Intervention: Educate parents about need for appropriate amounts of formula, feeding tips for discharge to home, appropriate rate of growth and weight change.

Monitoring and Evaluation: Weight records, decreased vomiting and episodes of GERD, normalized labs for K^+ and Cl^- and other labs.

INTERVENTION

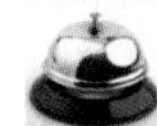

OBJECTIVES

- Increase energy intake to improve growth and respiratory functioning by correcting nutritional deficits (Lai et al, 2006).
- Correct gastroesophageal reflux. Position an infant carefully if formula fed.
- Avoid pareneral overfeeding, which may lead to PN-associated cholestasis (Robinson and Ehrenkranz, 2008).
- Achieve desirable growth. Infants with BPD tend to have delayed development (Bott et al, 2004). Energy needs are approximately 25–50% above normal. Correct malnutrition and anorexia from respiratory distress and ventilator support.
- Provide optimal protein for linear growth, development, and resistance to infection. Improve lean body mass if depleted.
- Spare protein by providing extra energy from fat and carbohydrate. However, excesses of carbohydrate can increase CO_2 production and prevent extubation; calculate needs carefully.
- Replace lost electrolytes, especially chloride, which may lead to death if uncorrected.
- Prevent EFA deficiency.
- Prevent complications, such as aspiration pneumonia or choking during feeding.
- Fluid restriction may be needed if fluid retention is noted; monitor closely.
- Prevent metabolic bone disease by including sufficient calcium and vitamin D intake.

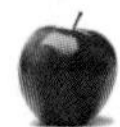

FOOD AND NUTRITION

- Energy requirements will be 25% above normal; provide 120–160 kcal/kg to achieve optimal weight.
- Within the first few days of life, TPN or tube feeding may be required. Initially: 70 (PN) or 95 (enteral) kcal/kg, increasing gradually to 130–180 kcal/kg after acuity subsides.

- Protein requirements may be slightly higher than usual. Careful formula management is needed; Trophamine is beneficial (Blau et al, 2007). Initially, use 2.0 g protein/kg, increasing to 2.5–3.5 g/kg.
- Decrease total carbohydrate (CHO) intake if glucose intolerance develops; monitor blood glucose levels.
- Provide at least the normal recommended allowances for antioxidant and other important nutrients. Include vitamins A, D, and E (use water-miscible sources if necessary); provide adequate calcium, phosphorus, and iron if needed. Nutrient or energy-enriched infant formulas may be needed for catch-up growth.
- Fluid intake (may be restricted to <150 cc/kg/d) and sodium levels may need to be restricted if there is pulmonary edema or hypertension.
- With decreased suck and swallowing ability, tube feeding may be better tolerated. Infants can tolerate most formulas. Nocturnal tube feeding may be useful, especially with growth failures. With gastroesophageal reflux (GERD) a gastrostomy feeding tube may be appropriate.
- Increase fat:CHO ratio with respiratory distress. To meet EFA needs, start with 0.5–1 g/kg and progress to 3 g/kg.
- Omega-3 fatty acids, selenium, inositol, vitamins A and E have been suggested for use with infants who have chronic pulmonary insufficiency (Biniwale and Ehrenkranz, 2006; Bott et al, 2004).
- When ready to progress to an oral diet, use of solids may be better tolerated than liquids. If necessary, thicken liquids or formula (e.g., with baby cereal or other thickeners). Use a supine position to avoid aspiration.

Common Drugs Used and Potential Side Effects

- Exogenous steroid therapy (dexamethasone or methylprednisone) is only used for pulmonary compliance in ventilated premature infants (Grier and Halliday, 2005). This may compromise vitamin A status and restrict bone growth. Sodium retention, anorexia, edema, hypertension, and potassium losses are side effects. Take with food to decrease GI effects. Use more protein and less sodium; enhance potassium if needed.
- Antibiotics are needed during infections; acidophilus and probiotic products may alleviate losses of intestinal bacteria.
- Bronchodilators or caffeine may be used for apnea of prematurity. Anorexia can occur.
- Diuretics may be needed to lessen pulmonary edema. Monitor those that deplete serum potassium, such as furosemide (Lasix). Magnesium, calcium, and folate may be also depleted; appetite may decline.
- Cysteine, N-aceyl cystiene, or cystine may be used in combination with chloride.

Herbs, Botanicals, and Supplements

- Herbs and botanicals should not be used for BPD because the lungs are not able to perform their role in oxygenation of cells.
- Use of acidophilus and probiotic products may be useful with chronic antibiotic therapy.

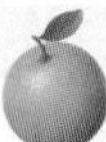

NUTRITION EDUCATION, COUNSELING, CARE MANAGEMENT

- Diet must be re-evaluated periodically to reflect growth and disease process. Assure adequacy of vitamins and related nutrients for lung health (for example, vitamin A).
- Ensure that all foods and beverages are nutrient dense.
- New foods may be introduced gradually; thicken as needed to avoid aspiration.
- Fluid intake should be adequate to meet needs but not excessive.
- Discuss signs of overhydration and dehydration with the parent/caregiver.
- Oral–motor skills may be delayed from long-term ventilator use; discuss how to make adjustments with caregiver.

Patient Education—Food Safety

- Hand washing with soap and hot water is recommended before preparing formula or meals. Use clean utensils and containers for mixing formula.
- Before using tap water for formula preparation or to give as a beverage, let cold tap water run for 2 minutes to remove any lead that may be in the pipes.
- Follow the 2-hour rule: discard any beverage or food that has been left at room temperature for 2 hours or longer.
- Do not use honey in the diets of infants to decrease potential risk of botulism.

For More Information

- American Lung Association
  http://www.lungusa.org/
- National Blood, Heart, and Lung Institute
  http://www.nhlbi.nih.gov/health/dci/Diseases/Bpd/Bpd_WhatIs.html

BRONCHOPULMONARY DYSPLASIA—CITED REFERENCES

Bancalari E, Claure N. Definitions and diagnostic criteria for bronchopulmonary dysplasia. *Semin Perinatol.* 30:164, 2006.

Biniwale MA, Ehrenkranz RA. The role of nutrition in the prevention and management of bronchopulmonary dysplasia. *Semin Perinatol.* 30:200, 2006.

Blau J, et al. Effects of protein/nonprotein caloric intake on parenteral nutrition associated cholestasis in premature infants weighing 600–1000 grams. *J Parenter Enteral Nutr.* 31:486, 2007.

Bott L, et al. Nutrition and bronchopulmonary dysplasia. *Arch Pediatr.* 11:234, 2004.

Cohen J, et al. Perturbation of gene expression of the chromatin remodeling pathway in premature newborns at risk for bronchopulmonary dysplasia. *Genome Biol.* 8:210, 2007.

D'Angio CT, Maniscalco WM. Bronchopulmonary dysplasia in preterm infants: pathophysiology and management strategies. *Paediatr Drugs.* 6:303, 2004.

Farhath S, et al. Pepsin, a marker of gastric contents, is increased in tracheal aspirates from preterm infants who develop bronchopulmonary dysplasia. *Pediatrics.* 121:e253, 2008.

Grier DG, Halliday HL. Management of bronchopulmonary dysplasia in infants: guidelines for corticosteroid use. *Drugs.* 65:15, 2005.

Lai N, et al. The role of nutrition in the prevention and management of bronchopulmonary dysplasia. *Semin Perinatol.* 30:200, 2006.

Robinson DT, Ehrenkranz RA. Parenteral nutrition-associated cholestasis in small for gestational age infants. *J Pediatr.* 152:59, 2008.

Spears K, et al. Low plasma retinol concentrations increase the risk of developing bronchopulmonary dysplasia and long-term respiratory disability in very-low-birth-weight infants. *Am J Clin Nutr.* 80:1589, 2004.

CARBOHYDRATE METABOLIC DISORDERS

NUTRITIONAL ACUITY RANKING: LEVEL 4

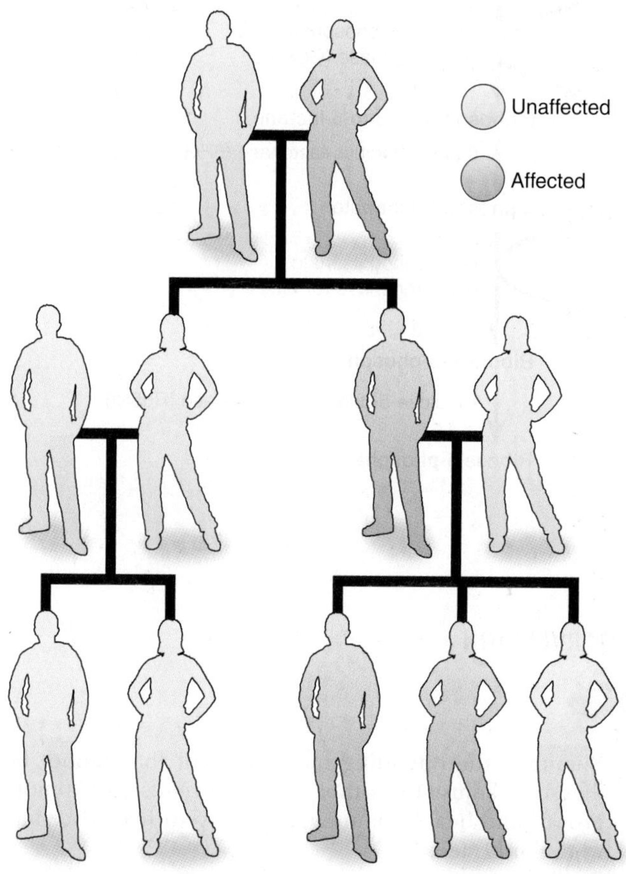

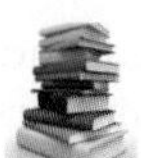

DEFINITIONS AND BACKGROUND

Abnormalities of glucose metabolism are the most common errors of carbohydrate metabolism; causes include both environmental and genetic factors and generally lead to one of the forms of diabetes (see chapter 9). Glucose is transported across cell membranes by active sodium-facilitated transport in the intestinal or renal cells; in all other cells, the GLUT family of glucose transporters are needed (Brown, 2000). Diagnosis of "carbohydrate malabsorption" occurs during infancy or childhood, with hypoglycemia, hepatomegaly, poor physical growth, and deranged biochemical profiles.

Congenital glucose–galactose malabsorption (congenital renal glycosuria) is an extremely rare, autosomal recessive trait. Watery, profuse diarrhea occurs from deficiency in the sodium-coupled cotransport of glucose and galactose in the intestinal mucosa. There is no cure, but removal of lactose, sucrose, and glucose lessons symptoms. **Glucose transporter type 1 (Glut1) deficiency syndrome** produces a seizure disorder with low glucose in the cerebrospinal fluid, developmental delay, and acquired microcephaly (Wang et al, 2004). **Glut2 deficiency** produces Fanconi–Bickel syndrome, which resembles type I glycogen storage disease (GSD; Brown, 2000).

Fructose intolerance results from a defect in the enzyme converting fructose to glucose (1-phosphofructaldolase). It is an autosomal recessive disease, as common as 1 in 20,000 persons in some European countries. Fructose intolerance causes GI discomfort, nausea, malaise, and growth failure. Ingesting fructose causes profound hypoglycemia; if left untreated, progressive liver disease results.

Galactosemia (galactose-1-phosphate uridylyltransferase deficiency or GALT deficiency) causes cataracts, hepatomegaly, and mental retardation. It occurs in one of 60,000 births. People with galactosemia are unable to fully metabolize the simple sugar galactose. The enzyme galactokinase may play a role (Holden et al, 2004). High levels of the sugar alcohol, galactitol, may be present. FTT, vomiting or diarrhea, jaundice, liver disease occur after milk ingestion. Bone density may decline over time (Panis et al, 2004). Cataracts, encephalopathy, or death from *E. coli* sepsis may occur (Berry, 2008). In females, serum FSH levels may be elevated and primary ovarian insufficiency (POI) may prevent successful pregnancy (Berry, 2008).

GSDs are rare genetic disorders in which glycogen cannot be metabolized to glucose in the liver because of enzyme deficits. Glycogen is the storage form of glucose and is found in the liver and muscles; a small amount is also found in the kidney and intestine. In severe cases of GSD, liver transplantation may be needed. Table 3-4 lists the various types of GSD.

Sucrose intolerance occurs rarely as a genetic defect or temporarily after GI flu or irritable bowel distress. Sucrase and maltase deficiency may occur simultaneously, with an osmotic diarrhea.

Lactose intolerance is discussed in chapter 7; the autosomal recessive trait deficit is encoded by the lactase gene on chromosome 2 with a frequency of 5% to 90% in humans.

TABLE 3-4 Signs of Cerebral Palsy

Struggles with fine motor skills: handling scissors, using crayons, buttoning a shirt, and any other movement that uses fingers and hands.
Struggles with gross motor skills: walking, riding a tricycle, kicking a ball, and other movements using legs and arms.
Trouble sitting upright; it takes a lot of muscle tone to sit up without toppling over.
Shakes a lot or has uncontrollable jerking of her legs, arms, or torso.
Muscles are weak.
Body tremors, drooling, weakened muscles in his face; may lose control of his tongue.
Trouble moving from one position to another.
Trouble sucking.

Source: http://www.cerebralpalsy.org/what-is-cerebral-palsy/symptoms/.

The Pentose Pathway and Glutathione Production
GSH & GSSG: glutathione

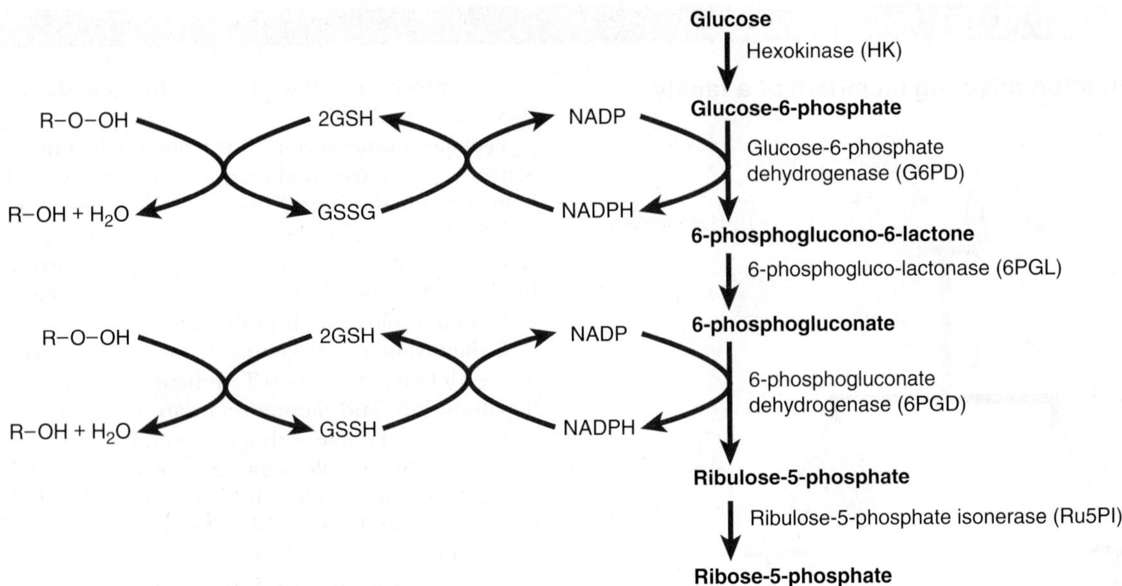

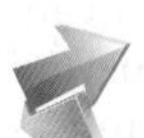

ASSESSMENT, MONITORING, AND EVALUATION

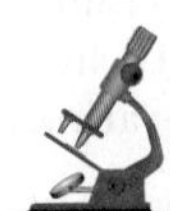

CLINICAL INDICATORS

Genetic Markers: The congenital defects relate to aberrant transporter genes: glucose–galactose malabsorption syndrome, *SGLT1*; glucose transporter 1 deficiency syndrome, *GLUT1*; Fanconi–Bickel syndrome, *GLUT2*; fructose intolerance, *fructose-1-phosphate aldolase*. The GSDs have deficiency in various types of microsomal *glucose-6-phosphatase (G6Pase)* activity.

Clinical/History

- Height or length
- Weight
- BMI
- Growth (%)
- Diet/intake history
- Infections
- Nausea and vomiting
- Jaundice
- Infantile seizures
- Acquired microcephaly
- Development delay or FTT?
- Edema
- Demyelinating neuropathy?

Lab Work

- Gluc (decreased in fructosemia)
- HgbA1 c (decreased erythrocyte glucose uptake)
- Hypoglycorrhachia (CSF glucose <40 mg/dL)
- Trig, Chol (elevated in Von Gierke's disease)
- LFTs: ALT, AST, CK
- Urinary and serum galactose or fructose
- Acetone
- Serum phosphate
- Serum lactate
- Serum ammonia
- Serum bilirubin
- Uric acid
- Alb

INTERVENTION

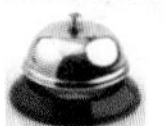

OBJECTIVES

- Eliminate the offending macronutrient that cannot be digested; adjust the other macronutrients to promote growth and health maintenance. Prevent hypoglycemia, where indicated.
- Read labels carefully.
- Fructose intolerance requires omission of fructose from the diet.
- For galactosemia, correct the diet to prevent physical and mental retardation, cataracts, portal hypertension, and cirrhosis. Vitamin E seems to have positive, protective effects. Read labels carefully; galactose is not always reported. Consider infant formulas containing glucose, without lactose and maltose; lactose-restricted diet products;

SAMPLE NUTRITION CARE PROCESS STEPS

Abnormal GI Function

Assessment Data: Weight and growth charts, nausea and vomiting, elevated LFTs, and frequent episodes of hypoglycemia.

Nutrition Diagnoses (PES): Abnormal GI function related to metabolic disorder and GSD as evidenced by nausea and vomiting.

Intervention: Educate parents about frequency and timing for meals and snacks, enhancing energy intake through six to eight small meals daily plus nightly gastrostomy feeding of a complete nutritional supplement with cornstarch, DHA, and special oil.

Monitoring and Evaluation: Weight records, growth, tolerance for various food consistencies, less nausea and vomiting.

rice-based milk substitutes; lactose-free products that contain glucose.
- For (Glut1) deficiency syndrome, a higher fat intake is useful. The ketogenic or a modified Atkins diet should be introduced early and continue into adolescence (Ito et al, 2008; Klepper, 2008).
- For the GSDs, maintain glucose homeostasis, prevent hypoglycemia, promote positive nitrogen balance and growth, and correct or prevent fatty liver. Prevent EFA deficiency (Abdel-Ghaffar et al, 2003). Consider carbohydrate-modified products such as cornstarch (as a low-release glucose source).
- Sucrose/maltose intolerance requires omission of sucrose and maltose from the diet.

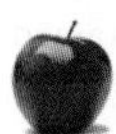

FOOD AND NUTRITION

Congenital Glucose–Galactose Malabsorption

- Use a diet free from sucrose, lactose, and glucose. Add fructose to a CHO-free formula incrementally as tolerated.
- Fructose may be used for older children; the other CHO sources should be avoided.

Fructosemia

- Diet must exclude fructose, sucrose, sorbitol, invert sugar, maple syrup, honey, and molasses.
- Read labels carefully. Tube feedings or intravenous solutions may contain sources of fructose.

Galactosemia

- Use a lactose and galactose-free diet—no milk, milk products, soybeans, peaches, lentils, liver, brains, or breads or cereals containing milk or cream cheese. Omit fresh blueberries and honeydew melon; fresh cherries, citrus, mango, red plums, and strawberries are allowed (Stepnick-Gropper et al, 2000).
- For infants, try Isomil or ProSobee, Elecare, Nutramigen, or formulas containing casein hydrolysate.
- Supplement with calcium, vitamin D, vitamin E, and riboflavin. In some disorders, galactose can often be reintroduced later in life.
- Read labels carefully; galactose is not reported on labels. Formulas labeled "low lactose" are *not* good substitutes; they contain lactose in amounts that can seriously harm patients with galactosemia.
- Be careful when using tube feedings or intravenous solutions; they may contain lactose.

Glycogen Storage Disorders

- Increase protein intake to improve muscle strength (Bembi et al, 2003).
- Use small, frequent feedings and, if steroids are used in treatment, a low-sodium diet. Long-term use of steroids can deplete stores of calcium and phosphorus and may elevate glucose, cause stunting, or cause weight gain.
- Avoid lactose and sucrose. Read all product labels.
- Glucose may be used. Concentrated sweets may be restricted unless made with pure glucose syrup.
- Cornstarch is used to prevent hypoglycemia.
- Sometimes, night feedings with additional daytime meals work effectively. Giving 4 tbsp cornstarch in 5 oz of fluid and 3 oz of juice, carnitine, DHA via gastrostomy (24 mL/h) at night may help the liver to maintain a normal blood glucose level (Isaacs and Zand, 2007).
- A multivitamin–mineral supplement with vitamin C, iron, and calcium may be needed because fruits and milk are limited. As necessary, replete nutrients such as vitamin B_{12}, folate, calcium, and iron.

Sucrose/Maltose Intolerance

- Omit sucrose and maltose from the diet.
- For the nongenetic form, gradually add these sugars back into the diet.
- Tube feedings or intravenous solutions may contain sources of sucrose or maltose; read labels.

Common Drugs Used and Potential Side Effects

- For persons with galactosemia, eliminate drugs containing lactose; supplement with calcium and riboflavin.
- Sucrose and maltose are added to many drugs; check carefully.
- All vitamin–mineral supplements must be free of the nontolerated carbohydrates.
- If liver transplantation is needed, support the immunosuppression with appropriate nutrition interventions. Changes in fluid or sodium or other nutrients may be required.
- In Pompe disease, Myozyme (alglucosidase alfa) may be prescribed.

Herbs, Botanicals, and Supplements

- Herbs and botanicals should not be used for these conditions because there are no controlled trials to prove efficacy.

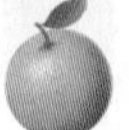

NUTRITION EDUCATION, COUNSELING, CARE MANAGEMENT

- Explain which sources of carbohydrate are allowed specific to the disorder.
- Read labels carefully. Many foods contain milk solids, galactose (e.g., luncheon meats, hot dogs), and other sugars; omit according to the disorder. Contact formula companies regarding product updates.

Patient Education—Food Safety

- Hand washing with soap and hot water is recommended before preparing formula or meals. Use clean utensils and containers for mixing formula.
- Before using tap water for formula preparation or to give as a beverage, let cold tap water run for 2 minutes to remove any lead that may be in the pipes.
- Follow the 2-hour rule: discard any beverage or food that has been left at room temperature for 2 hours or longer.
- Do not use honey in the diets of infants to decrease potential risk of botulism.

For More Information

- Association for Glycogen Storage Disease—United States
  http://www.agsdus.org/
- International Pompe Association
  http://www.worldpompe.org/
- March of Dimes
  http://www.marchofdimes.com

INBORN CARBOHYDRATE METABOLIC DISORDERS—CITED REFERENCES

Abdel-Ghaffar YT, et al. Essential fatty acid status in infants and children with chronic liver disease. *East Mediterr Health J.* 9:61, 2003.

Bembi EB, et al. Efficacy of multidisciplinary approach in the treatment of two cases of nonclassical infantile glycogenosis type II. *Inherit Metab Dis.* 26:675, 2003.

Berry GT. Galactosemia and amenorrhea in the adolescent. *Ann N Y Acad Sci.* 1135:112, 2008.

Brown GK. Glucose transporters: structure, function and consequences of deficiency. *J Inherit Metab Dis.* 23:237, 2000.

Bruno C, et al. Clinical and genetic heterogeneity of branching enzyme deficiency (glycogenosis type IV). *Neurology.* 63:1053, 2004.

Cabrera-Abreu J, et al. Bone mineral density and markers of bone turnover in patients with glycogen storage disease types I, III and IX. *J Inherit Metab Dis.* 27:1, 2004.

Holden HM, et al. Galactokinase: structure, function and role in type II galactosemia. *Cell Mol Life Sci.* 61:2471, 2004.

Isaacs JS, Zand DJ. Single-gene autosomal recessive disorders and Prader-Willi syndrome: an update for food and nutrition professionals. *J Am Diet Assoc.* 107:466, 2007.

Ito S, et al. Modified Atkins diet therapy for a case with glucose transporter type 1 deficiency syndrome. *Brain Dev.* 30:226, 2008.

Klepper J. Glucose transporter deficiency syndrome (GLUT1DS) and the ketogenic diet. *Epilepsia.* 49:46S, 2008.

Melis D, et al. Brain damage in glycogen storage disease type I. *J Pediatr.* 144:637, 2004.

Panis B, et al. Bone metabolism in galactosemia. *Bone.* 35:982, 2004.

Raben N, et al. Replacing acid alpha-glucosidase in Pompe disease: recombinant and transgenic enzymes are equipotent, but neither completely clears glycogen from type II muscle fibers. *Mol Ther.* 11:48, 2005.

Stepnick-Gropper S, et al. Free galactose content of fresh fruits and strained fruit and vegetable baby foods: more foods to consider for the galactose-restricted diet. *J Am Diet Assoc.* 100:573, 2000.

Wang D, et al. Functional studies of the T295M mutation causing Glut1 deficiency: glucose efflux preferentially affected by T295M. *Pediatr Res.* 64: 538, 2004.

CEREBRAL PALSY

NUTRITIONAL ACUITY RANKING: LEVEL 3

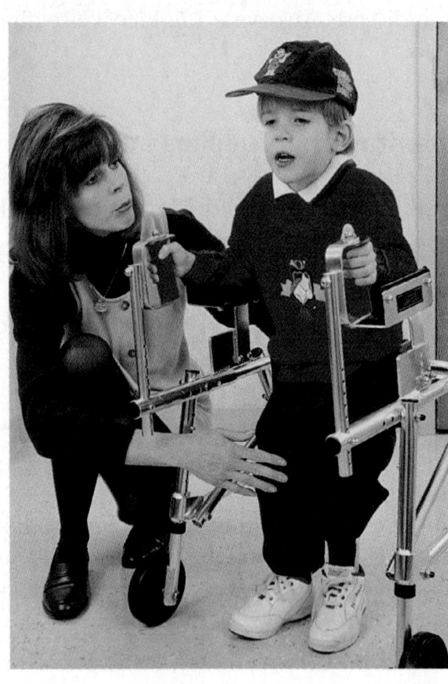

Adapted from: Weber J RN, EdD and Kelley J RN, PhD. *Health Assessment in Nursing,* 2nd ed. Philadelphia: Lippincott Williams & Wilkins, 2003.

DEFINITIONS AND BACKGROUND

Cerebral palsy (CP) results from brain damage to motor centers before, during, or after birth. Human epidemiological data suggest a relationship between CP and cytokines or inflammation (Gaudet and Smith, 2001). One of 500 live births may be affected. Each year, 1200 to 1500 preschool-age children in the United States are identified as having CP, which causes physical and mental disabilities that are nonprogressive.

Infants may present with early abnormal rolling, stiffness, irritability, and developmental delays (see Table 3-5). Seizures, mental retardation, hyperactive gag reflex, tongue thrust, poor lip closure, inability to chew properly, behavioral problems, visual or auditory problems may occur. Symptoms may be mild or severe, and vary from one person to the next. Skeletal maturation is frequently delayed.

Spastic (uncontrolled shaking or difficult, stiff movement) affects about 75%, **athetoid** (involuntary worm-like movement) affects 15%, **ataxic** (impaired coordination and balance) affects about 10%, and many individuals have a **mixed** form of CP. In many individuals, wasting of voluntary muscles contributes to reduced resting energy needs (Hogan, 2004). The potential for malnutrition exists, wherein indirect calorimetry is useful to assure adequacy of intake (Hogan, 2004).

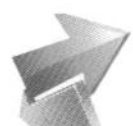

ASSESSMENT, MONITORING, AND EVALUATION

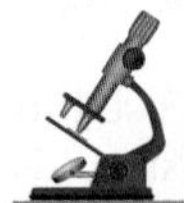

CLINICAL INDICATORS

Genetic Markers: The condition is not genetic in origin.

Clinical/History		
Low birth weight (LBW)	Low 5-minute Apgar score (below 7)	Height or length Weight and growth chart (%)

- Shaking, worm-like, or stiff movements
- Impaired balance and coordination
- Skull x-ray
- Chewing problems
- Diet/intake history
- Self-feeding problems
- Seizures
- GERD
- Constipation

Lab Work

- Gluc
- Alb
- Serum Ca^{++}, Mg^{++}
- Transferrin
- Alk phos
- H & H, serum Fe, ferritin

INTERVENTION

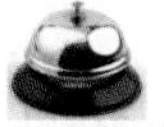

OBJECTIVES

- Alleviate malnutrition resulting from the patient's inability to close lips, suck, bite, chew, or swallow.
- Promote independence through use of adaptive feeding devices. Eye–hand coordination is often lacking, and grasp may not be strong.
- Assess appropriate energy and nutrient needs. When adequately nourished, children and adolescents with CP appear more tranquil and require decreased feeding time (Hogan, 2004). Promote mealtimes in a quiet, unhurried environment.

TABLE 3-5 Medications for Congenital Heart Disease

Generic Name	Brand Name	Concerns
Acebutol	Sectral	GI distress or nausea
Atenolol	Tenormin	GI distress or nausea
Azathioprine	Imuran	
Baby aspirin	Bayer	
Captopril	Capoten	GI distress or nausea
Cisapride	Propulsid	
Digoxin	Lanoxin	
Enalapril	Vasotec	
Furosemide	Lasix	GI distress or nausea; potassium, magnesium, calcium, and folate may be depleted
Hydrochlorothiazide	Hydrodiuril	GI distress or nausea; potassium, magnesium, calcium, and folate may be depleted
Lisinopril	Zestril	
Metoprolol	Lopressor	
Prednisone	Deltasone	Depletes calcium and phosphorus; may elevate glucose, cause stunting, or cause weight gain.
Propranolol	Inderal	
Spironolactone	Aldactone	
Warfarin	Coumadin	Need steady intake of vitamin K; no big fluctuations

SAMPLE NUTRITION CARE PROCESS STEPS

Difficulty with Feeding Self and Soy Allergy

Assessment Data: Weight and growth charts, medical history of aspiration, difficulty consuming adequate intake orally or by tube, soy allergy.

Nutrition Diagnosis (PES): NB 2.6. Self-feeding difficulty related to inability to bite properly and use utensils in CP as evidenced by weight loss of 4 lb in 6 months, current BMI of 13, ht and wt percentiles both <5%, history of aspiration when tube fed, allergy to soy.

Interventions:

Food and Nutrient Delivery

ND 1.2. Increase caloric intake through bolus feeding.

ND 1.3. Provide high-calorie, high protein formula free of soy.

Nutrition Education.

E 1.1. Discuss importance of nutrition and foods child is able to tolerate.

Counseling

C 2. RD to counsel mother and home nurse on importance of enhancing high calorie foods as necessary to prevent weight and muscle loss.

Care Management

RC 1.3. RD to collaborate with MD and home nurse for highest quality of care for patient, RD to collaborate with formula company to find high calorie high protein formula that is soy-free.

Monitoring and Evaluation: Weight records, improved intake of sufficient energy and protein to rebuild muscle mass and improve in growth percentiles; improved BMI for age.

- Correct nutritional deficits, altered growth rate, developmental delays, or retardation.
- Prevent or correct constipation, aspiration pneumonia, gastroesophageal reflux, pressure ulcers.

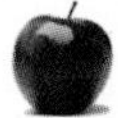

FOOD AND NUTRITION

- Energy requirements of children and adolescents will vary depending on functional capacity, degree of mobility, severity of disease, and level of altered metabolism (Hogan, 2004). Reduce energy intake for spastic patients or those with severely limited activity, 11 kcal/cm for ages 5–11. For moderately active patients, use 14 kcal/cm for ages 5–11. Increase energy intake (up to 45 kcal/kg) to accommodate for added movements of the athetoid patient over age 18.
- Breast milk is recommended for infants with CP (Vohr et al, 2006).
- Feeding gastrostomy tubes are a reasonable alternative for severe feeding and swallowing problems and poor weight gain (Rogers, 2004; Sullivan et al, 2004). Night feedings may allow more normal daytime routines. Daytime bolus feedings of high-calorie, high-protein formulas at scheduled times may also be needed to provide adequate nutrition in some cases.

- For chewing problems, eliminate coarse, stringy foods. Puree foods as needed.
- With frequent vomiting, assess actual intake; anti-emetic medications may be needed.
- For constant dribbling, add cereal or yogurt to fluids. Replace fluids, thickened if needed.
- For constipation, use laxative or high-fiber foods such as bran in the diet. Provide extra fluids. In younger children, too much fiber can displace intake of adequate nutrition.
- Supplement with a general multivitamin–mineral supplement, especially for B-complex vitamins, calcium, and vitamin D (Henderson et al, 2005).
- For pressure ulcers or skin breakdown from minimal positioning of the body, ensure adequate protein, vitamins C and A, and zinc. Work with caregivers to turn and reposition every 2 hours.

Common Drugs Used and Potential Side Effects

- Dantrolene (Dantrium) inhibits the release of calcium in muscle and skeletal tissue, preventing muscle cramping and spasms. Diarrhea, changes in BP, weight loss, and constipation may all occur.
- Klonopin (clonazepam) is a benzodiazepine used to slow down the central nervous system (CNS) for treatment of spasticity. Side effects may include constipation or diarrhea, dizziness, drowsiness, clumsiness, unsteadiness, a "hangover" effect, headache, nausea, and vomiting.
- Antibiotics such as baclofen may cause or aggravate diarrhea. Use of acidophilus and probiotic products may alleviate loss of intestinal bacteria.
- Laxatives may often be needed; monitor fiber and fluid needs. Milk of magnesia can be used safely in a pediatric dosage. Avoid using laxatives containing mineral oil.
- Anticonvulsants may increase risk of osteomalacia. Nutrient deficiencies are common: vitamins D, B_6, B_{12}, and K, folate, calcium, and biotin are often insufficient and should be replaced.

Herbs, Botanicals, and Supplements

- Herbs and botanicals should not be used; there are no controlled trials to prove efficacy.
- Probiotics may be used to alleviate loss of intestinal bacteria. Encourage natural sources such as yogurt or acidophilus milk, if tolerated.

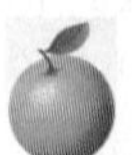

NUTRITION EDUCATION, COUNSELING, CARE MANAGEMENT

- Remind older patients to keep lips closed to avoid losing food from their mouths as they try to chew.
- Fortify the diet with dry or evaporated milk, wheat germ, and other nutrient enhancers when intake is inadequate.
- Allow extra time for feedings. Use of adaptive feeding equipment may be beneficial. Provide special training as needed for a specific feeding procedure (e.g., a preemie nipple for poor suck).
- Help parent or caretaker with problems related to dental caries, drugs, constipation, pica, or weight.
- Exercise can be beneficial, such as recreational sports, yoga, and hippotherapy.
- Tube feeding may be needed. Ensure proper positioning to avoid aspiration or GERD.

Patient Education—Food Safety

- Hand washing with soap and hot water is recommended before preparing formula or meals. Use clean utensils and containers.
- Before using tap water for formula preparation or to give as a beverage, let cold tap water run for 2 minutes to remove any lead that may be in the pipes.
- Follow the 2-hour rule: discard any beverage or food that has been left at room temperature for 2 hours or longer.
- Do not use honey in the diets of infants to decrease potential risk of botulism.

For More Information

- American Academy of Developmental Medicine and Dentistry http://www.aadmd.org
- American Association on Health and Disabilities http://www.aahd.us/
- American Cerebral Palsy Information Center http://www.cerebralpalsy.org
- CP Connection http://www.cpconnection.com/
- CP Resource Center http://twinenterprises.com/cp/
- Developmental Disabilities Nurses Association http://www.ddna.org/
- Disability Resource Network http://www.d-r-d.com/
- Easter Seals http://www.easter-seals.org
- Hemiplegic Cerebral Palsy http://www.hemikids.org/
- United Cerebral Palsy Association, Inc. http://www.ucpa.org/

CEREBRAL PALSY—CITED REFERENCES

Gaudet L, Smith G. Cerebral palsy and chorioamnionitis: the inflammatory cytokine link. *Obstet Gynecol Surv.* 56:433, 2001.

Henderson RC. Longitudinal changes in bone density in children and adolescents with moderate to severe cerebral palsy. *J Pediatr.* 146:769, 2005.

Hogan SE. Energy requirements of children with cerebral palsy. *Can J Diet Pract Res.* 65:124, 2004.

Rogers B. Feeding method and health outcomes of children with cerebral palsy. *J Pediatr.* 145:S28, 2004.

Sullivan PB, et al. Impact of gastrostomy tube feeding on the quality of life of carers of children with cerebral palsy. *Dev Med Child Neurol.* 46:796, 2004.

Vohr BR, et al. Beneficial effects of breast milk in the neonatal intensive care unit on the developmental outcome of extremely low birth weight infants at 18 months of age. *Pediatrics.* 118:115, 2006.

CLEFT LIP AND PALATE (OROFACIAL CLEFTS)

NUTRITIONAL ACUITY RANKING: LEVEL 3

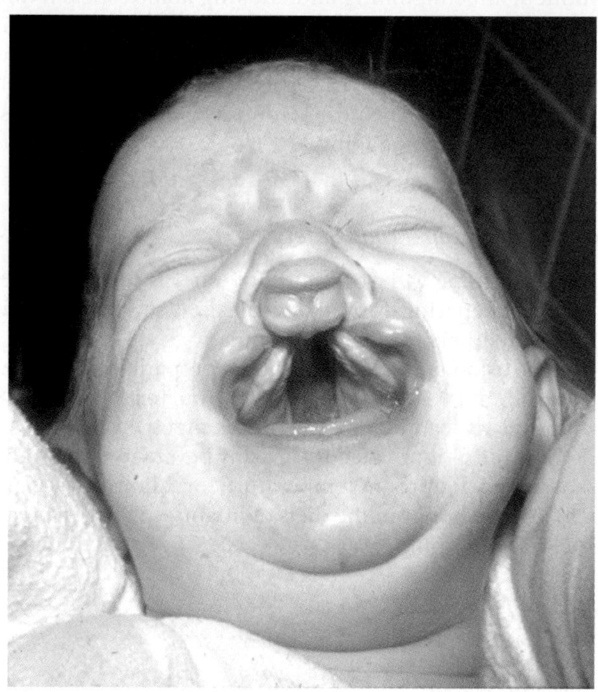

Adapted from: Rubin E MD and Farber JL MD. *Pathology,* 3rd ed. Philadelphia: Lippincott Williams & Wilkins, 1999.

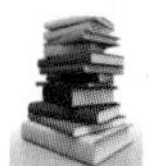

DEFINITIONS AND BACKGROUND

Cleft lip and palate are congenital malformations occurring during the embryonic period of development. They result in a fissure in the lip and roof of the mouth, which may be unilateral or bilateral. Incidence is approximately one in 700 births in Caucasians, or about 5000 births annually in the United States. Infants with cleft palate are often smaller in size and weight than other infants.

Periconceptional folate and folic acid intake prevents orofacial clefts (OFC; Krapels et al, 2004). Other nutrients also play a role, and many mothers who eat poorly risk having a baby with OFC. Sufficient preconceptual intake of macronutrients and key micronutrients may decrease OFC risk (Krapels et al, 2006; Mitchell et al, 2003). There is also a risk from inadequate zinc intake (Tamura et al, 2005).

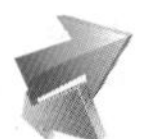

ASSESSMENT, MONITORING, AND EVALUATION

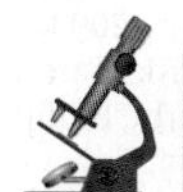

CLINICAL INDICATORS

Genetic Markers: Interferon regulatory factor 6 (IRF6) gene may be related.

Clinical/History
- Length (height)
- Growth (%)
- Weight
- Weight changes
- Diet/intake history
- Head circumference
- Cleft type (unilateral or bilateral; complete or incomplete)
- Otitis media (OM) or other infections
- Chewing difficulty

Lab Work
- Gluc
- Alb
- H & H
- Serum Ca^{++}, Mg^{++}

INTERVENTION

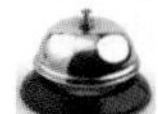

OBJECTIVES

- Cleft palate is more of a problem than cleft lip. Compensate for the patient's inability to suck because of the air space between the mouth and nose.
- Prevent choking, air swallowing, coughing, and fatigue as much as possible.
- Encourage breastfeeding where possible to protect against OM (Aniansson et al, 2002).
- Supply the child with energy to heal and to grow; offer tips for meal planning and resources because feeding will be a challenge (Redford-Badwal et al, 2003).
- For surgery, allow extra energy and protein for healing; use a multivitamin supplement. Before surgery, a custom retainer device may be placed in the mouth and is intended to gradually pull the edges of the cleft closer to achieve better lip repair. The device also aids in the feeding process.

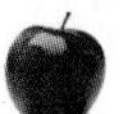

FOOD AND NUTRITION

- Provide a normal diet in accordance with the patient's age and dietary recommendations. Monitor diet carefully

SAMPLE NUTRITION CARE PROCESS STEPS

Inability to Bite or Chew

Assessment Data: Weight and growth charts, difficulty chewing and biting into foods.

Nutrition Diagnoses (PES): NC 1.2. Biting/chewing difficulty related to craniofacial malformations as evidenced by prolonged feeding time and decreased intake.

Intervention: Educate parents about texture changes, timing for meals, enhancing energy intake through high calorie foods and supplements, oral health and hygiene.

Monitoring and Evaluation: Weight records, growth, tolerance for various food consistencies.

because mother may have had a poor diet during preconceptual period and pregnancy.

- For infant feeding, use a medicine dropper or plastic bottle with a soft nipple and enlarged hole. The use of a squeezable, collapsible bottle with a longer nipple and a large crosscut opening, which allows parents to control the flow of milk, can help. Release formula or milk a little at a time, in coordination with the infant's chewing movements. Burp infant frequently to release swallowed air. Feed the infant in an upright position to prevent aspiration.
- When the infant is 4–6 months of age, begin to add solids in the diet. Pureed baby foods can be used, or the infant can be spoon fed with milk used to dilute the baby foods. Feed solids from a spoon and avoid use of a bottle or commercial syringe feeder, unless prescribed for unique circumstances.
- Avoid fruit peelings, nuts, peanut butter, leafy vegetables, heavy cream dishes, popcorn, grapes, biscuits, cookies, and chewing gum as they may get lodged in the palate. Avoid spicy, acidic foods if they cause irritation.

Common Drugs Used and Potential Side Effects

- No specific medicines are used for cleft lip and palate; surgery is the primary treatment. After surgery, there may be a need for antibiotics if infection sets in.
- Women who are taking valproate, lithium, carbamezine and other bipolar disorder medicines should discontinue use during pregnancy to reduce risk for cleft lip or palate.
- If genetic testing indicates an MTHFR allele, L-methylfolate (such as in Deplin) may be prescribed.

Herbs, Botanicals, and Supplements

- Herbs and botanicals are not required for cleft lip or palate.

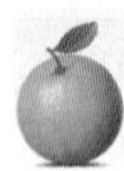

NUTRITION EDUCATION, COUNSELING, CARE MANAGEMENT

- Explain how to feed the infant with a special nipple as needed.
- Solids may be started at 4–6 months. Using thickened baby food or pureed items as tolerated.
- Supplement the diet with vitamin C if citrus juices are not taken well.
- Have the parents use only small amounts of liquid when they are feeding an infant. To prevent choking, slow swallowing should be encouraged and proper positioning should be taught.
- Discuss the impact of surgery and how to promote effective healing by using a nutrient-dense diet with adequate amounts of protein, energy, vitamins A and C, and zinc.
- Because of the types of problems that may occur (teeth in the area of the cleft may be missing or improperly positioned, affecting biting and chewing ability; speech difficulties; frequent colds, sore throats, OM, tonsillitis), assistance from a variety of therapists and professionals is needed. The dietitian can assist with nutrition and feeding-related issues. Nutrient density and texture assessments should be ongoing.

Patient Education—Food Safety

- Hand washing with soap and hot water is recommended before preparing formula or meals. Use clean utensils and containers for mixing formula.
- Before using tap water for formula preparation or to give as a beverage, let cold tap water run for 2 minutes to remove any lead that may be in the pipes.
- Follow the 2-hour rule: discard any beverage or food that has been left at room temperature for 2 hours or longer.
- Do not use honey in the diets of infants; this will decrease the risk of botulism.

For More Information

- AboutFace USA
  http://www.aboutfaceusa.org/
- About Smiles
  http://www.aboutsmiles.org/
- American Cleft Palate-Craniofacial Association
  http://www.cleftline.org/
- Center for Craniofacial Development and Disorders
  http://www.hopkinsmedicine.org/craniofacial/Home/Index.cfm
- Cleft Lip and Palate Resources
  http://www.widesmiles.org/
- Cleft Palate Foundation
  http://www.cleftline.org/aboutclp/
- FACES: The National Craniofacial Organization
  http://www.faces-cranio.org/
- Federation for Children with Special Needs
  http://www.faces-cranio.org/
- Forward Face: The Charity for Children with Craniofacial Conditions
  http://www.nffr.org/ForwardFace.htm
- Smile Train
  http://www.smiletrain.org/library/PublicLibrary.html

CLEFT LIP AND PALATE—CITED REFERENCES

Aniansson G, et al. Otitis media and feeding with breast milk of children with cleft palate. *Scand J Plast Reconstr Surg Hand Surg.* 36:9, 2002.

Krapels IP, et al. Nutrition and genes in the development of orofacial clefting. *Nutr Rev.* 64:280, 2006.

Mitchell LE, et al. Retinoic acid receptor alpha gene variants, multivitamin use, and liver intake as risk factors for oral clefts: a population-based case-control study in Denmark, 1991–1994. *Am J Epidemiol.* 158:69, 2003.

Redford-Badwal DA, et al. Impact of cleft lip and/or palate on nutritional health and oral-motor development. *Dent Clin North Am.* 47:305, 2003.

Tamura T, et al. Plasma zinc concentrations of mothers and the risk of nonsyndromic oral clefts in their children: a case-control study in the Philippines. *Birth Defects Res A Clin Mol Teratol.* 73:612, 2005.

- Congenital Heart Defects
  http://www.congenitalheartdefects.com/
- Congenital Heart Information Network
  http://www.tchin.org/
- Heart Center Encyclopedia
  http://www.cincinnatichildrens.org/health/heart-encyclopedia/default.htm
- Heart Institute for Children
  http://www.thic.com/Default.htm
- Kids with Heart, National Association for Children's Heart Disorders, Inc
  http://kidswithheart.org/
- United Hearts
  http://kidswithheart.org/

CONGENITAL HEART DISEASE—CITED REFERENCES

Barbas KH, Kelleher DK. Breastfeeding success among infants with congenital heart disease. *Pediatr Nurs.* 30:285, 2004.

Children's Hospital Boston. Accessed April 27, 2009, at http://www.childrenshospital.org/az/Site2116/mainpageS2116P0.html.

Feingold B, Law YM. Nesiritide use in pediatric patients with congestive heart failure. *J Heart Lung Transplant.* 23:1455, 2004.

Owens JL, Musa N. Nutrition support after neonatal cardiac surgery. *Nutr Clin Pract.* 24:242, 2009.

CYSTINOSIS AND FANCONI'S SYNDROME

NUTRITIONAL ACUITY RANKING: LEVEL 3

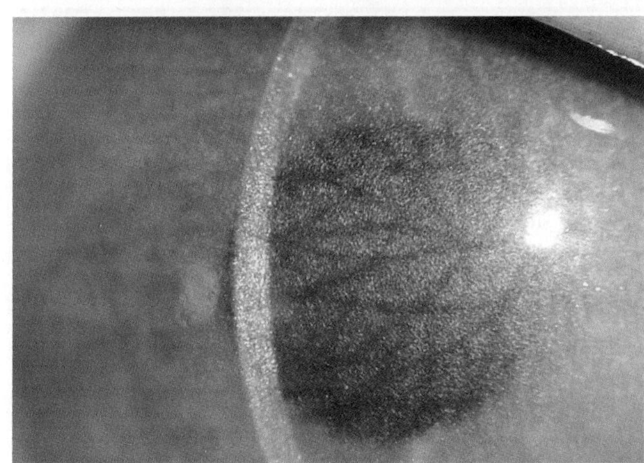

Adapted from: Tasman W, Jaeger E. *The Wills Eye Hospital Atlas of Clinical Ophthalmology,* 2nd ed. Lippincott Williams & Wilkins, 2001.

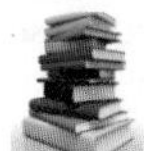

DEFINITIONS AND BACKGROUND

In cystinosis, crystals of cystine are deposited throughout the body. If left untreated, the disease may lead to kidney failure. Toxic accumulations of copper in the brain and kidney account for neurological symptoms. Cystinosis may be inherited or acquired, such as by lead poisoning. Manifestations are also seen in hereditary fructose intolerance. Myopathy leads to restrictive lung disease in adults who have not received long-term cystine depletion. Whether or not oral cystamine therapy can prevent this complication remains to be determined (Anikster et al, 2001).

Infantile nephropathic cystinosis, the most severe form, is a lysosomal membrane transport defect. FTT, rickets, metabolic acidosis, unexplained glucosuria of renal tubular origin, loss of color in the retina of the eyes, and severe photophobia can appear as early as 3–18 months of age. In **intermediate cystinosis**, kidney and eye symptoms become apparent during the teenage years or early adulthood. Polyuria, growth retardation, rickets, acidosis, and vomiting are present. In **benign or adult cystinosis**, crystalline cystine accumulates primarily in the cornea of the eyes and adults may present with acidosis, hypokalemia, polyuria, or osteomalacia.

Fanconi's syndrome, a generalized tubular dysfunction, can be either acquired or inherited. The hereditary form may accompany Wilson's disease, galactosemia or glycogen storage diseases. Nephrotoxic drugs, such as use of some chemotherapy agents, streptozocin, antiretrovirals, valproate, or outdated tetracycline, may cause the acquired form (Knorr et al, 2004). Vitamin D deficiency, myeloma, amlyoidosis, and heavy metal intoxication may also be triggers. Regardless of origin, Fanconi's syndrome results in multiple organ damage, with profound renal damage. Excessive urination (polyuria), excessive thirst (polydipsia), and severe hypokalemia occur. Renal transplantation may be needed.

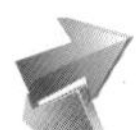

ASSESSMENT, MONITORING, AND EVALUATION

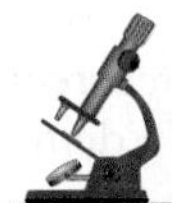

CLINICAL INDICATORS

Genetic Markers: The affected gene in the inherited form is *CTNS*, located on chromosome 17, which codes for cystinosin.

Clinical/History

Birth weight (infant or child)
Present weight
Length or Height
Growth (%), head circumference
Abnormal sensitivity to light (photophobia)
Loss of color in the retina
Rickets
Dehydration
Dysphagia
Patchy brown skin
Diet/intake history
Polydipsia, polyuria

Lab Work

Gluc
Ca^{++}, Mg^{++}
Aminoaciduria

Serum phosphorous (decreased)	K^+ (decreased)	I & O
	CO_2	Uric acid
	Alb	(decreased)
Phosphaturia	H & H	BUN, Creat
Aminoaciduria	Serum Fe	Ceruloplasmin
Na^+	Serum vitamin D	WBCs

INTERVENTION

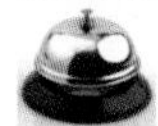

OBJECTIVES

- Remove the offending nephrotoxin in the acquired forms.
- Prevent bone demineralization and kidney failure. Correct hypokalemia, hypophosphatemia, and vitamin D insufficiency.
- Manage swallowing dysfunction.
- Support growth, which tends to be stunted in children.
- Prevent or delay corneal damage.
- Provide sufficient volumes of fluid and supplemental nutrients.
- Prepare for renal transplantation if needed. Postoperatively, promote wound healing and prevent graft rejection.

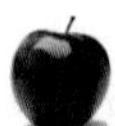

FOOD AND NUTRITION

- Use a diet low in cystine, with protein-free diet, PFD1 or PFD2 from Mead Johnson.
- Provide sufficient fluid intake. Input and output should be checked by standards for age.
- Supplement with vitamin D_3 (cannot convert 25-dihydroxycholecalciferol); give phosphate and calcium as appropriate. Bicarbonate is also needed.
- Provide sufficient sodium and potassium replacements.
- Alter consistency (liquids, solids) as needed.
- Prepare for wound healing with sufficient vitamins A, C, zinc, protein, and energy.

Common Drugs Used and Potential Side Effects

- Sodium bicarbonate or citrate should be used to correct acidosis. Take separately from iron supplements. Edema can occur.
- K depletion may require replacement therapy with a K-containing salt.
- Cysteamine (Cystagon), administered orally, halts glomerular destruction and decreases cystine content in cells. It mitigates morbidity and death (Gahl et al, 2007).
- Long-term GH treatment can be safe and effective; it should be started early in the course of the disease (Wuhl et al, 2001).

SAMPLE NUTRITION CARE PROCESS STEPS

Inadequate Vitamin and Mineral Intakes

Assessment Data: Weight and growth charts, lab reports showing losses of K^+ and phosphorus in the urine, evidence of rickets (bowed legs).

Nutrition Diagnoses (PES): Inadequate mineral intake (potassium and phosphorus) related to excessive urinary losses from cystinosis as evidenced by urine tests, insufficient vitamin D metabolism and rickets.

Intervention: Educate parents about sources of vitamin D, potassium and phosphorus from medications and diet.

Monitoring and Evaluation: Weight records, growth, labs for potassium, phosphorus, and vitamin D.

Herbs, Botanicals, and Supplements

- Herbs and botanicals should not be used for this condition because there are no controlled trials to prove efficacy.
- Use of Chinese herbs may be problematic, causing some forms of cystinosis in susceptible individuals. Discourage use.

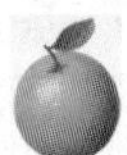

NUTRITION EDUCATION, COUNSELING, CARE MANAGEMENT

- Emphasize the importance of correcting fluid and electrolyte imbalances.
- Discuss any necessary changes in consistency to assist with dysphagia.
- Discuss diet for managing renal failure if necessary.
- If transplantation is needed, discuss guidelines for managing side effects such as graft–host resistance.

Patient Education—Food Safety

- Hand washing with soap and hot water is recommended before preparing formula or meals. Use clean utensils and containers for mixing formula.
- Before using tap water for formula preparation or to give as a beverage, let cold tap water run for 2 minutes to remove any lead that may be in the pipes.
- Follow the 2-hour rule: discard any beverage or food that has been left at room temperature for 2 hours or longer.
- Do not use honey in the diets of infants to decrease potential risk of botulism.

For More Information

- American Foundation for Urologic Disease http://www.afud.org
- Cystinosis Central http://medicine.ucsd.edu/cystinosis/Index.htm\
- Cystinosis Foundation http://www.cystinosisfoundation.org/
- Cystinosis Research Foundation http://www.cystinosis.org/

CYSTINOSIS AND FANCONI'S SYNDROME—CITED REFERENCES

Anikster Y, et al. Pulmonary dysfunction in adults with nephropathic cystinosis. *Chest.* 119:394, 2001.

Gahl WA, et al. Nephropathic cystinosis in adults: natural history and effects of oral cysteamine therapy. *Ann Int Med.* 144:242, 2007.

Knorr M, et al. Fanconi syndrome caused by antiepileptic therapy with valproic acid. *Epilepsia.* 45:868, 2004.

Wuhl E, et al. Long-term treatment with growth hormone in short children with nephropathic cystinosis. *J Pediatr.* 138:880, 2001.

DOWN SYNDROME

NUTRITIONAL ACUITY RANKING: LEVEL 2

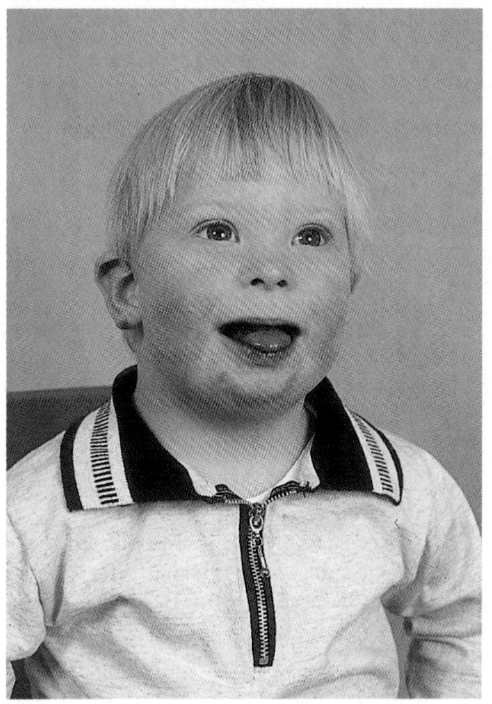

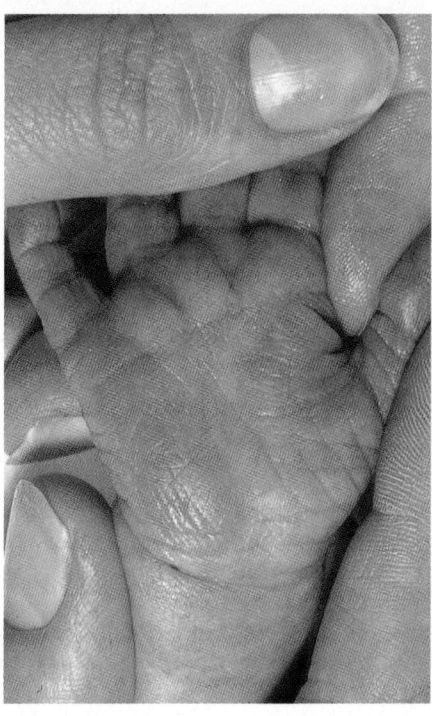

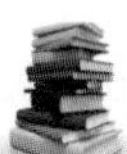

DEFINITIONS AND BACKGROUND

DS is a congenital defect in which patients carry an altered chromosome; trisomy patients have an extra chromosome 21. Children with DS have short stature, decreased muscle tone, constipation, intestinal defects, weight changes, and mental retardation. There is a higher risk for congenital heart disease, gum disease, celiac disease, Hirschsprung's disease, hypothyroidism, leukemia, respiratory problems, and gastroesophageal reflux. Incidence of the syndrome is often related to maternal age.

Chronic oxidative stress is a consideration; antioxidants, such as selenium, vitamins C and E, are important to include. Research also suggests that folate has a relationship. Women of childbearing age should consume 400 mg folic acid daily though food sources and/or supplementation. (Czeizel and Puho, 2005).

Compared with other individuals, those with DS may have lower levels of vitamin A, thiamin, folate, vitamin B_{12}, vitamin C, magnesium, manganese, selenium, zinc, carnitine, carnosine, and choline; excesses of copper, cysteine, phenylalanine (Phe), and superoxide dismutase are sometimes encountered (Thiel and Fowkes, 2004). Disorders of metabolism involving vitamin B_6, vitamin D, calcium, and tryptophan may play a role (Thiel and Fowkes, 2004).

The use of chromosome engineering to generate trisomic mouse models and large-scale studies of genotype–phenotype relationships in patients will contribute to the future understanding of DS (Wiseman et al, 2009). First-trimester screening is generally recommended.

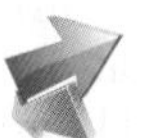

ASSESSMENT, MONITORING, AND EVALUATION

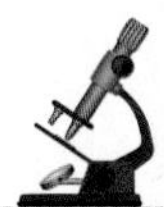

CLINICAL INDICATORS

Genetic Markers: DS is caused by trisomy of chromosome 21 (Hsa21). There are other alleles that may have an impact.

Clinical/History

- Length or height
- Birth weight
- Present weight
- BMI
- Diet/intake history
- Head circumference
- DS growth chart
- Growth (%)
- Hyperextensibility of joints
- History of prematurity?
- Large tongue, eye slant
- Endocardial defects
- Developmental delay
- Small nose with flat bridge
- Pica
- Skin prick test

Lab Work

- Gluc
- Uric acid (increased)
- Plasma zinc
- Chol, Trig
- Na^+, K^+
- Ca^{++}, Mg^{++}
- I & O
- Serum folate

SAMPLE NUTRITION CARE PROCESS STEPS

Overweight

Assessment Data: Weight and growth charts, BMI >normal range.

Nutrition Diagnoses (PES): NC 3.3. Overweight related to inadequate energy expenditure in DS as evidenced by BMI >28, limited activity levels, and frequent consumption of high fat foods and snacks.

Intervention: Discuss differing growth patterns from usual which may lead to excessive weight gain. Discuss optimal nutrition goals and physical activity, encouraging plenty of daily activity. Review foods to avoid because of risks for choking.

Monitoring and Evaluation: Weight records, growth and improved BMI levels, tolerance for various foods and consistencies.

INTERVENTION

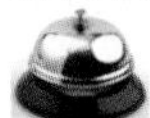

OBJECTIVES

- Provide adequate energy and nutrients for growth. Short stature is not caused by nutritional deficiencies; use appropriate DS growth charts.
- Monitor introduction of solid food, which may be delayed. Fruits and vegetables may not be consumed in adequate amounts.
- To avoid lowered intake of vitamins and minerals, treat obesity in children with DS with a balanced diet plus vitamin and mineral supplements; no energy restriction; and an increase in physical activity.
- Assist with feeding problems; tongue thrust and poor suck are common.
- Reduce emotional problems that lead to overeating. Overfeeding should be avoided. Use proper positioning.
- Manage constipation, diarrhea, gluten enteropathy, urinary tract infections (UTIs), gum and periodontal diseases, which are common. Prevent osteoporosis and bone disease.

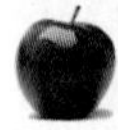

FOOD AND NUTRITION

- Supply adequate amounts of energy for age; for children aged 5–11 years, use 14.3 kcal/cm for girls and 16.1 kcal/cm for boys (Lucas, 2004, p. 41).
- Use protein according to age-dependent dietary reference intakes.
- Use a gluten-free diet if celiac disease is present (Hill et al, 2005).
- Monitor pica, overeating, and idiosyncrasies.
- Provide supplemental sources of folate, vitamin A, vitamin E, zinc, iron, and calcium if intake of fruits, vegetables, meats, dairy products, or whole grains is limited.
- Provide feeding assistance if needed. Tube feed if the patient is unable to eat orally; gradually wean to solids when possible.
- Provide extra fluid for drooling, diarrhea, or spillage.
- Encourage complex carbohydrates, prune juice, etc., if constipation is a problem.

Common Drugs Used and Potential Side Effects

- Aricept may have some benefit in individuals with DS. Nausea or diarrhea are sometimes side effects.
- For MTHFR alleles, products such as L-methylfolate (Deplin) may be given.

Herbs, Botanicals, and Supplements

- Herbs and botanicals should not be used; because there are no controlled trials to prove efficacy.

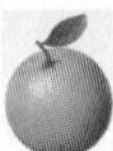

NUTRITION EDUCATION, COUNSELING, CARE MANAGEMENT

- Explain feeding techniques that may be beneficial. Discuss use of self-feeding utensils if needed.
- Help control energy intake and physical activity for appropriate levels.
- Never rush mealtime. Encourage socialization.
- Discuss how growth patterns differ from usual; FTT (Krugman and Dubowitz, 2003) or excessive weight gain may result as the child grows older.

Patient Education—Food Safety

- Hand washing with soap and hot water is recommended before preparing formula or meals. Use clean utensils and containers for mixing formula.
- Before using tap water for formula preparation or to give as a beverage, let cold tap water run for 2 minutes to remove any lead that may be in the pipes.
- Follow the 2-hour rule: discard any beverage or food that has been left at room temperature >2 hours.
- Do not use honey in the diets of infants to decrease potential risk of botulism.

For More Information

- Down Syndrome
  http://www.nas.com/downsyn/
- Down Syndrome Quarterly
  http://www.denison.edu/dsq
- Drexel University—Down Syndrome Growth Charts
  http://www.growthcharts.com/
  http://www.growthcharts.com/charts/DS/charts.htm
- National Association for Down Syndrome
  http://www.nads.org/
- National Down Syndrome Society
  http://www.ndss.org/content.cfm
- Special Olympics
  http://www.specialolympics.org/Special+Olympics+Public+Website/default.htm

DOWN SYNDROME—CITED REFERENCES

Czeizel AE, Puho E. Maternal use of nutritional supplements during the first month of pregnancy and decreased risk of Down's syndrome: case-control study. *Nutrition*. 21:698, 2005.

Hill ID, et al. Guideline for the diagnosis and treatment of celiac disease in children: recommendations of the North American Society for Pediatric Gastroenterology, Hepatology and Nutrition. *J Pediatr Gastroenterol Nutr.* 40:1, 2005.

Krugman SD, Dubowitz H. Failure to thrive. *Am Fam Physician.* 68:879, 2003.

Lucas B, ed. *Children with special care needs: nutrition care handbook.* Chicago: The American Dietetic Association, 2004.

Thiel RJ, Fowkes SW. Down syndrome and epilepsy: a nutritional connection? *Med Hypotheses.* 62:35, 2004.

Wiseman FK, et al. Down syndrome–recent progress and future prospects. *Hum Mol Genet.* 18:75, 2009.

FAILURE TO THRIVE

NUTRITIONAL ACUITY RANKING: LEVEL 4

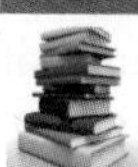

DEFINITIONS AND BACKGROUND

FTT is a diagnostic term used to describe infants and children who fail to grow and develop at a normal rate; it indicates protein, energy, vitamin, and mineral insufficiency. In many pediatric centers, one third of the referred children are malnourished. FTT is a complex problem that can be caused by many medical or social factors; without treatment, chronic illnesses or death may ensue.

Prompt diagnosis and intervention are important for preventing malnutrition and developmental delays. Careful attention must be paid to growth charts and medical histories (Krugman and Dubowitz, 2003). Food refusal, poor feeding, vomiting, gagging, irritability, and FTT are commonly found in both infantile feeding disorders (IFD) and common treatable medical conditions (Levy et al, 2009).

Weight is the most reliable marker for FTT. According to the American Academy of Pediatrics (2004), FTT is established when weight (or weight/height) is less than 2 standard deviations below the mean for sex and age and/or the weight curve has dropped more than 2 percentile lines on the National Center for Health Statistics growth charts after a previously stable pattern. Other indices include a small head circumference, muscular wasting, apathy, weight loss, or poor weight gain. Learning failure (e.g., slow to talk, behavior problems) can occur. Infants with DS, intrauterine growth retardation (IUGR), or premature birth follow different growth patterns than usual; monitor carefully to evaluate for FTT (Krugman and Dubowitz, 2003). About 25% of normal infants will shift to a lower growth percentile in the first 2 years of life and then remain at that percentile; this is not FTT (Krugman and Dubowitz, 2003).

Primary FTT originates from social/environmental deficits, inadequate feeding procedures, or caretaker behaviors. Adolescent mothers may need a lot of support and education. Proximity and touch are especially disturbed in feeding disorders (i.e., mothers provide less touch that supports growth), and children demonstrate signs of touch aversion (Feldman et al, 2004). Early interventions by trained home visitors may promote a more nurturing environment and reduce developmental delays.

Secondary FTT originates from some disease states (e.g., cancer, allergies, chronic infections, cystic fibrosis, cleft lip or palate, DS, or other physical or mental disability). Growth failure plus fever of unknown origin and anemia in older children or teens may suggest the onset of Crohn's disease; evaluation is recommended. About half of the causes of FTT are organic; the other 50% are from inorganic causes. The American Dietetic Association suggests at least five medical nutrition therapy visits for infants and children with FTT.

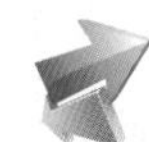

ASSESSMENT, MONITORING, AND EVALUATION

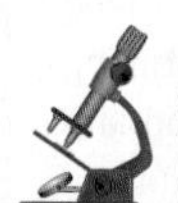

CLINICAL INDICATORS

Genetic Markers: Genes causing FTT would be related to the specific condition, such as s congenital heart defect, spina bifida, DS, cystic fibrosis.

Clinical/History

Height
Very low birth weight?
Apgar scores
Premature or small for gestational age (SGA)?
Current or goal weights
Growth grid
Percent height for age (actual height/expected height)
Head circumference; microcephaly?
Skinfold thickness
Diet and intake history
Feeding schedule and timing
Food allergy, especially milk allergy
GERD
Medical history
Breastfed or bottle fed?
Solid food introduction pattern
Diarrhea or vomiting?
Constipation
Dehydration
Inadequate access to food?
Infections, parasites?
Frequent UTIs
Maternal depression?

Lab Work

H & H
Serum Fe, ferritin
Anemia (iron, sickle cell, other)
Alb
Gluc
Chol, Trig
BUN
Thyroid function tests
I & O
Sweat test

INTERVENTION

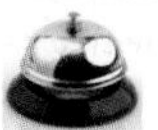

OBJECTIVES

- All children with FTT need additional calories for catch-up growth at about 150% of the energy requirement for

SAMPLE NUTRITION CARE PROCESS STEPS

FTT

Assessment Data: Weight and growth charts, medical conditions causing excessive energy expenditure or requirements, feeding methods used for the child, available financial resources to buy food or formula, access to safe and sufficient food supply.

Nutrition Diagnoses (PES): NI 2.1. Inadequate oral food/beverage intake related to minimal intake of formula and age-appropriate foods as evidenced by drop in more than 2 percentile lines on the National Center for Health Statistics growth chart after having achieved a previously stable pattern and medical Dx of FTT.

Interventions:

Food and Nutrition Delivery:

ND 5.7. Feeding environment to support growth in 12-month-olds.

ND 1.2. To follow increased caloric intake and frequent snacks.

Nutrition Education:

E 2.2. RD to provide nutrition counseling to support weight gain in patient and teach mother and caretaker how to properly feed according to infant's nutritional needs. Discuss adequate timing for feeding child. Educate and teach mother about appropriate feeding behaviors and practices for 12-month-olds.

Counseling:

C 2. Counsel mother/caretaker on how to provide nutritional needs for patient and environment to support those need. Goal is to achieve daily gains of weight, 30 g/d.

Coordination of Care:

RC 1.3. RD to collaborate with MD; RD will refer patient for in-home assessment and follow-through. Correct environmental causes of FTT. Refer to WIC or SNAP (food stamps) programs to help with financial challenges and food insecurity.

Monitoring and Evaluation: Weight records, growth, tolerance for various foods or formulas, financial access to food.

their expected, not actual, weight (Krugman and Dubowitz, 2003). Use calculations for determining needs from the most current *Pediatric Manual of Clinical Dietetics.*

- Identify and correct etiologies such as decreased energy intake, increased nutrient losses, increased metabolic demands. Determine if malnutrition is primary (from faulty feeding patterns or dietary inadequacy) or secondary (from disease process interfering with intake).
- Teach the parent or caretaker how to properly feed and how to determine needs. Advise parents to support nurturing during feeding.
- Provide the most optimal nutrition compatible with a normal growth pattern. Achieve daily gains of 30 g for young infants; extra may be desirable for catch-up. Nutrient-enriched formulas are probably not necessary (Henderson et al, 2007).
- Provide a schedule of feeding for infant's age to support catch-up growth and improved brain development (Powers et al, 2008). See Table 3-7 for more details.

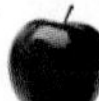

FOOD AND NUTRITION

- Conduct a thorough nutrition assessment and acquire actual intake records when possible. Evaluate the child's nutritional history and growth in comparison with the percentiles of other same-age children. If special growth charts are needed, use those instead (as for DS). Discuss findings with parent or caretaker.
- Calculate energy and protein needs carefully. While not easy to do, indirect calorimetry may be needed.
- Check recommended intakes for all nutrients. Provide adequate zinc and vitamin B_6, as determined by the infant's age; 120–130% is a common practice.
- Monitor growth (weight) weekly; feeding behaviors.
- If the infant is dehydrated, provide adequate amounts of fluids. However, FTT can be aggravated by excessive consumption of fruit juice and sweetened beverages (often 12–30 oz daily) which may replace other nutrient-dense foods. Limit to 4–6 oz daily until overall diet quality and growth rate have improved.
- Provide meals and snacks at scheduled times; support a comfortable social and emotional environment. Family meals and allowing children to be a part of meal preparation are also important.
- If FTT children are strictly vegan, monitor for vitamins B_{12}, D, B_6, iron, zinc, and calcium deficiencies.
- Tube feeding may be useful as a supplemental or alternative feeding method; nightly feeding is an effective recommendation if it can be managed by the caregiver.

Common Drugs Used and Potential Side Effects

- Evaluate medications given for any reason to determine if some or all affect nutritional intake. Adjust diet as needed.
- Endogenous cannabinoids or other appetite enhancers are being studied for their safety and effectiveness in FTT.

Herbs, Botanicals, and Supplements

- Herbs and botanicals should not be used for FTT; there are no controlled trials to prove efficacy.
- Probiotics are useful for their live micro-organisms with a health benefit for GI disorders, cancer, infant allergies, FTT, and infections (Brown and Valiere, 2004).
- Zinc supplementation may be needed during catch-up growth in malnourished children (Castillo-Duran and Weisstaub, 2003). Avoid prolonged or excessive doses.

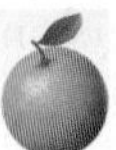

NUTRITION EDUCATION, COUNSELING, CARE MANAGEMENT

- Describe appropriate nutritional intake according to age and any predisposing medical conditions.
- Encourage the use of appropriate growth charts at home to monitor success. Develop a progress chart for developmental milestones. Growth spurts follow sustained weight gains; monitor growth frequently.

TABLE 3-7 Grading and Treatment for Hirschsprung's-Associated Enterocolitis

Grade	Clinical Symptoms
I	Mild explosive diarrhea, mild or moderate abdominal distention; no systemic manifestations
II	Moderate explosive diarrhea, moderate-to-severe abdominal distention; mild systemic symptoms
III	Severe explosive diarrhea, marked abdominal distention, and shock or impending shock
Fiber enhancement	
Breakfast	Whole wheat waffles with fresh fruit. Cereal choices: oatmeal, Frosted Mini Wheats, Kashi Mighty Bites, Raisin Bran, Wheat Chex. Whole wheat bagel, or whole wheat English muffin with chunky peanut butter. Bran muffins. Dried fruit to increase fiber content. Add fresh fruit
Lunch or dinner	Vegetable soup with whole wheat crackers. Whole wheat sandwich with leaf lettuce, tomato, meat of choice. Whole wheat macaroni and cheese with peas. Whole wheat spaghetti with sautéed zucchini and tomatoes in sauce. Fresh fruit. Whole wheat pizza with sauce, cheese, and vegetable toppings (green, red, yellow or orange peppers, mushrooms, tomatoes, olives). For tacos, use whole wheat tortillas, add vegetables (tomatoes, lettuce, olives, avocado). Brown rice, whole wheat pasta, legumes, beans; add a vegetable as a side. Green, red, yellow or orange peppers and cucumber slices with vegetable dip. Sliced pears, peaches, strawberries, or cantaloupe with fruit dip. Celery, 2 Tbsp peanut butter, raisins. Whole grain crackers

Fiber supplements:

Name	Active Ingredient	Serving Size	Amount of Fiber
Metamucil wafers	Psyllium 50% soluble	2 wafers	6 g
Metamucil powder	Psyllium 65% soluble	1 tbsp	3 g
Ground flax seed	45% insoluble, 55% soluble	1 tbsp	3 g
Benefiber	Wheat dextrin, 100% soluble	2 tbsp	3 g
Citrucil	Methocellulose, 100% soluble	1 scoop or 4 caplets	2 g
Pectin	100% soluble	1.75 oz package	4.3 g

Sources:
1. American Dietetic Association. *Fiber facts: soluble fiber and heart disease*. Chicago: American Dietetic Association, 2007.
2. Children's Hospital of Boston. Accessed April 27, 2009, at http://www.childrenshospital.org/az/Site2116/mainpageS2116P0.html.
3. Li BW, Andrews KW, Pehrsson PR. Individual sugars, soluble, and insoluble dietary fiber contents of 70 high consumption foods. *J Food Comp Anal.* 15:715–723, 2002.

- Offer simple, specific instructions when needed, such as mechanics of breastfeeding and typical intakes for children of same age. If formula is used, improper mixing of formula is common; help correct any misunderstandings.
- Discuss nutrient density (e.g., milk vs. sweetened carbonated beverages; whole fruit vs. juice).
- Explain proper use of over-the-counter vitamin–mineral supplements, age-appropriate for the child.
- Address any harmful or unusual dietary beliefs (Feld and Hyams, 2004).
- Practical suggestions should be offered regarding nurturing and emotional support for the child. Parenting classes may be beneficial.
- Coordinate referral to child welfare services where neglect is suspected (Block et al, 2005). Refer to WIC programs, La Leche League, SNAP (food stamps) whenever appropriate.
- Follow-up should be provided at outpatient clinics or by home visits.

Patient Education—Food Safety

- Hand washing with soap and hot water is recommended before preparing formula or meals. Use clean utensils and containers for mixing formula.
- Before using tap water for formula preparation or to give as a beverage, let cold tap water run for 2 minutes to remove any lead that may be in the pipes.
- Follow the 2-hour rule: discard any beverage or food that has been left at room temperature for 2 hours or longer.
- Do not use honey in the diets of infants; this will decrease the potential risk of botulism.

For More Information

- Kids Health
  http://kidshealth.org/parent/nutrition_fit/nutrition/failure_thrive.html
- Medline—FTT
  http://www.nlm.nih.gov/MEDLINEPLUS/ency/article/000991.htm

FAILURE TO THRIVE—CITED REFERENCES

American Academy of Pediatrics. *Pediatric nutrition handbook,* 5th ed. Elk Grove Village, IL: American Academy of Pediatrics, 2004.

Block RW, et al. Failure to thrive as a manifestation of child neglect. *Pediatrics.* 116:1234, 2005.

Brown AC, Valiere A. Probiotics and medical nutrition therapy. *Nutr Clin Care.* 7:56, 2004.

Castillo-Duran C, Weisstaub G. Zinc supplementation and growth of the fetus and low birth weight infant. *J Nutr.* 133:1494S, 2003.

Feld LG, Hyams JS, eds. *Growth assessment and growth failure. Consensus in pediatrics.* Evansville, IN: Mead Johnson & Company, 2004.

Feldman R, et al. Mother-child touch patterns in infant feeding disorders: relation to maternal, child, and environmental factors. *J Am Acad Child Adolesc Psychiatry.* 43:1089, 2004.

Henderson G, et al. Nutrient-enriched formula versus standard term formula for preterm infants following hospital discharge. *Cochrane Database Syst Res.* 17(4):CD004696, 2007.

Krugman SD, Dubowitz H. Failure to thrive. *Am Fam Physician.* 68:879, 2003.

Levy Y, et al. Diagnostic clues for identification of nonorganic vs organic causes of food refusal and poor feeding. *J Pediatr Gastroenterol Nutr.* 48:355, 2009.

Powers GC, et al. Postdischarge growth and development in a predominantly Hispanic, very low birth weight population. *Pediatrics.* 122:1258, 2008.

FATTY ACID OXIDATION DISORDERS

NUTRITIONAL ACUITY RANKING: LEVEL 4

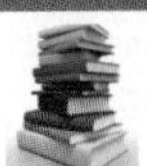

DEFINITIONS AND BACKGROUND

Fatty acid oxidation disorders disrupt mitochondrial energy generation and ketone production (Isaacs and Zand, 2007). Muscle protein breaks down and may lead to death if the heart muscle is involved. The fatty acid disorders with dietary implications include medium-chain acyl-CoA dehydrogenase deficiency (MCAD), long-chain 3-hydroxyacyl-CoA dehydrogenase (LCHAD) deficiency, and very long chain acyl-CoA dehydrogenase deficiency (Isaacs and Zand, 2007).

MCAD is caused by the lack of an enzyme required to convert fat to energy. Children with MCAD cannot use MCTs to make energy, so the body begins to malfunction when they fast (i.e., they have no more long-chain dietary fats available from the diet). MCAD occurs in approximately one in every 10,000 live births. MCAD occurs mostly among Caucasians of Northern European background. Symptoms typically begin in infancy or early childhood, often with simple lethargy. While some affected individuals have no symptoms at birth, disorders such as hypoglycemia, seizures, coma, brain damage, or cardiac arrest can occur very quickly with illness. If not detected and treated appropriately, MCAD can result in death. About 1 in 100 sudden infant death syndrome (SIDS) deaths are probably a result of undiagnosed MCAD (Nennstiel-Ratzel et al, 2005).

Early detection allows treatment and a normal life expectancy. Medical nutrition therapy to lower dietary fats does not decrease toxic metabolites because the body can make triglycerides from carbohydrates, proteins, or fats (Isaacs and Zand, 2007). The appropriate fatty acids must be omitted.

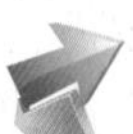

ASSESSMENT, MONITORING, AND EVALUATION

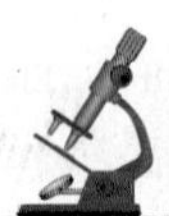

CLINICAL INDICATORS

Genetic Markers: MCAD involves medium-chain acyl-coenzyme A (CoA) dehydrogenase deficiency; adenosine replaces guanosine at position 985 of the MCAD gene.

Clinical/History
Length (height)
Birth weight
Present weight
Growth (%)
Diet/intake history
Seizures?
Retardation?

Lab Work
Gluc
Alb
Chol
Trig
Lipid Panel
H & H
Serum Fe

INTERVENTION

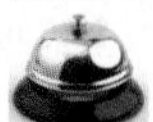

OBJECTIVES

- Avoid periods of fasting, day and night (Roe and Ding, 2001). Use IV glucose when food cannot be tolerated, such as with colds or flu.
- Customize protocol for the individual. LCHAD requires a severe dietary restriction of long-chain fats, to the lowest level that can deliver the EFAs and fat-soluble vitamins (Isaacs and Zand, 2007). MCT can be used in LCHAD but not in MCAD.
- Provide EFAs.

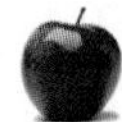

FOOD AND NUTRITION

- Restrict periods of fasting by offering small, frequent feedings (Oey et al, 2005).

SAMPLE NUTRITION CARE PROCESS STEPS

Excessive Intake of Types of Fats

Assessment Data: Weight and growth charts.

Nutrition Diagnoses (PES): Excessive intake of medium chain fatty acids related to MCAD deficiency as evidenced by signs of lethargy and elevated levels of triglycerides.

Intervention: Educate parents about avoiding sources of MCT; document in medical record about formulas to avoid.

Monitoring and Evaluation: Weight records, growth, improvement in lipid levels, reduced lethargy, normal mental development for age.

- A diet with avoidance of the specific, problematic fatty acids will be needed. For example, do not use enteral formulas that contain MCTs in MCAD.
- The diets will be higher in carbohydrates and fat-free protein foods.
- Supplement linoleic and a-linolenic acids; monitor by laboratory measurements of fatty acids.
- Supplemental carnitine has been recommended.
- Waking the child at least once during the night, or feeding by gastrostomy or NG tube overnight, is required for most of the fatty acid oxidation disorders (Isaacs and Zand, 2007).
- Monitor weight and growth closely to prevent obesity, but do not skip meals or feedings.

Common Drugs Used and Potential Side Effects

No specific drugs are used. Dietary alterations are the management.

Herbs, Botanicals, and Supplements

- Herbs and botanicals should not be used for MCADD because there are no controlled trials to prove efficacy for any related problems.

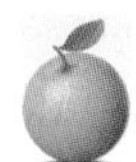

NUTRITION EDUCATION, COUNSELING, CARE MANAGEMENT

- Educate about the dangers of fasting, including periods during illness.
- Share information about frequent feedings and how to avoid the designated fatty acids from supplemental products, formulas, etc.

Patient Education—Food Safety

- Hand washing with soap and hot water is recommended before preparing formula or meals. Use clean utensils and containers for mixing formula.
- Before using tap water for formula preparation or to give as a beverage, let cold tap water run for 2 minutes to remove any lead that may be in the pipes.
- Follow the 2-hour rule: discard any beverage or food that has been left at room temperature for 2 hours or longer.
- Do not use honey in the diets of infants to decrease potential risk of botulism.

For More Information

- Fatty Oxidation Disorder
  http://www.fodsupport.org/
- MCAD
  http://www.mcadangel.com/mcad-links.html
- National Newborn Screening
  http://genes-r-us.uthscsa.edu/

FATTY ACID OXIDATION DISORDERS—CITED REFERENCES

Isaacs JS, Zand DJ. Single-gene autosomal recessive disorders and Prader-Willi syndrome: an update for food and nutrition professionals. *J Am Diet Assoc.* 107:466–478, 2007.

Nennstiel-Ratzel U, et al. Reduced incidence of severe metabolic crisis or death in children with medium chain acyl-CoA dehydrogenase deficiency homozygous for c.985 A_G identified by neonatal screening. *Mol Gen Metab.* 85:157, 2005.

Oey NA, et al. Long-chain fatty acid oxidation during early human development. *Pediatr Res.* 57:755, 2005.

Roe CR, Ding J. Mitochrondrial fatty acid oxidation disorders. In: Scriver C, Beaudet A, Sly W, Valle D, eds. *The metabolic and molecular bases of inherited disease.* New York, NY: McGraw-Hill, 2001:2297–2326.

FETAL ALCOHOL SYNDROME

NUTRITIONAL ACUITY RANKING: LEVEL 1–2

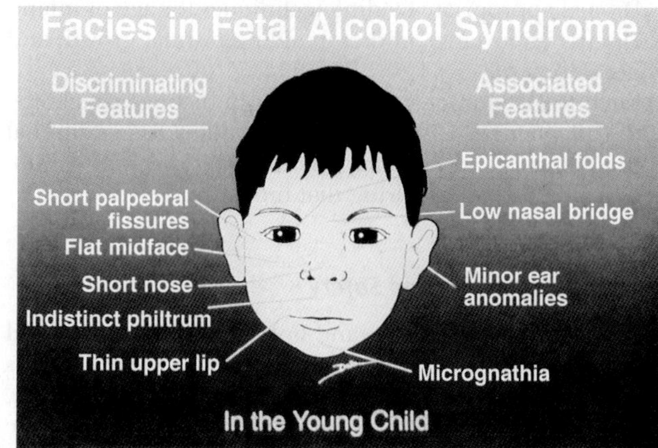

Adapted from: Sadler T, PhD. *Langman's Medical Embryology,* 9th ed. Image Bank. Baltimore: Lippincott Williams & Wilkins, 2003.

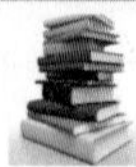

DEFINITIONS AND BACKGROUND

Generally noted shortly after birth, fetal alcohol syndrome (FAS) is a syndrome in infants with developmental delay, ocular anomalies, LBW, tremors, short stature, retarded intellect, seizures, and microcephaly. There is a continuum of FAS recognized as fetal alcohol spectrum disorders (FASD).

FAS is the third leading cause of mental retardation in the United States; it is the most preventable (Centers for Disease Control and Prevention, 2004).

No level of alcohol consumption during pregnancy is safe (Centers for Disease Control and Prevention, 2004). Exposure to alcohol during brain development can permanently alter the physiology of the hippocampal formation, thus promoting epileptic activity and depression (Bonthius et al, 2001). Disrupted cholesterol homeostasis may contribute to neurotoxicity; the developing brain requires cholesterol for proper cell proliferation (Guizzetti and Costa, 2005). Approximately 10% of pregnant women use alcohol and 2% engage in binge drinking or frequent use of alcohol (Centers for Disease Control and Prevention, 2004).

Acetaldehyde damages RNA (Eriksson, 2001; Wang et al, 2009). The steady concurrent use of tobacco and alcohol by young women emphasizes the need for enhanced efforts to reduce initial tobacco and alcohol use by young people. Women who report abuse of tobacco or alcohol should be evaluated for abuse of both substances, and interventions should address abuse of both substances, especially to prevent FAS (Ebrahim et al, 2000).

Early risk assessment is needed, though it may be difficult to find and treat children who have FASD. Using the combination of weight and head circumference below the 10th percentile at birth is useful for identifying children at substantial risk for growth and developmental delays (Weiss et al, 2004). Children with FAS may have more social and medical needs. They often have more facial dysmorphology, growth deficiency, central nervous system dysfunction, muscular problems, hospitalizations for OM, pneumonia, dehydration, and anemia (Kvigne et al, 2004).

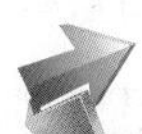

ASSESSMENT, MONITORING, AND EVALUATION

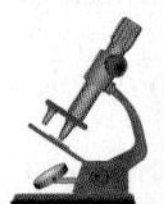

CLINICAL INDICATORS

Genetic Markers: FAS is considered to be environmental.

Clinical/History		Lab Work
Birth weight	Head circumference (<10th percentile)	Alb
Current weight (often below 10th percentile)	Seizures	Na^+, K^+
Length	Physical growth delay	Gluc
Growth (%)	Functional deficits (motor, social, memory, etc.).	H & H
Diet/intake history		Serum Fe
		Ca^{++}, Mg^{++}
		Serum folate

INTERVENTION

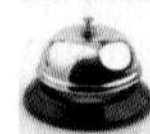

OBJECTIVES

- Promote effective family coping skills and effective parental bonding.
- Prevent additional retardation or developmental delays, blindness, other complications.
- Improve intake and nutritional status.
- Prevent or correct vomiting, cardiac symptoms, other problems.
- Encourage normal growth patterns; prevent FTT.

SAMPLE NUTRITION CARE PROCESS STEPS

Inadequate Energy Intake

Assessment Data: Weight and growth charts, head circumference below 10% tile.

Nutrition Diagnoses (PES): Inadequate energy intake related to increased energy demands from FAS as evidenced by microcephaly (head circumference below 10% tile) and slow growth rate for age.

Intervention: Educate parents about enhancing energy intake through nutrient-dense foods and supplements.

Monitoring and Evaluation: Weight records, growth, head circumference more closely normal for age.

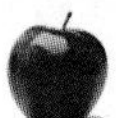

FOOD AND NUTRITION

- Provide a diet appropriate for age and status. Ensure adequate protein and energy for catch-up growth.
- If necessary, provide tube feeding or TPN while hospitalized. Some infants may require additional nutrition support in the home setting to promote better growth and development.

Common Drugs Used and Potential Side Effects

- Anticonvulsants may be needed to correct seizures. Monitor for depletion of vitamins C, D, B_6, B_{12}, and K, folic acid, and calcium.

Herbs, Botanicals, and Supplements

- Herbs and botanicals should not be used for FAS because there are no controlled trials to prove efficacy.

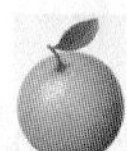

NUTRITION EDUCATION, COUNSELING, CARE MANAGEMENT

- Discuss appropriate feeding techniques for age of infant.
- Discuss importance of diet in aiding normal growth and development.
- Encourage mother's participation in alcohol rehabilitation if needed. Discuss her future plans for additional pregnancies and encourage counseling to avoid continued alcohol intake during that time.

Patient Education—Food Safety

- Hand washing with soap and hot water is recommended before preparing formula or meals. Use clean utensils and containers for mixing formula.
- Before using tap water for formula preparation or to give as a beverage, let cold tap water run for 2 minutes to remove any lead that may be in the pipes.

- Follow the 2-hour rule: discard any beverage or food that has been left at room temperature for 2 hours or longer.
- Do not use honey in the diets of infants; this will decrease potential risk of botulism.

For More Information

- CDC–Division of Birth Defects and Developmental Disabilities, FAS Site http://www.cdc.gov/ncbddd/fas/
- CDC Diagnosis and Referral Guide http://www.cdc.gov/ncbddd/fas/documents/FAS_guidelines_accessible.pdf
- Fetal Alcohol and Drug Unit http://depts.washington.edu/fadu
- Fetal Alcohol Syndrome Handbook http://www.usd.edu/cd/publications/fashandbook.cfm
- Fetal Alcohol Syndrome websites http://www.come-over.to/FAS/faslinks.htm
- FAS Community Resource Center http://www.come-over.to/FASCRC/
- National Center for Family Support http://www.familysupport-hsri.org/
- National Clearinghouse for Alcohol and Drug Information (NCADI) http://www.health.org/
- National Council on Alcoholism and Drug Dependence (NCADD) http://www.ncadd.org/
- National Organization of Fetal Alcohol Syndrome http://www.nofas.org/

FETAL ALCOHOL SYNDROME—CITED REFERENCES

Bonthius D, et al. Alcohol exposure during the brain growth spurt promotes hippocampal seizures, rapid kindling, and spreading depression. *Alcohol Clin Exp Res.* 25:734, 2001.

Centers for Disease Control and Prevention. Alcohol consumption among women who are pregnant or who might become pregnant—United States, 2002. *MMWR Morb Mortal Wkly Rep.* 53:1178, 2004.

Ebrahim S, et al. Combined tobacco and alcohol use by pregnant and reproductive-aged women in the United States. *Obstet Gynecol.* 96:767, 2000.

Eriksson C. The role of acetaldehyde in the actions of alcohol (update 2000). *Alcohol Clin Exp Res.* 25:15S, 2001.

Guizzetti M, Costa LG. Disruption of cholesterol homeostasis in the developing brain as a potential mechanism contributing to the developmental neurotoxicity of ethanol: an hypothesis. *Med Hypotheses.* 64:563, 2005.

Kvigne VL, et al. Characteristics of children who have full or incomplete fetal alcohol syndrome. *J Pediatr.* 145:635, 2004.

Wang LL, et al. Ethanol exposure induces differential microRNA and target gene expression and teratogenic effects which can be suppressed by folic acid supplementation. *Hum Reprod.* 24:562, 2009.

Weiss M, et al. The Wisconsin Fetal Alcohol Syndrome Screening Project. *WMJ.* 103:53, 2004.

HIRSCHSPRUNG'S DISEASE (CONGENITAL MEGACOLON)

NUTRITIONAL ACUITY RANKING: LEVEL 4

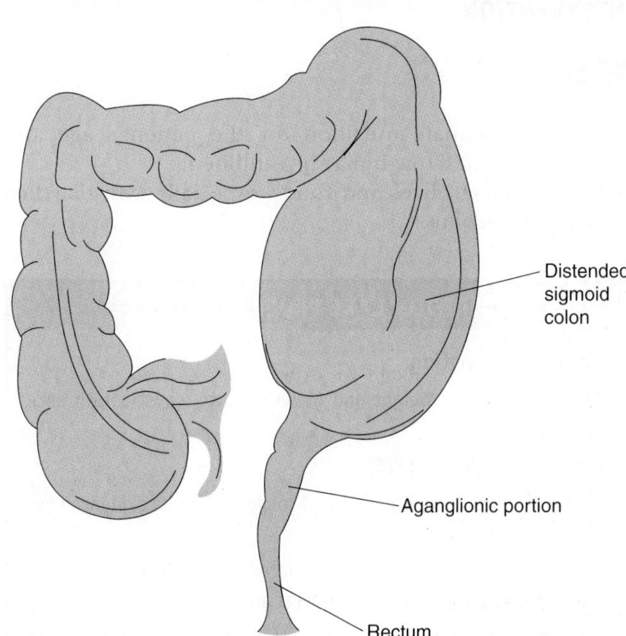

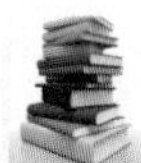

DEFINITIONS AND BACKGROUND

Hirschsprung's disease (HD) is characterized by the absence of ganglion cells and the presence of hypertrophic nerve trunks in the distal bowel. HD is also known as jejunal gangliosus or congenital megacolon. Its incidence is 1 in 5000 live births. HD may reoccur in other babies born to the same family with a child with HD (Stewart and von Allmen, 2003).

As a congenital malformation, HD interferes with normal mass peristalsis and functional obstruction. Normally, ganglia stimulate the gut and allow peristalsis to occur. In HD, the ganglia are missing, and segments of bowel become obstructed. This creates abdominal distention, failure to pass meconium stool, vomiting, and constipation. If diagnosed when older, growth failure may be a presenting sign.

Surgical removal may be required to alleviate bowel obstruction, followed by a temporary colostomy. Complications after a definitive pull-through procedure for HD include stricture formation, enterocolitis, and occasionally, wound infection (Finck et al, 2001). Often, removal of the affected area and reconnection of the colon occurs at age 6 months or older.

Over the long term, one in five patients will have continued constipation, occasional soiling, and incontinence, and one in 10 patients may have severe problems. A special type of enterocolitis, HD-associated enterocolitis (HAE), may also be a concern (Nofech-Mozes et al, 2004). The condition can be life threatening, and signs include hypoalbuminemia, diarrhea and vomiting, and anorexia and weight loss. See Table 3-8.

TABLE 3-8 Glycogen Storage Diseases (GSDs): Deficiency of a Glycogen Synthase That Normally Converts Glycogen to Glucose

Disease	Description
GSD1: glucose-6 phosphatase deficiency (G6PD), von Gierke disease	Slow or stunted growth, enlarged liver, delayed or absent pubertal development, gout, kidney failure, and a poor ability to withstand fasting due to low blood sugar occur. Patients with this condition are prone to frequent infections, hemolytic anemia, and inflammatory bowel disease. Brain damage can result from low glucose availability (Melis et al, 2004). Early death was common. Portacaval shunt may be considered in patients with height for age <3rd percentile (Corbeel et al, 2000).
GSD 2: alpha-glucosidase deficiency, Pompe disease	Onset in infancy is the most severe; most patients present with hypotonia and cardiomyopathy. Recombinant human GAA (rhGAA) can be tested for enzyme replacement (Raben et al, 2005).
GSD 3: debrancher enzyme deficiency, Cori disease or Forbes disease	There may be low bone density and a high risk for osteoporosis (Cabrera-Abreu et al, 2004).
GSD4: brancher enzyme deficiency, Andersen disease	Glycogen branching enzyme (GBE) deficiency results in the accumulation of an amylopectin-like polysaccharide and presents with liver disease, progressing to cirrhosis (Bruno et al, 2004).
GSD5: muscle glucagon phosphorylase deficiency, McArdle disease	X-linked liver glycogenosis (XLG) is one of the most common forms; onset is often in adults. Low levels of phosphorylase result in abnormal storage of glycogen in muscle tissue, muscle pain, cramping, stiffness, and poor exercise tolerance. Avoid strenuous exercise.
GSD6: liver phosphorylase deficiency, Hers disease	Gross hepatomegaly and hypoglycemia occur with reduced liver phosphorylase activity.
GSD7: muscle phosphofructokinase deficiency, Tarui disease	This syndrome presents often with exertional myopathy and hemolytic syndrome.
GSD9 a: liver glycogen phosphorylase kinase deficiency	Growth retardation, abdominal distention, and hepatomegaly may be present (Schippers et al, 2003). Liver transplantation results in normal fasting glucose production and normal glucose and insulin concentrations.
GSD9b: β-subunit phosphorylase kinase Fanconi-Bickel syndrome	Hepatorenal glycogenosis is abnormal.

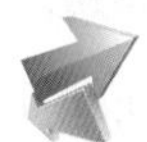

ASSESSMENT, MONITORING, AND EVALUATION

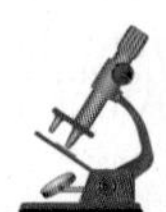

CLINICAL INDICATORS

Genetic Markers: HD develops before a child is born but is not thought to be genetic.

Clinical/History

- Birth weight
- Length
- Present weight
- FTT?
- Growth (slow)
- Diet/intake history
- Failure to pass meconium after birth (newborn)
- Watery diarrhea (newborn)
- Constipation
- Temperature (fever?)
- Vomiting
- Abdominal distention
- Rectal bleeding?
- Dehydration; I & O
- Abdominal x-ray
- Barium enema
- Malabsorption
- Enterocolitis?

Lab Work

- H & H
- Serum Fe, ferritin
- Alb
- Na^+, K^+
- Ca^{++}, Mg^{++}
- Gluc
- LFTs

INTERVENTION

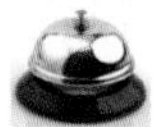

OBJECTIVES

- Provide adequate nutrition for the patient's age and development. Growth may be inhibited.
- Replace electrolytes and fluids, especially with diarrhea and enterocolitis.

SAMPLE NUTRITION CARE PROCESS STEPS

Altered GI Function

Assessment Data: Weight and growth charts, constipation and stool records.

Nutrition Diagnoses (PES):

NC 1.4. Altered GI function related to megacolon as evidenced by current complaints of constipation.

NB 1.7. Undesirable food choices related to lack of fruit and vegetable intake and increase in cookies and crackers in diet.

Intervention: Educate parents about high fiber foods and increased use of fruits, vegetables, whole grains and fluids.

Monitoring and Evaluation: Weight records, decreased symptoms of constipation, improved stooling pattern.

- Compensate for poor absorption of nutrients; water-miscible forms of fat-soluble vitamins may be needed.
- Prevent complications after surgery, especially constipation, incontinence, or enterocolitis.

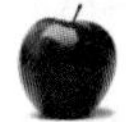

FOOD AND NUTRITION

- Use a high-energy/high-protein diet. Enteral products, oral supplements, or TPN can be used.
- Monitor serum electrolytes, especially potassium, if laxatives are used. Encourage a diet high in fiber and fluid to wean off medication if possible.
- Provide fluids adequate for the patient's age, hydration status, and extra fluid requirements.
- Use a laxative diet (Cincinnati Children's, 2009); see Table 3-8.
- Provide TPN if large sections of the bowel are removed. Advance infant feedings as tolerated using human milk or preterm or standard infant formulas, and then gradually progress to soft/bland foods.
- Monitor calcium, magnesium, and other nutrients if long-term TPN is needed.

Common Drugs Used and Potential Side Effects

- Antibiotics may be needed if perforation has occurred or when there is enterocolitis. Monitor for side effects.
- In constipation, laxatives can deplete numerous nutrient reserves; monitor carefully. Encourage a diet high in fiber and fluid to wean off medication if possible.

Herbs, Botanicals, and Supplements

- Herbs and botanicals should not be used for megacolon because there are no controlled trials to prove efficacy.

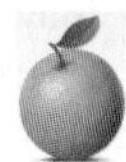

NUTRITION EDUCATION, COUNSELING, CARE MANAGEMENT

- Teach patient about sources of protein, energy, potassium, and other key nutrients from diet.
- Discuss wound healing or colostomy procedures after surgery.
- For constipation and bowel incontinence, a high-fiber diet may be useful; discuss signs and symptoms of obstruction to report immediately to a doctor. Initial suggestion: age plus 10, example 4 years + 10 = 14 g/d.
- Extra fluids will be needed with high-fiber intake.

Patient Education—Food Safety

- Hand washing with soap and hot water is recommended before preparing formula or meals. Use clean utensils and containers for mixing formula.
- Before using tap water for formula preparation or to give as a beverage, let cold tap water run for 2 minutes to remove any lead that may be in the pipes.
- Follow the 2-hour rule: discard any beverage or food that has been left at room temperature for 2 hours or longer.
- Do not use honey in the diets of infants to decrease potential risk of botulism.

For More Information

- Hirschsprung's & Motility Disorders Support Network
  http://www.hirschsprungs.info/index.html
- International Foundation for Functional Gastrointestinal Disorders
  http://www.iffgd.org/
- National Digestive Diseases Clearinghouse
  http://digestive.niddk.nih.gov/ddiseases/pubs/hirschsprungs_ez/index.htm
- United Ostomy Association
  http://uoa.org/

HIRSCHSPRUNG'S DISEASE—CITED REFERENCES

Cincinnati Children's. Laxative diet. Accessed April 27, 2009, at http://www.cincinnatichildrens.org/svc/alpha/c/colorectal/imperforate-anus/patients-families/bowel-manage/constipate/laxative-diet.htm.

Finck C, et al. Presentation of carcinoma in a patient with a previous operation for Hirschsprung's disease. *J Pediatr Surg.* 36:E5, 2001.

Nofech-Mozes Y, et al. Difficulties in making the diagnosis of Hirschsprung disease in early infancy. *J Paediatr Child Health.* 40:716, 2004.

Stewart DR, von Allmen D. The genetics of Hirschsprung disease. *Gastroenterol Clin North Am.* 32:819, 2003.

HIV INFECTION, PEDIATRIC

NUTRITIONAL ACUITY RANKING: LEVEL 4

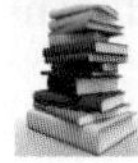

DEFINITIONS AND BACKGROUND

There are unique considerations related to HIV infection in infants, children, and adolescents. With the use of highly active antiretroviral therapy (HAART), there is minimal mother-to-child transmission of HIV infection in developed countries (i.e., 1–2% only) (King et al, 2004; Newell and Thorne, 2004). In developed nations, HIV infection is more of a chronic disease, with extensive medications, costs, and side effects to consider. A high proportion of HIV-infected individuals are African or African American.

Developing nations still have a battle to address. Infants who are breastfed by HIV-infected mothers have the risk of acquiring the infection. In addition, HIV-infected mothers may transmit opportunistic pathogens to their infants. FTT and protein–calorie malnutrition are common. Every child with HIV infection should be assessed at baseline and every 4–6 months thereafter to determine risk of nutritional compromise. Severity or degree of nutritional risk is measured with anthropometric, biochemical, dietary intake, and medical data. Salivary gland disease is a common finding related to HIV infection; gland enlargement or xerostomia may present, and the reduction in saliva must be addressed (Pinto and DeRossi, 2004).

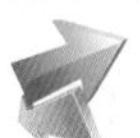

ASSESSMENT, MONITORING, AND EVALUATION

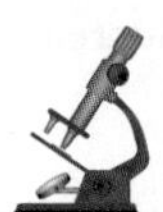

CLINICAL INDICATORS

Genetic Markers: HIV infection is not genetic but is transmitted prenatally by the infected mother, or by contaminated needles or blood transfusions.

Clinical/History		**Lab Work**
Height	Head circumference (infants)	H & H
Weight	Stunting	Serum Fe
Weight for height, BMI	FTT	Alb
Growth percentile and pattern	Mid-arm muscle circumference (MAMC)	Na^+, K^+
Diet/intake history; energy intake	Opportunistic infections	Ca^{++}, Mg^{++}
		Gluc
		Immunological status
		CD4+ T-cell counts
		Vitamin A level

SAMPLE NUTRITION CARE PROCESS STEPS

Inadequate Energy Intake

Assessment Data: Weight and growth charts, frequent infections.

Nutrition Diagnoses (PES): Inadequate energy intake related insufficient intake, diarrrheal losses, and high metabolic demand of HIV as evidenced by weight loss and frequent opportunistic infections.

Intervention: Educate parent/caregiver about use of tolerated high calorie foods and supplements.

Monitoring and Evaluation: Weight records, growth, tolerance of formulas or supplemental products.

INTERVENTION

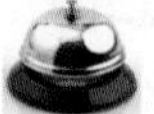

OBJECTIVES

- Maternal factors, including Vitamin A level and CD4+ T-cell counts during pregnancy, as well as infant viral load and CD4+ T-cell counts in the first several months of life, can help identify those infants at risk for rapid disease progression who may benefit from early aggressive therapy.
- Achieve a normal growth pattern; allow for catch-up growth and monitor growth patterns closely.
- Prevent opportunistic infections by improving or maintaining immune status with good nutrition.
- Alleviate wasting syndrome, diarrhea, malabsorption, enteric infections, malnutrition, and immune deficiency. Preserve lean body mass.
- Follow the CDC evidence-based guidelines (CDC, 2009):
    1. Emphasize the important role of effective antiretroviral therapy in augmenting immune function
    2. Support diagnosis and management of immune reconstitution inflammatory syndrome, a condition in which the immune system begins to recover, but then responds aggressively to a previously acquired opportunistic infection
    3. Prevent Hepatitis B and C, *Mycobacterium tuberculosis* infection, malaria
    4. Manage drug–drug interactions and drug–nutrient interactions

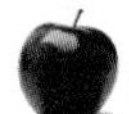

FOOD AND NUTRITION

- Use a high-protein diet. Enteral products, oral supplements, and frequent snacks should be used if required. Protein needs may be 1.5–2 times the usual for age and gender.
- Energy needs may vary from 50% to 200% of the usual requirements. Children with severe encephalopathy may be bed bound and require fewer total calories.
- Assure adequacy of fluid intake, especially with many medications to be taken each day.
- A multivitamin supplement is needed to provide at least 100% of the daily needs. Poor absorption may be a problem for vitamins A, C, B_6, and B_{12}, folate, iron, selenium, and zinc. Calcium is needed to prevent loss of bone mass (O'Brien et al, 2001).
- Naturally occurring antioxidants are safe when consumed in normal amounts. For example, include nuts for vitamin E and selenium and citrus fruits for vitamin C. Be aware of excesses from pills and other supplemental forms because excesses can deplete immunity. Mega doses are up to 10 times the RDA (American Academy of Pediatrics, 2004) and have not proven to be of benefit.
- Aggressive nutritional support is critical. Nocturnal, continuous feedings may be useful.

Common Drugs Used and Potential Side Effects

- Few HIV medicines are produced in pediatric formulations. Those drugs available as syrups have limitations, such as short shelf-life, objectionable taste, difficult measuring of correct doses, and expense. For a list of FDA-approved medications used in HIV infection, see Section 15.

- HIV-infected mothers may transmit opportunistic pathogens to their infants. There may be antibiotics or antiviral agents prescribed that should be closely monitored for nutritional and GI side effects. Adherence to complex antiretroviral (HAART) therapy requires addressing developmental, psychosocial, and family factors (Mellins et al, 2004). Early treatment saves lives.

Herbs, Botanicals, and Supplements

- Herbs and botanicals should not be used for HIV; there are no clinical trials proving efficacy.
- HIV-infected individuals may be attracted to the many possible supplements on the market. Carefully review all items and discuss their viability or potential for harm.
- Use of acidophilus and probiotic products may alleviate loss of intestinal bacteria.

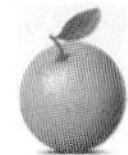

NUTRITION EDUCATION, COUNSELING, CARE MANAGEMENT

- There will be a need for medication management, a nutrient-dense diet, doctor visits, and other intervention and therapies. Provide support to the child and family or caregivers.
- Encourage formula feeding for mothers who has HIV infection.
- Discuss HIV infection prevention strategies, especially with noninfected teens. Researchers are working on a vaccine for HIV prevention.
- Children should receive all of their usual vaccinations to prevent other illnesses or complications.

Patient Education—Food Safety

- Hand washing with soap and hot water is recommended before preparing formula or meals. Use clean utensils and containers for mixing formula.
- Before using tap water for formula preparation or to give as a beverage, let cold tap water run for 2 minutes to remove any lead that may be in the pipes.
- Follow the 2-hour rule: discard beverages and foods that left at room temperature for 2+ hours.
- Avoid honey in the diets of infants to decrease the risk of botulism.

For More Information

- AIDS Pediatric guidelines
  http://www.aidsinfo.nih.gov/Guidelines/GuidelineDetail.aspx?GuidelineID=8
- AIDS Vaccine Advocacy Coalition (AVAC)
  www.avac.org
- American Foundation for AIDS Research (amFAR)
  www.amfar.org
- Baylor AIDS Curriculum
  http://bayloraids.org/curriculum/
- Baylor International Pediatric AIDS Initiative
  http://bayloraids.org/
- Johns Hopkins University School of Medicine AIDS Site
  www.hopkins-aids.edu/
- National Institute of Allergy and Infectious Diseases (NIAID)
  www.niaid.nih.gov/daids/
- National Institutes of Health. Pediatric guidelines
  http://aidsinfo.nih.gov/contentfiles/Pediatric_OI.pdf
- National Pediatric AIDS Network
  http://www.npan.org/
- Pediatric AIDS Foundation
  http://www.pedaids.org/
- U.S. Coalition for Child Survival
  www.child-survival.org

HIV INFECTION, PEDIATRIC—CITED REFERENCES

American Academy of Pediatrics. *Pediatric nutrition handbook.* 5th ed. Elk Grove Village, IL: American Academy of Pediatrics, 2004.

CDC. Centers for Disease Control and Prevention. Accessed April 27, 2009, at http://www.cdc.gov/mmwr/pdf/rr/rr5804.pdf.

King SM, et al. Evaluation and treatment of the human immunodeficiency virus-1–exposed infant. *Pediatrics.* 114:497, 2004.

Mellins CA, et al. The role of psychosocial and family factors in adherence to antiretroviral treatment in human immunodeficiency virus-infected children. *Pediatr Infect Dis J.* 23:1035, 2004.

Newell ML, Thorne C. Antiretroviral therapy and mother-to-child transmission of HIV-1. *Expert Rev Anti Infect Ther.* 2:717, 2004.

O'Brien K, et al. Bone mineral content in girls perinatally infected with HIV. *Am J Clin Nutr.* 73:821, 2001.

Pinto A, De Rossi SS. Salivary gland disease in pediatric HIV patients: an update. *J Dent Child.* 71:33, 2004.

HOMOCYSTINURIA

NUTRITIONAL ACUITY RANKING: LEVEL 3–4

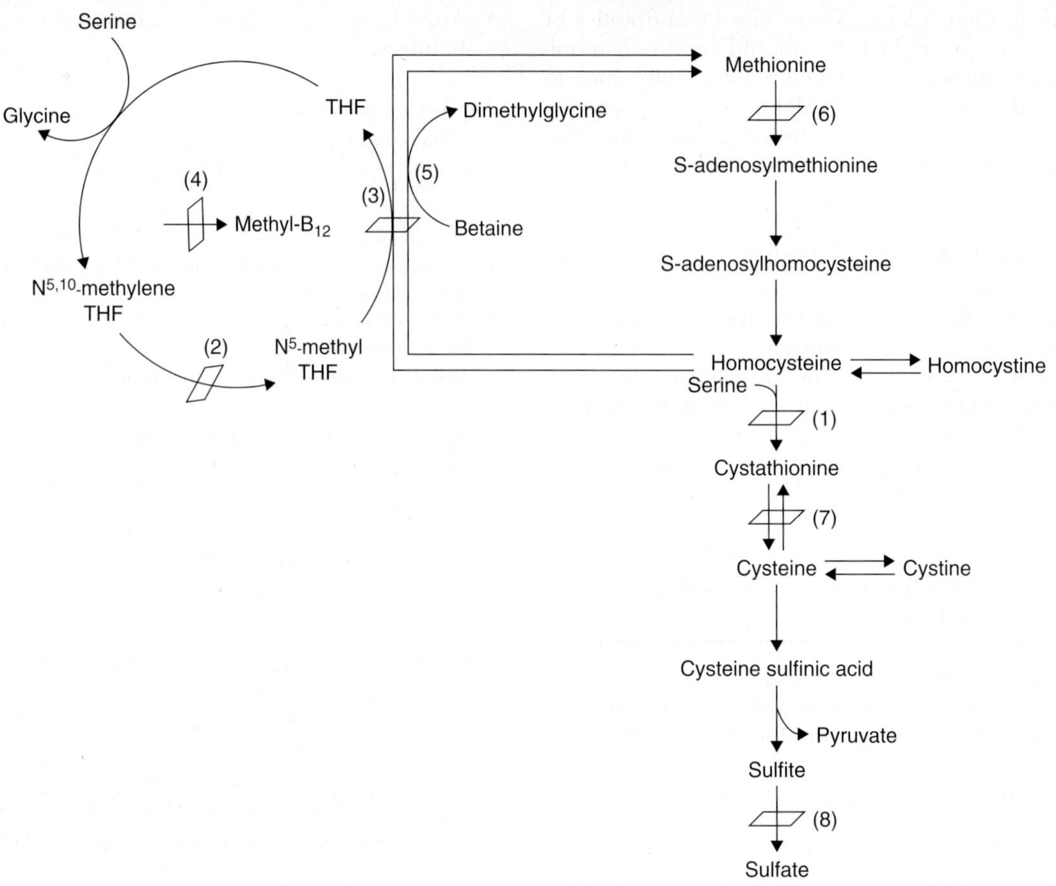

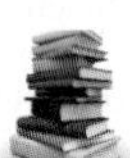

DEFINITIONS AND BACKGROUND

The significance of homocysteine (Hcy) in human disease was unknown until 1962, when cases of homocystinuria were correlated with vascular disease (McCully, 2007). Hcy is usually converted to cysteine and partly remethylated to methionine with the help of vitamin B_{12} and folate.

Homocystinuria (HCU) is a rare, autosomal recessive metabolic disorder of amino acid metabolism. In HCU type I from deficiency of cystathionine-beta-synthase (which requires vitamin B6 for activation). Hcy accumulates in the blood, methionine builds up, cysteine decreases, mental retardation and eye changes can occur from a lack of glutathione production (Ramakrishnan et al, 2006). In types II, III, and IV, methionine is decreased and no mental retardation occurs; here, treatment involves folate, vitamin B_{12} and avoiding excess of methionine (Ramakrishnan et al, 2006). Newborn screening is recommended (Refsum, Fredriksen et al, 2004).

HCU due to deficiency of CBS is inherited as an autosomal recessive trait. Human CBS is an *S*-adenosylmethionine–regulated enzyme that plays a key role in the metabolism of Hcy. HCU type 1 occurs in 1 in 200,000 births worldwide, with stronger prevalence in Ireland, Norway, and Qatar. Untreated, it leads to mental retardation, seizures, altered growth, hepatic disease, osteoporosis, thromboses, glaucoma, cataracts, and strokes. Individuals with HCU may be unusually tall in stature, with long arms and legs; this growth is directly mediated by Hcy.

Deranged vitamin B_6 metabolism or low levels of reductase enzyme may also cause HCU. A single biochemical test is not available; abnormal urinary tHcy response after methionine loading is the most sensitive test (Guttormsen et al, 2001). Urinary excretion of Hcy occurs but is unusual.

5,10-Methylene-tetrahydrofolate reductase deficiency (MTHFR) affects many enzyme systems. It can present with mental retardation, microcephaly, gait disturbance, psychiatric disturbances, seizures, abnormal EEG, and limb weakness. Therapy usually involves administration of folinic acid to enhance enzyme activity; 5-methyl-tetrahydrofolate to replace the missing end product; extra betaine, hydroxycobalamin, carnitine, and riboflavin to assist with related enzymatic actions.

For some patients, medications can reduce the excretion of Hcy in the urine, increase body weight, and improve mental function. Methionine may be given to correct low serum levels, and pyridoxine may lower serum Hcy levels if needed. If individuals do not respond to combinations of these drugs, supportive care is offered to reduce symptoms.

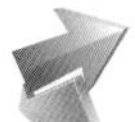

ASSESSMENT, MONITORING, AND EVALUATION

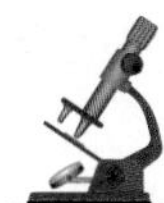

CLINICAL INDICATORS

Genetic Markers: Mutations in the cystathionine beta-synthase (CBS) on chromosome 21 are most common. Methylene-tetrahydrofolate reductase (MTHFR), 5-methyltetrahydrofolate-homocysteine methyltransferase (MTR), and 5-methyltetrahydrofolate-homocysteine methyltransferase reductase (MTRR) genes cause HCU less frequently. Patients with a cobalamin C (CblC) defect have combined methylmalonic aciduria and HCU (Heil et al, 2007).

Clinical/History

- Birth weight
- Present weight
- Length
- Growth (%); FTT?
- Scoliosis
- Diet/intake history
- Nearsightedness
- Lens dislocation
- Blood clots in veins
- Mental retardation
- Cognitive changes or psychiatric problems
- Osteopenia or osterporosis (DEXA)
- Marflan syndrome (long limbs, tall stature)

Lab Work

- ALT, AST
- Gluc
- Plasma methionine (fluctuates)
- Plasma cysteine
- Serum Hcy (elevated)
- Urinary methylmalonic acid
- Urinary tHcy after methionine load
- Serum folate
- Macrocytic anemia?
- MTHFR activity
- Serum B_{12}
- Serum B_6
- Serum Ca^{++}, Mg^{++}

SAMPLE NUTRITION CARE PROCESS STEPS

Inadequate Intake of Bioactive Substances

Assessment Data: Weight and growth chart showing long limbs, tall stature for age, lab tests showing HCU and low serum levels of vitamins B_6, B_{12}, and folate, myopia and hx of thrombotic clots in legs.

Nutrition Diagnoses (PES): Inadequate intake of bioactive substances related to genetic defect as evidenced by HCU and low serum levels of B_6, B_{12}, and folate.

Intervention: Educate parents about dietary enhancements for foods rich in B_6, B_{12}, and folate. Counseling about appropriate drug therapy and desirable nutritional outcomes.

Monitoring and Evaluation: Weight and growth records showing slower increments in added height; improved serum levels of vitamins; decreased or minimal Hcy in the urine.

INTERVENTION

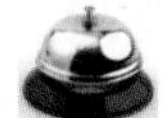

OBJECTIVES

- Prevent mental retardation, growth delays, fractures, lens changes. Fractures occur because of defective collagen formation. A lens may become dislocated in CBS deficiency.
- Prevent cardiovascular complications (arterial and venous thrombosis, stroke, hypertension). Note: Dramatic decline in cardiovascular mortality in the United States since 1950 may be attributable in part to voluntary fortification of the food supply with vitamin B_6 and folic acid (McCully, 2007). Supplement with essential nutrients. Low folic acid intake aggravate the symptoms.
- In **Type I HCU,** reduce methionine in the diet to prevent accumulation of Hcy.
- **Metabolic disorders of cobalamin** will require intramuscular vitamin B_{12}.
- **Alterations of the MTHFR alleles** may require use of L-methylfolate.

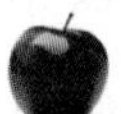

FOOD AND NUTRITION

- Increase fluid intake.
- **HCU type I** is treated with supplementation of vitamin B_6 and cystine (to supply sulfur). If nonresponsive to B_6, use a low-methionine diet with a supplement of cystine. Reduce intake of methionine from meat, poultry, fish, and eggs. Soy products (e.g., Isomil, ProSobee, Soyalac) can be used. XMET Maxamaid (SHS North America), Hominex 1 for infants or Hominex 2 for children (Ross Laboratories), or Product HOM 1 or HOM 2 (Mead Johnson) is also useful.
- **For cobalamin metabolic disorders:** Intramuscular vitamin B_{12} is needed; dietary or supplemental vitamin B_{12} is not effective.
- **For MTHFR:** Methylated folic acid, Vitamins B_6 and B_{12}, riboflavin, choline, and betaine are useful supplements.

Common Drugs Used and Potential Side Effects

- Dipyridamole may be used to decrease thrombosis.
- Pyridoxine therapy (vitamin B_6) for longer than 1 month is useful for some forms. The doctor may prescribe 100–500 mg or higher.
- Folic acid and vitamin B_{12} should be supplied in a methylated form if needed. For example, Cerefolin (Pan Am Labs) contains methylated folate and B_{12} plus *N*-acetylcysteine; Deplin contains 7.5 mg L-methylfolate.
- Choline and betaine may be useful (Alfthan et al, 2004; Busby et al, 2005).

Herbs, Botanicals, and Supplements

- Herbs and botanicals should not be used for HCU because there are no controlled trials to prove efficacy.

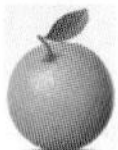

NUTRITION EDUCATION, COUNSELING, CARE MANAGEMENT

- Emphasize the importance of controlling diet, snacks, using proper forms of supplemental nutrients.
- Discuss good food sources of folic acid and other B-complex vitamins. Therapy with folic acid, vitamin B_6, l-carnitine, and intramuscular vitamin B_{12} often results in improvement of symptoms (Heil et al, 2007).
- Newborn screening of tHcy is useful to detect vitamin B_{12} deficiency or HCU (Refsum et al, 2004).
- Because of increased incidence of osteoporosis, high serum Hcy levels interfere with collagen cross-linking (McLean et al, 2004). Controlling serum Hcy is important for bone health.

Patient Education—Food Safety

- Hand washing with soap and hot water is recommended before preparing formula or meals. Use clean utensils and containers for mixing formula.
- Before using tap water for formula preparation or to give as a beverage, let cold tap water run for 2 minutes to remove any lead that may be in the pipes.
- Follow the 2-hour rule: discard any beverage or food that has been left at room temperature for 2 hours or longer.
- Do not use honey in the diets of infants to decrease potential risk of botulism.

For More Information

- Children Living with Inherited Metabolic Diseases
  http://www.climb.org.uk/
- NIH Genetics Home Reference
  http://ghr.nlm.nih.gov/condition=homocystinuria
- Save Babies
  http://www.savebabies.org/diseasedescriptions/homocystinuria.php

HOMOCYSTINURIA—CITED REFERENCES

Alfthan G, et al. The effect of low doses of betaine on plasma homocysteine in healthy volunteers. *Br J Nutr.* 92:665, 2004.

Busby MG, et al. Choline- and betaine-defined diets for use in clinical research and for management of trimethylaminuria. *J Am Diet Assoc.* 105:1836, 2005.

Guttormsen A, et al. Disposition of homocysteine in subjects heterozygous for homocystinuria due to cystathionine beta-synthase deficiency: relationship between genotype and phenotype. *Am J Med Genet.* 100:204, 2001.

Heil SG, et al. Marfanoid features in a child with combined methylmalonic aciduria and homocystinuria (CblC type). *J Inherit Metab Dis.* 30:811, 2007.

McCully KS. Homocysteine, vitamins, and vascular disease prevention. *Am J Clin Nutr.* 86:1563, 2007.

McLean RR, et al. Homocysteine as a predictive factor for hip fracture in older persons. *N Engl J Med.* 350:2042, 2004.

Ramakrishnan S, et al. Biochemistry of homocysteine in health and diseases. *Indian J Biochem Biophys.* 43:275, 2006.

Refsum H, et al. Screening for serum total homocysteine in newborn children. *Clin Chem.* 50:1769, 2004.

Refsum H, et al. Birth prevalence of homocystinuria. *J Pediatr.* 144:830, 2004.

LARGE FOR GESTATIONAL AGE INFANT (INFANT MACROSOMIA)

NUTRITIONAL ACUITY RANKING: LEVEL 1–3

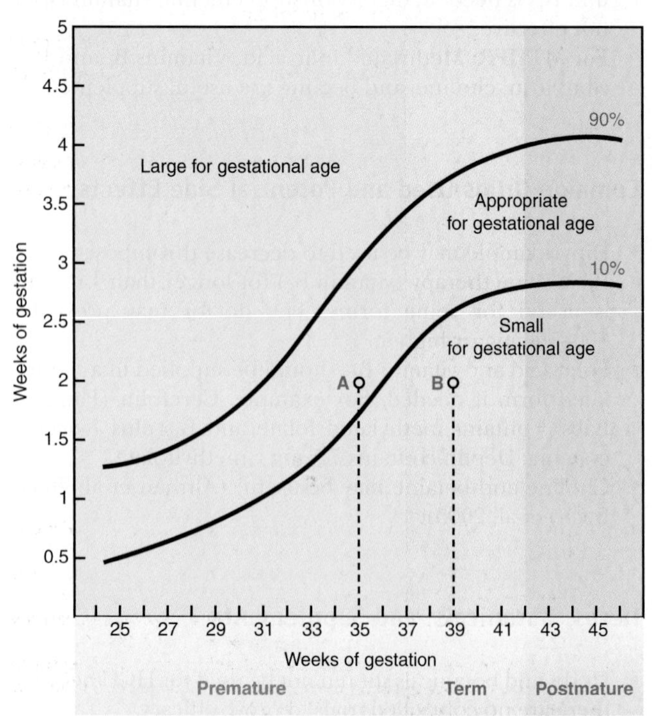

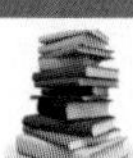

DEFINITIONS AND BACKGROUND

Infants whose weight is more than the 90th percentile for gestational age are classified as large for gestational age (LGA). Birth weight is high (3300–4000 g) at 40 weeks. Obesity and gestational diabetes increase the risk of an LGA delivery (Ehrenberg et al, 2004). LGA infants may also be born to mothers who are multiparous.

Macrosomia in newborns raises the risk for birth-related problems (Samaras et al, 2004). Problems may include hypoglycemia, respiratory distress, aspiration pneumonia, bronchial paralysis, or facial paralysis. LGA neonates usually have higher body fat and lower lean body mass than appropriate for gestational age (AGA) infants. Cord plasma adiponectin and leptin levels are very high in LGA infants; adiponectin is involved in regulating fetal growth (Tsai et al, 2004).

After birth, rapid adaptation is necessary for infants to be able to maintain independent glucose homeostasis; this process is compromised in LGA infants (Beardsall et al, 2008). Controlling maternal weight gain remains an important goal for successful pregnancy outcome. High birth weight may eventually promote impaired glucose tolerance, diabetes, obesity, or cancer (Samaras et al, 2004).

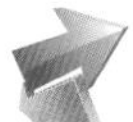

ASSESSMENT, MONITORING, AND EVALUATION

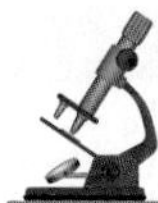

CLINICAL INDICATORS

Genetic Markers: Mitochondrial RNA deletions may be involved, but no specific gene has been identified.

Clinical/History	Neonatal Behavior Assessment Scale (motor maturity, autonomic stability, and withdrawal)	Lab Work
Head circumference	Respirations	Serum Gluc; hypoglycemia?
Length	pCO_2, pO_2 levels	Elevated serum insulin
Birth weight more than the 90th percentile for gestational age	BP	Chol, Trig
Neonatal Growth Assessment Scores	Diet/intake history	Alb
	I & O	Hemoglobin
		Hct (elevated)?
		Hyperbilirubinemia?
		Urinary acetone

INTERVENTION

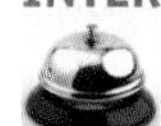

OBJECTIVES

- Allow adequate growth rate and development.
- Prevent rapid phase of hypoglycemia.
- Maintain energy intake at a desired level while allowing adequate growth in the infant. Prevent obesity and its consequences for the infant as much as possible.
- Monitor serum lipids or bilirubin as deemed necessary.

SAMPLE NUTRITION CARE PROCESS STEPS

Abnormal Nutritional Labs

Assessment Data: Abnormal labs for blood glucose, insulin, bilirubin, hematocrit in LGA infant.

Nutrition Diagnoses (PES): Abnormal nutritional lab values related to macrosomia as evidenced by neonatal hyperinsulinism after termination of maternal glucose at birth.

Interventions:

Prophylactic IV infusion of 10% dextrose in water until early frequent feedings can be established.

Educate mother about monitoring for signs of hypoglycemia, hyperbilirubinemia.

Monitoring and Evaluation:

Blood glucose levels should be closely monitored by bedside testing.

Evaluate over first few weeks for blood glucose control and normalization of serum insulin, bilirubin, hematocrit.

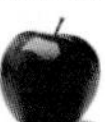

FOOD AND NUTRITION

- Feed the infant often, as indicated by infant's appetite and goal weight pattern. Control total glucose intake if infant shows signs of hyperglycemia.
- Alter intake of fat as determined by lipid profile.
- Maintain a sufficient level of protein if energy needs to be restricted from CHO or fat.

Common Drugs Used and Potential Side Effects

- Insulin may be necessary to control hyperglycemia. Beware of any excesses of insulin, which could aggravate hypoglycemia.

Herbs, Botanicals, and Supplements

- Herbs and botanicals should not be used for LGA infants because there are no controlled trials to prove efficacy for any related problems.

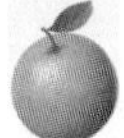

NUTRITION EDUCATION, COUNSELING, CARE MANAGEMENT

- Discuss normal growth patterns as appropriate for the infant, reviewed in concert with the pediatrician. Signs of hyperglycemia and hypoglycemia should be discussed.
- Review risks inherent in another pregnancy, especially if the mother has diabetes. Counseling may be beneficial.

Patient Education—Food Safety

- Hand washing with soap and hot water is recommended before preparing formula or meals. Use clean utensils and containers for mixing formula.
- Before using tap water for formula preparation or to give as a beverage, let cold tap water run for 2 minutes to remove any lead that may be in the pipes.
- Follow the 2-hour rule: discard any beverage or food that has been left at room temperature for 2 hours or longer.
- Do not use honey in the diets of infants to decrease potential risk of botulism.

For More Information

- American College of Obstetricians and Gynecologists http://www.acog.org
- Large for Gestational Age http://www.chp.edu/CHP/P02383

LARGE FOR GESTATIONAL AGE INFANT—CITED REFERENCES

Beardsall K, et al. Insulin and carbohydrate metabolism. *Best Pract Res Clin Endocrinol Metab.* 22:41, 2008.

Ehrenberg HM, et al. The influence of obesity and diabetes on the prevalence of macrosomia. *Am J Obstet Gynecol.* 191:964, 2004.

Samaras TT, et al. Is short height really a risk factor for coronary heart disease and stroke mortality? A review. *Med Sci Monit.* 10:63, 2004.

Tsai PJ, et al. Cord plasma concentrations of adiponectin and leptin in healthy term neonates: positive correlation with birthweight and neonatal adiposity. *Clin Endocrinol (Oxf).* 61:88, 2004.

LEUKODYSTROPHIES

NUTRITIONAL ACUITY RANKING: LEVEL 1

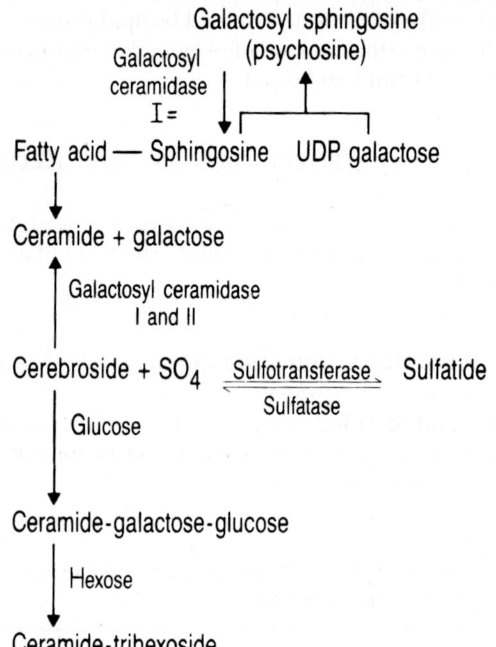

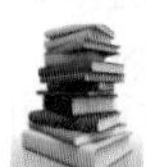

DEFINITIONS AND BACKGROUND

Leukodystrophies (peroxisome biogenesis disorders) are genetic disorders that affect the myelin sheath. While the genetic defect and biochemical abnormalities have been defined, there is a wide range of phenotypic expression (Moser et al, 2005). Neonatal adrenoleukodystrophy and infantile **Refsum's disease** are mild phenotypes. The most severe form is **Zellweger's syndrome**, which may be fatal and is characterized by an enlarged liver, high serum levels of iron and copper, and visual changes. Noninvasive and presymptomatic diagnosis and prenatal diagnosis are available; family screening and genetic counseling are important (Moser et al, 2005).

X-linked adrenoleukodystrophy (X-ALD) is one of the autosomal recessive disorders with an enzymatic defect in very long–chain fatty acid (VLCFA) oxidation, which is usually abundant in sphingomyelin. Ultimately, the myelin sheath surrounding the nerves is destroyed, causing demyelination and neurological problems. Adrenal gland malfunction causes Addison's disease (adrenal insufficiency). Accumulation of saturated VLCFA, especially hexacosanoate (C26:0), occurs because there is a missing or defective protein (ALD protein) to process that fatty acid. The incidence of X-ALD is estimated to be one in 17,000 in all ethnic groups (Moser et al, 2005).

Onset of X-ALD is usually in childhood, with a rapid, progressive demyelination, hypotonia, and psychomotor retardation. However, at least half of patients with X-ALD are adults with somewhat milder manifestations, and women who are carriers may become symptomatic (Moser et al, 2005). X-ALD is often misdiagnosed as ADHD in boys and as multiple sclerosis in men and women (Moser et al, 2005).

Prognosis is poor and death may occur up to a decade after onset.

The observation that dietary fatty acids affect membrane composition has led to the use of modified diets in these conditions. Lorenzo's oil is a mixture of oleic and erucic (rapeseed, or canola) oils, which reduces the production of VLCFA. Early oral administration helps infants and children with the neonatal form (Suzuki, 2001). In addition, the omega-3 fatty acid, DHA, is present in large amounts in infant brains but is often absent in infant formulas. Therefore, intake of omega-3 fatty acids is now recommended. Gene therapy of endogenous hematopoietic stem cells, pharmacological upregulation of other genes encoding proteins involved in peroxisomal beta-oxidation, reduction of oxidative stress, and possibly lovastatin are under study (Semmler et al, 2008).

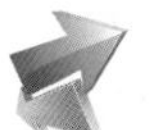

ASSESSMENT, MONITORING, AND EVALUATION

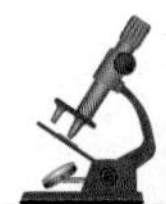

CLINICAL INDICATORS

Genetic Markers: Most of the leukodystrophies are genetic. X-linked adrenoleukodystrophy (X-ALD) is caused by defects of the ABCD1 gene on chromosome Xq28. See website http://www.ulf.org/types/types.html for details about the 34 known types.

Clinical/History

Height
Weight
Growth chart
Diet/intake history
Bronzing of skin (Addison's disease)
Cataracts or glaucoma?
Poor sucking; feeding problems

Lab Work

Plasma phosphatidylcholine
Fatty acid profile; VLCFA (elevated?)
Alb
Chol
Trig
Plasma sphingomyelin
H & H
Pipecolic acid testing

INTERVENTION

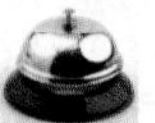

OBJECTIVES

- Decrease rapid progression of demyelination of CNS by offering sufficient fatty acids (DHA). Overall, maintain total VLCFA levels while altering fatty acid sources.
- Prevent or lessen complications of the disorder, including adrenal dysfunction.
- Support the physical therapy by maintaining strength with an adequate diet.

SAMPLE NUTRITION CARE PROCESS STEPS

Self-Feeding Difficulty

Assessment Data: Abnormal weight and growth, difficulty with self-feeding.

Nutrition Diagnoses (PES): Self-feeding difficulty related to low vision and limited mobility.

Intervention: Educate parents about DHA and appropriate fat ratios. Counsel about tips for self-feeding, including special adaptive equipment.

Monitoring and Evaluation: Weight records, growth, slower disease progression.

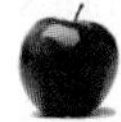

FOOD AND NUTRITION

- Increase endogenous VLCFA synthesis of monounsaturated fatty acids by restricting exogenous (dietary) VLCFA (C26:0) to less than 3 mg and by increasing oleic acid (C18:1). The typical American diet yields 35–40% total energy from fat with 12–40 mg C26:0 daily.
- Offer a low- to very low–fat diet, with supplementation of oleic and erucic acids (Lorenzo's oil), plus DHA (Deon et al, 2008). Include sources of omega-3 fatty acids, such as salmon, tuna, or mackerel, for older children and adults. Use good food sources of vitamins C, E, selenium, zinc for antioxidant properties.
- Lorenzo's oil is similar to olive oil (87% C18:1, 4.8% linoleic acid) but lacks measurable fatty acids with a chain length greater than C20. It can be used in cooking, as a supplement in juice, as an oil for salad dressings, or in food preparation instead of margarine, butter, mayonnaise, or shortening.
- If the patient requires tube feeding, a formula can be developed that contains nonfat milk, specialty oils, corn syrup or sugar, and a vitamin–mineral supplement.

Common Drugs Used and Potential Side Effects

- Hormone-replacement therapy is necessary in all patients with adrenal insufficiency (Semmler et al, 2008). Long-term prednisone and spironolactone may cause hyperglycemia and osteoporosis.
- Use of lovastatin is being tested.

Herbs, Botanicals, and Supplements

- Herbs and botanicals should not be used for this condition because there are no clinical trials proving efficacy.
- Studies suggest that vitamin E, selenium, and carnitine (antioxidants) should be considered.

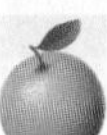

NUTRITION EDUCATION, COUNSELING, CARE MANAGEMENT

- The whole family can support the diet; it can be adapted for everyone. Discuss cooking methods using Lorenzo's oil.
- Restaurant dining can be a problem and special meals may have to be developed for travel.
- If nausea occurs, the oil can be taken in an emulsion.

Patient Education—Food Safety

- Hand washing with soap and hot water is recommended before preparing formula or meals. Use clean utensils and containers for mixing formula.
- Before using tap water for formula preparation or to give as a beverage, let cold tap water run for 2 minutes to remove any lead that may be in the pipes.
- Follow the 2-hour rule: discard any beverage or food that has been left at room temperature for 2 hours or longer.
- Do not use honey in the diets of infants to decrease potential risk of botulism.

For More Information

- Genetic Fairness
  http://www.geneticfairness.org/
- Myelin Project
  http://www.myelin.org/
- National Institute of Neurological Disorders and Stroke
  http://www.ninds.nih.gov/disorders/adrenoleukodystrophy/adrenoleukodystrophy.htm
- Rare Diseases
  http://www.rarediseases.org/
- United Leukodystrophy Foundation
  http://www.ulf.org/

LEUKODYSTROPHIES—CITED REFERENCES

Deon M, et al. Hexacosanoic and docosanoic acids plasma levels in patients with cerebral childhood and asymptomatic X-linked adrenoleukodystrophy: Lorenzo's oil effect. *Metab Brain Dis.* 23:43, 2008.

Moser HW, et al. Adrenoleukodystrophy: new approaches to a neurodegenerative disease. *JAMA.* 294:3131, 2005.

Semmler A, et al. Therapy of X-linked adrenoleukodystrophy. *Expert Rev Neurother.* 8:1367, 2008.

Suzuki Y. The clinical course of childhood and adolescent adrenoleukodystrophy before and after Lorenzo's oil. *Brain Dev.* 23:30, 2001.

LOW BIRTH WEIGHT OR PREMATURITY

NUTRITIONAL ACUITY RANKING: LEVEL 3–4

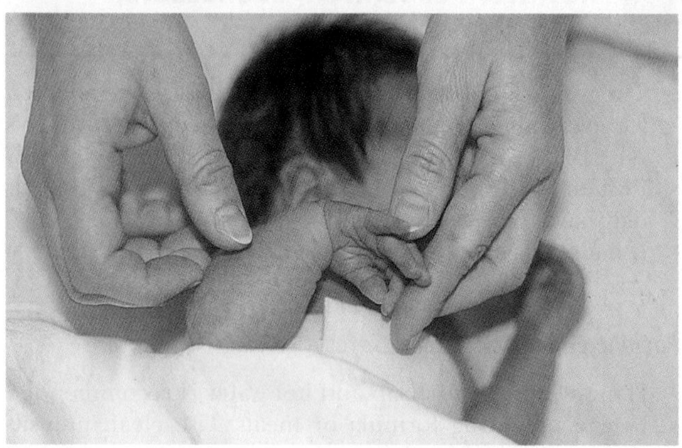

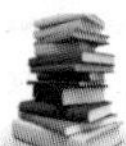

DEFINITIONS AND BACKGROUND

Every newborn is classified as one of the following: premature (<37 weeks of gestation), full-term (37–42 weeks of gestation), or postterm (>42 weeks of gestation). **Prematurity** is generally correlated with LBW. **LBW** infants may be small for date, have IUGR, or have dysmaturity. LBW infants weigh less than 2500 g or 5.5 lb (<10th percentile for gestational age) at birth. VLBW infants (<1300–1500 g) are especially prone to nutritional deficits. Infants who weigh 1000 g are called "micropreemies."

Low weight or BMI at conception or delivery, as well as poor weight gain during pregnancy, are associated with LBW, prematurity, and maternal delivery complications (Ehrenberg et al, 2003).

In the United States, infants born to mothers younger than 20 or older than 35 years are more likely to be preterm than infants born to mothers 20–35 years old (March of Dimes, 2009). Teens should be counseled to delay pregnancy until they are adults.

LBW infants have higher risk of mortality, morbidity, and poor growth. Typical problems of the LBW or premature infant include hypoglycemia, hypothermia, jaundice, dry skin, decreased subcutaneous fat, and anemia. Admission to neonatal intensive care units (NICUs) is common, especially for respiratory distress.

Adequate nutrition support almost immediately after birth is important to prevent growth restriction.

Undernutrition at critical stages of development (especially protein) produces long-term short stature, organ growth failure, neuronal deficits of number and dendritic connections, later behavioral and cognitive outcomes (Hay, 2008). Without nutrition starting immediately after birth, the infant enters a catabolic condition, which limits normal development and growth (Hay, 2008). During the first months after discharge, VLBW babies need to have nutrition support to help promote early catch-up growth and mineralization. Careful and frequent monitoring of growth patterns is needed to prevent developmental delays.

Premature breast milk has higher electrolyte, protein, and MCT levels than mature breast milk. Breastfeeding in the NICU is very beneficial and has long-term benefits for the child (Vohr et al, 2006). Feeding "on demand" is best (Crosson and Pickler, 2004). Preterm infants have lower energy expenditure when they are fed breast milk than when they are fed formula (Lubeztsky et al, 2003). Early feeding increases intestinal lactase activity, which is a marker of intestinal maturity and may influence clinical outcomes. Nearly all studies have shown that minimal enteral feeding approaches (e.g., "trophic feeds") promote the capacity to feed enterally (Hay, 2008).

Omega-3 fatty acids are important for healthy infants (Fewtrell et al, 2004). Maternal dietary intake of DHA is important. The brain, retina, and neural tissues are rich in DHA and arachidonic acid (ARA). Table 3-9 lists the nutritional deficits found in premature or LBW infants.

Milk has distinct advantages over formulas in avoiding necrotizing enterocolitis (NEC); minimal enteral feeding regimens produce less NEC than more aggressive enteral feeding (Hay, 2008). Caution must also be used in feeding as overfeeding has the potential to produce adipose tissue, or obesity, which then leads to insulin resistance, glucose intolerance, and diabetes (Hay, 2008).

Supplementation for premature infants remains controversial. Glutamine does not decrease sepsis (Poindexter et al, 2004), whereas selenium supplementation does (Darlow and Austin, 2003). Overall, the American Dietetic Association recommends at least five medical nutrition therapy visits for high-risk, premature infants.

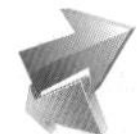

ASSESSMENT, MONITORING, AND EVALUATION

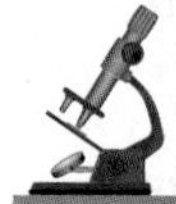

CLINICAL INDICATORS

Genetic Markers: There are no specific markers that predict LBW.

Clinical/History

- Birth weight
- Gestational age
- Birth length
- % weight/length (Olsen et al, 2009)
- Diet/intake history
- Swallowing reflex
- Temperature (often decreased)
- Sucking reflex
- Apgar scores
- I & O
- Hypotension?
- Infection?
- Respiratory distress?
- Retinopathy of prematurity (ROP)?

Lab Work

- Gluc
- H & H; No. of RBCs
- Anemia?
- Alb
- Ca^{++}, Mg^{++}
- Na^{+}, K^{+}
- Transthyretin
- ALT, AST
- Serum folic acid and vitamin B_{12}
- Serum phosphorus
- Lecithin to sphingomyelin ratio (L:S ratio)
- Bilirubin

TABLE 3-9 Nutritional Deficits in the Premature or Low Birth Weight Infant

Problem	Implication
Immaturity at the cellular level	Altered biochemical needs
Underdeveloped digestive/absorptive abilities	Malabsorption
Essential fatty acid deficiency	Slowed growth, renal and lung changes, fatty liver, impaired water balance, RBC fragility, and dermatitis
Delayed oral neuromuscular development and small gastric capacity	Limited ability to consume adequate amounts of nutrients
Marginal nutrient stores at birth	Fat, glycogen, and minerals such as calcium and phosphorus
Slow growth	Higher metabolic demands
Poor nutritional intake of the mother	Deficiencies such as folate

INTERVENTION

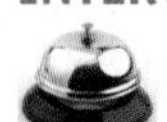

OBJECTIVES

- Begin feedings of distilled water or colostrum as soon as possible for infants without respiratory distress. Early feeding (3–5 days after birth) tends to allow babies to mature faster; they have fewer days of intolerance, a shorter hospital length of stay, and earlier tolerance of full feedings.
- Encourage the mother to breastfeed as long as possible. Taurine is an especially important nutrient in breastmilk (Verner et al, 2007). If tube feeding is needed, mother can express milk to be given to the infant; it can also be supplemented to meet special needs. Supplement with EFAs and DHA. Assure adequate intake of folate and vitamin B_{12} to prevent anemias.
- Provide glucose as soon after birth as possible; adjust according to frequent measurements of plasma glucose to achieve and maintain concentrations >45 mg/dL but <120 mg/dL to avoid hypoglycemia, and hyperglycemia respectively (Hay, 2008).

SAMPLE NUTRITION CARE PROCESS STEPS

Inadequate Protein-Energy Intake

Assessment Data: Low birth weight, inadequate growth, poor feeding skills.

Nutrition Diagnoses (PES): Inadequate intake of protein and energy related to prolonged feeding time and difficulty latching-on, as evidenced by premature birth, underweight (<3 percentile) and irritability after feeding.

Intervention: Educate staff and parents about nutritional requirements and appropriate formula choice if mother has discontinued breastfeeding.

Monitoring and Evaluation: Weight records, catch-up growth, tolerance of formula feedings, less irritability after feeding.

- When possible, use enteral feedings instead of parenteral to reduce onset of cholestasis and osteopenia.
- Gradually increase energy and protein to meet the needs of rapid growth. For protein, ensure a proper whey to casein ratio.
- With parenteral feeding, include amino acids in proper amounts, especially cysteine, taurine (Wharton et al, 2004), tyrosine, glycine, and arginine (Wu et al, 2004). Intravenous TrophAmine can be used. Be sure selenium is provided (Darlow and Austin, 2003).
- Promote catch-up growth and development. While long-term effects such as metabolic syndrome occur among LBW or premature infants later in life, effective nutrition support is needed (Greer, 2007).
- Prevent illness, rickets, respiratory distress, hypoglycemia or hyperglycemia, NEC, infections, obstructive jaundice, and tyrosinemia.

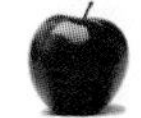

FOOD AND NUTRITION

- While in the radiant warmer, provide water at 60–80 mL/kg body weight/d; gradually increase to 150 mL/kg. Add electrolytes (sodium, potassium, and chloride) on at least the second day.
- Day 1: Breastfeed or give glucose at 6–8 mg/kg/min. Advance by no more than 20 mL/kg daily.
- Progress to special formulas such as Similac Special Care 24 or Enfamil Premature Formula (24 kcal/oz) to yield 120–150 mL/kg up to 180–200 mL/kg/d. NeoSure or Enfacare are helpful for transition to home (22 kcal/oz with added Ca^{++} and phosphorus).
- Within 7 days, the diet should provide 120–150 kcal/kg BW daily; carbohydrate should be 40–45% total kcal (10–30 g/kg). Protein should be age specific.
- Tube feeding initiation: Start at 10–15 mL/hr at one quarter strength. Progress as tolerated to desired rate. Specialty products have been developed for VLBW infants, such as Mead Johnson's Enfamil Human Milk Fortifier (Berseth et al, 2004). See Table 3-10 for estimated energy and macronutrient calculations.
- Use TPN if not feeding by day 3; glucose infusion rate is 15 mg/kg/min. TPN needs are similar to enteral needs. Crystalline amino acid infusions promote positive nitrogen balance by use of 1 g/kg/d as soon as possible. Use up to 3 g/kg/d of lipid infused continuously or early enteral feeding to prevent cholestatic liver disease. Monitor for carnitine deficiency. See Table 3-11 for recommended vitamin and mineral intakes.
- There may be subtle and delayed hunger cues from the infant. If poor sucking or swallowing instincts exist, the infant may need gavage feeding. Feed every 2 hours or use continuous drip feeding and change to bolus feedings when full strength is tolerated. If infant weighs 1000–1750 g, feed more vigorously; if infant weighs 1750 g or more, feed as a normal-term infant.
- The micronutrient needs of a stable, preterm LBW infant may be as follows: high levels of calcium 120–230 mg/kg; vitamin E (water soluble), 6.0–12.0 mg/kg; 2.5 mg iron/100 kcal in formula (necessary only if stores are depleted); vitamin D, 400 IU/d; folic acid, 25–50 µg/kg; sodium to avoid hyponatremia, 2–3 mEq/kg; vitamin C,

TABLE 3-10 Nutrient Needs of Preterm Infants

	Under 2.5 kg body weight	Over 2.5 kg body weight
Daily basal needs	60–80 kcal/kg	40–70 kcal/kg
+ Fecal losses	10–20 kcal/kg	10–20 kcal/kg
+ Growth (tissue synthesis, energy stores)	10 kcal/kg	10 kcal/kg
Total energy needs[a]	110–130 kcal/kg enteral	100–120 kcal/kg enteral
Parenteral needs (no fecal losses, no thermogenic effect of food)	90–110 kcal/kg	80–100 kcal/kg
Protein	3.5–4.0 g/kg enteral	3.6–4.0 g/kg enteral
Amino acids	2–3 g/kg parenteral	3.2–3.5 g/kg parenteral
Lipid	0.5 g/kg for essential fatty acids	0.5 g/kg for essential fatty acids
Fluid	80 mL/kg; increase 10–20 mL/kg daily to 120–160 mL/kg	60 mL/kg; increase 10–20 mL/kg daily to 120–150 mL/kg

[a]Add extra kilocals for fever (7% per 1-degree elevation); cardiac failure; sepsis; failure to thrive; major surgery; BPD.

REFERENCES

Hay WW Jr. Strategies for feeding the preterm infant. *Neonatology*. 94:245, 2008.

Pierro A. Metabolism and nutritional support in the surgical neonate. *J Ped Surg*. 37:811, 2002

Mirtollo J, et al. Safe practices for parenteral nutrition. *J Parenter Enteral Nutr.* 28:39S, 2004.

TABLE 3-11 Parenteral Vitamin and Mineral Needs in Preterm Infant

Nutrient	Recommended Intake for Infants <2.5 kg	Recommended Intake for Infants >2.5 kg
Vitamin A	280 μg	700 μg
Vitamin D	160 IU	400 IU
Vitamin E	2.8 mg	7 mg
Vitamin K	80 μg	200 μg
Vitamin C	32 mg	80 mg
Thiamin	0.48 mg	1.2 mg
Riboflavin	0.56 mg	1.4 mg
Niacin	6.8 mg	17 mg
Pyridoxine (B_6)	0.40 mg	1.0 mg
Folic acid	56 μg	140 μg
Vitamin B_{12}	0.40 μg	1 μg
Biotin	8 μg	20 μg
Pantothenate	2 mg	5 mg
Calcium	80–100 mg/kg	80–100 mg/kg
Phosphorus	43–62 mg/kg	43–62 mg/kg
Magnesium	6–10 mg/kg	6–10 mg/kg
Chromium	0.05–0.2 μg/kg	0.2 μg/kg
Copper	20 μg/kg	20 μg/kg
Iodide	1 μg/kg	1 μg/kg
Manganese	1 μg/kg	1 μg/kg
Molybdenum	0.25 μg/kg	0.25 μg/kg
Selenium	1.5–2 μg/kg	2 μg/kg
Zinc	400 μg/kg	50–250 μg/kg

Needs are estimated for use with a solution of 2.5 g/dL of amino acids infused at 120–150 mL/kg/dL.

Derived from: Hay WW Jr. Strategies for feeding the preterm infant. *Neonatology.* 94:245, 2008, and Mirtollo, et al. Safe practices for parenteral nutrition. *J Parenter Enteral Nutr.* 28:39S, 2004.

18–24 mg/kg; and phosphorus, 60–140 mg/kg. Monitor need for vitamins A and B_{12}, magnesium, zinc, selenium, and copper. Other nutrients should be provided according to DRI tables for the newborn.

- Total fat should be 5–7 g/kg to meet half of energy needs without excess carbohydrate. Soybean oil provides EFAs (1–2% kcals as EFA) in the form of linoleic acid. Exogenous carnitine may be needed to take EFAs into the mitochondria. Inositol may be needed in respiratory distress.

Common Drugs Used and Potential Side Effects

- With hyperkalemia and hyperglycemia, continuous intravenous insulin is needed.
- Sometimes, supplemental thyroid hormone or iodide may be prescribed.
- Other medications may be used for underlying disease states. Monitor for side effects.
- Use caution with vitamin supplements. Early vitamin supplementation may promote increased asthma, especially in black children (Milner et al, 2004).

Herbs, Botanicals, and Supplements

- Herbs and botanicals should not be used for LBW or premature infants because there may be allergic or asthmatic reactions.
- Glutamine supplementation does not seem to alleviate NEC.

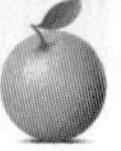

NUTRITION EDUCATION, COUNSELING, CARE MANAGEMENT

- Teach the caretaker or parent about increased nutrient needs of LBW or premature infant. Special formulas have

80 kcal/dL (usual is 67 kcal/dL) and have MCT, extra protein, calcium, phosphorus, and sodium.

- Emphasize progression of infant feeding for an adequate growth pattern and weight. Catch-up is common by 2–3 years of age in this population. VLBW infants experience catch-up growth and attain predicted genetic height during adolescence (Anderson, 2008).
- Emphasize the importance of nutrient density for growth (e.g., zinc, vitamin B_6, and vitamin E).
- Do not overfeed; excess nonprotein energy is stored as fat regardless of its source (fat or carbohydrate). High-energy or MCT intake in otherwise healthy, growing preterm infants should be avoided (Romero et al, 2004).
- Monitor for the tendency to aspirate, for lactose intolerance, and for other problems. Feed slowly to avoid NEC.
- The child may benefit from the WIC program if available.
- Follow-up clinic or home visits are recommended. Offer tips such as using small, frequent feedings; using a quiet, calm environment for feeding; supporting the jaw; and trying special feeding equipment if needed (angle-neck bottle).

Patient Education—Food Safety

- Hand washing with soap and hot water is recommended before preparing formula or meals. Use clean utensils and containers for mixing formula.
- Before using tap water for formula preparation or to give as a beverage, let cold tap water run for 2 minutes to remove any lead that may be in the pipes.
- Follow the 2-hour rule: discard any formula, beverage or food that has been left at room temperature for 2 hours or longer.
- Do not use honey because of the potential risk of botulism.

For More Information

- March of Dimes–Prematurity
  http://www.modimes.org/prematurity/
- Prematurity
  http://www.prematurity.org/
- UNICEF
  http://www.unicef.org

LOW BIRTH WEIGHT OR PREMATURITY—CITED REFERENCES

Anderson D. Nutrition in the care of the low-birth-weight infant. In: Mahan K, Escott-Stump S, eds. *Krause's food, nutrition, and diet therapy.* 12th ed. Philadelphia: WB Saunders, 2008.

Berseth CL, et al. Growth, efficacy, and safety of feeding an iron-fortified human milk fortifier. *Pediatrics.* 114:e699, 2004.

Crosson DD, Pickler RH. An integrated review of the literature on demand feedings for preterm infants. *Adv Neonatal Care.* 4:216, 2004.

Darlow BA, Austin NC. Selenium supplementation to prevent short-term morbidity in preterm neonates. *Cochrane Database Syst Rev.* 4:CD003312, 2003.

Ehrenberg HM, et al. Low maternal weight, failure to thrive in pregnancy, and adverse pregnancy outcomes. *Am J Obstet Gynecol.* 189:1726, 2003.

Fewtrell MS, et al. Randomized, double-blind trial of long-chain polyunsaturated fatty acid supplementation with fish oil and borage oil in preterm infants. *J Pediatr.* 144:471, 2004.

Greer FR. Long-term adverse outcomes of low birth weight, increased somatic growth rates, and alterations of body composition in the premature infant: review of the evidence. *J Pediatr Gastroenterol Nutr.* 45:S147, 2007.

Hay WW Jr. Strategies for feeding the preterm infant. *Neonatology.* 94:245, 2008.

Lubeztsky R, et al. Energy expenditure in human milk-versus formula-fed preterm infants. *J Pediatr.* 143:750, 2003.

March of Dimes. Born too soon and too small in the United States. Accessed May 1, 2009, at http://www.marchofdimes.com/.

Milner JD, et al. Early infant multivitamin supplementation is associated with increased risk for food allergy and asthma. *Pediatrics.* 114:27, 2004.

Olsen IE, et al. Use of a body proportionality index for growth assessment of preterm infants. *J Pediatr.* 154:486, 2009.

Poindexter BB, et al. Parenteral glutamine supplementation does not reduce the risk of mortality or late-onset sepsis in extremely low birth weight infants. *Pediatrics.* 113:1209, 2004.

Romero G, et al. Energy intake, metabolic balance and growth in preterm infants fed formulas with different nonprotein energy supplements. *J Pediatr Gastroenterol Nutr.* 38:407, 2004.

Verner A, et al. Effect of taurine supplementation on growth and development in preterm or low birth weight infants. *Cochrane Database Syst Rev.* 17(4):CD006072, 2007.

Vohr BR, et al. Beneficial effects of breast milk in the neonatal intensive care unit on the developmental outcome of extremely low birth weight infants at 18 months of age. *Pediatrics.* 118:115, 2006.

Wharton BA, et al. Low plasma taurine and later neurodevelopment. *Arch Dis Child Fetal Neonatal Ed.* 89:497, 2004.

Wu G, et al. Arginine deficiency in preterm infants: biochemical mechanisms and nutritional implications. *J Nutr Biochem.* 15:442, 2004.

MAPLE SYRUP URINE DISEASE

NUTRITIONAL ACUITY RANKING: LEVEL 3–4

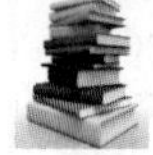

DEFINITIONS AND BACKGROUND

Maple syrup urine disease (MSUD) results from an autosomal recessive trait, causing an inborn error of metabolism of the BCAAs leucine, isoleucine, valine. Byproduct ketoacids become elevated and may cause life-threatening cerebral edema and dysmyelination (Riazi et al, 2004). The elevated BCAAs (leucinosis) cause an infant or child with MSUD to become symptomatic. Neurotransmitter deficiencies related to BCAA accumulation, and energy deprivation through Krebs cycle disruption from ketoacid accumulation, are mechanisms (Zinnanti et al, 2009).

In the United States, MSUD occurs in one in 225,000 births. The Mennonite population from eastern Pennsylvania has a high percentage of births with this disorder. MSUD also occurs in other populations throughout the world. Onset occurs in children between the ages of 1 and 8 years.

Symptoms in an infant include poor sucking reflex, anorexia, FTT, listlessness, irritability, and a characteristic odor (sweet, burnt maple syrup odor of the urine and sweat).

TABLE 3-12 Types and Nutrition Interventions for Maple Syrup Urine Disease (MSUD)

Type	Nutrition Intervention
Classic MSUD	Most common. Little or no enzyme activity (usually <2% of normal). Protein from branched-chain amino acids (BCAAs) must be severely restricted.
Intermediate MSUD	Higher level of enzyme activity (approximately 3–8% of normal). Tolerance for leucine is slightly better. Management is the same as for the classic form.
Intermittent MSUD	Milder form; greater enzyme activity (8–15% of normal). Few symptoms until 12–24 months of age, often in response to an illness or larger protein intake. During episodes of illness or fasting, the BCAA levels elevate, the characteristic odor becomes evident, and the child can go into a metabolic crisis.
Thiamin-responsive MSUD	Rare form. Giving large doses of thiamin to the thiamin-responsive child will increase the enzyme activity. Moderate protein restriction is needed.

Derived from: data available at http://www.msud-support.org/overv.htm, accessed January 2, 2005.

Afflicted infants have a high-pitched cry and may alternate between being limp or rigid. Without treatment, symptoms progress rapidly to seizures, coma, and death (Schonberger et al, 2004). With earlier diagnosis and treatment, there is a lower risk of peripheral neuropathy.

Nutrition therapy is lifelong. Supplemental isoleucine and valine are usually required (Chuang and Shih, 2001). The amino acid mixture contributes 30–40% of total energy, leaving 60–70% from food (Isaacs and Zand, 2007). Note that thiamin is the coenzyme for BCAAs and should be made available. There are four classifications for the types of MSUD: classic, intermediate, intermittent, and thiamin-responsive; these refer to the amount and type of enzyme activity present. See Table 3-12.

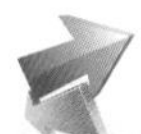

ASSESSMENT, MONITORING, AND EVALUATION

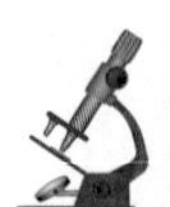

CLINICAL INDICATORS

Genetic Markers: The branched-chain alpha-keto acid dehydrogenase (BCKD) is missing.

Clinical/History

Length (height)
Birth weight
Present weight
Growth (%)
Diet/intake history
Perspiration with maple odor
Grand mal seizures?
Hypertonicity
Cerebral edema?

Lab Work

Plasma leucine, isoleucine, valine (therapeutic range of 100–300 µmol/L)
Plasma L-alloisoleucine 0.5 µmol/L (most specific and most sensitive for MSUD)
Urinary excretion of ketoacids
Urine odor of burnt maple syrup
Alb
Globulin
Uric acid (increased?)
H & H
Serum Fe
Serum osmolality

INTERVENTION

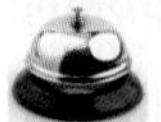

OBJECTIVES

- Prevent endogenous protein catabolism (Morton et al, 2002).
- Prevent toxic concentrations of BCAAs (Riazi et al, 2004) by using an appropriate medical formula, special intravenous feeding, or low-BCAA diet. Monitor serum levels of leucine frequently to determine current status.
- Support normal growth and development with adequate protein synthesis and prevention of essential amino acid deficiencies. Overcome any difficulty with feeding related to poor sucking reflex.
- Control intake of BCAAs for life. As the child grows, add BCAAs individually in a controlled manner.
- Maintain normal serum osmolality (Morton et al, 2002).
- In emergencies, hemodialysis is sometimes necessary (Hmiel et al, 2004).

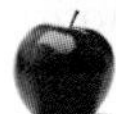

FOOD AND NUTRITION

- Restrict intake of BCAAs in the diet to 45–62 mg/d (Riazi et al, 2004). Use Mead Johnson's MSUD powder or Ross Laboratories' Maxamaid MSUD. Use the latter with PFD1 or PFD2 (Mead Johnson) because it contains no cholesterol or fat.
- When BCAA levels are high (during illness or fasting), it may be necessary to use a specific IV solution that allows the excess leucine, valine, and isoleucine to be used for protein synthesis in the body, thereby rapidly decreasing the elevated levels.

SAMPLE NUTRITION CARE PROCESS STEPS

Excessive Protein Intake

Assessment Data: Weight and growth charts, elevated serum leucine.

Nutrition Diagnoses (PES): Excessive protein intake related to MSUD and genetic inability to metabolize large amounts of dietary BCAAs as evidenced by high serum leucine and elevated urinary keto-acids.

Intervention: Educate parents about appropriate formula to manage MSUD. Counsel about appropriate formula and food sources of leucine and needed supplements, including thiamin.

Monitoring and Evaluation: Weight records, growth, improved appetite, improved serum and urinary lab test results.

- Provide adequate energy intake from CHO and fat to spare amino acids for building tissue, etc.
- Use small amounts of milk in the diet to support growth. Cow's milk contains 350 mg of leucine, 228 mg of isoleucine, and 245 mg of valine per 100 mL.
- Avoid eggs, meat, nuts, and other dairy products. Gelatin, a form of protein low in BCAAs, may be used in the diet.
- If hemodialysis is needed, monitor fluid, protein, and electrolytes carefully.

Common Drugs Used and Potential Side Effects

- Sometimes insulin or a similar agent is given to speed up the utilization of excess BCAAs.
- The doctor may prescribe large doses of thiamin for children who are thiamin-responsive.
- Avoid use of aspirin with MSUD; individuals with this condition are more prone to Reye's syndrome.
- Norleucine is being tested as a possible treatment for emergency management of MSUD crises.

Herbs, Botanicals, and Supplements

- Herbs and botanicals should not be used for MSUD because there are no controlled trials to prove efficacy.

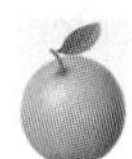

NUTRITION EDUCATION, COUNSELING, CARE MANAGEMENT

- Educate caregiver and patient that the diet must be maintained for life.
- Discuss the diet's total energy and protein intake that are appropriate for the patient's age and stage of development.
- Illness or infection can cause elevations of BCAAs. This can lead to vomiting, diarrhea, irritability, sleepiness, unusual breathing, staggering, hallucinations, and slurred speech. This is an emergency and must be treated immediately.
- With knowledge of the pathophysiology of MSUD and understanding of what to do for cerebral edema, fluid and electrolyte management, nutrition, and psychosocial issues, a full life is possible (Robinson and Drumm, 2001).

Patient Education—Food Safety

- Hand washing with soap and hot water is recommended before preparing formula or meals. Use clean utensils and containers for mixing formula.
- Before using tap water for formula preparation or to give as a beverage, let cold tap water run for 2 minutes to remove any lead that may be in the pipes.
- Follow the 2-hour rule: discard any beverage or food that has been left at room temperature for 2 hours or longer.
- Do not use honey in the diets of infants to decrease potential risk of botulism.

For More Information

- Cambrooke Foods
  http://www.cambrookefoods.com/
- MSUD Family Support Group
  http://www.msud-support.org/
- National Newborn Screening
  http://genes-r-us.uthscsa.edu/
- Nutrient Data
  http://www.nal.usda.gov/fnic/foodcomp/search/
- Save Babies
  http://www.savebabies.org/
- Screening
  http://www.msud-support.org/testing.htm

MAPLE SYRUP URINE DISEASE—CITED REFERENCES

Chuang DT, Shih VE. Maple syrup urine disease (branched-chain ketoaciduria). In: Scriver C, Beaudet A, Sly W, Valle D, eds. *The metabolic and molecular bases of inherited disease.* New York, NY: McGraw-Hill, 2001:1971–2006.

Hmiel SP, et al. Amino acid clearance during acute metabolic decompensation in maple syrup urine disease treated with continuous venovenous hemodialysis with filtration. *Pediatr Crit Care Med.* 5:278, 2004.

Morton DH, et al. Diagnosis and treatment of maple syrup disease: a study of 36 patients. *Pediatrics.* 109:999, 2002.

Riazi R, et al. Total branched-chain amino acids requirement in patients with maple syrup urine disease by use of indicator amino acid oxidation with L-[1–13 C]phenylalanine. *Am J Physiol Endocrinol Metab.* 287:142, 2004.

Robinson D, Drumm LA. Maple syrup disease: a standard of nursing care. *Pediatr Nurs.* 27:255, 2001.

Schonberger S, et al. Dysmyelination in the brain of adolescents and young adults with maple syrup urine disease. *Mol Genet Metab.* 82:69, 2004.

Zinnanti WJ, et al. Dual mechanism of brain injury and novel treatment strategy in maple syrup urine disease. *Brain.* 132:903, 2009.

NECROTIZING ENTEROCOLITIS

NUTRITIONAL ACUITY RANKING: LEVEL 4

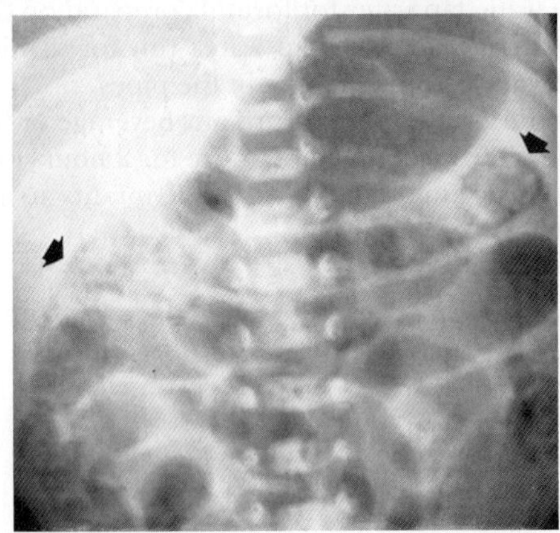

Adapted from: Ronald L. *Eisenberg, an Atlas of Differential Diagnosis,* 4th ed. Philadelphia: Lippincott Williams & Wilkins, 2003.

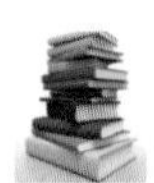

DEFINITIONS AND BACKGROUND

NEC involves ischemia of the intestinal tract and invasion of the mucosa with enteric pathogens. This is a common GI problem in preterm and SGA infants with tissue injury and inflammation, congenital heart disease, or with Hirschsprung's disease. Symptoms and signs include a distended abdomen, lethargy, respiratory distress, pallor, hyperbilirubinemia, vomiting, diarrhea, grossly bloody stools, and sepsis.

NEC is the leading cause of short bowel syndrome in infancy; it is a medical emergency. NEC affects about 1–8% of all admissions to NICUs. Thrombocytopenia within the first 3 days after a diagnosis of NEC suggests a higher likelihood of bowel gangrene, morbidity, and mortality (Kenton et al, 2005). Neonatal endotoxemia and release of proinflammatory cytokines are important contributors to NEC; gut barrier failure plays an important role in adverse outcomes (Sharma et al, 2007).

If feeding intolerance is significant, it is beneficial to use breast milk rather than formula. Milk has distinct advantages over formulas; minimal enteral feeding regimens produce less NEC than more aggressive enteral feeding (Hay, 2008). There is no conclusive evidence about the use of special formulas that include glutamine or arginine. Preventive strategies include amino acid or polyunsaturated fatty acid administration (Reber and Nankervis, 2004).

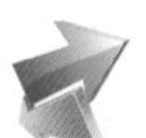

ASSESSMENT, MONITORING, AND EVALUATION

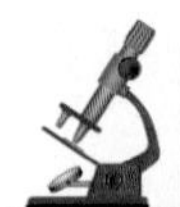

CLINICAL INDICATORS

Genetic Markers: NEC is not genetic in origin.

Clinical/History

- Height/length
- Weight/birth weight
- Diet/intake history
- Head circumference
- Vomiting
- Diarrhea?
- Distended abdomen
- Lethargy
- Respiratory distress
- Pallor
- Hyperbilirubinemia
- Grossly bloody stools
- Sepsis

Lab Work

- CBC; elevated WBCs
- Thrombocytopenia (low platelet count)
- Neutropenia
- Hemoglobin (decreased)
- Hct (altered?)
- Abdominal x-rays
- Pro time (prolonged), INR
- Guaiac test for blood in stools
- Na^+ (decreased)
- K^+ (increased)
- Platelets (decreased)
- Gluc
- Lactic acidosis
- pO_2, pCO_2

INTERVENTION

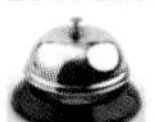

OBJECTIVES

- TPN is needed for 14–21 days while the intestine heals.
- Prevent or correct dehydration, hypoglycemia, and electrolyte imbalances.
- Correct diarrhea and further malnutrition.
- Prepare patient for bowel surgery, for wound healing, and for the possibility of ostomy feeding if surgery becomes necessary, as for perforation or after peritonitis.
- Because breastfeeding is more protective than formula feeding, promote maternal breastfeeding or use of donor milk after TPN (Updegrove, 2004).

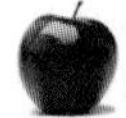

FOOD AND NUTRITION

- Acute: No oral feedings; use IVs to support circulation. TPN as appropriate with periods of extensive intestinal inflammation and peritonitis.
- Recovery: Use two times RDA of protein; 25% more kilocals than normal for age; frequent feedings. Where possible, offer donor milk if mother cannot breastfeed.

SAMPLE NUTRITION CARE PROCESS STEPS

Increased Energy Expenditure

Assessment Data: Weight loss, sepsis, diarrhea and vomiting, fever, stooling pattern.

Nutrition Diagnoses (PES): Increased energy expenditure related to NEC with losses from diarrhea and vomiting as evidenced by fever, bloody stools, distended abdomen, and altered lab values.

Intervention: Provide support for use of breastmilk, where possible.

Monitoring and Evaluation: Weight stabilization or gains in growth, cessation of bloody stools and diarrhea or vomiting, resolution of fever and sepsis, lab values returning to normal.

- Some partially elemental formulas are available, such as Pregestimil or Nutramigen, or more elemental nutrients may be required if the digestive tract has not recovered fully. Among infants between 1000 and 2000 g at birth, giving feedings at 30 mL/kg/d seems to be a safe practice and is faster than using 20 mL/kg/d (Caple et al, 2004).
- Ensure adequate iron, copper, and zinc. Iron-fortified products may reduce the need for blood transfusions in VLBW infants (Berseth et al, 2004). Copper seems to protect against TPN-related liver damage from intrauterine growth deficits (Zambrano et al, 2004).
- Occasionally, a colostomy or ileostomy must be performed, and tube feeding may be needed.

Common Drugs Used and Potential Side Effects

- Aggressive treatment of hyperglycemia may be needed, as with insulin (Hall et al, 2004). Monitor for side effects.
- Systemic antibiotics are started, usually a β-lactam antibiotic and an aminoglycoside. Some outbreaks may be infectious.

Herbs, Botanicals, and Supplements

- Studies suggest use of probiotics (Henry and Moss, 2004). A systematic Cochrane review promotes enteral feeding of probiotics in preterm infants >1000 g at birth but not for smaller infants (Alfaleh and Bassler, 2008). *Lactobacillus acidophilus* and *Bifudus infantis* may be beneficial.
- Herbs and botanicals should not be used for NEC.

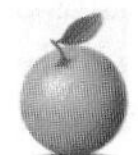

NUTRITION EDUCATION, COUNSELING, CARE MANAGEMENT

- Promote breastfeeding or use of donor milk.
- When formula is used, assure that the parent/caretaker understands the differences between ready-to-feed and concentrated formula related to, hypertonicity of the solution.
- If surgery and short-gut is the resolution, long-term TPN may be needed.
- Careful monitoring of growth is important. Besides bowel sequelae, VLBW infants who survive NEC are at risk for impairment of growth and neurodevelopment (Yeh et al, 2004).
- Monitor weight and stool changes; advise physician when necessary.

Patient Education—Food Safety

- Hand washing with soap and hot water is recommended before preparing formula or meals. Use clean utensils and containers for mixing formula.
- Before using tap water for formula preparation or to give as a beverage, let cold tap water run for 2 minutes to remove any lead that may be in the pipes.
- Follow the 2-hour rule: discard any beverage or food that has been left at room temperature for 2 hours or longer. Powdered infant formulas are not sterile and may contain pathogenic bacteria; milk products are also media for bacterial proliferation (Agostoni et al, 2004).
- Do not use honey in the diets of infants to decrease potential risk of botulism.

For More Information

- Merck Manual
  http://www.merck.com/mrkshared/mmanual/section19/chapter260/260n.jsp
- Necrotizing Enterocolitis
  http://www.pediatrie.be/NECROT_%20ENTEROCOL.htm

NECROTIZING ENTEROCOLITIS—CITED REFERENCES

Agostoni C, et al. Preparation and handling of powdered infant formula: a commentary by the ESPGHAN Committee on Nutrition. *J Pediatr Gastroenterol Nutr.* 39:320, 2004.

Alfaleh K, Bassler D. Probiotics for prevention of necrotizing enterocolitis in preterm infants. *Cochrane Database Syst Rev.* 23(1):CD005496, 2008.

Caple J, et al. Randomized, controlled trial of slow versus rapid feeding volume advancement in preterm infants. *Pediatrics.* 114:1597, 2004.

Hall NJ, et al. Hyperglycemia is associated with increased morbidity and mortality rates in neonates with necrotizing enterocolitis. *J Pediatr Surg.* 39:898, 2004.

Hay WW Jr. Strategies for feeding the preterm infant. *Neonatology.* 94:245, 2008.

Henry MC, Moss RL. Current issues in the management of necrotizing enterocolitis. *Semin Perinatol.* 28:221, 2004.

Kenton AB, et al. Severe thrombocytopenia predicts outcome in neonates with necrotizing enterocolitis. *J Perinatol.* 25:14, 2005.

Reber KM, Nankervis CA. Necrotizing enterocolitis: preventative strategies. *Clin Perinatol.* 31:157, 2004.

Sharma R, et al. Neonatal gut barrier and multiple organ failure: role of endotoxin and proinflammatory cytokines in sepsis and necrotizing enterocolitis. *J Pediatr Surg.* 42:454, 2007.

Updegrove K. Necrotizing enterocolitis: the evidence for use of human milk in prevention and treatment. *J Hum Lact.* 20:335, 2004.

Yeh TC, et al. Necrotizing enterocolitis in infants: clinical outcome and influence on growth and neurodevelopment. *J Formos Med Assoc.* 103:761, 2004.

Zambrano E. Total parenteral nutrition induced liver pathology: an autopsy series of 24 newborn cases. *Pediatr Dev Pathol.* 7:425, 2004.

NEURAL TUBE DEFECTS: SPINA BIFIDA AND MELOMENINGOCELE

NUTRITIONAL ACUITY RANKING: LEVEL 3

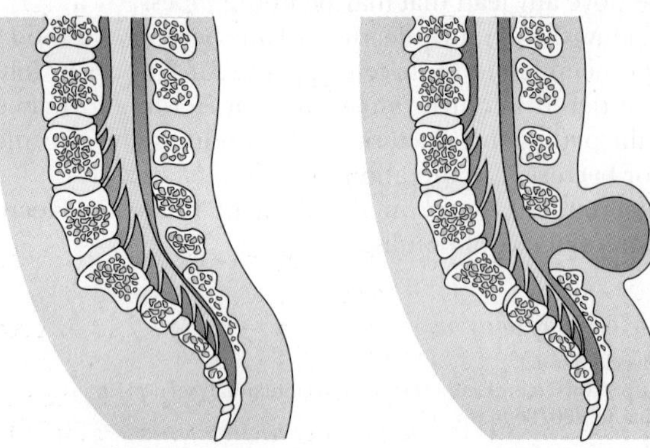

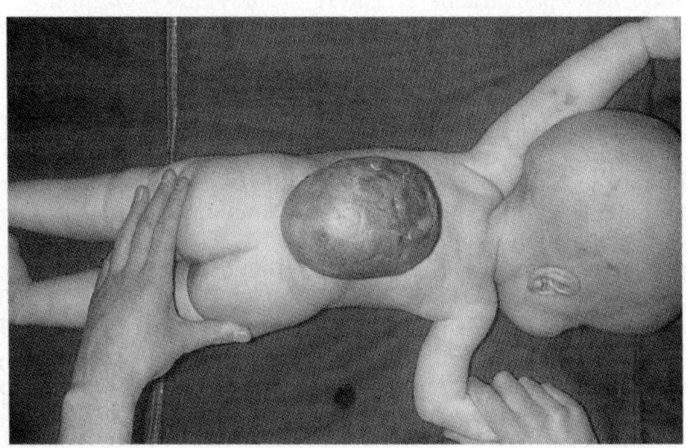

Reprinted with permission from: Pillitteri A. *Maternal and Child Health Nursing,* 4th ed. Philadelphia: Lippincott Williams & Wilkins, 2003.

The neural tube folds and closes during the third and fourth weeks of pregnancy to form the brain and spinal cord (Li et al, 2006). Neural tube defects (NTDs) are serious birth defects of the spine (spina bifida) and brain (anencephaly), affecting approximately 3000 pregnancies each year in the United States. Women at risk for having a baby with NTDs are of English/Irish ancestry or Hispanic ancestry, may have diabetes mellitus, are obese, have poor dietary habits, or take medications that are folate antagonists.

The natural folates are chemically unstable and poorly bioavailable in contrast to the chemical form, folic acid (Scott, 2009). Periconceptional consumption of folic acid (400 mg daily) reduces the occurrence of NTDs by 50–70% (Centers for Disease Control and Prevention, 2004; Hamner et al, 2009). No more than one fifth of women take supplements effectively, largely due to the fact that over half of pregnancies are unplanned (Scott, 2009).

A remarkable successes of epidemiology was the demonstration in the late twentieth century that spina bifida and anencephaly are caused primarily by folate deficiency (Oakley, 2009). The genetic MTHFR polymorphisms may cause congenital folate malabsorption, severe MTHFR deficiency, and formiminotransferase deficiency (Whitehead, 2006). In these cases, diets deficient in folate *do not* influence the incidence or severity of NTDs; folic acid and methionine cycle genes for SNP genotyping alter the effects of diet (Boyles et al, 2006).

Low levels of betaine-tHcy methyltransferase (BHMT) and choline may be associated with NTDs (Boyles et al, 2006; Innis et al, 2007; Shaw et al, 2004). Betaine (trimethylglycine) is formed from choline, or from the diet (seafood, wheat germ, bran, and spinach). Risks may be greater when vitamin B_{12} status is low (van der Linden et al, 2006). Because results vary from one population to another, studies are needed to clarify how different populations respond to betaine and choline from diet or supplements.

Spina bifida includes any congenital defect involving insufficient closure of the spine (usually laminae of the vertebrae). Most defects occur in the lower lumbar or sacral areas of the back (the lowest areas of the back) because this area is the last part of the spine to close. **Spina bifida occulta** involves the bones of the spine not closing completely while the spinal cord and meninges remain in place; skin covers the defect. **Spina bifida cystica** is more severe. **Anencephaly** forms when the brain does not close; the baby lacks parts of the brain, skull, or scalp, may be deaf, blind, and usually will not thrive.

In **meningoceles**, the meninges (the membranes covering the spinal cord) protrude through the vertebral defect but the spinal cord remains in place. Clubfoot, dislocated hip, scoliosis, and other musculoskeletal deformities may also be present. **Myelomeningocele (MMC)** is one of the most severe forms of birth defects of the brain and spinal cord. MMC accounts for about 75% of all cases of spina bifida, affecting 1 of every 800 infants. Pregnant women may show a positive alpha-fetoprotein level during prenatal testing in a triple screen. The spinal canal is incomplete. This causes decreased or lack of function of body areas controlled at or below the defect. Partial or complete paralysis of the legs, partial or complete lack of sensation, loss of bowel or bladder control, meningitis, hydrocephalus, and hip dislocation may also be present. Sometimes, surgery for the tethered cord or to repair the hydrocephaly improves quality of life. MMC patients are usually wheelchair bound, wear braces, or use crutches. Obesity can increase likelihood of pressure ulcers or make ambulation and surgery more difficult.

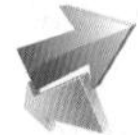

ASSESSMENT, MONITORING, AND EVALUATION

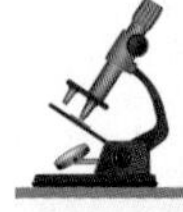

CLINICAL INDICATORS

Genetic Markers: Folate status is a significant determinant of NTD risk; genetic variation, folate nutriture, and specific metabolic, and/or genomic pathways are involved (Beaudlin and Stover, 2007). Women who have a methylenetetrahydrofolate reductase (MTHFR) allele tend to have a higher risk for giving birth to an infant with an NTD. Hispanic and Latina women,

women from the United Kingdom and Italy may have this allele and should be tested before pregnancy.

Clinical/History		
Height, weight	Spinal x-rays or computed tomography (CT) scan	H & H
Birth weight/length	Diarrhea or Constipation	Serum Fe
Growth percentile	Incontinence	Chol
Weight changes	Skin integrity	Na^+, K^+
Diet/intake history (folate, choline, B_{12}, betaine)	Hydrocephaly	Ca^{++}, Mg^{++}
Temperature	**Lab Work**	Serum folic acid
I & O	Gluc	MTHFR allele?
Vertebral defect	Alb, transthyretin	Hcy
		Serum B_{12}, Methylmalonic acid

INTERVENTION

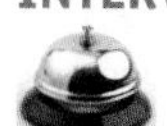

OBJECTIVES

- Manage feeding problems, which are common. Assure proper positioning for all feedings.
- Achieve and maintain ideal BMI for age. There are decreased energy needs because of short stature and limited mobility. Obesity is common.
- Reduce impact of the defect. Promote any and all possible ambulation or activity.

SAMPLE NUTRITION CARE PROCESS STEPS

Inadequate Folic Acid Intake

Assessment Data: Prenatal weight gain, dietary records, and nutrient analysis, MTHFR allele.

Nutrition Diagnoses (PES): NI 54.2. Inadequate vitamin (folic acid) intake related to diet history and increased needs during pregnancy as evidenced by diet recall with folate intake much lower than needs in pregnancy (600 mcg) and prior birth of an infant with NTD.

Interventions:

Food and Nutrient Delivery:

ND 1.3. Add natural sources of folate to diet—orange juice, carrots, green vegetables.

ND 1.3. Eat fortified cereal at breakfast and whole grains such as oatmeal, brown rice.

ND 3.2. Recommend folic acid supplement of 400 μg/d.

Education: Rich folate sources from food; importance of taking a daily multivitamin supplement.

Counseling: Investigate need for L-methylfolate during pregnancy related to genetic allele.

Monitoring and Evaluation: Weight and health records. Prenatal care and intake of supplemental folic acid. Note of willingness to comply with recommendations.

- Correct infections; prevent or correct sepsis and pressure ulcers.
- Correct nutrient deficiencies.
- Alter diet to prevent or correct constipation, obesity, and UTIs.
- Increase independence and self-care potentials.
- Preserve brain function as far as possible.
- Correct swallowing problems (from Arnold–Chiari malformation of the brain).
- Initiate treatment or surgical intervention as appropriate.

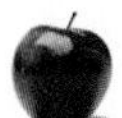

FOOD AND NUTRITION

- Individualize diet for proper nutrition to achieve a desirable weight and monitor carefully.
- Decrease energy to control weight. Use special growth charts. The standard CDC charts will be irrelevant. For children under age 8 who are minimally active, use 9–11 kcal/cm or 50% fewer calories than recommended for child of a similar age (Lucas, 2004, p. 41). For older teens or adults, 7 kcal/cm may be needed for weight loss; generally, needs are about 50% of normal.
- Provide adequate protein, folic acid, B-complex vitamins, choline, betaine, zinc, and other nutrients for age.
- Low-calorie snacks may be the only between-meal snacks allowed.
- Provide adequate nutrients for wound healing if surgery has been performed. For healing of any pressure ulcers, adequate zinc, vitamins A and C, and protein are required.
- For females of childbearing age, pay attention to folic acid, choline, vitamin B_{12}, betaine intakes. A multivitamin with minerals should be recommended for those who lack variety in their diets.
- Ensure adequate fiber intake and fluid to prevent or correct problems with diarrhea or constipation.
- Individuals with spina bifida are often allergic to latex; they may require a diet that limits use of apples, avocado, banana, bell pepper, cherries, chestnut, kiwi, nectarines, peach, plums, potato, and tomato.

Common Drugs Used and Potential Side Effects

- Antibiotics may be required if the patient develops sepsis. Use of acidophilus and probiotic products may alleviate loss of intestinal bacteria.
- Avoid zinc and iron with parenteral administration in sepsis; these are bacterial nutrients.
- Botulinum-A toxin injections have been used in cases of neurogenic detrusor overactivity to manage some bladder incontinence (Leippold et al, 2003). Otherwise, medications for managing urinary incontinence may be used; monitor for side effects.
- Medications prescribed may affect the utilization of folate: anticonvulsant medications (e.g., phenytoin), metformin, sulfasalazine, triamterene, and methotrexate. Other medications deplete important nutrients prenatally, such as antibiotics, antihypertensives, cathartics, corticosteroids, stimulants, sulfonamides, and tranquilizers. Vitamin and mineral supplements are needed to compensate for the specific nutrient alteration.

- Sulfonamides may crystallize vitamin C in the bladder; extra vitamin C, protein, iron, and folate may be needed.

Herbs, Botanicals, and Supplements

- Herbs and botanicals should not be used because there are no controlled trials to prove efficacy for any related problems.
- Use of low-calorie cranberry juice may help reduce UTIs.

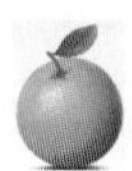

NUTRITION EDUCATION, COUNSELING, CARE MANAGEMENT

- Behavior modification, low-calorie food and snack preparation, rewards, and activity/exercise factors should be reviewed with the parent/caretaker. Food lists with green "go" foods, red "stop" foods, and yellow "caution" foods have been used with success in weight management.
- Discuss potential medical conditions, such as fractures, seizures, lazy eye, early puberty, and latex allergy. Bone health and allergies can be managed with some nutritional interventions.
- Family counseling may be needed in preparation for future pregnancies. Referral to a local chapter of the March of Dimes may be beneficial.
- Even with food fortification, women of childbearing age should be advised to take a folic acid–containing supplement on a daily basis (Schuaibi et al, 2008). Choline, betaine, and B_{12} should be included as well.

Patient Education—Food Safety

- Hand washing with soap and hot water is recommended before preparing formula or meals. Use clean utensils and containers for mixing formula.
- Before using tap water for formula preparation or to give as a beverage, let cold tap water run for 2 minutes to remove any lead that may be in the pipes.
- Follow the 2-hour rule: discard any beverage or food that has been left at room temperature for 2 hours or longer.
- Do not use honey in the diets of infants to decrease potential risk of botulism.

For More Information

- Association for Spina Bifida and Hydrocephalus
  www.asbah.org
- CDC—Spina Bifida
  http://www.cdc.gov/ncbddd/birthdefects/SpinaBifida.htm
- CDC Folic Acid National Campaign
  http://www.cdc.gov/ncbddd/Folicacid
- Management of Myelomenigocele Study
  http://www.spinabifidamoms.com/english/index.html
- NIH—Spina Bifida
  http://www.ninds.nih.gov/disorders/spina_bifida/spina_bifida.htm
- Pregnancy Planning
  http://www.cdc.gov/ncbddd/pregnancy/
- Spina Bifida Association
  http://www.sbaa.org

NEURAL TUBE DEFECTS—CITED REFERENCES

Beaudlin AE, Stover PJ. Folate-mediated one-carbon metabolism and neural tube defects: balancing genome synthesis and gene expression. *Birth Defects Res C Embryo Today.* 81:183, 2007.

Boyles AL, et al. Neural tube defects and folate pathway genes: family-based association tests of gene-gene and gene-environment interactions. *Environ Health Perspect.* 114(10):1547, 2006.

Centers for Disease Control and Prevention. Use of vitamins containing folic acid among women of childbearing age—United States, 2004. *MMWR Morb Mortal Wkly Rep.* 53:847, 2004.

Hamner HC, et al. Predicted contribution of folic acid fortification of corn masa flour to the usual folic acid intake for the US population: National Health and Nutrition Examination Survey 2001–2004. *Am J Clin Nutr.* 89: 305, 2009.

Leippold T, et al. Botulinum toxin as a new therapy option for voiding disorders: current state of the art. *Eur Urol.* 44:165, 2003.

Lucas B, ed. *Children with special care needs: nutrition care handbook.* Chicago: The American Dietetic Association, 2004.

Oakley GP Jr. The scientific basis for eliminating folic acid-preventable spina bifida: a modern miracle from epidemiology. *Ann Epidemiol.* 19:226, 2009.

Scott JM. Reduced folate status is common and increases disease risk. It can be corrected by daily ingestion of supplements or fortification. *Novartis Found Symp.* 282:105, 2009.

Schuaibi AM, et al. Folate status of young Canadian women after folic acid fortification of grain products. *J Am Diet Assoc.* 108:2090, 2008.

Shaw GM, et al. Periconceptional dietary intake of choline and betaine and neural tube defects in offspring. *Am J Epid.* 160(2):102, 2004.

Van Der Linden IJ, et al. The methionine synthase reductase 66 A>G polymorphism is a maternal risk factor for spina bifida. *J Mol Med.* 84(12): 1047, 2006.

Whitehead VM. Acquired and inherited disorders of cobalamin and folate in children. *Br J Hematol.* 134(2):125, 2006.

OBESITY, CHILDHOOD

NUTRITIONAL ACUITY RANKING: LEVEL 3–4 (COUNSELING)

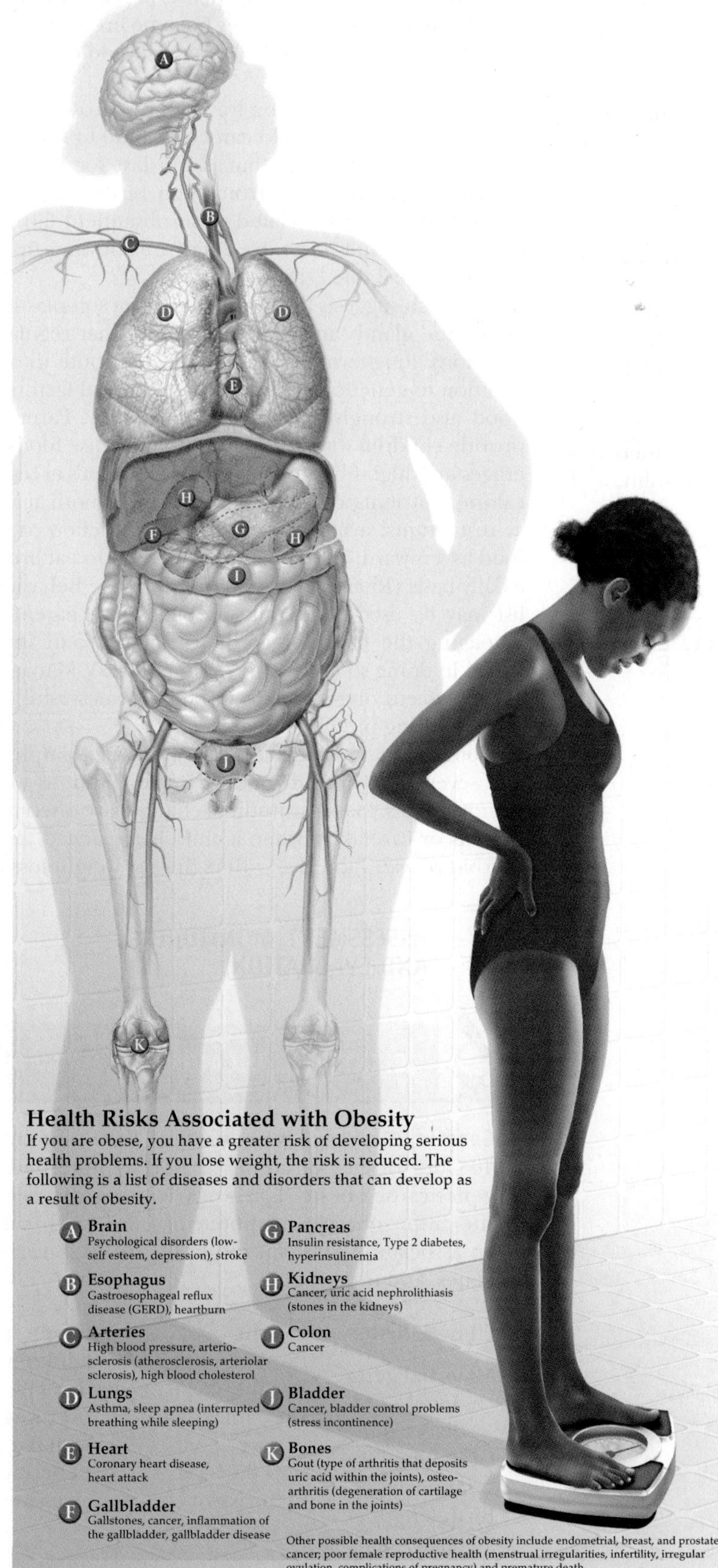

Health Risks Associated with Obesity
If you are obese, you have a greater risk of developing serious health problems. If you lose weight, the risk is reduced. The following is a list of diseases and disorders that can develop as a result of obesity.
A Brain
Psychological disorders (low-self esteem, depression), stroke
B Esophagus
Gastroesophageal reflux disease (GERD), heartburn
C Arteries
High blood pressure, arterio-sclerosis (atherosclerosis, arteriolar sclerosis), high blood cholesterol
D Lungs
Asthma, sleep apnea (interrupted breathing while sleeping)
E Heart
Coronary heart disease, heart attack
F Gallbladder
Gallstones, cancer, inflammation of the gallbladder, gallbladder disease
G Pancreas
Insulin resistance, Type 2 diabetes, hyperinsulinemia
H Kidneys
Cancer, uric acid nephrolithiasis (stones in the kidneys)
I Colon
Cancer
J Bladder
Cancer, bladder control problems (stress incontinence)
K Bones
Gout (type of arthritis that deposits uric acid within the joints), osteo-arthritis (degeneration of cartilage and bone in the joints)
Other possible health consequences of obesity include endometrial, breast, and prostate cancer; poor female reproductive health (menstrual irregularities, infertility, irregular ovulation, complications of pregnancy) and premature death.

Asset provided by Anatomical Chart Co.

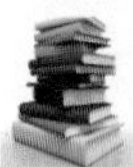

DEFINITIONS AND BACKGROUND

The prevalence of overweight is increasing for children and adolescents in the United States. "At risk for overweight" is defined by the sex- and age-specific ≥85th percentile cutoff points of the CDC growth charts or of BMI for age; overweight or obese is defined as ≥95th percentile of growth charts or BMI for age. BMI increases during the first year of life and then decreases; it begins to rise again at 6–6.5 years of age. BMI tables are not useful before age 2; they are a screening tool and do not reflect body composition well. While BMI tables have limitations, they are considered a reasonable place to begin; an increase in BMI of three to four units is a reason to investigate further.

The preferred weight gain pattern in childhood is as follows: infant doubles birth weight by 6 months and triples birth weight at 12 months. Tripling birth weight before 1 year is associated with increased risk of obesity. In year 2, gain is 8–10 lb (3.5–4.5 kg); in year 3, gain is 4.5–6.5 lb (2–3 kg); annually thereafter, the gain is about 4.5–6.5 lb (2–3 kg). Until 6 years of age, the number of fat cells increases (hyperplasia). After 6 years of age, the size of fat cells increases (hypertrophy). Hormones play a role. Leptin, insulin, and adiponectin regulate lipid metabolism.

TABLE 3-13 Complications of Childhood Obesity

Psychosocial	Poor self-esteem Anxiety Depression Eating disorders Social isolation Lower educational attainment
Neurologic	Pseudotumor cerebri
Endocrine	Insulin resistance Type 2 diabetes Precocious puberty Polycystic ovaries (girls) Hypogonadism (boys)
Cardiovascular	Dyslipidemia Hypertension Coagulopathy Chronic inflammation Endothelial dysfunction
Pulmonary	Sleep apnea Asthma Exercise intolerance
Gastrointestinal	Gastroesophageal reflux Steatohepatitis Gallstones Constipation
Renal	Glomerulosclerosis
Musculoskeletal	Slipped capital femoral epiphysis Blount's disease[a] Forearm fracture Back pain Flat feet

[a]Blount's disease is a growth disorder of the tibia that causes the lower leg to angle inward (tibia vara).

Obesity is an epidemic. Rates of unhealthy body weight among children and adolescents have tripled since the 1980s. Three critical periods for prevention of adult obesity are: ages 5–7 years, adolescence, and pregnancy. Interaction between genes in the fetus and maternal overnutrition or undernutrition are relevant; obese women should attempt healthy weight loss before they become pregnant (American Dietetic Association, 2009). Women should then be encouraged to breastfeed.

After birth, overfeeding for catch-up growth in a premature or underweight child can contribute to obesity; weight gain proceeds at a rate that is too fast for linear growth. Overnutrition, resulting from high birth weight or gestational diabetes, is associated with subsequent fatness in the child. Many adult-onset disorders are showing up in obese children; see Table 3-13.

Research suggests that phthalates from soft plastics disrupt endocrine glands and affect hormones that regulate bodily functions; long-term exposure may contribute to obesity. In addition to genetics and environment, social factors in childhood also strongly influence adult obesity. Parents should provide children with access to nutrient-dense foods and beverages and high-fiber foods; reduce children's access to high-calorie, nutrient-poor beverages and foods both at home and at restaurants; avoid excessive food restriction; do not use food as a reward; and encourage children to eat breakfast on a daily basis (Ritchie et al, 2005). A Lifestyle Behavior Checklist may be used to identify problems that parents have in managing the behavior of their children and their confidence in doing so (West and Sanders, 2009). Management of preadolescent obesity seems to be most successful when it is started during preschool years.

Counseling must distinguish between "simple obesity" and severe or "morbid" obesity in the child, as well as the comorbidities. Major attitudinal changes are often needed in parents or caretakers when a child has reached the severe/morbid phase. Table 3-14 offers tips for weight loss plans.

ASSESSMENT, MONITORING, AND EVALUATION

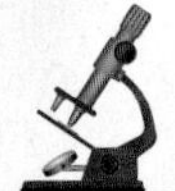

CLINICAL INDICATORS

Genetic Markers: Twin studies have shown that 40–70% of the variation in BMI is inherited. The genetics of obesity is a work in progress; see Web site http://obesitygene.pbrc.edu/. Research suggests an association between the FTO, MC3R, seven other genes, and overweight.

Clinical/History

Maternal gestational diabetes
Gestational age at birth
Birth length, birth weight
Height
Present weight
Weight hx
Diet/intake history
BMI 85–94% = at risk of continuing overweight into adulthood
BMI ≥95% = overweight with need for in-depth assessment

TABLE 3-14 When to Initiate Weight Loss Diets in Children

Children aged 2–7 years	BMI: 85th to 94th percentiles; BMI greater than the 95th percentile with no complications	Maintain weight
	BMI is above the 95th percentile with mild complications (mild hypertension, dyslipidemia, insulin resistance)	Gradual weight loss is recommended
	Patients with acute complications such as pseudotumor cerebri, sleep apnea, obesity hypoventilation syndrome, or orthopedic problems	Refer to a pediatric obesity center
Children 7 years of age and older	BMIs between the 85th and 94th percentiles with no complications	Maintain weight
	If the BMI is between the 85th and 94th percentiles with mild complications or the BMI is equal to or above the 95th percentile	Gradual weight loss is recommended

Source: Marcason W. At what age should an overweight child follow a calorie-restricted diet? *J Am Diet Assoc.* 104:834, 2004.

Family hx of CHD, diabetes mellitus, hypertension, overweight/obesity
Breastfed versus formula or other milk (young child)
BP
Acanthosis nigricans

Number of hours of TV watching per day
Inactive lifestyle?
Skipping meals?

Lab Work

H&H, Serum Fe
Chol, Trig (elevated)?
Serum Hcy
Gluc
Alk phos
Alb
Ca^{++}, Mg^{++}
Na^{+}, K^{+}
LFTs Serum insulin

INTERVENTION

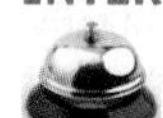

OBJECTIVES

Health Recommendations (American Academy of Pediatrics, 2009)

- Identify and track patients at risk by virtue of family history, birth weight, or socioeconomic, ethnic, cultural, or environmental factors. Calculate and plot BMI annually in all children and adolescents; use change in BMI to identify rate of excessive weight gain relative to linear growth. Develop a weight maintenance or weight loss plan that is individualized for the child.
- Encourage parents and caregivers to promote healthy eating patterns by offering nutritious snacks, such as vegetables and fruits, low-fat dairy foods, and whole grains; encouraging children's autonomy in self-regulation of food intake and setting appropriate limits on choices; and modeling healthy food choices.
- Routinely promote physical activity, including unstructured play at home, in school, in child care settings, and throughout the community. Limit television, computer, and video time to a maximum of 2 h/d.
- Recognize and monitor for risk factors such as hypertension, dyslipidemia, hyperinsulinemia, impaired glucose tolerance, metabolic syndrome, early puberty, liver disease, eating disorders, skin infections, food allergies, asthma, and sleep apnea.
- Discuss tips that are easily handled by the dietetics professional; refer complex cases to a behavioral specialist. Discourage the use of sweets and foods to reward behavior. Avoid the "clean plate" theory, but be wary about withholding food, which can have the opposite effect.

SAMPLE NUTRITION CARE PROCESS STEPS

Overweight

Assessment Data: Weight and growth charts, physical activity pattern showing sedentary lifestyle and minimal activity (no recess, outside activity swing use set only), BMI >85 percentile for age.

Nutrition Diagnoses (PES): Excessive energy intake (N1-1.5 or N1-2.2) related to low physical activity level and intake of high calorie snacks as evidenced by diet and activity records.

Interventions:

Food-nutrient delivery:

ND 1.1. General healthful diet; establishing regular meal patterns (three meals a day with two snacks) that follow healthy plate tool, incorporating fiber into the diet (more whole grains, more fruits and vegetables), increasing to about 26 g/d.

ND 1.3. Specific foods and beverages (healthy snacks and low-calorie beverages).

Education:

E 1. Initial/brief nutrition education on label reading, portion sizes of food, and fiber intake. Educate parents about how to increase activity levels with games, dancing, outside play, and healthier, lower calorie snacks and beverages.

Counseling:

C 2. Nutritional-related cognitive behavioral therapy using motivational interviewing to determine what parents and patient want to change and are willing to work on regarding high fat/sugary foods in the home, frequent fast food meals, and inadequate fiber intake.

Coordination of care

RC 1. Referral to an agency or dietitian who conducts grocery store tours to help choose foods more wisely.

Monitoring and Evaluation: Weight records, growth chart showing improved height for weight (below 85 percentile BMI) for age.

- Help the child "find" the right body for him or her. Encourage self-recognition of hunger cues (e.g., stop eating when feeling "full").

Advocacy Objectives

- Help parents, teachers, coaches, and others who influence youth to discuss health habits, not body build, as part of their efforts to control overweight and obesity.
- Enlist policy makers from local, state, and national organizations and schools to support a healthful lifestyle for all children, including a proper diet and adequate opportunity for a regular physical activity.
- Encourage organizations that are responsible for health care and health care financing to provide coverage for effective obesity prevention and treatment strategies.
- Encourage public and private sources to direct funding toward research on effective strategies to prevent overweight and obesity and to maximize limited family and community resources.
- Support social marketing that promotes healthful food choices and increased physical activity.

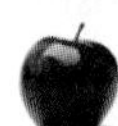

FOOD AND NUTRITION

- Support needs for the child according to age and sex of the child: protein at 10–35%, fat at 25–40%, and CHO at 45–65% (Institute of Medicine, 2002). Plan a diet with basal calories plus activity, and likelihood of growth spurts.
- Weight loss is typically recommended for children over age 7 or for younger children who have related health concerns; slow and steady—anywhere from 1 lb/wk to 1 lb/mo (Mayo Clinic, 2009).
- For family teaching, discuss easy behavioral changes. Place less emphasis on a specific calorie level than on portion sizes that are child-appropriate. Use MyPyramid for kids.
- Emphasize low-fat, low-cholesterol foods with elevated cholesterol. Use plant stanols and sterols in the diet.
- Reduce the energy intake by reducing the energy density of foods, increasing fresh fruits and nonstarchy vegetables low-calorie versions of products. Decrease the use of sweets as snack foods or dessert. Decrease the use of fatty or fried foods.
- Include sources of iron, B-complex vitamins, vitamin C, and protein, if needed to correct anemias.
- Limit milk to a reasonable daily amount for the age. Be sure others foods are consumed in addition to milk. Use low-fat or skim milk after 2 years of age.
- Limit juice to 6 oz for young children. Limit sugar-sweetened beverages in general.
- Added sugars in foods/beverages should comprise <25% of total calories consumed.
- Control between-meal snacks; offer fresh fruit or vegetables, plain crackers, pretzels, plain popcorn, cooked egg slices, unsweetened fruit or vegetable juices, and low-fat cheese cubes. Age-appropriate snacks are important; avoid popcorn and other foods that may cause choking in young children.
- Give small helpings at meals; allow more small helpings until "full." Discuss "hunger cues" and "satiety cues."
- Ensure that the family has adequate fluoridated water, as dental caries are common.

Common Drugs Used and Potential Side Effects

- Discourage the use of drugs for weight loss; no diet medicines are safe for children younger than 16 years. Sibutramine added to a comprehensive behavioral program for teens can induce significant weight loss.
- Antidepressants are sometimes prescribed for childhood depression, which is common. Side effects such as changes in metabolism and appetite can contribute to obesity in some children. Both childhood depression and anxiety are associated with increased BMI percentiles; childhood psychopathology is an important factor that should be carefully monitored (Rofey et al, 2009).

Herbs, Botanicals, and Supplements

- Herbs and botanicals should not be used for childhood obesity; there are no controlled trials to prove efficacy or safety.
- Physicians may ask dietitians to discuss herbs, botanicals, life cycle, and disease-specific and obesity guidance with their patients.

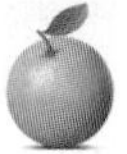

NUTRITION EDUCATION, COUNSELING, CARE MANAGEMENT

- Responsibilities should be shared. Parents are responsible for a proper emotional setting and for what is offered; the child is responsible for what and how much is eaten (Satter, 2009). Emphasis becomes *supporting each child's normal growth* (Satter, 2009). See Table 3-15 for more tips.
- Intervention should start early and focus on the family, not just the child. Educate parents about the dangers of medical complications.
- Discuss age-appropriate portions and snacks. Many parents innocently overfeed their children; show them child-sized plates and utensils with sample portion sizes.
- Try to alter intake of one "problem food" per visit (regular soda or sugar-sweetened fruit punch). Diluting juice, substituting lower calorie beverages, and calculating number of calories saved can be quite effective. Reading labels is a useful teaching tool.
- Tailor treatment and prevention efforts for each person. Interactive interventions and self-monitoring are keys to success for many individuals (Lombard et al, 2009). Internet-based coaching sessions may be quite helpful as they can be tailored to the individual's needs and concerns (Block et al, 2008).
- Integrate culturally appropriate approaches and strategies. Bilingual professionals might help with developing culturally sensitive programming.
- Encourage regular family meals whenever possible; limit unplanned or habitual snacking. Between meals, ice water can be offered as a special treat instead of sweetened beverages. Good role modeling by parents is essential. Maintain the child's self-image through positive reinforcement.
- Discuss the relationship of food, weight, and energy balance. Metabolic rates are low while watching television. When working with families to prevent and treat childhood

TABLE 3-15 Components of Successful Weight Loss for Children

Component	Comment
Reasonable weight loss goal	Initially, a rate of 1 lb per month if <95th or >85th percentile with comorbidity, based on age.
Dietary management	Guide family choices rather than dictating; encourage child to eat when hungry and to eat slowly. Encourage family meals. Avoid using food as reward or withholding as punishment. Drink plenty of water and limit sugar-sweetened beverages. Plan healthy snacks. Aim for five servings of fruits and vegetables each day. Promote healthy breakfast each day. Consume milk with dinner instead of soft drinks.
Physical activity	Begin according to child's fitness level, with ultimate goal of 60 minutes of moderate activity daily.
Behavior modification	Teach self-monitoring, nutritional education, control of cues, modification of eating habits, physical activity, attitude change, reinforcements, and rewards.
Family involvement	Review family activity and television viewing patterns; involve parents in nutrition counseling.

Adapted from: Mullen MC, Shield J. *Childhood and adolescent overweight: the health professional's guide to identification, treatment and prevention*. Chicago, IL: American Dietetic Association, 2004.

weight problems, one should attend to children's time spent with screen media, the frequency of family mealtimes, and parents' perceptions of neighborhood safety for children's outdoor play (Gable et al, 2007). Limit television and nonproductive computer time to <2 hours daily (American Academy of Pediatrics, 2009). Encourage activity, such as jogging, ball games, swimming, bike riding, and school-based physical activities, since many children who enter adolescence overweight will become overweight or obese adults. Dance videos are easy to do at home, especially for children who are self-conscious.

- Discourage potentially dangerous weight-control schemes or practices.
- A system for "traffic light" foods can be used for younger children: green for "go" foods, yellow for "caution" foods, and red for "stop" foods.
- Parents who practice restrained eating with their children tend to be overly indulgent later (fast/feast); the result is chronic anxiety. Eating can become very controlled, inconsistent, and emotional. Highlight nonfood-related achievements; avoid nagging about diet or food.
- In extreme obesity, bariatric surgery may be needed. Improved quality of life generally occurs for teens (Murray, 2008). However, there are profound implications and risks that differ from adults; they may have greater weight regain and may be noncompliant with treatment after surgery (Levitsky et al, 2009). Research on nonsurgical treatments is on-going.

Patient Education—Food Safety

- Hand washing with soap and hot water is recommended before preparing meals.
- Before using tap water as a beverage, let cold tap water run for 2 minutes to remove any lead that may be in the pipes.
- Follow the 2-hour rule: discard beverage or food that has been left at room temperature for 2+ hours.

For More Information

- Blueprint for Physical Activity
  http://movingtothefuture.org/frontpage_files/55/55_frontpage_file1.pdf
- CDP
  http://www.cdc.gov/nchs/products/pubs/pubd/hestats/overwght99.htm
- Center for Health and Health Care in Schools
  http://www.healthinschools.org/Health-in-Schools/Health-Services/Schools-and-Childhood-Overweight.aspx
- CDC Charts for BMI in Children and Teens
  http://apps.nccd.cdc.gov/dnpabmi/
- CDC Contributing Factors in Childhood Obesity
  http://www.cdc.gov/nccdphp/dnpa/obesity/childhood/contributing_factors.htm
- Ellyn Satter Institute
  http://www.ellynsatter.com/
- Healthy Youth
  http://www.cdc.gov/HealthyYouth/nutrition/facts.htm
- International Food Information Council
  http://ific.org/nutrition/obesity/index.cfm
- Maternal and Child Nutrition Center
  http://www.mchlibrary.info/KnowledgePaths/kp_overweight.html
- MyPyramid for Kids
  http://www.cnpp.usda.gov/MyPyramidforKids.htm
- NIDDK Weight Control Network
  http://win.niddk.nih.gov/publications/over_child.htm
- University of Minnesota Nutrition Curriculum
  http://www.epi.umn.edu/let/nutri/chobese/assess.shtm

OBESITY, CHILDHOOD—CITED REFERENCES

American Academy of Pediatrics. Overweight and obesity. Accessed May 5, 2009, at http://www.aap.org/healthtopics/overweight.cfm.

American Dietetic Association. Position of the American Dietetic Association and American Society for Nutrition: obesity, reproduction, and pregnancy outcomes. *J Am Diet Assoc.* 109:918, 2009.

Block G, et al. Development of Alive! (A Lifestyle Intervention Via Email), and its effect on health-related quality of life, presenteeism, and other behavioral outcomes: randomized controlled trial. *J Med Internet Res.* 10:e43, 2008.

Gable S, et al. Television watching and frequency of family meals are predictive of overweight onset and persistence in a national sample of school-aged children. *J Am Diet Assoc.* 107:53, 2007.

Institute of Medicine, Food and Nutrition Board. (2002). *Dietary reference intakes for energy, carbohydrate, fiber, fat, fatty acids, cholesterol, protein, and amino acids, vitamin a, vitamin k, arsenic, boron, chromium, copper, iodine, iron, manganese, molybdenum, nickel, silicon, vanadium, and zinc.* Washington, DC: National Academy Press, 2002.

Levitsky LL, et al. Adolescent obesity and bariatric surgery. *Current Opin Endocrinol Diab Obes.* 16:37, 2009.

Lombard CB, et al. Weight, physical activity and dietary behaviour change in a population of young mothers: short term results of the HeLP-her cluster randomized controlled trial. *Nutr J.* 8:17, 2009.

Mayo Clinic. Childhood obesity. Accessed May 5, 2009, at http://www.mayoclinic.com/health/childhood-obesity/DS00698/DSECTION=treatments-and-drugs.

Murray PJ. Bariatric surgery in adolescents: mechanics, metabolism, and medical care. *Adolesc Med State art Rev.* 19:450, 2008.

Ritchie LD, et al. Family environment and pediatric overweight: what is a parent to do? *J Am Diet Assoc.* 105:70S, 2005.

Rofey DL, et al. A longitudinal study of childhood depression and anxiety in relation to weight gain. *Child Psychiatry Hum Dev.* 40(4):517–526, 2009.

Satter E. Ellyn Satter Associates. Accessed May 4, 2009, at http://www.ellynsatter.com.

West F, Sanders MR. The Lifestyle Behaviour Checklist: a measure of weight-related problem behaviour in obese children. *Int J Pediatr Obesity.*12;1–8, 2009.

OTITIS MEDIA

NUTRITIONAL ACUITY RANKING: LEVEL 1

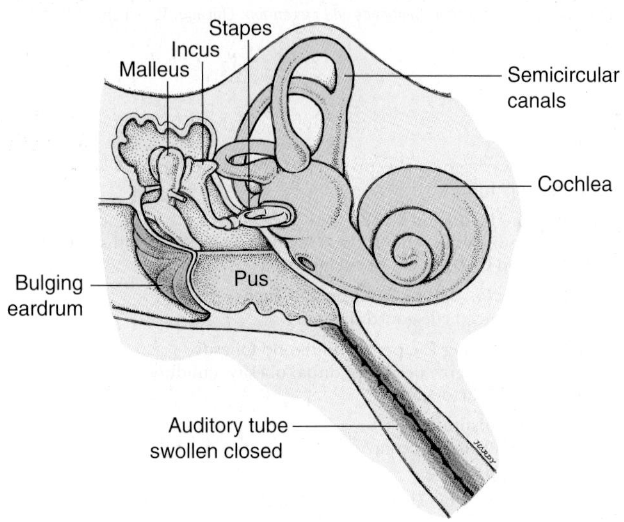

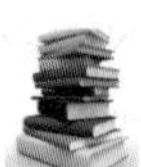

DEFINITIONS AND BACKGROUND

Acute OM (acute middle ear infection) occurs when there is a bacterial or viral infection of the fluid of the middle ear that leads to production of pus, excess fluid, or even bleeding in the middle ear. The Eustachian tube becomes clogged. Tubes of the ear of a child are shorter and less slanted than in adults, allowing bacteria and viruses to find their way into the middle ear more easily. Pressure from fluids associated with OM may cause the eardrum to rupture.

Ear infections often occur along with respiratory infections (such as *H. influenza*) or with blocked sinuses and Eustachian tubes caused by allergies. OM with effusions (OME) can lead to significant hearing loss in children if not properly treated. Recent illness of any type and lowered immunity; crowded or unsanitary living conditions; genetic factors; cold climate and high altitude; and bottle feeding of infants (can allow fluid to pool in the throat near the Eustachian tube) may be etiologies. LBW infants may be prone to repeated ear infections.

Breast milk is more protective than formula feeding (Ip et al, 2007). Breast milk contains lactoferrin and a number of other anti-inflammatory factors (Hanson, 2007). The prevalence of early-onset and repeated OM continues to increase among preschool children; an increase in prevalence of allergic conditions is a concern (Auinger et al, 2003).

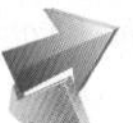

ASSESSMENT, MONITORING, AND EVALUATION

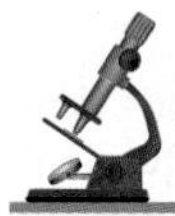

CLINICAL INDICATORS

Genetic Markers: Susceptibility to infections may run in families.

Clinical/History	I & O	Lab Work
Height Birth length Birth weight Present weight Diet/intake history Family history of asthma, allergies	Fever? Irritability, fussiness? Exposure to cigarette smoking? Audiometry	H & H Serum Fe Chol, Trig Gluc Alb Na^+, K^+ Serum IgE and allergy testing

INTERVENTION

OBJECTIVES

- Promote breastfeeding of newborns, especially for 6 months or longer.
- If formula fed, babies should be positioned in a semi-upright position so that the milk will flow downward into the baby's stomach and not wash up and into the baby's nasal passages and up through the Eustachian tubes. Always position the infant's head higher than the stomach.
- In older children, monitor nutrient density of the diet to maintain a healthy immune system. Inclusion of more fruit and a children's multivitamin–mineral supplement may be needed for poor eaters or during food jags.
- Prevent chronic suppurative OM and hearing loss.

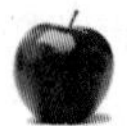

FOOD AND NUTRITION

- Determine the recommended allowances for the child's age group: kilocal, protein, and other nutrients. Plan a reasonable menu pattern accordingly.

SAMPLE NUTRITION CARE PROCESS STEPS

Intake of Unsafe Foods

Assessment Data: Diet and intake history, recent lab testing indicating allergy to milk and eggs, frequent ear infections, notation that infant was not breastfed after 3 weeks of age.

Nutrition Diagnoses (PES): Intake of unsafe foods related to recent identification of specific food allergies (milk, eggs) as evidenced by six ear infections in past 2 years.

Intervention: Educate parents about foods that are to eat/prepare; food labeling; choices at restaurants, schools. Counsel about adapting recipes and holiday meals that suit the family.

Monitoring and Evaluation: Alleviation of responses to food allergens, improvement or elimination of food allergy reactions at home, at school, and out at restaurants. Improved nutritional quality of life as observed by parent(s).

- Highlight foods that include sufficient levels of iron, vitamins A, D_3, and C, and zinc to support a healthy immune system to fight further infections. Studies are under way to determine if antioxidant-rich foods make any difference in healing.
- If child has food allergies, discuss options for maintaining a healthy diet, especially if large food group categories must be eliminated.

Common Drugs Used and Potential Side Effects

- Antibiotics such as penicillin are often prescribed for bacterial infections; side effects may include rash, vomiting, and diarrhea. Viral infections have to run their course.
- Vaccines may be available for some of the bacterial agents that cause OM.

Herbs, Botanicals, and Supplements

- Xylitol may have anti-adhesive factors for reducing infections, but no commonly available products have been tested.
- Probiotics in foods such as yogurt can help to replenish the gut and support healthy immunity.

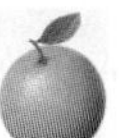

NUTRITION EDUCATION, COUNSELING, CARE MANAGEMENT

- Explain to parents that overfeeding can aggravate asthma, which is often triggered by bouts of OM. If needed, teach principles for managing food allergies and asthma.
- Toddlers should not be taking a bottle to bed.
- Discuss the role of nutrition and immunity.
- Chronic recurrence should be addressed with an ear-nose-throat specialist to prevent hearing loss and speech delay.
- Smoking around the child should be discontinued (Kuiper et al, 2007).
- Use of pacifiers, cow's milk allergy, environmental smoke or mold, and other issues may be problematic. More clinical trials are needed to determine the best advice.

For More Information

- Family Doctor
  http://familydoctor.org/055.xml
- I-tonsil
  http://www.itonsil.com/index.html
- National Speech and Hearing Association
  http://www.asha.org/public/hearing/disorders/causes.htm
- NIH Health and Hearing
  http://www.nidcd.nih.gov/health/hearing/otitism.asp

OTITIS MEDIA—CITED REFERENCES

Auinger P, et al. Trends in otitis media among children in the United States. *Pediatrics.* 112:514, 2003.

Hanson LA. Session 1: Feeding and infant development breast-feeding and immune function. *Proc Nutr Soc.* 66:384, 2007.

Ip S, et al. Breastfeeding and maternal and infant health outcomes in developed countries. *Evid Rep Technol Assess.* 153:1, 2007.

Kuiper S, et al. Interactive effect of family history and environmental factors on respiratory tract-related morbidity in infancy. *J Allergy Clin Immunol.* 120:388, 2007.

PHENYLKETONURIA

NUTRITIONAL ACUITY RANKING: LEVEL 4

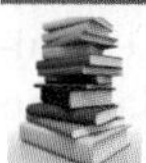

DEFINITIONS AND BACKGROUND

Phenylketonuria (PKU) is a rare, inherited condition that occurs in one in 10,000 births. Phenylalanine (Phe) is not metabolized to tyrosine because of a mutation in Phe hydroxylase. Infants are tested for this disorder after birth and after the first feeding and again if levels of Phe are above given cutoff levels (≥6 mg/dL). If very strict diets are followed early and continually, normal development and life span are possible. Children with PKU who follow their special diet for life have fewer intellectual and neurological deficits; do not discontinue at any age. Refer to a metabolic dietitian or special programs at the state level.

Desirable serum Phe levels are below 10 mg/dL; higher levels are associated with declining IQ. There is international consensus that patients with Phe levels <360 μM on a free diet do not need Phe-lowering dietary treatment, whereas patients with levels >600 μM do. In general, however, "diet for life" is the rule, especially for women with PKU who are considering pregnancy.

Tyrosine is an essential amino acid in patients with PKU because of the limited Phe converted to tyrosine. Treatment with large neutral amino acid supplements may help to correct low or deficient blood concentrations of both tyrosine and tryptophan, which are precursors for dopamine and serotonin (Koch et al, 2003). Individuals who follow diets low in natural proteins should be advised to take selenium and iron supplements (Acosta et al, 2004).

Serum lipids are usually under good control because of the vegetarian-type diet needed for PKU (Schulpis et al, 2003). However, micronutrient status of folic acid and vitamins B_6 and B_{12} can be low, and there may be a risk for coronary artery disease.

Tetrahydrobiopterin (BH4) is the natural cofactor that fuels the activity of the phenylalanine hydroxylase (PAH) enzyme. When BH4 is given orally to some people with PKU, the activity of mutated PAH improves; this is "BH4-responsive PKU" in which lowering of Phe by 30% has been seen (Michals-Matalon, 2008; Michals-Matalon et al, 2007). This gives an exciting new treatment for PKU for those who are responsive.

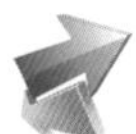

ASSESSMENT, MONITORING, AND EVALUATION

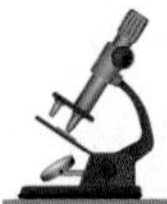

CLINICAL INDICATORS

Genetic Markers: Mutation in the phenylalanine hydroxylase (PAH) gene.

Clinical/History

Birth weight
Present weight
Growth (%)
Diet/intake history
Developmental delay
Retardation?
Musty odor in urine and sweat
Length/height
Dry skin or dermatitis
Blonder hair than siblings
Electroencephalograms (EEGs)
Seizures

Lab Work

Response to dose of 10 mg/kg BH4
Plasma Phe
Urinary Phe
Plasma tyrosine
H & H, serum Fe, ferritin
Serum pyridoxine, vitamin B_{12}, folic acid
Serum carnitine (may be low)
Serum zinc and selenium

INTERVENTION

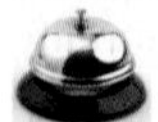

OBJECTIVES

- Prevent toxic buildup of abnormal metabolites to prevent mental retardation, and to promote normal intellectual and social development.
- Establish the child's daily requirement for Phe, protein, and energy according to age. The appropriate Phe intake for age is as follows: infants 0–3 months, 60–90 mg/kg; infants 4–6 months, 40 mg/kg; infants 7–9 months, 35 mg/kg; infants 10–12 months, 30 mg/kg; children 1–2 years, 25 mg/kg; and children 2+ years, 20 mg/kg of body weight.
- Provide a diet aiding growth and development with a high energy to protein ratio to spare protein.
- Introduce solids and textures at usual ages; encourage self-feeding when it is possible for the infant.
- Establish a positive attitude toward the modified diet for parents, caretakers, and the child.
- Monitor for deficiency in nutrients, such as DHA, vitamin B_{12}, folic acid, selenium, and iron.

SAMPLE NUTRITION CARE PROCESS STEPS

Inappropriate Intake of Types of Amino Acids

Assessment Data: Diet intake records, serum lab values of Phe, previous education on appropriate diet for PKU management; negative response to BH4 administration.

Nutrition Diagnosis: Inappropriate intake of amino acids related to low comprehension of nutrition care plan as evidenced by serum Phe level of 12 mg/dL, where >8 mg/dL indicates loss of dietary control in PKU.

Intervention: Counseling on Phe in diet, use of special formulas and products, referral to State Health Department for resources and financial support, referral to child health clinics.

Monitoring and Evaluation: Serum Phe reports, changes in mental health status and alertness.

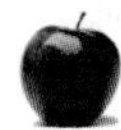

FOOD AND NUTRITION

- Use a diet low in Phe. Use special milk substitutes made from casein hydrolysate, corn oil, corn syrup, tapioca starch, minerals, and vitamins: Phenyl-free, or Maxamaid XP. Phenyl-free does not provide total nutritional needs. Phlexy-10 is available from SHS North America.
- Initially, the infant's tolerance must be assessed individually, and progress in treatment must develop accordingly. A small amount of milk and 85–100% from specialty formula are used to meet the infant's needs. Subtract Phe requirement in formula from total needs (the difference is that which is provided by solid foods).
- Glycomacropeptide (GMP), an intact protein formed from cheese whey, contains minimal Phe and can be supplemented with limiting AAs as a safe and highly acceptable alternative to synthetic AAs as the primary protein source in PKU (van Calcar et al, 2009). It is now recognized that the phenalalanine:tyrosine ratio affects executive function in PKU, so care must be taken to plan the diet properly (Sharman et al, 2009).
- Determine if serum iron, vitamin B_{12}, folic acid, selenium, or other nutrient levels are low and enhance diet or use a multivitamin–mineral supplement as needed.
- Introduce solids and textures at the appropriate ages. Omit meat, fish, poultry, bread, milk, cheese, legumes, and peanut butter from the diet of older children. Try

using low-protein bread, pasta, crackers, cookies, and muffin mixes.

- To add calories, try jam, jelly, sugar, honey, molasses, syrups, cornstarch, and oils that are Phe-free. Flavors can be added to the formula to continue its use as a beverage.
- Fish oil supplements may be used to replace the DHA missing from a standard Phe-free diet; this helps improve neurologic development and fine motor coordination (Beblo, 2007). The exact amount of DHA needed is not known (Koletzko et al, 2009).

Common Drugs Used and Potential Side Effects

- Kuvan (phenoptin) contains sapropterin dihydrochloride, a synthetic dihydrochloride salt of naturally occurring tetrahydrobiopterin (BH4). Individuals with PKU should be tested to determine if they could benefit from taking this medication (Michals-Matalon, 2008; Trefz et al, 2009).

Herbs, Botanicals, and Supplements

- Herbs and botanical products are not recommended for use in PKU.
- Fish oil supplements may be beneficial (Koletzko et al, 2009; Beblo, 2007).

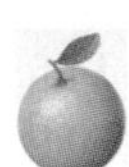

NUTRITION EDUCATION, COUNSELING, CARE MANAGEMENT

- Because initial acceptance of formula may be poor due to its strong taste, the mother should be careful not to express her own distaste. Recommend appropriate recipes and cookbooks.
- Monitor the calculation of Phe in the diet. Avoid items sweetened with aspartame (NutraSweet), including diet sodas.
- School challenges vary, but the diet provides good control for most cases (Filiano, 2006). Attention deficit disorder can present as the child grows older.
- Self-management should begin by 7–8 years of age, at least for formula preparation. By 12 years of age, the child should begin calculating his or her own intake of Phe from foods.
- Women who have PKU tend to give birth to children with microcephaly, mental retardation, congenital heart defects, and IUGR. Metabolic control by the end of the first trimester is, therefore, important as a goal. Treatment at any time during pregnancy may reduce the severity of delayed development. Referral to a metabolic dietitian is highly recommended.

Patient Education—Food Safety

- Hand washing with soap and hot water is recommended before preparing formula or meals. Use clean utensils and containers for mixing formula.
- Before using tap water for formula preparation or to give as a beverage, let cold tap water run for 2 minutes to remove any lead that may be in the pipes.
- Follow the 2-hour rule: discard any beverage or food that has been left at room temperature for 2 hours or longer.
- Do not use honey in the diets of infants to decrease potential risk of botulism.

For More Information

- Children's PKU Network
  http://www.kumc.edu/gec/support/pku.html
- Diet Tips for PKU
  http://www.pkunews.org/
- March of Dimes—PKU
  http://www.marchofdimes.com/professionals/14332_1219.asp
- National Coalition for PKU and Allied Disorders
  http://www.pku-allieddisorders.org/
- PKU News
  www.pkunews.org
- Save babies
  http://www.savebabies.org/diseasedescriptions/pku.php

PHENYLKETONURIA—CITED REFERENCES

Acosta P, et al. Iron status of children with phenylketonuria undergoing nutrition therapy assessed by transferrin receptors. *Genet Med.* 6:96, 2004.

Beblo S. Effect of fish oil supplementation on fatty acid status, coordination, and fine motor skills in children with phenylketonuria. *J Pediatr.* 150:479, 2007.

Filiano JJ. Neurometabolic diseases in the newborn. *Clin Perinatol.* 33:411, 2006.

Koletzko B, et al. Omega-3 LC-PUFA supply and neurological outcomes in children with phenylketonuria (PKU). *J Pediatr Gastroenterol Nutr.* 48:2S, 2009.

Michals-Matalon K. Sapropterin dihydrochloride, 6-R-L-erythro-5,6,7,8-tetrahydrobiopterin, in the treatment of phenylketonuria. *Expert Opin Investig Drugs.* 17:245, 2008.

Michals-Matalon K, et al. Response of phenylketonuria to tetrahydrobiopterin. *J Nutr.* 137:1564, 2007.

Sharman R, et al. Biochemical markers associated with executive function in adolescents with early and continuously treated phenylketonuria. *Clin Genet.* 75:169, 2009.

Trefz FK, et al. Efficacy of sapropterin dihydrochloride in increasing phenylalanine tolerance in children with phenylketonuria: a phase III, randomized, double-blind, placebo-controlled study. *J Pediatr.* 154:700, 2009.

van Calcar SC, et al. Improved nutritional management of phenylketonuria by using a diet containing glycomacropeptide compared with amino acids. *Am J Clin Nutr.* 89:1068, 2009.

PRADER-WILLI SYNDROME

NUTRITIONAL ACUITY RANKING: LEVEL 3–4

Prader-Willi Food Pyramid

FATS & SWEETS
Use sparingly

MEAT, POULTRY, FISH, DRY BEANS, EGGS
1–2 servings daily, 2 oz. each

MILK, YOGURT & CHEESE GROUP
2 servings daily

BREAD, CEREAL, RICE & PASTA GROUP
3–5 servings daily

RICE

FRUIT GROUP
4 servings daily

VEGETABLE GROUP
6–8 servings daily

Prader-Willi Food Pyramid http://www.pwsausa.org/syndrome/foodpyramid.htm.

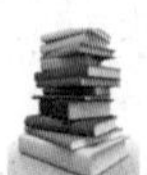

DEFINITIONS AND BACKGROUND

Prader-Willi syndrome (PWS) is a disorder caused by DNA abnormalities of chromosome 15. Major characteristics are infant hypotonia, hypogonadism, mental retardation (average IQ is around 70), small hands and feet, atypical facial features, and obesity because of insatiable appetite in early childhood. Short stature is part of the syndrome and is not nutritional in origin.

The incidence of PWS is 1 in 10,000–16,000 births in the United States. Onset occurs at birth, but symptoms begin by 1–4 years of age. PWS infants often present with absence of crying, poor suck, lethargy, and floppy muscle tone (hypotonia). Motor development is delayed. Hyperphagia results in marked obesity with high risk of metabolic and cardiovascular complications (Schmidt et al, 2008). Lifelong morbidities include osteoporosis, type 2 diabetes, respiratory disorders, and cardiorespiratory failure related to obesity and hypotonia (Allen and Carrel, 2004). Sexual development is incomplete; most PWS individuals are infertile.

Ghrelin levels are high in PWS (DelParigi et al, 2002). It is produced mostly by the stomach but also by the pituitary, hypothalamus, GI tract, lung, heart, pancreas, kidney, and testis. Ghrelin stimulates GH secretion, appetite and food intake, fat mass deposition, and weight gain gastric motility and acid secretion; exerts cardiovascular and anti-inflammatory effects; modulates cell proliferation; and influences endocrine and exocrine pancreatic secretion, as well as glucose and lipid metabolism.

Early dietary treatment starting at the second year of life and continued until the age of 10 years is effective in avoiding excessive weight gain in patients with PWS, but results in shorter stature; GH may be useful (Eiholzer and Whitman, 2004; Schmidt et al, 2008). Individuals with PWS are not able to control their food sneaking, stealing, and gorging behaviors. Because they are difficult to manage, approximately 75% of PWS patients live in group homes. Distinction of behavioral problems from psychiatric illness is important as well (Goldstone et al, 2008).

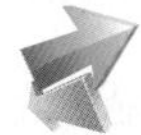

ASSESSMENT, MONITORING, AND EVALUATION

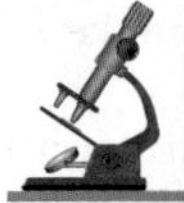

CLINICAL INDICATORS

Genetic Markers: The OCA2 gene is associated with PWS in the long arm of chromosome 15 (region 15q11–q13). In 99% of cases of PWS, the child has two chromosome regions that are both maternally inherited; DNA from the father is missing for chromosome 15 (Isaacs and Zang, 2007).

Clinical/History		
Height	FTT, then rapid weight gain between 1 and 6 years of age	BMI
Birth weight		Slow mental development
		Almond shaped eyes

Irregular areas of skin (bands, stripes, or lines)
Small head, hands, feet
Sleep apnea
Asthma?
Hypotonia, floppy limbs
Down-turned mouth
Hyperphagia
Light hair, eyes

Lab Work

DNA-based diagnostic testing of chromosome 15
Hyperghrelinemia
Gluc, Glucose tolerance test (GTT)
Alb
BP
Chol, Trig
LFTs pCO_2, pO_2
H & H
Serum Fe

INTERVENTION

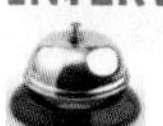

OBJECTIVES

- Reduce excess weight. Monitor weight weekly.
- In preschool children, prevent obesity.
- Maintain recommended dietary intakes for all nutrients, especially protein to promote growth and development.
- Provide feeding assistance if needed.
- Prevent complications including CHD, hypertension, diabetes, sleep apnea, dental problems, and pneumonia. Correct serum lipid levels if elevated.
- Minimize unusual food-seeking behaviors such as eating food from the trash or eating inappropriate or unpalatable food combinations. Correct pica and related nutritional deficits, especially iron.
- Promote an exercise program.

SAMPLE NUTRITION DIAGNOSES

PWS

Assessment Data: Diet, weight, and physical activity histories.

Nutrition Diagnosis: Obesity related to excessive nutrient intake as evidenced by BMI of 35 and nutrition history indicating consumption of 2900 kcal/d and sneaking of foods between meals.

Interventions:

Food and Nutrient Delivery:

ND 1.3. Use of the Prader-Willi food pyramid to plan meals.

ND 5.7. Adjust availability and locations of foods kept in the house to minimize food sneaking.

Education:

E 2.5. Teach portions based on the PW food pyramid. Give examples of meals and snacks based on total servings from food groups; provide examples of age-appropriate physical activities.

Counseling:

Appropriate nutrient intake, enhancing physical activity, and keeping logs. Use of "Go-Caution-No" foods in color-coded "stoplight" system.

Monitoring and Evaluation: Have patient return in 1 month to assess weight, diet, and activity logs.

FOOD AND NUTRITION

- Often, these children start with FTT and then become obese by age six; identify where the child is on this continuum. Gavage feeding may be needed for infants.
- Use 10–11 kcal/cm of height to maintain weight; 8.5 kcal/cm for slow weight loss (Lucas, 2004, p. 41). For older teens, reduce the total calorie level to 7–8 kcal/cm for weight loss, or 10–14 kcal/cm to maintain). Patients' needs are about 60% of those without PWS.
- Ensure that the diet provides adequate protein and nutrients with RDAs for age.

Common Drugs Used and Potential Side Effects

- Weight loss products have not proven to be useful in this population. Drugs may react differently and are, therefore, not recommended.
- GH may be used to correct short stature and hormone replacement therapy may be used to improve signs of osteopenia or osteoporosis (Allen and Carrel, 2004; Schmidt et al, 2008).
- Ghrelin antagonists are being developed. Ghrelin peaks are related to habitual meal patterns and tend to rise in anticipation of eating rather than eliciting feeding (Frecka and Mattes, 2008).

Herbs, Botanicals, and Supplements

- Persons with PWS may be more sensitive; small doses of herbs and drugs may cause a greater reaction than in other people (see http://www.pwsausa.org/syndrome/herbal.htm). Therefore, herbs and botanicals should not be used.

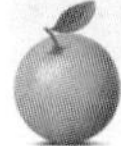

NUTRITION EDUCATION, COUNSELING, CARE MANAGEMENT

- Discuss feeding practices plus activity factors. Encourage daily activity.
- Behavior modification is an important part of treatment. Help the patient lose weight with specific behavior modification techniques; teach the green/yellow/red (go/caution/stop) method for food choices.
- Record keeping and calorie counting are useful. Control of excess intake is the main goal; locked refrigerators or cupboards may be needed.
- An interdisciplinary approach is useful (Eiholzer and Whitman, 2004). There is a need to reduce guilt and depression; self-monitoring is the eventual goal.

For More Information

- Heimlich Maneuver—for choking
  http://www.heimlichinstitute.org/howtodo.html#chokingAnchor
- NIH—Prader Willi
  http://ghr.nlm.nih.gov/condition=praderwillisyndrome/show/NIH+Publications
- Prader Willi Pyramid
  http://www.pwsausa.org/syndrome/foodpyramid.htm
- Prader-Willi Syndrome Association
  http://www.pwsausa.org/

PRADER-WILLI SYNDROME—CITED REFERENCES

Allen DB, Carrel AL. Growth hormone therapy for Prader-Willi syndrome: a critical appraisal. *J Pediatr Endocrinol Metab.* S17;1297S, 2004.

Eiholzer U, Whitman BY. A comprehensive team approach to the management of patients with Prader-Willi syndrome. *J Pediatr Endocrinol Metab.* 17:1153, 2004.

DelParigi A, et al. High circulating ghrelin: a potential calcium use for hyperphagia and obesity in Prader-Willi syndrome. *J Clin Endocrinol Metab.* 87:5461, 2002.

Frecka JM, Mattes RD. Possible entrainment of ghrelin to habitual meal patterns in humans. *Am J Physiol Gastrointest Liver Physiol.* 294:699, 2008.

Goldstone AP, et al. Recommendations for the diagnosis and management of Prader-Willi syndrome. *J Clin Endocrinol Metab.* 93:4183, 2008.

Lucas B, ed. *Children with special care needs: nutrition care handbook.* Chicago, IL: The American Dietetic Association, 2004.

Schmidt H, et al. Successful early dietary intervention avoids obesity in patients with Prader-Willi syndrome: a ten-year follow-up. *J Pediatr Endocrinol Metab.* 21:651, 2008.

RICKETS

NUTRITIONAL ACUITY RANKING: LEVEL 3

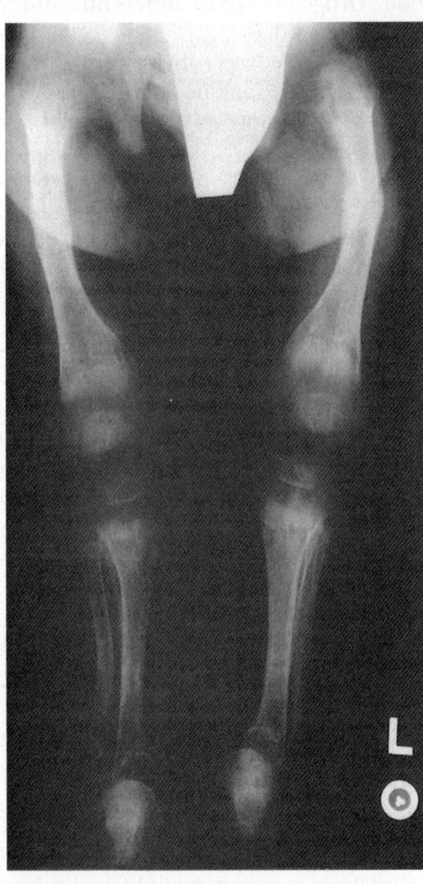

Adapted from: Becker KL, Bilezikian JP, Brenner WJ, et al. *Principles and Practice of Endocrinology and Metabolism,* 3rd ed. Philadelphia: Lippincott Williams & Wilkins, 2001.

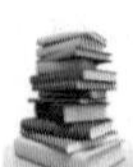

DEFINITIONS AND BACKGROUND

Rickets is generally caused by failure of osteoid to calcify during periods of growth. Vitamin D_3 (cholecalciferol) is formed in the skin from cholesterol with stimulation from ultraviolet-B light. Calcitriol is a steroid hormone that has impact on over 1000 genes in the human body (Edlich et al, 2009). Vitamin D insufficiency and deficiency during pregnancy may lead to lower maternal weight gain, disturbed skeletal homeostasis in the infant with reduced bone mineralization, rickets, and fractures (Pawley and Bishop, 2004). Less often, a deficiency of calcium or phosphorus may contribute to rickets. In adults, the condition is known as osteomalacia.

Because sunlight is important to skin production of vitamin D, where exposure is limited, deficiency is likely. Prevention and treatment of vitamin D deficiency is accomplished by regulated sun exposure as well as vitamin D supplementation (Edlich et al, 2009). Natural vitamin D levels, those found in humans living in a sun-rich environment, are between 40 and 70 ng/mL (Cannell and Hollis, 2008).

Rickets can be seen in 30–70% of premature, LBW and VLBW infants; it is also seen in breastfed children from multiple births, and infants with darker skin pigmentation living at higher latitudes. An increased number of children have rickets because more African American women are breastfeeding, fewer infants receive vitamin D supplements, and mothers and children are exposed to less sunlight.

Rickets may also occur in fat malabsorption syndrome, steatorrhea, anticonvulsant use, renal failure, or biliary cirrhosis. One detrimental consequence of untreated vitamin D-rickets is dilated cardiomyopathy (Brown et al, 2009). It is, therefore, important to identify and treat vitamin D deficiency.

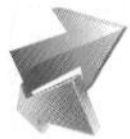

ASSESSMENT, MONITORING, AND EVALUATION

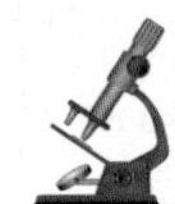

CLINICAL INDICATORS

Genetic Markers: X-linked hypophosphatemic rickets (XLH) is related to the PHEX gene and is the most common cause of vitamin D–resistant rickets.

Clinical/History		
Height	Decreased linear growth	Metabolic acidosis
Weight	Steatorrhea	DEXA scan for bone density
Growth (%)	Muscle spasm	Wrist radiographs
Diet/intake history	Chvostek's sign (facial spasm)	

	Lab Work	
Radiographs for fractures	25(OH) D levels: sufficient $\geq$30 ng/mL; deficient $\leq$20 ng/mL	Hypophosphatemia?
Leg bowing, inability to walk or stand	Urinary Ca^{++} (elevated)	Serum Ca^{++} (often low)
Seizures or irritability	Alk phos (increased)	Parathyroid hormone (elevated)
		Mg^{++}, Na^{+}, K^{+}

INTERVENTION

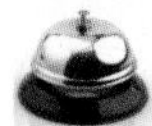

OBJECTIVES

- Correct body mineral status; prevent further problems and deformity. Vitamin D participates in mineral homeostasis, regulation of gene expression, and cell differentiation. Complement drug therapy with adequate diet.
- Prevent or correct hypocalcemia, dental caries, bone fractures.
- Promote growth; short stature can result if not treated early enough.

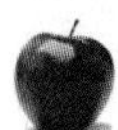

FOOD AND NUTRITION

- Use vitamin D–fortified milk if there are no milk allergies or lactose intolerance. Use calcium-containing foods such as cheeses, yogurt, fortified juice and ice cream, if fluid milk is not tolerated.
- Consuming vitamin D–fortified foods improves 25(OH)D concentrations. Fatty ocean fish are better sources than most other foods; hence, cod liver oil used to be given to children in past generations.
- If diet is inadequate in the specific nutrients, ensure intake of a supplement appropriate for age and sex. Avoid excesses of phytate from high fiber diets.
- Follow guidelines for sensible sun exposure and supplemental vitamin D; 800–1000 IU/d is reasonable (Holick, 2008). The skin forms vitamin D using 5-dihydrotachysterol, then hydroxylating in the liver to vitamin D_2 (calcidiol, or 25-hydroxycholecalciferol), which circulates in the plasma. The active form is hydroxylated in the kidney into cholecalciferol (calcitriol or 1,25-dihydroxycholecalciferol). Note that a healthy liver and kidney must be available to make the active form.

Common Drugs Used and Potential Side Effects

- A large dose of vitamin D is given upon a rickets diagnosis; 2000–7000 IU vitamin D per day should be sufficient (Cannell and Hollis, 2008).
- With steatorrhea, check serum levels of vitamin D and calcium and supplement appropriately.
- Rickets may occur secondary to prolonged antacid, anticonvulsant, or furosemide (Lasix) use; a vitamin D supplement will be needed.

Herbs, Botanicals, and Supplements

- Sunlight, artificial ultraviolet B (UVB) radiation, and vitamin D_3 supplementation are sources of vitamin D (Cannell and Hollis, 2008).
- Long- term harm from higher doses of vitamin D is not clear (Cranney et al, 2008). No more than the UL should be taken.

SAMPLE NUTRITION CARE PROCESS STEPS

Inadequate Vitamin Intake

Assessment Data: Low serum 25(OH) D_3, intake history for young child, X-rays.

Nutrition Diagnoses (PES): Inadequate vitamin D intake related to low intake of fortified foods including dairy products as evidenced by low serum levels, X-ray showing bowed legs and rickets.

Intervention: Educate mother about use of vitamin D_3 in fortified foods including milk and cereals daily. Discuss good sources of supporting nutrients (calcium, etc.).

Monitoring and Evaluation: X-rays, serum 25(OH) D_3, food diary and intake records showing improved intake of vitamins and minerals.

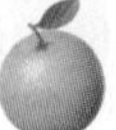

NUTRITION EDUCATION, COUNSELING, CARE MANAGEMENT

- Discuss needed alterations of the diet in conjunction with drug therapy.
- Good posture and positioning are important aspects of treatment.
- The recommended intakes for vitamin may not be enough, especially for dark-skinned children and those who live in northern latitudes (Misra et al, 2008; Ward et al, 2007). Discuss the role of sunlight in vitamin D metabolism.
- Infants who are given vegan diets may have low intakes of vitamin D.

Patient Education—Food Safety

- Hand washing with soap and hot water is recommended before preparing formula or meals. Use clean utensils and containers for mixing formula.
- Before using tap water for formula preparation or to give as a beverage, let cold tap water run for 2 minutes to remove any lead that may be in the pipes.
- Follow the 2-hour rule: discard any beverage or food that has been left at room temperature for 2 hours or longer.
- Do not use honey in the diets of infants to decrease potential risk of botulism.

For More Information

- American Academy of Family Physicians http://familydoctor.org/online/famdocen/home/children/parents/special/bone/902.printerview.html

- NIH—Medline
  http://www.nlm.nih.gov/medlineplus/rickets.html
- Vanderbilt—History of Rickets
  http://www.mc.vanderbilt.edu/biolib/hc/nh8.html

RICKETS—CITED REFERENCES

Brown J, et al. Hypocalcemic rickets and dilated cardiomyopathy: case reports and review of literature. [published online ahead of print April 23, 2009] *Pediatr Cardiol.* 30:818, 2009.

Cannell JJ, Hollis BW. Use of vitamin D in clinical practice. *Altern Med Rev.* 13:6, 2008.

Cranney A, et al. Summary of evidence-based review on vitamin D efficacy and safety in relation to bone health. *Am J Clin Nutr.* 88:513S, 2008.

Edlich R, et al. Modern concepts in the diagnosis and treatment of vitamin D deficiency and its clinical consequences. *J Environ Pathol Toxicol Oncol.* 28:1, 2009.

Holick MF. Vitamin D: a D-lightful health perspective. *Nutr Rev.* 66:182S, 2008.

Pawley N, Bishop NJ. Prenatal and infant predictors of bone health: the influence of vitamin D. *Am J Clin Nutr.* 80:1748S, 2004.

Ward LM, et al. Vitamin-D deficiency rickets among children in Canada. *CMAJ.* 177:161, 2007.

SMALL FOR GESTATIONAL AGE INFANT AND INTRAUTERINE GROWTH RETARDATION

NUTRITIONAL ACUITY RANKING: LEVEL 3

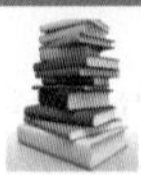

DEFINITIONS AND BACKGROUND

Infants whose weight is less than 10th percentile for gestational age are "small for gestational age" (SGA). Each year, about 40,000 infants born in the United States are SGA; they are at risk for preterm delivery, perinatal asphyxia, meconium aspiration, and hypoglycemia (Zaw et al, 2003). Another name for SGA infants is intrauterine growth restriction (IUGR). There is usually a wide range in weight gain after birth in SGA infants.

Nongenetic causes may retard intrauterine growth but are not often apparent before 32–34 weeks of gestation. Growth retardation due to nongenetic factors may cause malnutrition while sparing growth of the brain and long bones. Some other genetic disorders and congenital infections result in total growth retardation, in which height, weight, and head circumference are equally affected.

IUGR results from placental insufficiency. This insufficiency can result from maternal diseases (hyperemesis, preeclampsia, primary hypertension, renal disease, or diabetes); from infections such as cytomegalovirus, rubella virus, or *Toxoplasma gondii*; or if the mother is a narcotic or cocaine addict or heavy user of alcohol or tobacco (Dodds et al, 2006) (Table 3-16).

The fetus needs glucose, amino acids, and oxygen to grow normally. If IUGR was caused by chronic placental malnutrition, SGA infants may demonstrate remarkable catch-up growth within the first 2–3 years after delivery, if provided with adequate nutrition. The rates of catch-up growth vary according to many factors including birth weight, gestational age, parental size, adequacy of intrauterine growth, neurological impairment, clinical course, and nutrition (Carver, 2005). Insulin-like growth factor has a critical role in mediating fetal and postnatal growth (Randhawa and Cohen, 2005).

Common complications in SGA infants include hypoglycemia, perinatal asphyxia, meconium aspiration, polycythemia, respiratory distress syndrome, and NEC (Dodds et al, 2006). Prognosis is quite serious for infants who have perinatal asphyxia or congenital conditions.

TABLE 3-16 Risk Factors for Developing IUGR in Pregnancy

Pregnancies that have any of the following conditions may be at a greater risk for developing IUGR:

- Maternal weight of less than 100 lb
- Poor nutrition during pregnancy
- Birth defects or chromosomal abnormalities
- Use of drugs, cigarettes, and/or alcohol
- Pregnancy induced hypertension (PIH)
- Placental abnormalities
- Umbilical cord abnormalities
- Multiple pregnancy
- Gestational diabetes in the mother
- Low levels of amniotic fluid or oligohydramnios

Source: American Pregnancy Web site at http://www.americanpregnancy.org/pregnancycomplications/iugr.htm, accessed May 10, 2009.

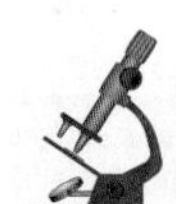

ASSESSMENT, MONITORING, AND EVALUATION

CLINICAL INDICATORS

Genetic Markers: SGA is not a genetically oriented condition.

Clinical/History		Lab Work
Prenatal ultrasound	Meconium aspiration?	Glucose
Length, Weight	I & O	BUN, creatinine
Growth (<10 percentile)	BP	Serum phosphorus
Decreased linear growth	Temperature	Serum Ca^{++}
	Thin, pale	Polycythemia?
	Loose skin?	

SAMPLE NUTRITION CARE PROCESS STEPS

Malnutrition

Assessment Data: Weight and growth charts, showing <10 percentile for gestational age.

Nutrition Diagnoses (PES): Malnutrition related to intrauterine growth retardation as evidenced by weight/length percentile at 9% and SGA birth.

Intervention: Educate mother about breastfeeding versus formula feeding, the need for gradual catch-up growth without overfeeding, and supporting healthy immunity.

Monitoring and Evaluation: Weight records, catch-up growth rate, health status (fewer infections, illnesses over time).

INTERVENTION

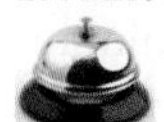

OBJECTIVES

- Correct body mineral status; prevent further problems and deformity.
- Complement any necessary drug therapy with adequate diet. Monitor carefully for side effects.
- Identify and treat underlying congenital problems.
- Promote catch-up growth, since short stature can result if not treated early enough. Compensatory catch-up growth may continue into adolescence and adulthood (Carver, 2005). If too rapid in the first 6 months, children may be obese at age 3 (Taveras et al, 2009).
- Prevent or correct hypoglycemia, perinatal morbidity, and other complications.
- Prevent long-term consequences, such as hypertension, insulin resistance and metabolic syndrome, type 2 diabetes mellitus, cardiovascular disease, short stature, and polycystic ovary syndrome (van Weissenbruch et al, 2005).

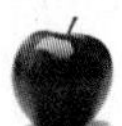

FOOD AND NUTRITION

- Promote exclusive breastfeeding whenever possible to promote cognitive development. At least 6 months is needed.
- While nutrient-enriched formulas that provide 22 kcal/oz are often prescribed for VLBW preterm infants after hospital discharge, for promoting greater rates of catch-up growth and increases in head circumference, studies are not as clear in SGA infants (Carver, 2005).
- Use a balanced diet appropriate for older children. Include reasonable snacks with high-quality nutritional value.
- If diet is inadequate in the specific nutrients, ensure intake of a sufficient level of vitamin D, calcium, and phosphorus for age and sex.

Common Drugs Used and Potential Side Effects

- GH therapy for improving height in these children has been approved by the FDA; it promotes growth acceleration and normalization of height during childhood. High doses can affect carbohydrate metabolism and cause hyperglycemia.

Herbs, Botanicals, and Supplements

- Herbs and botanicals should not be used in children.

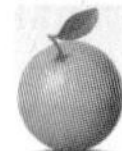

NUTRITION EDUCATION, COUNSELING, CARE MANAGEMENT

- Help families adjust to special requirements for their child. The child may have diabetes and other chronic consequences from being born SGA.
- Children born SGA without postnatal catch-up are shorter and have higher weight than children of similar age, height, and sex. In addition, insufficient nutrition during the first 3 years of life is correlated with poor neurodevelopmental outcomes (Belfort et al, 2008). Discuss the importance of good nutrition in infancy.
- Prepare for future pregnancies by discussing the need to avoid alcohol and tobacco.

Patient Education—Food Safety

- Hand washing with soap and hot water is recommended before preparing formula or meals. Use clean utensils and containers for mixing formula.
- Before using tap water for formula preparation or to give as a beverage, let cold tap water run for 2 minutes to remove any lead that may be in the pipes.
- Follow the 2-hour rule: discard any beverage or food that has been left at room temperature for 2 hours or longer.
- Do not use honey in the diets of infants to decrease potential risk of botulism.

For More Information

- Intrauterine Growth Retardation
  http://familydoctor.org/online/famdocen/home/women/pregnancy/fetal/313.html

SMALL FOR GESTATIONAL AGE—CITED REFERENCES

Belfort MB, et al. Infant growth and child cognition at 3 years of age. *Pediatrics.* 122:689, 2008.

Carver JD. Nutrition for preterm infants after hospital discharge. *Adv Pediatr.* 52:23, 2005.

Dodds L, et al. Outcomes of pregnancies complicated by hyperemesis gravidarum. *Obstet Gynecol.* 107:285, 2006.

Randhawa R, Cohen P. The role of the insulin-like growth factor system in prenatal growth. *Mol Genet Metab.* 86:84, 2005.

Taveras EM, et al. Weight status in the first 6 months of life and obesity at 3 years. *Pediatrics.* 123:1177, 2009.

van Weissenbruch MM, et al. Fetal nutrition and timing of puberty. *Endocr Dev.* 8:15, 2005.

TYROSINEMIA

NUTRITIONAL ACUITY RANKING: LEVEL 4

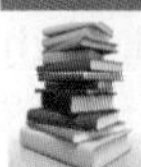

DEFINITIONS AND BACKGROUND

Hereditary tyrosinemia type I (HTI), a severe disease affecting primarily the liver, is caused by a deficiency of fumarylacetoacetate hydrolase (FAH). Tyrosine, Phe, and methionine build up. The condition is acute, often causing death within the first year of life. Type I needs to be treated with diet for life and is a much more severe disease than other types. This condition results in liver failure or severe nodular cirrhosis with renal tubular involvement. This form is common in Quebec, Canada; it affects 1 in 100,000 individuals.

Tyrosine accumulation can be aggravated by vitamin C deficiency, a high-protein diet, or liver immaturity. Prenatal diagnosis is possible and can be performed by measuring succinyl acetone in the amniotic fluid or FAH in amniotic fluid cells, allowing for genetic counseling. Liver transplantation may be needed.

Type II tyrosinemia is caused by a deficiency of the enzyme tyrosine aminotransferase (TAT) and affects the eyes with excessive tearing and photophobia; eye pain and redness; painful skin lesions on the palms and soles; and intellectual disability. Type III is caused by a deficiency of the enzyme 4-hydroxyphenylpyruvate dioxygenase (HPD) that presents with seizures, intermittent ataxia, and intellectual disorders.

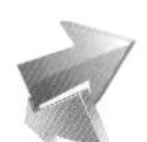

ASSESSMENT, MONITORING, AND EVALUATION

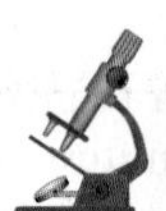

CLINICAL INDICATORS

Genetic Markers: Deficiency of FAH, the last enzyme of tyrosine catabolism, leads to accumulation of the toxic substrate fumarylacetoacetate (FAA) in hepatocytes and renal proximal tubular cells (Jacobs, 2006). Mutations in the HPD and TAT genes cause types I and II. The gene is mapped to band 15q23–q25. About 30 distinct mutations have been reported for Type I.

Clinical/History

- Birth weight, present weight
- Growth (%)
- Diet/intake history
- Abdominal distention
- Hyperpigmentation
- Dermatitis
- "Cabbage-like" odor
- Rancid butter–like odor (type I)
- FTT
- Irritability
- Jaundice
- Diarrhea, bloody stools
- Annual CT or MRI of liver

Lab Work

- Urinary succinyl acetoacetate levels (high)
- FAH (very low?)
- Plasma Phe
- Methionine
- H & H
- Serum Fe
- Plasma tyrosine
- LFTs (elevated)
- Bilirubin (elevated)
- Phosphate
- Gluc (low?)
- Alb (often low)
- Nitisinone level

INTERVENTION

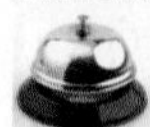

OBJECTIVES

- Restrict Phe and tyrosine from the diet to promote normal growth and intellectual development.
- Provide adequate vitamin C for conversion processes.
- Prevent severe liver, kidney and neurological, damage, or rickets (Jacobs, 2006).

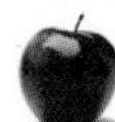

FOOD AND NUTRITION

- Initially, feed a Phe/tyrosine hydrolysate to infants, with small amounts of milk added to provide the minimum requirements of tyrosine and Phe. Mead Johnson product TYROS and 3200-AB; Ross product Maxamaid XPHEN, TYR; or TYROMEX-1 or TYREX from SHS can be used.
- If blood methionine levels are elevated, try PFD1 or PFD2 (Mead Johnson). Use carbohydrate supplements, vitamins, and minerals.
- Low-tyrosine/Phe diet limits foods such as cow's milk and regular formula; avoid meat, eggs and cheese. Regular flour, dried beans, nuts and peanut butter must also be limited. Focus on fruits and vegetables and the special formula.
- Supplement with vitamins C and D appropriate to the patient's age.

Common Drugs Used and Potential Side Effects

- Nitisinone (Orfadin) reduces the toxic effects of tyrosine in the body when used along with the dietary restrictions (Santra et al, 2008). Fortunately, with this medication,

SAMPLE NUTRITION CARE PROCESS STEPS

Abnormal GI Function

Assessment Data: Altered LFTs, anorexia, irritability, cabbage-like body odor, bloody diarrhea.

Nutrition Diagnoses (PES): Altered GI function related to missing FAH enzyme as evidenced by bloody diarrhea, poor appetite, altered LFTs.

Intervention: Educate parents about the special formula and diet for managing tyrosinemia. Refer to genetic counselor if they wish to have more children.

Monitoring and Evaluation: Normal weight and growth, LFTs, normal intellectual development after following the diet and taking the medicine. No sign of rickets.

liver transplantation may not be necessary and hepatic carcinoma may be delayed.
- Antibiotics may be needed to correct infections. Use of acidophilus and probiotic products may alleviate loss of intestinal bacteria.
- Vitamin D may be needed if the child has rickets.

Herbs, Botanicals, and Supplements

- Herbs and botanicals should not be used for tyrosinemia because there are no controlled trials to prove efficacy.

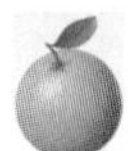

NUTRITION EDUCATION, COUNSELING, CARE MANAGEMENT

- Provide sources of tyrosine and Phe in the diet determined appropriately for age and body size.
- Adjust intake of energy and nutrients according to the patient's age.
- Discuss desirable intake of protein (avoid excesses) and encourage adequate intake of vitamin C to meet recommended levels.
- Genetic counseling is advised for the family members (Scott, 2006).

Patient Education—Food Safety

- Hand washing with soap and hot water is recommended before preparing formula or meals. Use clean utensils and containers for mixing formula.
- Before using tap water for formula preparation or to give as a beverage, let cold tap water run for 2 minutes to remove any lead that may be in the pipes.
- Follow the 2-hour rule: discard any beverage or food that has been left at room temperature for 2 hours or longer.
- Do not use honey in the diets of infants to decrease potential risk of botulism.

For More Information

- American Liver Foundation
  http://www.liverfoundation.org/
- Medscape—Tyrosinemia
  http://emedicine.medscape.com/article/949816-overview
- Save Babies
  http://www.savebabies.org/diseasedescriptions/tyrosinemia.php
- University of Washington
  http://depts.washington.edu/tyros/abouttyr.htm

TYROSINEMIA—CITED REFERENCES

Jacobs SM, et al. Kidneys of mice with hereditary tyrosinemia type I are extremely sensitive to cytotoxicity. *Pediatr Res.* 59:365, 2006.

Santra S, et al. Renal tubular function in children with tyrosinemia type I treated with nitisinone. *J Inherit Metab Dis.* 31:399, 2008.

Scott CR. The genetic tyrosinemias. *Am J Med Genet C Semin Med Genet.* 142:121, 2006.

UREA CYCLE DISORDERS

NUTRITIONAL ACUITY RANKING: LEVEL 2–4

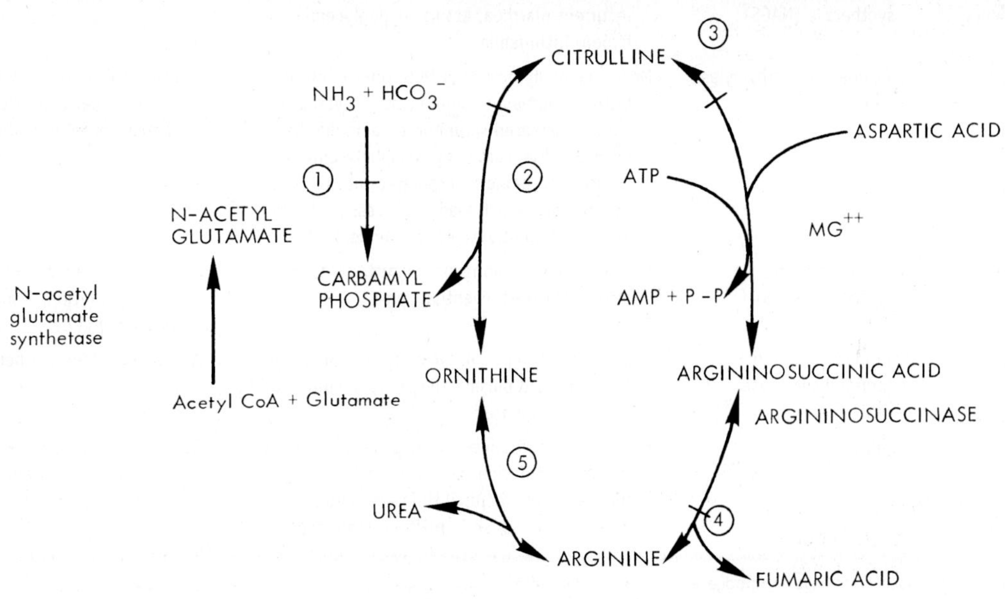

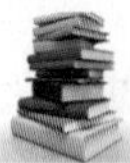

DEFINITIONS AND BACKGROUND

As a group, urea cycle disorders occur in one in 25,000 newborns. Table 3-17 describes the urea cycle disorders and their treatment. Ornithine transcarbamylase (OTC) deficiency is the most common disorder. Statewide newborn screening does not always include these conditions, but screening is important if there is any family history of these disorders.

The urea cycle disorders are manifested most often in the newborn between ages 1 and 5 days, when they are often initially thought to be septic. With later onset, patients have partial enzyme deficiencies and are recognized after a clinical episode months or years later. When they present in childhood, adolescence, and adulthood, there may be FTT, persistent vomiting, developmental delay, behavioral changes, hyperammonemia, irritability, somnolence, seizures, and coma; if not treated rapidly, they may cause irreversible neuronal damage. Diagnosis of urea cycle disorder should be considered in any child or adult with unexplained neurological and psychiatric disorders with anorexia, unexplained coma with cerebral edema, and respiratory alkalosis. Some cases of SIDS may be related to urea cycle disorders.

The hyperammonemia that occurs is a deadly neurotoxin. Chronic hyperammonemia results in increased L-tryptophan metabolites including serotonin. Ammonia levels above 60 μmol/L lead to anorexia, irritability, lethargy, vomiting, somnolence, disorientation, asterixis, cerebral edema, coma, and death (Cohn and Roth, 2004).

Diet is one of the main treatments of these disorders; protein intake should be adjusted according to the metabolic disorder, its severity, the patient's age, growth rate, and preferences (Wilcken, 2004). Poor appetite, nutritional problems, and chronic catabolism are common and difficult to treat (Wilcken, 2004).

Any patient on a low-protein diet should be monitored clinically, with appropriate laboratory tests and an emergency plan; hemodialysis may be needed. Most patients, except those with arginase deficiency, will need supplements of arginine, but the value of other supplements, including citrate and carnitine, is unclear (Wilcken, 2004). Gene therapy and liver transplantation are treatments that show promise.

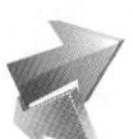

ASSESSMENT, MONITORING, AND EVALUATION

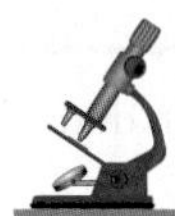

CLINICAL INDICATORS

Genetic Markers: Deficiencies of CPSI, ASS, ASL, NAGS, and ARG are inherited in an autosomal recessive manner. OTC deficiency is inherited in an X-linked manner. All are genetic diseases associated with lack of a protein or enzyme activity in the urea cycle.

TABLE 3-17 **Urea Cycle Disorders (UCD)**

UCD	Enzyme Deficiency	Symptoms/Comments	Treatment
Type I hyperammonemia	Carbamoylphosphate synthetase I (CPS I)	Within 24–72 hours after birth, infant becomes lethargic, needs stimulation to feed, vomiting, increasing lethargy, hypothermia and hyperventilation; without measurement of serum ammonia levels and appropriate intervention, infant will die	Arginine that activates *N*-acetylglutamate synthetase
N-acetylglutamate synthetase deficiency	*N*-acetylglutamate synthetase (NAGS)	Severe hyperammonemia, deep coma, acidosis, recurrent diarrhea, ataxia, hypoglycemia, hyperornithinemia	Carbamoyl glutamate to activate CPS I
Type 2 hyperammonemia	Ornithine transcarbamylase (OTC)	Most commonly occurring UCD, only X-linked UCD, ammonia and amino acids elevated in serum, increased serum orotic acid due to mitochondrial carbamoylphosphate entering cytosol and being incorporated into pyrimidine nucleotides, which leads to excess production and consequently excess catabolic products	High-carbohydrate, low-protein diet, ammonia detoxification with sodium phenylacetate or sodium benzoate
Classic citrullinemia	Argininosuccinate synthetase (ASS)	Episodic hyperammonemia, vomiting, lethargy, ataxia, seizures, eventual coma	Arginine administration to enhance citrulline excretion; also sodium benzoate for ammonia detoxification
Argininosuccinic aciduria	Argininosuccinate lyase (argininosuccinase) (ASL)	Episodic symptoms similar to classic citrullinemia, elevated plasma and cerebral spinal fluid argininosuccinate	Arginine and sodium benzoate
Hyperargininemia	Arginase	Rare UCD, progressive spastic quadriplegia and mental retardation, ammonia and arginine high in cerebral spinal fluid and serum arginine, lysine, and ornithine high in urine	Diet of essential amino acids excluding arginine, low-protein diet

Adapted from: http://themedicalbiochemistrypage.org/nitrogen-metabolism.html#clinical.

Clinical/History	Developmental delay	month of age; 35–50 μg/dL in older children and adults
Birth weight, present weight	**Lab Work**	Phos
Growth (%)	Plasma amino acid levels (specific to disorder)	Gluc
Diet/intake history	Hyperammonemia: 150 μg/dL in neonates; 70 μg/dL in infants to one	Alb
FTT		H & H
Vomiting		Blood gases
Irritability		Na^+, K^+, Cl^-
Somnolence		Ketonuria
Lethargy, seizures or coma		

INTERVENTION

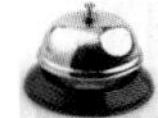

OBJECTIVES

- Restrict total protein from the diet to minimize endogenous ammonia production and protein catabolism. Limit one or more essential amino acids while providing adequate energy and nutrients (Trahms, 2008).
- Promote anabolism with normal growth and development for age; use energy from nonprotein sources in amounts to spare protein for other purposes.
- Normalize blood ammonia levels and reduce the effects of hyperammonemia to prevent neuronal damage. Elevated levels of ammonia can come from either muscle breakdown or diet; determine which process is the problem.
- Administer desired substrates of the urea cycles. If necessary, support dialysis if blood ammonia levels are three to four times above normal.

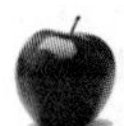

FOOD AND NUTRITION

- Use a protein-controlled diet (often 1.0–1.5 g/kg daily) with use of special amino acid formulas developed specifically for urea cycle disorders. These formulas provide approximately 50% of the daily dietary protein allowance; some patients may require individual BCAA supplementation.
- Pharmaceutical grade (not over-the-counter) L-citrulline (for OTC and CPS deficiency) or L-arginine free base (ASA and citrullinemia) is also required. These are not to be used in arginase deficiency.
- Add extra energy sources if needed to support growth and development. Weight gain is the best measure of success in infants and children. Metabolic nutritionists routinely prescribe calorie modules such as Prophree, Polycose and ModuCal. If dehydration occurs, intravenous fluids and glucose may be needed.
- Multiple vitamins and calcium supplements are recommended.

SAMPLE NUTRITION CARE PROCESS STEPS

Altered Nutrition-Related Lab Values

Assessment Data: Weight and growth charts showing FTT, anorexia, elevated serum ammonia.

Nutrition Diagnoses (PES): Altered nutrition-related labs related to hyperammonemia in urea cycle disorder as evidenced by anorexia, lethargy and sleepiness, FTT with weight/height at 3 percentile.

Intervention: Educate parents about low protein formula, enhancing energy intake through high calorie foods and supplements containing calcium.

Monitoring and Evaluation: Weight records, growth, improved appetite and intake, reduced serum ammonia levels, greater alertness.

Common Drugs Used and Potential Side Effects

- Protein restriction is used in conjunction with medications to remove ammonia from the blood. Medications are given by way of tube feedings, either via gastrostomy tube or NG tube. To provide alternative route for ammonia, what is given depends on where the defect in the urea cycle has occurred.
- Arginine is often supplemented (400–700 mg/d), except for arginine deficiency (Trahms, 2008). For argininosuccinate synthetase and argininosuccinate lyase deficiencies, 0.4–0.7 g arginine/kg/d is given; 0.17 g/kg/d of citrulline is given for carbamyl phosphate synthetase deficiency.
- Sodium phenylbutyrate (Buphenyl) is used to normalize serum ammonia by diverting nitrogen to alternative paths for excretion (Scaglia et al, 2004). It is administered three to four times daily to keep ammonia under control.

Herbs, Botanicals, and Supplements

- Herbs and botanicals should not be used for urea cycle disorders because there are no controlled trials to prove efficacy.

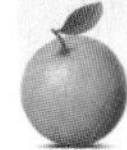

NUTRITION EDUCATION, COUNSELING, CARE MANAGEMENT

- Provide sources of all essential amino acids in the diet, determined appropriately for age and body size. There are tables available for these purposes (Trahms, 2008).
- Adjust intake of energy and nutrients according to the patient's age.
- Comprehensive newborn screening is recommended for families who have had the birth of one or more children with these disorders.

Patient Education—Food Safety

- Hand washing with soap and hot water is recommended before preparing formula or meals. Use clean utensils and containers for mixing formula.

- Before using tap water for formula preparation or to give as a beverage, let cold tap water run for 2 minutes to remove any lead that may be in the pipes.
- Follow the 2-hour rule: discard any beverage or food that has been left at room temperature for 2 hours or longer.
- Do not use honey in the diets of infants to decrease potential risk of botulism.

For More Information

- Children Living with Inherited Metabolic Disorders (Climb)
  http://www.climb.org.uk/
- My Special Diet
  http://www.myspecialdiet.com/
- National Urea Cycle Disorders Foundation
  http://www.nucdf.org
- Organic Acidemia Association
  http://www.oaanews.org/
- UCD Kids Network
  http://www.nucdf.org/

UREA CYCLE DISORDERS—CITED REFERENCES

Cohn RM, Roth KS. Hyperammonemia, bane of the brain. *Clin Pediatr (Phila).* 43:683, 2004.

Scaglia F, et al. Effect of alternative pathway therapy on branched chain amino acid metabolism in urea cycle disorder patients. *Mol Genet Metab.* 81:S79, 2004.

Trahms C. Metabolic disorders. In: Mahan K, Escott-Stump S, eds. *Krause's food, nutrition, and diet therapy.* 12th ed. Philadelphia: WB Saunders, 2008.

Wilcken B. Problems in the management of urea cycle disorders. *Mol Genet Metab.* 81:S86, 2004.

WILSON'S DISEASE (HEPATOLENTICULAR DEGENERATION)

NUTRITIONAL ACUITY RANKING: LEVEL 3

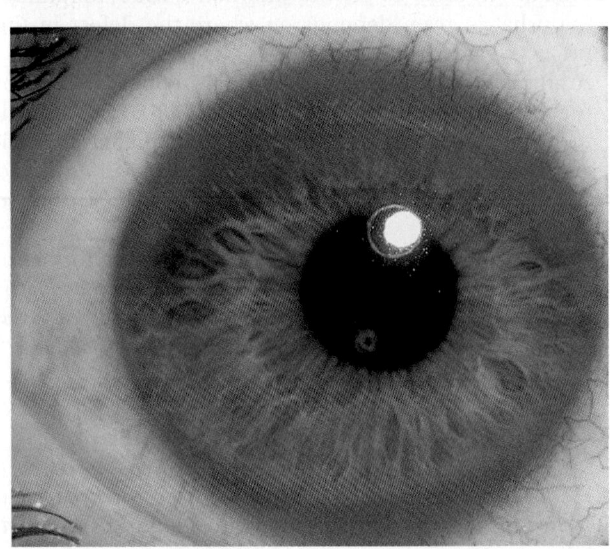

Adapted from: Gold DH, MD, and Weingeist TA, MD, PhD. *Color Atlas of the Eye in Systemic Disease.* Baltimore: Lippincott Williams & Wilkins, 2001.

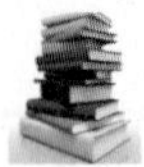

DEFINITIONS AND BACKGROUND

The major physiological role of copper is to serve as a cofactor to a number of key metabolic enzymes. Copper is a trace element essential for normal cell homeostasis, promoting iron absorption for hemoglobin synthesis and for formation of bone and myelin sheath. In hepatic tissues, 90% of the copper in the copper-albumin complex is converted to ceruloplasmin. Wilson's disease is a rare inborn disease related to copper storage (Merle et al, 2007). Tissue deposition occurs instead of formation of ceruloplasmin in Wilson's disease.

An autosomal recessive disorder, Wilson's disease results in hepatolenticular degeneration, cirrhosis, neurologic damage, damage to the kidney, brain, and cornea. Onset occurs at birth, but symptoms may appear from 5 to 40 years of age. The disease may lead to neurodegeneration and behavior abnormalities. Three types of neurological symptoms can occur: dystonic syndrome (dystonic postures and choreoathetosis); ataxic syndrome (postural and intentional tremor and ataxia of the limbs); and parkinsonian syndrome (hypokinesia, rigidity, and resting tremor). Shortened attention span, slurring of speech, and depression are early symptoms. Individuals who present with neuropsychiatric problems are often identified later in life and have poorer outcomes than those with hepatic symptoms (Merle et al, 2007).

A low-copper diet is seldom essential but implemented when other therapies are unsuccessful (e.g., copper-chelating agents). Other dietary treatments under study include the use of increased histidine, specific polyunsaturated fatty acids, low soy, and other plans. If not diagnosed until onset of fulminant liver failure, the patient will die by age 30. Liver transplantation is the best treatment. New ideas regarding the clinical management of this disorder will emerge with elucidation of the cellular basis of the disease (Fink and Schilsky, 2007).

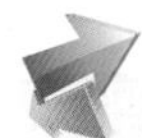

ASSESSMENT, MONITORING, AND EVALUATION

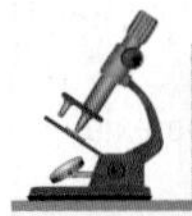

CLINICAL INDICATORS

Genetic Markers: Wilson disease involves two abnormal copies of the *ATP7B* gene, one from each parent. The alteration is on chromosome 13.

Clinical/History		
Height Weight BMI	Kayser–Fleischer ring (gold or gray–brown opacity of peripheral cornea)	Enlarged liver Swallowing difficulty Drooling? Easy bruising Jaundice?

Fixed pseudo-smile	**Lab Work**	Bilirubin (>300 μmol/L)
Postural tremor of arms	Ceruloplasmin (often low)	Alk phos, low (<600 IU/L)
Rigidity	Serum Cu (abnormal)	Serum zinc
Abrupt personality change	Liver copper levels	Alb
Splenomegaly, esophageal varices?	Urinary Cu	H & H
Hepatitis or cirrhosis?	ALT, AST [low transaminases (100–500 IU/L)]	BUN, Creat
		Serum P
		PT or INR

INTERVENTION

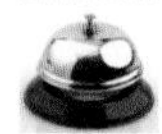

OBJECTIVES

- Keep optimal balance of copper in patient.
- Decrease serum copper levels, generally with drug chelation. Enhance urinary excretion of excesses.
- Prevent or reverse damage to body tissues and liver.
- Watch caloric intake to prevent obesity.
- Monitor changes in gag reflex or dysphagia.
- Provide sufficient zinc to chelate excess copper under doctor's supervision.
- Prepare for transplantation where possible.
- Prevent or correct bone demineralization (Selimoglu et al, 2008).

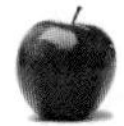

FOOD AND NUTRITION

- A normal diet provides 2–5 mg/d of copper. To lower copper in the diet (to 1–2 mg), use limited amounts of liver, kidney, shellfish, nuts, raisins and other dried fruits, dried legumes, brain, oysters, mushrooms, chocolate, poultry, and whole-grain cereals.
- A lacto–ovo–vegetarian diet may be useful to increase content of fiber and phytates; copper is less available in vegetarian diets.

SAMPLE NUTRITION CARE PROCESS STEPS

Excessive Mineral Intake

Assessment Data: Neurological symptoms, altered LFTs, changes in the eye, low ceruloplasmin and elevated serum copper.

Nutrition Diagnoses (PES): Excessive mineral (copper) intake related to Wilson's disease and disordered copper metabolism as evidenced by altered labs for copper and ceruloplasmin.

Intervention: Educate parents about the role of copper in the body, and how zinc interacts; discuss the medication effects and the need for possible transplantation.

Monitoring and Evaluation: Improved neurological symptoms and lab values posttransplantation.

- Control energy intake, food textures, and other nutrients if necessary.
- Increase fluid intake but avoid alcoholic beverages.
- Increase zinc from meat, poultry, fish, eggs, and milk if deemed appropriate for the patient.
- Assure adequate intake of calcium, vitamins D and K for bone health (Selimoglu et al, 2008).

Common Drugs Used and Potential Side Effects

- Zinc acetate may be used to chelate copper with fewer side effects than D-penicillamine. Doses of 75–150 mg are often prescribed. Oral zinc is a suitable alternative to penicillamine as long-term maintenance therapy.
- D-penicillamine (Cuprimine or Depen), a copper-chelating agent, should be taken orally before meals. A vitamin B_6 supplement is needed with this drug; usually a dose of 25 mg.
- Laxatives or stool softeners may be needed. Encourage a diet high in fiber and fluid to wean off medication if possible.
- Corticosteroids and immunosuppressive therapy are used for autoimmune hepatitis. Side effects can be significant, including hyperglycemia, osteopenia, and nutrient depletion.
- Tetrathiomolybdate is being tested for use in Wilson's disease (Brewer et al, 2006).

Herbs, Botanicals, and Supplements

- A neurological disorder has been noted after taking Chinese herbs; it is best to avoid them in Wilson's disease (Wang and Yang, 2003).

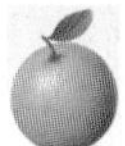

NUTRITION EDUCATION, COUNSELING, CARE MANAGEMENT

- Teach the patient about the copper and zinc content of foods. Explain that breast milk has higher copper levels than cow's milk to those individuals who need to know.
- Help the patient with feeding at mealtimes, if poor muscular control is demonstrated.
- Discuss effective coping mechanisms, community resources, and genetic counseling.
- Discuss the importance of maintaining prescribed drug therapy, which is essential for life.

Patient Education—Food Safety

- Hand washing with soap and hot water is recommended before preparing formula or meals. Use clean utensils and containers for mixing formula.
- Before using tap water for formula preparation or to give as a beverage, let cold tap water run for 2 minutes to remove any lead that may be in the pipes.
- Follow the 2-hour rule: discard any beverage or food that has been left at room temperature for 2 hours or longer.

- Do not use honey in the diets of infants to decrease potential risk of botulism.

For More Information

- National Institute of Neurological Disorders and Stroke
http://www.ninds.nih.gov/disorders/wilsons/wilsons.htm
- NIDDK
http://digestive.niddk.nih.gov/ddiseases/pubs/wilson/
- Wilson's Disease Association
http://www.wilsonsdisease.org/
- Wilson's Disease Center
http://www.wilsonsdiseasecenter.org/

WILSON'S DISEASE—CITED REFERENCES

Brewer GJ, et al. The use of tetrathiomolybdate in treating fibrotic, inflammatory, and autoimmune diseases, including the non-obese diabetic mouse model. *J Inorgan Biochem.* 100:927, 2006.

Fink S, Schilsky ML. Inherited metabolic disease of the liver. *Curr Opin Gastroenterol.* 23:237, 2007.

Merle U, et al. Clinical presentation, diagnosis and long-term outcome of Wilson's disease: a cohort study. *Gut.* 56:115, 2007.

Selimoglu MA, et al. Bone mineral density of children with Wilson disease: efficacy of penicillamine and zinc therapy. *J Clin Gastroenterol.* 42:194, 2008.

Wang XP, Yang RM. Movement disorders possibly induced by traditional Chinese herbs. *Eur Neurol.* 50:153, 2003.

S E C T I O N

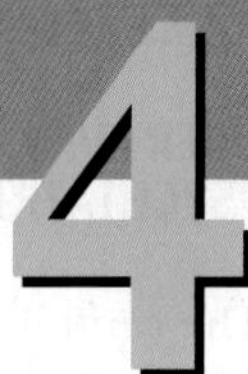

Neuro-psychiatric Conditions

CHIEF ASSESSMENT FACTORS

- Blunting of Emotions, Apathy, Egocentricity
- Bowel or Bladder Dysfunction
- Confusion, Memory Loss; Disorientation Regarding Place and Time
- Depression, Anxiety
- Disturbed Taste, Smell, Changes in Vision
- Dizziness, Vertigo, Drowsiness
- Dysphagia; Coughing or Choking While Eating/Swallowing
- Easy Aspiration of Food into Lungs
- Extremities: Coldness, Stiffness, Limited Movement, Discoloration, Pain
- Hallucinations, Tremors; Tics, Spasms, Ataxia
- Headaches, Pain
- Impulse Control Disorder
- Loss of Consciousness, Seizures
- Marked Disturbance in Eating Behaviors, Pica
- Mood Swings, Behavioral Changes, Psychotic Delusions
- Nervousness, Irritability
- Numbness, Paralysis, Sensory Pain
- Poor or Weaker Judgment; Difficulty Performing Familiar Tasks
- Problems with Abstract Thinking, Personality Changes
- Status of Food in Oral Cavity
- Stress (may speed up aging process because of protein kinase C)
- Weakness

OVERVIEW OF NEUROLOGICAL AND PSYCHIATRIC DISORDERS

The central nervous system (CNS) consists of the brain and spinal cord. The brain has three main sections: the cerebrum, the cerebellum, and the brainstem. The normal adult brain weighs 3 lb; it grows steadily until 20 years of age and then loses weight for the rest of life. Gray matter consists of CNS tissue rich in neuronal cell bodies, their dendrites, axons, and glial cells; it includes the cerebral cortex, the central spinal cord, the cerebellar cortex, and the hippocampal cortex. White matter refers to large axon tracts in the brain and spinal cord involved with the cerebral hemispheres, the cerebellum, and the hippocampus. Figure 4-1 shows the brain and the spinal cord.

This chapter provides an overview of neurological and psychiatric disorders that have nutritional implications. A few disorders are found in other relevant sections; autism in Section 3, dysphagia in Section 7, anesthesia in Section 14. The primary neurological disorders are separated from psychiatric disorders. The newest edition of the *Diagnostic and Statistical Manual of Mental Disorders* (*DSM*) is due in 2012; the American Psychiatric Association (APA) and NIMH worked together to expand the scientific basis for psychiatric diagnosis and classification.

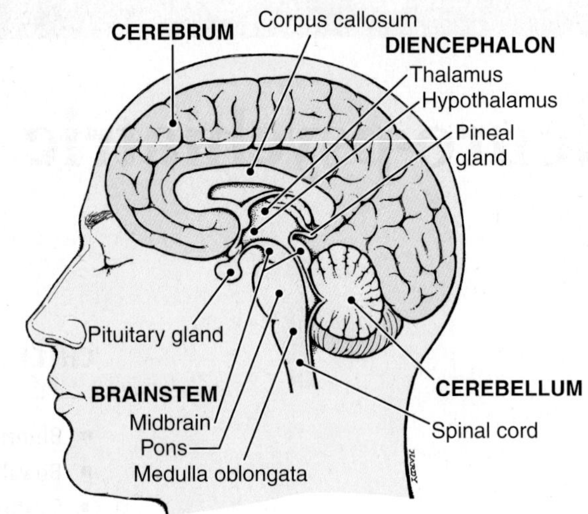

Figure 4-1

The brain and the gut work synergistically with each other and with other organs. Table 4-1 lists functions of the brain. Table 4-2 lists the cranial nerves and highlights those that affect chewing and swallowing. Nutrition influences the genetic onset and consequences of many chronic diseases.

TABLE 4-1 Brain Parts and Their Functions

Parts	Relevant Nerves	Functions
FOREBRAIN		
Cerebrum–temporal lobe	8th cranial nerve	Controls hearing, expressive language, music and rhythm. Contains the hippocampus. Diseases that affect this area include Alzheimer's disease, depression, and mania
Cerebrum–frontal lobe		Controls personality, mood, behavior, reasoning, emotional control, and cognition. Diseases affecting this area include Alzheimer's disease, depression, mania, and Huntington's disease
Cerebrum–parietal lobe		Comprehension of written language and oral speech; sensory stimulation such as pain, touch, smell, hearing, and heat; body position. Alzheimer's disease affects this area; epilepsy and stroke may also impact this area
Cerebrum–occipital lobe	2nd cranial nerve	Vision
Thalamus		Relays sensory information to the cerebral cortex
Hypothalamus		Lies beneath the thalamus. Secretes corticotropin-releasing hormone, affects metabolism by its influence on pituitary gland. Secretes vasopressin, which regulates sleep and wake cycles
Limbic system	System of nerve pathways	**Amygdala** affects depression **Hippocampus** may affect mania, depression, and Alzheimer's. Located inside the temporal lobe (humans have two hippocampi, one in each side of the brain). Part of the limbic system. Plays a part in memory, learning, and navigation
MIDBRAIN	3rd cranial nerve	Site between hindbrain and forebrain. Controls oculomotor nerve; eye movement. Affected in Parkinson's disease and some strokes
HINDBRAIN		
CEREBELLUM	3rd–5th cranial nerves	Found at bottom rear of the head. Posture and balance; voluntary movements such as sitting, standing, and walking. Directing attention and measuring time; other motor and cognitive functions. Stroke often affects this area
Pons	4th–7th cranial nerves	Connects brainstem with cerebellum. Receives information from visual areas to control eye and body movements. Controls patterns of sleep and arousal; coordination of muscular movements; helps maintain equilibrium. Affects sleep disorders
Medulla oblongata	8th–12th cranial nerves	Hearing, balance, some taste, some swallowing. Movement of the tongue. Involuntary functions such as heartbeat, circulation, muscle tone, and breathing. Stroke often affects this area
SPINAL CORD		Sends and receives messages to and from brain and body parts

Developed from: Brainexplorer, http://www.brainexplorer.org, accessed May 13, 2009.

TABLE 4-2 Cranial Nerves and Those Specifically Affecting Mastication and Swallowing

	Nerve	Function	Affected Part of Body
I	Olfactory	Smell	Olfactory bulbs
II	Optic	Vision	Retina
III	Oculomotor	Eyeball movement Lens accommodation	Four eyeball muscles and one eyelid muscle
	Oculomotor	Pupil constriction	
IV	Trochlear	Eyeball movement	Superior oblique muscles
V	Trigeminal[a]	Sensations General sensory from tongue Proprioception	Face, scalp, teeth, lips, eyeballs, nose and throat lining Anterior two thirds of tongue Jaw muscles for mastication
	Trigeminal	Chewing	Muscles of mastication
VI	Abducens	Eyeball movement	Lateral rectus muscle
VII	Facial[a]	Taste Proprioception	Anterior two thirds of tongue Face and scalp
	Facial	Facial expressions	Muscles of the face
	Facial	Salivation and lacrimation	Salivary and lacrimal glands via submandibular and pterygopalatine ganglia
VIII	Vestibulocochlear	Balance Hearing	Vestibular apparatus of internal ear Cochlear of internal ear
IX	Glossopharyngeal[a]	Taste Proprioception for swallowing Blood pressure receptors	Posterior two thirds of tongue Throat muscles Carotid sinuses
	Glossopharyngeal	Swallowing and gag reflex Tear production	Throat muscles Lacrimal glands
	Glossopharyngeal	Saliva production	Parotid glands
X	Vagus	Chemoreceptors Pain receptors Sensations Taste	Blood oxygen concentration, aortic bodies Respiratory and digestive tracts External ear, larynx, and pharynx Tongue
	Vagus	Heart rate and stroke volume Peristalsis Air flow Speech and swallowing	Pacemaker and ventricular muscles Smooth muscles of digestive tract Smooth muscles in bronchial tubes Muscles of larynx and pharynx
XI	Spinal Accessory	Head rotation	Trapezius and sternocleidomastoid muscles
XII	Hypoglossal[a]	Speech and swallowing	Tongue and throat muscles

Adapted from: http://www.teaching-biomed.man.ac.uk/resources/wwwcal/cranial_nerves/page2.asp, accessed January 16, 2005.
[a]Cranial nerves affecting chewing and swallowing.

One individual may have up to 500,000 single nucleotide polymorphisms (Ferguson, 2007). A steady stream of neurotransmitters is needed for good mental and neurological health, yet they are subject to dietary manipulation. Increases or decreases in dietary precursors of serotonin, dopamine, norepinephrine, and acetylcholine affect nerve functioning. Brain levels of tryptophan, tyrosine, or choline control the rates at which neurons synthesize serotonin, dopamine, or acetylcholine, respectively (Wurtman, 2008). "Brain foods" can be suggested to prevent or treat many stress-related mental disorders (Takeda, 2004).

Heritable abnormalities include major depressive disorder (MDD), attention deficit hyperactivity disorder (ADHD), bulimia nervosa (BN), dysthymic disorder, fibromyalgia, generalized anxiety disorder, irritable bowel syndrome, migraine, obsessive-compulsive disorder, panic disorder, posttraumatic stress disorder, premenstrual dysphoric disorder, and social phobia (Hudson et al, 2003). The biological link between psychiatric and metabolic disorders is now clear (Bazar et al, 2006). Insulin resistance, diabetes, hypertension, metabolic syndrome, obesity, attention-deficit disorders, depression, psychosis, sleep apnea, inflammation, autism, and schizophrenia (SCZ) operate through common pathways; treatments used for one may prove beneficial for others (Bazar et al, 2006). Melatonin (MT), for example, is a powerful antioxidant that protects mitochondrial DNA; it easily crosses blood–brain barrier and has a role in ADHD, Alzheimer's disease (AD), autism, Parkinson's disease, seasonal affective disorder (SAD), and bipolar disorders (BDs).

Lipids are also essential for brain and neuron functioning. Lipid peroxidation is the outcome of free radical-mediated injury to the brain, where it directly damages membranes and generates oxidized products. Brain lipid peroxidation is a therapeutic target early in Alzheimer's and Huntington's diseases (Montine et al, 2004; Wu and Meydani, 2004). Brain P-450 enzymes catalyze the formation of neurosteroids and eicosanoids and they metabolize substrates such as vitamins A and D, cholesterol, and bile acids (Liu et al, 2004).

Nutrient intake has long-range effects. Deficiencies of vitamins B_{12}, folic acid, B_6, C, or E, iron, or zinc mimic the effects of radiation on the body by damaging DNA through strand breaks and oxidative lesions; deficient iron or biotin causes mitochondrial decay and oxidant leakage, leading to accelerated aging and neural decay (Ames, 2004).

Micronutrient scarcity during periods of human evolution has altered DNA and promoted some of our modern, late-onset diseases (Ames, 2006). Dietetic professionals should consider the complexities of neuropsychiatric conditions as well as the influence of diet on both reproductive and adult health.

A multidisciplinary approach is most effective. Psychotherapy addresses the will to change, responsibility for self, and search for meaning and identity. Psychiatrists focus on the medical and chemical management of prescribed drugs. Social workers assist with family and relationship issues. Dietitians focus on overall health status, medical issues, prescribed medicines, alternative therapies, and appropriate nutritional treatments. Assessment must include careful review of medical and treatment histories. Interventions must apply a positive approach, prevention of malnutrition, use of the team concept, restoration of feeding abilities, and improved nutritional quality of life. Table 4-3 lists important disorders; Table 4-4 lists neurotransmitters and their nutritional relevance; and Table 4-5 describes nutrients and substances important for brain health.

CITED REFERENCES

Ames BN. A role for supplements in optimizing health: the metabolic tune-up. *Arch Biochem Biophys.* 423:227, 2004.

Ames BN. Low micronutrient intake may accelerate the degenerative diseases of aging through allocation of scarce micronutrients by triage. *Proc Natl Acad Sci USA.* 103:17589, 2006.

Bazar KA, et al. Obesity and ADHD may represent different manifestations of a common environmental oversampling syndrome: a model for revealing mechanistic overlap among cognitive, metabolic, and inflammatory disorders. *Med Hypotheses.* 66:263, 2006.

Ferguson LR, et al. Nutrigenomics and gut health. *Mutat Research.* 622:1, 2007.

Liu M, et al. Cytochrome P450 in neurological disease. *Curr Drug Metab.* 5:225, 2004.

MacKay-Sim A, et al. Schizophrenia, vitamin D, and brain development. *Int Rev Neurobiol.* 59:351, 2004.

Montine KS, et al. Isoprostanes and related products of lipid peroxidation in neurodegenerative diseases. *Chem Phys Lipids.* 128:117, 2004.

Wu D, Meydani SN. Mechanism of age-associated up-regulation in macrophage PGE2 synthesis. *Brain Behav Immun.* 18:487, 2004.

Wurtman RJ. Synapse formation and cognitive brain development: effect of docosahexaenoic acid and other dietary constituents. *Metabolism.* 57:6S, 2008.

TABLE 4-3 **Disorders of Mental Health (*DSM-IV*)**

Mental Health Disorders	Explanation or Relevance to Nutrition
Acute stress disorder	Development of anxiety and dissociative and other symptoms within 1 month following exposure to an extremely traumatic event; other symptoms include re-experiencing the event and avoidance of trauma-related stimuli.
Adjustment disorder	Maladaptive reaction to identifiable stressful life events.
Amnestic disorder	Mental disorder characterized by acquired impairment in the ability to learn and recall new information, sometimes accompanied by inability to recall previously learned information, and not coupled to dementia or delirium.
Anxiety disorders	A group of mental disorders in which anxiety and avoidance behavior predominate, including panic disorders, agoraphobia, specific phobia, social phobia, obsessive-compulsive disorder, posttraumatic stress disorder, acute stress disorder, generalized anxiety disorder, and substance abuse anxiety disorder.
Attention-deficit disorder	Mental disorder characterized by inattention (such as distractibility, forgetfulness, not finishing tasks, and not appearing to listen), by hyperactivity and impulsivity (such as fidgeting and squirming, difficulty in remaining seated, excessive running or climbing, feelings of restlessness, difficulty awaiting one's turn, interrupting others, and excessive talking). See Section 3 for details.
Autistic disorder	Severe pervasive developmental disorder with onset usually before 3 years of age and a biological basis related to neurological or neurophysiological factors. Characterized by qualitative impairment in reciprocal social interaction (e.g., lack of awareness of the existence of feelings in others, failure to seek comfort at times of distress, lack of imitation), in verbal and nonverbal communication, and in capacity for symbolic play. Restricted and unusual repertoire of activities and interests.
Binge eating disorder	An eating disorder characterized by repeated episodes of binge eating, as in bulimia nervosa, but not followed by inappropriate compensatory behavior such as purging, fasting, or excessive exercise.
Bipolar disorders	Mood disorders characterized by a history of manic, mixed, or hypomanic episodes, usually with concurrent or previous history of one or more major depressive episodes.
Body dysmorphic disorder	A mental disorder in which a normal-appearing person is either preoccupied with some imagined defect in appearance or is overly concerned about some very slight physical anomaly.
Catatonic disorder	Catatonia due to the physiological effects of a general medical condition and neither better accounted for by another mental disorder nor occurring exclusively during delirium.
Childhood disintegrative disorder	Pervasive developmental disorder characterized by marked regression in a variety of skills, including language skills, social skills or adaptive behavior, play, bowel or bladder control, and motor skills, after at least 2, but less than 10, years of apparently normal development.

(continued)

TABLE 4-3 Disorders of Mental Health (*DSM-IV*) *(continued)*

Mental Health Disorders	Explanation or Relevance to Nutrition
Circadian rhythm sleep disorder	Lack of synchrony between the schedule of sleeping and waking required by the external environment and that of a person's own circadian rhythm.
Conduct disorder	A type of disruptive behavior disorder of childhood and adolescence characterized by a persistent pattern of conduct in which rights of others or age-appropriate societal norms or rules are violated. Misconduct includes aggression toward people or animals, destruction of property, deceitfulness, theft, and serious violations of rules.
Conversion disorder	Mental disorder with loss or alteration of voluntary motor or sensory functioning suggesting physical illness (such as seizures, paralysis, dyskinesia, anesthesia, blindness, or aphonia) having no demonstrable physiological basis.
Delusional disorder	Mental disorder marked by well-organized, logically consistent delusions but lacking other psychotic symptoms. Most functioning is not markedly impaired, the criteria for schizophrenia have never been satisfied, and symptoms of a major mood disorder have been present only briefly if at all.
Depersonalization disorder	Dissociative disorder characterized by one or more severe episodes of depersonalization (feelings of unreality and strangeness in one's perception of the self or one's body image) not due to another mental disorder, such as schizophrenia. The perception of reality remains intact; patients are aware of their incapacitation. Episodes are usually accompanied by dizziness, anxiety, fears of going insane, and derealization.
Depressive disorders	Mood disorders in which depression is unaccompanied by manic or hypomanic episodes.
Disruptive behavior	Group of mental disorders of children and adolescents consisting of behavior that violates social norms, is disruptive, distressing others more than it does the person with the disorder.
Dissociative disorders	Mental disorders characterized by sudden, temporary alterations in identity, memory, or consciousness, segregating normally integrated memories or parts of the personality from the dominant identity of the individual.
Dissociative identity disorder	Multiple personality disorder; characterized by the existence in an individual of two or more distinct personalities, each having unique memories, characteristic behavior, and social relationships.
Dysthymic disorder	Mood disorder characterized by depressed feeling (sad, blue, low), by loss of interest or pleasure in one's usual activities, and by at least some of the following: altered appetite, disturbed sleep patterns, lack of energy, low self-esteem, poor concentration or decision-making skills, and feelings of hopelessness. Symptoms have persisted for more than 2 years but are not severe enough to meet the criteria for major depressive disorder.
Eating disorder	Any of several disorders (anorexia nervosa, bulimia nervosa, pica, and rumination disorder) in which abnormal feeding habits are associated with psychological factors.
Factitious disorder	Repeated, intentional simulation of physical or psychological signs and symptoms of illness for no apparent purpose other than obtaining treatment.
Generalized anxiety disorder	Excessive, uncontrollable anxiety and worry about two or more life circumstances, for 6 months or longer, accompanied by some combination of restlessness, fatigue, muscle tension, irritability, disturbed concentration or sleep, and somatic symptoms.
Impulse control disorders	Repeated failure to resist an impulse to perform some act harmful to oneself or to others.
Learning disorders	Academic functioning that is substantially below the level expected on the basis of the patient's age, intelligence, and education, interfering with academic achievement or other functioning. Included are reading disorder, mathematics disorder, and disorder of written expression.
Mental disorder	Any clinically significant behavioral or psychological syndrome characterized by the presence of distressing symptoms, impairment of functioning, or significantly increased risk of suffering pain, disability, loss of freedom or death. Mental disorders manifest a behavioral, psychological, or biological dysfunction in the individual.
Motor skills disorder	Inadequate development of motor coordination, severe enough to limit locomotion or restrict the ability to perform tasks, schoolwork, or other activities.
Obsessive-compulsive disorder	Anxiety disorder characterized by recurrent obsessions or compulsions, which are severe enough to interfere significantly with personal or social functioning. Performing compulsive rituals may release tension temporarily; resisting them causes increased tension.
Oppositional defiant disorder	Disruptive behavior characterized by a recurrent pattern of defiant, hostile, disobedient, and negativistic behavior directed toward those in authority, including such actions as defying the requests or rules of adults, deliberately annoying others, arguing, spitefulness, and vindictiveness that occur much more frequently than would be expected on the basis of age and developmental stage.
Pain disorder	A somatoform disorder characterized by a chief complaint of severe chronic pain that causes substantial distress or impairment in functioning; the pain is neither feigned nor intentionally produced, and psychological factors appear to play a major role in its onset, severity, exacerbation, and maintenance.
Panic disorder and agoraphobia	Recurrent panic attacks, episodes of intense apprehension, fear, or terror associated with somatic symptoms such as dyspnea, palpitations, dizziness, vertigo, faintness, shakiness; and psychological symptoms such as feelings of unreality, depersonalization, fears of dying, going crazy, or losing control. There is usually chronic nervousness and tension between attacks.

(continued)

TABLE 4-3 Disorders of Mental Health (*DSM-IV*) *(continued)*

Mental Health Disorders	Explanation or Relevance to Nutrition
Personality disorders	Enduring, inflexible, and maladaptive personality traits that deviate markedly from cultural expectations, are self-perpetuating, pervade a broad range of situations, and either generate subjective distress or result in significant impairments in social, occupational, or other functioning. Onset is by adolescence or early adulthood.
Pervasive developmental disorders	Impaired development in multiple areas, including the acquisition of reciprocal social interaction, verbal and nonverbal communication skills, and imaginative activity and by stereotyped interests and behaviors; included are autism, Rett's syndrome, childhood disintegrative disorder, and Asperger's syndrome.
Premenstrual dysphoric disorder	Premenstrual syndrome with signs of depression, lethargy.
Reading disorder	Learning disorder in which the skill affected is reading ability, including accuracy, speed, and comprehension.
Rumination disorder	Eating disorder seen in infants under 1 year of age. After a period of normal eating habits, the child begins excessive regurgitation and rechewing of food, which is then ejected from the mouth or reswallowed. If untreated, death from malnutrition may occur.
Schizoaffective disorder	A major depressive episode, manic episode, or mixed episode occurs along with prominent psychotic symptoms characteristic of schizophrenia, the symptoms of the mood disorder being present for a substantial portion of the illness, but not for its entirety, and not being due to the effects of a psychoactive substance.
Seasonal affective disorder	A cyclically recurring mood disorder characterized by depression, extreme lethargy, increased need for sleep, hyperphagia, and carbohydrate craving; it intensifies in specific seasons, most commonly winter. It is hypothesized to be related to melatonin levels. "Mood disorder with seasonal pattern."
Separation anxiety disorder	Excessive, prolonged, developmentally inappropriate anxiety and apprehension in a child concerning removal from parents, home, or familiar surroundings.
Shared psychotic disorder	A delusional system that develops in one or more persons as a result of a close relationship with someone who already has a psychotic disorder with prominent delusions.
Sleep disorders	Chronic disorders involving sleep. Primary sleep disorders comprise dyssomnias and parasomnias; causes of secondary sleep disorders may include a general medical condition, mental disorder, or psychoactive substance.
Speech disorder	Defective ability to speak, either psychogenic or neurogenic.
Substance-related disorders	A variety of behavioral or psychological anomalies resulting from ingestion of or exposure to a drug of abuse, medication, or toxin.

Adapted from: Merck Manual, http://www.mercksource.com/pp/us/cns/cns_home.jsp, accessed May 13, 2009.

TABLE 4-4 Neurotransmitters and Nutritional Relevance

Type	Neurotransmitter	Postsynaptic Effect	Functions and Nutritional Relevance
Amino acids	Gamma aminobutyric acid (GABA)	Inhibitory	Glutamate is a precursor. Pyridoxal phosphate is a cofactor for both synthesis and break-down.
	Glycine	Inhibitory	Glycine inhibits neurotransmitter signals in the CNS. Available from dietary proteins, but most contain only small amounts (exception is collagen). Unique role as a type of antioxidant.
	Glutamate	Excitatory	The most important neurotransmitter for normal brain function; >50% of the neurons in the brain release glutamate. Glutamate can be used to synthesize glutamine by taking up ammonia; this reduces excessive ammonia levels in the brain and is important in diseases such as hepatic encephalopathy. The "sodium salt" of glutamic acid, monosodium glutamate (MSG), is responsible for one of the five basic tastes of the human sense of taste, umami; MSG is extensively used as a food additive. No specific dietary precursors. Primarily synthesized in the brain from alpha-keto glutarate and glucose. Glutamate is a precursor of GABA.
	Aspartate	Excitatory	Acidic analog of asparagine. No specific dietary precursors. Synthesized primarily from glutamate.
Biogenic monoamines	Dopamine	Excitatory	A monoamine neurotransmitter, concentrated in the basal ganglia. It is widely distributed throughout the brain in the nigrostriatal, the mesocorticolimbic, and the tuberohypophyseal pathways. Decreased brain dopamine levels contribute to Parkinson's disease, while an increase in dopamine concentration has a role in psychosis. Synthesized from phenylalanine and tyrosine.
Biogenic amine	Acetylcholine	Excitatory	Main neurotransmitter in the parasympathetic nervous system that controls heart rate, digestion, secretion of saliva, and bladder function. Drugs that affect cholinergic activity produce changes in these body functions. Affected by choline from the diet (eggs, soybeans). Some antidepressants act by blocking cholinergic receptors; this anticholinergic activity is an important cause of dry mouth. Botulism suppresses release of acetylcholine, and nicotine increases receptors for acetylcholine. Alzheimer's disease seems to be related to a malfunction in this neurotransmitter.

(continued)

TABLE 4-4 Neurotransmitters and Nutritional Relevance *(continued)*

Type	Neurotransmitter	Postsynaptic Effect	Functions and Nutritional Relevance
	Epinephrine	Excitatory	Affects fight or flight reactions; secreted in greater quantity during anger and fear, with resulting increase in heart rate and hydrolysis of glycogen to glucose. Used as a stimulant in cardiac arrest, as a vasoconstrictor in shock, as a bronchodilator in asthma, and to lower intraocular pressure in glaucoma. Secreted by the adrenal medulla.
	Noradrenaline	Excitatory	Synthesized from phenylalanine and tyrosine. A monoamine neurotransmitter that affects "fight or flight," attention and arousal, and blood pressure.
	Serotonin	Excitatory	Synthesized from tryptophan in the diet. Affects mood control, regulation of sleep, pain perception, body temperature, blood pressure, and hormonal activity. Also affects gastrointestinal and cardiovascular systems.
	Histamine	Excitatory	A potent agent believed to be involved in sleep–wake cycles and allergy.

From: http://www.brainexplorer.org/neurological_control/Neurological_index.shtml, accessed May 13, 2009.

TABLE 4-5 Nutrients for Brain Health

Diets that provide adequate amounts of complex carbohydrates, essential fats, amino acids, vitamins and minerals, and water support a balanced mood. Diet is one part of the jigsaw in the promotion of good mental health (Mental Health Foundation, 2009).

Nutrient or Factor	Role in the Brain	Comments
PROTEINS		
Aromatic amino acids (tryptophan, tyrosine, and phenylalanine)	Precursors of serotonin, dopamine, and norepinephrine	Increase in brain tryptophan from eating a carbohydrate-rich/protein-poor meal causes parallel increases in the amounts of serotonin released into synapses. Tryptophan can induce sleep from high-carbohydrate meals; high-protein meals tend to increase alertness.
Corticotropin-releasing hormone	Disturbances occur in periods of stress in the hypothalamic–pituitary–adrenal axis	Eating is often suppressed during stress due to anorectic effects of corticotropin-releasing hormone and increased during recovery from stress due to appetite-stimulating cortisol. Night eating syndrome is related to cortisol levels.
Cytokines	Influence sleep and eating behaviors; involved in many infectious, inflammatory, neoplastic, metabolic, and degenerative illnesses	Implicated in depressive and anxiety disorders; schizophrenic disorders (chronic and acute); autistic disorder; eating disorders; and obsessive-compulsive disorder.
Dietary antioxidants	Improve cognitive functioning	Fruits, vegetables, coffee, and tea. Strong inverse relationship between coffee intake and risk of suicide (Takeda, 2004). Quercetin (in red apples with skins, onions, blueberries, cranberries, strawberries) seems to protect against brain-cell damage (Silva et al, 2004).
LIPIDS		
Endocannabinoids	A class of lipids including amides, esters, and ethers of long-chain polyunsaturated fatty acids (Battista et al, 2004). They are activated by a CB2 receptor agonist, arachidonoylglycerol, and by elevated endogenous levels of endocannabinoids (Van Sickle et al, 2005)	Anandamide (N-arachidonoylethanolamine; AEA) and 2-arachidonoylglycerol are the main endogenous agonists of cannabinoid receptors, able to mimic several pharmacological effects of delta(9)-tetrahydrocannabinol, the active principal component of *Cannabis sativa* preparations such as hashish and marijuana (Battista et al, 2004). Nonpsychotropic therapeutic interventions using enhanced endocannabinoid levels may be used in localized brain areas (Van Sickle et al, 2005).
Essential fatty acids (EFA)	Fluidity of neuronal membrane, synthesis and functions of brain neurotransmitters, immune system integrity (Yehuda et al, 2005)	The blood–brain barrier determines the bioavailability. The myelination process determines the efficiency of brain and retinal functions of EFA. Since they must be supplied from the diet, a decreased bioavailability is induces major disturbances (Yehuda et al, 2005).
Omega-3 fatty acids *DHA, EPA	Control inflammatory and autoimmune processes; part of the brain lipid membranes. DHA depletion leads to losses in neuronal function (Lim et al, 2005)	Helpful in depression, bipolar disorder, multiple sclerosis, and other neurological conditions. DHA and arachidonic acid (AA) may not distribute evenly in the brain. There are age-induced regional changes in fatty acid composition of brain phospholipids. DHA, uridine (as uridine monophosphate), and choline are all found in mother's milk, and included in most infant formulas; these substances are part of a regulatory mechanism through which plasma composition influences brain development (Wurtman, 2008).
Omega-6 polyunsaturated fatty acids ALA, GLA	Part of the brain lipid membranes	Useful in anorexia nervosa and several neurological conditions. May reduce risk for Parkinson's disease (de Lau et al, 2005).

(continued)

TABLE 4-5 Nutrients for Brain Health *(continued)*

Nutrient or Factor	Role in the Brain	Comments
MINERALS		
Iron	Normal amounts are required for normal functioning. 7% of the general population, and 19% of women between ages of 12–50 may be deficient (UC Davis, 2009)	Iron sufficiency prevents anemia. Deficiency causes DNA breaks (UC Davis, 2009).
Selenium	Parts of the United States and China have areas where soil is deficient in selenium	Antioxidant properties protect the brain and nerves from damage. Brazil nuts are a rich source.
Zinc	18% of the US population is deficient (UC Davis, 2009)	Zinc functions as part of the insulin molecule and hundreds of enzymes. Deficiency causes DNA damage with chromosome breaks; this leads to brain and immune dysfunction (UC Davis, 2009).
VITAMINS		
Niacin	2% of the general population may be deficient (UC Davis, 2009)	Deficiency disables DNA repair (poly ADP ribose); this leads to neurological damage and memory loss (UC Davis, 2009).
Vitamins B_6, B_{12}, and folic acid	Lower elevated amounts of homocysteine. 10% of the population may be deficient in these B_6; 4% may be deficient in B_{12} (UC Davis, 2009)	These play a role in many neurological conditions. Methylated forms may be needed in individuals who have the MTHFR genotype. B_{12} deficiency leads to neurological damage (UC Davis, 2009).
Vitamins C and E	Vitamins C and E function as antioxidants	Antioxidant properties are protective.
Vitamin D	Vitamin D has been found to delay onset of multiple sclerosis and effects of depression (especially seasonal affective disorder). It is being studied in schizophrenia	Vitamin D has nuclear hormone receptors that regulate gene expression and nervous system development.
OTHER		
[a]Uridine	A pyrimidine nucleoside that is formed when uracil is attached to a ribose ring	Component of RNA. Its nucleotides participate in the biosynthesis of polysaccharide compounds. Foods containing uridine may help to alleviate depression (Carlezon et al, 2005).
[a]Choline	A nutrient that improves the environment of the brain cells (Zeisel, 2004)	Choline is a nutrient found in egg yolks, milk, nuts, fish, liver and other meats, and human breast milk. It is the essential building block acetylcholine, and it plays a vital role in the formation of phospholipids in cell membranes. Pregnant women should include a good source in their daily diets.

[a]NOTE. A preparation containing uridine, docosahexaenoic acid (DHA,) and choline is being tested for improved cognition, and enhanced neurotransmitter release (Wurtman et al, 2009).

REFERENCES

Battista N, et al. Endocannabinoids and their involvement in the neurovascular system. *Curr Neurovasc Res.* 1:129, 2004.

Carlezon WA Jr, et al. Antidepressant-like effects of uridine and omega-3 fatty acids are potentiated by combined treatment in rats. *Biol Psychiatry.* 57:343, 2005.

de Lau LM, et al. Dietary fatty acids and the risk of Parkinson disease: the Rotterdam study. *Neurology.* 64:2040, 2005.

Lim SY, et al. N-3 fatty acid deficiency induced by a modified artificial rearing method leads to poorer performance in spatial learning tasks. *Pediatr Res.* 58:741, 2005.

Mental Health Foundation. Accessed May 13, 2009, at http://www.mentalhealth.org.uk/welcome.

Silva BA, et al. Neuroprotective effect of *H. perforatum* extracts on beta- amyloid-induced neurotoxicity. *Neurotox Res.* 6:119, 2004.

Takeda E. Stress control and human nutrition. *J Med Invest.* 51:139, 2004.

UC Davis. University of California-Davis NCMHD Center of Excellence for Nutritional Genomics. Accessed May 14, 2009, at http://nutrigenomics.ucdavis.edu/nutrigenomics/index.cfm?objectid=9688A280-65 B3-C1E7-02E9FCDABDD84C68.

Van Sickle MD, et al. Identification and functional characterization of brainstem cannabinoid CB2 receptors. *Science.* 310:329, 2005.

Wurtman RJ. Synapse formation and cognitive brain development: effect of docosahexaenoic acid and other dietary constituents. *Metabolism.* 57:6S, 2008.

Yehuda S, et al. Essential fatty acids and the brain: from infancy to aging. *Neurobiol Aging.* 26:98S, 2005.

Zeisel SH. Nutritional importance of choline for brain development. *J Am Coll Nutr.* 23:621, 2004.

For More Information

- American Academy of Neurology
  http://www.aan.com
- American Association of Neuroscience Nurses
  http://www.aann.org
- American Neurological Association
  http://www.aneuroa.org
- American Psychiatric Association—DSM-V
  www.dsm5.org
- American Society of Neurorehabilitation
  http://www.asnr.com
- Brain Research Foundation
  http://brainresearchfdn.org/
- Society for Neuroscience
  http://www.sfn.org

NEUROLOGICAL DISORDERS

ALZHEIMER'S DISEASE AND DEMENTIAS

NUTRITIONAL ACUITY RANKING: LEVEL 3

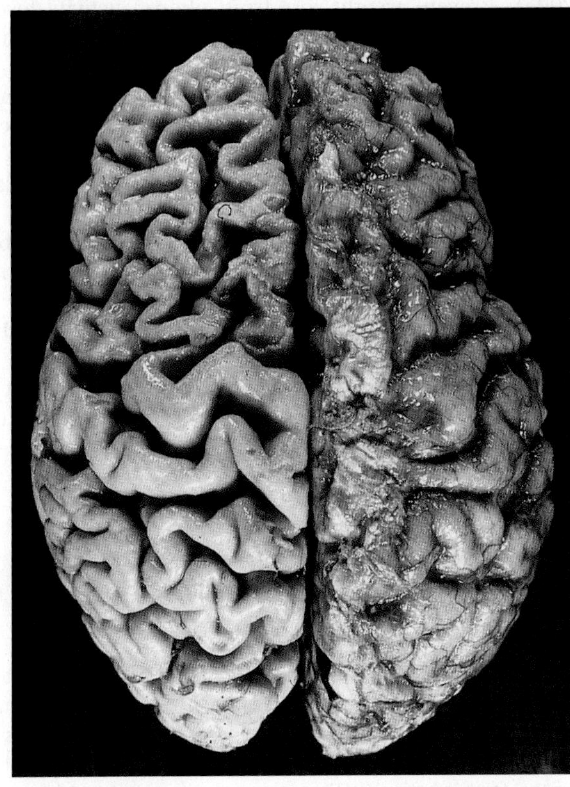

Adapted from: Raphael Rubin, David S. Strayer, *Rubin's Pathology: Clinicopathologic Foundations of Medicine,* 5th ed. Philadelphia: Lippincott Williams & Wilkins, 2008.

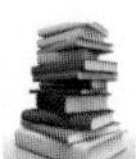

DEFINITIONS AND BACKGROUND

Dementias include multiple cognitive defects with memory loss; they often involve aphasia, apraxia, agnosia, and disturbed daily functioning. Risk factors include diabetes, cardiovascular disease, stroke, hypertension, head injury, aging, depression, and family history. Of over 50 dementias, **AD** is the most common, with progressive deterioration of intellect, memory, personality, and self-care. Other conditions should be ruled out by medical evaluation. Early stages of AD manifest with short-term memory loss; problems finding the appropriate word; asking the same questions over and over; difficulty making decisions and planning ahead; suspiciousness; changes in senses of smell and taste; denial; depression; loss of initiative; personality changes; and problems with abstract thinking.

AD is characterized by deposition of extracellular neuritic, beta-amyloid peptide-containing plaques in cerebral cortical regions and presence of intracellular neurofibrillary tangles in cerebral pyramidal neurons (Schliebs, 2005). Acetylcholine-containing neurons are especially affected. Acetylcholine normally triggers breakdown of the beta-amyloid precursor protein (APP) in brain cells. Impaired cerebral energy metabolism and pyruvate dehydrogenase activity are also found (Martin et al, 2005).

Insulin and associated signaling molecules begin to disappear from the brain during early AD, suggesting a form of "type 3 diabetes." Insulin deficiency and insulin resistance mediate AD-type neurodegeneration; indeed, experimental brain diabetes is treatable with drugs currently used to treat T2DM (de la Monte and Wands, 2008). Altered glycogen synthase kinase-3 (GSK-3) function, decreased serum insulin-like growth factor I (IGF-I) levels, and carotid atherosclerosis are independent risk factors for AD (Lester-Coll et al, 2006; Wantanabe et al, 2005).

Apolipoprotein E (ApoE) is an important determinant of lipoprotein metabolism and risk for oxidative damage (Dietrich et al, 2005). Because ApoE also influence cognitive function and decline, prevention of cardiovascular disease may slow the onset of AD (Kang et al, 2005). Because age-related proinflammattory cytokines are also involved, there is a reduced risk of AD in users of nonsteroidal anti-inflammatory drugs (Staehelin, 2008).

Mood instability and increased distractibility, irritability, agitation, and irregular sleep can be present. Behavioral changes, such as aggressive behavior, psychosis, and overactivity, occur frequently and determine the need for institutionalization or use of mood stabilizers. A lifetime of depression may actually precede AD and should be corrected (Ownby et al, 2006; Rapp et al, 2006).

Declining body mass over time is strongly linked to the risk of developing AD (Buchman et al, 2005). Metabolic acidosis promotes muscle wasting; diets that are rich in net acid-producing protein and cereal grains relative to their content of net alkali-producing fruit and vegetables may therefore contribute to a reduction in lean tissue mass in older adults (Dawson-Hughes et al, 2008).

Circadian patterns of food intake change and disturbed eating patterns occur, with altered macronutrient selection and preference for carbohydrates (Greenwood et al, 2005).

Numerous observational studies demonstrate a positive correlation between a high intake of antioxidants and better cognitive function in the elderly (Staehelin, 2008). Use of nutrients that increase the levels of brain catecholamines and protect against oxidative damage is critical: vitamins C and E, zinc, iron, copper, and selenium should be provided (Squitti et al, 2005). Antioxidants in foods such as blueberries, cranberries, strawberries, kale, and spinach may improve cognitive function; and coffee drinkers tend to have lower levels of AD later in life (Eskelinen et al, 2009). There is substantial epidemiological evidence from a number of recent studies that demonstrate a protective role of omega-3 fatty acids, such as docosahexaenoic acid (DHA), in AD and cognitive decline (Morris, 2009).

Finally, vitamins B_6 and B_{12} and folate should be used to lower homocysteine (tHcy) levels. Comprehensive treatment of AD requires thorough caregiver support and thoughtful use of medications for cognition enhancement, neuroprotection, and treatment of agitation. While the prognosis for

AD is improving, death most often occurs from renal, pulmonary, or cardiac complications between 2 and 20 years after onset of symptoms. Pneumonia is a common cause of morbidity and death, related to dysphagia, aspiration, altered mobility, decreased nutritional status, and lowered immune response.

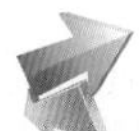

ASSESSMENT, MONITORING, AND EVALUATION

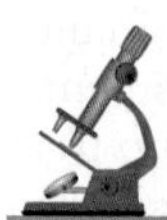

CLINICAL INDICATORS

Genetic Markers: ApoE epsilon4 allele is a primary gene that has been confirmed in AD. Hypomethylation of the amyloid A4 precursor gene and hyperhomocysteinemia may contribute to the pathophysiology of AD (Abdolmaleky et al, 2004; Aisen et al, 2008). Cerebrospinal-fluid biomarkers beta-amyloid 42 (Aß42), T-tau, and P-tau may identify early-stage AD (Mattsson et al, 2009).

Clinical/History

- Height, weight
- Subtle weight loss
- Current BMI,% change
- Dietary/intake history
- Intake and output (I & O)
- Anorexia and poor intake
- Nausea, vomiting
- Diarrhea
- Bowel incontinence
- Electroencephalogram (EEG)
- Loss of sense of smell
- Hx of Down syndrome or depression?
- Computed tomography (CT) scan
- Brain magnetic resonance imaging (MRI)
- Medial temporal lobe thickness (often thinned)
- Mini-Mental State Examination
- Severe Impairment Battery and Global Deterioration Scale
- Mattis Dementia Rating Scale
- Behavioral disturbances: Neuropsychiatric Inventory
- Behavioral function: London Psychogeriatric Rating Scale

Lab Work

- Cerebrospinal fluid biomarkers [Aβ42, T-tau, P-tau]
- Choline acetyltransferase activity (ChAT)
- C-reactive protein (CRP)
- Cholesterol (may be high)
- Glucose (gluc)
- Serum tHcy (elevated?)
- Serum folate; methyltetrahydrofolate reductase (MTHFR) levels
- Serum vitamin B_{12}
- Serum zinc
- Serum copper
- Alanine aminotransferase (ALT)
- Aspartate aminotransferase (AST)
- Dopamine (DA)
- Cerebral spinal fluid (CSF) pyruvate and lactate levels
- Na^+, K^+
- Blood urea nitrogen (BUN)
- Creatinine (creat)
- H & H
- Serum Fe
- Albumin or transthyretin

INTERVENTION

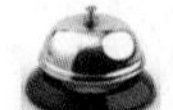

OBJECTIVES

- To effectively enhance intake, interventions must work with changing needs and intake patterns (Young et al, 2005). Prevent weight loss from altered activity levels, poor eating habits, depression, impaired memory, and self-feeding difficulty.
- Maintain activity to preserve function. Walking 90 minutes per week helps to maintain lean body mass and can possibly help alleviate anorexia.
- Avoid constipation or impaction; support bowel or bladder continence through proper scheduling.
- Encourage self-feeding at mealtimes as long as possible. Begin using finger foods and items easy to consume without utensils.
- Prevent or correct dehydration, pressure ulcers, and other signs of nutritional decline. Preserve muscle mass.
- Monitor dysphagia, pocketing of food, or aspiration. Use gastrostomy feeding, especially in early stages. While the

SAMPLE NUTRITION CARE PROCESS STEPS

Self-Feeding Difficulty

Assessment Data: Food records indicating poor intake; weight loss; forgetting how to feed self. Requires total feeding. Anorexia and complaints of taste changes, lost sense of smell. Lab results showing low albumin and transthyretin. Recent dehydration and urinary tract infection (UTI).

Nutrition Diagnoses (PES): Self-feeding difficulty related to inability to use utensils (fork, spoon) at advanced stage of Alzheimer's as evidenced by weight loss, I & O with recent dehydration, dietary intake records showing intake of about 25–50% of meals served.

Interventions:

Food and Nutrient Delivery:

ND 1.3 Specific foods/beverage—finger foods and nutrient-dense diet.

ND 3.1.1.Commercial beverage supplement 1 can twice daily.

ND 3.2.1 Supplement with multivitamin–mineral once daily.

ND 4.5 Feeding assistance—fed by staff.

Education: Educate caregivers about introducing finger foods items, reducing distractions at mealtime, scheduling of meals to give structure, use of frequent and portable snacks throughout the day to improve intake of nutrients and energy. Reinforce safe feeding strategies with caregivers to avoid aspiration.

Counseling: C-2.2 Goal setting: improve oral intake, prevent aspiration, regain lost weight. Avoid constipation, dehydration, and impaction.

Coordination of Nutrition Care: RC-1.1 Team meeting with nursing, social services, speech therapy, recreation therapy.

Monitoring and Evaluation: Improved weight, visceral protein levels; less agitation.

terminal stage of AD is generally indicated by the inability to swallow, the benefit of enteral feeding (EN) is limited at that point.
- Use creative feeding strategies. Offer frequent snacks, day and night if desired.
- Protect patient from injuries and provide emotional support for patient and family.
- To assist with eating-related behavioral problems, there are many tips. For example, for attention deficit, verbally direct the patient through the eating process; make food and fluids visible. Give one food at a time; offer small bites. Serve soft foods to reduce the need for chewing.
- Keep simple routines and a consistent environment. Minimize distractions at mealtime. Provide a quiet environment. If group dining is a concern, provide meals in room or with a single partner.
- Use finger foods and cups with cover/spout if the patient paces.

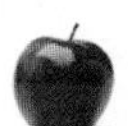

FOOD AND NUTRITION

- Ensure a healthy diet, including protein and increased calories for age, sex, and activity, especially for "wanderers" and those who pace. Persons with AD may need 35 kcal/kg of body weight or more.
- Adequate **vitamin E** (such as in nuts, creamy salad dressings). Include nutrient-dense foods that are high in antioxidants. Coffee, cocoa, and red wine contain flavonols that increase blood flow to the brain; one serving of wine daily can be included.
- Provide more oily fish (salmon, halibut, trout, and tuna) for **omega-3 fatty acids**. Fish oil capsules have not been shown to be quite as effective.
- **Omega 6 fatty acids** may also be beneficial, such as from vegetable oils.
- Extra **folic acid** may lessen decline of cognitive function; offer leafy greens, orange juice, broccoli. To lower tHcy levels, folic acid, vitamins B and B_{12} are important (Zhou and Practico, 2009). Avoid excesses of vitamin B_{12} from red meat and high-fat dairy products.
- Use color-rich fruits and vegetables (blueberries, cranberries, strawberries, spinach, kale, broccoli, oranges, and other citrus fruits). Higher intake of foods rich in potassium, such as fruit and vegetables, favors preservation of muscle mass (Dawson-Hughes et al, 2008).
- Foods high in copper include liver, kidney, oysters, nuts, dried beans and legumes, cocoa, eggs, prunes, and potatoes.
- Offer meals at regular and consistent times each day. Allow sufficient time for eating. Offer one course at a time (first salad, then entree, then fruit dessert) to prevent confusion. Avoid distractions; use calming background music. Cueing to eat is also useful.
- Use dishes without a pattern; white is a good choice.
- Use a simple place setting and a single eating utensil. Use a bowl for easier scooping and special spoons or adaptive equipment as needed. Serve soup in mugs.
- Finger foods, such as sandwiches cut into four, cheese cubes, pancakes or waffles cut in smaller pieces, hard cooked egg halves, chicken strips, julienne vegetables, and brownies (vs. pie), are easier to eat and help to maintain weight.
- Provide a high-carbohydrate meal for dinner to increase food intake during later stages of the disease; this reflects the preference for high-carbohydrate foods (Young et al, 2005). Plan menus accordingly; offer nutrient-dense desserts, such as fruit tarts, puddings topped with fruit, and custards.
- Tube feed or use texture-altered foods with thickened liquids as needed to compensate for dysphagia.
- Choline may be beneficial; use soybeans or eggs (Michel et al, 2006).
- Adequate fluid intake is essential. Offer regular drinks of water, juice, milk, and other fluids to avoid dehydration.
- Cut back on saturated fats, which increase brain beta-amyloid levels. Omit high-fat dairy products, fast food items, fried foods, and processed foods.

Common Drugs Used and Potential Side Effects

- See Table 4-6.

Herbs, Botanicals, and Supplements

- Allopregnanolone (APalpha, a metabolite of progesterone) is reduced in the serum, plasma, and brain of aged individuals and Alzheimer's patients; researchers are evaluating its possible use (Wang et al, 2008).
- Chinese medicines show promise in combinations; Huperzine A (Chinese club moss,) gingko biloba, and ginseng are under Study (Fu and Li, 2009).
- Coenzyme Q10 and choline supplements are under study.
- Curry, cumin, and turmeric may block beta-amyloid plaque formation in the brain and can be encouraged as seasonings.
- Folic acid, vitamins B_6, and B_{12} supplements do not slow cognitive decline in dementia but can lower tHcy levels (Aisen et al, 2008; Malouf et al, 2003). Cerefolin® contains N-acetylcysteine (NAC) and L-methylfolate. Where there are MTHFR polymorphisms, the active form of folate (methyltetrahydrofolate) may be needed (Mischoulon and Raab, 2007).
- Genetic risk factors for cognitive decline may remain latent pending age-related decline in nutrition, suggesting the importance of early intervention with key dietary supplements (including alpha-lipoic acid [ALA], DHA) to delay the progression of age-related cognitive decline (Suchy et al., 2009).
- Gingko biloba interacts with anticoagulants and antiplatelets such as aspirin, warfarin, and dipyridamole. Clinical trials have not shown effectiveness when used alone (Birks et al, 2009).
- Horse balm, rosemary, dandelion, procaine, sage, and lecithin have been suggested but long-term trials have not confirmed their usefulness.

TABLE 4-6 Medications for Alzheimer's Disease and Possible Side Effects

Medication	Side Effects
Antidepressants	Minimal improvements have been noted. Mirtazapine may be useful in the treatment of the comorbid symptoms of weight loss, insomnia, and anxiety, a reflection of its enhancement of brain serotonergic and noradrenergic neurotransmission. Large, randomized controlled trials (RCTs) are needed.
Atypical antipsychotics	The efficacy of risperidone and olanzapine for the treatment of psychotic symptoms has been demonstrated by large RCTs in Alzheimer's disease.
Cholinesterase inhibitors donepezil (Aricept®), galantamine (Reminyl® or Razadyne®), rivastigmine (Exelon®)	Can slow agitation and the progression of cognitive and functional deficits in Alzheimer's disease in early stages by blocking acetylcholine breakdown. They improve cognitive function, behavior, and daily functioning. Nausea, diarrhea, insomnia, fatigue and loss of appetite may occur.
Cerefolin®	Contains methylated B_{12} and folic acid, as well as N-acetylcysteine.
Coenzyme Q10	Studies are inconclusive at this time. Indivuduals who take statins may need a supplement to reduce side effects such as rhabdomyolysis.
Hydergine	Relieves symptoms of declining mental capacity. Nausea and gastrointestinal (GI) distress are common.
Ibuprofen and other nonsteroidal, anti-inflammatory drugs	May reduce the risk of development of Alzheimer's disease by reducing inflammatory processes.
Insulin	If Alzheimer's disease is related to diabetes, it may be important to assure that adequate levels of insulin are available to the brain.
Laxatives	To control constipation. Offer high-fiber foods and sufficient fluid.
Mood stabilizers (lithium)	Low doses may be useful when combined with antipsychotics. Lithium regulates amyloid-beta precursor protein processing (Su et al, 2004).
Memantine (Namenda)	This regulates the activity of glutamate, a messenger chemical involved in learning and memory.
Selegiline (Eldepryl)	Selegiline should not be used with ginseng, ma huang (ephedra), yohimbe, or St. John's wort.
Statins	People taking statin drugs may have lower blood cholesterol and less incidence of Alzheimer's disease. They may have the ability to break down plaque-building amyloid protein.
Tacrine (Cognex)	For use in mild-to-moderate AD. May cause nausea, vomiting, or liver damage. Used less often today.
Vitamin E	Use of alpha-tocopherol has had mixed results in the literature (Petersen et al, 2005).

http://www.alz.org/national/documents/topicsheet_treatments.pdf, accessed September 1, 2009.

- Omega-3 fatty acids are known to reduce cytokines and then lower the AD risk (Fotuhi et al, 2009; Morris, 2009; Staehelin, 2008).
- Panax ginseng has demonstrated efficacy in some studies (Lee et al, 2009).
    - SAM as a supplement can facilitate glutathione and acetylcholine utilization (Chan et al, 2008). Longer trials are needed.
    - Repeat testing of vitamin B_{12} every 2 years. Where deficiency occurs, treat and prevent neurological and hematological consequences by providing B_{12} (Prodan et al, 2009).

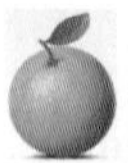

NUTRITION EDUCATION, COUNSELING, CARE MANAGEMENT

- A nutrition education program intended for caregivers of AD patients can yield positive effects on patient weights and cognitive function.
- There is growing evidence for possible dietary risk factors in the development of AD and cognitive decline with age, such as antioxidant nutrients, fish, dietary fats, and B-vitamins (Morris, 2009). Promote use of the Mediterranean or DASH diets. Encourage use of fruits such as blueberries and other berries. Exercise and an antioxidant-rich diet may be protective against further cognitive decline.
- Encourage routines such as regular mealtimes, and good mouth care. Reduce distractions at mealtime.
- Refer family or caretakers to support groups. Long-term care or home care may be needed at some point in time.
- Special feeding methods may be needed. If the patient must be spoon fed, gently holding his or her nose will force the mouth open.
- Liquid supplements can add extra calories and protein without excessive expense. Baking nutritious cookie bars or snacks enhances calorie intake and addresses the need for sensory stimulation.
- Use unbreakable dishes and utensils to avoid injury. Cutting and preparing foods for the patient are useful.
- Offspring of affected family members should be tested and treated for hypertension; pro-inflammatory cytokines and ApoE genes should also be assessed (van Exel et al, 2009).

Patient Education—Foodborne Illness

- Careful food handling will be important. The same is true for hand washing, especially with incontinence. Use of hand wipes before meals is recommended.

For More Information

- Alzheimer's Association
http://www.alz.org/
- Alzheimer's Disease Education and Referral (ADEAR) Center
http://www.alzheimers.org
- Alzheimer's Disease International
http://www.alz.co.uk/
- Alzheimer's Research Forum
http://www.alzforum.org/
- Web MD
http://www.webmd.com/alzheimers/default.htm

ALZHEIMER'S DISEASE AND DEMENTIAS—CITED REFERENCES

Abdolmaleky HM, et al. Methylomics in psychiatry: modulation of gene-environment interactions may be through DNA methylation. *Am J Med Genet B Neuropsychiatr Genet.* 127B:51, 2004.

Aisen PS, et al. High-dose B vitamin supplementation and cognitive decline in Alzheimer disease: a randomized controlled trial. *JAMA.* 300:1774, 2008.

Birks J, Grimley Evans J. Ginkgo biloba for cognitive impairment and dementia. *Cochrane Database Syst Rev.*1:CD003120, 2009.

Buchman AS, et al. Change in body mass index and risk of incident Alzheimer disease. *Neurology.* 65:892, 2005.

Chan A, et al. Dietary and genetic compromise in folate availability reduces acetylcholine, cognitive performance and increases aggression: critical role of S-adenosyl methionine. *J Nutr Health Aging.* 12:252, 2008.

Dawson-Hughes B, et al. Alkaline diets favor lean tissue mass in older adults. *Am J Clin Nutr.* 87:662, 2008.

de la Monte SM, Wands JR. Alzheimer's disease is type 3 diabetes-evidence reviewed. *J Diabetes Sci Technol.* 2:1101, 2008.

Dietrich M, et al. Associations between apolipoprotein E genotype and circulating F2-isoprostane levels in humans. *Lipids.* 40:329, 2005.

Eskelinin MH, et al. Midlife coffee and tea drinking and the risk of late-life dementia: a population-based CAIDE study. *J Alzheimers Dis.* 16:85, 2009.

Fotuhi M, et al. Fish consumption, long-chain omega-3 fatty acids and risk of cognitive decline or Alzheimer disease: a complex association. *Nat Clin Pract Neurol.* 5:140, 2009.

Fu LM, Li JT. A systematic review of single Chinese herbs for Alzheimer's disease treatment. [published online ahead of print September 21, 2009] *Evid Basec Complement Alternat Med.*

Greenwood CE, et al. Behavioral disturbances, not cognitive deterioration, are associated with altered food selection in seniors with Alzheimer's disease. *J Gerontol A Biol Sci Med Sci.* 60:499, 2005.

Kang JH, et al. Apolipoprotein E, cardiovascular disease and cognitive function in aging women. *Neurobiol Aging.* 26:475, 2005.

Lee ST, et al. Panax ginseng enhances cognitive performance in Alzheimer disease. *Alzheimer's Dis Assoc Disord.* 22:222, 2008.

Lester-Coll N, et al. Intracerebral streptozotocin model of type 3 diabetes: relevance to sporadic Alzheimer's disease. *J Alzheimers Dis.* 9:13, 2006.

Malouf M, et al. Folic acid with or without vitamin B_{12} for cognition and dementia. *Cochrane Database Syst Rev.* 4:CD004514, 2003.

Martin E, et al. Pyruvate dehydrogenase complex: metabolic link to ischemic brain injury and target of oxidative stress. *J Neurosci Res.* 79:240, 2005.

Mattsson N, et al. CSF biomarkers and incipient Alzheimer disease in patients with mild cognitive impairment. *JAMA.* 302:385, 2009.

Michel V, et al. Choline transport for phospholipid synthesis. *Exp Biol Med (Maywood).* 231:490, 2006.

Mischoulon D, Raab MF. The role of folate in depression and dementia. *J Clin Psychiatry.* 68:28, 2007.

Morris MC. The role of nutrition in Alzheimer's disease: epidemiological evidence. *Eur J Neurol.* 16:1S, 2009.

Ownby RL, et al. Depression and risk for Alzheimer disease: systematic review, meta-analysis, and metaregression analysis. *Arch Gen Psychiatry.* 63:530, 2006.

Petersen RC, et al. Vitamin E and donepezil for the treatment of mild cognitive impairment. *N Engl J Med.* 352:2379, 2005.

Poehlman E, Dvorak R. Energy expenditure, energy intake, and weight loss in Alzheimer disease. *Am J Clin Nutri.* 71:650S, 2000.

Prodan CI, et al. Cumulative incidence of vitamin B_{12} deficiency in patients with Alzheimer disease. [published online ahead of print May 21, 2009] *J Neurol Sci.* 284:144, 2009.

Rapp MA, et al. Increased hippocampal plaques and tangles in patients with Alzheimer disease with a lifetime history of major depression. *Arch Gen Psychiatry.* 63:161, 2006.

Schliebs R. Basal forebrain cholinergic dysfunction in Alzheimer's disease: interrelationship with beta-amyloid, inflammation and neurotrophin signaling. *Neurochem Res.* 30:895, 2005.

Squitti R, et al. Excess of serum copper not related to ceruloplasmin in Alzheimer disease. *Neurology.* 64:1040, 2005.

Staehelin HB. Neuronal protection by bioactive nutrients. *Int J Vitamin Nutr Res.* 78:282, 2008.

Su Y, et al. Lithium, a common drug for bipolar disorder treatment, regulates amyloid-beta precursor protein processing. *Biochemistry.* 43:6899, 2004.

Suchy J, et al. Dietary supplementation with a combination of alpha-lipoic acid, acetyl-L-carnitine, glycerophosphocoline, docosahexaenoic acid, and phosphatidylserine reduces oxidative damage to murine brain and improves cognitive performance. *Nutr Res.* 29:70, 2009.

van Exel E, et al. Vascular factors and markers of inflammation in offspring with a parental history of late-onset Alzheimer disease. *Arch Gen Psychiatry.* 66:1263, 2009.

Wang JM, et al. Regenerative potential of allopregnanolone. *Brain Res Rev.* 57:398, 2008.

Wantanabe T, et al. Relationship between serum insulin-like growth factor-1 levels and Alzheimer's disease and vascular dementia. *J Am Geriatr Soc.* 53:1748, 2005.

Wurtman RJ, et al. Use of phosphatide precursors to promote synaptogenesis. [published online ahead of print April 11, 2009] *Annu Rev Nutr.* 29:59, 2009.

Young KW, et al. A randomized, crossover trial of high-carbohydrate foods in nursing home residents with Alzheimer's disease: associations among intervention response, body mass index, and behavioral and cognitive function. *J Gerontol A Biol Sci Med Sci.* 60:1039, 2005.

Zhou JM, Practico D. Acceleration of brain amyloidosis in an Alzheimer's disease mouse model by a folate, vitamin B_6 and B_{12}-deficient diet. [published online ahead of print December 11, 2009] *Exp Gerontol.* 45:195.

AMYOTROPHIC LATERAL SCLEROSIS

NUTRITIONAL ACUITY RANKING: LEVEL 3

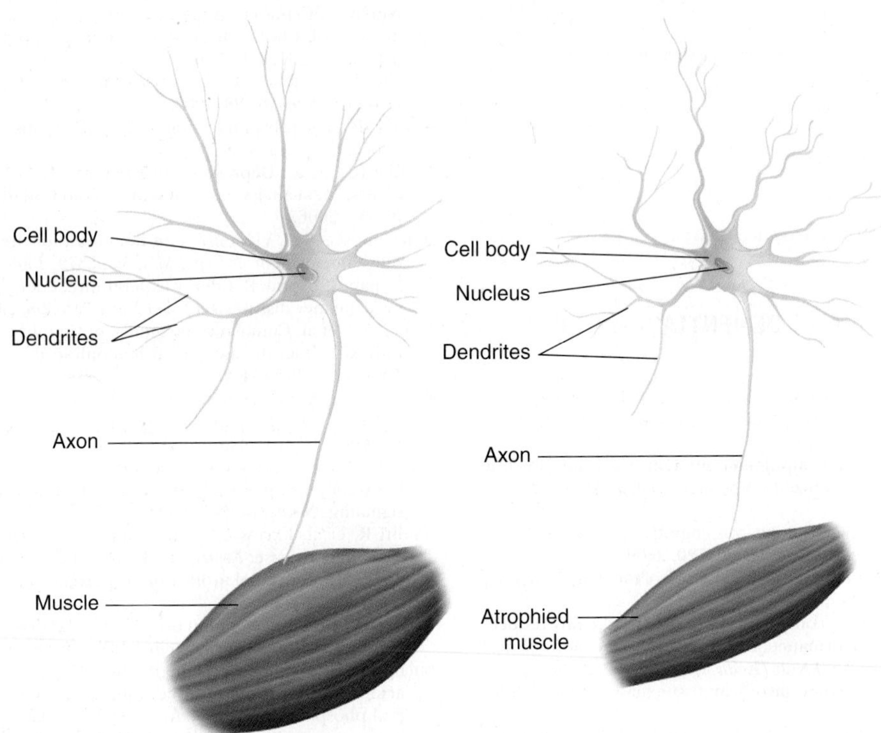

Asset provided by Anatomical Chart Co.

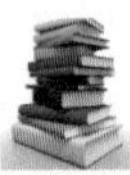

DEFINITIONS AND BACKGROUND

Amyotrophic lateral sclerosis (ALS) is a progressive motor neuron disease of adult life that destroys nerve cells from the spinal cord to muscle cells. The name "no muscle nourishment." Symptoms include muscular wasting and atrophy, drooling, loss of reflexes, respiratory infections or failure, spastic gait, and weakness. Respiratory failure occurs as a result of bulbar, cervical, and thoracic loss of motor neurons; inspiratory muscles are affected.

Men and women are affected equally, in about 20,000 people in the United States. ALS usually occurs after age 40; it is also known as progressive spinal muscular atrophy or Lou Gehrig's disease. Management of respiratory failure includes the use of strategies that limit aspiration pneumonia, the reduction in secretions, positioning of the patient to a maximal mechanical advantage, and use of noninvasive positive pressure ventilation.

Malnutrition is aggravated by elevated metabolic needs and swallowing dysfunction in the lower set of cranial nerves. The malnutrition produces neuromuscular weakness and adversely affects patients' quality of life. In later stages of the disease, percutaneous endoscopic gastrostomy (PEG) feeding may be needed. However, consider patient preferences and advance directives; individuals have the right to accept or refuse treatment (American Dietetic Association, 2008). Quality of life does not necessarily improve (Langmore et al, 2006).

Dietary factors have been suspected of being risk factors for ALS. Lycopene and magnesium are important nutrients (Oyanagi et al, 2006). Environmental exposure to arsenic depletes s-adenosyl-methionine (SAM) especially with folate insufficiency (Dubey and Shea, 2007). Elevated tHcy damages motor neurons and may be linked to faster progression of ALS (Zoccolella et al, 2008). However, there is no known cure at this time and ALS patients usually have respiratory distress, anxiety, pain, choking episodes, or pneumonia at the end of life.

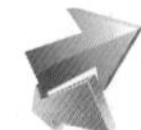

ASSESSMENT, MONITORING, AND EVALUATION

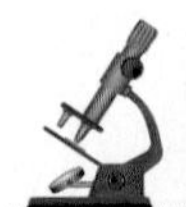

CLINICAL INDICATORS

Genetic Markers: Mutations in the c-1 (SOD-1) gene result in familial amyotrophic ateral sclerosis (FALS). Over 135 mutations have been identified in the various forms of ALS.

Clinical/History	Electromyogram (EMG)	Ca^{++}, Mg^{++}
Height	Gag reflex	Albumin (alb), transthyretin
Weight	ALS Functional Rating Scale (ALSFRS-R)	Transferrin
Weight changes	Ventilatory dependency?	BUN, Creat
BMI (<18.5 indicates undernutrition)	**Lab Work**	Nitrogen (N) balance
Dietary/intake history	H & H	Gluc
Swallowing difficulty	Serum Fe	CRP
Temperature, fever?	Na^+, K^+	tHcy
I & O		Serum folate, B_{12}, B_6
		pCO_2, pO_2

INTERVENTION

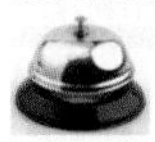

OBJECTIVES

- Maintain good nutrition to prevent further complications. Meet extra energy requirements (Vaisman et al, 2009).
- Reduce difficulties in chewing and swallowing. Monitor gag reflex.
- Reduce the patient's fear of aspiration; test swallowing reflexes with water and feed slowly.
- Minimize the possibility of UTI and constipation.
- Correct negative nitrogen balance and nutritional deficiencies.
- Ease symptoms to maintain independence as long as possible.
- Reduce fatigue from the eating process; provide a slow pace to avoid choking.

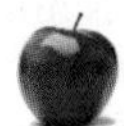

FOOD AND NUTRITION

- In initial stages, use a soft diet. Flaky fish, ground meats, and casseroles may be encouraged, along with foods moistened with gravies and sauces. Provide adequate fiber in the diet, perhaps Benefiber or psyllium when fibrous foods are no longer tolerated.
- The diet should include 2–3 L of water daily. Thicken liquids as needed with commercial thickeners, gelatin powder, or mashed potato flakes. Sips of liquid are best tolerated between bites of food.
- Place food at side of mouth and tilt head forward to facilitate swallowing, when possible.
- Enhance energy intake (Vaisman et al, 2009). Five to six small meals should be scheduled daily.
- Increase protein intake to counteract wasting.
- Diet and feedings should provide antioxidants such as vitamins E and C and selenium; zinc, magnesium, potassium, folate, omega-3 fatty acids, lycopene, and phosphorus.
- Foods should be moistened and not dry or crumbly. Cake and crackers should not be served plain; yogurt, applesauce, and pudding generally are acceptable.
- PEG or percutaneous endoscopic jejunostomy (PEJ) tube placement is well tolerated with dysphagia.

SAMPLE NUTRITION CARE PROCESS STEPS

Swallowing Difficulty

Assessment Data: Food records indicating poor intake; weight loss; paralysis of throat muscles with difficulty swallowing.

Nutrition Diagnoses (PES): Difficulty swallowing related to paralysis of throat muscles as evidenced by weight loss and dietary intake records showing 20–25% of meals consumed orally.

Interventions: Education of patient and family about structured meals, use of tolerated liquids and pureed foods to improve intake of nutrients and energy, prevent further weight loss.

Monitoring and Evaluation: Improved weight; delay of the need for tube feeding, or initiation early in the illness if patient wishes to have it.

Common Drugs Used and Potential Side Effects

- Ceftriaxone alters glutamate and has been found to prolong survival in animal models of ALS.
- Riluzole (a glutamate release inhibitor and membrane stabilizer) has been used to block nerve cell destruction. It seems to slow the disease but not curb its progress. Adding vitamin E to this therapy does not seem to cause any improvement (Graf et al, 2005).
- Studies suggest that recombinant erythropoietin, magnesium, lithium and valproate, lycopene, or anti-inflammatory drugs may be beneficial; however, more clinical trials are needed.

Herbs, Botanicals, and Supplements

- While no specific herbs and botanical products have demonstrated efficacy, supplement use is common in this population.

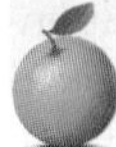

NUTRITION EDUCATION, COUNSELING, CARE MANAGEMENT

- Dietary counseling is important, but oral intake rapidly becomes insufficient and enteral nutritional support may be needed. Discuss care plan in front of patient; include the patient in the decision.
- In early stages, discuss adding fiber to the diet to prevent constipation and explain which foods have fiber.
- Encourage the planning of small, adequately balanced meals.
- Carefully monitor the patient's weight loss; 10% loss is common.
- Lightweight utensils are beneficial. A referral to an occupational therapist is recommended.
- Minimize chewing, but avoid use of baby food. Puree adult foods, especially preferred foods that are seasoned as usual for the individual.

- In later stages, decide if enteral nutrition will be used. If care will be given at home, teach family members what they can do to provide the feedings.

Patient Education—Foodborne Illness

- Careful food handling will be important. The same is true for sanitizing work area before and after preparing tube feedings to prevent contamination. Formula companies have good information on safe handling of formula in the home and institution.

For More Information

- ALS Association
  http://www.alsa.org/
- ALS Neurology Channel
  http://www.neurologychannel.com/als/index.shtml
- ALS Therapy Development Foundation
  http://www.als.net/

AMYOTROPHIC LATERAL SCLEROSIS—CITED REFERENCES

American Dietetic Association. Position of The American Dietetic Association: ethical and legal issues in nutrition, hydration and feeding. *J Am Diet Assoc.* 108:879, 2008.

Graf M, et al. High dose vitamin E therapy in amyotrophic lateral sclerosis as add-on therapy to riluzole: results of a placebo-controlled double-blind study. *J Neural Transm.* 112:649, 2005.

Langmore SE, et al. Enteral tube feeding for amyotrophic lateral sclerosis/motor neuron disease. *Cochrane Database Syst Rev.* 4:CD004030, 2006.

Oyanagi K, et al. Magnesium deficiency over generations in rats with special references to the pathogenesis of the Parkinsonism-dementia complex and amyotrophic lateral sclerosis of Guam. *Neuropathology.* 26:115, 2006.

Sherman MS, et al. Standard equations are not accurate in assessing resting energy expenditure in patients with amyotrophic lateral sclerosis. *J Parenter Enteral Nutr.* 28:442, 2004.

Vaisman N, et al. Do patients with amyotrophic lateral sclerosis (ALS) have increased energy needs? *J Neurol Sci.* 279:26, 2009.

Zoccolella S, et al, Elevated plasma homocysteine levels in patients with amyotrophic lateral sclerosis. *Neurology.* 70:222, 2008.

BRAIN TRAUMA

NUTRITIONAL ACUITY RANKING: LEVEL 4

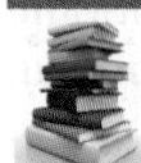

DEFINITIONS AND BACKGROUND

There are two types of brain injury: nontraumatic or traumatic. Nontraumatic head injury develops slowly, from arthritis, cancer, infections, or degeneration of the vertebrae. Traumatic brain injury (TBI) results from head injury after motor vehicle or industrial accidents, falls, fights, explosions, and gunshot wounds (40% involve alcohol use). The term TBI is not used for persons who are born with a brain injury or for injuries that happen during the birth process.

Any sudden impact or blow to the head (with or without unconsciousness) may cause a TBI, and two thirds of patients with TBI die before reaching a hospital. Low cerebral blood flow and cerebral perfusion pressure (CPP) are associated with poor outcome (White and Venkatesh, 2008).

Immediate signs of concussion (seen within seconds or minutes) include any loss of consciousness, impaired attention, vacant stare, delayed responses, inability to focus, slurred or incoherent speech, lack of coordination, disorientation, unusual emotional reactions, and memory problems. Classification is by location, effect, and severity. **Hypothalamic lesions** can promote hyperphagia. **Lateral lesions** can lead to aphasia and cachexia. **Frontal lobe damage** may result in loss of voluntary motor control and expressive aphasia. **Occipital lobe damage** impairs vision. **Temporal lobe damage** results in receptive aphasia and hearing impairments.

Hours, days, or even weeks after head injury, the patient may have persistent headache, dizziness with vertigo, poor attention or concentration, memory problems, nausea or vomiting, easy fatigue, irritability, intolerance for bright lights or loud noises, anxiety, depression, and disturbed sleep. Long-term TBI patients may exhibit dyspnea, vertigo, altered consciousness, seizures, vomiting, altered blood pressure (BP), weakness or paralysis, aphasia, and problems with physical control of hands, head, or neck with resulting difficulty in self-feeding. A brain injury often causes problems with understanding words, learning and remembering things, paying attention, solving problems, thinking abstractly, talking, behaving, walking, seeing, and hearing.

Brain trauma is accompanied by regional alterations of brain metabolism, overall reduction in metabolic rates, and persistent metabolic crisis (Vespa et al, 2005). Pyruvate dehydrogenase complex (PDHC) enzyme activity is lost with cerebral ischemia (Martin et al, 2005). Severe head injuries are also associated with negative nitrogen balances. With severe head injuries (Glasgow Coma Scale Score of 8), there is an increased tendency for gastric feeding to regurgitate into the upper airway; keeping the patient upright and checking residuals is important in such patients. Jejunal feedings are less apt to be aspirated. If the gastrointestinal (GI) tract cannot be used to reach nutritional goals within 3 days, total parenteral nutrition (TPN) is begun within 24–48 hours.

New neurons arise from progenitor cells that are maintained throughout adult life; they are enhanced by growth factors, drugs, neurotransmitters, and physical exercise and suppressed by aging, stress, glucocorticoids (Elder et al, 2006). Stem cell therapy has been studied for possible use in brain injuries.

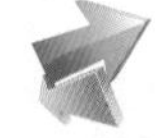

ASSESSMENT, MONITORING, AND EVALUATION

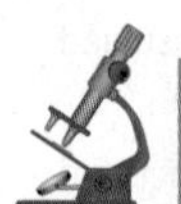

CLINICAL INDICATORS

Genetic Markers: Brain trauma is acquired.

Clinical/History	BMI	BP
Height	Dietary/intake history	Temperature
Weight		

Visual field examination	Lab Work	Total lymphocyte count (TLC)
Glasgow Coma Scale	pCO_2 and pO_2	Transferrin
Dysphagia?	Alb, transthyretin	H & H
Weight changes	Urinary urea nitrogen (UUN) excretion (24-hour specimens)	Serum Fe
Intracranial pressure	Gluc (increased with brain ischemia)	Na^+, K^+
CT scan	CRP	Ca^{++}, Mg^{++}
Skull x-rays	Folic acid	AST (increased with brain necrosis)
Brain scan	Complete blood count (CBC)	BUN, Creat
Cerebral angiography		Alkaline phosphatase (alk phos)
EEG		Serum ethanol (ETOH)
I & O		

INTERVENTION

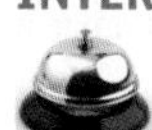

OBJECTIVES

- Prevent life-threatening complications, such as aspiration pneumonia, meningitis, sepsis, UTIs, syndrome of inappropriate antidiuretic hormone (SIADH), hypertension, pressure ulcers, Curling's ulcer, and GI bleeding.
- Assess regularly the substrate needs to prevent malnutrition, cachexia, or overfeeding. Indirect calorimetry to determine the respiratory quotient and resting energy expenditure should be determined twice weekly.
- Based on the level of nitrogen wasting and the nitrogen-sparing effect of feeding, full nutritional replacement is desirable by day 7.
- Prevent or correct hyperglycemia by carefully regulating glucose and insulin intake.
- Provide adequate protein for improving nitrogen balance (serum albumin tends to be low, especially if comatose, and urinary losses may be twice the normal).
- Monitor hydration; prevent either dehydration or overhydration.
- Correct self-feeding, breathing, and swallowing problems. Promote return to self-care where possible.

SAMPLE NUTRITION CARE PROCESS STEPS

Inadequate Oral Food and Beverage Intake

Assessment Data: Food records indicating poor intake; comatose; requiring tube feeding.

Nutrition Diagnoses (PES): Inadequate oral food and beverage intake related to coma following TBI as evidenced by requirement for tube feeding to meet elevated energy requirements.

Interventions: Provision of enteral nutrition to meet energy, protein, glucose, lipid and micronutrients requirements and prevent weight loss.

Monitoring and Evaluation: Tolerance of enteral nutrition; no physical signs of malnutrition; improvement in cognition or resolution of coma through recovery period.

- Prevent or reduce seizure activity, convulsions, intracranial edema, fluid overload (especially with TPN).
- After patient is stabilized, adapt to residual impairments.

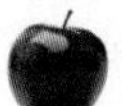

FOOD AND NUTRITION

- EN should begin as soon as the patient is hemodynamically stable, attempting to reach 35–45 kcal/kg and a protein intake of 2.0–2.5 g/kg as soon as possible. Tube feeding is preferable; if malabsorption persists, a short course of supplemental PN may help.
- The need for surgery or ventilation will have an effect on the ability to progress to any oral intake.
- Patients who are immobile for a long period of time may have a 10% decrease in weight from lowered metabolic rate. Energy intake will need to be varied accordingly.
- Increased urinary zinc losses can occur. Monitor potassium, phosphorus, and magnesium requirements as losses are often high. Otherwise, a general multivitamin–mineral supplement should suffice.
- Progress, when possible, to oral intake. A dysphagia may be needed.
- Use of probiotics (such as yogurt or buttermilk) can help to maintain GI integrity and immunity.
- Over time, a patient may gain excessive weight if the brain injury affected the hypothalamus. Some patients forget that they have eaten and state their constant hunger. Monitor energy intake carefully.

Common Drugs Used and Potential Side Effects

- Analgesics are used for pain. Antacids and Pepcid may then be needed to reduce the onset of stress ulcers.
- Anticonvulsants may be needed to reduce seizure activity; these may deplete folic acid levels and other nutrients. Presence of food reduces effectiveness of the liquid form of phenytoin (Dilantin). Adjust phenytoin dosage rather than holding feedings.
- Insulin is used when hyperglycemia occurs or persists.
- Reglan may be used as a promotility agent in tube-fed patients to assist in transit time and to decrease the risk of aspiration.
- Soluble or mixed fibers (Benefiber or other soluble fiber supplements) or laxatives (Metamucil) are often helpful in alleviating constipation. However, bloating, nausea, diarrhea, or vomiting may result.

Herbs, Botanicals, and Supplements

- Avoid using phenytoin (Dilantin) with evening primrose oil, gingko biloba, and kava.

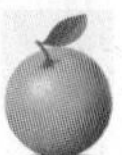

NUTRITION EDUCATION, COUNSELING, CARE MANAGEMENT

- Encourage the patient to chew and swallow slowly, if and when the patient is able to eat solids.
- Gradually relearn self-feeding techniques.
- Be wary of extreme food temperatures; patients may have become less sensitized to hot and cold.

- Serve colorful and attractive meals for better acceptance.
- The team approach is beneficial, with occupational therapists, speech therapists, psychologists, and physical therapists helping design treatment plans.
- Plate guards, long-handled utensils, and other adaptive feeding devices may be useful. Discuss with the occupational therapist.
- Discuss a healthy eating pattern and use of foods such as yogurt for probiotics.
- Emotional changes are common after a head injury. Family members should be prepared to address changes that relate to mealtimes, eating patterns, weight management, and the need for consistency and structure.
- Many brain injury patients do not receive counseling about the long-term effects of their injury. Provide written instructions for review later.

Patient Education—Foodborne Illness

- Careful food handling will be important.
- Sanitize work areas before and after preparing tube feedings to prevent contamination. Formula companies have good information on safe handling of formula in the home and institution.

For More Information

- Brain and Spinal Cord
  http://www.brainandspinalcord.org/
- Brain Injury Association
  http://www.biausa.org
- Brain Trauma Foundation
  http://www.braintrauma.org/
- National Institute of Neurological Disorders and Stroke
  http://www.ninds.nih.gov/

BRAIN TRAUMA—CITED REFERENCES

Elder GA, et al. Research update: neurogenesis in adult brain and neuropsychiatric disorders. *Mt Sinai J Med.* 73:931, 2006.

Martin E, et al. Pyruvate dehydrogenase complex: metabolic link to ischemic brain injury and target of oxidative stress. *J Neurosci Res.* 79:240, 2005.

Vespa P, et al. Metabolic crisis without brain ischemia is common after traumatic brain injury: a combined microdialysis and positron emission tomography study. *J Cereb Blood Flow Metab.* 25:763, 2005.

White H, Venkatesh B. Cerebral perfusion pressure in neurotrauma: a review. *Anesth Analog.* 107:979, 2008.

CEREBRAL ANEURYSM

NUTRITIONAL ACUITY RANKING: LEVEL 2–3

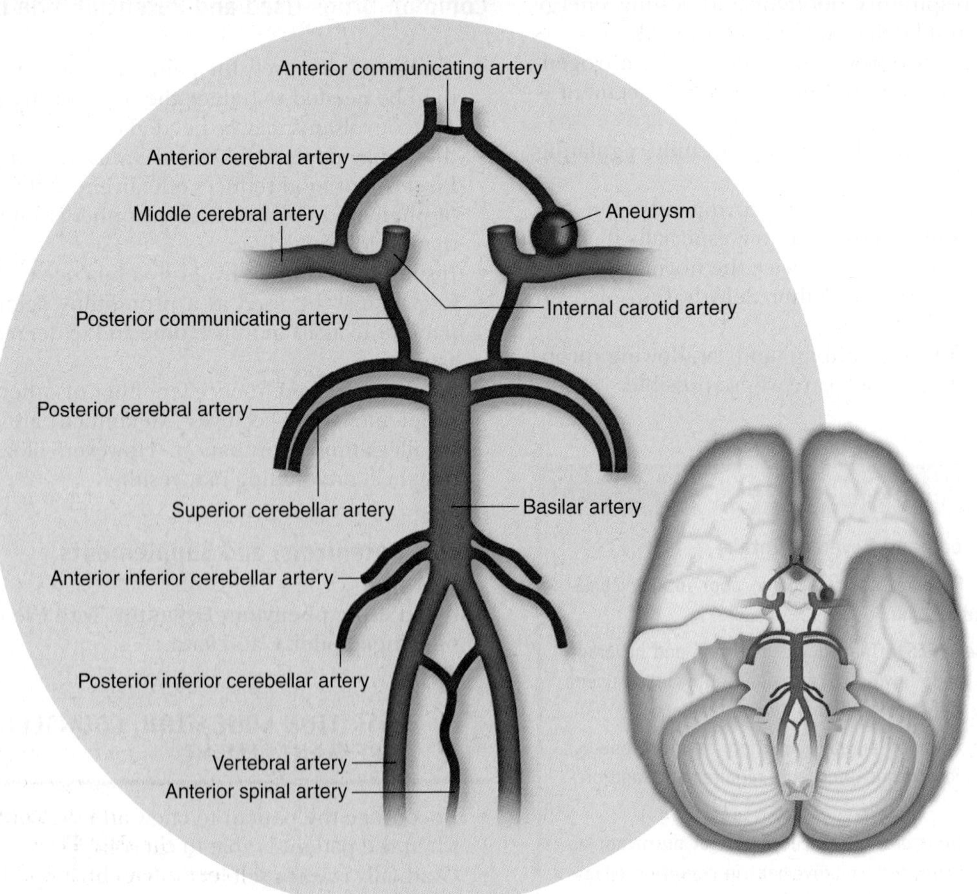

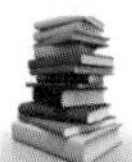

DEFINITIONS AND BACKGROUND

A cerebral aneurysm may involve the dilation of a cerebral artery resulting from a weakness of the blood vessel wall. Symptoms include altered consciousness, drowsiness, confusion, stupor or coma, headache, facial pain, eye pain, blurred vision, vertigo, tinnitus, hemiparesis, elevated BP, and dilated pupils. Aneurysms may burst and cause hemorrhage. Epidemiological evidence suggests that most intracranial aneurysms do not rupture. It is important to identify which unruptured intracranial aneurysms (UIAs) are at greatest risk of rupture when considering which to repair (Wiebers et al, 2004).

An **intracranial** hemorrhage is bleeding inside the skull, usually from head injury. Bleeding within the brain is **intracerebral**. Hemorrhages between the brain and the subarachnoid space are **subarachnoid hemorrhages**; those between the meninges are **subdural hemorrhages**; and those between the skull and covering of the brain are **epidural hemorrhages**. Hemorrhagic stroke may occur. After an aneurysmal subarachnoid hemorrhage, nearly half of patients die, and the half who survive suffer from irreversible cerebral damage (Chen et al, 2004).

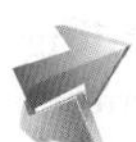

ASSESSMENT, MONITORING, AND EVALUATION

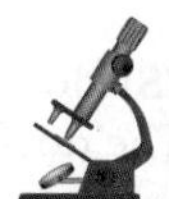

CLINICAL INDICATORS

Genetic Markers: Alagille syndrome (AGS) is a dominantly inherited multisystem disorder involving the liver, heart, eyes, face, and skeleton, caused by mutations in Jagged1; intracranial bleeding is a recognized complication and cause of mortality. Otherwise, most aneurysms are not genetic.

Clinical/History	CT scan results	Triglycerides (trig)
Height	Angiography	Alb, transthyretin
Weight	Cerebrospinal fluid analysis	Gluc
BMI	Pneumonia?	Na^+, K^+
Weight changes	Fever?	H & H
Dietary/intake history	**Lab Work**	Serum Fe
I & O	Chol (LDL, HDL)	pO_2, pCO_2
BP (increased)		
Brain MRI		

INTERVENTION

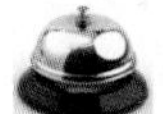

OBJECTIVES

- Limit fluids as necessary to reduce cerebral edema.
- Rest is essential. Avoid constipation and straining at stool.
- Decrease or manage hypertension.
- Prevent further complications and lingering neurological problems.

SAMPLE NUTRITION CARE PROCESS STEPS

Inadequate Oral Food and Beverage Intake

Assessment Data: Semi-concious state, inability to eat orally.

Nutrition Diagnoses (PES): Inadequate oral food and beverage intake related to recent TBI after a car accident as evidenced by cognitive deficits and high risk for aspiration and pneumonia.

Interventions: EN because oral feeding not safe or feasible. Calculate protein, energy, fluid requirements as well as rate and goal intake.

Monitoring and Evaluation: Tolerance of enteral nutrition; labs stable for glucose, prealbumin, electrolytes. Gradual return to oral diet if possible.

- Prepare for surgery if safe and possible. Reduce fever prior to surgery (Todd et al, 2009).
- Gradually encourage self-feeding.

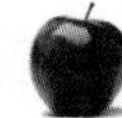

FOOD AND NUTRITION

- Nothing by mouth unless ordered; appropriate IVs are used. With cognitive progress, a tube feeding or diet will be prescribed.
- Restrict fluid, sodium, saturated fat and cholesterol if deemed necessary. Enhance potassium if necessary.
- Alter dietary fiber intake, as appropriate.
- Offer sufficient antioxidant foods and omega-3 fatty acids where appropriate.

Common Drugs Used and Potential Side Effects

- In some cases, aspirin may be given at levels of 150–300 mg daily.
- Cardiovascular drugs are usually ordered according to significant parameters. Adjust dietary intake accordingly.
- Diuretics may be used. Monitor potassium replacement if furosemide is prescribed.
- Nimodipine is used to treat symptoms resulting from hemorrhage by increasing blood flow to injured brain tissue.
- Papaverine is used to improve blood flow in patients with circulation problems by relaxing the blood vessels.

Herbs, Botanicals, and Supplements

- No specific herbs and botanical products have been used for cerebral aneurysm in any clinical trials.

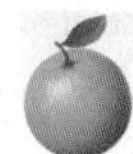

NUTRITION EDUCATION, COUNSELING, CARE MANAGEMENT

- If enteral nutrition must continue at home, the caregiver should be taught appropriate and safe techniques.
- Discuss fiber sources from the diet. Foods such as prune juice or bran added to cereal can be helpful in alleviating constipation.

- Counsel regarding self-feeding techniques.
- Discuss role of nutrition in preventing further cardiovascular or neurological problems.

Patient Education—Foodborne Illness

- Careful food handling will be important.
- Sanitize counters or work area before and after preparing tube feedings to prevent contamination. Formula companies have good information on safe handling of formula in the home and institution.

For More Information

- American Association of Neurological Surgeons http://www.aans.org/
- Brain Aneurysm Foundation http://www.bafound.org/
- National Institute of Neurological Disorders and Stroke http://www.ninds.nih.gov/disorders/cerebral_aneurysm/detail_cerebral_aneurysm.htm

CEREBRAL ANEURYSM—CITED REFERENCES

Chen PR, et al. Natural history and general management of unruptured intracranial aneurysms. *Neurosurg Focus.* 17:e1, 2004.

Todd MM, et al. Perioperative fever and outcome in surgical patients with aneurysmal subarachnoid hemorrhage. *Neurosurgery.* 64:897, 2009.

Uhl E, et al. Intraoperative computed tomography with integrated navigation system in a multidisciplinary operating suite. *Neurosurgery.* 64:651, 2009.

Wiebers DO, et al. Pathogenesis, natural history, and treatment of unruptured intracranial aneurysms. *Mayo Clin Proc.* 79:1572, 2004.

COMA OR PERSISTENT VEGETATIVE STATE

NUTRITIONAL ACUITY RANKING: LEVEL 4

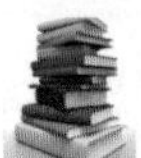

DEFINITIONS AND BACKGROUND

Coma is the unconscious state in which the patient is unresponsive to verbal or painful stimuli. Impaired consciousness or coma can occur from a stroke, head injury, meningitis, encephalitis, sepsis, lack of oxygen, epileptic seizure, toxic effects of alcohol or drugs, liver or kidney failure, high or low blood glucose levels, or altered body temperature. Coma usually only lasts for a few weeks and most people recover fully. Medical staff use the Glasgow Coma Scale to determine prognosis. Often, the 1-month performance on measures such as Disability Rating Scale (DRS) and Glasgow Outcome Scale (GOS) scores help predict status 6 months post injury (Pastorek et al, 2004). Nutritional support is associated with improved survival in coma patients. Most patients are tube fed because it is safer and more practical than hand feeding. Clinical care factors such as time delay for orders and enteral access are impediments to EN provision in the first week of neurocritical illness (Zarbock et al, 2008).

A patient in a **permanently vegetative state (PVS)** does not have the ability to request or refuse treatment. The doctor determines the diagnosis of PVS. According to the American Dietetic Association position (2008), the definition of brain death is central to the dilemma of feeding permanently unconscious patients. Dietitians play an integral role with other members of the team in developing and implementing ethical guidelines for feeding patients (American Dietetic Association, 2008). Table 4-7 lists the consequences of withholding food and fluid from patients whose advance directives indicate no "heroic measures."

TABLE 4-7 Consequences of Withholding Food and Fluid in Terminally Ill Patients

Neither nutrition nor hydration improves comfort or quality of life in terminally ill patients. Physiological adaptation allows patients not to suffer from the absence of food, as follows:

1. Two thirds of the patients who are not fed or hydrated at the end of life feel no hunger. They usually have loss of appetite and reduced enjoyment of food.
2. Thirst and dry mouth are common initially. Use ice chips, lubricating the lips, and small amounts of food and water to reduce the thirst sensations from dehydration.
3. Dehydration eventually results in hemoconcentration and hyperosmolality with subsequent azotemia, hypernatremia, and hypercalcemia. These changes produce a sedative effect on the brain just before death.
4. Withholding or minimizing hydration can reduce disturbing oral and bronchial secretions, the need for frequent urination, and coughing from diminished pulmonary congestion.

Adapted from: American Dietetic Association. Position of the American Dietetic Association: ethical and legal issues in nutrition, hydration, and feeding. *J Am Diet Assoc.* 108:879, 2008.

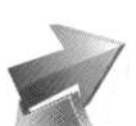

ASSESSMENT, MONITORING, AND EVALUATION

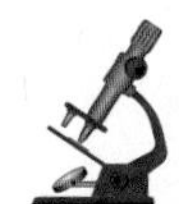

CLINICAL INDICATORS

Genetic Markers: Coma is generally a result of an accident or other head injury. Some genetic disorders may lead to coma if undiagnosed and untreated.

Clinical/History

Height
Weight
BMI
Weight change (using a bed scale)
Dietary/intake history
Unconsciousness
Glasgow Coma Scale score (>13 mild; <8 severe) for eye, motor, and verbal responses
BP
I & O
CT scan or MRI

Lab Work	Trig	Serum alcohol level
H & H	Alb	tHcy levels
Serum Fe	Gluc	Serum folic acid
pCO_2, pO_2	BUN, Creat	Serum vitamin B_{12}
Chol, full lipid profile (HDL, LDL)	Urine tests for chemicals, glucose	

INTERVENTION

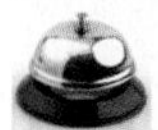

OBJECTIVES

- Maintain standards related to primary condition.
- When possible, elevate head to prevent aspiration during feeding process.
- Assess daily energy and fluid requirements. Adequate caloric intake is associated with improved outcome (Zarbock et al, 2008).
- Prevent or treat pressure ulcers, constipation, and other complications of immobility.
- For terminally ill patients, follow their wishes as directed by advance directives.

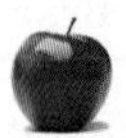

FOOD AND NUTRITION

- Immediately give intravenous glucose until etiology is clearly identified. Parenteral fluids may also be appropriate at this time.
- Tube feed for increased energy and protein requirements every 2–3 hours, or as ordered by the physician. If tube fed, a formula with fiber can be helpful in preventing or easing constipation; be sure sufficient fluid is included as well.
- TPN may be appropriate for some persons, following evaluation of the original disorder, sepsis, and other complicating factors.
- Progress, when or if possible, to oral feedings.
- For patients who are terminally ill, gradual withdrawal of food and fluid is appropriate if directed by the patient's advance directives.

SAMPLE NUTRITION CARE PROCESS STEPS

Inadequate Energy Intake

Assessment Data: Inability to eat orally, leading to poor intake. Weight changes; % usual body weight.

Nutrition Diagnoses (PES): Inadequate energy intake related to coma and inability to chew and swallow as evidenced by intake meeting less than 10% of estimated requirements.

Interventions: Enteral nutrition to meet estimated needs for energy and nutrients.

Monitoring and Evaluation: Weight status, stabilization of labs, and improved energy intake.

Common Drugs Used and Potential Side Effects

- Anticonvulsants, such as phenytoin (Dilantin), decrease folic acid over time. Avoid use with evening primrose oil, gingko biloba, and kava.
- Antacids may be needed to prevent stress ulcers.
- Cathartics are often used. Monitor for electrolyte imbalances.
- Steroids may be used. Side effects include sodium retention, increased losses of potassium and calcium and magnesium, and nitrogen depletion.

Herbs, Botanicals, and Supplements

- No specific herbs and botanical products have been used in comatose patients in any clinical trials.
- With phenytoin (Dilantin), avoid use with evening primrose oil, gingko biloba, and kava.

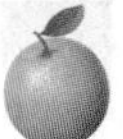

INTERVENTION: NUTRITION EDUCATION, COUNSELING, CARE MANAGEMENT

- Discuss with caretaker or family any necessary measures that are completed to provide adequate nourishment. Explain importance of prevention of complications such as aspiration.
- Evaluate potential for self-feeding over time.
- A Medic Alert bracelet or other ID is useful for persons with disorders that can lead to unconsciousness.

Patient Education—Foodborne Illness

- Careful food handling will be important. Caregivers must wash their hands before initiating tube feeding, TPN, or oral feeding process.
- Sanitizing work area before and after preparing tube feedings to prevent contamination. Formula companies have good information on safe handling of formula in the home and institution.

For More Information

- Coma
  http://www.neuroskills.com/coma.shtml
- Glasgow Coma Scale
  http://www.neuroskills.com/glasgow.shtml
- Neurology Channel
  http://www.neurologychannel.com/coma/index.shtml

COMA—CITED REFERENCES

American Dietetic Association. Position of the American Dietetic Association: ethical and legal issues in nutrition, hydration, and feeding. *J Am Diet Assoc.* 108:879, 2008.

Pastorek NJ, et al. Prediction of global outcome with acute neuropsychological testing following closed-head injury. *J Int Neuropsychol Soc.* 10:807, 2004.

Zarbock SD, et al. Successful enteral nutritional support in the neurocritical care unit. *Neurocrit Care.* 9:210, 2008.

EPILEPSY AND SEIZURE DISORDERS

NUTRITIONAL ACUITY RANKING: LEVEL 2

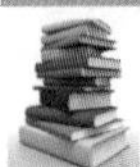

DEFINITIONS AND BACKGROUND

Epilepsy is a disturbance of the nervous system with recurrent seizures, loss of consciousness, convulsions, motor activity, or behavioral abnormalities. The seizures result from excessive neuronal discharges in the brain. A grand mal seizure involves an aura, a tonic phase, and a clonic phase. A petit mal seizure involves momentary loss of consciousness. A single seizure does not imply epilepsy. There are many forms of epilepsy, each with its own symptoms. In two thirds of cases, no structural abnormality is found. Incidence is two to six in 1000 people. Approximately 45,000 children under the age of 15 develop epilepsy each year, often those with cerebral palsy or spina bifida.

A ketogenic diet should be considered for refractory epilepsy (Papandreou et al, 2006; Vaisleib et al, 2004). Chronic ketosis modifies the tricarboxcylic acid cycle, increases GABA synthesis in brain, limits reactive oxygen species generation, and boosts energy production in brain tissue; these changes stabilize synaptic function and increase the resistance to seizures throughout the brain (Bough and Rho, 2007).

A ketogenic diet contains 70–90% fat with the remainder as protein and carbohydrates (CHO). A medium-chain triglyceride (MCT) diet alleviates some of the obstacles of compliance and acceptance. While overall caloric restriction may improve efficacy of the ketogenic diet (Cheng et al, 2004), the diet may slow growth (Peterson et al, 2005). An alternative diet that is not as strict uses a low–glycemic index treatment, with more liberal total carbohydrate intake (Pfeifer and Thiele, 2005).

Bone health, altered hepatic cytochrome P-450 enzymes, decreased metabolism of vitamin D, resistance to parathyroid hormone, inhibition of calcitonin secretion, and impaired calcium absorption are affected by use of antiepileptic drugs (Fitzpatrick, 2004).

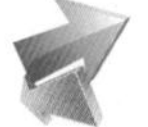

ASSESSMENT, MONITORING, AND EVALUATION

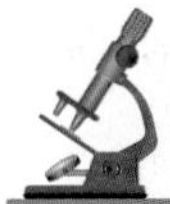

CLINICAL INDICATORS

Genetic Markers: In close relatives (parents, brothers, sisters, and children) of people with generalized epilepsy, the risk of epilepsy is about four times as high as in the general population. In the close relatives of people with partial epilepsy, the risk is twice as high as in the general population.

Clinical/History		
Height	BMI	BP
Weight	Dietary/intake history of fatty acids	I & O
		CT scan
		Skull x-ray

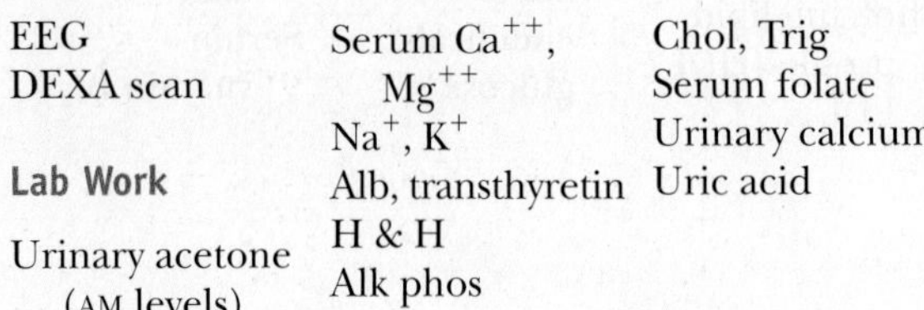

EEG	Serum Ca^{++}, Mg^{++}	Chol, Trig
DEXA scan	Na^{+}, K^{+}	Serum folate
Lab Work	Alb, transthyretin	Urinary calcium
Urinary acetone (AM levels)	H & H	Uric acid
	Alk phos	

INTERVENTION

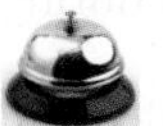

OBJECTIVES

- Minimize seizures via medications, ketogenic diet, or lesionectomy.
- If drug therapy does not work (as in the case of intractable myoclonic or akinetic seizures of infancy), a ketogenic diet may be used (Neal et al, 2008). Reverse the usual ratio of cholesterol and fat. Provide a diet that avoids excess of CHO. Beware of changing the diet abruptly; a gradual approach is preferred.
- With signs of hyperuricemia or hypercalciuria, increase fluid intake and consider use of diuretics.
- Correct nutritional deficits from long-term anticonvulsant medication use (disorders of vitamin D, calcium, and bone metabolism). Phenytoin therapy (PHT) decreases serum folate by half, thereby increasing risk of deficiency.
- Monitor for possible long-term cardiac problems or a decline in bone health.

SAMPLE NUTRITION CARE PROCESS STEPS

Inadequate Intake of Fatty Acids

Assessment Data: Frequent, treatment-refractable seizures in child; difficulty with self-feeding.

Nutrition Diagnoses (PES): Inadequate intake of fatty acids related to high CHO intake as evidenced by frequent seizures and use of regular diet.

Interventions: Food-Nutrient Delivery: Alter diet or tube feeding to increase ratio of lipid to CHO for ketogenic effect. Education of patient/caregiver about the role of lipids in brain health and preparation of the ketogenic diet; consequences of long-term use of anticonvulsants on bone health and folate status.

Monitoring and Evaluation: Decreased frequency of seizures, tolerance of ketogenic diet, sufficient growth or weight maintenance, adequate bone density.

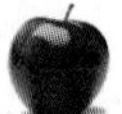

FOOD AND NUTRITION

- Provide a diet reflecting the patient's age and activity. Protein should meet needs; such as 0.8–1 g/kg body weight.
- The high-fat, high-protein, low-carbohydrate Atkins diet is somewhat ketogenic and may be useful in managing medically resistant epilepsy (Kossoff and Rho, 2009).
- The ketogenic diet is a low-carbohydrate, adequate-protein, high-fat diet that biochemically mimics the fasting state and has been used to successfully treat seizures for 85 years (Huffman and Kossoff, 2006). However, the diet may be unpalatable. The diet follows a ratio of 3:1 or 4:1 of fats to carbohydrate and protein.
- MCTs are more ketogenic, having more rapid metabolism and absorption. MCTs provide 60% of kcal (the rest of the diet would consist of 10% other fats, 10% protein, and 20% carbohydrates). Stimulants such as tea, coffee, colas, and alcohol are not usually recommended with the ketogenic diet. If the pure ketogenic diet is not tolerated, modify it with low–glycemic index foods (Pfeifer and Thiele, 2005).
- Supplements may be needed, especially calcium, vitamin D, folic acid, vitamins B_6 and B_{12}.
- Add sufficient fiber and fluid for relief of constipation.

Common Drugs Used and Potential Side Effects

- Cough syrups, laxatives, and other medications may contain a high CHO content; monitor for interactions with the diet.
- Common anticonvulsants and potential side effects are listed in Table 4-8. Anticonvulsant therapy interferes with vitamin D metabolism, leading to a calcium imbalance, rickets or osteomalacia. Therapy with D3 is recommended.

Herbs, Botanicals, and Supplements

- Vitamin B_6 is associated with neuronal function. Avoid high doses of pyridoxine with phenobarbital or phenytoin because seizure control might be compromised. If vitamin B_6 is added to either drug regimen, keep it at the lowest effective dose and monitor serum drug levels.
- St. John's wort should not be used with monoamine oxidase inhibitors (MAOI), selective serotonin reuptake inhibitors (SSRIs), cyclosporine, digoxin, oral contraceptives, HIV protease inhibitors, theophylline, warfarin, or calcium channel blockers such as amlodipine, diltiazem,

TABLE 4-8 Medications Used in Epilepsy

Generic Name	Trade Name	Possible Side Effects
Carbamazepine	Carbatrol, Tegretol XR, Tegretol	Dry mouth, vomiting, nausea, anorexia, low red blood cell and white blood cell counts.
Clonazepam	Klonopin	Anorexia, weight loss or gain, increased thirst.
Diazepam	Diazepam Intesol, Diastat, Valium	Anorexia, weight loss or gain, increased thirst.
Ethosuximide	Zarontin	Gastrointestinal upset, anemia, and weight loss. Take with food or milk.
Felbamate	Felbatol	Constipation, nausea, vomiting, and anorexia.
Fosphenytoin	Cerebyx	Water-soluble phenytoin. May need vitamin D, calcium, thiamin, magnesium.
Gabapentin	Neurontin	Weight gain and increased appetite occur. Take magnesium supplement separately by 2 hours.
Lamotrigine	Lamictal	Anorexia, weight loss, nausea and vomiting, abdominal pain.
Levetiracetam	Keppra	Anorexia, headache.
Oxcarbazepine	Trileptal	Restrict fluid with hyponatremia.
Phenobarbital	Luminal	Depletes vitamins D, K, B_{12}, B_6, folate, and calcium. Nausea, vomiting, constipation, sedation, and anorexia can occur. Limit caffeine and alcohol. May elevate serum cholesterol levels.
Phenytoin	Dilantin	Gum hyperplasia and carbohydrate intolerance. It binds serum proteins and decreases folate, vitamins B_{12} and C, and magnesium absorption. Be careful with vitamin B_6; excesses can reduce drug effectiveness. Stop tube feedings 30 minutes before and after administration of the medication; nutritional intake may need to be calculated over 21 versus 24 hours.
Primidone	Mysoline	Gastrointestinal upset, anemia, and weight loss. Take with food or milk. Primidone is similar to a barbiturate; vomiting may occur.
Tiagabine	Gabitril	Mouth ulcers, nausea and vomiting may occur.
Topiramate	Topamax	Weight loss and anorexia are common.
Valproate, valproic acid, divalproex sodium	Depacon, Depakote, Depakene, Depakote ER	Nausea, vomiting, anorexia, weight gain, or hair loss.
Vigabatrin	Sabril	Visual field loss can occur.
Zonisamide	Zonegran	Anorexia and weight loss are common.

or verapamil. Avoid use with benzodiazepines such as alprazolam, clonazepam, diazepam, and midazolam.
- Psyllium and ginseng should not be used with divalproex sodium (Depakote) or lithium.
- With phenytoin (Dilantin), avoid use with evening primrose oil, gingko biloba, and kava.

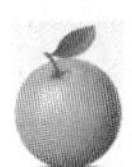

NUTRITION EDUCATION, COUNSELING, CARE MANAGEMENT

- Ketogenic diets cause nausea and vomiting; a small drink of fruit juice can help relieve the symptoms. Regular monitoring of the diet is crucial.
- An ID tag, such as Medic Alert, is recommended.
- To increase long-chain triglycerides (LCTs), add sour cream, whipped cream, butter, margarine, or oils to casseroles, desserts, or other foods. To use MCT, add it to salad dressings, fruit juice, casseroles, and sandwich spreads. Pseudo ice cream may be made with frozen, flavored whipped cream.
- Women who have epilepsy and wish to have children need advice about medications and possible side effects. Pregnancy itself can increase seizure frequency; infants can be born with low birth weight, developmental delay, or epilepsy (Yerby et al, 2004).
- Because of the potential for loss of bone mineral density, discuss use of more calcium and vitamin D-rich foods. A multivitamin–mineral supplement may be recommended.
- Alcohol should be avoided.

Patient Education—Foodborne Illness

- Careful food handling will be important. Hand washing is key as well.

For More Information

- American Epilepsy Society
  http://aesnet.org
- Epilepsy Foundation
  http://www.EpilepsyFoundation.org

EPILEPSY AND SEIZURE DISORDERS—CITED REFERENCES

Bough KJ, Rho JM. Anticonvulsant mechanisms of the ketogenic diet. *Epilepsia.* 48:43, 2007.

Cheng CM, et al. Caloric restriction augments brain glutamic acid decarboxylase-65 and -67 expression. *J Neurosci Res.* 77:270, 2004.

Fitzpatrick LA. Pathophysiology of bone loss in patients receiving anticonvulsant therapy. *Epilepsy Behav.* 5:S3, 2004.

Huffman J, Kossoff EH. State of the ketogenic diet(s) in epilepsy. *Curr Neurol Neurosci Rep.* 6:332, 2006.

Kossoff EH, Rho JM. Ketogenic diets: evidence for short-term and long-term efficacy. *Neurotherapeutics.* 6:406, 2009.

Neal EG, et al. The ketogenic diet for the treatment of childhood epilepsy: a randomised controlled trial. *Lancet Neurol.* 7:500, 2008.

Papandreou D, et al. The ketogenic diet in children with epilepsy. *Br J Nutr.* 95:5, 2006.

Peterson SJ. Changes in growth and seizure reduction in children on the ketogenic diet as a treatment for intractable epilepsy. *J Am Diet Assoc.* 105:718, 2005.

Pfeifer HH, Thiele EA. Low-glycemic-index treatment: a liberalized ketogenic diet for treatment of intractable epilepsy. *Neurology.* 65:1810, 2005.

Vaisleib II, et al. Ketogenic diet: out patient initiation, without fluid, or caloric restrictions. *Pediatr Neurol.* 31:198, 2004.

Yerby MS, et al. Risks and management of pregnancy in women with epilepsy. *Cleve Clin J Med.* 71:S25, 2004.

GUILLAIN–BARRÉ SYNDROME

NUTRITIONAL ACUITY RANKING: LEVEL 3

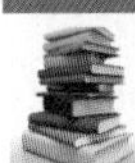

DEFINITIONS AND BACKGROUND

Guillain–Barré syndrome (GBS) is an acute inflammatory demyelinating polyneuropathy with rapidly increasing weakness, numbness, pain, and paralysis of the legs, arms, trunk, face and respiratory muscles. It often occurs after infection with influenza or *Campylobacter jejuni;* bloody diarrhea, fever, cramping, and headache are presenting symptoms. In general, the role of *C. jejuni* has been greatly underestimated (Schmidt-Ott et al, 2006). GBS may progress to respiratory failure; paralysis of lower extremities or quadriplegia; unstable BP; aspiration; dysphagia; difficulty with chewing; impaired speech; muscular pain; low-grade fever; tachycardia; weight loss, anorexia; UTIs. Sometimes ventilatory assistance is needed.

Most people recover fully from GBS, but some may need intensive care support followed by wheelchair assistance. There is no treatment that has been totally effective. Most people recover within a few weeks, but some may still have residual effects for years.

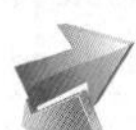

ASSESSMENT, MONITORING, AND EVALUATION

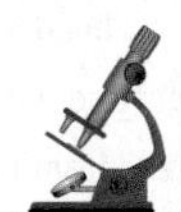

CLINICAL INDICATORS

Genetic Markers: It is believed that GBS results primarily after infection and not from genetic causes.

Clinical/History		Lab Work
Height	Vomiting	CBC
Weight	Bloody diarrhea?	H & H
BMI	Fatigue and weakness	Serum Fe
Weight changes	Nerve conduction velocity test	Alb
Dietary/intake history	Loss of reflexes (knee, etc.)	pO_2, pCO_2
BP		Lumbar puncture for CSF protein levels
Temperature		Gluc
Dysphagia		

SAMPLE NUTRITION CARE PROCESS STEPS

Intake of Unsafe Food

Assessment Data: Diet history revealing intake of undercooked chicken at a sporting event, followed by bloody diarrhea, fever, and vomiting.

Nutrition Diagnoses (PES): Intake of unsafe food related to *C. jejuni and* medical diagnosis of Guillan-Barre as evidenced by GI symptoms and bloody diarrhea, weakness, and fatigue.

Interventions: Education about proper food handling and consumption of foods properly cooked to desired internal temparture.

Monitoring and Evaluation: Improvement in symptoms and gradual improvement in quality of life; better understanding of food handling and issues related to food safety.

INTERVENTION

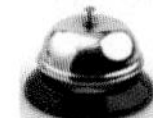

OBJECTIVES

- Meet added energy requirements from fever, weight loss.
- Adjust diet or method of feeding for chewing and swallowing problems.
- Wean, if possible, from ventilator dependency.
- Improve neurological functioning and overall prognosis.

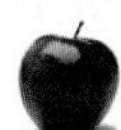

FOOD AND NUTRITION

- Acute: Intravenous fluids will be required. Tube feeding or TPN may be necessary while patient is acutely ill over a period of time. Increased energy intake and protein may be necessary; increase lipid intake to reduce CO_2 production while on the ventilator.
- Progression: a thick, pureed diet may be beneficial with dysphagia. When safe and tolerated, a soft or general diet may be used.
- Supplement oral intake with frequent snacks, such as shakes or eggnog, if unintentional weight loss has occurred. A vitamin–mineral supplement may be beneficial, especially if intake has been poor.

Common Drugs Used and Potential Side Effects

- Antibiotics may be needed for UTIs.
- Autoimmune globulin may be given.
- Analgesics are used to reduce pain and inflammation.
- Steroids are seldom used except for chronic relapsing polyneuropathy; their effects can be deleterious over time, especially for bone health.
- Vasopressors may be used.

Herbs, Botanicals, and Supplements

- High doses of pyridoxine (B_6) should not be taken with phenobarbital or phenytoin. Keep it at the lowest effective dose and monitor serum drug levels.
- No studies have been conducted for efficacy of herbs or botanical products in GBS.

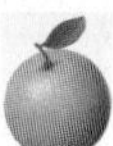

NUTRITION EDUCATION, COUNSELING, CARE MANAGEMENT

- Discuss adequacy of energy and protein intake to improve weight status and nutritional health.
- Avoid foodborne illnesses, upper respiratory infections, and exposure to other illnesses.
- Avoid constipation by use of fruits, vegetables, crushed bran, prune juice, and adequate fluid intake.
- Encourage self-feeding where possible. Arrange for special feeding utensils if needed.

Patient Education—Foodborne Illness

- *C. jejuni* is the most frequently diagnosed bacterial cause of human gastroenteritis in the United States. Avoid drinking raw milk; eating raw or undercooked meat, shellfish, and poultry; eating tofu or unwashed raw vegetables.
- Hand washing is important. Wash hands with soap before handling raw foods.
- Prevent cross-contamination in the kitchen. Proper refrigeration and sanitation are also essential.

For More Information

- CDC: Seasonal Flu and GBS
  http://www.cdc.gov/FLU/about/qa/gbs.htm
- Guillain-Barré Foundation International
  http://gbs-cidp.org/
- NINDS Information Page
  http://www.ninds.nih.gov/disorders/gbs/gbs.htm

GUILLAIN–BARRÉ SYNDROME—CITED REFERENCE

Schmidt-Ott R, et al. Improved serological diagnosis stresses the major role of *Campylobacter jejuni* in triggering Guillain-Barré syndrome. *Clin Vaccine Immunol.* 13:779, 2006.

HUNTINGTON'S DISEASE

NUTRITIONAL ACUITY RANKING: LEVEL 3

DEFINITIONS AND BACKGROUND

Huntington's disease (HD) is a genetic, autosomal-dominant, neurodegenerative disorder. There is a defective gene that leads to microscopic death of selected neurons (Arrasate et al, 2004; Zhang et al, 2008). Normally, huntingtin's protein is cleared away through the Ubiquitin Proteosome System (UPS) in which proteins that are not needed or that have misfolded are tagged for degradation by ubiquitin (HDSA, 2009). Transglutaminase (TGase) activity is increased in affected regions of the brain.

HD develops in middle to late life, with involuntary, spasmodic, irregular movements (chorea), cerebral degeneration, cognitive decline, and speech difficulties. HD differs from AD in that there is loss of control of voluntary movements. Behavioral changes begin 10 years before the movement disorder, which may begin between age 35 and 40 years.

Nutritional intake plays an important role. Folic acid affects DNA methylation; coenzyme Q10 and unsaturated fatty acids are important for neuroprotection (Bonelli and Wenning, 2006).

Remotivation therapy leads to increased self-awareness, increased self-esteem, and improved quality of life. Duration of HD is generally 13–15 years before death, which often results from pneumonia or a fall. Stem cell transplantation shows promise for treatment; the therapy uses small cell ribonucleic acid (siRNA) to prevent the mutant proteins from being reproduced.

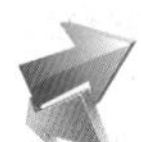

ASSESSMENT, MONITORING, AND EVALUATION

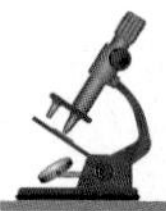

CLINICAL INDICATORS

Genetic Markers: The defective gene on the short arm of chromosome 4 causes abnormal polyglutamine expansion within the protein huntingtin (HTT).

The DNA segment known as a CAG trinucleotide repeats with three DNA building blocks (cytosine, adenine, and guanine) that appear multiple times in a row, usually 10–35 times; the CAG segment is repeated 36–120 times in HD (NIH, 2009).

Clinical/History
- Height
- Weight
- BMI
- Weight changes
- Dietary/intake history
- Ability to self-feed
- Chewing and swallowing difficulties
- I & O
- Brain CT scan
- Depressed mood, irritability
- Obsessive and compulsive
- Dementia
- Grimacing
- Involuntary movements (chorea)
- Unified Huntington's Disease Rating Scale

Lab Work
- BUN/Creat
- Serum glucose
- H & H
- CRP
- Acetylcholine and dopamine levels
- Alb, transthyretin
- tHcy levels
- Serum folate
- Vitamin B_{12}
- PLP levels or serum vitamin B_6

INTERVENTION

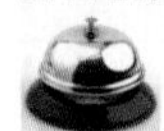

OBJECTIVES

- Promote normal nutritional status, despite tissue degeneration. Extra energy intake is important (Trejo et al, 2004).
- Encourage the patient to self-feed until this is no longer possible.
- Swallowing problems are significant (see Dysphagia, Section 7). Avoid aspiration of solids and liquids.
- Manage gluten intolerance if celiac disease is present.

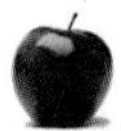

FOOD AND NUTRITION

- Provide a diet that gives sufficient energy and protein to prevent pressure ulcers and other sequelae. Usually 1–1.5 g/kg protein is needed. A patient with HD may need up to 5000 kcals/d. In later stages, if weight gain is a problem, change diet as needed.
- Use a thick, pureed, or chopped diet as appropriate. Feed slowly to prevent choking. Small, frequent meals are suggested.
- Include adequate liquid as dehydration is common.
- Tube feed when necessary; bolus feedings are usually tolerated.
- Provide adequate fiber (e.g., prune juice or tube feedings that contain fiber) for normal elimination.
- Supplement with a multivitamin–mineral supplement; folic acid and other B-complex vitamins may be especially important.

SAMPLE NUTRITION CARE PROCESS STEPS

Swallowing Difficulty

Assessment Data: Weight changes and eating difficulty, dysphagia, and lack of muscle coordination.

Nutrition Diagnoses (PES): NC 1.1 Swallowing difficulty related to dysphagia and lack of muscle coordination as evidenced by choking at mealtime and with thin liquids and recent loss of 10 lb.

Interventions: Education of caregiver about thickening liquids for safer swallowing and the possible use of percutaneous gastrostomy feeding tube as needed.

Monitoring and Evaluation: No choking episodes; tolerance of thickened liquids or enteral nutrition. Improved weight status.

- If gluten intolerance occurs, omit gluten from the diet from wheat, barley, rye and oat products, and flours. Label reading is essential.

Common Drugs Used and Potential Side Effects

- Supplement with vitamin E, antioxidants, and omega-3 fatty acids to reduce inflammation; folic acid, vitamins B_{12} and B_6 to lower serum tHcy levels if elevated.
- Minocycline may slow the disease process by blocking caspases from entering the brain.
- Riluzole has been used with some success and few side effects as a membrane stabilizer and glutamate-release inhibitor.
- Tetrabenazine (Xenazine) reduces chorea, and was approved in 2008 in the United States. It can cause insomnia or nausea. Neuroleptics and benzodiazepines may also be used.
- Antiparkinsonian medications such as Sinemet help with hypokinesia and rigidity.
- A new drug is being tested; called ACR16, it stabilizes brain levels of dopamine for motor, cognitive, and psychiatric changes.

Herbs, Botanicals, and Supplements

- Avoid large doses of vitamin B_6.
- No clinical trials have proved efficacy for use of herbs and botanicals.

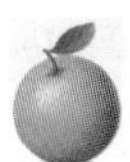

NUTRITION EDUCATION, COUNSELING, CARE MANAGEMENT

- Semisolid foods may be easier to swallow than thin liquids. Teach family or caretakers about the Heimlich maneuver to manage episodes of choking.
- Adding protein and calories through supplements or nutritionally dense foods may be essential.
- If the patient or family wishes to forego tube feeding and hydration, the dietitian should discuss all possible consequences of malnutrition that may occur including dehydration and pressure ulcers.
- Encourage genetic counseling; each child of an affected parent has a 50% chance of inheriting the disease.

Patient Education—Foodborne Illness

- Careful food handling will be important.
- Sanitize counters or work area before and after preparing tube feedings to prevent contamination. Formula companies have good information on safe handling of tube feeding formula in the home and institution.

For More Information

- Huntington's Disease Society of America http://www.hdsa.org/
- Huntington's National Research Roster http://hdroster.iu.edu/index.asp

HUNTINGTON'S DISEASE—CITED REFERENCES

Arrasate M, et al. Inclusion body formation reduces levels of mutant huntingtin and the risk of neuronal death. *Nature.* 431:805, 2004.

Bonelli RM, Wenning GK. Pharmacological management of Huntington's disease: an evidence-based review. *Curr Pharm Des.* 12:2701, 2006.

HDSA. Accessed May 21, 2009, at http://www.hdsa.org/research/news/acetylation.html.

NIH. Accessed May 21, 2009, at http://ghr.nlm.nih.gov/condition=huntingtondisease.

Trejo A, et al. Assessment of the nutrition status of patients with Huntington's disease. *Nutrition.* 20:192, 2004.

Zhang H, et al. Full length mutant huntingtin is required for altered Ca^{2+} signaling and apoptosis of striatal neurons in the YAC mouse model of Huntington's disease. *Neurobiol Dis.* 31:80, 2008.

MIGRAINE HEADACHE

NUTRITIONAL ACUITY RANKING: LEVEL 1

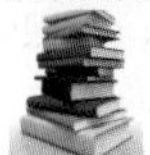

DEFINITIONS AND BACKGROUND

Migraine is a neurological process of the trigeminovascular system. Migraine involves paroxysmal attacks of headache, vasospasm, and increased coagulation, often preceded by visual disturbances. Nausea, vomiting, and acute sensitivity to light or sound may occur. These headaches affect 12% of the adult population (28 million people) in the United States and cause a significant economic loss in productivity. Women may be affected as a result of hormones (Martin et al, 2006). Lack of food or sleep, MT disturbances, exposure to light, anxiety, stress, fatigue, or hormonal irregularities can set off a migraine attack. In addition, a drop in serotonin or estrogen, or intake of vasodilators in some foods may cause blood vessels to swell and aggravate migraines. Studies have linked migraine with epilepsy, sleep disorders, ear problems, and vertigo (Eggers, 2007). In addition, elevated tHcy levels may contribute. A B-complex vitamin containing riboflavin, folic acid, vitamins B_6 and B_{12} is recommended.

Reactions to food are often within 24 hours after consuming the offending food or beverage. Treatment begins with a headache-food diary and the selective avoidance of foods presumed to trigger attacks; omission of all potential triggers is not recommended. Immunoglobulin E–mediated food allergy is infrequent.

Celiac disease may present with neurological symptoms, including migraines. Migraine may also arise because of disruption in neurovascular endothelia caused by elevated tHcy (Lea et al, 2009). Lowering tHcy through vitamin supplementation reduces migraine disability in some individuals (Lea et al, 2009).

Vascular-amine toxicity causes a rapid increase in BP when high-tyramine foods such as cheese, wine, beer, fava beans, and sauerkraut are eaten in combination with medications such as MAOIs. Limit tyramine to 25 mg/d; provide instructions for patients on MAOIs.

Exercise, relaxation, massage therapy, biofeedback, and other therapies limit discomfort in migraine treatment. Migraines may be reduced with intake of omega-3 fatty acids from fish oil and from intake of olive oil. Long-term prophylactic drug therapy is appropriate after exclusion of headache-precipitating trigger factors, including dietary factors. Improved sleep hygiene, moderation of caffeine intake, regular exercise, and identification of provocative influences such as stress, foods, and social pressures are essential. People who are prone to migraines are at risk for stroke and should be monitored carefully.

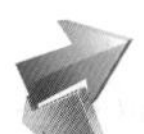

ASSESSMENT, MONITORING, AND EVALUATION

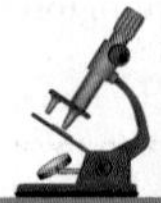

CLINICAL INDICATORS

Genetic Markers: Migraine may be caused by inherited abnormalities. Elevated tHcy promotes migraine disability in a subgroup of patients who have the MTHFRC677 T genotype (Lea et al, 2009).

Clinical/History

- Height
- Weight
- BMI
- Dietary/intake history
- Headache symptoms and duration
- Foods eaten in past 24 hours; diary
- History of similar reactions
- Recent illnesses
- Dehydration or edema?
- Migraine Disability Assessment Score
- Migraine with aura?

Lab Work

- Serum histamine
- Prothrombin time (PT) or international normalized ratio (INR)
- Serum Na^+, K^+ Ca^{++}, Mg^{++}
- Gluc
- Serum tissue transglutaminase IgA (tTGA) antibodies

INTERVENTION

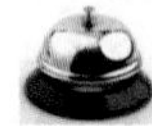

OBJECTIVES

- Eliminate stressors and triggers (crowds, bright lights, noises). Reduce or eliminate use of foods that cause migraines for the individual.

SAMPLE NUTRITION CARE PROCESS STEPS

Poor Food Choices

Assessment Data: Food records indicating poor intake of fruits and vegetables, fish, and olive oils while using high amounts of bacon and lard; frequent migraine headaches.

Nutrition Diagnoses (PES): Poor food choices related to nutrient density as evidenced by frequent migraine headaches (>2 weekly) and daily intake of bacon and lard while avoiding use of fish, olive oil, fruits, and vegetables.

Interventions: Education about nutrient density in foods and encouragement to increase fruits, vegetables, fish, and olive oils and reduce use of other fats.

Monitoring and Evaluation: Fewer migraine headaches, better quality of life, reduction in use of migraine medicines.

- Encourage a well-balanced diet, with adequate meal spacing to prevent fasting or skipping of meals.
- Obesity is a factor in some chronic daily headaches; weight loss may be indicated.
- Improve quality of life. Reduce migraine intensity and duration.
- Reduce frequency of migraines and increase responsiveness to therapy.
- Prevent complications, such as ischemic stroke.

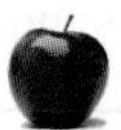

FOOD AND NUTRITION

- Promote regular mealtimes, regular exercise, and adequate relaxation.
- Data surrounding the role of certain foods and substances in triggering headaches are controversial, but certain patients may be sensitive to phenylethylamine, tyramine, aspartame, monosodium glutamate, nitrates, nitrites, alcohol, and caffeine (Sun-Edelstein and Mauskop, 2009). Limit sensitive foods specific to the individual (see Table 4-9).

Common Drugs Used and Potential Side Effects

- Antiemetics may be prescribed if there is nausea or frequent vomiting.
- Botulinum toxin type A (BoNTA; BOTOX) treatment may be a useful option for headache patients demonstrating poor compliance with oral prophylactic regimens (Cady and Screiber, 2008).
- Medicines can be used to relieve pain and restore function during attacks. Drugs such as almotriptan, eletriptan, naratriptan, rizatriptan, sumatriptan, and zolmitriptan may be used to enhance the effects of serotonin with few side effects.
- Drugs designed to lower BP also may prevent headaches, such as thiazides, beta-blockers, angiotensin-converting enzyme (ACE) inhibitors, and angiotensin II receptor agonists.
- If effective medicines are not found to treat headache at its onset, daily preventive medicines are sometimes used.

TABLE 4-9 Foods Implicated in Various Types of Headaches

Food	Description
Alcohol	Champagne and red wine contain both phenols and tyramine; sulfites may also be involved as a trigger. Beer may be another problem. Alcoholic beverages: limit to two normal size drinks of choices such as Cutty Sark scotch, Seagram's VO whisky, Riesling wine (National Headache Foundation, 2010).
Caffeine-containing products	Coffee, tea, and cola can trigger caffeine-withdrawal headache from methyl xanthines (18 hours after withdrawal); taper withdrawal gradually. Coffee is the major source of caffeine in adults; soft drinks are the major source for children and teens (Frary et al, 2005).
Cheese and tyramine	Aged cheese that contains tyramine has been implicated. Ripened cheeses: cheddar, emmentaler, stilton, brie, and camembert.
Chocolate	Chocolate contains phenylethylamine (no clear relationship to migraine).
Fermented foods	Chicken livers, aged cheese such as cheddar, red wine, pickled herring, chocolate, broad beans, and beer contain tyramine (no clear relationship to migraine).
Fruits	Bananas, figs, raisins; some citrus fruits.
Gluten	Celiac disease has been associated with migraine (Bushara, 2005).
Histamine-containing foods	Scombroid fish (slightly spoiled).
Ice cream	Some individuals are sensitive to the cold.
Nuts, peanuts	Some contain vasodilators. Avoid nuts and peanut butter if necessary.
Processed meats	Hot dogs, bacon, ham, and salami contain nitrites.
Sulfites	Some people respond to the sulfites in shrimp, packaged potato products.
Vegetables	Onions, pea pods, lima beans.

This may include anticonvulsants; nonsteroidal anti-inflammatory drugs (NSAIDs) such as Ibuprofen; tricyclic antidepressants (TCAs), and serotonergic agents.

- MT may be useful in migraine headaches (Masruha et al, 2008; Vogler et al, 2006).
- Avoid using aspirin in children younger than 15 because of the potential for Reye's syndrome.

Herbs, Botanicals, and Supplements

- While capsaicin from hot chili peppers may be used as a source of relief for cluster headache pain, it does not relieve migraines.
- The following supplements may help in the preventative treatment of migraines, in a decreasing order of preference: magnesium, Petasites hybridus, feverfew, coenzyme Q10, riboflavin, and alpha lipoic acid (Sun-Edelstein and Mauskop, 2009).
- Feverfew and riboflavin have not shown strong efficacy (Tepper, 2008). Side effects of feverfew include decreased platelet aggregation if used with warfarin, aspirin, and ticlopidine. NSAIDs (ibuprofen, indomethacin, advil) decrease the herb's anti-inflammatory action; do not use together.
- Where food-plant sensitivities exist (melon/ragweed, carrot/potato, apple/birch, wheat/grasses, ragweed/dandelion greens) bee pollen and echinacea may cause an allergic reaction.
- Evening primrose, red pepper, willow, and ginger have been recommended; no studies prove efficacy. Counsel about avoiding herbal teas, especially if they contain toxic ingredients.

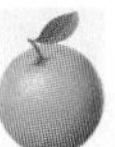

NUTRITION EDUCATION, COUNSELING, CARE MANAGEMENT

- Fasting can increase likelihood of a headache. Regular mealtimes are important.
- Encourage the patient to identify various, individual triggers. Teach the patient how to keep an accurate food diary for food sensitivities. Read food labels and avoid items containing ingredients that are problematic.
- Monitor drugs taken for underlying conditions such as asthma, reactive airway disease, hypertension, glaucoma, and ear problems. Discuss the possibility of "medication overuse headache" or rebound headaches after caffeine from the diet or medicines.
- Psychotherapy may be useful for mental and emotional stress. Regular sleeping patterns are needed; evaluate for insomnia and sleep apnea.
- Evidence-based behavioral medicine treatments include patient education, cognitive behavioral therapy (CBT), biofeedback, relaxation training, and stress management (Andrasik et al, 2009). Some authorities may also recommend acupuncture.

Patient Education—Food Safety

- Food storage is a major issue. Extended holding times, especially in high-protein foods, is a concern.
- Teach safe food handling, handwashing, and other practices.

For More Information

- American Council for Headache Education http://www.achenet.org

- American Headache Society
  http://www.ahsnet.org
- Medline: Headache
  http://www.nlm.nih.gov/medlineplus/headache.html
- National Headache Foundation—Food
  http://www.headaches.org/education/Headache_Topic_Sheets/Diet_and_Headache_-_Foods
- National Migraine Association
  http://www.migraines.org/
- Neurology Channel
  http://www.neurologychannel.com/migraine/index.shtml
- Tyramine-Restricted Diet
  http://www.headaches.org/pdf/Diet.pdf
- World Headache Alliance
  http://www.w-h-a.org

MIGRAINE HEADACHE—CITED REFERENCES

Andrasik F, et al. Behavioral medicine for migraine and medication overuse headache. *Curr Pain Headache Rep.* 13:241, 2009.

Bushara KO. Neurologic presentation of celiac disease. Neurologic presentation of celiac disease. *Gastroenterology.* 128:92S, 2005.

Cady R, Schreiber C. Botulinum toxin type A as migraine preventive treatment in patients previously failing oral prophylactic treatment due to compliance issues. *Headache.* 48:900, 2008.

Condo M, et al. Riboflavin prophylaxis in pediatric and adolescent migraine. *J Headache Pain.* 10:361, 2009.

Eggers SD. Migraine-related vertigo: diagnosis and treatment. *Curr Pain Headache Rep.* 11:217, 2007.

Eli R, Fasciano JA. A chronopharmacological preventive treatment for sleep-related migraine headaches and chronic morning headaches: nitric oxide supersensitivity can cause sleep-related headaches in a subset of patients. *Med Hypotheses.* 66:461, 2006.

Frary C, et al. Food sources and intakes of caffeine in the diets of persons in the United States. *J Am Diet Assoc.* 105:110, 2005.

Honaker J, Samy RN. Migraine-associated vestibulopathy. *Curr Opin Otolaryngol Head Neck Surg.* 16:412, 2008.

Lea R. The effects of vitamin supplementation and MTHFR (C677 T) genotype on homocysteine-lowering and migraine disability. *Pharmacogenet Genomics.* 19:422, 2009.

Martin VT, et al. Symptoms of premenstrual syndrome and their association with migraine headache. *Headache.* 46:125, 2006.

Masruha MR, et al. Low urinary 6-sulphatoxymelatonin concentrations in acute migraine. *J Headache Pain.* 9:221, 2008.

Millichap JG, Yee MM. The diet factor in pediatric and adolescent migraine. *Pediatr Neurol.* 28:9, 2003.

National Headache Foundation. accessed October 3, 2010, at http://www.headaches.org/education/Headache_Topic_Sheets/Diet_and_Headache_-_Foods

Sun-Edelstein C, Mauskop A. Foods and supplements in the management of migraine headaches. *Clin J Pain.* 25:446, 2009.

Tepper SJ. Complementary and alternative treatments for childhood headaches. *Curr Pain Headache Rep.* 12:379, 2008.

Vogler B, et al. Role of melatonin in the pathophysiology of migraine: implications for treatment. *CNS Drugs.* 20:343, 2006.

MULTIPLE SCLEROSIS

NUTRITIONAL ACUITY RANKING: LEVEL 2

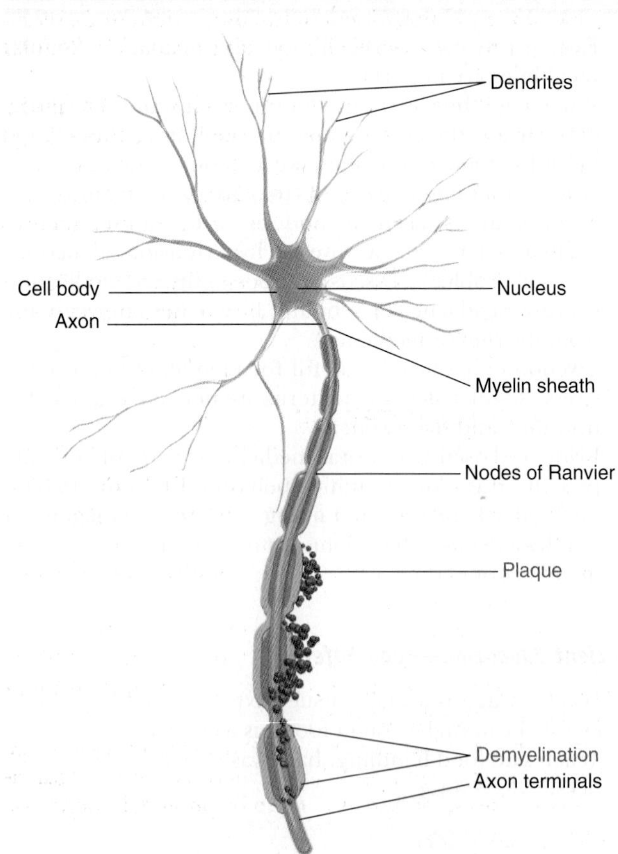

Asset provided by Anatomical Chart Co.

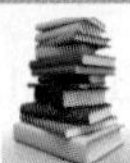

DEFINITIONS AND BACKGROUND

Multiple sclerosis (MS) involves scarring and the loss of myelin sheath, the insulating material around nerve fibers. The disease causes progressive or episodic nerve degeneration and disability. Insufficient vitamin D_3 plays a role; persons living in colder climates and those with less sun exposure are more prone (Kantarci and Wingerchuk, 2006). MS has a much higher incidence among Caucasians than in any other race and affects women two to three times as often as men. MS affects over 400,000 people in the United States and 2.5 million people worldwide.

MS is an autoimmune disease. Proinflammatory cytokines such as tumor necrosis factor-alpha (TNF-α) instruct the adaptive immune system (T and B cells and other cells and proteins) to launch an attack to suppress the "invader." Th17 T-cells are a type of immune cell known to play a role in the onset of MS. Onset is usually between 20 and 40 years of age (average age, 27 years). Symptoms include tingling; numbness in arms, legs, trunk, or face; double vision; fatigue; weakness; clumsiness; tremor; stiffness; sensory impairment; loss of position sense; and respiratory problems. Dysphagia can occur. Spasticity and bladder dysfunction are also common.

After diagnosis, 70% of persons with MS are as active as previously. Relapsing-remitting MS shows clear relapses with some amount of recovery in between; it affects about 80% of all people with MS. Ten percent of individuals with MS have primary progressive MS, without relapses. A description of the types of MS is in Table 4-10.

TABLE 4-10 Types of Multiple Sclerosis

Name	Characteristics
Relapsing-Remitting Multiple Sclerosis (RRMS)	Symptom flare-ups followed by recovery; stable between attacks
Secondary-Progressive Multiple Sclerosis (SPMS)	Second phase of RRMS; progressive worsening of symptoms with or without superimposed relapses; treatments may delay this phase
Primary-Progressive Multiple Sclerosis (PPMS)	Gradual but steady accumulation of neurological problems from onset
Benign	Few attacks and little or no disability after 20 years
Progressive-Relapsing Multiple Sclerosis (PRMS)	Progressive course from the onset, sometimes combined with occasional acute symptom flare-ups
Malignant of Fulminant Multiple Sclerosis	Rapidly progressive disease course

Multiple Sclerosis Association of America, http://www.msassociation.org/about_multiple_sclerosis/commontypes, accessed May 25, 2009.

During chronic CNS inflammation, nicotinamide adenine dinucleotide (NAD) concentrations are altered by T-helper Th1-derived cytokines; use of pharmacological doses of nontryptophan NAD precursors have been suggested (Penberthy and Tsunoda, 2009).

Magnesium, vitamin B_6, vitamin B_{12}, zinc, vitamin D_3, vitamin E, selenium, and omega-3 fatty acids have been suggested. Vitamin B_{12} is important for proper myelination of the spinal cord (Montanha-Rojas et al, 2005).

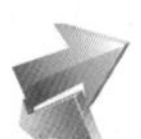

ASSESSMENT, MONITORING, AND EVALUATION

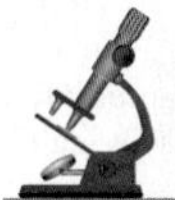

CLINICAL INDICATORS

Genetic Markers: MS tends to run in families. Altered human leukocyte antigen (HLA) genes in chromosome 6; IL2RA and IL7RA as receptors for interleukins; and the gene that encodes kinesin (KIF1B) may enhance the onset of MS.

Clinical/History	Lab Work	
Height	Alb	H & H
Weight	Chol	Serum Fe
BMI	Trig (may be low in autoimmune disorders)	Gluc
Dietary/intake history	Na⁺, K⁺	MRI scan
BP	Serum D_3	Evoked potentials test
I & O	Alk phos	CSF (WBC, γ-globulin are increased)
Edema		EEG
Temperature		L:S ratio

SAMPLE NUTRITION CARE PROCESS STEPS

Self-Feeding Difficulty

Assessment Data: Difficulty with self-feeding, loss of strength in hands, dependent on assistants.

Nutrition Diagnoses (PES): Self-feeding difficulty related to poor hand strength and MS as evidenced by inability to use standard meal utensils.

Interventions: Alteration of food consistency and use of adaptive feeding utensils to adjust and enhance ability to feed self; finger foods where possible, such as julienne vegetables, sandwiches cut into strips, soup in a mug.

Monitoring and Evaluation: Ability to grasp items at mealtime as evidenced by increased ability to do some self-feeding with finger foods and less dependency on staff for assistance.

INTERVENTION

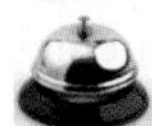

OBJECTIVES

- During the chronic phase of the disease, treatment goals are to reduce the incidence of respiratory infections, UTIs, bowel problems, muscle spasms, contractures, pressure ulcers, constipation or fecal impactions.
- Adjust energy intake to avoid excessive weight gain, if this becomes a problem.
- Maintain good nutritional status. Since vitamin D_3 seems to play a role in autoimmunity, supplement with 800 IU daily.
- Reduce fatigue associated with mealtimes. Frequent, small meals may be better tolerated than three large ones.
- During the active phase of the disease, corticosteroids may be used to decrease symptoms. Alter diet accordingly.
- Prevent chronic diseases such as coronary heart disease or osteoporosis, which may occur with immobilization.

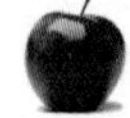

FOOD AND NUTRITION

- Normal protein and adequate carbohydrate intakes are recommended. Use olive oil and fish oil (omega-3 fatty acids) more often.
- Provide adequate intake of multivitamins, especially vitamins D_3 and B_{12}.
- Laxative foods and liquids may ease constipation.
- Control sodium intake during steroid therapy. Otherwise, sodium plays an important role in lipid/protein transport in myelin tissues.
- Small, frequent meals may be better tolerated than large meals. If swallowing difficulties increase and coordination decreases, foods may need to be pureed, liquefied or fed by tube.
- To prevent UTIs, cranberry juice is quite effective (Raz et al, 2004).

Common Drugs Used and Potential Side Effects

- A man-made retinoid (AM80) prevents early symptoms of the autoimmune disease by blocking the function of Th17 T-cells.
  - Immune-modifying drugs must have FDA approval. Interferon injections are useful. Interferon-β1 a (Avonex or Rebif) may cause nausea, diarrhea, liver damage, flu-like symptoms, headache, infections, or anemia. Interferon-β1b (Betaseron) may cause weight changes, abdominal pain, diarrhea, constipation, fever, headache, hypertension, or tachycardia.
  - Corticosteroids are not FDA-approved for use in MS. If used, they require controlled sodium intake. Glucose intolerance, negative nitrogen balance, and decreased serum zinc, calcium, and potassium may occur.
  - A combination of CT and a subtherapeutic dose of $1,25(OH)(2)D_3$ suppresses autoimmune encephalitis (EAE) without causing hypercalcemia (Becklund et al, 2009). Further studies are needed.
  - Antispasticity drugs such as baclofen (Lioresal) may cause nausea, diarrhea, and constipation. If Sinemet (L-dopa) is used, avoid large doses of vitamin B_6.
  - The immunosuppressant azathioprine (Imuran) reduces new brain lesions in relapsing-remitting MS (Massacesi et al, 2005). Its use is still experimental.
  - Cannabinoids are potent immunosuppressive and anti-inflammatory agents; cannabinoid receptor 1 (CB1) is expressed on the cells of the CNS and cannabinoid receptor 2 (CB2) is expressed on immune cells; they affect apoptosis, and suppress cytokine and chemokine production (Rieder et al, 2009).
  - A complete list of medications is available at: http://www.msassociation.org/about_multiple_sclerosis/medications/types/

Herbs, Botanicals, and Supplements

- Many patients with MS seek alternative therapies for their pain, fatigue, and stress. Diet, essential fatty acid (EFA) supplements, vitamin–mineral supplements, homeopathy, botanicals (Shinto et al, 2004) as well as exercise, herbal therapy, cannabis, massage, and acupuncture (Olsen, 2009).
- Based on available evidence, the prophylactic use of vitamin D is a viable option as an adjunct to conventional medicine (Kimball et al, 2007; Namaka et al, 2008).
- St. John's wort should not be used with MAO inhibitors, SSRI antidepressants, cyclosporine, digoxin, oral contraceptives, HIV protease inhibitors, theophylline, warfarin, or calcium channel blockers such as amlodipine, diltiazem, or verapamil. No studies have been conducted for efficacy in MS patients.
- Stinging nettle, pineapple, black currant, and purslane have been recommended for MS; no clinical trials have proven efficacy.
- Despite beneficial reports regarding nonherbal supplements such as ALA, luteolin, evening primrose oil and vitamins such as B_{12}, the lack of evidence does not support their prophylactic use (Namaka et al, 2008).

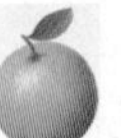

NUTRITION EDUCATION, COUNSELING, CARE MANAGEMENT

- Teach the patient how to control energy intake, especially if inactive.
- Discuss the role of fat and vitamin E in myelin sheath formation and maintenance, and where to find sources of linoleic acid and omega-3 fatty acids from the diet.
- Teach the patient about foods high in fiber.
- Avoid total inactivity. Physical therapy may be beneficial.
- Encourage moderate exposure to sunlight for vitamin D.
- Use tabletop cooking methods and equipment to avoid lifting. Utensils with large handles may be useful in food preparation and self-feeding. Foods may need to be cut before serving.
- Allergen-free, gluten-free, pectin-free, fructose-restricted, raw foods diets, and liquid diets are ineffective.
- Avoid smoking.

Patient Education—Foodborne Illness

- Careful food handling will be important. The same is true for sanitizing work area before and after preparing tube feedings to prevent contamination. Formula companies have good information on safe handling of formula in the home and institution.

For More Information

- Consortium of Multiple Sclerosis Centers
  http://www.mscare.org
- Multiple Sclerosis Association of America
  http://www.msaa.com/
- National MS Society
  http://www.nmss.org/

MULTIPLE SCLEROSIS—CITED REFERENCES

Becklund BR, et al. Enhancement of 1,25-dihydroxyvitamin D_3-mediated suppression of experimental autoimmune encephalomyelitis by calcitonin. *Proc Natl Acad Sci USA*. 106:5276, 2009.

Kantarci O, Wingerchuk D. Epidemiology and natural history of multiple sclerosis: new insights. *Curr Opin Neurol.* 19:248, 2006.

Kimball SM, et al. Safety of vitamin D_3 in adults with multiple sclerosis. *Am J Clin Nutr.* 86:645, 2007.

Massacesi L, et al. Efficacy of azathioprine on multiple sclerosis new brain lesions evaluated using magnetic resonance imaging. *Arch Neurol.* 62:1843, 2005.

Montanha-Rojas EA, et al. Myelin basic protein accumulation is impaired in a model of protein deficiency during development. *Nutr Neurosci.* 8:49, 2005.

Namaka M, et al. Examining the evidence: complementary adjunctive therapies for multiple sclerosis. *Neurol Res.* 30:710, 2008.

Olsen SA. A review of complementary and alternative medicine (CAM) by people with multiple sclerosis. *Occup Ther Int.* 16:57, 2009.

Penberty WT, Tsunoda I. The importance of NAD in multiple sclerosis. *Curr Pharm Des.* 15:64, 2009.

Raz R, et al. Cranberry juice and urinary tract infection. *Clin Infect Dis.* 38:1413, 2004.

Rieder SA, et al. Cannabinoid-induced apoptosis in immune cells as a pathway to immunosuppression. [published online ahead of print May 18, 2009] *Immunobiology.* 215:598, 2009.

Shinto L, et al. Complementary and alternative medicine in multiple sclerosis: survey of licensed naturopaths. *J Altern Complement Med.* 10:891, 2004.

MYASTHENIA GRAVIS AND NEUROMUSCULAR JUNCTION DISORDERS

NUTRITIONAL ACUITY RANKING: LEVEL 2

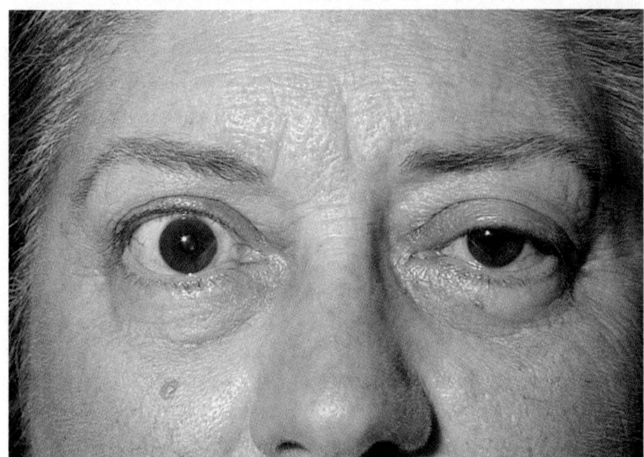

Adapted from: Tasman W, Jaeger E. *The Wills Eye Hospital Atlas of Clinical Ophthalmology*, 2nd ed. Lippincott Williams & Wilkins, 2001.

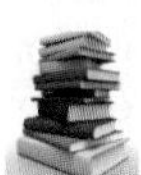

DEFINITIONS AND BACKGROUND

Myasthenia gravis (MG) is an autoimmune disorder caused by autoantibodies against the nicotinic acetylcholine receptor on the postsynaptic membrane at the neuromuscular junction (Thanvi and Lo, 2004). The neuromuscular junction lies beyond the protection of the blood–brain barrier and is particularly vulnerable to antibody-mediated attack. Individuals with seronegative MG have autoantibodies to acetylcholine receptors and muscle-specific kinase (MuSK protein) for cell signaling (NINDS, 2009).

Few types are congenital, most are acquired. Acquired neuromuscular junction disorders include botulism, autoimmune MG, and drug-induced MG. General immunosuppression is primary. Treatments that reduce complement-mediated damage or inhibit the binding of pathogenic antibodies are under development (NINDS, 2009). The disease frequently is associated with thymic morphologic abnormalities; removal of the thymus gland works for about 70% of cases (Juel and Massey, 2005).

Symptoms and signs of MG include drooping eyelids (ptosis), double vision (diplopia), fatigue, general weakness, dysphagia, weak voice, inability to walk on heels, pneumonia or respiratory arrest. Diabetes, sleep apnea, and thyroid problems are common in persons who have MG and should be closely monitored.

MG occurs in approximately 18,000 affected people in the United States. Incidence begins with the first peak in the third decade and a second peak in the sixth decade (Thanvi and Lo, 2004). Plasmapheresis can be used during a crisis to remove the abnormal antibodies. A myasthenic crisis is defined as the need for mechanical ventilatory support, usually following progressive weakness and oropharyngeal symptoms (Bershad et al, 2008).

When MG is suspected, a tensilon test involves insertion of a small intravenous catheter through which tensilon is given; this very short-acting drug blocks the degradation of acetylcholine. The short-term availability of acetylcholine results in improved muscle function, often in the eye area.

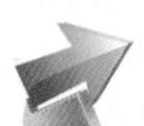

ASSESSMENT, MONITORING, AND EVALUATION

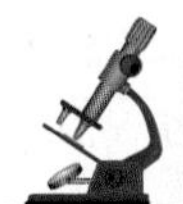

CLINICAL INDICATORS

Genetic Markers: In MG, the expression of acetylcholine receptors (AChRs) in the thymus is under the control of the autoimmune regulator protein (AIRE). Polymorphisms in the AChR promote early onset of disease. Congenital myasthenia and congenital myasthenic syndrome are caused by defective genes.

Clinical/History
- Height
- Weight
- BMI
- Dietary/intake history
- I & O
- Weight changes
- Ptosis
- Diplopia
- Tensilon test
- Chest CT scan for thymoma
- Sleep apnea?

Lab Work
- Na^+, K^+
- BP
- CRP
- Acetylcholine antibodies test
- EMG
- Gluc
- Mg^{++}, Ca^{++}
- Alb
- H & H
- Serum Fe
- T3, T4, TSH

SAMPLE NUTRITION CARE PROCESS STEPS

Dysphagia

Assessment Data: Swallowing study, weight changes, BMI 17.

Nutrition Diagnoses (PES): Difficulty swallowing related to neuromuscular disorder (MG) as evidenced by aspiration of food and liquids into lung on swallowing evaluation and weight loss (BMI now 17).

Interventions: Thickened liquids and pureed foods as tolerated; PEG tube placement and enteral nutrition at night to regain lost weight.

Monitoring and Evaluation: Weight gain, no further incidents of aspiration, tolerance of thickened liquids and pureed foods and/or enteral nutrition when necessary.

INTERVENTION

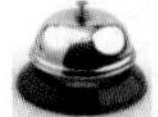

OBJECTIVES

- Increase the likelihood of obtaining adequate nutrition by altering the consistency of foods. This is necessary when muscles used in chewing and swallowing are weakened. Work with Speech Therapist accordingly.
- Feedings should be small to reduce fatigue. Allow adequate time to complete meals.
- Prevent permanent structural damage to the neuromuscular system during crises.
- Prevent or manage respiratory failure.
    - Encourage participation in rehabilitation programming.

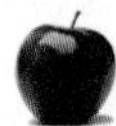

FOOD AND NUTRITION

- Diet should include frequent, small feedings of easily masticated foods.
- Provide tube feeding when needed.
- If corticosteroids are part of treatment, use a low-sodium diet. Provide adequate potassium supplements.
- Use a high-energy diet if weight loss occurs, which is common.
- Avoid giving medications with thin liquids such as coffee or juice; give with milk and crackers or bread.

Common Drugs Used and Potential Side Effects

- Prednisone is usually started at a high dose every day, then reduced to every other day. In the event of intolerable side effects or failure of treatment, other immunosuppressants may be used, most commonly azathioprine (Imuran). GI distress, nausea, vomiting, and anorexia may occur.
- Transient symptomatic control can be achieved by the initiation of pyridostigmine (Mestinon) that blocks the degradation of acetylcholine at the neuromuscular junction, increasing the level of acetylcholine with better muscle response to stimulation by the nerve. Mestinon is a temporary symptomatic treatment and does not reverse the course of the illness. Limit sodium intake. Anorexia, abdominal cramps, diarrhea, and weakness may result. Long-acting capsules may be needed if morning weakness persists.
- Long-term use of antacids negatively affects calcium and magnesium metabolism.

Herbs, Botanicals, and Supplements

- No studies have been conducted for efficacy of herbs or botanicals in MG patients.

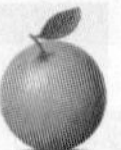

NUTRITION EDUCATION, COUNSELING, CARE MANAGEMENT

- Show the patient how to prepare foods and nutrient-dense beverages with the use of a blender, if necessary.
- Indicate how to take medication with food or milk. Discuss potential side effects.
- Avoid alcohol.
- Food and utensils should be arranged within easy reach of the patient; lightweight items are preferable.
- The International Classification of Functioning (ICF), Disability and Health rehabilitation practitioners is a worldwide accepted model providing a universal language for the description and classification of functioning (Rauch et al, 2008).

Patient Education—Foodborne Illness

- Careful food handling will be important. The same is true for sanitizing work area before and after preparing tube feedings to prevent contamination. Formula companies have good information on safe handling of formula in the home and institution.

For More Information

- Myasthenia Gravis Foundation of America
  http://www.myasthenia.org/
- National Institute of Neurological Disorders and Stroke
  http://www.ninds.nih.gov/disorders/myasthenia_gravis/detail_myasthenia_gravis.htm
- Neuromuscular Junction Disorders
  http://www.neuro.wustl.edu/neuromuscular/synmg.html

MYASTHENIA GRAVIS AND NEUROMUSCULAR JUNCTION DISORDERS—CITED REFERENCES

Bershad EM, et al. Myasthenia gravis crisis. *South Med J.* 101:63, 2008.

Juel VC, Massey SM. Autoimmune myasthenia gravis: recommendations for treatment and immunologic modulation. *Curr Treat Options Neurol.* 7:3, 2005.

NINDS. Accessed May 26, 2009, at http://www.ninds.nih.gov/disorders/myasthenia_gravis/detail_myasthenia_gravis.htm.

Rauch A, et al. How to apply the International Classification of Functioning, Disability and Health (ICF) for rehabilitation management in clinical practice. *Eur J Phys Rehabil.* 44:329, 2008.

Thanvi BR, Lo TC. Update on myasthenia gravis. *Postgrad Med J.* 80:690, 2004.

PARKINSON'S DISEASE

NUTRITIONAL ACUITY RANKING: LEVEL 2

Dopamine levels

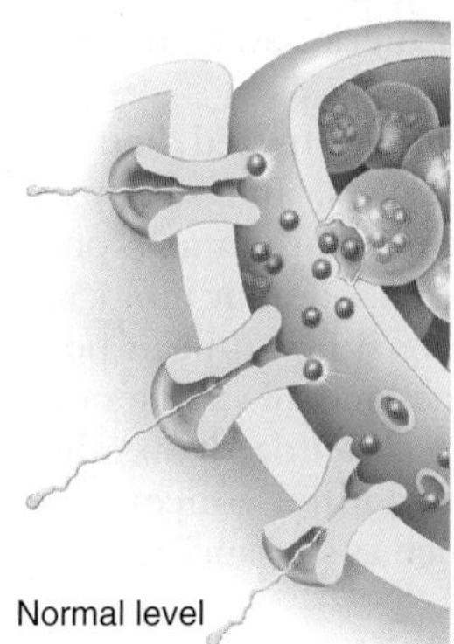

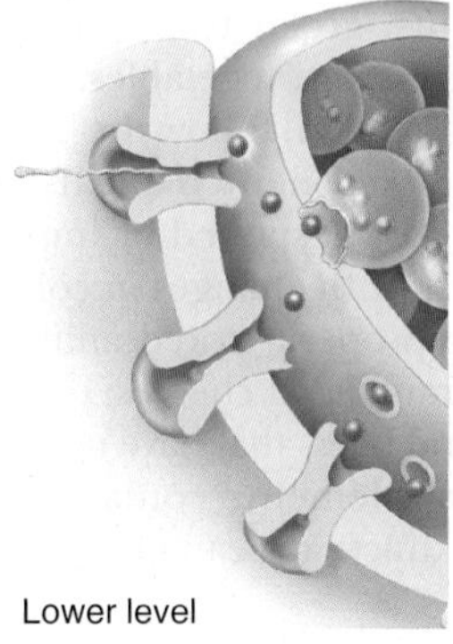

Asset provided by Anatomical Chart Co.

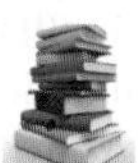

DEFINITIONS AND BACKGROUND

Parkinson disease (PD) is an age-related neurodegenerative disorder that affects 1–2% of persons aged 60 years and older (Olanow et al, 2009). There are diminished levels of dopamine at the basal ganglia of the brain, causing tremor of hands, arms, legs, jaw, and face; rigidity of limbs and trunk; slowness of gait; coordination difficulty; chewing problems; dysphagia; problems with speech. A test for PD progression includes a decline in ability to smell and the speed of wrist movements. Depression and dementia-related symptoms may also occur. Levodopa must be provided. Although levodopa continues as the gold standard for efficacy, its chronic use is associated with potentially disabling motor complications (Poewe, 2009).

Approximately 24 conditions are categorized as PDs. Between 1–1.5 million people are affected, men slightly more often than women. Life expectancy is 12.5 years after diagnosis. Yet, causes and pathophysiology are poorly understood. Oxidative stress contributes to apoptotic death of dopamine neurons (Bournival et al, 2009). Long-term exposure to manganese, herbicides, pesticides, or high intake of iron with high manganese may promote PD symptoms (Ascherio et al, 2006; Fitsanakis et al, 2006). Some medications such as major tranquilizers or metoclopramide can also cause PD-like symptoms.

Esophageal motor abnormalities and constipation are common. Constipation appears about 10–20 years prior to motor symptoms (Ueki and Otsuka, 2004). Unintentional weight loss is frequent, resulting in increased morbidity and mortality. Weight loss occurs from increased energy expenditure due to tremor, dyskinesias, and rigidity; reduced energy intake due to olfactory dysfunction, cognitive impairment, depression, dysphagia, and disability; and medication-related side effects, including dry mouth, nausea/vomiting, appetite loss, anorexia, insomnia, fatigue, and anxiety. PD is progressive. Advancing disease is associated with the emergence of freezing, falling, and dementia which are not adequately controlled with dopaminergic therapies (Olanow et al, 2009).

Increased plasma tHcy accelerates the selective dopaminergic cell death underlying PD (De Lau et al, 2005). Adequate B-complex intake and measurement of serum levels of B_{12} may be important. Higher serum vitamin B_{12} levels are associated with lower dyskinesia risk (Camicioli et al, 2009), whereas folate therapy does not seem to be singularly protective (Chen et al, 2004).

Overall, neuroprotection is desirable. Oxidative stress initiates or promotes degeneration of neurons; antioxidant therapy may be protective. Resveratrol in grape juice and red wine, and quercetin in green tea are two natural polyphenols that have preventive qualities in PD (Bournival et al, 2009). Drinking 4–5 cups of coffee daily and foods rich in vitamin E and vitamin D_3 may also be protective (Evatt et al, 2008).

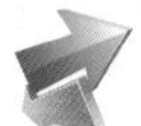

ASSESSMENT, MONITORING, AND EVALUATION

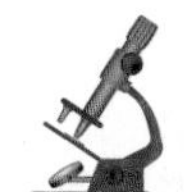

CLINICAL INDICATORS

Genetic Markers: There is significant variation in the prevalence of PD between different populations. Rates are highest in populations of European origin. Melanocortin 1 receptor (MC1R) genes are associated with red hair and fair skin (Han et al, 2006); risk for PD seems to be highest among those with this Cys/Cys genotype (Gao et al, 2009). There are many other candidate genes for PD: alpha-synuclein, DJ-1, PINK-1 (kinase), and UCHL-1. Two mutated copies of the Parkin gene are needed for the rare, autosomal recessive form of PD, with early onset in the fourth decade.

Clinical/History

Height
Weight
BMI
Dietary/intake history
BP
I & O
Dysphagia
Tremors
Bradykinesia
Difficulty arising from a chair
Slowed activities of daily living
Depression, anorexia
Constipation
Micrographia
Reduced arm swing
Postural instability
DEXA for bone mineral density
Insomnia
Stooped, shuffling gait
Urinary frequency and urgency
Skin evaluation; melanoma?
Unified Parkinson Disease Rating Scale (UPDRS)

Lab Work

Plasma 25-hydroxyvitamin D (25[OH]D)
Na^+, K^+
N balance
H & H
Serum Fe
Alb, transthyretin
Dopamine
Norepinephrine
BUN, Creat
ALT, AST
Gluc
Plasma urate
Ca^{++}, Mg^{++}
Serum manganese
Serum tHcy
Serum folate and B_{12}

> **SAMPLE NUTRITION CARE PROCESS STEPS**
>
> **Dehydration**
>
> ***Assessment Data:*** Weight loss, poor intake of food and fluids, swallowing difficulty, easy fatigue at mealtimes and early satiety, coughing after swallowing, poor skin turgor.
>
> ***Nutrition Diagnoses (PES):*** Inadequate fluid intake related to swallowing difficulty and poor intake as evidenced by I & O records showing consumption of 25% of estimated needs and decreased intake of thin liquids because of coughing and early satiety.
>
> ***Interventions:*** Swallowing evaluation (Speech Therapy) with selection of appropriate thickened liquids or pureed foods and ways in which fluids can be added to foods; use of IV fluids as needed.
>
> ***Monitoring and Evaluation:*** Improvement in I & O related to fluids from food and beverages; improved skin turgor; return to previous weight.

INTERVENTION

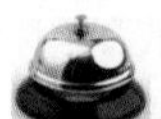

OBJECTIVES

- Supply dopamine to the brain; monitor diet therapy accordingly.
- Maintain optimal physical and emotional health. Exercise may be protective, especially for men (Carne et al, 2005).
- Improve the ability to eat. Use semisolid foods rather than fluids when sucking/swallowing reflexes are reduced. Drooling may be a problem. Request a swallow evaluation from a speech therapist to determine proper consistency of foods, and (See Dysphagia entry in Section 7).
- Provide adequate energy to prevent weight loss, and avoid gaining excessive weight as well.
- Provide adequate hydration, especially when thickened liquids are needed. Coffee is a good choice.
- Correct alterations in GI function (i.e., increased transit time, heartburn, and constipation).
- Preserve functioning; delay disability as long as possible.
- When used MAOIs, use a tyramine-restricted diet to prevent severe headaches, blurred vision, difficulty thinking, seizures, chest pain or symptoms of a stroke.
- Lower elevated tHcy levels where needed (Caccamo et al, 2007).

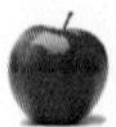

FOOD AND NUTRITION

- A high intake of protein diminishes the effectiveness of levodopa; use 0.5 g/kg of body weight. If unplanned weight loss occurs, up to 1–1.5 g/kg plus extra energy may be needed. For some, a protein redistribution diet is used (i.e., low-protein breakfast and lunch with high-protein dinner and snack). This diet is not always effective, and often provides insufficient protein. Timing of levodopa should be monitored to avoid conflicting responses to protein at mealtimes.
- Plan diet according to results of swallowing evaluation. Cut, mince, or soften foods as required. Use small, frequent meals if needed.
- To increase fiber, add crushed bran to hot cereal or try prune juice.
- A multivitamin–mineral supplement may be beneficial, especially for vitamins C, E, and the B-complex vitamins. Folate, vitamins B_6 and B_{12} will be important to lower elevated tHcy levels (Biselli et al, 2007; Grimble, 2006).
- Highlight foods such as vegetable oils, salad dressings, nuts, green tea, coffee, turmeric, and antioxidant-rich fruits and vegetables.
- If needed, follow the Tyramine-restricted diet: avoid aged and fermented meats, sausages, and salamis; pickled herring; spoiled or improperly stored meat, poultry and fish with changes in coloration, odor, or mold; spoiled or improperly stored animal livers; broad bean pods; sauerkraut; aged cheeses; red wines and all varieties of tap beer and beers that have not been pasteurized; over-the-counter supplements containing tyramine; concentrated yeast extract; soybean products such as soy sauce and tofu.

Common Drugs Used and Potential Side Effects

- Elevated plasma tHcy levels have been observed in PD patients treated with levodopa. New approaches may be needed for management of PD in persons who have MTHFR alleles (Caccamo et al, 2007; Camicioli et al, 2009; Todorovic et al, 2006).
- See Table 4-11 for specific medications used in PD.

Herbs, Botanicals, and Supplements

- Because creatine kinase/phosphocreatine system plays a significant role in the CNS with the high and fluctuating energy demand, exogenous creatine supplementation tends to reduce neuronal cell loss (Andres et al, 2008).
- Coenzyme Q10 may be beneficial, but more research is needed.
- Other forms of CAM therapy are common, but patients do not always tell their health providers. Because of potential interactions with medications and excess costs, patients should be encouraged to discuss their use with their doctor before taking any forms of alternative medicine. Use of evening primrose, St. John's wort, passionflower, velvet bean, or gingko have not been proven effective.
- Kava should not be taken by patients with PD; it decreases effectiveness of medications.
- Ginseng, ma huang (ephedra), yohimbe, and St. John's wort should not be used with MAOIs, including selegiline (Eldepryl).

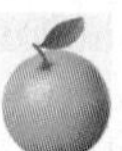

NUTRITION EDUCATION, COUNSELING, CARE MANAGEMENT

- Education for the patient and family, access to support groups, regular exercise, and good nutrition are essential. Provide tips on antioxidant foods such as blueberries, green tea, coffee.
- Explain how to blenderize food or how to make food and beverages more nutrient dense, as needed.

TABLE 4-11 Medications for Parkinson's Disease and Possible Side Effects

Medication	Side Effects
Antidepressants	Weight gain, dry mouth, or nausea can result.
Anticholinergics Cogentin (benztropine), Artane (trihexyphenidyl), Ethopropazine	Confusion, agitation, dizziness, sedation, euphoria, tachycardia, hypotension, dry mouth, constipation, nausea, urinary retention and blurred vision.
Antiviral agent Symmetrel (amantadine)	Possible adverse effects include anorexia, dry mouth, nausea, constipation, dizziness, insomnia, blurred vision, depression, ataxia, confusion, fatigue, leg/ankle edema, hallucinations, anxiety, and livedo reticularis (skin discoloration).
Catechol-O-methyltransferase (COMT) inhibitors Tasmar (tolcapone), Comtan (entacapone)	These drugs slow the breakdown of dopamine. Diarrhea, orthostatic hypotension, hallucinations, sleep disturbances, dyskinesias, muscle cramping, and vivid dreams may occur with use. Liver function testing should be scheduled regularly while on these medications.
Dopamine agonists Parlodel (bromocriptine), Mirapex (pramipexole), Requip (ropinirole)	These stimulate dopamine receptors. Edema, psychosis, nausea, headache, fatigue, confusion, somnolence and "sleep attacks." With ropinirole, fewer side effects, such as dyskinesia, have been identified. Some studies suggest that dopamine agonists, rather than levodopa, should be the initial symptomatic therapy in Parkinson's disease.
Apokyn (apomorphine hydrochloride)	Approved for the treatment of acute, intermittent hypomobility episodes associated with advanced Parkinson's disease.
Ibuprofen	Users of ibuprofen are less likely to develop Parkinson's disease than nonusers.
Levodopa/carbidopa Sinemet, Sinemet CR, Atamet, Madopar	Nausea, vomiting, weakness, hallucinations, mental confusion, orthostatic hypotension, fatigue, sudden daytime sleep onset, insomnia, elevated serum glucose and homocysteine, and anemia. Large neutral amino acids block levodopa absorption, both from the gut and at the blood–brain barrier. Levodopa preparations should be taken 30–60 minutes prior to meals; intake of vitamin B_6 should be limited to DRI levels. Up to 15 mg of vitamin B_6 can be taken daily in either food or supplement form. Today's preparations combine levodopa with carbidopa. Increase intake of foods rich in vitamin B_{12}, folate, and vitamin C.
MAO type B inhibitors Eldepryl (selegiline), Azilect (rasagiline)	Insomnia, dry mouth, confusion, hypertension, abdominal pain, and weight loss. Selegiline should not be used with ginseng, ma huang (ephedra), yohimbe, or St. John's wort. A low tyramine diet should be used with rasagiline.

- Help patient to control weight, which may fluctuate from either reduced mobility or the inability to ingest sufficient quantities.
- Place all foods within easy reach of the patient. Braces may help the patient control severe tremors at mealtime.
- Music therapy, Tai Chi, and yoga help to relieve depression and improve balance.
- Discuss how to resolve issues such as weight loss, constipation, osteopenia, gastroesophageal reflux disease (GERD), side effects of medications, xerostomia, and dehydration.
- Deep brain stimulation of the subthalamic nucleus shows promise. Medtronic has two new devices that can be used with PD patients to help control tremors: Activa RC and Activa PC.
- Maintain bone mineral density, as hip fractures are common. BMD is related to leg muscle strength (Pang and Mak, 2009).

Patient Education—Foodborne Illness

- Careful food handling will be important. The same is true for sanitizing work area before and after preparing tube feedings to prevent contamination. Formula companies have good information on safe handling of formula in the home and institution.

For More Information

- American Parkinson's Disease Association
  http://www.apdaparkinson.org/
- Michael J. Fox Foundation for Parkinson's Research
  http://www.MichaelJFox.org/
- National Parkinson's Foundation
  http://www.parkinson.org/
- Nutrition for Parkinson's
  http://www.nutritionucanlivewith.com/index.html
- Parkinson's Disease Foundation, Inc.
  http://www.pdf.org/
  http://www.pdf.org/pdf/FactSheet_Nutrition.pdf
- Parkinson's Genetic Research Group
  http://depts.washington.edu/pgrgroup/
- Society for Neuroscience
  http://web.sfn.org/
- We Move
  http://www.wemove.org/par/
- Young Parkinson's
  http://www.youngparkinsons.org/pages/index/siteindex.htm

PARKINSON'S DISEASE—CITED REFERENCES

Adihetty P, Beal MF. Creatine and its potential therapeutic value for targeting cellular energy impairment in neurodegenerative diseases. *Neuromolecular Med.* 10:275, 2008.

Andres RH, et al. Functions and effects of creatine in the central nervous system. *Brain Res Bull.* 76:329, 2008.

Ascherio A, et al. Pesticide exposure and risk for Parkinson's disease. *Ann Neurol.* 60:197, 2006.

Biselli PM, et al. Effect of folate, vitamin B6, and vitamin B12 intake and MTHFR C677 T polymorphism on homocysteine concentrations of renal transplant recipients. *Transplant Proc.* 39:3163, 2007.

Caccamo D, et al. Effect of MTHFR polymorphisms on hyperhomocysteinemia in levodopa-treated Parkinsonian patients. *Neuromolecular Med.* 9:249, 2007.

Camicioli RM, et al. Homocysteine is not associated with global motor or cognitive measures in nondemented older Parkinson's disease patients. *Mov Disorders.* 24:176, 2009.

Carne W, et al. Efficacy of a multidisciplinary treatment program on one-year outcomes of individuals with Parkinson's disease. *Neurorehabilitation.* 20:161, 2005.

Chen H, et al. Folate intake and risk of Parkinson's disease. *Am J Epidemiol.* 160:368, 2004.

de Lau LM, et al. Dietary fatty acids and the risk of Parkinson disease: the Rotterdam study. *Neurology.* 64:2040, 2005.

Etminan M, et al. Intake of vitamin E, vitamin C, and carotenoids and the risk of Parkinson's disease: a meta-analysis. *Lancet Neurol.* 4:362, 2005.

Evatt ML, et al. Prevalence of vitamin D insufficiency in patients with Parkinson disease and Alzheimer disease. *Arch Neurol.* 65:1348, 2008.

Fitsanakis VA, et al. The use of magnetic resonance imaging (MRI) in the study of manganese neurotoxicity. *Neurotoxicology.* 27:798, 2006.

Gao X, et al. Genetic determinants of hair color and Parkinson's disease risk. *Ann Neurol.* 65:76, 2009.

Grimble RF. The effects of sulfur amino acid intake on immune function in humans. *J Nutr.* 136:1660S, 2006.

Han J, et al. Melanocortin 1 receptor variants and skin cancer risk. *Int J Cancer.* 119:1976, 2006.

Klein AM, Ferrante RJ. The neuroprotective role of creatine. *Subcell Biochem.* 46:205, 2007.

Mosharov EV, et al. Interplay between cytosolic dopamine, calcium, and alpha-synuclein causes selective death of substantia nigra neurons. *Neuron.* 62:218, 2009.

Olanow CW, et al. The scientific and clinical basis for the treatment of Parkinson disease (2009). *Neurology.* 72:1S, 2009.

Pang MY, Mak MK. Muscle strength is significantly associated with hip bone mineral density in women with Parkinson's disease: a cross-sectional study. *J Rehabil Med.* 41:223, 2009.

Poewe W. Treatments for Parkinson disease–past achievements and current clinical needs. *Neurology.* 72:65S, 2009.

Ueki A, Otsuka M. Life style risks of Parkinson's disease: association between decreased water intake and constipation. *J Neurol.* 251:II18, 2004.

SPINAL CORD INJURY

NUTRITIONAL ACUITY RANKING: LEVEL 3

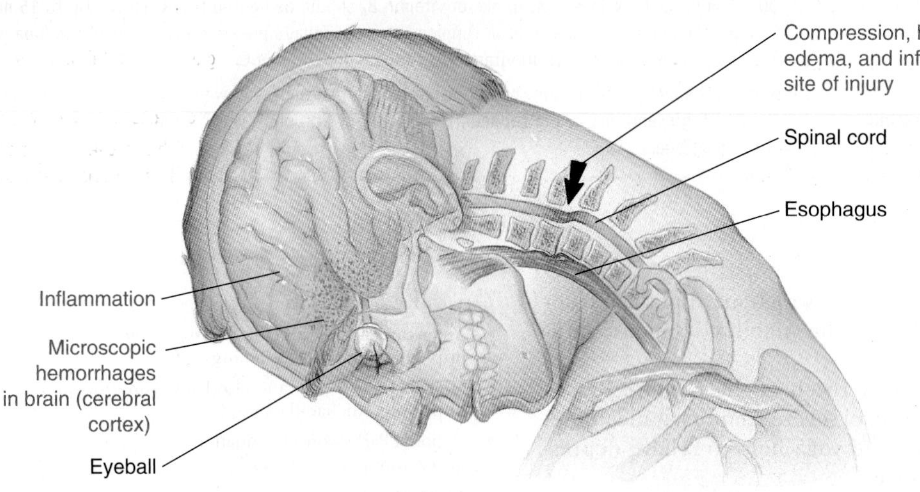

Asset provided by Anatomical Chart Co.

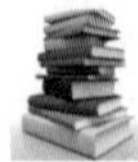

DEFINITIONS AND BACKGROUND

Spinal cord injury (SCI) is often caused by traffic accidents, falls, diving accidents, sports injury, or gunshot wounds. Partial versus total self-care deficits depend on resulting paralysis or loss of sensation below the site of the injury. Classification usually includes the cause, direction of injury, level of injury, stability of vertebral column, and degree of cord involvement. See Table 4-12.

Most injury causes permanent disability or loss of movement (paralysis) and sensation below the site of the injury. Paralysis that involves the majority of the body, including the arms and legs, is called quadriplegia or tetraplegia because of injuries to one of the eight cervical segments of the spinal cord. Those with paraplegia have lesions in the thoracic, lumbar, or sacral regions of the spinal cord.

The nervous system of a patient with neurological trauma is vulnerable to variations in oxygen, glucose, and other nutrients. Indirect calorimetry is the best method for identifying energy requirements (Shepherd, 2009). Pressure ulcers are very common in this population; see Section 2.

SCI patients with a BMI of $>$22 should be considered at risk for obesity (Laughton et al, 2009). After long-term immobility, SCI patients may require weight loss, using varied psychosocial, behavioral, and dietary interventions (Chen et al, 2006).

Treatment using fetal stem cells has profound implications for recovery in the SCI population. More research is forthcoming.

TABLE 4-12 Expected Functional Level of Spinal Cord Disruption

Quadriplegia	Paraplegia
C1-C3 Vagus domination of heart, respiration, blood vessels, all organs below injury. Movement in neck and above, loss of innervation to diaphragm, absence of independent respiratory function. Ability to drive power wheelchair equipped with portable respirator by using chin control or sip and puff, lack of bowel and bladder control.	**T1–T6** Sympathetic innervation to heart, vagus domination of the rest. Full innervation of upper extremities, back, essential intrinsic muscles of hands; full strength and dexterity of grasp; decreased trunk stability; decreased respiratory reserve. Full independence in self-care and in a wheelchair, ability to drive a car with hand controls (in most clients), ability to use full body brace for exercise but not for functional ambulation, lack of bowel and bladder control.
C4 Vagus domination of heart, respiration, and all vessels and organs below injury. Sensation and movement above neck. Ability to drive power chair using chin control or sip and puff, lack of bowel and bladder control.	**T6–T12** Vagus domination only of leg vessels, gastrointestinal, and genitourinary organs. Full, stable thoracic muscles and upper back; functional intercostals, resulting in increased respiratory reserve. Full independent use of wheelchair; ability to stand erect with full body brace, ambulate on crutches with swing (though gait is difficult); inability to climb stairs; lack of bowel and bladder control.
C5 Vagus domination of heart, respiration, and all vessels and organs below injury. Full neck, partial shoulder, back, biceps; gross elbow, inability to roll over or use hands; decreased respiratory reserve. Ability to drive power chair with mobile hand supports, ability to use hand splints (in some clients), lack of bowel and bladder control.	**L1–L2** Vagus domination of leg muscles. Varying control of legs and pelvis, instability of lower back. Good sitting balance, full use of wheelchair.
C6 Vagus domination of heart, respiration, and all vessels and organs below injury. Shoulder and upper back abduction and rotation at shoulder, full biceps to elbow flexion, wrist extension, weak grasp of thumb, decreased respiratory reserve. Ability to assist with transfer and perform some self-care, feed self with hand devices, push a wheelchair on smooth, flat surface; lack of bowel and bladder control.	**L3–L4** Partial domination of leg vessels, gastrointestinal, and genitourinary organs. Quadriceps and hip flexors, absence of hamstring function, flail ankles. Completely independent ambulation with short leg braces and canes, inability to stand for long periods, bladder and bowel continence.
C7 Vagus domination of heart, respiration, and all vessels and organs below injury. All triceps to elbow extension, finger extensors and flexors, good grasp with some decreased strength, decreased respiratory reserve. Ability to transfer self to a wheelchair, roll over and sit up in bed, push self on most surfaces, perform most self-care; independent use of wheelchair; ability to drive a car with hand controls (in some clients); lack of bowel and bladder control.	

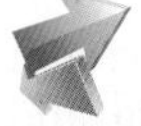

ASSESSMENT, MONITORING, AND EVALUATION

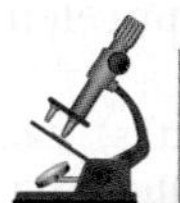

CLINICAL INDICATORS

Genetic Markers: A SCI is not usually genetic.

Clinical/History
- Height
- Weight
- BMI
- Indirect calorimetry (rest 30 minutes prior)
- Dietary/intake history
- I & O
- BP (tends to be elevated)
- Cervical x-rays
- Somatosensory-evoked potentials
- Myelogram
- MRI or CT scan
- DEXA
- Triceps skinfold
- Mid-arm circumference
- Pulmonary edema
- Pneumonia

Lab Work
- H & H (decreased)
- Serum Fe
- Alb
- Serial transthyretin levels
- Na^+, K^+
- Creat (eventually decreased)
- BUN
- Gluc
- pCO_2, pO_2
- RQ (if over 1.0, evaluate for overfeeding)
- PT or INR
- Ca^{++}, Mg^{++}
- Hypercalciuria
- Parathormone (may be low)
- 25-hydroxyvitamin D_3
- N balance
- Erythrocyte sedimentation rate (ESR)
- CRP (elevated)
- Serum B_{12}

SAMPLE NUTRITION CARE PROCESS STEPS

Inadequate Protein Intake

Assessment Data: SCI 6 months ago; poor intake of protein foods.

Nutrition Diagnoses (PES): Inadequate protein related to poor intake of protein-rich foods as evidenced by dietary recall and early skin breakdown.

Interventions: Change diet order to provide protein-enhanced foods that are nutrient dense. Educate patient about rationale for the protein to protect the skin integrity.

Monitoring and Evaluation: Improved protein intake; better quality of life by increased ability to participate in physical and occupational therapies.

INTERVENTION

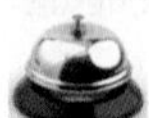

OBJECTIVES

Immediate

- Monitor for acid–base and electrolyte imbalances. Assess needs on admission and then daily thereafter.
- Maintain blood glucose at or below 140 mg/dL in critical phase (ADA, 2009). If on a ventilator, keep blood glucose levels between 80 and 110 mg/dL.
- Reduce the danger of aspiration by avoiding oral feedings in supine patients. Initiate tube feeding within 24–48 hours after admission to intensive care (Shepherd, 2009). Early EN is desirable because of the demands of the brain and nerves.
- If needed, use parenteral nutrition if there is intolerance of EN, such as high gastric residuals or aspiration.
- Ensure adequate fluid and calcium intake to prevent renal stones.
- Slow down weight loss and any progressive muscle wasting by maintaining protein and energy sufficiency.
- Increase opportunities for rehabilitation by monitoring weight changes; loss of 10–30% in the first month is common.
- Prevent UTIs, paralytic ileus, pneumonia, malnutrition, pressure ulcer, constipation, stress ulcer, and fecal impaction. Note that elevated CRP is associated with UTIs or pressure ulcers within a year (Gibson et al, 2008; Morse et al, 2008).

Long Term

- Mobilize, prevent complications, and regain as much independence as possible. Participate in muscle vibration stimulation and other therapies whenever possible.
- Monitor weight gain since excessive weight gain can lead to pressure ulcers and make patient transfers more difficult. Maintain an ideal body weight with a BMI of 18–22 (Laughton et al, 2009).
- Promote neuronal growth and survival, encourage the formation of synapses, enhance the production of myelin, and restore conduction capabilities and thus restore the compromised circuitry in the injured spinal cord.
- Prevent osteoporosis and risk of fractures.
- Manage long-term problems with bowel motility with fiber, fluid and laxatives (Shepherd, 2009).
- Prevent heart disease. While women with paraplegia tend to maintain healthier diets (i.e., lower calorie and fat intakes, more nutrient density, less overweight,) individuals with tetraplegia tend to be overweight or obese (Groah et al, 2009).

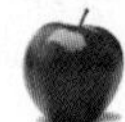

FOOD AND NUTRITION

- Provide patient with intravenous solutions as soon as possible after injury. Check blood gas measurements and chemistries. Once peristalsis returns, patient may be tube fed. Elevate head of bed 45°, if possible, to prevent aspiration (ADA, 2009).
- Determine energy needs by indirect calorimetry. Patients with paraplegia need 28 kcal/kg/d and those with quadriplegia need 23 kcal/kg/d (Shepherd, 2009).
- Paraplegics initially need 1.5–1.7 g protein/kg. Progress to more normal intake, such as 0.8 g/kg, when nitrogen balance returns after several weeks. Patients with large pressure ulcers will need an increase in protein back to 1.5 g/kg.
- Ensure adequate CHO and fat intake, including at least 1–2% EFAs.
- Encourage adequate fluid (1 mL/kcal/d); use more with fever or pressure ulcers.
- Include adequate fiber (15 g/d). Be careful with gas-forming foods; monitor tolerance.
- Ensure adequate intake of thiamin, niacin, vitamins B_6, B_{12}, and C, and amino acids. Monitor iron stores and adjust diet as needed.
- Provide adequate vitamin D_3 and calcium intake.
- With hypertension, the DASH diet may be useful (increases in calcium, potassium, and magnesium are beneficial).
- Increase intake of antioxidant-rich foods and omega-3 fatty acids (DHA) for neuroprotection (King et al, 2006).
- Tube feeding should be used over parenteral nutrition where possible (ADA, 2009). An immune-enhancing formula may be recommended but is not always essential. Do not recommend use of blue dye to detect aspiration (ADA, 2009).

Common Drugs Used and Potential Side Effects

- Corticosteroids such as prednisone are used to prevent swelling. Long-term use can cause hyperglycemia and nitrogen, calcium, and potassium losses. Sodium retention occurs.
- Analgesics for pain relief (e.g., aspirin/salicylates) can prolong bleeding time. GI bleeding may eventually result.
- Laxatives may be used; encourage fiber and fluid instead.
- For a bowel regimen, use of erythromycin, metoclopramide, a stool softener and a stimulant laxative may be prescribed (Shepherd, 2009). There are no contraindications to the use of promotility agents (ADA, 2009).
- Anabolic steroids (oxandrolone) help alleviate anorexia and may be helpful in managing pressure ulcers.
- To protect against fractures, bisphosphonates may help prevent acute bone loss; use IV rather than oral route to reduce reflux.

Herbs, Botanicals, and Supplements

- Studies have found usefulness in pretreatment of patients with creatine for neuroprotection before spinal surgery.

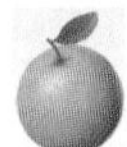

NUTRITION EDUCATION, COUNSELING, CARE MANAGEMENT

- Help promote a structured feeding routine. Feed slowly (over 30–45 minutes) using small bites of food.
- The majority of people with SCI would benefit from nutritional counseling to prevent emerging secondary conditions (Groah et al, 2009; Tomey et al, 2005).
- Provide weight control measures for successful rehabilitation (Chen et al, 2006).
- Teach patient about good sources of iron and other minerals, vitamins, and protein.
- Discuss long-term risks of heart disease.
- Encourage participation in weight-bearing exercise to reduce calcium loss and risk of fracture or osteoporosis.

Patient Education—Foodborne Illness

- Careful food handling will be important. The same is true for sanitizing work area before and after preparing tube feedings to prevent contamination. Formula companies have good information on safe handling of formula in the home and institution.

For More Information

- American Spinal Injury Association (ASIA)
  http://www.asia-spinalinjury.org/
- Children and Spinal Cord Injury
  http://www.childrenshospital.org/az/Site1150/mainpageS1150P0.html
- Christopher and Dana Reeve Paralysis Foundation
  http://www.christopherreeve.org/
- Cure Paralysis Now
  http://www.cureparalysisnow.org/
- Dermatome Chart
  http://www.asia-spinalinjury.org/publications/2006_Classif_worksheet.pdf
- Foundation for Spinal Cord Injury Prevention, Care, & Cure
  http://www.fscip.org/
- International Spinal Cord Society
  http://www.iscos.org.uk/
- Model Spinal Cord Injury System Dissemination Center
  http://www.mscisdisseminationcenter.org/
- National Spinal Cord Injury Association
  http://www.spinalcord.org/
- NIH—Medline
  http://www.nlm.nih.gov/medlineplus/spinalcordinjuries.html
- NINDS Spinal Cord Injury
  http://www.ninds.nih.gov/disorders/sci/sci.htm
- Paralyzed Veterans of America
  http://www.pva.org
- Spinal Cord Centers
  http://www.sci-recovery.org/sci-centers.htm
- Spinal Cord Injury Information Network
  http://www.spinalcord.uab.edu/
- Spinal Cord Recovery
  http://www.sci-recovery.org/

SPINAL CORD INJURY—CITED REFERENCES

ADA. Evidence analysis library. Accessed May 31, 2009, at http://www.adaevidencelibrary.com/topic.cfm?cat=3016.

Chen Y, et al. Obesity intervention in persons with spinal cord injury. *Spinal Cord.* 44:82, 2006.

Gibson AE, et al. C-Reactive protein in adults with chronic spinal cord injury: increased chronic inflammation in tetraplegia vs paraplegia. *Spinal Cord.* 46:616, 2008.

Groah SL, et al. Nutrient intake and body habitus after spinal cord injury: an analysis by sex and level of injury. *J Spinal Cord Med.* 32:25, 2009.

King VR, et al. Omega-3 fatty acids improve recovery, whereas omega-6 fatty acids worsen outcome, after spinal cord injury in the adult rat. *J Neurosci.* 26:4672, 2006.

Laughton GE, et al. Lowering body mass index cutoffs better identifies obese persons with spinal cord injury. [published online ahead of print April 9, 2009] *Spinal Cord.* 47:757, 2009.

Morse LR, et al. Association between mobility mode and C-reactive protein levels in men with chronic spinal cord injury. *Arch Phys Med Rehabil.* 89:726, 2008.

Shepherd E. Nutrition care for the spinal cord injured patient. *Support Line.* 30(6):25, 2009.

Tomey KM, et al. Dietary intake and nutritional status of urban community-dwelling men with paraplegia. *Arch Phys Med Rehabil.* 86:664, 2005.

STROKE (CEREBROVASCULAR ACCIDENT)

NUTRITIONAL ACUITY RANKING: LEVEL 3

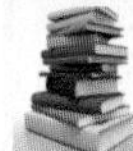

DEFINITIONS AND BACKGROUND

A cerebrovascular accident (CVA) (stroke) is caused by damage to a portion of the brain resulting from loss of blood supply due to a blood vessel spasm, clot, or rupture. Sporadic strokes can occur, but most have a genetic, polygenic component. Eighty percent of strokes are ischemic. Transient ischemic attacks (TIAs) are brief episodes of blood loss to the brain from a clot or an embolism; 10% of victims will have a major CVA within a year. Stroke patients need to be seen medically within 60 minutes to begin appropriate treatment. Some people recover completely; others may be seriously disabled or die. The urgent presenting symptoms are listed in Table 4-13.

Hypertension, smoking, diabetes mellitus, atrial fibrillation, and oral contraceptive use are key risk factors for strokes. Unconsciousness, paralysis, and other problems may occur depending on the site and extent of the brain damage. Left CVA affects sight and hearing most commonly, including the ability to see where foods are placed on a plate or tray. Patients with a right-hemisphere, bilateral, or brainstem CVA have significant problems with feeding and swallowing of food; speech problems also occur.

TABLE 4-13 Most Common Stroke Symptoms

- Sudden numbness or weakness of face, arm, or leg, especially on one side of the body
- Sudden confusion, trouble speaking or understanding
- Sudden trouble seeing in one or both eyes
- Sudden trouble walking, dizziness, loss of balance or coordination
- Sudden severe headache with no known cause

Neurogenic deficits may include motor deficits with muscle weakness of the tongue and lips; nerve damage with resulting lack of coordination; apraxia; sensory deficits with an inability to feel food in the mouth. Cognitive deficits include difficulty sustaining attention, poor short-term memory, visual field problems, impulsiveness, aphasia, and judgment problems such as not knowing how much food to take or what to do with the food once it reaches the mouth. Strokes cause 10% of all fatalities in the United States.

A dietary pattern with high intakes of red and processed meats, refined grains, sweets and desserts may increase stroke risk, whereas a diet higher in fruits and vegetables, fish, and whole grains may protect against stroke. Intake of cruciferous and green leafy vegetables, citrus fruits, and carotenoids seem to be protective. Among elderly individuals, consumption of tuna or other broiled or baked fish is associated with lower risk of ischemic stroke, while intake of fried fish is associated with higher risk (Mozaffarian et al, 2005). Both fish and omega-3 fatty acids seem to prevent thrombotic strokes.

Individualized dietary advice to those with coronary heart disease can reduce stroke mortality and morbidity, yet this is often overlooked by physicians (Spence, 2006). Risk reduction from controlled trials with supplemental vitamins C or E has not been consistent. Vitamin E influences the activity of enzymes PKC, PP2 A, COX-2, 5-lipooxygenase, nitric oxide synthase, NADPH-oxidase, superoxide dismutase, and phospholipase A2 and modulates gene expression. Vitamin C levels tend to be lower among stroke patients, probably due to the relationship to inflammation and oxidative stress.

Lowering elevated serum tHcy is also important. For example, homocystinuria is a metabolic disorder that is a known life-threatening risk factor for ischemic stroke. Folate deficiency and hyperhomocysteinemia increase oxidative DNA damage and ischemic lesion size in stroke patients (Endres et al, 2005). Intake of folate, vitamins B_6 and B_{12} should be maintained in high-risk groups.

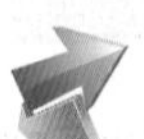

ASSESSMENT, MONITORING, AND EVALUATION

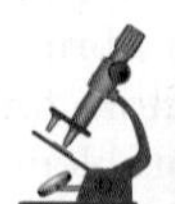

CLINICAL INDICATORS

Genetic Markers: Pro-inflammatory gene polymorphisms are related to both coronary heart disease and stroke. Alterations in the 9p21 chromosome relate to atherosclerotic stroke (Gschwendtner et al, 2009), whereas MTHFR C677 T, beta-Fg—455 A/G, beta-Fg—48 T/C, PAI-1 4G/5G, and ApoE epsilon2–4 are associated with ischemic stroke (Xu et al, 2008).

Clinical/History

Height
Weight
BMI
Waist to hip ratio
Dietary/intake history
Positron emission tomography (PET) scan
Sleep apnea
Chewing ability
Hand to mouth coordination
Gag reflex absent?
BP
Temperature
Visual field scan
EEG
Carotid ultrasound
CT scan or MRI
I & O

Lab Work

CRP
PT
INR: 2.0–4.0 desirable
Na^+, K^+
Ca^{++}, Mg^{++}
Chol (total, HDL, LDL)
Trig
tHcy
Serum folate
Ferritin
H & H
Gluc (often increased)
Creatine phosphokinase (CPK)
Serum uric acid

SAMPLE NUTRITION CARE PROCESS STEPS

Imbalance of Nutrients

Assessment Data: Food records indicating high sodium intake and limited use of fruits and vegetables for calcium, magnesium, and potassium.

Nutrition Diagnoses (PES): Imbalance of nutrients related to dietary intake of mostly processed, high sodium foods and few fruits, vegetables, or dairy as evidenced by diet history.

Interventions: Education about use of the DASH diet (enhanced fruits, vegetables, low fat dairy) and whole grains.

Monitoring and Evaluation: Improved BP; no more TIAs or strokes; improved balance between sodium and other minerals (calcium, potassium, magnesium).

Difficulty Swallowing

Assessment Data: Results of swallow study and x-rays, food diary, and problems noted with specific types of liquids/foods; swallow studies and conferences with speech therapist; patient is also aphasic.

Nutrition Diagnoses (PES): Swallowing difficulty related to consumption of general diet after CVA as evidenced by coughing after intake of thin liquids.

Intervention: Alter diet to thicken liquids with all meals, snacks, medication passes, special events, dining out. Provide recipes for use of thickened liquids in daily meals.

Monitoring and Evaluation: Reduced incidence of coughing after drinking beverages; no hospital admissions for pneumonia. Able to communicate in spite of aphasia using head nod and eyes to communicate preferences and choices.

INTERVENTION

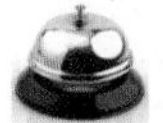

OBJECTIVES

- **Immediate treatment:** Maintain fluid-electrolyte balance for lifesaving measures.
- **Ongoing treatment:** Improve residual effects such as dysphagia, hemiplegia, and aphasia. Correct side effects such as, constipation, UTIs, pneumonia, renal calculi, and pressure ulcers.
- If the patient is excessively overweight, weight reduction is necessary to lower elevated BP or lipids and to lessen the workload of the cardiovascular system.
- Chewing should be minimized with dysphagia; prevent choking. Avoid use of straws if there is dysphagia.
- Lower elevated serum lipids; try to improve HDL cholesterol levels.
- Promote self-help, self-esteem, and independence.
- Prevent additional strokes, which are common. See Table 4-14. Since inflammation may be caused by a response to oxidized low-density lipoproteins, chronic infection, or other factors, monitor CRP.

TABLE 4-14 Strategies Used to Prevent Strokes

GOAL: Lower or Less	Blood pressure at 120/80 or below. Smoking; quitting is best. Limit sodium from salt shaker, processed meats, pickles, and olives. Maintain serum cholesterol levels of 200 or lower; LDL of 100 or lower; triglycerides of 150 or less Energy intake: avoid obesity.
GOAL: Higher or More	Exercise moderately each day for at least 30–60 minutes. Brisk walking (about 3 mph) is most protective; but any walking is good. High-dose statin, low to standard doses of antihypertensive therapy, aspirin, cardiac rehabilitation (Robinson and Maheshwari, 2005). Eat a balanced diet including fruits, vegetables, whole grains, low fat dairy products for more potassium, vitamin C, calcium, magnesium. Include omega-3 fatty acids in foods regularly (fatty fish, flaxseed, and walnuts). May use omega-3 fish oil. Include natural sources of fatty acids and vitamin E, such as mayonnaise, creamy salad dressings, margarine, and nuts. Vitamin K may curtail vascular calcification; 500 μg may be needed. Take a multivitamin–mineral supplement daily, especially for folic acid, vitamins B_6, and B_{12}, to reduce homocysteine levels and to help lower blood pressure. Achieve and maintain body weight within BMI range for height. Maintain or elevate HDL to >60. Drink alcoholic beverages in moderation only (one drink for women, two for men per day). Alcohol boosts HDL and may reduce clot formation.

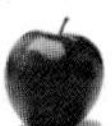

FOOD AND NUTRITION

- **Initial treatment:** Nothing by mouth (NPO) with intravenous fluids for 24–48 hours. Avoid overhydration. Tube feeding may be needed, especially gastrostomy or jejunostomy. If the patient is comatose, tube feeding definitely is required, and the head of the bed should be elevated at least 30°–45° during feeding to prevent aspiration.
- **Recovery:** Treatment should progress from NPO to liquids. Sip feeding may improve nutrient intake and nutritional status of stroke patients who do not have swallowing difficulties with liquids.
- Provide adequate energy intake (patient's weight should be checked frequently). Monitor the patient's activity levels. From 25–45 kcal/kg and 1.2–1.5 g protein/kg may be needed, depending on weight status and loss of lean body mass.
- Texture modification to compensate for dysphagia should be made to reduce risk of choking and/or aspiration. Thick pureed liquids or a mechanical soft diet may be needed. Liquids can be thickened with gels.
- Always start with small amounts of food. Use easy-to-chew foods and spoon rather than fork foods. Progress slowly.
- With dysphagia, avoid foods that cause choking or that are hard to manage (e.g., tart juices and foods, dry or crisp foods, fibrous meats, unboned fish, chewy or stringy meats, sticky peanut butter or bananas, thinly pureed foods that are easily aspirated, mixed foods with varying consistency, excessively sweet drinks or tart fruits that aggravate drooling, raw vegetables). Mashed potatoes or soft breads for some patients may be hard to swallow.
- With decreased salivation, moisten foods with small amounts of liquid. Use thickener products to make semisolids out of soup, beverages, juices, and shakes. Test swallowing periodically. When ready, use of a syringe or training cup is beneficial.
- The amount of saturated and trans fatty acids in the planned diet should be <10% of total calories, and the dietary cholesterol intake should be <300 mg/d. A useful recommendation is to reduce the quantity of fat by 20–25%, reduce animal fats, and decrease the amount of salt added to foods in cooking and at the table.
- Replace saturated fat with monounsaturated sources; use more olive, soybean or canola oils and nuts such as walnuts, almonds, macadamias, pecans, and pistachios. Walnuts contain alpha linolenic acid; almonds are a good source of vitamin E. Nuts also contain flavonoids, phenols, sterols, saponins, elegiac acid, folic acid, magnesium, copper, potassium, and fiber. The Mediterranean diet is a useful diet to follow; in this diet, unsaturated fats replace most of the saturated fat, and fruits and vegetables are highlighted (Spence, 2006).
- Use plant sterols and stanols, as from margarines and related products.
- Increase omega-3 fatty acids from fish.
- Use skim milk products whenever possible. Milk fat is negatively correlated with certain cardiovascular disease risk factors.
- Increase potassium to reduce risk of additional strokes. Avoid use of potassium-sparing diuretics or with end-stage

renal disease. Fruits and vegetables are the best sources (oranges, bananas, prunes, baked potatoes); milk is another good source. Magnesium, vitamin E, folic acid, and vitamins B_{12} and B_6 should be included in sufficient quantities to meet at least minimum daily requirements. Use the DASH diet plan (see Section 6).

- Fluid should be given in sufficient quantity if tolerated; estimate needs at 30 mL/kg and increase to 35 mL/kg if dehydration occurs. Give oral beverages at the end of the meal to increase solid food intake in patients who have early satiety or fatigue with meals.
- The diet should provide adequate fiber from prune juice, bran, whole grain breads and cereals, oatmeal, bran, wheat germ, popcorn, brown rice.
- Use caution with supplemental vitamin C; excesses may act as a pro-oxidant.
- Flavonoids such as grape juice, green tea, and red wine are useful if the patient can tolerate thin liquids.

Common Drugs Used and Potential Side Effects

- Angiotensin-converting enzyme inhibitors/angiotensin receptor blockers may cause diarrhea or GI distress. Atacand, Teveten, Avapro, Cozaar, Benicar, Micardis, or Diovan should be used with a low sodium, low calorie diet. They may cause anemia or hyperkalemia. Be careful with salt substitutes; read contents carefully.
- Anticoagulants used to prevent thromboembolism, such as warfarin (Coumadin), require a controlled amount of vitamin K. Monitor tube feeding products and supplements. Many patients who are taking warfarin can safely monitor their INR levels at home and adjust their medications accordingly. Monitor supplements containing vitamins A, C, and E with these drugs because of potential side effects. Avoid taking with dong quai, fenugreek, feverfew, excessive garlic, ginger, gingko, and ginseng.
- Aspirin is often used to prevent future strokes as a blood thinner (generally 1 tablet per day). Monitor for GI bleeding or occult blood loss. Aspirin is safer than warfarin and just as effective for treating blocked arteries in the brain (Koroshetz, 2005).
- Grapefruit juice decreases drug metabolism in the gut (via P450-CYP3A4 inhibition) and can affect medications up to 24 hours later. Avoid taking with alprazolam, buspirone, cisapride, cyclosporine, statins, tacrolimus, and many others.
- Products containing phenylpropanolamine (PPA) are a risk for stroke. PPA has been pulled from the shelves but may still be in some cough medicines in the home.
- Statins (Lipitor, Lescol, Mevacor, Pravachol, Crestor, and Zocor) are commonly prescribed. Nausea, abdominal pain, and other GI effects are common. Do not take with grapefruit juice or St. John's wort. Monitor liver enzymes.
- Stool softeners may be used. Tube feeding containing a mix of soluble and insoluble fiber can be used. If a low-residue formula is used, a fiber supplement such as Benefiber can be mixed with water and administered via Y-port.
- Thiazide diuretics, such as Lasix, may be used and can deplete potassium.

Herbs, Botanicals, and Supplements

- The patient should not take herbals and botanicals without discussing with the physician.
- Coenzyme Q10 should not be used with gemfibrozil, TCAs, or warfarin. Coenzyme Q10 may act similarly to vitamin K.
- Niacin (nicotinic acid) should not be taken with statins, antidiabetic medications, and carbamazepine because of potentially serious risks of myopathy and altered glucose control.
- Large doses of vitamin E should not be taken with warfarin because of possible increased bleeding. Avoid doses greater than 400 IU/d.
- Garlic, willow, pigweed, gingko, or evening primrose have been recommended; no clinical trials have proven efficacy.

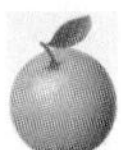

NUTRITION EDUCATION, COUNSELING, CARE MANAGEMENT

- Help the patient simplify meal preparation. Arrange food and utensils within reach. Discuss the use of appropriate assistive devices.
- Explain which sources of adequate nutrition do not aggravate the patient's condition. Discuss fat, cholesterol; sodium, potassium, calcium, magnesium, specific vitamins, and other nutrients in the DASH diet. Correlate with drug therapy.
- Help the patient make mealtime safe and pleasant. Encourage small bites of food and slow, adequate chewing.
- Discuss ways to prevent future strokes; linolenic acid from walnut, canola, and soybean oils may be protective. Increased fruit and vegetable intake is also protective.
- Physical therapy is very important in early stages after a stroke, especially to regain use of limbs such as hands and arms.
- Manage depression, which is common after a stroke. Treatments may include patient and family counseling and education, reestablishment of sleep pattern, improving diet, regular physical activity, or medication.
- Future prevention strategies should be taught to stroke patients and their families. Modifiable risk factors include hypertension, exposure to cigarette smoke, diabetes, atrial fibrillation and certain other cardiac conditions, dyslipidemia, carotid artery stenosis, sickle cell disease, postmenopausal hormone therapy, poor diet, physical inactivity, and obesity and body fat distribution (Goldstein et al, 2006). Potentially modifiable risk factors include the metabolic syndrome, alcohol use, oral contraceptive use, migraine headache, hyperhomocysteinemia, inflammation (Goldstein et al, 2006).
- The American Heart Association, American Cancer Society, and American Diabetes Association agree that lifestyle changes are essential for prevention of stroke and associated disability.

Patient Education—Foodborne Illness

- Careful food handling will be important. If tube feeding is needed, discuss proper sanitation of work counters during preparation.

- Hand washing is important, especially for caregivers if the patient is unable to feed himself or herself.

For More Information

- American Academy of Physical Medicine and Rehabilitation http://www.aapmr.org/
- American Stroke Association http://www.strokeassociation.org/
- National Aphasia Association http://www.aphasia.org
- National Institute of Neurological Disorders and Stroke http://www.ninds.nih.gov/
- National Rehabilitation Awareness Foundation http://www.nraf-rehabnet.org/
- National Rehabilitation Hospital http://www.nrhrehab.org/
- National Stroke Association http://www.stroke.org/
- North Carolina Stroke Association http://www.ncstroke.org/
- UCLA Stroke Center http://www.stroke.ucla.edu/

STROKE—CITED REFERENCES

Endres M, et al. Folate deficiency increases postischemic brain injury. *Stroke.* 36:321, 2005.

Goldstein LB, et al. Primary prevention of ischemic stroke: a guideline from the American Heart Association/American Stroke Association Stroke Council: cosponsored by the Atherosclerotic Peripheral Vascular Disease Interdisciplinary Working Group; Cardiovascular Nursing Council; Clinical Cardiology Council; Nutrition, Physical Activity, and Metabolism Council; and the Quality of Care and Outcomes Research Interdisciplinary Working Group. *Circulation.* 113:e873, 2006.

Gschwendtner A, et al. Sequence variants on chromosome 9p21.3 confer risk for atherosclerotic stroke. *Ann Neurol.* 65:531, 2009.

Koroshetz W. Warfarin, aspirin, and intracranial vascular disease. *N Engl J Med.* 352:1368, 2005.

Mozaffarian D, et al. Fish consumption and stroke risk in elderly individuals: the cardiovascular health study. *Arch Intern Med.* 165:200, 2005.

Robinson JG, Maheshwari N. A "poly-portfolio" for secondary prevention: a strategy to reduce subsequent events by up to 97% over five years. *Am J Cardiol.* 95:373, 2005.

Spence JD. Nutrition and stroke prevention. *Stroke.* 37:2430, 2006.

Xu X, et al. Meta-analysis of genetic studies from journals published in China of ischemic stroke in the Han Chinese population. *Cerebrovasc Dis.* 26:48, 2008.

TARDIVE DYSKINESIA

NUTRITIONAL ACUITY RANKING: LEVEL 2

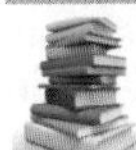

DEFINITIONS AND BACKGROUND

Tardive dyskinesia (TD) is a movement disorder characterized by involuntary oro-facial, limb, and truncal movements (Tsai et al, 2009). It is usually caused by the use of drugs that block dopamine receptors (dopamine receptor antagonists [DRAs]). When used in the classic sense, TD is produced by the long-term use of drugs to treat SCZ that act by blocking dopamine receptors. TD occurs in 20–40% of all patients receiving long-term antipsychotic drugs. Patients are often elderly and chronically institutionalized.

Phenylalanine sensitivity has been speculated as the cause of TD. Amine-depleting agents such as reserpine (Serpalan, Serpasil) and tetrabenazine (Nitoman) deplete dopamine, norepinephrine, and serotonin. Tarvil, a medical food with high branched-chain amino acids, targets excess phenylalanine and has few side effects.

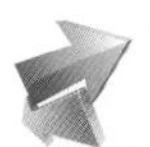

ASSESSMENT, MONITORING, AND EVALUATION

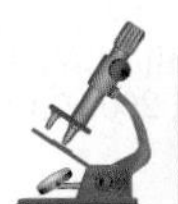

CLINICAL INDICATORS

Genetic Markers: There have been a sizeable number of candidate gene studies. A total of 128 candidate genes were studied in 710 subjects—2580 SNPs in 118 candidate genes selected from the literature (e.g., dopamine, serotonin, glutamate, and GABA pathways) and composite genotypes for 10 drug-metabolizing enzymes. No single marker or haplotype association reached statistical significance after adjustment for multiple comparisons (Tsai et al, 2009).

Clinical/History

Height
Weight
BMI
Dietary/intake history
BP
Chorea, athetosis, dystonia
Tics or facial grimacing
Abnormal Involuntary Movement Scale
Tremors

Lab Work

CRP
BUN, Creat
H & H
Serum Fe
Serum tHcy
Serum folate
Serum prolactin (often increased)
Acetylcholine levels
Gluc
Alb, transthyretin
Ceruloplasmin
Serum Cu
Serum phenylalanine

INTERVENTION

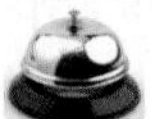

OBJECTIVES

- Prevent or correct malnutrition, weight loss, and other problems.
- Identify and assist with problems, such as puckering of the lips, difficulty sucking and eating.
- Restore capacity for eating orally as far as possible.
- Alter textures as necessary (eating problems are rare or occur late in the condition).

SAMPLE NUTRITION CARE PROCESS STEPS

Self-Feeding Difficulty

Assessment Data: Food intake sporadic because of difficulty feeding self; weight loss.

Nutrition Diagnoses (PES): Self-feeding difficulty related to dyskinesia as evidenced by food intake <75% desirable amount and weight loss of 10 lb in past 3 months and BMI 18.

Interventions: Enhance nutrient intake and offer easy to handle finger foods at frequent intervals. Educate about nutrient density. Counsel about ways to increase energy intake to improve weight.

Monitoring and Evaluation: Improved weight status. Increased ability to eat sufficient amounts of kilocals and nutrient-dense choices using finger foods and frequent meals or snacks.

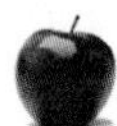

FOOD AND NUTRITION

- Offer the usual diet with soft textures to reduce chewing as needed.
- Decrease energy intake if obese; increase intake if underweight.
- Carbohydrate craving is common. Watch overall intake of sweets or offer nutrient-dense varieties to reduce hyperglycemia.
- Increase dietary choline from foods such as eggs, soybeans, peanuts, and liver.
- Moisten foods with gravy, sauces, and liquids if dry mouth is a problem.
- Alter fiber intake if needed to prevent or correct constipation.
- Ensure adequate intake of antioxidants and omega-3 fatty acids (colorful fruits and vegetables, nuts, fish and seafood).

Common Drugs Used and Potential Side Effects

- Psychiatric conditions are often treated with phenothiazines, butyrophenones, dibenzodiazepines, indolones, diphenylbutylpiperidines, and thioxanthenes. These are more likely to cause TD than the newer antipsychotic agents.
  - Incidence of TD with the use of newer atypical antipsychotic agents such as clozapine (Clozaril), olanzapine (Zyprexa), risperidone (Risperdal), and quetiapine (Seroquel) is minimal (Casey, 2006). Risperidone (Risperdal) appears to bring out the symptoms of TD more frequently, as compared to the other newer atypical antipsychotic agents.
  - Drugs other than those used to treat psychiatric illnesses can also block the dopamine receptors. These include anticholinergics and SSRIs, which are used to treat depression. Whether MAOIs and tricyclics cause TD is not known.
  - Reduction in the use of the drugs that caused TD is desirable. Changing to a different medication, such as an atypical antipsychotic, is recommended. Patients on antipsychotics should be checked regularly.
- TD has also been known to develop in patients who have been treated for digestive and GI disorders with medications such as metoclopramide (Reglan).
- Tetrabenzine, a medication that reduces levels of dopamine, has been of some use in treating TD symptoms.
- "Anti-Parkinsonian" drugs such as Aricept and Miraplex appear to offer some benefit.

Herbs, Botanicals, and Supplements

- No studies have been conducted for efficacy of herbs or botanicals in TD.

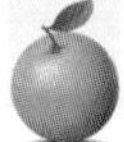

NUTRITION EDUCATION, COUNSELING, CARE MANAGEMENT

- Diet instructions should be offered directly to the patient unless this is not possible.
- Discuss major issues related to nutrition, self-feeding practices, moistening of foods, use of adaptive equipment as needed.
- Discuss sources of foods that contain branched-chain amino acids and how to obtain medical foods that may be used.

Patient Education—Foodborne Illness

- Careful food handling will be important. The same is true for hand washing.

For More Information

- NIMH
  http://www.nimh.nih.gov/index.shtml
- NINDS—Tardive Dyskinesia
  http://www.ninds.nih.gov/disorders/tardive/tardive.htm
- Tardive Dyskinesia
  http://www.tardivedyskinesia.com/
- We Move—Tardive Dyskinesia
  http://www.wemove.org/td/

TARDIVE DYSKINESIA—CITED REFERENCES

Casey DE. Implications of the CATIE trial on treatment: extrapyramidal symptoms. *CNS Spectr.* 11(suppl 7):25, 2006.

Tsai HT, et al. A candidate gene study of tardive dyskinesia in the CATIE schizophrenia trial. [published online ahead of print May 27, 2009] *Am J Med Genet B Neuropsychiatr Genet.* 153B:336, 2010.

TRIGEMINAL NEURALGIA

NUTRITIONAL ACUITY RANKING: LEVEL 1–2

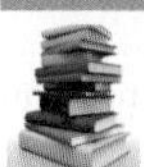

DEFINITIONS AND BACKGROUND

Trigeminal neuralgia (TN) or tic douloureux manifests as a disorder of the fifth cranial nerve and is characterized by paroxysms of excruciating pain of a burning nature. The painful periods alternate with pain-free periods. The frequency of the paroxysms ranges from a few to hundreds of attacks a day; remission can last for months to years, but tend to shorten over time (Zakrewska and Linskey, 2009).

The disorder is rare before 40 years of age and is more common in elderly women. The right side of the face is affected more often; the pain can be incapacitating. Dentists often play a role in identifying this condition (Bagheri et al, 2004). Loss of taste after surgery can occur. Recent use of radiosurgery or a gamma knife procedure has shown promise.

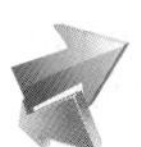

ASSESSMENT, MONITORING, AND EVALUATION

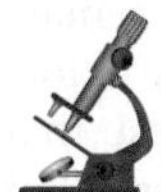

CLINICAL INDICATORS

Genetic Markers: Whether TN is related to celiac disease has yet to be determined.

Clinical/History		
Height	Temperature	Na^+, K^+
Weight	EEG	Folate
BMI	Carotid ultrasound	Ca^{++}, Mg^{++}
Dietary/intake history	CT scan or MRI	Chol (total, HDL, LDL)
PET scan	I & O	Trig
Chewing ability	**Lab Work**	Ferritin
BP	CRP	H & H
		Gluc

SAMPLE NUTRITION CARE PROCESS STEPS

Difficulty Chewing

Assessment Data: Problems with weight loss, pain with eating meals, difficulty chewing solids.

Nutrition Diagnoses (PES): Inadquate oral food and beverage intake related to difficulty chewing as evidenced by diagnosis of TN with excruciating pain, especially with solids.

Interventions: Education of patient about pureed foods and liquefying meal items to reduce chewing; nutrient-dese food and beverage choices.

Monitoring and Evaluation: Regain of lost weight, no further complaints of pain with chewing, improved nutrient intake.

INTERVENTION

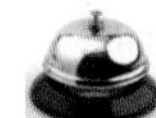

OBJECTIVES

- Control pain with medications, especially before meals.
- Provide appropriate counseling and assistance with consistency of meals (foods and beverages).
- Individualize for preferences and tolerances.
- Maintain body weight within a desirable range.
- Manage celiac disease if present.

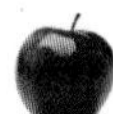

FOOD AND NUTRITION

- Use a normal diet as tolerated, perhaps altering to soft or pureed foods as needed. Omit gluten if celiac disease is diagnosed.
- Small, frequent feedings may be better tolerated than large meals.
- Liquids may be preferred if given by straw. Individualize.
- Avoid extremes in temperature.
- Use nutrient-dense foods if weight loss occurs.

Common Drugs Used and Potential Side Effects

- Anticonvulsants such as topiramate, phenytoin (Dilantin) or carbamazepine (Tegretol) are used. Diarrhea, nausea, and vomiting are common (He et al, 2006). Ensure adequate intake of folate.
- Nonsteroidal anti-inflammatory medications or narcotics may be used to reduce pain.
- Opiate-based analgesics offer the best relief. In some cases, Botox has been used.
- Baclofen may help patients eat when jaw movement tends to aggravate the symptoms.

Herbs, Botanicals, and Supplements

- No studies have been conducted for efficacy of herbs or botanicals in TN.
- With anticonvulsants such as phenytoin (Dilantin), avoid use with evening primrose oil, gingko biloba, and kava.

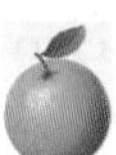

NUTRITION EDUCATION, COUNSELING, CARE MANAGEMENT

- The importance of oral and dental hygiene should be stressed, even with pain. Use pain medications as directed.
- The patient should be encouraged to avoid eating when tense or nervous.
- Relaxation therapy, yoga, tai chi, and biofeedback may be beneficial.

Patient Education—Foodborne Illness

- Careful food handling will be important. The same is true for hand washing.

For More Information

- Mayo Clinic—Trigeminal Neuralgia
  http://www.mayoclinic.com/health/trigeminal-neuralgia/DS00446
- NIH—Trigeminal Neuralgia
  http://www.ninds.nih.gov/disorders/trigeminal_neuralgia/detail_trigeminal_neuralgia.htm
- Neuropathic Facial Pain
  http://www.endthepain.org/

TRIGEMINAL NEURALGIA—CITED REFERENCES

Bagheri SC, et al. Diagnosis and treatment of patients with trigeminal neuralgia. *J Am Dent Assoc.* 135:1713, 2004.

He L, et al. Non-antiepileptic drugs for trigeminal neuralgia. *Cochrane Database Syst Rev.* 3:CD004029, 2006.

Zakrewska JM, Linskey ME. Trigeminal neuralgia. *Clin Evid (online).* Pii:1207, 2009.

PSYCHIATRIC DISORDERS—EATING DISORDERS

ANOREXIA NERVOSA

NUTRITIONAL ACUITY RANKING: LEVEL 3

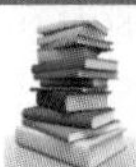

DEFINITIONS AND BACKGROUND

Anorexia nervosa (AN) is an eating disorder (ED) in which the patient severely rejects food, causing extreme weight loss, low basal metabolic rate, and exhaustion. About 6–15% of the population is affected. AN is more common in girls, especially just after, peaking at 12–13 and 19–20 years of age. But AN can occur at any age.

Signs include relentless pursuit of thinness, misperception of body image, and restrained eating, binge eating, or purging (see Bulimia and Binge Eating Disorder entries). Generally, cases are separated into "restricting" or "binge-purging" types: anorectic restrictor (AN-R) and anorectic bulimics (AN-B). Fear of fatness and a codependent focus outside of one's self are common in AN. The intense fear of becoming fat (not diminishing as weight loss progresses) has no known physical cause. Patients with EDs may have dermatologic manifestations secondary to starvation; recognition of these signs can lead to early diagnosis and treatment.

Weight is 85% or less of former weight; there is usually amenorrhea. Length of amenorrhea, estrogen exposure (age minus age at menarche minus years of amenorrhea), and body weight have independent effects on bone densities; therefore, osteopenia is common. Long-term sequelae may include Cushing's disease and osteoporosis. Without treatment, death may occur, usually from cardiac arrhythmias.

Problems include perfectionism, denial, impulse control, manipulative behavior, trust issues, power and misinformation within the family, low tolerance for change and new situations, fear of growing up and assuming adult responsibilities. Individuals with AN are overly dependent on parents or family, obsessive-compulsive, meticulous, introverted, emotionally reserved, socially insecure, overly rigid in thinking, self-denying, and overly compliant. Individuals with AN have high constraint, constriction of affect and emotional expressiveness, ahendonia and asceticism; restricting food intake becomes powerfully reinforcing because it provides a temporary respite from dysphoria (Kaye, 2009).

Because patients deny the severity of their illness, they delay seeking psychiatric treatment. Teens with ED often use subterfuge to give the impression that they are cooperating with treatment plans, when they in fact are not. These behaviors prolong treatment and can lead to malnutrition. Group parenting education may be quite helpful (Zucker et al, 2006).

Some careers promote a thin body for success (e.g., fashion, air travel, entertainment, and athletics). Many female athletes struggle with an ED. The main concern is inadequate energy intake (Gabel, 2006). Studies suggest that individuals with AN have lower than optimal levels of polyunsaturated fatty acids (including ALA and GLA). Two or more consecutive spontaneous menses implies resumption of menses; this depends on body weight but not on body fat. Weight regain in subjects with AN is associated with an increase in serum leptin concentrations (Mauler et al, 2009). Insulin-like growth factor I (IGF-I) is a biochemical marker of malnutrition and a sensitive index of nutritional repletion in patients with EDs. Fortunately, the majority of patients with EDs make a full recovery.

Dietitians must be able to identify and refer patients with EDs. Death by suicide occurs in a disproportionate percentage of individuals with AN (Zucker et al, 2007). Yet, evidence for successful treatment is weak (Bulik et al, 2007). Tube feeding, when accepted, helps to increase weight and improve cognitive and physical functioning. Medical nutrition therapy for EDs is a specialization that requires training beyond entry level. The American Dietetic Association has recommended eight medical nutrition therapy visits by a trained professional for persons who have EDs.

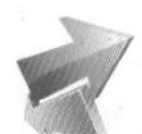

ASSESSMENT, MONITORING, AND EVALUATION

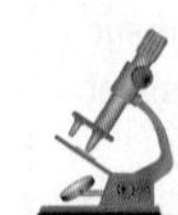

CLINICAL INDICATORS

Genetic Markers: A genetic component may play a role in determining a person's susceptibility to anorexia. Researchers are currently attempting to identify the particular gene or genes that might affect a person's tendency to develop this disorder. The agouti gene may play a role in AN.

Clinical/History	EKG	Alb, transthyretin, N balance
Height	Arrthymias?	Chol (low?)
Present weight	Parental Authority Questionnaire (PAQ)	Trig
Usual weight	Eating Disorders Inventory-2 (EDI-2)	Gluc
Recent weight	Eating Attitudes Test (EAT-26)	BUN (low?)
Percentage of weight changes	Perfectionism, compulsiveness	H & H
BMI (often <17.5)		Serum Fe
Weight goal/timing	**Lab Work**	Thyroid-stimulating hormone (TSH)
Dietary/intake history	Luteinizing hormone (LH) response to gonadotropin-releasing hormone (GnRH)	TLC; Leukopenia?
Bulimia or vomiting?	Follicle-stimulating hormone (FSH)	Na^+, Cl^-
Tooth erosion or decay	IGF-I	K^+ (hypokalemia?)
Laxative or diuretic abuse?	Serum estradiol (low)	Serum amylase (with vomiting)
BP; hypotension?	Serum cortisol (high)	Serum Ca^{++}, Mg^{++}
Amenorrhea	Urinary cortisol (high)	Serum phosphorus
Blotchy or yellow skin	Sex hormone–binding globulin (SHBG)	Liver function tests
Lanugo hair		Leptin levels
Muscle wasting		*Ghrelin levels
Edema		* Plasma levels of ghrelin increase before meals and decrease strongly after meals.
Blood in stool?		
MRI or CT scan for ventricular enlargement from malnutrition		
DEXA (after 6 months underweight)		

SAMPLE NUTRITION CARE PROCESS STEPS

Harmful Beliefs About Food And Nutrition

Assessment Data: BMI charts and current versus desirable weight for height; body fat measurements.

Nutrition Diagnosis (PES): Disordered eating pattern related to complaints of being "too fat" as evidenced by current weight of 82 lb and self-limited dietary intake of 450 kcals daily on nutrient analysis.

Intervention: Provide meals appropriate for refeeding protocol; education and counseling about appropriate body size, weight, BMI; goal setting for self-management.

Monitoring and Evaluation: Improved weight and height for age; intake records; discussion about perceptions of mealtimes and eating, body image.

INTERVENTION

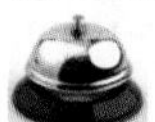

OBJECTIVES

- Restore normal physiological function by correcting starvation and its associated changes, including electrolyte imbalance, bradycardia, and hypotension.
- Check weight or growth charts to determine difference and to set goals. Promote weight gain of 1–3 lb weekly (in-patient) and 0.5–1 lb weekly (outpatient) to reach a weight closer to a healthy BMI.
- Promote adequate psychotherapy and use of medications to protect the heart, fluid, and electrolytes, which are the most important.
- Obtain diet history to assess bulimia, vomiting, and use of diuretics or laxatives.
- Do not force feedings; rejection of food is part of the illness. Promote normal eating behavior instead.
- Gradually increase intake to a normal or high-energy intake to lessen likelihood of edema and other consequences of malnutrition.
- For young women, promote normal menstrual cycles. Estrogen seems to be correlated with cognitive function (Chui et al, 2008).
- Reduce preoccupation with weight and food. Erroneous perceptions of "normal" should be alleviated. Promote adequate self-esteem.
- Refer to appropriate care for psychiatric maladies and comorbid conditions, especially insulin-dependent diabetes mellitus.
- Coordinate nutrition education and counseling with the overall team plan. Table 4-14 shows how average women compare with "fashion women"; counseling will need to be adjusted according to the individual's self-perception.

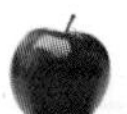

FOOD AND NUTRITION

- Serve attractive, palatable meals in small amounts, observing food preferences. Small, frequent meals are useful. Encourage variety.
- Limit bulky foods during the early stages of treatment; GI intolerance may persist for a long time. Assure the patient that constipation will be alleviated.
- Diet should be called a "low-calorie diet for AN" to convince the patient of the counselors' good intentions.
- According to the standards set by the APA (2005): start at 30–40 kcal/kg (about 1000–1600 kcals/d) and increase as possible. Promote weekly weight gain by gradually attaining intake of up to 70–100 kcal/kg for some patients. Weight maintenance may need to be 40–60 kcal/kg.
- Protein refeeding takes a long time. Repletion may not be complete until weight has returned to normal. Monitor for improved biochemical results (BUN, albumin).
- Monitor serum cholesterol levels; low levels have been correlated with suicidality (Favaro et al, 2004).
- While not a preferred method, use tube feeding if necessary (i.e., only if the patient weighs 40% of lower end of BMI range for normal). Nocturnal tube feeding may be especially helpful.

- Help the patient resume normal eating habits. Have the patient measure and record food intake at first; then, gradually lessen the emphasis on food.
- A "no added salt" diet may reduce fluid retention.
- It may be useful to avoid caffeine because of stimulant/diuretic effect.
- A vitamin–mineral supplement may be needed for zinc and other nutrients.

Common Drugs Used and Potential Side Effects

- Pharmacotherapy is not always successful in AN. Olanzapine may have some benefit with reductions in depression and anxiety. Dry mouth and constipation are the most common side effects.
- Antidepressants may be prescribed; nutritional side effects should be monitored carefully. SSRIs are considered to be more effective. However, fluoxetine has failed to demonstrate protection against relapse in AN (Walsh et al, 2006).
- Antiepileptic drugs (AEDs) may be used. Carbamazepine and valproate may be effective in treating patients with AN when used to treat an associated mood or seizure disorder (McElroy et al, 2009).

Herbs, Botanicals, and Supplements

- No specific herbs and botanical products have been used for AN in clinical trials.

NUTRITION EDUCATION, COUNSELING, CARE MANAGEMENT

- Most treatments are based on consensus rather than evidence (Gowers, 2008). At this time, the evidence base is strongest for family therapy for AN (Keel and Haedt, 2008).
- The RD is uniquely qualified to provide medical nutrition therapy for the normalization of eating patterns and nutritional status (American Dietetic Association, 2006).
- See Table 4-15.

TABLE 4-15 Average Woman Versus "Fashion Woman"

	Average Woman	Barbie Doll	Store Mannequin
Height	5′4″	6′0″	6′0″
Weight	145 lbs	101 lbs	Not available
Dress size	11–14	4	6
Bust	36–37″	39″	34″
Waist	29–31″	19″	23″
Hips	40–42″	33″	34″

Anorexia Nervosa and Related Eating Disorders. "Statistics: How many people have eating disorders?"http://www.anred.com/stats.html *ANRED*. 2005, accessed July 1, 2008.

Patient Education—Foodborne Illness

- Careful food handling will be important. The same is true for sanitizing work area before and after preparing tube feedings to prevent contamination. Formula companies have good information on safe handling of formula in the home and institution.

For More Information

- Academy for Eating Disorders
  http://www.aedweb.org
- Anorexia Nervosa and Related Eating Disorders (ANRED)
  http://www.anred.com/
- Eating Disorders Anonymous
  http://www.eatingdisordersanonymous.org/
- Eating Disorder Recovery
  http://www.addictions.net/
- International Association of Eating Disorders Professionals (IAEDP)
  http://www.iaedp.com/
- National Association of Anorexia Nervosa and Associated Disorders (ANAD)
  http://www.anad.org/
- Practice Guideline for Eating Disorders
  http://www.psych.org/psych_pract/treatg/pg/prac_guide.cfm

ANOREXIA NERVOSA—CITED REFERENCES

American Dietetic Association. Position of The American Dietetic Association: nutrition intervention in the treatment of anorexia nervosa, bulimia nervosa, and eating disorders not otherwise specified (EDNOS). *J Am Diet Assoc.* 106:2073, 2006.

American Psychiatric Association. Treatment of patients with eating disorders, third edition. American Psychiatric Association. *Am J Psychiatry.* 163: 4S, 2006.

Bulik CM, et al. Anorexia nervosa treatment: a systematic review of randomized controlled trials. *Int J Eat Disord.* 40:310, 2007.

Chui HT, et al. Cognitive function and brain structure in females with a history of adolescent-onset anorexia nervosa. *Pediatrics.* 122:426, 2008.

Favaro A, et al. Total serum cholesterol and suicidality in anorexia nervosa. *Psychosom Med.* 66:548, 2004.

Field AE, et al. Family, peer, and media predictors of becoming eating disordered. *Arch Pediatr Adolesc Med.* 162:574, 2008.

Gabel KA. Special nutritional concerns for the female athlete. *Curr Sports Med Rep.* 5:187, 2006.

Gowers SG. Management of eating disorders in children and adolescents. *Arch Dis Child.* 93:331, 2008.

Kaye W. Neurobiology of anorexia and bulimia nervosa. *Physiol Behav.* 94:121, 2009.

Keel PK, Haedt A. Evidence-based psychosocial treatments for eating problems and eating disorders. *J Clin Child Adolesc Psychol.* 37:39, 2008.

Low KG, et al. Effectiveness of a computer-based interactive eating disorders prevention program at long-term follow-up. *Eat Disord.* 14:17, 2006.

Mauler B, et al. Hypercaloric diets differing in fat composition have similar effects on serum leptin and weight gain in female subjects with anorexia nervosa. *Nutr Res.* 29:1, 2009.

McElroy SL, et al. Role of antiepileptic drugs in the management of eating disorders. *CNS Drugs.* 23:149, 2009.

Walsh BT, et al. Fluoxetine after weight restoration in anorexia nervosa: a randomized controlled trial. *JAMA.* 295:2605, 2006.

Wilfrey DE, et al. Classification of eating disorders: toward DSM-V. *Int J Eating Disord.* 40:123, 2007.

Zucker NL, et al. A group parent-training program: a novel approach for eating disorder management. *Eat Weight Disord.* 11:78, 2006.

Zucker NL, et al. Anorexia nervosa and autism spectrum disorders: guided investigation of social cognitive endophenotypes. *Psycholol Bull.* 133:976, 2007.

BINGE EATING DISORDER

NUTRITIONAL ACUITY RANKING: LEVEL 3–4

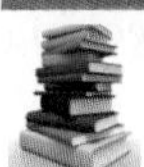

DEFINITIONS AND BACKGROUND

Food intake and energy balance are regulated by two complementary drives: the homeostatic pathway increases motivation to eat following depletion of energy stores, and the hedonic (reward-based) pathway increases the desire to consume foods that are highly palatable during periods of abundance (Lutter and Nestler, 2009). Binge eating disorder (BED) involves recurrent episodes of eating in a discrete period of time an amount of food larger than most people would eat in the same time, a sense of lack of control over the eating episodes, rapid or secretive eating, guilt, and shame. BED is far more prevalent than AN and BN. The DSM-V will make BED an official diagnosis with frequency and duration at once per week for 3 months (Wilfrey et al, 2007).

Episodes may involve three or more of the following behaviors: eating more rapidly than normal, eating until uncomfortable, eating when not physically hungry, eating these foods alone, and feeling disgusted, guilty, or depressed. Adolescent and young adult vegetarians may be at increased risk for binge eating with loss of control (Robinson-O'Brien, 2009).

Binge eating is a serious problem among a subset of the obese. Weight cycling involves weight loss followed by weight regain along with psychological distress. Chronic dieting may predispose vulnerable individuals to binge eating, alcoholism, or drug abuse.

Many individuals with this problem have a personal or parental history of substance abuse. Persons with BED tend to be depressed and overweight. A single traumatic event, several years of unusual stress or pain, an extended period of emotional pain, or a mood disorder may be involved. Regardless of actual weight, there are high degrees of psychological distress in this group of individuals (Didie and Fitzgibbon, 2005). "Clinical" perfectionism involves both the determined pursuit of self-imposed standards and extremely vulnerable self-evaluation.

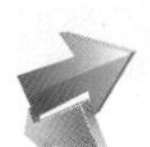

ASSESSMENT, MONITORING, AND EVALUATION

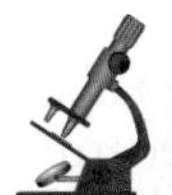

CLINICAL INDICATORS

Genetic Markers: People who have this disorder may be genetically predisposed to weigh more than the cultural ideal, so they may eat little, get hungry, and then binge in response to that hunger.

Clinical/History

Height
Weight
BMI
% Weight changes
Dietary/intake history
Binge pattern and frequency
Socially Prescribed Perfectionism Scale
Parental Authority Questionnaire (PAQ)
Eating Disorders Inventory-2 (EDI-2)
Eating Attitudes Test (EAT-26)

Lab Work

Serum cortisol (high?)
Na^+, K^+, Cl^-
BUN, Creat
Gluc
Urinary acetone
Chol, Trig

INTERVENTION

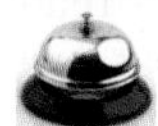

OBJECTIVES

- Support the individual's counseling and therapy to identify the causes of binges. Help them follow a step-wise plan using self-monitoring records; regular patterns of eating to displace binge eating; alternative behaviors to help resist urges.
- Educate about food, eating, body shape, and weight patterns. Eliminate all aspects of restrained eating.
- Develop skills for dealing with difficulties that triggered past binges. Identify and challenge problematic ways of thinking.
- Consider the origins of the binge eating problem and then evaluate family and social factors that can be changed.
- Plan for the future. Have realistic expectations and strategies ready for when problems occur.
- Encourage a return to eating that is under the control of the individual.
- Correct any imbalances that have occurred as a result of the binges (e.g., weight, electrolyte imbalances).
- Support therapy, especially if there is a dual diagnosis, such as substance abuse.

SAMPLE NUTRITION CARE PROCESS STEPS

Excessive Oral Food and Beverage Intake

Assessment Data: Food records indicating periods of binge eating twice a week for the past 8 months.

Nutrition Diagnoses (PES): Excessive oral food and beverage intake related to binge episodes as evidenced by food diary and intake records showing emotional binges when under stress.

Interventions: Education about the hazards of purging and the benefits of eating healthy portions and nutrient-dense foods. Coordination of care with psychotherapist to manage stress through yoga, CBT, and appropriate levels of physical activity.

Monitoring and Evaluation: Reports of fewer episodes of binge-purge cycles; improved quality of life; weight within desirable BMI range.

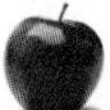

FOOD AND NUTRITION

- A balanced diet, using principles of the dietary guidelines and the Food Guide Pyramid, should be planned according to age, sex, and goals for BMI.
- A slightly higher protein intake than usual helps to reduce binge eating, provide more satiety, and lower overall food intake.
- Alter diet according to medications, therapies, medical recommendations, and interdisciplinary care plan. This may include restriction of CHO, protein, fat, sodium, or other nutrients accordingly.

Common Drugs Used and Potential Side Effects

- Pharmacotherapy is often beneficial in addition to psychotherapy. Antidepressants may be useful; monitor their specific effects.
- Topiramate (Topamax) may be an effective BED treatment; it has mild side effects, such as weight loss, that may be desirable.
- Sibutramine significantly reduces binge eating behavior and body weight in BED.

Herbs, Botanicals, and Supplements

- No specific herbs and botanical products have been used for binge eating in any clinical trials.

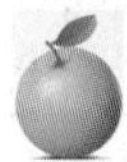

NUTRITION EDUCATION, COUNSELING, CARE MANAGEMENT

- Encourage use of a food diary to record time, place, foods eaten, cues, binge feelings, and other comments.
- Discuss exercise and its effect on sense of well-being; shopping, holidays, and stressors.
- Discuss not skipping breakfast and lunch. This may lead to bingeing late into the evening or night.
- Focus on self-efficacy and proper assertiveness for coping with stressors.

Patient Education—Foodborne Illness

- Careful food handling will be important. The same is true for hand washing.
- Note any unusual behaviors, such as pica, and discuss food safety issues if relevant.

For More Information

- Academy for Eating Disorders
  http://www.aedweb.org
- Mayo Clinic
  http://www.mayoclinic.com/health/binge-eating-disorder/DS00608
- National Eating Disorders Association
  http://www.edap.org/

BINGE EATING DISORDER—CITED REFERENCES

Didie ER, Fitzgibbon M. Binge eating and psychological distress: is the degree of obesity a factor? *Eat Behav.* 6:35, 2005.

Lutter M, Nestler EJ. Homeostatic and hedonic signals interact in the regulation of food intake. *J Nutr.* 139:629, 2009.

Robinson-O'Brien R, et al. Adolescent and young adult vegetarianism: better dietary intake and weight outcomes but increased risk of disordered eating behaviors. *J Am Diet Assoc.* 109:648, 2009.

Sigel E. Eating disorders. *Adolesc Med State Art Rev.* 19:547, 2008.

Wilfrey DE, et al. Classification of eating disorders: toward DSM-V. *Int J Eating Disord.* 40:123, 2007.

BULIMIA NERVOSA

NUTRITIONAL ACUITY RANKING: LEVEL 3–4

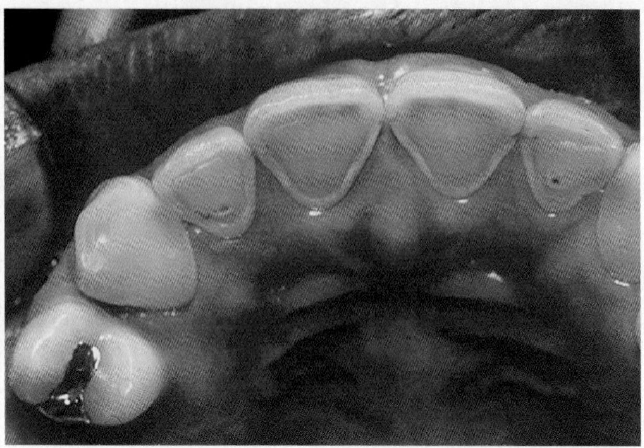

Adapted from: Langlais RP, Miller CS. *Color Atlas of Common Oral Diseases.* Philadelphia: Lea & Febiger, 1992.

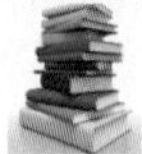

DEFINITIONS AND BACKGROUND

BN is an ED with food addiction as the primary coping mechanism. Criteria for diagnosis include recurrent episodes of binge eating, sense of lack of control, self-evaluation unduly influenced by weight or body shape, recurrent and inappropriate compensating behavior two times weekly for 3 months or longer (vomiting, use of laxatives or diuretics, fasting, excessive exercise). In BN, repeated binge episodes increase gastric capacity, which delays emptying, blunts cholecystokinin (CCK) release, and impairs satiety response.

Of the 5–30% of the population with bulimia, 85% are college-educated women. Weight may be normal or near-normal. When not bingeing, individuals with BN tend to be dieting; when hungry, they may binge and purge again. Their self-worth tends to be associated with thinness. The most restrained patients with BN have the greatest desire to lose weight (Lowe et al, 2007).

Pathogenesis of BN suggests functional abnormalities within a neural system for self-regulatory control, which may contribute to binge eating and other impulsive behaviors (Marsh et al, 2009). Individuals with BN may experience loneliness, irritability, passivity, sadness, addictive behavior patterns, or suicidal behavior. Individuals with BN may shoplift, be promiscuous, and abuse alcohol, drugs, or credit cards. Disordered eating may occur for some time before drug or alcohol problems. Because disturbances in neuronal systems modulate feeding, mood, and impulse control, altered serotonin levels contribute to the disordered eating.

Significantly, the drive for thinness and body dissatisfaction relate to the patient's perception of father as "authoritarian" (Enten and Golan, 2009). Bulimics use food as a coping mechanism. Codependency is a dysfunctional pattern of relating to feelings. Individuals with BN focus on others or on things outside of themselves and deny their feelings. Fear, shame, despair, anger, rigidity, denial, and confusion are integral. Because of the low self-esteem, cognitive dysfunction, use of food or substance to relieve anxiety or depression, secretiveness, social isolation, and denial, psychotherapy is of primary importance. The team approach is best coordinated with the physician, a nutritionist, and a mental health professional.

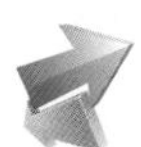

ASSESSMENT, MONITORING, AND EVALUATION

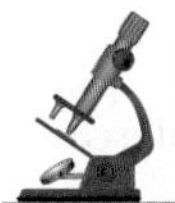

CLINICAL INDICATORS

Genetic Markers: Alterations in the serotonin (5-HT) 2A receptor are associated with behavioral impulsiveness and BN. Disturbances of 5-HT function occur when people are ill, and persist after recovery (Kaye, 2009).

Clinical/History

Height
Weight, current
Usual weight
BMI
Percentage of weight changes
Hx of laxative and diuretic abuse
BP
Dietary/intake history
Oral and dental concerns
Tooth enamel erosion (perimolysis)
Knuckles with rough skin
Broken blood vessels in the eye
Salivary gland swelling
Excessive bathroom use (to vomit)
Perfectionism, obsessive-compulsiveness, dysphoria
Parental Authority Questionnaire (PAQ)
Eating Disorders Inventory-2 (EDI-2)
Eating Attitudes Test (EAT-26)

Lab Work

Serum amylase (high)
Chol, Trig
Gastrin
LH, FSH (may be low)
Gluc
Alb
Na^+, K^+, Cl^-
Serum cortisol
Serum folate
BP
H & H

SAMPLE NUTRITION CARE PROCESS STEPS

Disordered Eating Pattern

Assessment Data: Food records; binge-purging behaviors as indicated in food diaries.

Nutrition Diagnosis (PES): Disordered eating pattern related to harmful belief about food and nutrition (i.e., that kcals are not available after using vomiting or use of laxatives) as evidenced by purging behaviors after a binge.

Intervention: Educate and counsel about food and absorption after meals, dangers of vomiting and laxatives for weight control. Counsel about stress management and coping mechanisms using biofeedback, yoga or other techniques besides use of food.

Monitoring and Evaluation: Improved food records; decreased use of vomiting and laxatives as a weight-control measure; improved self-esteem and quality of life.

INTERVENTION

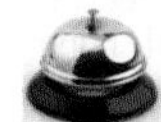

OBJECTIVES

- Stabilize fluid and electrolyte imbalances.
- Individualize care plan to address weight history, dieting and binge eating episodes, purging behaviors, meal and exercise patterns.
- Promote effective weight control along with stress management. Establish a target weight in accordance with present weight, desirable BMI, reasonable time frame for recovery, and related factors. Modest energy restriction does not promote disordered eating (Wadden et al, 2004).
- Correct or prevent edema.
- Counteract lowered metabolic rate with balanced diet and exercise.
- Prevent oral health problems from vomiting and poor eating habits. About one third of persons with this condition will have erosion. Table 4-16 elaborates the oral manifestations and issues of concern in BN.

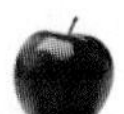

FOOD AND NUTRITION

- Use controlled portions of a regular diet, usually with three meals and two snacks.
- Provide basal energy needs plus 300–400 calories as a beginning stage.
- Decrease sugar and alcohol intake, stressing the importance of other key nutrients. Highlight nutrient density and impact on health, appearance, and stamina.
- Encourage exercise along with diet and psychotherapy. Exercise decreases negative mood, improves EDs, and leads to more overall weight loss (Fossati et al, 2004).

Common Drugs Used and Potential Side Effects

- The anticonvulsant Topiramate has shown good results in both binge and purge symptoms; it causes anorexic symptoms and weight loss.

TABLE 4-16 **Tips for Helping Patients with Eating Disorders (EDs)**

Goal	Suggested Action
Full participation, especially in-patient	Manage anxiety disorders, which may precede onset of the ED. Patients with the binge eating/purging type of anorexia nervosa are significantly less likely to complete in-patient treatment.
Manage avoidant personality style	Persons with anorexia nervosa and avoidant personality style may discontinue therapy early.
Become an effective, independently functioning person	Convey principles rather than rigid "rules" to avoid reinforcing the patient's compulsive rituals, preoccupation with food, and perfectionism.
Positive, regular habits	Behavioral contracting is useful.
Balanced diet	Discuss how a balanced diet affects weight goals. Encourage healthy snacks. Medical nutrition therapy and education are cornerstones of therapy.
Identify hunger cues	Discuss signs of hunger and satiety.
Positive family relationships and healthy conflict management	Family dynamics play a role. Include family members in education and counseling sessions. Conflict management, support for individuality and personal opinions, and discussion of emotions will be part of therapy.
Healthy assertiveness and self-efficacy	Codependent behavior generally is a problem. Help the individual develop healthy reconnections and assertiveness. Computer-based psychosocial counseling may be helpful (Low et al, 2006).
Address social pressure for thinness	Preventive actions during middle school years may be helpful. For older individuals, open discussion of these issues may be useful as well.
Prevent relapse, which is common	Starvation and self-imposed dieting may lead to binges once food is available. Preoccupation with food and eating, emotional lability, dysphoria, and distractibility are common.
Monitor patients who have type 1 diabetes	Monitor for poor control, bulimia, skipping meals, hypoglycemia, hyperglycemia, and complications. Eating disorders are common in type 1 DM.
Support healthy pregnancies	Successful treatment includes appropriate pattern of weight gain, decreases in bingeing and purging behaviors, and normal infant birth weight. Special guidance is needed to achieve positive fetal outcomes. Use a team approach.
Promote healthy levels of physical activity	Discuss goals for the individual. Sometimes exercise is a goal in itself; therapy may be needed to address this issue along with eating patterns. Excessive exercise and hyperactivity are common.

- Antidepressants such as sertraline may be used (O'Reardon et al, 2004). Monitor side effects such as glucose changes, dry mouth, constipation, increased BP, abdominal cramps, and weight changes. Avoid use with ma huang (ephedra), St. John's wort, and gingko biloba because they may enhance the effects and cause restlessness.
- Fluoxetine can help reduce binge eating and purging behaviors (Shapiro et al, 2007).
- Laxative and diuretic abuse can cause cardiac arrest and other problems. Discourage this practice.

Herbs, Botanicals, and Supplements

- Alternative medicines are frequently used in this population; many products are available with potentially significant toxicities, especially diet pills and diuretics.
- Ma huang (ephedra), St. John's wort, and gingko biloba may enhance the effects of antidepressants and cause restlessness.
- With anticonvulsants, avoid use with evening primrose oil, gingko biloba, and kava.

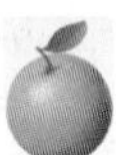

NUTRITION EDUCATION, COUNSELING, CARE MANAGEMENT

- Use of a biopsychosocial approach offers a means of working toward healing the whole person (Kreipe, 2006).

The four elements of successful treatment in adolescents are (Kreipe and Yussman, 2003):

- Recognizing the disorder and restoring physiological stability early in its course.
- Establishing a trusting, therapeutic partnership with the adolescent.
- Involving the family in treatment.
- Using an interdisciplinary team approach.

- The combination of cognitive-behavioral therapy (CBT) with a nutritional education and a physical activity program helps to decrease depression and anxiety (Fossati et al, 2004).
- Help the patient rediscover the ability to be alone without giving in to the urge to binge. Assertiveness training may be of great benefit.
- Information, as from basic nutrition texts, can also encourage improved habits.
- Discuss the outcomes of electrolyte imbalance, such as muscle spasms, kidney problems, or cardiac arrest.
- Assert that there is "no such thing as a forbidden food." Discuss how to handle the cycle of bulimia: hopelessness or anxiety leading to gorging, leading to fear of fatness, leading to vomiting or drug abuse, leading to release from fear, leading to guilt, etc.
- Stringent oral hygiene after vomiting may reduce dental erosion.
- Self-help groups are often beneficial.
- Table 4-17 describes other disordered eating patterns and some tips.

TABLE 4-17 Assessment of Oral Manifestations in Bulimia Nervosa

Condition	Issues of Concern
Enamel erosion (perimolysis)	Thermal sensitivity and pain
Salivary gland swelling (sialadenosis)	Hypertrophy from regurgitation of acidic contents; malnutrition
Dry mouth (xerostomia)	From vomiting, laxative, or diuretic abuse
Increased serum amylase	Two to four times increased levels occur after binging and vomiting; a marker for bulimia
Mucosal trauma	Abrasions and bleeding from rapid, forceful regurgitation
Gingival recession	From frequent and rigorous tooth brushing
Dental caries	From increased intake of junk foods, candy, sweets

Patient Education—Foodborne Illness

- Careful food handling and hand washing are important. If constant hand washing is a concern, referral to a mental health provider may be useful.

For More Information

- Academy for Eating Disorders http://www.aedweb.org
- Eating Disorders Anonymous http://www.eatingdisordersanonymous.org/
- National Association of Anorexia Nervosa and Associated Disorders (ANAD) http://www.anad.org/
- National Eating Disorders Association http://www.edap.org/
- Women's Health—Bulimia Nervosa http://www.womenshealth.gov/FAQ/bulimia-nervosa.cfm

BULIMIA NERVOSA—CITED REFERENCES

Enten RS, Golan M. Parenting styles and eating disorder pathology. *Appetite.* 52:784, 2009.

Fossati M, et al. Cognitive-behavioral therapy with simultaneous nutritional and physical activity education in obese patients with binge eating disorder. *Eat Weight Disord.* 9:134, 2004.

Kaye W. Neurobiology of anorexia and bulimia nervosa. *Physiol Behav.* 94:121, 2009.

Kreipe RE. The biopsychosocial approach to adolescents with somatoform disorders. *Adolesc Med Clin.* 17:1, 2006.

Kreipe RE, Yussman SM. The role of the primary care practitioner in the treatment of eating disorders. *Adolesc Med.* 14:133, 2003.

Lowe MR, et al. The relationship of weight suppression and dietary restraint to binge eating in bulimia nervosa. *Int J Eating Disord.* 40:640, 2007.

O'Reardon JP, et al. Clinical trial of sertraline in the treatment of night eating syndrome. *Int J Eat Disord.* 35:16, 2004.

Shapiro JR, et al. Bulimia nervosa treatment: a systematic review of randomized controlled trials. *Int J Eat Disord.* 40:321, 2007.

Wadden TA, et al. Dieting and the development of eating disorders in obese women: results of a randomized controlled trial. *Am J Clin Nutr.* 80(3):560, 2004.

MENTAL DISORDERS–OTHER

BIPOLAR DISORDER

NUTRITIONAL ACUITY RANKING: LEVEL 1–2

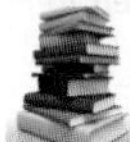

DEFINITIONS AND BACKGROUND

Abnormalities in brain biochemistry and circuits are responsible for the extreme shifts in mood, energy, and functioning that characterize BD. Bipolar affective disorders are characterized by mood swings from mania (exaggerated feeling of well-being, stimulation, and grandiosity in which a person can lose touch with reality) to depression (overwhelming feelings of sadness, anxiety, and low self-worth, which can include suicidal thoughts and suicide attempts). The disorders affect men and women equally. Children are rarely diagnosed. See Table 4-18.

The old name for BD is manic-depressive illness. The spectrum involves depression with varying degrees of excitatory signs and symptoms. Genetics seem to be involved. Relatives of people with bipolar affective disorder and depression are more likely to be affected. In general, the less severe the case, the later the onset of clinically observable mood disorder.

According to the DSM-IV, BD is a severe, recurrent, lifelong illness that affects up to about 7% of Americans. Lifetime prevalence rates for bipolar I and II disorder range up to 2%; for cyclothymia, a milder form of BD, prevalence ranges from 3% to 5%. More recent prevalence estimates are even higher. The World Health Organization reports that BD is the sixth leading cause of years lived with disability, worldwide.

For doctors working in a primary care setting, it is important to recognize the signs and symptoms of BD; it is commonly misdiagnosed as unipolar depression. Patients with bipolar depression are significantly more likely to report hallucinations, current suicidal ideation, and low self-esteem than patients with unipolar depression but less likely to report disturbed appetite (Das et al, 2005; Olfson et al, 2005).

The cyclical nature of the disorder poses challenges and barriers. Mood swings significantly impair the ability to function in social situations and to hold down a job. Patients often need to take days off from work either due to worsening clinical symptoms or hospitalization. When at work, problems may result from mood episodes such as poor concentration or low motivation during depression and inappropriate behavior during mania.

In mania, a person's behavior is often reckless and self-damaging. During mania, patients may spend excessive amounts of money or may have excessive urges to drive fast.

TABLE 4-18 Other Disordered Eating Patterns

Disorder	Description
Anorexia athletica (compulsive exercising)	The person repeatedly exercises beyond the requirements for good health and is a fanatic about weight and diet. Not a formal diagnosis; behaviors are usually a part of anorexia nervosa, bulimia, or obsessive-compulsive disorder. Focuses on challenge and does not savor victory; proud of being an "elite athlete." Rarely satisfied with athletic achievements or performance. Needs a team approach for therapeutic intervention.
Body dysmorphic disorder (BDD)	BDD is thought to be a subtype of obsessive-compulsive disorder. It is not a variant of anorexia nervosa or bulimia nervosa. The person feels "ugly" and suffers from shyness and acts withdrawn in new situations or with unfamiliar people. Often strikes before age 18; affecting 2% of people in the United States. Sufferers are excessively concerned about appearance, in particular perceived flaws of face, hair, and skin. They are convinced these flaws exist despite reassurances from friends and family members who usually can see nothing to justify such intense worry and anxiety. High risk for despair and suicide; may undergo unnecessary expensive plastic surgery. BDD is treatable and begins with an evaluation by a physician and mental health care provider. Treatments include medication that adjusts serotonin levels in the brain and cognitive-behavioral therapy. A clinician makes the diagnosis and recommends treatment based on the needs and circumstances of each person.
Cyclic vomiting syndrome	Cycles of frequent vomiting, usually (but not always) found in children, often related to migraine headaches. Careful medical assessment is needed. Not a true eating disorder.
Eating disorders not otherwise specified (ED-NOS)	Official diagnosis describing atypical eating disorders where a person meets some but not all criteria for one specific eating disorder. Food behaviors are not normal and healthy; for example, behavior that resembles bulimia nervosa because of purging but without binge eating.
Gourmand syndrome	Person is preoccupied with fine food, including its purchase, preparation, presentation, and consumption. Exceedingly rare; thought to be caused by injury to the right side of the brain (as from tumor, concussion, or stroke). Relationship to addictions or obsessive-compulsive disorder possible. Had normal relationship with food prior to injury. Start with a neurologist evaluation.
Muscle dysmorphic disorder (bigorexia)	Sometimes called bigorexia, muscle dysmorphia is the opposite of anorexia nervosa. People with this disorder obsess about being small and undeveloped. They worry that they are too little and too frail. Even if they have good muscle mass, they believe their muscles are not big enough or are inadequate. Depression is the underlying concern. May understand the risks of steroid use but continue anyway. This condition results in disordered eating with very high protein and very low fat and often very low carbohydrate, often combined with excessive supplements.
Night eating syndrome	Affects 1–2% of general population. Likely that over one quarter of all morbidly obese persons may have this condition. This disorder is being considered for next psychiatric diagnostic classification manual. The person has little or no appetite for breakfast, delays first meal for several hours after waking up, and is often upset about how much was eaten the night before. Most calories are eaten late in the day or during the night. Sertraline, a selective serotonin reuptake inhibitor, may be beneficial in the treatment of night eating syndrome (O'Reardon et al, 2004). Psychotherapy is recommended. Self-help groups such as Overeaters Anonymous or group therapy can help.
Nocturnal sleep-related eating disorder	More of a sleep disorder than a true eating disorder. Individual eats while asleep and may sleep walk. No conscious memory of eating when they awaken again. Much guilt and confusion ensues.
Orthorexia nervosa	Eating the "right" food becomes an important, or even the primary, focus of life. One's worth or goodness is seen in terms of what one does or does not eat. Personal values, relationships, career goals, and friendships become less important than the quality and timing of what is consumed. May be a type of obsessive-compulsive disorder.
Pica	A craving for nonfood items such as dirt, clay, plaster, chalk, or paint chips. Pica may occur in pregnancy, in people whose diets are deficient in minerals found in the substances, in people with psychiatric conditions or developmental disabilities, or in people with family history of similar customs. Sometimes people who diet become hungry and ease their hunger with nonfood substances. May cause a medical emergency if obstruction or severe constipation occurs or if electrolyte imbalances occur.
Rumination syndrome	Person eats, swallows, and then regurgitates food back into the mouth where it is chewed and swallowed again. Process may be repeated several times or for several hours per episode. Process may be voluntary or involuntary. Ruminators report that regurgitated material does not taste bitter and that it is returned to the mouth with a gentle burp, not violent gagging or retching, not even nausea. Consequences range from minor inconveniences to life-threatening crises and include bad breath, indigestion, chapped lips and chin, damage to dental enamel and tissues in the mouth, aspiration pneumonia, failure to grow (children), weight loss, electrolyte imbalance, and dehydration.

From: O'Reardon RP, Stunkard AJ, 2004. Anorexia Nervosa and Related Eating Disorders, Inc., http://www.anred.com/defslesser.html, accessed January 18, 2005.

During the depressive phase of the illness, patients may try to self-medicate themselves with alcohol or other substances, leading to problems with abuse or dependence. A series of four or more manic or depressive episodes in 12 months is known as "rapid cycling," a condition that can be more difficult to treat. Patients with bipolar I disorder are ill nearly half the time and have a high probability of relapse; bipolar II is more chronic, more depressive, and associated with more neuroticism and emotional instability between episodes than bipolar I (Keller, 2004).

Magnetic resonance spectroscopy imaging (MRSI) of the brains of patients (before starting medication) shows different patterns in the chemical fingerprint in more severe cases than patients with mild-to-moderate disease. Severe BD requires more aggressive treatment. Cholesterol levels are lower during manic and depressive phases. Individuals treated with omega-3 fatty acids (in combination with their usual mood stabilizing medications) for 4 months experience fewer mood swings (Keck et al, 2006).

For treatment of resistant BD, high-dose thyroid hormones, calcium channel blockers, electroconvulsant therapy, omega-3 fatty acids, vitamin D_3, and psychosocial strategies have been investigated. Comorbid conditions are almost always involved. Anxiety, substance use, and conduct disorders are the most common; overeating, hypersexuality, attention-deficit hyperactivity, impulse control, autism spectrum disorders, and Tourette's syndrome are less common (McElroy, 2004). For these "dual diagnoses," both psychotherapy and appropriate medications are important (Levin and Hennessey, 2004).

The most common medical comorbidities include migraine, thyroid illness, obesity, type 2 diabetes, cardiovascular disease, chronic fatigue syndrome, asthma, chronic bronchitis, multiple chemical sensitivities, hypertension, and gastric ulcer tend to be significantly higher in bipolar patients (McElroy, 2004; McIntyre et al, 2006). Painful physical symptoms are common. Treatment of both physical and emotional symptoms associated with mood disorders may increase a patient's chance of achieving remission; abnormalities of serotonin and noradrenaline are strongly associated (Wise et al, 2005).

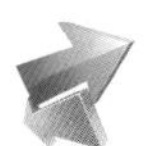

ASSESSMENT, MONITORING, AND EVALUATION

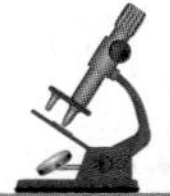

CLINICAL INDICATORS

Genetic Markers: BD and severe major depression are highly heritable, but differ from single-gene (Mendelian) diseases in that they are the end products of multiple causes (Cannon and Keller, 2006).

Clinical/History
Height
Weight
BMI
Dietary/intake history
BP
I & O
Constipation
Food pica?
Disordered eating?
Bipolar symptoms
Mood Disorder Questionnaire
Sheehan Disability Scale
Clinical Global Impression Severity and Improvement Scores for Bipolar Disorder (CGI-BP)
DEXA scan

Lab Work
H & H
Serum Fe
Alb
Chol with full profile
Trig
Serum tHcy
CRP
Serum Ca^{++}, Mg^{++}
Gluc
Serotonin
Thyroid tests (T3, T4, TSH)
Na^+, K^+

SAMPLE NUTRITION CARE PROCESS STEPS

Inadequate Intake of Certain Types of Fats

Assessment Data: Low serum cholesterol (LDL and HDL); cycling BD with little or no intake during manic and depressive phases; low weight for height.

Nutrition Diagnoses (PES): Inadequate intake of omega-3 fatty acids related to cycling BD with poor appetite and low fat intake as evidenced by total cholesterol <140 (low LDL and HDL) and BMI of 17.5.

Interventions: Food and nutrient delivery related to change in diet to include more omega 3 fatty acids and total kilocals. Education about the role of lipid in proper brain functioning. Counseling about healthy "brain foods" such as salmon, tuna, antioxidant foods.

Monitoring and Evaluation: Dietary intake records showing improved intake of omega-3 fatty acids, energy, and regular meals; BMI improving and closer to low normal (18.5).

INTERVENTION

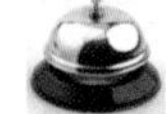

OBJECTIVES

- Support efforts at maintaining a balance between nutritional intake, physical activity, medications, and well-being.
- Monitor energy intake; counsel appropriately and offer tips for reducing kilocals from meals, snacks, and beverages. Metabolic syndrome can result.
- Monitor for medical problems related to weight gain, such as low HDL and high LDL cholesterol levels, elevated triglyceride levels, hyperglycemia or diabetes, and cardiovascular problems.
- Seek stable periods that are relatively normal ("euthymia"). Reduce stress, which elevates protein kinase C levels in the brain.
- Manage comorbid conditions that occur, such as diabetes, obesity, cardiovascular disease, and thyroid disorders.
- Maintain bone density since losses are common with use of various medications.

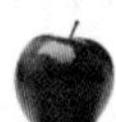

FOOD AND NUTRITION

- Persons with BD may need an energy-controlled diet if their medications cause weight gain or obesity. Those who eat poorly will need a change in habits to gain weight.
- Snacks that are low in energy or fat may be useful between meals. Offer suggestions on what to keep on hand.
- During episodes of depression, keep prepared meals such as frozen dinners or packaged meals on hand.
- Discuss fluid and fiber if constipation is a problem.
- Include sufficient to higher levels of calcium and vitamin D intake from diet; a multivitamin–mineral supplement may be beneficial.
- Include omega-3 fatty acids. Fish oil–enriched diets increase omega-3 fatty acids in tissue phospholipids; flax oil increases circulating 18:3ω-3, thereby presenting tissue with this EFA for further elongation and desaturation (Barcelo-Coblijn et al, 2005).

Common Drugs Used and Potential Side Effects

- Because of the risks of treating BD with antidepressant monotherapy, physicians should assess their depressed patients for mania before prescribing antidepressants (Olfson et al, 2005).
- The APA guideline for the treatment of BD recommends optimizing individual medications before switching to combination therapy, especially preventing discontinuation of therapy because of side effects (Bowden, 2004). Depressive symptoms of BD have a more negative impact on a patient's life than manic symptoms (Gao and Calabrese, 2005).
- **New antipsychotics** are effective for acute mania, and some may ultimately prove effective in acute depression (e.g., olanzapine combined with fluoxetine, quetiapine) and maintenance (Gao and Calabrese, 2005). Some antipsychotics, particularly olanzapine, clozapine, chlorpromazine, and thioridazine, result in serious weight gain. Energy expenditure is lower in people taking atypical antipsychotics; weight management programs may need to offer 280 kcals less per day (Sharpe et al, 2005). Aripiprazole (Abilify) is effective and has fewer side effects than some of the other atypical antipsychotics (Perlis et al, 2006).
- **Mood stabilizers**, such as lithium carbonate (Lithane, Lithobid, Lithotabs) and valproate, stabilize mood by significantly decreasing the manic, hypomanic, and depressive symptoms. Lithium causes weight gain; up to 25% of lithium users become clinically obese. Lithium requires constancy in sodium intake and limits on caffeine. Metallic taste, nausea, vomiting, and diarrhea may also occur. Valproate increases testosterone levels in teenage girls and may lead to polycystic ovary syndrome; careful monitoring is needed. These medications are contraindicated in pregnancy and lactation; lithium is associated with cardiac malformations, and valproate has been associated with neural tube defects.
- **New anticonvulsants** may be useful for aspects of BDs. Lamotrigine is used for maintenance or for acute bipolar depression. Compared with lithium and divalproex, lamotrigine is more effective in preventing bipolar depression (Gao and Calabrese, 2005). Topiramate may be used for problems related to obesity, bulimia, alcohol dependence, and migraine.
- **Multinutrient combinations** of vitamins, minerals, herbals, and the omega-3 fatty acids eicosapentaenoic acid (EPA) and DHA have been found to be somewhat effective (Kidd, 2004). Pramipexole, a dopamine D2/D3 receptor agonist, and omega-3 fatty acidsare used to augment mood stabilizers and are excellent in reducing depressive symptoms (Gao and Calabrese, 2005).
- Treatment of comorbid conditions may include use of gabapentin for anxiety or pain and zonisamide for obesity.
- **Medicines that can cause mania** include: amphetamines, Antabuse, anticholinergics, baclofen, benztropine, bromocriptine, bupropion, captopril, cimetidine, corticosteroids, cyclosporine, hydralazine, isoniazid, levodopa, MAOIs such as Nardil or Parnate, Ritalin, Synthroid, opioids, procarbazine, and yohimbe.
- **Medicines that can cause depression** include: acyclovir, alcohol, anticonvulsants, asparaginase, baclofen, barbiturates, benzodiazepines, beta-blockers, bromocriptine, calcium channel blockers, corticosteroids, cycloserine, dapsone, estrogens, fluoroquinolone, histamine H_2–receptor antagonists, interferon, isotretinoin, mefloquine, methyldopa, metoclopramide, narcotics, progestins, statins, sulfonamides.

Herbs, Botanicals, and Supplements

- Ginger, licorice, purslane, rosemary, and ginseng have been suggested; no clinical trials have proven efficacy in BDs.
- Ginseng and yohimbe should not be used with MAO inhibitors.
- Gingko biloba interacts with anticoagulants and antiplatelets such as aspirin, warfarin, and dipyridamole.
- L-tryptophan may be tried for insomnia or depression. Do not use with MAO inhibitors, SSRI antidepressants, or serotonin receptor antagonists.
- Ma huang (ephedra) and kava should not be taken by patients with depression.
- Omega-3 fatty acids have a benefit in managing depression. Supplementation may improve symptoms of depression in children and BD in adults; 360 mg/d EPA and 1560 mg/d DHA for 6 weeks show good results (Clayton et al, 2009).
- Psyllium and ginseng should not be used with divalproex or lithium.
- St. John's wort is used as a natural antidepressant. Do not use with MAO inhibitors, SSRI antidepressants, cyclosporine, digoxin, oral contraceptives, HIV protease inhibitors, theophylline, warfarin, or calcium channel blockers such as amlodipine, diltiazem, or verapamil.

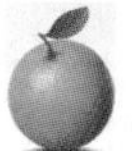

NUTRITION EDUCATION, COUNSELING, CARE MANAGEMENT

- Teach creative menu planning and food preparation methods that address the side effects and symptoms the patient is experiencing.
- Teach the patient how to moisten foods for dry mouth syndrome resulting from certain medications. Sugar-free candy may help.
- Limit caffeine-containing foods and beverages in the late evening to improve sleep.
- Individuals who are prone to bouts of depression or mania may find it difficult to eat properly. Simple meals and snacks should be readily available.
- Since there is a higher risk for suicide, individuals with BD should be carefully monitored for signs of severe depression and should seek help from a mental health professional immediately.
- Functional outcomes are reliable measure of response to treatment. Changes in circadian rhythm and sleep patterns may predict onset of relapse. Patients and families may benefit from education and therapy.

Patient Education—Foodborne Illness

- Careful food handling will be important. The same is true for hand washing.

For More Information

- Bipolar Disorder
  http://www.cmellc.com/topics/bdfaq.html
- Depression and Bipolar Support Alliance
  http://www.dbsalliance.org/
- Food and Mood
  http://www.dbsalliance.org/pdfs/foodmoode2.pdf
- JAMA Patient Page
  http://jama.ama-assn.org/cgi/reprint/301/5/564.pdf
- Medline—Bipolar Disorder
  http://www.nlm.nih.gov/medlineplus/bipolardisorder.html
- Mental Health Links
  http://mentalhealth.samhsa.gov/links/default2.asp
- NIMH—Bipolar Disorder
  http://www.nimh.nih.gov/health/publications/bipolar-disorder/complete-index.shtml
- National Mental Health Information Center
  http://www.mentalhealth.samhsa.gov/

BIPOLAR DISORDER—CITED REFERENCES

Barcelo-Coblijn G, et al. Dietary alpha-linolenic acid increases brain but not heart and liver docosahexaenoic acid levels. *Lipids.* 40:787, 2005.

Bowden CL. Making optimal use of combination pharmacotherapy in bipolar disorder. *J Clin Psychiatry.* 15:21S, 2004.

Cannon TD, Keller MC. Endophenotypes in the genetic analyses of mental disorders. *Annu Rev Clin Psychol.* 2:267, 2006.

Clayton EH. Reduced mania and depression in juvenile bipolar disorder associated with long-chain omega-3 polyunsaturated fatty acid supplementation. [published online ahead of print January 21, 2009] *Eur J Clin Nutr.* 63(8):1037, 2009.

Das AK, et al. Screening for bipolar disorder in a primary care practice. *JAMA.* 293:956, 2005.

Gao K, Calabrese JR. Newer treatment studies for bipolar depression. *Bipolar Disord.* 7:13S, 2005.

Keck PE Jr, et al. Double-blind, randomized, placebo-controlled trials of ethyl-eicosapentanoate in the treatment of bipolar depression and rapid cycling bipolar disorder. *Biol Psychiatry.* 60:1020, 2006.

Keller MB. Improving the course of illness and promoting continuation of treatment of bipolar disorder. *J Clin Psychiatry.* 15:10S, 2004.

Kidd PM. Bipolar disorder and cell membrane dysfunction. Progress toward integrative management. *Altern Med Rev.* 9:107, 2004.

Levin FR, Hennessey G. Bipolar disorder and substance abuse. *Biol Psychiatry.* 56:738, 2004.

McElroy SL. Diagnosing and treating comorbid (complicated) bipolar disorder. *J Clin Psychiatry.* 15:35S, 2004.

McIntyre RS, et al. Medical comorbidity in bipolar disorder: implications for functional outcomes and health service utilization. *Psychiatr Serv.* 57: 1140, 2006.

Olfson M, et al. Bipolar depression in a low-income primary care clinic. *Am J Psychiatry.* 162:2146, 2005.

Perlis RH, et al. Atypical antipsychotics in the treatment of mania: a meta-analysis of randomized, placebo-controlled trials. *J Clin Psychiatry.* 67:509, 2006.

Sharpe JK, et al. Resting energy expenditure is lower than predicted in people taking atypical antipsychotic medication. *J Am Diet Assoc.* 105:612, 2005.

Wise TN, et al. Management of painful physical symptoms associated with depression and mood disorders. *CNS Spectr.* 10:1S, 2005.

DEPRESSION

NUTRITIONAL ACUITY RANKING: LEVEL 1 (MILD); LEVEL 2 (NUMEROUS MEDICATIONS)

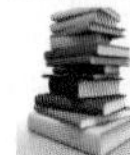

DEFINITIONS AND BACKGROUND

Depression involves changes in body chemistry (neurotransmitters) because of genetics or after a traumatic event, hormonal changes, altered health habits, the presence of another illness, or substance abuse. Persons with major depressive disorder (MDD) have had at least one major depressive episode over a 14-day period or longer. It may be recurrent throughout their lives. MDD is debilitating and has a high morbidity rate (Farah, 2009).

The lifetime risk for depression is 10–25% in women, 5–12% in men (Fava, 2007). Depression frequently develops between the ages of 25 and 44. Approximately 20 million adult Americans experience depression every day. Diagnosis of depression is indicated by four of eight of the following symptoms: SIGECAPS—Sleep changes, loss of Interest, inappropriate Guilt (hopelessness), Energy decline, Concentration changes, Appetite changes, Psychomotor changes, and Suicidal tendencies. In addition, prolonged sadness and unexplained crying spells, chronic irritability and agitation or anxiety, chronic pessimism or indifference, indecisiveness, social withdrawal, and unexplained aches and pains may also be present.

Folate seems to have a causal relationship in depression (Lewis et al, 2006). When there are lower red blood cell folate levels, episodes of depression are longer and more severe (Fava, 2007). Deplin® contains 7.5 mg L-methylfolate and may help in managing depressive episodes. It unmasks vitamin B_{12} anemia whereas folic acid masks vitamin B_{12} anemia. After 4-week trials of Deplin®, if patients are not feeling better, psychiatrists often recommend doubling the dose to 15 mg/d (Zajecka, 2007).

Depression is a leading cause of disability in the United States. Careful assessment is needed to determine the specific type of depression and its most effective treatments. **Dysthymia** is a chronic, moderate type of depression expressed as poor appetite or overeating, insomnia or oversleeping, low energy, fatigue, irritability, and high stress. Children and teens who experience depression may experience frequent headaches and absences from school. Men often mask signs of depression by working long hours or drinking too much. Women may have depression during times of hormonal change (menstruation, pregnancy, miscarriage, the postpartum period, and menopause). **Postpartum depression** negatively affects both mother and child; early detection and treatment are needed.

Older individuals may experience depression along with a chronic disease such as heart disease, diabetes, or hypertension. CRP tends to be elevated in depression and may contribute to heart disease (Ford and Erlinger, 2004). Elevated tHcy levels should be treated. In nursing homes, it is expected that about 50% of individuals will have some form of depression for which medication should be prescribed.

Many persons with depression have a deficiency of brain serotonin. A mixed diet of protein/CHO should provide tryptophan, a precursor of serotonin. Intake of dietary protein high in tryptophan increases the ratio of tryptophan to large neutral amino acids (LNAA). Antidepressants that are serotonin reuptake modulators actually promote growth of serotonin innervation in the forebrain (Zhou et al, 2006). Painful physical symptoms commonly exist comorbid with depressive disorders; abnormalities of serotonin and noradrenaline are strongly associated and play a role in pain perception (Wise et al, 2005).

Psychotherapy can change brain chemistry after cognitive restructuring. For some persons for whom medications and therapy are not effective, electroconvulsive therapy (ECT) may also be helpful. A pacemaker-like device that sends electrical stimulations into the vagus nerve of the neck may help to alleviate depressive symptoms. And, recent studies show that vitamin D is an important component for alleviating depression. SAD increases with latitude, so vitamin D and sunlight or light therapy may be beneficial.

Monitoring physical health, including nutrition, is an important adjunct to medication or psychotherapy. Adequate intake of the omega-3 fatty acids may reduce depression (Casper, 2004). The omega-3 fatty acids are important components of nerve cell membranes and help nerve cells communicate with each other. In medicated patients, added treatment with omega-3 fatty acids, particularly EPA, may ameliorate symptoms of MDD (Casper, 2004). Finally, use of fresh versus highly processed foods should be considered. A highly processed food dietary pattern is a risk factor for depression years later, whereas a whole food pattern is protective (Akbaraly et al, 2009).

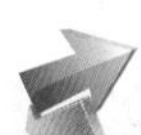

ASSESSMENT, MONITORING, AND EVALUATION

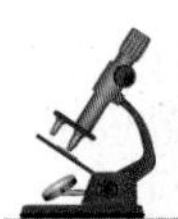

CLINICAL INDICATORS

Genetic Markers: About 40% of risk for major depression is inherited; 60% is from environmental factors such as substance abuse. Multiple genes play a role in depression (Psychiatric GWAS Consortium, 2009). Individuals with the C>T type of MTHFR allele are at high risk for depression (Almeida et al, 2008). Testing for MTHFR levels and augmenting therapy with methylfolate and omega-3 fatty acids is suggested (Fava, 2007; Shelton, 2007). Research has identified some genetic mutations found only in women, related to female hormone regulation; these biological differences are being clarified.

Clinical/History
Height
Weight
BMI
Weight changes
Dietary/intake history
BP
Food pica
I & O
Constipation
DEXA scan

Lab Work
H & H
Serum Fe
Alb
Ca^{++}, Mg^{++}
Gluc
Serotonin
Thyroid tests (T3, T4, TSH)
Na^{+}, K^{+}
N balance
MTHFR
Serum tHcy
Serum folate and B_{12}
CRP

SAMPLE NUTRITION CARE PROCESS STEPS

Altered Nutrient Utilization

Assessment Data: Altered methyltetrahydrofolate reductase (MTHFR) with C>T allele; signs of severe depression with insomnia and poor dietary intake; elevated tHcy levels.

Nutrition Diagnoses (PES): Altered nutrient utilization of folate related to MTHFR allele as evidenced by lab test, diagnosis of MDD, and poor intake from oral diet.

Interventions: Education about the role of folate in depression; discussion about genetics and how the C>T allele can aggravate depression. Counseling about use of L-methylfolate and dietary sources of folate, vitamins B_6 and B_{12}.

Monitoring and Evaluation: Improved lab results for tHcy; fewer episodes of prolonged depression; improved quality of life.

INTERVENTION

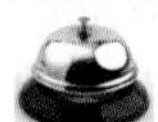

OBJECTIVES

- Provide adequate nutritional intake (e.g., excessive weight loss or shock therapy requires increased energy intake). Monitor weight at least twice monthly to evaluate status and changes.
- Assess usual eating habits and related problems, which may include loneliness, difficulty in activities of daily living, boredom, lack of hobbies and interests, and poor sleep habits. Adequate drug therapy usually helps appetite improve.
- Monitor for consequences from certain antidepressants, such as weight gain.
- Assure adequate intake of amino acids, omega-3 fatty acids, folic acid, vitamins D_3 and B_{12}.
- Reduce stress, which elevates protein kinase C levels in the brain.

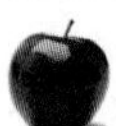

FOOD AND NUTRITION

- Use a diet providing high-quality protein. Inadequate protein intake may reflect decreased intake of iron, thiamine, riboflavin, niacin, and vitamins B_6 and B_{12} as well.
- Increase intake of omega-3 fatty acids and uridine from foods such as fish, walnuts, molasses, and sugar beets (Carlezon et al, 2005). Supplements may also be used, but dietary change is beneficial.
- Low serum folate is common in many depressed adults, especially women (Ramos et al, 2004; Tolmunen et al, 2004). Intake of 400 μg is needed daily. Use L-methylfolate where MTHFR alleles have been identified.
- Vitamin D_3 and calcium should be supplemented (Mussolino et al, 2004; Payne et al, 2008).
- If serum tHcy levels are high, include vitamins B_6 and B_{12} in addition to folate.
- Use a tyramine-restricted diet for patients given MAOI drugs. Such a diet excludes aged cheese, beer, red wine, ale, chicken livers, broad bean pods, sausage, salami,

pepperoni, commercial gravies, ripe avocado, fermented soy sauce, and pickled or smoked herring.

- If overeating, limit access to food and provide low-calorie diet information.
- Encourage increased physical activity, which often helps to lift depressed moods.
- Sometimes a craving for carbohydrates occurs; monitor if weight gain is a problem or if overall nutrient density decreases.
- Liquid supplements may be useful when preparing meals seems overwhelming.
- TPN is not advised for patients who are suicidal.

Common Drugs Used and Potential Side Effects

- SSRIs and TCAs do not always provide symptom relief. Yet, the SSRIs increase the density of nerve-impulse carrying axons in the brain, thus rewiring the neocortex and limbic system (Zhou et al, 2006). Their use may be more beneficial than previously anticipated.
- Some serotonergic antidepressants (e.g., fluoxetine, Prozac) can reduce hyperglycemia, normalize glucose homeostasis, and increase insulin sensitivity, whereas some noradrenergic antidepressants (e.g., desipramine) exert opposite effects (McIntyre et al, 2006).
- L-methylfolate may be needed to help alleviate depression (Mischoulon and Raab, 2007; Stahl, 2007).
- See Table 4-19 for more details.

Herbs, Botanicals, and Supplements

- Ginseng and yohimbe should not be used with MAO inhibitors.
- Licorice, ginger, purslane, rosemary, and ginseng have been suggested for depression; no clinical trials prove efficacy.
- L-tryptophan may be tried for insomnia or depression. Do not use with MAO inhibitors, SSRI antidepressants, or serotonin receptor antagonists.
- Ma huang (ephedra) and kava should not be used with antidepressants.
- Omega-3 fatty acids (EPA and DHA) may be taken in capsule form; usually 1000 mg several times a day will be needed.
- St. John's wort is used as a natural antidepressant. Do not use with MAO inhibitors, SSRI antidepressants, cyclosporine, digoxin, oral contraceptives, HIV protease inhibitors, theophylline, warfarin, or calcium channel blockers such as amlodipine, diltiazem, or verapamil.

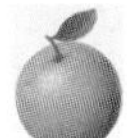

NUTRITION EDUCATION, COUNSELING, CARE MANAGEMENT

- Encourage full involvement with psychotherapy, CBT, or interpersonal therapy (IPT). These are helpful adjuncts for medication. Hopefulness and resilience are also important.

TABLE 4-19 The Bipolar Spectrum and Symptoms

Bipolar type I	Depression and varying degrees of excitatory signs and symptoms up to full mania	Onset during teens and early adulthood; 60% will have problems with substance abuse
Bipolar type II	Discrete hypomanic episodes; may appear to have just depression, but mood stabilizers seem to help more than antidepressants	50% will have problems with substance abuse
Bipolar type III	Hypomania associated with antidepressants and/or psychostimulants	
Bipolar type IV	Hyperthymic temperament	Onset during 4th or 5th decade of life
Bipolar type V	Recurrent depressions without discrete irritability, hypomania, but mixed hypomanic episodes with agitation, and racing thoughts during depression	
Bipolar type VI	Alzheimer's type	Onset in the 6th or 7th decade
Manic symptoms	Severe changes in mood, either extremely irritable or overly silly and elated Overly inflated self-esteem, grandiosity Increased energy Decreased need for sleep, ability to go with very little or no sleep for days without tiring Increased talking, talks too much, too fast; changes topics too quickly; cannot be interrupted Distractibility, attention moves constantly from one thing to the next Hypersexuality, increased sexual thoughts, feelings, or behaviors; use of explicit sexual language Increased goal-directed activity or physical agitation Disregard of risk, excessive involvement in risky behaviors or activities	
Depressive symptoms	Persistent sad or irritable mood Loss of interest in activities once enjoyed Significant change in appetite or body weight Difficulty sleeping or oversleeping Physical agitation or slowing Loss of energy Feelings of worthlessness or inappropriate guilt Difficulty concentrating Recurrent thoughts of death or suicide	

- Teach creative menu planning and food preparation methods that address the side effects and symptoms the patient is experiencing.
- Promote the use of whole foods (fruits, vegetables, fish) and discourage processed foods (fried foods, sweetened desserts, processed meats; Akbarahly et al, 2009).
- Teach the patient how to moisten foods for dry mouth syndrome resulting from certain medications. Sugar-free candy may help.
- Promote exercise, which seems to help reduce symptoms of depression. Teens may be especially vulnerable to depression, and exercise may help improve other health-related behaviors, including eating better (Fulkerson et al, 2004).
- Limit caffeine-containing foods and beverages in the late evening to promote better sleep.
- Nicotine dependence and major depression are often related; treat mutually (Manley et al, 2009).
- After giving birth, postpartum "blues," postpartum depression, or postpartum psychosis may occur. Maternal depression in the perinatal period may lead to poor growth for infants (Rahman et al, 2004). Education is needed for new mothers.
- In the elderly, "failure to thrive" usually includes impaired physical function, malnutrition, depression, and cognitive impairment (Robertson and Montagnini, 2004). Treatment of depression may help to improve appetite. Adding breakfast to homebound meals is a good start (Gollub and Weddle, 2004).

Patient Education—Foodborne Illness

- Careful food handling will be important. The same is true for hand washing.

For More Information

- Academy of Cognitive Therapy
http://www.academyofct.org
- American Mental Health Counselors Association
http://www.amhca.org/
- American Psychiatric Association
http://www.psych.org/
- American Society of Geriatric Psychiatry
http://www.aagpgpa.org/
- Anxiety Disorders of America
http://www.adaa.org/
- Depression
http://www.depression.com/
- National Depression Screening
http://www.mentalhealthscreening.org/infofaq/depression.aspx
- NIMH—Depression
http://www.nimh.nih.gov/health/publications/depression/complete-index.shtml

DEPRESSION—CITED REFERENCES

Akbaraly TN, et al. Dietary pattern and depressive symptoms in middle age. *Brit J Psychiatry.* 195:408, 2009.

Almeida OP, et al. Homocysteine and depression in later life. *Arch Gen Psychiatry.* 65:1286, 2008.

Carlezon WA Jr, et al. Antidepressant-like effects of uridine and omega-3 fatty acids are potentiated by combined treatment in rats. *Biol Psychiatry.* 57:343, 2005.

Casper RC. Nutrients, neurodevelopment, and mood. *Curr Psychiatry Rep.* 6:425, 2004.

Colangelo LA, et al. Higher dietary intake of long-chain omega-3 polyunsaturated fatty acids is inversely associated with depressive symptoms in women. [published online ahead of print February 3, 2009] *Nutrition.* 25:1011, 2009.

Farah A. The role of L-methylfolate in depressive disorders. *CNS Spectr.* 14:2, 2009.

Fava M. Augmenting antidepressants with folate: a clinical perspective. *J Clin Psychiatry.* 68:4S, 2007.

Ford DE, Erlinger TP. Depression and C-reactive protein in US adults: data from the Third National Health and Nutrition Examination Survey. *Arch Intern Med.* 164:1010, 2004.

Fulkerson JA, et al. Depressive symptoms and adolescent eating and health behaviors: a multifaceted view in a population-based sample. *Prev Med.* 38:865, 2004.

Gollub EA, Weddle DO. Improvements in nutritional intake and quality of life among frail homebound older adults receiving home-delivered breakfast and lunch. *J Am Diet Assoc.* 104:1227, 2004.

Lewis SJ, et al. The thermolabile variant of MTHFR is associated with depression in the British Women's Heart and Health Study and a meta-analysis. *Mol Psychiatry.* 11:352, 2006.

Manley MJ, et al. Association of major depression with subtypes of nicotine dependence found among adult daily smokers: a latent class analysis. [published online ahead of print June 6, 2009] *Drug Alcohol Depend.* 104:126, 2009.

McIntyre RS, et al. The effect of antidepressants on glucose homeostasis and insulin sensitivity: synthesis and mechanisms. *Expert Opin Drug Saf.* 5:157, 2006.

Mischoulon D, Raab MF. The role of folate in depression and dementia. *J Clin Psychiatry.* 68:28S, 2007.

Mussolino ME, et al. Depression and bone mineral density in young adults: results from NHANES III. *Psychosom Med.* 66:533, 2004.

Payne ME, et al. Calcium and vitamin D intakes may be positively associated with brain lesions in depressed and nondepressed elders. *Nutr Res.* 28:285, 2008.

Rahman A, et al. Impact of maternal depression on infant nutritional status and illness: a cohort study. *Arch Gen Psychiatry.* 61:946, 2004.

Ramos MI, et al. Plasma folate concentrations are associated with depressive symptoms in elderly Latina women despite folic acid fortification. *Am J Clin Nutr.* 80:1024, 2004.

Robertson RG, Montagnini M. Geriatric failure to thrive. *Am Fam Physician.* 70:343, 2004.

Shelton RC. Augmentation Strategies to Increase Antidepressant Efficacy. *J Clin Psychiatry.* 68:18S, 2007.

Stahl SM. Novel therapeutics for depression: L-methylfolate as a trimonoamine modulator and antidepressant-augmenting agent. *CNS Spectrum.* 12:739, 2007.

Todorovic Z, et al. Homocysteine serum levels and MTHFR C677 T genotype in patients with Parkinson's disease, with and without levodopa therapy. *J Neurol Sci.* 248:56, 2006.

Tolmunen T, et al. Dietary folate and the risk of depression in Finnish middle-aged men. A prospective follow-up study. *Psychother Psychosom.* 73:334, 2004.

Wise TN, et al. Management of painful physical symptoms associated with depression and mood disorders. *CNS Spectr.* 10:1S, 2005.

Zajecka JM. Augmentation strategies to increase antidepressant tolerability. *J Clin Psychiatry.* 68(10):23S, 2007.

Zhou L, et al. Evidence that serotonin reuptake modulators increase the density of serotonin innervation in the forebrain. *J Neurochem.* 96:396, 2006.

SCHIZOPHRENIA

NUTRITIONAL ACUITY RANKING: LEVEL 1–2

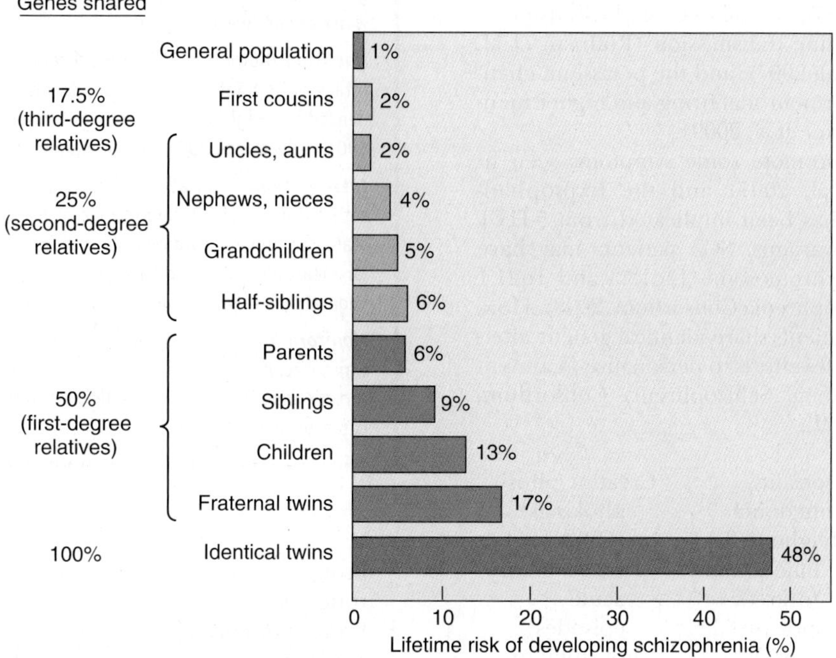

Adapted from: Gottesman, 1991, p. 96.

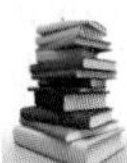

DEFINITIONS AND BACKGROUND

SCZ is a group of disorders manifested by disordered thinking, hallucinations, delusions, apathy, social withdrawal, and mood or behavioral disturbances (delusional, catatonic, or paranoid). In the resulting psychosis, the individual loses contact with reality. SCZ has a heritability estimated at 73–90% (International Schizophrenia Consortium, 2008).

SCZ can be either episodic or chronic. When patients are at risk of self-harm or harm to others, hospital treatment is appropriate. Delusions may involve control, persecution, grandiosity, or abnormal fears. Hallucinations are perceptions of an external stimulus without a source in the external world.

Nearly 1% of the population develops SCZ, with onset generally between ages 15 and 25 years (earlier in males). SCZ has been thought to have a genetic component and is associated with reduced dopamine signaling and executive function impairment (Roffman et al, 2007). However, there are many structural DNA copy number variants (CNVs) in the brains of individuals with SCZ; these rare deleterious variants may be more important in SCZ predisposition than common polymorphisms (Need et al, 2009).

Molecular mechanisms critical for adolescent brain development are disturbed in SCZ patients from genes associated with energy metabolism and protein and lipid synthesis (Harris et al, 2009). Oxidative stress, oxidative injury, and abnormal membrane phospholipid metabolism suggest that PUFA fatty acid depletion occurs (duBois et al, 2005). Similar to diabetes, conversion of ALA to EPA or DHA is inefficient in SCZ. Supplementation with antioxidants and omega-3 fatty acids is recommended. Otherwise, effective serum lipid control is difficult to attain (Weiss et al, 2006).

Low vitamin D availability during brain development interacts with susceptibility genes to alter brain development. Vitamin D supplementation during the first year of life is important, especially in families with a history of SCZ.

Folate, cobalamin (B_{12}), tHcy, and MTHFR polymorphisms are also found in SCZ. Patients with SCZ who have the MTHFR A>C genotype have a slight correlation with positive symptoms such as hallucinations and hearing voices, whereas the C>T allele promotes negative symptoms (depression, dysthymia) but actually protects against positive symptoms (Roffman et al, 2007; Zintzaras, 2006). Both folate and cobalamin deficiencies should be identified (Miller, 2008). Supplementation with S-adenosylmethionine (SAM) may be useful (Frankenburg, 2007; Gilbody et al, 2007).

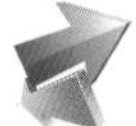

ASSESSMENT, MONITORING, AND EVALUATION

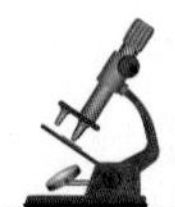

CLINICAL INDICATORS

Genetic Markers: No single gene has been identified. Reelin (a secretory protease that manages neuronal migration, dopamine signaling, and synaptogenesis) is heavily methylated in SCZ (Guidotti et al, 2009; Roffman et al, 2007; Suzuki et al, 2008). Viral infections reduce reelin levels and may trigger SCZ. If the reelin-VLDLR/ApoER2 signaling pathway is significant, peripheral VLDLR mRNA levels may be biological markers of SCZ (Suzuki et al, 2008). Other susceptibility genes are neuregulin 1 (NRG1); DISC-1 genes (Lipska et al, 2006); catechol-O-methyltransferase (COMT) for dopamine transmission (Roffman et al, 2008; Woodward et al, 2007); and the potassium channel KCNH2 gene, for neuronal firing and higher mental functions (Huffaker et al, 2009).

MTHFR alleles promote some symptoms seen in SCZ (Roffman et al, 2007) and the tryptophan-serotonin pathway has been implicated from 5-HTT gene polymorphic variants. SCZ patients may have large deletions on chromosome 15q13.3 and 1q21.1 (International Schizophrenia Consortium, 2008). However, very few SCZ patients share identical genetic alterations; this complicates efforts to personalize treatment regimens (International Schizophrenia Consortium, 2008; Need et al, 2009).

Clinical/History

Height
Weight
Weight changes
BMI
Dietary/intake history
I & O
BP
Global Assessment of Functioning Scale (GAF)
Positive and Negative Syndrome Scale (PANSS)
Delusions, auditory hallucinations
Blunted speech
Flat affect
Lack of motivation
Asociality
Anhedonia
Heightened emotionality to stress
Disorganized speech and thought disorder
EEG and brainwave patterns
MRI with hippocampus reduction (Velakoulis et al, 2006)
PET scans

Lab Work

Peripheral VLDLR mRNA levels
Gluc
Creatine phosphokinase (CPK) (elevated in acute episodes)
Chol (total profile)
Trig
Alb, transthyretin
Na^+, K^+
H & H
Serum Fe
tHcy
Methylmalonic acid
MTHFR polymorphisms
Serum folate and B_{12}
CRP
Serum insulin
Serum D_3
Ca^{++}, Mg^{++}

INTERVENTION

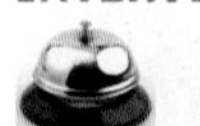

OBJECTIVES

- Develop a trusting relationship; make expectations clear to the patient.
- Provide adequate nourishment to prevent significant weight changes; gain is common with many antipsychotic medications.
- Correct any nutritional deficits in folate, vitamins B_6 and B_{12}, and vitamin D. Use L-methylfolate with MTHFR alleles.

SAMPLE NUTRITION CARE PROCESS STEPS

Poor Food Choices

Assessment Data: Food records indicating poor intake; weight gain; elevated serum LDL and triglycerides; hypertension; high waist circumference.

Nutrition Diagnoses (PES): Poor food choices related to regular intake of high fat, fast foods and few fruits and vegetables as evidenced by weight gain while on antipsychotics, BP of 170/95, LDL 190, triglycerides 300, waist circumference 42 and BMI 32.

Interventions: Education about better food choices to lower serum lipids and BP; importance of managing weight and health status to prevent cardiovascular disease. Counseling about regular mealtimes, ways to increase fiber, antioxidant-rich fruit and vegetable intake. Use motivational interviewing.

Monitoring and Evaluation: Improved weight status (lower BMI, waist circumference); lipids closer to normal for age and sex; no further weight gain with medicines; better food choices as indicated on food records.

- Promote a normal pattern of dietary intake and exercise routines.
- Prevent or correct constipation or impaction.
- Manage diabetes and coronary heart disease, which tend to be common and often under-diagnosed (Henderson, 2005). Metabolic syndrome is—two to four times higher in SCZ than in the general population (Ellingrod et al, 2008; McEvoy et al, 2005). Both decreased MTHFR activity (in C>T allele carriers) and elevated tHcy can increase risk of cardiovascular disease (Ellingrod et al, 2008).
- Reduce stress, which increases protein kinase C in the brain, increases forgetfulness, and speeds up the aging process.

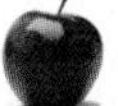

FOOD AND NUTRITION

- A balanced diet for age and sex should be used. Reduce sugars and saturated fats if diabetes or metabolic syndrome are present.
- Adjust calories according to goal weight for patient and medications.
- Reduce potential accidents by avoiding glass containers and serving dishes.
- Vitamins C, D, B_6, and B_{12}, folate, and selenium levels may be low in persons with SCZ; encourage improved intake accordingly.
- Highlight the use of antioxidant-rich foods (berries, nuts, green tea) and omega-3 fatty acids (salmon, tuna, sardines).
- Suggest use of the DASH diet if BP is high.

Common Drugs Used and Potential Side Effects

- Some drugs can cause psychiatric symptoms. Anxiety, mania, hallucinations, suicidal thoughts, and bizarre behavior may result from various medications, and a doctor should be contacted if these occur:

Confusion: acyclovir, propoxyphene (Darvon), and cimetidine (Tagamet)
Depression: oral contraceptives, ibuprofen, metronidazole (Flagyl), barbiturates, cimetidine, and diazepam (Valium)
Excitement or agitation: alprazolam, amphetamines, barbiturates, metronidazole, and diazepam Insomnia: acyclovir and alprazolam
Paranoia: amphetamines, cannabis, ibuprofen, cimetidine, and TCAs

- Try offering a beverage or snack to reduce anxiety before adding new medications (Ativan, Xanax, Klonopin, Paxil).
- To reduce hypermethylation of GABAergic promoters, COX-2 inhibitors or valproate may be used along with atypical antipsychotics (Table 4-20).
- What works for one person may not work for another. See Table 4-21 for more guidance on medications.

Herbs, Botanicals, and Supplements

- Ginseng should not be used with CNS stimulants, caffeine, hormones, steroids, antipsychotics, MAO inhibitors, lithium.
- Gingko biloba interacts with anticoagulants and antiplatelets such as aspirin, warfarin, and dipyridamole.
- Indian snakeroot is used for mental illness in some cultures. Do not use with digoxin, phenobarbital, levodopa, albuterol, furosemide, thiazide diuretics, MAO inhibitors, beta-blockers such as atenolol or propranolol, or tranquilizers. Problems include potential sedation, increased BP, arrhythmias, and CNS excitation.
- Kava and valerian should not be taken with anxiety-reducing drugs (e.g., alprazolam, diazepam, lorazepam).
- Tryptophan metabolism may be altered by proinflammatory cytokines; this affects serotonin production and functioning. If L-tryptophan is taken, avoid use with MAO inhibitors, SSRI antidepressants, or serotonin receptor antagonists. Deaths have been related to the use of L-tryptophan in the past.
- Ma huang (ephedra) and kava should not be taken in patients with depression.
- Psyllium should not be used with divalproex or lithium.
- St. John's wort should not be used with MAO inhibitors, SSRI antidepressants, cyclosporine, digoxin, oral contraceptives, HIV protease inhibitors, theophylline, warfarin, or calcium channel blockers such as amlodipine, diltiazem, or verapamil.
- Yohimbe should not be used with MAO inhibitors.

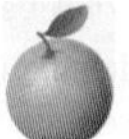

NUTRITION EDUCATION, COUNSELING, CARE MANAGEMENT

- Teach nutrition principles to the patient or the caregiver.
- Encourage self-care. Successfully terminate client relationship when independence is possible.
- Provide follow-up, especially with regression. If daily medications are a problem, monthly injectable medications may be useful.
- Trauma, pain, endocrine disorders, infection, and metabolic disorders may cause agitation (Marco and Vaughan, 2005). A quiet environment is needed, especially for meals.
- Weight gain is common (Patel et al, 2009). Weight loss programs, cholesterol-lowering (TLC) plans, or the DASH diet may be needed.

TABLE 4-20 Antipsychotic Medications and Possible Side Effects

Medication	Side Effects
Tranquilizers	Triavil combines an antidepressant with a tranquilizer. Nausea, diarrhea, and vomiting may result.
Typical antipsychotics: clozapine (Clozaril),butyrophenone (Haldol), thiothixene (Navane)	May cause dizziness, drowsiness, dry mouth, weight gain, edema, nausea, constipation, or vomiting. They help to quiet symptoms and help when the patient is resistant to other drugs and alternatives.
Phenothiazines: perphenazine (Trilafon), fluphenazine (Prolixin), prochlorperazine (Compazine), chlorpromazine (Thorazine)	Chlorpromazine (Thorazine) contains sulfites. It may cause dry mouth, constipation, and weight gain.
Atypical antipsychotics (aAPs): aripiprazole (Abilify), quetiapine (Seroquel), risperidone (Risperdal), olanzapine (Zyprexa), ziprasidone (Geodon)	The phospholipids in the neuronal membranes of the brain are rich in highly unsaturated essential fatty acids (EFAs). With a beneficial effect on dyskinesia as well, EPA is an effective adjunct to antipsychotics. Aripiprazole exhibits high affinity for dopamine, serotonin, and histamine receptors. Ziprasidone is not as likely to cause weight gain as some other antipsychotics. Olanzapine performs modestly better than most other medications, but weight gain can be significant. Long-acting risperidone injection may increase adherence and lead to improved clinical and economic outcomes for individuals with schizophrenia (Edwards et al, 2005). Typical doses may be: olanzapine (schizophrenia: 15 mg; mania: 20 mg); quetiapine (schizophrenia: 750 mg; mania: 800 mg); ziprasidone (schizophrenia and mania: 160 mg); aripiprazole (schizophrenia and mania: 30 mg).
SSRIs and obsessive-compulsive disorder medications	Prozac, Anafranil, Luvox, and Zoloft have been used with some success. Avoid use with ma huang (ephedra) and St. John's wort. Fluvoxamine (Luvox) is an SSRI that may cause anorexia, dry mouth, nausea, diarrhea, and constipation.

TABLE 4-21 Medications for Depression and Mood Disorders and Possible Side Effects

Medication	Side Effects
Dual-mechanism antidepressants: Cymbalta (duloxetine), Effexor (venlafaxine)	Approved for the treatment of major depressive disorder in 2004, these are serotonin and norepinephrine reuptake inhibitors. Dual-mechanism antidepressants do not appear to disrupt glucose homeostatic dynamics. Brain-derived neurotrophic factor, which is increased with antidepressant treatment, appears to influence regulation of mood and perception of pain; evidence indicates that dual-acting agents may have an advantage in modulating pain over those agents that increase either serotonin or noradrenaline alone (Wise et al, 2005).
Other antidepressants	Clomipramine (Anafranil) is used in obsessive-compulsive disorders. Dry mouth is common; hard sugar-less candy or chewing gum may be useful. Anorexia and abdominal pain are also common. Norpramin (desipramine) may cause abdominal cramps, altered blood glucose levels, and vomiting. Avoid use with ma huang (ephedra), St. John's wort, and ginkgo biloba. Nortriptyline (Aventyl, Pamelor) may cause increased appetite for sweets, GI distress, vomiting, and diarrhea. Wellbutrin (bupropion) tends to have a stimulating effect but may also cause weight loss, dry mouth, nausea, and vomiting. It may be used to help with smoking cessation.
Monoamine oxidase inhibitors: Parnate (tranylcypromine), Nardil (phenelzine), Marplan (isocarboxazid)	Nonselective hydrazine monoamine oxidase inhibitors (e.g., phenelzine) are associated with hypoglycemia and an increased glucose disposal rate (McIntyre et al, 2006). Tyramine is a pressor amine. Tyramine-restricted diet to prevent hypertensive crisis: spoiled, overripe, and aged products are the most problematic. Beware of Chianti wines, beer, fava beans, and sauerkraut. Constipation, weight gain, and GI distress are common side effects. Avoid ginseng, L-tryptophan, yohimbe, St. John's wort, kava, and ma huang (ephedra).
SAMe (S-5-adenosyl-methionine)	Useful for mild depression but may trigger coronary problems. A positive side effect is that it may actually help with degenerative joint disease symptoms.
Selective serotonin reuptake inhibitors (SSRIs): Paxil (paroxetine), Prozac (fluoxetine), Zoloft (sertraline)	May cause abdominal pain, anorexia, diarrhea, and weight changes; SSRIs are used to treat despair and helplessness. Prozac may also cause nausea, vomiting, glucose changes, and decreased sodium. Do not use in pregnancy; neurobehavioral effects have been noted in otherwise healthy infants. Fetal exposure to a mother's antidepressants during pregnancy may leave her newborn in withdrawal, known as neonatal abstinence syndrome (Levinson-Castiel et al, 2006). Zoloft can cause dry mouth and diarrhea; avoid use with St. John's wort and ma huang (ephedra).
Tranquilizers, benzodiazepines: Halcion (triazolam), Versed (midazolam), Serax (oxazepam), Librium (chlordiazepoxide), Xanax (alprazolam), Restoril (temazepam), Ativan (lorazepam), Klonopin (clonazepam), Tranxene (clorazepate) Valium (diazepam), Dalmane (flurazepam)	The main use of the short-acting benzodiazepines is in insomnia, while anxiety responds better to medium- to long-acting substances that will be required all day. Benzodiazepines may cause either weight loss or gain and GI distress. Avoid use with sedatives or chamomile. Increased thirst is common.
Tricyclic antidepressants: Tofranil (imipramine), Elavil (amitriptyline), Asendin (amoxapine), Doxepin (sinequan)	May cause dry mouth, increase in appetite, weight gain, nausea, vomiting, syndrome of inappropriate antidiuretic hormone (SIADH), constipation, anorexia, or stomatitis.

- Osteoporosis may be a problem with long-term medication use; monitor carefully (Hummer et al, 2005).
- Breastfeeding mothers should avoid use of medications as much as possible. Should psychiatric medication be necessary, available information regarding the effects of these medications on the infant should be provided.
- Nicotine addiction is much higher in the SCZ population. Cigarette smoke contains many pro-oxidants that contribute directly to oxidative stress. Support efforts to quit, but make sure the patient is aware that psychotic symptoms may be heightened during that time.
- Substance abuse reduces the effectiveness of treatment; amphetamines, cocaine, PCP, and marijuana may make the symptoms of SCZ worse.

Patient Education—Foodborne Illness

- Careful food handling will be important. The same is true for hand washing.

For More Information

- CATIE study
  http://www.nimh.nih.gov/health/trials/practical/catie/index.shtml
- Mayo Clinic—Schizophrenia
  http://www.mayoclinic.com/health/schizophrenia/DS00196
- Medline—Schizophrenia
  http://www.nlm.nih.gov/medlineplus/schizophrenia.html
- NIMH—Schizophrenia
  http://www.nimh.nih.gov/health/publications/schizophrenia/complete-index.shtml
- Schizophrenia
  http://www.schizophrenia.com/

SCHIZOPHRENIA—CITED REFERENCES

duBois TM, et al. Membrane phospholipid composition, alterations in neurotransmitter systems and schizophrenia. *Prog Neuropsychopharmacol Biol Psychiatry.* 29:878, 2005.

Edwards NC, et al. Cost effectiveness of long-acting risperidone injection versus alternative antipsychotic agents in patients with schizophrenia in the USA. *Pharmacoeconomics.* 23:75S, 2005.

Ellingrod VL, et al. Metabolic syndrome and insulin resistance in schizophrenia patients receiving antipsychotics genotyped for the methylenetetrahydrofolate reductase (MTHFR) 677 C/T and 1298 A/C variants. *Schizophr Res.* 98:47, 2008.

Frankenburg FR. The role of one-carbon metabolism in schizophrenia and depression. *Harv Rev Psychiatry.* 15(4):146, 2007.

Gilbody S, et al. Methylenetetrahydrofolate reductase (MTHFR) genetic polymorphisms and psychiatric disorders: a HuGE review. *Am J Epidemiol.* 165:1, 2007.

Guidotti A, et al. Characterization of the action of antipsychotic subtypes on valproate-induced chromatin remodeling. *Trends Pharmacol Sci.* 30:55, 2009.

Harris LW, et al. Gene expression in the prefrontal cortex during adolescence: implications for the onset of schizophrenia. *BMC Med Genomics.* 2:28, 2009.

Henderson DC. Schizophrenia and comorbid metabolic disorders. *J Clin Psychiatry.* 66:11S, 2005.

Huffaker SJ, et al. A primate-specific, brain isoform of KCNH2 affects cortical physiology, cognition, neuronal repolarization and risk of schizophrenia. *Nat Med.* 15:509, 2009.

Hummer M, et al. Osteoporosis in patients with schizophrenia. *Am J Psychiatry.* 162:162, 2005.

International Schizophrenia Consortium. Rare chromosomal deletions and duplications increase risk of schizophrenia. *Nature.* 455:237, 2008.

Levinson-Castiel R, et al. Neonatal abstinence syndrome after in utero exposure to selective serotonin reuptake inhibitors in term infants. *Arch Pediatr Adolesc Med.* 160:173, 2006.

Lipska BK, et al. Functional genomics in postmortem human brain: abnormalities in a DISC1 molecular pathway in schizophrenia. *Dialogues Clin Neurosci.* 8:353, 2006.

Marco CA, Vaughan J. Emergency management of agitation in schizophrenia. *Am J Emerg Med.* 23:767, 2005.

McEvoy JP, et al. Prevalence of the metabolic syndrome in patients with schizophrenia: baseline results from the Clinical Antipsychotic Trials of Intervention Effectiveness (CATIE) schizophrenia trial and comparison with national estimates from NHANES III. *Schizophr Res.* 80:19, 2005.

Miller AL. The methylation, neurotransmitter, and antioxidant connections between folate and depression. *Altern Med Rev.* 13:216, 2008.

Need AC, et al. A genome-wide investigation of SNPs and CNVs in schizophrenia. [published online ahead of print February 6, 2009] *PLoS Genet.* 2009 Feb; 5(2):e1000373.

Patel JK, et al. Metabolic profiles of second-generation antipsychotics in early psychosis: findings from the CAFE study. *Schizophr Res.* 111:9, 2009.

Roffman JL, et al. Contribution of methylenetetrahydrofolate reductase (MTHFR). Polymorphisms to negative symptoms in schizophrenia. *Biol Psychiatry.* 63:42, 2007.

Roffman JL, et al. MTHFR 677C –> T genotype disrupts prefrontal function in schizophrenia through an interaction with COMT 158Val –> *Met. Proc Natl Acad Sci USA.* 105:17573, 2008.

Roffman JL, et al. Neuroimaging-genetic paradigms: a new approach to investigate the pathophysiology and treatment of cognitive deficits in schizophrenia. *Harv Rev Psychiatry.* 14:78, 2006.

Suzuki K, et al. Decreased expression of reelin receptor VLDLR in peripheral lymphocytes of drug-naive schizophrenic patients. *Schizophr Res.* 98: 148, 2008.

Velakoulis D, et al. Hippocampal and amygdala volumes according to psychosis stage and diagnosis. *Arch Gen Psychiatry.* 63:139, 2006.

Weiss AP, et al. Treatment of cardiac risk factors among patients with schizophrenia and diabetes. *Psychiatr Serv.* 57:1145, 2006.

Woodward ND, et al. COMT val108/158met genotype, cognitive function, and cognitive improvement with clozapine in schizophrenia. *Schizophr Res.* 90:86, 2007.

Zintzaras E. C677 T and A1298 C methylenetetrahydrofolate reductase gene polymorphisms in schizophrenia, bipolar disorder and depression: a meta-analysis of genetic association studies. *Psychiatr Genet.* 16:105, 2006.

SLEEP AND CIRCADIAN RHYTHM DISORDERS

NUTRITIONAL ACUITY RANKING: LEVEL 1

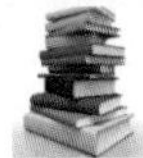

DEFINITIONS AND BACKGROUND

Primary insomnia is described as difficulty getting to sleep or staying asleep over a time period of at least one month; it occurs in 10% of the population. This equals about 70 million people. The prevalence of insomnia is high among older adults; 44% of older persons experience nighttime symptoms of insomnia at least a few nights per week (National Sleep Foundation, 2009).

Circadian rhythm sleep disorders have wake–sleep cycles differ from the typical pattern. Delayed sleep phase syndrome involves a longer time to get to sleep with periods of alertness during the night. The irregular sleep–wake pattern causes the individual to sleep at irregular times, with wakefulness at night and naps during the day. Other sleep disorders include sleep apnea, where breathing is interrupted during sleep, daytime sleepiness (narcolepsy), and restless legs syndrome.

Sleep affects energy balance. Short sleep duration may be related to high BP, depression and obesity in children and teens (Javaheri et al, 2008; Landhuis et al, 2008; Liem et al, 2008; Shaikh et al, 2008).

MT is an indole formed from L-trytophan that plays a major role in sleep and circadian rhythm (Konturek et al, 2007).

MT is produced primarily in the GI tract, but it is also found in the pineal gland, retina, lens, bone marrow, and skin (Pandi-Perumal et al, 2008). Its production increases with darkness and drops again with light, including artificial lighting. Production also decreases with age.

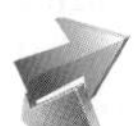

ASSESSMENT, MONITORING, AND EVALUATION

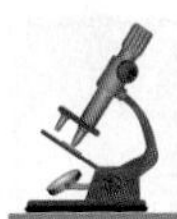

CLINICAL INDICATORS

Genetic Markers: Sleep disorders with an established genetic basis include fatal familial insomnia, familial advanced sleep-phase syndrome, chronic primary insomnia, and narcolepsy with cataplexy. Recent gene association studies have identified multiple gene mutations in several other sleep disorders.

Clinical/History

Height
Weight
BMI
Obesity?
EEG
EMG
Wake (W), nonrapid eye movement (NREM) sleep
Rapid eye movement (REM) sleep

BP	Lab Work	Gluc
Loud snoring?	Ca^{++}, Mg^{++}	Chol (total profile)
Restless leg syndrome	Na^{+}, K^{+}, Cl^{-}	
Depression or anxiety	H & H	
	Serum Fe	

INTERVENTION

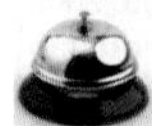

OBJECTIVES

- Improve nutritional status and outcome.
- Calculate energy requirements and promote a weight loss program if obesity is a problem.
- Manage intake of bioactive substances that affect sleep (i.e., caffeine, alcohol).
- Teach principles related to good health: balanced diet without excessive energy intake, adequate physical activity, routine sleeping habits.

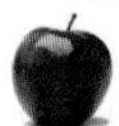

FOOD AND NUTRITION

- Adequate intake of thiamin and other B-complex vitamins, zinc, protein, vitamin A, and any other depleted nutrients will be important.
- An energy controlled plan may be needed. The DASH diet may also be beneficial with hypertension.
- Limit caffeine and alcohol, especially later in the evening.

Common Drugs Used and Potential Side Effects

- Benzodiazepines are commonly used. They may cause dry mouth or dehydration.
- MT analogues have a rapid onset of action, improve sleep quality, and enhance mood. Agomelatine has 5-HT(2c) antagonist properties that may be used in treating patients with major depression, insomnia, and some other sleep disorders (Pandi-Perumal et al, 2008). Ramelteon is another MT agonist recently approved for long-term treatment of insomnia.

SAMPLE NUTRITION CARE PROCESS STEPS

Excessive Bioactive Substance Intake

Assessment Data: Sleep problems; no hx of medical conditions that cause insomnia; diet hx with high caffeine intake.

Nutrition Diagnoses (PES): Excessive bioactive substance intake (caffeine) related to consumption of 10–12 cups of coffee throughout the day as evidenced by insomnia, chronic fatigue, and heartburn.

Interventions: Education about the need to reduce caffeine intake to promote healthier sleep.

Monitoring and Evaluation: Fewer complaints about heartburn; better sleeping habits and less chronic fatigue; intake of two to three cups of coffee per day and increased intake of other beverages.

- MT, when taken with calcium, acts as an immunostimulator. Because this could aggravate conditions such as rheumatoid arthritis, use these supplements with caution.
- As appropriate, antidepressants or anti-anxiety medications may be prescribed. Side effects vary.
- Pain may cause insomnia. Cancer, arthritis, and other conditions may be present. Adequate pain medication will be needed.

Herbs, Botanicals, and Supplements

- Valerian is a popular botanical used for insomnia. Side effects may include pruritis, headache, or GI distress.

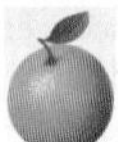

NUTRITION EDUCATION, COUNSELING, CARE MANAGEMENT

- CBT and family, group, and self-help therapies are all recommended.
- Many people benefit from relaxation training.
- If the individual is obese, a weight management program, sleep enhancement, and exercise plan will be needed.
- Avoid alcohol, nicotine, and caffeine for 3–4 hours before bedtime.
- Exercise in the afternoon rather than too close to bedtime.

Patient Education—Foodborne Illness

- Basic food handling and handwashing techniques are important.

For More Information

- American Academy of Sleep Medicine
  http://www.aasmnet.org/
- Medline—Sleep Disorders
  http://www.nlm.nih.gov/medlineplus/sleepdisorders.html
- National Center on Sleep Disorders Research
  http://www.nhlbi.nih.gov/about/ncsdr/
- National Sleep Foundation
  http://www.sleepfoundation.org
- National Institutes of Health—Sleep Tutorial
  http://www.nlm.nih.gov/medlineplus/tutorials/sleepdisorders/htm/index.htm
- Valerian
  http://ods.od.nih.gov/factsheets/valerian.asp
- Your Guide to Healthy Sleep
  http://www.nhlbi.nih.gov/health/public/sleep/healthy_sleep.pdf

SLEEP DISORDERS—CITED REFERENCES

Javaheri S, et al. Sleep quality and elevated blood pressure in adolescents. *Circulation.* 118:1034, 2008.

Konturek SJ, et al. Localization and biological activities of melatonin in intact and diseased gastrointestinal tract (GIT). *J Physiol Pharmacol.* 58:381, 2007.

Landhuis CE, et al. Childhood sleep time and long-term risk for obesity: a 32-year prospective birth cohort study. *Pediatrics.* 122:955, 2008.

Liem ET, et al. Association between depressive symptoms in childhood and adolescence and overweight in later life: review of the recent literature. *Arch Pediatr Adolesc Med.* 162:981, 2008.

Pandi-Perumal SR, et al. The effect of melatonergic and non-melatonergic antidepressants on sleep: weighing the alternatives. *World J Biol Psychiatry.* 4:1, 2008.

Shaikh MG, et al. Reductions in basal metabolic rate and physical activity contribute to hypothalamic obesity. *J Clin. Endocrinol. Metab.* 93:2588, 2008.

SUBSTANCE USE DISORDERS AND ADDICTION

NUTRITIONAL ACUITY RANKING: LEVEL 1 (WITHDRAWAL/REHABILITATION)

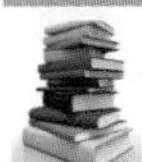

DEFINITIONS AND BACKGROUND

Substance use often leads to addiction. Addiction is a brain disorder, a chronic disorder with compulsive and relapsing behavior. Three predisposing factors exist: constitutional liability (biochemical), personality factor (psychological vulnerability), and social factors (environmental conditioning). Sensitivity to reward (STR) seems to play a role (Davis et al, 2004). The master "pleasure" molecule of addiction is dopamine (D2 receptor gene). Heroin, amphetamines, marijuana, alcohol, nicotine, and caffeine all trigger the release of dopamine. Abnormalities in the metabolism of dopamine, serotonin, and norepinephrine contribute to substance dependency. In some cases, use of antidepressant medications alleviate the dependency.

Abuse of chemical substances may be chronic or acute and may involve abuse of alcohol, prescription or over-the-counter drugs, or illicit drugs. Initial use of drugs of abuse converge on the mesolimbic dopamine pathway from the ventral tegmental area (VTA); these drugs modulate glutamatergic transmission activating the dopamine neurons, a critical early stage in the development of addiction (Heikkinen et al, 2009; Xiao et al, 2009). Physiological problems that result are definite, specific to the abused substance. Social, emotional, vocational, and legal problems may arise.

Persons with substance dependency tend to have type A personalities and are prone to perfectionism and depression. Substance abusers are codependent, neglecting their own feelings and emotions. EDs and substance disorders may represent different expressions of the same underlying problem, with cognitive dysfunction, use of food or substance to relieve negative affect (anxiety or depression), secretiveness about the problem, and social isolation. Addiction to food may also be a reality; brain circuits can also be deranged with natural rewards such as food (Davis et al, 2004). Overweight individuals may use food as a reward, just as substance abusers use pharmacological substances for a reward for the dopamine-specific part of the brain.

Alcoholism is a chronic relapsing disease that is frequently unrecognized and untreated; approximately one third of patients remain abstinent, and one third are fully relapsed 1 year after withdrawal from alcohol (Oroszi and Goldman, 2004). Many alcoholics are malnourished; nutritional interventions are needed to prevent liver disease. Antioxidants as precursors of endogenous glutathione show promise (Lieber, 2003). Protein calorie malnutrition (PCM) is predictive of mortality in alcoholic liver disease; deficiencies of folate, thiamine, pyridoxine, and vitamin A promote anemia, altered cognitive states, and night blindness (Halsted, 2004).

Addictions share some of the same biological pathways. Because polydrug use may alter food intake, taste preferences, and nutrient metabolism and because denial is common, psychotherapy along with substance withdrawal is recommended. Dysfunctional eating patterns and excessive weight gains have been observed during recovery from drug and alcohol addictions; food deprivation during active addiction may contribute (Cowan and Devine, 2008). Assertive outreach is effective in engaging and linking persons to substance abuse treatment services, even if they are homeless (Fisk et al, 2006). Giving up should not be an option (Table 4-22).

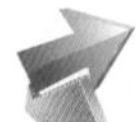

ASSESSMENT, MONITORING, AND EVALUATION

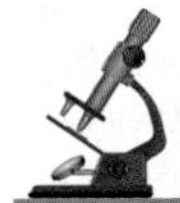

CLINICAL INDICATORS

Genetic Markers: The collaborative study on genetics of alcoholism (COGA) supports the premise that alcohol dependence is inherited in 50–60% of cases (Dick et al, 2008). Alcohol dehydrogenases, catechol-O-methyltransferase (COMT), opioid receptors, and HTTLPR (which alters serotonin transport) all affect the process of addiction and relapse (Oroszi and Goldman, 2004). In addition, the gamma-amino-butyric acid (GABA) neurotransmitter mediates actions of alcohol.

Clinical/History	Lab Work	
Height	Prolactin levels	Serum folate
Weight	Serotonin levels	Serum B_{12}
BMI	Ca^{++}, Mg^{++}	Serum tHcy
Weight changes	Na^{+}, K^{+}, Cl^{-}	CRP
Dietary/intake history	H & H	Liver function tests
I & O	Serum Fe	
BP	Alb or transthyretin	
Tremors, delirium?	Gluc	
Multidimensional Addictions and Personality Profile (MAPP)	Chol (total profile)	
	Trig (often very high in alcoholics)	
	Serum thiamin	

INTERVENTION

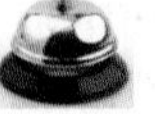

OBJECTIVES

- Normalize brain levels of neurotransmitters.
- Correct fluid and electrolyte imbalances or dehydration.
- Protect during withdrawal (e.g., alcohol detoxification may cause tremors, hallucinations, seizures, and delirium tremens). Of persons with delirium tremens, 20% may die, even with therapy; monitor closely.
- Modify diet for medical conditions. Alcoholics experience problems such as liver failure, cirrhosis, pancreatitis, GI

TABLE 4-22 **Common Addictions and Issues**

Substance	Issues
Alcohol	The most consistent predictor of alcohol dependency is alcoholism in a biological parent. Alcoholics are more likely to diet from stroke or cirrhosis. An estimated 3 million children between 14 years and 17 years of age are problem drinkers; the earlier the exposure, the more likely dependency will occur. To assess for problems, C-A-G-E questions include: Have you tried to cut back? Has anybody ever annoyed you regarding this behavior? Have you ever felt guilty about it? Have you ever needed an early morning eye opener? With two or more yes answers, a problem should be addressed.
Caffeine	Caffeine and nicotine are the most common psychostimulant drugs used worldwide. Caffeine affects the brain in ways that are similar to cocaine and other stimulants, but it is not as addictive overall.
Chocolate	Chocolate may be used as self-medication for low magnesium levels and to balance low neurotransmitters for mood (serotonin and dopamine). Chocolate contains methylxanthines, biogenic amines, and cannabinoid-like fatty acids. Chocolate cravings may occur (Smit et al, 2004), especially related to menses in women.
Club drugs: LSD (acid), MDMA (Ecstasy), GHB, GBL, ketamine (special K), Fentanyl, Rohypnol, amphetamines, methamphetamine	"Club drug" is a vague term that refers to a wide variety of drugs including MDMA (ecstasy), GHB, Rohypnol, ketamine, methamphetamine, and LSD. Uncertainties about the drug sources, pharmacological agents, chemicals used to manufacture them, and possible contaminants make it difficult to determine toxicity, consequences, and symptoms. Serious health problems may result from their use.
Cocaine	The pure chemical, cocaine hydrochloride, has been an abused substance for more than 100 years, and coca leaves, the source of cocaine, have been ingested for thousands of years. Use has increased, and now over 1.5 million Americans are users. Young adults aged 18–25 are most likely to initiate use. Years later, cocaine use may be linked to Parkinson's disease. A herbal supplement can reduce the cravings associated with chronic cocaine use. N-acetylcysteine (NAC) is a potential agent to modulate the effects of cocaine addiction, heroin addiction, and possibly alcoholism.
Heroin	Heroin is processed from morphine, a naturally occurring substance extracted from the seedpod of the Asian poppy plant. Heroin usually appears as a white or brown powder. Street names for heroin include smack, H, skag, and junk. Other names may refer to types of heroin produced in a specific geographical area, such as Mexican black tar. Use of heroin may be fatal. Use during pregnancy may cause spontaneous abortion.
Marijuana	Marijuana is the most commonly used illicit drug in the United States. The main active chemical in marijuana is THC (delta-9-tetrahydrocannabinol). The membranes of certain nerve cells in the brain contain protein receptors that bind to THC. Once in place, THC kicks off a series of cellular reactions that ultimately lead to the high that users experience.
Nicotine	Along with directly stimulating the brain's reward system, nicotine stimulates it indirectly by altering the balance of inputs from two types of neurons that help regulate its activity level.
Prescription medications	Pain relievers, tranquilizers, stimulants, and sedatives are very useful treatment tools. When people do not take them as directed, they may become addicted. Inappropriate or nonmedical use of prescription medications is a serious public health concern. Nonmedical use of prescription medications like opioids, central nervous system (CNS) depressants, and stimulants can lead to abuse and addiction, which are characterized by compulsive drug seeking and use.
Steroids, anabolic	Anabolic-androgenic steroids are man-made substances related to male sex hormones. They are available legally only by prescription to treat conditions that occur when the body produces abnormally low amounts of testosterone, such as in delayed puberty and impotence. They are also prescribed to treat body wasting in patients with AIDS and other diseases that result in loss of lean muscle mass. Athletes may abuse anabolic steroids to enhance performance and also to improve physical appearance. Anabolic steroids are taken orally or injected, typically in cycles of weeks or months (referred to as "cycling"), rather than continuously.

Sources: http://www.nida.nih.gov/Drugpages/, accessed June 15, 2009; Smit HJ, et al. Methylxanthines are the psycho-pharmacologically active constituents of chocolate. *Psychopharmacology*. 176:412, 2004.

bleeding, esophageal varices, renal impairment, ascites, and edema. Intravenous drug users are at risk for contracting hepatitis C or HIV infection. See appropriate entries.

- Reorient to reality; develop trusting relationships between patient and care providers. Promote abstinence and long-term treatment.
- Improve nutritional status and outcome. Dietitians can provide nutrition education and can help in drug treatment and rehabilitation programs (Grant et al, 2004).
- Prevent or correct EDs, present in approximately 50% of this population. Avoid major changes in food choices and intake during recovery to prevent drastic weight fluctuations.
- Use motivational interviewing to work through problems, such as resistance and ambivalence for making life changes (Westra, 2004).

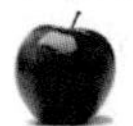

FOOD AND NUTRITION

- According to I & O values, adjust fluid intake. Offer beverages that are nonalcoholic favorites. Reductions in the use of caffeine are often suggested.
- Encourage nutrient-dense foods. Fruits, vegetables, whole grains, and fish are important inclusions.
- Adequate intake of protein will be essential.

SAMPLE NUTRITION CARE PROCESS STEPS

Excessive Alcohol Intake

Assessment Data: Food recall/diet history; alcohol intake; assessment of access to food and resources (money, family support, social service agencies, alcohol counseling or therapy).

PES: Excessive alcohol intake related to social anxiety as evidenced by patient report, admission with alcohol intoxication, and history of rehabilitation for alcohol dependence.

Intervention: Provide nourishing foods and beverages. Counsel about the role of nutrient-dense foods and how alcohol provides only heat and kilocals. Coordinate with social services for additional rehab if appropriate.

Monitoring and Evaluation: Report of improved food and beverage intake; alcohol-free lifestyle changes; improved self esteem and quality of life; reduced social anxiety after rehab program.

- Include adequate calories, especially because patients often become hypoglycemic. Feed several times daily to help regulate blood glucose.
- Adequate intake of thiamin, other B-complex vitamins, zinc, protein, vitamin A, or other depleted nutrients is important during recovery.
- Adjust diet, as appropriate, to reduce excess sweets; many chemical abusers tend to substitute CHO for their dependency drug.
- Adequate fiber intake may be useful to correct or prevent constipation.

Common Drugs Used and Potential Side Effects

- Antabuse, when mixed with alcohol, can cause severe nausea, vomiting, low BP, and flushing.
- Bromocriptine (Parlodel) may also be used for some drug-recovery patients. Nausea, vomiting, or constipation may occur.
- Methadone maintenance therapy continues to be one of the major effective forms of addiction pharmacotherapy and underscores the importance of biological factors in the physiology and treatment of the addictive diseases (Kreek et al, 2004).
- Naltrexone decreases the pleasurable sensation of alcohol; it is used for narcotic dependency after detoxification. Anorexia, weight loss, nausea, vomiting, and abdominal cramping or pain may occur.
- Subutex/Suboxone (buprenorphine/naloxone) are oral tablets used for the treatment of opiate dependence.
- Stool softeners may be beneficial if constipation results after withdrawal, as with cocaine abuse.
- TCAs (imipramine, desipramine) are often beneficial with some side effects such as dry mouth.

Herbs, Botanicals, and Supplements

- No studies have been conducted for efficacy of herbs or botanicals in substance abuse patients.
- St John's wort should not be taken with antidepressants.

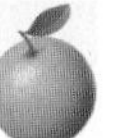

NUTRITION EDUCATION, COUNSELING, CARE MANAGEMENT

- Help the patient accept responsibility for his or her own actions. CBT and family, group, and self-help therapies are all recommended.
- Treatment should focus on sufficient duration and intensity, family support, after-care and follow-up, self-help groups, collaboration with social services, and a drug-free lifestyle. One of five individuals will be drug free or sober after 5 years. New studies will include new, effective medications and evaluations of the changes that occur in the brain.
- Help to maintain abstinence. Avoid discussion of unanswerable questions such as "why" substances have been abused.
- In recovery, simple guidelines are useful: eat breakfast and regular meals daily; eat a variety of foods; make mealtimes pleasant and unhurried; choose healthy snacks; drink decaffeinated coffee.
- Discuss issues regarding personal "control." Coping skills will be needed to reduce helplessness. Include patient in decision making to increase self-esteem and confidence.
- Discuss the dangers of diet pills and starvation to control appetite and weight.
- Long-term alcohol abuse can specifically target beta cells of the pancreas, increasing risk of diabetes. Heroin use can cause glucose intolerance, but unlike in alcohol abuse, this usually resolves with abstinence.
- Heavy drinkers tend to have higher total and HDL cholesterol levels than controls. Moderate alcohol intake does not seem to be protective against coronary heart disease through lipid reduction alone; resveratrol may be one protective factor.
- Sports teams can provide peer-led education about healthy lifestyles and reduction in disordered eating patterns or substance abuse (Elliott et al, 2004).
- If a person smokes cigarettes, having smoking cessation interventions seems to help long-term sobriety for other addictions (Prochaska et al, 2004).
- Help plan adequate discharge planning, follow-up, and family therapy or other support group interactions.

Patient Education—Foodborne Illness

- Careful food handling will be important. The same is true for hand washing.

For More Information

- Addictions
  http://www.addiction.com/
- Alcoholics Anonymous
  http://www.alcoholics-anonymous.org
- American Society of Addiction Medicine
  http://www.asam.org/
- National Clearinghouse for Alcohol and Drug Information
  http://ncadi.samhsa.gov/
- National Council on Alcoholism and Drug Dependence
  http://www.ncadd.org
- National Institute on Drug Abuse (NIDA)
  http://www.nida.nih.gov/
- NIDA Statistics
  http://www.nida.nih.gov/drugpages/stats.html

- Recovery Month
  http://www.recoverymonth.gov/
- Substance Abuse and Mental Health Services
  http://www.icpsr.umich.edu/SAMHDA/

SUBSTANCE USE DISORDERS—CITED REFERENCES

Cowan J, Devine C. Food, eating, and weight concerns of men in recovery from substance addiction. *Appetite.* 50:33, 2008.

Davis C, et al. Sensitivity to reward: implications for overeating and overweight. *Appetite.* 42:131, 2004.

Dick DM, et al. A Systematic single nucleotide polymorphism screen to fine-map alcohol dependence genes on chromosome 7 identifies association with a novel susceptibility gene ACN9. *Biol Psychiatry.* 63:1047, 2008.

Elliott DL, et al. Preventing substance use and disordered eating: initial outcomes of the ATHENA (Athletes Targeting Healthy Exercise and Nutrition Alternatives) program. *Arch Pediatr Adolesc Med.* 158:1043, 2004.

Fisk D, et al. Assertive outreach: an effective strategy for engaging homeless persons with substance use disorders into treatment. *Am J Drug Alcohol Abuse.* 32:479, 2006.

Grant LP, et al. Nutrition education is positively associated with substance abuse treatment program outcomes. *J Am Diet Assoc.* 104:604, 2004.

Halsted CH. Nutrition and alcoholic liver disease. *Semin Liver Dis.* 24:289, 2004.

Heikkinen AE, et al. Long-lasting modulation of glutamatergic transmission in VTA dopamine neurons after a single dose of benzodiazepine agonists. *Neuropsychopharmacology.* 34:290, 2009.

Kreek MJ, et al. Evolving perspectives on neurobiological research on the addictions: celebration of the 30th anniversary of NIDA. *Neuropharmacology.* 47:324S, 2004.

Lieber CS. Relationships between nutrition, alcohol use, and liver disease. *Alcohol Res Health.* 27:220, 2003.

Oroszi G, Goldman D. Alcoholism: genes and mechanisms. *Pharmacogenomics.* 5:1037, 2004.

Prochaska JJ, et al. A meta-analysis of smoking cessation interventions with individuals in substance abuse treatment or recovery. *J Consult Clin Psychol.* 72:1144, 2004.

Smit HJ, et al. Methylxanthines are the psycho-pharmacologically active constituents of chocolate. *Psychopharmacology.* 176:412, 2004.

Westra HA. Managing resistance in cognitive behavioural therapy: the application of motivational interviewing in mixed anxiety and depression. *Cogn Behav Ther.* 33:161, 2004.

Xiao C, et al. Ethanol facilitates glutamatergic transmission to dopamine neurons in the ventral tegmental area. *Neuropsychopharmacology.* 34:307, 2009.

SECTION 5

Pulmonary Disorders

CHIEF ASSESSMENT FACTORS

- Altered Respirations
- Anorexia
- Blood Gases: Partial Pressure of Oxygen (pO_2); Partial Pressure of Carbon Dioxide (pCO_2)
- Clubbing of Nail Beds
- Confusion, Somnolence
- Cough, Especially with Chest Pain
- Cyanosis of Lips, Nail Beds
- Dizziness
- Elevated Blood Pressure (BP)
- Engorged Eye Veins
- Fever or Chills
- Flaring Nostrils; Red, Swollen Nose
- Hemoptysis (Coughing Up Blood)
- Hoarseness
- Orthopnea, Tachypnea
- Pain (Chest, Abdominal)
- Pallor; Ashen or Gray Coloring
- Poor Exercise or Activity Tolerance
- Rapid Breathing, Excessive Perspiration
- Restlessness, Irritability
- Shortness of Breath (Dyspnea)
- Stridor (Crowing Sound on Inhalation)
- Wheezing (Whistling, Musical Sound from Obstructed Airways)

PULMONARY NUTRITION NOTES

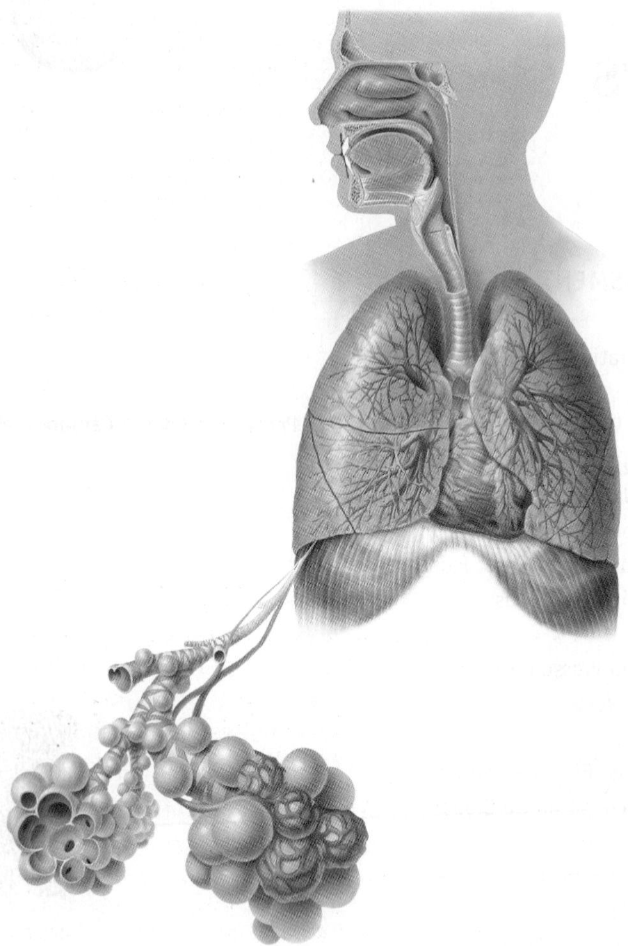

Asset provided by Anatomical Chart Co.

TABLE 5-1 Causes of Malnutrition in Patients with Pulmonary Disease

Aerophagia and rapid breathing
Anemia (low oxygen-carrying capacity)
Anorexia of chronic illness
Cellular hypoxia
Chronic debility
Decreased lung immunity
Decreased lung surfactant and elasticity
Depression, anxiety with anorexia
Difficulty in eating with continuous dyspnea
Fever
Gastric hypomotility
Hypermetabolism, as in chronic obstructive pulmonary disease (COPD)
Increased mechanical work of breathing
Increased workload of the heart
Inflammation
Lung cancer
Malabsorption, as in cystic fibrosis
Medications causing nausea and anorexia
Pneumonia
Polypharmacy
Poor respiratory muscle strength and endurance
Restricted diet
Right-sided heart failure
Vitamin deficiency, leading to poor epithelial integrity and weak lung muscles

NOTE. Death in patients with COPD is typically due to acute respiratory failure, pneumonia, lung cancer, cardiac disease, or pulmonary embolism.
Adapted from: Merck Manual: Chronic obstructive pulmonary disease; Accessed January 28, 2006, at http://www.merck.com/mrkshared/mmg/sec10/ch78/ch78a.jsp.

Pulmonary surfactant is a complex and highly active material composed of lipids and proteins that is found in the fluid lining the alveolar surface of the lungs. It protects the lungs from injuries and infections caused by inhaled particles and micro-organisms (Wright, 2005a). The role for surfactant was first studied in premature infants with respiratory distress syndrome (RDS), which is now routinely treated with an exogenous replacement (Stevens et al, 2004). Biochemical surfactant abnormalities have been described in asthma, bronchiolitis, chronic obstructive pulmonary disease, lung transplantation; infectious and suppurative lung diseases (cystic fibrosis [CF], pneumonia;) adult RDS, pulmonary edema, chronic lung disease of prematurity, interstitial lung diseases. Surfactant replacement therapy has been tested with positive outcomes. In acute respiratory syndrome, exogenous surfactant does not improve survival, but patients who received surfactant had a greater improvement in gas exchange during 24-hour treatment (Spragg et al, 2004).

The evidence for the role of diet in pulmonary disease is clear. Intake of fruit, fish, antioxidant vitamins, fatty acids, sodium or magnesium, helps to alleviate symptoms of asthma and Chronic obstructive pulmonary disease. Because antioxidant nutrients are positively corrected with lung function, vitamin C, vitamin E, beta-carotene, and selenium are important. Flavonoids, such as quercetin and resveratrol, in apples, onions, oranges, berries, and red wine support lung health (Arts and Hollman, 2005; Donnelly et al, 2004; Neuhouser, 2004). Vitamin D helps to maintain healthy lung function (Wright, 2005b). Vitamin E helps to stave off upper respiratory infections; 200 IU daily gives better response to vaccines for diseases such as flu, ear infections, pneumonia, bronchitis, sinusitis, and other pathological conditions (Meydani et al, 2004). Almonds, mango, sunflower seeds, vegetable oils, and whole grains are good sources. Table 5-1 lists factors that contribute to malnutrition with pulmonary disease.

Omega-3 fatty acids can calm inflamed airways; include salmon, respiratory quotients (RQs) tuna, mackerel, walnuts, and flaxseed oil more often. Table 5-2 lists the RQs for fats, protein, and carbohydrates (CHO). In general, it is assumed that fats decrease CO_2 output more than CHO.

TABLE 5-2 Respiratory Quotient (RQ) and Nutrients

RQ = VO_2/VCO_2
RQ from fat = 0.7
RQ from protein = 0.8
RQ from carbohydrates (CHO) = 1.0

For More Information

- American Lung Association
  http://www.lungusa.org/
- Canadian Lung Association
  http://www.lung.ca/
- National Heart, Lung, and Blood Institute
  http://www.nhlbi.nih.gov/health/public/lung/index.htm
- National Jewish Health
  http://www.nationaljewish.org/healthinfo/index.aspx

CITED REFERENCES

Arts IC, Hollman PC. Polyphenols and disease risk in epidemiologic studies. *Am J Clin Nutr.* 81:317S, 2005.

Donnelly LE, et al. Anti-inflammatory effects of resveratrol in lung epithelial cells: molecular mechanisms. *Am J Physiol Lung Cell Mol Physiol.* 287:774, 2004.

Meydani SN, et al. Vitamin E and respiratory tract infections in elderly nursing home residents: a randomized controlled trial. *JAMA.* 292:828, 2004.

Neuhouser ML. Dietary flavonoids and cancer risk: evidence from human population studies. *Nutr Cancer.* 50:1, 2004.

Spragg RG, et al. Effect of recombinant surfactant protein C-based surfactant on the acute respiratory distress syndrome. *N Engl J Med.* 351:884, 2004.

Stevens TP, et al. Early surfactant administration with brief ventilation vs selective surfactant and continued mechanical ventilation for preterm infants with or at risk for respiratory distress syndrome. *Cochrane Database Syst Rev.* 3:CD003063, 2004.

Wright JR. Immunoregulatory functions of surfactant proteins. *Nat Rev Immunol.* 5:58, 2005a.

Wright JR. Make no bones about it: increasing epidemiologic evidence links vitamin D to pulmonary function and COPD. *Chest.* 128:3781, 2005b.

ASTHMA

NUTRITIONAL ACUITY RANKING: LEVEL 1

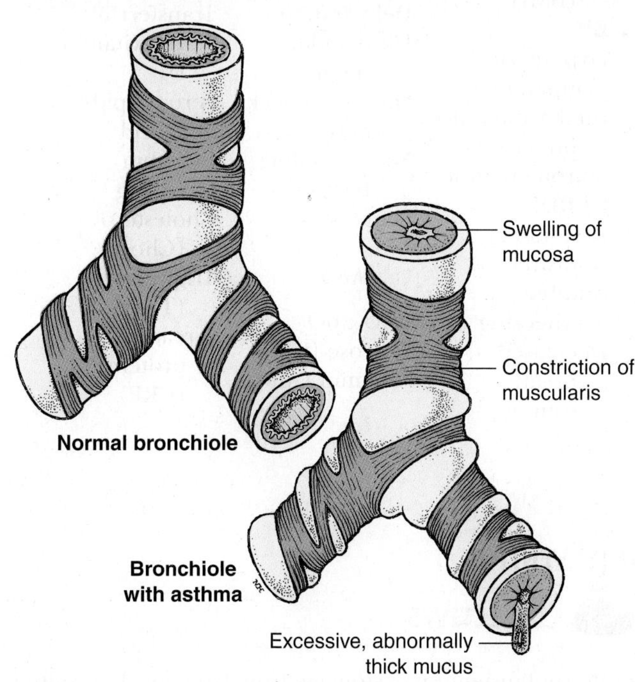

Adapted from: Neil O. Hardy. Wesport, CT. *Stedman's Medical Dictionary*, 27th ed. Baltimore: Lippincott Williams & Wilkins, 2000, p. 158.

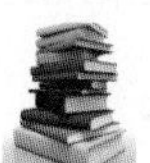

DEFINITIONS AND BACKGROUND

Bronchial asthma involves paroxysmal dyspnea accompanied by wheezing and is caused by spasm of the bronchial tubes or swelling of their mucous membranes. Bronchial asthma differs from wheezing caused by cardiac failure (cardiac asthma), in which an x-ray shows fluid in the lung. Asthma involves inflammation of the lining of the airways, obstruction, and increased sensitivity of the airways. Table 5-3 provides a checklist for signs and symptoms of asthma.

Between 10 and 15 million Americans are affected by asthma, including about 5% of children. Asthma seems to be inherited in two thirds of cases. Two main types of bronchial asthma are recognized: allergic (extrinsic) and nonallergic (intrinsic or infectious). Exercise-induced bronchospasm is much less common.

Children who are exposed to second-hand smoke may have chronic cough or symptoms of asthma. Chronic poor control can lead to a serious condition, status asthmaticus, which generally requires hospitalization and can be life threatening. Brittle asthma is a rare form of asthma with repeated attacks; food intolerance is common. Many infants with wheezing have transient conditions that resolve. The common cold virus and rhinovirus (RV) are major triggers; this pattern continues for adults with allergic asthma (Tan, 2005).

Breastfeeding provides immunological protection when the infant's immune system is immature and a modest protective effect against wheeze in early childhood (Kim et al, 2009; Oddy et al, 2004). Longer duration of breastfeeding seems to be more protective. Supplementation of maternal diet with fish oil is associated with altered neonatal immune responses to allergens (Devereux, 2009). Reduced maternal

TABLE 5-3 Early Warning Signs of Asthma

Head/eyes	Glassy eyes; dark circles; watery eyes; headache; feverish; pale
Nose	Stuffy nose; runny nose; sneezing
Mouth/throat	Chin or throat itches; change in sputum; dry mouth; funny feeling in chest
Chest/lungs	Fast heartbeat; coughing; changes in breathing; downward trend in peak flow numbers
Behavior/mood	Easily upset or irritable; weak; slowing down; feeling sad; more quiet, excited or restless than usual; desire to be alone; insomnia
Exercise tolerance	Poor tolerance for exercise; sweaty; easy fatigue

intake of vitamins D and E, zinc during pregnancy seems to be associated with increased asthma and wheezing outcomes in children up to the age of 5 years (Devereux, 2009).

Nutritional status is important for healthy lungs. Intravenous treatment with multiple nutrients may be of considerable benefit; pulmonary function improves progressively with longer treatment (Schrader, 2004). Diet affects the pathophysiology of asthma by altered immune or antioxidant activity with consequent effects on airway inflammation. Maternal intake of vitamins D and E and zinc can modify fetal lung development (Devereux, 2009). Low serum vitamin D has been shown to be a marker for severity of childhood asthma (Brehm et al, 2009).

Overall, dietary modification may help patients manage their asthma and their overall health. A multidisciplinary approach is required to move forward and understand the complexity of the interaction of dietary factors and asthma (Kim et al, 2009). Obesity and overweight may lead to less-effective therapy from inhaled corticosteroid treatments (Sutherland et al, 2009). While there is currently no conclusive evidence about the role of specific nutrients, food types, or dietary patterns past early childhood on asthma prevalence (Kim et al, 2009); Table 5-4 lists various nutrients and their potential effects on asthma.

TABLE 5-4 Nutrients and Their Potential Mechanisms in Asthma

Nutrient(s)	Activity and Potential Mechanisms of Effect
Vitamins A (carotenoids), C, and E	Antioxidants for protection against endogenous and exogenous oxidant inflammation
Vitamin C	Prostaglandin inhibition (Harik-Kahn et al, 2004)
Vitamin D	Vitamin D modulates T-cell responses (Devereux, 2009)
Vitamin E	Membrane stabilization, inhibition of immunoglobulin E (IgE) production. Modulation of T-cell responses (Devereux, 2009)
Flavones and flavonoids	Antioxidants; mast cell stabilization
Magnesium	Smooth muscle relaxation, mast cell stabilization (Schrader, 2004)
Selenium	Antioxidant cofactor in glutathione peroxidase
Copper, zinc	Antioxidant cofactors in superoxide dismutase. Zinc modulates T-cell responses (Devereux, 2009)
Omega-3 fatty acids	Leukotriene substitution, stabilization of inflammatory cell membranes (Wong, 2005). PUFA modulate T-cell responses (Devereux, 2009)
Omega-6 polyunsaturated/trans fatty acids	Increased eicosanoid production (Nagel and Linseisen, 2005)
Sodium	Increased smooth muscle contraction; reductions can increase airway responsiveness (Mickleborough and Gotshall, 2004)

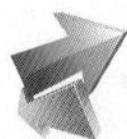

ASSESSMENT, MONITORING, AND EVALUATION

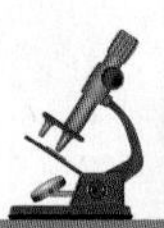

CLINICAL INDICATORS

Genetic Markers: Tobacco smoke and genetic susceptibility are risk factors for wheezing and asthma (Sadeghnejad et al, 2008). Interleukin 6 (IL6) IL6 receptor (IL6R), and IL13 are candidate genes. Maternal diet plays an epigenetic role by sensitizing fetal airways to respond abnormally to environmental insults (Devereux, 2009; Kim et al, 2009). In addition, beta2-adrenergic receptor (beta2AR) gene polymorphisms are associated with asthma in different racial or ethnic populations.

Clinical/History

- Height
- Weight
- Body mass index (BMI)
- BP
- Hypotension?
- Temperature
- Intake and output (I & O)
- Spirometry test
- GERD?
- Respiratory distress
- Audible wheezing
- Decreased breath sounds
- Tachycardia
- Cyanosis
- Anxiety
- Pulmonary edema
- Dehydration
- Hard and dry cough
- Distended neck veins
- Food or sulfite allergies?
- Skin testing

Lab Work

- pCO_2, pO_2
- Glucose (Gluc)
- Albumin (Alb)
- Hemoglobin and hematocrit (H & H)
- Serum Fe, ferritin
- Transferrin
- Serum vitamin D_3
- Serum lipids
- Uric acid
- Bilirubin
- Ca^{++}, Mg^{++}
- Cholesterol (Chol)
- Triglycerides (Trig)
- C-reactive protein (CRP)

INTERVENTION

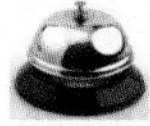

OBJECTIVES

- Prevent distention of stomach from large meals, resulting in distress, GERD, or aggravation of asthma.
- Prevent lung infection and inflammation. Promote improved resistance against infections.
- For allergic asthma, identify and control allergens in the environment.
- Promote adequate hydration to liquefy secretions.
- Optimize nutritional status. Sufficient vitamins C, B_6, D, and E, selenium and magnesium are important. Reduce intake of oleic acid, but increase omega-3 fatty acids if tolerated.
- Encourage a health maintenance program, including physical activity where possible.
- Caffeine relaxes muscles and opens the airways; 2–3 cups of coffee daily may be useful in adults.

SAMPLE NUTRITION CARE PROCESS STEPS

Overweight

Assessment Data: BMI >90%tile for age; complaints of heartburn and GERD after meals; asthma triggered by allergies; diet hx showing frequent intake of high sugary snacks between meals.

Nutrition Diagnoses (PES): Overweight related to excessive intake of energy as CHO with asthma as evidenced by BMI >90%tile for age, GERD, and diet hx revealing intake of high CHO snacks throughout the day.

Interventions: Education about the role of weight management and asthma; review of any known food allergies; discussion about appropriate energy intake for age and activity. Counseling about alternative snacks with a mix of protein-CHO-fats.

Monitoring and Evaluation: BMI closer to desirable range; fewer complaints of GERD; better tolerance of drug therapy for asthmatic episodes; improved quality of intake for meals and snacks.

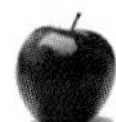

FOOD AND NUTRITION

- Infants should be exclusively breastfed to reduce the risk of asthma in susceptible families.
- Provide balanced, small meals that are nutrient dense (high-quality protein, vitamins, and minerals), to reduce risk of infections.
- Lose weight by following a lower energy intake if needed (Oddy et al, 2004; Sutherland et al, 2009).
- Encourage extra fluids unless contraindicated. Theobromine in cocoa tends to increase blood flow to the brain and to reduce coughing; use often.
- Use less sodium (Mickleborough and Gotshall, 2004).
- Highlight foods rich in vitamins A and C, magnesium, and zinc. Use more broccoli, grapefruit, oranges, sweet peppers, kiwi, tomato juice, and cauliflower for vitamin C.
- Quercetin in apples, pears, onions, oranges, and berries should be encouraged (5 or more servings per week). Other nutrients that support immunocompetence should be included.
- Omit specific food allergens for children if identified: as milk, eggs, seafood, tree nuts, peanuts, fish, wheat or soy. For adults, tree nuts, peanuts, fish and shellfish allergies tend to persist.
- Sulfites salicylates may aggravate asthma in 5% of this population, especially adults with severe disease. Sulfite-containing foods or beverages should be avoided.
- Salicylate sensitivity is common in 5–20% of asthmatics who are hypersensitive to aspirin. Many fruits and some vegetables contain salicylates.
- If fish is tolerated, consumption of fish two to three times weekly may help reduce leukotriene synthesis (Wong, 2005). If nuts are tolerated, include selenium from Brazil nuts and vitamin E from most nuts.
- Omega-3 fatty acids from fish oils, walnuts, and flaxseed have been suggested. Some studies suggest that EPA is more useful than DHA (Mickleborough et al, 2009) whereas others suggest the opposite (Weldon et al, 2007). The evidence is not yet clear.
- Saturated fatty acids (SFAs) and oleic acid (from margarine) may contribute to clinical onset of asthma; limit their use (Nagel and Linseisen, 2005).

Common Drugs Used and Potential Side Effects

- An airway renin–angiotensin system is triggered by release of mast-cell renin; ANG II is a critical factor for new therapeutic targets in the management of airway disease (Kano et al, 2008; Reid et al, 2007).
- See Table 5-5.

Herbs, Botanicals, and Supplements

- Many patients with asthma use alternative therapies. Antioxidant and natural anti-inflammatory and immunomodulatory remedies may prove beneficial.
- In China, a combination of three herbal extracts (ASHMI) may be used in anti-asthma intervention (Wen et al, 2005). Seaweed may be used to treat asthma in Vietnamese and oriental cultures (Dang and Hoang, 2004).
- Dietary fatty acids such as gamma linolenic acid (GLA; borage oil) modulate endogenous inflammatory mediators without side effects (Ziboh et al, 2004).
- Ephedra (ma huang) is an effective bronchodilator, but it increases BP significantly. Problems with blood glucose, arrhythmias, increased heart rate, and central nervous system (CNS) stimulation can also occur. The Food and Drug Administration (FDA) has removed it from the market, but some forms are still available.
- Stinging nettle, licorice, gingko, and anise have not shown efficacy; side effects must be evaluated.
- St. John's wort can inhibit theophylline's effectiveness.

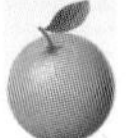

NUTRITION EDUCATION, COUNSELING, CARE MANAGEMENT

- Mild, chronic asthma can be a warning; if untreated, it can lead to an acute exacerbation.
- Waiting to introduce solids to an infant does not necessarily protect against onset of asthma and allergy (Zutavern et al, 2004).
- Early multivitamin–mineral supplementation may trigger asthma in susceptible children; the exact reasons are not clear (Milner et al, 2004). A healthy, nutrient-dense diet should be consumed instead.
- All medications should be taken as directed by the physician. An emergency pack should be carried at all times containing a rescue inhaler and, if needed, epinephrine injection device and a chewable antihistamine tablet.
- Work with the patient/family to avoid precipitating triggers. Reduce exposure to triggers such as pet dander, food allergens, second-hand smoke. Discuss exercise, rest, and nutrition.
- Massage therapy enhances relaxation, decreases anxiety, and promotes better lung function.

TABLE 5-5 **Medications Used in Asthma**

Medication	Description
Antibiotics	Long-term use can cause diarrhea and other problems. Penicillin should not be taken with fruit juices.
Anticholinergics (Atrovent, Combivent)	Quick-relief asthma medications. Dry mouth is common side effect.
Beta-agonists (metaproterenol albuterol; levalbuterol; salbumol)	Relaxes smooth muscle around airways. Side effects include shakiness, rapid heart rate, nervousness and elevated blood glucose. Metaproterenol (Metaprel, Alupent) may alter taste and cause nausea or vomiting. Albuterol (Ventolin, Proventil) may have cardiac side effects or may cause nausea or diarrhea.
Bronchodilators: theophylline (Theo-Dur, Slo-BID, Slo-Phyllin, Theolair, Uniphyl)	No longer first choice of asthma medication. Nausea, vomiting, and sleeplessness can be a problem Theophylline metabolism is affected by protein and CHO availability; avoid extreme changes in protein and CHO intake. Because it is a methylxanthine, avoid extreme changes in usual intakes of caffeine-containing foods. Theophylline depresses levels of vitamin B_6. In addition, lipid levels (cholesterol, HDL, and LDL) are higher in children who take theophylline.
Corticosteroids (methylprednisolone [Medrol], Deltasone, Orapred, Prelone)	Many side effects such as fluid retention, low serum potassium, GI distress, retaining excess sodium, causing hyperglycemia, and other problems. Monitor carefully, especially if needed over a long period of time. AeroBid contains an anti-inflammatory steroid and is inhaled; it may cause nausea, vomiting, or diarrhea. Bone mineral density is often decreased after long-term use of inhaled corticosteroids.
Epinephrine	May be required for emergencies. Intravenous (IV) administration of epinephrine results in a prolonged increase in resting energy expenditure (REE) as measured by respiratory quotient (RQ); fuel for this is increased CHO oxidation.
Expectorants	Potassium iodide may affect existing thyroid problems.
Long-term control medications	Anti-immunoglobulin E: Reduces histamine release; may be useful with allergic form of asthma. Combination therapy (Advair): Combining an inhaled corticosteroid and a long-lasting beta$_2$-agonist seems to provide consistent relief for people with asthma. Intal (cromolyn) and Tilade (nedocromil) are inhaled medications useful for asthma triggered by cold weather, exercise, and allergies. Inhaled nasal steroids: AeroBid (flunisolide), Azmacort (triamcinolone), Flovent (fluticasone), Pulmicort (budesonide), and Qvar (beclomethasone HFA). These prevent inflammation and reduce swelling inside airways; they also reduce mucus production. Leukotriene modifiers: Accolate, Singulair, Zyflo. These relax the smooth muscle around the airways and reduce inflammation. Serevent (salmeterol xinafoate), Advair (fluticasone propionate and salmeterol inhalation powder), and Foradil or Tubuhaler Aerolizer (formoterol fumarate); these medications can worsen asthma or cause death. Formoterol may deplete potassium levels and cause heart palpitations.
Omega-3 fatty acid supplements	Omega-3 fatty acid supplements may decrease inflammation and improve lung function in adults with asthma, but there is no conclusive evidence. Omega-6 fatty acids tend to increase inflammation and worsen respiratory function.

Patient Education—Foodborne Illness

- Careful food handling will be important. Hand washing is key as well.

For More Information

- Allergy and Asthma Advocate
  http://www.aaaai.org/
- Allergy and Asthma Network—Mothers of Asthmatics
  http://www.aanma.org/
- Asthma and Allergy
  http://allergy.healthcentersonline.com/allergyasthmabasics/
- National Asthma Center
  http://www.nationaljewish.org/healthinfo/conditions/asthma/index.aspx
- National Asthma Education and Prevention Program (NAEPP)
  http://aspe.hhs.gov/sp/asthma/
- Salicilate allergy
  http://www.webmd.com/allergies/guide/salicylate-allergy

ASTHMA—CITED REFERENCES

Brehm JM, et al. Serum vitamin D levels and markers of severity of childhood asthma in Costa Rica. *Am J Respir Crit Care Med.* 179:765, 2009.

Dang DH, Hoang TM. Nutritional analysis of Vietnamese seaweeds for food and medicine. *Biofactors.* 22:323, 2004.

Devereux G. Early life events in asthma—diet. *Pediatr Pulmonol.* 42:663, 2009.

Kano S, et al. Immediate hypersensitivity elicits renin release from cardiac mast cells. *Int Arch Allergy Immunol.* 146:71, 2008.

Kim JH, et al. Diet and asthma: looking back, moving forward. *Respir Res.* 10:49, 2009.

Mickleborough T, Gotshall RW. Dietary salt intake as a potential modifier of airway responsiveness in bronchial asthma. *J Altern Complement Med.* 10:633, 2004.

Mickleborough T, et al. Eicosapentaenoic acid is more effective than docosahexaenoic acid in inhibiting proinflammatory mediator production and transcription from LPS-induced human asthmatic alveolar macrophage cells. *Clin Nutr.* 28:71, 2009.

Milner JD, et al. Early infant multivitamin supplementation is associated with increased risk for food allergy and asthma. *Pediatrics.* 114:27, 2004.

Nagel G, Linseisen J. Dietary intake of fatty acids, antioxidants and selected food groups and asthma in adults. *Eur J Clin Nutr.* 59:8, 2005.

Oddy WH, et al. The relation of breastfeeding and body mass index to asthma and atopy in children: a prospective cohort study to age 6 years. *Am J Public Health.* 94:1531, 2004.

Reid AC, et al. Renin: at the heart of the mast cell. *Immunol Rev.* 217:123, 2007.

Sadeghnejad A, et al. IL13 gene polymorphisms modify the effect of exposure to tobacco smoke on persistent wheeze and asthma in childhood, a longitudinal study. *Respir Res.* 10:92, 2008.

Schrader WA Jr. Short and long term treatment of asthma with intravenous nutrients. *Nutr J.* 3:6, 2004.

Sutherland ER, et al. Body mass index and phenotype in subjects with mild-to-moderate persistent asthma. *J Allergy Clin Immunol.* 126:1328, 2009.
Tan WC. Viruses in asthma exacerbations. *Curr Opin Pulm Med.* 11:21, 2005.
Wen MC, et al. Efficacy and tolerability of anti-asthma herbal medicine intervention in adult patients with moderate-severe allergic asthma. *J Allergy Clin Immunol.* 116:517, 2005.
Weldon SM, et al. Docosahexaenoic acid induces an anti-inflammatory profile in lipopolysaccharide-stimulated human THP-1 macrophages more effectively than eicosapentaenoic acid. *J Nutr Biochem.* 18:250, 2007.
Wong KW. Clinical efficacy of n-3 fatty acid supplementation in patients with asthma. *J Am Diet Assoc.* 105:98, 2005.
Ziboh VA, et al. Suppression of leukotriene B4 generation by ex-vivo neutrophils isolated from asthma patients on dietary supplementation with gammalinolenic acid-containing borage oil: possible implication in asthma. *Clin Dev Immunol.* 11:13, 2004.
Zutavern A, et al. The introduction of solids in relation to asthma and eczema. *Arch Dis Child.* 89:303, 2004.

BRONCHIECTASIS

NUTRITIONAL ACUITY RANKING: LEVEL 1

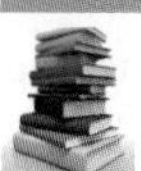

DEFINITIONS AND BACKGROUND

Bronchiectasis (BX) is an irreversible widening of portions of the bronchi resulting from damage to the bronchial wall with chronic dilation. It may be present with recurrent bronchitis or pneumonia. The most common acquired cause is acute respiratory illness in patients with COPD. Other causes include measles, whooping cough, tuberculosis (TB), fungal infection, inhaled object, lung tumor, CF, ciliary dyskinesia, immunoglobulin deficiency syndromes, rheumatoid arthritis, ulcerative colitis, human immunodeficiency virus (HIV) infection, and heroin abuse.

BX secondary to primary immunodeficiency in childhood is not always progressive; it is possible to slow or prevent disease progression with appropriate treatment (Haidopoulou et al, 2009). In non-CF BX, airway obstruction deteriorates over time; precaution must be taken to prevent significant morbidity and mortality (Twiss et al, 2006).

Relapse can be controlled with antibiotics, chest physiotherapy, inhaled bronchodilators, proper hydration, and good nutrition. Surgical resection or bilateral lung transplantation may be an option for improving quality of life that has few complications.

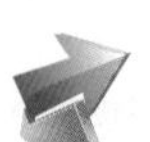

ASSESSMENT, MONITORING, AND EVALUATION

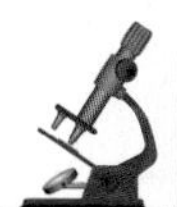

CLINICAL INDICATORS

Genetic Markers: Congenital BX usually affects infants and children related to problems with lung development in a fetus but is not genetic in origin.

Clinical/History

Height
Weight
BMI
Weight loss?
Diet history
BP
I & O
Chest high-resolution computed tomography (HRCT)
Altered respiratory rate
Chronic cough
Early morning paroxysmal cough
Decreased breath sounds
Weight loss, anorexia
Pneumonia?
Fever?
Shortness of breath (SOB)
Fatigue
Bluish skin or paleness
Coughing up blood
Chest x-ray
Sputum culture: profuse, foul, or purulent

Lab Work

Transthyretin
Retinol-binding protein (RBP)
Gluc
Na^+, K^+
Ca^{++}, Mg^{++}
Chol
Trig
H & H
Serum Fe
Transferrin
Blood urea nitrogen (BUN)
pO_2, pCO_2

INTERVENTION

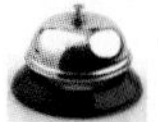

OBJECTIVES

- Promote recovery and prevent relapse of symptoms. Prevent lung collapse or atelectasis.
- Avoid fatigue associated with mealtimes.
- Prevent or correct dehydration.
- Improve weight status, when necessary.
- Reduce fever and inflammation.
- Support lung function with higher antioxidant intake.
- Prepare patient for surgery if needed.

SAMPLE NUTRITION CARE PROCESS STEPS

Unintentional Weight Loss

Assessment Data: Fever, anorexia, fatigue, chronic cough with purulent sputum, weight loss of 15 lb in past 2 months.

Nutrition Diagnoses (PES): Unintentional weight loss related to fever, fatigue and poor appetite as evidenced by loss of 15 lb in 2 months.

Interventions: Food and nutrient enhancement through nutrient-dense, energy-rich foods and beverages. Education about recipes and beverages to replace weight that are easy to prepare and consume.

Monitoring and Evaluation: Regain of lost weight; improved appetite; more destable BMI.

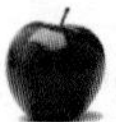

FOOD AND NUTRITION

- Use a diet with 1.0–1.25 g protein/kg and sufficient calories to meet elevated metabolic requirements appropriate for age and sex.
- Small, frequent feedings may be better tolerated.
- Fluid intake of 2–3 L daily may be offered, unless contraindicated.
- Intravenous fat emulsions may be indicated (eicosanoids are inflammatory modulators, and thromboxanes and leukotrienes tend to be potent mediators of inflammation). Omega-3 fatty acids should be enhanced in the oral diet by including salmon, tuna, sardines, walnuts, and flaxseed. Supplements may also be useful.
- Adequate antioxidant use with vitamins C and E and selenium may be beneficial. Ensure adequate potassium intake, depending on medications used.

Common Drugs Used and Potential Side Effects

- Antibiotics are used if the condition is bacterial. Aerosol administration of high-dose tobramycin in non-CF bronchiectatic patients is safe (Drobnic et al, 2005).
- Expectorants help bring up the mucus. Mucus thinners help make it easier to cough.
- Bronchodilators help open up the airways and corticosteroids help reduce airway swelling and inflammation. Monitor side effects according to the specific drugs used.

Herbs, Botanicals, and Supplements

No clinical trials have proven efficacy for use of herbs or botanicals in BX.

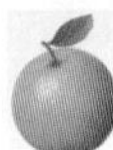

NUTRITION EDUCATION, COUNSELING, CARE MANAGEMENT

- Discuss the role of nutrition in health and recovery; emphasize quality proteins and nutrient-dense foods, especially if the patient is anorexic.
- A flu shot or pneumonia shot may be needed annually.
- Emphasize fluid intake, perhaps juices or calorie-containing beverages instead of water.
- Discuss desirable sources of fatty acids, such as omega-3 foods.

Patient Education—Foodborne Illness

- Careful food handling will be important. Hand washing is key as well.

For More Information

- Bronchiectasis
  http://www.lung.ca/diseases/bronchiectasis.html
- Merck Manual
  http://www.merck.com/mmhe/sec04/ch047/ch047a.html

BRONCHIECTASIS—CITED REFERENCES

Drobnic ME, et al. Inhaled tobramycin in non-cystic fibrosis patients with bronchiectasis and chronic bronchial infection with *Pseudomonas aeruginosa*. *Ann Pharmacother.* 39:39, 2005.

Haidopoulou K, et al. Bronchiectasis secondary to primary immunodeficiency in children: longitudinal changes in structure and function [epub ahead of print Jun 9, 2009]. *Pediatr Pulmonol.* 44:669, 2009.

Twiss J, et al. Longitudinal pulmonary function of childhood bronchiectasis and comparison with cystic fibrosis. *Thorax.* 61:414, 2006.

BRONCHITIS (ACUTE)

NUTRITIONAL ACUITY RANKING: LEVEL 1

DEFINITIONS AND BACKGROUND

Bronchitis is caused by inflammation of the air passages. Acute bronchitis is an acute respiratory infection that is manifested by cough and sputum production that lasts for no more than 3 weeks (Braman, 2006). The acute form may follow a cold or other upper respiratory infection, producing hemoptysis, sore throat, nasal discharge, slight fever, cough, and back and muscle pain.

Causes include *Mycoplasma pneumoniae, Chlamydia, or* exposure to strong acids, ammonia, or chlorine fumes, air pollution ozone, or nitrogen dioxide. The chronic form from cigarette smoking and air pollution can produce breathing difficulty, wheezing, blueness, fits of coughing, and sputum production. (See Chronic Obstructive Pulmonary Disease entry.)

Risks for acute bronchitis are much higher in smokers. Mental patients and homeless persons tend to smoke more than other individuals and are at higher risk for acute bronchitis (Himelhoch et al, 2004; Snyder and Eisner, 2004). In addition, smoking has negative consequences for maternal health as well as fetal health during pregnancy; the risk of bronchitis is 15 times higher for smokers than for nonsmokers (Roelands et al, 2009).

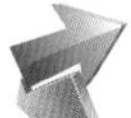

ASSESSMENT, MONITORING, AND EVALUATION

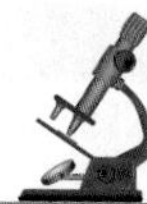

CLINICAL INDICATORS

Genetic Markers: Tachykinins NK receptors, substance P, T lymphocytes, and neurokinin A appear to influence human airway health and susceptibility to bronchitis.

Clinical/History

Height
Weight
BMI
I & O
Hydration status
Edema
Productive cough longer than 3 weeks
Green or yellow sputum
Breathing difficulty
Chest x-ray

Lab Work

Gluc
Na^+, K^+
Ca^{++}, Mg^{++}
Serum lipids (decreased?)
H & H, serum Fe
Alb, transthyretin
Oxygen saturation
CRP

INTERVENTION

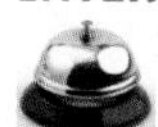

OBJECTIVES

- Normalize body temperature when there is fever.
- Replenish nutrients used in respiratory distress.
- Prevent complications such as dehydration and otitis media; avoid further infections.
- Allow ample rest before and after feedings.
- Prevent dehydration. Extra fluids are needed.
- Relieve discomfort.
- Support lung function through high antioxidant foods.

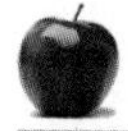

FOOD AND NUTRITION

- Provide a regular or high-calorie diet, specific to the patient's needs.
- If milk gives a sensation of thickening mucus secretions, skim milk may be better tolerated and is important for adequate calcium consumption.
- Provide adequate amounts of vitamins C and E, selenium, and potassium.
- Increase the intake of fluids (2–3 L), unless contraindicated.
- Appropriate fatty acid intake may be beneficial to reduce inflammation.
- A low energy intake may be needed after the acute phase to promote weight loss, improve BMI, and promote a healthier level of respiratory functioning (Canoy et al, 2004).

Common Drugs Used and Potential Side Effects

- Bronchodilators can cause gastric irritation. They should be taken with milk, food, or an antacid.
- Theophylline can be toxic if a diet high in CHO and low in protein is used. Avoid large amounts of stimulant beverages, namely, coffee, tea, cocoa, and cola, unless the physician permits.
- Use of antibiotics for the treatment of acute bronchitis is not justified (Braman, 2006).

Herbs, Botanicals, and Supplements

- No clinical trials have proven efficacy for eucalyptus, mullein, horehound, stinging nettle, or marshmallow.
- Belladonna leaf and root are respiratory antispasmodic agents. They should not be used with tricyclic antidepressants, some antihistamines, phenothiazines, or quinidine. Sedation, dry mouth, and difficult urination may occur.

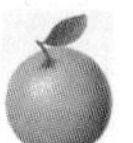

NUTRITION EDUCATION, COUNSELING, CARE MANAGEMENT

- Explain to patient that adequate hydration is one of the best ways to liquefy secretions.
- Maintain body weight within a healthy range.
- Promote healthy diet that includes a balance of nutrients, with anti-oxidant-rich foods.

Patient Education—Foodborne Illness

- Careful food handling will be important. Hand washing is key as well.

For More Information

- Medline—Bronchitis
  http://www.nlm.nih.gov/medlineplus/bronchitis.html
- Web-MD—Bronchitis
  http://www.webmd.com/a-to-z-guides/acute-bronchitis-topic-overview

SAMPLE NUTRITION CARE PROCESS STEPS

Inadequate Fluid Intake

Assessment Data: Poor skin turgor, low I & O, frequent cough making drinking difficult, weight loss.

Nutrition Diagnoses (PES): Inadequate fluid intake related to frequent coughing spells and difficulty drinking beverages as evidenced by poor skin turgor, loss of 2 kg fluid, and low I & O.

Interventions: Food and nutrient delivery enhancement with nutrient and calorie-dense beverages such as shakes or nutritional supplements. Education about recipes for calorie-rich beverages.

Monitoring and Evaluation: Improved I & O and skin turgor; improved fluid intake, and recovery of lost weight.

BRONCHITIS—CITED REFERENCES

Braman SS. Chronic cough due to acute bronchitis: ACCP evidence-based clinical practice guidelines. *Chest.* 129:95S, 2006.

Canoy D, et al. Abdominal obesity and respiratory function in men and women in the EPIC-Norfolk Study, United Kingdom. *Am J Epidemiol.* 159:1140, 2004.

Himelhoch S, et al. Prevalence of chronic obstructive pulmonary disease among those with serious mental illness. *Am J Psychiatry.* 161:2317, 2004.

Roelands J, et al. Consequences of smoking during pregnancy on maternal health. *J Womens Health.* 18:867, 2009.

Snyder LD, Eisner MD. Obstructive lung disease among the urban homeless. *Chest.* 125:1719, 2004.

CHRONIC OBSTRUCTIVE PULMONARY DISEASE

NUTRITIONAL ACUITY RANKING: LEVEL 3

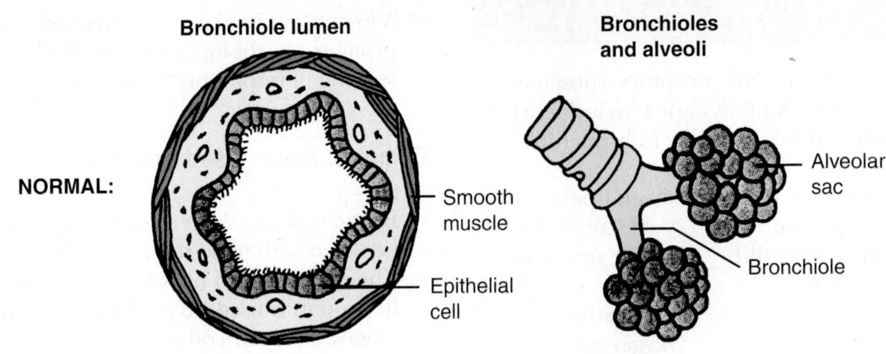

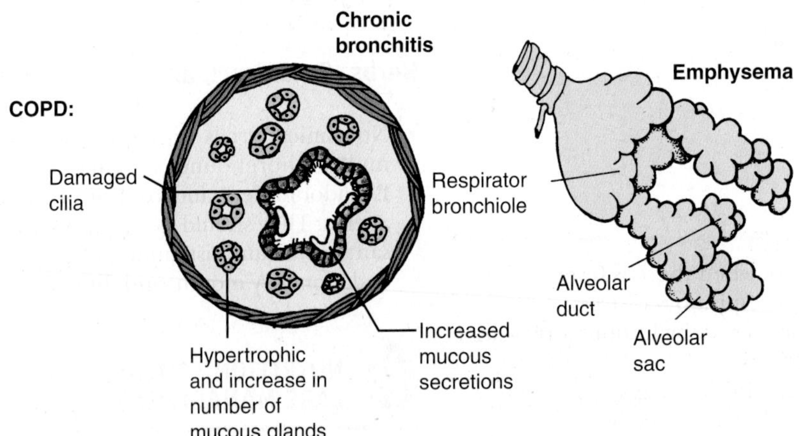

Adapted from: Nettina, Sandra M., MSN, RN, CS, ANP, *The Lippincott Manual of Nursing Practice*, 7th ed. Lippincott, Williams & Wilkins, 2001.

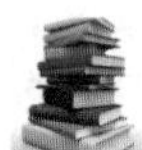

DEFINITIONS AND BACKGROUND

Chronic obstructive pulmonary disease (COPD) may result from a history of emphysema, asthma, or chronic bronchitis with persistent lower airway obstruction. COPD is the fourth leading cause of death in the United States. Smoking is the most common cause. According to the Centers for Disease Control and Prevention (CDC), approximately 440,000 persons die each year of a cigarette smoking–attributable illness in the United States. Nonsmoking causes of COPD include alpha-1 antitrypsin deficiency, connective tissue diseases, HIV infection, and some metabolic disorders.

COPD is associated with muscular impairment, nutritional depletion, and systemic inflammation. Symptoms and signs of COPD include dyspnea on exertion, frequent hypoxemia, decreased forced expiratory volume in 1 second (FEV_1), and destruction of the alveolar capillary bed. In COPD, total air quantity is blown out much sooner. COPD is a leading cause of death in the United States.

Chronic bronchitis ("blue bloater") patients have inflamed bronchial tubes, excess mucus production, chronic cough (for 3 months each year), SOB, and no weight loss. Cardiac enlargement with failure is common.

Emphysema ("pink puffer") patients have weight loss and thinness without heart failure. It is characterized by tissue destruction, distention, and destruction of pulmonary air spaces by smoking and air pollution. Wheezing, SOB, and chronic mild cough result. Nutritional depletion is significantly greater in patients who have emphysema than in those who have chronic bronchitis. Serious weight loss occurs from anorexia, secondary to significant SOB and gastrointestinal (GI) distress. Malnutrition, tissue wasting, and oxidative stress play a role.

Approximately 75% of patients with COPD suffer from weight loss, where chronic mouth breathing, dyspnea, aerophagia, certain medications, and depression often act in concert. Low body weight or recent weight loss and, in particular, depleted lean body mass (LBM) in patients with COPD are predictors of mortality, outcomes after acute exacerbations, hospital admission rates, and need for mechanical ventilation (Mallampalli, 2004). Risk of respiratory mortality is high.

Elevated resting and activity-related energy expenditure, reduced dietary intake relative to resting energy expenditure, accelerated negative nitrogen balance, medication effects, and an elevated systemic inflammatory response contribute to weight loss (Mallampalli, 2004).

Nutritional supplementation may have a role in the management of COPD when provided as part of an integrated rehabilitation program incorporating a structured exercise component.

The pathological mechanisms of COPD involve neutrophil granulocytes, cytotoxic T cells, macrophages, and mast cells (Ekberg-Jansson et al, 2005). Interventions aimed at controlling cytokine production may be required to reverse cachexia. Starvation, as in anorexia nervosa, can cause emphysema, even without smoking (Coxson et al, 2004).

Recommendations for fats, CHO, proteins, and water must be individualized. For patients with acute exacerbations of COPD in the intensive care unit (ICU), serum total protein is associated with hospital mortality; therefore, protein intake must be carefully monitored (Yang et al, 2004).

Nutritional support is a mainstay of the comprehensive therapeutic approach to patients with COPD because of progressive malnutrition, due to reduced energy intake, increased energy expenditure, and impaired anabolism (Anker et al, 2009).

Fruit and vegetable intake is important and protective. Foods such as meats, vegetables, and coffee may be more bland to the patient than he or she remembers; recognition of this may be important in planning meals.

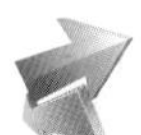

ASSESSMENT, MONITORING, AND EVALUATION

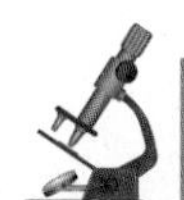

CLINICAL INDICATORS

Genetic Markers: Copeptin is a prognostic marker for short-term and long-term prognoses in patients with COPD requiring hospitalization (Stolz et al, 2007). In addition, glutathione-S transferase omega (GSTO) is a candidate gene for COPD (Wilk et al, 2007) and the vitamin D endocrine system is being studied (Janssen et al, 2009).

Clinical/History

Height
Weight
BMI
Diet history
Temperature
I & O
Pulmonary function tests
Spirometry
Expiratory airflow limitation
Excessive mucus production
Wheezing
SOB
Morning headache
Anorexia, depression
BP
Chest x-ray
Electrocardiogram (ECG)
Respirations
Ascites
Edema

Lab Work

Gluc
Na^+, K^+
Ca^{++}, Mg^{++}
Serum Fe
Hemoglobin
Hct >48% may reflect chronic hypoxemia
Serum vitamin D_3
TLC
pH
pO_2 <50 mm Hg
$PaCO_2$ >50 mm Hg
Alb, transthyretin
BUN
CRP
Chol
Trig

SAMPLE NUTRITION CARE PROCESS STEPS

Early Satiety and COPD

Assessment: Food intake records, weight, preferred foods. Early satiety and problems with coordination of breathing and swallowing.

Nutrition Diagnosis (PES): Involuntary weight loss related to early satiety, problems with breathing and swallowing, and inadequate intake of calorie-dense foods as evidenced by 20-lb weight loss and fatigue at mealtimes.

Intervention: Frequent small meals of easily digested foods with added fats and calorie-dense oral supplements.

Monitoring and Evaluation: Weight changes, improvement in calorie intake, less fatigue while eating.

INTERVENTION

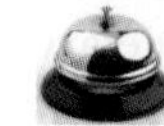

OBJECTIVES

- Screen early and correct any malnutrition. Because there is less oxygen available for energy production, the patient is less active, and there is less blood flow to the GI tract and muscles. Malnutrition increases likelihood of infections. Provide medical nutrition therapy (MNT) focusing on prevention and treatment of weight loss and related conditions, especially in underweight patients (ADA, 2009).
- Promote intake of a nutrient-dense diet rich in antioxidant foods.
- Overcome anorexia resulting from slowed peristalsis and digestion. Patient lethargy, poor appetite, and gastric ulceration resulting from inadequate oxygen to the gut.
- Improve ventilation before meals with intermittent positive-pressure breathing and overall physical conditioning to strengthen respiratory muscles. Lessen work efforts by losing excess weight, if needed.
- Prevent respiratory infections or respiratory acidosis from decreased elimination of CO_2.
- Alleviate difficulty in chewing or swallowing related to SOB. Patients with COPD have disrupted coordination of breathing and swallowing and may be at risk for aspiration (Gross et al, 2009). Breathe carefully, eat slowly, and rest when the meal is finished.
- Prevent or correct dehydration, which thickens mucus.
- Avoid constipation and prevent straining with defection at stool.
- Avoid distention from large meals or gaseous foods. Eat while sitting up to lessen discomfort.
- Ensure adequate flavor of foods because taste is often minimized (Wardwell et al, 2009).
- Consider nutritional support to prevent progressive weight loss, since restoration of lean and fat body mass may not be achievable (Anker et al, 2009). Medical food supplements should be influenced more by the patient's preference than nutritional factors such as percentage of fat or CHO, as there is limited evidence to support consumption of a particular macronutrient composition (ADA, 2009).
- Assess and help improve quality of life of people with COPD, especially as it relates to their ability to obtain,

prepare, and consume food to meet nutritional needs; impairment with activities of daily living is common (ADA, 2009).

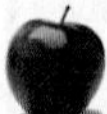

FOOD AND NUTRITION

- A high-protein/high-calorie diet is necessary to correct malnutrition. Use 1.2–1.7 g protein/kg and sufficient kilocals for anabolism (start with 30–35 kcal/kg, depending on current weight). Use BMI and weight change to assess weight status, body composition, and calorie needs (ADA, 2009).
- A diet without tough or stringy foods and an antireflux regimen are useful. Gas-forming vegetables may cause discomfort for some patients.
- Increased use of omega-3 fatty acids in foods such as salmon, haddock, mackerel, tuna, and other fish sources may be beneficial (ADA, 2009; Romieu et al, 2005).
- Encourage a diet that meets Recommended Dietary Allowances for antioxidant vitamins A, C, and E (ADA, 2009). To enrich the diet with antioxidants, use more citrus fruits, whole grains, and nuts. There is a protective effect of fruit and possibly vitamin E.
- Fluid intake should be high, especially if the patient is febrile. Use 1 mL/kcal as a general rule. This may translate to eight or more cups of fluid daily. For discomfort, consume liquids between meals to increase ability to consume nutrient-dense foods at mealtimes.
- Limit salt intake. Too much sodium can cause fluid retention or peripheral edema, which may interfere with breathing.
- Fiber should be increased gradually, perhaps through use of psyllium, crushed bran, prune juice, or extra fruits and vegetables.
- Use small, concentrated feedings at frequent intervals to lessen fatigue. For example, eggnogs and shakes may be helpful between meals.
- Morning may be the best meal of the day for many patients with COPD. See Tables 5-6 and 5-7 for ways to add extra protein or calories to the diet.
- Parenteral nutrition (PN) is reserved for patients in whom malabsorption has been documented where enteral nutrition has failed (Anker et al, 2009).

Common Drugs Used and Potential Side Effects

- Bronchodilators (Atrovent, Theo-Dur, etc). are used to liquefy secretions, treat infections, and dilate the bronchi. They can cause gastric irritation and ulceration.
- Antibiotics, steroids, expectorants, antihistamines, diuretics, anticholinergics, and other drugs may be used. Monitor side effects accordingly.
- Oral or parenteral corticosteroids significantly reduce treatment failure and the need for additional medical treatment; adverse drug reactions may occur (Wood-Baker et al, 2005).

Herbs, Botanicals, and Supplements

- No clinical trials have proven efficacy for use of mullein, camu-camu, licorice, red pepper, peppermint, or eucalyptus.
- Ephedra (ma huang) is an effective bronchodilator, but it increases BP significantly. Avoid taking with digoxin, hypoglycemic agents for diabetes, monoamine oxidase inhibitor (MAOI) antidepressants, antihypertensive medications, oxytocin, theophylline, caffeine, and dexamethasone steroids. Problems with BP, blood glucose, arrhythmias, increased heart rate, and CNS stimulation can occur.
- Vitamin D supplementation may be beneficial to prevent upper respiratory infections (Ginde et al, 2009).

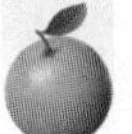

NUTRITION EDUCATION, COUNSELING, CARE MANAGEMENT

- Early detection, prevention, and early treatment of involuntary weight loss means putting more emphasis on dietary change (Brug et al, 2004; Weekes et al, 2009). Explain how to concentrate protein and calories in five to six small meals a day rather than three large ones.
- To conserve energy while preparing meals at home, choose foods that are easy to prepare. Try having the main meal early in the day to have more energy later.

TABLE 5-6 Tips for Adding Calories to a Diet

Food	Tip
Fats	Butter or margarine, cream, sour cream, gravies, salad dressings, and shortening. Mix butter into hot foods such as soups and vegetables, mashed potatoes, cooked cereals, and rice. Serve hot bread with lots of melted butter. Mayonnaise can be added to salads or sandwiches. Sour cream or yogurt can be used on vegetables such as potatoes, beans, carrots, and squash. Try sour cream or yogurt in gravy or salad dressings for fruit. Whipping cream has 60 kcal per tablespoon; add it to pies, fruits, pudding, hot chocolate, gelatin, eggnog, and other desserts. Fry the entree (e.g., chicken, meat, fish) and sauté vegetables in butter or oil.
Sweets	Spread jelly or honey on toast or cereal; mix honey in tea. Add marshmallows to hot chocolate.
Snacks	Have snacks ready to eat, such as nuts, dried fruits, candy, buttered popcorn, crackers and cheese, granola, ice cream, and popsicles.
Beverages	Drink milk shakes with lots of ice cream added; these will be high in calories and protein. Use sugar-sweetened beverages such as carbonated beverages, coffees with whipped cream and sugar, and sugar-sweetened ades.

TABLE 5-7 Tips for Adding Protein to a Diet[a]

Food	Tip
Meats and meat substitutes	Add diced or ground meat to soups and casseroles. Serve a chef salad with cheese, ham, turkey, and sliced egg. Peanut butter can be spread on crackers, apples, celery, pears, and bananas. Nuts are a good snack with both fat and protein.
Dairy products	Add milk powder to hot or cold cereals, scrambled eggs, mashed potatoes, soups, gravies, ground meats (e.g., meat patties, meatballs, meatloaf), casserole dishes, and baked goods. Use milk or half and half instead of water when making soups, cereals, instant puddings, cocoa, and canned soups. Add grated cheese or cheese chunks to sauces, vegetables, soups, casseroles, hot crab dip, and mashed potatoes. Add extra cheese to pizza. Use yogurt as a fruit dip, or add yogurt to sauces and gravies.
Milk powder	Add skim milk powder to the regular amount of milk used in recipes or for a beverage. For double-strength milk, add 1 cup of dry powder to 1 quart of fluid milk, let it sit overnight for 286 kcals and 15 g of protein.
Beverages	Add protein powder to casseroles, soups, sauces, gravies, milkshakes, and eggnogs. One scoop may have 4 or 5 g of protein, depending on the brand. Some do not stir in as well as others; some dissolve better in hot foods. Buy instant breakfast mixes and use them instead of milk with meals or as snacks; one 8-oz glass provides 280 kcal. Formula products that are high in protein may be useful as supplements with or between meals or with medication pass in an institution.
Desserts	Choose dessert recipes that contain egg such as sponge or angel food cake, egg custard, bread pudding, and rice pudding.

[a]Protein can be added to many foods without having to increase the number of foods eaten.

Encourage slow eating and rest periods before and after meals.

- Encourage the patient to make small, attractive meals.
- Explain that excessively hot or cold foods may cause coughing spells for some individuals.
- Limit fluid intake with meals to decrease early satiety and subsequent decreased food intake.
- Schedule treatments to mobilize mucus (postural drainage, aerosol treatment) 1 hour before and after meals to prevent nausea.
- Improve physical conditioning with planned exercises, especially strengthening exercises and dancing. Consumption of an oral supplement may be beneficial to support exercise.
- If using oxygen, be sure the cannula is worn during and after meals. Eating and digestion require energy and oxygen.
- Maintain a relaxed atmosphere to make meals enjoyable.
- Promote good oral hygiene; periodontal disease is common.
- MNT should be coordinated with the team of clinical professionals to integrate rehabilitative elements into a system of patient self-management and regular exercise (ADA, 2009).

Patient Education—Foodborne Illness

- Careful food handling will be important. Hand washing is key as well.

For More Information

- AARC—COPD
  http://www.aarc.org/patient_education/tips/copd.html
- American Thoracic Society
  http://www.thoracic.org/
- National Emphysema Treatment Trial (Nett)
  http://www.nhlbi.nih.gov/health/prof/lung/nett/lvrsweb.htm
- Stages of COPD
  http://www.yourlunghealth.org/lung_disease/copd/stages/Stages_of_COPD.pdf
- Your Lung Health
  http://www.yourlunghealth.org/lung_disease/copd/decrease/index.cfm

CHRONIC OBSTRUCTIVE PULMONARY DISEASE—CITED REFERENCES

American Dietetic Association. Chronic Obstructive Pulmonary Disease Evidence-Based Nutrition Practice Guideline for adults. Accessed June 22, 2009, at http://www.adaevidencelibrary.com/topic.cfm?cat=3708.

Anker SD, et al. ESPEN guidelines on parenteral nutrition: cardiology [epub ahead of print June 9, 2009]. *Clin Nutr.* 28:455, 2009.

Brug J, et al. Dietary change, nutrition education and chronic obstructive pulmonary disease. *Patient Educ Couns.* 52:249, 2004.

Coxson HO, et al. Early emphysema in patients with anorexia nervosa. *Am J Respir Crit Care Med.* 170:748, 2004.

Ekberg-Jansson A, et al. Bronchial mucosal mast cells in asymptomatic smokers relation to structure, lung function and emphysema. *Respir Med.* 99:75, 2005.

Ginde AA, et al. Association between serum 25-hydroxyvitamin D level and upper respiratory tract infection in the Third National Health and Nutrition Examination Survey. *Arch Intern Med.* 23:169, 2009.

Gross RD, et al. The coordination of breathing and swallowing in chronic obstructive pulmonary disease. *Am J Respir Crit Care Med.* 179:559, 2009.

Janssens W, et al. Vitamin D beyond bones in chronic obstructive pulmonary disease: time to act. *An J Respir Crit Care Med.* 179:630, 2009.

Mallampalli A. Nutritional management of the patient with chronic obstructive pulmonary disease. *Nutr Clin Pract.* 19:550, 2004.

Romieu I, et al. Omega-3 fatty acid prevents heart rate variability reductions associated with particulate matter. *Am J Respir Crit Care Med.* 172:1534, 2005.

Stolz D, et al. Copeptin, C-reactive protein, and procalcitonin as prognostic biomarkers in acute exacerbation of COPD. *Chest.* 131:1058, 2007.

Wardwell L, et al. Effects of age, gender and chronic obstructive pulmonary disease on taste acuity. *Int J Food Sci Nutr.* 19:1, 2009.

Weekes CE, et al. Dietary counselling and food fortification in stable COPD: a randomised trial. *Thorax.* 64:326, 2009.

Wilk JB, et al. Framingham Heart Study genome-wide association: results for pulmonary function measures. *BMC Med Genet.* 8:8S, 2007.

Wood-Baker RR, et al. Systemic corticosteroids for acute exacerbations of chronic obstructive pulmonary disease. *Cochrane Database Syst Rev.* 1:CD001288, 2005.

Yang S, et al. Acute exacerbation of COPD requiring admission to the intensive care unit. *Respirology.* 9:543, 2004.

CHYLOTHORAX

NUTRITIONAL ACUITY RANKING: LEVEL 2–4

DEFINITIONS AND BACKGROUND

Chylothorax involves accumulation of clear lymph (chyle) in the pleural or thoracic space. It may be spontaneous or caused by amyloidosis, congenital chylothorax, coronary artery bypass grafting (CABG), violent vomiting, lymphoma, thoracic cage compression after cardiopulmonary resuscitation (CPR), thoracic duct trauma or surgery, sarcoidosis, or TB. Chylothorax is caused by surgical procedures in about half of all cases (Maldonado et al, 2009).

Chylous effusions look like milk. Since chyle represents direct absorption of fat from the small intestine lacteals, it is rich in triglycerides. Management of chylothorax may include use of total parenteral nutrition (TPN), low-fat enteral nutrition, thoracentesis to remove the chylous fluid, or surgical ligation of the thoracic duct (Suddaby and Schiller, 2004).

In the congenital form, breast milk and/or regular infant feeding formula should be used before proceeding to medium-chain triglyceride (MCT)–rich formula. Surgery may be considered if conservative management fails. Surgery is needed in the care of small babies with massive chylothorax, such as daily output exceeding 50 mL/kg per day (Cleveland et al, 2009).

> **SAMPLE NUTRITION CARE PROCESS STEPS**
>
> **Inappropriate Intake of Types of Fats**
>
> ***Assessment Data:*** Chylothorax with high pleural triglyceride levels in infant.
>
> ***Nutrition Diagnoses (PES):*** Inappropriate intake of types of fatty acids related to chylothorax as evidenced by pleural triglyceride levels of 120 mg/dL.
>
> ***Interventions:*** Use of breast milk or MCT oil formula in the infant.
>
> ***Monitoring and Evaluation:*** Reduced pleural triglycerides and signs of chylohorax.

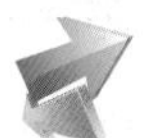

ASSESSMENT, MONITORING, AND EVALUATION

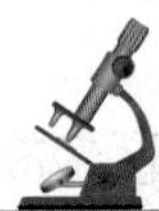

CLINICAL INDICATORS

Genetic Markers: Congenital chylothorax is the leading cause of pleural effusion in newborns but is not genetic in origin.

Clinical/History

- Height
- Weight
- BMI
- Weight changes
- Temperature
- I & O
- Lung x-ray
- Pleural fluid analysis for triglyceride >110 mg/dL
- Dyspnea
- Tachypnea
- Decreased breath sounds

Lab Work

- Alb, transthyretin
- Chol
- Trig
- TLC (decreased)
- Gluc
- Ca^{++}, Mg^{++}
- Na^+, K^+
- CRP
- BUN, creatinine (Creat)
- pCO_2, pO_2

INTERVENTION

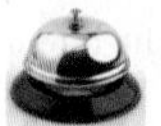

OBJECTIVES

- Offer continuous chest-tube drainage to decrease pleural chyle.
- Drainage of chyle from the chest or abdomen results in rapid weight loss and profound cachexia. Lessen consequences of a nutritional or immunological nature from drainage (e.g., sepsis, protein–calorie malnutrition, decreased lymphocytes).
- Replace fat, protein, and micronutrient losses from exudates.
- Achieve a positive nitrogen balance.
- Support involvement of a surgical nutrition support team, which is associated with better patient management and a reduction in inappropriate TPN orders (Saalwachter et al, 2004).

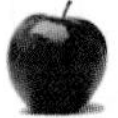

FOOD AND NUTRITION

- Decrease enteral fat intake for patients who are tube fed. For patients who are fed orally, reduce total fat intake until condition is resolved; also for these patients, a low-fat diet may be used alone or with an elemental product.
- Some patients may be able to tolerate a low long-chain fatty acid formula given as a tube feeding (TF) (Cormack et al, 2004).
- For patients without sepsis, TPN may be indicated; care is needed to avoid aggravating the condition.
- Replace exudate losses of nutrients such as vitamin A and zinc. Check serum levels and replace with higher levels of the recommended intakes if necessary.

Common Drugs Used and Potential Side Effects

- Octreotide (Sandostatin) may be given as conservative medical management (Paget-Brown et al, 2006; Suver et al, 2004). Nausea, vomiting, abdominal pain, diarrhea, and flatulence can occur. Use with the low-fat diet to decrease GI side effects.

- Medications are given, as appropriate, for the etiology. Monitor side effects accordingly, especially in conditions such as TB or cancer in which numerous side effects are created from drug therapies.
- Bronchodilators may be used. Some nausea and vomiting may occur.

Herbs, Botanicals, and Supplements

- No clinical trials have proven efficacy for use of herbs or botanicals in chylothorax.

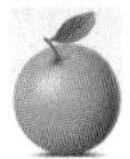

NUTRITION EDUCATION, COUNSELING, CARE MANAGEMENT

- Discuss the importance of adequate nutrition in recovery.
- Discuss interventions that are appropriate for the conditions and diagnoses involved.

Patient Education—Foodborne Illness

- Careful food handling will be important. Hand washing is key as well.

For More Information

- E-medicine
  http://www.emedicine.com/med/topic381.htm
- Medscape
  http://emedicine.medscape.com/article/172527-overview

CHYLOTHORAX—CITED REFERENCES

Cleveland K, et al. Massive chylothorax in small babies. *J Pediatr Surg.* 44:546, 2009.

Cormack BE, et al. Use of Monogen for pediatric postoperative chylothorax. *Ann Thorac Surg.* 77:301, 2004.

Maldonado F, et al. Pleural fluid characteristics of chylothorax. *Mayo Clin Proc.* 84:129, 2009.

Paget-Brown A, et al. The use of octreotide to treat congenital chylothorax. *J Pediatr Surg.* 41:845, 2006.

Saalwachter AR, et al. A nutrition support team led by general surgeons decreases inappropriate use of total parenteral nutrition on a surgical service. *Am Surg.* 70:1107, 2004.

Suddaby EC, Schiller S. Management of chylothorax in children. *Pediatr Nurs.* 30:290, 2004.

Suver DW, et al. Somatostatin treatment of massive lymphorrhea following excision of a lymphatic malformation. *Int J Pediatr Otorhinolaryngol.* 68:845, 2004.

COR PULMONALE

NUTRITIONAL ACUITY RANKING: LEVEL 2–4

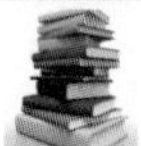

DEFINITIONS AND BACKGROUND

Acute cor pulmonale (right ventricular failure) occurs when relevant increases in pulmonary vascular resistance overwhelm compensatory mechanisms. Cor pulmonale may be acute, subacute, or chronic. The acute form is generally caused by acute respiratory failure (RF) or pulmonary embolism. A heart disease that follows disease of the lung (such as end-stage emphysema, silicosis), chronic cor pulmonale creates hypertrophy and eventual failure.

The body secretes B-type natriuretic peptide (BNP) from the cardiac ventricles in response to ventricular stretch and pressure overload; this counteracts vasoconstriction that occurs as a compensatory mechanism (Prahash and Lynch, 2004).

Long-term exposure to combustion-related fine particulate air pollution is a risk factor. Pulmonary hypertension (PH) and cor pulmonale may affect patients with COPD or CF. Children who have Prader-Willi syndrome may also experience obesity-related cor pulmonale (Stevenson et al, 2004).

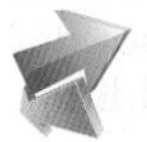

ASSESSMENT, MONITORING, AND EVALUATION

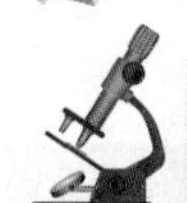

CLINICAL INDICATORS

Genetic Markers: Genes important in early lung development are also important in determining adult risk for COPD and its consequences (Bush, 2008). Glucocorticoid resistance may be related to cytokines, excessive activation of the transcription factor activator protein 1, reduced histone deacetylase-2 (HDAC2) expression, and increased P-glycoprotein-mediated drug efflux (Barnes and Adcock, 2009).

Clinical/History		
Height	Diet history	Echocardiography
Weight	I & O	BP (hypertension?)
BMI	Edema of feet, ankles	
Obesity?	Chest x-ray	

Right upper quadrant (RUQ) pain	Clubbing of fingers and toes	Na^+
SOB	Sleep apnea?	K^+
Distended neck veins	Cyanosis	Ca^{++}, Mg^{++}
Hypoxia	Hepatomegaly	H & H
Wheezing, cough	**Lab Work**	Serum Fe
Fatigue, weakness	BNP	BUN, Creat
	Alb	pCO_2 (increased)
		pO_2 (decreased)
		CRP

INTERVENTION

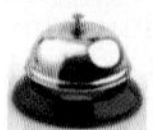

OBJECTIVES

- Improve the patient's capacity to eat meals without straining the diaphragm.
- Correct malnourished status but avoid weight gain that stresses the heart.
- Reduce or prevent fluid retention and edema to lessen cardiac workload.
- Prevent additional damage to cardiac and respiratory tissues.
- Improve energy levels and stamina. Oxygen may be needed, even at mealtimes.
- Support adequate lung function with higher antioxidant intake.

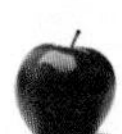

FOOD AND NUTRITION

- Recommend small, frequent meals or oral supplements rather than three large meals (Anker et al, 2006).
- Use a nutrient-dense diet with concentrated protein sources. Double-strength milk, foods with milk powder added to them, high-calorie supplements, and addition of extra gravies or sauces to meals are useful when quantity of food must be kept minimal because of dyspnea.
- Restrict sodium or adjust fluid restriction as needed.
- Use foods that reduce likelihood of gastric irritation and reflux. For example, use low-acidic fruits, vegetables, and juices.
- Provide adequate potassium and magnesium intake with the Dietary Approaches to Stop Hypertension (DASH) diet.
- Include adequate levels of vitamins C, D, and E and selenium for antioxidant properties (Barnes and Adcock, 2009).
- Control CHO if needed. Insulin resistance is also common (Zamanian et al, 2009).
- Oral nutritional supplements or TF enables nutritional intake to be maintained or increased when usual intake is inadequate (Anker et al, 2006).

SAMPLE NUTRITION CARE PROCESS STEPS

Excessive Sodium Intake

Assessment Data: Diet history revealing intake of 8–10 g sodium daily, low intake of potassium, calcium and magnesium; ankle and foot edema; SOB.

Nutrition Diagnoses (PES): Excessive sodium intake related to dietary habits and long-term hypertension as evidenced by BP 212/100, elevated BNP, and dietary intake low in potassium, calcium and magnesium.

Interventions: Offer DASH diet education and alter diet to enhance fruits and vegetables and low-fat dairy products. Monitor sodium intake and offer alternatives for recipes and menu planning. Counsel about dining out and traveling. Evaluate medications for nutritional side effects.

Monitoring and Evaluation: Improved BP and fewer incidents of SOB; alleviation of edema. Improved BNP levels and fewer signs of heart failure.

Common Drugs Used and Potential Side Effects

- Bosentan or sildenafil may be given by mouth
- Calcium channel blockers and anticoagulants may be used. Monitor specific medicines for side effects.
- Thiazide diuretics can cause potassium depletion.
- Anabolic pharmacotherapy has the potential to improve nutritional status and function (Anker et al, 2006).
- To reverse glucocorticoid resistance, vitamin D may restore interleukin-10 response and use of antioxidants may be recommended (Barnes and Adcock, 2009).

Herbs, Botanicals, and Supplements

- No clinical trials have proven efficacy for use of herbs or botanicals in cor pulmonale.

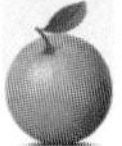

NUTRITION EDUCATION, COUNSELING, CARE MANAGEMENT

- Plan small, attractive meals that are nutrient dense. If fluid and sodium must be limited, provide tips.
- Recommend snacks that are nutrient dense and protein-rich but do not provide excessive sodium.
- Emphasize the importance of eating slowly to reduce SOB.
- Weight loss may be needed (Olson and Zwillich, 2005).
- Monitor heart murmurs in children to identify potential risks or need for surgery. If untreated, cor pulmonale can lead to right-sided heart failure and death.

Patient Education—Foodborne Illness

- Careful food handling will be important. Hand washing is key as well.

For More Information

- Medline
  http://www.nlm.nih.gov/MEDLINEPLUS/ency/article/000129.htm
- Merck Manual
  http://www.merck.com/mmpe/sec07/ch074/ch074c.html

COR PULMONALE—CITED REFERENCES

Anker SD, et al. ESPEN Guidelines on Enteral Nutrition: cardiology and pulmonology. *Clin Nutr.* 25:311, 2006.

Barnes PJ, Adcock IM. Glucocorticoid resistance in inflammatory diseases. *Lancet.* 373:1905, 2009.

Bush A. COPD: a pediatric disease. *COPD.* 5:51, 2008.

Olson AL, Zwillich CH. The obesity hypoventilation syndrome. *Am J Med.* 118:948, 2005.

Prahash A, Lynch T. B-type natriuretic peptide: a diagnostic, prognostic, and therapeutic tool in heart failure. *Am J Crit Care.* 13:46, 2004.

Stevenson DA, et al. Unexpected death and critical illness in Prader-Willi syndrome: report of ten individuals. *Am J Med Genet A.* 124:158, 2004.

Zamanian RT, et al. Insulin resistance in pulmonary arterial hypertension. *Eur Respir J.* 33:318, 2009.

CYSTIC FIBROSIS

NUTRITIONAL ACUITY RANKING: LEVEL 3

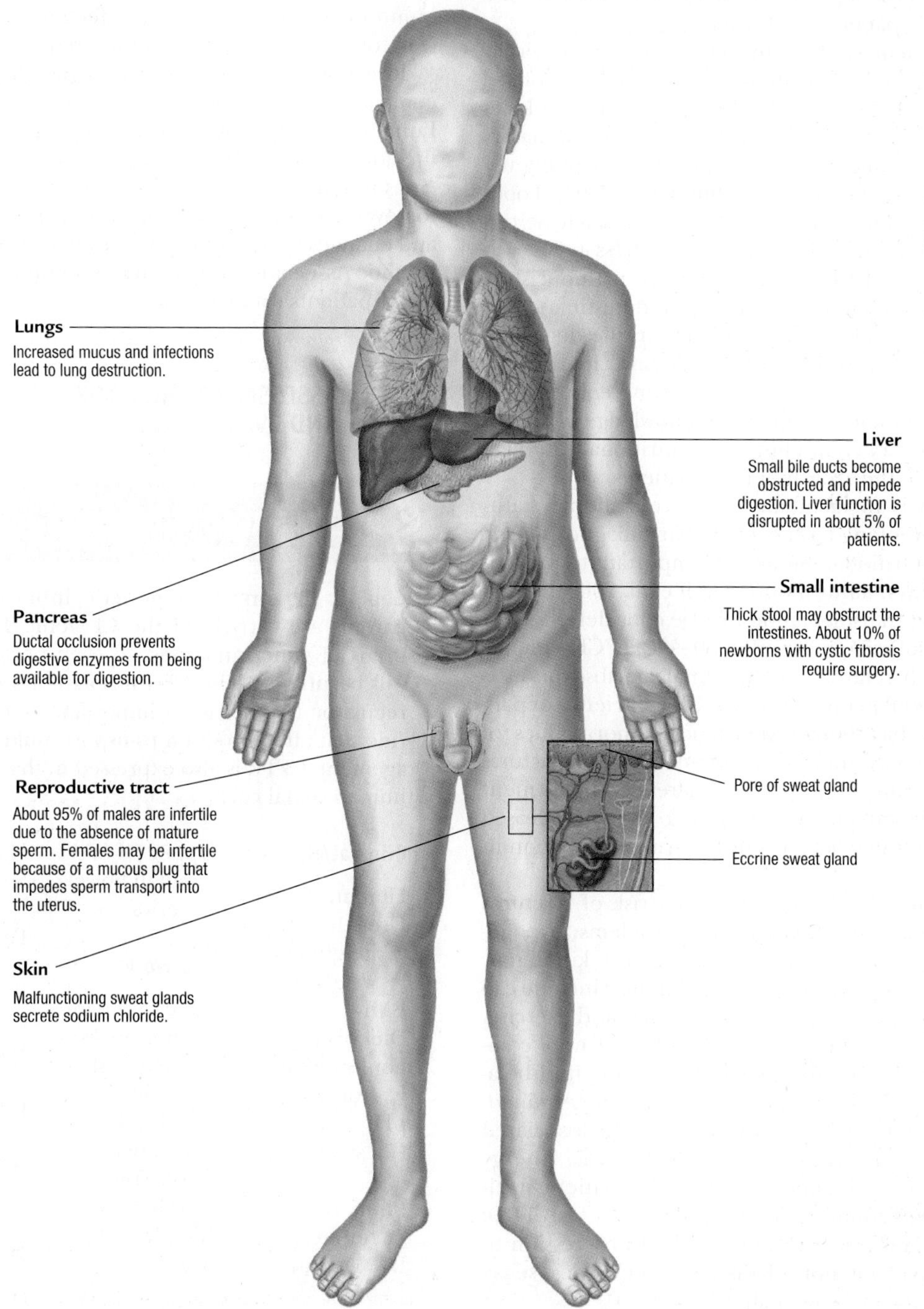

Lungs
Increased mucus and infections lead to lung destruction.
Liver
Small bile ducts become obstructed and impede digestion. Liver function is disrupted in about 5% of patients.
Small intestine
Thick stool may obstruct the intestines. About 10% of newborns with cystic fibrosis require surgery.
Pancreas
Ductal occlusion prevents digestive enzymes from being available for digestion.
Reproductive tract
About 95% of males are infertile due to the absence of mature sperm. Females may be infertile because of a mucous plug that impedes sperm transport into the uterus.
Pore of sweat gland
Eccrine sweat gland
Skin
Malfunctioning sweat glands secrete sodium chloride.

Asset provided by Anatomical Chart Co.

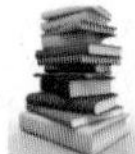

DEFINITIONS AND BACKGROUND

CF is a life-limiting, autosomal recessive inherited disease characterized by thick mucus and frequent pulmonary infections. There is general dysfunction of mucus-producing exocrine glands; high levels of sodium and chloride in the saliva, tears, and sweat; and highly viscous secretions in the pancreas, bronchi, bile ducts, and small intestine. Meconium ileus is a classic sign in newborn infants with CF; it is thicker than usual and passes more slowly.

CF affects approximately 30,000 children and adults in the United States. About one in 3200 Caucasians is affected; 2–5% of Caucasians carry the CF gene. The majority of CF patients have been diagnosed by age 3, but about 10% are not diagnosed until age 18 or older. The median life expectancy for CF patients is 33 years.

The CFTR system controls the efflux of physiologically important anions, such as glutathione (GSH) and bicarbonate, as well as chloride (Hudson, 2004). Interleukin-8 and cytokines also play a role in CF (Augarten et al, 2004). Anti-inflammatory and antioxidant treatments are recommended, including use of omega-3 fatty acids and selenium (Innes et al, 2007). Foods rich in lecithin, choline, betaine, and DHA can safely be recommended to reduce the effects of oxidative stress in CF.

The percentage of CF children who are malnourished varies; weight-based indicators greatly underestimate the extent. A link has been established between the degree of malnutrition and the severity of the disease. Inadequate intake, malabsorption, and increased energy requirements are common. Careful follow-up, better knowledge of energy requirements, dietary counseling, and nutritional intervention help optimize the growth of these patients.

A major goal is to maintain a good nutritional status because it improves long-term survival. Early diagnosis of CF and aggressive nutritional therapy are important to prevent growth failure and malnutrition (Farrell et al, 2005). When appropriate, lung transplantation may be considered.

Pancreatic insufficiency occurs in 80–90% of CF patients; 85% show growth retardation. Intestinal malabsorption is severe in virtually all people who have CF. Deficiency of pancreatic enzymes, bicarbonate deficiency, abnormalities of bile salts and mucosal transport, and anatomical structural changes are relevant. Appropriate pancreatic replacement therapy, combined with pharmacotherapy to address increased acidity of the intestines, achieves near-normal absorption in many patients.

Decreased bone density and increased risk of fractures are seen in patients with CF. Nutrition problems, hypogonadism, inactivity, corticosteroid use, and cytokines may contribute to the low bone mass. Treatment may include calcium, vitamin D_3, vitamin K, bisphosphonates, and exercise.

Diabetes may also occur in persons with CF (more commonly in older individuals), reflecting impairment of beta-cell function, which is probably genetically determined. Onset of CF-related diabetes (CFRD) is often associated with a decline in health and nutritional status. Energy requirements may be higher than usual for patients with CF. Microvascular complications are common in CFRD; microalbuminuria is a sensitive indicator of progression to diabetic nephropathy in non-CF diabetes, but it is less sensitive for CF patients (Dobson et al, 2005).

Some patients are diagnosed in adulthood; patients diagnosed as adults differ distinctly from long-term CF survivors diagnosed as children (Nick and Rodman, 2005). While respiratory symptoms are not as severe and prognosis is more favorable, pancreatitis is more common (Nick and Rodman, 2005).

Progressive pulmonary disease associated with chronic bacterial infection and inflammation is the major cause of morbidity and mortality; CRP and IgG levels are indicators of severity (Levy et al, 2007). With anemia from chronic inflammation, treat the underlying inflammation rather than using supplemental iron (Fischer et al, 2007).

Overall, patients with CF who receive optimal nutrition have better growth, maintain better nutritional reserves, and have better pulmonary function than patients with CF who have poor nutrition (Hart et al, 2004). Metabolic and immunological response to infection and the increased work of breathing escalate calorie requirements.

Research supports the potential benefits of gene therapy; compacted DNA is used to get healthy genes into CF cells. Lung transplantation may be needed. Other treatments include use of antibiotics for infections and inhaled medicines to open the airways. Because no single strategy works for every patient, close monitoring of growth, symptoms, and changes in respiratory status must occur. The American Dietetic Association recommends a minimum of 4 MNT visits for patients who have CF.

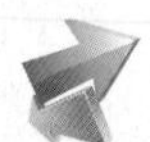

ASSESSMENT, MONITORING, AND EVALUATION

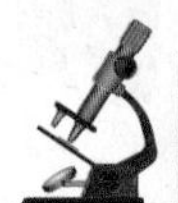

CLINICAL INDICATORS

Genetic Markers: CF is genetic, inherited when both parents are carriers of the CF gene. There are hundreds of gene mutations, so each person's symptoms will be unique. The CF transmembrane conductance regulator (CFTR) is an important molecule for chloride that affects sodium transport, fluid, and ion management. CFTR is also expressed in the neurons of the human spinal cord.

Clinical/History

- Height, weight
- Growth chart for height and weight
- BMI
- Diet history
- Foul smelling stools
- pH
- Chest x-ray or CT scan
- Pulmonary function test
- DEXA scan
- Upper GI or small bowel series

Lab Work

- Pilocarpine iontophoresis sweat test (>60 mEq/L)
- pCO_2, pO_2
- Chol, Trig (elevated?)
- Na^+, K^+, CL^-
- Alb
- H & H
- Serum Fe, ferritin
- Pancreatic enzymes (amylase, lipase)
- White blood cell count (WBC)
- Prothrombin time (PT)
- International normalized ratio (INR)
- Serum vitamin K

Gluc	Secretin stimulation test	Fecal elastase-1 in stool
CRP	Trypsin or chymotrypsin in stool	Serum copper (Cu)
Serum carotene levels		
Ca^{++}, Mg^{++}		

INTERVENTION

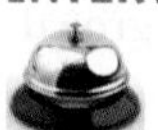

OBJECTIVES

- Determine current level of care needed (Table 5-8). Effective treatment should allow a normal diet, symptom control, malabsorption correction, and attainment of a normal nutritional state and growth.
- Achieve or maintain desirable BMI. BMI percentile is a better evaluation than % ideal body weight (IBW) in CF patients; %IBW underestimates the severity of malnutrition in children with short stature and overestimates the severity of malnutrition in children with tall stature (Zhang and Lai, 2004).
- Correct anorexia from respiratory distress.
- Provide optimal amounts of protein for growth, development, and resistance to infection. Increase LBM if depleted. Spare protein by providing up to twice the normal amount of calories from CHO and fat as in usual diet plans. Stunting may require extra protein, as from TF (Geukers et al, 2005).
- Decrease electrolyte losses in vomiting and steatorrhea. Replace lost electrolytes.
- Achieve adequate enzyme replacement to bring about near-normal digestion. Reduce excessive nutrient losses from maldigestion and malabsorption.
- Provide essential fatty acids in a tolerated form. Reduce arachidonic acid use to lessen inflammatory cascade. Include omega-3 fatty acids and antioxidants such as selenium and vitamins C and E. Vitamin E may be especially important for improving cognitive function (Koscik et al, 2004).
- Promote adequate bone mass, as serum levels of vitamins D and K may be low (Grey et al, 2008).
- Correct edema, diarrhea, anemia, azotorrhea, and steatorrhea.

SAMPLE NUTRITION CARE PROCESS STEPS

Poor Nutritional Quality of Life

Assessment Data: Low BMI, anorexia, polypharmacy, depression.

Nutrition Diagnoses (PES): Poor nutritional quality of life related to GI distress with meals and polypharmacy as evidenced by depression, low BMI and anorexia.

Interventions: Offer nutrient dense foods. Collaborate with medical team to address depression and polypharmacy. Assure intake of pancreatic enzymes with meals to reduce GI distress.

Monitoring and Evaluation: Improved appetite and intake; BMI closer to normal range; improved nutritional quality of life.

TABLE 5-8 Nutritional Management for Cystic Fibrosis (CF)

Routine care	Within desired BMI
Anticipatory guidance	At 90–95% desired BMI
Supportive intervention	At 85–90% desired BMI
Rehabilitative care	At 75–85% desired BMI
Resuscitative or palliative care	Below 75% desired BMI

- Prevent progressive pulmonary disease or complications such as glucose intolerance, intestinal obstruction, cirrhosis, and pancreatic or cardiac diseases.
- Improve lung function outcomes from better nutrition and fewer chronic infections (McPhail et al, 2008).

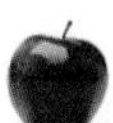

FOOD AND NUTRITION

- Energy expenditure may be as high as 199% of predicted in CF patients. CF patients may need to be given 120–150% more calories than for age-matched and gender-matched controls; this may mean 3000–4000 kcal for teens.
- Design the plan for 45–65% CHO and 20–30% fat. For persons with acute disease, starch and fat will not be well tolerated unless adequate levels of pancreatic enzymes are provided. Calorie intake should be about 150 kcal/kg for children and 200 kcal/kg for infants. Specific interventions for increasing total energy intake in CF patients are the role of the dietitian (Powers et al, 2004). Many supplements are available at little or no cost to the patient.
- Manage glucose levels if CF diabetes mellitus (CFDM) develops. Intensive insulin therapy and CHO counting will be important.
- Protein should be 10–35% of total calories. This may translate into 4 g/kg for infants, 3 g/kg for children, 2 g/kg for teens, and 1.5 g/kg for adults.
- Increase fat:CHO ratio with respiratory distress. Special respiratory formulas may be useful during those times, or use of MCTs and safflower oil may be beneficial. Be sure to time intake according to the use and type of pancreatic enzymes.
- Encourage intake of omega-3 fatty acids (DHA and EPA), selenium, betaine, and choline to reduce inflammation and enhance immunity.
- Supplement the diet with two times the normal RDAs for fat-soluble vitamins A, D, and E (use water-miscible sources such as "ADEKS" brand).
- Replace vitamin K as needed; check levels regularly. Either 1 mg or 5 mg doses of vitamin K will help replenish low levels (Drury et al, 2008).
- Use extra riboflavin if there is cheilosis; include the other B-complex vitamins and vitamin C at recommended levels.
- Be sure that iron, zinc, copper, selenium intakes meet recommended levels.
- Use liberal amounts of salt to replace perspiration losses.
- Lactose intolerance is common. Omit milk during periods of diarrhea if lactose intolerance persists.
- Intolerance for gas-forming foods and concentrated sweets may occur; alter dietary plans accordingly.

- Soft foods may be useful if chewing causes fatigue.
- Fluid intake should be liberal unless contraindicated.
- Use of turmeric and cumin in foods may be beneficial for CF patients (Berger et al, 2005). Research is ongoing to determine overall practicality of uses.
- Infants can tolerate most formulas (may need 24 kcal/oz) and commercial products that include some MCT oil. Do not add pancreatic enzymes to formula because desired amounts may not be totally consumed or enzymes may block the opening of the nipple.
- Nocturnal TF may be appropriate with growth failure. With reflux, a gastrostomy feeding tube may be well tolerated (Oliver et al, 2004). PN is not recommended due to high risk of infection.

Common Drugs Used and Potential Side Effects

- Growth hormone may be used to bring onset of puberty in prepubescent children who have CF (Vanderwel and Hardin, 2006).
- New areosol treatments show promise. See Table 5-9 for alternative therapies.

Herbs, Botanicals, and Supplements

- Interesting studies suggest that curcumin may directly stimulate CFTR Cl^- channels (Berger et al, 2005). Use of turmeric and cumin in foods served to this population may have therapeutic benefits.
- Dietary supplement use is prevalent among CF children. Identify use of nonprescribed supplements because of unknown effects on growth and development and the potential for adverse drug interactions (Ball et al, 2005).
- The individual with CF should work with the CF nutritionist to maintain a healthy diet before considering adding herbal therapies. Each label on any supplement should be read carefully; some ingredients that can be toxic to people with CF.

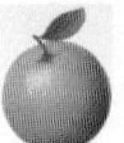

NUTRITION EDUCATION, COUNSELING, CARE MANAGEMENT

- Diet must be periodically reevaluated to reflect growth and disease process.
- New foods may be introduced gradually.
- A behavioral and nutrition intervention can be used with children to enhance weight and height velocities (Powers et al, 2005).
- To liquefy secretions, adequate fluid intake should be ensured. Discuss signs of dehydration and how to prevent or correct.
- Bronchopulmonary drainage, three times daily, may be required. Plan meals to be 1 hour before or after therapy.
- Ensure that all foods and beverages are nutrient dense.
- As needed, discuss issues related to fertility (most males with CF are infertile, but females are not).
- In adults with CF, 40% have glucose intolerance. Discuss how to manage diabetes in those cases.
- Discuss reimbursement issues for TFs and pumps.
- Depression is common and should be adequately managed (Quittner et al, 2008). Hypnosis may be useful in reducing pain from frequent intravenous injections or other treatments.

Patient Education—Foodborne Illness

- Careful food handling will be important. Hand washing is key as well.

TABLE 5-9 Medications Used in Cystic Fibrosis (CF) and Potential Side Effects

Medication	Description and Side Effects
Aerosolized antibiotics	TOBI (tobramycin solution for inhalation) can be delivered in a more concentrated dose directly to the site of CF lung infections and is preservative free.
Antibiotics	Antibiotics are needed during infections. Monitor for magnesium depletion.
Azithromycin	Azithromycin is an antibiotic that is effective in people with CF whose lungs are chronically infected with the common *Pseudomonas aeruginosa* bacteria.
Bisphosphonates	Bisphosphonates may be used to increase bone density.
Bronchodilators	Bronchodilators are used to open breathing passages. Monitor for side effects.
Glutathione (GSH)	Buffered GSH has been tested in some CF patients. Nebulized buffered GSH may ameliorate CF disease; longer and larger studies of inhaled GSH are warranted (Bishop et al, 2005).
L-arginine	Oral L-arginine (200 mg) may reduce nitric oxide levels, which can be detrimental (Grasemann et al, 2005). More studies are needed.
Mucolytics	Mucolytics, such as potassium iodide, liquefy secretions.
Pancreatic enzymes (pancrelipase)	Pancreatic granules (Viokase or Cotazym) are used to help improve digestion/absorption. Enteric preparations (Pancreas) act in the duodenum, so give before meals; for nocturnal feedings, give before, during, and after feedings. Avoid mixing with milk or ice cream. If too much is given, anorexia and constipation may result. Return of a voracious appetite and increase in stool bulk suggest an inadequate dosage. Dosing should be based on stool tests for malabsorption.
Pulmozyme	A mucus-thinning drug shown to reduce the number of lung infections and improve lung function.
Ursodeoxycholic acid	Used for meconium ileus and liver disease associated with CF (Lamireau et al, 2004).

NOTE. The need to take up to 40–60 pills daily is common in CF.

For More Information

- Cystic Fibrosis
  http://www.cysticfibrosis.com/
- Cystic Fibrosis Foundation
  http://www.cff.org/
- Cystic Fibrosis Research
  http://www.cfri.org/indexframes.htm
- Medline
  http://www.nlm.nih.gov/medlineplus/ency/article/000107.htm
- NHLBI—Cystic Fibrosis
  http://www.nhlbi.nih.gov/health/dci/Diseases/cf/cf_what.html
- NIH
  http://ghr.nlm.nih.gov/condition=cysticfibrosis
- Nutrition for CF
  http://www.nlm.nih.gov/medlineplus/ency/article/002437.htm

CYSTIC FIBROSIS—CITED REFERENCES

Augarten A, et al. Systemic inflammatory mediators and cystic fibrosis genotype. *Clin Exp Med.* 4:99, 2004.

Ball SD, et al. Dietary supplement use is prevalent among children with a chronic illness. *J Am Diet Assoc.* 105:78, 2005.

Berger AL, et al. Curcumin stimulates CFTR Cl-channel activity. *J Biol Chem.* 280:5221–5226, 2005.

Bishop C, et al. A pilot study of the effect of inhaled buffered reduced glutathione on the clinical status of patients with cystic fibrosis. *Chest.* 127:308, 2005.

Dobson L, et al. Microalbuminuria as a screening tool in cystic fibrosis-related diabetes. *Pediatr Pulmonol.* 39:103, 2005.

Drury D, et al. Efficacy of high dose phylloquinone in correcting vitamin K deficiency in cystic fibrosis. *J Cyst Fibros.* 7:457, 2008.

Farrell PM, et al. Evidence on improved outcomes with early diagnosis of cystic fibrosis through neonatal screening: enough is enough! *J Pediatr.* 147:30S, 2005.

Fischer R, et al. Lung disease severity, chronic inflammation, iron deficiency, and erythropoietin response in adults with cystic fibrosis. *Pediatr Pulmonol.* 42:1193, 2007.

Geukers VG, et al. Short-term protein intake and stimulation of protein synthesis in stunted children with cystic fibrosis. *Am J Clin Nutr.* 81:605, 2005.

Grasemann H, et al. Oral L-arginine supplementation in cystic fibrosis patients: a placebo-controlled study. *Eur Respir J.* 25:62, 2005.

Grey V, et al. Prevalence of low bone mass and deficiencies of vitamins D and K in pediatric patients with cystic fibrosis from 3 Canadian centers. *Pediatrics.* 122:1014, 2008.

Hart N, et al. Nutritional status is an important predictor of diaphragm strength in young patients with cystic fibrosis. *Am J Clin Nutr.* 80:1201, 2004.

Hudson VM. New insights into the pathogenesis of cystic fibrosis: pivotal role of glutathione system dysfunction and implications for therapy. *Treat Respir Med.* 3:353, 2004.

Innes SM, et al. Choline-related supplements improve abnormal plasma methionine-homocysteine metabolites and glutathione status in children with cystic fibrosis. *Am J Clin Nutr.* 85:702, 2007.

Koscik RL, et al. Cognitive function of children with cystic fibrosis: deleterious effect of early malnutrition. *Pediatrics.* 113:1549, 2004.

Lamireau T, et al. Epidemiology of liver disease in cystic fibrosis: a longitudinal study. *J Hepatol.* 41:920, 2004.

Levy H, et al. Inflammatory markers of lung disease in adult patients with cystic fibrosis. *Pediatr Pulmonol.* 42:256, 2007.

McPhail GL, et al. Improvements in lung function outcomes in children with cystic fibrosis are associated with better nutrition, fewer chronic pseudomonas aeruginosa infections, and dornase alfa use. *J Pediatr.* 153:752, 2008.

Nick JA, Rodman DM. Manifestations of cystic fibrosis diagnosed in adulthood. *Curr Opin Pulm Med.* 11:513, 2005.

Oliver MR, et al. Factors affecting clinical outcome in gastrostomy-fed children with cystic fibrosis. *Pediatr Pulmonol.* 37:324, 2004.

Powers SW, et al. A comparison of food group variety between toddlers with and without cystic fibrosis. *J Hum Nutr Diet.* 17:523, 2004.

Powers SW, et al. Randomized clinical trial of behavioral and nutrition treatment to improve energy intake and growth in toddlers and preschoolers with cystic fibrosis. *Pediatrics.* 116:1442, 2005.

Quittner AL, et al. Prevalence and impact of depression in cystic fibrosis. *Curr Opin Pulm Med.* 14:582, 2008.

Vanderwel M, Hardin DS. Growth hormone normalizes pubertal onset in children with cystic fibrosis. *J Pediatr Endocrinol Metab.* 19:237, 2006.

Zhang Z, Lai HJ. Comparison of the use of body mass index percentiles and percentage of ideal body weight to screen for malnutrition in children with cystic fibrosis. *Am J Clin Nutr.* 80:982, 2004.

INTERSTITIAL LUNG DISEASE

NUTRITIONAL ACUITY RANKING: LEVEL 1–2

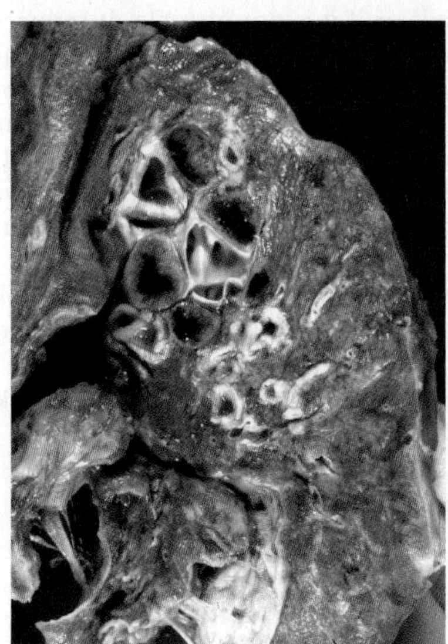

Adapted from: Cagle PT, MD. *Color Atlas and Text of Pulmonary Pathology.* Philadelphia: Lippincott WIlliams & Wilkins, 2005.

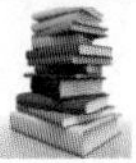

DEFINITIONS AND BACKGROUND

Interstitial lung disease (ILD) is a general term that includes a variety of chronic lung disorders, sometimes also known as "interstitial pulmonary fibrosis." In ILD, the lung tissue is damaged; the walls of the air sacs in the lung become inflamed; and, finally, scarring (fibrosis) occurs in the interstitium (tissue between the air sacs). The lung becomes stiff.

Although the histologic patterns of ILD in children and adults share similar features, important differences exist in etiology, clinical manifestations, and outcome (Young et al, 2008). Causes of adult ILD include environmental exposure to inorganic dust (such as silica) or organic dust (such as animal or bacterial proteins); exposure to gases, fumes, or poisons; or medical conditions such as sarcoidosis, scleroderma, rheumatic arthritis, and lupus. Agricultural workers also can be affected, with moldy hay causing allergic reactions in a disorder known as Farmer's Lung.

Breathlessness during exercise and dry cough can be the first symptoms. Other symptoms vary in severity. Further testing is usually recommended to identify the specific type of ILD a person has; some have known causes and some have unknown causes (idiopathic). The course of these diseases is unpredictable.

Some ILDs improve with medication if treated when inflammation occurs. Inflammation of these parts of the lung may heal or may lead to permanent scarring of the lung tissue. Fibrosis results in scarring and permanent loss of that tissue's ability to transport oxygen. The level of disability that a person experiences depends on the amount of scarring of the tissue. Oxygen may be needed; some patients need it all of the time, and others need it only during sleep and exercise.

A pulmonary rehabilitation program is often recommended for education, exercise conditioning, breathing retraining, energy-saving techniques, respiratory therapy, nutritional counseling, and psychosocial support. Lung transplantation has become an option for some patients.

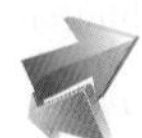

ASSESSMENT, MONITORING, AND EVALUATION

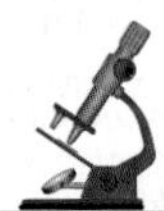

CLINICAL INDICATORS

Genetic Markers: Prevalence of ILDs is low in children. A total of 10–16% may be familial, with mutations in surfactant proteins or the SFTPC and ABCA3 gene (Nogee, 2006).

Clinical/History	Chest x-ray or CT scan	Lab Work
Height, weight	Pulmonary function test	pCO_2, pO_2
Growth chart for height and weight	Exercise function test	Chol, Trig
BMI	Clubbing of fingers	Na^+, K^+, Cl^-
Diet history	Dry cough	Alb
Fecal fat study	Cyanosis	H & H
pH		Serum Fe
Bronchoalveolar lavage (BAL)		WBC count
Lung biopsy		PT or INR
		Gluc
		Ca^{++}, Mg^{++}

SAMPLE NUTRITION CARE PROCESS STEPS

Underweight

Assessment Data: Poor dietary intake, underweight for height.

Nutrition Diagnoses (PES): Underweight (NC 3.1) related to inadequate energy intake as evidenced by low percentile height, weight 30%tile on growth chart and estimated intake approximately 500 calories below estimated needs.

Interventions: Enhance intake through adding protein and calories to casseroles and foods served. Educate about nutrient density and increasing calories. Counsel with tips about eating slowly and frequently.

Monitoring and Evaluation: Weight gain closer to desired BMI; improved intake of energy and nutrients.

INTERVENTION

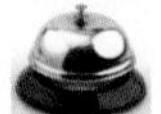

OBJECTIVES

- Early identification and aggressive treatment are needed to lessen inflammation and prevent further lung damage.
- Remove the source of the problem, if known.
- Lessen the effect of complications.
- Maintain nutritional immunity as far as possible. Improve poor status.
- Provide nutritional repletion before surgery, if surgery is scheduled.

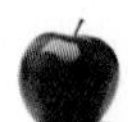

FOOD AND NUTRITION

- If not contraindicated, offer 3–3.5 L fluid daily to liquefy secretions and to help lower temperature.
- A high-calorie, soft diet is recommended, especially if oxygen is used. Frequent, small meals may be beneficial.
- Discuss how to make mealtimes relaxed, especially if oxygen is required at the same time. Plan for longer mealtimes accordingly.
- A multivitamin–mineral supplement may be beneficial, especially for vitamins A, C, and E. Vitamin E reduces the extent of pulmonary damage in some types of ILD (Card et al, 2003).
- Ensure adequate potassium intake, as from fruits and juices.
- When possible, add more fiber to prevent constipation.
- TF at night may be beneficial if intake is poor during the day. A gastrostomy or transpyloric feeding tube may be desirable.

Common Drugs Used and Potential Side Effects

- Oral prednisone or methylprednisone is frequently the first medication used to help decrease inflammation.
- Cyclophosphamide (Cytoxan) may be used if steroid therapy fails or if it is not possible. It reduces inflammation by killing some inflammatory cells and suppressing their function. Response to therapy may require up to 6 months or longer. In some cases, a combination of prednisone and cyclophosphamide is used with good results. Side effects include GI irritation, bladder inflammation, bone marrow suppression, infection, and blood disorders.
- Azathioprine (Imuran) is used if there are problems tolerating the side effects of the above medications. It is not as effective as cyclophosphamide, but side effects are more tolerable. Side effects include fever, skin rash, GI irritation, and blood disorders.
- Interferon has been tested in clinical trials with some promising results.

Herbs, Botanicals, and Supplements

- Herbs and botanicals should not be used for ILD because there are no controlled trials to prove efficacy.

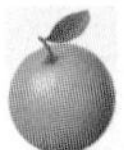

NUTRITION EDUCATION, COUNSELING, CARE MANAGEMENT

- Discuss how a balanced diet supports overall immunity and health status. Teach principles of the Food Guide Pyramid and the Dietary Guidelines.
- Teach how to incorporate antioxidants and related nutrients in the diet, especially if energy intake is low because of poor appetite.
- Influenza vaccine and pneumococcal pneumonia vaccine are both recommended for people with ILD.
- Rehabilitation and education programs may help some people. Local support groups have benefited people with ILD and their family members and friends.

Patient Education—Foodborne Illness

- Careful food handling will be important. Hand washing is key as well.

For More Information

- Children's Interstitial Lung Disease
  http://emedicine.medscape.com/article/1003631-treatment
- Interstitial Lung Disease Program
  http://www.nationaljewish.org/a4.html
- Medicine Net
  http://www.medicinenet.com/interstitial_lung_disease/article.htm

INTERSTITIAL LUNG DISEASE—CITED REFERENCES

Card JW, et al. Attenuation of amiodarone-induced pulmonary fibrosis by vitamin E is associated with suppression of transforming growth factor-beta1 gene expression but not prevention of mitochondrial dysfunction. *J Pharmacol Exp Ther.* 304:277, 2003.

Nogee LM. Genetics of pediatric interstitial lung disease. 18:287, 2006.

Young LR, et al. Usual interstitial pneumonia in an adolescent with ABCA3 mutations. *Chest.* 134:192, 2008.

PNEUMONIA

NUTRITIONAL ACUITY RANKING: LEVEL 1–2

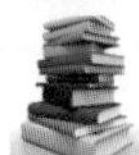

DEFINITIONS AND BACKGROUND

Pneumonia involves acute inflammation of the alveolar spaces of the lung. Lung tissue is consolidated as alveoli fill with exudate, usually after a cold or the flu. To protect against pneumonia, dental and oral health care are important. Dental plaque germs may be inhaled and may lead to onset of pneumonia; regular tooth brushing, flossing, and dental check-ups are recommended (El-Solh et al, 2004).

A productive cough that is painful and incessant (generally with green/yellow sputum that progresses to pink, brown, or rust color) may be indicative. Pneumonia may be classified as community acquired, hospital acquired, or atypical. Table 5-10 describes the common types of pneumonia. The most common form is community-acquired pneumococcal pneumonia. With treatment, most types of bacterial pneumonia can be cured within 1–2 weeks; viral pneumonia may last longer. Mycoplasmal pneumonia resolves in 4–6 weeks. Before antibiotics, pneumonia caused many deaths in elderly individuals; it now ranks sixth among causes of death in the United States.

People at high risk for pneumonia include the elderly; the very young; those with COPD, diabetes mellitus, congestive heart failure, sickle cell anemia, AIDS, or asthma; and people undergoing cancer therapy or organ transplantation. Nursing home residents have chronic medical conditions that gradually lead to "decompensation" in functional status, nutritional status, and pulmonary clearance. Elderly patients with low body weight and hypoalbuminemia are more likely to die from pneumonia than healthy patients.

Inflammation may cause low serum albumin levels in many pneumonia patients. GSH is the primary antioxidant that lines alveolar space; selenium, vitamins E and C may be beneficial. However, supplementation alone will not prevent pneumonia in well-nourished older individuals (Merchant et al, 2004).

Enteral feeding provides nutrients for patients who require endotracheal tubes and mechanical ventilation. There is a presumed increase in the risk of ventilator-associated pneumonia (VAP) with TF, but this is not always true.

Pneumonia due to immune system suppression and membrane damage induced by oxidative stress suggest that sufficient fatty acid intake may be useful in the nutritional repletion of such patients with pneumonia. The American Dietetic Association previously recommended 3 MNT visits for persons who have pneumonia.

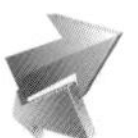

ASSESSMENT, MONITORING, AND EVALUATION

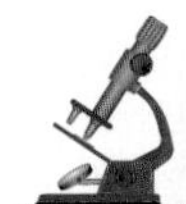

CLINICAL INDICATORS

Genetic Markers: Genes that have inflammatory molecules such as tumor necrosis factor, interleukin-10, and angiotensin-converting enzyme may play a role in susceptibility to pneumonia. Population studies are needed.

Clinical/History
Height
Weight
BMI
I & O
Diet history
BP
Chills, fever (102–106°F), delirium
Pleuritic pain

TABLE 5-10 Types of Pneumonia

Type	Description
Allergic	From sensitivity to dust or pollen.
Aspiration	From swallowing a foreign substance. The gastric volume predisposing to aspiration is larger than 30 mL (Kalinowski and Kirsch, 2004). Just a few hours with "nothing by mouth" helps prepare for surgery because risk of aspiration is lower than previously believed. Ventilator-associated pneumonia, a common and serious complication in critically ill patients who require a ventilator, results from pneumonia occurring >48 hours after endotracheal intubation (Parker and Heyland, 2004). It is caused by microaspiration of contaminated oropharyngeal or gastrointestinal secretions into the airways (Parker and Heyland, 2004).
Bacterial	From bacteria normally present in mouth/throat. Quick onset with high fever and rapid breathing. Several bacteria may be relevant. *Streptococcus pneumoniae* causes about 25% of bacterial types. *Mycoplasma* causes walking pneumonia, notorious for sore throat and headache in addition to the usual symptoms; causes about 20% of all kinds of pneumonia. When pneumonia is due to pertussis (whooping cough), long coughing spells, turning blue from lack of air, and making a classic "whoop" sound when trying to take a breath will occur. *Haemophilus influenzae* type b (Hib) is America's most common cause of bacterial meningitis; it is also an agent of pneumonia.
Chemical	From accidental inhalation of toxic fumes and chemicals, often in the workplace or when using cleaning agents such as bleach in a closed space.
Healthcare-associated pneumonia	Pneumonia in any patient who has been hospitalized in an acute care hospital for 2 or more days within the past 90 days; residents of a nursing home or long-term care facility; recipients of recent intravenous antibiotic therapy, chemotherapy, or wound care within the past 30 days; or patients who have attended a dialysis clinic.
Hypostatic	In bedridden persons, usually elderly individuals.
Pneumocystis carinii pneumonia	Caused by a fungus, primarily in AIDS patients.
Viral	More common; leads to about 50% of pneumonia cases. Symptoms appear more gradually; less severe than bacterial form. Wheezing is common in this type. Adenoviral infections often affect infants and young children. Other viruses that can cause pneumonia include rhinovirus, influenza, respiratory syncytial virus, and parainfluenza virus (croup).

Difficult, painful respirations
SOB, rales, rhonchi
Bronchoscopy
Productive cough (purulent, green, or rust)
Respiratory rate (increase)
Fatigue, weakness
Tachypnea, tachycardia
Anorexia, malaise
Abdominal distention
Anxiety, restlessness
Cyanosis of nail beds

Lab Work

WBCs (increased)
pCO_2, pO_2
Na^+, K^+
Ca^{++}, Mg^{++}
Alb, transthyretin
CRP
H & H
Serum Fe, ferritin
Transferrin
Gluc
BUN, Creat

INTERVENTION

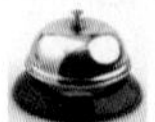

OBJECTIVES

- Prevent or correct dehydration.
- Relieve breathing difficulty and discomfort. Oxygenate all tissues.
- Prevent weight loss from a hypermetabolic state.
- Support diet with adequate antioxidants and nutrient-dense foods.
- Avoid additional infections; prevent sepsis and multiple organ dysfunction syndrome.
- In convalescent stage, avoid constipation.

FOOD AND NUTRITION

- If not contraindicated, offer 3 L or more of fluid daily to liquefy secretions and to help lower elevated temperature.
- Progress, as tolerated, to a high-calorie diet. If overweight, allow normal calorie intake for age and sex.
- Early enteral nutrition, properly administered, can decrease upper GI intolerance and nosocomial pneumonia (Kompan et al, 2004).
- Frequent, small meals and a soft diet may be tolerated better.
- A multivitamin–mineral supplement may be beneficial, especially including selenium and vitamins E and C. Vitamin A is needed to keep mucous membranes healthy.

SAMPLE NUTRITION CARE PROCESS STEPS

Inadequate Fluid Intake

Assessment Data: Dehydration, rapid breathing, poor skin turgor, I & O records.

Nutrition Diagnoses (PES): Inadequate fluid intake related to fever of 103°F, and pneumonia as evidenced by signs of dehydration and low I & O.

Interventions: Encourage intake of fluids at all meals and between meals as well. Keep water or a beverage on hand within easy reach.

Monitoring and Evaluation: Improved I & O records; reduction of fever; normal skin turgor.

- When possible, add more fiber to prevent constipation.
- Ensure adequate potassium intake, as from fruits and juices.

Common Drugs Used and Potential Side Effects

- A 7-day course of low-dose hydrocortisone infusion speeds recovery from community-acquired pneumonia (CAP) and prevents complications due to sepsis (Confalonieri et al, 2005).
- Antibiotics, such as clarithromycin (Biaxin), are used in bacterial pneumonia. Nausea, diarrhea, and abdominal pain can occur.
- Telithromycin (Ketek) is used for the treatment of infections caused by bronchitis, bacterial sinusitis, and CAP.
- Analgesics are used to reduce pain and antipyretics are used to lessen fever.
- Cephalosporins are often useful for nursing home-acquired pneumonia (Muder et al, 2004). Ceftobiprole may be used against MRSA, *Enterococcus faecalis, Enterobacteriaceae,* and *Pseudomonas aeruginosa.*

Herbs, Botanicals, and Supplements

- No clinical trials have proven efficacy for use of herbs or botanicals, such as echinacea, honeysuckle, garlic, dandelion, astragalus, and baikal skullcap in pneumonia patients.

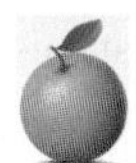

NUTRITION EDUCATION, COUNSELING, CARE MANAGEMENT

- Discuss the role of diet and fluid intake in recovery.
- Loss of swallowing function can lead to dehydration, malnutrition, pneumonia, and reduced quality of life for senior citizens; increasing strength of head and neck musculature can be recommended (Ney et al, 2009). In hypostatic pneumonia, occupational or physical therapy may be beneficial.
- Fruit and vegetable juices add calories, fluid, and sometimes fiber to the diet and can be available at bedside.
- Routine immunizations are available against *Haemophilus influenzae* and pertussis beginning at 2 months of age pertussis immunization is the "P" part of the routine DtaP or DTP.
- Vaccines are now also given against the pneumococcus organism (PCV), a common cause of bacterial pneumonia. Although the polysaccharide pneumococcal vaccine (PPV) does not prevent CAP, it might still improve outcomes in those who develop pneumonia (Johnstone et al, 2007).
- Flu vaccines are recommended for individuals with chronic illnesses such as heart and lung disorders, including asthma. Premature infants may need protection against respiratory syncytial virus (RSV). Individuals who have HIV infection may need protection against *Pneumocystis carinii.*
- Protect people who have pneumonia from others who have respiratory tract infections, such as the common cold.

Patient Education—Foodborne Illness

- Careful food handling will be important.
- Hand washing is key as well, especially after sneezing and coughing and before eating.

For More Information

- American Lung Association—Pneumonia
  http://www.lungusa.org/diseases/lungpneumoni.html
- KidsHealth
  http://kidshealth.org/kid/ill_injure/sick/pneumonia.html
- Medicine Net
  http://www.medicinenet.com/pneumonia/article.htm

PNEUMONIA—CITED REFERENCES

Confalonieri M, et al. Hydrocortisone infusion for severe community-acquired pneumonia: a preliminary randomized study. *Am J Respir Crit Care Med.* 171:242, 2005.

El-Solh AA, et al. Colonization of dental plaques: a reservoir of respiratory pathogens for hospital-acquired pneumonia in institutionalized elders. *Chest.* 126:1575, 2004.

Johnstone J. Effect of pneumococcal vaccination in hospitalized adults with community-acquired pneumonia. *Arch Intern Med.* 167:1938, 2007.

Kalinowski CP, Kirsch JR. Strategies for prophylaxis and treatment for aspiration. *Best Pract Res Clin Anaesthesiol.* 18:719, 2004.

Kompan L, et al. Is early enteral nutrition a risk factor for gastric intolerance and pneumonia? *Clin Nutr.* 23:527, 2004.

Merchant AT, et al. Vitamin intake is not associated with community-acquired pneumonia in U.S. men. *J Nutr.* 134:439, 2004.

Muder RR, et al. Nursing home-acquired pneumonia: an emergency department treatment algorithm. *Curr Med Res Opin.* 20:1309, 2004.

Ney DM, et al. Senescent swallowing: impact, strategies, and interventions. *Nutr Clin Pract.* 24:395, 2009.

Parker CM, Heyland DK. Aspiration and the risk of ventilator-associated pneumonia. *Nutr Clin Pract.* 19:597, 2004.

PULMONARY EMBOLISM

NUTRITIONAL ACUITY RANKING: LEVEL 1–2

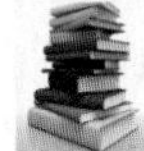

DEFINITIONS AND BACKGROUND

A pulmonary embolism is caused by a partial or complete occlusion of a pulmonary artery from a blood clot from another part of the body that has found its way to the lung. The condition can be life-threatening. Sudden, sharp substernal pain, SOB, cyanosis, pallor, faintness, fever, hypotension, and wheezing can occur, sometimes followed by right heart failure. Approximately 10% of patients suffer some form of tissue death or pulmonary infarction.

Venous thrombosis most often starts in the calf veins and moves on to the lung. Thrombosis in the veins is triggered by venostasis, hypercoagulability, and vessel wall inflammation (the Virchow triad).

Common causes include recent surgery, fractures, immobility, burns, obesity, chemotherapy, old age, heart failure, polycythemia, ulcerative colitis, homocystinemia, and even pregnancy. It is actually one of the primary concerns during pregnancy (Stone and Morris, 2005). Hormone replacement therapy (HRT) is no longer recommended for women after menopause because of the increased risk for pulmonary embolism (Hillman et al, 2004).

Massive pulmonary embolism causes hypotension, with a systolic arterial pressure less than 90 mm Hg; mortality ranges from 30% to 60%. Nonmassive pulmonary embolism presents with systolic arterial pressure greater than or equal to 90 mm Hg and is much more common. Oxygen therapy is always initiated, and fibrinolytic therapy is the primary mode of treatment.

Interesting studies have been conducted to evaluate the role of diet on embolism. In the Iowa cohort study of older women, greater intake of alcohol was associated with a lower risk of incident thromboembolism; no associations were seen with "Western" or "Prudent" dietary patterns, fruit, vegetables, dairy, meat, refined grains, whole grains, regular soda, vitamins E, vitamin B_6, vitamin B_{12}, folate, omega-3 fatty acids, or saturated fat (Lutsey et al, 2009). In the Longitudinal Investigation of Thromboembolism Etiology study, greater intake of fish, fruit, and vegetables were noted as beneficial (Steffen et al, 2007). Clearly, more research is needed.

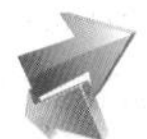

ASSESSMENT, MONITORING, AND EVALUATION

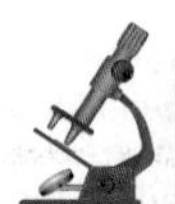

CLINICAL INDICATORS

Genetic Markers: Hereditary factors that may produce a hypercoagulable state include Antithrombin III deficiency, Protein C or Protein S deficiency, Factor V Leiden, plasminogen or fibrinogen abnormalities.

Homocysteine, factor VIII and von Willebrand factor levels are risks for embolism and they are influenced by dietary intake (Steffen et al, 2007).

Clinical/History

Height
Weight
BMI
Sudden SOB
Hemoptysis with pink, foamy mucus
Tachypnea (respiratory rate >16/min)
Tachycardia (heart rate >100/min)
Arterial blood gases
Diaphoresis
Temperature (fever)
I & O
Sharp chest pain
ECG
Echocardiography
Doppler ultrasound
Cardiac murmur
Palpitations
Low oxygen saturation (hypoxia)
Perfusion scans
CT pulmonary angiography
Cyanosis

Lab Work

Alb, transthyretin
Na^+, K^+
Ca^{++}, Mg^{++}
PT or INR
WBCs (increased)
Troponin (high?)
H & H, Serum Fe
Elevated BNP?
Liver function tests
Homocysteine
Folic acid and B_{12} levels

INTERVENTION

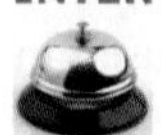

OBJECTIVES

- Prevent right-sided heart failure, atelectasis, and bleeding.
- Stabilize PT and INR if warfarin (Coumadin) is used.
- Maintain lung function through higher antioxidant intake.
- Normalize body temperature where there is fever.
- Replenish nutrients depleted by respiratory distress.
- Oxygenate tissues.
- Eliminate edema when present.

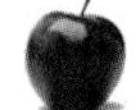

FOOD AND NUTRITION

- Use a regular or high-calorie diet; use a low-sodium diet for patients with edema.
- Increase fluid intake as tolerated.
- Control vitamin K in diet when PT cannot be stabilized.
- Small meals may be needed.

SAMPLE NUTRITION CARE PROCESS STEPS

Involuntary Weight Loss

Assessment Data: Poor oral intake and weight loss of 15 lb in 6 months; swallowing difficulty; decreased appetite and frequent coughing during meals.

Nutrition Diagnoses (PES): Involuntary weight loss related to poor oral intake, coughing at meals and swallowing difficulty as evidenced by 15 lb weight loss in 6 months.

Interventions:

ND 4.5 Patient to use oxygen via nasal cannula during meals to assist with breathing and swallowing and to improve energy levels.

E2.2 Basic education tips on managing discomfort related to SOB by using—five to six small meals throughout the day that are easily prepared; consume main meal early in the day; drink fluids between meals; add protein and calories into meal items.

RC2.2 Refer to local meals on wheels program for home-delivered meals 5 days per week.

Monitoring and Evaluation: Improvement in oral intake and weight status; fewer complaints of fatigue at mealtime; better appetite.

- Provide sufficient antioxidants such as vitamins C and E and selenium. A diet including more plant foods, alcohol, and fish and less red and processed meat may be suggested (Lutsey et al, 2009; Steffen et al, 2007).

Common Drugs Used and Potential Side Effects

- Rivaroxaban is a novel oral direct factor Xa inhibitor for prophylaxis in total knee and hip replacements, with few side effects and low potential for drug–food interactions (Chen and Lam, 2009). Liver enzymes should be checked during use.
- Heparin slows down clot progression and reduces risk of further clots. Warfarin (Coumadin) increases clotting times by thinning the blood. If problems in stabilizing the PT exist, controlled vitamin K may be needed. Use stable amounts of green leafy vegetables and fish.
- Fibrinolytic therapy is a primary treatment. Alteplase is generally infused over several hours. Tissue plasinogen activator (tPA) is also available for thrombolysis.
- Estrogen-containing contraceptives and hormone replacements may promote an embolism in susceptible women. Close medical monitoring is advised.

Herbs, Botanicals, and Supplements

- No clinical trials have proven efficacy for use of herbs or botanicals in pulmonary embolism.

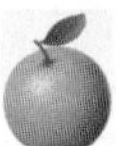

NUTRITION EDUCATION, COUNSELING, CARE MANAGEMENT

- Explain sources of vitamin K in the diet. Therapy often continues for 3–6 months.
- Individuals on long airline flights should try to obtain some physical activity to prevent embolism.

Patient Education—Foodborne Illness

- Careful food handling will be important. Hand washing is key as well.

For More Information

- E-medicine
  http://www.emedicine.com/EMERG/topic490.htm
- Mayo Clinic
  http://www.mayoclinic.com/health/pulmonary-embolism/DS00429/
- Web MD
  http://www.webmd.com/a-to-z-guides/pulmonary-embolism-topic-overview

PULMONARY EMBOLISM—CITED REFERENCES

Chen T, Lam S. Rivaroxaban: an oral direct factor xa inhibitor for the prevention of thromboembolism. *Cardiol Rev.* 17:192, 2009.

Hillman JJ, et al. The impact of the Women's Health Initiative on hormone replacement therapy in a Medicaid program. *J Womens Health (Larchmt).* 13:986, 2004.

Lutsey PL, et al. Diet and incident venous thromboembolism: the Iowa Women's Health Study. *Am Heart J.* 157:1081, 2009.

Steffen LM, et al. Greater fish, fruit, and vegetable intakes are related to lower incidence of venous thromboembolism: the Longitudinal Investigation of Thromboembolism Etiology. *Circulation.* 117:188, 2007.

Stone SE, Morris TA. Pulmonary embolism during and after pregnancy. *Crit Care Med.* 33:294S, 2005.

RESPIRATORY DISTRESS SYNDROME

NUTRITIONAL ACUITY RANKING: LEVEL 3–4

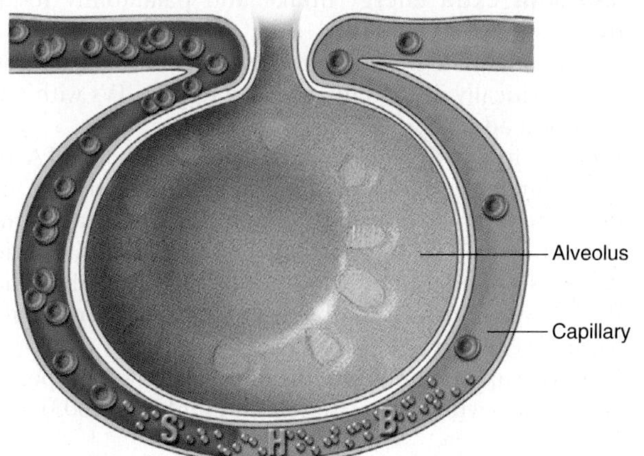

Phase 1. Injury reduces normal blood flow to the lungs. Platelets aggregate and release histamine (H), serotonin (S), and bradykinin (B).

Asset provided by Anatomical Chart Co.

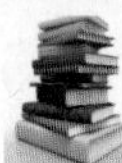

DEFINITIONS AND BACKGROUND

RDS may occur as part of systematic inflammatory response syndrome (SIRS), affecting approximately 70% of patients in the ICU. Acute respiratory distress syndrome (ARDS) develops within 24–48 hours in patients who have sepsis or who are critically ill, in shock, or severely injured. Other causes include infectious pneumonia, aspiration of food into the lung, several blood transfusions, pulmonary embolism, chest injury, burns, near drowning, cardiopulmonary bypass surgery, pancreatitis, overdose of drugs such as heroin, methadone, or aspirin.

ARDS has three pathologic stages: exudative, proliferative, and fibrotic. Patients often have pulmonary edema but have normal left atrial and pulmonary venous pressures.

In infants, RDS occurs in premature or low birth weight babies as hyaline membrane disease. Such babies are often born to mothers who have diabetes. Surfactant treatment may be of significant benefit in newborn infants with respiratory compromise (Finer, 2004).

One of the most common causes of ARDS in adults is sepsis. Here, a high-fat diet or formula with EPA may be beneficial. In ARDS, an overwhelming inflammatory response damages the endothelial-alveolar units, reducing oxygen diffusion and increasing pulmonary workload (Singer and Shapiro, 2009). Specialized enteral formulas may be beneficial adjunctive therapy by reducing lung inflammation and improving oxygenation (Malik and Zaloga, 2010; Priestley and Helfaer, 2004).

Indirect calorimetry (IC) accurately estimates a patient's energy expenditure; this helps the health care team when there is weaning failure.

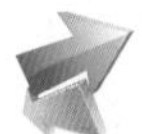

ASSESSMENT, MONITORING, AND EVALUATION

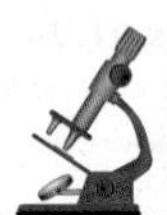

CLINICAL INDICATORS

Genetic Markers: ARDS may have a relationship with tumor necrosis factor-a (TNF-a), interleukin-b (IL-b), interleukin 10 (IL-10), and soluble intercellular adhesion molecule 1 (sICAM-1).

Clinical/History	**Lab Work**	
Height	Complete blood count (CBC)	Transferrin
Weight	Low blood pH (acidic)	pCO_2, pO_2
BMI	H & H	Transthyretin
Growth profile	Serum Fe, ferritin	Na^+, K^+
Diet history		Ca^{++}, Mg^{++}
IC		Serum phosphorus
I & O		BUN, Creat
BP		
Temperature		
RQ		

SAMPLE NUTRITION CARE PROCESS STEPS

Excessive Enteral Nutrition

Assessment Data: Ventilator dependency for acute respiratory distress, ICU admission, inability to consume oral food and beverages, IC indicates energy needs as 1400 kcals/d; current TF order for 2000 kcals

Nutrition Diagnoses (PES): Excessive enteral nutrition related to overfeeding with order for 2000 kcals as evidenced by IC results suggesting 1400 kcals as sufficient.

Interventions: Nutrition prescription should change to match energy needs. Educate nutrition support team about results of IC (1400 kcals vs. current order for 2000 kcals). Suggest immunomodulating diet (IMD) formula supplemented with fructo-oligosaccharieds (FO).

Monitoring and Evaluation: Improved arterial blood gases; enteral nutrition formula tolerated; able to gradually wean from ventilator.

INTERVENTION

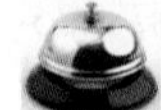

OBJECTIVES

- Identify the cause and remove the ongoing insult. Promote rapid recovery and oxygenation of tissues; support ventilator management.
- Prevent relapse. Avoid secondary insults through aggressive immune surveillance, complete nutrition, and adequate oxygen delivery.
- Counteract side effects of medications as ordered.
- Replace essential fatty acids, carnitine, and other nutrients.
- Prevent malnutrition, which depresses CNS output for ventilatory drive. Starvation decreases the desire to breathe, causing an abnormal breathing pattern, pneumonia, and atelectasis. Muscle mass (including diaphragm) varies with body weight, and refeeding may take 2–3 weeks.
- Prevent overfeeding (hepatic dysfunction, fatty liver, and CO_2 overproduction) and underfeeding (morbidity, mortality, and decreased response to therapy). Avoid refeeding syndrome.
- Prevent fluid overload.
- Support lung function, which is found to be better with higher antioxidant intake levels (Singer et al, 2006).
- An IMD that is supplemented with FO improves the outcome of medical ICU patients with SIRS/sepsis and ARDS (Marik and Zaolga, 2010).

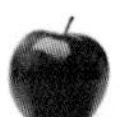

FOOD AND NUTRITION

- Provide parenteral fluids and oxygen as needed.
- Progress, when possible, to oral feedings. Use TPN only if GI tract is nonfunctional. TPN-induced changes in CO_2 production occur if overfed (Plurad et al, 2009).
- For calories, use 30–35 kcal/kg. Nonprotein calories should come from 50% glucose and 50% lipid.
- Increased fat may be required to normalize the RQ. Fat also adds extra energy intake and palatability to the diet.
- Ensure adequate provision of EFA. Low linoleic acid status in critically ill RDS infants may require IVs with a fat emulsion added.
- Increase intake of omega-3 fatty acids, especially EPA and GLA (Singer et al, 2006). Enteral administration of fish oil, antioxidants and arginine improves oxygenation and clinical outcomes (Singer and Shapiro, 2009). Provide vitamins C and E and selenium at slightly higher than RDA levels, and fat-soluble vitamins in water-miscible form if necessary.
- Inositol supplementation promotes survival of premature infants with RDS (Howlett and Ohlsson, 2003).

Common Drugs Used and Potential Side Effects

- Heparin or warfarin (Coumadin) may be used as a blood thinner.

- Ventilator-dependent surgical patients receiving oxandrolone have prolonged courses of mechanical ventilation; oxandrolone may enhance collagen deposition and fibrosis in the later stages of ARDS and thus delay recovery (Bulger et al, 2004).

Herbs, Botanicals, and Supplements

- Use of n-3 PUFA targets the inflammatory response in ARDS (Singer and Shapiro, 2009).

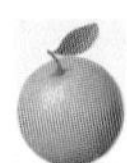

NUTRITION EDUCATION, COUNSELING, CARE MANAGEMENT

- Discuss the role of fat intake on respiratory requirements. Fat decreases CO_2 production.
- Small, frequent feedings may be beneficial.
- Tight glucose control is needed.
- Prone positioning, especially for meals, is recommended.

Patient Education—Foodborne Illness

- Careful food handling will be important. Hand washing is key as well.

For More Information

- Acute Respiratory Distress Clinical Network
http://www.ardsnet.org/
- ARDS Support
http://www.ards.org/
- Medscape
http://emedicine.medscape.com/article/803573-overview
- Respiratory Distress Syndrome
http://www.nhlbi.nih.gov/health/dci/Diseases/Ards/Ards_WhatIs.html

RESPIRATORY DISTRESS SYNDROME—CITED REFERENCES

Bulger EM, et al. Oxandrolone does not improve outcome of ventilator dependent surgical patients. *Ann Surg.* 240:472, 2004.

Finer NN. Surfactant use for neonatal lung injury: beyond respiratory distress syndrome. *Paediatr Respir Rev.* 5:S289, 2004.

Howlette A, Ohlsson A. Inositol for respiratory distress syndrome in preterm infants. *Cochrane Database Syst Rev.* 4:CD000366, 2003.

Marik PE, Zaloga GP. Immunonutrition in high-risk surgical patients: a systematic review and analysis of the literature. *JPEN J Parenter Enteral Nutr.* 34:378, 2010.

Plurad D, et al. A 6-year review of total parenteral nutrition use and association with late-onset acute respiratory distress syndrome among ventilated trauma victims. *Injury.* 40:511, 2009.

Priestley MA, Helfaer MA. Approaches in the management of acute respiratory failure in children. *Curr Opin Pediatr.* 16:293, 2004.

Singer P, et al. Benefit of an enteral diet enriched with eicosapentaenoic acid and gamma-linolenic acid in ventilated patients with acute lung injury. *Crit Care Med.* 34:1033, 2006.

Singer P, Shapiro H. Enteral omega-3 in acute respiratory distress syndrome. *Curr Opin Clin Nutr Metab Care.* 12:123, 2009.

RESPIRATORY FAILURE AND VENTILATOR DEPENDENCY

NUTRITIONAL ACUITY RANKING: LEVEL 4

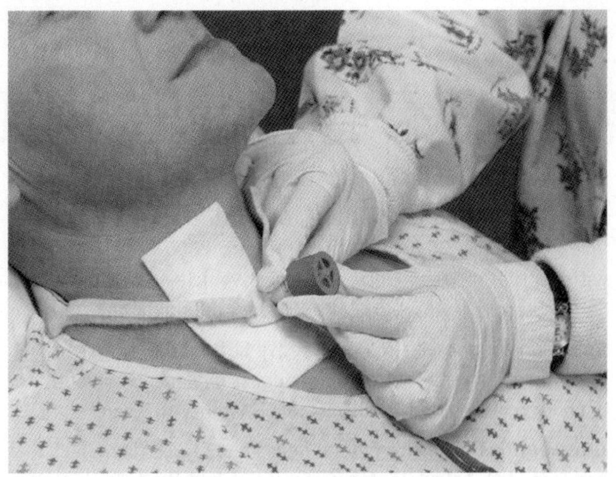

Adapted from: Springhouse. *Lippincott's Visual Encyclopedia of Clinical Skills*. Philadelphia: Wolters Kluwer Health, 2009.

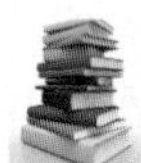

DEFINITIONS AND BACKGROUND

RF involves ineffective gas exchange across the lungs by the respiratory system. Arterial blood gases should be used to determine the presence of RF and Table 5-11 lists common causes. Acute respiratory failure (ARF) involves sudden absence of respirations, with confusion or unresponsiveness and failure of pulmonary gas exchange mechanism. Chronic pulmonary disease or an acute injury can cause ARF, which requires mechanical ventilation.

TABLE 5-11 Causes of Respiratory Failure

Symptom	Cause
Airway obstruction	Chronic bronchitis, emphysema, bronchiectasis, cystic fibrosis, asthma, bronchiolitis, inhaled particles, subglottic stenosis, tumor, laryngeal edema
Poor breathing	Obesity, sleep apnea, drug intoxication, trauma, hypothyroidism
Neuromuscular disease	Myasthenia gravis, muscular dystrophy, polio, Guillain-Barré syndrome, botulism, polymyositis, stroke, amyotrophic lateral sclerosis, spinal cord injury
Abnormality of lung tissue	Acute respiratory distress, drug reaction, pulmonary fibrosis, fibrosing alveolitis, widespread tumors, radiation therapy, sarcoidosis, burns
Abnormality of chest wall	Kyphoscoliosis, chest wound

Mechanical ventilation can be delivered with a plastic tube inserted through the nose or mouth into the trachea. A tracheostomy is safer and more comfortable for long-term ventilation for either pure oxygen or a mixture of oxygen and air.

Anabolic and catabolic hormones, muscle work, and nutritional status affect skeletal muscle mass and muscle strength. Substrate plus muscle work help to stimulate protein synthesis. Randomized controlled trials comparing early aggressive use of enteral nutrition with delayed, less-aggressive use of enteral nutrition suggest that providing early, aggressive enteral nutrition promotes improved clinical outcomes (Stapleton et al, 2007). In starvation, respiratory muscles are catabolized to meet energy needs; refeeding helps ventilatory response. Enteral feedings started within 24–48 hours may reduce length of time on a ventilator.

Daily screening of ventilator patients is recommended, followed by trials of spontaneous breathing. The process of weaning takes a few days and requires proper refeeding. Table 5-12 identifies ventilator-dependency feeding stages. The length of ventilator dependency time relates to energy and CHO intake. Aggressive immune surveillance, nutritional support, and fluid management are critical (Michaels, 2004).

Older patients are more at risk for RF and may be harder to wean (Sevransky and Haponik, 2003). Attention must be paid to factors such as electrolytes, infections, anemia, heart failure, medications, or hypothyroidism (Datta and Scalise, 2004). Use of an evidence-based nutrition support protocol improves the likelihood of meeting nutritional requirements (Mackenzie et al, 2005). Patients with RF often have 30% or higher increase in oxygen requirements. Too much oxygen can be damaging, though, so careful monitoring is needed. Lung function is found to be better with higher antioxidant levels.

TABLE 5-12 Ventilatory-Dependency Feeding Stages

Stage	Objectives and Actions
Intubation/ Acute Phase	Replenish muscle glycogen stores and reverse catabolism. Enteral nutrition by day 3; parenteral by day 7 if GI tract not functioning.
Preweaning	Maintain positive nitrogen balance, improve visceral protein stores, improve lean body mass, and promote weight gain. Evaluate albumin or prealbumin levels.
Weaning 1–4 weeks	Provide energy substrates to cover needs of respiratory muscles that are working harder; minimize CO_2 production. Be careful not to overfeed. Check prealbumin levels and monitor fatigue. Get a Speech evaluation for swallowing. Assess for gastrostomy if needed.
Rehabilitation	Maintain nutrient needs despite anorexia or dysphagia; support anabolism. Maintain enteral nutrition at night until oral intake meets needs. If aspiration risk remains, continue gastrostomy.

Sources: Delmore BA. Levine's framework in long-term ventilated patients during the weaning course. *Nurs Sci Q.* 19:247, 2006.
Matarese LE, Gottschlich M. Contemporary nutrition support practice: *a clinical guide.* St Louis: Elsevier, 2003:398–399.

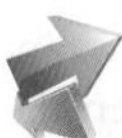

ASSESSMENT, MONITORING, AND EVALUATION

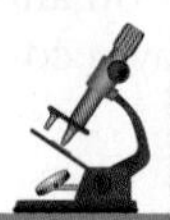

CLINICAL INDICATORS

Genetic Markers: Mutations in the ABCA3 transporter have been associated with childhood respiratory disease; there is a role for surfactant, a mixture of phospholipids, cholesterol, and hydrophobic proteins (Fitzgerald et al, 2007; Shulenin et al, 2004).

Clinical/History

Height
Weight
BMI
Resting energy expenditure (REE) from IC
Diet history
I & O
$PaO_2 < 60$ mm Hg
$PaCO_2 > 50$ mm Hg
Respiratory rate
RQ
BP
Temperature (fever?)
Forced vital capacity (FVC)
Skinfold thickness

Lab Work

Hypophosphatemia (can cause ARF)
Gluc
Urinary Gluc
Transthyretin (decreased)
TLC (decreased)
H & H
Serum Fe, ferritin
Na^+, K^+
Ca^{++}, Mg^{++}
WBC (elevated)
Chol, Trig
Transferrin
Thyroid tests
CRP
pH (acidemia below 7.4, alkalemia above 7.4)

SAMPLE NUTRITION CARE PROCESS STEPS

Excessive CHO Intake

Assessment Data: IC indicates need for 1675 kcals daily. TF provides 65% CHO, 20% lipid, 15% protein; 2300 kcals total. ARF with ventilator dependency post motor vehicle accident. BMI 24. Serum glucose levels 350, 250, 301 on 3 days.

Nutrition Diagnoses (PES): Excessive CHO intake related to high CHO and energy content of TF formula as evidenced by ventilator dependency, elevated CO_2 levels, and inability to wean.

Interventions: Evaluate enteral needs and select TF product that has less CHO. Calculate energy, protein, and fluid needs with a new product and provide rate and amount using continuous drip equal to 1675 kcals daily. Monitor use of insulin and adjust according to serum glucose levels.

Monitoring and Evaluation: Gradual weaning from ventilator dependency. Improved blood gases and lower CO_2 production. Weight maintenance; BMI remaining at 24. Serum glucose within acceptable range.

INTERVENTION

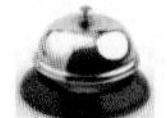

OBJECTIVES

- Promote normalized nutritional intake despite hypermetabolic status of the patient and the prohibition of oral intake due to endotracheal tubes.
- Oxygenate tissues and relieve breathlessness; decrease CO_2 production.
- Monitor sensations of hunger when patients are unable to communicate their hunger and thirst.
- Prevent respiratory muscle dysfunction by ensuring that the patient is properly nourished.
- Provide intensive metabolic support with insulin therapy, an appropriate blood glucose target, nutrition risk assessment, early or combined enteral nutrition and PN, and close nutritional monitoring (Mechanick and Chiolero, 2008).
- Counteract hypotension caused by positive-pressure ventilation, acidosis, or both.
- Provide nutritional substrates that will maintain surfactant production and LBM. Achieve or maintain weight; note that not all patients are malnourished.
- Prevent atelectasis, pulmonary infection, sepsis, glucose or lipid intolerance, multiple organ dysfunction syndrome, and aspiration.
- Alleviate GI complications, which are a concern with mechanical ventilation. Hypomotility and diarrhea are common.
- Protocol-driven weaning reduces use of mechanical ventilation (Dries et al, 2004; Graham and Kirbey, 2006). Adjust goals as appropriate.
- Maintain flexible approaches to patient requirements. Nutritional supplements containing selenium, vitamins, and antioxidants may provide needed support to shift from catabolic to anabolic, reduce free radicals, and quiet inflammation (Meltzer and Moitra, 2008).

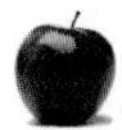

FOOD AND NUTRITION

- Begin nourishing the patient as soon as possible to wean the patient from the ventilator. Start a TF of low osmolality slowly to avoid gastric retention or diarrhea. Advance gradually and use continuous administrations unless contraindicated. Do not add blue food coloring to feedings to detect aspirate in tracheal secretions (Kattelman et al, 2006).
- Ambulatory adults need about 30 kcal/kg daily. In ICU, the goal of 20–25 kcal/kg is sought; if it cannot be met, then combined enteral and PN should be considered to reduce the risk of complications and longer length of stay (Scurlock and Mechanick, 2008).
- Increased needs occur from labored breathing; monitor using IC. Use of specialty products such as Pulmocare or Respalor may be recommended, but they are not always necessary. Include 2% of total fat as essential fatty acids with some omega-3 fatty acids.
- Provide 1.2–1.5 g protein/kg/d (Mechanick and Chiolero, 2008).
- While hypermetabolism and malnutrition are common, there is no need for supplemental PN to increase caloric delivery in the early phase of critical illness (Stapleton et al, 2007). Monitor TPN carefully for complications such as pneumonia, refeeding syndrome from high-calorie loading, and increased CO_2 production.
- Patients with pulmonary edema should have their sodium intake reduced if needed. Include adequate protein in the diet to prevent additional fluid retention from lowered colloidal osmotic pressure.
- Supplement diet with a multivitamin supplement. Include antioxidant-rich foods for vitamins E, selenium, carotenoids, and vitamin C. Phosphorus and magnesium may be needed if stores are depleted.

Common Drugs Used and Potential Side Effects

- Bronchodilators, antibiotics, diuretics, or corticosteroids may be needed. Monitor side effects.
- For diarrhea, treatment depends on the cause. For *Clostridium difficile* infection, antibacterial therapy should be discontinued, if possible, and treatment with oral metronidazole should be initiated (Mutlu et al, 2003).

Herbs, Botanicals, and Supplements

- No clinical trials have proven efficacy for use of herbs or botanicals in RF.

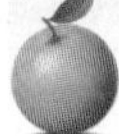

NUTRITION EDUCATION, COUNSELING, CARE MANAGEMENT

- A daily calorie count may be needed to assess the patient's nutritional status.
- The greatest danger in using enteral nutrition is aspiration. Low-osmolarity products are essential, as well as elevation of the head of the bed.
- Discuss early satiety, bloating, fatigue, dyspnea as related to food or TF intake.
- Delivery of enteral nutrition in patients receiving mechanical ventilation is interrupted by practices required for the care of these patients (O'Meara et al, 2008). Discharge planning for the ventilator patient to return home is ideal.

Patient Education—Foodborne Illness

- Careful food handling will be important. Hand washing is key as well.

For More Information

- Merck Manual—Respiratory Failure
  http://www.merck.com/mmhe/sec04/ch055/ch055a.html
- Medicine Net
  http://www.medterms.com/script/main/art.asp?articlekey=10698
- Respiratory Failure
  http://www.med-help.net/AcuteRespiratoryFailure.html

RESPIRATORY FAILURE AND VENTILATOR DEPENDENCY—CITED REFERENCES

Datta D, Scalise P. Hypothyroidism and failure to wean in patients receiving prolonged mechanical ventilation at a regional weaning center. *Chest.* 126:1307, 2004.

Delmore BA. Levine's framework in long-term ventilated patients during the weaning course. *Nurs Sci Q.* 19:247, 2006.

Dries DJ, et al. Protocol-driven ventilator weaning reduces use of mechanical ventilation, rate of early reintubation, and ventilator-associated pneumonia. *J Trauma.* 56:943, 2004.

Fitzgerald ML, et al. ABCA3 inactivation in mice causes respiratory failure, loss of pulmonary surfactant, and depletion of lung phosphatidylglycerol. *J Lipid Res.* 48:621, 2007.

Graham AS, Kirby AL. Ventilator management protocols in pediatrics. *Respir Care Clin N Am.* 12:389, 2006.

Kattelman K, et al. Preliminary evidence for a medical nutrition therapy protocol: enteral feedings for critically ill patients. *J Am Diet Assoc.* 106:1226, 2006.

Mackenzie SL, et al. Implementation of a nutrition support protocol increases the proportion of mechanically ventilated patients reaching enteral nutrition targets in the adult intensive care unit. *JPEN J Parenter Enteral Nutr.* 29(2):74, 2005.

Matarese L, Gottschlich M. *Contemporary nutrition support practice: a clinical guide,* 2nd ed. St Louis: Elsevier, 2003:398–400.

Mechanick JI, Chiolero R. Special commentary: a call for intensive metabolic support. *Curr Opin Clin Nutr Metab Care.* 11:666, 2008.

Meltzer JS, Moitra VK. The nutritional and metabolic support of heart failure in the intensive care unit. *Curr Opin Clin Nutr Metab Care.* 11:140, 2008.

Michaels AJ. Management of post traumatic respiratory failure. *Crit Care Clin.* 20:83, 2004.

Mutlu GM, et al. Prevention and treatment of gastrointestinal complications in patients on mechanical ventilation. *Am J Respir Med.* 2:395, 2003.

O'Meara D, et al. Evaluation of delivery of enteral nutrition in critically ill patients receiving mechanical ventilation. *Am J Crit Care.* 17:53, 2008.

Scurlock C, Mechanick JI. Early nutrition support in the intensive care unit: a US perspective. *Curr Opin Clin Nutr Metab Care.* 11:152, 2008.

Sevransky JE, Haponik EF. Respiratory failure in elderly patients. *Clin Geriatr Med.* 19:205, 2003.

Shulenin S, et al. ABCA3 gene mutations in newborns with fatal surfactant deficiency. *N Engl J Med.* 350:1296, 2004.

Stapleton RD, et al. Feeding critically ill patients: what is the optimal amount of energy? *Crit Care Med.* 35:535S, 2007.

SARCOIDOSIS

NUTRITIONAL ACUITY RANKING: LEVEL 1–2

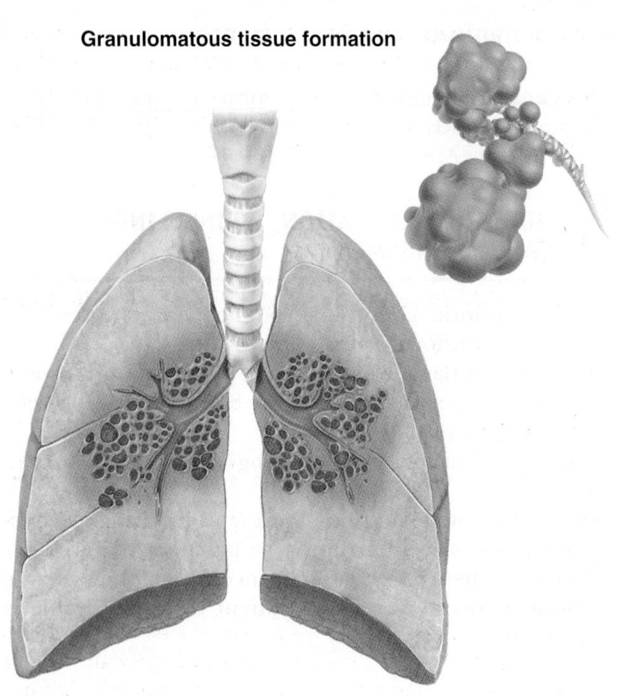

Asset provided by Anatomical Chart Co.

DEFINITIONS AND BACKGROUND

Sarcoidosis is a disease of undetermined origin with tiny patches of inflammation (granulomas) occurring in almost any organ. Pulmonary effects are most common. It develops most often between ages 20 years and 40 years, more often among women than men, and more commonly among Swedes, Danes, and African Americans. Sarcoidosis is more common among nonsmokers than among smokers.

In children, renal impairment of sarcoidosis usually is caused by either hypercalcemia leading to nephrocalcinosis or interstitial nephritis with or without granulomata (Thumfart et al, 2005). Lofgren's syndrome is a classic set of signs and symptoms involving fever, enlarged lymph nodes, arthritis in the ankles, or erythema nodosum. Overall, prognosis is good for most cases, and most sarcoidosis subsides on its own within 3 years. In 10% of cases, the condition becomes chronic. Sarcoidosis leads to organ damage in about one third of the people diagnosed; the lungs, heart, or brain may be affected.

Hypercalcemia can occur in patients with granulomatous disorders such as sarcoidosis, often related to high serum 1,25-dihydroxyvitamin D (OHD) concentrations (Falk et al, 2007). Endogenous antioxidant defense is significantly reduced, and oxidative stress underlies the pathology of this disease (Boots et al, 2009).

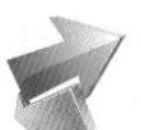

ASSESSMENT, MONITORING, AND EVALUATION

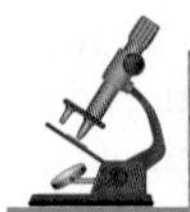

CLINICAL INDICATORS

Genetic Markers: Sarcoidosis CD4+ T cells are primarily responsible for the systemic responses. The 1-alpha-hydroxylase gene affects alveolar macrophages and disturbances in calcium metabolism.

Clinical/History		
Height	BMI	BP
Weight	Weight loss?	Fever
	Diet history	

Tender red lumps on shins or ankles	PH cor pulmonale	Alkaline phosphatase (Alk phos)
Lupus pernio (painful sores on face)	Clubbing of fingers, hypoxemia	Nitrogen (N) balance
Granulomas	Iritis, glaucoma, blindness	Transferrin
Enlarged liver or spleen	Chest pain, even heart failure	Globulin (increase common)
Uveitis	Chest x-ray	Serum Ca^{++} (increased)
SOB, cough	Biopsy	Ca^{++} in urine (increased?)
Night sweats	Gallium scan	Serum vitamin D_3
Bone or joint pain	TB test (rule out tuberculosis)	Na^+, K^+
Anorexia, weakness, aching joints	Pulmonary function tests	Mg^{++}
Abdominal pain, lymphadenopathy	**Lab Work**	Uric acid (increased)
Bone cysts in hands and feet	H & H (anemia common)	PO_4
	Serum Fe, ferritin	Kveim test
	Alb (decreased)	Erythrocyte sedimentation rate (ESR)
	CRP (elevated)	

INTERVENTION

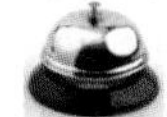

OBJECTIVES

- Reduce heart failure, BX, and related problems.
- Correct weight loss, anorexia, fever, and abdominal pain.
- Improve ability to breathe and eat normally.
- Prevent further deterioration of organ functions with any and all affected organ systems.
- Prevent or correct fluid retention.

SAMPLE NUTRITION CARE PROCESS STEPS

Imbalance of Nutrients

Assessment Data: Altered lab values, elevated uric acid, and ESR; uveitis, wheezing, coughing, Dx of sarcoidosis; diet hx showing minimal intake of vitamins and minerals.

Nutrition Diagnoses (PES): Imbalance of nutrients related to minimal intake of omega-3 fatty acids, vitamins, and minerals as evidenced by chronic inflammation and altered labs (uric acid, ESR, CRP).

Interventions: Modify dietary intake to increase antioxidants from fruits, vegetables, whole grains, and nuts as well as omega-3 fatty acids from salmon/tuna/sardines. Provide multivitamin—mineral supplement. Educate about the natural role of diet in reducing inflammation.

Monitoring and Evaluation: Improved balance of nutrients from diet and supplementation; normalized labs including CRP, ESR, uric acid.

- High levels of calcium may accumulate in the blood and urine. Monitor for related nausea, anorexia, vomiting, thirst, excessive urination, or renal failure.

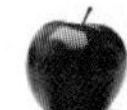

FOOD AND NUTRITION

- Restrict salt if necessary for heart failure or for use of corticosteroids. A 2- to 3-g sodium diet may be beneficial.
- Use a diet containing adequate to high potassium (unless medications are used).
- Patients might benefit from antioxidants such as quercetin (Boots et al, 2009). More fruits and vegetables should be consumed.

Common Drugs Used and Potential Side Effects

- Prednisone is used to suppress severe symptoms such as SOB. Watch electrolytes, nitrogen balance, and other changes. Treatment may require several years.
- Methotrexate works best for treating sarcoidosis that affects lungs, eyes, skin, or joints. Folic acid depletion can occur (Low et al, 2008).
- Calcium-chelating agents may be used if hypercalcemia persists.
- Sarcoid granulomatous interstitial nephritis may respond to infliximab therapy (Thumfart et al, 2005). The drug seems to work against elevated TNF.
- For pain or fever, nonsteroidal anti-inflammatory drugs (NSAIDs) such as ibuprofen may help.

Herbs, Botanicals, and Supplements

- No clinical trials have proven efficacy for use of herbs or botanicals in sarcoidosis.

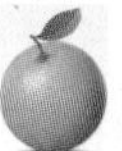

NUTRITION EDUCATION, COUNSELING, CARE MANAGEMENT

- If the patient is using steroids, antacids could also be taken to reduce GI side effects. Check with the doctor.
- Discuss the role of diet in maintaining immunocompetence and in improving tolerance for other therapies.
- Follow regarding calcium and vitamin D supplements to avoid prolonged hypercalcemia and hypercalciuria. If needed, avoid intake of fish oils and excessive sun exposure.

Patient Education—Foodborne Illness

- Careful food handling will be important. Hand washing is key as well.

For More Information

- Mayo Clinic—Sarcoidosis
  http://www.mayoclinic.com/health/sarcoidosis/ds00251
- National Heart, Lung, and Blood Institute—Sarcoidosis
  http://www.nhlbi.nih.gov/health/public/lung/other/sarcoidosis/index.htm

- National Sarcoidosis Resources Center
http://www.nsrc-global.net/
- Sarcoidosis Center
http://www.sarcoidcenter.com/
- Sarcoidosis Family Aid and Research Foundation Hotline
http://www.medicinenet.com/sarcoidosis/page10.htm
- Sarcoidosis Research Institute
http://www.sarcoidcenter.com/sricontents.htm

SARCOIDOSIS—CITED REFERENCES

Boots AW, et al. Antioxidant status associated with inflammation in sarcoidosis: a potential role for antioxidants. *Respir Med.* 103:364, 2009.

Falk S, et al. Hypercalcemia as a result of sarcoidosis with normal serum concentrations of vitamin D. *Med Sci Monit.* 13:113, 2007.

Low PS, et al. Discovery and development of folic-acid-based receptor targeting for imaging and therapy of cancer and inflammatory diseases. *Acc Chem Res.* 41:120, 2008.

Thumfart J, et al. Isolated sarcoid granulomatous interstitial nephritis responding to infliximab therapy. *Am J Kidney Dis.* 45:411, 2005.

SLEEP APNEA

NUTRITIONAL ACUITY RANKING: LEVEL 2–3

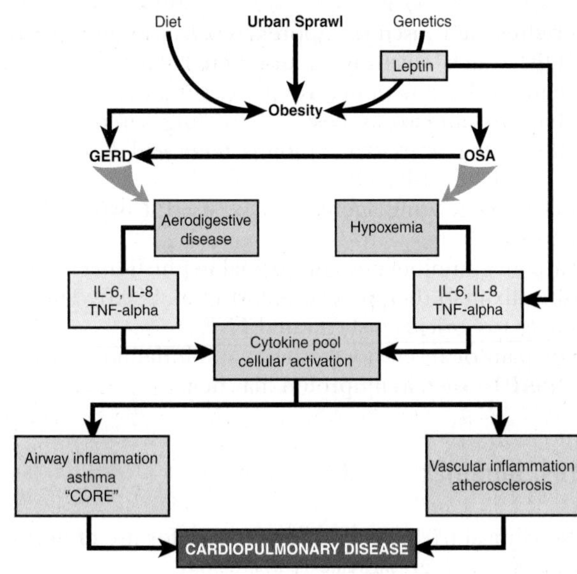

Obstructive sleep apnea (OSA) can lead to chronic disease, such as cardiopulmonary disease.

DEFINITIONS AND BACKGROUND

Approximately 4% of middle-aged men and 2% of middle-aged women suffer from obstructive sleep apnea (OSA). OSA affects 12–18 million Americans and is associated with irritability, excessive daytime sleepiness, an inability to concentrate, depression, morning headaches, and decreased job performance in adults. Untreated sleep apnea also can increase an individual's risk of heart attack, high BP, diabetes, stroke, and automobile accidents. OSA is often undiagnosed and is a major contributing factor in the development of essential hypertension.

Sleep apnea occurs in both genders and in all ages, weights, and ethnicities. Certain risk factors are associated with a higher incidence, such as excess weight or obesity (BMI >25); family history of sleep apnea; male sex; large neck (greater than 17 inches in men, greater than 16 inches in women); recessed chin; physical abnormality in the nose, throat, or upper airway structure; older age; smoking; use of alcohol or sleeping pills; ethnicity (African Americans, Pacific Islanders, and Hispanics seem to be at an increased risk); and snoring.

Sleep apnea may develop in any patient who has an endocrine disorder or is receiving certain hormonal therapies. Increases in habitual sleep duration is associated with elevations in CRP and IL-6 while reduced sleep duration is associated with elevated TNFa levels; activation of proinflammatory pathways may represent a mechanism by which extreme sleep habits affect health (Patel et al, 2009). IL-6, TNF*a*, and insulin levels are elevated in sleep apnea independently of obesity; visceral fat is the primary parameter linked with sleep apnea (Vgontzas, 2008).

Effective assessment and management of OSA may lead to a reduction in insulin resistance and hypertension as well as other markers of vascular risk in patients with metabolic syndrome (Yee et al, 2004). Untreated severe OSA results in elevated CRP levels and cardiovascular risks. Clinicians should be aware. Both atherosclerosis and OSA are associated with endothelial dysfunction; increased CRP, interleukin-6, fibrinogen, and plasminogen activator inhibitor; and reduced fibrinolytic activity. OSA has also been associated with enhanced platelet activity and aggregation and leukocyte adhesion on endothelial cells (Parish and Somers, 2004).

Obstructive sleep–disordered (OSD) breathing is common in children (3–12% of children snore); mild sleep apnea affects 1–10% of children (Chan et al, 2004). Risk factors of children who are more at risk for OSA are physical abnormalities of the face or skull, cerebral palsy, muscular dystrophy, Down syndrome, sickle cell disease, obesity, and mouth breathing. Consequences of untreated OSA include failure to thrive, enuresis, attention-deficit disorder, behavior problems, poor academic performance, and cardiopulmonary disease (Chan et al, 2004). Sleep deprivation and sleep apnea may even be related to some sudden infant death syndrome (SIDS) cases; upper airway obstruction and depressed arousability from sleep may contribute (Franco et al, 2004).

Treatment includes the use of continuous positive airway pressure (CPAP), weight loss in obese children, or adenotonsillectomy. Use of a CPAP device can be worn while sleeping. This device works to keep the airway open by continuously blowing air through the nasal passages at a high pressure. CPAP may help medically treated patients with heart failure and other cardiovascular conditions. In addition, some dental appliances may reposition the tongue or lower jaw so that the airway remains open while the patient sleeps, thus preventing the apnea. Surgical treatments may also be done, such as septoplasty, tonsillectomy, uvulopalatopharyngoplasty (UPPP, also known as UP3), and laser-assisted uvulopalatopharyngoplasty (LAUP).

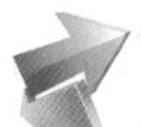

ASSESSMENT, MONITORING, AND EVALUATION

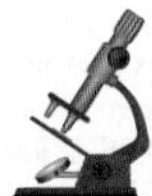

CLINICAL INDICATORS

Genetic Markers: IL-6, TNF*a*, and insulin levels are elevated in sleep apnea.

Clinical/History

- Height
- Weight
- BMI
- Abdominal adiposity?
- PCOS?
- Diet history
- BP
- Chest x-ray
- Polysomnography (sleep study)
- Hypopnea (less than normal breath)
- Apnea–hypopnea index (AHI)
- Respiratory disturbance index (RDI)
- Epworth Sleepiness Scale (ESS)

Lab Work

- Gluc
- Serum insulin
- CBC
- H & H (anemia common)
- Serum Fe, ferritin
- CRP
- Homocysteine
- Alb, transthyretin
- Ca^{++}, Mg^{++}
- Na^{+}, K^{+}
- pCO_2, pO_2

INTERVENTION

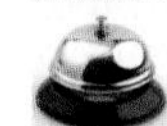

OBJECTIVES

- If obese, weight loss will be beneficial. Obesity is associated with comorbidities such as PH, hypoventilation, and sleep apnea that may lead to disability or death (Poirier et al, 2009).
- In children with sleep apnea and failure to thrive, medical or surgical treatments may help to alleviate the problem so catch-up growth can occur. These children may have reduced upper airway muscle tone, evident mostly during REM sleep stages (Eckert et al, 2009).
- Lessen insulin resistance, where possible.
- Manage other medical and health complications that are present in the individual; cardiovascular disease, hypertension, or metabolic syndrome may coexist with OSA.

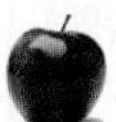

FOOD AND NUTRITION

- Lower energy intake to promote weight loss of 1–1.5 lb weekly if possible.
- Alter diet plan if needed to manage diabetes, sickle cell anemia, or other underlying conditions.
- The DASH diet or a calorie-controlled diet may be useful.

> **SAMPLE NUTRITION CARE PROCESS STEPS**
>
> **Obesity and Metabolic Syndrome**
>
> ***Assessment Data:*** Divorced male, age 45, BMI 31, chronic hypertension, central adiposity, hx of sleep apnea with snoring, HDL 40, LDL 210, diet hx shows eating away from home six to eight times weekly, no cooking skills or interest, drinks two to three alcoholic beverages daily.
>
> ***Nutrition Diagnoses (PES):*** Obesity related to excessive intake of energy-dense foods as evidenced by BMI 31, hypertension, sleep apnea, and central adiposity (waist 46").
>
> ***Interventions:*** Educate about simpler meals that are nutrient-dense and less energy-dense, lower in fat and alcohol; good choices from grocery store or dining at restaurants. Materials from Cooperative Extension or Health Department on "eating for one." Referral go to Sleep Disorder Clinic if interested.
>
> ***Monitoring and Evaluation:*** Meal and food choices; improvement in BMI, BP, lipids; less problem with snoring and sleep apnea. Participation in Sleep Disorder Clinic evaluation.

Common Drugs Used and Potential Side Effects

- OSA can be induced, unmasked, or exacerbated by the effects of sedative, analgesic, and anesthetic agents (Jain and Dhand, 2004). Sleeping agents are not generally recommended.
- Treatment of depression or mood disorders may be needed. In patients who are on chronic neuroleptic drugs for schizophrenia, weight management will be very important.

Herbs, Botanicals, and Supplements

- No clinical trials have proven efficacy for use of herbs or botanicals in sleep apnea.

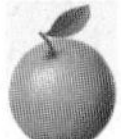

NUTRITION EDUCATION, COUNSELING, CARE MANAGEMENT

- Typically, patients diagnosed with sleep apnea are advised to avoid tobacco, alcohol, sedatives, and medications that relax the airway and/or reduce respiratory function.
- Regular exercise and weight reduction can help some patients with mild or moderate sleep apnea minimize their symptoms.
- Sleep apnea sufferers are advised to avoid sleeping on their back, if possible. Using pillows and other devices that help the patient sleep in a side position may help.
- The relationship of OSA with hypertension, stroke, and cardiovascular disease should be discussed.
- Help with obesity if needed, especially central adiposity (Schwartz et al, 2008).
- Patients who have a cough, OSA, rhinosinusitis, and esophageal reflux clustered together can be categorized as having CORE syndrome (Arter et al, 2004).

Patient Education—Foodborne Illness

- Careful food handling will be important. Hand washing is key as well.

For More Information

- Narcolepsy Network
  http://www.websciences.org/narnet/
- National Sleep Foundation
  http://www.sleepfoundation.org/
- Sleep Apnea Association
  http://www.sleepapnea.org/

SLEEP APNEA—CITED REFERENCES

Arter JL, et al. Obstructive sleep apnea, inflammation, and cardiopulmonary disease. *Front Biosci.* 9:2892, 2004.

Chan J, et al. Obstructive sleep apnea in children. *Am Fam Physician.* 69:1147, 2004.

Eckert DJ, et al. The influence of obstructive sleep apnea and gender on genioglossus activity during rapid eye movement sleep. *Chest.* 135:954, 2009.

Franco P, et al. Decreased arousals among healthy infants after short-term sleep deprivation. *Pediatrics.* 114:192, 2004.

Jain SS, Dhand R. Perioperative treatment of patients with obstructive sleep apnea. *Curr Opin Pulm Med.* 10:482, 2004.

Parish JM, Somers VK. Obstructive sleep apnea and cardiovascular disease. *Mayo Clin Proc.* 79:1036, 2004.

Patel SR, et al. Sleep duration and biomarkers of inflammation. *Sleep.* 32:200, 2009.

Poirier P, et al. Cardiovascular evaluation and management of severely obese patients undergoing surgery. A Science Advisory From the American Heart Association [epub ahead of print June 15, 2009.]. *Circulation.* 120:86, 2009.

Schwartz AR, et al. Obesity and obstructive sleep apnea: pathogenic mechanisms and therapeutic approaches. *Proc Am Thorac Soc.* 5:185, 2008.

Vgontzas AN. Does obesity play a major role in the pathogenesis of sleep apnoea and its associated manifestations via inflammation, visceral adiposity, and insulin resistance? *Arch Physiol Biochem.* 114:211, 2008.

Yee B, et al. Neuroendocrine changes in sleep apnea. *Curr Opin Pulm Med.* 10:475, 2004.

THORACIC EMPYEMA

NUTRITIONAL ACUITY RANKING: LEVEL 2

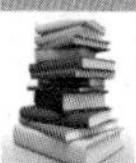

DEFINITIONS AND BACKGROUND

Thoracic empyema involves accumulation of pus in the pleural cavity, sometimes as a complication of pneumonia. Complications may include septic shock, multiple organ failure, cardiac insufficiency, and end-stage renal failure. A chest tube may be placed (thoracentesis) to drain the infection.

In diaphragmatic injury, empyema is a rare but serious complication that can lead to prolonged hospital or ICU lengths of stay; gastric trauma is often associated (Bramparas et al, 2009). Use of prophylactic antibiotics may be prescribed.

An increase in the incidence of thoracic empyema in children has been noted, and the causative pathogen is often unknown (Saglani et al, 2005). *Staphylococcus aureus* is a common micro-organism isolated from the bacterial cultures, as is *Mycobacterium tuberculosis* (Ozel et al, 2004). With an increasing incidence of *S. aureus*, particularly MRSA, the use of video-assisted thoracoscopy (VATS) results in a decreased duration of fever and length of hospitalization (Schultz et al, 2004).

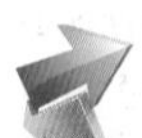

ASSESSMENT, MONITORING, AND EVALUATION

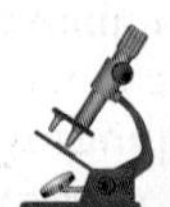

CLINICAL INDICATORS

Genetic Markers: Most empyema is from pneumonia or trauma. The noted virulence of invasive pneumococcal disease (IPD) after the initiation of vaccine has led to speculation about antibiotic resistance in some individuals.

Clinical/History		Lab Work
Height	Productive cough	Alb, transthyretin
Weight	I & O	H & H
BMI	Dyspnea, orthopnea	Serum Fe
Weight loss?	Constant localized chest pain	Gluc
Anorexia, fatigue	Tachycardia, tachypnea	Na^+, K^+
Diet history	CT scan	Ca^{++}, Mg^{++}
BP	Ultrasound	pO_2 (often decreased)
Temperature (fever?)	Tachycardia?	pCO_2
Pleural examination		Transferrin
		CRP

SAMPLE NUTRITION CARE PROCESS STEPS

Inadequate Oral Food and Beverage Intake

Assessment Data: Chronic cough and chest pain, fatigue and anorexia with weight loss of 12 lb in past month. Fever 102°F for past 3 days.

Nutrition Diagnoses (PES): Inadequate oral food and beverage intake related to anorexia, fever, tachcardia, chronic cough and chest pain from thoracic empyema as evidenced by weight loss of 12 lb in past month.

Interventions: Educate about simple, nutrient and energy-dense meals and snacks. Counsel about ways to lessen fatigue with mealtime preparation. Coordinate care with home-delivered meals or shopping assistance when discharged.

Monitoring and Evaluation: Improved oral food and beverage intake as per patient food diary and weight gain of 5 lb in 3 weeks after returning home. Fewer complaints of anorexia or poor nutrition quality of life.

INTERVENTION

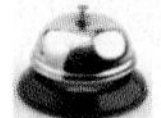

OBJECTIVES

- Lessen fatigue; promote improved well-being.
- Reduce fever. Prevent sepsis, organ failure, and other complications.
- Correct weight loss.
- Control and reduce anorexia.
- Support the capacity for wound healing if surgery is needed.

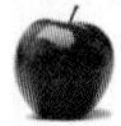

FOOD AND NUTRITION

- Provide diet as ordered. Patient may need high-calorie/ high-protein foods served at frequent intervals.
- Two or more liters of fluid may be needed daily, unless contraindicated.
- Meals should be served in an attractive manner to stimulate appetite.
- A multivitamin–mineral supplement may be useful.

Common Drugs Used and Potential Side Effects

- Antibiotics such as streptokinase are common (Cameron and Davies, 2004). Monitor side effects accordingly.
- Monitor effects of other medications as prescribed.

Herbs, Botanicals, and Supplements

- No clinical trials have proven efficacy for use of herbs or botanicals in thoracic empyema.

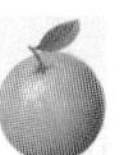

NUTRITION EDUCATION, COUNSELING, CARE MANAGEMENT

- Discuss the role of nutrition in illness and recovery, especially as it relates to immunocompetence.
- With family, discuss signs to observe for future problems or relapses.

Patient Education—Foodborne Illness

- Careful food handling will be important. Hand washing is key as well.

For More Information

- Empyema
  http://emedicine.medscape.com/article/355892-overview
- NIH—Empyema
  http://www.nlm.nih.gov/MEDLINEPLUS/ency/article/000123.htm
- Thoracic Empyema
  http://www.encyclopedia.com/html/e1/empyema.asp

THORACIC EMPYEMA—CITED REFERENCES

Bramparas G, et al. Risk factors for empyema after diaphragmatic injury: results of a National Trauma Databank analysis. *J Trauma.* 66:1672, 2009.

Cameron R, Davies HR. Intra-pleural fibrinolytic therapy versus conservative management in the treatment of parapneumonic effusions and empyema. *Cochrane Database Syst Rev.* 2:CD002312, 2004.

Ozel SK, et al. Conservative treatment of postpneumonic thoracic empyema in children. *Surg Today.* 34:1002, 2004.

Saglani S, et al. Empyema: the use of broad range 16 S rDNA PCR for pathogen detection. *Arch Dis Child.* 90:70, 2005.

Schultz KD, et al. The changing face of pleural empyemas in children: epidemiology and management. *Pediatrics.* 113:1735, 2004.

TRANSPLANTATION, LUNG

NUTRITIONAL ACUITY RANKING: LEVEL 3–4

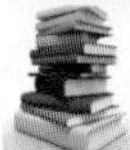

DEFINITIONS AND BACKGROUND

Lung transplantation (LTX) is an accepted treatment for end-stage pulmonary parenchymal and vascular diseases. LTX is a well-tolerated, effective therapy for RF with interstitial lung disease, CF or COPD. The International Society for Heart and Lung Transplantation and the Cystic Fibrosis Foundation have uniform guidelines for transplantation candidate selection. Over 13,000 LTXs have occurred worldwide (Tynan and Hasse, 2004).

Proper nutrition plays a key role in preparing for LTX. Therefore, the LTX dietitian plays an important role and meets with the patient for an initial interview. Weight and weight history, foods typically eaten, and appetite are reviewed. Being at ideal body weight range for height helps assure good physical condition for pretransplantation pulmonary rehabilitation and for the transplantation itself. Certain patients with advanced pulmonary disease are unable to eat enough to maintain ideal body weight because of increased metabolic demands and breathlessness with eating. In such situations, it may be recommended that a percutaneous endoscopic gastrostomy (PEG) feeding tube be placed.

Proper nutrition is critical to maximize the chances of a successful transplantation. Occasionally, listing for transplantation will be delayed until the patient's nutritional status improves. LBM depletion may be associated with more severe hypoxemia, reduced walking distance, and a higher mortality. Both undernutrition and obesity should be carefully managed before surgery. Diabetes is a common problem after LTX in CF patients even though quality of life is dramatically improved (Hadjiliadis, 2007).

As with other types of transplantations, graft–host resistance and sepsis are the major concerns after LTX. Infections are the most common cause of morbidity and mortality in LTX recipients. Immunosuppressive therapy with glucocorticoids contributes to protein degradation.

Nitrogen balance after LTX is negative because of high glucocorticoid requirements; aggressive nutritional intervention and increased nitrogen intake are needed to reduce protein losses in these patients. Chronic infection (bronchiolitis obliterans syndrome) is the most common cause of death after transplantation (Quattrucci et al, 2005).

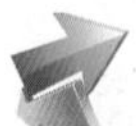

ASSESSMENT, MONITORING, AND EVALUATION

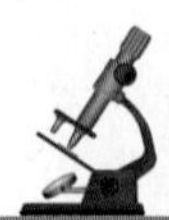

CLINICAL INDICATORS

Genetic Markers: Organ transplant researchers are increasingly using microarrays to identify specific patterns of gene expression that predict and characterize acute and chronic rejection. Increased expression of genes involved in inflammation, apoptosis, and T-cell activation and proliferation may play a role in organ rejection (Lande et al, 2007).

Clinical/History	Lab Work	
Height	Alb, transthyretin	BUN, Creat
Weight	CRP	Na^+, K^+
BMI	Transferrin	Ca^{++}, Mg^{++}
Weight changes	Chol, Trig	PO_4
Diet history	H & H	AST, ALT
RQ	Serum Fe, ferritin	Lactate
Ventilator support	Gluc	TLC
I & O		CRP
		pCO_2, pO_2

INTERVENTION

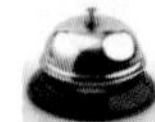

OBJECTIVES

Preoperative

- Because nutritional depletion in LTX candidates is highly prevalent, it should be precisely assessed both before and after LTX. Attempts should be made to increase LBM and reverse cachexia and vitamin and mineral deficiencies before LTX.
- Prepare for a surgical procedure. Most patients will require sodium or fluid restrictions; monitor serum potassium as well.
- Allow for mild weight loss with a planned diet if the patient is obese and has time to do this.

Postoperative

- Prevent infection, surgical complications, organ rejection, and organ failure.
- Promote wound healing.
- Support ideal body weight and LBM maintenance.
- Reduce protein losses, support nitrogen balance, and correct hypoalbuminemia.

SAMPLE NUTRITION CARE PROCESS STEPS

Inadequate Protein Intake

Assessment Data: BMI 18, recent weight loss of 20 lb, lung failure with planned Tx surgery, low serum albumin.

Nutrition Diagnoses (PES): Inadequate protein intake related to loss of LBM and insufficient oral intake as evidenced by albumin 2.1 and diet history showing low meat and milk consumption.

Interventions: Enhance meals by adding dry milk powder to recipes such as mashed potatoes and casseroles; offer puddings, eggnog and oral supplements between meals; add protein powder scoops to milkshakes or soups. Educate patient and family about the importance of protein for maintaining LBM and wound healing.

Monitoring and Evaluation: Improved intake of protein-rich foods. Successful wound healing after surgery. Improvement in weigh and BMI over several months.

- Prevent aspiration.
- Wean from ventilator or oxygen when possible.
- Treat comorbid conditions such as cardiovascular disease (CVD), osteoporosis, dyslipidemia, diabetes, hyperglycemia, metabolic syndrome, and hyperkalemia (Tynan and Hasse, 2004).

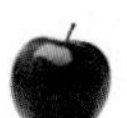

FOOD AND NUTRITION

Preoperative

- Prepare patient nutritionally to alleviate malnutrition in advance (Inouye et al, 2004). Home enteral or PN may be useful.
- Promote adequate intake of kcal (25–30 kcal/kg) and protein (1 g/kg body weight).
- Manage coexisting problems such as diabetes, heart disease, and hypertension with an appropriate diet such as the DASH diet.

Postoperative

- Return to oral intake by 48–72 hours postoperatively, when possible. Limit simple CHO when there are signs of hyperglycemia (Tynan and Hasse, 2004).
- Promote adequate intake of kcal (30–35 kcal/kg) and protein of 1.3–1.5 g/kg body weight (Tynan and Hasse, 2004). Use high nitrogen TF when needed, but do not overfeed, and monitor for needed changes in electrolytes according to lab values. Discontinue TF when intake meets >60% of estimated needs (Tynan and Hasse, 2004).
- Parenteral solutions may be used if the gut is nonfunctioning (Tynan and Hasse, 2004).
- Calorie-dense options should be considered if fluid restriction is required. Use caution with high-caloric loads because of RQ; maintain sufficient fat intake to prevent excess CO_2 production from a high-CHO intake.
- Restrict sodium and potassium if needed to improve cardiac or renal status.

TABLE 5-13 Medications Used for Lung Transplant Patients

Medication	Description
Azathioprine (Imuran)	May cause leukopenia, thrombocytopenia, oral and esophageal sores, macrocytic anemia, pancreatitis, vomiting, diarrhea, and other side effects that are complex. Folate supplementation and other dietary modifications (liquid or soft diet, use of oral supplements) may be needed. The drug works by lowering the number of T cells; it is often prescribed along with prednisone for conventional immunosuppression.
Corticosteroids (such as prednisone, hydrocortisone)	Used for immunosuppression. Side effects include increased catabolism of proteins, negative nitrogen balance, hyperphagia, ulcers, decreased glucose tolerance, sodium retention, fluid retention, and impaired calcium absorption and osteoporosis. Cushing's syndrome, obesity, muscle wasting, and increased gastric secretion may result. A higher protein intake and lower intake of simple CHOs may be needed.
Cyclosporine	Does not retain sodium as much as corticosteroids do. Intravenous doses are more effective than oral doses. Nausea, vomiting, and diarrhea are common side effects. Hyperlipidemia, hypertension, and hyperkalemia also may occur; decrease sodium and potassium as necessary. Elevated glucose and lipids may occur. The drug is also nephrotoxic; a controlled renal diet may be beneficial.
Immunosuppressants	Less nephrotoxic than cyclosporine but can cause nausea, anorexia, diarrhea, and vomiting. Monitor carefully. Fever (muromonab [Orthoclone OKT3] and stomatitis also may occur; alter diet as needed and antithymocyte globulin).
Diuretics	Diuretics such as furosemide may cause hypokalemia. Low-sodium/low-calorie diets may be indicated. If spironolactone is used, it spares potassium.
Tacrolimus (Prograf, FK506)	Suppresses T-cell immunity; it is 100 times more potent than cyclosporine, thus requiring smaller doses. Side effects include GI distress, nausea, vomiting, hyperkalemia, and hyperglycemia. Tacrolimus therapy has aided in success of lung transplantation and has become the primary immunosuppressant agent used (Fan et al, 2009; Garrity and Mehra, 2004). A low-potassium diet may be needed to prevent cardiac arrhythmia (Tynan and Hasse, 2004).

- Reduce energy intake and increase activity if weight gain or diabetes occurs after long-term corticosteroid use (Tynan and Hasse, 2004).
- Prevent osteoporosis by using adequate calcium and vitamin D. Provide sufficient magnesium and vitamins to heal and promote adequate nutritional status.

Common Drugs Used and Potential Side Effects

- Using tacrolimus as primary immunosuppressant for lung transplant recipient results in comparable survival and reduction in acute rejection episodes when compared with cyclosporine (Fan et al, 2009). See Table 5-13 for more information.

Herbs, Botanicals, and Supplements

- No clinical trials have proven efficacy for use of herbs or botanicals after LTX.

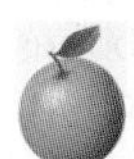

NUTRITION EDUCATION, COUNSELING, CARE MANAGEMENT

- Discuss appropriate calorie and protein levels. Protein helps to heal after surgery.
- Drink plenty of water until restriction is prescribed.
- Decreased saturated fat and cholesterol intakes may be useful to decrease cardiac risks and to prevent unwanted weight gain, which is common. Read food labels and monitor portions carefully. Choose condiments such as mustard rather than mayonnaise or salad dressing. Choose healthy cooking methods. Instead of frying, try baking, grilling, broiling, or steaming foods; instead of oil, use nonstick, fat-free spray or sauces.
- Adequate fiber (from fresh fruits, vegetables, and whole grains) is important.
- A gradual return to activity will be important.
- Eat a minimum amount of salt, processed foods, and snacks. Use herbs and spices to add flavor instead of salt.
- Add calcium by eating calcium-rich foods, such as low-fat dairy products and green, leafy vegetables, or by using calcium supplements.
- Avoid alcohol and do not use drugs that are not prescribed.

Patient Education—Foodborne Illness

- Preventing infection is very important after transplantation surgery. Hand washing is critically important.
- Careful food handling will be important.

For More Information

- Cystic Fibrosis—Transplantation
  http://www.cff.org/treatments/LungTransplantation/
- Fast Facts about Transplants
  http://www.ustransplant.org/csr/current/fastfacts.aspx
- International Society for Heart and Lung Transplantation
  http://www.ishlt.org/
- Lung Transplantation
  http://www.nlm.nih.gov/medlineplus/lungtransplantation.html
- Organ Procurement and Transplantation Network
  http://www.optn.org/
- Transplant Terms
  http://www.transplantliving.org/Community/glossary.aspx
- Trans Web
  http://www.transweb.org/

TRANSPLANTATION, LUNG—CITED REFERENCES

Fan Y, et al. Tacrolimus versus cyclosporine for adult lung transplant recipients: a meta-analysis. *Transplant Proc.* 41:1821, 2009.
Garrity ER Jr, Mehra MR. An update on clinical outcomes in heart and lung transplantation. *Transplantation.* 77:S68, 2004.
Hadjiliadis D. Special considerations for patients with cystic fibrosis undergoing lung transplantation. *Chest.* 131:1224, 2007.
Inouye Y, et al. Benefits of home parenteral nutrition before lung transplantation: report of a case. *Surg Today.* 34:525, 2004.
Lande JD, et al. Novel insights into lung transplant rejection by microarray analysis. *Proc Am Thorac Soc.* 4:44, 2007.
Quattrucci S, et al. Lung transplantation for cystic fibrosis: 6-year follow-up. *J Cyst Fibros.* 4:107, 2005.
Tynan C, Hasse JM. Current nutrition practices in adult lung transplantation. *Nutr Clin Pract.* 19:587, 2004.

TUBERCULOSIS

NUTRITIONAL ACUITY RANKING: LEVEL 1–2

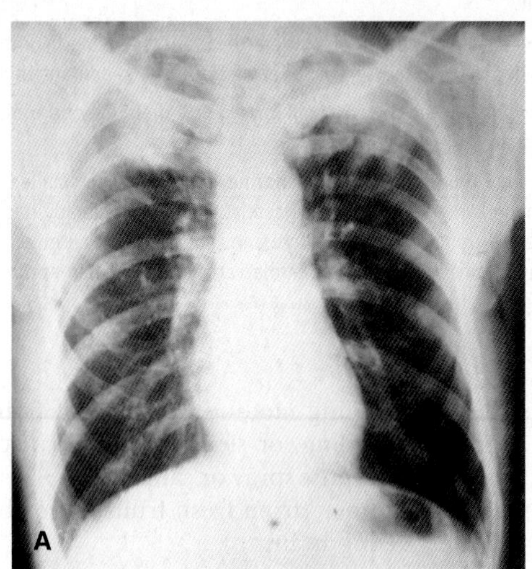

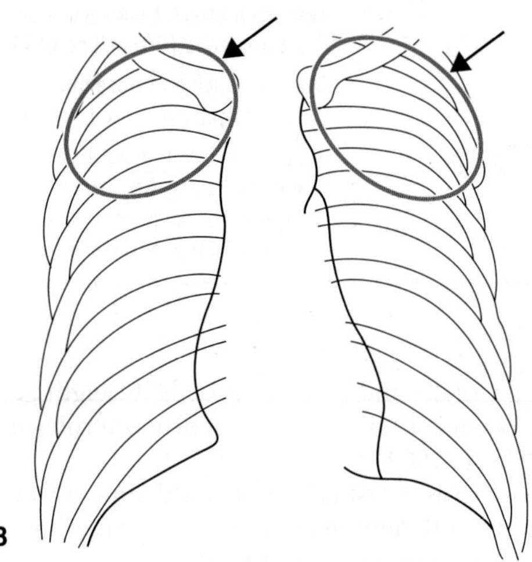

A is an X-ray of tubercular lungs. **B** shows the presence of TB by circled areas.
Adapted from: Engleberg NC, Dermody T, DiRita V. *Schaecter's Mechanisms of Microbial Disease,* 4th ed. Baltimore: Lippincott Williams & Wilkins, 2007.

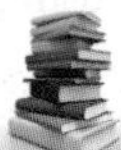

DEFINITIONS AND BACKGROUND

TB is caused by a tubercle bacillus (*Mycobacterium tuberculosis*) invading the lungs and setting up an inflammatory process. Healing occurs with a calcification of the tubercular cavity. TB causes loss of appetite, constant fatigue, tissue wasting, exhaustion, hemoptysis, cough lasting 3 weeks or longer with occasional blood-tinged sputum, fever or chills, profuse night sweats, and weight loss. The acute form resembles pneumonia; the chronic form causes low-grade fever.

Nearly one third of the world's population is infected with *M. tuberculosis* (Pai et al, 2006). More than 9 million new cases were reported in 2007, many of them in Africa. An increase in TB in the United States may be related to inadequate compliance with prescribed drug therapy or to recently acquired or reactivated latent infections. Among U.S. born citizens, non-Hispanic African American, Mexican Americans, and individuals living in poverty have the highest risk for TB (Bennett et al, 2008). Immunocompromised persons are more vulnerable to the effects of TB, especially those persons who have HIV infection. Hypermetabolism appears to play a role in the wasting process in patients infected with both HIV and TB. HIV infection is associated with a significant downregulation of whole-body protein flux, adding to the nutritional decline if TB is also present (Paton et al, 2003).

Vitamin D signaling within macrophages enables them to respond to and kill *Mycobacterium tuberculosis* organisms (Bikle, 2008; Shapira et al, 2009). This is an intracrine–autocrine–paracrine system for vitamin D that is just being recognized (Adams et al, 2007).

Active TB begins in the lungs but often spreads through the bloodstream as extrapulmonary TB. Fatigue, abdominal tenderness, painful urination, headache, SOB, arthritis-like symptoms, kidney damage, and pain in the spine and bones can occur. TB meningitis is a very dangerous complication, especially for the elderly.

Many TB patients have early, unplanned readmission and often need assistance with activities of daily living. They may have drug complications, the need to use a nonstandard drug regimen, and other illnesses. With a high prevalence of malnutrition, a relatively low utilization rate of nutritional services, and the potential effect of adverse reactions to therapeutic drugs, careful attention is needed for this patient population.

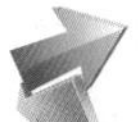

ASSESSMENT, MONITORING, AND EVALUATION

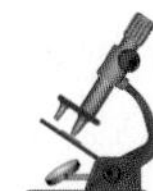

CLINICAL INDICATORS

Genetic Markers: It is suspected that TB has connections with allergy. There are higher levels of specific IgE, interleukin (IL)-6, and interferon (IFN) gamma to different inhalant allergens in TB patients; successful treatment lowers these levels (Ellertsen, 2009). In addition, polymorphisms in the gene that encodes the vitamin D receptor (VDR) influence host response to *Mycobacterium tuberculosis* (Roth et al, 2004).

Bioconversion of 25-hydroxyvitamin D_3 (25D3) into bioactive 1,25D3, leading to VDR activation and antimicrobial activity against intracellular TB (Krutzik et al, 2008).

Clinical/History

- Height
- Weight
- BMI
- Diet history
- BP
- Mantoux skin test
- QuantiFERON®-TB Gold test (QFT-G)
- T-SPOT® TB test
- Chest x-rays (irregular white areas on dark background)
- Bronchoscopy
- Blood-tinged sputum
- Biopsy or sputum test for *M. tuberculosis*
- Temperature, fever or chills
- Night sweats
- Anorexia
- Spinal tap for polymerase chain reaction (PCR)
- I & O

Lab Work

- Alb, transthyretin
- CRP
- RBP
- TLC
- Lymphopenia?
- H & H
- Serum Fe, ferritin
- Normocytic anemia?
- Serum pyridoxine
- N balance
- Chol (decreased)
- Na^+, K^+
- Ca^{++}, Mg^{++}
- Serum folate
- Transferrin
- BUN, Creat
- Liver function tests (from medication use)

INTERVENTION

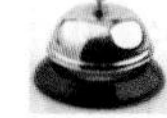

OBJECTIVES

- Maintain or prevent losses in weight. Reduce fever. The basal metabolic rate is 20–30% above normal to counteract fever of 102°F or higher.
- Normalize serum calcium and vitamin D_3 levels; either hypocalcemia or hypercalcemia may occur.
- TB often coincides with nutritional deficiencies; micronutrient supplementation may improve the outcome in patients undergoing TB treatment (Villamor et al, 2008).

SAMPLE NUTRITION CARE PROCESS STEPS

Involuntary Weight Loss

Assessment Data: Analysis of estimated oral intake below estimated needs.

Nutrition Diagnosis (PES): Involuntary weight loss related to insufficient intake and frequent coughing spells, medication-related GI symptoms as evidenced by 15-lb weight loss since TB diagnosis months ago.

Intervention: Food and nutrient delivery with careful timing of meals and snacks in relation to medication administration and coughing episodes. Small, frequent meals and oral supplements.

Monitoring and Evaluation: Monitor and evaluate changes in intake and weight; tolerance for medications; and nutritional quality of life.

- Replace nutrient losses from lung hemorrhage, if present.
- Promote healing of the cavity.
- Counteract neuritis from isoniazid (INH) therapy, when used.
- Stimulate appetite, which is generally poor.
- Prevent dehydration.
- Prevent lung inflammation, infections, and complications.

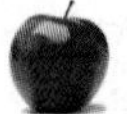

FOOD AND NUTRITION

- Use a well-balanced diet containing liberal amounts of protein and adequate calories. It may be useful to calculate needs as 35–45 kcal/kg if weight loss has been significant.
- Use adequate fluids (35 cc/kg) unless otherwise contraindicated.
- Add more omega-3 fatty acids; they may improve food intake, restore normal eating patterns, and prevent body weight loss (Ramos et al, 2004).
- Ensure that the diet provides sufficient levels of calcium and vitamin D.
- Iron and vitamin C are needed for proper hemoglobin formation and wound healing.
- B-complex vitamins, especially vitamin B_6, are needed to counteract INH therapy.
- Use supplemental vitamin A as carotene as it is poorly converted.
- Alcohol should not be used as a calorie replacement or appetite enhancer.

Common Drugs Used and Potential Side Effects

- Current anti-TB chemotherapies, although effective, are associated with side effects and are limited in treating drug-resistant strands (Shapira et al, 2009).
- See Table 5-14 for more drug therapies.

TABLE 5-14 **Medications Used for Tuberculosis (TB)**

Medication	Description
Aminosalicylic acid	Interferes with vitamin B_{12} and folate absorption. Nausea and vomiting are common.
Chemotherapy	Chemotherapy can increase serum calcium levels.
Ethionamide (Trecator-SC)	Requires a vitamin B_6 supplement. It may cause anorexia, metallic taste, nausea, vomiting, diarrhea, weight loss, and hypoglycemia.
Ethambutol (Myambutol)	May cause GI distress, nausea, or anorexia. It should not be used longer than 2 months because it can harm the eyes.
Immunotherapy	According to the Centers for Disease Control and Prevention (2004): TB disease is a potential adverse reaction from treatment with tumor necrosis factor-alpha (TNF-α) antagonists infliximab (Remicade), etanercept (Enbrel), and adalimumab (Humira). These products block TNF-α, an inflammatory cytokine, and are approved for treating rheumatoid arthritis and other selected autoimmune diseases. Blocking TNF-α can allow TB disease to emerge from latent *Mycobacterium tuberculosis* infection. Health care providers should take steps to prevent TB in immunocompromised patients and remain vigilant for TB as a cause of unexplained fever.
Isoniazid (INH)	May cause neuritis by depleting vitamin B_6; usual dose is 300 mg INH with 50 mg pyridoxine. Bad taste can be disguised in pureed fruit or jam to make it palatable, especially for pediatric patients. Niacin, calcium, and vitamin B_{12} are also depleted. Nausea, jaundice, vomiting, stomach cramping, and dry mouth are common. INH must be taken for 9 months to eradicate the condition completely.
Pyrazinamide (PZA)	May cause anorexia, nausea, and vomiting. It can be hepatotoxic.
Rifampin (Rifadin, Rimactane)	Has side effects such as anorexia and GI distress.
Streptomycin	One of the first drugs used to treat TB. It is given by injection. Use of longer than 3 months can affect balance and hearing.

NOTE. Therapy always involves two or more drugs because of the long-term treatment period required.

Herbs, Botanicals, and Supplements

- No clinical trials have proven efficacy for use of eucalyptus, echinacea, garlic, licorice, honeysuckle, or forsythia in TB management.
- Deficiencies of multiple micronutrients (MMN) are common in developing countries or where TB is common; outcomes are better using MMN than when providing just one to two micronutrients (Allen et al, 2009). Vitamins D, E, and selenium are supplements that should be highlighted.

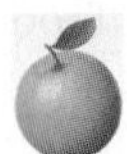

NUTRITION EDUCATION, COUNSELING, CARE MANAGEMENT

- Add protein powders or nonfat dry milk to beverages, casseroles, soups, and desserts to increase protein and calcium intake, unless contraindicated for other medical reasons.
- Encourage preparation of small, appetizing meals. Plan rest periods before and after meals.
- Discuss tips for managing anxiety related to weight loss, night sweats, loss of strength, high fever, and abnormal chest x-rays.
- Discuss communicability of TB. Family members and those living in proximity should have x-rays and other tests. About 5% of exposures result in TB within 1 year; others may be dormant until another condition sets in such as HIV infection, diabetes, or leukemia.
- Promote adequate rehabilitation if the patient is an alcoholic.
- Promote as much quality of life as possible; this is often overlooked (Marra et al, 2004).
- A TB vaccine is available. The BCG (bacille Calmette-Guérin) vaccine for TB disease is not widely used in the United States, but it is often used in other countries where TB is common.

Patient Education—Foodborne Illness

- Careful food handling will be important. Foodservice employees who are exposed to those at risk for active TB should be tested regularly. People are at risk and may need to be tested if they:
  - Have symptoms of active TB disease
  - Have been exposed to someone (family member, friend, or coworker) who has active TB
  - Have HIV infection, diabetes, or chronic kidney failure
  - Take steroids or other immune-suppressing drugs for chronic medical conditions
  - Live or work in a homeless shelter, prison, hospital, nursing home, or other group setting
  - Have recently moved from a region with active TB (Africa, Asia, the Caribbean, Eastern Europe, and Latin America).
- When preparing food:
  - Separate raw meat from cooked or ready-to-eat foods. Do not use the same chopping board or the same knife for preparing raw meat and cooked or ready-to-eat foods.
  - Do not handle either raw or cooked foods without washing hands in between.
  - Do not place cooked meat back on the same plate or surface it was on before it was cooked.
  - All foods from poultry should be cooked thoroughly, including eggs. Egg yolks should not be runny or liquid. Because influenza viruses are destroyed by heat,

the cooking temperature for poultry meat should reach 70°C (158°F).

- Wash egg shells in soapy water before handling and cooking, and wash hands afterwards.
- Do not use raw or soft-boiled eggs in foods that will not be cooked.
- After handling raw poultry or eggs, wash hands and all surfaces and utensils thoroughly with soap and water.
- Do not eat uncooked or undercooked poultry or poultry products, including food with uncooked poultry blood.

For More Information

- CDC
  http://www.cdc.gov/tb/links/default.htm
- JAMA—Patient page for TB
  http://jama.ama-assn.org/cgi/reprint/300/4/464.pdf
- Joint HIV/TB Interventions
  http://www.who.int/hiv/topics/tb/tuberculosis/en/
- Lung Association of Canada
  http://www.lung.ca/diseases-maladies/tuberculosis-tuberculose_e.php
- National Tuberculosis Curriculum Consortium
  http://ntcc.ucsd.edu/
- National TB Center
  http://www.nationaltbcenter.edu/
- NIH—Medline
  http://www.nlm.nih.gov/medlineplus/tuberculosis.html
- Travelers Health Website
  http://www.cdc.gov/travel
- World Health Organization
  http://www.who.int/tb/en/

TUBERCULOSIS—CITED REFERENCES

Adams JS, et al. Vitamin D in defense of the human immune response. *Ann N Y Acad Sci.* 1117:94, 2007.

Allen LH, et al. Provision of multiple rather than two or fewer micronutrients more effectively improves growth and other outcomes in micronutrient-deficient children and adults. *J Nutr.* 139:1022, 2009.

Bennett DE, et al. Prevalence of tuberculosis infection in the United States population: the national health and nutrition examination survey, 1999–2000. *Am J Respir Crit Care Med.* 177:348, 2008.

Bikle DD. Vitamin D and the immune system: role in protection against bacterial infection. *Curr Opin Nephrol Hypertens.* 17:348, 2008.

Centers for Disease Control and Prevention. Tuberculosis associated with blocking agents against tumor necrosis factor-alpha—California, 2002–2003. *MMWR Morb Mortal Wkly Rep.* 53:683, 2004.

Ellertsen LJ. Allergic sensitization in tuberculosis patients at the time of diagnosis and following chemotherapy. *BMC Infect Dis.* 9:100, 2009.

Krutzik SR, et al. IL-15 links TLR2/1-induced macrophage differentiation to the vitamin D-dependent antimicrobial pathway. *J Immunol.* 181:7115, 2008.

Marra CA, et al. Factors influencing quality of life in patients with active tuberculosis. *Health Qual Life Outcomes.* 2:58, 2004.

Pai M, et al. New tools and emerging technologies for the diagnosis of tuberculosis. Part I. Latent tuberculosis. *Expert Rev Mol Diagn.* 6:413, 2006.

Paton NI, et al. Effects of tuberculosis and HIV infection on whole-body protein metabolism during feeding, measured by the [15 N]glycine method. *Am J Clin Nutr.* 78:319, 2003.

Ramos EJ, et al. Effects of omega-3 fatty acid supplementation on tumor-bearing rats. *J Am Coll Surg.* 199:716, 2004.

Roth DE, et al. Association between vitamin D receptor gene polymorphisms and response to treatment of pulmonary tuberculosis. *J Infect Dis.* 190: 920, 2004.

Shapira Y, et al. Mycobacterium tuberculosis, autoimmunity, and vitamin D [epub ahead of print Jun 20,. 2009]. *Clin Rev Allergy Immunol.* 38:169, 2010.

Villamor E, et al. A trial of the effect of micronutrient supplementation on treatment outcome, T cell counts, morbidity, and mortality in adults with pulmonary tuberculosis. *J Infect Dis.* 197:1499, 2008.

S E C T I O N 6

Cardiovascular Disorders

CHIEF ASSESSMENT FACTORS

- Age: Males ≥45 Years of Age and Females ≥55 Years of Age
- Alcohol Use (none, moderate, excessive)
- Angiograms, ECG, Echocardiograms
- Ascites, Edema
- Blood Pressure
- Cardiogenic Shock: Low Systolic Blood Pressure (BP), Cool and Moist Skin, Decreased Urinary Output, Pulmonary Edema, Tachycardia, Weak Pulse
- Chest Pain
- Cholesterol and Lipid Profiles (higher HDL is protective, small dense LDL is atherogenic)
- Contraceptive Use or Menopause
- C-Reactive Protein (CRP) and CoQ10 serum levels
- Decreased Cardiac Output: Arrhythmias, Fatigue, Labored Respirations, Pallor, Rales, Vertigo
- Diabetes
- Dietary Pattern with High Saturated Fat Intake
- Electrolyte Balance
- Exercise Patterns
- Family Hx (Use ATP III Guidelines) or Sibling Cardiovascular Disease
- Herbs or Botanical Product Use
- Homocysteinemia and Genetic Alleles Predisposing to Heart Diseases
- International Normalized Ratio (INR) Coagulation Index
- Lactic Acid Dehydrogenase (LDH), Creatine Phosphokinase (CPK) Levels
- Medications
- Obesity
- Smoking and Tobacco Use
- Type A Personality, Stressful Lifestyle
- Serum Vitamin D_3 levels
- Xanthomas

OVERVIEW: DIET IN HEART DISEASE

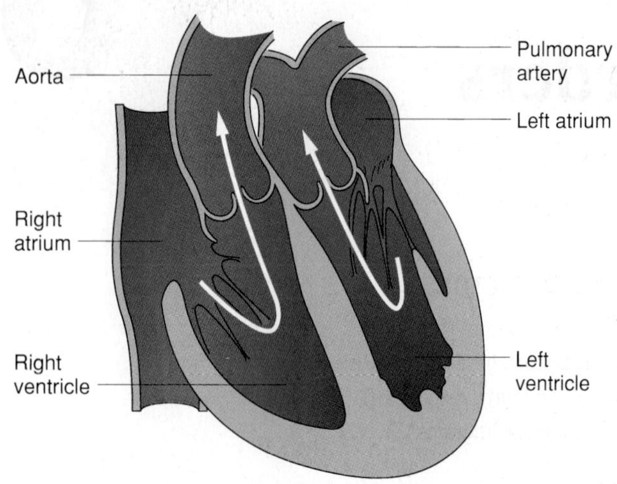

Adapted from: Michael W. Mulholland, Ronald V. Maier et al. *Greenfield's Surgery Scientific Principles And Practice,* 4th ed. Philadelphia: Lippincott Williams & Wilkins, 2006.

LIPIDS

Cardiovascular disease (CVD) includes hypertension, coronary heart disease (CHD), heart failure (HF), congenital heart defects, and stroke; CHD accounts for thousands of deaths annually. CVD accounts for almost 50% of all deaths in industrialized nations. Estimates for the year 2006 are that 80,000,000 people in the United States have one or more forms of CVD (American Heart Association, 2009). Despite a dramatic decline in mortality over the past three decades, CHD remains a leading cause of death and disability. Death rates for women have not declined as much as those for men.

Classic cardiovascular risk factors are common but largely undertreated and undercontrolled in many regions of the world (Bhatt et al, 2006). Seventy percent of CVD can be prevented or delayed with dietary choices and lifestyle modifications (Forman and Bulwer, 2006). There are 12 modifiable dietary, lifestyle, and metabolic risk factors: high blood glucose, low-density lipoprotein (LDL) cholesterol (Chol), and blood pressure (BP); overweight-obesity; high dietary trans fatty acids and salt; low dietary polyunsaturated fatty acids, omega-3 fatty acids (seafood), and fruits and vegetables; physical inactivity; alcohol use; and tobacco smoking (Danaei et al, 2009). Of these factors, tobacco smoking and high BP are responsible for the most causes of death in the United States.

Many patients with classic CVD risk factors can achieve risk-reduction goals without medications within 3 months after initiating therapeutic lifestyle changes (TLCs). TLC includes exercise training, nutrition counseling, and other appropriate lifestyle interventions based on several well-established behavior change models. The benefits of primary prevention of CVD are greatest for people who have multiple risk factors. Secondary prevention is beneficial for high-risk and low-risk patients. The Adult Treatment Panel (ATP III) report provides scientific evidence for dyslipidemia management. While dyslipidemia with small dense LDL molecules is atherogenic, dietary Chol is only one of many factors to play a role in the etiology of heart disease. Chol is readily made from acetate in all animal tissues and has many roles in the body. In children and teens, widespread Chol screening is not warranted, except where there is early cardiovascular morbidity and mortality in immediate family members. There is a strong, independent relationship of vitamin D_3 [25(OH)D] deficiency (levels <20 ng/mL) with prevalent CVD in a large sample of the U.S. adult population; this has implications for both angina and myocardial infarction (MI, Kendrick et al, 2009). Other nutrients also play a role. Studies show a link between intake of fruit, vegetables, and whole grains and protection against CHD due to fiber, vitamin, mineral, and phytochemical content. Folate, vitamins B_6, B_{12}, E, and C, flavonoids, phytoestrogens, and a wholesome total dietary pattern may be protective.

In a specific analysis of "low-fat" diets, there were no significant effects on the incidence of stroke and CHD, but there were small reductions in LDL and total Chol (TC) levels, diastolic BP, and factor VIIc levels (Howard et al, 2006). There are indirect benefits of a diet with a lower intake of saturated and trans fats, higher intake of vegetable and fruits, use of specific types of fats including fish oils, as well as fish, and perhaps energy restriction (Anderson, 2006). Epidemiologic data suggest that omega-3 fatty acids derived from fish oil reduce CVD (Marik and Valon, 2009).

An Elderly Dietary Index (EDI) is useful for assessing risk factors for CVD in older adults (Kourlaba et al, 2009). Because kidney disease is a risk factor for mortality and CVD in older adults, elevated cystatin C and albuminuria are independent, graded risk factors for CVD and mortality (Rifkin et al, 2009).

Nutrition counseling should receive high priority, both in medical training and in patient care for both men and women (Krummel, 2008). The American Dietetic Association estimates cost savings per cardiovascular case to be nearly $2500 annually with nutrition counseling, thereby reducing the need for many medications. Key components of counseling include: (1) reduced caloric intake; (2) reduced total fat, saturated fat, trans fat, and Chol with proportional increases in monounsaturated, omega-3, and omega-6 fatty acids; (3) increased dietary fiber, fruit, and vegetables; (4) increased micronutrients (e.g., folate and vitamins B_6 and B_{12}); (5) increased plant protein in lieu of animal protein; (6) reduced portions of highly processed foods; (7) adopting a Mediterranean dietary pattern; (8) adding physical activity; and smoking cessation (Forman and Bulwer, 2006). See Table 6-1 regarding evidence for dietary recommendations in heart disease.

The Women's Nutrition Intervention Study used a low-fat eating plan that serves as a model for implementing a long-term dietary intervention in clinical practice (Hoy et al, 2009). Table 6-2 lists other influential factors on diet and its relationship to heart disease. In the future, the development of functional foods that contain ingredients that have preventive benefits will be important. Products that contain green tea wth Epigallocatechin-3-gallate (EGCG), omega-3 fatty acids, folate, vitamins C and E, flavonoids such as quercertin, eritadenine in mushrooms will be popular (Ferguson, 2009). Table 6-3 provides a list of commonly used herbs and botanical products in heart disease.

TABLE 6-1 Levels of Best Evidence in Dietary Recommendations for Heart Disease[a]

Dietary Recommendation	Evidence Level
Antioxidants	
Supplemental beta-carotene (60–200 mg/d) does not decrease the risk for cardiovascular death or nonfatal myocardial infarction (MI) in primary and secondary prevention patients.	I
Supplemental vitamin E, given in both natural and synthetic forms, in doses of 30–600 mg/d or 400–800 IU/d, alone or in combination with other antioxidants, is not harmful but has not been shown to decrease the risk for cardiovascular death or MI.	II
Supplemental vitamin E (100–1200 IU/d) alone or in combination with other antioxidants has not been shown to have a favorable or unfavorable effect on serum lipids.	II
Supplemental vitamin C (50–1000 mg/d) in combination with other antioxidants (vitamin E, beta-carotene, selenium) has not been shown to have any effect on cardiovascular death or MI.	II
Supplemental beta-carotene (60–120 mg/d) is associated with an increase in all-cause mortality and cardiovascular death in patients at increased risk for lung cancer.	II
Supplemental vitamins C and E, beta-carotene, and selenium should not be taken with simvastatin–niacin drug combinations because this may lower HDL2 cholesterol, a beneficial subfraction of HDL cholesterol.	II
Hypertension	
Consuming a diet rich in fruits and vegetables and low-fat dairy products and low in sodium and saturated fat will decrease blood pressure. Reductions have been 4–12 mm Hg in systolic and 1–3 mm Hg in diastolic blood pressure. This dietary pattern is enhanced by weight loss and increased physical activity.	I
Fiber	
Consuming diets high in total fiber (17–30 g/d) and soluble fiber (7–13 g/d) as part of a diet low in saturated fat and cholesterol can further reduced total cholesterol by 2–3% and LDL by up to 7%.	I
Diets high in total dietary fiber (>25 g/d) are associated with decreased risk for coronary heart disease (CHD) and Cardiovascular disease (CVD).	II
LDL Cholesterol Reduction	
A diet consisting of 25–35% total fat, <7% saturated and trans fat, and <200 mg dietary cholesterol lowers serum total and LDL cholesterol 9–16% and decreases the risk of CHD.	I
Isocalorically replacing saturated fatty acids with MUFA and PUFA is associated with reductions in LDL cholesterol.	I
Omega-3 Fatty Acids	
Approximately 1 g/d of eicosapentaenoic acid (EPA) and docosahexaenoic acid (DHA) from a supplement or fish decreases the risk of death from cardiac events in patients with heart disease.	II
Regular consumption of an average of two servings of fatty fish per week (about 3.5 oz per serving; high in EPA and DHA) is associated with a 30–40% reduced risk of death from cardiac events.	II
Increased plasma levels and adipose tissue and cholesterol ester concentrations of alpha linolenic acid, EPA, and DHA have been associated with reduced risk of mortality.	II
Nuts	
Consumption of 50–113 g (1/2 to 1 cup) of nuts daily with a diet low in saturated fat may decrease total cholesterol by 4–21% and LDL cholesterol by 6–29% when weight is not gained.	II
Consumption of 5 oz of nuts per week is associated with reduced risk of CVD.	II
Soy Protein	
Studies varied greatly in their estimation of the effect of diets low in saturated fat and cholesterol containing ~26–50 g of soyprotein either as food or as a soy supplement, with 0–165 mg of isoflavones. Studies of individuals with normal or elevated total cholesterol >200 mg/dL and individuals with diabetes varied, showing either 0–20% lower serum total cholesterol; 0–22% lower triglycerides; 4–24% lower LDL cholesterol.	II
Diets containing up to 30 g of soy protein (as supplements) per day are well tolerated.	II
Statins, Stanols, and Sterols	
Plant sterols and stanols are potent hypocholesterolemic agents. Daily consumption of 2–3 g (through margarine, low-fat yogurt, orange juice, breads, and cereals) lowers total cholesterol concentrations in a dose-dependent manner without changing HDL cholesterol or triacylglycerol concentrations.	I
For patients receiving statin therapy, plant stanols further reduce LDL and total cholesterol.	I
The total and LDL cholesterol-lowering effects of stanols and sterols are evident even when sterols and stanols are consumed as part of a cholesterol-lowering diet.	I
Sterols lower total cholesterol by 6–11% and LDL cholesterol by 7–15%. Stanols lower total cholesterol by 4–10% and LDL cholesterol by 7–14%.	II
An intake of 2–3 g of plant sterols and stanols per day generally appears to be safe.	II

Adapted from: American Dietetic Association, Evidence analysis library. Web site accessed July 1, 2009, at http://www.adaevidencelibrary.org/. Key: Level I evidence = strong evidence from randomized controlled trials; level II evidence = moderate evidence.

TABLE 6-2 **Key Influences and Factors Related to Heart Disease**

Influence	Description
Alcohol	Moderate red wine consumption may be associated with desirable changes in HDL cholesterol. The "French paradox" suggests that wine intake and type of fat consumed are protective.
Alpha linolenic acid (ALA)	ALA in flaxseed, walnuts, and canola oil may protect against sudden cardiac death and cardiac arrhythmias.
Aspirin and salicylates	Aspirin (usually 80 mg/d) and other salicylates inhibit production of enzymes that influence platelet release and aggregation, vasoconstriction, and vasodilation. Salicylates have analgesic, antipyretic, and anti-inflammatory properties. They occur naturally in many foods, including herbs, spices, fruits, and tomatoes.
Apolipoprotein (Apo) E phenotype	ApoE genotype modifies the serum lipid response to changes in dietary fat and cholesterol intake. Inherited hypercholesterolemias are common disorders characterized by elevated LDL cholesterol levels and premature coronary heart disease.
Carbohydrate	High glycemic index foods should be studied further for their effects on heart disease.
C-reactive protein (CRP)	Inflammation is important in atherosclerosis. CRP is one of the acute phase proteins that increase during systemic inflammation. Dietary/lifestyle factors that decrease CRP levels are: weight loss, alpha linolenic acid, vegetarian diet, and moderate alcohol intake.
Cholesterol, total serum	The NHLBI promotes <200 mg/dL as desirable; 200–239 mg/dL is borderline high; >240 mg/dL is high. Age, lifestyle habits (smoking high BMI), and high serum cholesterol levels are consistently associated with CHD mortality. The ATP III report found that even older persons with established CHD can show benefit from LDL-lowering therapy.
Cholesterol, HDL	Low levels of HDL cholesterol are an independent risk factor for cardiovascular death; HDL <40 mg/dL is low and not desirable; >60 mg/dL is high and better. In women, changes in HDL cholesterol and triglyceride levels are good predictors of coronary risk.
Cholesterol, LDL (see Table 6-1)	Initiate therapeutic lifestyle changes (TLC) if LDL is above goal; this is a primary target of therapy. LDL <100 mg/dL is optimal; 100–129 mg/dL is near-optimal; 130–159 mg/dL is borderline high; 160–189 mg/dL is high; and >190 mg/dL is very high. Statins can help lower LDL levels.
Copper	Elevated serum copper levels are strong pro-oxidants. Supplementation is not recommended; the relationship of copper and zinc is complex and excesses are not desirable.
Dairy products	Low fat dairy products provide a major source of vitamins and minerals.
Diabetes	Elevated systolic and diastolic blood pressure, high serum cholesterol level, high body mass index, presence of diabetes, and smoking status are key risks for CHD. Replace saturated fat with monounsaturated fat.
Eggs	Limit intake to no more than 1 whole egg daily, especially with diabetes.
Erythrocyte sedimentation rate (ESR)	ESR is a marker of inflammation but whether this signifies an independent marker for heart disease remains to be seen.
Estrogen	High plasma triglycerides are an independent risk factor for CHD. Hormone replacement therapy may protect younger more than older women.
Exercise	Low fitness in adolescents and adults is common in the U.S. population and is associated with an increased prevalence of CVD. Increased exercise is associated with a lower waist circumference and higher HDL cholesterol levels. Inactive individuals benefit by even slightly increasing activity, such as walking.
Fats, monounsaturated (MUFA) (see Table 6-1)	Nuts are a good source of MUFA. Substitution of extra virgin olive oil for saturated fats will not only decrease SFA but provide phytochemicals.
Fats, saturated (SFA)	SFA is more important than total cholesterol intake in affecting total and LDL cholesterol levels, and risk of CHD, in women especially.
Fiber and whole grains (see Table 6-1)	Whole grains and high fiber from cereals, vegetables, and fruits are protective against CHD. Fiber may protect against CHD by lowering blood cholesterol (soluble fibers), attenuating blood triglyceride levels (mostly soluble fibers), decreasing hypertension (all fibers), and normalizing postprandial blood glucose levels (all fibers). Total fiber is important.
Flavonoids	There are over 6000 so far. Chocolate decreases blood pressure and enhances blood flow. Dark chocolate also improves insulin sensitivity. Soy isolate protein and green tea tend to be helpful in lowering CVD risks. Flavonoids in red wine, grape juice, grapefruit, tea, onions, apples, cloves, licorice, and sage are beneficial.
Folic acid	Diets that are low in folate and carotenoids (beta-carotene, lutein, zeaxanthin) contribute to increased coronary risk mortality.
Glycemic load, high	High glycemic load due to high intake of refined carbohydrates is positively related to CAD risk, independent of other known risk factors.
Homocysteine (tHcy)	Elevated tHcy levels are associated with increased risk of cardiac disease, stroke, and peripheral artery disease. Therapy with folic acid and vitamins B_6 and B_{12} can reduce plasma tHcy levels. Fortified breakfast cereals that contain 200 μg folic acid are useful. The Dietary Approaches to Stop Hypertension (DASH) diet also reduces tHcy; the diet includes high quantities of fruits, vegetables, low-fat dairy products, whole grains, poultry, fish, and nuts.

(continued)

TABLE 6-2 Key Influences and Factors Related to Heart Disease *(continued)*

Influence	Description
Iron	High heme iron intake may increase risks of coronary heart disease (CHD) while anemia is damaging to the heart. A carefully balanced iron intake is a safe recommendation.
Mediterranean diet	A Mediterranean diet is protective. Mediterranean diets have a healthier balance between omega-3 and omega-6 fatty acids. The Mediterranean diet does not include much meat (high omega-6 fatty acids;) it emphasizes whole grains, fresh fruits and vegetables, fish, olive oil, garlic, and wine.
Metabolic syndrome	Atherogenic dyslipidemia is characterized by three lipid abnormalities: elevated triglycerides, small LDL particles, and reduced HDL cholesterol. Dyslipidemia, elevated blood pressure, impaired glucose tolerance, and central obesity comprise the metabolic syndrome. Prevention includes (1) correcting overweight by reducing energy density of the diet and (2) improving insulin sensitivity and associated metabolic abnormalities through a reduction of dietary saturated fat, partially replaced with MUFA and PUFA. Mild-to-moderate alcohol intake is protective while excessive intake is detrimental.
Methionine	Found in red meats, methiomine may contribute to fatty plaque buildup by its relationship to elevated homocysteine.
Nicotinic acid	Niacin has a potent effect on high-denisty lipoprotein (HDL) cholesterol levels. Data on cardiovascular event rate reductions are limited.
Nuts and seeds (see Table 6-1)	Nuts and seeds provide monounsaturated fat, natural vitamin E, magnesium, and other heart-healthy nutrients Walnuts and almonds are especially effective for reducing lipids.
Obesity	Individuals who are obese in middle age have a higher risk of hospitalization and mortality from CHD. A major goal of dietary prevention and treatment is to attain and maintain weight within a healthy body weight range. Decreasing excess calories, reducing total fat intake, adding fiber, reducing excess intake of refined carbohydrates, and increasing exercise can help achieve this goal.
Omega-3 fatty acids (see Table 6-1)	Both eicosapentaenoic acid (EPA) and docosahexaenoic acid (DHA) in foods and supplements decrease production of inflammatory mediators. Omega-3 s may reduce CHD events. Japan has the lowest heart disease rate in the world; fish is a common part of that diet. RBC ^{15}N is a biomarker of EPA and DHA intake; it is rapid and inexpensive (O'Brien et al, 2009).
Oral health	Poor oral health may be a risk factor for CHD; improvement of periodontal status may influence the related systemic inflammation.
Phytosterols and stanols (see Table 6-1)	Plant stanol or sterol esters are phytosterols found in plant foods such as corn, soy, and other vegetable oils. Plant stanol esters block intestinal absorption of dietary and biliary cholesterol. Fat-soluble vitamins are not significantly affected. Sunflower kernels, pistachio nuts, sesame seeds and wheat germ are good sources.
Plasma lipoprotein (a) [Lp(a)]	Elevated plasma Lp(a) is an independent risk factor of heart disease. Ethnicity-related differences in Lp(a) levels exist.
Quercetin and antioxidants from fruits and vegetables	Vegetables, citrus fruits, seeds, olive oil, tea, and spices are antioxidant foods to include in the diet. Fruits are more protective than vegetables. Quercetin (in apples, onions) protects against CHD and hypertension. Pomegranate can lower cholesterol synthesis and spices and herbs can suppress inflammatory pathways.
Smoking	Both active smoking and secondary exposure are associated with the progression of atherosclerotic heart disease. Smoking is of greater concern among persons who also have diabetes mellitus and hypertension, or who drink a lot of alcohol (Culllen et al, 2009).
Soy protein (see Table 6-1)	The FDA permits labeling of products high in soy protein as helpful in lowering heart disease risk; products must contain at least 6.25 g per serving. Tofu contains 13 g of soy protein in one 4-oz serving; one soy burger contains 10–12 g of protein; 1/4 cup of soy nuts and 1/2 cup of tempeh contain 19 g of protein each.
Trans fatty acids (TFAs)	TFAs are strongly associated with systemic inflammation in patients with heart disease. Food labels must list the amount of TFAs.
Triglycerides	High levels of triglycerides are an independent risk factor of cardiovascular death. A low-fat diet can help.
Vitamin C (see Table 6-1)	Vitamin C has a role in cholesterol metabolism and affects levels of LDL cholesterol. Men, smokers, elderly individuals, and persons with diabetes or hypertension tend to have lower levels of serum ascorbic acid and higher risks for heart disease.
Vitamin E (see Table 6-1)	Alpha-tocopherol decreases lipid peroxidation and platelet aggregation and functions as a potent anti-inflammatory agent. Prospective human clinical trials with alpha-tocopherol have not shown effectiveness in lowering CHD risk.
Vitamin K	Vitamin K influences vascular health. Use darker greens or red leaf lettuce to increase vitamins A and K.

Cullen MW, et al. No interaction of body mass index and smoking on diabetes mellitus risk in elderly women. *Prev Med.* 48:74, 2009.

TABLE 6-3 **Commonly Used Herbs and Botanical Products in Heart Disease**

Chromium	Chromium is sometimes used for dyslipidemia. Do not use excesses of chromium with insulin or hypoglycemic agents because chromium may lower glucose levels excessively.
Coenzyme Q10 (CoQ10; ubiquinone)	Statins block production of farnesyl pyrophosphate, an intermediate in the synthesis of ubiquinone. Because CoQ10 and statins share a similar pathway, they can be taken simultaneously (Mabuchi et al, 2005; Strey et al, 2005). While there is insufficient evidence to prove the role of CoQ10 deficiency in statin-associated myopathy, there are no specific risks for this supplement. Do not take with gemfibrozil, tricyclic antidepressants, or warfarin.
L-arginine	Arginine appears to reduce endothelin, a protein that causes blood vessel constriction and is found in high amounts in HF patients; avoid use after an MI (Schulman et al, 2006).
Danshen	Used for ischemic heart disease. Avoid large amounts with warfarin, aspirin, and other antiplatelet drugs as it can increase risk of bleeding or bruising.
Fenugreek	This product may improve serum lipid levels slightly. Do not take with diuretics.
Garlic	Garlic may have short-term effects on blood lipids. Avoid use in large amounts with warfarin, aspirin, and other antiplatelet drugs because of increased risks of bleeding or bruising. It may also increase insulin levels with hypoglycemic results; monitor carefully in patients with diabetes.
Grapefruit	Grapefruit juice decreases drug metabolism in the gut (via P-450–CYP3A4 inhibition) and can affect medications up to 24 hours later. Consistency of use is more important than total quantity. Avoid taking with alprazolam, buspirone, cisapride, cyclosporine, statins, tacrolimus, and other cardiac drugs.
Guggul; Gugulipid	This yellowish resin from mukul myrrh tree is used in Indian Ayurveda medicine. It lowers low-density lipoprotein (LDL) and increases high-density lipoprotein (HDL) because of its plant sterols; it also stimulates the thyroid, is an anti-inflammatory, and works like an antioxidant. Gugulipid is the safest form, but a high dose is needed. Gastrointestinal discomfort may occur. Do not take with Inderal or Cardizem, and do not use during pregnancy or lactation.
Hawthorn	This is used for heart failure in Germany. Hawthorn should not be taken with digoxin, angiotensin-converting enzyme (ACE) inhibitors, and other cardiovascular drugs.
Niacin (nicotinic acid)	Do not take with statins, antidiabetic medications, or carbamazepine because of potentially serious risks of myopathy and altered glucose control.
Omega-3 fatty acids	Some studies support the role of DHA and EPA in preventing heart failure, but not with a high-fat diet (Shah et al, 2009). Fish oil capsules can cause hypervitaminosis A and D if taken in large doses. Avoid use in pregnant or lactating women. Avoid taking with warfarin, aspirin, and other antiplatelet medications because of the risk of increased bruising or bleeding.
Psyllium (metamucil)	Used to lower total and LDL cholesterol levels; evidence is slim.
Vitamin C and E, beta-carotene, and selenium	Do not take with simvastatin–niacin drug combinations because the combination of these antioxidants may lower HDL2 cholesterol, a beneficial subfraction of HDL cholesterol.
Vitamin E	Do not take with warfarin because of the possibility of increased bleeding. Avoid doses greater than 400 IU/d.

REFERENCES

Mabuchi H, et al. Reduction of serum ubiquinol-10 and ubiquinone-10 levels by atorvastatin in hypercholesterolemic patients. *J Atheroscler Thromb.* 12:111, 2005.

Schulman SP, et al. L-arginine therapy in acute myocardial infarction: the Vascular Interaction with Age in Myocardial Infarction (VINTAGE MI) randomized clinical trial. *JAMA.* 295:58, 2006.

Shah KB, et al. The cardioprotective effects of fish oil during pressure overload are blocked by high fat intake. role of cardiac phospholipid remodeling [published online ahead of print Jul 13, 2009]. *Hypertension.* 54:65, 2009.

Strey CH, et al. Endothelium-ameliorating effects of statin therapy and coenzyme Q10 reductions in chronic heart failure. *Atherosclerosis.* 179:201, 2005.

SODIUM AND OTHER MINERALS

A majority of Americans over age 60 have high BP with a shortened life expectancy. High BP affects over 73,600,000 in the United States (American Heart Association, 2009). Hypertension increases the risk for coronary artery disease (CAD), MI, stroke, renal failure, and HF. Careful attention to hypertension is essential in all ages and both sexes. African Americans and Hispanics of Caribbean descent tend to have a high prevalence of hypertension. Vitamin D plays a role in heart health (Martins et al, 2007). Increasing sun exposure or using a supplement may be indicated (Scragg et al, 2007). There are also many benefits in reducing sodium intake while increasing intakes of potassium, calcium, magnesium, and whole grains. Table 6-4 highlights key nutrients (folic acid, potassium, magnesium, and calcium) and provides heart healthy food choices based on the Dietary Approaches to Stop Hypertension (DASH) diet principles.

Excessive alcohol intake is one of the major causes of magnesium loss from various tissues, including the heart; magnesium loss may represent a predisposing factor to the onset of alcohol-induced pathologies including stroke and cardiomyopathy (Romani, 2008). Rich sources of magnesium include nuts and seeds, soybeans, tofu, chocolate, dark-green vegetables, legumes, yogurt, wheat germ and dairy products. Although supplement use can help meet DRI levels for calcium, vitamin C and magnesium, supplementation may not work for potassium and may be too high for some other nutrients (Burnett-Hartman et al, 2009). In 2004, The Institute of Medicine of the National Academy of Sciences issued recommendations for intake of water and electrolytes that include the following suggestions:

- **CHLORIDE:** 2300 mg daily for adults to replace losses in perspiration.
- **POTASSIUM:** 4700 mg is needed to lower BP and reduce the risk of kidney stones and bone loss for most adults. No upper limit is set. African Americans may benefit. Natural sources are best.
- **SODIUM:** 1500 mg for adults aged 19–50; 1300 mg for adults aged 50–70; 1200 mg for adults aged 71 and over.

TABLE 6-4 Key Sources of Folate, Potassium, Calcium, and Magnesium and the DASH Diet Principles

Folate Sources	Micrograms (μg)	Folate Sources	Micrograms (μg)
Breakfast cereals fortified with 100% of the daily value (DV), 3/4 cup	400	Avocado, raw, all varieties, sliced, 1/2 cup sliced	45
Beef liver, cooked, braised, 3 oz	185	Peanuts, all types, dry roasted, 1 ounce	40
Cowpeas (blackeyes), immature, cooked, boiled, 1/2 cup	105	Lettuce, romaine, shredded, 1/2 cup	40
Breakfast cereals, fortified with 25% of the DV, 3/4 cup	100	Wheat germ, crude, 2 tablespoons	40
Spinach, frozen, cooked, boiled, 1/2 cup	100	Tomato juice, canned, 6 oz	35
Great Northern beans, boiled, 1/2 cup	90	Orange juice, chilled, includes concentrate, 3/4 cup	35
Asparagus, boiled, 4 spears	85	Turnip greens, frozen, cooked, boiled, 1/2 cup	30
Rice, white, long-grain, parboiled, enriched, cooked, 1/2 cup	65	Orange, all commercial varieties, fresh, 1 small	30
		Bread, white, 1 slice	25
Vegetarian baked beans, canned, 1 cup	60	Bread, whole wheat, 1 slice	25
Spinach, raw, 1 cup	60	Egg, whole, raw, fresh, 1 large	25
Green peas, frozen, boiled, 1/2 cup	50	Cantaloupe, raw, 1/4 medium	25
Broccoli, chopped, frozen, cooked, 1/2 cup	50	Papaya, raw, 1/2 cup cubes	25
Egg noodles, cooked, enriched, 1/2 cup	50	Banana, raw, 1 medium	20
Broccoli, raw, 2 spears (each 5-in long)	45		

From: U.S. Department of Agriculture, Agricultural Research Service. USDA national nutrient database for standard reference, Release 16. 2003. Nutrient Data Laboratory Home Page, accessed July 7, 2009, at http://www.nal.usda.gov/fnic/cgi-bin/nut_search.pl.

Potassium Sources	Milligrams (mg)	Potassium Sources	Milligrams (mg)
Apricots, 3 medium	272	Orange juice, 8 oz	473
Artichoke, 1 cup, raw	644	Papaya, 1 whole	781
Avocado, Jerusalem, 1 medium	976	Potato, baked with skin, medium	1081
Banana, 1 cup	537	Pumpkin, 1 cup, cooked	564
Beans, canned white, 1 cup	1189	Prunes (dried plums), 1 cup, stewed	796
Beet greens, boiled, 1/2 cup	653	Prune juice, 1 cup	707
Broccoli, 1 cup chopped	457	Raisins, 1/3 cup	362
Cantaloupe, 1 cup	427	Refried beans, canned, 1 cup	673
Grapefruit juice, sweetened, 1 cup	405	Spinach, 1 cup, cooked	574
Halibut, cooked, 1/2 fillet	916	Sweet potato, canned, 1 cup	796
Kidney beans, 1 cup	713	Tomato, 1 medium	426
Kiwifruit, 1 medium	252	Tomato juice, 6 oz	417
Lima beans, cooked, 1 cup	955	Tomato puree, 1/2 cup	1328
Milk, 1 cup, skim	382	Tomato sauce, 1 cup	940
Milk, 1 cup, chocolate	425	Tropical trail mix, 1 cup	993
Milkshake, 16 oz, vanilla	579	Vegetable juice cocktail, 1 cup, canned	467
Nectarine, 1 medium	273	Winter squash, 1 cup	896
Orange, 1 medium	237	Yogurt, 8 oz, low fat	443

For other sources. Web site accessed July 7, 2009, at http://www.nal.usda.gov/fnic/foodcomp/Data/SR17/wtrank/sr17w306.pdf.

Calcium Sources	Milligrams (mg)	Calcium Sources	Milligrams (mg)
Broccoli, cooked, 1 cup	156	Collards, 1 cup, cooked	266
Cheddar cheese, 1 oz	204	Eggnog, 1 cup	330
Cheese sauce, 1 cup	756	Enchilada with cheese, 1	324
Cheese, Swiss, 1 oz	224	Milk, canned evaporated, 1 cup	742
Clam chowder, New England, 1 cup	186	Milk, fluid, 1%, 1 cup	290
Milk, fluid, chocolate, low fat, 1 cup	288	Tofu made with calcium, 1/4 block	164

(continued)

TABLE 6-4 Key Sources of Folate, Potassium, Calcium, and Magnesium and the DASH Diet Principles *(continued)*

Calcium Sources	Milligrams (mg)	Calcium Sources	Milligrams (mg)
Milkshake, thick, vanilla, 11 oz	457	Total brand cereal, 3/4 cup	1104
Molasses, blackstrap, 1 tablespoon	172	Sardines, canned with bones, 3 oz	325
Pudding, chocolate, 4 oz, ready to serve	102	Spinach, canned, 1 cup	272
Ricotta cheese, part skim, 1 cup	669	Turnip greens, frozen, cooked, 1 cup	249
Soybeans, green, cooked, 1 cup	261	Yogurt, low fat with fruit, 1 cup	345

For a more specific list, Web site accessed July 7, 2009, at http://www.nal.usda.gov/fnic/foodcomp/Data/SR17/wtrank/sr17w301.pdf.

Magnesium Sources	Milligrams (mg)	Magnesium Sources	Milligrams (mg)
Barley, pearled, raw 1 cup	158	Plantain, raw, 1 medium	66
Beans, canned white, 1 cup	134	Seeds, pumpkin or squash seed kernels, 1 oz (142 seeds)	151
Broccoli, cooked, 1 cup	33	Soybeans, mature, cooked, 1 cup	148
Cereal, All-Bran, 1/2 cup	109	Spinach, cooked, 1 cup	163
Chocolate candy, semisweet, 1 cup	193	Tomato paste, 1 cup	110
Halibut, cooked, 1/2 fillet	170	Trail mix, with chocolate chips, nuts, seeds, 1 cup	235
Nuts, Brazil, 6–8	107	Whole-grain wheat flour, 1 cup	166
Oat bran, 1 cup	221		
Okra, cooked, 1 cup	94		

For a more specific list, Web site accessed July 7, 2009, at http://www.nal.usda.gov/fnic/foodcomp/Data/SR17/wtrank/sr17w304.pdf.

DASH Diet Principles	Food
Vegetables, choose 4–5 servings daily	Carrots, sweet potatoes, pumpkin, winter squash
	Green leafy vegetables (broccoli, kale, cabbage, etc.), green beans
	Tomato salsas, 6-oz servings of tomato juice or other vegetable juices
Fruits, choose 4–5 servings daily	Fresh fruits, including apples, bananas, cantaloupe, melons, berries
	Red or black grapes; grape juice (1 cup per day)
	Grapefruit, especially pink (40% more beta-carotene)
	Dried fruits, especially apricots, dates, prunes
	Pomegranates and other antioxidant juices (blueberry juice, red wine, orange juice, cranberry juice, green tea)
Protein-rich foods, choose 2 or less	Lean chicken and turkey breast
	Salmon and other fish
	Meats that are lean or have fat trimmed away
Low-fat dairy, 2–3 servings daily	Skim milk and yogurt (8 oz)
	Low-fat cheeses (1-1/2 oz per serving)
Low-fat foods	Tomato sauces with pasta
	Homemade pizza with low-fat toppings (chicken, vegetables, low-fat cheese)
Grains, choose 7–8 servings daily	Oatmeal, shredded wheat; high-fiber, low-sugar cereals
	Baked whole-wheat chips and tortillas
	Whole-grain breads and pastas, wheat germ
Nuts, seeds, and dry beans, 4–5 servings per week	Peanuts, walnuts, almonds, pistachios, other nuts in moderation
	Pumpkin seeds, sunflower seeds, sesame seeds
	Bean and chickpea dishes and dips
Oils, 2–3 servings	Olive oil and canola oil substituted for other oils
	Salad dressings and dips with nonfat sour cream or homemade yogurt

NOTE: Most of these foods are recommended in both the DASH and Mediterranean diets.
For more information, see Web site accessed July 7, 2009, at http://www.nhlbi.nih.gov/health/public/heart/hbp/dash/new_dash.pdf.

Highly active people may need more. If sodium sensitive, intake may need to be lower. Upper limit (UL) is set at 2.3 g sodium/d; over 95% of the American public consumes sodium above the UL level on a regular basis.

- **WATER:** 91 oz daily for women, 125 oz daily for men; more in hot climates or with physical activity. Drinking fluids with and between meals according to thirst is usually sufficient, although seniors may lose their thirst sensation. Beverages provide 80% of daily intake, 20% comes from food.

For More Information

- American Association of Cardiovascular Pulmonary Rehabilitation http://www.aacvpr.org/
- American Heart Association http://www.americanheart.org/

LIPIDS—CITED REFERENCES

American Heart Association. Accessed June 7, 2009, at http://www.americanheart.org.

Anderson C. Dietary modification and CVD prevention: a matter of fat. *JAMA*. 295:693, 2006.

Bhatt DL, et al. International prevalence, recognition, and treatment of cardiovascular risk factors in outpatients with atherothrombosis. *JAMA*. 295:180, 2006.

Burnett-Hartman AN, et al. Supplement use contributes to meeting recommended dietary intakes for calcium, magnesium, and vitamin C in four ethnicities of middle-aged and older Americans: the Multi-Ethnic Study of Atherosclerosis. *J Am Diet Assoc*. 109:422, 2009.

Danaei G, et al. The preventable causes of death in the United States: comparative risk assessment of dietary, lifestyle, and metabolic risk factors. *PLoS Med*. 6(4):e1000058, 2009.

Ferguson LR. Nutrigenomics approaches to functional foods. *J Am Diet Assoc*. 109:452, 2009.

Forman D, Bulwer BE. Cardiovascular disease: optimal approaches to risk factor modification of diet and lifestyle. *Curr Treat Options Cardiovasc Med*. 8:47, 2006.

Howard BV, et al. Low-fat dietary pattern and risk of cardiovascular disease: the Women's Health Initiative Randomized Controlled Dietary Modification Trial. *JAMA*. 295:655, 2006.

Hoy MK, et al. Implementing a low-fat eating plan in the Women's Intervention Nutrition Study. *J Am Diet Assoc*. 109:688, 2009.

Kendrick J, et al. 25-Hydroxyvitamin D deficiency is independently associated with cardiovascular disease in the Third National Health and Nutrition Examination Survey. *Atherosclerosis*. 205:255, 2009.

Kourlaba G, et al. Development of a diet index for older adults and its relation to cardiovascular disease risk factors: the Elderly Dietary Index. *J Am Diet Assoc*. 109:1022, 2009.

Krummel D. Nutrition in cardiovascular disease. In: Mahan K, Escott-Stump S, eds. *Krause's food, nutrition, and diet therapy*. 12th ed. Philadelphia, PA: WB Saunders, 2008.

Marik PE, Varon J. Omega-3 dietary supplements and the risk of cardiovascular events: a systematic review. *Clin Cardiol*. 32:365, 2009.

Martins D, et al. Prevalence of cardiovascular risk factors and the serum levels of 25-hydroxyvitamin D in the United States: data from the Third National Health and Nutrition Examination Survey. *Arch Intern Med*. 167:1159, 2007.

Rifkin DE, et al. Albuminuria, impaired kidney function and cardiovascular outcomes or mortality in the elderly [published online ahead of print 2009]. *Nephrol Dial Transplant*. 25:1560, 2010.

Romani AM. Magnesium homeostasis and alcohol consumption. *Magnes Res*. 21:197, 2008.

Scragg R, et al. Serum 25-hydroxyvitamin D, ethnicity, and blood pressure in the Third National Health and Nutrition Examination Survey. *Am J Hypertens*. 20:713, 2007.

ANGINA PECTORIS

NUTRITIONAL ACUITY RANKING: LEVEL 1

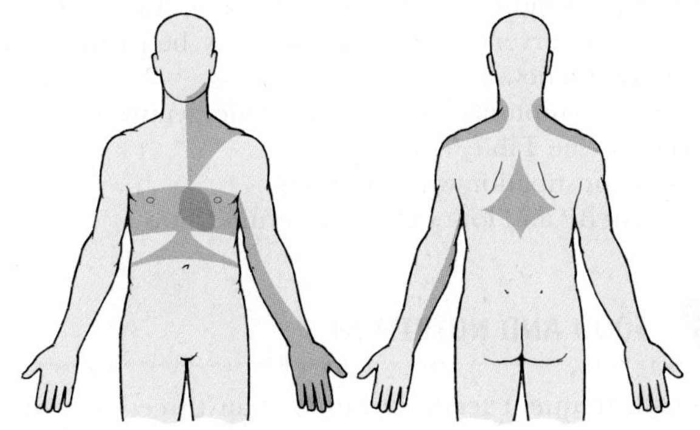

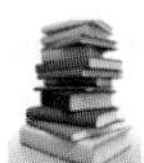

DEFINITIONS AND BACKGROUND

Angina pectoris involves retrosternal chest pain or discomfort from decreased blood flow to the myocardium from decreased oxygen supply (often during exertion). Traditional risk factors include tobacco use, hypertension, diabetes mellitus, dyslipidemia, obesity, sedentary lifestyle, atherogenic diet; high-sensitivity C-reactive protein (hsCRP), lipoprotein (a), and elevated homocysteine (tHcy). Angina can also occur from anemia, hyperthyroidism, aortic stenosis, or vasospasm. In hypertrophic cardiomyopathy (HCM), an area of abnormally thick heart muscle impairs the heart's pumping action and causes angina during or shortly after exercise.

Stable (classic) angina occurs after exertion and is relieved by rest and vasodilation; it lasts 3–5 minutes. Intractable (progressive) angina causes chronic chest pain that is not relieved by medical treatment. Variant angina is a mixed condition. If diagnosed early, the chance of living longer than 10–12 years is at least 50%. A very low–fat diet (i.e., 10% fat calories) has a substantial impact (Griel and Kris-Etherton, 2006). In addition, vitamin D provision through sun exposure or supplementation may be indicated when serum levels are below 20 ng/L (Kendrick et al, 2009).

An "ABCDE" approach is effective: "A" for antiplatelet therapy, anticoagulation, angiotensin-converting enzyme (ACE) inhibition, and angiotensin receptor blockade; "B" for beta-blockade and BP control; "C" for Chol treatment and cigarette-smoking cessation; "D" for diabetes management and diet; and "E" for exercise (Gluckman et al, 2005). Management of factors leading to the metabolic syndrome is also recommended (see Table 6-5). Cardiac rehabilitation helps to improve aerobic exercise capacity, physical functioning, and mental depression. Invasive treatments for chronic stable angina are only needed in a small number of patients (Kirwan et al, 2005). Currently, use of percutaneous coronary intervention (PCI) improves quality of life by relieving angina in patients with stable CAD (Brar and Stone, 2009).

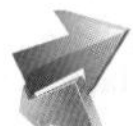

ASSESSMENT, MONITORING, AND EVALUATION

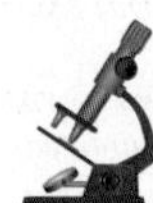

CLINICAL INDICATORS

Genetic Markers: There are shared genetic pathways for angina pectoris (AP) and CHD death among both sexes; AP is important as a risk factor for CHD death (Zdravkovic et al, 2007).

Clinical/History
Height
Weight
Body mass index (BMI)
Waist circumference
Recent weight changes (e.g., gain)
Diet history
Chest pain
Shortness of breath
Sweating, nausea, vertigo
Ache in neck or jaw, earache
Numbness or burning sensations
Pulse (NL = 60–100 beats/min)
BP
Intake and output (I & O)
Electrocardiogram (ECG)
Radionucleotide imaging
Exercise stress test
Coronary angiography

Lab Work
Chol—LDL, HDL, total
Advanced lipid testing—lipoprotein particle size
Triglycerides (TGs)
Lactate dehydrogenase (LDH)
tHcy
C-reactive protein (CRP)
CoQ10 serum levels
Serum folate
Glucose (Gluc)
Hemoglobin and hematocrit (H & H)
Serum Fe, ferritin
Total iron-binding capacity (TIBC)
Aspartate aminotransferase (AST)
Alanine aminotransferase (ALT)
Transferrin
Na^+, K^+
Ca^{++}, Mg^{++}
Alkaline phosphatase (Alk phos)

SAMPLE NUTRITION CARE PROCESS STEPS

Overweight

Assessment Data: BMI >90 percentile for age; complaints of heartburn and chest pain; diet hx shows intake of energy about 600 kcals extra per day and BMI 28.

Nutrition Diagnoses (PES): Overweight related to excessive energy intake as evidenced by BMI of 28 and limited physical activity.

Interventions: Education about the role of weight and heart disease, including angina. Counseling about desirable energy intake for age and activity level; ways to gradually increase physical activity.

Monitoring and Evaluation: BMI closer to desirable range; tolerance of physical activity; adequate drug therapy for angina.

TABLE 6-5 Signs of the Metabolic Syndrome (Any Three of the Following)

Risk Factor	Defining Level
Abdominal obesity[a]	Waist circumference[b]
Men	>102 cm (>40 in)
Women	>88 cm (>35 in)
Triglycerides	≥150 mg/dL
HDL cholesterol	
Men	<40 mg/dL
Women	<50 mg/dL
Blood pressure	≥130/≥85 mm Hg
Fasting glucose	≥110 mg/dL

From: National Heart, Lung, and Blood Institute. Web site accessed July 7, 2009, at http://www.nhlbi.nih.gov/guidelines/cholesterol/atglance.htm#Step1.
[a]Overweight and obesity are associated with insulin resistance and the metabolic syndrome. Abdominal obesity is more highly correlated with the metabolic risk factors than is an elevated BMI. Simple measure of waist circumference is recommended to identify the body weight component.
[b]Some male patients can develop multiple metabolic risk factors when the waist circumference is only marginally increased, e.g., 94–102 cm (37–39 in). Such patients may have a strong genetic contribution to insulin resistance. They should benefit from changes in life habits.

INTERVENTION

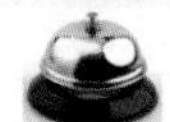

OBJECTIVES

- Relieve chest pain. Improve circulation to the heart.
- Increase activity as tolerated. Gradually increase exercise, especially through programs in cardiac rehabilitation.
- Maintain adequate rest periods.
- Maintain weight or lose weight if obese. A conventional dietetic intervention with weight loss helps to reduce pain frequency.
- Reduce symptoms of the metabolic syndrome where present (see Table 6-5).
- Avoid constipation with straining.
- Control BP and lower elevated serum Chol.

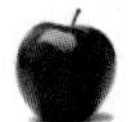

FOOD AND NUTRITION

- Small, frequent feedings rather than three large meals are indicated.
- Increase fiber as tolerated; include an adequate fluid intake. Increase intake of fruits.
- Restrict saturated fats, dietary Chol, and sodium as necessary according to the individual profile. A very low–fat diet can be quite effective (Griel and Kris-Etherton, 2006).
- Limit stimulants such as caffeine to less than 5 cups of coffee or the equivalent daily. Energy drinks may contain 50–500 mg of caffeine.
- Promote calorie control if overweight; modify by age and sex.
- If tHcy levels are high, add more foods with folic acid, vitamins B_6 and B_{12} to the diet.

- A Mediterranean diet that is rich in alpha linolenic acid (ALA) is effective (Estruch et al, 2006). It is prudent to increase intake of olive, soybean, and canola oils, seeds and nuts, including walnuts, almonds, macadamias, pecans, peanuts, and pistachios. Walnuts contain ALA; almonds are a good source of vitamin E. Nuts also contain flavonoids, phenols, phytosterols, saponins, elegiac acid, folic acid, magnesium, copper, potassium, and fiber. Pistachios, sunflower kernels, sesame seeds, and wheat germ are highest in phytosterols; use often.
- Beta-carotene supplements actually seem to increase angina. Dietary sources of carotenoids are a healthier choice.

Common Drugs Used and Potential Side Effects

- Relief comes from use of tricyclic agents, beta-blockers, statins, or ACE inhibitors (Bugiardini and Bairey Mertz, 2005). Isosorbide (Isordil or Imdur) may cause nausea, vomiting, or dizziness; take on an empty stomach. Nadolol (Corgard) is a beta-blocker; it may cause weakness. Disopyramide (Norpace) may cause abdominal pain, nausea, or constipation.
- Antiplatelet therapy or anticoagulation therapy will be prescribed. Monitor for vitamin K intake with warfarin.
- Calcium channel blockers (verapamil [Calan], nicardipine, or diltiazem [Cardizem]) are used to dilate coronary arteries and slow down nerve impulses through the heart, thereby increasing blood flow. Nausea, edema, or constipation may be side effects. Take on an empty stomach. These drugs may also cause HF or dizziness; avoid taking with aloe, buckthorn bark and berry, cascara, and senna leaf. With nifedipine (Procardia), nausea, weakness, dizziness, and flatulence may occur; take after meals.

Herbs, Botanicals, and Supplements

- The patient should not take herbals and botanicals without discussing with the physician. See Table 6-3.

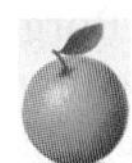

NUTRITION EDUCATION, COUNSELING, CARE MANAGEMENT

- The patient will require stress management, activity, and education about proper eating habits.
- Discuss the role of nutrition in maintenance of wellness and in CVD. Discuss in particular: fiber, total fat intake, potassium and sodium, calcium and other nutrients, and caffeine.
- Discuss the importance of weight control in reduction of cardiovascular risks.
- Elevate the head of the bed 30–45° for greater comfort.
- Unstable angina is dangerous and should be treated as a potential emergency; new, worsening, or persistent chest discomfort should be evaluated in a hospital emergency department or "chest pain unit" and monitored carefully for acute MI (heart attack), severe cardiac arrhythmia, or cardiac arrest leading to sudden death. Dyspnea is a key factor and should be addressed (Arnold et al, 2009).

Patient Education—Foodborne Illness

- Careful food handling will be important. Hand washing is key as well.

For More Information

- American Heart Association—Angina
  http://www.americanheart.org/presenter.jhtml?identifier=4472
- Medicine Net—angina
  http://www.medicinenet.com/angina/article.htm
- NHLBI—angina
  http://www.nhlbi.nih.gov/health/dci/Diseases/Angina/Angina_WhatIs.html

ANGINA PECTORIS—CITED REFERENCES

Arnold SV, et al. The impact of dyspnea on health-related quality of life in patients with coronary artery disease: results from the PREMIER registry. *Am Heart J.* 157:1042, 2009.

Brar SS, Stone GW. Advances in percutaneous coronary intervention. *Curr Cardiol Rep.* 11:245, 2009.

Bugiardini R, Bairey Mertz CN. Angina with "normal" coronary arteries: a changing philosophy. *JAMA.* 293:477, 2005.

Estruch R, et al. Effects of a Mediterranean-style diet on cardiovascular risk factors: a randomized trial. *Ann Intern Med.* 145:1, 2006.

Gluckman TJ, et al. A simplified approach to the management of non-ST-segment elevation acute coronary syndromes. *JAMA.* 293:349, 2005.

Griel AE, Kris-Etherton PM. Beyond saturated fat: the importance of the dietary fatty acid profile on cardiovascular disease. *Nutr Rev.* 64:257, 2006.

Kirwan BA, et al. Treatment of angina pectoris: associations with symptom severity. *Int J Cardiol.* 98:299, 2005.

Zdravkovic S, et al. Genetic influences on angina pectoris and its impact on coronary heart disease. *Eur J Hum Genet.* 15:872, 2007.

ARTERITIS

NUTRITIONAL ACUITY RANKING: LEVEL 1

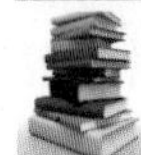

DEFINITIONS AND BACKGROUND

Arteritis involves inflammation of artery walls with decreased blood flow. **Cranial arteritis** (temporal or giant-cell arteritis) yields chronically inflamed temporal arteries with a thickening of the lining and a reduction in blood flow; this condition is linked to polymyalgia rheumatica (PMR). Women older than 55 years of age are twice as likely to have the condition compared with other people. The greatest danger is permanent blindness or stroke.

Buerger's disease involves an arteritis that causes limb pain and numbness. **Periarteritis nodosa** is an autoimmune disease that can affect any artery in the body. A rare form, **Takayasu's arteritis**, affects the mesenteric artery and creates local ischemia; IL-8 may be involved. Patients with **giant cell arteritis** (GCA) are at risk for developing extra-cranial large vessel inflammation. GCA is a medical emergency with neuro-ophthalmic complications and permanent vision loss in up to a fifth of patients (Borg and Dasgupta, 2009).

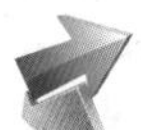

ASSESSMENT, MONITORING, AND EVALUATION

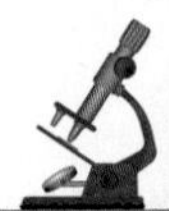

CLINICAL INDICATORS

Genetic Markers: Tumor necrosis factor appears to influence susceptibility and interleukin (IL)-1 receptor antagonist seems to play a role in the pathogenesis. Other genetic markers are being studied.

Clinical/History

- Height
- Weight
- BMI
- Diet history
- BP
- Temperature (mild fever?)
- Severe, throbbing headache (temples, back of the head)
- Red, swollen, painful temporal artery
- Anorexia, weight loss
- Scalp tenderness
- Dysphagia
- Hearing problems or vision changes
- Jaw pain
- Muscular aches
- Abnormal arterial biopsy (necrotizing vasculitis with granulomatous proliferation)
- Ultrasonography

Lab Work

- White blood cell count (WBC) (increased)
- Erythrocyte sedimentation rate (ESR) >50 mm/h
- CRP
- CoQ10 serum levels
- Na^+, K^+
- Ca^{++}, Mg^{++}
- Gluc
- Albumin (Alb) or transthyretin
- Creatinine kinase (CK)
- Transferrin
- Chol—total, HDL, LDL
- Trig
- H & H (often decreased)
- Serum Fe, ferritin
- tHcy level
- Serum folate and B_{12}

INTERVENTION

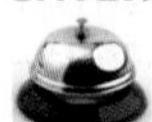

OBJECTIVES

- Prevent stroke and blindness, which are potential complications.
- Reduce inflammation.
- Promote increased blood flow through the affected vessels.
- Modify intake according to requirements and coexisting problems such as hypertension.

SAMPLE NUTRITION CARE PROCESS STEPS

Dysphagia

Assessment Data: Weight loss, dysphagia and jaw pain, throbbing headache.

Nutrition Diagnoses (PES): Dysphagia related to arteritis with jaw pain as evidenced by weight loss, complaints of difficulty swallowing solids, choking on thin liquids.

Interventions: Education about blending foods and simplifying meal planning to increase intake. Swallowing evaluation for determination of appropriate textures and thickening of liquids. Counseling on positioning at mealtime to reduce likelihood of aspiration.

Monitoring and Evaluation: Improved intake for meals and snacks; fewer complaints of difficulty swallowing. No further weight loss.

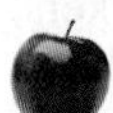

FOOD AND NUTRITION

- Follow usual diet, with increased calories if patient is underweight or decreased calories if the patient is obese.
- Reduce excess sodium and total fat intake; monitor regularly. Increase intake of fruits.
- Patient may need to include carnitine in the diet. Although not yet proven, it may be reasonable to include in the diet more sources of vitamins E, B_6, and B_{12}, riboflavin, and folic acid or to use a multivitamin supplement that includes sufficient amounts.
- With steroids, decreased sodium intake with higher potassium intake may be needed. Adequate to high protein may also be necessary. Monitor for glucose intolerance.
- Omega-3 fatty acids may be used to reduce inflammation. Include salmon, tuna, sardines, mackerel, walnuts, and related foods.
- Treat with supplements of folic acid, vitamins B_6 and B_{12} to reduce elevated tHcy concentrations.

Common Drugs Used and Potential Side Effects

- The mainstay of therapy remains corticosteroids (Borg and Dasgupta, 2009). High-dose prednisone successfully controls the inflammatory process. Side effects include elevated glucose and decreased nitrogen levels, especially with long-term use.
- Methotrexate is being evaluated but more research is needed.
- Low-dose aspirin is sometimes recommended.

Herbs, Botanicals, and Supplements

- The patient should not take herbals or botanicals without discussing with the physician. See Table 6-3.

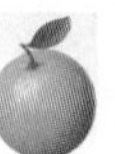

NUTRITION EDUCATION, COUNSELING, CARE MANAGEMENT

- Discuss the role of nutrition in the maintenance of health for CVD.

- Discuss the effects of medications on nutritional status and appetite.
- If dysphagia is present, discuss ways to alter texture or liquid consistencies.
- With long-term use of prednisone, monitor for osteoporosis, cataracts, easy bruising, elevated glucose levels.

Patient Education—Foodborne Illness

- Careful food handling will be important. Hand washing is key as well.

For More Information

- American Autoimmune Association
  http://www.aarda.org/
- Emedicine: Temporal arteritis
  http://emedicine.medscape.com/article/809492-overview
- Giant Cell Arteritis
  http://www.mayoclinic.com/health/giant-cell-arteritis/DS00440
- Takayasu Arteritis Foundation
  http://www.takayasus.org/

ARTERITIS—CITED REFERENCE

Borg FA, Dasgupta B. Treatment and outcomes of large vessel arteritis. *Baillieres Best Pract Res Clin Rheumatol.* 23:325, 2009.

ATHEROSCLEROSIS, CORONARY ARTERY DISEASE, DYSLIPIDEMIA

NUTRITIONAL ACUITY RANKING: LEVEL 3

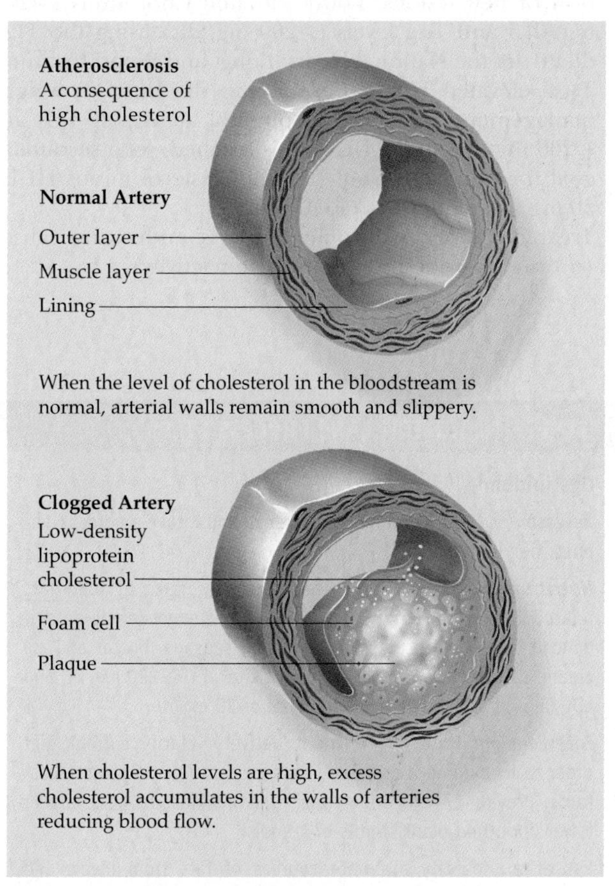
Atherosclerosis
A consequence of high cholesterol
Normal Artery
Outer layer
Muscle layer
Lining
When the level of cholesterol in the bloodstream is normal, arterial walls remain smooth and slippery.
Clogged Artery
Low-density lipoprotein cholesterol
Foam cell
Plaque
When cholesterol levels are high, excess cholesterol accumulates in the walls of arteries reducing blood flow.

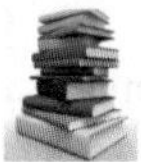

DEFINITIONS AND BACKGROUND

Atherosclerosis involves progressive narrowing of the arterial tree, giving rise to collateral vessels. Fat-deposit accumulations occur; the heart, brain, and leg arteries are most often affected. Metabolic syndrome is prevalent (see Table 6-5). Obesity leads to a proinflammatory and prothrombotic state that potentiates atherosclerosis (Moller and Kaufman, 2005). Vascular lipid accumulation and inflammation are hallmarks of atherosclerosis. As precursors to prostaglandins, thromboxanes, leukotrienes, lipoxins, and resolvins, essential fatty acids (EFAs) have significant clinical implications in hypertension, CHD and atherosclerosis (Das, 2006). The initial insult in adipose inflammation is mediated by macrophage recruitment and endogenous activation of Toll-like receptors, perpetuated through chemokine secretion, adipose retention of macrophages, and elaboration of pro-inflammatory adipocytokines (Shah et al, 2009). Then, paracrine and endocrine adipose inflammatory events induce a local and systemic inflammatory, insulin-resistant state promoting dyslipidemia and CVD (Shah et al, 2009).

CAD occurs when the coronary arteries that supply blood to the heart muscle become hardened and narrowed due to the buildup of plaque on the inner walls or lining of the arteries. Blood flow to the heart is reduced as plaque narrows the coronary arteries and diminishes oxygen supply to the heart muscle. CAD is common and is most often caused by smoking, high BP, low HDL Chol, family history of early CHD, and age (see Tables 6-1 and 6-2 for a long list of dietary and other relevant factors). Obesity, diabetes, and insulin resistance are also risks. Elevated plasma tHcy is an independent risk factor and a strong predictor of mortality in patients with CAD (Ntaios et al, 2010). Angioplasty is safe and as effective as bypass surgery for treatment of CAD.

Ischemia is a local and temporary deficiency of blood caused by obstruction, as from thrombosis. People with ischemic heart disease benefit from diets high in monounsaturated fatty acids (MUFA), omega-3 fatty acids, whole grains, vitamin E, wine, vegetables, and fruits.

Dyslipidemia involves hypertriglyceridemia and low levels of high-density lipoprotein Chol. These imbalances in individual lipid components contribute to the increased risk of CAD. Serum lipid reductions decrease CAD risk; for each 1% reduction in serum Chol, there is a 2% reduction in CAD risk.

Chol screening is recommended, even for older adults. When treated, risks decrease significantly; therefore, early nutritional intervention is beneficial. In addition to BMI, use waist circumference or waist-to-hip ratio (WHR) to assess obesity and CVD risk since BMI alone is not a good predictor of CVD risk in persons over 65 years of age (ADA Evidence Analysis Library, 2009). In addition, correction of dyslipidemia in patients after coronary artery bypass graft (CABG) surgery prevents progression of atherosclerosis.

A therapeutic lifestyle modification program is effective. Nutrition and physical activity interventions have the potential to dramatically reduce the risks. Dietary counseling and education by a registered dietitian are associated with improved diet-related outcomes, and sufficient time to consult with a dietitian should be planned in cardiac rehabilitation (Locklin Holmes et al, 2005). Referral to a registered dietitian for medical nutrition therapy (MNT) is recommended whenever an individual has an abnormal lipid profile or CHD, with a planned initial visit lasting from 45–90 minutes and at least two to six planned follow-up visits of 30–60 minutes each (ADA Evidence Analysis Library, 2009).

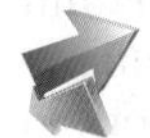

ASSESSMENT, MONITORING, AND EVALUATION

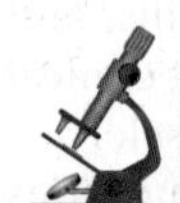

CLINICAL INDICATORS

Genetic Markers: Lipid alterations have a polygenic basis. Family history is the most significant independent risk factor for CAD. In the Multi-Ethnic Study of Atherosclerosis (MESA) the lipid-related HMG-CoA reductase (HMGCR) variations differed greatly among ethnicities (Chen et al, 2009). Another study identified 30 distinct loci with lipoprotein concentrations variants (Kathiresan et al, 2009). ApoE and lipoprotein lipase (LPL) genes have been known for some time. In addition, elevated plasma tHcy can result from genetic errors, including methylenetetrahydrofolate reductase (MTHFR) C677T and A1298C polymorphisms (Freitas et al, 2008). Genetic testing is needed in high-risk population groups (Olthof and Verhoef, 2005).

Clinical/History		
Height	Waist circumference >102 cm (40 in) in men and >88 cm (35 in) in women	Diet history
Weight		BP
BMI		Pancreatitis?
		Xanthomas?

Lab Work		
CRP	LDL Chol: Goal <100 mg/dL	Serum B_6
CoQ10 serum levels	Advanced lipid testing—small particle size	H & H
Trig: Goal below 150 mg/dL	tHcy: serum and urinary	Serum Fe
TC (often increased)	Serum and urinary folate	Na^+, K^+
HDL: Goal >40 mg/dL in men and >50 mg/dL in women	Serum and urinary B_{12}	Ca^{++}, Mg^{++}
		Gluc
		AST, ALT
		Serum copper

INTERVENTION

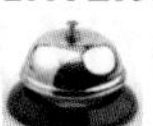

OBJECTIVES

- Use a team approach to support the best possible outcomes: doctors, nurses, dietitians, other therapists.
- Improve LDL and HDL Chol levels to prevent formation of new lesions. Lower elevated Chol levels (>200 mg/dL) and Trig levels (>200 mg/dL) using the TLC diet from the National Heart, Lung, and Blood Institute.
- Treat elevated TGs if over 150 mg/dL. Intensify weight management and increase physical activity. If TGs are ≥200 mg/dL after LDL goal is reached, set a secondary goal for non-HDL Chol (total cholesterol minus HDL) 30 mg/dL higher than LDL goal.
- Treat metabolic syndrome. Address underlying causes (overweight/obesity and physical inactivity).

SAMPLE NUTRITION CARE PROCESS STEPS

Dyslipidemia

Assessment Data: Food frequency recall and intake records; computer nutrient analysis.

Nutrition Diagnosis (PES): Inappropriate intake of food fats related to food and nutrition-related knowledge deficit as evidenced by daily consumption of bacon, sausage, butter and ice cream, saturated fat intake of 15% of kilocal, TC 220 mg/Dl, and LDL Chol of 165 mg/dL and HDL Chol of 30 mg/dL.

Intervention: Food and Nutrient Delivery: Clarify current diet order to include no fried foods, bacon, sausage, and creams/custards. Provide Cheerios or oatmeal for breakfast to help further lower Chol. Add plant sterols or stanols.

Education: identify alternate sources of fats from meals and snacks that are more desirable.

Monitoring and Evaluation: Repeat lab values after 3–6 months; dietary recall. Goal = TC below 200 mg/dL.

- Initiate and maintain weight loss if overweight. Obesity with a high waist circumference is especially important to correct in both men and women.
- Moderate carbohydrate restriction and weight control can improve dyslipidemia.
- Correct elevated levels of tHcy (>6 μmol/L).
- Use more flavonoids, phytochemicals, soy products, and fruits and vegetables.
- Treat hypertension; use aspirin for CAD patients to reduce prothrombotic state if appropriate.
- Monitor for effects of MTHFR genotype (Ilhan et al, 2008). This may be useful in predicting the development of premature coronary artery disease, especially in hypertensive adolescents (Koo et al, 2008) and those who have type 1 diabetes (Wiltshire et al, 2008).

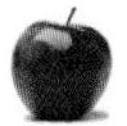

FOOD AND NUTRITION

- There is no "one size fits all" guideline; combine diet with exercise and other lifestyle changes. The Mediterranean diet tends to be quite acceptable to most people and works well in lowering coronary risk factors; it encourages use of olive oil, red wine, fish, fruits, and vegetables.
- The Evidence Analysis Library of the American Dietetic Association recommends the "Therapeutic Lifestyle" diet consisting of 25–35% total fat, <7% saturated and trans fat, and <200 mg dietary Chol (NHLBI, 2009). To keep fat at about 3 g/100 kcal, examples include:

25% of kilocals	30% of kilocals	35% of kilocals
28 g in 1000 kcals	33 g in 1000 kcals	39 g in 1000 kcals
33 g in 1200 kcals	40 g in 1200 kcals	47 g in 1200 kcals
42 g in 1500 kcals	50 g in 1500 kcals	59 g in 1500 kcals
50 g in 1800 kcals	60 g in 1800 kcals	70 g in 1800 kcals
56 g in 2000 kcals	67 g in 2000 kcals	78 g in 2000 kcals
67 g in 2400 kcals	80 g in 2400 kcals	93 g in 2400 kcals

- Use isocaloric replacement of saturated fatty acids (SFA) with MUFA and polyunsaturated fatty acids (PUFA); include olive oil and canola oil in cooking and salad dressings.
- A diet rich in fruits, vegetables, low-fat dairy products, and low in sodium and saturated fat can decrease BP, an effect that is enhanced by weight loss and increased physical activity.
- Consume 1/2 cup of nuts daily or 5 oz per week with a diet low in saturated fat and Chol to decrease TC. Nuts contain flavonoids, phenols, sterols, saponins, elegiac acid, folic acid, magnesium, copper, potassium, and fiber. Almonds are a very good source of vitamin E; walnuts contain ALA.
- Consume antioxidants from dietary sources. Vitamin E foods include asparagus, spinach, wheat germ, nuts, salad oils, and creamy salad dressings. Vitamin C foods should be consumed in amounts that meet DRI levels. Supplemental antioxidants alone or in combination with other antioxidants may act as pro-oxidants and have no protection for CVD events (ADA Evidence Analysis Library, 2009).
- Use flavonoids from tea, blueberries, yellow onions, red wine, grape juice, apples, cocoa, dark chocolate, products such as CocoaVia. Pomegranate increases antioxidant consumption and lowers LDL Chol (Arias and Ramon-Laca, 2005). Cinnamon, cloves, licorice, and sage are recommended as well.
- Consume a diet high in total fiber (17–30 g/d) and soluble fiber (7–13 g/d) as part of a diet low in saturated fat and Chol. Soluble fiber may include oatmeal, high fiber cereal, prunes, oat bran, corn bran, apples, and legumes as good sources. Risk factors associated with **BP**, lipoprotein subclasses and particle sizes, insulin resistance, postprandial glucose, fatal and non-fatal MI, or stroke are decreased as dietary fiber intake increases (ADA Evidence Analysis Library, 2009).
- Consume 2–3 g of plant sterols and stanols (through margarine, low-fat yogurt, orange juice, breads, and cereals) daily to lower total and LDL Chol, even with statins. Stanol-containing margarines may be consumed for at least 3 weeks before reassessment. Consume one extra carotenoid-rich fruit or vegetable per day to maintain plasma carotenoid levels when consuming sterol-enriched spreads.
- Pistachios, sunflower kernels, sesame seeds, and wheat germ are high in natural phytosterols; use often.
- Intake of approximately 1 g/d of EPA and DHA from a supplement or fish may decrease the risk of death from cardiac events in patients with heart disease. Regular consumption of an average of two servings of fatty fish per week (about 3.5 oz per serving) reduces risk of death from cardiac events. However, a low-to-moderate fat diet is also needed (Shah et al, 2009).
- Diets containing soy are well tolerated but soy will produce varied results based on initial Chol level and conditions such as diabetes.
- Use fewer animal proteins and more legumes or vegetable protein sources. Fish and shellfish may be used three to four times weekly, especially sources rich in omega-3 fatty acids. Remove chicken skin before cooking or just before serving. Lean beef and chicken are considered to be comparable.
- Trans fatty acids should be avoided; read labels.
- Provide chromium, copper, vitamin K in recommended amounts.
- A diet rich in folic acid, vitamins B_6 and B_{12}, betaine and choline might benefit cardiovascular health through a tHcy-lowering effect (da Costa et al, 2005; Olthof and Verhoef, 2005). Betaine is widely distributed in animals and plants, especially seafood, wheat germ, bran, and spinach; intake from foods is estimated at 0.5–2 g/d (Olthof and Verhoef, 2005).
- The DASH diet is useful; see Table 6-4. This diet will include 9–12 servings of fruits and vegetables, 2–3 servings of low-fat dairy products, less than 2.3 g sodium, weight loss if necessary, and increased physical activity with moderate intensity three times per week (ADA Evidence Analysis Library, 2009).

Common Drugs Used and Potential Side Effects

- Reduced progression of atherosclerosis is associated with intensive statin treatment which reduces both atherogenic lipoproteins and CRP (Nissen et al, 2005). Try "Diet First, Then Drugs": see Table 6-6.
- If anticoagulants (warfarin) are used, limit vitamin K–containing foods to 1 per day. Foods high in vitamin K include mayonnaise, canola and soybean oils, Brussels sprouts, collards, endive, spinach, watercress, red bibb lettuce, cabbage, broccoli, kale, and parsley.
- Aspirin may decrease serum ferritin by increasing occult blood loss if used over a long time.
- Digitalis and digoxin (Lanoxin) require the patient to avoid excessive amounts of vitamin D, natural licorice, fiber, and potassium. Take these drugs 30 minutes before meals. Do not take with herbal teas, Siberian ginseng, milkweed, hawthorn, guar gum, or St. John's wort.
- Gemfibrozil (Lopid) is used for elevated TGs when there is a risk of pancreatitis; taste changes or abdominal pain may occur. Probucol (Lorelco) may cause vomiting or anorexia.
- Statins reduce Chol production by the liver. They may lower coenzyme Q10 to the point of deficiency. Simvastatin may cause constipation; fluvastatin may cause nausea and abdominal cramps; pravastatin can elevate AST and ALT levels or cause nausea, vomiting, and diarrhea. Interestingly, statins support bone health. Increase omega-3 fatty acids and reduce the omega-6 to omega-3 ratio to allow statins to work more effectively.
- Thiazides, propranolol, estrogens, and oral contraceptives may increase lipid levels or may lower folate levels. Monitor for specific side effects.
- Colesevelam HCl (WelChol) can be used with statins; it is not absorbed into the bloodstream and has few side effects.

Herbs, Botanicals, and Supplements

- In one small clinical trial, red yeast rice and TLC decreased LDL Chol level without increasing CPK levels; this may be a treatment option for dyslipidemic patients who cannot tolerate statin therapy (Becker et al, 2009).

TABLE 6-6 Drugs Affecting Lipoprotein Metabolism

Drug Class	Agents and Daily Doses	Lipid/Lipoprotein Effects	Side Effects and Comments	Contraindications
Statins—HMG-CoA reductase inhibitors	Lovastatin (20–80 mg) Pravastatin (20–40 mg) Simvastatin (20–80 mg) Fluvastatin (20–80 mg) Atorvastatin (10–80 mg)	LDL-C, ↓18–55% HDL-C, →5–15% TG, ↓7–30%	Muscle pain and tenderness; myopathy Severe cases: rhabdomyolysis and release of myoglobin into the bloodstream Increased liver enzymes	Absolute: Active or chronic liver disease Relative: Concomitant use of certain drugs[a]
Bile acid sequestrant	Cerivastatin (0.4–0.8 mg) Cholestyramine (4–16 g) Colestipol (5–20 g) Colesevelam (2.6–3.8 g)	LDL-C, ↓15–30% HDL-C, →3–5% TG, No change or increase	GI distress Constipation; use more fiber Decreased absorption of other drugs Add folate and fat-soluble vitamins; mix with liquids	Absolute: Dysbetalipoproteinemia TG >400 mg/dL Relative: TG >200 mg/dL
Nicotinic acid (Nico-Bid, Nico-400)	Immediate-release (crystalline) nicotinic acid (1.5–3 g), extended-release nicotinic acid (Niaspan) (1–2 g), sustained-release nicotinic acid (1–2 g)	LDL-C, ↓5–25% HDL-C, →15–35% TG, ↓20–50%	Flushing Hyperglycemia Hyperuricemia (or gout) Upper GI distress Hepatotoxicity or altered LFTs Vomiting, diarrhea	Absolute: Chronic liver disease Severe gout Relative: Diabetes Hyperuricemia Peptic ulcer disease
Fibric acids	Gemfibrozil (600 mg BID) Fenofibrate (200 mg) Clofibrate (1000 mg BID)	LDL-C, ↓5–20% (may be increased in patients with high TG) HDL-C, →10–20% TG, ↓20–50%	Dyspepsia Gallstones Myopathy Weight gain Diarrhea, nause	Absolute: Severe renal disease Severe hepatic disease

HDL-C, high-density lipoprotein cholesterol; LDL-C, low-density lipoprotein cholesterol; TG, triglycerides; LFT, liver function test; GI, gastrointestinal.
Adapted from National Heart, Lung, and Blood Institute. Web site accessed July 7, 2009, at http://www.nhlbi.nih.gov/guidelines/cholesterol/atp3full.pdf.
[a]Cyclosporine, macrolide antibiotics, various antifungal agents, and cytochrome P-450 inhibitors (fibrates and niacin should be used with appropriate caution).

- Folic acid lowers plasma tHcy by 25% maximally, because 5-methyltetrahydrofolate is a methyl donor in the remethylation of tHcy to methionine (Olthof and Verhoef, 2005). In the NORVIT trial, researchers concluded that folic acid supplements could cause more harm than good if given with B_{12} supplements (Bonaa et al, 2006). However, betaine given in high doses (6 g/d and higher) acutely reduces increased tHcy after methionine loading by up to 50%, whereas folic acid has no effect (Olthof and Verhoef, 2005). This fact may have played a role in the outcome of recent folic acid trials where Albert et al (2008) and Ebbing (2008) and their colleagues reported that long-term studies for lowering tHcy with folic acid, B_{12} and B_6 supplements failed to prevent cardiac events.
- Herbs and botanicals such as angelica, hawthorn, canola, cinchona, valerian, willow, grape, pigweed, and chicory have proven efficacy. Discuss herbs and botanicals with the physician; see Table 6-3.

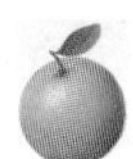

NUTRITION EDUCATION, COUNSELING, CARE MANAGEMENT

- Discuss the roles of heredity, exercise, and lifestyle habits. BP, Chol, obesity, and diabetes are affected by dietary patterns; some control is possible.
- Adherence with the 2005 Dietary Guidelines for Americans (DGA) is significantly associated with slower atherosclerosis progression and less metabolic syndrome (Fogli-Cawley et al, 2007; Imamura et al, 2009).
- There is no Chol in foods of plant origin. Encourage use of a plant-based diet.
- Explain which foods are sources of saturated fats and trans fatty acids. Identify foods that are sources of polyunsaturated fats and monounsaturated fats (olive and peanut oils). An easy first step is changing to skim milk products instead of whole milk.
- Diets low in fat have different tastes and textures. If one changes diet too quickly, the diet may seem dry and unpalatable. Suggest changing gradually. Teach new ideas for moistening foods without adding excess fat (e.g., using applesauce instead of oil in some baked goods). Provide lists of resources such as cookbooks, newsletters, product samples, or coupons.
- Describe food sources of saturated MUFAs and PUFAs and Chol; discuss olive, soybean, walnut, and peanut oil uses. Help the patient make suitable substitutions. Although egg yolks contain Chol, they can be planned into the diet three to four times weekly.
- Use of red wine appears to be protective, but more studies are needed to verify effects on hemodynamics (Karatzi et al, 2009).
- Fish should be included several times weekly. Omega-3 fatty acids are found in fatter fish such as salmon, herring, tuna, mackerel, and other seafood.
- Sources of soluble fiber (guar gum, pectin) include apples, legumes, oat and corn brans. Include other whole-grain foods for insoluble fiber as both types of fiber are beneficial.
- Encourage reading of food labels, including how to identify various ingredients such as "free, low, reduced" Chol.
- Aerobic exercise, weight loss, smoking cessation, and lifestyle changes are needed. Provide ideas, coping skills, motivational factors, and environmental barriers. Cardiac Rehabilitation programs that use a mind–body approach are useful.
- For individuals have MTHFR genetic allele, it is prudent to discuss dietary or supplemental measures (Klerk et al, 2002; Koo et al, 2008; Wiltshire et al, 2008). Sources of vitamin B_6 include eggs, meats, fish, vegetables, yeast, whole-wheat grains, and milk. Sources of vitamin B_{12} include liver, meat, eggs, dairy products, and fish. See Table 6-4 for good sources of folate.
- Discuss low-fat cooking methods, such as baking, broiling, flame cooking, grilling, marinating, poaching, roasting, smoking, or steaming.
- Olestra, a fat substitute, decreases absorption of dietary fat. Use in moderate amounts to prevent diarrhea.
- Routine periodic fasting has been shown to have merit in reducing risk of CAD (Horne et al, 2008).
- Intensive lifestyle changes maintained for 5 years or longer may be needed. A strict low fat diet can help reverse athersclerosis. Check serum lipids at least annually.

Patient Education—Foodborne Illness

- Careful food handling will be important. Hand washing is key as well.

For More Information

- American Heart Association—Atherosclerosis
  http://www.americanheart.org/presenter.jhtml?identifier=4440
- Dyslipidemia
  http://www.merck.com/mmpe/sec12/ch159/ch159b.html
- NCEP Guidelines
  http://www.nhlbi.nih.gov/about/ncep/index.htm
- NHLBI—ATP Guidelines, 2004 update
  http://www.nhlbi.nih.gov/guidelines/cholesterol/atp3upd04.htm
- Your LDL and You
  http://nhlbisupport.com/chd1/treatment.htm

ATHEROSCLEROSIS, CORONARY ARTERY DISEASE, DYSLIPIDEMIA—CITED REFERENCES

ADA Evidence Analysis Library. American Dietetic Association. Chicago, IL. Accessed November 7, 2009, at http://www.adaevidencelibrary.com/topic.cfm?cat=3015.

Albert CM, et al. Effect of folic acid and B vitamins on risk of cardiovascular events and total mortality among women at high risk for cardiovascular disease: a randomized trial. *JAMA.* 299;2027, 2008.

Arias BL, Ramon-Laca L. Pharmacological properties of citrus and their ancient and medieval uses in the Mediterranean region. *J Ethnopharmacol.* 97:89, 2005.

Becker DJ, et al. Red yeast rice for dyslipidemia in statin-intolerant patients. *Ann Intern Med.* 150:830, 2009.

Bonaa KH, et al. Homocysteine lowering and cardiovascular events after acute myocardial infarction. *New Engl J Med.* 354:1578, 2006.

Chen YC, et al. The HMG-CoA reductase gene and lipid and lipoprotein levels: the Multi-Ethnic Study of Atherosclerosis [published online ahead of print Jun 25, 2009]. *Lipids.* 44:733, 2009.

da Costa KA, et al. Choline deficiency in mice and humans is associated with increased plasma homocysteine concentration after a methionine load. *Am J Clin Nutr.* 81:440, 2005.

Das UN. Essential fatty acids—a review. *Curr Pharm Biotechnol.* 7:467, 2006.

Fogli-Cawley JJ, et al. The 2005 Dietary guidelines for Americans and risk of the metabolic syndrome. *Am J Clin Nutr.* 86:1193, 2007.

Freitas AI, et al. Methylenetetrahydrofolate reductase gene, homocysteine and coronary artery disease: the A1298 C polymorphism does matter. *Thromb Res.* 122:648, 2008.

Horne BD, et al. Usefulness of routine periodic fasting to lower risk of coronary artery disease in patients undergoing coronary angiography. *Am J Cardiol.* 102:814, 2008.

Ilhan N, et al. The 677 C/T MTHFR polymorphism is associated with essential hypertension, coronary artery disease, and higher homocysteine levels. *Arch Med Res.* 39:125, 2008.

Imamura F, et al. Adherence to 2005 Dietary guidelines for Americans is associated with a reduced progression of coronary artery atherosclerosis in women with established coronary artery disease. *Am J Clin Nutr.* 90:193, 2009.

Kathiresan S, et al. Common variants at 30 loci contribute to polygenic dyslipidemia. *Nat Genet.* 41:56, 2009.

Karatzi K, et al. Red wine, arterial stiffness and central hemodynamics. *Curr Pharm Des.* 15:321, 2009.

Klerk M, et al. MTHFR 677 C–>T polymorphism and risk of coronary heart disease: a meta-analysis. *JAMA.* 288:2023, 2002.

Koo HS, et al. Methylenetetrahydrofolate reductase tt genotype as a predictor of cardiovascular risk in hypertensive adolescents. *Pediatr Cardiol.* 29:136, 2008.

Locklin Holmes A, et al. Dietitian services are associated with improved patient outcomes and the MEDFICTS dietary assessment questionnaire is a suitable outcome measure in cardiac rehabilitation. *J Am Diet Assoc.* 105:1533, 2005.

Moller DE, Kaufman KD. Metabolic syndrome: a clinical and molecular perspective. *Annu Rev Med.* 56:45, 2005.

Ntaios G et al. Iatrogenic hyperhomocysteinemia in patients with metabolic syndrome: A systematic review and metaanalysis. [published online ahead of print August 19, 2010]. *Atherosclerosis.*

Nissen SE, et al. Statin therapy, LDL cholesterol, C-reactive protein, and coronary artery disease. *N Engl J Med.* 352:29, 2005.

Olthof MR, Verhoef P. Effects of betaine intake on plasma homocysteine concentrations and consequences for health. *Curr Drug Metab.* 6:15, 2005.

Shah KB, et al. The Cardioprotective effects of fish oil during pressure overload are blocked by high fat intake. role of cardiac phospholipid remodeling [published online ahead of print Jul 13, 2009]. *Hypertension.* 54:605, 2009.

Wiltshire EJ, et al. Methylenetetrahydrofolate reductase and methionine synthase reductase gene polymorphisms and protection from microvascular complications in adolescents with type 1 diabetes. *Pediatr Diabetes.* 9:348, 2008.

CARDIAC CACHEXIA

NUTRITIONAL ACUITY RANKING: LEVEL 4

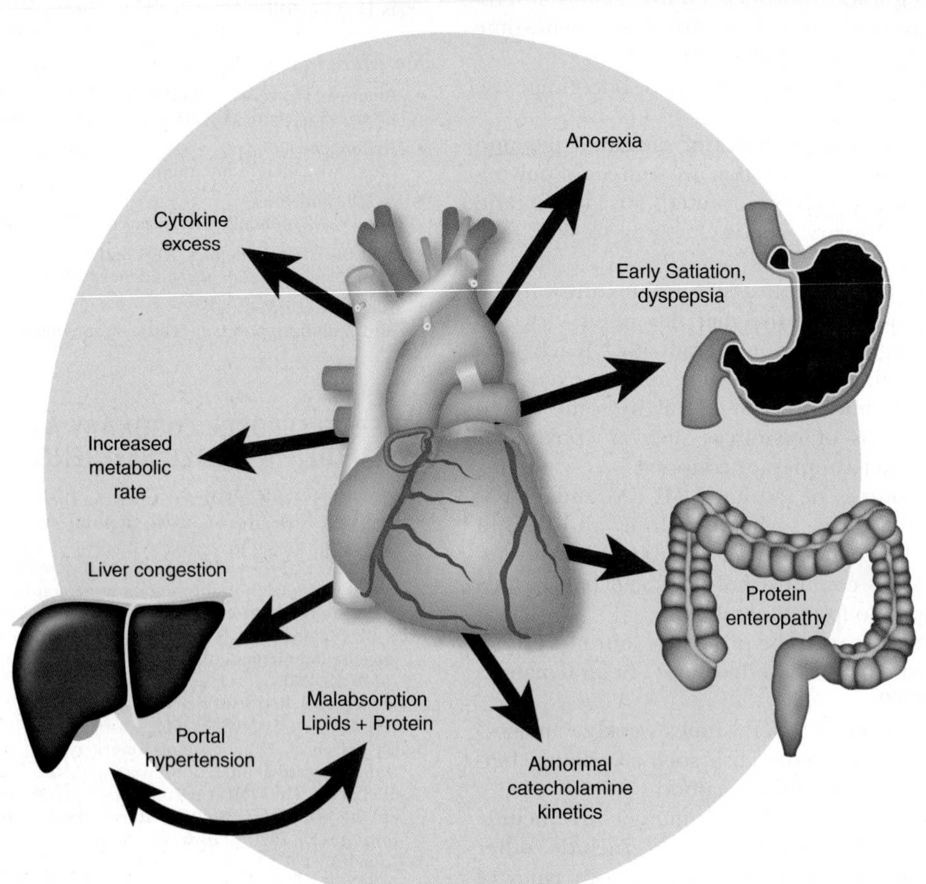

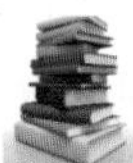

DEFINITIONS AND BACKGROUND

Cardiac cachexia is concurrent with HF of such severity that patients cannot eat adequately to maintain weight. It involves a loss of more than 10% of lean body mass and can clinically be defined as a body weight loss of 7.5% of previous dry body weight over 6 months or longer. The condition usually follows HF (moderate to severe), with some valvular heart disease. Nutritional insults generally affect the heart muscle severely, and the insult may be significant. While the pathophysiological alterations leading to cardiac cachexia are unclear, metabolic, neurohormonal and immune abnormalities may play a role. Cachectic HF patients show raised plasma levels of epinephrine, norepinephrine, cortisol, renin, and aldosterone. Patients with cardiac cachexia suffer from a general loss of fat tissue, lean tissue, and bone tissue. Lower, rather than higher, Chol levels are associated with poor clinical outcome in patients with chronic HF.

Chronic HF (CHF) is increasingly recognized as a multisystem disease with alterations in intestinal morphology, permeability, and absorption that lead to chronic inflammation (Sandek et al, 2009). The wasting associated with chronic HF is an independent predictor of mortality. A loss of body weight or skeletal muscle mass is common in older persons and precedes a poor outcome; starvation results in a loss of body fat and nonfat mass due to inadequate intake of protein and energy and sarcopenia is associated with a reduction in muscle mass and strength (Thomas, 2007). Cardiac cachexia as a terminal stage of chronic HF carries a poor prognosis (von Haehling et al, 2009).

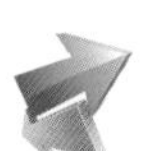

ASSESSMENT, MONITORING, AND EVALUATION

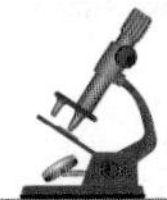

CLINICAL INDICATORS

Genetic Markers: Ghrelin (the growth-hormone-releasing peptide in the stomach) may play a role in cachexia; more studies are needed. Tumor necrosis factor may be involved (Anker et al, 2004). In addition, adiponectin seems to have a role in the wasting process.

Clinical/History

Height
Weight, current
Dry weight
BMI
Waist circumference; ascites?
Anorexia, weight loss?
Edema
BP
Fatigue
Shortness of breath (dyspnea)
Steatorrhea or diarrhea
Loss of muscle mass
Supraclavicular and temporal muscle wasting

Lab Work

Chol—total (low?)
Trig
CRP (elevated?)
CoQ10 serum levels
Gluc
Fecal fat (in steatorrhea)
H & H
Serum Fe, ferritin
Liver function tests
Thyroid-stimulating hormone (TSH)
Total lymphocyte count (TLC)
Serum insulin
Alb, transthyretin
Serum thiamin
Transferrin
Na^+, K^+
Ca^{++}, Mg^{++}
tHcy
Serum folate and vitamin B_{12}
Blood urea nitrogen (BUN)
Creatinine (Creat)

SAMPLE NUTRITION CARE PROCESS STEPS

Unintentional Weight Loss

Assessment Data: BMI <18, HF and shortness of breath, weight loss of 20 lb in 12 months.

Nutrition Diagnoses (PES): Unintentional weight loss related to low oral intake as evidenced by weight loss of 20 lb in past year and BMI 17.5.

Interventions: Education about ways to enhance energy and nutrient density in meals and snacks.

Monitoring and Evaluation: BMI now >19 in 3 months; better intake of energy-dense foods and beverages.

INTERVENTION

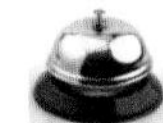

OBJECTIVES

- Improve hypoxic state and heart functioning.
- Correct malnutrition, wasting, malabsorption, and steatorrhea. Patients with HF have breathing difficulties, fatigue, nausea, loss of appetite, early feeling of fullness, or ascites that tend to decrease intake.
- Optimize heart function through balance of medications, antioxidants, fluids, and electrolytes.
- Reduce impact of inflammatory cytokines. Meet hypermetabolic state with adequate energy intake.
- Prevent infection or sepsis, especially if tracheostomy is required.
- Provide gradual repletion to prevent overloading in a severely depleted patient.
- Treat constipation or diarrhea as necessary.

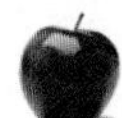

FOOD AND NUTRITION

- Energy needs may be calculated as high as 50% above basic needs.
- Protein should be estimated at a rate of 1.0–1.5 g/kg, increasing or decreasing depending on renal or hepatic status.
- Offer tube feeding (TF) or parenteral nutrition if appropriate. Sometimes, TFs are not well tolerated because of access to the thoracic cavity and reduced blood flow to the gastrointestinal (GI) tract. High-calorie, low-volume products have a high density of calories; they are appropriate for persons with a fluid limitation but must be monitored with renal or hepatic insufficiency.
- Provide small, frequent meals to prevent overloading with high glucose or fat. A diet high in saturated fat may actually be beneficial (Berthiaume et al, 2010).
- Provide as many preferred foods as feasible to improve appetite and intake.

- Antioxidants may benefit. Nutrient-dense foods containing omega-3 fatty acids can be safely recommended. Use more foods such as fish, fruits, cinnamon, cocoa, green tea, berries, nuts and foods that contain flavonols. Use the DASH diet as much as possible (Levitan et al, 2009).
- Sodium may need to be restricted to 1–2 g daily. In older patients, a more lenient 4–6 g may suffice. Modify potassium intake as appropriate. The DASH diet is useful.
- Diet may need to be high in folate, magnesium, zinc, iron (depending on serum levels), vitamins E, B_6, and B_{12}. Thiamin should be included to alleviate cardiac beri-beri, which is common.

Common Drugs Used and Potential Side Effects

- Therapeutic approaches include appetite stimulants such as megestrol acetate, medroxyprogesterone acetate, and cannabinoids (von Haehling et al, 2009).

Herbs, Botanicals, and Supplements

- Discuss herbs and botanicals with the physician. See Table 6-3.

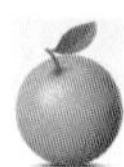

NUTRITION EDUCATION, COUNSELING, CARE MANAGEMENT

- Balance medications, fluid, and electrolytes carefully.
- Supplements may be beneficial between meals to improve total calorie intake (e.g., sherbet shakes).
- The importance of diet in cardiovascular health should be addressed, but rapid weight loss should be prevented. Patients with low BMI are at higher risk after cardiac surgery than obese patients.
- Exercise, with supervised guidance, can be beneficial to rebuild lean body mass.

Patient Education—Foodborne Illness

- Careful food handling will be important. Hand washing is key as well.

For More Information

- Cardiac Cachexia
  http://www.heartfailure.org/
- Heart Hope
  http://www.hearthope.com/
- Merck Manual—Heart Failure
  http://www.merck.com/mmpe/print/sec07/ch074/ch074a.html

CARDIAC CACHEXIA—CITED REFERENCES

Anker SD, Berthiaume JM, et al. The myocardial contractile response to physiological stress improves with high saturated fat feeding in heart failure. *Am J Physiol Heart Circ Physiol.* 299:410, 2010.

Hunt SA, et al. 2009 Focused update incorporated into the ACC/AHA 2005 Guidelines for the diagnosis and management of heart failure in adults. *J Am Coll Cardiol.* 53:e1, 2009.

Levitan EB, et al. Relation of consistency with the dietary approaches to stop hypertension diet and incidence of heart failure in men aged 45 to 79 years. *Am J Cardiol.* 104:1416, 2009.

Sandek A, et al. Nutrition in heart failure: an update. *Curr Opin Clin Nutr Metab Care.* 12:384, 2009.

Thomas DR. Loss of skeletal muscle mass in aging: Examining the relationship of starvation, sarcopenia and cachexia. *Clin Nutr.* 26:389, 2007.

von Haehling S, et al. Cardiac cachexia: a systematic overview. *Pharmacol Ther.* 121:227, 2009.

CARDIOMYOPATHIES

NUTRITIONAL ACUITY RANKING: LEVEL 3

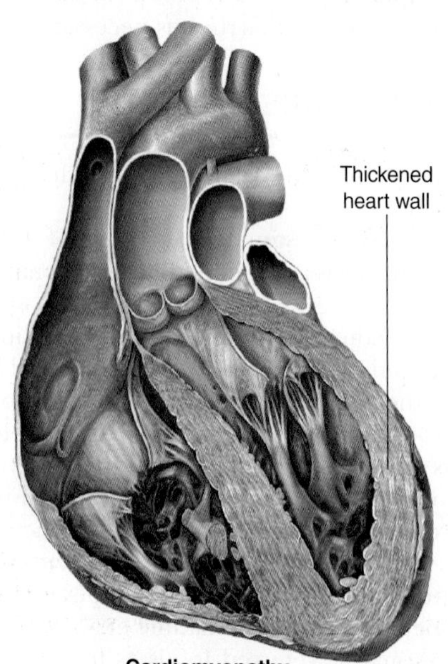

Cardiomyopathy

Asset provided by Anatomical Chart Co.

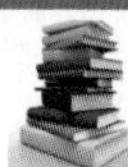

DEFINITIONS AND BACKGROUND

Cardiomyopathies may be caused by many known diseases or have no specific known cause. They are progressive disorders that impair the structure or function of the muscular wall of the lower chambers of the heart. Echocardiography is useful in demonstrating cardiac abnormalities.

In **restrictive cardiomyopathy**, the heart chambers are unable to properly fill with blood because of stiffness in the heart. Amyloidosis or scleroderma are common causes.

Dilated congestive cardiomyopathy (DCC) is most commonly caused by CHD in the United States. DCC may also occur from a viral infection such as coxsackievirus B, from diabetes or thyroid disease, or from excessive alcohol, cocaine, or antidepressant use. Rarely, pregnancy or rheumatory arthritis can also trigger DCC. Because prenatal dilated cardiomyopathy (DCM) can also be the presenting sign of cblC (cobalamin C deficiency) inborn errors of metabolism should be considered in view of the possible impact on treatment and future reproductive options (De Bie et al, 2009).

The first symptoms of DCC are shortness of breath on exertion and easy fatigability; sometimes, a fever and flu-like symptoms occur if triggered by a virus. Calcium and potassium irregularities have been noted (Olson et al, 2005). Remaining heart muscle stretches to compensate for lost pumping action, and when the stretching no longer compensates, DCC occurs. Blood may pool in the swollen heart, and clots may form on the chamber walls. Seventy percent of patients with DCC die within 5 years of the beginning of their symptoms, and the prognosis worsens as the walls become thinner and the heart valves begin to leak. Because of this, DCC is the most common cause for heart transplantation.

HCM may occur as a birth defect or as a result of acromegaly (excessive growth hormone in the blood), a pheochromocytoma, or a neurofibromatosis. Glycogen storage disease may also present with some cardiomyopathy (Arad et al, 2005). Thickening of the heart wall causes high BP, pulmonary hypertension, and chronic shortness of breath. Faintness, chest pain, irregular heartbeats and palpitations, and HF with dyspnea will occur. Hyperhomocysteinemia chelates copper and impairs copper-dependent enzymes; therefore, copper supplementation may be needed (Hughes et al, 2008).

HCM is a possible cause of sudden death; it is largely confined to young people but can occur suddenly at any stage of life. Most patients with mild hypertrophy are at low risk. Treatment options for patients with obstructive HCM include medical therapy, pacemaker insertion, percutaneous transluminal septal myocardial ablation, mitral valve replacement, and surgical resection of the obstructing muscle. Nonsurgical septal reduction therapy is also an effective therapy for symptomatic patients with obstructive HCM. A heart transplant may be indicated.

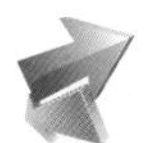

ASSESSMENT, MONITORING, AND EVALUATION

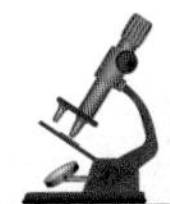

CLINICAL INDICATORS

Genetic Markers: About 90% of cases of HCM are familial with mutations in the MYBPC3 gene, encoding cardiac myosin-binding protein C (van Dijk et al, 2009). Genetic factors also may be responsible for half of DCM cases.

Clinical/History	ECG	CRP
Height	Cardiac catheterization	CoQ10 serum levels
Weight, current	Temperature	Prothrombin time (PT)
Dry weight	Dyspnea	INR
BMI	Fatigue and poor exercise tolerance	Na^+, K^+
Waist circumference	Ascites or edema	Ca^{++}, Mg^{++}
Diet history	**Lab Work**	Gluc
Heart murmur	Chol—total, HDL, LDL	H & H
Atrial fibrillation?	Trig	Serum Fe, ferritin
BP (normal or low)		Serum copper
Echocardiography		Serum insulin
Alb, transthyretin	Low serum vitamin D or rickets?	Homocystinuria?
Transferrin	Urinary methylmalonic acid	Serum tHcy
BUN, Creat		Serum folate and B_{12}

INTERVENTION

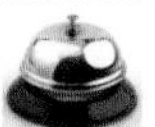

OBJECTIVES

- Improve hypoxic state and heart functioning.
- Correct malnutrition, malabsorption, and steatorrhea.
- Growth failure is a significant clinical problems of children with cardiomyopathy; nearly one third of these children manifest some degree of growth failure (Miller et al, 2007).
- Optimize heart function through balance of medications, fluids, and electrolytes.
- Meet hypermetabolic state with adequate calories.
- Provide gradual repletion to prevent overloading in a severely depleted patient.
- Treat constipation or diarrhea as necessary.
- Prepare for surgery, if planned.

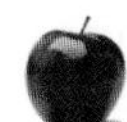

FOOD AND NUTRITION

- Energy may be calculated as much as 50% above usual needs. Optimal intake of macronutrients and antioxidants that can protect against free radical damage are needed (Miller et al, 2007).
- Protein should be calculated at a rate of 1.0–1.5 g/kg, increasing or decreasing depending on renal or hepatic status.
- Provide small, frequent meals to prevent overloading with high glucose or with rapid fat infusion. Provide as

SAMPLE NUTRITION CARE PROCESS STEPS

Excessive Intake of Fluids

Assessment Data: Dietary intake records; I & O records. Presence of 1+ pitting edema. Signs of cardiac failure with lung crackles.

Nurition Diagnosis (PES): Excessive intake of fluids related to food choices and preference for primarily soups and liquids on most days of the week as evidenced by edema, low BP and easy fatigue.

Intervention: Education and counseling about fluid limits using a food diary, fluid calculation chart, I & O records.

Monitoring and Evaluation: Weight maintenance versus fluctuations; improved intake records and food diaries reflecting successful management of fluid intake. Fewer symptoms of HF and improved breathing.

many preferred foods as feasible to improve appetite and intake.

- Follow TLC diet interventions. Pistachios, sunflower kernels, sesame seeds, and wheat germ are high in phytosterols; use often.
- The DASH diet is useful. Diet may need to be high in calcium and potassium (Olson et al, 2005); folate, magnesium, copper, zinc, and iron may also be needed, depending on serum levels. Increasing vitamins E, B_6, and B_{12} may be beneficial. Thiamin should also be included because of likelihood of cardiac beriberi.
- Sodium may need to be restricted to 2–4 g daily; modify potassium intake as appropriate for serum levels.
- Offer TF or parenteral nutrition if appropriate. Sometimes, TFs are not well tolerated because of proximity to the thoracic cavity and because of reduced blood flow to the GI tract. High-calorie, low-volume products are useful for their high density of calories. They are appropriate for persons with a fluid limitation but must be monitored in patients with renal or hepatic difficulty.

Common Drugs Used and Potential Side Effects

- Anticoagulant therapy is needed to prevent clots from causing heart attacks, strokes, and other problems. With warfarin (Coumadin), use a controlled amount of vitamin K; check TF products and supplements. Limit foods high in vitamin K to 1 serving per day. Foods high in vitamin K include mayonnaise, canola and soybean oils, Brussels sprouts, collards, endive, spinach, watercress, red bibb lettuce, cabbage, broccoli, kale, and parsley.
- Blood-thinning medications: Omega-3 fatty acids may increase the blood-thinning effects of aspirin or warfarin. While the combination of aspirin and omega-3 fatty acids may actually be helpful under certain circumstances (such as heart disease), they should only be taken together under the guidance and supervision of a health care provider. Be wary of using supplements containing vitamins A and C with these drugs; side effects may be detrimental. Vitamin E should not be taken with warfarin because of the possibility of increased bleeding; avoid doses greater than 400 IU/d. Avoid taking with dong quai, fenugreek, feverfew, excessive garlic, ginger, ginkgo, and ginseng because of their effects.
- Beta-blockers and calcium channel blockers may be used to reduce the force of heart contractions.
- Diuretics: Side effects may include potassium depletion; review types used and alter diet accordingly. Some diuretics spare calcium and protect bone health.
- Digoxin: Monitor potassium intake or depletion carefully, especially when combining with diuretics. Avoid excessive intakes of fiber and wheat bran. Avoid use with hawthorn, milkweed, guar gum, and St. John's wort.
- Insulin may be needed if patient has diabetes or becomes hyperglycemic. Alter mealtimes accordingly.

Herbs, Botanicals, and Supplements

- Table grape powder contains important phytochemicals; a diet with grape powder may reduce cardiac oxidative damage, increase cardiac glutathione, lower BP, improve cardiac function, reduce systemic inflammation, reduce cardiac hypertrophy and fibrosis (Seymour et al, 2008).
- Discuss herbs and botanicals with the physician. See Table 6-3. CoQ10 may be protective.
- Ephedra and adderol have been associated with cardiomyopathy and should be avoided.

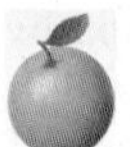

NUTRITION EDUCATION, COUNSELING, CARE MANAGEMENT

- Adequate rest is essential. Avoidance of stress is also important.
- Balance medications, fluid, and electrolytes carefully.
- Supplements may be beneficial between meals to improve total calorie intake (e.g., sherbet shakes).
- The importance of diet in cardiovascular health should be addressed. A moderate calorie restriction may be beneficial.
- Because of the high risk for sudden death in HCM patients, they should be advised against participation in highly competitive sports.
- For inherited forms of HCM, genetic counseling may be beneficial if planning a family.

Patient Education—Foodborne Illness

- Careful food handling will be important. Hand washing is key as well.

For More Information

- Cardiomyopathy
  http://www.americanheart.org/presenter.jhtml?identifier=4468
- Cardiomyopathy in the Young
  http://www.cardiomyopathy.org/Cardiomyopathy-in-the-Young.html
- Hypertrophic cardiomyopathy
  http://www.cardiomyopathy.org/

CARDIOMYOPATHIES—CITED REFERENCES

Arad M, et al. Glycogen storage diseases presenting as hypertrophic cardiomyopathy. *N Engl J Med.* 352:362, 2005.

De Bie I, et al. Fetal dilated cardiomyopathy: an unsuspected presentation of methylmalonic aciduria and hyperhomocystinuria, cblC type. *Prenat Diagn.* 29:266, 2009.

Hughes WM, et al. Role of copper and homocysteine in pressure overload heart failure. *Cardiovasc Toxicol.* 8:137, 2008.

Miller TL, et al. Nutrition in Pediatric Cardiomyopathy. *Prog Pediatr Cardiol.* 24:59, 2007.

Olson TM, et al. Sodium channel mutations and susceptibility to heart failure and atrial fibrillation. *JAMA.* 293:447, 2005.

Seymour EM, et al. Chronic intake of a phytochemical-enriched diet reduces cardiac fibrosis and diastolic dysfunction caused by prolonged salt-sensitive hypertension. *J Gerontol A Biol Sci Med Sci.* 63:1034, 2008.

van Dijk SJ, et al. Cardiac myosin-binding protein C mutations and hypertrophic cardiomyopathy: haploinsufficiency, deranged phosphorylation, and cardiomyocyte dysfunction. *Circulation.* 119:1473, 2009.

HEART FAILURE

NUTRITIONAL ACUITY RANKING: LEVEL 3

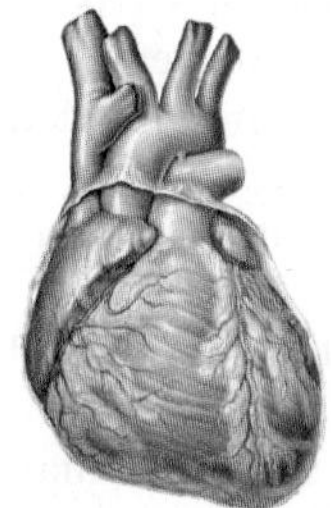

- **Heart Failure**
  Carbohydrates maintain sodium and fluid balance. A carbohydrate deficiency promotes loss of sodium and water, which can adversely affect blood pressure and cardiac function if not corrected.

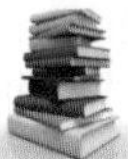

DEFINITIONS AND BACKGROUND

HF is the leading cause of CVD and related death, with nearly 5 million cases in the United States. HF results in reduced heart pumping efficiency in the lower two chambers, with less blood circulating to body tissues, congestion in lungs or body circulation, ankle swelling, abdominal pain, ascites, hepatic congestion, jugular vein distention, and breathing difficulty. The ability of mitochondria to oxidatively synthesize ATP from ADP and inorganic phosphate is compromised in the myocardium of HF patients.

Left ventricular failure will cause shortness of breath and fatigue; right ventricular failure causes peripheral and abdominal fluid accumulation. HF is a common diagnosis in hospitalized patients and four stages have been identified (Hunt et al, 2005):

- Stage A has mild symptoms and no limitation on physical activity.
- Stage B shows structural heart disease but no signs or symptoms of HF.
- Stage C demonstrates signs and symptoms of structural HF.
- Stage D shows refractory HF requiring specialized interventions.

HF can be caused by CHD, previous heart attack, history of cardiomyopathy, lung disease such as chronic obstructive pulmonary disease (COPD), severe anemia, excessive alcohol consumption, or low thyroid function. Male sex, lower education, physical inactivity, cigarette smoking, overweight, diabetes, hypertension, valvular heart disease, and CHD are all independent risk factors. The leading cause of HF in Western countries is ischemic heart disease. Therefore, aggressive therapy to halt progression of coronary atherosclerosis can have a major impact on controlling or curing HF.

B-type natriuretic peptide (BNP) is secreted by ventricles when pressure goes up in the heart. CoQ10 has been identified as a factor to consider. Patients with HF have low plasma levels of CoQ10, an essential cofactor for mitochondrial electron transport and myocardial energy supply (Molyneux et al, 2008). Low plasma TC concentrations have also been associated with higher mortality in HF; the relationship between CoQ10 and LDL-C levels may contribute to this association (Molyneux et al, 2008).

Decreased renal flow is common; BUN may be increased. Early adaptations to mild HF show susceptibility to sodium excess. Evidence suggests that advanced HF is a multifactorial metabolic syndrome that can lead to cardiac cachexia, which then carries a very poor prognosis. The mechanisms underlying this association are poorly understood. Inflammatory cytokines may play a pathogenic role. HF is associated with elevated levels of angiotensin II in the blood, causing vessel contraction and high BP in addition to muscle wasting. Studies are reviewing the role of other factors.

Dairy nutrients (calcium, potassium and magnesium) have a BP lowering effect, as shown by studies showing the effectiveness of the DASH diet (Levitan et al, 2009). Low calcium increases intracellular calcium concentrations, thereby increasing 1,25-dihydroxyvitamin D(3) and parathyroid hormone (PTH), causing calcium influx into vascular smooth muscle cells and greater vascular resistance (Kris-Etherton et al, 2009). Dairy peptides may act as ACE inhibitors, thereby inhibiting the renin-angiotensin system with consequent vasodilation (Kris-Etherton et al, 2009). While sodium restriction and diuretics are basic treatments, treatment may also include implantation of a pacemaker or even cardiac transplantation. Joint efforts of cardiologists, endocrinologists, immunologists, and registered dietitians are required to develop effective therapeutic strategies. Referral to a registered dietitian is needed for MNT. For a person with HF, one planned initial visit and at least one to three planned follow-up visits can lead to improved dietary pattern and quality of life, decreased edema and fatigue, more optimal pharmacological management, and fewer hospitalizations (American Dietetic Association, 2009).

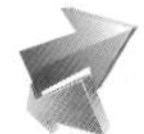

ASSESSMENT, MONITORING, AND EVALUATION

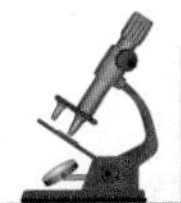

CLINICAL INDICATORS

Genetic Markers: Nuclear factor kappa B (NF-kappaB) is chronically activated in cardiac myocytes; the NFKB1 -94 insertion/deletion ATTG polymorphism is associated with DCM (Zhou et al, 2009).

Clinical/History

Height
Weight
BMI
Waist–hip ratio
Weight changes?
Diet history
BP
Shortness of breath
Dry, hacking cough or wheezing
Skin, cyanotic or pale
Abnormal breath sounds
Increased heart rate; pulse >80 beats/min
Temperature
Pitting edema, fatigue (right-sided HF)
Pulmonary edema, rales, dyspnea (left-sided HF)
Glomerular filtration rate (GFR)
Oliguria
Confusion, impaired thinking
Chest x-ray
Echocardiography

ECG	Partial pressure of oxygen (pO_2)	Ca^{++}, Mg^{++}
Cardiac catheterization	Specific gravity (increased)	Gluc
	Chol—total, HDL, LDL	Serum zinc
Lab Work	Trig	Alk phos
CRP	H & H	Alb, transthyretin
Serum CoQ10	Serum Fe, ferritin	BUN, Creat
BNP or NT-pro-BNP levels	tHcy	PT or INR
Uric acid	Serum folate	LDH (increased)
Oximetry	Serum B_{12}	Nitrogen (N) balance
Partial pressure of carbon dioxide (pCO_2)	Na^+, K^+	AST, ALT

INTERVENTION

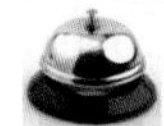

OBJECTIVES

- Lessen demands on the heart and restore hemodynamic stability.
- Prevent cardiogenic shock, thromboembolism, and renal failure.
- Maintain BP <140/90 mm Hg in all patients or <130/80 mm Hg in those with diabetes or chronic kidney disease (Khan et al, 2009).
- Eliminate or reduce edema.
- Avoid distention and elevation of diaphragm, which reduces vital capacity. Avoid overfeeding in cachexic patients to prevent refeeding syndrome.
- Attain desirable BMI and WHR to decrease oxygen requirements and tissue nutrient demands. Replenish lean body mass (LBM) when needed.

SAMPLE NUTRITION CARE PROCESS STEPS

Herb and Drug–Nutrient Interactions

Assessment Data: Food frequency recall and intake records; medical prescription for warfarin. Taking large doses of vitamin K supplement randomly, and St John's wort (300 mg BID) for "the blues."

Nutrition Diagnosis (PES): Excessive bioactive substance intake (N1-4.2) related to knowledge deficit as evidenced by subtherapeutic INR of 1.2.

Intervention: Education about supplement-drug interaction and effects of vitamin K while using warfarin. Counseling to discontinue use of St. John's wort and consider psychological counseling. Coordinate care and referral for counseling.

Monitoring and Evaluation: Repeat INR weekly until therapeutic dose is achieved. Assess compliance with discontinuation of St John's wort and random use of vitamin K supplements. Assess understanding of risks of use of herbs or supplements while taking warfarin.

- Prevent or correct cardiac cachexia, low BP, listlessness, weak pulse from potassium-depleting diuretics, anorexia, nausea and vomiting, and sepsis.
- Correct nutrient deficits. Assure adequate intake of dairy products, as tolerated (Kris-Etherton et al, 2009).
- Because anemia is associated with an increased risk of mortality in both systolic and diastolic HF, strategies to increase hemoglobin levels should be used when needed (Groenveld et al, 2008).
- Encourage use of omega-3 fatty acids with a low-to-moderate fat intake (Shah et al, 2009).
- Prevent pressure ulcers from reduced activity levels and poor circulation.
- Promote use of the DASH diet and whole grains (Levitan et al, 2009; Nettleton et al, 2009). In addition, promote weight reduction, physical activity, restriction of dietary sodium, and excessive alcohol intake as methods for lowering BP.

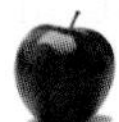

FOOD AND NUTRITION

Evidence-based recommendations for Registered Dietitians (RDs) to follow in providing nutrition treatment for people with HF include (American Dietetic Association, 2009):

- Appropriate daily intake of protein for clinically stable patients; HF patients have significantly higher protein needs than those without HF.
- Fluid intake between 48 and 64 oz/d, depending on fatigue or shortness of breath.
- Sodium intake less than 2 g/d to improve clinical symptoms and quality of life.
- Consume folate through food and/or a combination of B_6, B_{12}, and folate supplementation.
- Promote the DASH diet, with adequate potassium, calcium, and magnesium (Gums, 2004). Table 6-7 lists the sodium content of common foods. Table 6-8 provides some alternative tips for lowering sodium in the diet. For TF, use a low-sodium product and increase volume gradually.
- With total parenteral nutrition, ensure adequate intake of all micronutrients as well as macronutrients.
- Provide antioxidants, such as vitamin E, at DRI levels; there is no evidence that more is better. It is safe to consume more pomegranate, blueberry, and grape products.
- If patient is obese, a calorie-controlled diet can be recommended. A vegan pattern may be helpful with five to six small meals daily.
- Limit caffeine only if needed. The evidence is not definitive in this area (Ahmed et al, 2009).
- Beans, cabbage, onions, cauliflower, and Brussels sprouts may cause heartburn or flatulence; avoid if needed.
- Whole grains cut the risk for HF while eggs and high-fat dairy products contribute to it, according to the ARIC study (Nettleton et al, 2009). Add soluble fiber to the diet from apples or oat bran.
- Pistachios, sunflower kernels, sesame seeds, and wheat germ are high in phytosterols; use often.
- Thiamin levels tend to be low. Cardiovascular problems may be associated with beri-beri.
- Limit alcohol intake; for women, 1 drink per day and for men, 2 drinks or less a day.

TABLE 6-7 Sodium Content of Typical Food Items

Food Item	Milligrams (mg)	Food Item	Milligrams (mg)
Meat, poultry, and fish		**Dairy products**	
Sirloin steak (3 oz)	53	Butter, salted (1 tbsp)	116
Baked salmon (3 oz)	55	Milk (1 cup)	122
Chicken breast (3 oz)	64	Sour cream (1 cup)	123
Ground beef patty (4 oz)	87	Margarine (1 tbsp)	134
Chicken leg, fried (2.5 oz)	194	Chocolate pudding (1 cup)	180
Tuna, canned (3 oz)	468	Baked custard (1 cup)	209
Hot dog (1)	504	Buttermilk (1 cup)	257
Salami (2 slices)	607	Parmesan cheese (1/4 cup)	465
Fast food hamburger (4 oz)	763	Cheddar cheese (1 cup)	701
Corned beef (3 oz)	802	Cottage cheese, creamy (1 cup)	911
Ham, canned (3 oz)	908	Cheese sauce, prepared from recipe (1 cup)	1198
Fast foods, shrimp, breaded and fried (6–8 shrimp)	1446	**Snacks, drinks, condiments, desserts**	
Submarine sandwich (one 6″ roll, cold cuts)	1651	Orange juice (1 cup)	2
Smoked salmon (3 oz)	1700	Peanuts, unsalted (1 cup)	22
Soups, Vegetables, Fruit		Chocolate fudge (1 oz)	54
Apple (1)	0	Diet cola, with Saccharin	75
Banana (1)	1	Club soda (12 oz)	78
Mixed vegetables, frozen (1 cup)	64	Potato chips (10)	94
Mixed vegetables, canned (1 cup)	243	Mustard (1 tbsp)	129
Chicken noodle soup, canned (1 cup)	1106	Ketchup (1 tbsp)	156 (1 cup)
Tomato sauce, canned (1 cup)	1482	Hard pretzel (1)	258
Sauerkraut (1 cup)	1560	Shortbread cookies (2)	300
Breads and grains		Apple pie (1 slice)	476
Wheat bread (1 slice)	106	Peanuts, salted (1 cup)	626
Oatmeal, cooked (1 cup)	2	Vegetable juice (1 cup)	883
Italian bread (1 slice)	176	Dill pickle (1)	928
Bagel (1)	245	Pretzel twists (10)	966
English muffin (1)	378	Pie crust, 1 shell	976
Bread crumbs (1 cup)	3180	Beef bouillon (1 packet)	1019

REFERENCE

USDA Nutrient Database. Web site accessed July 7, 2009, at http://www.nal.usda.gov/fnic/foodcomp/Data/SR14/wtrank/sr14w307.pdf.

TABLE 6-8 Tips for Lowering Sodium in the Diet

Choose More Often

- Fresh, plain frozen, or canned "with no salt added" vegetables
- Fresh poultry, fish, and lean meat, rather than canned or processed types
- Rice, pasta, and hot cereals cooked without salt. Cut back on instant or flavored rice, pasta, and cereal mixes, which usually have added salt.
- "Convenience" foods that are lower in sodium. Cut back on frozen dinners, pizza, packaged mixes, canned soups or broths, and salad dressings; these often have a lot of sodium
- Canned foods, such as tuna, drained and rinsed to remove some sodium
- Low- or reduced-sodium or no salt added versions of foods
- Ready-to-eat breakfast cereals that are lower in sodium, such as shredded wheat
- Rinse canned beans before using
- Herbs, spices, and salt-free seasoning blends in cooking and at the table. To make a spice blend, mix together 1 tablespoon each: ground cumin, onion powder, ground celery seed, ground basil, ground marjoram, ground oregano, ground thyme, ground coriander, crushed rosemary, garlic powder and paprika. One teaspoon contains 10 mg sodium and 46 mg potassium

Choose Less Often

- Hogmaws, ribs, and chitterlings
- Smoked or cured meats like bacon, bologna, hot dogs, ham, corned beef, luncheon meats, and sausage
- Canned fish like tuna, salmon, sardines, and mackerel
- Buttermilk
- Most cheese spreads and cheeses
- Salty chips, nuts, pretzels, and pork rinds
- Some cold (ready to eat) cereals highest in sodium, instant hot cereals
- Quick cooking rice and instant noodles, boxed mixes like rice, scalloped potatoes, macaroni and cheese, and some frozen dinners, pot pies, and pizza
- Regular canned vegetables
- Pickled foods such as herring, pickles, relish, olives, and sauerkraut
- Regular canned soups, instant soups
- Butter, fatback, and salt pork
- Soy sauce, steak sauce, salad dressing, ketchup, barbecue sauce, garlic salt, onion salt, seasoned salts like lemon pepper, bouillon cubes, meat tenderizer, and monosodium glutamate (MSG)

From: National Heart, Lung, and Blood Institute. Reduce salt and sodium in your diet. Accessed July 7, 2009, at http://www.nhlbi.nih.gov/hbp/prevent/sodium/sodium.htm.

- The following Figure provides a suggested interdisciplinary nutrition care plan:

INTERDISCIPLINARY NUTRITION CARE PLAN
Congestive Heart Failure (CHF)

Client Name: ________ **#:** ________ **Initiated by:** ________ **Date:** ________

SCREEN
Nutrition Screen diagnosis: CHF
Signed: ________ Date: ________

GOALS (Check any/all):

❑ Maintain or improve nutritional status in ____ (goal time).

❑ Eat meals/snacks without experiencing shortness of breath (SOB) in ____ (goal time).

❑ Perform Activities of Daily Living (ADLs) with minimal SOB in ____ (goal time).

ASSESS *(Check any/all)*
Shortness of breath (SOB) while
❑ Eating ❑ Performing ADLs
Weight/BMI
❑ BMI <20 (High Risk)
❑ BMI <27
❑ Fluctuations ≥ 3–5 lb/wk
Hydration status
❑ Edema ❑ 1+ ❑ 2+ ❑ 3+
❑ Fluid restriction
Exercise tolerance
❑ Fatigue ❑ Restlessness
❑ **Medications**
❑ **Pre- or postsurgery**
Poor Oral Intake Symptoms
❑ Complex diet order
❑ Nausea/vomiting
❑ Poor appetite/early satiety
❑ Problems chewing/swallowing
❑ Depression/anxiety
❑ GI distress
❑ Anorexia
Signed: ________ Date: ________

None →

MODERATE RISK INTERVENTIONS
(Check any/all)
❑ **Eating Well With CHF** provided and explained
❑ **Food Record** provided and explained
❑ **How to read labels for sodium content explained and encouraged**
Obtain Dr. orders as needed:
❑ RD chart consult
❑ Monitor weight q:_____
❑ BID/TID supplements
❑ **Other:**________
(See notes for documention.)
Signed: ________ Date: ________

Next visit ↓

ASSESS RESPONSE *(Check any/all)*
SOB while
❑ Eating ❑ Performing ADLs
❑ Weight fluctuations
❑ Exercise tolerance declining
❑ Fatigue increasing
Hydration status
❑ Edema ❑ Dehydration
❑ **Other:**________
(See notes for documention.)
Signed: ________ Date: ________

None →

OUTCOMES ACHIEVED
❑ SOB decreased
❑ Weight stabilized or improved
❑ Exercise tolerance maintained or improved
❑ Hydration status maintained or improved
❑ Nutritional status maintained or improved
❑ **Other:**________
(See notes for documention.)
❑ Repeat Nutrition Risk Screen in ____ days
Signed: ________ Date: ________

1 or more ↓ (from ASSESS); ← 1 or more (from ASSESS RESPONSE)

HIGH-RISK INTERVENTIONS *(Check any/all)*
❑ **Eating Well With CHF** provided and explained
❑ **Food Record** provided and explained
❑ **How to read labels and track sodium intake stressed**
Obtain Dr. orders as needed:
❑ RD referral for home visit(s)
❑ Monitor weight q:_____
❑ Monitor I & O q:_____
❑ Multiple vitamin/mineral supplement
❑ BID/TID supplements
❑ **Other:**________
(See notes for documention.)
Signed: ________ Date: ________

Next visit ↓

ASSESS RESPONSE *(Check any/all)*
SOB while
❑ Eating ❑ Performing ADLs
❑ Continued weight fluctuation
Hydration status
❑ Continued or increased edema
❑ Dehydration
❑ Exhibiting poor oral intake symptoms
❑ **Other:**________
(See notes for documention.)
Signed: ________ Date: ________

None →

OUTCOMES ACHIEVED
❑ SOB decreased
❑ Weight maintained or improved
❑ Exercise tolerance maintained or improved
❑ Hydration status maintained or improved
❑ Nutritional status maintained or improved
❑ **Other:**________
(See notes for documention.)
❑ Repeat Nutrition Risk Screen in ____ days
Signed: ________ Date: ________

1 or more ↓

OUTCOMES NOT ACHIEVED
Reassess/evaluate need for EN/PN (refer to Tube Feeding Nutrition Care Plan). Document on Nutrition Variance Tracking form.

Adapted with permission from www.RD411.com, Inc.

Common Drugs Used and Potential Side Effects

- Most patients with HF require combination therapy that includes a diuretic, an ACE inhibitor, an angiotensin II receptor blocker, beta-blockers, aldosterone antagonists, specialized implantable pacemakers. Once BP is controlled, acetylsalicylic acid therapy should be considered (Kahn et al, 2009).
- Nesiritide, a recombinant form of BNP may be used with acute HF (Waldo et al, 2008). Because obesity is associated with lower BNP levels in healthy individuals and patients with chronic congestive HF, use caution for interpretation of BNP levels (Krauser et al, 2005).
- Teach how to manage vitamin K intake if on warfarin. See Table 6-9.

TABLE 6-9 Medications Used in Heart Failure

Medication	Description	Medication	Description
Angiotensin-converting enzyme (ACE) inhibitors Benazepril (*Lotensin*) Captopril (*Capoten*) Enalapril (*Vasotec*) Fosinopril (*Monopril*) Lisinopril (*Zestril/Prinivil*) Moexipril (*Univasc*) Perindopril (*Aceon*) Quinapril (*Accupril*) Ramipril (*Altace*) Trandolapril (*Mavik*)	ACE inhibitors block angiotensin II and decrease aldosterone output, thereby decreasing sodium and water retention. Monitor for hyperkalemia, nausea, vomiting, dizziness, and abdominal pain.	**Adrenergic system blockers** **Beta-blockers** Atenolol (*Tenormin*) Bisoprolol (*Zebeta*) Carvedilol (*Coreg*) Metoprolol (*Toprol XL*) Propranolol (*Inderal*)	Beta-adrenergic blockers reduce cardiac output in competing for available receptor sites; they decrease sympathetic stimulation of the heart. At first use, they may cause fatigue and fluid retention.
		Cardiac glycosides **Digitalis** Lanoxin (Digoxin)	Digitalis can deplete potassium, especially when taken with furosemide. Beware of excesses of wheat bran, which can decrease serum drug levels. Anorexia or nausea may occur.
Angiotensin receptor blockers Candesartan (*Atacand*) Eprosartan (*Teveten*) Irbesartan (*Avapro*) Losartan (*Cozaar*) Olmesartan (*Benicar*) Telmisartan (*Micardis*) Valsartan (*Diovan*)	Common adverse effects include hypotension and dizziness, a concern when there is also blurred vision or worsening renal function.	**Diuretics** Hydrochlorothiazide (*Microzide*); Eplerenone (*Inspra*); Furosemide (*Lasix*); Spironolactone (*Aldactone*)	Avoid use with fenugreek, ginkgo, and yohimbe. Some diuretics spare calcium and protect bone health.
Aldosterone blockers Eplerenone, Spironolactone		**Loop diuretics** Bumetanide, Furosemide (Lasix), Torsemide	Most loop diuretics deplete potassium and magnesium; calcium levels also decline. Glucose tolerance may be decreased; anorexia, nausea, or vomiting may occur. Use a low-sodium diet. Avoid use with Nonsteroidal anti-inflammatory drugs (NSAIDs).
Anticoagulants Warfarin (Coumadin)	Consume foods high in vitamin K no more than once per day. Foods with high vitamin K content include: spinach, broccoli, Brussels sprouts, green raw cabbage, turnip greens, mustard greens, collard greens, parsley, green scallions, lettuce, endive, watercress, cucumber peels, kale, canola oil, soybean oil, raw chives, green onions, seaweed, green peas, liver, Swiss chard. Avoid taking with dong quai, fenugreek, feverfew, ginger, ginkgo, ginseng, excesses of ginger, aniseed, celery, cranberry juice, dandelion, licorice, onion, passion flower, or willow bark. Coenzyme Q10, green tea, goldenseal, St. John's wort, and yarrow will decrease the effectiveness of warfarin.	**Thiazide diuretics** Hydrochlorothiazide (*Microzide*) Chlorthalidone Indapamide Metolazone	Most thiazide diuretics deplete potassium, which must be replaced, either orally or by medication. Hyperkalemia can occur with use of potassium-sparing diuretics if lab values are not carefully monitored. Use potassium-rich foods and juices such as orange juice, bananas, potatoes. Monitor for signs of dehydration.
		Potassium-sparing diuretics Amiloride Spironolactone (Aldactone) Triamterene (Dyrenium)	No extra K^+ is needed.
		Salt substitutes	Salt substitutes generally contain KCl. Use could lead to hyperkalemia if potassium-sparing diuretics are part of treatment.
		Statins	Statins may be used if the underlying problem is related to coronary artery disease or dyslipidemia.

REFERENCE

Hunt et al, 2005. Cleveland Clinic, website accessed 10/11/10 at: http://www.clevelandclinic.org/health/health-info/docs/1800/1822.asp?index=8121

Hunt SA, et al. ACC/AHA 2005 guideline update for the diagnosis and management of chronic heart failure in the adult: a report of the American College of Cardiology/American Heart Association Task Force on Practice Guidelines (Writing Committee to Update the 2001 Guidelines for the Evaluation and Management of Heart Failure). *J Am Coll Cardiol.* 46:e-1, 2005.

Herbs, Botanicals, and Supplements

- The patient should not take herbals and botanicals without discussing with the physician. It is important to stress that no supplement or diet can cure HF. Taurine, hawthorn, magnesium, and other supplements have not been documented as effective at this time. See Tables 6-3 and 6-9 for more details.
- CoQ10 deficiency is detrimental to the long-term prognosis of HF (Molyneux et al, 2008). Supplementation of both CoQ10 and creatine may prove to be useful in HF; more controlled trials are needed.
- Supplementation with eicosapentaenoic acid (EPA) and docosahexaenoic acid (DHA) from fish oil may prevent HF through lowering proinflammatory fatty acid arachidonic acid and urine thromboxane B2; high-fat diets (60% fat) block these effects in the chronically stressed myocardium.
- Pomegranate (*Punica granatum*) berries, grape and other antioxidant-rich juices can be safely consumed.

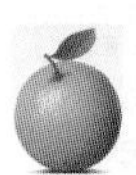

NUTRITION EDUCATION, COUNSELING, CARE MANAGEMENT

- Identify the stage of readiness for change in the patient. The most difficult lifestyle changes include smoking cessation, weight loss, and restriction of dietary sodium (Paul and Sneed, 2004). Supervised nutrition intervention is of great importance (Colin Ramirez et al, 2004).
- Help patient plan fluid intake; usually 75% with meals and 25% with medications or between meals.
- A congested feeling may cause a poor appetite. Offer small, appetizing, frequent snacks, or meals. Use high-calorie, low-volume supplements to increase nutrient density when needed.
- Never force the patient to eat; rest before and after meals. Naps are good for heart health. Even bed rest may be required. To reduce congestion in the lungs, the patient's upper body should be elevated. For most patients, resting in an armchair is better than lying in bed. Relaxing and contracting leg muscles are important to prevent blood clots. As the patient improves, progressively more activity will be recommended.
- HF is associated with sleep apnea, in which tissues at the back of the throat periodically collapse and become blocked, causing the sleeper to gasp for air. Sleep apnea is associated with poorer survival in patients with HF. A continuous positive airway pressure (CPAP) device appears to improve ejection fraction; see Section 5.
- Teach label reading and tips for easy meal preparation. Choose items that state: sodium free, very low sodium, low sodium, reduced sodium, light in sodium, or unsalted. Avoid excessive use of canned soups, cured or smoked meats, and commercial sauces. Many frozen dinners are high in sodium; choose healthier brands.
- Check the water supply for use of softening agents. Monitor sodium-containing medications, toothpastes, and mouthwashes. Discuss spices and seasonings as salt alternatives.
- Freeze small meal portions to simplify meal preparation. Refer to local congregate meal programs or inquire about home-delivered meals if needed; many will provide low-sodium meals upon request.
- Implantation of circulatory assist devices as a permanent alternative to heart transplantation (destination therapy) is used with patients with HF who are not responding to medications. The HeartMate Left Ventricular Assist System is FDA-approved.

Patient Education—Foodborne Illness

- Careful food handling will be important. Hand washing is key as well.

For More Information

- Heart Failure
  http://www.hearthope.com/learn.html
- National Heart, Lung, and Blood Institute
  http://www.nhlbi.nih.gov/hbp/hbp/effect/heart.htm
  http://www.nhlbi.nih.gov/hbp/prevent/h_eating/h_eating.htm
- Spices and Seasonings
  http://www.nhlbi.nih.gov/hbp/prevent/sodium/flavor.htm

HEART FAILURE—CITED REFERENCES

Ahmed HN, et al. Coffee consumption and risk of heart failure in men: an analysis from the Cohort of Swedish Men. *Am Heart J.* 158:667, 2009.

American Dietetic Association. Heart Failure Evidence-Based Nutrition Practice Guideline. Accessed July 13, 2009, at http://www.adaevidencelibrary.com/topic.cfm?cat=3249.

Colin Ramirez E, et al. Effects of a nutritional intervention on body composition, clinical status, and quality of life in patients with heart failure. *Nutrition.* 20:890, 2004.

Groenveld HF, et al. Anemia and mortality in heart failure patients a systematic review and meta-analysis. *J Am Coll Cardiol.* 52:818, 2008.

Gums JG. Magnesium in cardiovascular and other disorders. *Am J Health Syst Pharm.* 61:1569, 2004.

Kahn NA, et al. The 2009 Canadian Hypertension Education Program recommendations for the management of hypertension: Part 2—therapy. *Can J Cardiol.* 25:287, 2009.

Krauser DG, et al. Effect of body mass index on natriuretic peptide levels in patients with acute congestive heart failure: a ProBNP Investigation of Dyspnea in the Emergency Department (PRIDE) substudy. *Am Heart J.* 149:744, 2005.

Kris-Etherton P, et al. Milk products, dietary patterns and blood pressure management. *J Am Coll Nutr.* 28:103S, 2009.

Levitan EB, et al. Consistency with the DASH diet and incidence of heart failure. *Arch Intern Med.* 169:851, 2009.

Molyneux SL, et al. Coenzyme Q10: an independent predictor of mortality in chronic heart failure. *J Am Coll Cardiol.* 52:1435, 2008.

Nettleton JA, et al. Incident heart failure is associated with lower whole-grain intake and greater high-fat dairy and egg intake in the Atherosclerosis Risk in Communities (ARIC) study. *J Am Diet Assoc.* 108:1881, 2009.

Paul S, Sneed NV. Strategies for behavior change in patients with heart failure. *Am J Crit Care.* 13:305, 2004.

Schulman SP, et al. L-arginine therapy in acute myocardial infarction: the Vascular Interaction with Age in Myocardial Infarction (VINTAGE MI) randomized clinical trial. *JAMA.* 295:58, 2006.

Shah KB, et al. The cardioprotective effects of fish oil during pressure overload are blocked by high fat intake. Role of cardiac phospholipid remodeling [published online ahead of print Jul 13, 2009]. *Hypertension.* 54:65, 2009.

Waldo SW, et al. Pro-B-type natriuretic peptide levels in acute decompensated heart failure. *J Am Coll Cardiol.* 51:1874, 2008.

Zhou B, et al. Functional polymorphism of the NFKB1 gene promoter is related to the risk of dilated cardiomyopathy. *BMC Med Genet.* 10:47, 2009.

HEART TRANSPLANTATION OR HEART–LUNG TRANSPLANTATION

NUTRITIONAL ACUITY RANKING: LEVEL 4

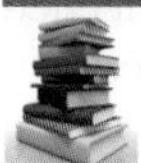

DEFINITIONS AND BACKGROUND

Heart transplantation (HTx) is usually performed for terminal HF, often with cardiomyopathy. Usually, the transplantation will be a Jarvik-7 or a live donor heart. Screening includes evaluations for chronic, coexisting illness, psychosocial stability, and normal or reversible cardiac status. The best candidates are younger than 55 years of age with normal hepatic and renal functioning and are free of diabetes mellitus and pulmonary problems, peptic ulcers, and peripheral heart disorders.

Heart–lung transplantation is rare, as for complex cases of cystic fibrosis, pulmonary fibrosis, emphysema, Eisenmenger's syndrome, and primary pulmonary hypertension. Graft–host resistance and sepsis are the major concerns.

Survival rates after transplantation are getting better. Pre-HTx diabetes, donor age, and incidences of infection and rejection within 2 years of HTx predict long-term (>10 years) survival (Radovancevic et al, 2005). Main causes of death early after transplantation are rejection, nonspecific graft failure, and right ventricular failure due to pulmonary hypertension (Bauer et al, 2005).

Implantation of circulatory assist devices as a permanent alternative to HTx is an option for patients who are not candidates for HTx (Lietz and Miller, 2005). Ventricular assist devices (VADs) are now quite common. More recently, cell-based cardiac repair using human embryonic stem cells (hESCs) represent an attractive source for obtaining cardiomyocytes (Zhu et al, 2009).

Traditional risk factors, high oxidative stress, and reduced antioxidant defenses play a role in the pathogenesis of atherosclerosis, especially in transplanted hearts. Dietary measures are important. Flavonoid-rich dark chocolate induces coronary vasodilation, improves coronary vascular function, and decreases platelet adhesion (Flammer et al, 2007). Omega-3 fatty acids lower Chol levels, improve endothelial function, and can reduce the risk of sudden death in HTx recipients (Harris et al, 2004; Wenke, 2004). Finally, obesity, dyslipidemia, hypertension, and diabetes mellitus are common after HTx. Therefore, dietary intervention to obtain weight and metabolic control after HTx is needed to decrease TC, TGs, glucose plasma level, and weight loss (Guida et al, 2009).

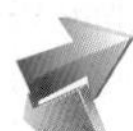

ASSESSMENT, MONITORING, AND EVALUATION

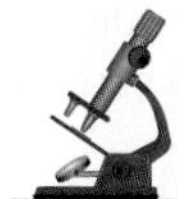

CLINICAL INDICATORS

Genetic Markers: Cardiac transplantation may be required for idiopathic DCM, which is inherited in approximately one third of cases. In addition, recipient renin–angiotensin–aldosterone system (RAAS) polymorphisms are associated with a higher risk of rejection, graft cytokine expression, graft dysfunction, and a higher mortality after cardiac transplantation (Auerbach et al, 2009).

Clinical/History

Height
Weight
BMI
Waist circumference
Diet history
Edema
BP
Stress test
Chest x-ray
ECG
Coronary angiogram
Echocardiogram
Cardiopulmonary test
Ultrasound of abdomen and blood vessels
Cardiac catheterization

Lab Work

Urinary Na^+
Na^+, K^+
Ca^{++}, Mg^{++}
CRP
H & H
Serum Fe
Transferrin
Complete blood cell count (CBC)
BUN, Creat
AST, ALT
ECG
pCO_2, pO_2
Alb, transthyretin
Chol—HDL, LDL, total
Trig
Gluc
tHcy
Serum folate and B_{12}

INTERVENTION

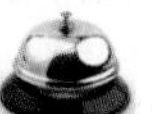

OBJECTIVES

- Promote adequate wound healing; prevent or correct wound dehiscence.
- Normalize heart functioning; prevent morbidity and death. Control infection and rejection during the first 2 years after HTx to improve survival.

SAMPLE NUTRITION CARE PROCESS STEPS

Inadequate Intake of Bioactive Substances

Assessment Data: Food frequency recall and intake records; computer nutrient analysis showing no intake of omega 3 fatty acid-rich foods or chocolate. Consumes meals only at fast food restaurants. Low HDL and elevated LDL levels. Recent HTx surgery for ASHD and hypertension.

Nutrition Diagnosis (PES): Inadequate intake of bioactive substances (flavonols) related to poor diet as evidenced by diet history and daily fast food intake.

Intervention: Education about the role of antioxidant-rich foods and omega-3 fatty acids in heart disease, especially after transplantation. Counseling about food choice options besides eating daily at fast food restaurants and how to include chocolate, cocoa, nuts and seeds as easy snack items.

Monitoring and Evaluation: Repeat lab values after 3–6 months; dietary recall indicating use of bioactive substances at least once daily and fewer meals at fast food restaurants.

- Control side effects of steroid and immunosuppressive therapy.
- Prevent complications such as hepatic or renal failure and diabetes mellitus.
- Maintain or improve nutritional status and fluid balance.
- Protect against posttransplantation hyperlipidemia, hypertension, and graft coronary vasculopathy (GCV). GCV is an accelerated form of atherosclerosis in transplanted hearts that is one of the most important late complications of HTx and is the single most limiting factor for long-term survival (Wenke, 2004).

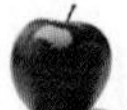

FOOD AND NUTRITION

Pretranplantation

- Control calories, protein, sodium, potassium, fat, and Chol as appropriate for specific underlying condition (see appropriate sections). Keep in mind the role of nutrients needed for wound healing, including adequate energy intake.
- Fluid overload must be avoided; limit to 1 L daily, using a nutrient-dense product if needed.
- Avoid alcohol, which can aggravate cardiomyopathies.
- Reduce cardiac stimulants (such as caffeine) until fully recovered.

Posttransplantation

- Increase diet as tolerated and as appropriate for status. Alter as needed. Include appropriate levels of calcium, magnesium, potassium, and fiber; the DASH diet is beneficial.
- Increase use of omega-3 fatty acids from fish and fish oils.
- Increase use of cardioprotective agents such as vitamins E, B_6, and B_{12} and folic acid. It is also prudent to use olive, soybean, and canola oils.

TABLE 6-10 Medications Used after Transplantation

Medication	Description
Analgesics	Analgesics are used to reduce pain. Long-term use may affect such nutrients as vitamin C and folacin; monitor carefully for each specific medication.
Cardiac medications	Antihypertensives, antilipemics, diuretics, and potassium supplements may be used. Monitor side effects accordingly. Some diuretics spare calcium and protect bone health.
Azathioprine (Imuran)	Azathioprine may cause leukopenia, thrombocytopenia, oral and esophageal sores, macrocytic anemia, pancreatitis, vomiting, diarrhea, and other complex side effects. Folate supplementation and other dietary modifications (liquid or soft diet, use of oral supplements) may be needed. The drug works by lowering the number of T cells; it is often prescribed along with prednisone for conventional immunosuppression.
Corticosteroids (prednisone, hydrocortisone [Solu-Cortef])	Corticosteroids such as prednisone and hydrocortisone are used for immunosuppression. Side effects include increased catabolism of proteins, negative nitrogen balance, hyperphagia, ulcers, decreased glucose tolerance, sodium retention, fluid retention, and impaired calcium absorption and osteoporosis. Cushing's syndrome, obesity, muscle wasting, and increased gastric secretion may result. A higher protein intake and lower intake of simple CHOs may be needed.
Cyclosporine	Cyclosporine does not retain sodium as much as corticosteroids do. Intravenous doses are more effective than oral doses. Nausea, vomiting, and diarrhea are common side effects. Hyperlipidemia, hypertension, and hyperkalemia may also occur; decrease sodium and potassium as necessary. Elevated glucose and lipids may occur. The drug is also nephrotoxic; a controlled renal diet may be beneficial. Taking omega-3 fatty acids during cyclosporine therapy may reduce the toxic side effects (such as high blood pressure and kidney damage) associated with this medication in transplantation patients.
Diuretics	Diuretics such as furosemide may cause hypokalemia. Aldactone actually spares potassium; monitor drug changes closely. In general, avoid use with fenugreek, yohimbe, and ginkgo.
Immunosuppressants	Immunosuppressants such as muromonab (Orthoclone OKT3) and antithymocyte globulin (ATG) are less nephrotoxic than cyclosporine but can cause nausea, anorexia, diarrhea, and vomiting. Monitor carefully. Fever and stomatitis also may occur; alter diet as needed.
Statins	Statins may be used to manage coronary artery disease or dyslipidemia.
Tacrolimus (Prograf, FK506)	Tacrolimus suppresses T-cell immunity; it is 100 times more potent than cyclosporine, thus requiring smaller doses. Side effects include GI distress, nausea, vomiting, hyperkalemia, and hyperglycemia.

- Nuts contain flavonoids, phenols, sterols, saponins, elegiac acid, folic acid, magnesium, copper, potassium, and fiber. Walnuts contain ALA; almonds are a good source of vitamin E. Macadamias, pecans, and pistachios are also beneficial.
- Include chocolate and cocoa frequently.
- For TF, use a product low in sodium and advance gradually.

Common Drugs Used and Potential Side Effects

- See Table 6-10.

Herbs, Botanicals, and Supplements

- The patient should not take herbals and botanicals without discussing with the physician.

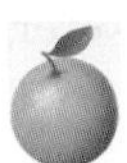

NUTRITION EDUCATION, COUNSELING, CARE MANAGEMENT

- Discuss the role of nutrition in wound healing, immunocompetence, and cardiovascular health. Specify nutrients that are known to be protective.
- Discuss how exercise affects the use of calories.
- Discuss, as appropriate, fiber intake and sources of fat and Chol. Highlight the importance of maintaining an adequate diet to reduce risks of further heart disease and complications. Transplant CAD proceeds at an accelerated rate; this procedure is not a permanent cure.
- To improve quality of life in transplantation patients, web-based counseling and support may play a vital role in follow-up care and in patient and family adjustments (Dew et al, 2004). This type of support is helpful, especially in rural areas where access to MNT is limited.

Patient Education—Foodborne Illness

- Careful food handling will be important. Hand washing is key as well.

For More Information

- American Heart Association
  http://www.americanheart.org/
- Heart Transplantation
  http://www.pbs.org/wgbh/nova/eheart/transplant.html

HEART TRANSPLANTATION OR HEART–LUNG TRANSPLANTATION—CITED REFERENCES

Auerbach SR, et al. Recipient genotype is a predictor of allograft cytokine expression and outcomes after pediatric cardiac transplantation. *J Am Coll Cardiol.* 53:1909, 2009.

Bauer J, et al. Perioperative management in pediatric heart transplantation. *Thorac Cardiovasc Surg.* 53:S155, 2005.

Dew MA, et al. An internet-based intervention to improve psychosocial outcomes in heart transplant recipients and family caregivers: development and evaluation. *J Heart Lung Transplant.* 23:745, 2004.

Flammer AJ, et al. Dark chocolate improves coronary vasomotion and reduces platelet reactivity. *Circulation.* 116:2376, 2007.

Guida B, et al. Role of dietary intervention and nutritional follow-up in heart transplant recipients. *Clin Transplant.* 23:101, 2009.

Harris WS, et al. Omega-3 fatty acids in cardiac biopsies from heart transplantation patients: correlation with erythrocytes and response to supplementation. *Circulation.* 110:1645, 2004.

Lietz K, Miller LW. Will left-ventricular assist device therapy replace heart transplantation in the foreseeable future? *Curr Opin Cardiol.* 20:132, 2005.

Radovancevic B, et al. Factors predicting 10-year survival after heart transplantation. *J Heart Lung Transplant.* 24:156, 2005.

Wenke K. Management of hyperlipidaemia associated with heart transplantation. *Drugs.* 64:1053, 2004.

Zhu WZ, et al. Human embryonic stem cells and cardiac repair. *Transplant Rev.* 23:53, 2009.

HEART VALVE DISEASES

NUTRITIONAL ACUITY RANKING: LEVEL 2

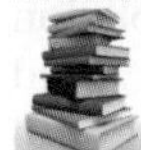

DEFINITIONS AND BACKGROUND

The heart has four valves (tricuspid, pulmonary, aortic, and mitral). Inflammation of any or several of these valves can cause stenosis with thickening (which narrows the opening) or incompetence (with distortion and inability to close fully). If the mitral valve is not functioning properly, due to injury or disease, blood leaks back into the left atrium (regurgitates) when the left ventricle contracts and backs up into the lungs. Because some of the blood being pumped by the left ventricle flows back into the left atrium, less blood is pumped into the aorta and throughout the body. The heart compensates for this by increasing the size of the left ventricle to increase the amount of blood it is pumping and to maintain an adequate forward flow of blood throughout the body. Unfortunately, compensation eventually leads to impairment of the left ventricle's ability to contract, which leads to further backup of blood into the lungs.

Mitral valve prolapse is the most common cause of severe mitral regurgitation in the United States. Overall prognosis of patients is excellent, but a small subset will develop serious complications, including infective endocarditis or sudden cardiac death (Hayek et al, 2005). Echocardiography is used for diagnosing this condition, and mitral valve repair is the treatment. With advancements in PCIs, some patients benefit from a hybrid approach involving initial planned PCI followed by valve surgery, rather than conventional CABG/valve surgery (Byrne et al, 2005).

Mitral stenosis (stiffening) can cause lung congestion, breathlessness after exercise or while lying down, hemoptysis, bronchial infections, chest pains, and right HF. Most people who have had rheumatic heart disease later have primarily mitral stenosis. **Aortic stenosis** can cause symptoms of angina, vertigo, fainting on exertion, and left HF. **Tricuspid stenosis** increases the risk of HF. **Pulmonary stenosis** is rare and occurs in only 2% of all valve disorders.

Patients at high risk for valvular disease should be screened for hyperhomocysteinemia; for prevention, a multivitamin supplement with vitamins B_6 and B_{12} and folate should be taken.

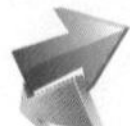

ASSESSMENT, MONITORING, AND EVALUATION

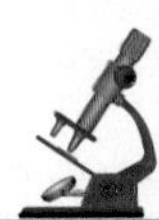

CLINICAL INDICATORS

Genetic Markers: Congenital heart defects are a cause of some valve disorders, but most are acquired.

Clinical/History

Height
Weight
BMI
Waist–hip ratio
Diet history
Weight changes
Edema in belly, ankles, feet
Pulse
Cool, moist skin
BP
Urinary output (decreased)
I & O
Cardiac catheterization
ECG
Vertigo
Fainting
Breathlessness after exertion?
Heart palpitations
Shortness of breath

Lab Work

CRP
Alb, transthyretin
H & H
Serum ferritin
Chol—total, HDL, LDL
Trig
BUN, Creat
Na^+, K^+
Ca^{++}, Mg^{++}
Gluc
tHcy
Serum folate
Serum B_{12}

INTERVENTION

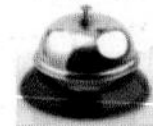

OBJECTIVES

- Prevent HF (right- or left-sided), bacterial endocarditis, emboli or atrial fibrillation, and sudden death. Prevent stroke; mitral annular calcification is an independent predictor of stroke.
- Prepare, if necessary, for valve replacement surgery.
- Prevent or correct cardiogenic shock with tachycardia and other symptoms.
- Correct or manage atherosclerosis.

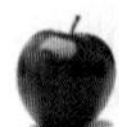

FOOD AND NUTRITION

- Avoid excesses of calories, sodium, and fluid (as appropriate for the patient). In some patients with vertigo, fluid and sodium restrictions may actually be detrimental.
- If weight loss has taken place, add extra calories and snacks to return to a more desirable body weight.
- Use adequate vitamins E, B_6, and B_{12} and folic acid.
- The DASH diet is useful. Encourage use of flavonoids such as chocolate, cocoa, pomegranate, or grape juices, apples, onions, tea, or red wine when feasible. Flavonoids may help to reduce blood clot formation.

> **SAMPLE NUTRITION CARE PROCESS STEPS**
>
> **Excessive Vitamin K Intake**
>
> ***Assessment Data:*** Food intake records; computer nutrient analysis showing intake of vitamin K from multivitamin supplement and fortified nutritional beverages exceeding 150% of recommended levels while on warfarin; INR 1.0–1.5 range.
>
> ***Nutrition Diagnosis (PES):*** Excessive vitamin K intake related to intake of oral supplements and multivitamin preparation as evidenced by low INR while on anticoagulant therapy.
>
> ***Intervention:*** Educate patient and family about appropriate levels of vitamin K. Counsel about an appropriate supplement and oral beverage choice with less vitamin K content.
>
> ***Monitoring and Evaluation:*** Intake from multivitamin and oral supplements in lower range of daily vitamin K requirements; improved INR and bleeding times.

- Ensure adequate intake of omega-3 fatty acids. However, avoid high fat diets as the benefits of omega-3 s are reduced with those diets (Shah et al, 2009).
- Control intake of vitamin K while on warfarin. Changes in dietary vitamin K (phylloquinone) intake may contribute to marked variations in the INR in patients receiving oral warfarin anticoagulant therapy, with potentially serious adverse outcomes (Couris et al, 2006).

Common Drugs Used and Potential Side Effects

- Anticoagulants are commonly used. Monitor vitamin K–rich foods carefully; use no more than 1 per day (especially green leafy vegetables).
- If aspirin is used, monitor for GI side effects or occult blood loss if used for a long time.
- Diuretics may be used with fluid overload. Monitor potassium and sodium intake carefully. Some diuretics spare calcium and protect bone health.
- Because fenfluramine-phentermine (Fen-Phen) weight reduction drugs promoted valvular heart disease and pulmonary hypertension, they were removed from the market.
- Digoxin may be needed to strengthen the heart's pumping action after surgery. Monitor potassium intake or depletion carefully, especially when combining with diuretics. Avoid excessive intakes of fiber and wheat bran. Avoid use with hawthorn, milkweed, guar gum, and St. John's wort.
- Statins may be used to manage CAD or dyslipidemia. See Table 6-6.

Herbs, Botanicals, and Supplements

- See Table 6-3 for details.

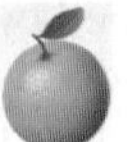

NUTRITION EDUCATION, COUNSELING, CARE MANAGEMENT

- Careful use of all prescribed medications will be essential, with adequate return visits to the physician at appropriate intervals.
- Alternative food preparation methods may be suggested to reduce sodium or energy intake.

- Persons with a history of heart valve abnormalities may require antibiotic therapy to prevent infections, especially before surgery or dental work.
- After surgery, the patient should receive information about nutrition in wound healing. Some procedures are more invasive than others and will require longer healing time.

Patient Education—Foodborne Illness

- Careful food handling will be important. Hand washing is key as well.

For More Information

- Heart and Valvular Diseases
  http://www.nhlbi.nih.gov/health/public/heart/index.htm
- Heart Murmur
  http://www.nhlbi.nih.gov/health/dci/Diseases/heartmurmur/hmurmur_what.html
- Heart Valve Disease
  http://www.americanheart.org/presenter.jhtml?identifier=4598
- Medicine Net—Valve Disease
  http://www.medicinenet.com/heart_valve_disease/article.htm
- Medline Plus
  http://www.nlm.nih.gov/medlineplus/heartvalvediseases.html
- Texas Heart Institute—Heart Anatomy
  http://www.texasheartinstitute.org/HIC/Anatomy/Anatomy.cfm

HEART VALVE DISEASES—CITED REFERENCES

Byrne JG, et al. Staged initial percutaneous coronary intervention followed by valve surgery ("hybrid approach") for patients with complex coronary and valve disease. *J Am Coll Cardiol.* 45:14, 2005.

Couris R, et al. Dietary vitamin K variability affects International Normalized Ratio (INR) coagulation indices. *Int J Vitam Nutr Res.* 76:65, 2006.

Hayek E, et al. Mitral valve prolapse. *Lancet.* 365:507, 2005.

Shah KB, et al. The Cardioprotective effects of fish oil during pressure overload are blocked by high fat intake. Role of cardiac phospholipid remodeling [published online ahead of print Jul 13, 2009]. *Hypertension.* 54:65, 2009.

HYPERTENSION

NUTRITIONAL ACUITY RANKING: LEVEL 3

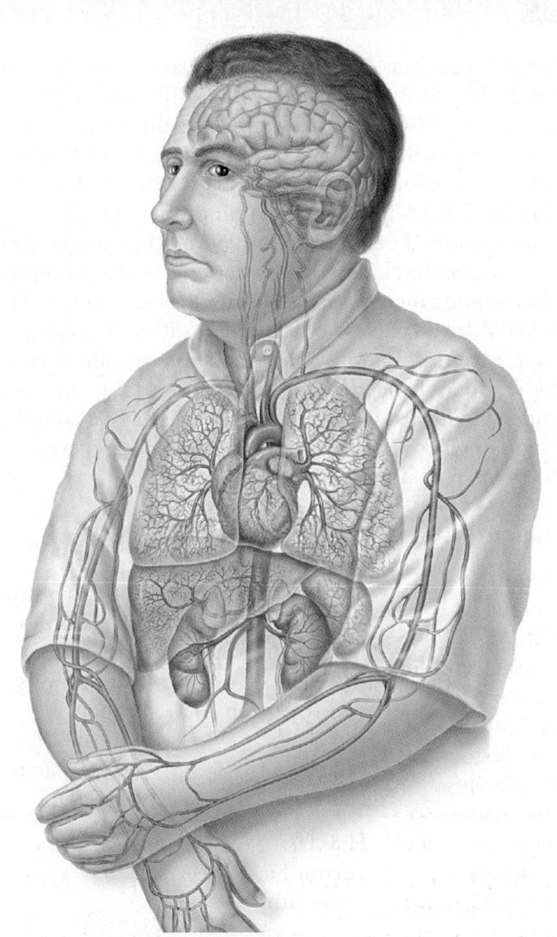

Asset provided by Anatomical Chart Co.

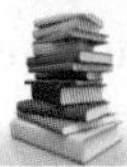

DEFINITIONS AND BACKGROUND

Hypertension is defined as having a sustained systolic and diastolic BP greater than 140 and 90 mm Hg, respectively. See Table 6-11. It affects about 600 million people worldwide and about 27% of the U.S. adult population.

Hypertension nearly doubles the risk for heart attack, stroke, and HF, especially for people over age 65. BP often increases with age and is highly prevalent in elderly individuals. Symptoms of hypertension include frequent headaches, impaired vision, shortness of breath, nose bleeds, chest pain, dizziness, failing memory, snoring and sleep apnea, and GI distress.

TABLE 6-11 Categories for Blood Pressure Levels in Adults (Ages 18 years and Older)

	Blood Pressure Level (mm Hg)		
Category	**Systolic**		**Diastolic**
Normal	<120	and	<80
Prehypertension	120–139	or	80–89
High blood pressure:			
Stage 1 hypertension	140–159	or	90–99
Stage 2 hypertension	≥160	or	≥100

From: National Heart, Lung, and Blood Institute. Accessed July 16, 2009, at http://www.nhlbi.nih.gov/hbp/detect/categ.htm.

Identifiable causes of high BP include sleep apnea, drug-related causes, CKD, Cushing's syndrome, steroid therapy, pheochromocytoma, primary aldosteronism, thyroid and parathyroid diseases, and reno-vascular disease. Untreated hypertension can result in stroke, HF, renal failure, MI, accelerated bone loss and risk of fractures, and long-term memory problems. The Joint National Committee on Prevention, Detection, Evaluation, and Treatment of High Blood Pressure, the JNC 7 Report (NHLBI, 2009) identified following priority concerns:

- In persons over age 50, systolic BP >140 mm Hg is a more important CVD risk factor than diastolic BP. Those who are normotensive at age 55 have a 90% lifetime risk of developing hypertension. Beginning at 115/75 mm Hg, CVD risk doubles for each increment of 20/10 mm Hg.
- Prehypertensive individuals (systolic BP of 120–139 mm Hg or diastolic BP of 80–89 mm Hg) require health-promoting lifestyle modifications to prevent the progressive rise in BP and CVD. However, patients must be motivated to stay on their treatment plans.

Endothelial activation, oxidative stress, and vascular smooth muscle dysfunction (hypertrophy, hyperplasia, remodeling) can promote inflammation and stiffened blood vessels (Houston, 2005). Elevated CRP is a marker of reduced production of nitric acid in the blood vessels. CRP over 3.5 represents endothelial dysfunction, the earliest event in atherosclerosis (Streppel et al, 2005). With endothelial dysfunction, diet greatly affects vascular reactivity.

Fish oil, antioxidants, folic acid, soy protein, and the Mediterranean diet (high consumption of vegetables, fish, and olive oil and moderate wine consumption) may have a positive effect. Increasing intake of fiber in populations where intake is far below recommended levels may help to prevent hypertension (Streppel et al, 2005). Weight loss is also important; abdominal adiposity promotes high CRP levels.

There is increasing evidence for use of nutrients such as omega-3 PUFA, vitamin C, folic acid, and potassium. The DASH eating plan is rich in fiber, vegetables, fruit, and nonfat dairy products and significantly lowers BP. The decreases are often comparable to those achieved with BP-lowering medication.

For patients with CKD who have hypertension; it is critical to control BP to reduce negative consequences. Current National Kidney Foundation guidelines recommend reducing sodium intake to less than 2.4 g/d; reducing potassium in patients with a GFR of <60 mL/min. Black populations benefit most from reduced salt intake, increased potassium intake, and the DASH diet (Appel et al, 2006).

Because nutrient–gene interactions determine a broad array of consequences such as vascular problems and hypertension, consuming optimal nutrition, nutraceuticals, vitamins, antioxidants, and minerals and moderately restricting alcohol may prevent, delay the onset, reduce the severity, treat, or control hypertension (Houston, 2005). For example, Vitamin D deficiency activates the rennin–angiotensin–aldosterone system and can predispose to hypertension and left ventricular hypertrophy; it can also increase parathyroid hormone that is associated with insulin resistance and hypertension (Lee et al, 2008).

Malignant hypertension, which occurs in only 1% of those with essential hypertension (EH), has medical urgency. In this condition, there is accelerated hypertension (systolic >220 mm Hg or diastolic >120 mm Hg) with no evidence of target organ damage. This differs from a medical emergency, such as a stroke, where it is important to lower elevated BP immediately. African Americans are at higher risk than individuals with European heritage.

Long-term sodium reductions of 400 mg in those with uncontrolled hypertension would eliminate about 1.5 million cases, potentially increasing productivity by $2.5 billion annually and more aggressive diet changes of 1100 mg of sodium reductions yield potential productivity benefits of $5.8 billion annually (Dall et al, 2009). Therefore, clinicians are encouraged to work closely with patients to agree on BP goals and develop a treatment plan. Reduced salt intake, weight loss, moderate alcohol consumption among those who drink, increased potassium intake, and use of the DASH diet are among the most effective strategies (Appel et al, 2006). The American Dietetic Association recommends at least three MNT visits for patients with hypertension.

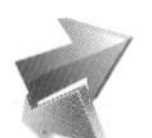

ASSESSMENT, MONITORING, AND EVALUATION

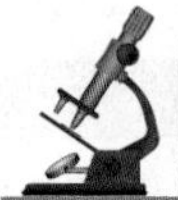

CLINICAL INDICATORS

Genetic Markers: A genome-wide association study of systolic BP (SBP) and diastolic BP (DBP) and hypertension in the CHARGE Consortium, identified significance in four SNPs for SBP (ATP2B1, CYP17A1, PLEKHA7, SH2 B3), six for DBP (ATP2B1, CACNB2, CSK-ULK3, SH2 B3, TBX3-TBX5, ULK4), and one (ATP2B1) for hypertension (Levy et al, 2009). Severe mutations often result in the development of hypertension at a young age while subtle mutations may take decades to manifest. The MTHFR folate alleles are associated with EH because of their relationship with tHcy metabolism (Ilhan et al, 2008). Identifying genes associated with BP advances understanding of BP regulation and highlights potential drug targets for the prevention or treatment (Levy et al, 2009; Mein et al, 2004; Wang et al, 2009).

Clinical/History

Height
Weight
BMI
Waist circumference
BP pattern
Diet history
Headaches, dizziness
Snoring or sleep apnea?
Polysomnogram
I & O
Renal arteriography
Chest x-ray
Renal ultrasound
Intravenous pyelogram
ECG

Lab Work

H & H
Serum Fe, ferritin
CRP
Alb, transthyretin
Urinary Alb to Creat ratio (high levels impair arterial dilatory capacity)
Chol—HDL, LDL
Trig
LDH

BUN	Parathormone (PTH)	Serum folate and B_{12}
Creat, GFR	AST, ALT	Plasma ascorbic acid
Uric acid	Alk phos	Urinary Ca^{++}
Plasma renin	Serum vitamin D	Urinary cortisol
Na^+, K^+	PT or INR	
Chloride	Gluc	
Serum Ca^{++}, Mg^{++}	tHcy	

INTERVENTION

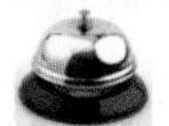

OBJECTIVES

- Assess medical risk factors, comorbidities, and identifiable causes of the hypertension. For example, essential hypertension affects 1 billion people worldwide and has a genetic basis (Mein et al, 2004).
- Reduce cardiovascular (HF, stroke) and renal morbidity and mortality (ADA, 2009) by lowering high BP. The DASH dietary pattern reduces SBP by 8–14 mm Hg (ADA, 2009).
- For individuals with hypertension and diabetes or renal disease, maintain BP goal of <130/80 mm Hg (ADA, 2009).
- Increase vascular and lymphocyte beta-adrenergic responsiveness. Dietary sodium intake should be limited to no more than 2300 mg sodium (100 mmol) per day; this level can lowers SBP by approximately 2–8 mm Hg (ADA, 2009).
- Achieve and maintain an optimal body weight (BMI 18.5–24.9); weight reduction lowers SBP by 5–20 mm Hg per 22 lb (10 kg) body weight loss (ADA, 2009).
- Increase magnesium, calcium, vitamins D, E, and K where serum levels or dietary intake is low.
- Encourage adequate intake of fluids unless contraindicated. Avoid excesses of alcohol that may increase BP.
- Dietitians should encourage individuals to engage in aerobic physical activity for at least 30 min/d on most days of the week, as it reduces systolic BP by approximately 4–9 mm Hg (ADA, 2009).

SAMPLE NUTRITION CARE PROCESS STEPS

Hypertension (HTN)

Assessment: Diet history and food records, BP records.

Nutrition Diagnosis (PES): Excessive intake of sodium related to high intake of commercially prepared and packaged foods as evidenced by BP s of 160/105 mm Hg and lack of knowledge about sources of sodium.

Intervention: Initial/brief nutrition education (E-1) to communicate the relationship between nutrition and HTN. Discuss lower sodium food choices, label reading, and options to reduce BP. Discuss choices for healthier meals and snacks. Promote use of BP monitoring records, easy preparation meals made from scratch, recipe alterations, shopping tips, tips for dining away from home.

Monitoring and Evaluation: BP reports, food records showing improved intake of sodium in daily diet.

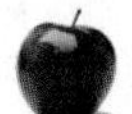

FOOD AND NUTRITION

- The DASH diet works within 14 days of initiation. This diet is rich in fruits, vegetables, and low-fat dairy foods; it is low in SFA and total fat. Adequate amounts of potassium from skim milk, baked potatoes, grapefruit, oranges, bananas, lima beans, and other fruits and vegetables should be planned daily.
- Tips on eating the DASH way: Start small; make gradual changes in eating habits. Organize meals around carbohydrates such as pasta, rice, beans, or vegetables. Carbohydrates such as beans, whole grains, oat bran, and fruits (apples, blueberries) and vegetables should make up 50% of the diet.
- Treat meat as one part of the whole meal, instead of the main focus. Use fruits or low-fat, low-calorie foods such as sugar-free gelatin for desserts and snacks.
- Increase fruits and vegetables (5–10 servings daily) for their flavonoid, phytochemical, potassium content and properties (ADA, 2009). Besides the DASH diet, Mediterranean and vegetarian diet patterns tend to lower BP and can be beneficial.
- Limit sodium intake. Only 20–50% of patients with hypertension are sodium sensitive. Patients with EH are more sodium sensitive than patients whose conditions are secondary to other disorders (Houben et al, 2005).
- Read labels carefully. If some thing is sodium free, it has 5 mg or less per serving. Something that is light in sodium has 50% less than the usual recipe. A food that is labeled low sodium must be 149 mg or less per serving. About 77% of salt in the diet comes from processed foods, 12% naturally, and the remainder is either added during cooking or at the table. Table 6-12 lists common salts, salt substitutes, and their content.
- Use an energy-controlled diet if weight loss is needed.
- Olive, soybean, and canola oils can be substituted for some saturated fats in cooking. Pistachios, sunflower kernels, sesame seeds, and wheat germ are good sources of phytosterols; use often.
- Limit alcoholic beverages to one drink for women and to two drinks for men.
- Use sources of omega-3 fatty acids, such as mackerel, haddock, sardines, and salmon, several times weekly. Tuna should be used less often because potential mercury content could elevate BP.
- Higher intake of dairy products seems to reduce serum uric acid levels; high uric acid levels are often correlated with BP and stroke (Choi et al, 2005).
- Increase food sources of folic acid, vitamins B_{12}, and B_6 for overall cardiovascular health. Vitamin D is also important. Vitamin D deficiency is associated with increased risk of developing incident hypertension or sudden cardiac death in individuals with preexisting CVD (Judd and Tangpricha, 2009).
- Caffeine from habitual coffee intake is not problematic (Winkelmayer et al, 2005). Hibiscus tea, green tea, cocoa and chocolate should be encouraged.

TABLE 6-12 Sodium and Potassium in Salt, Salt Substitutes, Herbal Seasonings

Type	Milligrams (mg) of Sodium per 1/4 tsp	Milligrams (mg) of Potassium per 1/4 tsp
Morton's table salt	590	0
Morton sea salt	560	0
Morton's salt balance	440	200
Diamond crystal salt sense	390	0
Lawry's seasoned salt	380	0
Morton's lite salt	290	350
Papa dash	240	0
Baking soda	205	0
Monosodium glutamate	123	0
Sterling lo-salt mixture	115	150
Baking powder	85	0
Nu salt	0	795
Nosalt	0	650
Morton salt substitute	0	610
Also salt	0	300
Mrs, dash salt-free seasoning blends	0	5–15
Benson's gourmet salt free seasonings	<5	minimal
Durkee smart seasons	0	0–15
McCormick salt-free seasoning blends	1	20–40

Derived from: Edwards A. Salt, salt substitutes, and seasoning alternatives. *J Renal Nutr.* 18:e23, 2008.

Common Drugs Used and Potential Side Effects

- Dietitians should assess food/nutrient-medication interactions in patients that are on pharmacologic therapy for hypertension, as many antihypertensive medications interact with food and nutrients (ADA, 2009). See Table 6-13.
- In uncomplicated stage 1 hypertension, dietary changes are the initial treatment, then drug therapy. In hypertensive patients already on drug therapy, lifestyle modification and reduced salt intake, can further lower BP (Appel et al, 2006).
- Use of a diuretic is part of the treatment plan in most patients. For stage 1, thiazide diuretics may suffice; in stage 2, two-drug combinations may be needed. Drug classes that have been shown to be effective in reducing hypertension's cardiovascular complications include ACE inhibitors, angiotensin receptor blockers, beta-blockers, and calcium channel blockers. Most persons will need multiple medications to lower BP to a desired level.
- Note that use of estrogens and oral contraceptives can increase BP.
- Antihypertensive therapy is challenging in the elderly because of metabolic and physiological alterations, comorbidities, polypharmacy, and biological variability. For example, ACE inhibitors and beta-blockers may provide beneficial therapeutic effects to the EH patients by decreasing tHcy levels, while thiazide diuretics increase tHcy (Poduri et al, 2009).

Herbs, Botanicals, and Supplements

- Green coffee bean extract, oolong, and moderate-strength green teas may be beneficial in lowering BP (Kozuma et al, 2005). Hibiscus tea may also be beneficial.
- While vitamin D supplementation is simple, safe, and inexpensive, large randomized controlled trials are needed to identify how much is needed to prevent hypertension (Lee et al, 2008).
- Use of 1000 mg of a specific olive leaf extract EFLA943 has been shown to lower BP in twins (Perrinjacquet-Moccetti et al, 2008). Larger population studies are suggested.
- See Table 6-3 for more information.

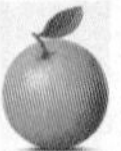

NUTRITION EDUCATION, COUNSELING, CARE MANAGEMENT

- Encourage patience; it takes 2 weeks to see the results while following the DASH diet.
- Remove the salt shaker from the table. Have the patient taste food before salting. Avoid excesses of processed and

TABLE 6-13 Medications for Hypertension

Medication	Description
Angiotensin-converting enzyme (ACE) inhibitors (benzepril/Lotensin, captopril/Capoten, enalapril/ Vasotec, fosinopril/Monopril, lisinopril/Prinivil or Zestril, moexipril/Univasc, perindopril/Aceon, quinipril/Accupril, ramipril/Altace, trandolapril/Mavik)	ACE inhibitors prevent angiotensin I from conversion; they are useful in heart failure. Ramipril has been noted to prevent diabetes in hypertensive patients. Nausea, vomiting, and abdominal pain may occur; do not take with potassium supplements. Captopril (Capoten) can alter BUN/creatinine; take 1 hour before meals and reduce calories and sodium. Loss of taste can occur. Patients who take captopril and enalapril may develop zinc deficiency.
Angiotensin II receptor antagonists (candesartan/Atacand, eprosartan/Teveten, irbesartan/Avapro, losartan/Cozaar, olmesatran/Benicar, telmiartan/Micardis, valsatran/Diovan)	Use with low-sodium, low-calorie diet. GI distress can occur. Some are mixed with thiazide diuretics; monitor for potassium depletion.
Direct renin inhibitors (DRIs) (aliskiren/Tekturna)	
Beta-blockers (atenolol/Tenormin, pindolol/Visken, propranolol/Inderal, acebutolol/Sectral, bisoprolol/Zebeta, metoprolol/Lopressor, timolol/Blocadren, prazosin/Minipress)	Beta-blockers decrease the force and rate of heart contractions, thereby decreasing blood pressure. Dizziness and nausea are common side effects. Low-calorie, low-sodium diet may be useful. Metoprolol (Lopressor) should be taken with a low-calorie, low-sodium diet. Diarrhea, nausea, vomiting, or abdominal cramps may occur. Prazosin (Minipress) may cause nausea, weight gain, anorexia, diarrhea, or constipation.
Calcium channel blockers (amlodipine/Norvasc; diltiazem/Cardizem; felodipine/Plendil)	Use with low-sodium, low-calorie diet. Avoid natural licorice.
Diuretics Thiazides (furosemide/Lasix, indapamide/Lozol, chlorthalidone/Clorpres, hydrochlorothiazide/ Hydrodiuril Microzide)	Thiazides deplete potassium and may require supplementation; diarrhea or GI bleeding can occur. Avoid natural licorice. Chlorthalidone may alter blood glucose or potassium levels; it may cause anorexia, vomiting, constipation, and nausea. In general, avoid use with fenugreek, yohimbe, and ginkgo.
Diuretic-antihypertensives (amiloride/Moduretic)	A low-calorie, low-sodium diet is important. Potassium loss is minimized. Avoid use with alcohol.
Melatonin	The nocturnal decline of blood pressure (BP) coincides with the elevation of melatonin, which may exert vasodilatating and hypotensive effects; prolonged administration of melatonin may improve the day–night rhythm of BP.

canned foods. The normal adult needs only 1/2 teaspoon of sodium (200 mg) per day. Greater amounts of salt are required only in hot, humid conditions, during lactation, or with other salt-losing states. In such conditions, 2000 mg of salt is sufficient.

- Low fat dairy products have been linked with lower risk for hypertension; include often.
- Interesting food flavors are often hidden by salt. Discuss use of other seasonings and recipes. Monitor potassium in salt substitutes and medications to prevent hyperkalemia; read all labels carefully.
- Obesity leads to a proinflammatory and prothrombotic state that potentiates hypertension. Work on a weight loss program if needed.
- In children, an assessment of psychological and psychosocial factors that lead to obesity and hypertension should be undertaken (Kiessling et al, 2008).
- Increase physical activity when possible. Encourage use of pedometers for daily feedback.
- Omit or reduce alcohol intake severely, if needed.
- Assure adequate sleep; adverse changes to BP are noted with shorter duration.

Patient Education—Foodborne Illness

- Careful food handling will be important. Hand washing is key as well.

For More Information

- DASH Diet
  http://www.nih.gov/news/pr/apr97/Dash.htm
- JNC 7
  http://www.nhlbi.nih.gov/guidelines/hypertension/jnc7full.htm
- Malignant hypertension
  http://www.nlm.nih.gov/medlineplus/ency/article/000491.htm
- National High Blood Pressure Education Program
  http://www.nhlbi.nih.gov/about/nhbpep/index.htm
  http://www.nhlbi.nih.gov/hbp/index.html
- World Hypertension League
  http://www.mco.edu/whl/

HYPERTENSION—CITED REFERENCES

ADA. American Dietetic Association Evidence Analysis Library. Accessed July 15, 2009, at http://www.adaevidencelibrary.com/template.cfm?key=1947&cms_preview=1.

Appel LJ, et al. Dietary approaches to prevent and treat hypertension: a scientific statement from the American Heart Association. *Hypertension.* 47:296, 2006.

Choi HK, et al. Intake of purine-rich foods, protein, and dairy products and relationship to serum levels of uric acid: the Third National Health and Nutrition Examination Survey. *Arthritis Rheum.* 52:283, 2005.

Dall TM, et al. Predicted national productivity implications of calorie and sodium reductions in the American diet. *Am J Health Promot.* 23:423, 2009.

Houben AJ, et al. Microvascular adaptation to changes in dietary sodium is disturbed in patients with essential hypertension. *J Hypertens.* 23:127, 2005.

Houston MC. Nutraceuticals, vitamins, antioxidants, and minerals in the prevention and treatment of hypertension. *Prog Cardiovasc Dis.* 47:396, 2005.

Ilhan N, et al. The 677 C/T MTHFR polymorphism is associated with essential hypertension, coronary artery disease, and higher homocysteine levels. *Arch Med Res.* 39:125, 2008.

Judd SE, Tangpricha V. Vitamin D deficiency and risk for cardiovascular disease. *Am J Med Sci.* 338:40, 2009.

Kiessling SG, et al. Obesity, hypertension, and mental health evaluation in adolescents: a comprehensive approach. *Int J Adolesc Med Health.* 20:5, 2008.

Kozuma K, et al. Antihypertensive effect of green coffee bean extract on mildly hypertensive subjects. *Hypertens Res.* 28:711, 2005.

Lee JH, et al. Vitamin D deficiency an important, common, and easily treatable cardiovascular risk factor? *J Am Coll Cardiol.* 52:1949, 2008.

Levy D, et al. Genome-wide association study of blood pressure and hypertension [published online ahead of print May 10, 2009]. *Nat Genet.* 41:677, 2009.

Mein CA, et al. Genetics of essential hypertension. *Hum Mol Genet.* 13:169, 2004.

NHLBI. Seventh Report of the Joint National Committee on Prevention, Detection and Treatment of High Blood Pressure. Website Accessed July 16, 2009, at http://www.nhlbi.nih.gov/guidelines/hypertension/jnc7full.htm.

Perrinjacquet-Moccetti T, et al. Food supplementation with an olive (Olea europaea L). leaf extract reduces blood pressure in borderline hypertensive monozygotic twins. *Phytother Res.* 22:1239, 2008.

Poduri A, et al. Effect of ACE inhibitors and beta-blockers on homocysteine levels in essential hypertension. *J Hum Hypertens.* 22:289, 2009.

Streppel MT, et al. Dietary fiber and blood pressure: a meta-analysis of randomized placebo-controlled trials. *Arch Intern Med.* 165:150, 2005.

Wang Y, et al. From the cover: whole-genome association study identifies STK39 as a hypertension susceptibility gene. *Proc Natl Acad Sci USA.* 106:226, 2009.

Winkelmayer WC, et al. Habitual caffeine intake and the risk of hypertension in women. *JAMA.* 294:2330, 2005.

MYOCARDIAL INFARCTION

NUTRITIONAL ACUITY RANKING: LEVEL 3

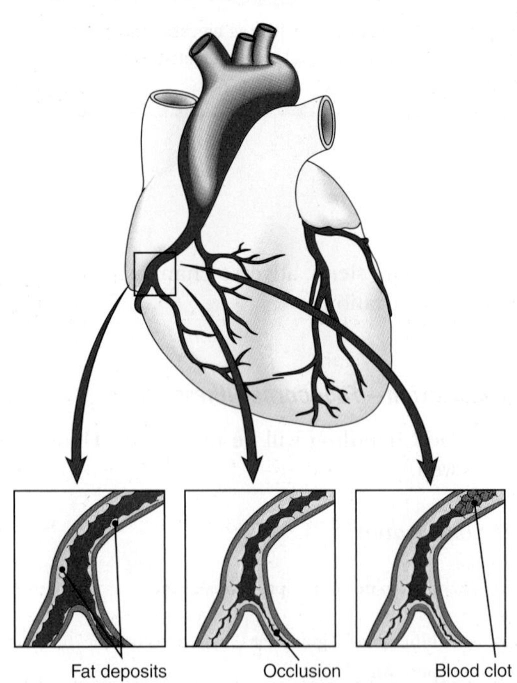

Adapted from: Cohen BJ, Wood DL. *Memmler's The Human Body in Health and Disease.* 9th ed. Philadelphia: Lippincott Williams & Wilkins, 2000.

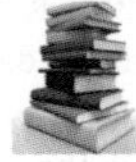

DEFINITIONS AND BACKGROUND

MI is necrosis in the heart muscle caused by prolonged inadequate blood supply or oxygen deficit. A **coronary occlusion** (heart attack) is the closing of a coronary artery feeding heart muscle by fatty deposits or a blood clot; it manifests with heavy squeezing pain radiating to the jaw or back, nausea, vomiting, diaphoresis, anxiety, and weakness. Abnormal lipids, smoking, hypertension, diabetes, abdominal obesity, psychosocial factors, inadequate consumption of fruits and vegetables, alcohol consumption, and lack of regular physical activity account for most of the risk factors for MI worldwide; Table 6-14 provides a complete list.

Women have symptoms of an MI that differ from men. Prodromal symptoms include unusual fatigue, shortness of breath, and pain in the shoulder blade/upper back; medical practitioners must develop an awareness of and a more comprehensive approach to treating women.

Stages after an MI include critical (first 48 hours), acute (3–14 days), and convalescent (15–90 days). Treatment with Chol-lowering medications and antioxidants may decrease MI and may reduce adverse coronary events. Table 6-15 lists potential complications after an MI. CVDs cause 12 million deaths worldwide, and MI is a significant problem.

TABLE 6-14 Risk Factors for Myocardial Infarction

- Family history of heart disease
- Patient history of heart disease
- Diabetes or elevated blood glucose, even in nondiabetics
- Hypertension
- Advanced age
- High lipoprotein (a) lipids
- African American ethnicity
- Stress, smoking, sedentary lifestyle, compulsive personality
- Poor diet (high sodium, high fat, high intake of alcohol; low intake of B-complex vitamins, calcium, magnesium, and potassium; low intake of fruits and vegetables)
- Obesity

Fruit and vegetable intake should be encouraged. Platelet aggregation is central in acute coronary syndromes, including MI and unstable angina. Effects of flavonoids on endothelial and platelet function might explain their protective benefits on cardiac risk (Vita, 2005). Studies relate wine/resveratrol with reduction in myocardial damage.

An **arrhythmia** is a variation from normal heartbeat rhythm. Among its many forms is a slowing of the heartbeat to less than 60 beats per minute (bradycardia), a speedup to more than 100 beats per minute (tachycardia), and premature or "skipped" beats. Post-MI patients will need to monitor themselves for arrhythmias.

On the basis of the ECG, a distinction is made between ST-elevation (where thrombolysis, PCI, angioplasty or stent insertion are used), versus non-ST elevation where medications suffice. In some cases, coronary artery bypass surgery (CABG) is an option.

TABLE 6-15 Complications After Myocardial Infarction

- Arrhythmias with risk of sudden death
- Cardiogenic shock
- Cardiac tamponade
- Cholesterol emboli due to cardiac catheterization or during CABG
- Heart failure with pulmonary edema
- Left ventricular free wall rupture
- Pericarditis
- Re-infarction
- Renal failure
- Splenic infarction with fever, tachycardia, left upper quadrant abdominal pain
- Thrombosis or CVA with ischemic bowel or renal infarct
- Valve insufficiency
- Ventricular septal defect

Sources: O'Keefe JH Jr, et al. Thromboembolic splenic infarction. *Mayo Clin Proc.* 61:967, 1986; Puletti M, et al. Incidence of systemic thromboembolic lesions in acute myocardial infarction. *Clin Cardiol.* 9:331, 1986; Prieto A, et al. Nonarrhythmic complications of acute MI. *Emerg Med Clin North Am.* 19:397, 2001.

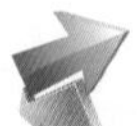

ASSESSMENT, MONITORING, AND EVALUATION

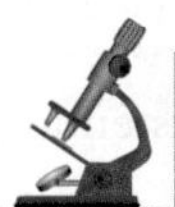

CLINICAL INDICATORS

Genetic Markers: Genetic factors and interactions between multiple genes and environmental factors indicate an association with MI or CHD of polymorphisms in MTHFR, LPL, APOE, and those in LTA and at chromosomal region 9p21.3 by genome-wide scans (Yamada et al, 2008).

Clinical/History

Height
Weight
BMI
Waist circumference
Diet history
Temperature (low grade fever?)
Pulse (NL = 60–100 beats/min)
Tightness in the chest
Nausea, anxiety
Syncope
Wheezing, diaphoresis
Chest pain, radiating
Severe fatigue
Migraine headaches?
BP
I & O
Radionucleotide imaging
Echocardiography
ECG
Chest X-ray

Lab Work

Creatine kinase-MB (CK-MB)
Troponin I (TnI) or troponin T (TnT) levels
CRP
Gluc (elevated levels will increase risk)
AST
Serum Cu (increased)
LDH (increased)
WBC count (increased)
Na^+, K^+
Ca^{++}, Mg^{++}
pCO_2, pO_2
PT or INR
Chol—total, HDL, LDL
Trig (often increased)
BUN, Creat, GFR
Cystacin C (elevated with low GFR)
tHcy
Serum folate and B_{12}
H & H
Serum Fe, ferritin

SAMPLE NUTRITION CARE PROCESS STEPS

Myocardial Infarction (MI)

Assessment: Diet history and food records, lipid profile, review of current and previous medications used for heart disease.

Nutrition Diagnosis (PES): Inappropriate intake of types of food fats due to nutrition-related knowledge deficit as evidenced by LDL Chol of 155 mg/dL and use of large meat portions at lunch and dinner meals.

Intervention: Easy meal preparation and recipe adaptations, shopping and dining away from home tips, one-on-one counseling and goal setting for making changes in choices of food fats.

Monitoring and Evaluation: Lipid profile, food diary and records, goal achievement.

INTERVENTION

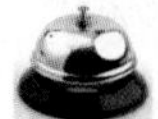

OBJECTIVES

- Promote rest to reduce heart strain. Avoid the distention of heavy meals.
- Prevent arrhythmias by serving food at body temperature.
- Avoid both constipation and flatulence.
- Avoid excessive heart stimulation from caffeine. Energy drinks may contain 50–500 mg of caffeine.
- Reduce elevated levels of lipids: keep Chol below 200 mg/dL, TGs below 200 mg/dL, HDL between 40 and 60 mg/dL, and LDL between 100 and 129 mg/dL.
- Decrease energy required to chew, prepare meals, perform activities of daily living during convalescence.
- Identify modifiable risk factors and complications; reduce risks when possible (see Tables 6-14 and 6-15). For example, lose weight if obese.
- Consume more fish and a diet rich in ALA to reduce the risk of fatal heart attack.

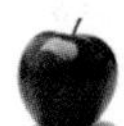

FOOD AND NUTRITION

- Initially, use liquids to promote rest while reducing the dangers of aspiration or vomiting. Reduce fluid and caffeine intake to that recommended by the physician. As treatment progresses, diet should include soft, easily digested foods that are low in saturated fats, Chol, and gas-forming foods.
- Limit diet to 2 g of sodium, or remove salt from the table. Schedule three to six small meals daily.
- If needed, use an energy-controlled diet to reduce the heart's workload.
- The DASH diet and Mediterranean diet are useful. Increase intake of fish, whole grains, and olive oil. Onions, tea, apples, grape juice, and pomegranate contain flavonoids and should be used often. Red wine is recommended, if approved by the physician.
- Adequate calcium, magnesium and potassium will be needed, but not in excess. Consuming micronutrients at levels exceeding those provided by a dietary pattern consistent with American Heart Association (AHA) Dietary Guidelines will not confer additional CVD risk reduction (Kris-Etherton et al, 2004).
- Decrease intake of whole-milk products, red meats, visible fat on meat/poultry, and commercial baked goods. Limit egg yolks to four to five times weekly if lipids are elevated.
- Increase food sources of vitamins E and K, folic acid, and vitamins B_6 and B_{12}.
- Fiber is especially important; choose vegetables, fruits, and cereal grains.
- Include judicious use of nuts, such as walnuts, almonds, macadamias, pecans, and pistachios. Walnuts contain ALA; almonds are a good source of vitamin E. Nuts also contain flavonoids, phenols, sterols, saponins, elegiac acid, folic acid, magnesium, copper, potassium, and fiber.
- Pistachios, sunflower kernels, sesame seeds, and wheat germ are highest in phytosterols; use often.

Common Drugs Used and Potential Side Effects

- Appropriate drugs are provided according to needs established by the profile (elevated BP or lipids). Review specific drugs given to the patient and treat accordingly. Nitrates, beta-blockers, calcium channel blockers, statins, and related drugs are given according to the cause and risk factors for the patient.
- Anticoagulants such as warfarin (Coumadin) may be given where bleeding tendencies are not present. Limit to one vitamin K–rich food per day (green leafy vegetables such as kale, broccoli, spinach, and turnip greens). Avoid taking with dong quai, fenugreek, feverfew, excessive garlic, ginger, ginkgo, and ginseng.
- Aspirin is often recommended later to prevent recurrent MIs. Watch for GI bleeding or other side effects such as occult blood loss.
- Mexiletine (Mexitil) and propafenone (Rythmol) are used to treat arrhythmias. Nausea, vomiting, or constipation may occur. Procainamide (Procan) may result in a bitter taste, nausea, anorexia, or diarrhea.
- Morphine is used for relief of pain but should be given in minimal amounts to prevent hypotension and other side effects.

Herbs, Botanicals, and Supplements

- Dietary supplementation with omega-3 fatty acids should be considered in the secondary prevention of cardiovascular events (Marik and Valon, 2009). Study of the associations between EPA and DHA intake and disease requires a valid biomarker of dietary intake; RBC delta(15)N as a biomarker of EPA and DHA intake is rapid and inexpensive (O'Brien et al, 2009).
- At this time, the scientific data do not justify the use of antioxidant vitamin supplements.
- See Table 6-3 for more guidance on herbs and botanical products.

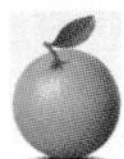

NUTRITION EDUCATION, COUNSELING, CARE MANAGEMENT

- Position patient and arrange utensils to avoid or lessen fatigue. Encourage relaxation, especially at mealtimes.
- If needed, use a weight-control diet.
- Discuss roles of fats, Chol, sodium, potassium, calcium, magnesium, and fiber in the diet. Encourage use of the DASH or Mediterranean diets (see Table 6-4). A vegetarian diet may also be beneficial (Craig et al, 2009).
- Monitor for changes in renal status. A GFR of <60 mL/min may indicate high risk for cardiac death in women (Kurth et al, 2009).
- Avoid excesses of carbohydrate and alcohol, especially with diabetes or elevated BP.
- Individuals continue to have multiple risk factors for CAD that place them at high risk for future events. Discuss convalescence and prevention of HF.
- The patient should stop smoking, follow the recommended diet, and manage other risk factors. A positive attitude toward the modified diet is essential for changing food behaviors.

- The reduction of exposure to second-hand smoke is also beneficial (Glantz et al, 2008; Pell et al, 2008).
- Management of anxiety is an important feature for recovery (Kuhl et al, 2009).
- Discuss a gradual increase in activity. Cardiac rehabilitation programs are very helpful (Lisspers et al, 2005). Aerobic physical activities, such as exercise or walking at work, seem to reduce the risk of MI, whereas anaerobic activities, such as heavy lifting, may increase risk of MI (Fransson et al, 2004).
- A comprehensive management plan uses the "ABCDE" approach: "A" for antiplatelet therapy, anticoagulation, ACE inhibition, and angiotensin receptor blockade; "B" for beta-blockade and BP control; "C" for Chol treatment and cigarette smoking cessation; "D" for diabetes management and diet; and "E" for exercise (Gluckman et al, 2005).

Patient Education—Foodborne Illness

- Careful food handling will be important. Hand washing is key as well.

For More Information

- Heart Attack
  http://www.heartpoint.com/mi.html
- JAMA Patient Page
  http://jama.ama-assn.org/cgi/reprint/299/4/476.pdf
- Medicine Net
  http://www.medicinenet.com/heart_attack/article.htm
- Myocardial Infarction
  http://www-medlib.med.utah.edu/WebPath/TUTORIAL/MYOCARD/MYOCARD.html

MYOCARDIAL INFARCTION—CITED REFERENCES

Craig WJ, et al. Position of the American Dietetic Association: vegetarian diets. *J Am Diet Assoc.* 109:1266, 2009.

Fransson E, et al. The risk of acute myocardial infarction: interactions of types of physical activity. *Epidemiology.* 15:573, 2004.

Glantz S. Meta-analysis of the effects of smoke free laws on acute myocardial infarction: an update. *Prev Med.* 47:452, 2008.

Gluckman TJ, et al. A simplified approach to the management of non-ST-segment elevation acute coronary syndromes. *JAMA.* 293:349, 2005.

Kris-Etherton PM, et al. Antioxidant vitamin supplements and cardiovascular disease. *Circulation.* 110:637, 2004.

Kuhl EA, et al. Relation of anxiety and adherence to risk-reducing recommendations following myocardial infarction. *Am J Cardiol.* 103:1629, 2009.

Kurth T, et al. Kidney function and risk of cardiovascular disease and mortality in women: a prospective cohort study. *BMJ.* 338:2392, 2009.

Lisspers J, et al. Long-term effects of lifestyle behavior change in coronary artery disease: effects on recurrent coronary events after percutaneous coronary intervention. *Health Psychol.* 24:41, 2005.

Marik PE, Varon J. Omega-3 dietary supplements and the risk of cardiovascular events: a systematic review. *Clin Cardiol.* 32:365, 2009.

O'Brien DM, et al. Red blood cell delta15 N: a novel biomarker of dietary eicosapentaenoic acid and docosahexaenoic acid intake. *Am J Clin Nutr.* 89:913, 2009.

Pell JP, et al. Smoke-free legislation and hospitalizations for acute coronary syndrome. *N Engl J Med.* 359:482, 2008.

Vita JA. Polyphenols and cardiovascular disease: effects on endothelial and platelet function. *J Clin Nutr.* 81:292S, 2005.

Yamada Y, et al. Molecular genetics of myocardial infarction. *Genomic Med.* 2:7, 2008.

PERICARDITIS AND CARDIAC TAMPONADE

NUTRITIONAL ACUITY RANKING: LEVEL 2

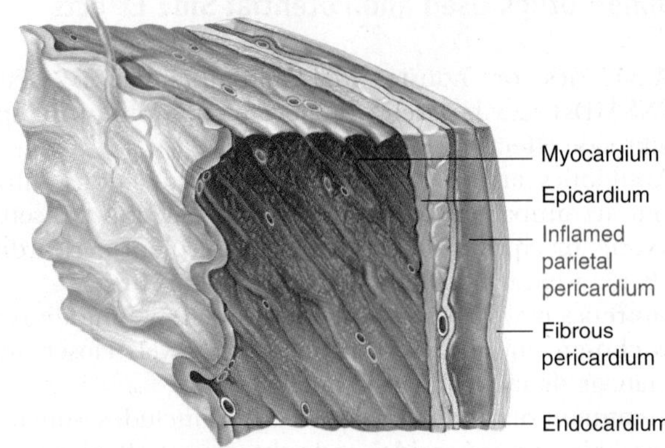

Asset provided by Anatomical Chart Co.

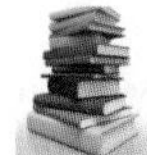

DEFINITIONS AND BACKGROUND

Pericarditis is inflammation of the pericardium due to human immunodeficiency virus (HIV)/acquired immunodeficiency syndrome (AIDS), MI, rheumatic diseases, radiation treatment, viral infection, trauma, neoplasm, chronic renal failure, or lupus. Bacterial pericarditis occurs by direct infection during trauma, thoracic surgery or catheter drainage, spread from *Staphylococcus, Streptococcus, Haemophilus,* and *Mycobacterium tuberculosis* (Pankuweit et al, 2005).

Severe substernal chest pain, dyspnea, shortness of breath, fever, chills, diaphoresis, nausea, fatigue, and anxiety are common in the acute stage. The chronic stage of pericarditis often results from tuberculosis and may involve ascites, edema of the extremities, HF, shrinkage of the pericardium, shortness of breath, coughing, fatigue, ascites, and leg edema.

Although pericarditis usually is not a life-threatening condition, other life-threatening conditions may cause chest pain and should be ruled out. These include MI, dissection of the aorta, pulmonary embolus, collapsed lung, and perforation or rupture of parts of the esophagus or stomach. Control of symptoms through diuretics is the usual treatment.

The most serious complication is **cardiac tamponade**, with accumulation of fluid or blood within the pericardial sac. If uncontrolled, this condition may lead to HF, arrest, or shock (Meltzer and Karia, 2005). Decreased heart sounds, distended neck veins with inspiratory rise in venous pressure (Kussmaul's sign), decreased BP, and abdominal pain may occur. In children, cases of cardiac tamponade have occurred as a complication of malignancies, cardiac surgery, trauma, infections, central venous catheter placement, rheumatologic and autoimmune diseases (Cousineau and Savitsky, 2005). Pericardial effusions causing tamponade are rare in patients with lupus, but high-dose corticosteroids are often needed (Rosenbaum et al, 2009).

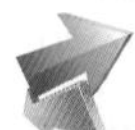

ASSESSMENT, MONITORING, AND EVALUATION

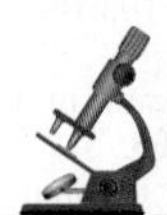

CLINICAL INDICATORS

Genetic Markers: A deficiency in the interleukin-1 receptor activated kinase 4 (IRAK-4) has recently been associated with severe recurrent, Gram-positive bacterial infections and related heart infections (Comeau et al, 2008). In addition, Familial Mediterranean fever is an autosomal recessive disease that presents with recurrent Peritonitis. More studies of the genetics of pericardial diseases are needed.

Clinical/History

- Height
- Weight
- Weight changes (loss?)
- BMI
- Waist circumference
- Diet history
- Low-grade intermittent fever?
- High fever?
- I & O
- Ascites or hepatomegaly?
- Tachypnea, dyspnea
- Cyanosis?
- Cough
- Dysphagia
- Pericardial friction rub
- ECG
- Cardiac catheterization
- Magnetic resonance imaging (MRI)
- Computed tomography (CT)

Lab Work

- CRP
- Gluc
- Alb, transthyretin
- BP
- BUN, Creat, GFR
- H & H
- Serum Fe
- Transferrin
- Na^+, K^+
- Ca^{++}, Mg^{++}
- WBC
- tHcy
- Serum folate and B_{12}

INTERVENTION

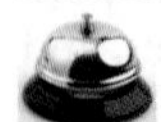

OBJECTIVES

- It is critical for anyone who experiences chest pain to seek immediate medical attention to determine the cause and receive prompt, appropriate treatment to improve cardiac functioning.
- Maintain bed rest during acute stages.
- Prevent sepsis, HF, and shock, especially if cardiac tamponade occurs.
- Decrease fever and inflammation, which may last 10–14 days in the acute form.
- Reduce nausea and anorexia.
- Prevent fluid overload if CPN is administered.

SAMPLE NUTRITION CARE PROCESS STEPS

Malnutrition

Assessment Data: Diet history and food records indicating intake of about 60% of usual intake; dyspnea, anorexia, nausea, recent fevers up to 103°F. BMI 17; usual BMI 20.

Nutrition Diagnosis (PES): Malnutrition related to pericarditis and chronically poor intake as evidenced by BMI of 17 and weight loss over the past year of 15 lb.

Intervention: Add protein powder to mixed dishes that are served. Educate about nutrient density and ways to add calories and protein. Review medications and suggest ways to increase appetite; discuss with medical team.

Monitoring and Evaluation: Improved intake and appetite; BMI closer to usual. Fewer complaints of fever, nausea, anorexia.

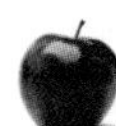

FOOD AND NUTRITION

- Maintain an adequate diet as needed for any underlying conditions; increase protein and calories if tolerated and if needed to prevent loss of LBM.
- Alter sodium and fluids intake if necessary.
- Small, frequent feedings to reduce nausea may be indicated.
- Monitor diet and supplements adequately. Thiamin for the heart muscle and potassium may be especially necessary; vitamins B_6 and B_{12} and folic acid may be needed if tHcy levels are elevated. It may also be prudent to increase vitamin E levels.
- The DASH diet, TLC diet, and Mediterranean diet are good choices.

Common Drugs Used and Potential Side Effects

- Analgesics or nonsteroidal anti-inflammatory drugs (NSAIDs) may be used to relieve pain. Monitor for specific side effects.
- Antibiotics are needed for bacterial infections. Intravenous antibacterial therapy, such as vancomycin, ceftriaxone, or ciprofloxacin, is used in purulent pericarditis (Pankuweit et al, 2005). Monitor for side effects.
- Diuretics may be used. If a potassium-depleting diuretic is chosen, monitor serum potassium levels closely and manage dietary changes if needed.
- Treatment of tuberculous pericarditis includes isoniazid, rifampin, pyrazinamide, and ethambutol (Pankuweit et al, 2005). Prednisone is given and then progressively reduced in 6–8 weeks; GI distress, hyperglycemia, and calcium and nitrogen depletion may result.
- Some medications can trigger an immune response that causes pericarditis. These medications include isoniazid (Nydrazid), hydralazine (Apresoline), penicillin, antiarrhythmic agents such as procainamide (Procanbid or Pronestyl), and seizure medications such as phenytoin (Dilantin).

Herbs, Botanicals, and Supplements

- See Table 6-3 for guidance.

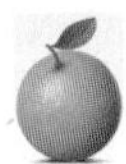

NUTRITION EDUCATION, COUNSELING, CARE MANAGEMENT

- Discuss the importance of avoiding fatigue.
- The patient should plan rest periods before and after activities and meals.
- Highlight the importance of nutrition in immunocompetence.
- Discuss any drug–nutrient interactions that are possible according to the treatment plan.

Patient Education—Foodborne Illness

- Careful food handling will be important. Hand washing is key as well.

For More Information

- Cardiac Tamponade
  http://www.nlm.nih.gov/medlineplus/ency/article/000194.htm
- Medline—Pericarditis
  http://www.nlm.nih.gov/medlineplus/ency/article/000182.htm
- Merck Manual—Pericarditis
  http://www.merck.com/mmpe/sec07/ch078/ch078a.html
- Mount Sinai
  http://www.mssm.edu/cvi/pericarditis.shtml
- Pericarditis
  http://cardiologychannel.com/pericarditis/
- Pericarditis and Cardiac Tamponade
  http://www.emedicine.com/emerg/topic412.htm

PERICARDITIS AND CARDIAC TAMPONADE—CITED REFERENCES

Comeau JL, et al. Staphylococcal pericarditis, and liver and paratracheal abscesses as presentations in two new cases of interleukin-1 receptor associated kinase 4 deficiency. *Pediatr Infect Dis J.* 27:170, 2008.

Cousineau A, Savitsky E. Cardiac tamponade presenting as an apparent life-threatening event. *Pediatr Emerg Care.* 21:104, 2005.

Meltzer H, Karia VG. Cardiac tamponade. *Catheter Cardiovasc Interv.* 64:245, 2005.

Pankuweit S, et al. Bacterial pericarditis: diagnosis and management. *Am J Cardiovasc Drugs.* 5:103, 2005.

Rosenbaum E, et al. The spectrum of clinical manifestations, outcome and treatment of pericardial tamponade in patients with systemic lupus erythematosus: a retrospective study and literature review. *Lupus.* 18:608, 2009.

PERIPHERAL ARTERY DISEASE

NUTRITIONAL ACUITY RANKING: LEVEL 2

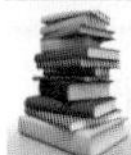

DEFINITIONS AND BACKGROUND

Peripheral vascular disease (PVD) can affect the arteries, the veins, or the lymph vessels. The most common and important type of PVD is **peripheral artery disease (PAD)**. PAD, defined as atherosclerosis in the lower extremities, affects nearly 8.5 million people in the United States (Dobesh et al, 2009). Prevalence increases dramatically with age; by age 70, about 20% of the population has PAD. PAD disproportionately affects Mexican Americans and nonhispanic blacks. People with PAD face a six to seven times higher risk of heart attack or stroke. Occlusion of an artery occurs from a clot or by plaque buildup in the extremities, such as the hands and feet numbness, tingling in lower extremities, pain, difficult ambulation, gangrene with potential amputation. See Table 6-16.

Causes of PAD include heavy smoking, arterial embolism, obesity, diabetes mellitus, real insufficiency, poor circulation, atherosclerosis, or exposure to heavy metals. Urinary cadmium, tungsten, and possibly antimony have been associated with PAD (Navas-Acien et al, 2005). Modifiable risk factors such as smoking, dyslipidemia, hypertension, and diabetes should be addressed (Aronow, 2005; Nijm et al, 2005).

Elevated levels of fibrinogen and CRP may indicate that there is inflammation. PAD is a red flag that the same process may be going on elsewhere; PAD is often associated with other life-threatening vascular diseases. Exercise is the first-line treatment for intermittent claudication with symptoms of aching pain, numbness, weakness, or fatigue (Dobesh et al, 2009).

TABLE 6-16 Sites Where Peripheral Arterial Disease Produces Symptoms

Arteries supplying blood to the brain	Stroke is a serious complication.
Arteries supplying blood to the kidneys	Renal artery stenosis is one of the causes of high blood pressure and renal failure.
Arteries supplying blood to the legs	Diminished ability to walk can occur; worst-case scenario leads to amputation.
Arteries supplying blood to the intestines	Mesenteric arterial disease is less frequent but can cause severe pain, weight loss, and death from intestinal gangrene.

Endothelial dysfunction may reduce functional capacity via attenuations in peripheral blood flow; dietary decosahexaenoic acid (DHA) may improve this dysfunction (Stebbens et al, 2008). When National Health and Nutrition Examination Survey (NHANES) data were evaluated to determine specific nutrients that are associated with PAD, it was found that higher consumption of antioxidants (vitamin A, C, and E), vitamin B_6, fiber, folate, and omega-3 fatty acids have a significant protective effect (Lane et al, 2008). Because hypovitaminosis D is more common in blacks than Hispanics or whites, check serum levels of serum 25-hydroxyvitamin D (25[OH]D) and supplement as needed (Reis et al, 2008). Dietary supplementation may protect against PAD (Lane et al, 2008).

Angioplasty may be needed to clear obstruction, relieve symptoms, heal ulcers, and prevent amputation. Indications for lower extremity angioplasty, preferably with stenting, or bypass surgery are (1) incapacitating claudication in persons that interferes with work or lifestyle; (2) limb salvage in persons with limb-threatening ischemia as manifested by rest pain, nonhealing ulcers, and/or infection or gangrene; and (3) vasculogenic impotence (Aronow, 2005). If the limb cannot be salvaged, amputation would be needed.

Buerger's disease is the obstruction of small- and medium-sized arteries by inflammation triggered by smoking and is usually found among men aged 20–40 years. Skin ulcers or gangrene may result if smoking is not discontinued. Walking is beneficial, unless the person has gangrene, sores, or pain at rest.

Raynaud's syndrome allows small arterioles in the fingers and toes to go into spasm, and the skin turns pale or patchy red to blue. Sometimes the underlying cause is not known. Approximately 60–90% of cases occur in young women. Scleroderma, rheumatoid arthritis, atherosclerosis, nerve disorders, hypothyroidism, injury, and reactions to certain drugs are causes. Some people also have migraine headaches and pulmonary hypertension. These individuals must protect their extremities from the cold or take mild sedatives for pain.

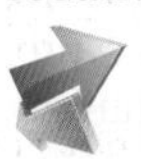

ASSESSMENT, MONITORING, AND EVALUATION

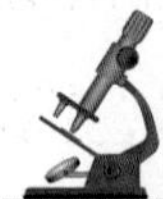

CLINICAL INDICATORS

Genetic Markers: Adipokine angiopoietin-like 4 gene (ANGPTL4[E40K]) variant appears to confer reduced genetic risk for CHD and other conditions, including PAD (Folsom et al, 2008). These common alleles are correlated with low TG and high HDL-C (Nettleton et al, 2009). Dietary fat intake modifies relations between HDL-C and polymorphisms in hepatic lipase (LIPC-514 C—>T), cholesteryl ester transfer protein (CETP TaqIB), and lipoprotein lipase (LPL S447X) genes (Nettleton et al, 2007).

Clinical/History
Height
Weight
BMI
Waist–hip ratio
Diet history
BP
Smoking history
Ankle brachial index (ABI) test <0.9
Exercise tolerance, stress testing
Ulcerations
Gangrene
ECG
Cardiac catheterization
MRI or CT scan

Lab Work
CRP
Chol—total, HDL, LDL
Trig
BUN, Creat
Uric acid
tHcy
Serum folate and B_{12}
Gluc
Serum insulin
Na^+, K^+
Ca^{++}, Mg^{++}
Serum 25-hydroxyvitamin D (25[OH]D)

INTERVENTION

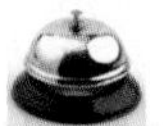

OBJECTIVES

- Treatment goals are aimed at decreasing cardiovascular risk, as well as improving quality of life (Dobesh et al, 2009). Reduce complications such as angina, HF, heart attack, stroke, renal failure, ulcerative disease, gangrene of lower extremities or toes.
- Prevent sepsis, pressure ulcers, or the need for amputation.
- Correct high levels of tHcy.
- Attain desired body weight if obese.
- Reduce the inflammatory process, as possible. CRP and other inflammatory markers offer risk prediction (Haugen et al, 2007).
- Modify carbohydrate and fat intakes (Nettleton, 2009).
- Correct hypovitaminosis D if needed.

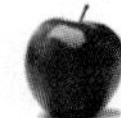

FOOD AND NUTRITION

- If patient is obese, use a low-calorie diet with high fiber.
- Diet should provide adequate protein intake for wound healing with ulcers or surgery.
- Vitamin E in almonds, filberts, avocados, sunflower seeds, vegetable oils, margarine, mayonnaise, and wheat germ are the best sources. Pistachios, sunflower kernels, sesame seeds, and wheat germ are high in phytosterols and should be used frequently.

SAMPLE NUTRITION CARE PROCESS STEPS

Inadequate Intake of Fatty Acids

Assessment: Diet history and food records, BP records. Labs with elevated LDL Chol.

Nutrition Diagnosis (PES): Inadequate intake of omega-3 fatty acids related to poor diet and peripheral circulation as evidenced by elevated LDL Chol intake.

Intervention: Education about the role of omega-3 fatty acids in cardiovascular health and reduction of inflammation.

Monitoring and Evaluation: Improved dietary records showing use of omega-3 fatty acids from diet and supplements.

- Increase folic acid, riboflavin, and vitamins B_6 and B_{12} if serum tHcy levels are elevated.
- The DASH, TLC, and Mediterranean diet patterns are useful.
- Olive oil consumption along with a dietary supplement of fish oil may be helpful in the management of PVD. Avoid use of butter and saturated fats.
- Correct vitamin D deficiency as needed.

Common Drugs Used and Potential Side Effects

- Antiplatelet drugs such as aspirin or clopidogrel may be helpful.
- Antibiotics may be used to control infections.
- ACE inhibitors are an important risk-reduction therapy for patients with PAD. Beta-blockers should be given if CAD is present (Aronow, 2005).
- Anticoagulants such as warfarin may be used. Use no more than one high–vitamin K food source daily. Avoid taking with dong quai, fenugreek, feverfew, excessive garlic, ginger, ginkgo, or ginseng because of their effects.
- Isoxsuprine (Vasodilan) may be used to dilate the vessels. If niacin is used as a vasodilator, do not use large doses without monitoring by a physician.
- Pentoxifylline (Trental) improves blood flow. GI distress, nausea, and anorexia may occur; take with meals.
- Statins reduce the incidence of intermittent claudication and improve exercise duration (Aronow, 2005).

Herbs, Botanicals, and Supplements

- Coenzyme Q10, ginger, purslane, and gingko have been recommended for PAD, but no clinical trials have proven efficacy. Use a vitamin D supplement if serum levels are low.
- See Table 6-3 for more information.

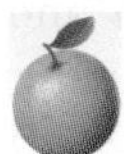

NUTRITION EDUCATION, COUNSELING, CARE MANAGEMENT

- Emphasize the importance of weight control and exercise.
- Reduce excess alcohol consumption if TGs are elevated.
- Fish and meatless meals should be used three to four times weekly.
- Hyperbaric oxygen treatments may be needed to heal lesions. Here, oxygen permeates the flesh, and anaerobic bacteria cannot survive.
- Encourage a smoking cessation program.

Patient Education—Foodborne Illness

- Careful food handling will be important. Hand washing is key as well.

For More Information

- American Heart Association
  http://www.americanheart.org/presenter.jhtml?identifier=4692
- Amputee Coalition
  http://www.amputee-coalition.org/
- Peripheral Artery Disease
  http://www.nhlbi.nih.gov/health/dci/Diseases/pad/pad_what.html
- Vascular Web
  http://www.vascularweb.org/patients/NorthPoint/Leg_Artery_Disease.html

PERIPHERAL ARTERY DISEASE—CITED REFERENCES

Aronow WS. Management of peripheral arterial disease. *Cardiol Rev.* 13:61, 2005.

Dobesh PP, et al. Pharmacologic therapy for intermittent claudication. *Pharmacotherapy.* 29:526, 2009.

Folsom AR, et al. Variation in ANGPTL4 and risk of coronary heart disease: the Atherosclerosis Risk in Communities Study. *Metabolism.* 57:1591, 2008.

Haugen S, et al. Risk assessment in the patient with established peripheral arterial disease. *Vasc Med.* 12:343, 2007.

Lane JS, et al. Nutrition impacts the prevalence of peripheral arterial disease in the United States. *J Vasc Surg.* 48:897, 2008.

Navas-Acien A, et al. Metals in urine and peripheral arterial disease. *Environ Health Perspect.* 113:164, 2005.

Nettleton JA, et al. Associations between HDL-cholesterol and polymorphisms in hepatic lipase and lipoprotein lipase genes are modified by dietary fat intake in African American and White adults. *Atherosclerosis.* 194:e131, 2007.

Nettleton JA, et al. Carbohydrate intake modifies associations between ANGPTL4[E40 K] genotype and HDL-cholesterol concentrations in White men from the Atherosclerosis Risk in Communities (ARIC) study. *Atherosclerosis.* 203:214, 2009.

Nijm J, et al. Circulating levels of proinflammatory cytokines and neutrophil-platelet aggregates in patients with coronary artery disease. *Am J Cardiol.* 95:452, 2005.

Reis JP, et al. Differences in vitamin D status as a possible contributor to the racial disparity in peripheral arterial disease. *Am J Clin Nutr.* 88:1469, 2008.

Stebbens CL, et al. Effects of dietary decosahexaenoic acid (DHA) on eNOS in human coronary artery endothelial cells. *J Cardiovasc Pharmacol Ther.* 13:261, 2008.

THROMBOPHLEBITIS

NUTRITIONAL ACUITY RANKING: LEVEL 1

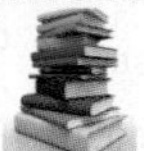

DEFINITIONS AND BACKGROUND

Phlebitis is inflammation of a vein that usually is caused by infection or injury. Blood flow may be disturbed, with blood clots (thrombi) adhering to the wall of the inflamed vein. This condition usually occurs in leg veins, especially in varicose veins. Blood clots in the thigh veins are usually more serious than those in the lower leg and are usually deep vein thromboses (DVTs).

Fatty acids have been implicated in the etiology of thrombophlebitis, but there is no clearly demonstrated mechanism. Blood tHcy levels are an important, independent,

TABLE 6-17 Causes of Thrombophlebitis

- Age: Over age 60 is more common, but it can occur any time
- Cancer and its treatment; especially in recently diagnosed patients, patients with cancer that has spread to distant sites (metastases), and those with certain genetic mutations (Blom et al, 2005)
- Central venous catheters
- Inherited conditions that cause increased risk for clotting; factor V Leiden, the genetic defect underlying resistance to activated protein C, is one factor that causes inherited thrombophilia
- Low blood flow in a deep vein due to injury, surgery, or immobilization
- Obesity or overweight
- Oral contraceptives or hormone replacement therapy; both estrogen and progesterone affect the condition
- Pregnancy and postpartum, especially the first 6 weeks after giving birth
- Sitting for a long period of time (long trips in a car or airplane)
- Varicose veins, which are enlarged, twisted, painful superficial veins resulting from poorly functioning valves, usually in the legs. They affect women more commonly than men.

and frequent risk factor for venous thrombosis. The VITRO (VItamins and ThROmbosis) trial was the first multicenter, randomized, double-blind and placebo-controlled study to evaluate the effect of tHcy-lowering therapy by means of 5 mg folic acid, 0.4 mg vitamin B_{12} and 50 mg vitamin B_6; it did not prevent recurrences (den Heijer et al, 2007).

Venous thromboembolism (VTE) is a major cause of morbidity and mortality worldwide, and the annual incidence of VTE is 1 per 1000 (Bramlage et al, 2005). Table 6-17 lists common causes of thrombophlebitis.

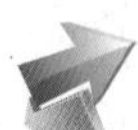

ASSESSMENT, MONITORING, AND EVALUATION

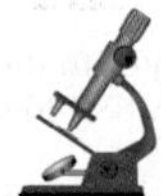

CLINICAL INDICATORS

Genetic Markers: Venous thrombosis is one of the leading causes of maternal morbidity and mortality; it is highly increased in carriers of factor V Leiden or the prothrombin 20210 A mutation (Pomp et al, 2008). It has also been noted with folate MTHFR alleles.

Clinical/History

Height
Weight
BMI
Waist–hip ratio
Diet history
Recent weight changes
Temperature
I & O
BP
Pain, redness, warmth, tenderness, itching
Hard or cordlike swelling along the affected vein
Venography
Duplex ultrasound
Doppler study
Ankle BP measurements

Lab Work

CRP
Factor V Leiden kit
Alb, transthyretin
Chol—total, HDL, LDL
Trig
BUN, Creat
Uric acid
WBC
H & H
Gluc
TLC
Na^+, K^+
Ca^{++}, Mg^{++}
tHcy
Serum folate and B_{12}
Sex hormone–binding globulin (SHBG)—for oral contraceptive users

INTERVENTION

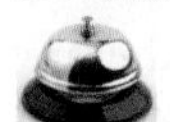

OBJECTIVES

- Stop the clot from getting bigger.
- Reduce inflammation and swelling.
- Prevent septicemia, pulmonary embolism (with chest pain and shortness of breath), and related complications.
- Lower elevated plasma tHcy, which increases the risk of VTE.

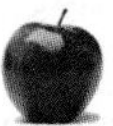

FOOD AND NUTRITION

- Weight control diet may be needed if the patient is obese. The DASH, TLC, and Mediterranean diets may be beneficial.
- Sodium restriction may be beneficial for persons with a generally high salt or sodium intake. Monitor carefully.
- For general cardiovascular health, adequate vitamins B_6 and B_{12} and folic acid intakes should be included. Intake of B vitamins through diet, supplementation, and fortified foods effectively reduces tHcy concentration and thus may reduce the risk.
- Thiamin and vitamin E are also beneficial for heart health at levels meeting but not exceeding daily requirements.
- Encourage use of omega-3 fatty acids from fish and other foods.
- Pistachios, sunflower kernels, sesame seeds, and wheat germ are high in phytosterols; use often.
- Flavonoids (including tannins, quercetin, and phenols) in grapes, strawberries, blueberries, apples, kale, broccoli, onions, garlic tea, beer, and red wine may reduce platelet activity and prevent clots.

SAMPLE NUTRITION CARE PROCESS STEPS

Assessment: Diet history and food records, BP records.

Nutrition Diagnosis (PES): Inadequate intake of types of fat

Intervention: Nutrition education about food and supplemental sources of EPA and DHA.

Monitoring and Evaluation: No clotting problems. BP improved or controlled.

- Foods that contain vitamin K can change how well warfarin (Coumadin) will work. Eat a balanced diet that does not vary in usual content of these vitamin K–rich foods so that the medication can be regulated.

Common Drugs Used and Potential Side Effects

- The anticoagulant warfarin (Coumadin) may be used, with side effects that alter use of vitamin K. Monitor intake carefully. Avoid supplements that are high in vitamins E, C, or A during use. Avoid taking with dong quai, fenugreek, feverfew, excessive garlic, ginger, ginkgo, and ginseng because of their effects.
- Another anticoagulant drug, ximelagatran (Exanta), may be useful as well (O'Brien and Gage, 2005). It is an oral direct thrombin inhibitor (DTI) that binds noncovalently and reversibly to both fibrin-bound and freely circulating thrombin (Petersen, 2005).
- Antibiotics are used in bacterial infections.
- Aspirin or acetaminophen may be used to reduce fever or pain. Chronic use of aspirin may decrease serum ferritin by increasing occult blood loss.
- Thrombolytics may be given to quickly dissolve blood clots that cause symptoms during life-threatening situations. Thrombin inhibitors may be used to interfere with the clotting process.

Herbs, Botanicals, and Supplements

- See Table 6-3 for guidance.

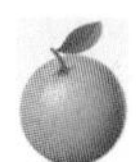

NUTRITION EDUCATION, COUNSELING, CARE MANAGEMENT

- Bedrest may be important during acute stages of DVT. Leg and foot elevation may be required. Monitor side effects of immobility if patient will be immobilized for a long period of time.
- Zinc ointment may relieve itching.
- The DASH diet plan should be taught. Discuss flavonoids and other nutrients.
- For overall improvement of venous health, encourage patient to stop smoking, increase exercise, lower elevated lipids, and wear compression stockings if needed.
- Discuss sources of the B vitamins, and suggest a supplement if appropriate, especially for individuals with MTHFR mutations (Varga et al, 2005).

Patient Education—Foodborne Illness

- Careful food handling will be important. Hand washing is key as well.

For More Information

- Coumadin—Interactive Tutorial
  http://www.nlm.nih.gov/medlineplus/tutorials/coumadinintroduction/htm/index.htm
- JAMA Patient Page
  http://jama.ama-assn.org/cgi/reprint/296/4/468.pdf
- Mayo Clinic
  http://www.mayoclinic.com/health/thrombophlebitis/DS00223
- Medline
  http://www.nlm.nih.gov/medlineplus/ency/article/001108.htm
- National Institutes of Health—Thrombophlebitis
  http://www.nlm.nih.gov/medlineplus/deepveinthrombosis.html

THROMBOPHLEBITIS—CITED REFERENCES

Blom JW, et al. Malignancies, prothrombotic mutations, and the risk of venous thrombosis. *JAMA.* 293:715, 2005.

Bramlage P, et al. Current concepts for the prevention of venous thromboembolism. *Eur J Clin Invest.* 35:4S, 2005.

den Heijer M, et al. Homocysteine lowering by B vitamins and the secondary prevention of deep vein thrombosis and pulmonary embolism: a randomized, placebo-controlled, double-blind trial. *Blood.* 109:139, 2007.

O'Brien CL, Gage BF. Costs and effectiveness of ximelagatran for stroke prophylaxis in chronic atrial fibrillation. *JAMA.* 293:699, 2005.

Petersen P. Ximelagatran: a promising new drug in thromboembolic disorders. *Curr Pharm Des.* 11:527, 2005.

Pomp ER, et al. Pregnancy, the postpartum period and prothrombotic defects: risk of venous thrombosis in the MEGA study. *J Thromb Haemost.* 6:632, 2008.

Varga EA, et al. Cardiology patient pages. Homocysteine and MTHFR mutations: relation to thrombosis and coronary artery disease. *Circulation.* 111:289, 2005.

SECTION 7

Gastrointestinal Disorders

CHIEF ASSESSMENT FACTORS

- Abdominal Pain or Distention
- Appetite, Anorexia
- Ascites, Jaundice
- Bezoars (Undigested Foreign Matter, Usually in Stomach)
- Change in Eating or Bowel Habits
- Change in Stools, Consistency, and Frequency; Fecal Incontinence
- Constipation
- Dentition
- Diarrhea (bloody, explosive)
- Dysphagia
- Easy Fatigue
- Edema of Extremities
- Feeding Method for Digestive or Absorptive Problems
- Hemorrhoids, Rectal Bleeding or Polyps
- Indigestion, Heartburn, Reflux
- Nausea, Vomiting, Regurgitation
- Painful or Cramping Abdomen, Flatulence
- Painful Oral Tissues, Tongue
- Use of Antacids, Stool Softeners, Diuretics, Laxatives, Histamine Blockers
- Weight Loss

INTRODUCTION AND BACKGROUND FOR GASTROINTESTINAL DISORDERS

Digestion

Digestion is a process that physically and chemically breaks down food in preparation for absorption. It begins with mastication and mixing of food with salivary fluid and enzymes (oral phase). In the gastric phase, pepsin and gastric acid begin to work. Chyme is then delivered to the small intestine for mixing with pancreatic and biliary juices. The pancreatic phase involves pancreatic amylase and lipase, proteases, and phospholipase. The intestinal phase involves disaccharidases (maltase, lactase, and sucrase), peptidases, and cholecystokinin for bile salts. *Maldigestion* involves the interference at any of these stages, including abnormal emptying of the stomach and pancreatic insufficiency.

Absorption

Passage of molecular nutrients into the bloodstream from the intestinal cells, starts primarily in the duodenum, with monosaccharides, amino acids and small peptides, monoglycerides, and free fatty acids. Water is also absorbed to maintain isotonicity of blood and cells. Bile and fat are needed to absorb fat-soluble vitamins A, D, E, and K. Water-soluble vitamins C and B-complex are usually absorbed in the intestinal mucosa with some storage in the liver. *Malabsorption* can result from dysfunction from any of the above steps.

Small Intestine

It is approximately 3.8 cm in diameter and 4.8-m long, covered with villi projections to increase absorptive surface. Villi cells have a rapid turnover rate of 2–5 days. Fecal fat is a valuable test of lipid digestion/absorption.

Large Intestine

It is approximately 5 cm in diameter and 1.5-m long, with two sections (colon and rectum) forming a frame around a highly convoluted small intestine. A diet high in whole and unrefined foods (whole grains, dark green and yellow/orange vegetables and fruits, legumes, nuts, and seeds) is high in antioxidant phenolic compounds, fibers, and other phytochemicals, all of which are beneficial.

Rectum

It is approximately 12-cm long. The area is susceptible to polyps and tumors.

The entire process of digestion/absorption takes about 24 hours, with large variations among individuals.

Digestive problems such as abdominal pain, diarrhea, nausea, and vomiting result in approximately millions of physician visits, billions in direct U.S. medical costs annually, and frequent use of prescription medications. Table 7-1 lists gastrointestinal (GI) conditions that may lead to malnutrition. The enteric nervous system (ENS) consists of many different types of enteric neurons forming complex reflex circuits that underlie or regulate many gut functions (Young, 2008). The identification of the genetic, molecular, and cellular mechanisms responsible for the colonization of the gut by enteric neuron precursors provides an exciting future management for GI disorders.

The GI tract does not respond well to inflammation where digestion, absorption, and gut barrier protection is impaired (Tappenden, 2008). Arachidonic acid (AA) is the precursor of inflammatory eicosanoids-like prostaglandin E(2) and leukotriene B(4); the n-3 PUFAs eicosapentaenoic acid (EPA) and docosahexaenoic acid (DHA) are anti-inflammatory. Fish oil supplementation in patients with inflammatory bowel diseases (IBD) results in n-3 PUFA incorporation into gut mucosal tissue with the potential for modified inflammation, improved gut histology, decreased disease activity, reduced use of corticosteroids (Calder, 2008), and decreased risk of colorectal cancer (Habermann et al, 2009). Glutamine (an amino acid needed in stress or

TABLE 7-1 Gastrointestinal Conditions That May Lead to Malnutrition

Malabsorption	
Celiac disease	Pancreatic insufficiency
Crohn's disease	Short bowel syndrome
Disaccharidase deficiencies	Ulcerative colitis
Dumping syndrome	
HIV infection or AIDS	
Mechanical Function	
Achalasia or esophageal hypomotility	Esophageal obstruction
Adynamic ileus	Hirschsprung's disease
Bezoar formation after gastric surgery	Pyloric stenosis
Bowel obstruction	Tracheoesophageal fistula
Esophageal stricture	
Conditions that May Cause Fear of Eating	
Aspiration risk	Crohn's disease
Bloating/obstruction/distension/pain	Dental disease
Cholelithiasis and other biliary diseases	Diarrhea
Diverticulitis	Irritable bowel syndrome
Dumping syndrome	Lactose intolerance
Dysphagia	Pancreatitis (acute or chronic)
Esophageal spasm	Peptic ulcer
Flatulence	Proctitis
Food allergies	Rectal fissures
Gastritis	Reflux esophagitis
Ill-fitting dentures	Ulcerative colitis

TABLE 7-2 Enteral Nutrition, Prebiotics, Probiotics, and Synbiotics in Gastrointestinal Tract Function

When an oral diet is not feasible, **enteral nutrition (EN)** is needed to avoid prolonged starvation, to prevent deterioration of intestinal integrity, and to avoid translocation of gut bacteria. One or two basic formulas can meet most patients' needs.

Prebiotics: Low-digestible carbohydrates that are not digested in the upper GI tract become fermented in the large intestine. They have physiological benefits similar to those of dietary fiber. Short-chain fatty acids (SCFAs) are produced from fermentation of fiber; the SCFAs are fuel for mucosal cells, so they benefit the gut tissue. Fermentation leads to the selective stimulation and growth of beneficial gut bacteria such as *bifidobacteria* (prebiotics). Carbohydrates that offer desirable physiological properties are resistant starch (RS), oligofructose, and polydextrose.

Probiotics are live microbial food supplements; they support balance in the intestinal tract. Probiotics have the ability to modify gut pH, antagonize pathogens, produce lactase, and stimulate immunomodulatory cells. Functional foods such as yogurt with live cultures may decrease the incidence of cancer, allergic reactions, and lactose intolerance. Probiotics also have immunomodulating properties and enhance the mucosal barrier in inflammatory bowel disease, pancreatitis, liver transplantation, and diarrhea (Jenkins et al, 2005).

Synbiotics are combinations of prebiotics and probiotics. By combining specific prebiotics and plant fibers into multifiber synbiotics, immunosupportive effects are possible (Bengmark and Martindale, 2005). The use of these products may become common practice in intensive care and GI units. Crohn's disease and ulcerative colitis are caused by overly aggressive immune responses to a nonpathogenic enteric bacteria in genetically predisposed individuals; administration of probiotics, prebiotics, or synbiotics can restore a predominance of beneficial *Lactobacillus* and *Bifidobacterium*. They may be protective against colon cancer as well (Pool-Zobel, 2005).

REFERENCES

Bengmark S, Martindale R. Prebiotics and synbiotics in clinical medicine. *Nutr Clin Pract.* 20:244, 2005.

Jenkins B, et al. Probiotics: a practical review of their role in specific clinical scenarios. *Nutr Clin Pract.* 20:262, 2005.

Pool-Zobel BL. Inulin-type fructans and reduction in colon cancer risk: review of experimental and human data. *Br J Nutr.* 93:S73, 2005.

TABLE 7-3 Conditions That May Benefit from Use of Intestinal Fuels[a]

Bowel resection
Constipation
Diarrhea
Diverticulosis
Dumping syndrome
Inflammatory bowel disease (IBD)
Irritable bowel syndrome (IBS)
Parenteral nutrition–induced bowel atrophy
Radiation/chemotherapy damage to the GI tract
Tube feeding

[a]Glutamine, short-chain fatty acids, soy, fermentable fiber, prebiotics, probiotics

sepsis) requires GI processing to become effective; this is likely true for other nutrients. Threonine is an essential amino acid that is abundantly present in intestinally produced glycoproteins; studies in infants suggest a high obligatory visceral need for it in protein synthesis (van der Schoor et al, 2007). Lysine, arginine, and other amino acids are also used in intestinal health, providing support for early enteral feeding whenever possible. Table 7-2 gives details about the role of enteral nutrition, prebiotics, probiotics, and synbiotics in GI health. The right product and the right ingredients can make a big difference. Therefore, it is beneficial to employ a nutrition support specialist or team in facilities where many patients need enteral or parenteral support. Table 7-3 lists GI conditions that may benefit from nutritional enhancements and Table 7-4 describes the role of dietitians in the GI specialty area.

TABLE 7-4 Knowledge and Skills of Dietitians in Gastrointestinal Specialty

The GI dietetics practitioner:

Knows sites of digestion and absorption of macronutrients and micronutrients
Understands normal digestion, nutrient secretion, and absorption
Identifies key nutritional screening factors for persons with GI disease
Explains the association between diet and other therapies in treating GI disorders
Knows the value and limitations of enteral and parenteral nutrition formulas and common functional food ingredients
Knows how to handle complex GI problems in conditions as diverse as cystic fibrosis (Mascarenhas, 2003) and celiac disease (Niewinski, 2008)
Recognizes extremes of dietary intake and the effects of diet on GI function and symptoms
Understands how GI dysfunction, surgical resections, and diseases affect nutritional status
Understands how other diseases and conditions can affect GI function, such as diabetes and gastroparesis, postanesthetic ileus, neurological injury, and hormonal changes
Understands the consequences of eating patterns in both healthy persons and in those who have GI disease

REFERENCES

Beyer PL. Gastrointestinal disorders: roles of nutrition and the dietetics practitioner. *J Am Diet Assoc.* 98:272, 1998.

Mascarenhas MR. Treatment of Gastrointestinal Problems in Cystic Fibrosis. *Current Treat Options Gastroenterol.* 6:427, 2003.

Niewinski MM. Advances in celiac disease and gluten-free diet. *J Am Diet.* 108:661, 2008.

For More Information

- American College of Gastroenterology
  http://www.acg.gi.org/
- American Digestive Health Foundation
  http://www.fdhn.org/
- American Gastroenterological Association
  http://www.gastro.org
- American Society of Gastrointestinal Endoscopy
  http://www.asge.org
- Cleveland Clinic Foundation
  http://www.clevelandclinic.org/gastro/
- National Institute of Diabetes and Digestive and Kidney Diseases (NIDDK)
  http://www.niddk.nih.gov/
- Society of American Gastrointestinal Endoscopic Surgeons
  http://www.sages.org
- Society of Gastroenterology Nurses and Associates
  http://www.sgna.org
- World Organization for Digestive Endoscopy
  http://www.omed.org

CITED REFERENCES

Calder PC. Polyunsaturated fatty acids, inflammatory processes and inflammatory bowel diseases. *Mol Nutr Food Res.* 52:885, 2008.

Habermann N, et al. Modulation of gene expression in eicosapentaenoic acid and docosahexaenoic acid treated human colon adenoma cells. *Genes Nutr.* 4:73, 2009.

Tappenden KA. Inflammation and intestinal function: where does it start and what does it mean? *JPEN J Parenter Enter Nutr.* 32:648, 2008.

van Der Schoor SR, et al. The gut takes nearly all: threonine kinetics in infants. *Am J Clin Nutr.* 86:1132, 2007.

Young HM. Functional development of the enteric nervous system—from migration to motility. *Neurogastroenterol Motil.* 20:20S, 2008.

UPPER GI: ESOPHAGUS

DYSPHAGIA

NUTRITIONAL ACUITY RANKING: LEVEL 3–4

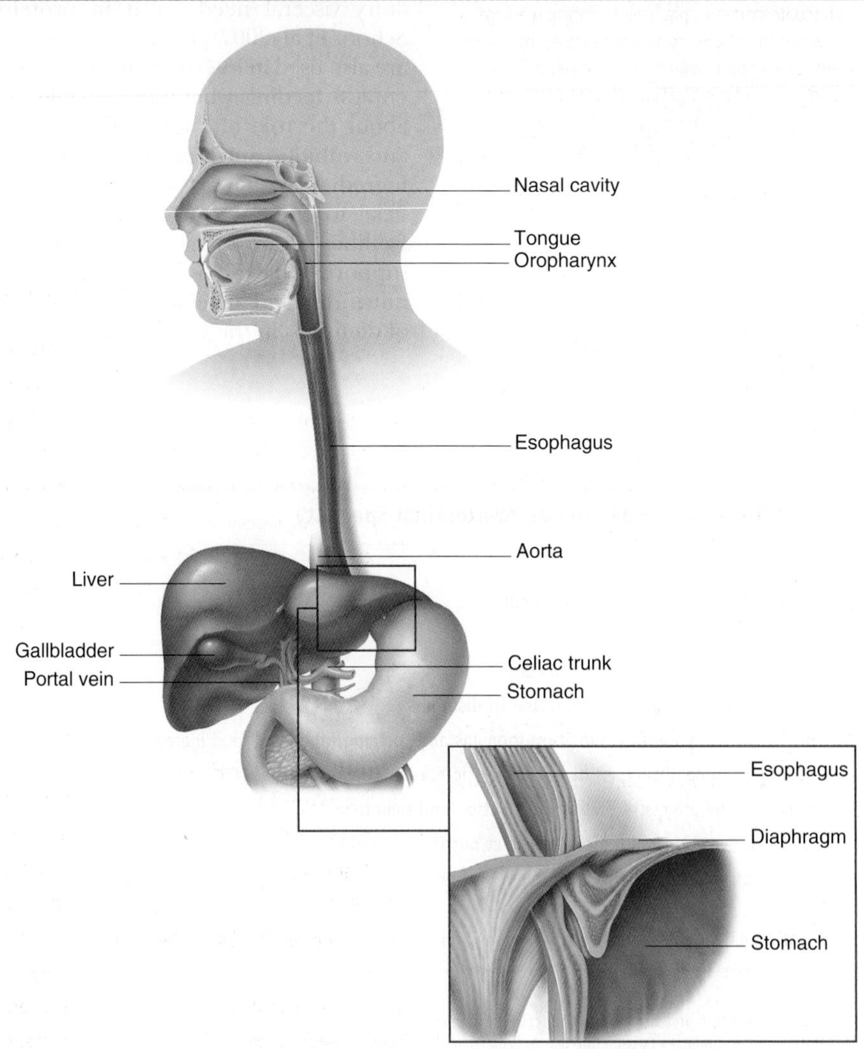

Asset provided by Anatomical Chart Co.

TABLE 7-5 Standard Questions in the Evaluation of Dysphagia

Describe any difficulty swallowing that you have.
Is the swallowing difficulty greater for solids or liquids?
How long have you had this swallowing difficulty?
Do you have heartburn along with this difficulty swallowing?
Is swallowing painful?
Do you get chest pain?
Does food get stuck when you swallow?
Do you choke or cough with swallowing?
Do you have temperature sensitivity (especially cold foods and beverages)?
Has there been any weight loss?

Adapted from: http://www.ncbi.nlm.nih.gov/bookshelf/br.fcgi?book=cm&part=A2747, accessed July 25, 2009.

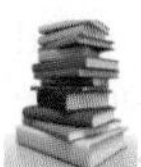

DEFINITIONS AND BACKGROUND

Anatomic or physiological swallowing problems of dysphagia create a disturbance in the normal transfer of food from the oral cavity to the stomach. Swallowing requires 5–10 seconds and three phases for completion—oral phase, pharyngeal phase, and esophageal phase. All must be adequate to prevent choking and/or aspiration into the lung. Signs of possible dysphagia include coughing with meals, choking, drooling, or pocketing of foods. Consult speech therapist for a full evaluation; a barium swallow may reveal silent aspiration. Videofluoroscopy (VF) is the gold standard. Questions to ask about swallowing difficulty are listed in Table 7-5.

Progress diet when possible, under guidance of the therapist. Inadequate dietary intake, weight loss, nutrient deficiencies, protein-energy malnutrition, and dehydration may result from prolonged dysphagia. In children with developmental disabilities, diagnosis-specific treatment of feeding disorders results in significantly improved energy consumption and nutritional status.

Dysphagia is classified into oropharyngeal dysphagia due to malfunction of the pharynx and upper esophageal sphincter, or esophageal dysphagia due to malfunction of the esophagus. Common causes of dysphagia are listed in Table 7-6.

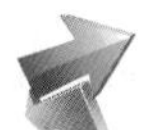

ASSESSMENT, MONITORING, AND EVALUATION

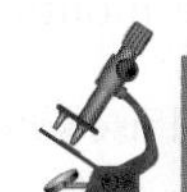

CLINICAL INDICATORS

Genetic Markers: Mutations in the PABPN1 gene can cause an oculopharyngeal muscular dystrophy.

Clinical/History

Height
Weight
Body mass index (BMI)
Weight changes
Diet history and swallowing problems—current, history, duration
Fiberoptic endoscopic evaluation of swallowing (FEES)
Videofluoroscopic swallowing study
Esophagoscopy
Barium swallow
Cookie swallow test
Pocketing of food under tongue or in cheeks
Spitting food out of mouth
Facial weakness
Slow oral transit time
Choking
Coughing before, during, or after swallowing
Excessive eating time
Wet, gurgly voice after drinking or eating
Slurred speech
Poor tongue control or excessive movement
Hoarseness, breathy voice
Recurrent pneumonia
Mealtime resistance—clenching teeth or throat
Regurgitation of food through nose or mouth
Upper GI bleeding
Blood pressure (BP)

Lab Work

Hemoglobin and hematocrit (H & H)
Blood urea nitrogen (BUN)
Albumin (Alb)
C-reactive protein (CRP)
Na^+, K^+, Cl^-
Ca^{++}, Mg^{++}
Other labs specific for the disorder

TABLE 7-6 Common Causes of Dysphagia

Achalasia	Head trauma
Aging	Hiatal hernia
Alzheimer's disease	Huntington's disease
Amyotrophic lateral sclerosis	Lung cancer
Cerebral palsy	Meningitis
Cerebrovascular accident (stroke)	Multiple sclerosis
Chronic obstructive lung disease	Muscular dystrophy
Cleft lip or palate	Myasthenia gravis
Closed head injury	Myotonic dystonia
Dehydration from medications	Parkinson's disease
Diabetes, type 1 (long term)	Pneumonia with aspiration history
Encephalopathy	Poliomyelitis
Esophageal inflammation	Prematurity
Esophageal fistula	Pulmonary disorders
Esophageal obstruction or stricture	Radiation treatment to head/neck
Esophageal trauma	Sjögren's disease
Gastroparesis	Spinal cord injury
Gastroesophageal reflux (GERD)	Throat cancer or injury
Goiter	Tongue cancer
Guillain-Barré syndrome	Tracheoesophageal fistula
Head or neck cancer	Zenker's diverticulum

SAMPLE NUTRITION CARE PROCESS STEPS

Dysphagia

Assessment Data: Weight loss, dysphagia and jaw pain, throbbing headache

Nutrition Diagnoses (PES): Dysphagia related to progression of Parkinson's disease as evidenced by weight loss, difficulty swallowing solids, and choking on thin liquids.

Interventions: Education about blending foods and simplifying meal planning to increase intake. Swallowing evaluation for determination of appropriate textures and thickening of liquids. Counseling on positioning at mealtime to reduce likelihood of aspiration.

Monitoring and Evaluation: Improved intake for meals and snacks; fewer complaints of difficulty swallowing. No further weight loss.

INTERVENTION

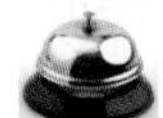

OBJECTIVES

- Prevent choking and aspiration of foods and beverages.
- Promote weight maintenance or gain if losses have occurred. In head and neck cancer patients, anorexia and dysphagia are factors that adversely affect outcome of treatments (Kubrak et al, 2010).
- Individualize diet based on patient needs and preferences. Refer to speech therapist, who will help to determine the level of consistency that is required (e.g., nectar or syrup, honey, pudding). Monitor for pocketing of food.
- For some patients, thin liquids may be needed. Modify levels of dysphagia diets as impairment level changes; upgrade when and if safe for the patient.
- Support independence in eating whenever possible. Provide foods that stimulate the swallowing reflex.
- For persons who have viscous oral secretions or dry mouth, liquefy foods before serving by adding broth, juice, or water. Provide moistened foods or thickened beverages for adequate hydration.
- Correct any nutrient deficits. Prevent pressure ulcers, if relevant.

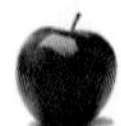

FOOD AND NUTRITION

- The patient may be fed enterally if needed. Results from the FOOD (Feed or Ordinary Food) Collaboration Trials showed that nasogastric (NG) tube feeding (TF) was favored over percutaneous endoscopic gastrostomy (PEG) as the early route of feeding in dysphagic stroke patients (Prosser-Loose and Paterson, 2006).
- If needed, jejunostomy feedings may be more appropriate for the patient's condition. Home TF may be needed, depending on the medical condition and cause of dysphagia.
- If central parenteral nutrition (CPN) is needed, monitor closely for ability to progress back to TF or oral diet.
- Following a protocol, clinical guideline, or algorithms improves dysphagia management.
- Calculate needs at 30–35 kcal/kg. Use a 1- to 1.5-g protein intake per kilogram to assure adequacy and to prevent loss of lean body mass. Monitor cardiac, hepatic, and renal status accordingly.
- Prevent aspiration by careful selection of foods and beverages, such as thick, soft, pureed foods instead of thin liquids. Thickening may be at honey, nectar, or pudding consistency; the label on the thickener will indicate the amount required for the differing levels. When a thickened liquid diet is ordered, foods such as gelatin should not be used because they liquefy at body temperature. Thicken foods and beverages with special products such as Thick-It, Thicken-Up, and Thick 'n Easy; these products use thickeners to make semisolids out of coffee, soup, beverages, juices, and shakes.
- It is possible to use mashed potato flakes to thicken some meat and casserole dishes. Baby rice cereal is an inexpensive thickener as well. Fruit purees are also helpful in thickening juices and some desserts.
- Progress over time to a soft diet.
- With a decreased saliva production, moisten foods with small amounts of liquid and use extra fats, mild sauces, and gravies.
- Monitor for deficiencies in fiber, vitamins A and C if whole grains, fruits, and vegetables are not consumed.
- Avoid alcoholic and extremely hot or cold liquids and beverages.
- Avoid foods that cause choking or are hard to manage: tart juices and foods, dry or crisp foods such as crackers and chips, bony fish, chewy meats such as steak, sticky foods such as peanut butter or bananas, thinly pureed foods that are easily aspirated, foods with varying consistency, excessively sweet drinks that aggravate drooling, carbonated beverages, dry bread in sandwiches.
- Avoid foods that are easily aspirated: popcorn, bran cereals, nuts, dry mashed potatoes, cottage cheese, corn, celery, pineapple, other fruits or vegetables with skins or fibrous pulp.
- Where there is reduced oral sensation, position food in the most sensitive area and use cold foods.
- To form a more cohesive bolus of food in the mouth, serve semisolid consistencies.
- For a severely sore mouth, avoid acidic foods and use soft foods at moderate temperatures.
- For delayed or absent swallowing reflex, temperature extremes and spicy foods may help excite the nerves necessary to function better. Some thickened liquids may actually be beneficial. Use cohesive foods that do not fall apart.
- Finely crushed bran on cereal, powdered fiber, or high-fiber tube-feeding products can help alleviate constipation.
- An interdiscplinary care plan is available for use.

INTERDISCIPLINARY NUTRITION CARE PLAN
Dysphagia

Client Name: ______________ **#:** ________ **Initiated by:** ________ **Date:** ________

SCREEN
Nutrition Screen diagnosis: Dysphagia
Signed: ____________ Date: ______

GOALS (Check any/all):

❑ Safely eat and drink without risk in ____ (goal time).

❑ Swallow efficiently to maintain nutrition and hydration in ____ (goal time).

❑ Advance to normal texture of food in ____ (goal time).

Weight ❑ maintained, or ❑ loss/ ❑ gain of ____ lb in ____ (goal time).

ASSESS *(Check any/all)*
❑ **Food/liquid texture modification**
Weight/BMI
- ❑ Weight loss >3 lb/wk or >5%/mo or >10%/6 mo
- ❑ BMI <20 (High risk)
- ❑ BMI <27

❑ **Medications**
❑ **Infection (e.g., pneumonia)**
❑ **Pressure ulcers/wounds**
Poor oral intake symptoms
- ❑ Complex diet order
- ❑ Nausea/vomiting
- ❑ Poor appetite/early satiety
- ❑ Problems chewing/swallowing
- ❑ Depression/anxiety
- ❑ GI distress

Signed: ____________ Date: ______

None →

MODERATE RISK INTERVENTIONS
(Check any/all)
❑ **Foods that are easy to swallow** provided and explained
❑ **Food record** provided and explained
Obtain Dr. orders as needed:
- ❑ RD chart consult
- ❑ SLP chart consult
- ❑ OT chart consult
- ❑ Monitor weight q:_____
- ❑ Monitor I & O q:_____
- ❑ BID/TID supplements

❑ **Other:**________________
(See notes for documention.)

Signed: ____________ Date: ______

Next visit ↓

ASSESS RESPONSE *(Check any/all)*
❑ Further food/liquid texture modification required
❑ Weight change not appropriate per goal
❑ Dehydration
❑ Onset of pulmonary infection
❑ Exhibiting Poor Oral Intake Symptoms
❑ **Other:**________________
(See notes for documention.)

Signed: ____________ Date: ______

None →

OUTCOMES ACHIEVED
❑ Food/liquid texture advanced toward normal
❑ Weight maintained or improved
❑ Hydration status maintained or improved
❑ **Other:**________________
(See notes for documention.)
❑ Repeat Nutrition Risk Screen in ____ days

Signed: ____________ Date: ______

← 1 or more

1 or more ↓

HIGH-RISK INTERVENTIONS *(Check any/all)*
❑ **Foods that are easy to swallow** provided and explained
❑ **Food record** provided and explained
Obtain Dr. orders as needed:
- ❑ RD referral for home visit(s)
- ❑ SLP referral for home visit(s)
- ❑ OT referral for home visit(s)
- ❑ Monitor weight q:_____
- ❑ Monitor I & O q: _____
- ❑ BID/TID supplements

❑ **Medication adjustment**
❑ **Other:**________________
(See notes for documention.)

Signed: ____________ Date: ______

Next visit ↓

ASSESS RESPONSE *(Check any/all)*
❑ Further food/liquid texture modification required
❑ Continued poor oral intake symptoms
❑ Weight change not appropriate per goal
❑ Dehydration
❑ Onset of pulmonary infection
❑ **Other:**________________
(See notes for documention.)

Signed: ____________ Date: ______

None →

OUTCOMES ACHIEVED
❑ Food/liquid texture advanced toward normal
❑ Weight maintained or improved
❑ Hydration status maintained or improved
❑ **Other:**________________
(See notes for documention.)
❑ Repeat Nutrition Risk Screen in ____ days

Signed: ____________ Date: ______

1 or more ↓

OUTCOMES NOT ACHIEVED
Reassess/evaluate need for EN/PN (refer to Tube Feeding Nutrition Care Plan). Document on Nutrition Variance Tracking form.

Common Drugs Used and Potential Side Effects

- For thick saliva and gagging, artificial saliva such as lemon glycerin may be useful.
- Papain or citrus juices may be useful for thinning secretions.

Herbs, Botanicals, and Supplements

- Herbs and botanical supplements should not be used without discussing with the physician.
- It is important to stress that no supplement or diet can cure dysphagia.

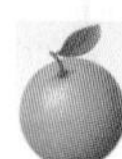

NUTRITION EDUCATION, COUNSELING, CARE MANAGEMENT

- Follow meals by brushing teeth to reduce dental caries; encourage optimal mouth care.
- Offer suggestions for specific changes in food preparation (e.g., adding moistening sauces, gravies, etc.) and cutting or mincing foods to increase control of the swallowing process.
- Encourage regular review of changes in swallowing abilities to identify early decline or to lessen restrictions when possible.
- Monitor for quality of life factors and adjust where possible.

Patient Education—Foodborne Illness

- If home TF is needed, teach appropriate sanitation and food-handling procedures.

For More Information

- Dysphagia On-Line (Nestle)
  http://www.dysphagiaonline.com/en/pages/01_what_is_dysphagia.aspx
- E-medicine
  http://emedicine.medscape.com/article/324096-overview
- NIH—Dysphagia
  http://www.nidcd.nih.gov/health/voice/dysph.asp

DYSPHAGIA—CITED REFERENCES

Kubrak C, et al. Nutrition impact symptoms: key determinants of reduced dietary intake, weight loss, and reduced functional capacity of patients with head and neck cancer before treatment [published online ahead of print July 22, 2009]. *Head Neck.* 32:290, 2010.

Prosser-Loose EJ, Paterson PG. The FOOD Trial Collaboration: nutritional supplementation strategies and acute stroke outcome. *Nutr Rev.* 64:289, 2006.

ESOPHAGEAL STRICTURE OR SPASM, ACHALASIA, OR ZENKER'S DIVERTICULUM

NUTRITIONAL ACUITY RANKING: LEVEL 3, STRICTURE; LEVEL 2 ACHALASIA

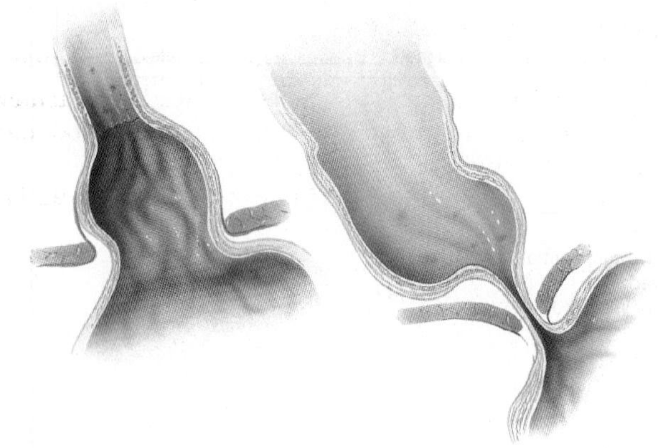

Asset provided by Anatomical Chart Co.

DEFINITIONS AND BACKGROUND

Esophageal stricture is caused by injury or chemical ingestion (such as lye), sliding hiatal hernia, esophageal cancer, reflux esophagitis (RE), peptic ulcer disease, or prolonged use of an NG tube. Another cause is eosinophilic esophagitis, with solid food dysphagia on presentation. Scar tissue builds up and prevents normal swallowing.

In **esophageal spasm**, segmented, concentric contractions occur simultaneously in the lower two thirds of the esophagus. Barium and manometric studies are useful in the evaluation. Achalasia and diffuse esophageal spasm are associated with hypertrophy of circular and longitudinal muscle layers (Mittal et al, 2005). Chemical denervation with *Clostridium botulinum* toxin (Botox) is effective in relieving spasm.

Achalasia is failure of the cardiac sphincter to relax, with obstruction of food passage into the stomach. In addition, the esophagus does not demonstrate normal waves of contraction after swallowing. The mechanisms remain poorly understood (Kraichely and Farrugia, 2006; Sonnenberg, 2009). Esophageal dilatation or surgical myotomy is common. Laparoscopic procedures are preferred (Pastor et al, 2009).

Zenker's diverticulum (ZD, or pharyngeal pouch) generally presents after 60 years of age, but patients may have years of dysphagia symptoms. Regurgitation of undigested food when patient bends over or lies down may occur. Serious complications include aspiration and malnutrition (Ferreira et al, 2008). Diagnosis is by barium swallow, and treatment is open surgical diverticulectomy. Minimally invasive (endoscopic stapling) devices are often used. Oral feeding is usually possible the day after surgery as general anesthesia is not needed.

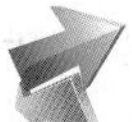

ASSESSMENT, MONITORING, AND EVALUATION

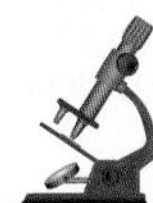

CLINICAL INDICATORS

Genetic Markers: Achalasia is usually of idiopathic origin but may be secondary to cancer or mast cell disorders.

Esophageal stricture secondary to radiation treatment may show signs of altered interleukin or tumor necrosis factor (TNF).

Clinical/History		Lab Work
Height	Regurgitation, halitosis	Glucose (Gluc)
Weight	Heartburn or other specific symptoms	Alb
Weight loss?	Endoscopy	CRP
BMI	Esophageal manometry	Gastrin
Diet history	Esophagoscopy	H & H
Intake and output (I & O)	Cineesophagography	Na^+, K^+, Cl^-
Dysphagia	BP	Ca^{++}, Mg^{++}
Substernal pain after meals		

INTERVENTION

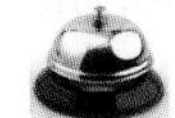

OBJECTIVES

- **Esophageal stricture:** Avoid large boluses of food. Provide adequate nutrition. Prevent weight loss. Remove cause or dilate, if necessary.
- **Esophageal spasm:** Avoid either very cold or very hot foods or beverages. Monitor dysphagia.
- **Achalasia:** Individualize diet according to patient tolerances and preferences. Monitor chronic dysphagia. Avoid aspiration.

SAMPLE NUTRITION CARE PROCESS STEPS

Dysphagia and Esophageal Stricture

Assessment Data: Weight loss, choking after swallowing, regurgitation, heartburn and chest pain after eating.

Nutrition Diagnoses (PES): Dysphagia related to altered GI function and esophageal stricture as evidenced by difficulty swallowing, abnormal barium swallow, and weight loss of 10 lb in last month.

Interventions: Education about blending foods and simplifying meal planning to increase intake. Swallowing evaluation for determination of appropriate textures and thickening of liquids. Counseling on positioning at mealtime; preparation for surgery

Monitoring and Evaluation: Improved intake of meals and snacks. Resolution of esophageal structure after surgery with no further weight loss.

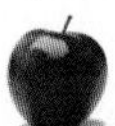

FOOD AND NUTRITION

- **Esophageal stricture:** Begin with liquid diet and progress to soft diet as tolerance increases. Adequate calories are needed. Gastrostomy may be needed. Antireflux regimen (no alcohol, weight loss) may be helpful. Avoid sticky and dry foods. Use thin liquids and pureed or soft foods.
- **Esophageal spasm:** Use diet as tolerated with modified temperatures for foods and beverages.
- **Achalasia:** Patients should take smaller bites of food, chew well, and eat slowly. Provide large volumes of fluids with each meal, unless dysphagia prevents appropriate swallowing of liquids. Tube feed if needed; may need to use gastrostomy TF.

Common Drugs Used and Potential Side Effects

- Antacids: Check the label for aluminum, calcium, magnesium, or sodium if other medical problems exist. Beware of long-term side effects.
- Isosorbide dinitrate and calcium channel blockers such as nifedipine may be needed 30 minutes before meals.
- Nitroglycerin often helps spasm. Headache is one possible side effect.

Herbs, Botanicals, and Supplements

- Herbs and botanical supplements should not be used without discussing with the physician.

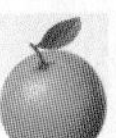

NUTRITION EDUCATION, COUNSELING, CARE MANAGEMENT

- Emphasize the importance of spacing meals and achieving relaxation. Recommend intake of food at moderate temperature only.
- Elevate head of bed for 30–45 minutes after meals and at bedtime.
- Encourage fluids at mealtimes.
- Avoid foods that aggravate dysphagia.
- Bland foods are not clearly beneficial and not required.

Patient Education—Foodborne Illness

- If home TF is needed, teach appropriate sanitation and food-handling procedures.

For More Information

- Achalasia
  http://www.medicinenet.com/achalasia/article.htm
- Baylor College of Medicine—Zenker's diverticulum
  http://www.bcm.edu/oto/grand/05_06_04.htm
- Esophagitis
  http://chorus.rad.mcw.edu/doc/00858.html

ESOPHAGEAL STRICTURE OR SPASM, ACHALASIA, AND ZENKER'S DIVERTICULUM—CITED REFERENCES

Ferreira LE, et al. Zenker's diverticula: pathophysiology, clinical presentation, and flexible endoscopic management. *Dis Esophagus.* 21:1, 2008.

Kraichely RE, Farrugia G. Achalasia: physiology and etiopathogenesis. *Dis Esophagus.* 19:213, 2006.

Mittal RK, et al. Sensory and motor function of the esophagus: lessons from ultrasound imaging. *Gastroenterology.* 128:487, 2005.

Pastor AC, et al. A single center 26-year experience with treatment of esophageal achalasia: is there an optimal method? *J Pediatr Surg.* 44:1349, 2009.

Sonnenberg A. Hospitalization for achalasia in the United States 1997–2006. *Dig Dis Sci.* 54:1680, 2009.

ESOPHAGEAL TRAUMA

NUTRITIONAL ACUITY RANKING: LEVEL 3–4

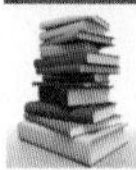

DEFINITIONS AND BACKGROUND

Esophageal trauma is a major traumatic condition that affects the esophagus; it is often caused by chemical burns, ingestion of foreign bodies, or injury. Diagnosis of penetrating pharyngeal and esophageal injuries is difficult when the patient has severe facial injuries, is obese, intubated, or hemodynamically unstable (Ahmed et al, 2009).

Boerhaave syndrome involves complete laceration of the esophagus, sometimes spontaneously from alcohol abuse with retching or secondary to endoscopy or vagotomy. **Mallory–Weiss syndrome** involves a mucosal gastric tear that can occur at the gastroesophageal (GE) junction or proximal stomach; it is also associated with retching or alcohol abuse.

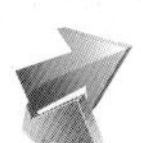

ASSESSMENT, MONITORING, AND EVALUATION

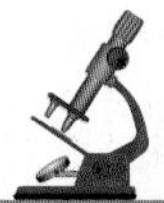

CLINICAL INDICATORS

Genetic Markers: Esophageal trauma is acquired, not genetic.

Clinical/History
- Height
- Weight
- BMI
- Weight changes
- Videoendoscopy
- I & O
- Nausea, vomiting
- Loss of consciousness
- Respiratory distress
- Esophageal perforation?
- Dysphagia
- Temperature

Lab Work
- Gluc
- BUN, creatinine (Creat)
- Na^+, K^+
- TLC
- H & H
- Serum Fe, ferritin, ferritin
- Alb or transthyretin
- Transferrin
- Ca^{++}, Mg^{++}

INTERVENTION

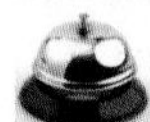

OBJECTIVES

- Emergency care, such as adequate ventilation, is given as needed.
- Allow the esophagus to rest and heal. Prepare for esophageal surgery if necessary.
- Keep the patient adequately hydrated.
- Improve swallowing capacity as rapidly as possible; prevent aspiration.
- Prevent malnutrition, weight loss, sepsis, constipation, fluid loss from exudates, and other complications.
- For serious injuries with permanent damage, it may be necessary for a gastrostomy TF to be used.

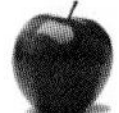

FOOD AND NUTRITION

- Nothing by mouth (NPO) as needed. Provide CPN, gastrostomy, or jejunostomy feedings as appropriate for the patient's condition.
- Calculate needs with extra protein, if applicable. Monitor cardiac, hepatic, and renal status.
- Progress over time to a soft diet. Avoid alcoholic beverages, extremely hot liquids and beverages, caffeine, and spicy foods if not tolerated.

SAMPLE NUTRITION CARE PROCESS STEPS

Unintentional Weight Loss

Assessment: Prior gunshot wound to the neck that required esophageal repair. Loss of 10 lb this year even though eating "a lot."

Nutrition Diagnosis (PES): Inability to digest/absorb nutrients (NC-1.4) related to surgical alteration in GI anatomical structure as evidenced by weight loss, albumin indicative of malnutrition.

Interventions: Food and Nutrient Delivery: ND 1.2—Alter diet as tolerated. ND 32.3 and 32.4—Initiate vitamin and mineral supplementation.

Education: E-1.2—Discuss ways to increase energy and nutrient density in food choices.

Counseling: C-2.3—Keep a food diary for 1 month. C-2.2—Set goal of only nutrient and energy-dense meals for 1 month if tolerated.

Monitoring and Evaluation: Review food diary after 1 month. Monitor weight for resolution of unintentional weight loss; goal is gain of 1–2 lb weekly.

- Provide adequate fluids but avoid overhydration.
- When able to eat orally, monitor for signs of dysphagia. Work with a speech therapist for proper consistency evaluations. Use appropriately thickened or thinned liquids and pureed foods until swallowing ability returns.
- Home TF may be needed, for which either a gastrostomy or jejunostomy will be used, depending on location and extent of injury and surgical repair.

Common Drugs Used and Potential Side Effects

- Liquid topical anesthetizing agents (such as lidocaine) may be used before meals to reduce pain.
- Antibiotics may be used in bacterial infections.

Herbs, Botanicals, and Supplements

- Herbs and botanical supplements should not be used without discussing with the physician.

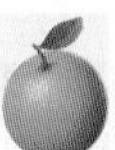

NUTRITION EDUCATION, COUNSELING, CARE MANAGEMENT

- When the patient can swallow, discuss the need to chew well and swallow carefully. The patient should also learn to eat slowly to prevent aspiration.
- Discuss the appropriate food textures for different stages of progress. This plan will be developed in accordance with the speech therapist and the physician.

Patient Education—Foodborne Illness

- If home TF is needed, teach appropriate sanitation and food-handling procedures.

For More Information

- Esophageal trauma
  http://emedicine.medscape.com/article/775165-overview

ESOPHAGEAL TRAUMA—CITED REFERENCES

Ahmed N, et al. Diagnosis of penetrating injuries of the pharynx and esophagus in the severely injured patient. *J Trauma.* 67:152, 2009.

ESOPHAGEAL VARICES

NUTRITIONAL ACUITY RANKING: LEVEL 2–3

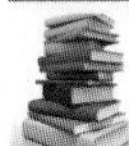

DEFINITIONS AND BACKGROUND

Acute bleeding from esophageal varices due to portal hypertension is a frequent and severe complication of liver cirrhosis (Lata et al, 2006). Esophageal varices occur in about half of all people with alcoholic cirrhosis and one third of these will experience variceal hemorrhage, a life-threatening event (Smith, 2010). Portal hypertension is defined as a portal pressure gradient exceeding 5 mm Hg where portosystemic collaterals decompress the portal circulation and give rise to varices (Toubia and Sanyal, 2008). Small esophageal veins become distended and may rupture due to increased pressure in the portal system. Thrombocytopenia and splenomegaly are independent predictors of large esophageal varices.

All cirrhotic patients should undergo endoscopic screening to detect varices. Severe fibrosis and esophageal varices may be diagnosed through a prothrombin index of less than 60%, alkaline phosphatase activity greater than 110 IU/L, and hyaluronate greater than 100 g/L in alcoholic patients (Vanbiervliet et al, 2005). Maintenance of a good renal function is essential in these patients (Lata et al, 2006). Fortunately, great strides have been made because of noninvasive imaging and pressure measurement. Mortality has been substantially reduced. Band ligation is the first-line endoscopic treatment. If this fails, the more invasive surgical shunt may be needed.

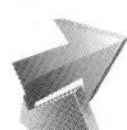

ASSESSMENT, MONITORING, AND EVALUATION

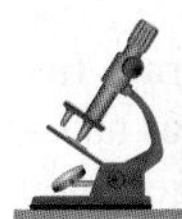

CLINICAL INDICATORS

Genetic Markers: Cirrhotic patients have an increased risk for thrombosis because of portal blood flow stasis; known risk factors include G20210 A mutation of prothrombin or factor V Leiden (Amitrano et al, 2007).

Clinical/History

Height
Weight
BMI
Diet history
Weight changes
Esophagoscopy
Edema
Melena
Upper GI bleeding
BP
Respiratory distress
Aspiration of emesis
Confusion
Abdominal distention,
Jaundice or hepatic coma

Lab Work

H & H
Serum Fe, ferritin
Ammonia (NH_3)
BUN
Alb (<4.0 g/dL)
Ascites
Na^+, K^+, Cl^-
Ca^{++}, Mg^{++}
Transferrin
Bilirubin (>20 mg/dL)
Platelet count (<200,000/mm^3)
Prothrombin index (<60%)
Hyaluronate (>100 g/L)
Alkaline phosphatase (Alk phos) (>110 IU/L)

SAMPLE NUTRITION CARE PROCESS STEPS

Excessive Alcohol Intake

Assessment: Intake history revealing poor intake of nutrient-dense foods and frequent meal skipping with use of one fifth of rum daily for 12+ years. Lab results showing elevated ammonia level, blood in stool, low H & H with documented anemia.

Nutrition Diagnoses (PES): Excessive alcohol intake related to intake of rum instead of meals as evidenced by bleeding and varices, diet history, altered hepatic labs.

Interventions: Enhance oral intake, or offer PEG TF as needed. Remove access to alcohol and coordinate care for referral to rehabilitation center when feasible.

Monitoring and Evaluation: No rebleeding. Adequate intake from TF and slow progression back to oral diet. Improved intake of all macro- and micronutrients, and improvement in labs. Corrected anemia.

INTERVENTION

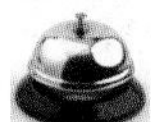

OBJECTIVES

- Promote healing and recovery.
- Prevent variceal rebleeding, which is a very frequent and severe complication in cirrhotic patients (Kravetz, 2007).
- Avoid constipation or straining with stool.
- Prevent or correct hepatic encephalopathy or coma; see Section 8.

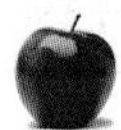

FOOD AND NUTRITION

- Generally, unless comatose, the patient can tolerate five to six small meals of soft foods. Avoid foods such as tacos, tortilla chips, or large pieces of raw fruits and vegetables.
- Alter carbohydrate, protein, and fat intake according to hepatic function and state of consciousness. Monitor micronutrient needs, such as iron if patient is anemic.
- Provide adequate fluid as allowed or controlled.
- To prevent constipation and straining, use foods such as prune juice or formulas with added fiber.
- Consider use of branched-chain amino acid formula for cirrhosis.

Common Drugs Used and Potential Side Effects

- Antacids may be beneficial to buffer gastric acidity. Extended use can cause problems with pH, altered mineral and nutrient use, and other imbalances.
- Beta-blockers; propranolol reduces the risk of bleeding, especially in cirrhosis (Suzuki et al, 2005). However, the combination of beta-blockers with mononitrate of isosorbide is superior to beta-blockade alone (Kravetz, 2007).
- Vasoactive agents, such as somatostatin analog and terlipressin, are useful.
- Vitamin K may be needed to help with clotting.

Herbs, Botanicals, and Supplements

- Herbs and botanical supplements should not be used without discussing with the physician.

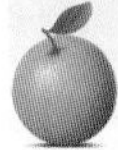

NUTRITION EDUCATION, COUNSELING, CARE MANAGEMENT

- The importance of good nutrition with proper consistency should be addressed. Avoid rough or crunchy foods that are fibrous or sharp; chew all foods well before swallowing.
- If gastrostomy is needed, discuss how to manage the process.
- If relevant, discuss the role of alcohol in contributing to the disease process with the patient and family. Advise the patient to avoid mouthwashes, cough syrups, and other products that contain alcohol.

Patient Education—Foodborne Illness

- If home TF is needed, teach appropriate sanitation and food-handling procedures.

For More Information

- Esophageal Varices
  http://www.nlm.nih.gov/medlineplus/ency/article/000268.htm

ESOPHAGEAL VARICES—CITED REFERENCES

Amitrano L, et al. Coagulation abnormalities in cirrhotic patients with portal vein thrombosis. *Clin Lab.* 53:583, 2007.

Kravetz D. Prevention of recurrent esophageal variceal hemorrhage: review and current recommendations. *J Clin Gastroenterol.* 41:318S, 2007.

Lata J, et al. Factors participating in the development and mortality of variceal bleeding in portal hypertension—possible effects of the kidney damage and malnutrition. *Hepatogastroenterology.* 53:420, 2006.

Smith MM. Emergency: Variceal hemorrhage from esophageal varices associated with alcoholic liver disease. *Am J Nurs.* 110:32, 2010.

Suzuki A, et al. Diagnostic model of esophageal varices in alcoholic liver disease. *Eur J Gastroenterol Hepatol.* 17:307, 2005.

Toubia N, Sanyal AJ. Portal hypertension and variceal hemorrhage. *Med Clin North Am.* 92:551, 2008.

Vanbiervliet G, et al. Serum fibrosis markers can detect large oesophageal varices with a high accuracy. *Eur J Gastroenterol Hepatol.* 17:333, 2005.

ESOPHAGITIS, GASTROESOPHAGEAL REFLUX DISEASE AND HIATAL HERNIA

NUTRITIONAL ACUITY RANKING: LEVEL 2–3

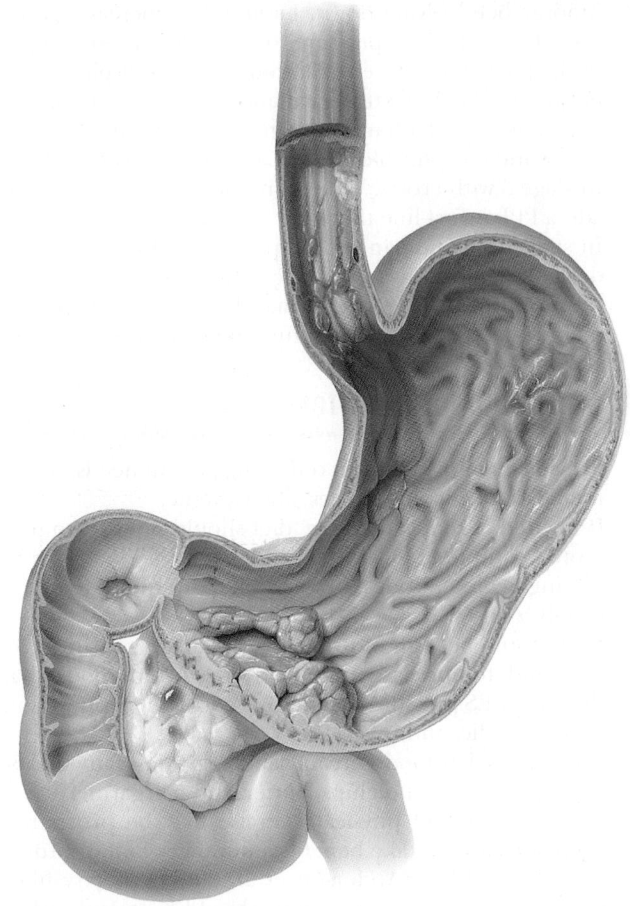

Asset provided by Anatomical Chart Co.

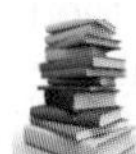

DEFINITIONS AND BACKGROUND

Esophagitis results from gastric juice being forced into the esophagus from the stomach. Pill-induced esophageal injury may occur from use of aspirin, tetracycline, vitamin C, ferrous sulfate, potassium chloride, or nonsteroidal anti-inflammatory drugs (NSAIDs). Take these with plenty of liquid.

Eosinophilic esophagitis (EoE or EE) is a disorder characterized by a severe, isolated eosinophilic infiltration of the esophagus that is unresponsive to aggressive acid blockade but responsive to the removal of dietary antigens (Liacouras et al, 2005). Adult patients usually present with dysphagia, food impaction and reflux-like symptoms (Gupte and Draganov, 2009). Known causes of tissue eosinophilia include GE reflux disease (GERD), infections, malignancy, collagen vascular diseases, hypersensitivity, and IBD (Gupte and Draganov, 2009). It is highly associated with atopic disease.

Barrett's esophagus is a condition that affects men more than women, and length of impact is greater in men than in women (Falk et al, 2005). It is also more common in Caucasians and in persons older than age 50. Symptoms are similar to GERD, but Barrett's esophagus is more likely to precede esophageal adenocarcinoma. Upper endoscopy and surveillance biopsies may be needed (Liu and Saltzman, 2006). Antioxidants (vitamins C, E, and beta-carotene) are important protective factors (Kubo et al, 2008), whereas obesity and the western diet may be promoters of cancer.

GERD and peptic ulcer disease are common in elderly individuals. GERD affects approximately 19 million Americans; prevalence is as high as 80% among asthma patients. There is a significantly higher prevalence of RE in an *Helicobacter pylori*-infected individuals of any age or sex (Moon et al, 2009). Distal esophageal cancer is associated with symptomatic GI reflux disease and Barrett's esophagus; surveillance programs are identifying patients early for curable esophageal adenocarcinoma (Demeester, 2006).

GERD may occur in infants but usually resolves by 6–12 months of age. Management involves thickened feedings and positioning. The recommended approach for infants with uncomplicated regurgitation is the reassurance of the parents about the physiological nature of excessive regurgitation and dietary recommendations for formula feeding. Symptoms of pediatric GERD include colic, inconsolable crying, frequent spitting up or vomiting, food refusal, failure to thrive, heartburn, stomach pains, chronic sore throat, chronic respiratory problems, asthma, and apnea. GERD diagnosis in older children warrants review for upper GI tract disorders, cow's milk allergy, or metabolic, infectious, renal, or central nervous system diseases.

Treatment guidelines address lifestyle changes, patient-directed (over the counter) therapy, acid suppression, promotility therapy, maintenance therapy, and antireflux surgery (DeVault and Castell, 2005). Intractable GERD may require minor surgery to strengthen a weak sphincter. Laparoscopic antireflux surgery is highly effective as a long-term treatment for severe GERD.

Hiatal hernia is caused by protrusion of part of the stomach through the diaphragm muscle, which separates the chest from the abdomen. This causes an enlarged diaphragm opening (hiatus) through which the esophagus passes to join the stomach. An increase in BMI is associated with the increased prevalence of hoatal hernia, esophageal mucosal injury, and complications because of increased intragastric pressure and increased GE pressure gradient (Fass, 2008). Hiatal hernia may show no symptoms or may contribute to heartburn, swallowing difficulty, reflux, or vomiting. Hiatal hernia surgery has evolved from anatomic repair to physiological restoration (Stylopoulos and Rattner, 2005).

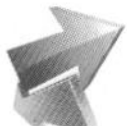

ASSESSMENT, MONITORING, AND EVALUATION

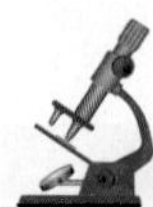

CLINICAL INDICATORS

Genetic Markers: Proton pump inhibitors (PPIs), such as omeprazole, lansoprazole, and rabeprazole are metabolized by CYP2C19 in the liver; there are genetic differences in the activity of this enzyme (Furuta et al, 2010). These genotypic differences influence the healing and eradication rates for GERD and *H. pylori* infection (Furuta et al, 2010). The pathogenesis of EE involves multiple tissues, cell types, and genes, and derives from complex genetic and environmental factors (Blanchard and Rothenberg, 2008).

Clinical/History

Height
Weight
BMI
Diet history
Weight changes
Upper GI endoscopy
Esophagoscopy
PillCAM (noninvasive visualization)
Manometry
Feeding difficulties in children
Recurrent vomiting
Reactive airway disease or nocturnal asthma
Choking attacks
Dental erosion or caries

Lab Work

H & H
Mean cell volume (MCV)
Na^+, K^+
Ca^{++}, Mg^{++}
Gluc
Gastrin
Alb, transthyretin
CRP
H. pylori infection?
Cholesterol (Chol)
Triglycerides (Trig)
Transferrin
Total iron-binding capacity (TIBC)
Bernstein test: HCl solution is dripped into the distal esophagus; positive test mimics patient symptoms

SAMPLE NUTRITION CARE PROCESS STEPS

Gastroesophageal Reflux Disease (GERD)

Assessment: Knowledge about the role of diet in GERD; food diary; timing of meals and related symptoms. Use of antacids with every meal and at bedtime.

Nutrition Diagnosis (PES): Undesirable food choices related to lack of knowledge regarding role of diet in GERD symptoms and complications as evidenced by frequent consumption of large, high-fat meals and alcoholic beverages.

Intervention: Teach about dietary changes that will alleviate GERD symptoms and possibly prevent complications. Counsel about lifestyle changes, such as weight loss, loose clothing, and upright posture during and after eating.

Monitoring and Evaluation: Report of relief from symptoms. No complications from GERD. Gradual reduction in need for antacids and medication.

INTERVENTION

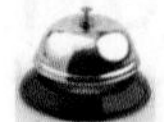

OBJECTIVES

- In stage 1, simple lifestyle modifications may be successful: elevate head of the bed, decrease fat intake, stop smoking, lose excess weight, avoid eating large meals, and do not eat 3 hours before lying down. Large meals increase gastric pressure and alter pressure on the lower esophageal sphincter (LES), thereby allowing reflux or aspiration to occur. Avoid tightly fitted garments around the abdomen.
- In stage 2, add pharmacological treatments, such as histamine-receptor blockers or antacids.
- In stage 3 with erosive esophagitis, it may be necessary to add a PPI as first-line therapy.
- In stage 4, maintenance therapy, use the lowest possible dose of medications to manage symptoms.
- In severe stage 5, surgery may be needed. This may include laparoscopic Nissan fundoplication.

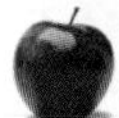

FOOD AND NUTRITION

- Provide an individual diet reflecting patient needs. Assess intake of fat, alcohol, spices, and caffeine.
- If needed, a reduced-energy diet should be used to promote weight loss.
- During acute episodes, provide small, frequent feedings of soft foods.
- Diet should be high in protein to stimulate gastrin secretion and to increase LES pressure. Avoid foods that decrease LES pressure, including chocolate, peppermint, onions, garlic, and spearmint.
- Use fewer fried foods, cream sauces, gravies, fatty meats, pastries, nuts, potato chips, butter, and margarine.
- Dietary fiber and physical exercise may be protective. Increased fiber intake benefits a number of GI disorders including GERD (Anderson et al, 2009). Dietary fiber intakes for children and adults should be calculated as 14 g/1000 kcal.
- Avoid foods that may irritate the esophagus, such as citrus juices, tomatoes, and tomato sauce. Other spicy foods are to be eliminated according to individual experience.
- If there is EoE, try a dietary elimination diet and add back foods one at a time to identify potential allergens (Liacouras et al, 2005).
- Fluids can be taken between meals to reduce abdominal distention and discomfort.
- Preterm infants may benefit from transpyloric feedings if they show signs suggestive of reflux and apnea (Malcolm et al, 2009).

Common Drugs Used and Potential Side Effects

- Antacids neutralize gastric contents. They destroy thiamin and may provide excess sodium for the body; check labels carefully. If the antacid contains calcium (e.g., Tums, which contains calcium carbonate), excess calcium may decrease levels of magnesium and phosphorus. Aluminum hydroxide (Maalox) depletes phosphorus, which is acceptable for patients with certain types of renal diseases, but otherwise this is not desirable for the long term. When used as an antacid, sodium bicarbonate can decrease iron absorption and causes sodium retention; use with caution.

- Calcium glycerophosphate (Prelief) is somewhat useful for relief of heartburn by neutralizing the acid in foods; it is available over the counter.
- PPIs, such as lansoprazole (Prevacid), omeprazole (Prilosec), and esomeprazole (Nexium) are popular treatments. When clarithromycin-resistant *H. pylori* (CRHP) occur, PPIs tend to inhibit the growth and motility of CRHP. Omeprazole is useful for refractory RE. Because CYP2C19 genotypes affect the recurrence rate of GERD symptoms during PPI maintenance therapy, genotype-based tailored therapy is needed (Furuta et al, 2010; Saitoh et al, 2009).

Herbs, Botanicals, and Supplements

- Herbs and botanical supplements should not be used without discussing with the physician.
- Chamomile, fennel, cardamom, cinnamon, dill, and licorice have been recommended for this condition, but no clinical trials have proven efficacy.

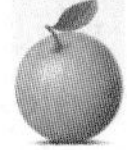

NUTRITION EDUCATION, COUNSELING, CARE MANAGEMENT

- Encourage the patient to avoid late evening meals and snacks and to avoid lying down or sleeping or swimming soon after a meal to guard against reflux.
- Teach the proper measures for controlling weight, including small, frequent feedings.
- Instruct the patient about lifestyle modifications listed in the Objectives. Patients with heartburn probably should not sleep in a waterbed.
- Chewing sugarless gum after meals may reduce reflux somewhat because of the saliva production.
- More effective communication and consumer education is required to enhance fiber consumption from foods or supplements (Anderson et al, 2009).

Patient Education—Foodborne Illness

- Careful food handling and washing hands before eating are useful recommendations.
- If home TF is needed, teach appropriate sanitation and food-handling procedures.

For More Information

- International Foundation for Gastrointestinal Disorders
  http://www.aboutgerd.org/
- Heartburn and Regurgitation Algorithm
  http://www.uwgi.org/guidelines/ch_03/ch03.htm
- National Institute of Diabetes and Digestive and Kidney Diseases (NIDDK)
  http://digestive.niddk.nih.gov/ddiseases/pubs/gerd/
- Prelief
  http://www.akpharma.com/prelief/preliefindex.html

HIATAL HERNIA, ESOPHAGITIS, AND GERD—CITED REFERENCES

Anderson JW, et al. Health benefits of dietary fiber. *Nutr Rev.* 67:188, 2009.

Blanchard C, Rothenberg ME. Basic pathogenesis of eosinophilic esophagitis. *Gastrointest Endosc Clin N Am.* 18:133, 2008.

Demeester SR. Adenocarcinoma of the esophagus and cardia: a review of the disease and its treatment. *Ann Surg Oncol.* 13:12, 2006.

DeVault K, Castell D. Updated guidelines for the diagnosis and treatment of gastroesophageal reflux disease. *Am J Gastroenterol.* 100:190, 2005.

Falk GW, et al. Barrett's esophagus in women: demographic features and progression to high-grade dysplasia and cancer. *Clin Gastroenterol Hepatol.* 3:1089, 2005.

Fass R. The pathophysiological mechanisms of GERD in the obese patient. *Dig Dis Sci.* 53:2300, 2008.

Furuta T, et al. Influences of different proton pump inhibitors on the antiplatelet function of clopidogrel in relation to CYP2C19 genotypes. *Br J Clin Pharmacol.* 70:383, 2010.

Gupte AR, Draganov PV. Eosinophilic esophagitis. *World J Gastroenterol.* 15:17, 2009.

Kubo A, et al. Dietary antioxidants, fruits, and vegetables and the risk of Barrett's esophagus. *Am J Gastroenterol.* 103:1614, 2008.

Liacouras CA, et al. Eosinophilic esophagitis: a 10-year experience in 381 children. *Clin Gastroenterol Hepatol.* 3:1198, 2005.

Liu JJ, Saltzman JR. Management of gastroesophageal reflux disease. *South Med J.* 99:735, 2006.

Malcolm WF, et al. Transpyloric tube feeding in very low birthweight infants with suspected gastroesophageal reflux: impact on apnea and bradycardia. *J Perinatol.* 29:372, 2009.

Moon A, et al. Positive association between helicobacter pylori and gastroesophageal reflux disease in children [published online ahead of print 9 June 2009]. *J Pediatr Gastroenterol Nutr.* 49:283, 2009.

Saitoh T, et al. Influences of CYP2C19 polymorphism on recurrence of reflux esophagitis during proton pump inhibitor maintenance therapy. *Hepatogastroenterology.* 56:703, 2009.

Stylopoulos N, Rattner DW. The history of hiatal hernia surgery: from Bowditch to laparoscopy. *Ann Surg.* 241:185, 2005.

STOMACH

DYSPEPSIA/INDIGESTION OR BEZOAR FORMATION

NUTRITIONAL ACUITY RANKING: LEVEL 1–2

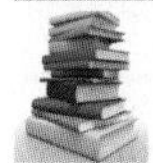

DEFINITIONS AND BACKGROUND

Indigestion (dyspepsia) may be secondary to other systemic disorders such as atherosclerotic heart disease, hypertension, liver disease, or renal disease. It may have psychogenic causes as well, such as during periods of anxiety. Symptoms may be graded from mild to severe for the individual patient. Gastric hypersensitivity is an important factor.

In rare cases, a patient may exhibit signs of **bezoar formation**, such as after gastric surgery or chronic use of medications that do not dissolve easily for that individual. A bezoar (foreign matter accumulation) may be made of plant material, medications, or swallowed foreign objects. The patient complains of vague abdominal pain or indigestion and may experience nausea or vomiting. An x-ray of the GI tract may be useful for a clarifying diagnosis.

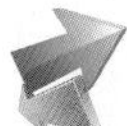

ASSESSMENT, MONITORING, AND EVALUATION

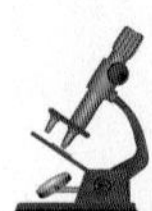

CLINICAL INDICATORS

Genetic Markers: Genetic factors in indigestion would be related to the primary disorder.

Clinical/History		Lab Work
Height	Anorexia	Gluc
Weight	Nausea or vomiting	*H. pylori* infection
Weight changes	Epigastric pain or burning	H & H
BMI	Postprandial fullness, early satiation	Serum Fe, ferritin
Diet history	Gastric barostat tests	MCV
Gastric burning sensation	Endoscopy	Alb, transthyretin
Bloating, heartburn, nausea	I & O	CRP
Burping, vomiting	Bezoar formation?	BUN, Creat
Early satiety, postprandial fullness		Na^+, K^+
		Ca^{++}, Mg^{++}

INTERVENTION

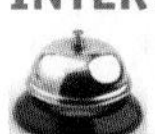

OBJECTIVES

- Determine whether the problem is psychogenic or organic in etiology. Do not oversimplify the patient's discomfort.
- If the patient has a bezoar, alter food and beverage consistencies.
- If the patient has irritable bowel or other GI condition, work closely with the medical team to manage dietary changes and reduce excessive use of medications.

SAMPLE NUTRITION CARE PROCESS STEPS

Dyspepsia

Assessment Data: Weight, BMI; recent GI surgery for extensive peptic ulcer disease; positive hx of *H. pylori* infection; heartburn with every meal and complaints of indigestion.

Nutrition Diagnoses (PES): Inadequate oral food and beverage intake related to frequent bouts of indigestion after GI surgery as evidenced by unplanned weight loss, reports of heartburn and indigestion with meals.

Interventions: Alter foods served to decrease use of acidic foods or stimulants such as caffeine and alcoholic beverages. Educate about simplifying meals and small snacks to increase intake. Counseling on food choices and lifestyle changes to improve intake and decrease discomfort.

Monitoring and Evaluation: Improved intake for meals and snacks. Fewer complaints of dyspepsia. No further weight loss. Reduced need for use of antacids for heartburn.

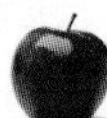

FOOD AND NUTRITION

- Diet should make use of well-cooked foods that are adequate in amount but not overly seasoned.
- Evaluate for any undetected food allergies and manage accordingly.
- A relaxed atmosphere is helpful, and small meals may be better tolerated.
- If the dyspepsia is organic in etiology, a soft, low-fat diet may be helpful.
- If there is irritable bowel as well, discuss fiber from fruits and vegetables (American Dietetic Association, 2008). Bran is not always well tolerated.
- If the patient has an obstruction or bezoar, a liquid diet may be useful until resolved.

Common Drugs Used and Potential Side Effects

- Antacids: Beware of nutritional side effects resulting from chronic use or dependency.
- Antisecretory drugs are useful (Suzuki et al, 2006). PPIs may be used, especially if reflux also exists. Lansoprazole (Prevacid), omeprazole (Prilosec), and esomeprazole (Nexium) are commonly used.
- NSAIDs are nonselective cyclooxygenase-1 (COX-1) and COX-2 inhibitors and may be associated with dyspepsia. Other anti-inflammatory medicines such as ibuprofen, aspirin, and naproxen (Aleve) can irritate the stomach. Acetaminophen (Tylenol) is a better choice for pain.

Herbs, Botanicals, and Supplements

- Herbs and botanical supplements should not be used without discussing with the physician.
- Ginger is often used as an antinauseant. Do not use large doses with warfarin, aspirin, other antiplatelet drugs, antihypertensive drugs, and hypoglycemic drugs. Additive effects can cause unpredictable changes in BP and decreases in blood glucose levels and may decrease platelet aggregation and thus increase bleeding. Ginger ale has few side effects.
- Chamomile, peppermint, red pepper, angelica, and coriander have been recommended, but no clinical trials have proven efficacy.

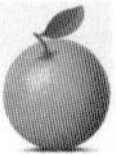

NUTRITION EDUCATION, COUNSELING, CARE MANAGEMENT

- Encourage the patient to eat in a relaxed atmosphere.
- Yoga and other stress-relieving lifestyle changes may be beneficial.
- Discuss the role of fiber in maintaining bowel regularity.
- Discuss tips for preparing meals that are lower in acid, stimulants, or other irritants.

Patient Education—Food Safety

- Careful food handling and hand washing are important to prevent introduction of foodborne pathogens to the diet of the individual. Preparation and storage techniques are also essential.
- If home TF is needed, teach appropriate sanitation and food handling procedures.

For More Information

- Dyspepsia
  http://familydoctor.org/474.xml
- Dyspepsia Algorithm
  http://www.uwgi.org/guidelines/ch_02/ch02.htm

DYSPEPSIA/INDIGESTION—CITED REFERENCES

American Dietetic Association. Position of the American Dietetic Association: health implications of dietary fiber. *J Am Diet Assoc.* 108:1716, 2008.

Suzuki H, et al. Therapeutic strategies for functional dyspepsia and the introduction of the Rome III classification. *J Gastroenterol.* 41:513, 2006.

GASTRECTOMY AND VAGOTOMY

NUTRITIONAL ACUITY RANKING: LEVEL 3–4

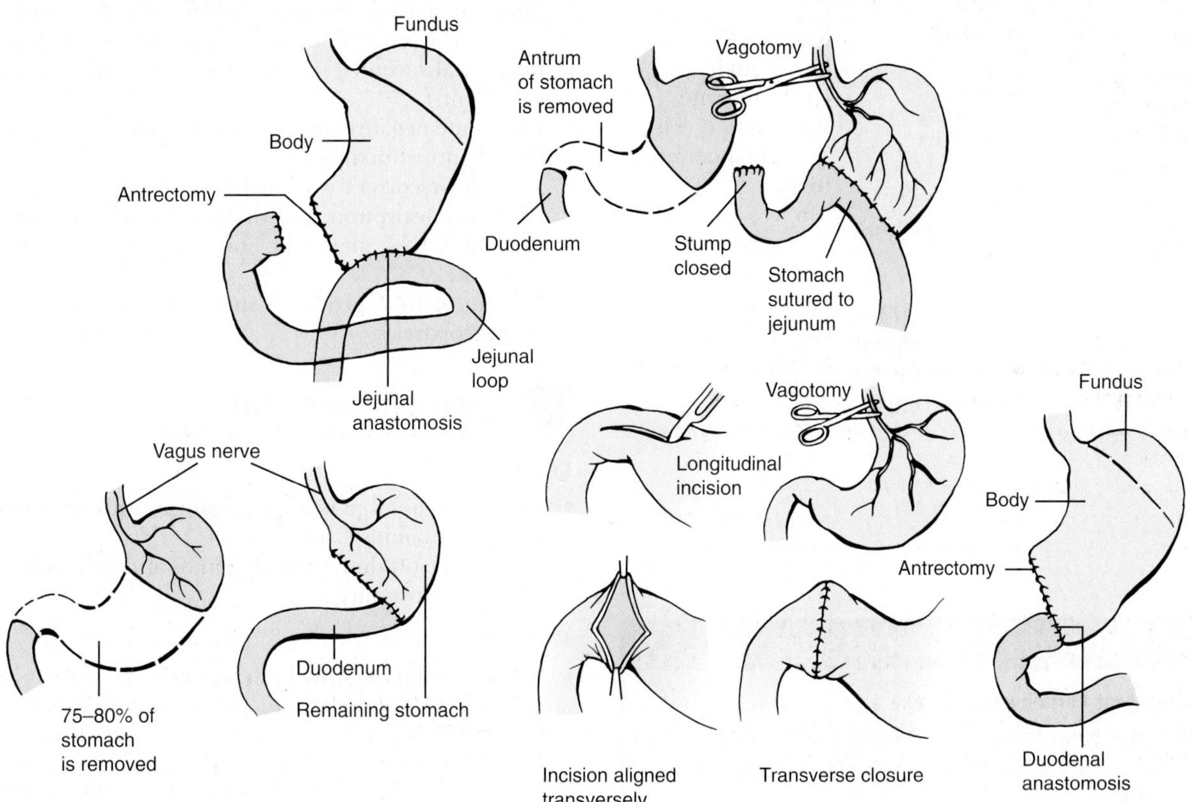

Adapted from: Nettina, Sandra M., MSN, RN, CS, ANP, The Lippincott Manual of Nursing Practice, 7th ed. Lippincott, Williams & Wilkins, 2001.

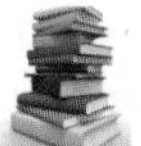

DEFINITIONS AND BACKGROUND

Gastrectomy and **vagotomy** are surgical procedures that are used for gastric cancer, when medical management for peptic ulcer has failed, or for perforation. The frequency with which elective gastric surgeries are performed has decreased in the past 20 years as drugs have become increasingly effective in treating ulcers. Laparoscopic-assisted gastrectomy is an increasingly common procedure for gastric cancer, with fewer side effects (Mochiki et al, 2005).

Billroth I (gastroduodenostomy) is an anastomosis between the stomach and duodenum after removal of the distal portion of the stomach. Billroth II (gastrojejunostomy) is an anastomosis between the stomach and jejunum after removal of two thirds to three fourths of the stomach; iron loss can occur. While the Billroth I and Billroth II operations have been used for reconstruction after a distal gastrectomy for gastric cancer, a Roux-en-Y reconstruction is increasingly performed to prevent duodenogastric reflux (Hoya et al, 2009).

Vagotomy is a procedure in which the vagus nerve is cut to reduce pain; much less nutritional intervention is required. Gastrectomy or vagotomy may lead to reactive hypoglycemia, which may drop plasma glucose levels to as low as 30–40 mg/dL due to rapid digestion and absorption of food, especially carbohydrates. Gastric emptying rate for solids may increase in some patients. In most of them, however, there is a normal to decreased emptying rate.

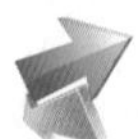

ASSESSMENT, MONITORING, AND EVALUATION

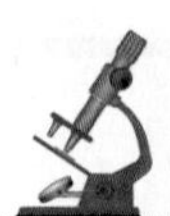

CLINICAL INDICATORS

Genetic Markers: Gastrectomy and vagotomy are surgical procedures. Any genetic relationships would be from the original problem.

Clinical/History	Lab Work	
Height	H & H	Na^+, K^+, Cl^-
Weight	Serum Fe, ferritin	Blood guaiac
BMI	Gluc	Urine acetone
Diet history	Glucose tolerance test (GTT)	White blood cell (WBC) count
BP	Chol, Trig	BUN
Temperature, fever	Pro-time (PT) or International Normalized Ratio (INR)	Alb, transthyretin
Electrogastrogram (EGG)		Serum amylase
Dual-energy x-ray absorptiometry (DEXA) scan		Serum B_{12}
		Ca^{++}, Mg^{++}
		Serum folate
		TIBC

SAMPLE NUTRITION CARE PROCESS STEPS

Inconsistent Carbohydrate Intake

Assessment Data: Weight loss, frequent emesis after meals, irregular blood glucose levels with reactive hypoglycemia several times weekly.

Nutrition Diagnoses (PES): Inconsistent carbohydrate intake related to lack of knowledge about nutrition after gastrectomy as evidenced by weight loss, complaints of profuse sweating, diarrhea, and vomiting after meals high in carbohydrate, and blood glucose levels that vary with bouts of reactive hypoglycemia.

Interventions: (ND-1) Order diet that is low fat, high protein, no concentrated sweets (NCS). Educate about foods that are high in simple carbohydrate and those that are complex. Counsel on eating slowly and drinking beverages between meals.

Monitoring and Evaluation: Improved intake for meals and snacks; fewer complaints of dumping syndrome. No further weight loss.

INTERVENTION

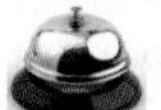

OBJECTIVES

Preoperative

- Empty the stomach and upper intestines.
- Ensure high-calorie intake for glycogen stores and weight maintenance or weight gain if needed. Ensure adequate nutrient storage to promote postoperative wound healing.
- Maintain normal fluid and electrolyte balance.

Postoperative

- Prevent distention and pain. Reduce the likelihood of the dumping syndrome: nausea, vomiting, abdominal distention, diarrhea, malaise, profuse sweating, hypoglycemia, hypotension, increased bowel sounds, and vertigo. Additional use of soy and fermentable fiber may be useful; liquid pectin may prolong gastric emptying time and reduce the onset of dumping.
- Compensate for loss of storage/holding space and lessen dumping of large amounts of chyme into the duodenum/jejunum at one time. Overcome effects of decreased hormonal output (secretin, pancreozymin, and cholecystokinin).
- Overcome negative nitrogen balance after surgery; restore healthy nutritional status.
- Prevent or correct iron malabsorption; steatorrhea, calcium malabsorption, and vitamin B_{12} or folacin anemias.
- Prevent or treat metabolic bone disease, which can occur over time.
- Prevent or treat problems such as bezoars, gastric stasis, or gastroparesis.

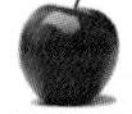

FOOD AND NUTRITION

Preoperative

- Use a soft diet that is high in calories with adequate protein and vitamins C and K.
- Regress to soft diet with full liquids and then NPO about 8 hours before surgery.

Postoperative

- Within a total quantity limit, intake of complex carbohydrates such as bread, rice, and vegetables should be liberal (50–60%). To lessen the hyperosmolar load, use only 0–15% of diet from foods made with sucrose, fructose, and glucose. Initial diet may need to be 20 mL of liquid nutritional supplement every few hours, progressing as tolerated. Gastrectomy patients will be limited by the size of the remaining stomach as well.
- A protein-rich food should be consumed with each meal. Include eggs, cheese, dried beans or peas, tender meat or poultry, boneless fish, yogurt, peanut butter, nuts, tofu, and cottage cheese.
- Lactose intolerance is common in patients with these conditions; use less milk or omit if needed. Monitor calcium intake carefully.
- Use a moderate fat intake (about one third of energy intake). If needed, medium-chain triglycerides (MCTs) may be beneficial with fat maldigestion, and pancreatic enzymes may also be needed in some cases.

- The diet should also provide adequate chromium, vitamin B_{12}, riboflavin, iron, folacin, calcium, and vitamin D. A liquid multivitamin–mineral supplement may be needed.
- If weight loss becomes a problem, a liquid supplemental beverage may be useful between meals and can be sipped throughout the day and evening.
- Diet should provide a moderate sodium intake; excess salt draws fluid into the duodenum. If there is diarrhea, losses of sodium in the stool may occur.
- Fluids should be taken 1 hour before or after meals, rather than with meals; assure adequate fluid intake overall.
- Sit upright while eating. Encourage slow eating and adequate chewing for all meals and snacks.
- Diet should provide frequent, small meals. Avoid extremes in food temperature.

Common Drugs Used and Potential Side Effects

- Antibiotics may be used to control bacterial overgrowth.
- Antidiarrheals such as Kaopectate and loperamide may be useful. Dry mouth, nausea, vomiting, and bloating may occur. Use plenty of fluids.
- For reactive hypoglycemia, use of an alpha-glucosidase inhibitor, acarbose, may be beneficial. GI side effects are common.
- Pancreatic enzymes may be useful; the usual dose provides two to three capsules with meals.
- If vitamin B_{12} deficiency occurs, shots may be needed.
- If bone density loss occurs, the use of calcium, vitamin D, or bisphosphonates may be prescribed, and these should be taken as directed.

Herbs, Botanicals, and Supplements

- Herbs and botanical supplements should not be used without discussing with the physician.

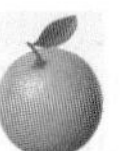

NUTRITION EDUCATION, COUNSELING, CARE MANAGEMENT

- Stress the importance of self-care and optimal functioning—what to do for illness, episodes of vomiting, eating away from home, and how to read labels for carbohydrate (CHO) content.
- Discuss the use of artificial sweeteners.
- Instruct the patient to eat slowly in an upright position and to remain upright for awhile after meals.
- Help the patient to overcome reluctance and the fear of eating. Discuss the dumping syndrome and its effects on nutrient absorption if untreated.

Patient Education—Foodborne Illness

- If home TF is needed, teach appropriate sanitation and food-handling procedures.

For More Information

- Anti-Dumping Syndrome Diet
  http://www.gicare.com/Diets/Dumping.aspx
- Gastrectomy—Surgical Channel
  http://www.surgerychannel.com/gastrectomy/index.shtml
- Medline
  http://www.nlm.nih.gov/medlineplus/ency/article/002945.htm

GASTRECTOMY AND VAGOTOMY—CITED REFERENCES

Hoya Y, et al. The advantages and disadvantages of a Roux-en-Y reconstruction after a distal gastrectomy for gastric cancer. *Surg Today.* 39:647, 2009.

Mochiki E, et al. Laparoscopic assisted distal gastrectomy for early gastric cancer: Five years' experience. *Surgery.* 137:317, 2005.

GASTRITIS AND GASTROENTERITIS

NUTRITIONAL ACUITY RANKING: LEVEL 3

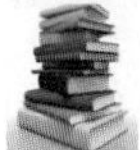

DEFINITIONS AND BACKGROUND

Gastritis involves inflammation of the stomach. Types of gastritis include bacterial (from *H. pylori*), autoimmune gastritis with pernicious anemia, erosive gastritis (from aspirin or NSAID use), alcohol-induced gastritis, bile reflux gastritis, or atrophic gastritis. The treatment of gastritis will depend on its cause; reduction of stomach acid by medication is often most helpful.

Helicobacter pylori infects half the world's population, causing **chronic gastritis** (Shanks and El-Omar, 2009). Bacterial, environmental and host genetic factors combine to define the degree of gastric damage in gastritis (Shanks and El-Omar, 2009). **Hemorrhagic gastritis** may result from chronic intake of alcohol or medications, Crohn's disease or HIV infection. **Atrophic gastritis** is chronic inflammation of the gastric mucosa without erosion but with hypochlorhydria or achlorhydria; it is important to monitor vitamin B_{12}, calcium, and ferric iron intake.

Gastroenteritis (GE) is an inflammation of the stomach and intestinal lining that may occur from eating chemical toxins in food (such as seafood, mushrooms, arsenic, or lead), drinking excessive alcohol, foodborne illness and viruses, cathartics or other drugs. GE produces malaise, nausea, vomiting, intestinal rumbles, diarrhea with or without blood and mucus, fever and prostration.

Viral gastroenteritis is contagious. Many different viruses can cause gastroenteritis, including rotaviruses or adenoviruses. Norovirus infection is associated with 90% of nonbacterial acute gastroenteritis (Sala et al, 2005).

Contaminated shellfish and raw oysters are major contributors. People who get viral gastroenteritis almost always recover completely if they consume adequate fluids to replace what they lose through vomiting or diarrhea.

Because the intestinal epithelium constitutes the largest and most important barrier against intraluminal toxins, antigens, and enteric flora, its dysfunction is a major factor contributing to the predisposition to inflammatory diseases (Groschwitz and Hogan, 2009). Post-infectious irritable bowel syndrome (PI-IBS) is a disorder where symptoms begin after an episode of acute GE with persistent subclinical inflammation, changes in intestinal permeability and alteration of gut flora (Thabane and Marshall, 2009). Some children acquire functional GI disorders after an episode of acute bacterial gastroenteritis (AGE) from *Salmonella* (54%), *Campylobacter*, or *Shigella* (Saps et al, 2008). Other issues related to intestinal dysfunction include food allergy, IBD, and celiac disease (Groschwitz and Hogan, 2009).

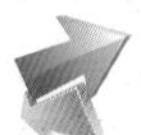

ASSESSMENT, MONITORING, AND EVALUATION

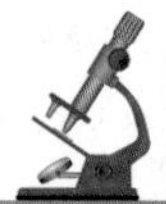

CLINICAL INDICATORS

Genetic Markers: Gastroenteritis is acquired and not genetic. Host genetic factors define the severity and extent of Helicobacter-induced gastritis; interleukin-1 and TNF-A gene clusters are involved (Shanks and El-Omar, 2009).

Clinical/History

Height
Weight
BMI
Diet history
Anorexia, nausea
Upset stomach
Hiccups
I & O
Signs of dehydration?
Fever?
Esophageal manometry
Barium swallow study
Upper GI endoscopy
Gastric biopsy
Diarrhea
Stool culture
Blood in stool?

Lab Work

Na^+, K^+, Cl^-
H & H
Serum Fe, ferritin
MCV
Serum folate
Serum B_{12}
Gluc
Alb, transthyretin
Ca^{++}, Mg^{++}
Hydrogen breath test
BUN, creatinine

INTERVENTION

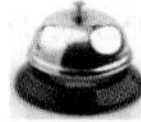

OBJECTIVES

- Prevent or correct dehydration, shock, hypokalemia, and hyponatremia.
- If hemorrhage occurs, consider a medical emergency.
- Allow the stomach and GI tract to rest. Empty stomach to permit mucous lining to heal.
- Omit lactose if not tolerated during bouts of gastroenteritis.

SAMPLE NUTRITION CARE PROCESS STEPS

Abnormal GI Function—Diarrhea

Assessment Data: Diarrhea, GI pain, slight fever; recent intake of undercooked beef and sushi while traveling.

Nutrition Diagnoses (PES): Altered GI function (NC-1.4) with foodborne illness as evidenced by diarrhea, slight fever (100°F) for 7 days and stool culture positive for *Escherichia coli* 0157:H7.

Interventions: Alter diet as tolerated; soft diet or liquids may be accepted. Provide oral rehydration products. Educate about foodborne illness related to *E. coli* 0157:H7 including food sources. Counseling about safe food-handling procedures and better choices at restaurants while traveling.

Monitoring and Evaluation: Resolution of diarrhea. Stool cultures free from *E. coli* 0157:H7. Improved knowledge about food safety as documented by correct responses to questions.

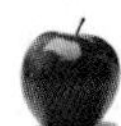

FOOD AND NUTRITION

- **Gastritis:** Omit foods that are poorly tolerated. Provide adequate hydration. If chronic, mucosal atrophy can lead to nutritional deficits (e.g., pernicious anemia, achlorhydria). Alter diet accordingly.
- **Acute gastroenteritis:** Patient will be NPO or on partial parenteral nutrition (PPN) for the first 24–48 hours to rest stomach. Use crushed ice to relieve thirst. Oral rehydration therapy may be useful. Progress to a soft diet, if desired. Alcohol is prohibited. Omit lactose if needed. Gradually add fiber-containing foods as tolerance improves. Rehydration solutions may be effective.
- **Chronic gastritis:** Use small, frequent feedings of easily tolerated foods. Progress with larger amounts and greater variety of foods, as tolerated. Restrict fat intake, which depresses food motility, and alcohol intake. Monitor lactose intolerance. Add fiber-containing foods as tolerated.

Common Drugs Used and Potential Side Effects

- Antacids: Watch for constipation caused by aluminum and calcium agents. Watch for diarrhea caused by magnesium agents.
- Antibiotics are used for infection. If used in excess over a long period of time, they may cause or aggravate gastroenteritis. Monitor carefully and suggest use of probiotics such as yogurt with live and active cultures.
- Sucralfate may be useful. Take separately from calcium or magnesium supplements by 30 minutes. Constipation may occur.
- Early postoperative medication with a PPI is effective in preventing gastritis after open-heart surgery (Hata et al, 2005). Lansoprazole (Prevacid), omeprazole (Prilosec), and esomeprazole (Nexium) are commonly used.
- Eliminate use of aspirin and other agents that may aggravate gastritis.
- If the gastritis is caused by pernicious anemia, B_{12} vitamin shots will be given.

Herbs, Botanicals, and Supplements

- Herbs and botanical supplements should not be used without discussing with the physician. Products such as ginger and ginger ale may alleviate some nausea.
- The Polynesian traditional food, poi, is a starchy paste made from taro plants (Brown et al, 2005). It may be useful as a probiotic.

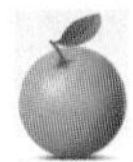

NUTRITION EDUCATION, COUNSELING, CARE MANAGEMENT

- Omit offenders in chronic conditions: alcohol, caffeine, and aspirin.
- Patients with chronic gastritis should be assessed for folate and vitamin B_{12} status. Atrophy of the stomach and intestinal lining interferes with folate and vitamin B_{12} absorption.
- Discuss calcium and riboflavin food sources if dairy products must be omitted.
- Discuss the role of fiber in achieving or maintaining bowel integrity.
- Discuss foodborne illness and its prevention (e.g., avoiding raw shellfish).
- Oral rehydration therapy (ORT) is recommended as first-line therapy for both mildly and moderately dehydrated children with gastroenteritis (Spandorfer et al, 2005).

Patient Education—Foodborne Illness

- If home TF is needed, teach appropriate sanitation and food-handling procedures.
- Careful food handling will be important. To prevent gastroenteritis, cook all foods to proper temperatures; wash all produce before cutting or eating; use careful hand washing.

For More Information

- Gastritis
  http://digestive.niddk.nih.gov/ddiseases/pubs/gastritis/
- Gastroenteritis
  http://www.cdc.gov/ncidod/dvrd/revb/gastro/faq.htm
- Merck manual
  http://www.merck.com/mmpe/sec02/ch013/ch013c.html

GASTRITIS AND GASTROENTERITIS—CITED REFERENCES

Brown AC, et al. A non-dairy probiotic's (poi) influence on changing the gastrointestinal tract's microflora environment. *Altern Ther Health Med.* 11:58, 2005.

Groschwitz KR, Hogan SP. Intestinal barrier function: molecular regulation and disease pathogenesis. *J Allergy Clin Immunol.* 124:3, 2009.

Hata M, et al. Prospective randomized trial for optimal prophylactic treatment of the upper gastrointestinal complications after open heart surgery. *Circ J.* 69:331, 2005.

Sala MR, et al. An outbreak of food poisoning due to a genogroup I norovirus. *Epidemiol Infect.* 133:187, 2005.

Saps M, et al. Post-infectious functional gastrointestinal disorders in children. *J Pediatr.* 152:812, 2008.

Shanks AM, El-Omar EM. *Helicobacter pylori* infection, host genetics and gastric cancer. *J Dig Dis.* 10:157, 2009.

Spandorfer PR, et al. Oral versus intravenous rehydration of moderately dehydrated children: a randomized, controlled trial. *Pediatrics.* 115:295, 2005.

Thabane M, Marshall JK. Post-infectious irritable bowel syndrome. *World J Gastroenterol.* 15:3591, 2009.

GASTROPARESIS AND GASTRIC RETENTION

NUTRITIONAL ACUITY RANKING: LEVEL 2–3

Etiologies of Gastroparesis

36%
31%
14%
8%
5%
6%

Post-surgical
Diabetes
Idiopathic
Miscellaneous
Pseudo-obstruction
Parkinsons Disease

DEFINITIONS AND BACKGROUND

Phases of normal digestion include: phase I (45–60 minutes of inactivity), phase II (30–45 minutes of intermittent peristaltic contractions), phase III (10 minutes of intense, regular contractions), and phase IV (brief transition between cycles). **Gastric retention** is caused by a partial obstruction at the outlet of the stomach into the small bowel. Gastric retention may result from diabetes, prolonged hyperglycemia, vagal autonomic neuropathy, scleroderma, Parkinson's disease, hypothyroidism, postviral syndromes, gastric surgery, or vascular insufficiencies.

Gastroparesis is a chronic disorder of gastric motility that is characterized by delayed emptying of either solids or liquids from the stomach in the absence of any mechanical obstruction; diabetes mellitus and postsurgical states cause the majority of these problems Complications include ketoacidosis, infection, and bezoar formation (Feigenbaum, 2006). Bezoars further obstruct the flow from the stomach to the small intestine. Gastroparesis may occur as a complication of end-stage liver disease and portal hypertension. Idiopathic gastroparesis is characterized by severely delayed gastric emptying of solids without obvious underlying organic cause (Karamanolis et al, 2007).

Because ghrelin is produced by enteroendocrine cells in the gastric mucosa, vagal function and regulation of ghrelin are impaired in gastroparesis (Gaddipati et al, 2006; Levin et al, 2006). Severe gastroparesis can result in recurrent hospitalizations, malnutrition, and even death (McKenna et al, 2008).

Gastroparesis can be difficult to treat. Prokinetic drugs are commonly used. Treatment may involve use of an implantable gastric electrical stimulation (GES) device or endoscopic botolinium toxin injection (Gumaste and Baum, 2008; Monnikes and van der Voort, 2006; Vittal and Pasricha, 2006). The surgical procedure has been found to be effective in reducing symptoms within 6 weeks (McKenna et al, 2008).

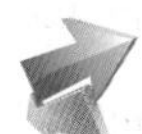

ASSESSMENT, MONITORING, AND EVALUATION

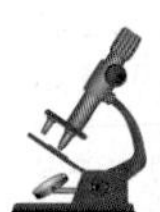

CLINICAL INDICATORS

Genetic Markers: No specific genetic disorder predicts the onset of gastric retention or gastroparesis.

Clinical/History

- Height
- Weight
- Weight changes
- BMI
- Diet history
- I & O
- Nausea, vomiting
- Abdominal pain after eating
- Heartburn
- Belching, bloating
- Flatulence
- Early satiety
- Gastric x-rays–EGG
- Gastric emptying test (slow emptying of liquids and/or solids)

Lab Work

- Gluc (poorly controlled, over 200 mg/dL?)
- H & H
- BUN, Creat
- Alb, transthyretin
- CRP
- Gastrin
- Ghrelin levels
- Na^+, K^+, Cl^-
- Ca^{++}, Mg^{++}
- Serum folate and B_{12}

INTERVENTION

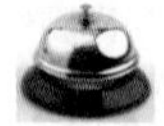

OBJECTIVES

- Decrease volume of meals served. Use liquids or foods that liquefy at body temperature so they are able to pass by a partial obstruction before or during digestion. Bypass or correct obstruction or other causes of retention.
- If diabetes is present, manage control of blood glucose. Differentiate from ketoacidosis, which has similar symptoms of nausea and vomiting. Pernicious vomiting may occur; distinguish from bulimia.
- Correct dehydration and electrolyte abnormalities.
- Reduce or control pain, diarrhea, or bouts of constipation.
- Ensure adequate intake of diet as prescribed to prevent weight loss and control malnutrition.
- Prevent or correct bezoar formation of indigestible solids.

> **SAMPLE NUTRITION CARE PROCESS STEPS**
>
> **Phytobezoar**
>
> ***Assessment Data:*** Weight loss. Abdominal pain. Swallowing evaluation showing gastroparesis and GI obstruction from phytobezoar.
>
> ***Nutrition Diagnoses (PES):*** Altered GI function (NC-1.4) related to phytobezoar as evidenced by delayed gastric emptying, abdominal pain and vomiting, and labs showing glucose levels of 250–300 mg/dL.
>
> ***Interventions:*** Food and Nutrient Delivery: Use a liquid, low residue diet until bezoar is resolved. Educate: Blending foods to improve intake. Coordinate care: insulin as needed to improve serum glucose control; try doses of coca cola to dissolve phytobezoar.
>
> ***Monitoring and Evaluation:*** Improved intake for meals and snacks. Improved glucose management. No further abdominal pain or vomiting. Resolution of phytobezoar.

- Monitor use of, or avoid where possible, medications that cause gastric stasis.

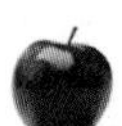

FOOD AND NUTRITION

- A soft-to-liquid diet lower in fat may be useful to prevent delay in gastric emptying. Isotonic liquids empty more quickly than hypertonic liquids.
- Six small meals may be better tolerated than large meals.
- Calculate protein and energy requirements according to underlying medical condition(s).
- Alter fiber intake according to needs (more to alleviate diarrhea, constipation; less with a history of bezoar formation).
- If patient complains of dry mouth, add extra fluids and moisten foods with broth or allowed sauces or gravies.
- For patients with a lesser obstruction of the stomach, progress to a mechanical soft diet.
- For patients with greater obstruction of the stomach, use a low-fiber diet or tube feed, checking residuals frequently.
- A jejunostomy TF may be indicated for persistent problems, even temporarily if needed to correct malnutrition. Consider if there is a history of significant weight loss, cyclical nausea and vomiting, or repeated hospitalizations for gastroparesis.
- Ensure that the patient sits upright during meals.

Common Drugs Used and Potential Side Effects

- Medications that may cause or aggravate gastric emptying include: alcohol, antacids containing aluminum, anticholinergics, calcitonin, calcium channel blockers, glucagon, interleukin-1, levodopa, lithium, octreotide, narcotics, nicotine, potassium salts, progesterone, sucralfate, tricyclic antidepressants, selective serotonin reuptake inhibitors (SSRIs) including Celexa, Paxil, Prozac, and Zoloft.
- Dopamine antagonists, such as metoclopramide and domperidone, and the motilin receptor agonist erythromycin have been the cornerstones in drug treatment of severe gastroparesis for more than a decade (Abrahamsson, 2007).

These drugs are less than ideal (Gumaste and Baum, 2008). Give metoclopramide (Reglan) 30 minutes before meals to increase gastric contractions and to relax the pyloric sphincter. Dry mouth, sleepiness, anxiety, and nausea can be side effects.
- If there is hyperglycemia, oral agents or insulin may be needed.
- Ghrelin receptor agonists may have a role as prokinetic agents (Levin et al, 2006).

Herbs, Botanicals, and Supplements

- Products such as ginger and ginger ale may alleviate some nausea. Use of herbal remedies is common in the Hispanic population. Herbs and botanical supplements should not be used without discussing with the physician.
- *Cuminum cyminum* is widely used in Ayurvedic medicine for the treatment of dyspepsia.
- Adolph's Meat Tenderizer (1 teaspoonful in 8 oz of water before each meal for 7 days) provides papain, a proteolytic enzyme that is a safe treatment for bezoars (Baker et al, 2007). Other studies suggest the use of coca cola.

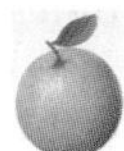

NUTRITION EDUCATION, COUNSELING, CARE MANAGEMENT

- Help the patient determine a specific dietary regimen. If there is diabetes, optimize glycemic control.
- Discuss methods for liquefying foods as needed.
- Bezoar formation may occur after eating oranges, coconuts, green beans, apples, figs, potato skins, Brussels sprouts, broccoli, and sauerkraut in a vulnerable individual.

Patient Education—Foodborne Illness

- If home TF is needed, teach appropriate sanitation and food-handling procedures.

For More Information

- Association of Gastrointestinal Motility Disorders, Inc. http://www.agmd-gimotility.org
- Cyclic Vomiting Association http://www.cvsaonline.org
- Gastroparesis and Dysmotilities Association http://gpda.net
- International Foundation for Functional Gastrointestinal Disorders http://www.iffgd.org

GASTROPARESIS AND GASTRIC RETENTION—CITED REFERENCES

Abrahamsson H. Severe gastroparesis: new treatment alternatives. *Best Pract Res Clin Gastroenterol.* 21:645, 2007.

Baker EL, et al. Resolution of a phytobezoar with Aldoph's Meat Tenderizer. *Pharmacotherapy.* 27:299, 2007.

Feigenbaum K. Update on gastroparesis. *Gastroenterol Nurs.* 29:239, 2006.

Gaddipati KV, et al. Abnormal ghrelin and pancreatic polypeptide responses in gastroparesis. *Dig Dis Sci.* 51:1339, 2006.

Gumaste V, Baum J. Treatment of gastroparesis: an update. *Digestion.* 78:173, 2008.

Karamanolis G, et al. Determinants of symptom pattern in idiopathic severely delayed gastric emptying: gastric emptying rate of proximal stomach dysfunction. *Gut.* 56:29, 2007.

Levin F, et al. Ghrelin stimulates gastric emptying and hunger in normal weight humans. *J Clin Endocrinol Metab.* 91:3296, 2006.

McKenna D, et al. Gastric electrical stimulation is an effective and safe treatment for medically refractory gastroparesis. *Surgery.* 144:566, 2008.

Monnikes H, Van Der Voort IR. Gastric electrical stimulation in gastroparesis: where do we stand? *Dig Dis.* 24:260, 2006.

Vittal H, Pasricha PF. Botulinum toxin for gastrointestinal disorders: therapy and mechanisms. *Neurotox Res.* 9:149, 2006.

GIANT HYPERTROPHIC GASTRITIS AND MÉNÉTRIER'S DISEASE

NUTRITIONAL ACUITY RANKING: LEVEL 3

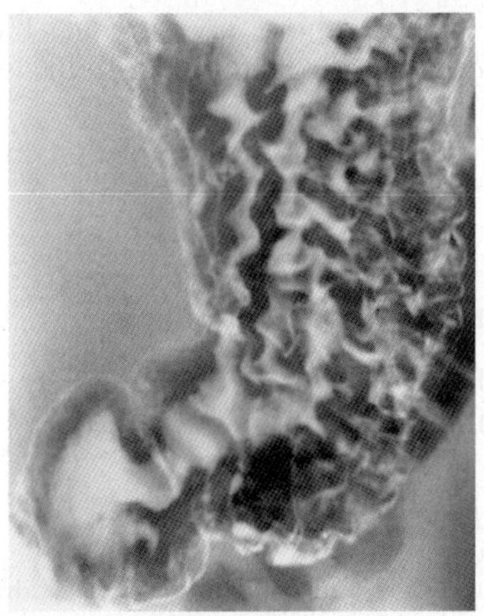

Adapted from: Ronald L. Eisenberg, *An Atlas of Differential Diagnosis.* 4th ed. Philadelphia: Lippincott Williams & Wilkins, 2003.

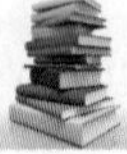

DEFINITIONS AND BACKGROUND

Giant hypertrophic gastritis (GHG) is a pathological condition with increased loss of plasma proteins, resulting in hydrolysis by the proteolytic enzymes of the gut. The hydrolyzed proteins are then reabsorbed as amino acids. Ascites or edema occur if the liver cannot produce sufficient albumin rapidly enough. The condition may precede stomach cancer. The disease is rare and diagnosed in patients with giant gastric folds, dyspeptic symptoms, and hypoalbuminemia due to GI protein loss.

Ménétrier's disease is a form of hyperplastic gastropathy and not a form of gastritis because inflammation is minimal. Overexpression of transforming growth factor (TGF)-alpha results in selective expansion of surface mucous cells in the body and fundus of the stomach. Ménétrier's disease is often associated with *H. pylori* infection. Most patients with

Ménétrier's disease are treated nonoperatively with nutritional support, antacids, and pain medications (Sanchez et al, 2007). Gastric resection provides permanent relief if needed.

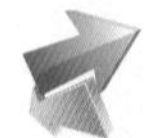

ASSESSMENT, MONITORING, AND EVALUATION

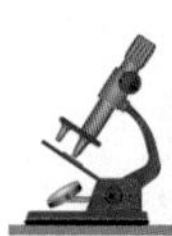

CLINICAL INDICATORS

Genetic Markers: The *H. pylori* strain with Ménétrier's disease has high hepatocyte growth factor (HGF) and TNF-alpha mRNA expressions from gastric fibroblasts (Ishikawa et al, 2008).

Clinical/History		
Height	Fecal occult blood test	CRP
Weight	Steatorrhea	Gluc
BMI	Generalized edema	Na^+, K^+
Diet history	Stomach ulcers?	Ca^{++}, Mg^{++}
Weight changes		Nitrogen (N) balance
Abdominal pain	**Lab Work**	Transferrin
Blood in vomit	Pepsin levels	H & H
Gastroscopy	*H. pylori* bacteria	Serum Fe, ferritin
Gastric biopsy	Alb, transthyretin	Serum folate and B_{12}
Abdominal ultrasound	Globulin	BUN, Creat
	A:G ratio	

INTERVENTION

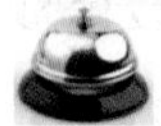

OBJECTIVES

- Replace protein; maintain adequate nitrogen balance.
- Reduce edema.
- Spare protein for tissue synthesis and repair.
- Promote normal dietary intake with a return to wellness.
- Delay or prevent onset of stomach cancer if possible.

SAMPLE NUTRITION CARE PROCESS STEPS

Inadequate Protein Intake

Assessment Data: Diagnosis of GHG with giant gastric folds, dyspepsia, hypoalbuminemia (serum levels <2.0).

Nutrition Diagnoses (PES): Inadequate protein intake (NI-52.1) related to GI protein loss as evidenced by serum albumin <2.0 g/dL.

Interventions: Alter diet to increase protein intake orally, or tube feed if necessary. Educate patient and family about the role of protein in alleviating edema and correcting low albumin levels.

Monitoring and Evaluation: Improvements in serum albumin from diet or transfusion (if needed). Transthyretin levels showing improvement over several weeks. Resolution of edema and improved quality of life.

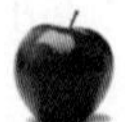

FOOD AND NUTRITION

- Use a high-protein/high-calorie diet. The protein level should be approximately 20% of total kilocal unless contraindicated for renal or hepatic problems.
- Omit any food intolerances.
- Include adequate sources of micronutrients in the diet; a basic supplement may be warranted.

Common Drugs Used and Potential Side Effects

- Ménétrier disease patients have been effectively treated with a specific blocking monoclonal antibody (Coffey et al, 2007). This reduces the frequency of nausea and vomiting, improves serum albumin concentration, and improves abnormalities of the stomach.
- For eradication of *H. pylori*, 2 weeks of treatment with an acid-suppressing drug (one time daily), Pepto-Bismol (four times daily), and antibiotics (three to four times daily) are prescribed. This therapy often must be used more than once. Other combinations may include the antibiotics omeprazole, clarithromycin, and ranitidine bismuth (Tritec).
- Lansoprazole (Prevacid), omeprazole (Prilosec), and esomeprazole (Nexium) may be prescribed.
- If prednisone is used for a long period of time, monitor for changes in glucose levels.

Herbs, Botanicals, and Supplements

- Herbs and botanical supplements should not be used without discussing with the physician.

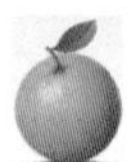

NUTRITION EDUCATION, COUNSELING, CARE MANAGEMENT

- Eliminate aggravating foods specific to the patient.
- Teach the patient about use of high biological value (HBV) proteins to replenish protein levels from GI losses.
- During recovery, the use of probiotics such as yogurt with live and active cultures may be helpful.

Patient Education—Foodborne Illness

- If home TF is needed, teach appropriate sanitation and food-handling procedures.

For More Information

- Giant hypertrophic gastritis
  http://www.cancer.gov/templates/db_alpha.aspx?CdrID=589414
- Medical terms on line
  http://www.medicaltermsonline.org/index.php?section=pages&item=Giant-hypertrophic-gastritis

GIANT HYPERTROPHIC GASTRITIS AND MÉNÉTRIER'S DISEASE—CITED REFERENCES

Coffey RJ, et al. Ménétrier disease and gastrointestinal stromal tumors: hyperproliferative disorders of the stomach. *J Clin Invest.* 117:70, 2007.

Ishikawa T, et al. Helicobacter pylori isolated from a patient with Ménétrier's disease increases hepatocyte growth factor mRNA expression in gastric fibroblasts: comparison with Helicobacter pylori isolated from other gastric diseases. *Dig Dis Sci.* 53:1785, 2008.

Sanchez C, et al. Laparoscopic total gastrectomy for Ménétrier's disease. *J Laparoendosc Adv Surg Tech A.* 17:32, 2007.

PEPTIC ULCER DISEASE

NUTRITIONAL ACUITY RANKING: LEVEL 2

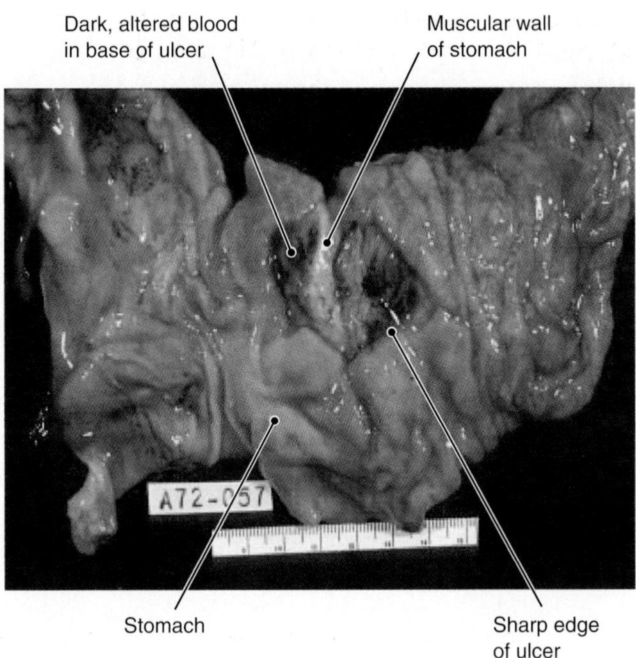

Adapted from: Thomas H. McConnell, *The Nature Of Disease Pathology for the Health Professions,* Philadelphia: Lippincott Williams & Wilkins, 2007.

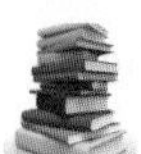

DEFINITIONS AND BACKGROUND

A peptic ulcer suggests an imbalance between digestive fluids in the stomach and duodenum, with erodion by gastric acid and pepsin and exposed nerves. Most ulcers are duodenal, within the first 25–30 cm.

One of 10 Americans suffers from peptic ulcer disease. *H. pylori* bacteria play a role in the etiology of 75% or more of peptic ulcers. *Helicobacter pylori* can be transmitted from person to person through close contact, exposure to vomit, or fecal–oral contamination. It can also be found in well water. Because the bacterium is one of the most genetically diverse bacterial species, more than half of the world population in both developed and developing countries are infected (Dube et al, 2009). It has been implicated in stomach cancer.

Hand washing is an important preventive measure. In addition, sulforaphane (SF) from broccoli is a powerful bactericidal agent against *H. pylori* (Yanaka et al, 2009) and intake of soy products may help reduce the effects of inflammation-related IL-10 genetic polymorphisms (Ko et al, 2009).

Individuals who have cirrhosis, chronic obstructive pulmonary disease, renal failure, and organ transplantation tend to have a higher risk for peptic ulcer disease (PUD). Bland diets neither heal ulcers nor cause a decrease in gastric acid secretion. Drug therapy is most effective in preventing ulcer recurrence and primarily consists of antibiotics and antacids. A vaccine to prevent *H. pylori* infection is being developed. In the meantime, vitamin B_{12} tends to be lower in patients who have peptic ulcers; anemia should be monitored.

The decline in duodenal ulcer disease and the established relation of peptic ulcer to *H. pylori* have eliminated the need for elective ulcer surgery. Options for refractory and complicated PUD include vagotomy and pyloroplasty, vagotomy and antrectomy with gastroduodenal reconstruction (Billroth I) or gastrojejunal reconstruction (Billroth II).

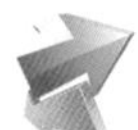

ASSESSMENT, MONITORING, AND EVALUATION

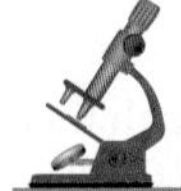

CLINICAL INDICATORS

Genetic Markers: *H. pylori* infection tends to run in families. This pathogen has been shown to follow the routes of human migration; the global *H. pylori* population has been divided into six ancestral populations, three from Africa, two from Asia, and one from Europe (Tay et al, 2009). In addition, the interleukin 1B gene has been identified as a factor, especially inflammation-related IL-10 genetic polymorphisms.

Clinical/History
- Height
- Weight
- BMI
- Diet history
- Weight and appetite changes
- Sharp and sudden abdominal pain
- Burning or gnawing pain (better with meals but returns)
- GI bleeding or black, tarry stools
- Nausea, vomiting
- Frequent bloating
- Chronic idiopathic urticaria or atopic dermatitis
- Stool test for *H. pylori*
- Endoscopy

Lab Work
- Red blood cell (RBC) count
- Anti-*H. pylori* immunoglobulin G antibody titer
- C-Urea breath test for *H. pylori*
- Chol, Trig
- BUN, Creat
- Alb, transthyretin

Alanine aminotransferase (ALT)	perforated ulcers)	Serum folate
Aspartate aminotransferase (AST)	Serum gastrin	PT or INR
Blood guaiac	(increased)	Transferrin
Amylase (increased in	Alk phos (increased)	Ca^{++}, Mg^{++}
	H & H	Serum B_{12}
	Serum Fe, ferritin	TIBC
		Na^{+}, K^{+}, Cl^{-}
		Ca^{++}, Mg^{++}

INTERVENTION

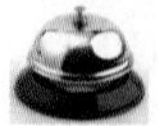

OBJECTIVES

- Eradicate any *H. pylori* infection where present. Take medications as directed. Rest during healing stages.
- Reduce pain. Avoid distention from large meals.
- Dilute stomach contents and provide buffering action.
- Correct anemia, if present. Vitamin B_{12} deficiency may be corrected after effective *H. pylori* treatment.
- Monitor and prevent steatorrhea, bone disease, dumping syndrome, and complications such as perforation and obstruction.

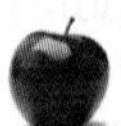

FOOD AND NUTRITION

- Use small feedings, frequently if preferred. Include high-protein foods and vitamin C to speed healing.
- Avoid personal intolerances. Citrus and acidic juices may cause pain during exacerbations. If a particular food bothers an individual, it should be avoided.
- Use broccoli and cruciferous vegetables often to enhance chemoprotection of the gastric mucosa against *H. pylori*-induced oxidative stress (Yanaka et al, 2009).
- Encourage soybean intake (Ko et al, 2009).
- Limit gastric stimulants if not tolerated, such as caffeine, alcohol, peppermint, black pepper, garlic, cloves, and chili powder. This is a "liberal bland" diet. See Table 7-7 regarding caffeine in beverages and medications.

SAMPLE NUTRITION CARE PROCESS STEPS

Undesirable Food Choices

Assessment: Food and symptoms diary. Positive stool guaic test. Altered GI lab results. No *H. pylori* present.

Nutrition Diagnosis (PES): Undesirable food choices related to chronic alcohol intake (beer and wine, 10 drinks/wk) as evidenced by nausea, sharp stomach pains, abdominal discomfort, black tarry stools and altered GI labs.

Intervention: Teach about role of alcohol in GI mucosal damage. Counsel about alternative lifestyle changes that will help alleviate GI pain. Encourage intake of broccoli for its chemoprotective effects.

Monitoring and Evaluation: Report of decreased alcohol consumption and less GI discomfort and pain. Resolution of peptic ulcer symptoms; improved lab results. No further tarry stools.

TABLE 7-7 Typical Caffeine Content of Beverages and Medications

Beverages/Medications	Measure	Caffeine (mg)
Coffee, brewed	5 oz	65–120 (average, 85)
Coffee, instant	5 oz	60–85 (average, 75)
Coffee, Starbucks Frappucino	8 oz	83
Espresso coffee	1 oz	30–50 (average, 40)
Decaffeinated coffee	5 oz	2–4
Black tea, brewed (most U.S. brands)	5 oz	20–50
Black tea, brewed (imported)	5 oz	25–60
Tea, instant	6 oz	28–30
Mountain Dew	12 oz	54
Cola drinks	12 oz	36–47
Coffee ice cream	4 oz	28
Baker's chocolate	1 oz	26
Dark chocolate	1 oz	5–35 (average, 20)
Milk chocolate	1 oz	1–15 (average, 6)
Cocoa beverage	8 oz	3–32 (average, 6)
Chocolate milk	8 oz	2–7 (average, 5)
Analgesic	1 tablet	30–66
Cold preparation	1 tablet	30
Chocolate syrup	1 oz	4
7-Up or Sprite	12 oz	0
Ovaltine	8 oz	0

Data from Leonard T, et al. The effects of caffeine on various body systems: a review. *J Am Diet Assoc.* 87:1048, 1987.

- Use fewer saturated fats and more polyunsaturated fats if increased lipid levels are found. AA metabolites may play a role in peptic ulcer disease.
- Monitor water supply as a potential source of *H. pylori*.

Common Drugs Used and Potential Side Effects (see Table 7-8)

- Most patients with PUD should avoid NSAIDs. Analgesics and corticosteroids, when taken over a long time, may cause GI bleeding and ulceration and should be taken with food. High doses of Advil or Motrin (ibuprofen), even for a few days, can significantly increase the risk of GI bleeding.
- For eradication of *H. pylori*, 2 weeks of treatment with an acid-suppressing drug (once daily), Pepto-Bismol (four times daily), and antibiotics (three to four times daily) are prescribed. A 1- to 2-week course of *H. pylori* eradication therapy is an effective treatment (Ford et al, 2006); triple therapy often must be used more than once. Quadruple therapy is also being tested (Feng et al, 2005). Some FDA-approved combinations include the antibiotics omeprazole, clarithromycin, and ranitidine bismuth (Tritec). Other antibiotics include amoxicillin, metronidazole, and tetracycline. Suggest use of probiotics, such as yogurt with live and active cultures.

TABLE 7-8 Medications Used in Peptic Ulcer Disease

Medication Type	Description	Specific Drugs
Antacids	Aluminum-containing and magnesium-containing antacids can be helpful in relieving symptoms of gastritis by neutralizing gastric acids. These agents are inexpensive and safe. Aluminum ions inhibit smooth muscle contraction, thus inhibiting gastric emptying. Use aluminum-containing antacids cautiously with upper GI hemorrhage. Magnesium and aluminum antacid mixtures are used to avoid bowel function changes.	Gaviscon contains magnesium as well as aluminum and may decrease absorption of thiamine, phosphate, and vitamin A. Gelusil contains magnesium, aluminum, and simethicone; it may have side effects similar to those of Gaviscon. Mylanta and Amphogel (aluminum hydroxide) may cause nausea, vomiting, and lowered vitamin A, calcium, and phosphate absorption. Take between meals, followed by water. Milk of magnesia (magnesium hydroxide) is a laxative–antacid and can deplete phosphorus and calcium over time. Magaldrate (Riopan) decreases serum vitamin A but can be used on a low-sodium diet.
H_2-receptor antagonists	These drugs inhibit the action of histamine on the parietal cell, which inhibits acid secretion. The drugs in this class are all equally effective and are available over the counter in half prescription strength for heartburn treatment. Histamine H_2 blockers should be taken with food. Since acid secretion and ulcer pain are most prevalent at night, taking Zantac or Tagamet before bed may be helpful. These drugs can elevate AST/ALT and creatinine, cause confusion in elderly individuals, and cause diarrhea, constipation, or urticaria.	Cimetidine (Tagamet) inhibits histamine at H_2 receptors of the gastric parietal cells, resulting in reduced gastric acid secretion, gastric volume, and hydrogen ion concentrations. Famotidine (Pepcid) competitively inhibits histamine at the H_2 receptor of the gastric parietal cells, resulting in reduced gastric acid secretion, gastric volume, and reduced hydrogen concentrations. Nizatidine (Axid) competitively inhibits histamine at H_2 receptors of gastric parietal cells, resulting in reduced gastric acid secretion, gastric volume, and reduced hydrogen concentrations. Ranitidine (Zantac) competitively inhibits histamine at the H_2 receptors of gastric parietal cells, resulting in reduced gastric acid secretion, gastric volume, and hydrogen concentrations. Ranitidine can cause nausea, constipation, and vitamin B_{12} malabsorption; may alter serum levels of serum iron.
Proton pump inhibitors (PPIs)	PPIs bind to the proton pump of parietal cell, inhibiting secretion of hydrogen ions into gastric lumen. PPIs relieve pain and heal peptic ulcers more rapidly than H_2 antagonists do. Drugs in this class are equally effective. All PPIs decrease serum concentrations of drugs that require gastric acidity for absorption, such as ketoconazole or itraconazole. PPIs are used for up to 4 weeks to treat and relieve symptoms of active duodenal ulcers. Physicians may prescribe for up to 8 weeks to treat all grades of erosive esophagitis.	Lansoprazole (Prevacid) decreases gastric acid secretion by inhibiting the parietal cell H^+/K^+ ATP pump. Omeprazole (Prilosec) decreases gastric acid secretion by inhibiting the parietal cell H^+/K^+ ATP pump. Omeprazole is now available over the counter. Esomeprazole (Nexium) is the S-isomer of omeprazole. It decreases gastric acid secretion by inhibiting the parietal cell H^+/K^+ ATP pump. May increase absorption of digoxin; may decrease absorption of iron. Rabeprazole (Aciphex, Alfence, Pariet) decreases gastric acid secretion by inhibiting the parietal cell H^+/K^+ ATP pump. It is used for short-term (4–8 weeks) treatment and symptomatic relief of gastritis. Pantoprazole (Protonix) decreases gastric acid secretion by inhibiting the parietal cell H^+/K^+ ATP pump. It is used for short-term (4–8 weeks) treatment and symptomatic relief of gastritis.
Gastrointestinal agents	These agents are effective in the treatment of peptic ulcers and in preventing relapse. Their mechanism of action is not clear. Multiple doses are required, and they are not as effective as the other options.	Sucralfate (Carafate) binds with positively charged proteins in exudates and forms a viscous adhesive substance that protects the GI lining against pepsin, peptic acid, and bile salts. Used for short-term management of ulcers. Sucralfate may cause constipation as one side effect.
Stomach acid protector	Bismuth subsalicylate	Bismuth is a component of Pepto-Bismol and is used to protect the stomach lining from acid; it kills *Helicobacter pylori*.

Adapted from: Shayne P. Gastritis and peptic ulcer disease, http://www.emedicine.com/emerg/topic820.htm, accessed February 28, 2005.

Herbs, Botanicals, and Supplements

- Herbs and botanical supplements should not be used without discussing with the physician.
- Ginger may be used as an antinauseant. Do not use large doses with warfarin, aspirin, or other antiplatelet drugs, antihypertensive drugs, and hypoglycemic drugs. Additive effects can cause unpredictable changes in BP and decreases in blood glucose levels and may decrease platelet aggregation and thus increase bleeding. Ginger ale is commonly used with few side effects.
- Licorice root may be recommended for gastric and duodenal ulcers. Do not take with digoxin, because it may cause potassium loss and digoxin toxicity. Licorice root may potentiate the effects of steroids, especially hydrocortisone, progesterone, and estrogens. Also avoid taking with thiazide diuretics and antihypertensive medications because of increased sodium and water retention, along with potential hypokalemia; spironolactone is especially antagonized by licorice root.
- Banana, garlic, cabbage, and yellow root have no clinical trials proving efficacy. Broccoli and soy products may be beneficial.

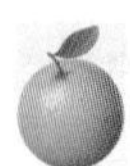

NUTRITION EDUCATION, COUNSELING, CARE MANAGEMENT

- As needed by the individual, offer guidance about dietary alterations that may be useful.
- Discuss the need to complete treatments for eradication of *H. pylori* bacteria, where present. One treatment is usually not sufficient. Suggest increasing intake of broccoli and soy products.
- Reduce intake of alcoholic beverages; stop smoking; and monitor any family history of ulcer disease to address it as quickly as possible.
- As a preventive measure, recommend endoscopy early in patients older than 45–50 years who have dysphagia, recurrent vomiting, weight loss, or bleeding.

Patient Education—Foodborne Illness

- Careful food handling will be important. Hand washing is important to reduce the spread of *H. pylori*. Always wash hands after using the bathroom and before eating.
- If home TF is needed, teach appropriate sanitation and food handling procedures.

For More Information

- Centers for Disease Control and Prevention—Peptic Ulcer
  http://www.cdc.gov/ulcer/md.htm
- Foundation for Digestive Health
  http://www.fdhn.org/html/education/ulcer/facts.html
- Helicobacter Foundation
  http://www.helico.com/
- Medline—Peptic Ulcer
  http://www.nlm.nih.gov/medlineplus/pepticulcer.html
- Web MD—Peptic Ulcer
  http://www.webmd.com/digestive-disorders/digestive-diseases-peptic-ulcer-disease

PEPTIC ULCER DISEASE—CITED REFERENCES

Dube C, et al. Helicobacter pylori in water sources: a global environmental health concern. *Rev Environ Health.* 24:1, 2009.

Feng LY, et al. Effects of killing *Helicobacter pylori* quadruple therapy on peptic ulcer: a randomized double-blind clinical trial. *World J Gastroenterol.* 11:1083, 2005.

Ford AC, et al. Eradication therapy for peptic ulcer disease in *Helicobacter pylori* positive patients. *Cochrane Database Syst Rev.* 2:CD003840, 2006.

Ko KP, et al. Soybean product intake modifies the association between interleukin-10 genetic polymorphisms and gastric cancer risk. *J Nutr.* 139: 1008, 2009.

Tay CY, et al. Population structure of Helicobacter pylori among ethnic groups in Malaysia: recent acquisition of the bacterium by the Malay population. *BMC Microbiol.* 9:126, 2009.

Yanaka A, et al. Dietary sulforaphane-rich broccoli sprouts reduce colonization and attenuate gastritis in Helicobacter pylori-infected mice and humans. *Cancer Prev Res.* 2:353, 2009.

VOMITING, PERNICIOUS

NUTRITIONAL ACUITY RANKING: LEVEL 3 (LONGER THAN 7 DAYS)

DEFINITIONS AND BACKGROUND

Pernicious, uncontrolled vomiting may occur in any of several disorders, including concussion or brain trauma, meningitis or encephalitis, intestinal blockage, migraine headaches, brain tumor or other forms of cancer, foodborne illness, gastroparesis, and pregnancy (hyperemesis gravidarum, see Pregnancy in Section 1). Hyperemesis gravidarum involves pregnancy-induced hormonal changes, often associated with concurrent *H. pylori* infection. The presence of weight loss, GI bleeding, persistent fever, chronic severe diarrhea, and significant vomiting is associated with a higher prevalence of organic disease in children and should be carefully assessed (American Academy of Pediatrics, 2005).

The biggest immediate risk with pernicious vomiting is dehydration, where losses of water, potassium, and sodium can affect the brain, kidneys, and heart. Watch for signs such as dry mouth membranes, dry lips, sunken eyes, rapid but weak pulse, rapid breathing, cold hands and feet, confusion, and difficulty with arousal. Nutritional deficits are possible when the vomiting is prolonged.

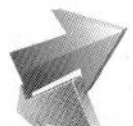

ASSESSMENT, MONITORING, AND EVALUATION

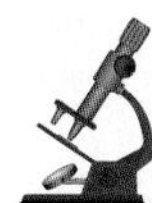

CLINICAL INDICATORS

Genetic Markers: Pernicious vomiting in itself is a symptom of an underlying condition and is not genetic.

Clinical/History		
Height	Orthostatic hypotension?	N balance
Weight	GI bleeding?	Gluc
Weight changes	**Lab Work**	H & H
BMI	Na^+, K^+, Cl^-	Serum Fe, ferritin
Diet history	Ca^{++}, Mg^{++}	Serum folate or B_{12}
Temperature (fever?)	Alb, transthyretin	Gastric emptying tests
Dehydration?	BUN, Creat	

INTERVENTION

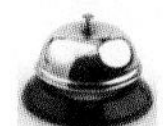

OBJECTIVES

- Correct electrolyte and fluid imbalances and unintentional weight loss
- Modify oral intake until vomiting resolves.
- Distinguish symptoms that could be related to bulimia nervosa.
- If there is hyperglycemia or diabetes, return to normal blood glucose levels as quickly as possible; insulin may be needed.
- For cancer patients, depending on the type of treatment (either curative or palliative) and on the patient's nutritional status, provide patient-tailored nutritional intervention such as oral supplementation, enteral or total PN (Marin Caro et al, 2007).

SAMPLE NUTRITION CARE PROCESS STEPS

Abnormal GI Function—Vomiting

Assessment: Food records, I & O reports, chemotherapy schedule and frequency. Uncontrollable vomiting three to four times daily for past week. Signs of dehydration.

Nutrition Diagnosis (PES): Inadequate food and beverage intake related to intolerance to oral diet and chemotherapy treatment as evidenced by dehydration and vomiting after meals, with weight loss of 5 lb over past week.

Intervention: Coordinate care: Alter meal pattern according to chemotherapy medications and timing, review timing of fluid intake related to meals. Offer sips of fluid every 1–2 hours while awake.

Monitoring and Evaluation: Food records, I & O reports, weight recovery. Resolution of vomiting episodes.

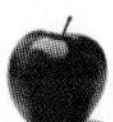

FOOD AND NUTRITION

- For patients with an acute condition, NPO for 24 hours with intravenous (IV) glucose is common. Oral rehydration solution may be needed. (See Diarrhea entry.)
- When tolerated, gastrostomy TF or jejunostomy may be warranted. An isotonic formula is desirable to reduce imbalances between solute and solvent. CPN may also be a consideration if the condition is prolonged.
- As the patient progresses to an oral diet, clear liquids such as cranberry juice or boullion may be helpful. Gradually add toast, crackers, jelly, and simple carbohydrates in small, frequent meals.
- Give fluids between meals (a "dry diet"). Avoid acidic fruit and vegetable juices if not tolerated.
- Consider avoiding foods that delay gastric emptying (high-fat, hypertonic, or highly fibrous foods).
- Gradually have the patient resume a normal diet. Decrease fatty foods if not tolerated.

Common Drugs Used and Potential Side Effects

- Anti-emetic agents may be indicated for some conditions. Meclizine or cyclizine may be prescribed; they are antihistamines and powerful antinausea agents.
- Selective serotonin 5-hydroxytryptamine-3 (5-HT3) receptor antagonists have proven to be safe and effective for postoperative nausea and vomiting; these include dolasetron, granisetron, ondansetron, and tropisetron, which bind to 5-HT3 receptors, blocking serotonin binding at vagal afferents in the gut and in the regions of the CNS involved in emesis (Gan, 2005).
- Insulin or oral agents may be needed if diabetes is also present.
- Peristaltic agents may be used in cases of gastroparesis.
- Chronic use of cannabinoids can lead to hyperemesis; this includes oral use of marijuana for cancer, multiple sclerosis, or social purposes.

Herbs, Botanicals, and Supplements

- Herbs and botanical supplements should not be used without discussing with the physician.
- Ginger is often used as an antinauseant. Do not use large doses with warfarin, aspirin, other antiplatelet drugs, antihypertensive drugs, and hypoglycemic drugs. Additive effects can cause unpredictable changes in BP, blood glucose levels, platelet aggregation, and bleeding.
- Ginger ale has few side effects and may help.

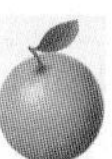

NUTRITION EDUCATION, COUNSELING, CARE MANAGEMENT

- Explain why fluids should be taken between meals. Identify adequate amounts of fluids to be consumed every day. Sips of 1–2 oz every few hours can be tolerated; this may include water, sports drinks, gelatin, and clear broth.
- There are many suitable oral rehydration products available from a pharmacy; discuss appropriate products with

the pharmacist. If needed, share the ingredient recipe if it is to be made at home.
- Do not force eating. Eat and drink slowly; stop when full. Make up lost calories at another time.
- Eat meals in a well-ventilated area free from odors.
- Do not lie down for 2 hours after eating. Do not overeat.
- Discuss the role of carbohydrates and fiber in maintaining blood glucose levels.
- Discuss reasons to seek immediate medical attention, including severe abdominal pain, severe headache, stiff neck, fever over 101°F, vomiting of blood, rapid breathing or pulse.
- In palliative care, nutritional support aims at improving patient's quality of life by controlling symptoms such as nausea, vomiting, and pain related to food intake (Marin Caro et al, 2007).

Patient Education—Food Safety

- Careful food handling and hand washing are important to prevent introduction of foodborne pathogens to the diet of the individual.
- If home TF is needed, teach appropriate sanitation and food-handling procedures.

For More Information

- Medicine Net
  http://www.medicinenet.com/nausea_and_vomiting/article.htm
- Nausea and Vomiting Algorithm
  http://www.uwgi.org/guidelines/ch_01/ch01txt.htm

VOMITING, PERNICIOUS—CITED REFERENCES

American Academy of Pediatrics. Subcommittee on Chronic Abdominal Pain; North American Society for Pediatric Gastroenterology Hepatology, and Nutrition. Chronic abdominal pain in children. *Pediatrics.* 115:370, 2005.

Gan TJ. Selective serotonin 5-HT(3) receptor antagonists for postoperative nausea and vomiting: are they all the same? *CNS Drugs.* 19:225, 2005.

Marin Caro MM, et al. Nutritional intervention and quality of life in adult oncology patients. *Clin Nutr.* 26:289, 2007.

LOWER GI: INTESTINAL DISORDERS

CARCINOID SYNDROME

NUTRITIONAL ACUITY RANKING: LEVEL 3

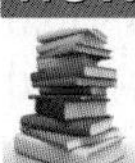

DEFINITIONS AND BACKGROUND

Carcinoid tumors are part of a group of GI and pancreatic endocrine tumors that secrete hormones, 5-HT, tachykinins, and other mediators (Druce et al, 2009). The rare neuroendocrine growth develops in the wall of the intestine and is usually discovered in x-rays or during surgery performed for other reasons. GI carcinoid tumors are difficult to diagnose (Gore et al, 2005). Carcinoid cancer patients often have elevated levels of serotonin or its precursor 5-hydroxytryptophan (Shah et al, 2005). Octreotide scanning has a sensitivity of primary tumor detection of 90% (Northrup and Lee, 2007). GI carcinoids comprise 90% of all carcinoid tumors and all carcinoids have malignant potential (Northrup and Lee, 2007). Sometimes, the growth occurs in the appendix area. The growths can be large enough to cause intestinal obstruction. Some growths metastasize to the liver, creating hormone-producing tumors with flushing of the head and neck (usually triggered by alcohol or exercise). Flushing symptoms can last for several hours from the release of vasoactive serotonin, histamine, and prostaglandins.

Other symptoms include swollen or watery eyes, explosive diarrhea, abdominal cramps, wheezing, breathlessness, and symptoms similar to heart failure. Cardiac lesions are also seen; up to one third of patients develop cardiac valvulopathy. Patients may benefit from a valve replacement. If liver involvement occurs, liver resection or transplantation may be needed.

Diversion of tryptophan to 5-HT synthesis occurs, resulting in less tryptophan for protein and nicotinamide synthesis. Pellagra and psychiatric symptoms result from depletion of tryptophan, which is consumed by the tumor for serotonin synthesis (van der Horst-Schrivers et al, 2004). Psychiatric symptoms should be evaluated carefully.

The malignant carcinoid syndrome is caused by circulating neuroendocrine mediators produced by the tumor and occurs in less than 10% of patients (Bell et al, 2005). Surgery is combined with continuous biotherapy with long-acting somatostatin analogs and interferon, which may alleviate symptoms and slow the disease progression (Akerstrom et al, 2005). Survival ranges from 3 to 20 years after diagnosis.

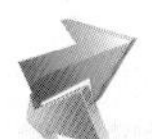

ASSESSMENT, MONITORING, AND EVALUATION

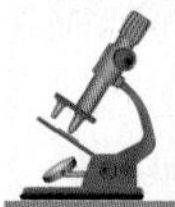

CLINICAL INDICATORS

Genetic Markers: Carcinoid tumor fibrosis is a CTGF/TGFbeta1-mediated stellate cell-driven fibrotic response (Kidd et al, 2007).

Clinical/History

- Height
- Weight
- BMI
- Diet history
- Diarrhea, flushing, wheezing (carcinoid syndrome)
- Breathlessness
- Number of stools, consistency
- Biopsy
- Endoscopy
- Octreotide scanning
- X-rays of GI tract
- Skin changes (scleroderma, pellagra)?
- Psychiatric symptoms?

Magnetic resonance imaging (MRI)	Serum histamine	TLC
	Serum serotonin (elevated)	H & H
Lab Work	Alb, transthyretin	Serum Fe, ferritin
5-HIAA test (urine 5-HIAA)	Transferrin	Na^+, K^+
		Ca^{++}, Mg^{++}

INTERVENTION

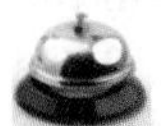

OBJECTIVES

- Ease symptoms of secretory diarrhea and reduce any pain.
- Slow progression of the disease, which is not cured by surgery.
- Control side effects of medications.
- Replenish electrolyte and fluid losses.
- Correct niacin deficiency. Biochemical niacin deficiency is prevalent among newly diagnosed carcinoid syndrome patients (Shah et al, 2005).

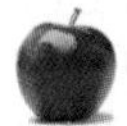

FOOD AND NUTRITION

- Decrease fiber intake during acute stages of diarrhea. Add pectin and ensure adequate fluid intake during those periods.
- Avoid alcoholic beverages. Limit caffeine intake to a controlled amount.
- During testing, omit foods that contain 5-HIAA: avocados, pineapple, bananas, kiwi fruit, plums, eggplant, walnuts, hickory nuts, and pecans.
- Omega-3 fatty acids may used for their role in reduction of inflammation; include fish such as salmon, sardines, tuna, and herring often.
- Since tryptophan is not adequately converted to niacin, a daily supplement with DRI levels may be suggested. Avoid excesses.

SAMPLE NUTRITION CARE PROCESS STEPS

Altered GI Function

Assessment Data: Explosive diarrhea, flushing, fear of eating.

Nutrition Diagnoses (PES): Altered GI function related to release of vasoactive substances as evidenced by explosive diarrhea and altered labs with diagnosis of carcinoid syndrome.

Interventions: Education about foods or alcohol that may aggravate symptoms. Counseling about postsurgical wound healing, if required. Discuss use of probiotics, adequate fluid, omega-3 fatty acid sources. Avoid alcohol if symptoms are aggravated by intake.

Monitoring and Evaluation: Fewer complaints of diarrhea, flushing, GI discomfort, and fear of eating.

Common Drugs Used and Potential Side Effects

- Subcutaneous injections of the somatostatin analog octreotide are used. This is expensive, and treatment may be for many years. Newer somatostatin analogs (such as lanreotide) are being tested. Vasoconstricting interleukin or cytotoxic drugs may control side effects.
- If kaolin (Kaopectate) and other medications are used to control diarrhea, constipation is a possible side effect.
- Bronchodilators may be used to control wheezing. Evaluate for potential side effects.

Herbs, Botanicals, and Supplements

- Herbs and botanical supplements should not be used without discussing with the physician.
- Monitor side effects if large doses of niacin are taken.

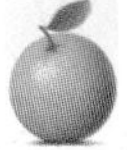

NUTRITION EDUCATION, COUNSELING, CARE MANAGEMENT

- Discuss measures specifically designed for the patient's status and tolerance levels.
- Suggest ways to make meals more appetizing if appetite is poor.
- Describe techniques for management of diarrhea, abdominal pain, or cramping by reducing fiber and fat intake during those times of flare.
- Probiotics such as acidophilus milk and yogurt with live and active cultures may be useful in the diet.

Patient Education—Foodborne Illness

- If home TF is needed, teach appropriate sanitation and food-handling procedures.

For More Information

- Carcinoid Syndrome
  http://www.emedicine.com/med/topic2649.htm

CARCINOID SYNDROME—CITED REFERENCES

Akerstrom G, et al. Management of midgut carcinoids. *J Surg Oncol.* 89:161, 2005.

Bell HK, et al. Cutaneous manifestations of the malignant carcinoid syndrome. *Br J Dermatol.* 152:71, 2005.

Druce M, et al. Fibrosis and carcinoid syndrome: from causation to future therapy. *Nat Rev Endocrinol.* 5:276, 2009.

Gore RM, et al. GI carcinoid tumours: appearance of the primary and detecting metastases. *Best Pract Res Clin Endocrinol Metab.* 19:245, 2005.

Kidd M, et al. CTGF, intestinal stellate cells and carcinoid fibrogenesis. *World J Gastroenterol.* 13:5208, 2007.

Northrup JA, Lee JH. Large bowel carcinoid tumors. *Curr Opin Gastroenterol.* 23:74, 2007.

Shah GM, et al. Biochemical assessment of niacin deficiency among carcinoid cancer patients. *Am J Gastroenterol.* 100:2307, 2005.

Van Der Horst-Schrivers AN, et al. Complications of midgut carcinoid tumors and carcinoid syndrome. *Neuroendocrinology.* 80:28S, 2004.

CELIAC DISEASE

NUTRITIONAL ACUITY RANKING: LEVEL 4

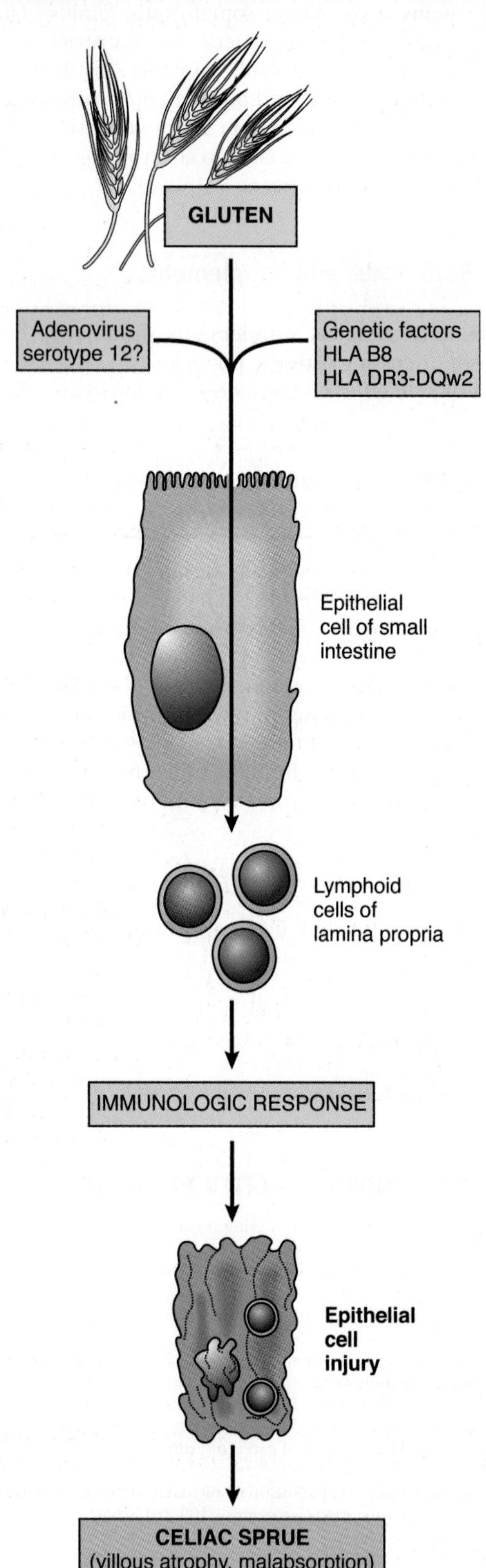

Adapted from: Rubin E MD and Farber JL MD. *Pathology,* 3rd ed. Philadelphia: Lippincott Williams & Wilkins, 1999.

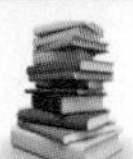

DEFINITIONS AND BACKGROUND

Celiac disease (CD) is a common, lifelong, genetically based autoimmune disorder that causes inflammation of the proximal small intestine (See and Murray, 2006). CD is characterized by inappropriate T cell–mediated immune response to ingested gluten from wheat, rye, and barley that leads to inflammation, villous atrophy, and crypt hyperplasia in the small intestine. Intestinal villi decrease in number, with less absorptive surface and fewer enzymes. Crypts are markedly elongated, causing mucosal malabsorption.

Other names for this disorder include celiac sprue, gluten enteropathy, or nontropical sprue. A major consensus panel determined that 1% of Caucasians (upwards of 3 million people) may have CD (See and Murray, 2006). While screening suggests that one in 133 people have it, the frequency may be closer to one in 100; undiagnosed CD seems to have increased dramatically in the United States during the past 50 years (Rubio-Tapia et al, 2009).

Diagnosis can occur at any age (infancy through old age) and often occurs after stress, pregnancy, or viral infections. Infants may present with impaired growth, diarrhea, pica, abdominal distention, pallor, edema, or vomiting. Children may have frequent, strong-smelling stools that are pale and foamy, diarrhea, irritability, a distended abdomen, easy fatigue, pallor, weight loss, vomiting, and anemia.

Increased intestinal permeability plays a pathogenic role in various autoimmune diseases including CD and type 1 diabetes (T1D) (Visser et al, 2009). Gliadin may also be involved in the pathogenesis of T1D (Visser et al, 2009). All persons with GI symptoms should be tested for CD, as should individuals with type 1 diabetes (T1D), unexplained iron deficiency anemia, elevated levels of transaminases, thyroid disorders, short stature, delayed puberty, fetal loss, and in relatives of patients who have CD (Thompson, 2005). Screening studies have revealed that CD may be asymptomatic in adults (Niewinski, 2008), or they may have episodic or nocturnal diarrhea, flatulence, intestinal bloating that mimics IBS, steatorrhea, weight loss, recurrent stomatitis, anemias or peripheral neuropathy.

Tissue transglutaminase is the main antigen for the antiendomysial antibodies used to diagnose CD. Deamidated gliadin antibodies (DGP) have shown promising results as serological markers for CD (Setty et al, 2008). False-negative test results can occur in children under age 2 years or in patients who have followed a gluten-free (GF) diet for a month or longer. The diagnostic criteria for CD need re-evaluation; endomysial antibody positivity without atrophy belongs to the spectrum of genetic gluten intolerance, and warrants dietary treatment (Kurppa J, et al. 2010).

Early diagnosis and treatment, together with regular follow-up visits with a dietitian, are necessary to ensure nutritional adequacy and to prevent malnutrition while adhering to the GF diet for life (Niewinski, 2008). Longer duration of exposure to gluten can increase the risk of other autoimmune diseases, including non-Hodgkin's or intestinal lymphoma, squamous cell cancer of the esophagus, type 1 diabetes, autoimmune thyroid disease, Addison's disease, lupus, primary biliary cirrhosis, osteoporosis, psoriasis, Sjogren's syndrome, and rheumatoid arthritis (National Institutes of Health, 2004).

Dermatitis herpetiformis (DH) is the skin manifestation, with intensely pruritic lesions that occur over the surface of the elbows, knees, legs, buttocks, trunk, neck, or scalp. Abnormal biopsy is evident, but GI symptoms are not always present. There may be immunoglobulin (IgA) deposits around the lesions, and large intake of iodine may trigger flares of DH.

When wheat, rye, and barley grains are consumed, they damage the mucosa of the small intestine, eventually leading to nutrient malabsorption. Moderate amounts of pure oats can be consumed. However, since much of the commercially available oat flour may be contaminated with wheat gluten, caution is advised for new patients.

Response to GF diets in children with autism may be related to amelioration of nutritional deficiency resulting from undiagnosed gluten sensitivity. Therefore, it is recommended that all children with neurodevelopmental problems be assessed for CD (Genius and Bouchard, 2009). Children and adolescents with symptoms of or an increased risk for CD should have the blood test for antibody to tissue transglutaminase (TTG). Those with an elevated TTG should be referred to a pediatric gastroenterologist for an intestinal biopsy. If tests prove positive, a GF diet is needed. Then, a gastroenterologist should follow all patients with CD.

Because oxidative stress plays an important role in the inflammatory process of CD, increased use of lycopene, quercertin, and tyrosol can be recommended (DeStefano et al, 2007). New forms of treatment propose the use of gluten-degrading enzymes to be ingested with meals, the development of GF grains by genetic modification, the use of substrates regulating intestinal permeability to prevent gluten entry across the epithelium, and different forms of immunotherapy (Setty et al, 2008).

Since the defect is permanent, the GF diet is curative and must be a permanent change. Surface cells of the mucosa are replaced within 5 days; swelling is reduced within 14 days; and villi improve within 6 months or up to 5 years. Consultation with a dietetics professional knowledgeable in CD is essential. An individualized, team approach is best because symptoms change over time.

ASSESSMENT, MONITORING, AND EVALUATION

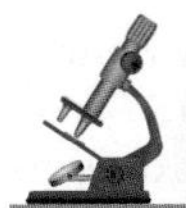

CLINICAL INDICATORS

Genetic Markers: Like an IBD, gliadin peptides are presented on the Human Leukocyte Antigen DQ2 or DQ-8 molecules of antigen-presenting cells to T helper cells, provoking a T helper 1 response that leads to damage by pro-inflammatory cytokines and interleukins (Festen et al, 2009; Visser et al, 2009). CD is more common among people with other genetic disorders including Down syndrome.

Single-nucleotide polymorphisms (SNPs) in the chromosome 4q27 region containing IL2 and IL21 are associated with CD; this is similar to other autoimmune diseases such as rheumatoid arthritis, type 1 diabetes, Graves' disease, psoriatic arthritis, and ulcerative colitis (UC, Glas et al, 2009).

Clinical/History

Height
Weight
BMI
Diet history
Failure to thrive or weight loss
Aphthous stomatitis
Fatigue, lassitude, depression
Recurrent abdominal pain, bloating
Strong-smelling stools that are pale and foamy
Distended abdomen
Irritability, pallor
Steatorrhea, chronic diarrhea
DH
Enamel defects of permanent teeth
Headaches?
Osteopenia, bone pain?
Infertility, frequent miscarriages?
Short stature?
Multiple small bowel biopsies showing flat villi
Abdominal computed tomography (CT) or MRI scan
Capsule endoscopy
Small bowel biopsy

Lab Work

Anti-TTG antibodies (tTG)—IgA and IgG (95–100% sensitive and specific)
Anti-endomysium antibodies-IgA (EMA)–100% specificity, >90% sensitivity
HLA-DQ2 and HLA-DQ8 haplotype
H & H
Serum Fe, ferritin (anemia is common)
Macrocytic anemia (low vitamin B_{12} or folate?)
Serum homocysteine (tHcy)
Serum carotene for vitamin A
Serum vitamins D, E, and K
Serum copper (decreased)
Serum phosphorus (decreased)
Serum zinc (decreased)
Ca^{++} (often low)
Na^{+}, K^{+}
Mg^{++}
Alb, transthyretin
CRP
Transferrin, TIBC
Lactic acid dehydrogenase (increased)
Xylose absorption
DEXA scan
Fecal chymotrypsin level
Fecal fat study
Liver function tests (mildly abnormal)

INTERVENTION

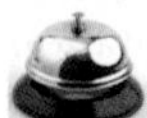

OBJECTIVES

There are six elements required for the management of CD (Thompson, 2005):

1. Consult a skilled dietetics professional. Medical nutrition therapy (MNT) to promote provided by a registered dietitian is strongly recommended improved self-management (American Dietetic Association, 2009).
2. Educate about the disease.
3. Adhere to a GF diet. Remove the offending protein (gliadin fraction) from the diet; glutenin is harmless. Improvement is noted within 4–5 days.

SAMPLE NUTRITION CARE PROCESS STEPS

Altered Nutrient Utilization—Celiac Disease

Assessment Data: Weight loss over the past year. I & O records; stool patterns and frequency; abdominal distention and bloating; DH. GI biopsies reveal CD; positive tTG test.

Nutrition Diagnosis (PES): Altered nutrient utilization related to flattened intestinal villi from CD as evidenced by positive biopsies and tTG test, presence of DH, frequent bouts of abdominal distention, bloating, diarrhea and weight loss.

Intervention: Education about the sources of gluten from diet and food and nonfood products. Provision of recipes for managing the GF diet. Supplier sources of GF foods and flours or grain products. Counseling about fluid sources and ways to incorporate fluids into meals and nourishments. Meal planning tips for the family.

Monitoring and Evaluation: Improved I & O records and weight gain. Normalized stool patterns and frequency. Fewer complaints of GI distress, bloating and diarrhea associated with meals. No signs of protein-energy malnutrition.

4. Identify and treat nutritional deficiencies:
   - Deficiencies of iron, folate, calcium, and vitamin D may be found.
   - Replace nutrients lost from diarrhea and steatorrhea.
   - Reverse bone demineralization, hypoalbuminemia, and hypoprothrombinemia where present.
   - Whole-body protein breakdown is common in CD, contributing to a high level of protein–calorie malnutrition.
   - Glutamine is an important fuel for the health of intestinal epithelial cells. Replenish as needed.
5. Provide access to an advocacy group. A local celiac support chapter is most helpful.
6. Provide continuous long-term follow-up care by a multidisciplinary team.

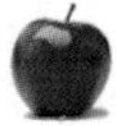

FOOD AND NUTRITION

- A GF diet excludes wheat, rye, and barley. Avoid products such as breading, stuffing, croutons, graham, bulgur, matzo, broth, breading or coating mixes, communion wafers, pastas, cracked wheat, semolina, farina, malt, malt flavoring, brown rice syrup, commercial soups, imitation bacon, imitation seafood, marinades, processed meats, roux, sauces, seasonings, self-basting poultry, soups and soup bases, thickeners, vegetarian meat substitutes, and commercial potato and rice mixes. Soy sauce, white or nonmalt vinegars, and wheat starch must be pure; read labels.
- Plan a diet that includes acceptable grains and starches; see Table 7-9.
- A Greek-Mediterranean dietary pattern with olive oil, nuts, fruits, and vegetable intake can be recommended. Lycopene, quercetin, and tyrosol may control the proinflammatory genes involved in CD (DeStefano et al, 2007). Tyrosol is found in wine and extra virgin olive oil; lycopene in tomato products, watermelon, pink grapefruit; quercetin in apples, citrus fruit, tea, capers, buckwheat, red grapes, broccoli, and red onions. Buckwheat contains rutin (quercetin-3-O-rutinoside) which produces a catabolite (3,4-dihydroxyphenylacetic acid) with significant reducing power, free-radical scavenging activity and enhanced antioxidant capacity of the colonic lumen (Jaganath et al, 2009).
- Because oats are sometimes contaminated with wheat during processing, avoid in initial stages of treatment. Include small-to-moderate amounts if tolerated after the first few months.
- Diet for adults should provide 1–2 g of protein/kg body weight from fresh meat, fresh fish, milk, cheese, and eggs. Examine processed items carefully since there is often gluten added.
- Diet should provide 35–40 kcal/kg body weight for adults.
- For infants with diarrhea, provide fluids, electrolytes, and a formula that is not high in fat content. Infants may tolerate banana powder; adults and children can eat starchy-type carbohydrates, bananas, leans meats, and fish. Rehydrate with oral rehydration solution or other fluids.
- Initially, the diet should include low amounts of fiber because of flattened mucosal villi; increase as tolerated. Fruits and vegetables are naturally low in gluten and should be included regularly.
- If TF is used, a glutamine-enriched product may be useful. Monitor ingredients carefully to avoid gluten.
- Lactose intolerance may be either temporary or permanent. Initially, dairy products (primarily milk and products made with milk) should be avoided. After 3–6 months of treatment, dairy products may be gradually reintroduced.
- GF products are often low in B vitamins, calcium, vitamin D, iron, zinc, magnesium, and fiber. Few GF products are enriched or fortified, adding to the risk of nutrient deficiencies. Correction of vitamin and mineral deficiencies is important. Supplements to the diet should include water-miscible vitamins A, D, E, and K, iron, calcium,

TABLE 7-9 Grains and Starches to Use Freely in Celiac Disease

Amaranth	Nut flours
Arrowroot	Quinoa
Beans (black, garbanzo, kidney, northern, pinto)	Poha flakes
Black-eyed peas, lentils, split peas	Potato
Buckwheat	Potato starch, potato flour
Cassava	Rice
Corn, corn bran, hasa marina	Sorghum
Gluten-free bread	Soy
Hominy, grits	Tapioca
Indian rice grass	Tef
Montina	Wild rice

folic acid, vitamin B_{12}, thiamine, and other B-complex vitamins.

- Products containing MCTs are often used when fat malabsorption is present, especially in adults.
- Foods that often are not allowed include commercial cream soups, creamed vegetables, ice cream (labels should be checked for thickening agents), cakes, cookies, and breads unless made with rice, corn, or potato flours. For toddlers, mixed infant dinners and junior dinners that contain flour thickeners, spaghetti, macaroni, and other pastas should not be used.

Common Drugs Used and Potential Side Effects

- No drug therapy has been proven to suppress the disease.
- Check all labels *each time* for gluten-containing ingredients. GF laxatives include psyllium seed laxatives (Metamucil, Naturacil), docusate sodium (Surfak), and bisacodyl (Dulcolax). Gliadins are often impurities in medications, including acetaminophen; check carefully.
- Corticosteroids may be used with numerous side effects. Take with food. Monitor for negative nitrogen or calcium balances, and for weight gain.

Herbs, Botanicals, and Supplements

- Herbs and botanical supplements should not be used without discussing with the physician.
- Avoid aloe, cascara, senna, and yellow dock because of enhancing effects when using bisacodyl.
- A B-complex supplement may be warranted if serum tHcy levels are elevated (Hadithi et al, 2009; Hallert et al, 2009). A general multivitamin–mineral supplement may be beneficial.
- With antibiotics, quercertin may interfere with fluroquinolones. Advise the physician if used in large amounts.
- Studies are ongoing about the need for carnitine supplementation in CD.

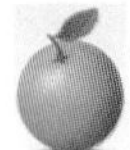

NUTRITION EDUCATION, COUNSELING, CARE MANAGEMENT

- **Strict lifelong elimination of gluten** and dietary adherence are essential (Chand and Mihas, 2006). If strictly followed, improvement will occur in most patients within 2 weeks. If results are not seen after 6–9 months of diet therapy, a new diagnosis should be sought.
- Endomysial antibodies are specific in predicting villous atrophy; patients with endomysial antibodies benefit from a GFD regardless of the degree of enteropathy (Kurppa et al, 2010).
- Intense expert dietary counseling is needed for all patients with CD because the diet is complex (American Dietetic Association, 2009; Niewinski, 2008). An effective plan requires extensive, repeated counseling and instruction of the patient by a skilled dietitian.
- Instruct the patient or family to read food labels *each time* for cereal, starch, flour, thickening agents, emulsifiers, gluten, stabilizers, hydrolyzed vegetable proteins, semolina, durum, triticale, bulgur, farina, couscous, broth, caramel coloring and monosodium glutamate (MSG).
- The Food Allergen Labeling and Consumer Protection Act (FALCPA) requires food labels to clearly identify wheat and other common food allergens in the list of ingredients. A GF symbol is now widely used by food manufacturers. Contact the manufacturer if there are questionable ingredients.
- "Wheat free" is not the same as gluten free; products may contain rye or barley.
- Because of possible contamination with wheat, oats should be avoided in new patients.
- "Wheat starch" is acceptable because the gliadin/gluten has been removed.
- Toothpaste, mouthwash, lipstick or chapstick, glue on envelopes or teabags, boxed candy, chewing gum wrappers, utensils in buffet lines, toasters, bulk food bins, jars used for various purposes, and other related items should be checked carefully and avoided if gluten is present.
- A Greek–Mediterranean dietary pattern high in olive oil, nuts, fruits and vegetable may be recommended.
- For children at school, it may be necessary to educate the staff, nurses and teachers about the GF diet to enhance compliance.
- Quality of life improves for most individuals with CD who follow the GF diet for at least a year (American Dietetic Association, 2009).

Patient Education—Foodborne Illness

- Careful food handling and hand washing are important to prevent introduction of foodborne pathogens to the individual who may be experiencing diarrhea and related GI discomfort.
- If home TF is needed, teach appropriate sanitation and food handling procedures.

For More Information

- Celiac Disease and Gluten-Free Diet Support Group
  http://www.celiac.com/
- Celiac Disease Foundation
  http://www.celiac.org
- Celiac Sprue Association
  http://www.csaceliacs.org/
- Children's Digestive Health and Nutrition Foundation
  http://www.cdhnf.org/wmspage.cfm?parm1=40
- Freeda Vitamins
  http://www.freedavitamins.com
- Gluten-Free Diet by Shelley Case
  http://www.glutenfreediet.ca
- Gluten Free Guide
  http://www.cdhnf.org/user-assets/documents/pdf/GlutenFreeDietGuideWeb.pdf
- Gluten-Free Pantry
  http://www.glutenfree.com/
- Gluten Intolerance Group of North America
  http://www.gluten.net/
- Guidelines for a Gluten-Free Lifestyle
  http://www.celiac.org/newsEvents.php
- National Celiac-Sprue Society
  http://www.csaceliacs.org
- NIDDK
  http://digestive.niddk.nih.gov/ddiseases/pubs/celiac/

CELIAC DISEASE—CITED REFERENCES

American Dietetic Association. Evidence analysis library: Celiac disease. Web site accessed November 8, 2009. at, http://www.adaevidencelibrary.com/topic.cfm?cat=3677&library=EBG.

Chand N, Mihas AA. Celiac disease: current concepts in diagnosis and treatment. *J Clin Gastroenterol.* 40:3, 2006.

DeStefano D, et al. Lycopene, quercetin and tyrosol prevent macrophage activation induced by gliadin and IFN-gamma. *Eur J Pharmacol.* 566:192, 2007.

Festen EA, et al. Inflammatory bowel disease and celiac disease: overlaps in the pathology and genetics, and their potential drug targets. *Endocr Metab Immune Disord Drug Targets.* 9:199, 2009.

Genius SJ, Bouchard TP. Celiac Disease Presenting as Autism [published online ahead of print 29 June 2009]. *J Child Neurol.* 25:114, 2009.

Glas J, et al. Novel genetic risk markers for ulcerative colitis in the IL2/IL21 region are in epistasis with IL23R and suggest a common genetic background for ulcerative colitis and celiac disease. *Am J Gastroenterol.* 104:1737, 2009.

Hadithi M, et al. Effect of B vitamin supplementation on plasma homocysteine levels in celiac disease. *World J Gastroenterol.* 15:955, 2009.

Hallert C, et al. Clinical trial: B vitamins improve health in patients with coeliac disease living on a gluten-free diet. *Aliment Pharmacol Ther.* 29:811, 2009.

Jaganath IB, et al. In vitro catabolism of rutin by human faecal bacteria and the antioxidant capacity of its catabolites [published online ahead of print 30 July 2009]. *Free Radic Biol Med.* 47:1180, 2009.

Kurppa J, et al. Celiac disease without villous atrophy in children: a prospective study. *J Pediatr.* 157:373, 2010.

National Institutes of Health. National Institutes of Health Consensus Development Conference Statement: Celiac disease, 2004. Accessed July 22, 2009 at http://consensus.nih.gov/2004/2004CeliacDisease118html. htm.

Niewinski MM. Advances in celiac disease and gluten-free diet. *J Am Diet Assoc.* 108:661, 2008.

Rubio-Tapia A, et al. Increased prevalence and mortality in undiagnosed celiac disease. *Gastroenterology.* 137:88, 2009.

See J, Murray JA. Gluten-free diet: the medical and nutrition management of celiac disease. *Nutr Clin Pract.* 21:1, 2006.

Setty M, et al. Celiac disease: risk assessment, diagnosis, and monitoring. *Mol Diagn Ther.* 12:289, 2008.

Thompson T. National Institutes of Health consensus statement on celiac disease. *J Am Diet Assoc.* 105:194, 2005.

Visser J, et al. Tight junctions, intestinal permeability, and autoimmunity: celiac disease and type 1 diabetes paradigms. *Ann N Y Acad Sci.* 1165:195, 2009.

CONSTIPATION

NUTRITIONAL ACUITY RANKING: LEVEL 1–2

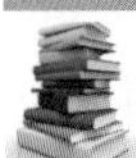

DEFINITIONS AND BACKGROUND

Constipation occurs when the fecal mass remains in the colon longer than the normal 24–72 hours after meal ingestion or when the patient strains to defecate. Stool type and frequency could be used to determine another problem, such as IBS. Constipation and fecal incontinence are common symptoms in patients with cerebral palsy, traumatic spinal cord injuries, spina bifida, multiple sclerosis, diabetic polyneuropathy, Parkinson's disease, and stroke. Intestinal obstruction, tumors and diverticulosis may narrow the intestine, which can also lead to constipation.

Atonic constipation ("lazy bowel") occurs when musculature of the bowel no longer functions properly, sometimes from laxative overuse or poor bowel habits. **Spastic constipation** entails increased narrowing of the colon with small, ribbon-like stools caused by inactivity, immobility, or obstruction; increasing physical activity may be useful. **TF constipation** occurs with use of low-fiber products, medications, or other products.

In infants and children, chronic constipation is a concern, with **encopresis** from poor bowel habits and poor fiber intake. There may be food allergies, such as to milk or wheat, which should also be addressed.

Treatment modalities for constipation include prokinetic agents, enemas administered through the enema continence catheter, and biofeedback. For chronic problems, bowel retraining may be necessary.

There is limited evidence that constipation can successfully be treated by increasing fluid intake unless there is dehydration (Muller-Lissner et al, 2005). Increasing physical activity may be helpful (Muller-Lissner et al, 2005). Some patients may be helped by a fiber-rich diet (American Dietetic Association, 2008). Water-soluble fibers (e.g., pectins, gums, mucilages, and some hemicelluloses) slow down intestinal transit while insoluble fibers from lignin, cellulose, and hemicellulose accelerate intestinal transit. Patients with more severe constipation may get increased bloating or distention when increasing dietary fiber intake; proceed slowly when making a change in fiber intake. Fiber supplements may also help.

Conservative therapies focus on a holistic approach in tandem with evolving drug therapies that target intestinal secretion and transit (Chatoor and Emmanuel, 2009). Chronic constipation decreases quality of life. A Constipation-Related Quality of Life measure is available but should be validated with different treatment methods used for chronic constipation (Wang et al, 2009). Surgical correction of rectocele and intussusception benefit those with anatomical symptoms; for those with predominantly functional features, surgery is best avoided (Chatoor and Emmanuel, 2009).

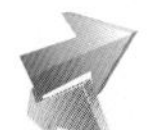

ASSESSMENT, MONITORING, AND EVALUATION

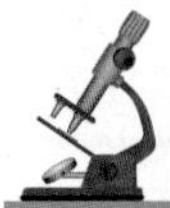

CLINICAL INDICATORS

Genetic Markers: Chronic constipation may have a genetic basis; research is underway.

Clinical/History

- Height
- Weight
- Recent weight changes
- BMI
- Diet history
- Defecation longer than every 3 days
- Bowel habits
- Stool color and number
- Hard, lumpy stools
- I & O
- BP
- Headaches
- Abdominal distention, pain, spasms
- Gas pain, flatulence
- Heartburn, indigestion
- Straining at stool
- Feeling of obstruction or incomplete evacuation

Colorectal transit study	Constipation Severity Index	H & H
Anorectal function test		Serum Fe, ferritin
Colonoscopy or sigmoidoscopy	**Lab Work**	Gluc
	Alb, transthyretin	Na^+, K^+
	BUN, Creat	Ca^{++}, Mg^{++}
		Stool guaiac

INTERVENTION

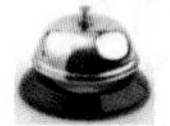

OBJECTIVES

- **Atonic constipation ("lazy bowel"):** Stimulate peristalsis, provide bulk, and retain water in the feces.
- **Spastic constipation:** Undue distention and stimulation of the bowel should be prevented during exacerbations. After the patient is well, fiber should be increased.
- **TF constipation:** Check for obstruction (nausea, vomiting, distention, and dehydration). Record I & O, along with activity levels.
- **Pediatric constipation and encopresis:** Provide laxatives and lubricants initially, followed by improved fiber and fluid intakes.

SAMPLE NUTRITION CARE PROCESS STEPS

Altered GI Function—Constipation

Assessment Data: Fluid intake records (I & O), medication history and recent changes, stool patterns and frequency. No food allergies or intolerances noted. Limited fluid intake recently.

Nutrition Diagnosis (PES): Altered GI function related to very low fluid intake and use of constipating medications as evidenced by patient complaints of hard, dry, infrequent stools, low intake of fluids, and poor nutritional quality of life.

Intervention: Food-Nutrient Delivery: Incorporate more fluids into meals and nourishments, discussion of fluid tracking with staff or family as well as patient. Offer hot or caffeinated beverages, such as coffee or hot tea. Try prune juice mixed with bran and applesauce, especially for the elderly.

Education: Discuss role of fiber, fluid and physical activity in maintenance of normal bowel activity.

Counseling: Discuss food sources and ways to increase fiber content in recipes and meals.

Coordination of Care: Discuss need for stool softener with doctor or nursing staff. Avoid mineral oil that interferes with nutrient absorption.

Monitoring and Evaluation: Fluid intake records, stool patterns and frequency records. Review medication changes or addition of stool softener. Note fewer complaints of incidents of hard, dry, and infrequent stools or straining. Note more GI comfort and improved nutritional quality of life.

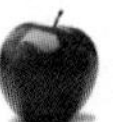

FOOD AND NUTRITION

- In general, it may be helpful to consume more fruits and vegetables and more servings from the bread/cereal group each day, especially whole grains, root vegetables such as carrots or potatoes, stewed dried fruit, and cabbage. Gradually increase fiber, maintain an adequate fluid intake, and exercise regularly.
- **Atonic constipation:** The diet should contain 20–35 g of fiber, with liberal use of whole grains, fruits, and vegetables. Adding a few carrots and whole-grain breads and cereal may be an easy solution. Use adequate fluid (30–35 mL/Kg).
- **Spastic constipation:** Decrease fiber during painful episodes. Then, increase use of prune juice, dried fruits, raw fruits and vegetables, nuts, and whole grains. If wheat allergy is a concern for a patient, do not promote use of bran.
- **TF constipation:** Use a fiber-containing formula if appropriate. Use adequate flushes.
- **Pediatric constipation and encopresis:** Add more fruits and vegetables to the diet; increase whole-grain fiber and fluid intake.

Common Drugs Used and Potential Side Effects

- There is limited evidence about efficacy of treatments used for constipation. Good evidence supports the use of polyethylene glycol and tegaserod. Moderate evidence supports the use of psyllium and lactulose. Limited-quality data exist for milk of magnesia, senna, bisacodyl, and stool softeners (Kamm et al, 2005; Ramkumar and Rao, 2005).
- Discourage overuse or dependence on laxatives and cathartics; see Table 7-10.
- Prescription medications that may cause constipation include opiates, anticholinergics, tricyclic antidepressants, calcium channel blockers, antiparkinsonian drugs, antipsychotics, diuretics and antihistamines.
- Over the counter drugs that can cause constipation include calcium-containing antacids, calcium supplements, iron supplements, NSAIDs, and antidiarrheal agents.

Herbs, Botanicals, and Supplements

- Herbs and botanical supplements should not be used without discussing with the physician.
- Flax, aloe (anthraquinones), fenugreek, and rhubarb have been recommended for constipation, but no clinical trials have proven efficacy.
- With use of bisacodyl, avoid aloe, cascara, senna, and yellow dock because of enhancing effects.
- A herbal tea (Smooth Move) increases bowel movements naturally (Bub et al, 2006).
- More studies on probiotic products are needed, but they have possibility.

TABLE 7-10 Medications for Constipation

Medication	Description
Bulking agents Psyllium (Metamucil, Effersyllium, Perdiem Fiber), Benefiber (with guar gum), methylcellulose (Citrucel), calcium polycarbophil (FiberCon), Fiberall, Fiber-Lax,Equilactin, Konsyl, Serutan	Fiber supplements that retain water and are safe choices. Take with plenty of water or juice (8 oz per teaspoonful). Results may require 1–4 teaspoons of the product.
Chloride channel activators Lubiprostone (Amitiza)	Activators increase intestinal motility and fluid to ease passage of stool. Not recommended for use longer than 12 months without doctor's evaluation.
Lubricant laxatives (Fleet Mineral Oil, Zymenol)	Lubricant laxatives coat the intestinal lining to allow easier passage of stool but may also interfere with absorption of calcium and fat-soluble vitamins.
Osmotic or Hyperosmolar laxatives (Cephulac, Fleet Phospho-Soda, Milk of Magnesia or MOM, Kristalose) or Lactulose (Chronulac) or Polyethylene Glycol 3350 (Miralax, Glycolax)	Osmoticsand saline laxatives draw fluid, cause bowel distention, and may be useful for idiopathic constipation. "The wetter the better." Take with plenty of fluid. Monitor for electrolyte imbalances. Use caution in diabetes. Miralax is safe and effective in pediatrics and pregnancy.
Prebiotics and probiotics	Use of probiotics such as yogurt with active cultures, lactobacilli and bifidobacteria, and prebiotics (nondigestible oligosaccharides) may be beneficial for gut integrity.
Stimulant laxatives Bisacodyl (Fleet Stimulant Laxative, Correctol, Dulcolax) Ex-Lax or Senokot (with senna) Herbal Authority Aloe Vera, Purge, Feen-a-Mint. Prunes (dried plums) are a natural stimulant laxative.	Stimulant laxatives irritate the intestine, causing bowel contractions. They can cause severe cramping, diarrhea, nausea, and electrolyte imbalances. Avoid using bisacodyl (Dulcolax) with dairy products; take with a high-fiber diet. Not recommended for daily or regular use as they can deplete vitamin D and calcium.
Stool softeners **(Emollient laxatives)** Docusate sodium (Colace, Fleet Sof-lax, Peri-Colace, Surfak)	Stool softeners are short-term solutions; they allow more water to penetrate stool and to facilitate elimination. Docusate sodium (Colace) should be taken with milk or juice. Long-term use can deplete electrolytes.
Tegaserod (Zelnorm)	Tegaserod was removed from the market in 2007.

See also: Drug Class Review on constipation Drugs at http://www.ncbi.nlm.nih.gov/books/bv.fcgi?rid=constip, accessed August 11, 2009.

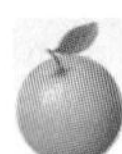

NUTRITION EDUCATION, COUNSELING, CARE MANAGEMENT

- Explain that proper diet can produce relief but cannot cure the condition. A normal bowel routine is needed, but daily fecal evacuation is not needed by everyone.
- Specifically identify foods that have a laxative effect for the patient. Explain why fiber should be increased on a gradual basis only and that items such as prune juice may help. For every gram of cereal fiber, stool weight increases by 3–9 g. For some, a cup of hot prune juice may be useful.
- Have the patient drink 8–10 glasses of water daily, as permitted. Warm fluids are especially useful.
- Exercise may be beneficial in maintaining regularity, especially abdominal-strengthening exercises.
- Discuss foods that have caused constipation, flatus, and GI distress; offer relevant suggestions.
- Medical assistance is needed for diarrhea, bleeding, infection, or other changes in bowel habits.
- Bowel retraining programs may be helpful and may include increasing exercise, including more fiber in the diet, drinking more liquids, and setting aside 15 minutes to spend on the toilet after breakfast. Regular practices may help reestablish a healthy pattern.
- In a pediatric population, dietary changes, corn syrup, or both may resolve constipation in 25% of children. Laxatives such as milk of magnesia and polyethylene glycol are efficient and safe for almost all cases (Loening-Baucke, 2005).

Patient Education—Foodborne Illness

- If home TF is needed, teach appropriate sanitation and food-handling procedures.
- Hand washing is extremely important after toileting.

For More Information

- Constipation
  http://digestive.niddk.nih.gov/ddiseases/pubs/constipation/
- Constipation Algorithm
  http://www.uwgi.org/guidelines/ch_05/AlgA.htm
- Emedicine
  http://www.emedicine.com/med/topic2833.htm
- International Foundation for Functional Gastrointestinal Disorders
  http://www.aboutconstipation.org/
- Med Info
  http://www.medinfo.co.uk/conditions/constipation.html
- Web MD—Chronic Constipation
  http://www.webmd.com/digestive-disorders/chronic-constipation-7/default.htm

CONSTIPATION—CITED REFERENCES

American Dietetic Association. Position of the American Dietetic Association: health implications of dietary fiber. *J Am Diet Assoc.* 108:1716, 2008.
Bub S, et al. Efficacy of an herbal dietary supplement (Smooth Move) in the management of constipation in nursing home residents: a randomized, double-blind, placebo-controlled study. *J Am Med Dir Assoc.* 7:556, 2006.
Chatoor D, Emmanuel A. Constipation and evacuation disorders. *Best Pract Res Clin Gastroenterol.* 23:517, 2009.
Kamm MA, et al. Tegaserod for the treatment of chronic constipation: a randomized, double-blind, placebo-controlled multinational study. *Am J Gastroenterol.* 100:362, 2005.
Loening-Baucke V. Prevalence, symptoms and outcome of constipation in infants and toddlers. *J Pediatr.* 146:359, 2005.
Muller-Lissner SA, et al. Myths and misconceptions about chronic constipation. *Am J Gastroenterol.* 100:232, 2005.
Ramkumar D, Rao SS. Efficacy and safety of traditional medical therapies for chronic constipation: systematic review. *Am J Gastroenterol.* 100:936, 2005.
Wang JY, et al. A valid and reliable measure of constipation-related quality of life. *Dis Colon Rectum.* 52:1434, 2009.

DIARRHEA, DYSENTERY, AND TRAVELER'S DIARRHEA

NUTRITIONAL ACUITY RANKING: LEVEL 2

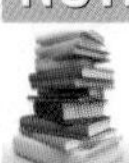

DEFINITIONS AND BACKGROUND

Diarrhea (acute enteritis) is a symptom of many disorders in which there is usually an increased peristalsis with decreased transit time through the GI tract. In Table 7-11, etiologies and comments related to diarrhea are given. Reduced reabsorption of water and watery stools result; see Table 7-12.

Bacterial diarrhea is caused from food or water contaminated with *Campylobacter, Salmonella, Shigella, and E. coli.* Chronic diarrhea involves production of loose stools with or without increased frequency for more than a month. An individualized approach, knowledge of GI physiology, and awareness of the physiological effects of foods or medications are best used to design an effective dietary plan (Schiller, 2006). Dehydration is a common problem; watch for decreased skin turgor, dry mucous membranes, thirst, 2% weight loss or more, low BP, postural hypotension, increased BUN and hematocrit, and decreased urinary output.

Early childhood diarrhea can come from or lead to malnutrition. Diarrhea is the leading cause of death in children younger than 5 years of age, especially in developing countries. Early rehydration may prevent many deaths in high-risk infants if mothers seek medical attention and offer proper rehydration solutions as soon as diarrhea begins. Oral rehydration solutions (ORS) are well tolerated and shorten illness and decrease fluid losses. Diarrhea can be prevented by breastfeeding, by immunizing all children

TABLE 7-11 Diarrhea: Etiologies, Comments and Bristol Stool Chart

Diarrhea Type	Cause	Comments
Antibiotic-induced	*Clostridium difficile* is the gram-positive anaerobic bacterium most often responsible.	Clindamycin or cephalosporin often causes diarrhea.
Chronic diarrhea	Celiac disease, cow's milk allergy, bacterial and parasitic factors, cystic fibrosis, or post-infectious gastroenteritis	Manage the underlying condition and often the diarrhea resolves. Celiac disease or food allergy should be considered.
Dysentery	**Dysentery is from poor sanitation; causes range from contact with feces to contamination by houseflies.**	**Dysentery may involve diarrhea, with blood and mucus, intestinal rumbling, cramps, fever, and pus in stools.**
Functional	From irritation or stress	Often resolves on its own
Organic	From intestinal lesion	May require further medical evaluation
Osmotic	From carbohydrate intolerance	Lactose, fructose, or sorbitol malabsorption may be a cause
Secretory	From bacteria, viruses, bile acids, laxatives, or hormones	This is typically a more serious condition. *Rotavirus* and *Norwalk virus* commonly affect infants and school-aged children; vomiting and watery diarrhea may occur. Norwalk-like viruses may also affect the frail elderly.
Traveler's diarrhea (TD)	**TD is from contaminated food or water.**	**TD is usually caused by enterotoxic bacteria (*E. coli, Campylobacter, Shigella, Salmonella,* or *Yersinia*) or viruses or protozoa, *Giardia* is less common.**

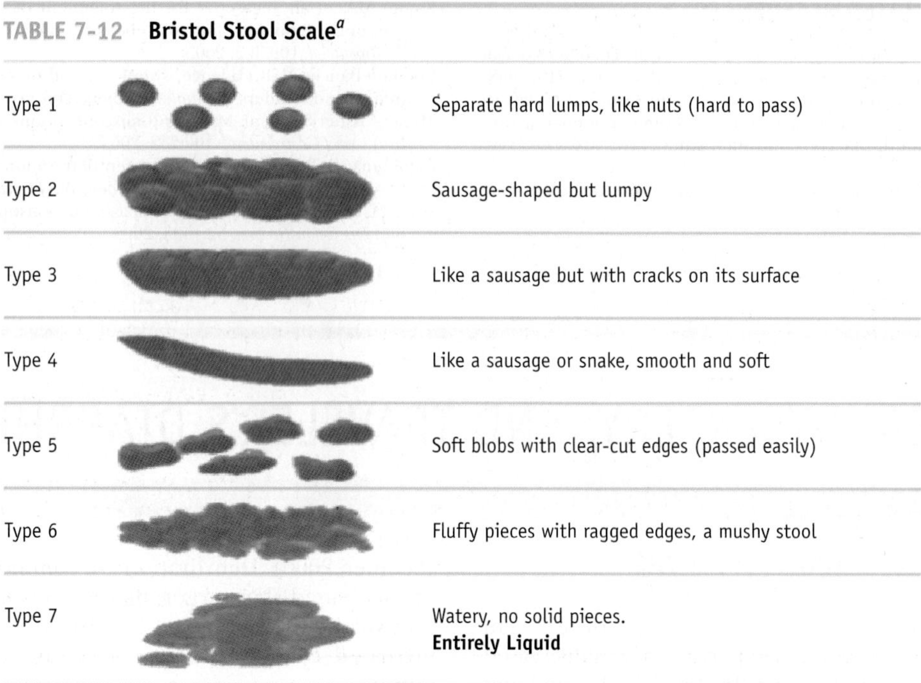

TABLE 7-12 Bristol Stool Scale[a]

	Description
Type 1	Separate hard lumps, like nuts (hard to pass)
Type 2	Sausage-shaped but lumpy
Type 3	Like a sausage but with cracks on its surface
Type 4	Like a sausage or snake, smooth and soft
Type 5	Soft blobs with clear-cut edges (passed easily)
Type 6	Fluffy pieces with ragged edges, a mushy stool
Type 7	Watery, no solid pieces. **Entirely Liquid**

[a]This medical aid was designed to classify feces into seven groups, developed by Heaton and Lewis at the University of Bristol, and first published in the *Scandinavian Journal of Gastroenterology* in 1997. The form of the stool depends on the time it spends in the colon. For more information, see www.continence.org.au. Accessed August 1, 2009.

against measles, by keeping food safe and water clean, and by washing hands before touching food.

***Clostridium difficile* infection (CDI)** diarrhea can be caused by use of most antibiotics. There may be profuse watery diarrhea that may be foul smelling; abdominal pain, cramping, and tenderness; stools that may be guaiac positive and grossly bloody; and fever or WBC count of 12,000–20,000/μL. In severe cases, toxic megacolon, colonic perforation, peritonitis, hypovolemic shock, sepsis, and hemorrhage might occur. Symptoms may develop within a few days or even 6–10 weeks after antibiotic therapy is completed. Because *C. difficile* may be a normal bowel organism (especially in children), simply culturing the organism does not mean that diarrhea is caused by *C. difficile.* In mild cases, symptoms will usually resolve spontaneously once the causative antibiotic is withdrawn. More severe cases warrant therapy with vancomycin and metronidazole for 10 days. Tapered-dose oral vancomycin followed by a pulsed-dose regimen, probiotic approaches, restoration of the normal flora, immunological approaches, toxin-binding approaches, and serial therapy with vancomycin followed by rifaximin may be needed for recurrent infections (Johnson, 2009). See Section 15 for more information.

Dysentery involves severe diarrhea containing mucus or blood. Vomiting of blood occurs. If left untreated, it may be fatal. Oral rehydration therapy is needed, and medication to treat any parasitic or bacterial infection.

For **traveler's diarrhea (TD)**, high-risk destinations include most countries in Latin America, Africa, the Middle East, and Asia. Both cooked and uncooked foods are a concern if they have been improperly handled. Risky foods include raw or undercooked meat and seafood and raw fruits and vegetables. Tap water, ice, and unpasteurized milk and dairy products can be associated with increased risk. Daily doses of rifaximin (Xifaxan) appear to significantly decrease the incidence of TD from *E. coli.*

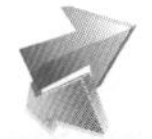

ASSESSMENT, MONITORING, AND EVALUATION

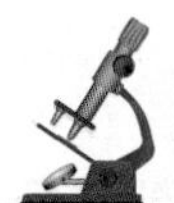

CLINICAL INDICATORS

Genetic Markers: Diarrhea is a symptom rather than a disease. Identify the cause and whether or not there is a genetic origin.

Clinical/History

Height
Weight
Weight changes
BMI
Diet history
Number of stools daily
Stool consistency (see Stool Chart)
BP
I & O; dehydration?
Temperature
Abdominal pain

Lab Work

Na^+ (decreased)
K^+, Cl^-
Ca^{++}, Mg^{++}
H & H
Serum Fe, ferritin
Lactose tolerance test
Hydrogen breath test
Stool culture such as for *C. difficile*
BUN:Creat ratio
Gluc
Alb, transthyretin
CRP
Serum copper
N balance

SAMPLE NUTRITION CARE PROCESS STEPS

Altered GI Function with Diarrhea

Assessment: Food diary, bowel patterns. Medical history or genetic etiology of diarrheal disorders.

Nutrition Diagnosis (PES): Altered GI function related to excessive intake of poorly absorbed CHOs as evidenced by frequent intake of apple juice and sorbitol-containing dietetic products with cramping and loose stools.

Intervention: Food and Nutrient Delivery: change diet as needed. Educate about impact of poorly absorbed CHO on bowel function.

Monitoring/Evaluation: Reports of less abdominal cramping and loose stools.

INTERVENTION

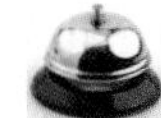

OBJECTIVES

- Determine cause and apply an appropriate treatment.
- Prevent or alleviate dehydration, electrolyte imbalances, anemia, weight loss, and hypoglycemia.
- Avoid refeeding syndrome. CPN may lead to reduction in nutrient intake and atrophy of the gut.
- Restore normal bowel motility. Alter stool consistency and quantity; up to 200 g of stool per day is normal.
- Avoid extremes in food and beverage temperatures, which may stimulate extra colonic activity.
- Correct intolerances for CHO and protein. Ensure adequate fat intake. Short-chain fatty acids enhance sodium reabsorption; include adequate fiber (American Dietetic Association, 2008).
- Probiotic foods may be useful, such as yogurt with live and active cultures.

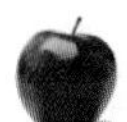

FOOD AND NUTRITION

- It may be useful to hold food for 12 hours with use of IV fluids and electrolytes. Start oral fluids as soon as allowed. Use oral rehydration therapy, shown in Table 7-13, or prepared products such as CeraLyte.
- **Infants:** Use rehydration solutions if allowed. Breastfeeding may be continued, or return to lactose-containing formula when feasible. Cut back on use of sorbitol (as in apple juice).
- **Adults:** Start with broth, tea, toast, and gradually add foods to a normal diet as tolerance progresses. Three to four small meals may be better tolerated. Products such as Gatorade may be useful. Banana flakes may be a safe, cost-effective treatment for diarrhea in critically ill patients on TFs. Use products containing probiotics. For potassium, include bananas, orange juice, fruits, and vegetables in the diet. Cocoa beans contain a large amount of flavonoids; dark chocolate may offer mild relief from diarrhea (Schuier et al, 2005).
- If TF is used, check tube placement and medications, presence of bloody stools, and endoscopic exams. Treatment includes changing medications, decreasing rate of feeding, changing to a high formula, antibiotic therapy, or using antidiarrheal medications. A jejunal placement may be too far for some patients and may actually cause some diarrhea.
- Use CPN only for intractable diarrhea. Osmotic diarrhea abates with NPO. Short-chain fatty acids from high-fiber sources may be useful.
- Use multivitamin–mineral supplements to replace vitamins A and C, zinc, iron, and other nutrients.

Common Drugs Used and Potential Side Effects

- Every patient should receive a careful medication review. Magnesium-containing antacids, digoxin, broad-spectrum antibiotics, antifungal agents, colchicine, thiazide diuretics and other antihypertensives, Azulfidine, methotrexate and other anticancer agents, cholinergic stimulants, antiemetics such as metoclopramide, and laxatives such as mineral oil or methylcellulose may cause drug-induced diarrhea. Sorbitol may cause diarrhea; it is found in many medications. Megadoses of vitamin C (>1 g daily) may cause diarrhea.
- Antibiotics are used if shigellae or amoebae are causing the problem. Suggest use of probiotics with antibiotic therapy. Intestinal flora modifiers (e.g., *Lactobacillus acidophilus*, Lactinex, Bacid) also help recolonize normal intestinal flora. A common prescription is three to four packages every day for 3 days in adults. Modifiers may be mixed with water for tube-fed patients.
- Antidiarrheal drugs are used to slow peristalsis or thicken stools. Kaolin (Kaopectate) has no major side effects but

TABLE 7-13 UNICEF/WHO Oral Rehydration Therapy[a]

Ingredients	Original ORS	New Reduced Osmolarity ORS
Sodium chloride	3.5 g/L	2.6 g/L
Potassium chloride	1.5 g	1.5 g/L
Sodium	2.5 g sodium bicarbonate	2.9 g/L trisodium citrate
Glucose	20 g /L of clean drinking water	13.5 g/L of clean drinking water

[a]Where ORS is not available, home-prepared solutions may use 1 teaspoon of salt, 8 teaspoons of sugar, and 4 oz of orange juice mixed into 1 L of water. From WHO Rehydration Project. Accessed August 1, 2009, at http://www.rehydrate.org/ors/ort_how_it_works.htm.

is not useful with infants. Lomotil should be taken with food; it may cause bloating, constipation, dry mouth, swollen gums, dizziness, nausea, and vomiting. Avoid using it with alcohol. Psyllium ingestion reduces stool looseness.
- Cholestyramine (Questran) may be used for bile acid diarrhea. Nausea, belching, or constipation may result. Replace fat-soluble vitamins.
- Ciprofloxacin is used for TD; one dose is often sufficient. It is a quinolone-class antibiotic. Avoid milk or yogurt. Nausea is one side effect.
- Vancomycin is used for treating *C. difficile.* Anorexia, GI distress, diarrhea, and nausea may result.
- Daily doses of rifaximin (Xifaxan) may significantly decrease TD from *E. coli.* It is not known yet if this same treatment is effective against TD from *Salmonella* and other bacteria.

Herbs, Botanicals, and Supplements

- Herbs and botanical supplements should not be used without discussing with the physician. Apple, carrot, blackberry, carob, bilberry, and tea have been recommended, but no clinical trials have proven efficacy.
- Probiotic medications may be helpful: for children, *Lactobacillus* GG or Culturelle; and for adults, *Saccharomyces boulardii.* Probiotics in foods can help to maintain good bacteria in the GI tract of those taking antibiotics. Yogurt may help to reculture the GI tract; check labels for live and active cultures. Acidophilus milk is also useful.

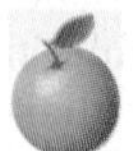

NUTRITION EDUCATION, COUNSELING, CARE MANAGEMENT

- Describe the effects of pectin as a thickening agent (as in apples and bananas), and inform about yogurt or acidophilus milk or other specific probiotic foods/supplements.
- Avoid sweetened carbonated beverages because their electrolyte content is low and osmolality is high. Caffeine, apple juice, and milk can aggravate diarrhea; omit until resolved.
- Limit fruit juice to 6 oz daily in children.
- Partially hydrolyzed guar gum (Benefiber) added to a diet ferments in the colon and produces short-chain fatty acids. This improves intestinal function, including colonic salt and water absorption (Alam et al, 2005). It may be a useful addition until diarrhea resolves.
- Newly formulated oral rehydration salts contain lower concentrations of glucose, and salt and zinc supplementation can drastically reduce the number of child deaths.
- Teach about the prevention and treatment of dehydration with appropriate fluids, breastfeeding of infants, and selective use of antibiotics to reduce the duration and severity of diarrheal episodes.
- Signs of dehydration include increased thirst, dark urine, light headedness, dry skin and less-frequent urination. Children may have no tears when crying, dry mouth and tongue, sunken abdomen or eyes.

Patient Education—Foodborne Illness

- The World Health Organization (2009) states the following facts:

  A total of 1.8 million people die every year from diarrheal diseases (including cholera); 90% are children under 5 who live in developing countries.

  Nearly all diarrheal disease is attributed to unsafe water supply, inadequate sanitation, and poor hygiene.

  Improved water supply reduces diarrhea morbidity by 21%, improved sanitation by 37.5%.

  Simply washing hands at critical times can reduce diarrheal cases by up to 35%. Improvement of drinking water quality, such as point of use disinfection, would lead to a reduction of diarrheal episodes by half.
- To prevent TD, follow these guidelines:

  Use safe, bottled water for drinking and brushing teeth.

  Wash hands before eating, using antiseptic gel or hand wipes.

  Avoid ice in drinks.

  Do not eat raw vegetables or salads, raw fruits, or unpasteurized dairy products.

  Avoid swimming in streams and lakes.

  Use only cooked foods and bottled beverages (e.g., water, juices, beer, etc.).

  Brush teeth with bottled water only.

  Use caution with fresh foods that may have been washed in contaminated water and foods prepared with unheated water (e.g., jello) or ice cubes made with contaminated water.

  If symptoms persist, medical attention should be sought.

For More Information

- CeraLyte
  http://www.ceraproductsinc.com/productline/ceralyte.html
- Centers for Disease Control and Prevention (CDC) Division of Parasitic Diseases
  http://www.cdc.gov/ncidod/dpd/
- Diarrhea
  http://digestive.niddk.nih.gov/ddiseases/pubs/diarrhea/
- Medicine Net—Diarrhea
  http://www.medicinenet.com/diarrhea/article.htm
- Diarrhea Algorithm
  http://www.uwgi.org/guidelines/ch_04/ch04.htm
- Giardiasis
  http://www.cdc.gov/ncidod/dpd/parasites/giardiasis/factsht_giardia.htm
- Rehydration Formula
  http://www.rehydrate.org/
- Travelers' Health (CDC)
  http://www.cdc.gov/travel/diarrhea.htm
- World Health Organization—Dysentery
  http://www.who.int/topics/dysentery/en/

DIARRHEA, DYSENTERY, AND TRAVELER'S DIARRHEA—CITED REFERENCES

Alam NH, et al. Partially hydrolysed guar gum supplemented comminuted chicken diet in persistent diarrhoea: a randomised controlled trial. *Arch Dis Child.* 90:195, 2005.

American Dietetic Association. Position of the American Dietetic Association: health implications of dietary fiber. *J Am Diet Assoc.* 108:1716, 2008.

Johnson S. Recurrent Clostridium difficile infection: causality and therapeutic approaches. *Int J Antimicrob Agents.* 33:33S, 2009.

Schiller LR. Nutrition management of chronic diarrhea and malabsorption. *Nutr Clin Pract.* 21:34, 2006.
Schuier M, et al. Cocoa-related flavonoids inhibit CFTR-mediated chloride transport across T84 human colon epithelia. *J Nutr.* 135:2320, 2005.
World Health Organization. Rehydration Project. Accessed August 1, 2009, at http://rehydrate.org/diarrhoea/index.html.

DIVERTICULAR DISEASES

NUTRITIONAL ACUITY RANKING: LEVEL 2–3

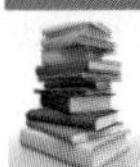

DEFINITIONS AND BACKGROUND

Diverticular disease results from formation of small pouches (diverticula) in the colon wall and lining due to chronic constipation. Diverticular disease occurs in Westernized countries because of low-fiber diets but is rare in societies that subscribe to high-fiber patterns. Lower GI bleeding from diverticulosis is a common reason for hospital admission, particularly in the elderly (Strate, 2005).

A high-fiber diet is the mainstay of management for diverticulosis (American Dietetic Association, 2008). Diverticulitis (inflammation) develops when bacteria or other irritants are trapped in the pouches, causing spasm and pain in the lower left side of the abdomen, as well as distention, nausea, vomiting, constipation or diarrhea, chills, and fever. Bowel cancer has been associated with the presence of diverticular disease.

Serotonin is widely distributed throughout the gut in both the enteric nerves and enterochromaffin cells, where they act as signal transducers and respond to bacterial or dietary substances with an inflammatory response and associated diarrheal symptoms respond well to 5-HT(3) receptor antagonists (Spiller, 2008). Probiotics and prebiotics are being tested for relief of pain and inflammation. Prebiotics such as guar gum are fermented into short chain fatty acids in the colon, where they stimulate water and sodium absorption. Probiotics are used to prevent or treat diarrhea; they are live organisms that eliminate toxins and inhibit proliferation of pathogens.

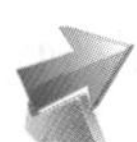

ASSESSMENT, MONITORING, AND EVALUATION

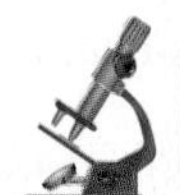

CLINICAL INDICATORS

Genetic Markers: Altered motility is an important feature of the pathogenesis of diverticular disease, and serotonin (5-HT) release is a primary trigger of gut motility (Costedio et al, 2008).

Clinical/History

Height
Weight
BMI
Diet history
Obesity?
Physical inactivity?
Stool number, frequency
BP
Abdominal pain
Blood in stool?
Sigmoidoscopy
Abdominal ultrasound
CT scan
Barium enema

Lab Work

H & H
Serum Fe, ferritin
Transferrin, TIBC
CRP
Erythrocyte sedimentation rate (increased)
Alb, transthyretin
Na^+, K^+
Ca^{++}, Mg^{++}
WBC (increased)

INTERVENTION

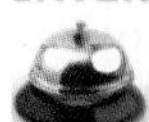

OBJECTIVES

Diverticulitis (Inflamed State)

- Allow complete bowel rest to prevent perforation by avoiding the laxative effect of excess fiber.
- Eliminate food particles that accumulate in sacs as they may cause bacterial contamination.

SAMPLE NUTRITION CARE PROCESS STEPS

Inadequate Fiber Intake

Assessment: Dietary recall of food intake with calculation of average fiber intake <8 g based on 24-hour recall and food frequency.

Nutrition Diagnoses (PES): Inadequate fiber intake (NI 5.8.5) related to nutrition-related knowledge deficit as evidenced by inability to list five foods high in fiber and average daily fiber intake less than 3 g/d. Altered GI function (NC 1.4) related to diarrhea for 3 days, frequent pain, and increased flatus over 3 months.

Interventions: Food-Nutrient Delivery—ND 1.2—soft diet, low-fiber foods until pain subsides.

Education—E 2.2—current diet order for soft, low fiber. Education on gradual introduction of fiber to diet to goal daily amount of 25–35 g; adequate fluid intake; increasing physical activity if possible. Provide list of high-fiber foods for inclusion in the diet, discuss the importance of fiber in diverticulosis.

Counseling: Discuss foods to avoid when there is discomfort.

Monitoring and Evaluation: Reassess dietary intake of fiber at next visit in 3 months; goal is to increase intake to 25–35 g/d. Evaluate daily dietary fiber intake using food recall/diary. Fewer complaints of pain, flatus, or diarrhea.

- Prevent peritonitis and abscess.
- Correct any GI bleeding, hypoalbuminemia, or anemia.
- Each person differs in the amounts and types of foods they can eat; keep a food diary to identify any foods that may cause symptoms or discomfort.

Diverticulosis (Convalescent State)

- Improve stool quality and increase volume, mostly from fiber.
- Relieve intraluminal pressure; decrease the contractions of colonic circular smooth muscle.
- Distend the bowel wall to prevent development of high-pressure segments and inflammation.
- Elimination of specific foods is not necessary.

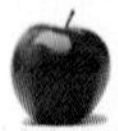

FOOD AND NUTRITION

Diverticulitis (Inflamed State)

- As treatment begins, use a soft diet with low fiber. Gradually add fiber as inflammation and pain decrease.
- Ensure adequate intake of protein and iron sources.
- A low-fat diet may be better tolerated.

Diverticulosis (Convalescent State)

- Diet should be high in fiber; 25–35 g/d is desirable. Whole grains, stewed or dried fruits, potato skins, raw carrots, or celery may be used; see Table 7-14. No evidence supports the common advice to avoid nuts and seeds (Strate et al, 2008). Eating nuts, corn, and popcorn does not increase the risk; in fact, nuts and popcorn may have a protective effect (Weisberger and Jamieson, 2009). Increase fiber gradually; avoid large excesses of fiber that may interfere with mineral absorption. Seeds in fruits or vegetables, and sunflower, pumpkin, caraway, poppy and sesame seeds do not enter, block, or irritate the diverticula and may be consumed.
- Adequate fluid is recommended.
- A vegetarian, plant-based diet is beneficial (Leitzmann, 2005) and a low-fat diet may reduce intracolonic pressure.

TABLE 7-14 **How to Eat More Fiber**

- To get adequate fiber in the diet, follow the U.S. Department of Agriculture Food Guidance System (MyPyramid), which recommends eating 2–4 servings of fruit, 3–5 servings of vegetables, and 6–11 servings of cereal and grain foods each day.
  1. Be smart by eating a whole-grain cereal that contains at least 5 g of fiber per serving. 1/2 cup of bran cereal contains 10 g of fiber.
  2. Beans, peas, and lentils contain 6–9 g per 1/2 cup portion. Add them to soups, stews, and salads.
  3. Eat raw vegetables as much as possible because cooking may reduce fiber content. A baked potato with skin, broccoli, shredded carrots, and cauliflower are great choices.
  4. Eat the peel on fruits (such as apples, pears), and vegetables (such as cucumbers) because much of the fiber is found in the skin.
  5. Eat fresh and dried fruits as snacks. Pears, apples, oranges, strawberries, other berries, prunes, bananas, and figs are all good choices.
  6. Read food labels. Select foods that contain fiber whenever possible.

Sources: U.S. Department of Agriculture Nutrient Database, Release 17, 2004; and Medline Plus. Dietary fiber. 2009. Accessed at http://www.nlm.nih.gov/medlineplus/dietaryfiber.html

Common Drugs Used and Potential Side Effects

- Antibiotics: For patients with severe and complicated diverticulitis, ampicillin, gentamicin, metronidazole, piperacillin, and tazobactam are used. Ciprofloxacin, metronidazole, and rifaximin are used for uncomplicated diverticular disease. Side effects may include nausea, vomiting, stomatitis, and other GI effects.
- There is not enough evidence to recommend the anti-inflammatory drug mesalamine or a polybacterial lysate for immunostimulation (Weisberger and Jamieson, 2009).
- Pain medicine may be needed when cramping or bloating is significant.
- Overusing laxatives may result in dependence on them.
- Probiotics seem to be beneficial.

Herbs, Botanicals, and Supplements

- Herbs and botanical supplements should not be used without discussing with the physician.
- Flax, wheat, wild yam, slippery elm, and chamomile have been recommended for this condition, but no clinical trials have proven efficacy.

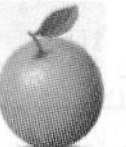

NUTRITION EDUCATION, COUNSELING, CARE MANAGEMENT

- Instruct patient concerning dietary fiber:

  Some ingested plant material is not digested by GI enzymes, including cellulose, pectin, lignin, and hemicelluloses.

  Some dietary fibers (whole grains) resist intestinal disintegration, whereas others (fruits and vegetables) are more or less disintegrated. In general, increased fiber increases stool volume, frequency, and transit rate and decreases intracolonic pressure (American Dietetic Association, 2008).

  Increased stool volume and decreased intracolonic pressure improve transit time.

  Take a fiber product such as methylcellulose (Citrucel) or psyllium (Metamucil) one to three times a day with at least 8 oz of water.
- Instruct patient to chew slowly and to avoid constipation and straining.
- If flatulence is a problem, advise that approximately 6 weeks will be needed to allow bacterial flora to adapt to increased fiber intakes.
- Adequate physical activity is beneficial.

Patient Education—Foodborne Illness

- Careful food handling and hand washing are important to prevent introduction of foodborne pathogens to the individual who may be experiencing diarrhea and related discomfort.
- If home TF is needed, teach appropriate sanitation and food-handling procedures.

For More Information

- Diverticular Diseases
  http://emedicine.medscape.com/article/774922-overview
- International Foundation for Functional Gastrointestinal Disorders
  http://www.iffgd.org/
- Merck Manual—Diverticular disease
  http://www.merck.com/mmhe/sec09/ch128/ch128c.html
- NIDDK
  http://digestive.niddk.nih.gov/ddiseases/pubs/diverticulosis/
- Web MD
  http://www.webmd.com/digestive-disorders/diverticular-disease

DIVERTICULAR DISEASES—CITED REFERENCES

American Dietetic Association. Position of the American Dietetic Association: health implications of dietary fiber. *J Am Diet Assoc.* 108:1716, 2008.

Costedio MM, et al. Serotonin signaling in diverticular disease. *J Gastrointest Surg.* 12:1439, 2008.

Leitzmann C. Vegetarian diets: what are the advantages? *Forum Nutr.* 57:147, 2005.

Spiller R. Serotonin and GI clinical disorders. *Neuropharmacology.* 55:1072, 2008.

Strate LL. Lower GI bleeding: epidemiology and diagnosis. *Gastroenterol Clin North Am.* 34:643, 2005.

Strate LL, et al. Nut, corn, and popcorn consumption and the incidence of diverticular disease. *JAMA.* 300:907, 2008.

Weisberger L, Jamieson B. Clinical inquiries: How can you help prevent a recurrence of diverticulitis? *J Fam Pract.* 58:381, 2009.

FAT MALABSORPTION SYNDROME

NUTRITIONAL ACUITY RANKING: LEVEL 3

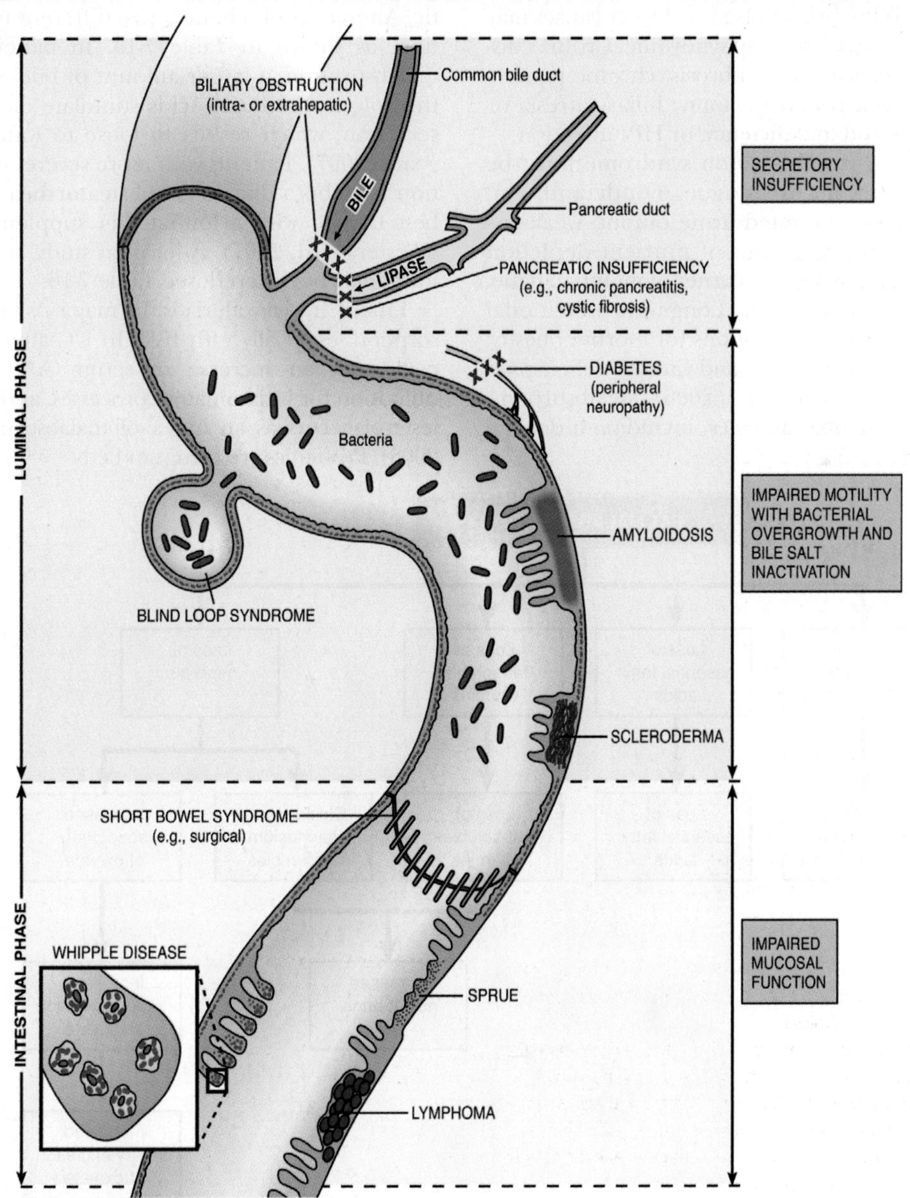

Adapted from: Rubin E MD and Farber JL MD. *Pathology,* 3rd ed. Philadelphia: Lippincott Williams & Wilkins, 1999.

TABLE 7-15 Altered Stools and Related Disorders

Characteristic	Disorder
Yellow or silver color	Fat malabsorption
Pale, foamy, mushy, or floating	Pan malabsorption
Formed in morning	Diarrhea
Formed in evening	Bile salt malabsorption

TABLE 7-16 Fecal Fat Study

Fat absorption is tested by quantitative measurement of total fat in the stool.

Preparation:	Consume 100 g of long-chain triglycerides (LCT) over 3 days
Normal excretion:	Less than 7 g (5% of a 60–100 g intake)
Mild malabsorption:	7–25 g (defects in micelle formation)
Moderate malabsorption:	25–30 g (intestinal mucosal disease)
Severe malabsorption:	More than 40 g (massive ileal resection or pancreatic disease)

Adapted from Hermann-Zaidins M. Malabsorption. *J Am Diet Assoc.* 86:1171, 1986.

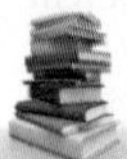

DEFINITIONS AND BACKGROUND

Fat malabsorption syndrome is caused by functional or organic causes. There may be fatigue, weight changes, steatorrhea, abdominal distention with cramps and gas, explosive diarrhea with foul-smelling stools, malnutrition and weight loss, and biochemical abnormalities. Exocrine pancreatic insufficiency is the principal cause. Other causes may include: postgastrectomy, blind loop syndrome, Crohn's disease, small bowel resection; cystic fibrosis, chronic pancreatitis, pancreatic cancer, pancreatectomy; biliary atresia or steatorrhea; CD, lipoprotein deficiency, or HIV infection.

The individual with malabsorption syndrome must be monitored for dehydration (dry tongue, mouth, and skin; increased thirst; low, concentrated urine output; weakness or dizziness when standing). Signs of nutrient depletion include nausea, vomiting, fissures at corner of mouth, fatigue, weakness, and dry, pluckable hair. Long-term nutritional monitoring is necessary after operations for morbid obesity, which can lead to fat malabsorption and vitamin deficiencies for vitamins A, D, and K (Malinowski, 2006). Malabsorption can have severe clinical consequences, including a decline in bone health.

To avoid nutritional deterioration, early screening for fat malabsorption should be recommended. Low total cholesterol (<120 mg/dL) or low serum carotene levels may be typical of fat malabsorption but are not necessarily diagnostic. Altered stools characterize different types of malabsorption, as shown in Table 7-15. In patients with bile acid malabsorption, a larger amount of bile acids is spilled into the colon, where the acids stimulate electrolyte and water secretion, which results in loose to watery stools (Westergaard, 2007). Patients with more severe bile acid malabsorption have both diarrhea and steatorrhea; these patients are best treated with a low-fat diet supplemented with MCTs (Westergaard, 2007). A fecal fat study, though now uncommon, may be ordered; see Table 7-16.

Enteric hyperoxaluria is the major risk factor for fat malabsorption, especially with IBD. In UC after restorative proctocolectomy, an increase of serum AA occurs with lower utilization for inflammatory processes, and reduced LDL cholesterol occurs as an index of malabsorption (Scarpa et al, 2008). Probiotics are being studied.

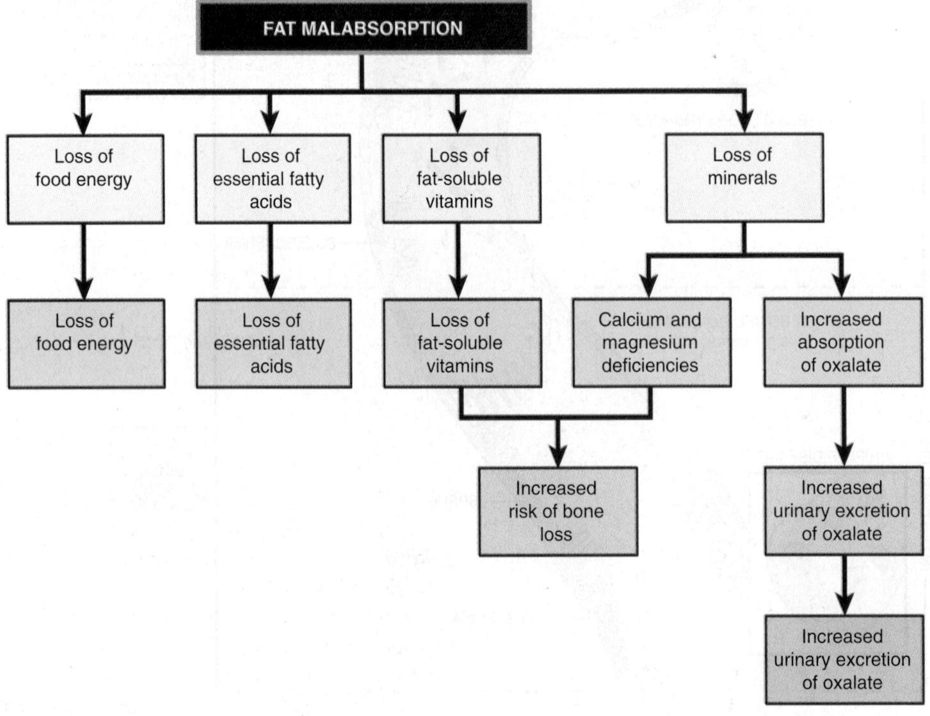

Adapted from: Merck Manual. Malabsorption syndromes. http://www.merck.com/media/mmpe/pdf/Figure_ 017-1.pdf. Website accessed 9/1/09.

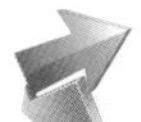

ASSESSMENT, MONITORING, AND EVALUATION

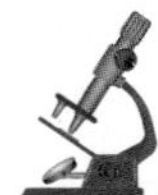

CLINICAL INDICATORS

Genetic Markers: Fat malabsorption is typically a symptom of an underlying disorder that may be either genetic or acquired.

Clinical/History

- Height
- Weight
- BMI
- Diet history
- BP (may be low)
- Signs of dehydration?
- Failure to thrive in children
- Perianal itching or soreness
- Frequent, foul-smelling stools
- Small intestine biopsy
- CT scan or MRI
- Barium enema or x-rays

Lab Work

- Tryptophan load test for vitamin B_6
- Fecal Ca^{++}
- Acid steatocrit
- Malabsorption blood test
- ^{14}C-triolein breath test
- Fecal fat study: 72-hour stool collection
- Labeled carbon breath test
- Sudan stain test
- Serum carotene, vitamin A (may be low)
- D-xylose test (decreased excretion?)
- Serum vitamin E
- Schilling test for vitamin B_{12}
- Na^+, K^+, Cl^- (may be low from diarrhea)
- Ca^{++}, Mg^{++} (may be low)
- Chol (may be decreased)
- Trig
- H & H
- Serum Fe, ferritin
- Gluc
- Alb, transthyretin (may be low)
- CRP

INTERVENTION

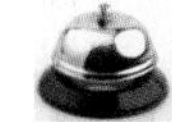

OBJECTIVES

- Monitor for malabsorption of fat-soluble vitamins (A, D, E, and K). Long-term consequences of vitamin deficiency results if fat malabsorption is not corrected.

SAMPLE NUTRITION CARE PROCESS STEPS

Abnormal Nutrient (FAT) Utilization

Assessment: I & O, abnormal nutritional labs for cholesterol, albumin, electrolytes. Fecal fat test results showing excesses of 20 g fat in stool; stools of yellowish hue. Abdominal pain.

Nutrition Diagnoses (PES): Abnormal fat utilization related to malabsorption as evidenced by fecal fat study showing fat in stool of >20 g/d, yellowish stools, and abdominal pain.

Interventions: Food and nutrient delivery: alter diet to include products containing MCT oil until condition can be resolved.

Education: Discuss how fat malabsorption affects metabolism and absorption of nutrients. Counseling: Inclusion of water-miscible forms of fat-soluble vitamins, more calcium and water-soluble vitamins.

Monitoring and Evaluation: Improvement in nutritional labs; fewer yellowish or abnormal stools. Fecal fat study showing less than 7 g fat. Less abdominal discomfort.

TABLE 7-17 Medium-Chain Triglycerides (MCTs)

- Many products now contain MCTs as the primary fat source.
- MCTs use portal (albumin-free fatty acids) rather than lymphatic system transport and absorption (using less lipase and bile).
- MCTs have an 8- to 10-carbon source of fat and are useful when longer chain fatty acids (16–18 carbons) cannot be efficiently digested or absorbed.
- MCTs have concentrated calories made from coconut oil for adjunct therapy.
- MCT oil has 230 kcal/30 mL (6–7 kcal/g). Use instead of vegetable oil in recipes.

- Prevent calcium oxalate stone formation, or correct where present.
- Correct all other nutrient deficiencies.
- Alleviate steatorrhea and reduce intake of fat sources that are not tolerated. MCTs are useful. See Table 7-17.

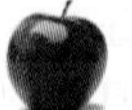

FOOD AND NUTRITION

- Initial treatment should consist of parenteral solutions or liquid formulas that contain MCT. MCTs alleviate steatorrhea in some cases; start with 20–60 g and increase gradually in an adult.
- For mild cases, oral feeding is preferred because it stimulates brush-border activity. For moderate-to-severe cases, tube feed if necessary (50 mL/hr full strength initially; advance gradually).
- Dietary fat may be limited to one egg and 4–6 oz of meat, poultry, or fish. Gradually check tolerance for long-chain triglycerides (LCTs) and work up to 30–40 g.
- Increase intake of protein, which may be in the form of skim milk, egg white, cereals, or legumes.
- Complex carbohydrates may be better tolerated than simple sugars. Lactose may not be tolerated.
- A multivitamin–mineral supplement may be necessary to offset fecal losses of nutrients, vitamins, and water in patients with malabsorption syndromes—especially zinc, folate, vitamin B_{12}, calcium, magnesium, iron, and fat-soluble vitamins (A, D, E, and K).
- Monitor or decrease dietary oxalate intake to prevent renal stones. Use of probiotics may be helpful.

Common Drugs Used and Potential Side Effects

- Antibiotics are used for bacterial overgrowth. Suggest use of yogurt with live and active cultures with antibiotic therapy. Intestinal flora modifiers (e.g., *Lactobacillus acidophilus*, Lactinex, Bacid) also help recolonize normal intestinal flora, perhaps three to four packages every day for 3 days in adults. They may be mixed with water for TFs.
- Antidiarrheals may be used, such as kaolin (Kaopectate). Cholestyramine may be needed for bile salt diarrhea; fat-soluble vitamins can be depleted.
- Cholylsarcosine (CS) is a semisynthetic bile salt replacement. If used properly, no side effects occur.
- Orlistat inhibits pancreatic lipase and blocks the absorption of 30% of ingested fat in patients seeking weight loss.

By its nature, it has the potential to create fat malabsorption syndrome, and use should be carefully monitored to assure that nutrient deficiencies do not occur.

- Pancreatic enzymes may be needed if there is pancreatic insufficiency.
- Patients with mild-to-moderate bile acid malabsorption present with watery diarrhea and generally respond very well to treatment with bile acid binders such as cholestyramine (Westergaard, 2007).

Herbs, Botanicals, and Supplements

- Herbs and botanical supplements should not be used without discussing with the physician.

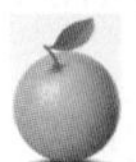

NUTRITION EDUCATION, COUNSELING, CARE MANAGEMENT

- Caution the patient about a rapid consumption of MCTs. If they are consumed too rapidly, hyperosmolar diarrhea may result. Abdominal discomfort, flatulence, diarrhea, or steatorrhea may indicate continued malabsorption; the physician should be contacted.
- Encourage several small, frequent meals throughout the day, avoiding fluids and foods that promote diarrhea. Monitor I & O of fluids, along with the number, color, and consistency of stools.
- Remember that a source of essential fatty acids may be needed if MCTs are used with a low-fat diet.

Patient Education—Foodborne Illness

- Careful food handling and hand washing are important to prevent introduction of foodborne pathogens to this individual who may be experiencing diarrhea and related discomfort.
- If home TF is needed, teach appropriate sanitation and food-handling procedures.

For More Information

- Fat Malabsorption Syndrome
  http://www.merck.com/mrkshared/mmanual/section3/chapter30/30a.jsp
- E-medicine
  http://www.emedicine.com/PED/topic1356.htm
- Merck manual—malabsorption
  http://www.merck.com/mkgr/mmg/sec13/ch111/ch111a.jsp

FAT MALABSORPTION SYNDROME—CITED REFERENCES

Malinowski SS. Nutritional and metabolic complications of bariatric surgery. *Am J Med Sci.* 331:219, 2006.

Scarpa M, et al. Restorative proctocolectomy for ulcerative colitis: impact on lipid metabolism and adipose tissue and serum fatty acids. *J Gastrointest Surg.* 12:279, 2008.

Westergaard A. Bile Acid malabsorption. *Curr Treat Options Gastroenterol.* 10:28, 2007.

INFLAMMATORY BOWEL DISEASE: CROHN'S DISEASE

NUTRITIONAL ACUITY RANKING: LEVEL 3–4

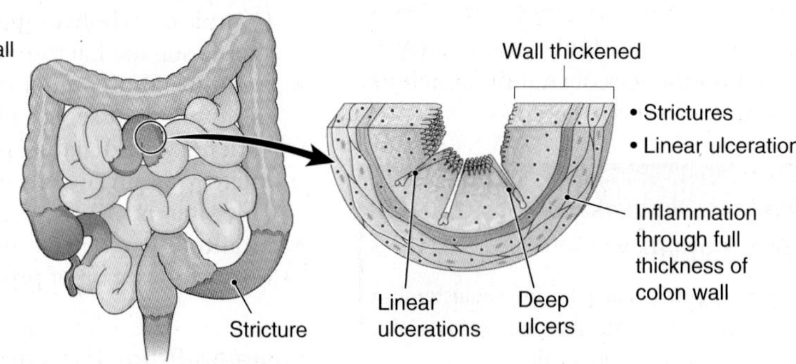

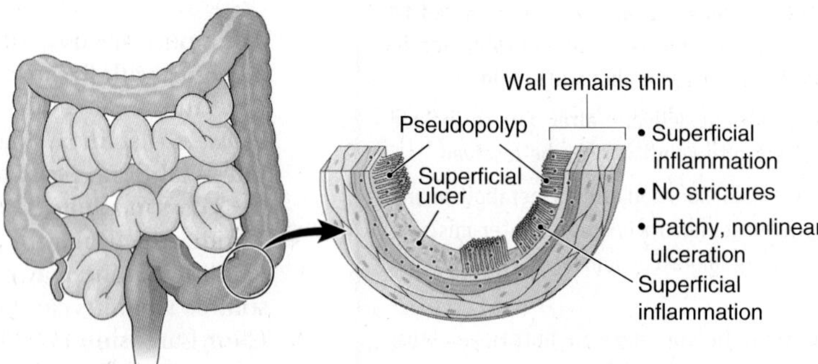

Adapted from: Thomas H. McConnell, *The Nature Of Disease Pathology for the Health Professions,* Philadelphia: Lippincott Williams & Wilkins, 2007.

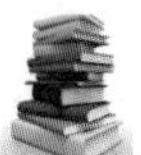

DEFINITIONS AND BACKGROUND

Crohn's disease involves acute and chronic granulomatous, IBD with a cobblestone effect. Onset is generally between 15 and 30 years of age. Crohn's disease differs from UC by affecting mucosal tissue of GI tract from oral cavity to rectum. In 33%, only the ileum is involved; in 45%, both the ileum and the large intestine are affected.

As many as 1.4 million persons in the United States and 2.2 million persons in Europe suffer from with IBD. Macroscopic cobblestoning, segmental colitis, ileal stenosis and ulceration, perianal disease, and multiple granulomas in the small bowel or colon strongly suggest a diagnosis of CD. The causative antigen in IBD is the microflora in the intestinal lumen, facilitated by an impaired innate immune system; these provoke T helper 1 and T helper 17 responses in Crohn's disease and a T helper 2 response in UC, resulting in pro-inflammatory cytokines and interleukins (Festen et al, 2009). Increased numbers of mucosa-associated *E. coli* are observed (Willing et al, 2009). Patients with CD exhibit a profound systemic failure of the acute inflammatory response that results in markedly delayed clearance of bacteria from the tissues, leading to local chronic granulomatous inflammation and compensatory adaptive changes (Sewell et al, 2009).

Environmental triggers include smoking, northern geographic residence, allergic and autoimmune responses. Both passive and active smoke exposure in childhood predisposes children to IBD (Mahid et al, 2007). In addition, the pathways for amino acids, fatty acids, bile acids and AA are altered (Jansson et al, 2009).

The intestinal lumen decreases; peristalsis from food intake causes cramping pain, especially in the right lower quadrant. Only 25% of Crohn's disease cases present with the classic triad of abdominal pain, weight loss, and diarrhea (Beattie et al, 2006). Chronic watery diarrhea results from edema, bile salt malabsorption, bacterial overgrowth, and ulceration. Children may present with growth failure, inflammation, fever, pallor, and anemia. Stricture may precipitate bowel obstruction. Fever, weight loss, nausea, mouth sores, anal fissures, vomiting, abdominal pain, intestinal bleeding, arthritis, iritis or uveitis, conjunctivitis, jaundice, or pruritus may also be present. Elevated plasma tHcy is common. Nutritional therapy is an essential adjunctive treatment. In cases of short bowel syndrome (SBS), long-term CPN may be essential.

Anti-TNF alpha (anti-TNFα) therapies have been used. Complications associated with Crohn's disease include arthritis, skin problems, inflammation in the eyes or mouth, kidney stones, gallstones, or other diseases of the hepatobiliary system. If medical management fails, surgery may be indicated for continuous bleeding; recurrent ileus, abscesses, or fistulae. After total proctocolectomy, patients have less morbidity and are more likely to be weaned off all Crohn's-related medications (Fichera et al, 2005).

Persons with Crohn's disease are at increased risk for colon cancer, obstruction, anorectal fistulas, and abscesses. Chronic inflammatory processes cause overproduction of reactive oxygen and nitrogen species, overproduction or activation of key AA metabolites and cytokines/growth factors, and immunity system dysfunction (Yang et al, 2009). Researchers are looking at genetically altering *Bacteroides ovatus*, naturally in the gut, to secrete human growth factor KGF-2 protein when exposed to xylan sugar and to heal the damage caused by inflammation (Hamady et al, 2008).

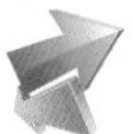

ASSESSMENT, MONITORING, AND EVALUATION

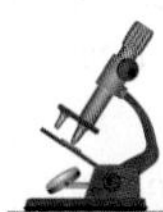

CLINICAL INDICATORS

Genetic Markers: Crohn's disease is associated with multiple mutations in the CARD15, the interleukin 23 receptor (IL23R) and autophagy-related 16-like 1 (ATG16L1) genes. The G allele of SNP rs2241880 confers strong risk for CD with a coding variant, threonine-to-alanine substitution at amino acid position 300 of the ATG16L1 protein (Grant et al, 2008).

Clinical/History
- Height
- Weight
- BMI
- Weight loss?
- Stunted growth?
- Diet history
- BP (fever?)
- Temperature
- Rectal bleeding
- Diarrhea
- Number of bowel movements, frequency
- Barium upper GI series with small bowel follow-through
- Abdominal CT
- Upper endoscopy
- Colonoscopy with biopsies

Lab Work
- WBC, ESR (increased)
- Crohn's disease activity factor (CDAI)
- CRP
- H & H
- Serum Fe, ferritin (decreased)
- Na^+, K^+
- Alb, transthyretin (low)
- Transferrin, TIBC
- N balance
- Serum tHcy
- Serum folate
- Serum B_{12} and Schilling test
- Ca^{++}, Mg^{++}
- Serum B_{12}
- Total protein
- BUN, Creat
- Serum carotene
- Serum zinc (decreased)
- TLC
- Serum Cu
- Hydrogen breath test

INTERVENTION

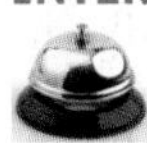

OBJECTIVES

- Replace fluid and electrolytes lost through diarrhea and vomiting. Lessen mechanical irritation and promote rest, especially with diarrhea.
- Replenish nutrient reserves; correct malabsorption or anemia. Poor nutritional status may be related to decreased intake from anorexia, nausea or vomiting, abdominal pain, restrictive diets, side effects of medications, protein losses from ulcerated mucosal lesions, blood loss or wound-healing requirements, bacterial overgrowth, and malabsorption.
- Monitor lactose and gluten intolerances, which may be present.
- Promote healing; rest bowel from offending agents. Provide foods that contain short-chain fatty acids and glutamine to promote healing.
- Prevent peritonitis, obstruction, renal calculi, and fistulas.

SAMPLE NUTRITION CARE PROCESS STEPS

Food and Nutrition Knowledge Deficit

Assessment: Food diary, x-ray reports, biopsy.

Nutrition Diagnosis (PES): Food and nutrition-related knowledge deficit (NB 1.1) related to management of Crohn's as evidenced by new diagnosis and request for information from patient and family.

Altered GI function (NC 1.4) related to inflammation in newly diagnosed Crohn's disease as evidenced by diarrhea for 2 weeks; abdominal pain and cramping after meals.

Involuntary weight loss (NC 3.2) related to diarrhea and inability to consume and digest adequate daily kilocal as evidenced by weight loss of 15 lb in last 60 days.

Interventions: Food and Nutrient Delivery: ND 3.2.1 Multivitamin/mineral supplement. Clear liquids advancing to low residue diet prior to discharge.

Educate on low residue diet as needed, use of probiotic foods, and small frequent meals with lactose-free foods as needed.

Coordinate Care: Refer to gastroenterology dietitian specialist for outpatient follow-up.

Monitoring and Evaluation: Improved intake and type of foods; symptoms resolved or improved. Monitor Hgb, Alb, Na^+, K^+ for improvements while inpatient; weight for maintenance and eventual regain to usual body weight; bowel health with regard to decreased cramping and diarrhea after meals.

- Promote weight gain or prevent losses from exudates or inadequate intake.
- Prepare for surgery if necessary after failed medical management, obstruction, fistula, or peritonitis. A total colectomy or a right-sided ileocolectomy may be necessary.
- In a child, promote growth. Growth spurts follow sustained weight gain.
- Reduce inflammatory process; fish oil intake may reduce severity of symptoms.
- Monitor mineral and trace element levels carefully to ensure adequacy. Iron tends to be low. Antioxidant intake should be increased.
- Prevent or correct metabolic bone disease (e.g., osteopenia, arthropathies) caused by disease itself, nutrient malabsorption, side effects of medications, or lifestyle factors.
- Because tHcy production within the intestinal mucosa may contribute to the inflammatory response and endothelial cell dysfunction, treat folate and vitamin B_{12} deprivation as well as methylenetetrahydrofolate reductase (MTHFR) polymorphisms (Peyrin-Biroulet et al, 2007). Prevent thrombotic events.

FOOD AND NUTRITION

- For adult energy requirements, estimate needs according to current BMI. A low BMI (<15) may require 35–45 kcal/kg; a BMI of 15–19 may require 30–35 kcal/kg; a BMI of 20–29 may require 25–30 kcal/kg; and a high BMI (>30) may only require 15–25 kcal/kg. Estimate needs at the high end of normal for growth and repair in infants or children.
- With strictures or fistulas, use a low-fiber diet that is high in energy with a high protein content of 1–1.5 g/kg.
- For some patients, TF with added glutamine may be useful. Polymeric formulas are acceptable; elemental products are not required. Randomized controlled trials show that enteral nutrition is effective.
- Perioperative PN may reverse malnutrition and facilitate rehabilitation (Yao et al, 2005). If CPN is needed after total colectomy, use indirect calorimetry to estimate needs.
- A diet relatively high in fat may improve energy balance. Limit fat intake only if steatorrhea is present, in which case MCTs may be better tolerated. Omega-3 fatty acids may be indicated.
- Supplement the diet with multivitamins and minerals, especially thiamine, folacin, vitamin B_{12}, vitamin E, zinc, vitamin D, calcium, magnesium, and iron. Vitamins A and K should be given every other day. With resection greater than 200 cm, selenium may become deficient; monitor carefully.
- Reduce lactose intake if not tolerated. Check for wheat and gluten tolerances.
- Monitor progress carefully; patients may be finicky. Small, frequent meals may be better tolerated.

Common Drugs Used and Potential Side Effects

- Therapies for CD typically include aminosalicylates and antibiotics (for mild mucosal disease), nutritional therapy (including elemental or polymeric formulas), corticosteroids (for moderate disease), and infliximab for corticosteroid-resistant or fistulizing disease (Rufo and Bousvaros, 2006). Standard treatments with 5-aminosalicylic acid, antibiotics, corticosteroids, and immunosuppressives have serious and potentially adverse events (Krygier et al, 2009).
- Anti-inflammation drugs are first-line treatments, with mesalamine in 5-ASA agents (Asacol, Canasa, Pentasa) or sulfasalazine (Azulfidine). Side effects include nausea, vomiting, heartburn, diarrhea, headache, folate depletion.
- Antibiotics reduce bacterial overgrowth and vitamin K may be needed for fistulas. Ampicillin, sulfonamide, cephalosporin, tetracycline, or metronidazole are common choices. Metronidazole may be used when there is anal involvement; nausea, vomiting, anorexia, or diarrhea may occur.
- Anti-diarrheal agents are needed, such as diphenoxylate, loperamide, and codeine.
- Corticosteroids such as Budesonide (Entocort) are used in large doses at first. They are most effective with colon involvement. Patients will need a diet that provides sodium restriction, with extra protein, calcium, and potassium. Corticosteroids are more effective than enteral nutrition (Zachos et al, 2007).

- Anti-TNFα therapy is beneficial. Infliximab (Remicade) was the first treatment approved specifically to reduce inflammation in Crohn's disease. The anti–TNF alpha agents are effective in the induction and maintenance of remission in luminal and fistulizing Crohn's disease; early use with immunosuppressives may alter progression of the disease and prevent late complications (Krygier et al, 2009).
- Some neuroregulatory peptides act as endogenous immune factors with anti-inflammatory effects; selective peptide analogs are being developed as novel therapeutic strategies for IBD patients (Motilva et al, 2008).
- Retinoic acid and vitamin D are being studied for their possible effects in gut immunity and Crohn's disease (O'Sullivan, 2009).
- In MTHFR polymorphisms, use of L-methylfolate may be useful; Deplin is one prescription drug.

Herbs, Botanicals, and Supplements

- Use of complementary medicine is common in this population (Langhorst et al, 2005). Omega-3 fatty acids help to reduce symptoms of Crohn's disease. Alpha linoleic acid (ALA) works better at decreasing bowel inflammation than EPA and DHA. Fish oil supplements can cause side effects such as flatulence and diarrhea.
- Phytochemicals such as turmeric (curcumin), red pepper (capsaicin), cloves (eugenol), ginger (gingerol), cumin, anise, and fennel (anethol), basil and rosemary (ursolic acid), garlic (diallyl sulfide, *S*-allylmercaptocysteine, ajoene), and pomegranate (ellagic acid) can suppress some inflammatory pathways (Aggarwal and Shishodia, 2004).
- Probiotics may be beneficial; clinical studies are needed to verify the specific bacteria to be recommended. Studies have been performed with a variety of antioxidants, glutamine, short-chain fatty acids and prebiotics.

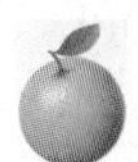

NUTRITION EDUCATION, COUNSELING, CARE MANAGEMENT

- Encourage patient to eat. Discuss fiber, fluid, and supplements.
- Periodic assistance or reevaluation by a qualified dietitian may be helpful. Alleviate fears associated with mealtimes.
- Ensure that sources of potassium are increased during periods of diarrhea.
- Instruct patient to chew foods well and avoid swallowing air.
- Bone density should be monitored yearly (Sylvester et al, 2007). Highlight calcium and vitamin D and discuss alternate sources when milk cannot be used. Promote exercise as well.
- Nocturnal TFs have been useful to regain weight or to promote growth. Total enteral nutrition with a liquid formula can suppress gut inflammation and induce remission in active Crohn's disease (Johnson et al, 2006; Newby et al, 2005).

Patient Education—Foodborne Illness

- Careful food handling and hand washing are important to prevent introduction of foodborne pathogens to the individual who may be experiencing diarrhea and related discomfort.
- If home TF is needed, teach appropriate sanitation and food-handling procedures.

For More Information

- Colon Cancer Screening
  http://www.uwgi.org/guidelines/ch_08/ch08txt.htm
- Crohn's Disease
  http://digestive.niddk.nih.gov/ddiseases/pubs/crohns/
- Crohn's and Colitis Foundation of America
  http://www.ccfa.org/
- HealingWell Crohn's Disease Resource Center
  http://www.healingwell.com/ibd/
- National Association for Colitis and Crohn's Disease
  http://www.nacc.org.uk/content/home.asp
- Reach Out for Youth with Ileitis and Colitis
  http://www.reachoutforyouth.org/

CROHN'S DISEASE—CITED REFERENCES

Aggarwal BB, Shishodia S. Suppression of the nuclear factor-kappaB activation pathway by spice-derived phytochemicals: reasoning for seasoning. *Ann N Y Acad Sci.* 1030:434, 2004.

Beattie RM, et al. Inflammatory bowel disease. *Arch Dis Child.* 91:426, 2006.

Festen EA, et al. Inflammatory bowel disease and celiac disease: overlaps in the pathology and genetics, and their potential drug targets. *Endocr Metab Immune Disord Drug Targets.* 9:199, 2009.

Fichera A, et al. Long-term outcome of surgically treated Crohn's colitis: a prospective study. *Dis Colon Rectum.* 48:963, 2005.

Grant SF, et al. Classification of genetic profiles of Crohn's disease: a focus on the ATG16L1 gene. *Expert Rev Mol Diagn.* 8:199, 2008.

Hamady ZZ, et al. Identification and use of the putative Bacteroides ovatus xylanase promoter for the inducible production of recombinant human proteins. *Microbiology.* 154:3165, 2008.

Jansson J, et al. Metabolomics reveals metabolic biomarkers of Crohn's disease. *PLoS One.* 4:e6386, 2009.

Johnson T, et al. Treatment of active Crohn's disease in children using partial enteral nutrition with liquid formula: a randomised controlled trial. *Gut.* 55:356, 2006.

Krygier DS, et al. How to manage difficult Crohn's disease: optimum delivery of anti-TNFs. *Expert Rev Gastroenterol Hepatol.* 3:407, 2009.

Langhorst J, et al. Amount of systemic steroid medication is a strong predictor for the use of complementary and alternative medicine in patients with inflammatory bowel disease: results from a German national survey. *Inflamm Bowel Dis.* 11:287, 2005.

Mahid SS, et al. Active and passive smoking in childhood is related to the development of inflammatory bowel disease. *Inflamm Bowel Dis.* 13:431, 2007.

Motilva V, et al. Intestinal immunomodulation. Role of regulative peptides and promising pharmacological activities. *Curr Pharm Des.* 14:71, 2008.

Newby EA, et al. Interventions for growth failure in childhood Crohn's disease. *Cochrane Database Syst Rev.* 3:CD003873, 2005.

O'Sullivan M. Symposium on 'The challenge of translating nutrition research into public health nutrition'. Session 3: Joint Nutrition Society and Irish Nutrition and Dietetic Institute Symposium on 'Nutrition and autoimmune disease'. Nutrition in Crohn's disease. *Proc Nutr Soc.* 68:127, 2009.

Peyrin-Biroulet L, et al. Vascular and cellular stress in inflammatory bowel disease: revisiting the role of homocysteine. *Am J Gastroenterol.* 102:1108, 2007.

Rufo PA, Bousvaros A. Current therapy of inflammatory bowel disease in children. *Pediatr Drugs.* 8:279, 2006.

Sewell GW, et al. The immunopathogenesis of Crohn's disease: a three-stage model [published online ahead of print 7 Aug 2009]. *Curr Opin Immunol.* 21:506, 2009.

Sylvester FA, et al. Natural history of bone metabolism and bone mineral density in children with inflammatory bowel disease. *Inflamm Bowel Dis.* 13:42, 2007.

Willing B, et al. Twin studies reveal specific imbalances in the mucosa-associated microbiota of patients with ileal Crohn's disease. *Inflamm Bowel Dis.* 15:653, 2009.

Yang GY, et al. Inflammatory bowel disease: a model of chronic inflammation-induced cancer. *Methods Mol Biol.* 511:193, 2009.

Yao GX, et al. Role of perioperative parenteral nutrition in severely malnourished patients with Crohn's disease. *World J Gastroenterol.* 11:5732, 2005.

Zachos M, et al. Enteral nutritional therapy for induction of remission in Crohn's disease. *Cochrane Database Syst Rev.* (1):CD000542, 2007.

INFLAMMATORY BOWEL DISEASE: ULCERATIVE COLITIS

NUTRITIONAL ACUITY RANKING: LEVEL 4

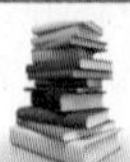

DEFINITIONS AND BACKGROUND

UC is a chronic inflammatory disease of the mucosa of the colon. Complications can include arthritis, severe skin rashes, endocarditis, cirrhosis, splenomegaly, and stomatitis. Patients with UC may have histological features such as microscopic inflammation of the ileum, histological gastritis, periappendiceal inflammation, patchiness, and relative rectal sparing at the time of diagnosis (North American Society for Pediatric Gastroenterology, 2007).

UC usually begins in the rectum or sigmoid colon. When UC affects only the rectum, it is called **ulcerative proctitis**. If the disease affects only the left side of the colon, it is called **distal colitis**; and if it permeates the entire colon, it is termed **pancolitis**. The condition is often a relentless, continuous lesion of the colon with some involvement of the terminal ileum. It does not affect full thickness of the intestine and never affects the small intestine. UC may be acute, mild, or chronic. **Indeterminate colitis** may be diagnosed with features of both UC and Crohn's disease; this is called **colitis of uncertain type or etiology** (Geboes et al, 2008).

The pathogenesis is complex and involves environmental, genetic, microbial, and immune factors. Onset of UC is usually between 15 and 35 years of age. There is a second, lesser peak of onset between ages 50 and 70 years. Intestinal microvascular ischemia usually precedes the onset of UC (Ibrahim et al, 2009). Blood in the stool is the most common symptom (Beattie et al, 2006) but children who present with UC may also have growth failure. Remissions occur, and there may be long periods between exacerbations. Flares often involve non-GI symptoms such as arthritis, uveitis, and ankylosing spondylitis. Because increased risk of colon cancer exists for the more extensive disease, patients with UC should be enrolled in a colonoscopy surveillance program after 8–10 years of disease duration (Rufo and Bousvaros, 2006).

Probiotic bacterial mixtures provide relief in mild-to-moderate UC by reducing the number of "bad" bacteria, reducing the amount of inflammation, increasing the mucus layer of the gut, and increasing the number of anti-inflammatory molecules in the intestine (Bibiolni et al, 2005). Researchers are looking at genetically altering *Bacteroides ovatus*, naturally in the gut, to secrete human growth factor KGF-2 protein when exposed to xylan sugar (Hamady et al, 2008). This may help to heal the damage caused by inflammation.

Both nutritional deficiencies and nutritional excesses impair GI responses and alter susceptibility to inflammation and other diseases. Enhancement of micronutrient nutrition is an important determinant of immunity and treatment of side effects in UC (Scrimgeour and Condlin, 2009).

Approximately 15% of patients with UC will develop a severe exacerbation requiring hospitalization (Doherty and Cheifiz, 2009). If medical management fails, surgical colectomy to remove the colon and rectum is curative. The ileocecal valve should be preserved where possible. Colectomy with creation of an ileal pouch anal anastomosis (J pouch) is standard for patients with severe or refractory colitis, resulting in an improved quality of life in most patients (Rufo and Bousvaros, 2006).

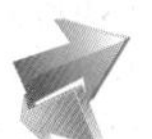

ASSESSMENT, MONITORING, AND EVALUATION

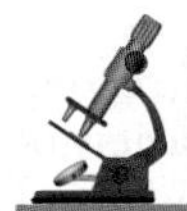

CLINICAL INDICATORS

Genetic Markers: IBD is associated with inheritance of several specific SNPs and gene variants that disrupt bacterial homeostasis mechanisms (Ferguson et al, 2007) and promote venous thrombosis (Bernstein et al, 2006). The ECM1 gene is found in UC (Jung and Hugit, 2009). Methionine synthase and MTHFR C677 T are also associated with extent of UC (Chen et al, 2008). Microflora in the intestinal lumen and an impaired innate immune system provoke a T helper 2 response, resulting in pro-inflammatory cytokines and interleukins (Festen et al, 2009). The IL-12-related cytokine, designated IL-23, establishes chronic inflammation and in the development of a Th cell subset producing IL-17, designated Th17 (Boniface et al, 2008; Shih and Targan, 2008).

Clinical/History		
Height	Temperature	Pus or mucus discharged between stools
Weight	Stool sample	Anemia, fatigue
BMI	Bloody or explosive diarrhea	Anorexia
Diet history	Crampy abdominal pain	

Biopsy
Sigmoidoscopy
Colonoscopy
Capsule endoscopy to rule out Crohn's

Lab Work

CRP
ESR
Perinuclear anti-neutrophilic cytoplasmic antibody (pANCA)
Anti-Saccharomyces cerevisiae antibody (ASCA)
Bilirubin
Chol, Trig
Na^+, K^+, Cl
BUN, Creat
Alb, RBP
Ca^{++}, Mg^{++}
Serum phosphorus, Alk phos
PT or INR
Transferrin, TIBC
N balance
Serum tHcy
Serum folate
Serum B_{12} and Schilling test
Genetic testing for ECM1 and MTHFR
H & H
Serum Fe, ferritin
Gluc
Complete blood count (CBC), ESR
WBC
Hydrogen breath test
Fecal fat study

INTERVENTION

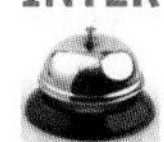

OBJECTIVES

- In acute stages, allow the bowel to heal and use products that include short-chain fatty acids and glutamine to prevent a decline in nutritional status. Correct fluid and electrolyte imbalance.
- Develop an optimal regimen of pharmacologic therapies, nutritional management, psychologic support, and properly timed surgery (when necessary) to maintain disease remission, minimize disease and drug-induced adverse effects, and optimize growth and development (Rufo and Bousvaros, 2006).

SAMPLE NUTRITION CARE PROCESS STEPS

Inadequate Nutrient Intake

Assessment Data: BMI 19, recent weight loss of 10 lb in 3 months, abdominal pain and bloody diarrhea at least once daily for 2 weeks. Diet hx reveals intolerance for high fiber fruits and vegetables and poor intake of protein-rich foods.

Nutrition Diagnoses (PES): Inadequate nutrient intake related to GI discomfort and maldigestion as evidenced by weight loss 10 lb in 3 months, intolerance of fruits and vegetables, poor intake of protein-rich foods.

Interventions: Food and nutrient delivery—change diet to low residue during flare. Educate about the role of diet in reducing inflammation; add omega-3 fatty acids and a multivitamin-mineral supplement once daily. Counsel about fiber-rich foods and when to avoid them (such as during times of GI distress). Discuss use of frequent small meals and intake of fruit and vegetable juices. Provide tips for adding protein and kilocals into the diet to regain lost weight. Discuss the option of using probiotic food sources.

Monitoring and Evaluation: Weight status; diet hx revealing improved intake from all food groups; fewer incidents of GI distress with use of the low residue diet, omega-3 fatty acid supplements, and appropriate medicines.

- Replenish depleted stores and correct poor nutritional status. Poor nutritional status may be related to decreased intake from anorexia, nausea or vomiting, abdominal pain, restrictive diets, side effects of medications, protein losses from ulcerated mucosal lesions, blood loss or wound-healing requirements, bacterial overgrowth, or malabsorption.
- Avoid further irritation of the bowel by managing fiber intake. Large fecal volume distends the bowel and could create obstruction. Correct for diarrhea, steatorrhea, obstruction, and related anemias.
- Provide sufficient dietary antioxidants and omega-3 fatty acids, which play a role in inflammatory processes. UC patients may be able to reduce steroid doses and achieve good symptom control by drinking a nutritionally balanced cocktail of fish oil, soluble fiber, and antioxidants daily.
- Prolonged use of corticosteroids, calcium and vitamin D deficiency, and a low BMI are some of the possible contributing factors to bone disease. Replenish as needed.
- Production of tHcy within the intestinal mucosa may contribute to the inflammatory response and endothelial cell dysfunction; treat folate and vitamin B_{12} deprivation as well as MTHFR polymorphisms, history of intestinal resection, or treatment with methotrexate (Peyrin-Biroulet et al, 2007). Prevent thrombotic events.

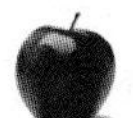

FOOD AND NUTRITION

- For adult energy requirements, estimate needs according to current BMI. A low BMI (<15) may require 35–45 kcal/kg; a BMI of 15–19 may require 30–35 kcal/kg; a BMI of 20–29 may require 25–30 kcal/kg; and a high BMI (>30) may only require 15–25 kcal/kg.
- Estimate needs at the high end of normal for growth and tissue repair in infants or children.
- To treat the condition in its acute state, a low-fiber diet is needed to minimize fecal volume. A nutritional supplement that contains fish oil, soluble fiber, and antioxidants reduces reliance on traditional therapies and lessens the need to start on corticosteroid therapy (Seidner et al, 2005).
- Persons with this condition often have lactose, wheat, or gluten intolerance. Alter diet accordingly.
- Dietary changes that have been suggested include use of less red meat, dairy products, artificial sweeteners, and caffeine. Controlled trials are needed to confirm efficacy of these changes.
- Diet should limit nuts, seeds, legumes, and coarse whole grains during a flare. Fresh fruits and vegetables may not be tolerated if they are highly fibrous; monitor carefully. A low-residue diet is useful during exacerbations.
- CPN is useful when needed, often for 2 weeks or longer during acute stages. CPN may be needed in long term if there is short-gut syndrome.
- As the patient progresses, a high-protein diet (1–1.5 g/kg) with high energy intake, given in six small feedings, is recommended. Protein may have to be restricted in patients with renal disease.
- Vitamin–mineral supplementation may be needed. Supplement the diet with multivitamins and minerals,

especially zinc, thiamin, folic acid, vitamin B_{12}, vitamin E, vitamin D, calcium, magnesium, and iron. Vitamins A and K can be given every other day. With resection greater than 200 cm, selenium may become deficient; monitor carefully.

- MCTs may be helpful. Use omega-3 fatty acid sources, such as salmon, mackerel, and tuna; supplements also may be beneficial.
- **After colectomy with ileostomy:** IV feeding should continue for 1–2 days. Diet should progress slowly to a low-fiber, high-protein regimen with high energy, vitamins, and minerals (especially sodium and potassium). The patient will need vitamin B_{12} injections and adequate fluid. CPN may be needed if progress is slow. Once liberalized, foods are added one at a time. Avoid gas-forming foods that may cause increased peristalsis; products to reduce flatulence may be helpful.

Common Drugs Used and Potential Side Effects

- The principal medical therapies used to induce disease remission in patients with UC are aminosalicylates for mild disease, corticosteroids for moderate disease, and cyclosporine for severe disease (Rufo and Bousvaros, 2006). Maintenance therapies that are used to prevent disease relapse include aminosalicylates, mercaptopurine, and azathioprine (Rufo and Bousvaros, 2006).
- Aminosalicylates (mesalamine, olsalazine, and sulfasalazine) contain 5-aminosalicylic acid (5-ASA) and reduce inflammation. Extra fluid intake is needed to avoid renal stone formation. anorexia, nausea, vomiting, and GI distress may occur. Folic acid supplements also may be required.
- Antibiotics such as metronidazole and ciprofloxacin reduce intestinal bacteria and directly suppress the intestine's immune system. They should be used with probiotics such as yogurt containing live and active cultures.
- Corticosteroids (prednisone, methylprednisolone, and budesonide) are used for patients with moderate-to-severe disease to reduce inflammation also. Although steroids can be quite effective for short-term control of acute episodes of colitis (flare-ups), they are not recommended for long-term use due to side effects. Negative nitrogen and calcium balances may result. Monitor the need for extra vitamins and minerals.
- Immunomodulatory medicines including azathioprine, 6-mercaptopurine (6-MP), 6-thioguanine (6-TG), and cyclosporine alter the immune cell interaction with the inflammatory process. They are used for patients when aminosalicylates and corticosteroids have been ineffective. Azathioprine and 6-MP may be useful in reducing dependence on corticosteroids and in maintaining remission in some patients. These medications take several months before their beneficial effects begin to work.
- Psyllium laxatives (Metamucil) can help with constipation and diarrhea. Long term use alters electrolytes. Flatulence or steatorrhea may occur.
- TNF-neutralizing agent infliximab (Remicade) appears to be an effective option for patients with UC that are not responding to conventional treatment.
- Therapies under investigation include tacrolimus and novel biologic drugs. However, there is the challenge of addressing potential safety issues, while more traditional drugs should be further developed to facilitate patient compliance (Pastroelli et al, 2009). The delivery system and frequency of medication administration should be resolved (Tindall, 2009).

Herbs, Botanicals, and Supplements

- Probiotics may be beneficial. Inulin and oligofructose have been suggested to increase the number of natural intestinal flora.
- Use of complementary medicine is common in this population (Langhorst et al, 2005). Further study is needed to evaluate whether glutathione or coenzyme Q10 affects prevention or treatment of IBD.
- Herbs and botanical supplements should not be used without discussing with the physician. Onion, cat's claw, boswellia, honeysuckle, peppermint, valerian, and tea have been recommended for this condition, but no clinical trials have proven efficacy.
- Omega-3 fatty acids may help to reduce symptoms of UC. ALA works better at decreasing bowel inflammation than EPA and DHA. Fish oil supplements may cause flatulence and diarrhea.

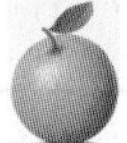

NUTRITION EDUCATION, COUNSELING, CARE MANAGEMENT

- Ensure that the patient avoids foods that are known to cause diarrhea. Avoid extremes in food or beverage temperatures.
- Pleasant mealtimes are an important part of treatment. Frequent, small meals may increase the total nutritional intake. Discontinue eating 2–3 hours before bedtime.
- Avoid iced or carbonated beverages, which may stimulate peristalsis in times of discomfort.
- Instruct the patient to eat slowly and chew foods well. Discuss fears related to eating.
- Frequent counseling by a dietitian may be helpful.
- It has been noted that women with IBD tend to be childless or have fewer children. However, fears should be discussed, as adverse reproductive problems are not common (Mountifield et al, 2009).

Patient Education—Foodborne Illness

- Careful food handling and hand washing are important to prevent introduction of foodborne pathogens to this individual who may be experiencing diarrhea and related discomfort.
- Avoid excessive use of hand sanitizers, as a healthy gut contains some bacteria.
- If home TF is needed, teach appropriate sanitation and food-handling procedures.

For More Information

- Crohn's and Colitis Foundation of America
http://www.ccfa.org/research/info/aboutcd
http://www.ccfa.org/info/diet?LMI=4.2

- FACSR
  http://www.fascrs.org/patients/conditions/ulcerative_colitis/
- National Institute of Diabetes and Digestive and Kidney Diseases (NIDDK)
  http://digestive.niddk.nih.gov/ddiseases/pubs/colitis/index.htm
- National Institutes of Health—Ulcerative Colitis
  http://www.nlm.nih.gov/medlineplus/ulcerativecolitis.html

ULCERATIVE COLITIS—CITED REFERENCES

Beattie RM, et al. Inflammatory bowel disease. *Arch Dis Child.* 91:426, 2006.

Bernstein CN, et al. Mutations in clotting factors and inflammatory bowel disease. *Am J Gastroenterol.* 102:338, 2006.

Bibiolni R, et al. VSL#3 probiotic-mixture induces remission in patients with active ulcerative colitis. *Am J Gastroenterol.* 100:1539, 2005.

Boniface K, et al. From interleukin-23 to T-helper 17 cells: human T-helper cell differentiation revisited. *Immunol Rev.* 226:132, 2008.

Chen M, et al. Methionine synthase A2756G polymorphism may predict ulcerative colitis and methylenetetrahydrofolate reductase C677 T pancolitis, in Central China. *BMC Med Genet.* 9:78, 2008.

Doherty GA, Cheifiz AZ. Management of acute severe ulcerative colitis. *Expert Rev Gastroenterol Hepatol.* 3:395, 2009.

Ferguson LR, et al. Nutrigenomics and gut health. *Mutat Res.* 622:1, 2007.

Festen EA, et al. Inflammatory bowel disease and celiac disease: overlaps in the pathology and genetics, and their potential drug targets. *Endocr Metab Immune Disord Drug Targets.* 9:199, 2009.

Geboes K, et al. Indeterminate colitis: a review of the concept—what's in a name? *Inflamm Bowel Dis.* 14:850, 2008.

Hamady ZZ, et al. Identification and use of the putative Bacteroides ovatus xylanase promoter for the inducible production of recombinant human proteins. *Microbiology.* 154:3165, 2008.

Ibrahim CB, et al. On the role of ischemia in the pathogenesis of IBD: A review [published online ahead of print 14 August 2009]. *Inflamm Bowel Dis.* 16:696, 2009.

Jung C, Hugit JP. Inflammatory Bowel Diseases: the genetic revolution. *Gastroenterol Clin Biol.* 33:123S, 2009.

Langhorst J, et al. Amount of systemic steroid medication is a strong predictor for the use of complementary and alternative medicine in patients with inflammatory bowel disease: results from a German national survey. *Inflamm Bowel Dis.* 11:287, 2005.

Mountifield R, et al. Fear and fertility in inflammatory bowel disease: a mismatch of perception and reality affects family planning decisions. *Inflamm Bowel Dis.* 15:720, 2009.

North American Society for Pediatric Gastroenterology. Differentiating ulcerative colitis from Crohn disease in children and young adults: report of a working group of the North American Society for Pediatric Gastroenterology, Hepatology, and Nutrition and the Crohn's and Colitis Foundation of America. *J Pediatr Gastroenterol Nutr.* 44:563, 2007.

Pastorelli L, et al. Emerging drugs for the treatment of ulcerative colitis [published online ahead of print 5 August 2009]. *Expert Opin Emerg Drugs.* 14:505, 2009.

Peyrin-Biroulet L, et al. Vascular and cellular stress in inflammatory bowel disease: revisiting the role of homocysteine. *Am J Gastroenterol.* 102:1108, 2007.

Rufo PA, Bousvaros A. Current therapy of inflammatory bowel disease in children. *Pediatr Drugs.* 8:279, 2006.

Scrimgeour AG, Condlin ML. Zinc and micronutrient combinations to combat gastrointestinal inflammation [published online ahead of print 13 August 2009]. *Curr Opin Clin Nutr Metab Care.* 12:653, 2009.

Seidner DL, et al. An oral supplement enriched with fish oil, soluble fiber, and antioxidants for corticosteroid sparing in ulcerative colitis: a randomized, controlled trial. *Clin Gastroenterol Hepatol.* 3:358, 2005.

Shih DQ, Targan SR. Immunopathogenesis of inflammatory bowel disease. *World J Gastroenterol.* 14:390, 2008.

Tindall WH. New approaches to adherence issues when dosing oral aminosalicylates in ulcerative colitis. *Am J Health Syst Pharm.* 66:451, 2009.

INTESTINAL FISTULA

NUTRITIONAL ACUITY RANKING: LEVEL 4

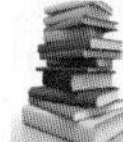

DEFINITIONS AND BACKGROUND

An intestinal fistula is an unwanted pathway from intestines to other organs (e.g., the bladder). External fistulas are between the small intestine and the outside (e.g., skin). Internal fistulas are between two internal organs. Most fistulas occur secondary to abdominal surgery, and a high proportion occurs in association with IBD, intestinal cancer, or trauma. In patients with a suspected fistula, CT followed by a colonoscopy helps to rule out malignancy.

Nutrition support may support spontaneous fistula closure. If spontaneous (nonoperative) closure does not occur in 5–6 weeks, it is unlikely to occur and an operation will be required (Osborn and Fischer, 2009).

GI cutaneous fistulas are among the more complex surgical conditions, with mortalities between 6% and 20%, and even up to 40% (Osborn and Fischer, 2009). Substantial morbidity is related to large fluid and electrolyte losses and metabolic disturbances; mortality is most often related to sepsis and malnutrition (Slater, 2009). Hypertriglyceridemia (266 mg/dL) is commonly observed with enterocutaneous fistulas; it is associated with sepsis, a high output small bowel fistula, nutrition by the parenteral route, and primary diseases with inflammatory etiology (Visschers et al, 2009).

Laparoscopic surgery may be a safe and effective procedure (Laurent et al, 2005), but surgery is performed only after 4–6 months of medical therapy. Fistuloclysis is a procedure in which nutrition is provided via an enteral feeding tube placed directly into the distal lumen of a high output fistula (Slater, 2009). The primary determinant of mortality after enterocutaneous fistula (ECF) repair is a failed operation leading to recurrence of the fistula, especially with IBD, fistula located in the small intestine, an interval of 36 weeks or longer between diagnosis and operation, and resection with stapled anastomosis (Brenner et al, 2009).

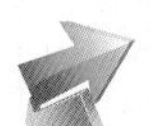

ASSESSMENT, MONITORING, AND EVALUATION

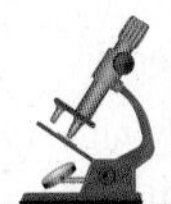

CLINICAL INDICATORS

Genetic Markers: A fistula is acquired in most cases.

Clinical/History		
Height	BMI	I & O
Weight	Diet history	Pain, tenderness
Weight loss	Temperature (Fever?)	Malaise
		CT scan

Fistulagram	Serum Fe, ferritin	RBP
Colonoscopy	Serum folate	BUN, Creat
Endosonography	N balance	Na^+, K^+, Cl^-
Lab Work	Alb, transthyretin	Transferrin
H & H		Ca^{++}, Mg^{++}

INTERVENTION

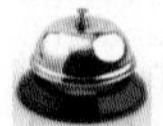

OBJECTIVES

- Promote rest and healing, minimize drainage from fistula, and prevent organ failure from sepsis.
- Monitor the type of dietary regimen according to the location of the fistula and surgical or medical treatment. Adjunctive steps following the operation usually include a gastrostomy and a catheter jejunostomy (Osborn and Fischer, 2009).
- Replace fluid and electrolyte imbalances.
- Decrease malnutrition and infections through aggressive nutritional support. Promote positive nitrogen balance. Additional surgery may be needed to drain infection.

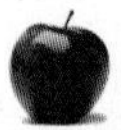

FOOD AND NUTRITION

- A jejunostomy may help a duodenal fistula. A higher protein intake than usual may be needed. Use of an elemental formula diet also may be beneficial for an extended period of time to support GI tract recovery.
- Use CPN for jejunal fistulas. Monitor closely for hypertriglyceridemia.
- Progress to a low-residue, soft or normal diet as tolerated.

SAMPLE NUTRITION CARE PROCESS STEPS

Excessive Parenteral Nutrition

Assessment Data: High output small bowel fistula, elevated triglycerides (>300 mg/dL), CPN for 10 days, 15 lb weight loss from Crohn's disease and poor intake over past year. BMI 19.

Nutrition Diagnoses (PES): Excessive intake from PN related to attempt to resolve high output small bowel fistula with CPN as evidenced by elevated triglycerides and use of CPN exceeding needs for 10 days.

Interventions: Calculation of current needs for protein, kilocals, and lipids to lower TG level without compromising fistula repair.

Monitoring and Evaluation: Weights, lab values (especially glucose and TG), gradual healing of fistula over 4–6 weeks without surgery, BMI improving slowly.

Common Drugs Used and Potential Side Effects

- Antibiotics commonly are used. Metronidazole and ciprofloxacin are useful.
- Infliximab has been used with some success for healing fistulas in IBD.
- Octreotide (somatostatin analog) inhibits endocrine/exocrine secretions and excessive GI motility. It is only used parenterally and can cause nausea, vomiting, abdominal pain, diarrhea, or flatulence.

Herbs, Botanicals, and Supplements

- Herbs and botanical supplements should not be used without discussing with the physician.
- Probiotic and prebiotic therapy may be useful.

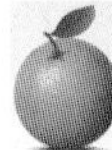

NUTRITION EDUCATION, COUNSELING, CARE MANAGEMENT

- Defined formula diets can help support spontaneous closure in approximately 4–6 weeks. If closure has not occurred, surgery is aided by better nutritional status.
- Instruct the patient regarding the fiber content of foods. Discuss how much to include during periods of flare-up and how to gradually increase fiber to achieve the goal set individually for that person.

Patient Education—Foodborne Illness

- Careful food handling and hand washing are important to prevent introduction of foodborne pathogens to this individual.
- If home TF is needed, teach appropriate sanitation and food-handling procedures.

For More Information

- American Society of Colon and Rectal Surgeons http://www.fascrs.org/patients/conditions/anal_abscess_fistula/
- Anal fissure http://www.gicare.com/diseases/Anal-fissure.aspx
- Fistula http://www.nlm.nih.gov/medlineplus/ency/article/002365.htm

INTESTINAL FISTULA—CITED REFERENCES

Brenner M, et al. Risk factors for recurrence after repair of enterocutaneous fistula. *Arch Surg.* 144:500, 2009.

Laurent SR, et al. Laparoscopic sigmoidectomy for fistulized diverticulitis. *Dis Colon Rectum.* 48:148, 2005.

Osborn C, Fischer JE. How I Do It: Gastrointestinal Cutaneous Fistulas [published online ahead of print 9 June 2009]. *J Gastrointest Surg.* 13:2068, 2009.

Slater R. Nutritional management of enterocutaneous fistulas. *Br J Nurs.* 18:225, 2009.

Visschers RG, et al. Development of hypertriglyceridemia in patients with enterocutaneous fistulas. *Clin Nutr.* 28:313, 2009.

INTESTINAL LYMPHANGIECTASIA

NUTRITIONAL ACUITY RANKING: LEVEL 3

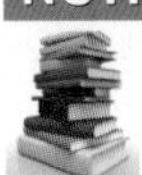

DEFINITIONS AND BACKGROUND

Intestinal lymphangiectasia (IL) is a rare protein-losing enteropathy (PLE). It occurs most often in children, with 11 years as the average age of onset. IL can also occur secondary to conditions such as Crohn's disease, scleroderma, sclerosing mesenteritis, CD, lupus, lymphenteric fistula, constrictive pericarditis, or pancreatitis. IL is potentially fatal if not recognized and properly treated (McDonald and Bears, 2009). Increased intestinal lymphatic pressure with vessel dilatation occurs, discharging fluid into the bowel lumen. The fluid is then digested by intestinal enzymes and is reabsorbed. Massive fluid retention occurs from obstructed lymph vessels, especially in the abdomen and pleural cavities. While malabsorption and PLE occur, only marginal loss of protein occurs in most cases.

The main clinical features of this disorder include edema, fat malabsorption, lymphopenia, and hypoalbuminemia. Nausea, vomiting, nonbloody diarrhea, and abdominal pain result. Long-range problems may include lymphoma, osteomalacia or osteoporosis.

A low-fat diet associated with MCT supplementation is the cornerstone of medical management (Vignes and Bellanger, 2008). The need for dietary control appears to be permanent, because clinical and biochemical findings re-appear after low-fat diet withdrawal (Vignes and Bellanger, 2008).

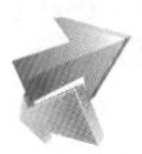

ASSESSMENT, MONITORING, AND EVALUATION

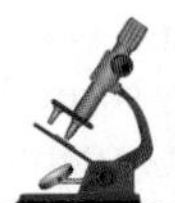

CLINICAL INDICATORS

Genetic Markers: Primary intestinal lymphangiectasia (PIL) is a rare disorder, generally diagnosed before 3 years of age; is it also called Waldman's disease (Vignes and Bellanger, 2008). Three genes, FLT4 (VEGFR3), FOXC2, and SOX18, cause varying forms of primary lymphedema (Finegold et al, 2008).

Clinical/History
Height
Weight
BMI
Weight loss, inability to gain weight
Stunting?
Diet history
Fatigue
Abdominal pain
Steatorrhea
Peripheral edema
Diarrhea
Chylous ascites?
Double-contrast radiographs of the small bowel
Ultrasound or CT scans
Jejunal biopsy

Lab Work
Fecal concentration of alpha-1 antitrypsin (>56 cc/d with diarrhea)
Jejunal biopsy (dilated lymphatic lacteal vessels)
Alb (decreased)
Transthyretin
Serum 25-OH-vitamin D and fat-soluble vitamins (low?)
Trace metal deficiency
Chol (normal or low)
Trig
Na^+, K^+
H & H
Serum Fe, ferritin
Transferrin (decreased)
TLC (Lymphocytopenia)
Hypogammaglobulinemia
Gluc
Ca^{++} (low)
Mg^{++}
BUN, Creat

INTERVENTION

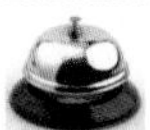

OBJECTIVES

- Identify and correct the underlying cause (e.g., constrictive pericarditis).
- Decrease symptoms and promote recovery. Minimize peripheral edema.
- Decrease intake of long-chain fatty acids because they form chylomicrons and stimulate lymphatic flow into the gut. Use MCTs because they are more water-soluble and can be absorbed through the portal vein instead of the lymphatic system.
- Meet all nutritional needs for age and sex. Monitor absorption of fat-soluble vitamins; ensure adequacy from dietary or supplemental sources.

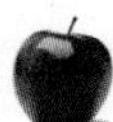

FOOD AND NUTRITION

- Reduce intake of long-chain fatty acids. A formula or low-fat diet using a high concentration of MCTs is useful.
- Adequate protein and calories are needed, according to the individual's needs.
- Fat-soluble vitamins may be required in water-miscible form for adequate absorption.
- A calcium supplement may also be needed.

SAMPLE NUTRITION CARE PROCESS STEPS

Inappropriate Intake of Types of Fats

Assessment Data: Peripheral edema, weight loss, diarrhea, fecal alpha-1 antitrypsin >60 cc/d, low albumin (3.0 g/dL)

Nutrition Diagnoses (PES): Inappropriate intake of fatty acids (long-chain) related to intolerance of long-chain fatty acids and IL as evidenced by diarrhea, weight loss, altered labs (albumin, alpha-1 antitrypsin).

Interventions: Food-Nutrient Delivery—reduce intake of long-chain fatty acids and use MCTs instead. Education—teach diet principles. Counseling about the diet for managing the life-long condition.

Monitoring and Evaluation: Improvements in edema, lab values, and diarrhea after following the diet and taking appropriate medication.

Common Drugs Used and Potential Side Effects

- Octreotide (Sandostatin) may be used. It is a potent inhibitor of growth hormone, glucagons, and insulin; it also suppresses gastrin, motilin, secretin, and pancreatic polypeptide.
- Over-the-counter remedies (bulking agents, drugs to control diarrhea) may be useful.

Herbs, Botanicals, and Supplements

- Herbs and botanical supplements should not be used without discussing with the physician.
- Supplements of vitamins and calcium are generally prescribed.

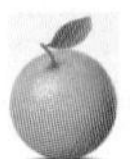

NUTRITION EDUCATION, COUNSELING, CARE MANAGEMENT

- Discuss the role of fat in digestion, along with the need for MCT oils in the daily diet.
- Discuss fat-soluble vitamins and their sources in the diet.
- To minimize peripheral edema, elevation of extremities above the head may be recommended to decrease cellulitis and lymphangitis. In addition, use of a recliner or elastic support stockings is suggested.
- It is not helpful to reduce salt intake or to use diuretics in this condition.

Patient Education—Foodborne Illness

- If home TF is needed, teach appropriate sanitation and food-handling procedures.

For More Information

- Intestinal Lymphangiectasia
  http://www.emedicine.com/med/topic1178.htm
- Medscape
  http://emedicine.medscape.com/article/1086917-overview
- Merck Manual
  http://www.merck.com/mmhe/sec09/ch125/ch125f.html

INTESTINAL LYMPHANGIECTASIA—CITED REFERENCES

Finegold DN, et al. HGF and MET mutations in primary and secondary lymphedema. *Lymphat Res Biol.* 6:65, 2008.

McDonald KQ, Bears CM. A preterm infant with intestinal lymphangiectasia: a diagnostic dilemma. *Neonatal Netw.* 28:29, 2009.

Vignes S, Bellanger J. Primary intestinal lymphangiectasia (Waldmann's disease). *Orphanet J Rare Dis.* 3:5, 2008.

INTESTINAL TRANSPLANTATION

NUTRITIONAL ACUITY RANKING: LEVEL 4

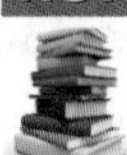

DEFINITIONS AND BACKGROUND

Intestinal transplantation (ITx) represents a difficult lifesaving intervention reserved for patients with irreversible intestinal failure (Varga et al, 2009). Intestinal failure leads to the inability to maintain protein energy, fluid, electrolyte, or micronutrient balance due to GI disease when on a normal diet. Transplantation is an effective therapy for the treatment of patients with end-stage intestine failure who cannot tolerate PN (Grant et al, 2005). The procedure should be considered before the development of PN failure (Matarese et al, 2007). PN-associated liver disease, recurrent catheter-related sepsis, and threatened loss of central venous access are the major reasons for transplantation. SBS, cancers, radiation enteritis, trauma, Crohn's disease, or other major intestinal diseases may also warrant ITx.

Transplantation of the small bowel restores quality of life for recipients who have functioning grafts. ITxs should be considered early in intestinal failure patients who develop liver injury to prevent irreversible liver disease that would mandate a simultaneous liver transplantation (Fryer, 2005). Medicare pays for ITx in patients who fail PN therapy in specific cases. Living-related donor transplantation is an option if a potential donor is available. The donor should have no history of liver disease or major intestinal pathology.

The carbohydrate and amino acid absorptive capacity of the transplanted intestine normalize within the first several months whereas fat absorption is impaired for several months. Morbidity and mortality following ITx are greater than that following liver or kidney transplantation, but long-term survival is improving. Infectious enteritis can occur in recipients after ITx; viral agents are the cause in most cases (Ziring et al, 2005). With newer immune-suppressive protocols, 1-year graft and patient survival rates have improved. Surgery and high-dose immunosuppression must be managed. Radiation to the small bowel before transplanting the organ, then administration of donor's bone marrow stem cells may reduce organ rejection. A loop ileostomy is often created for future endoscopy. Patients with ITx will require regular expert follow-up care and careful attention.

A serious complication of ITx is jejunal graft (JG) damage (Varga et al, 2009). Induction therapy, combined with advancements on surgical technique and clinical management, has improved patient and graft survival (Vianna and Mangus, 2009). An organized multidisciplinary approach is recommended for long-term follow-up.

Early and progressive enteral feeding using a complex polymeric formula is safe and effective after successful transplantation, eventually followed by unrestricted oral diet (Matarese et al, 2007). This modality of treatment is an alternative to PN, especially for those patients who have a poor quality of life as a result of PN (Middleton, 2007).

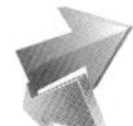

ASSESSMENT, MONITORING, AND EVALUATION

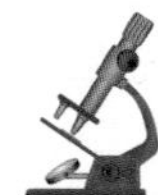

CLINICAL INDICATORS

Genetic Markers: Transplantation is a surgical procedure for a variety of conditions, some of which may be genetic.

Clinical/History

Height
Dry weight, present weight
BMI
Diet history
BP
I & O
Temperature
Wireless capsule endoscopy (CE)
Colonoscopy
CT scan to monitor for fistula or obstruction
Doppler ultrasonography
Liver biopsy

Lab Work

Alb, transthyretin
CRP
CBC count
Coagulation profile
Human leukocyte antigen (HLA) status
Ca^{++}, Mg^{++}
Na^+, K^+
H & H
Serum Fe, ferritin
Serum folacin
BUN, Creat
Glomerular filtration rate (GFR)
WBC, TLC
Gluc
Chol, Trig
N balance
Alk phos, phosphorus
AST, ALT
Bilirubin
Serum pH and lactate

INTERVENTION

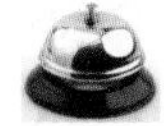

OBJECTIVES

- Timely nutrition assessment and intervention may improve outcomes. Recovery of normal motility and absorptive capacity are the goals after surgery.
- Prevent infection and promote wound healing.
- Replenish lost nutrient stores as malnutrition compromises posttransplantation survival.
- Meet metabolic demands and support recovery.
- Control complications. Diarrhea and high stomal output are common problems and can lead to nutrient deficits, especially electrolytes.
- Supplement enteral feedings with MCTs for several months posttransplantation.
- Supplement the diet with IV fats and fat-soluble vitamins (vitamin D, E, A, and K) until the intestinal lymphatics are reestablished.

SAMPLE NUTRITION CARE PROCESS STEPS

Altered GI Function

Assessment Data: Recent ITx following failure to tolerate PN; hx Crohn's disease; unintentional weight loss over past year.

Nutrition Diagnoses (PES): Altered GI function related to intestinal surgery as evidenced by intolerance of oral, enteral and PN with poor nutrition quality of life.

Interventions: Food and nutrient delivery—clear liquids, progressing slowly to enteral feedings that contain MCT. Progress gradually to oral diet. Educate about the transition period from enteral to oral diet. Counsel about potential problems, such as diarrhea, electrolyte depletion, vitamin and mineral deficiencies; teach about products or medications that may be needed.

Monitoring and Evaluation: Tolerance of enteral feedings post surgery. Resolution of diarrhea, high stomal output, abnormal labs. Achievement of desirable body weight range.

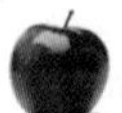

FOOD AND NUTRITION

- When GI function is re-established, as indicated by decreasing G-tube returns and increasing gas and enteric contents in the ileostomy, a diet can be initiated. Advance as tolerated to provide full nutritional support. Monitor fluid status and adjust as needed.
- Daily intake of protein should be appropriate for age and sex; 1.5 g/kg while on steroids may be recommended. Calories should be calculated as 30–35 kcal/kg.
- Control CHO intake and encourage use of whole grains, vegetables, and fruits in cases of hyperglycemia.
- To avoid the development of chylous ascites, a no-fat or low-fat diet can be initially used. Gradually increase fat intake to 25–30% of total kilocal.
- Daily intake of sodium should be 2–4 g until the drug regimen is reduced. Adjust potassium levels as needed.
- Daily intake of calcium should be 1–1.5 times the DRI levels to offset poor absorption. Children especially need adequate calcium for growth. Daily intake of phosphorus should be equal to calcium intake.
- Supplement diet with vitamin D, magnesium, and thiamin if needed.
- Reduce gastric irritants as necessary if GI distress or reflux occurs.
- The special diet may be discontinued when drug therapy is reduced to maintenance levels. Encourage exercise and a weight control plan thereafter.

Common Drugs Used and Potential Side Effects

- See Table 7-18.

Herbs, Botanicals, and Supplements

- Herbs and botanical supplements should not be used without discussing with the physician.
- Grapefruit juice decreases drug metabolism in the gut (via P-450–CYP3A4 inhibition). One glass can affect medications up to 24 hours later. Avoid taking with cyclosporine and tacrolimus.

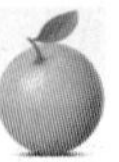

NUTRITION EDUCATION, COUNSELING, CARE MANAGEMENT

- Indicate which foods are sources of protein, calcium, and other key nutrients in the diet.

TABLE 7-18 Medications Used after Intestinal Transplantation

Education	Description
Antibiotics	Broad-spectrum intravenous antibiotics are administered for about 1 week after the transplant.
Antiviral prophylaxis	Ganciclovir and/or cytomegalovirus (CMV) immunoglobulin (CytoGam) may be used.
Corticosteroids (prednisone or Solu-Cortef)	Corticosteroids such as prednisone and Solu-Cortef are used for immunosuppression. Side effects include increased catabolism of proteins, negative nitrogen balance, hyperphagia, ulcers, decreased glucose tolerance, sodium retention, fluid retention, and impaired calcium absorption and osteoporosis. Cushing's syndrome, obesity, muscle wasting, and increased gastric secretion may result. A higher protein intake and lower intake of simple CHOs may be needed.
Cyclosporine	Cyclosporine does not retain sodium as much as corticosteroids do. Intravenous doses are more effective than oral doses. Nausea, vomiting, and diarrhea are common side effects. Hyperlipidemia, hypertension, and hyperkalemia may also occur; decrease sodium and potassium as necessary. Elevated glucose and lipids may occur. The drug is also nephrotoxic; a controlled renal diet may be beneficial. Taking omega-3 fatty acids during cyclosporine therapy may reduce the toxic side effects (such as high blood pressure and kidney damage) associated with this medication in transplantation patients.
Immunosuppressants	Immunosuppressants such as muromonab (Orthoclone OKT3) and antithymocyte globulin (ATG) are less nephrotoxic than cyclosporine but can cause nausea, anorexia, diarrhea, and vomiting. Monitor carefully. Fever and stomatitis also may occur; alter diet as needed.
Induction Therapy	Monoclonal (alemtuzumab, basiliximab, daclizumab) or polyclonal (Thymoglobulin) antibody preparations are often administered intraoperatively or preoperatively.
Probiotics, Prebiotics	Although research is still preliminary, the use of probiotics and prebiotics may become common practice in the future.
Prostaglandin E_1	Prostaglandin E_1 is given to improve the small bowel microcirculation.
Tacrolimus (Prograf, FK506)	Tacrolimus suppresses T-cell immunity; it is 100 times more potent than cyclosporine, thus requiring smaller doses. Side effects include GI distress, nausea, vomiting, hyperkalemia, and hyperglycemia.

- If the patient does not drink milk or use dairy products, discuss other sources of calcium.
- Alcohol should be avoided unless permitted by the doctor.
- Discuss control of hyperglycemia when appropriate. Discuss long-term problems such as obesity and dyslipidemia.
- Encourage moderation in diet; promote adequate exercise.
- Financial constraints can be a burden. Home care has evolved, but many disciplines are needed to keep everything in order.

Patient Education—Foodborne Illness

- Careful food handling and hand washing are important to prevent introduction of foodborne pathogens to the individual who may be experiencing graft–host rejection.
- Prevent infections from foodborne illness; patients who have undergone transplantation may be prone to increased risk more than other individuals.
- If home TF or CPN is needed, teach appropriate sanitation and food-handling procedures.

For More Information

- Intestinal Transplantation
http://www.emedicine.com/ped/topic2845.htm
- Intestinal Transplant Centers
http://www.intestinaltransplant.org/centres.htm
- Intestinal Transplant Registry
http://www.intestinaltransplant.org/

INTESTINAL TRANSPLANTATION—CITED REFERENCES

Fryer JP. Intestinal transplantation: an update. *Curr Opin Gastroenterol.* 21:162, 2005.

Grant D, et al. 2003 Report of the Intestine Transplant Registry: a new era has dawned. *Ann Surg.* 241:607, 2005.

Matarese LE, et al. Therapeutic efficacy of intestinal and multivisceral transplantation: survival and nutrition outcome. *Nutr Clin Pract.* 22:474, 2007.

Middleton SJ. Is intestinal transplantation now an alternative to home parenteral nutrition? *Proc Nutr Soc.* 66:316, 2007.

Varga J, et al. Development of jejunal graft damage during intestinal transplantation. *Ann Transplant.* 14:62, 2009.

Vianna RM, Mangus RS. Present prospects and future perspectives of intestinal and multivisceral transplantation. *Curr Opin Clin Nutr Metab Care.* 12:281, 2009.

Ziring D, et al. Infectious enteritis after intestinal transplantation: incidence, timing, and outcome. *Transplantation.* 79:702, 2005.

IRRITABLE BOWEL SYNDROME

NUTRITIONAL ACUITY RANKING: LEVEL 3

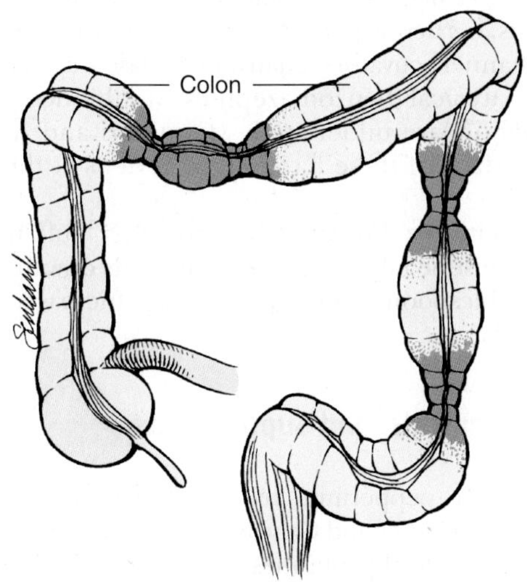

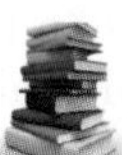

DEFINITIONS AND BACKGROUND

Irritable bowel syndrome (IBS) is a functional GI disorder affecting up to 3–15% of the general population in western countries (Camilleri and Andresen, 2009). The pathophysiology of IBS involves disturbances of the brain–gut axis (Camilleri and Andresen, 2009). Stimulated 5-HT3 receptors promote intestinal motility, secretion, and sensation. Approximately one in ten patients with IBS believe their IBS began with an infectious illness (Spiller and Garsed, 2009). Prospective studies have shown that 3–36% of enteric infections lead to persistent new IBS symptoms; bacterial enteritis, protozoan, and helminth infections are often followed by prolonged postinfective IBS (Spiller and Garsed, 2009). Rome III Diagnostic criteria for IBS include at least 3 months of continuous or recurrent symptoms of abdominal pain or discomfort relieved with defecation or associated with change in frequency of stool or changed consistency of stool. Individuals with IBS often have had a prolonged initial illness, a toxic infecting bacterial strain, history of smoking, mucosal markers of inflammation, female gender, depression and adverse life events in the preceding 3 months (Spiller and Garsed, 2009).

Because 95% of the body's serotonin is located in the GI tract, it is important to note that people with IBS have diminished receptor activity. There are several subgroups of IBS: alternating bowel habits (IBS-A), constipation-predominant IBS (IBS-C), and diarrhea-predominant IBS (IBS-D). Signs that IBS patients require medical attention include anemia, fever, persistent diarrhea, rectal bleeding, weight loss, and nocturnal symptoms. In addition, a family history of IBD, CD, or colorectal cancer requires further diagnostic work-up.

Up to 65% of IBS patients attribute their symptoms to food allergies (Zar et al, 2005). However, this finding has not been confirmed (Brant et al, 2009). Some IBS sufferers may have a mild form of CD and should be tested for gluten intolerance. Others may have lactose maldigestion. A food diary is useful to note symptoms and specific foods or practices that cause problems.

Therapies focus on specific GI dysfunctions (e.g., constipation, diarrhea, pain), and medications should only be used when nonprescription remedies do not work or when symptoms are severe. In some IBS patients, there is *H. pylori* infection; appropriate antibiotics may relieve symptoms. Therapies focus on nerve–gut communication dysfunction and antibiotics. Probiotics are another important therapy. Symptoms may also be improved by diets supplemented with probiotics such as hydrolyzed guar gum (Hadley and Gaardner, 2005) or bifidobacteria. Where carbohydrate malabsorption (lactose, fructose, or sorbitol) occurs, restrict the offending sugar(s). Overall, there is a reduction in quality of life (Brant et al, 2009). The American Dietetic Association has recommended three MNT visits for patients who have IBS.

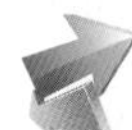

ASSESSMENT, MONITORING, AND EVALUATION

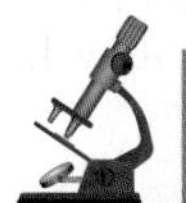

CLINICAL INDICATORS

Genetic Markers: Genetic modeling has identified a genetic link for IBS in twin studies (Lembo et al, 2007). However, the heritable components are poorly understood (Camilleri and Andresen, 2009).

Clinical/History		Lab Work
Height	Change in form of stool	tTG testing to rule out CD
Weight	Belching, flatulence, heartburn	Hydrogen breath test for lactose tolerance
Weight changes	Nausea	CRP
BMI	Mucus in stool?	H & H
Diet history	Polycystic ovarian syndrome?	Serum Fe, ferritin
Family history of GI disorders	Urgency for defecation	Alb, transthyretin
Recurrent abdominal pain or discomfort	Lower GI x-rays	Gluc
Change in frequency of stool	Colonoscopy or sigmoidoscopy	Na^+, K^+
		Ca^{++}, Mg^{++}

INTERVENTION

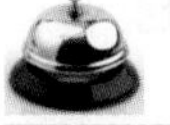

OBJECTIVES

- Encourage regular eating patterns, regular bowel hygiene, adequate rest, and relaxation.

> **SAMPLE NUTRITION CARE PROCESS STEPS**
>
> **Undesirable Food Choices**
>
> ***Assessment:*** Diet history with analysis of fiber, caffeine, fluid, and CHOs; family history and medication/food allergies; bowel patterns.
>
> ***Nutrition Diagnosis (PES):*** Undesirable food choices related to excessive intake of colas and coffee as evidenced by abdominal pain each day, symptoms of IBS-D, and poor nutritional quality of life.
>
> ***Intervention:*** Educate about better fluid choices, probiotics, prebiotics, fiber, reduction in gas-forming foods.
>
> ***Monitoring and Evaluation:*** Dietary and fluid intake changes; changes in abdominal pain, bowel patterns, frequency of diarrhea. Improved enjoyment of meals and a variety of foods and beverages.

- Avoid constipation by increasing physical activity and consuming adequate fluids and fiber (American Dietetic Association, 2008).
- Monitor for food intolerances to gluten in wheat, rye, barley; chocolate; lactose or milk products; caffeine; alcohol. Omit offending agents.
- Individualize diet management to the patient's symptoms. Alleviate pain, symptoms, and flatulence. Production of colonic gas, especially hydrogen, may be uncomfortable.
- Improve nutritional quality of life.

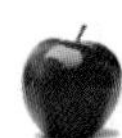

FOOD AND NUTRITION

- Fiber is marginally beneficial; insoluble fiber may worsen symptoms but soluble fiber may help to alleviate constipation (Heizer et al, 2009). In acute phases, a low-fiber diet may be better tolerated. As treatment progresses, use adequate but not excessive fiber and ensure adequate fluid intake (30–35 mL/kg).
- Avoid high-fat foods, which may increase cholecystokinin release. Avoid high sugar intake, which increases osmolarity.
- Liberal amounts of fruits and vegetables are useful. Omit gas-forming oligosaccharides (beans, barley, Brussels sprouts, cabbage, nuts, figs, and soybeans), if not tolerated. Limit or omit spicy foods if poorly tolerated.
- A modified exclusion diet and stepwise reintroduction of foods or trials of eliminating classes of food may be useful (Heizer et al, 2009). Omit milk products if lactose is not tolerated; add calcium in other forms.
- In patients with CD, omit gluten and supplement with B-complex vitamins if needed.

Common Drugs Used and Potential Side Effects

- 5-HT is a key modulator of GI sensorimotor function and this has led to the development of 5-HT(3) antagonists and 5-HT(4) agonists; alosetron (Lotronex), cilansetron, and tegaserod are all effective in the treatment of IBS (Ford et al, 2009). If constipation results, a lower dose may be needed (Krause et al, 2007).
- Antidepressants, novel selective anticholinergics, alpha-adrenergic agonists, opioid agents, cholecystokinin-antagonists, neurokinin-antagonists, somatostatin receptor agonists, corticotropin releasing factor antagonists, chloride channel activators, guanylate cyclase-c agonists, melatonin, atypical benzodiazepines, antibiotics, immune modulators are under study (Camilleri and Andresen, 2009). Many of these have mixed reviews at the present time.
- Methylcellulose (Metamucil) and other bulking agents always must be taken with large amounts of water. Generally, 1 tablespoon is sufficient per day. Increased peristalsis occurs.

Herbs, Botanicals, and Supplements

- Daily use of peppermint oil is effective in relieving IBS symptoms (Hadley and Gaardner, 2005; Heizer et al, 2009).
- The usefulness of probiotics in the form of foods such as live-culture yogurt and buttermilk for IBS symptoms is not established (Heizer et al, 2009). Two double-blind, randomized, placebo-controlled studies identified that *Bifidobacterium infantis* provides relief from IBS (Brenner and Chey, 2009; Spiller, 2005). Yogurt and other cultured foods may not be as effective as specific probiotics with high concentrations of microbes, but they are good sources of nutrients.
- To prevent intestinal gas from forming, try Beano and other products available on the market.
- Twice-weekly Acupuncture/Moxabustion treatment improves average daily abdominal pain and discomfort (Anastasi et al, 2009).

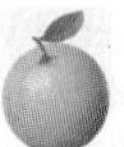

NUTRITION EDUCATION, COUNSELING, CARE MANAGEMENT

- Slowly increase dietary fiber by 2–3 g/d to prevent discomfort and to promote soft, painless stools. Large servings of bran may aggravate IBS; assess individually.
- IBS does not harm the intestines and does not lead to cancer; it is unrelated to IBD.
- Drink six to eight glasses of water or fluids per day. Avoid carbonated beverages, chewing gum, or eating quickly, which may promote gas production.
- Regular times for bowel evacuation should be planned.
- Ensure the patient has adequate food intake and is not afraid to eat because of potential pain.
- A food diary may help to identify any food sensitivities.
- Large meals can cause cramping and diarrhea; smaller meals or smaller portions eaten more often may help IBS symptoms. Meals that are low in fat and high in carbohydrates such as pasta, rice, whole-grain breads and cereals (except with CD), fruits, and vegetables may help.
- Refer the patient for stress management. Patients with rapidly cycling symptoms may need further counseling and support (Tillisch et al, 2005). Cognitive behavioral therapy is beneficial.

- Family members may need to flexible and help to create regularity in the home. Avoid disorganization, overscheduling, lack of planning.
- Regular exercise is important, such as walking, swimming, or yoga. Adequate sleep is important as well.

Patient Education—Foodborne Illness

- Careful food handling and hand washing are important to prevent introduction of foodborne pathogens to the individual who may be experiencing diarrhea and related discomfort.

For More Information

- American College of Gastroenterology—IBS
  http://www.acg.gi.org/patients/ibsrelief/
- E-Medicine Health
  http://www.emedicinehealth.com/irritable_bowel_syndrome/article_em.htm
- IBS Treatment Matrix
  http://www.acg.gi.org/patients/ibsrelief/treatmentmatrix/index.asp
- International Foundation for Functional GI Disorders
  http://www.iffgd.org/
- Living with IBS
  http://www.iamibs.org/
- Mayo Clinic
  http://www.mayoclinic.com/health/irritable-bowel-syndrome/DS00106
- National Digestive Diseases Information Clearinghouse
  http://digestive.niddk.nih.gov/ddiseases/pubs/ibs_ez/
  http://digestive.niddk.nih.gov/ddiseases/pubs/ibs_ez/IBS.pdf
- Web MD—IBS
  http://www.webmd.com/ibs/default.htm

IRRITABLE BOWEL SYNDROME—CITED REFERENCES

American Dietetic Association. Position of the American Dietetic Association: health implications of dietary fiber. *J Am Diet Assoc.* 108:1716, 2008.

Anastasi JK, et al. Symptom management for irritable bowel syndrome: a pilot randomized controlled trial of acupuncture/moxibustion. *Gastroenterol Nurs.* 32:243, 2009.

Brant LJ, et al. An evidence-based systematic review on the management of irritable bowel syndrome American College of Gastroenterology Task Force on IBS. *Am J Gastroenterol.* 104:1S, 2009.

Brenner DM, Chey WD. Bifidobacterium infantis 35624: a novel probiotic for the treatment of irritable bowel syndrome. *Rev Gastroenterol Disord.* 9:7, 2009.

Camilleri M, Andresen V. Current and novel therapeutic options for irritable bowel syndrome management [published online ahead of print 7 August 2009]. *Dig Liver Dis.* 41:854, 2009.

Ford AC, et al. Efficacy of 5-HT3 antagonists and 5-HT4 agonists in irritable bowel syndrome: systematic review and meta-analysis. *Am J Gastroenterol.* 104:1831, 2009.

Hadley SK, Gaardner SM. Treatment of irritable bowel syndrome. *Am Fam Physician.* 72:2501, 2005.

Heizer WD, et al. The role of diet in symptoms of irritable bowel syndrome in adults: a narrative review. *J Am Diet Assoc.* 109:1204, 2009.

Krause R, et al. A randomized, double-blind, placebo-controlled study to assess efficacy and safety of 0.5 mg and 1 mg alosetron in women with severe diarrhea-predominant IBS. *Am J Gastroenterol.* 102:1709, 2007.

Lembo A, et al. Influence of genetics on irritable bowel syndrome, gastro-oesophageal reflux and dyspepsia: a twin study. *Aliment Pharmacol Ther.* 25:11, 2007.

Spiller RC. Probiotics: an ideal anti-inflammatory treatment for IBS? *Gastroenterology.* 128:783, 2005.

Spiller R, Garsed K. Postinfectious irritable bowel syndrome. *Gastroenterol.* 136:1979, 2009.

Tillisch K, et al. Characterization of the alternating bowel habit subtype in patients with irritable bowel syndrome. *Am J Gastroenterol.* 100:896, 2005.

Zar S, et al. Food-specific serum IgG4 and IgE titers to common food antigens in irritable bowel syndrome. *Am J Gastroenterol.* 100:1550, 2005.

LACTOSE MALDIGESTION

NUTRITIONAL ACUITY RANKING: LEVEL 2–3

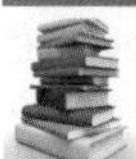

DEFINITIONS AND BACKGROUND

Lactose is a disaccharide (glucose-l galactose) found in milk. If lactase enzyme is missing, lactose passes into the colon, where it is fermented to gases and organic acids by colonic bacteria, resulting in bloating, cramping, nausea, or diarrhea.

A limited proportion of the human adult population retains intestinal lactase-phlorizin hydrolase (LPH) activity during adulthood, the lactase persistence phenotype (Robayo-Torres and Nichols, 2007). Lactase persistence is an autosomal-dominant trait that is common in European-derived populations (Smith et al, 2009). A staggering 4000 million people cannot digest lactose properly (Campbell et al, 2005). As many as 75% of all African American, Jewish, Native American, and Mexican American adults and 90% of Asian American adults are lactose intolerant. A total of 95% of all adults have adult-type hypolactasia (ATH) and have difficulty digesting milk sugar (Robayo-Torres and Nichols, 2007). Table 7-19 describes the various types of this condition.

CD can lead to lactase deficiency (Ojetti et al, 2005). An increased prevalence of lactose intolerance is also seen in patients with IBS. In addition, fructose intolerance may be unrecognized, and testing should clarify which disaccharide

TABLE 7-19 Types of Lactose Maldigestion

Type	Description	Incidence
Congenital, primary, or genetic	Rare, present at birth	Low incidence in children
Lactase "nonpersistence" or hypolactasia	Lactase decline, often to about 10% of neonatal values	Occurs after weaning; more common in adults
Secondary or acquired	From gastrointestinal disease, food allergy, antibiotics, or intestinal trauma	May occur in children after diarrhea or giardiasis. Common with HIV infection, inflammatory bowel disease.

is poorly tolerated. Children with suspected lactose intolerance can be assessed clinically by dietary lactose elimination or by tests including noninvasive hydrogen breath testing or invasive intestinal biopsy determination of lactase (and other disaccharidase) concentrations. (Heyman and Committee on Nutrition, 2006).

Lactose maldigesters can consume up to 1 cup (8 oz) of milk without experiencing symptoms; tolerance can be improved by consuming the milk with a meal, choosing yogurt or hard cheeses, or using products that aid in the digestion of lactose such as lactase supplements or lactose-reduced milks (Byers and Savaiano, 2005). Symptoms caused by lactose maldigestion need not hinder ingestion of a diet rich in dairy products that supplies around 1500 mg calcium daily (i.e., 2 cups of milk, 1 cup of yogurt, and several ounces of cheese). Bloating, abdominal pain, diarrhea, and overall symptom severity are often tolerable.

Pregnant women, children and teens who are lactose intolerant should be given appropriate counseling about intake of calcium from nonlactose sources. Individuals who are self-described as lactose intolerant may restrict dairy and calcium intake and are at greater risk of osteoporosis and bone fractures. The American Dietetic Association recommends at least three MNT visits for adults who have lactose maldigestion.

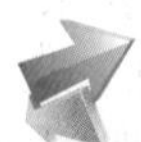

ASSESSMENT, MONITORING, AND EVALUATION

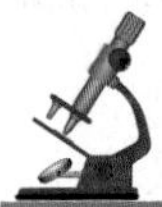

CLINICAL INDICATORS

Genetic Markers: Congenital lactase deficiency (CLD) occurs because of an SNP upstream from the lactase (C-13910 > T) gene (Ingram 2009).

Clinical/History	Stool acidity test	Mg^{++}
Height	**Lab Work**	Alk phos
Weight	Alb, transthyretin	Gluc
BMI	BUN, Creat	H & H
Weight changes	Ca^{++} (better absorption can occur over time)	Serum Fe, ferritin
Lactose challenge test		Na^+, K^+
Hydrogen breath test (3–5 hours)		

INTERVENTION

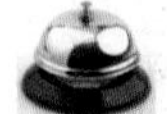

OBJECTIVES

- Manage pain and discomfort related to lactose ingestion that is caused by flatulence and bloating or diarrhea. Control lactose intake, which comprises 10% of the carbohydrate found in the American diet.
- Regular consumption of milk by lactase-deficient persons may improve colonic tolerance. Check for actual tolerance by monitoring intake.

> **SAMPLE NUTRITION CARE PROCESS STEPS**
>
> **Excessive Cho (Lactose) Intake**
>
> ***Assessment:*** Food diary and records with analysis of grams of lactose consumed on average day, stool frequency, and GI complaint reports.
>
> ***Nutrition Diagnosis (PES):*** Excessive CHO (lactose) intake related to poor food choices as evidenced by frequent use of liquid dairy products, ice cream and milkshakes with resulting abdominal pain and diarrhea.
>
> ***Intervention:*** Counseling on lactose-restricted diet, use of Lact-Aid and lactose-reduced products in meals and in cooking.
>
> ***Monitoring and Evaluation:*** Food records and reports of GI distress or diarrhea after diet alterations have been implemented consistently for at least 7 days.

- Offer calcium and riboflavin from other foods and sources besides lactose-containing dairy products.

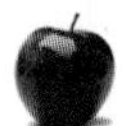

FOOD AND NUTRITION

- Most people can tolerate up to 6 g of lactose, which is found in ½ cup (4 oz) of fluid milk. If small amounts are gradually added over approximately 3 months, most adults can ultimately adapt to 12 g lactose, equal to one 8-oz glass of regular milk.
- Dairy foods contain approximately 1–8% lactose by weight (milk, 4–5%; yogurt, 4%; ice cream, 3–4%; milk chocolate, 8%; cottage cheese, 1–2%). Because symptoms are related to dose, consume no more than 8 oz of lactose-containing milk at a time after other foods have been consumed to slow down transit time. See Table 7-20.
- Provide lactase enzyme supplements (e.g., Lactaid, Lactrase, Dairy Ease) 30 minutes before the consumption of a lactose-containing product. Two capsules provide enough lactase to hydrolyze the lactose in an 8-oz glass of whole milk. Lactose-hydrolyzed milk is generally tolerated. Note that not all preparations are equally effective.
- Persons on a lactose-free diet can use lactate, casein (curds), lactalbumin, and calcium. If the patient is highly sensitive, check labels of foods for fillers, whey protein, milk, whey solids, and milk solids; most people can tolerate small amounts in mashed potatoes, breads, and medications. Processed cheese or cheese foods may have nonfat dry milk solids; use in moderate amounts.
- Fermented products (buttermilk, natural or aged cheese, yogurt with live and active cultures, cottage cheese, or sour cream) may be better tolerated than milk by many individuals.
- Frozen yogurt has little or no lactase activity. It may be tolerated in small amounts.
- For infants with the condition, try milk-free formulas; gradually introduce foods that contain milk or lactose to test for tolerance. Distinguish milk allergy (usually early in life) from lactose maldigestion (more often in adults).
- Secondary lactase deficiency results from injury to the small intestine that occurs with severe diarrheal illness, CD, Crohn's disease, or chemotherapy; this is more common in infancy.

TABLE 7-20 **Lactose and Substitutes in Common Foods**

Food and Portion	Portion	Lactose (g)
Evaporated milk	1 cup	24
Sweetened condensed milk	1/2 cup	20
Milk, reduced fat	1 cup	11–14
Acidophilus Milk	1 cup	11
Yogurt, whole milk	1 cup	10–12
Buttermilk	1 cup	10
Ice cream	1/2 cup	6
Yogurt, plain, low fat	1 cup	5
Sour cream or light cream	1/2 cup	4
Cottage cheese	1/2 cup	3 creamed, 2 dry
Cheese, hard	1 oz	1–2
Swiss cheese	1 oz	1
Cream cheese	1 oz	1
Butter or margarine	1 tsp	Trace

Recipe Substitutes for Dairy Products

- 1 cup whole milk = mix 1/2 cup water with 1/2 cup nondairy cream or use 1 cup soy or rice milk
- 1 cup skim milk = 1/4 cup nondairy cream plus 3/4 cup water
- 1 cup evaporated milk = 1 cup nondairy cream or soy milk
- 1 cup buttermilk = 1/2 cup nondairy cream plus 1/2 cup water + 1 tbsp lemon juice or vinegar
- 1 cup whipped cream = 1 cup nondairy whipped topping
- 1 tbsp cream cheese = 1 tbsp mayonnaise
- 1/2 cup cottage cheese = 1/2 cup tofu
- 1 tbsp butter = 1 tbsp milk-free margarine or 1 tbsp vegetable oil
- 1 cup sour cream = 1/4 cup cornstarch in 3/4 cup water plus 1/4 cup vinegar

Common Drugs Used and Potential Side Effects

- Many drugs contain lactose but seldom over 500 mg; most should be well tolerated. For example, some types of birth pills, as well as tablets for stomach acid and gas may contain lactose.
- Antidiarrheal agents such as loperamide (Imodium A-D) help reduce symptoms of lactose intolerance.

Herbs, Botanicals, and Supplements

- Probiotics (such as lactobacilli and bifidobacteria) and prebiotics (nondigestible oligosaccharides) assist in alleviating lactose intolerance and improving calcium absorption (Doron and Gorbach, 2006).
- Take calcium supplements containing calcium carbonate with meals because stomach acid enhances absorption. Calcium citrate can be taken with meals or on an empty stomach. Take calcium in doses of 500 mg several times a day rather than all at once.
- Herbs and botanical supplements should not be used without discussing with the physician.

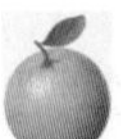

NUTRITION EDUCATION, COUNSELING, CARE MANAGEMENT

- Identify foods that are lactose free and foods that are lactose-free sources of calcium.
- Reading labels is helpful. Store-bought cookies, cakes, bread, baked goods, cereals, instant potatoes, soups, margarine, lunch meat, salad dressings, pancakes, biscuits, nondairy creamers or whipped toppings, and candy may contain lactose.
- The patient must read labels, looking for and avoiding "milk," "lactose," butter, cheese, cream, milk solids, powdered milk, and whey.
- Home-cooked meals and lactose-free recipes are useful. Recipes are available for use of lactose-free formulas in products such as meat loaf. Advise that heating of milk does not change lactose.
- If dairy products are eliminated, other dietary sources of calcium or calcium supplements need to be provided, especially for infants, children, teens (Heyman and Committee on Nutrition, 2006), and pregnant women. Calcium-fortified soy milk, broccoli, leafy greens, canned salmon, almonds, oranges, certain kinds of tofu and soy milk, and calcium-fortified breads and juices can be used.
- Kosher foods are often acceptable if they are pareve (nonmilk, nonmeat).
- Discuss how to use LactAid drops to allow the enzyme to hydrolyze the lactose. Five to 15 drops per quart of milk will reduce lactose by 70–99%.
- Drink milk with meals rather than alone to decrease symptoms.

Patient Education—Foodborne Illness

- Careful food handling and hand washing are important to prevent introduction of foodborne pathogens to the individual who may be experiencing diarrhea and related discomfort.

For More Information

- Dairy-Ease
  http://www.dairyease.com/benefits/
- Lactose-Free Diet
  http://www.gicare.com/pated/edtgs05.htm
- Lactose Intolerance
  http://digestive.niddk.nih.gov/ddiseases/pubs/lactoseintolerance/
- Lactose Intolerance Glossary
  http://www.medicinenet.com/lactose_intolerance/glossary.htm
- Lactose Diet
  http://www.cpmc.org/advanced/pediatrics/patients/topics/lactosefree.html
- LactAid (McNeil Consumer Products)
  http://www.lactaid.com/
- LactAid recipes
  http://lactaid.allrecipes.com/
- National Institute of Diabetes and Digestive and Kidney Diseases (NIDDK)
  http://digestive.niddk.nih.gov/ddiseases/pubs/lactoseintolerance_ez/#food

LACTOSE MALDIGESTION—CITED REFERENCES

Byers KG, Savaiano DA. The myth of increased lactose intolerance in African-Americans. *J Am Coll Nutr.* 24:569S, 2005.

Campbell AK, et al. The molecular basis of lactose intolerance. *Sci Prog.* 88:157, 2005.

Doron S, Gorbach SL. Probiotics: their role in the treatment and prevention of disease. *Expert Rev Anti Infect Ther.* 4:261, 2006.

Heyman MB, Committee on Nutrition. Lactose intolerance in infants, children, and adolescents. *Pediatrics.* 118:1279, 2006.

Ingram CJ. Lactose digestion and the evolutionary genetics of lactase persistence. *Hum Genet.* 124:579, 2009.

Ojetti V, et al. High prevalence of celiac disease in patients with lactose intolerance. *Digestion.* 71:106, 2005.

Robayo-Torres CC, Nichols BL. Molecular differentiation of congenital lactase deficiency from adult-type hypolactasia. *Nutr Rev.* 65:95, 2007.

Smith GD, et al. Lactase persistence-related genetic variant: population substructure and health outcomes. *Eur J Hum Genet.* 17:357, 2009.

MEGACOLON

NUTRITIONAL ACUITY RANKING: LEVEL 3

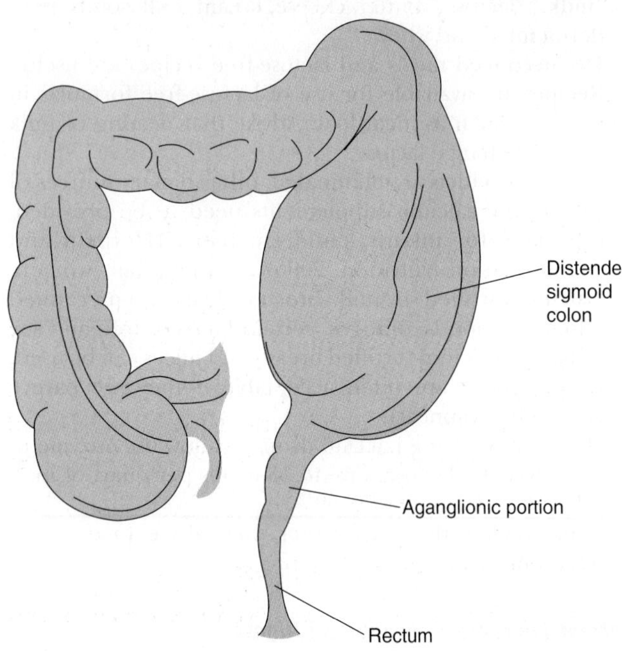

Adapted from: Pillitteri, A. *Maternal and Child Nursing,* 4th ed. Philadelphia: Lippincott, Williams & Wilkins, 2003.

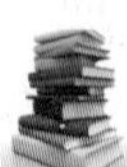

DEFINITIONS AND BACKGROUND

Megacolon may come in three forms: acute (before age 1), chronic (after age 10), or toxic. Acquired megacolon is associated with chronic constipation. The enlarged bowel results from an abnormal colonic dilatation often reaching 8–10 cm in diameter. It may occur in elderly persons who have a long history of elimination problems created by laxative abuse or constipation. Persons with diabetes, hypothyroidism, scleroderma, spinal cord injury, Parkinson's, multiple sclerosis, electrolyte imbalances, tumor, strictures, and other conditions may be affected. Worldwide, infection with *Trypanosoma cruzi* (Chagas disease) is the major cause of megacolon.

Normal urges to defecate are affected by physical activity, neurological status, chemical/drug use, and bowel condition. Normal reflexes are needed for muscular and sphincter control. Family physicians must be alert for the presence of uncommon but serious megacolon (Biggs and Dery, 2006). Signs and symptoms of megacolon involve abdominal distention, flatus, absence of stool, smearing or bowel incontinence, nausea, anorexia, fatigue, and headache. Note that the colon provides reabsorption of water and electrolytes as well as elimination of waste and regulation of bacterial homeostasis; motility is crucial for these roles.

The ENS is the intrinsic segment of the GI tract that controls essential functions such as motility, secretion, and blood flow; it is organized into neurons and glial cells that are distributed throughout the entire length of the gut wall (Burns and Pachnis, 2009). Enteric nervous system stem cells (ENSSCs) provide potential tools to replenish absent ganglia in the congenital form of megacolon, Hirschsprung's disease (Metzger et al, 2009). IBD is associated with a host of intestinal disease–related complications including toxic megacolon (Scherer, 2009). Subtotal colectomy with ileostomy remains the procedure of choice (Ausch et al, 2006; Gladman et al, 2005). Colectomy is complicated by considerable morbidity, while rates have improved over the past several decades (Teeuwen et al, 2009).

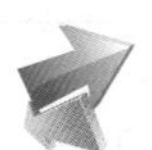

ASSESSMENT, MONITORING, AND EVALUATION

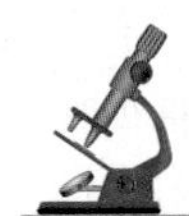

CLINICAL INDICATORS

Genetic Markers: Hirschsprung's disease is caused by a single gene mutation of the *RET* proto-oncogene on band 10q11.2. Megacolon can occur in multiple endocrine neoplasia type 2A (MEN 2A) or 2B (MEN 2B).

Clinical/History
Height
Weight
BMI
Diet history
BP
I & O
Stool pattern
Stool consistency
Endoscopy
Barium x-rays
Abdominal girth

Lab Work
BUN, Creat
Gluc
H & H
Serum Fe, ferritin
Na^+, K^+, Cl^-
Ca^{++}, Mg^{++}
Thyroid function
Stool guaiac

INTERVENTION

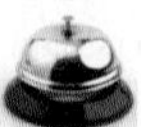

OBJECTIVES

- Prevent complications such as lung atelectasis from distention, sepsis, ulceration with hemorrhage or perforation, or sigmoid volvulus.

SAMPLE NUTRITION CARE PROCESS STEPS

Inadequate Fluid Intake

Assessment Data: Height, Weight, BMI normal. Hx chronic constipation and Parkinson's disease. Recent identification of megacolon. Minimal intake of fluids without prompting. Signs of early dementia.

Nutrition Diagnoses (PES): Inadequate fluid intake related to cognitive changes and forgetting to drink as evidenced by I & O records with chronic constipation and megacolon.

Interventions: Increase fluid intake to meet estimated needs (30 mL/kg). Offer beverages every 2 hours. Educate staff and family about cueing to drink and offering beverages often. Review effects of laxatives, stool softeners, and other prescribed medications on constipation.

Monitoring and Evaluation: Improvement in signs of chronic constipation; relief from megacolon. Improved fluid intake to meet estimated needs.

- Empty the bowel as needed, with osmotic laxatives, enemas, suppositories, cathartics, or digital disimpaction.
- Normalize bowel function as much as possible. Evaluate bowel pattern by history and at present, including drug use and laxative abuse. Exclude underlying cause if possible, such as calcium channel antagonists, narcotics, anticholinergics.
- Identify and correct any nutrient deficiencies, electrolyte imbalances, or protein-energy malnutrition.
- Assure adequate hydration.

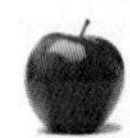

FOOD AND NUTRITION

- Use adequate fluid and fiber, pending status, and other conditions (such as heart failure). Prune juice added to hot cereal may help normalize bowel function. If raw fruits and vegetables are not tolerated at first, add over time. For some people, excessive bran will not be tolerated.
- Avoid excesses of refined foods and concentrated sweets to the exclusion of desirable foods.
- Fiber-rich TF may be needed for selected patients.

Common Drugs Used and Potential Side Effects

- Osmotic agents, such as magnesium salts, sorbitol, or lactulose are often used; some may increase flatulence.
- Stimulant laxatives (senna and bisacodyl) may decrease the ability of the colon to evacuate; they are not as helpful in this condition.
- Suppositories and stool softeners may be used or may have been used excessively. Monitor specific medications accordingly and their side effects.
- Anticholinergics, opiates, and antidepressants may increase or aggravate constipation. Limit use.

Herbs, Botanicals, and Supplements

- Herbs and botanical supplements should not be used without discussing with the physician.
- Many patients take natural herbal laxatives that contain cascara.

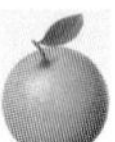

NUTRITION EDUCATION, COUNSELING, CARE MANAGEMENT

- Discuss the role of exercise in maintaining normal bowel function.
- Discuss the role of fluid and fiber in bowel regularity (American Dietetic Association, 2008). For example, drinking a cup of hot prune juice may be effective for some patients.
- Include probiotic foods such as yogurt with live and active cultures, lactobacilli and bifidobacteria, and prebiotics (nondigestible oligosaccharides) for gut integrity.

Patient Education—Foodborne Illness

- If home TF is needed, teach appropriate sanitation and food-handling procedures.

For More Information

- Acquired Megacolon
  http://www.emedicine.com/med/byname/megacolon-chronic.htm
- NIH—Megacolon
  http://www.nlm.nih.gov/medlineplus/ency/article/000248.htm

MEGACOLON—CITED REFERENCES

American Dietetic Association. Position of the American Dietetic Association: health implications of dietary fiber. *J Am Diet Assoc.* 108:1716, 2008.

Ausch C, et al. Aetiology and surgical management of toxic megacolon. *Colorectal Dis.* 8:195, 2006.

Biggs WS, Dery WH. Evaluation and treatment of constipation in infants and children. *Am Fam Physician.* 73:469, 2006.

Burns AJ, Pachnis V. Development of the enteric nervous system: bringing together cells, signals and genes. *Neurogastroenterol Motil.* 21:100, 2009.

Gladman MA, et al. Systematic review of surgical options for idiopathic megarectum and megacolon. *Ann Surg.* 241:562, 2005.

Metzger M, et al. Enteric nervous system stem cells derived from human gut mucosa for the treatment of aganglionic gut disorders. *Gastroenterology.* 136:2214, 2009.

Scherer JR. Inflammatory bowel disease: complications and extraintestinal manifestations. *Drugs Today.* 45:227, 2009.

Teeuwen PH, et al. Colectomy in patients with acute colitis: a systematic review. *J Gastrointest Surg.* 13:676, 2009.

OSTOMY: COLOSTOMY

NUTRITIONAL ACUITY RANKING: LEVEL 2–3

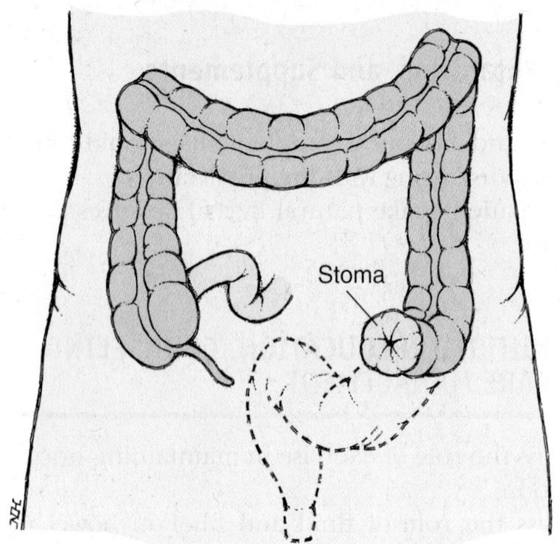

Adapted from: Neil O. Hardy. Wesport, CT. *Stedman's Medical Dictionary*, 27th ed. Baltimore: Lippincott Williams & Wilkins, 2000, p. 383.

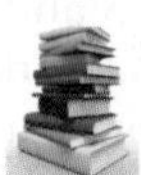

DEFINITIONS AND BACKGROUND

The colon functions primarily to absorb water and sodium and to excrete potassium and bicarbonate. A colostomy is an artificial outlet for intestinal wastes created surgically by bringing a portion of the colon through the abdominal wall, resulting in a stoma. Colostomy can be permanent or temporary. It may be indicated for intestinal cancer, diverticulitis, perforated bowel, radiation enteritis, obstruction, and Hirschsprung's disease. It may also be indicated for spinal cord–injured patients where bowel management (bowel care and defecation time) averages 6 hours/wk prior to stoma formation, but decreases to 1.5 hours/wk after a left colostomy, thus improving quality of life (Munck et al, 2009).

Abdominoperineal resection, with iliac colostomy, remains a standard treatment (Portier et al, 2005). With proper patient selection, laparoscopic colorectal surgery can be performed. Video-assisted, double barreled wet colostomy is minimally invasive. Table 7-21 lists the common types of colostomies.

Colostomy output is generally more formed than ileostomy output. Some colostomates can "irrigate," using a procedure similar to an enema to clean stool directly out of the colon through the stoma. This requires special irrigation appliances: an irrigation bag and a connecting tube (or catheter), a stoma cone, and an irrigation sleeve. A special lubricant is sometimes used on the stoma in preparation for irrigation. Following irrigation, some colostomates can use a stoma cap, a one- or two-piece system that simply covers and protects the stoma. This procedure is usually done to avoid the need to wear an appliance.

TABLE 7-21 Common Types of Colostomies

Colostomy Type	Description
Temporary Colostomy	Allows the lower portion of the colon to rest or heal. It may have one or two openings (if two, one will discharge only mucus).
Permanent Colostomy	Usually involves the loss of part of the colon, most commonly the rectum. The end of the remaining portion of the colon is brought out to the abdominal wall to form the stoma.
Sigmoid or Descending Colostomy	The most common type of ostomy surgery, in which the end of the descending or sigmoid colon is brought to the surface of the abdomen. It is usually located on the lower left side of the abdomen.
Transverse Colostomy	The surgical opening created in the transverse colon resulting in one or two openings. It is located in the upper abdomen, middle or right side.
Loop Colostomy	Usually created in the transverse colon. This is one stoma with two openings; one discharges stool, the second discharges mucus.
Ascending Colostomy	A relatively rare opening in the ascending portion of the colon. It is located on the right side of the abdomen.

Source: United Ostomy Association, Inc. What is ostomy? at http://www.uoa.org/ostomy_main.htm, accessed March 31, 2005.

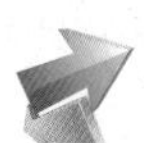

ASSESSMENT, MONITORING, AND EVALUATION

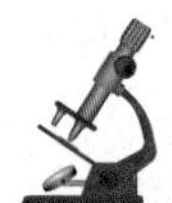

CLINICAL INDICATORS

Genetic Markers: Colostomy is a surgical procedure, occasionally used for a congenital condition.

Clinical/History
- Height
- Weight
- BMI
- Diet history
- I & O, hydration status
- Diarrhea or constipation
- Renal stones?

Lab Work
- H & H
- Serum Fe, ferritin
- Na^+, K^+
- Gluc
- Alb, transthyretin
- Ca^{++}, Mg^{++}
- Chol, Trig
- Transferrin, TIBC
- Serum B_{12}
- Serum folate
- PT or INR

INTERVENTION

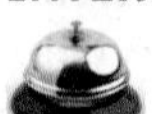

OBJECTIVES

- To avoid major problems of blockage, increased flatulence, and problems with certain foods, preoperative teaching and postoperative follow-up must include food selection guidance.

SAMPLE NUTRITION CARE PROCESS STEPS

Poor Nutritional Quality of Life—Ostomy

Assessment: I & O records or food diary; weight fluctuations. Complaints of abdominal discomfort and unplanned ostomy output of large quantity.

Nutrition Diagnosis (PES): Poor nutritional quality of life related to fear and frequent ostomy output as evidenced by weight fluctuations and reports of GI discomfort after meals.

Intervention: Educate about how to meet estimated nutritional needs using tolerated foods; how to track GI symptoms and food tolerances using a food diary.

Monitoring and Evaluation: Improved I & O records; stabilized weight. Fewer or no GI distress following meals when foods poorly tolerated are omitted from the diet. Ostomy output more predictable and normal.

- Speed wound healing and recovery.
- Correct weight loss or malnutrition from GI blood loss, anemia, protein malabsorption, steatorrhea.
- Prevent watery or unscheduled bowel movements. Correct or prevent dehydration.
- Individualize the diet: Eat regularly, avoid odor-causing foods, and monitor food preferences. Normalize nutritional quality of life as much as possible.
- Avoid infection and skin irritants.

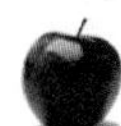

FOOD AND NUTRITION

- Early oral feeding in the patients undergoing colorectostomy is feasible, safe, and associated with reduced postoperative discomfort; it can accelerate the return of bowel function and improve rehabilitation (Zhou et al, 2006). Most people can resume oral diet 2 days after surgery.
- Progress from a liquid to a low-residue diet. To speed healing, the formula or diet should also be high in protein, energy, vitamins, and minerals.
- Diet should provide normal or increased salt intake. One to two quarts of fluid, taken between meals, should be ingested daily.
- Gradually introduce new foods; if done slowly, offending foods can be identified and obstruction can be controlled or prevented. Foods that may not be tolerated include:
  1. **Foods that may cause loose stools or diarrhea:** apple juice, prune juice, dried beans, chocolate, green beans, raw fruits and raw vegetables, fried foods, highly spiced foods, broccoli, and leafy green vegetables.
  2. **Gas or odor-causing foods:** alcohol (beer), beans, onions, cabbage, broccoli, cauliflower, Brussels sprouts, fish, eggs, asparagus, and garlic. Fresh parsley is a natural deodorizer.
  3. Foods that cause **urinary odor** include asparagus and seafood.
  4. Beets and red gelatin can cause **abnormal stool coloration.**
  5. Avoid **high fiber foods:** granola, bean sprouts, bamboo shoots, bran, whole-kernel corn, mushrooms, celery, nuts, pineapple, popcorn, coleslaw, apple skins, seeds, or coconut.
  6. Foods **most often avoided** because of an ostomy include fresh fruits and vegetables such as cabbage, beans, onions, hot dogs, sausages and other meats with casings.
- Foods that thicken stool include applesauce, bananas, marshmallows, rice, pasta, peanut butter, tapioca, and yogurt.
- Progress to a high-fiber diet with short-fibered foods.
- If calcium oxalate stones develop after the colostomy, diet should provide a high-fluid intake. Restrict intake of oxalates from spinach, rhubarb, wild greens, coffee and tea, and chocolate.
- Signs of blockage include: almost constant spurt of highly watery stool, bloating, cramping, swelling around stoma, strong odor of stool, nausea, vomiting, and pain. Avoid eating solid food, and do not take any laxatives or stool softeners. Drink a hot, caffeinated beverage; try a hot bath; gently massage the abdomen; and apply a pouch that has a larger opening.

Common Drugs Used and Potential Side Effects

- Probiotics and prebiotics may be useful for return of gut immunity.
- Polyethylene glycol solution may be used as an alternative fluid regimen for colostomy irrigation.
- Patients with electrolyte concerns should be carefully monitored if sodium phosphate preparations (Osmoprep, Visicol) are used for colonscopy preparation (Lichtenstein, 2009).
- Prednisone: Restrict excessive sodium intake. Monitor nitrogen, calcium, and potassium losses when used over a long period of time.
- Lomotil is a stool thickener and deodorizer; use plenty of fluids.
- Bulk-forming agents such psyllium (Metamucil) may be useful. Increased peristalsis occurs.

Herbs, Botanicals, and Supplements

- Herbs and botanical supplements should not be used without discussing with the physician.

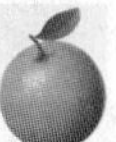

NUTRITION EDUCATION, COUNSELING, CARE MANAGEMENT

- Approximately 6 weeks are required to acclimate the bowel to new procedures of irrigation. Enemas are used to wash the bowel up to the ileocecal valve (with 1000 mL of tap water). Constipation can occur with dehydration; therefore, adequate intake of fluid and fiber is important.
- Use of a commercial deodorant in the colostomy bag is preferred for eliminating highly flavored or nutrient-dense foods.

- Instruct the patient to eat slowly, chew foods well, and avoid swallowing air.
- Irrigations should not be performed when there is vomiting or diarrhea. Working with an enterostomal therapist can be helpful for more suggestions.
- Regular mealtimes should be encouraged.
- Reassurance is needed, without misleading the patient. Some colostomies are permanent (Riansuwan et al, 2009). Quality of life may decrease after the procedure (Yau et al, 2009).
- If a temporary colostomy is performed, a patient may be evaluated for a reversal of the colostomy where the remaining colon and rectum must be examined for normalcy.

Patient Education—Foodborne Illness

- Careful food handling and hand washing are important to prevent introduction of foodborne pathogens to the individual who may be experiencing diarrhea and related discomfort.
- Proper ostomy care requires careful and constant hand washing.
- If home TF or CPN is needed, teach appropriate sanitation and food-handling procedures.

For More Information

- Colostomy—Medicine Net
  http://www.medicinenet.com/colostomy_a_patients_perspective/article.htm
- Colostomy Guide
  http://www.cancer.org/docroot/CRI/content/CRI_2_6x_Colostomy.asp
- Medline Plus
  http://www.nlm.nih.gov/MEDLINEPLUS/ency/article/002942.htm
- United Ostomy Association (UOA)
  http://www.uoa.org/ostomy_main.htm

OSTOMY: COLOSTOMY—CITED REFERENCES

Lichtenstein G. Bowel preparations for colonoscopy: a review. *Am J Health Syst Pharm.* 66:27, 2009.

Munck J, et al. Intestinal stoma in patients with spinal cord injury: a retrospective study of 23 patients. *Hepatogasterenterology.* 55:2125, 2009.

Portier G, et al. Use of malone antegrade continence enema in patients with perineal colostomy after rectal resection. *Dis Colon Rectum.* 48:499, 2005.

Riansuwan W, et al. Nonreversal of Hartmann's procedure for diverticulitis: derivation of a scoring system to predict nonreversal. *Dis Colon Rectum.* 52:1400, 2009.

Yau T, et al. Longitudinal assessment of quality of life in rectal cancer patients with or without stomas following primary resection. *Dis Colon Rectum.* 52:669, 2009.

Zhou T, et al. Early removing gastrointestinal decompression and early oral feeding improve patients' rehabilitation after colorectostomy. *World J Gastroenterol.* 2:2459, 2006.

OSTOMY: ILEOSTOMY

NUTRITIONAL ACUITY RANKING: LEVEL 3

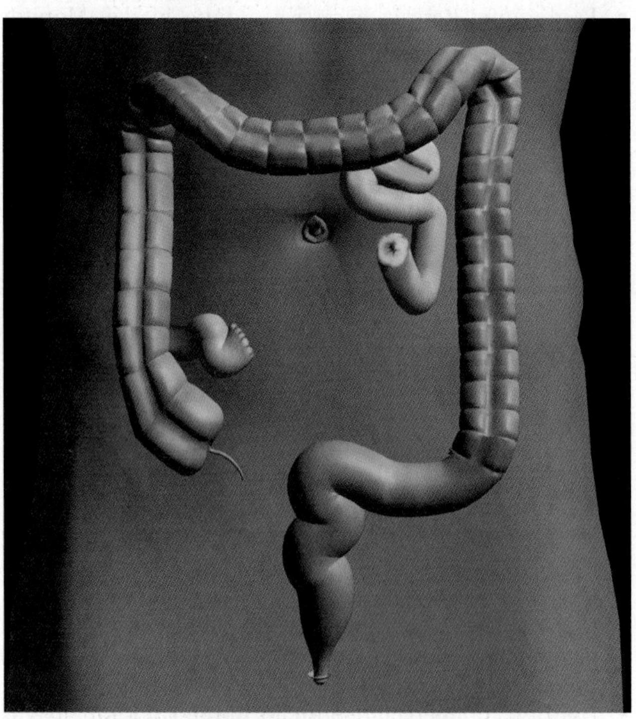

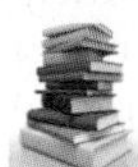

DEFINITIONS AND BACKGROUND

Used to treat intractable cases of ulcerative disease, Crohn's disease, polyposis, and colon cancer, an ileostomy is a surgical procedure (stoma/opening formation) that brings the ileum through the abdominal wall. It may be temporary or permanent. This procedure causes a decrease in fat, bile acid, and vitamin B_{12} absorption, as well as greater losses of sodium and potassium.

Patients will be incontinent of gas and stool. Ideally, the ileocecal valve can be kept to decrease bacterial influx into the small intestine. Of these patients, 50–70% will have recurrent disease. Effective ostomy management is important and involves establishment of an effective system for managing altered dietary and fluid intake, maintaining fluid and electrolyte balance, and preventing food blockage (Doughty, 2005).

Subtotal colectomy with ileostomy is a safe and effective treatment for patients requiring urgent surgery (Hyman et al, 2005). Interval ileal pouch–anal anastomosis reconstruction without a stoma after colectomy equals the more traditional protocol in terms of clinical outcome but yields lower hospital costs and probably a shorter length of hospital stay (Swenson et al, 2005). Table 7-22 describes the procedures for ileostomy.

TABLE 7-22 Ileostomy Procedures

Procedure	Description
Ileoanal Anastomosis	This is now the most common alternative to the conventional ileostomy. Technically, it is not an ostomy since there is no stoma. In this procedure, the colon and most of the rectum are surgically removed, and an internal pouch is formed out of the terminal portion of the ileum. An opening at the bottom of this pouch is attached to the anus such that the existing anal sphincter muscles can be used for continence. This procedure should only be performed on patients with ulcerative colitis or familial polyposis and who have not previously lost their rectum or anus. It is also called J-pouch, pull-thru, endorectal pullthrough, pelvic pouch, or a combination of these terms.
Continent Ileostomy	This surgical variation of the ileostomy is also called a **Kock pouch**. A reservoir pouch is created inside the abdomen with a portion of the terminal ileum. A valve is constructed in the pouch, and a stoma is brought through the abdominal wall. A catheter or tube is inserted into the pouch several times a day to drain feces from the reservoir. This procedure has generally been replaced in popularity by the ileoanal pouch. A modified version of this procedure called the Barnett continent ileal reservoir is performed at a limited number of facilities.

Source: United Ostomy Association, Inc. What is ostomy? at http://www.uoa.org/ostomy_main.htm, accessed March 31, 2005.

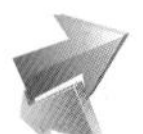

ASSESSMENT, MONITORING, AND EVALUATION

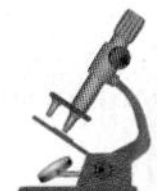

CLINICAL INDICATORS

Genetic Markers: Ileostomy is a surgical procedure, occasionally used for a congenital condition.

Clinical/History	Lab Work	
Height	H & H	Transferrin
Weight	Serum Fe, ferritin	TIBC
BMI	BUN, Creat	Gluc
Diet history	Na^+, K^+	WBC
Stool (occult blood)	Alb, transthyretin	Ca^{++}, Mg^{++}
BP		Serum B_{12}
		Schilling test if needed
		Serum folate

SAMPLE NUTRITION CARE PROCESS STEPS

Inadequate Fluid Intake

Assessment Data: I & O, weight changes, signs of dehydration, high output from ileostomy.

Nutrition Diagnoses (PES): Inadequate fluid intake related to losses from ileostomy and insufficient intake as evidenced by I & O records (intake 1200 mL, output 1600 mL/d).

Interventions: Food and nutrient delivery: Calculate needs, provide extra liquids with meals, offer a beverage every few hours. Educate: Discuss the need for extra fluids when ileostomal losses are increased, during febrile periods, when there is vomiting.

Monitoring and Evaluation: I & O records, weight records, fewer signs of dehydration (poor skin turgor, sunken eyeballs, etc).

INTERVENTION

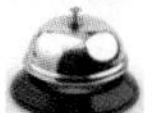

OBJECTIVES

- Modify the diet to counteract malabsorption of nutrients secondary to diarrhea, protein, and fluid losses, negative nitrogen balance from nutrient loss, and anorexia.
- Correct any anemia caused by inadequate intake or blood losses.
- Counteract weakness and muscle cramping from potassium losses.
- Provide increased energy intake during periods of fever or infection.
- Replenish calcium to reverse losses caused by steatorrhea and bone density loss if steroid therapy is used.
- Prevent gallstones, renal oxalate stones, bacterial overgrowth, and fatty acid malabsorption.

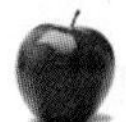

FOOD AND NUTRITION

- **Preoperatively:** Fiber and lactose intolerances are common; alter diet accordingly. With strictures, avoid popcorn, nuts, seeds, mushrooms, celery, fruit skins, and vegetable skins. Have the patient chew thoroughly.
- **Postoperatively:** Provide a high-energy, high-protein diet for wound healing that is low in excess insoluble fiber. Avoid the high-fiber foods suggested for preoperative care for about 4 weeks. Pectin in apples and oligosaccharides in oatmeal may be beneficial to add back first. Spinach or parsley are natural intestinal deodorizers, but beware of excesses of oxalate-rich foods.
- The patient needs an adequate intake of protein (provided by low-fat sources such as lean meats and egg white), vitamin B_{12} (provided by liver, fish, and eggs), folacin, calcium, magnesium, iron, sodium, vitamin C, and potassium.
- Diet should provide an adequate amount of fluids, especially in hot weather. Add salt if needed.
- Apple juice has chemoprotective properties for human colon cells. Intake of apple juice results in bioavailable polyphenols in the gut lumen, which could contribute

to reduced genotoxicity, enhanced antigenotoxicity and favorable modulation of GSTT2 gene expression (Veeriah et al, 2008).
- Since obesity can cause more discomfort, a weight management plan may be useful.

Common Drugs Used and Potential Side Effects

- Corticosteroids: With prednisone, restrict excessive sodium intake and monitor nitrogen and calcium losses. The corticosteroid budesonide (Entocort) may be administered to increase the absorptive capacity of the intestinal mucosa in patients with ileostomies (Ecker et al, 2005). Side effects may include increased appetite and weight gain, hypokalemia, and elevated CRP.
- Lomotil is a stool thickener and deodorizer. Plenty of fluids should be used.
- Probiotics and prebiotics may be useful to help with recovery of gut immunity. Research is underway for the use of a special form of *Bacteroides ovatus* (Hamady et al, 2008).
- Psyllium (Metamucil) is used as a bulk-forming agent. Increased peristalsis will occur.

Herbs, Botanicals, and Supplements

- Herbs and botanical supplements should not be used without discussing with the physician.
- Use of fish oil may be beneficial during periods of inflammation.

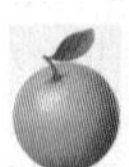

NUTRITION EDUCATION, COUNSELING, CARE MANAGEMENT

- Explain which foods are common sources of the needed nutrients in a diet or suggest supplementation with multivitamins and minerals. Encourage use of apple juice and other protective foods as tolerated.
- Monitor individual tolerance to offending foods such as gas-forming or fried foods, highly seasoned foods, nuts, raisins, and pineapple. Foods that may cause rapid intestinal transit or discomfort may include dried fruits, prune juice, fresh strawberries or peaches, coconut, nuts, seeds, cabbage, celery, bamboo shoots, corn, and milk.
- An enterostomal therapist may be of assistance.
- Discuss replacement of fluid and sodium, especially during hot weather.
- Eating before bedtime should be avoided to lessen discomfort.
- More than half of patients operated with proctocolectomy will need surgical intervention within 20 years; the failure rate is more than 10% and complications must be addressed (Wasmuth et al, 2009).

Patient Education—Foodborne Illness

- Careful food handling and hand washing are important to prevent introduction of foodborne pathogens to the individual who may be experiencing diarrhea and related discomfort.
- Proper ostomy care requires careful and constant hand washing.
- If home TF or PN is needed, teach appropriate sanitation and food-handling procedures.

For More Information

- Continent Ileostomy
  http://www.medicinenet.com/caring_for_a_continent_ileostomy/article.htm
- Ileostomy
  http://digestive.niddk.nih.gov/ddiseases/pubs/ileostomy/
- Ilesotomy Guide—American Cancer Society
  http://www.cancer.org/docroot/CRI/content/CRI_2_6x_Ileostomy.asp
- Jackson Gastroenterology
  http://www.gicare.com/pated/ecdgs11.htm
- Mayo Clinic—Ostomy
  http://www.mayoclinic.com/health/ostomy/SA00072
- United Ostomy Association
  http://www.uoa.org/ostomy_facts_ileostomy.htm

OSTOMY: ILEOSTOMY—CITED REFERENCES

Doughty D. Principles of ostomy management in the oncology patient. *J Support Oncol.* 3:59, 2005.

Ecker KW, et al. Long-term treatment of high intestinal output syndrome with budesonide in patients with Crohn's disease and ileostomy. *Dis Colon Rectum.* 48:237, 2005.

Hamady ZZ, et al. Identification and use of the putative Bacteroides ovatus xylanase promoter for the inducible production of recombinant human proteins. *Microbiology.* 154:3165, 2008.

Hyman NH, et al. Urgent subtotal colectomy for severe inflammatory bowel disease. *Dis Colon Rectum.* 48:70, 2005.

Swenson BR, et al. Modified two-stage ileal pouch-anal anastomosis: equivalent outcomes with less resource utilization. *Dis Colon Rectum.* 48:256, 2005.

Veeriah S, et al. Intervention with cloudy apple juice results in altered biological activities of ileostomy samples collected from individual volunteers. *Eur J Nutr.* 47:226, 2008.

Wasmuth HH, et al. Long-term surgical load in patients with ileal pouch-anal anastomosis. *Colorectal Dis.* 11:711, 2009.

PERITONITIS

NUTRITIONAL ACUITY RANKING: LEVEL 2

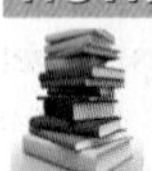

DEFINITIONS AND BACKGROUND

In peritonitis, inflammation of the peritoneal cavity due to infiltration of intestinal contents occurs. Contents from such conditions as ruptured appendix, gastric or intestinal perforation such as in diverticulitis, trauma, fistula, anastomotic leaks, or failed peritoneal dialysis (PD) may initiate the problem.

Bacterial peritonitis is a major cause of morbidity in pediatric PD patients and can lead to catheter removal, hospitalizations, peritoneal membrane dysfunction, and sepsis (Chand et al, 2009). Spontaneous bacterial peritonitis is also common in patients with cirrhosis and ascites because of bacterial translocation. The diagnostic evaluation of ascites involves an assessment of its cause by determining the serum-ascites albumin gradient and the exclusion spontaneous bacterial peritonitis (Hou and Sanyal, 2009). Peritonitis in liver transplant patients may suggest organ rejection (Macedo et al, 2005). Prophylactic antibiotics and omentectomy at catheter insertion are useful (Chand, 2009). Aggressive nutritional supplementation pre- and postoperatively is suggested (De Frietas et al, 2008). It is important to avoid refeeding syndrome.

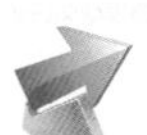

ASSESSMENT, MONITORING, AND EVALUATION

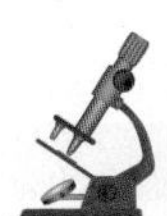

CLINICAL INDICATORS

Genetic Markers: Peritonitis is the result of infection and not genetic origins.

Clinical/History		
Height	Ileus	BUN, Creat
Weight	Sepsis?	Gluc
BMI	X-rays	Alb, transthyretin
Diet history	Paracentesis (>250 polymorphonucleate cells)	CRP
Abdominal pain, tenderness	Laparoscopy	Na^+, K^+
Abdominal rigidity (washboard appearance)	**Lab Work**	Ca^{++}, Mg^{++}
Fever?	H & H	TLC
BP	Serum Fe, ferritin	
I & O	WBC	

SAMPLE NUTRITION CARE PROCESS STEPS

Inadequate Energy Intake

Assessment Data: I & O records, weight, severe abdominal pain, intake <25% in past 24 hours, fever 102°F.

Nutrition Diagnoses (PES): Inadequate energy intake related to inability to eat orally and abdominal pain as evidenced by intake <25% in past day and fever demands about 21% higher energy needs than normal.

Interventions: IV fluids with dextrose until able to eat orally. Monitor for readiness to eat again, based on drop in fever, return of bowel sounds, tolerance for soft or bland foods.

Monitoring and Evaluation: Gradual return to oral diet with improved I & O records; weight returning to usual. No fever or signs of abdominal pain or peritonitis No signs of refeeding.

INTERVENTION

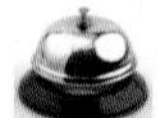

OBJECTIVES

- Correct fluid/electrolyte imbalances when present. Vigorous IV rehydration is needed.
- Provide bowel rest and recovery. PN may be better than NG feeding but further studies into dualenteral nutrition and PN are needed (De Frietas et al, 2008).
- Improve nutritional status, especially if patient has been malnourished over a period of time or if there is anorexia or ileus.
- Avoid high risk for refeeding syndrome (De Frietas et al, 2008).

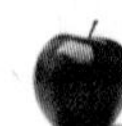

FOOD AND NUTRITION

- Patient generally is NPO with IV feedings for at least 24 hours. Progress as tolerated to a soft or general diet appropriate for the condition that caused the peritonitis originally.
- Increase protein intake to correct catabolic state. Increase calories because basal energy expenditure is generally elevated by 10–17%.

Common Drugs Used and Potential Side Effects

- Ciprofloxacin is effective in the treatment. Other antibiotics may be used for bacterial peritonitis. Monitor for specific side effects.
- Probiotics may be useful; research continues in this area.
- PPIs suppress gastric acid secretion, allowing bacterial colonization of the upper GI tract, this may predispose to bacterial overgrowth, translocation and peritonitis (Bajaj et al, 2009). Research is needed in this area.

Herbs, Botanicals, and Supplements

- Herbs and botanical supplements should not be used without discussing with the physician.

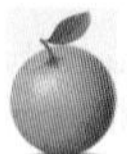

NUTRITION EDUCATION, COUNSELING, CARE MANAGEMENT

- With patients on CAPD, diet may need to be altered similar to the diet typical for renal patients.
- Discuss diet appropriate for the illness of origin (such as diabetes, hypertension, toxemia, or renal disease).

Patient Education—Foodborne Illness

- Careful food handling and hand washing are important to prevent introduction of foodborne pathogens to the individual.
- If home TF or CPN is needed, teach appropriate sanitation and food-handling procedures.

For More Information

- Mayo Clinic
  http://www.mayoclinic.com/health/peritonitis/DS00990/DSECTION%3Dcauses
- NIH—Peritonitis
  http://www.nlm.nih.gov/medlineplus/ency/article/001335.htm
- Peritonitis
  http://www.nlm.nih.gov/medlineplus/ency/article/001335.htm

PERITONITIS—CITED REFERENCES

Bajaj JS, et al. Association of proton pump inhibitor therapy with spontaneous bacterial peritonitis in cirrhotic patients with ascites. *Am J Gastroenterol.* 103;1130, 2009.

Chand DH, et al. Multicenter study of effects of pediatric peritoneal dialysis practices on bacterial peritonitis [published online ahead of print 25 August 2009]. *Pediatr Nephrol.* 25:149, 2009.

De Frietas D, et al. Nutritional management of patients undergoing surgery following diagnosis with encapsulating peritoneal sclerosis. *Perit Dial Int.* 28:271, 2008.

Hou W, Sanyal AJ. Ascites: diagnosis and management. *Med Clin North Am.* 93:801, 2009.

Macedo C, et al. Sclerosing peritonitis after intestinal transplantation in children. *Pediatr Transplant.* 9:187, 2005.

SHORT BOWEL SYNDROME

NUTRITIONAL ACUITY RANKING: LEVEL 4

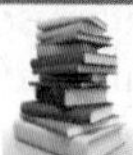

DEFINITIONS AND BACKGROUND

SBS is the predominant cause of intestinal failure, with a high degree of morbidity and mortality. Intestinal failure involves reduction of gut mass below the minimal amount needed for nutrient absorption. SBS involves surgical resection of a portion of the small bowel, compromising the absorptive surface and resulting in malabsorption (especially if more than 50% of the small intestine has been removed). Malnutrition from maldigestion, malabsorption diarrhea, and steatorrhea may result.

A bowel resection that results in SBS may be due to Crohn's disease, intestinal cancer, scleroderma, or fistula in adults; or it may be due to necrotizing enterocolitis, intestinal atresia, or mesentery artery occlusion in infants. If only 30% of the small intestine remains in an adult (or <30 cm in infants), the resulting malabsorption may be life threatening. Problems are significant when more than 70% of the bowel is resected, unless the terminal ileum and ileocecal valve remain. Every attempt should be made to keep the ileocecal valve to prevent contamination of the small intestine. See Table 7-23 regarding the implications of bowel resections.

Normal bowel length is about 600 cm. SBS generally leaves less than 150 cm of small intestine. A total of 100 cm is necessary to completely absorb bile salts; 50–70 cm of jejunum–ileum maintains minimal intestinal autonomy. The minimal length of functional bowel needed for enteral feeding is over 100 cm in the absence of an intact colon and over 60 cm in continuity with the colon.

Patients with SBS require long-term PN. After massive intestinal resection, the intestine undergoes adaptation, and nutritional autonomy may be obtained if the adaptive process is supported by both nutritive and nonnutritive factors (Weale et al, 2005). Length of small intestine remaining after resection is the best predictor of the final success in terminating PN. Home PN may cost between $400+ a day; most insurance companies cover up to $1 million, about 10 years of reimbursement.

Aggressive nutritional intervention is necessary for resolution of nutritional deficits and recovery of health. Early oral feeding after colorectal surgery is safe. Bowel adaptation takes about 1 year. Assessment must include oral intake, stool and urine output, serum electrolytes and visceral proteins, and body weight (DiBaise et al, 2006). Diarrhea and high stomal output are common problems and can lead to dehydration; hypokalemia; deficiencies of calcium, magnesium, and zinc; carbohydrate and lactose malabsorption; protein malabsorption; renal oxalate stone formation; cholesterol biliary stones; gastric acid hypersecretion; vitamin B_{12} or iron deficiency; fat-soluble vitamin deficiency; and diarrhea. See Table 7-24 for malabsorption concerns in SBS.

Patient education and motivation are key factors in successful weaning from PN, where possible (DiBaise et al, 2006).

TABLE 7-23 Implications of Bowel Resections

Loss of jejunum. Ileum undergoes hyperplasia; length and absorption per centimeter increases.

Loss of ileum. This is more serious than loss of jejunum because vitamin B_{12} and bile salts will be reabsorbed poorly as a result. The ileocecal valve keeps colonic bacteria out of the small intestine and regulates chyme flow. Some colonic adaptation occurs during the next 2–5 years.

Loss of colon. Overall, with removal of the colon versus the small intestine, fewer malabsorption problems occur. Loss of electrolyte and water-absorbing capacity occurs, as well as loss of salvage absorption of CHO and other nutrients. Most oxalate absorption occurs here.

In short bowel syndrome (SBS), short-chain triglycerides have a precursor in pectin; oligosaccharides increase O_2 uptake in the colon, thereby maintaining gut integrity. Early refeeding (i.e., free fatty acids, sugars, proteins) stimulates mucosal growth. Hyperphagia can increase enterocyte production. Adaptation requires adequate nutrition, intraluminal nutrients, and bile and pancreatic secretions. Enhancers of the adaptive process seem to include gastrin, glutamine, growth hormone, insulin, short-chain fatty acids, fats, some dietary fibers, cholecystokinin (CCK), glucagon, insulin-like growth factor I, neurotensin, and glucose.

TABLE 7-24 Malabsorption Concerns in Short Bowel Syndrome

Bacterial overgrowth, if ileocecal valve is absent
Decreased bile acid concentration (with loss of ileum and bacterial overgrowth)
Decreased surface area and lessened fluid reabsorption
Dumping syndrome from rapid transit and reduced bowel length
Gastric acid oversecretion with resulting damage to duodenal cells and altered pH, thus affecting pancreatic enzyme and bile activity
Maladaptive remaining small bowel, especially from original bowel disease, lactase deficiency
Pancreatic enzyme activity loss from duodenum, with malnutrition

The use of trophic substances may increase the absorptive function of the remaining gut. Glucagon-like peptide 2 (GLP-2) has been shown to improve intestinal absorption in SBS patients; it reduces fecal weight and enables SBS patients to maintain their intestinal fluid and electrolyte absorption at lower oral intakes (Jeppesen et al, 2009). Current guidelines, however, suggest that the use of growth hormone, glutamine and GLP-2 should not be recommended in patients with short bowel syndrome (Van Gossum et al, 2009).

Serial transverse enteroplasty (STEP) procedure is a safe way to lengthen the small bowel in patients with SBS (Ehrlich et al, 2007). Surgical bowel lengthening should be considered in any chronically PN-dependent patient when there is substantial bowel dilation, regardless of remnant bowel length (Thompson and Sudan, 2008). ITx may also restore quality of life by recovery of normal motility and absorptive capacity. While high-dose immunosuppression is a potential problem, advances in transplantation hold promise as an alternative to intestinal failure and chronic dependence on CPN.

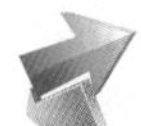

ASSESSMENT, MONITORING, AND EVALUATION

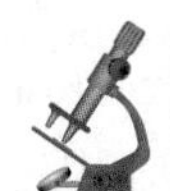

CLINICAL INDICATORS

Genetic Markers: SBS is a surgical procedure.

Clinical/History	Lab Work	
Height	H & H	Alk phos
Weight	Serum Fe, ferritin	Na^+ (serum, urine, stool)
BMI	Transferrin	K^+ (serum, urine, stool)
Diet history	CRP, ESR	Fecal nitrogen
Weight changes	D-xylose absorption	GTT
I & O	Serum gastrin (increased)	Gluc
Steatorrhea	Ca^{++}, Mg^{++}	RBP
Stool output	25-hydroxyvitamin D level	N balance
Dehydration?	Barium follow-through (BaFT) examination	Serum oxalate
Urinary output	Schilling test	Alb, transthyretin
DEXA bone density scan	Serum B_{12}	Serum amylase, lipase
		Serum copper
		Bile acid breath test
		Lactose tolerance test
		Hydrogen breath test
		Fecal fat test

INTERVENTION

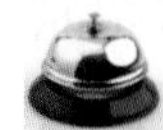

OBJECTIVES

- Determine the location and amount of the intestine that was resected to predict likelihood of diarrhea, malabsorption, and malnutrition (see Table 7-24). Provide nutrient replacements, dependent on area of resection (proximal jejunum—calcium, iron, magnesium, protein, CHO, and fat; terminal ileum—bile acids and intrinsic factor-bound vitamin B_{12}).
- Manage post surgical phases. The first phase lasts 1–3 months, massive diarrhea and limited absorption; the second phase: 4–12 months where weight gain begins and absorption improves. In the last phase between 13 and 24 months, maximal adaptation occurs, with possible discontinuation of PN when fluid is >7 L daily and when energy intake is sufficient for desired weight goal.
- Support hyperphagia, in which the amount of protein absorbed increases relative to the amount of remnant small bowel length. Try weaning off PN without trophic factors. If this is unsuccessful, a trophic factors should be attempted (Steiger et al, 2006).
- Prevent and correct fluid and electrolyte imbalances and dehydration. Oral intake could aggravate already massive losses of fluid (3–10 L/d is common). Immediately postoperatively, NPO with IV fluid replacement is likely. Eventually switch to oral intake as tolerated.
- Use remaining bowel surface and maximize efficacy. Prevent atrophy of small bowel mucosa, catheter sepsis, metabolic bone disease, and liver disease with long-term use of CPN. Carefully monitor for signs and symptoms of these problems and manage accordingly.

SAMPLE NUTRITION CARE PROCESS STEPS

Excessive Parenteral Infusion

Assessment Data: Calculations of energy needs showing PN infusion at a rate exceeding goal by 25%; hypophosphatemia, hypokalemia and signs of refeeding syndrome.

Nutrition Diagnoses (PES): Excessive parenteral infusion (NI 2.4) related to order for CPN solution that exceeds estimated needs by 25% (200 kcal/d) as evidenced by signs of refeeding syndrome with hypophosphatemia and hypokalemia.

Interventions: Reduction in CPN infusion to meet rather than exceed requirements Intervention code.

Monitoring and Evaluation: Consistent monitoring of labs until resolution of refeeding syndrome; tolerance of CPN solution with no further complications.

- Correct symptoms of deficiency and malabsorption, when possible, for vitamins B_{12}, A, D, E, and K and for the minerals zinc, potassium, and magnesium.
- Minimize weight loss (approximately 10 lb monthly until adaptation occurs). Maximize energy intake from fats and carbohydrates without worsening the diarrhea.
- Omit lactose if not tolerated; provide adequate calcium replacements.
- Decrease oxalate from the diet to reduce renal stone formation. Excess bile in the colon from decreased ileal absorption enhances absorption of free oxalate (normally only 10–15% is absorbed).
- Control or prevent gallstone formation (increased risk of two to three times normal), anemia, PLE, peptic ulcer from increased gastric acid secretion, and liver disease (often from home CPN). Parenteral fish-oil lipid or olive-oil emulsions are now more available.
- Allow remaining intestine to compensate over time by hypertrophy of villi and increased diameter. Home CPN is expensive but can be lifesaving for months or years. Transitional feedings may be needed over several months from PN to oral diet. For care of colostomy or ileostomy, see appropriate entries.

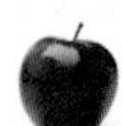

FOOD AND NUTRITION

- **First Postoperative Phase:** IV nutrition or CPN may be appropriate immediately before and approximately 5 days after surgery to allow rest. Determine whether the patient has problems with bloating. The first phase involves extensive diarrhea greater than 2 L daily; advance CPN slowly to avoid refeeding syndrome. At the end of this time, if diarrhea continues to be greater than 2 L, CPN may be lifelong.
- **Second Postoperative Phase:** Diarrhea is lessened and intestinal adaptation begins; CPN may be slowly reduced and polymeric TF started at a slow, continuous rate according to stomal output or stool output. Provide 40–60 kcal/kg and 1.2–1.5 g protein/kg. Providing patients with enteral nutrition, glutamine, dietary fiber, and r-hGH during bowel rehabilitation therapy allows weaning from CPN. If weight loss is greater than 1 kg/wk, CPN may need to be restarted.
- Nocturnal enteral rehydration is an intervention using ORS through PEG tubes at night; this allows for earlier discontinuation of CPN and improved fluid absorption.
- **Third Postoperative Phase:** Complete bowel adaptation begins as TF is tolerated and oral diet is slowly resumed (from 2 months to 1 year). Six small feedings that are high CHO and low fat may be tolerated (60% CHO, 20% protein, 20% fat, with a limit on MCT of 40 g/d). With no colon, the jejunostomy feeding may need to be 40–50% CHO, 20% protein, 30–40% fat. PN reductions can be made by either decreasing the days of PN infusion per week or decreasing the PN infusion volume equally across all days of the week.
- Supplemental zinc, potassium, liquid magnesium, oral calcium (600–1000 mg), manganese, iron, vitamin C, selenium, B-complex vitamins (especially folic acid), and other nutrients may be needed. Determine needs based on site of resection and signs of malnutrition.
- Monitor for needs for vitamins A, E, and D; use water-miscible forms. Patients with SBS are depleted in diet-derived carotenoids despite oral and IV multivitamin supplementation; reduction of PN lipid infusion may improve serum alpha-tocopherol concentrations (Luo et al, 2009). With antibiotic use, the patient will need extra vitamin K.
- Lactose-restricted and oxalate-restricted diets may be needed for an extended period of time. Rhubarb, spinach, beets, cocoa and chocolate, sweet potatoes, strawberries, celery, and peanuts are high-oxalate foods. Nuts and nut butters, berries, Concord grapes, sweet potatoes and potatoes, and most vegetables have smaller amounts.
- Omit alcoholic beverages and caffeine unless physician permits small quantities.
- Taking fluids between instead of with meals may be helpful to reduce dumping. Restrict at first to 1500 mL; progress as tolerated.
- With osmotic diarrhea, a reduction in simple carbohydrates and an increase in complex carbohydrates may be needed. Sorbitol, mannitol, and xylitol are usually poorly absorbed.
- Restricted foods such as lactose may be attempted and added back to the diet if they are tolerated. Bowel adaptation occurs over time and may eventually lead the patient back to an unrestricted diet.

Common Drugs Used and Potential Side Effects (see Table 7-25)

- **Note: Most oral medications are poorly tolerated in this condition!** Accelerated intestinal luminal transit time causes a reduction in absorption of certain antimicrobial agents, digoxin, hydrochlorothiazide, cyclosporine, cimetidine, mesalazine (5-aminosalicylic acid), oral contraceptives, and levothyroxine.
- Dietary glutamine (GLN) or oral antibiotics (ABX) can blunt gut barrier dysfunction (Tian et al, 2009). Antibacterial drugs, antimotility drugs, antidiarrheal agents, H_2 antagonists and PPIs, pancreatic enzymes, somatostatin analogs, antimicrobials, and trophic factors have been quite helpful in addition to nutritional therapy (Matarese and Steiger, 2006).

Herbs, Botanicals, and Supplements

- Herbs and botanical supplements should not be used without discussing with the physician.
- Probiotics and foods such as acidophilus or yogurt are useful aids in bowel adaptation phases. Not all probiotic bacteria have similar therapeutic effects. Research is available for probiotic supplementation for children with SBS (Wallace, 2009).

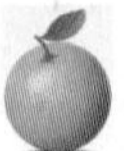

NUTRITION EDUCATION, COUNSELING, CARE MANAGEMENT

- Importance of nutrition and supplementation must be discussed to prevent or correct malnutrition and

TABLE 7-25 Medications Used in Short Bowel Syndrome

Medication	Description
Antibiotics	Tetracycline, Flagyl, Septra, or Cipro may be needed for bacterial overgrowth. Monitor hydrogen breath tests (especially with blind loop).
Antidiarrheals	Antidiarrheals such as Lomotil, Imodium, and codeine are useful. Liquid preparations often are better tolerated. If dehydration occurs, use oral rehydration therapy but not sports drinks, which do not have the adequate electrolyte replacements.
Bile salt replacements	Cholylsarcosine (CS) is a semisynthetic bile salt that may be useful in bile salt replacement therapy of short bowel syndrome (Furst et al, 2005).
Calcium supplements	Oral calcium supplements (OsCal or Tums four times daily) often are used to bind oxalate excesses and to decrease diarrhea. Do not take with a bulk-forming laxative or with an iron supplement. Increase water intake.
Cholestyramine	Cholestyramine may be used for choleraic diarrhea when less than 100 cm is resected and when the colon is in continuity; prevent excessive use. Take before meals. Nausea, vomiting, or constipation may occur.
Cimetidine or omeprazole	Cimetidine and omeprazole may be needed to decrease gastric hypersecretion; parenteral administration may be needed. Serum gastrin levels should be monitored. A dose two to three times higher than normal may be needed because of gastric hypersecretion; lack of sufficient time with intestinal mucosa leads to insufficient absorption. Vitamin B_{12} absorption decreases with use of these medications.
Clonidine	Clonidine can effectively reduce intestinal fluid and electrolyte losses and should be considered in patients with short bowel syndrome.
Growth hormone	Growth hormone increases water/sodium transport. It is useful in combination with glutamine and a modified diet, but results have been mixed.
Minerals	Liquid potassium and intravenous or intramuscular magnesium may be needed.
Pancreatic enzymes	Pancrelipase may improve fat and protein absorption after jejunal resection; results are variable.
Peptides	Glucagon-like peptide-2 (GLP-2) is an enteroendocrine peptide that is released in response to luminal nutrients; it seems to help support the adaptive response to resection (Martin et al, 2005).
Probiotics and prebiotics (synbiotics)	This type of therapy might be a potent modulator of intestinal flora and a promising strategy to treat short bowel patients with enterocolitis.
Vitamins	Vitamins that are chewable or in liquid form may be better tolerated. Parenteral vitamin B_{12} may be necessary. Add extra fat-soluble vitamins A, E, D, and K if deficiency occurs. Do not use vitamin C in excessively large quantities; some links with oxalate stones have been noted.

malabsorption. After adaptation, significant energy intakes will be needed to maintain desired weight.

- Provide recipes or food-preparation tips to support the specific dietary regimen and to evaluate tolerances over time.
- Progression in diet is allowed when the small intestine adapts over several months. Use yogurt with live and active cultures.
- Discuss the need for free water.
- The use of home CPN is beneficial in many cases. Judicious use of home CPN in this setting requires careful clinical assessment on a patient-by-patient basis (Hoda et al, 2005). A supportive attitude from family and caregivers is essential.
- There are potential benefits of a multidisciplinary intestinal rehabilitation program. Interventions can help decrease incidence and economic impact of intestinal failure.
- Exercise, such as resistance training, can help regenerate lean body mass.

Patient Education—Foodborne Illness

- Careful food handling and hand washing are important to prevent introduction of foodborne pathogens to the individual.
- If home TF or CPN is needed, teach appropriate sanitation and food-handling procedures.

For More Information

- E-medicine
  http://www.emedicine.com/ped/topic2088.htm
- Short Bowel Syndrome
  http://digestive.niddk.nih.gov/ddiseases/pubs/shortbowel/
- Short Bowel Syndrome—Pediatrics
  http://depts.washington.edu/growing/Assess/SBS.htm

SHORT BOWEL SYNDROME—CITED REFERENCES

DiBaise JK, et al. Strategies for parenteral nutrition weaning in adult patients with short bowel syndrome. *J Clin Gastroenterol.* 40:S94, 2006.

Ehrlich PF, et al. The 2 STEP: an approach to repeating a serial transverse enteroplasty. *J Pediatr Surg.* 42:819, 2007.

Furst T, et al. Enteric-coated cholylsarcosine microgranules for the treatment of short bowel syndrome. *J Pharm Pharmacol.* 57:53, 2005.

Hoda D, et al. Should patients with advanced, incurable cancers ever be sent home with total parenteral nutrition? A single institution's 20-year experience. *Cancer.* 103:863, 2005.

Jeppesen PB, et al. Short bowel patients treated for two years with glucagon-like Peptide 2: effects on intestinal morphology and absorption, renal function, bone and body composition, and muscle function. *Gastroenterol Res Pract.* 2009:616054, 2009.

Luo M, et al. Prospective analysis of serum carotenoids, vitamin A, and tocopherols in adults with short bowel syndrome undergoing intestinal rehabilitation. *Nutrition.* 25:400, 2009.

Martin GR, et al. Nutrient-stimulated GLP-2 release and crypt cell proliferation in experimental short bowel syndrome. *Am J Physiol Gastrointest Liver Physiol.* 288:431, 2005.
Matarese L, Steiger E. Dietary and medical management of short bowel syndrome in adult patients. *J Clin Gastroenterol.* 40:S85S, 2006.
Steiger E, et al. Indications and recommendations for the use of recombinant human growth hormone in adult short bowel syndrome patients dependent on parenteral nutrition. *J Clin Gastroenterol.* 40:S99S, 2006.
Thompson J, Sudan D. Intestinal lengthening for short bowel syndrome. *Adv Surg.* 42:49, 2008.
Tian J, et al. Dietary glutamine and oral antibiotics each improve indexes of gut barrier function in rat short bowel syndrome. *Am J Physiol Gastrointest Liver Physiol.* 296:348, 2009.
Van Gossum A, et al. ESPEN Guidelines on Parenteral Nutrition: gastroenterology. *Clin Nutr.* 28:415, 2009.
Wallace B. Clinical use of probiotics in the pediatric population. *Nutr Clin Pract.* 24:50, 2009.
Weale AR, et al. Intestinal adaptation after massive intestinal resection. *Postgrad Med J.* 81:178, 2005.

TROPICAL SPRUE

NUTRITIONAL ACUITY RANKING: LEVEL 4

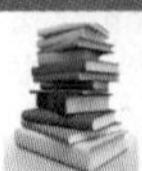

DEFINITIONS AND BACKGROUND

Tropical sprue is an acquired disorder that presents with chronic diarrhea, anorexia, weight loss, megaloblastic anemia (folic acid deficiency), light-colored stools, diarrhea, weight loss, pallor, sore tongue (vitamin B_{12} deficiency), and easy bruising (vitamin K deficiency). Etiology is often bacterial, viral, or parasitic infection or toxins in spoiled food. *Giardia intestinalis* is a common culprit. Tropical sprue may occur after traveling to the Caribbean, southern India, and Southeast Asia.

Tropical sprue causes progressive villus atrophy in the small intestine, similar to CD ("nontropical" sprue). Villi of the small intestinal mucosa become blunted, or obliterated. Treatment of tropical sprue includes folic acid and vitamin B_{12} replacement. However, even prolonged treatment fails to resolve malabsorption. While tropical sprue is less common than it was decades ago (Nath, 2005), sporadic tropical sprue is still an important cause of malabsorption in adults and in children in South Asia (Ramakrishna, 2007).

Biomarker (13)C-sucrose breath test (SBT) to measure enterocyte sucrase activity can be used as a marker of small intestinal villus integrity and function (Ritchie et al, 2009). Enhanced magnification endoscopy can help identify patchy areas of partial mucosal atrophy, potentially reducing the need for blind biopsies (Lo et al, 2007).

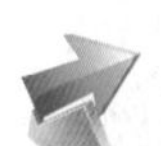

ASSESSMENT, MONITORING, AND EVALUATION

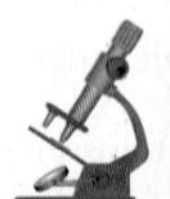

CLINICAL INDICATORS

Genetic Markers: An infectious cause is suspected in tropical sprue.

Clinical/History

Height
Weight
BMI
Diet history
Weight loss?
I & O; dehydration?
Malabsorption, especially for xylose
Glossitis
Cramps, nausea
Gas, indigestion
Paleness
Biopsy
Enhanced magnification endoscopy (EME)

Lab Work

Gluc
SBT
Na^+, K^+
H & H, Serum Fe, ferritin (decreased)
Alb, transthyretin (decreased)
Serum B_{12} (decreased)
Serum folate (decreased)
Ca^{++} (decreased)
Mg^{++}
PT or INR (altered)

INTERVENTION

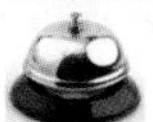

OBJECTIVES

- Provide fluids and electrolytes.
- Differentiate between tropical sprue and CD. Control diarrhea, which leads to malabsorption and malnutrition over time.
- Improve or correct folic acid, vitamin B_{12}, and vitamin K deficiencies. Treat tropical sprue with folate and vitamin B_{12} cures the macrocytic anemia and the accompanying glossitis.
- Avoid fatty foods that can cause oily, foul-smelling stools.

SAMPLE NUTRITION CARE PROCESS STEPS

Abnormal GI Function

Assessment Data: Diarrhea, fever, macrocytic anemia, biopsy showing flattened villi and diagnosis of tropical sprue.

Nutrition Diagnoses (PES): Abnormal GI function related to infectious process as evidenced by diarrhea, macrocytic anemia, and flattened villi on biopsy.

Interventions: Provide folic acid and vitamin B_{12} in supplemental form along with antibiotic therapy; extra fluids, sodium and potassium as needed. Progress to low-fat diet.

Monitoring and Evaluation: Improvement in macrocytic anemia; resolution of diarrhea.

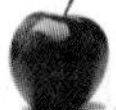

FOOD AND NUTRITION

- Use a regular diet with supplements of vitamin B_{12} and folic acid. Good sources of folacin include liver, kidney, yeast, leafy greens, lean beef, and eggs. Good sources of vitamin B_{12} include meat, poultry, fish, dairy products, and eggs.
- Avoid meals with fatty foods.
- Diet should provide sufficient amounts of energy intake, protein, calcium, iron, and vitamins.
- Extra fluid may be needed for dehydration.
- No gluten restriction is needed.

Common Drugs Used and Potential Side Effects

- Tetracycline may be used; do not take within 2 hours of a calcium-containing supplement or meal as calcium makes the drug less effective.
- Vitamin supplements are required, especially for vitamin B_{12}, folate, and vitamin K. Calcium may also be needed. Avoid excesses of any single nutrient for an extended time period.
- Suggest use of probiotics such as yogurt with live and active cultures during antibiotic therapy. Intestinal flora modifiers (e.g., *Lactobacillus acidophilus*, Lactinex, Bacid) also help recolonize normal intestinal flora in people on antibiotics. A common order is three to four packages every day for 3 days in adults. They may be mixed with water for TFs.

Herbs, Botanicals, and Supplements

- Herbs and botanical supplements should not be used without discussing with the physician.

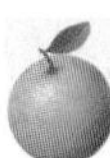

NUTRITION EDUCATION, COUNSELING, CARE MANAGEMENT

- Explain to the patient which foods are good sources of folic acid and vitamin B_{12}.
- Describe good sources of protein and calories from the diet.
- Describe how to follow a low-fat diet and how to use MCT oil in cooking.

Patient Education—Foodborne Illness

- Careful food handling and hand washing are important to prevent introduction of foodborne pathogens to the individual.
- If home TF or CPN is needed, teach appropriate sanitation and food-handling procedures.

For More Information

- NIH—Tropical Sprue
  http://www.nlm.nih.gov/MEDLINEPLUS/ency/article/000275.htm
- Tropical Sprue
  http://www.intelihealth.com/IH/ihtIH/WSIHW000/9339/10902.html

TROPICAL SPRUE—CITED REFERENCES

Lo A, et al. Classification of villous atrophy with enhanced magnification endoscopy in patients with celiac disease and tropical sprue. *Gasdtrointest Endosc.* 66:377, 2007.

Nath SK. Tropical sprue. *Curr Gastroenterol Rep.* 7:343, 2005.

Ramakrishna BS. Tropical malabsorption. *Postgrad Med J.* 82:779, 2007.

Ritchie BK, et al. 13 C-sucrose breath test: novel use of a noninvasive biomarker of environmental gut health. *Pediatrics.* 124:620, 2009.

WHIPPLE'S DISEASE (INTESTINAL LIPODYSTROPHY)

NUTRITIONAL ACUITY RANKING: LEVEL 3–4

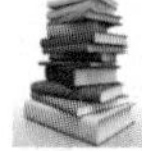

DEFINITIONS AND BACKGROUND

Whipple's disease is a chronic systemic inflammatory disease caused by *Tropheryma whipplei*. The hallmark of Whipple's disease is invasion of the intestinal mucosa with macrophages incompetent to degrade *T. whipplei* (Moos et al, 2010). This condition presents with weight loss, arthralgias, and diarrhea that involves infiltration of the small intestine with glycoprotein-laden macrophages in varying body tissues (Muller et al, 2005). Endocarditis and heart murmur are common. Infection may spread to the central nervous system, which may lead to loss of memory, confusion, or disturbed gait. Treatment is antibiotic therapy.

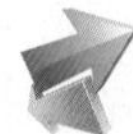

ASSESSMENT, MONITORING, AND EVALUATION

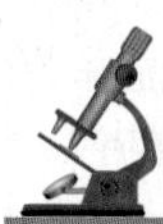

CLINICAL INDICATORS

Genetic Markers: Decreased production of Interleukin (IL)-12, IL-2 and Interferon (IFN)-g accompanied by an increased secretion of IL-4 may predispose patients for an infection with *T. whipplei* (Deriban and Marth, 2006).

Clinical/History

Height
Weight
BMI
Weight loss?
Wasting?
Diet history
Fever
I & O
Malabsorption, cholestasis
Gray to brown skin pigmentation
Lymphadenopathy
Confusion, memory loss
Edema?
Duodenal biopsy; villous blunting
Skin biopsy

Lab Work

Alk phos
Na^+, K^+
Ca^{++}, Mg^{++}
Alb (decreased)
CRP (elevated?)
Acid-Schiff (PAS)-positive foamy macrophages
T whipplei DNA—polymerase chain reaction (PCR) assays
H & H (decreased)
Serum Fe, ferritin
Transferrin

INTERVENTION

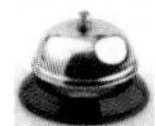

OBJECTIVES

- Reduce fever and inflammatory processes.
- Correct malnutrition and malabsorption.
- Correct anemia, iron overloading, or hypoproteinemia when present.
- Prevent or correct dehydration and electrolyte imbalances.

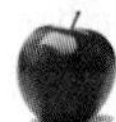

FOOD AND NUTRITION

- Use a high-protein/high-calorie diet appropriate for the patient's age and sex.
- Ensure that the diet includes sufficient vitamins and minerals, especially for vitamin D and calcium, when steatorrhea is a problem. Vitamins A, B-complex, and K may also be needed.
- Provide adequate fluid intake to reduce fever and replenish tissues.
- If edema is a problem, control excess sodium.

SAMPLE NUTRITION CARE PROCESS STEPS

Weight Loss

Assessment Data: I & O, weight loss, BMI, fever; low albumin, elevated CRP

Nutrition Diagnoses (PES): Involuntary weight loss (NC-3.2) related to fever and infection as evidenced by BMI below usual range and inflammatory process with elevated CRP.

Interventions: Offer frequent small meals and snacks with nutrient dense, calorie-rich foods. Educate about the role of nutrition in maintaining healthy immune system.

Monitoring and Evaluation: Weight gain back to usual weight; no further fever or weight loss. Maintain adequate hydration.

Common Drugs Used and Potential Side Effects

- Antibiotic treatment is mandatory and leads to a rapid clinical improvement and remission in most patients: 2-week parenteral cephalosporins followed by long-term therapy with trimethoprim-sulfamethoxazole. Trimethoprim-sulfamethoxazole (Bactrim) combinations may have numerous side effects; monitor closely for anorexia, nausea, vomiting, and diarrhea.

Herbs, Botanicals, and Supplements

- Use probiotic or prebiotic foods when possible to replenish "good" gut bacteria.
- Herbs and botanical supplements should not be used without discussing with the physician.

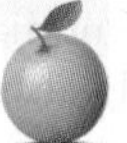

NUTRITION EDUCATION, COUNSELING, CARE MANAGEMENT

- Discuss inclusion of high-quality proteins in the diet. Frequent snacks may be beneficial if large meals are not tolerated.
- Provide lists for nutrient-dense foods rich in specific and needed nutrients (e.g., iron, calcium, etc).

Patient Education—Foodborne Illness

- Careful food handling and hand washing are important to prevent introduction of foodborne pathogens to the individual.
- If home TF or CPN is needed, teach appropriate sanitation and food-handling procedures.

For More Information

- NIH—Medline
  http://www.nlm.nih.gov/medlineplus/ency/article/000209.htm
- Whipple's Disease
  http://www.whipplesdisease.net/
- Whipple's Disease Info
  http://www.whipplesdisease.info/

WHIPPLE'S DISEASE—CITED REFERENCES

Deriban G, Marth T. Current concepts of immunopathogenesis, diagnosis and therapy in Whipple's disease. *Curr Med Chem.* 13:2921, 2006.

Moos V. Impaired immune functions of monocytes and macrophages in Whipple's disease [published online ahead of print 4 August 2009]. *Gastroenterology.* 138:210, 2010.

Muller SA, et al. Deadly carousel or difficult interpretation of new diagnostic tools for Whipple's disease: case report and review of the literature. *Infection.* 33:39, 2005.

Rectal Disorders

FECAL INCONTINENCE

NUTRITIONAL ACUITY RANKING: LEVEL 1

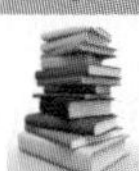

DEFINITIONS AND BACKGROUND

Fecal incontinence is the inability to control bowel movements, and stool may leak from the rectum unexpectedly. More than 5.5 million Americans have fecal incontinence, affecting both children and adults, especially seniors. Fecal incontinence is more common in women than in men (Novi and Mulvihill, 2005); see Table 7-26. Fecal incontinence affects up to 20% of community-dwelling adults and more than 50% of nursing home residents, and is one of the major risk factors for elderly persons in the nursing home (Leung and Rao, 2009).

Bowel training helps some people relearn how to control their bowels. In some cases, it involves strengthening muscles; in others, it means training the bowels to empty at a specific time of day. Biofeedback and sacral nerve stimulation may be useful in refractory patients and should be considered before colostomy (Leung and Rao, 2009; Jarrett et al, 2005). Biofeedback helps strengthen and coordinate the muscles. Kegel exercises may be used to strengthen the muscles in the pelvic floor, including those involved in controlling stool. This condition is often correlated with the presence of stroke and diabetes, or use of certain psychoactive medications (Quander et al, 2005). Treatment depends on the cause and severity of fecal incontinence; it may include dietary changes, medication, bowel training, and/or surgery. Surgery may be needed if fecal incontinence occurs in severe cases where injury has taken place. In patients with functional bowel disorders not responding to maximal medical treatment, bowel lavage or biofeedback therapy, can nowadays be treated by sacral nerve neuromodulation (Govaert et al, 2009).

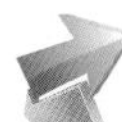

ASSESSMENT, MONITORING, AND EVALUATION

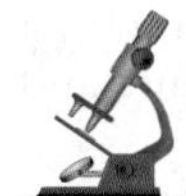

CLINICAL INDICATORS

Clinical/History		
Height	BMI	BP
Weight	Diet history	History of diarrhea
	I & O	

TABLE 7-26 Fecal Incontinence: Causes and Comments

Cause	Comments
Constipation	One of the most common causes of fecal incontinence, constipation causes large, hard stools to become lodged in the rectum. Watery stool can then leak out around the hardened stool. Constipation also causes the muscles of the rectum to stretch, which weakens the muscles so they cannot hold stool in the rectum long enough for a person to reach a bathroom. In children, early toilet training or some developmental disorders can cause or aggravate constipation. Consult the doctor for specific management techniques.
Damage to the anal sphincter muscles	Fecal incontinence can be caused by injury to one or both of the ring-like muscles at the end of the rectum called the anal internal and/or external sphincters. The sphincters keep stool inside. When damaged, the muscles are not strong enough to do their job, and stool can leak out. In women, the damage often happens when giving birth. The risk of injury is greatest if the doctor uses forceps to help deliver the baby or does an episiotomy, which is a cut in the vaginal area to prevent it from tearing during birth. Hemorrhoid surgery can damage the sphincters as well.
Damage to the nerves of the anal sphincter muscles or the rectum	Fecal incontinence can also be caused by damage to the nerves that control the anal sphincters or to the nerves that sense stool in the rectum. If the nerves that control the sphincters are injured, the muscle does not work properly, and incontinence can occur. If the sensory nerves are damaged, they do not sense that stool is in the rectum. The individual will not feel the need to use the bathroom until stool has leaked out. Nerve damage can be caused by childbirth, a long-term habit of straining to pass stool, stroke, and diseases that affect the nerves, such as diabetes and multiple sclerosis.
Loss of storage capacity in the rectum	Normally, the rectum stretches to hold stool until a person can get to a bathroom. But rectal surgery, radiation treatment, and inflammatory bowel disease can cause scarring that makes the walls of the rectum stiff and less elastic. The rectum then cannot stretch as much and cannot hold stool, and fecal incontinence results. Inflammatory bowel disease also can make rectal walls very irritated and thereby unable to contain stool.
Diarrhea	Diarrhea, or loose stool, is more difficult to control than solid stool that is formed. Even people who do not have fecal incontinence can have an accident when they have diarrhea.
Pelvic floor dysfunction	Abnormalities of the pelvic floor can lead to fecal incontinence. Examples of some abnormalities are decreased perception of rectal sensation, decreased anal canal pressures, decreased squeeze pressure of the anal canal, impaired anal sensation, a dropping down of the rectum (rectal prolapse), protrusion of the rectum through the vagina (rectocele), and/or generalized weakness and sagging of the pelvic floor. Often the cause of pelvic floor dysfunction is childbirth, and incontinence does not show up until the midforties or later (Bharucha et al, 2005).

Constipation	**Lab Work**	Stool (occult blood)
Anal manometry	H & H	Na^+, K^+
Anorectal ultrasonography	Serum Fe, ferritin	Ca^{++}, Mg^{++}
Proctography	BUN	
Proctosigmoidoscopy	Transferrin, TIBC	
Anal electromyography tests for nerve damage	PT	
	Alb, transthyretin	

INTERVENTION

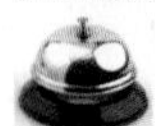

OBJECTIVES

- Timely assessment and intervention are needed to manage constipation and incontinence of stool. Maintain a food diary to determine when incontinence occurs and to identify changes that may be helpful.
- Establish a bowel training regimen to develop a regular pattern of bowel movements; some people train themselves to have bowel movements at specific times during the day, such as after every meal.
- Identify and treat underlying causes, such as diet- or medication-induced diarrhea, constipation, and fecal impaction (Leung and Rao, 2009).
- Prepare for surgery if needed.

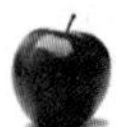

FOOD AND NUTRITION

- Daily intake of protein should be appropriate for age and sex. Calories should be calculated as 30–35 kcal/kg.
- Foods that may make the problem worse are drinks containing caffeine, such as coffee, tea, and chocolate, which relax the internal anal sphincter muscle. Other foods that have been implicated are cured or smoked meats such as sausage, ham, or turkey; spicy foods; alcohol; dairy products such as milk, cheese, and ice cream; fruits such as apples, peaches, or pears; fatty and greasy foods; sweeteners, such as sorbitol, xylitol, mannitol, and fructose, which are found in diet drinks, sugarless gum and candy, chocolate, and fruit juices.
- Serve smaller meals more frequently.
- Since liquid helps move food through the digestive system, drink half an hour before or after meals.
- Foods that contain soluble, digestible fiber slow the emptying of the bowels. Bananas, rice, tapioca, bread, potatoes, applesauce, cheese, smooth peanut butter, yogurt, pasta, and oatmeal may be helpful.
- High-fiber foods will add bulk and make stool easier to control. Fiber is found in fruits, vegetables, and grains. 20–30 g of fiber a day is needed; add it slowly.
- Too much fiber all at once can cause bloating, gas, or even diarrhea. If fiber intake makes diarrhea worse, cut back to two servings each of fruits and vegetables and remove skins and seeds. Increase fluid intake when fiber intake is increased to prevent fecal obstruction.

SAMPLE NUTRITION CARE PROCESS STEPS

Inadequate Physical Activity

Assessment Data: I & O, constipation and fecal incontinence, bedridden with no transfer from bed to chair; no walking.

Nutrition Diagnoses (PES): Inadequate physical activity related to nonambulatory status as evidenced by being bedridden for 5 months after hip replacement leading to fecal incontinence.

Interventions: Ensure adequate fluid and fiber intake; prune juice once daily as tolerated. Coordinate with physical therapy to enhance strengthening exercises; with nursing to offer bowel training.

Monitoring and Evaluation: Improvement in fecal continence; resident more compliant with bed exercises for strengthening lean body mass.

Common Drugs Used and Potential Side Effects

- If diarrhea is causing the incontinence, medication may help. Sometimes doctors recommend using bulk laxatives to help people develop a more regular bowel pattern. Antidiarrheal medicines, such as loperamide or diphenoxylate, may be used to slow down the bowel activity.
- Use of probiotic or prebiotic therapy is under study for this condition.

Herbs, Botanicals, and Supplements

- Herbs and botanical supplements should not be used without discussing with the physician.

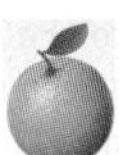

NUTRITION EDUCATION, COUNSELING, CARE MANAGEMENT

- The key to a successful bowel management program rests in tailoring the type of enema, medication, and diet to the specific type of colon (Bischoff et al, 2009).
- The skin around the anus is delicate and sensitive. Constipation and diarrhea or contact between skin and stool can cause pain or itching. To relieve discomfort, wash the area with water, but not soap, after a bowel movement; wash in the shower with lukewarm water or use a sitz bath. Premoistened, alcohol-free towelettes are a better choice than toilet paper. Let the area air dry after washing. Use a moisture-barrier cream. Wear loose clothing, absorbent pads and special undergarments (Leung and Rao, 2009).
- Ensure that the patient adequately exercises, rests, and maintains regular bowel habits.
- Indicate which foods are sources of fiber and other key nutrients in the diet. See Table 7-27.

TABLE 7-27 Fiber Content of Common Foods

Fruits	Amount	Grams of Fiber
Figs	2 dried	4.6
Pear	1 pear	4.0
Raspberries	1/2 cup	4.0
Strawberries, raw	1 cup, sliced	3.8
Apple, large with skin	1 apple	3.7
Apple, medium	1 apple	3.3
Prunes, dried	5 prunes	3.0
Orange	1 orange	3.1
Banana	1 banana	2.8
Tangerine	1 medium	1.9
Peach	1 medium	1.8
Peaches, canned	1/2 cup	1.3
Raisins	1 miniature box (14 g)	0.6
Vegetables		
Peas, split, cooked	1/2 cup	8.1
Lentils, cooked	1/2 cup`	7.8
Beans, kidney, canned	1/2 cup	4.5
Lima beans, cooked	1/2 cup	4.5
Black eyed peas	1/2 cup	4.0
Peas, green, canned	1/2 cup	3.5
Cauliflower	1 cup raw	2.5
Spinach, cooked	1/2 cup	2.2
Cabbage, raw	1 cup	2.0
Brussels sprouts	1/2 cup	2.0
Squash, acorn	1 cup raw	2.1
Carrots, raw	1/2 cup	1.8
Potatoes, boiled	1/2 cup	1.6
Zucchini, raw	1 cup	1.4
Broccoli, raw	1/2 cup	1.3
Celery, raw	1/2 cup	1.0
Lettuce, iceberg	1 cup shredded	0.8

Fruits	Amount	Grams of Fiber
Grains		
All Bran	1/2 cup	9.6
Raisin bran	1 cup	7.5
Shredded wheat	2 biscuits	5.0
Wheat bran flakes	3/4 cup	4.6
Rice, brown, cooked	1 cup	3.5
Total cereal	3/4 cup	3.4
Oatmeal, cooked	3/4 cup	3.0
Wheatena, cooked	1 packet	3.0
Oat bran muffin	One muffin	2.6
Bread, whole wheat	1 slice	1.9
Bread, whole grain (check label)	1 slice	1.7–2
Rye crisp wafer	1 wafer	1.7
Crackers, graham	2 squares	0.4
Bread, white wheat	1 slice	0.6
Other		
Nuts, mixed, dry roast	1 oz	2.6
Apple pie, sliced	1 slice	1.9
Chocolate cake, sliced	1 slice	1.8
Yellow cake, sliced	1 slice	0.2

Source: U.S. Department of Agriculture Nutrient Database for Standard Reference, Release 14 http://www.nal.usda.gov/fnic/foodcomp/Data/SR14/sr14.html, accessed September 1, 2009.

Patient Education—Foodborne Illness

- Careful food handling and hand washing are important to prevent introduction of foodborne pathogens to the individual.
- If home TF or CPN is needed, teach appropriate sanitation and food-handling procedures.

For More Information

- Mayo Clinic
  http://www.mayoclinic.com/health/fecal-incontinence/DS00477
- Medicine Net
  http://www.medicinenet.com/fecal_incontinence/article.htm
- NIDDK—Fecal incontinence
  http://digestive.niddk.nih.gov/ddiseases/pubs/fecalincontinence/

FECAL INCONTINENCE—CITED REFERENCES

Bharucha AE, et al. Relationship between symptoms and disordered continence mechanisms in women with idiopathic faecal incontinence. *Gut.* 54:546, 2005.

Bischoff A, et al. Treatment of fecal incontinence with a comprehensive bowel management program. *J Pediatr Surg.* 44:1278, 2009.

Govaert B, et al. Neuromodulation for functional bowel disorders. *Best Pract Res Clin Gastrointest.* 23:545, 2009.

Jarrett ME, et al. Sacral nerve stimulation for fecal incontinence following surgery for rectal prolapse repair: a multicenter study. *Dis Colon Rectum.* 48:1243, 2005.

Novi JM, Mulvihill BH. Fecal incontinence in women: a review of evaluation and management. *Obstet Gynecol Surv.* 60:261, 2005.

Quander CR, et al. Prevalence of and factors associated with fecal incontinence in a large community study of older individuals. *Am J Gastroenterol.* 100:905, 2005.

HEMORRHOIDS

NUTRITIONAL ACUITY RANKING: LEVEL 1

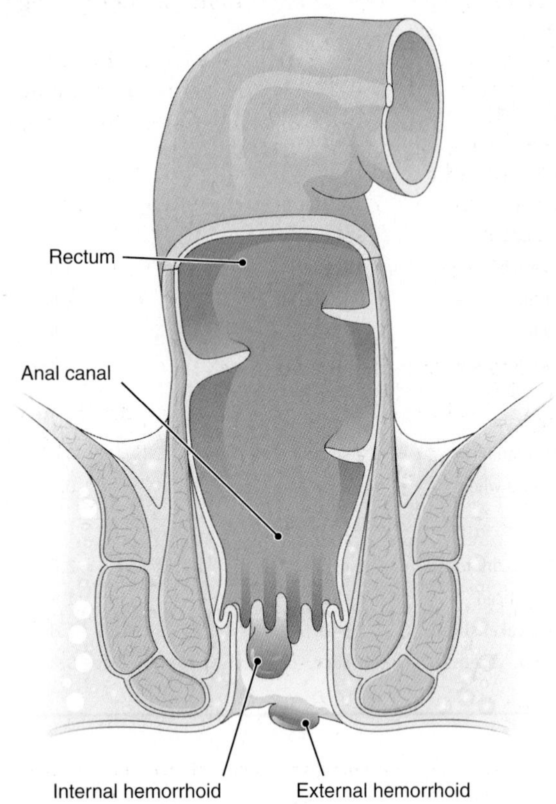

Adapted from: Thomas H. McConnell, *The Nature Of Disease Pathology for the Health Professions,* Philadelphia: Lippincott Williams & Wilkins, 2007.

DEFINITIONS AND BACKGROUND

Chronic constipation is believed to be the main cause of hemorrhoids. The disorder is common in Americans (50% of Americans older than 50 years of age will have suffered at least once, especially if obese). Causes include increased abdominal pressure secondary to straining during bowel movements, heavy lifting, childbirth, and benign prostatic hypertrophy.

Internal hemorrhoids are normal anatomical structures and rarely are painful (they may only bleed). External hemorrhoids are usually from excessive diarrhea or from constipation; they are tender, painful, bluish, localized swellings of varicose veins at the anal margin. Bleeding, pain, soiling, and prolapse are the classic symptoms in hemorrhoid disease (Johannsson et al, 2005). Although some patients fear that rectal bleeding signifies colorectal cancer, most patients with the primary diagnosis of symptomatic hemorrhoids do not need further investigative procedures (Tang et al, 2005).

Techniques that fix the cushions back in position can be performed in outpatients with reasonable success rates. Sclerotherapy—Used to treat varicose veins, in this procedure a chemical solution is injected into the vein, which causes the hemorrhoid to collapse. Surgery should be aimed at symptomatic hemorrhoids. Stapled hemorrhoidectomy is safe and effective for acute thrombosed hemorrhoids (Wong et al, 2009). Patients have reduced pain, shorter length of stay, and earlier return to work (Chung et al, 2005). Transanal hemorrhoidal dearterialization is also a potential treatment option for second-degree and third-degree hemorrhoids (Giordano et al, 2009).

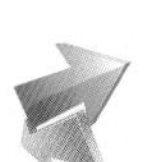

ASSESSMENT, MONITORING, AND EVALUATION

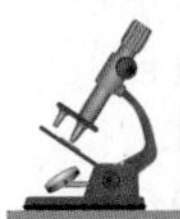

CLINICAL INDICATORS

Genetic Markers: Hemorrhoids are not likely to have a genetic origin.

Clinical/History

- Height
- Weight
- BMI
- Diet history
- I & O
- Anal itching
- Bright red blood on toilet tissue
- Pain during bowel movements
- One or more hard tender lumps near the anus
- Anoscope or sigmoidoscopy
- History of diarrhea
- Constipation

Lab Work

- H & H
- Serum Fe, ferritin
- BUN
- Transferrin, TIBC
- Alb, transthyretin
- Stool (occult blood)
- Na^+, K^+
- Ca^{++}, Mg^{++}

INTERVENTION

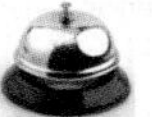

OBJECTIVES

- Provide comfort. Prevent prolapse and thrombosis.
- Avoid constipation, infection, and anemia.

SAMPLE NUTRITION CARE PROCESS STEPS

Inadequate Fiber Intake

Assessment Data: I & O and diet history revealing low fiber intake (<10 g daily).

Nutrition Diagnoses (PES): Inadequate fiber intake related to poor dietary intake as evidenced by recurrent hemorrhoids.

Interventions: Food and Nutrient Delivery—provide high fiber foods and extra fluids. Education—high fiber diet and how to assure adequate hydration; increasing physical activity such as walking.

Monitoring and Evaluation: Fewer complaints of hemorroids, straining during deification at stool, dry stool consistency.

- Reduce possible irritation from excessive amounts of fiber. Avoid irritants, such as laxatives.
- After surgery, reduce irritation while patient heals. Promote rapid healing. Prevent future recurrence.

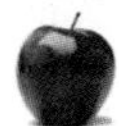

FOOD AND NUTRITION

- Diet should be low in fiber only when the patient is in pain. Otherwise, a high-fiber diet (25–35 g) should be used.
- Fluids should be increased to 8–10 glasses daily.
- After surgery, a low-fiber/soft diet should be used until full recovery occurs. Eventually, adequate fiber (25–35 g) should be taken.
- Omit lactose and highly seasoned foods only if not tolerated by the individual.

Common Drugs Used and Potential Side Effects

- Hemorrhoid creams with lidocaine, over-the-counter, can reduce pain.
- Laxatives and enemas may have caused faulty bowel function. Avoid use unless prescribed by the doctor.
- Troxerutin and carbazochrome are used as a combination therapy. Monitor for any untoward side effects.
- Lubrication with glycerin suppositories may help to reduce symptoms.
- Medicated suppositories such as Anusol HC (contains hydrocortisone) may help to decrease inflammation. Limit steroid-containing medications to less than 2 weeks of continuous use to avoid atrophy of anal tissues.
- Psyllium laxatives (Metamucil) can help with constipation; long-term use alters electrolytes. Flatulence or steatorrhea may occur.

Herbs, Botanicals, and Supplements

- Herbs and botanical supplements should not be used without discussing with the physician.
- Comfrey, plantain, butcher's broom, horse chestnut, and witch hazel have been recommended for this condition, but no clinical trials have proven efficacy.

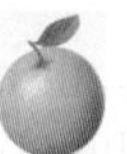

NUTRITION EDUCATION, COUNSELING, CARE MANAGEMENT

- Ensure that the patient adequately exercises, rests, and maintains regular bowel habits. Limit the time sitting on the toilet. Avoid straining.
- Teach the patient about the role of fiber in the diet.
- Persistent or recurrent bleeding requires medical attention, especially to monitor vitamin K, iron, and B-complex vitamin levels and to prevent additional losses.
- It is important to keep the anal skin area dry.
- Over-the-counter products may aggravate an allergic response.
- Warm sitz baths may help to reduce symptoms.

Patient Education—Foodborne Illness

- Careful food handling and hand washing are important to prevent introduction of foodborne pathogens to the individual.
- If home TF or CPN is needed, teach appropriate sanitation and food-handling procedures.

For More Information

- Ano-Rectal Algorithm
  http://www.uwgi.org/guidelines/ch_10/ch10.htm
- Hemorrhoids
  http://digestive.niddk.nih.gov/ddiseases/pubs/hemorrhoids/
- Web MD
  http://www.webmd.com/a-to-z-guides/hemorrhoids-topic-overview

HEMORRHOIDS—CITED REFERENCES

Chung CC, et al. Stapled hemorrhoidopexy vs. harmonic scalpel hemorrhoidectomy: a randomized trial. *Dis Colon Rectum.* 48:1213, 2005.

Giordano P, et al. Transanal hemorrhoidal dearterialization: a systematic review. *Dis Colon Rectum.* 52:1665, 2009.

Johannsson HO, et al. Bowel habits in hemorrhoid patients and normal subjects. *Am J Gastroenterol.* 100:401, 2005.

Tang T, et al. An approach to haemorrhoids. *Colorectal Dis.* 7:143, 2005.

Wong JC, et al. Stapled technique for acute thrombosed hemorrhoids: a randomized, controlled trial with long-term results. *Dis Colon Rectum.* 51:397, 2009.

PROCTITIS

NUTRITIONAL ACUITY RANKING: LEVEL 1

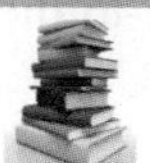

DEFINITIONS AND BACKGROUND

Proctitis is inflammation of the lining of the rectal mucosa and may be acute or chronic. Proctitis may be a side effect of medical treatments such as radiation therapy or antibiotics. It may also be caused by UC, rectal injury, bacterial infection, allergies, malfunction of the nerves in the rectum, Crohn's disease, or sexually transmitted diseases.

Proctitis is most common in UC patients at diagnosis, and younger patients are more likely than older patients to have extensive disease (Tarrant et al, 2008). For this form of proctitis, 5-aminosalicyclic acid (5-ASA) or corticosteroids may be applied directly to the area or taken in a pill form. Ileal pouch rectal anastomosis (IPRA) preserves bowel continuity and provides a good function (Kariv et al, 2009). There may also be a role for appendectomy in ulcerative proctitis (Bolin et al, 2009).

Antibiotics are used for proctitis caused by bacterial infection. Lymphogranuloma venereum (LGV) L2b proctitis may cause proctitis in HIV-positive men who have sex with men (MSM); doxycycline is the drug of choice (White, 2009).

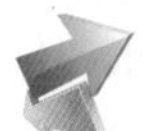

ASSESSMENT, MONITORING, AND EVALUATION

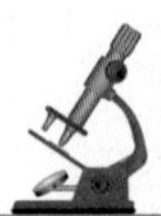

CLINICAL INDICATORS

Clinical/History		
Height	Frequent or continuous urge to defecate	Gluc
Weight	Constipation	BUN, Creat
BMI	Rectal fullness	Transferrin, TIBC
Diet history	Proctoscopy	Alb, transthyretin
I & O	Sigmoidoscopy	CRP
BP	**Lab Work**	Na^+, K^+
Bowel habits	Stool (occult blood)	Ca^{++}, Mg^{++}
Abdominal pain	HPV testing	Serum folate, vitamin B_{12}
Rectal bleeding	H & H	
Mucus in stool	Serum Fe, ferritin	
Left-sided abdominal pain		

SAMPLE NUTRITION CARE PROCESS STEPS

Inadequate Mineral (Iron) Intake

Assessment Data: I & O, abdominal pain, mucus and blood in stool, constipation, poor oral intake, medical diagnosis of anemia, labs indicative of anemia (low H & H, ferritin, Fe).

Nutrition Diagnoses (PES): Inadequate mineral (iron) intake related to blood loss and rectal bleeding in proctitis as evidenced by labs (low Fe, ferritin, H & H).

Interventions: Food and Nutrient Delivery—enhance food choices with iron-rich food choices. Educate about food choices that are rich in iron; discuss heme and nonheme sources. Counseling about use of medications and dietary changes that may be needed with abdominal pain.

Monitoring and Evaluation: Improvement in serum labs, less abdominal pain, fewer incidents of rectal bleeding.

INTERVENTION

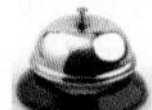

OBJECTIVES

- Manage symptoms and alleviate pain. Prepare for surgery if needed.
- Reduce inflammation and promote healing.
- Correct anemia from blood loss where present.

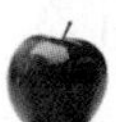

FOOD AND NUTRITION

- Diet therapy depends on the cause of proctitis. Identify appropriate etiology and review entries in this text for dietary management.
- Some patients find that avoidance of caffeine, red meat, dairy products, and artificial sweeteners can be beneficial.
- Use of omega-3 fatty acids may be helpful to reduce inflammation.

Common Drugs Used and Potential Side Effects

- Ulcerative proctitis patients with frequent relapses may need a longer duration of topical therapy. Prolonged oral mesalazine treatment period protects against the proximal spread of rectal inflammation (Pica et al, 2004).
- 5-ASA or corticosteroids may be needed if IBD is the cause. Monitor for numerous side effects.
- Antibiotics are the best treatment for proctitis caused by a specific bacterial infection. When proctitis is caused by use of an antibiotic that destroys normal intestinal bacteria, a doctor may prescribe metronidazole (Flagyl) or vancomycin (Vancocin), which should destroy the harmful bacteria.

Herbs, Botanicals, and Supplements

- Herbs and botanical supplements should not be used without discussing with the physician.

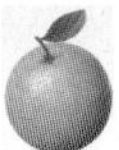

NUTRITION EDUCATION, COUNSELING, CARE MANAGEMENT

- Teach the patient about the role of fiber in the diet.
- It is important to keep the anal skin area dry. Over-the-counter products may aggravate an allergic response.

Patient Education—Foodborne Illness

- Careful food handling and hand washing are important to prevent introduction of foodborne pathogens to the individual.
- If home TF or CPN is needed, teach appropriate sanitation and food-handling procedures.

For More Information

- Ano-Rectal Algorithm
  http://www.uwgi.org/guidelines/ch_10/ch10.htm

- Mayo Clinic—Proctitis
  http://www.mayoclinic.com/health/proctitis/DS00705
- Proctitis
  http://digestive.niddk.nih.gov/ddiseases/pubs/proctitis/

PROCTITIS—CITED REFERENCES

Bolin TD, et al. Appendectomy as a Therapy for Ulcerative Proctitis [published online ahead of print 7 July 2009]. *Am J Gastroenterol.* 104:2476, 2009.

Kariv Y, et al. Ileal pouch rectal anastomosis: a viable alternative to permanent ileostomy in Crohn's proctocolitis patients. *J Am Coll Surg.* 208:390, 2009.

Pica R, et al. Oral mesalazine (5-ASA) treatment may protect against proximal extension of mucosal inflammation in ulcerative proctitis. *Inflamm Bowel Dis.* 10:731, 2004.

Tarrant KM, et al. Perianal disease predicts changes in Crohn's disease phenotype-results of a population-based study of inflammatory bowel disease phenotype. *Am J Gastroenterol.* 103:3082, 2008.

White JA. Manifestations and management of lymphogranuloma venereum. *Curr Opin Infect Dis.* 22:57, 2009.

S E C T I O N 8

Hepatic, Pancreatic, and Biliary Disorders

CHIEF ASSESSMENT FACTORS

Clinical Factors

- Abnormal Liver MRI, Ultrasound, or Biopsy
- Abdominal or Radiating Pain
- Anorexia, Malaise, Fatigue
- Ascites, Large Abdominal Girth, Pot Belly
- Brownish spots or blemishes on the skin
- Darkened urine
- Depression or mood swings
- Diabetes, Hyperglycemia, Hypoglycemia
- Diarrhea, Steatorrhea
- Edema in feet or ankles
- Encephalopathy?
- Flushed facial appearance
- Gastrointestinal (GI) Bleeding
- Hepatomegaly or Shrunken Liver (in cirrhosis)
- Itchy skin
- Hypoglycemia
- Jaundice
- Light colored stools
- Malnutrition, Subjective Global Assessment (SGA) Score
- Offensive body odor
- Red, swollen or itchy eyes
- Unusual Weight Loss or Gain
- Varices
- Vomiting, Nausea

Laboratory Assessment

A "liver panel" usually includes tests for alanine aminotransferase (ALT), aspartate aminotransferase (AST), bilirubin, and alkaline phosphatase. Liver Function is best measured by the prothrombin time (PT), international normalized ratio (INR) and albumin (see below).

- Bilirubin (total or indirect) is released from destroyed red blood cells and passed on to the liver where it is excreted through bile.
- Bleeding/clotting times: PT, INR measure how long it takes blood to form a clot in seconds; a normal PT/INR indicates that a normal amount of blood-clotting protein is available.

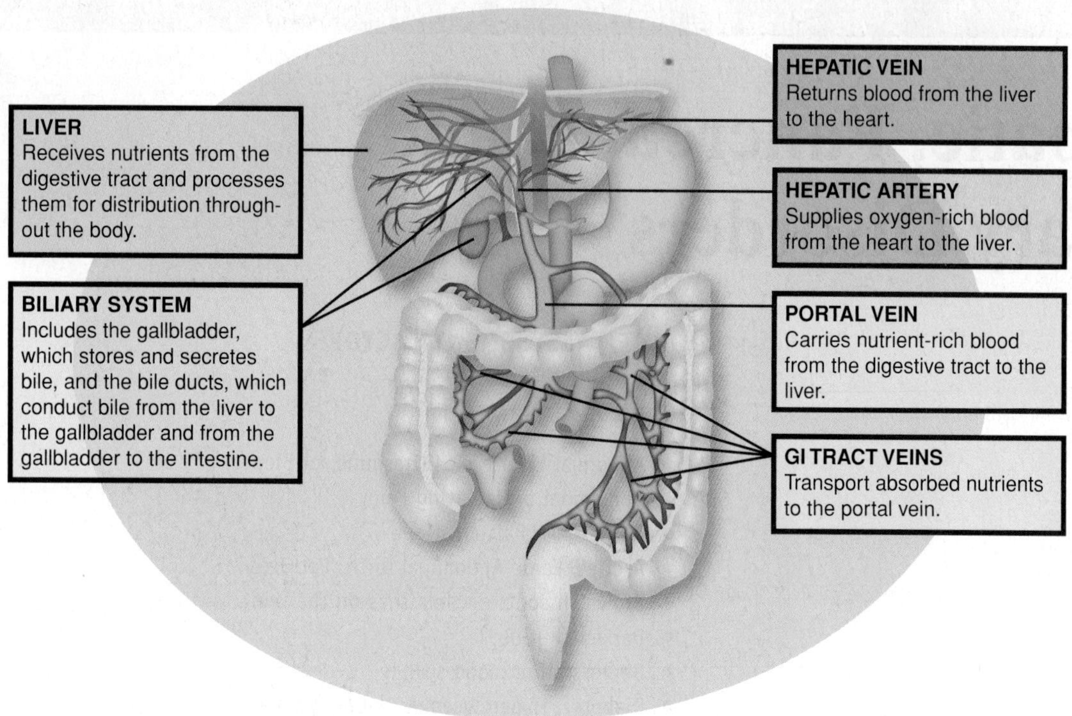
LIVER
Receives nutrients from the digestive tract and processes them for distribution throughout the body.
BILIARY SYSTEM
Includes the gallbladder, which stores and secretes bile, and the bile ducts, which conduct bile from the liver to the gallbladder and from the gallbladder to the intestine.
HEPATIC VEIN
Returns blood from the liver to the heart.
HEPATIC ARTERY
Supplies oxygen-rich blood from the heart to the liver.
PORTAL VEIN
Carries nutrient-rich blood from the digestive tract to the liver.
GI TRACT VEINS
Transport absorbed nutrients to the portal vein.

- Blood product transfusions.
- Cholestasis tests: Serum alkaline phosphatase (Alk Phos), Gamma-glutamyltransferase (GGT). High alk phos level occurs when there is a blockage of flow in the biliary tract or a buildup of pressure in the liver, often from a gallstone.
- Family history of liver diseases.
- Glucose levels: poorly controlled diabetes can lead to fatty liver.
- Intake of medications, vitamins, herbs, drugs, and alcohol.
- Liver enzymes: ALT (SGPT), AST (SGOT). The AST level is not as helpful as the ALT level for checking the liver.
- Neutrophils: role in inflammation, formation of pus, and destruction of bacteria; check ANC regularly while on interferon treatment. Total white blood cell (WBC) count includes neutrophils plus the four other types (eosinophils, basophils, monocytes, and lymphocytes).
- Pancreatic enzyme levels.
- Serum proteins: PT, INR, albumin, globulin, mitochondrial antibodies, antinuclear and smooth muscle antibodies. A normal INR is 1.0. Low levels of total protein (TP) may indicate impaired liver function.
- Serum ammonia.
- Subjective global assessment (SGA:) evaluation of protein-energy malnutrition (PEM) based on evidence of edema, ascites, muscle wasting, subcutaneous fat loss, decreased functional capacity, and GI symptoms of diarrhea, nausea, and vomiting.
- Specific markers: serum ferritin, ceruloplasmin, alpha-fetoprotein (tumor marker), alpha-1 antitrypsin.
- Thyroid tests: thyroid stimulating hormone (TSH) is produced by the pituitary gland in the brain and causes the thyroid gland to produce thyroid (T4 and T3). TSH may be high if using interferon treatments.
- Viral hepatitis tests (hepatitis A, B, and C serologies).

BACKGROUND: HEPATOBILIARY DISORDERS

Nutrition and the liver are interrelated since everything is refined and detoxified by the liver. The liver is the largest organ in the body, and it performs many complex and essential functions (see Table 8-1). As the body's internal chemical power plant, one cannot live without a liver. Mild elevations in liver chemistries such as ALT and AST can reveal serious underlying conditions, such as viral hepatitis, alcohol use, medication use, steatosis, fatty liver disease, nonalcoholic steatohepatitis (NASH), cirrhosis, or more chronic health conditions, such as diabetes, heart disease, or thyroid disease (Giboney, 2005). Serotonin is a mediator of several hepatic functions; in the diseased liver, it can promote hepatic fibrosis and steatohepatitis (Lesurtel et al, 2008).

Jaundice is a yellowish discoloration of the skin, mucous membranes, and some body fluids from accumulation of bile or bilirubin. Jaundice may be classified as *hemolytic* (from excessive red blood cell destruction), *hepatic* (from an immature liver or from damage), or *obstructive* (from obstructed biliary ducts or gallstones). In neonatal jaundice, there is a somewhat normal pattern of hyperbilirubinemia that is generally not detrimental. In obstructive jaundice, no bile pigment

TABLE 8-1 Liver, Gallbladder, and Pancreatic Functions

Liver

The largest single organ of the body; it is the central biochemical organ of the body. Functionally, it:

1. Converts galactose and fructose to glucose; makes glycogen; degrades glycogen upon demand.
2. Converts proteins into glucose; synthesizes albumin, globulin, fibrinogen, prothrombin, and transferrin; removes nitrogenous wastes (ammonia); provides transamination; synthesizes purines and pyrimidines; forms amines by decarboxylation.
3. Synthesizes triglycerides; forms very low-density lipoproteins (VLDLs); oxidizes fatty acids for energy and ketones.
4. Synthesizes cholesterol from acetate; makes high-density lipoproteins (HDLs).
5. Stores vitamins A, D, E, and K and some vitamin B_{12} and C.
6. Hydroxylates vitamin D for renal activation; activates folic acid to tetrahydrofolic acid (THFA).
7. Stores minerals (e.g., iron, copper, zinc, magnesium).
8. Detoxifies drugs.
9. Produces bile.

Gallbladder

Stores bile, which helps counteract stomach acidity and aids in fat digestion through emulsification.

Pancreas

1. Produces pancreatic juice when stimulated by secretin. Pancreatic juice contains bicarbonate, which helps neutralize acid chyme.
2. Secretes insulin and glucagon hormones.
3. Secretes metabolic/digestive enzymes involved in protein, carbohydrate, and fat metabolism. Pancreatic secretion has gastric, cephalic, and intestinal phases. The islets secrete insulin (b) and glucagon (a). The acini secrete lipase, amylase, trypsin, chymotrypsin, ribonuclease, and carboxypolypeptidase. The pancreas secretes enzymes (trypsin, lipase, and amylase) into the collecting duct as stimulated by cholecystokinin (also called pancreozymin), which is produced by the duodenum.

is present; stools become pale and clay colored, indicating fat maldigestion or malabsorption. Obstructive jaundice leads to bacterial translocation by disruption of the gut barrier, intestinal microecology, and impaired host immune defense. Anorexia is common in obstructive jaundice; biliary drainage improves appetite. Oral administration of an arginine, omega-3 fatty acids, glutamine, and an RNA-supplemented enteral diet for immunonutrition may be useful.

Nonalcoholic fatty liver disease is accumulation of fat in the liver of people who drink little or no alcohol. It may have only symptoms of fatigue, or it may progress to hepatosteatosis (NASH) or liver failure. NASH may occur in obese individuals and may have an inflammatory origin.

Oxidative stress contributes to hepatic cell damage when there is an excess of reactive species derived from oxygen (ROS) and nitrogen (RNS), or a defect of antioxidant molecules (Leung and Chan, 2009). This cell damage aggravates alcoholic liver disease, chronic viral hepatitis, autoimmune liver diseases and nonalcoholic steatohepatitis. Antioxidants in S-adenosylmethionine (SAMe), vitamin E, polyenylphosphatidylcholine, or silymarin have a protective effect on the liver and continue to be studied.

Malnutrition is often a problem in liver diseases. Oral nutritional supplements and tube feeding (TF) can be used to supplement intake when needed. TF improves nutritional status and liver function, reduces the rate of complications, and prolongs survival in cirrhosis and in acute liver failure (ALF). Long-term PN still promotes hepatobiliary dysfunction and steatosis and is used less often.

Use herbs and alternative therapies with caution. Use of glycyrrhizin, phyllanthin, silibinin, milk thistle, and sho-saiko to show merit. However, some herbs are hepatotoxic and should be avoided; this includes comfrey, chaparral, germander, and Chinese herbal mixtures.

BACKGROUND: PANCREATIC AND GALLBLADDER DISORDERS

In the United States, acute pancreatitis, chronic pancreatitis, and pancreatic cancer are the most common pancreatic disease states. Pancreatic cancer is responsible for nearly 30,000 deaths annually. Excessive consumption of alcohol is the major risk factor for pancreatic disease, and smoking causes pancreatic cancer (Lowenfels et al, 2005). To reduce the burden of pancreatic disease, focus on the control of three lifestyle factors: smoking, drinking, and obesity.

Bile is the greenish-yellow fluid made of bile salts and waste products such as bile pigments. Bile flows through small bile ducts inside the liver, then into the common bile duct outside of the liver. Some flows directly to the duodenum, and the rest is stored in the gallbladder. After a meal, the gallbladder releases some bile into the small intestine to help digest fats. Gallbladder disease is also strongly associated with obesity.

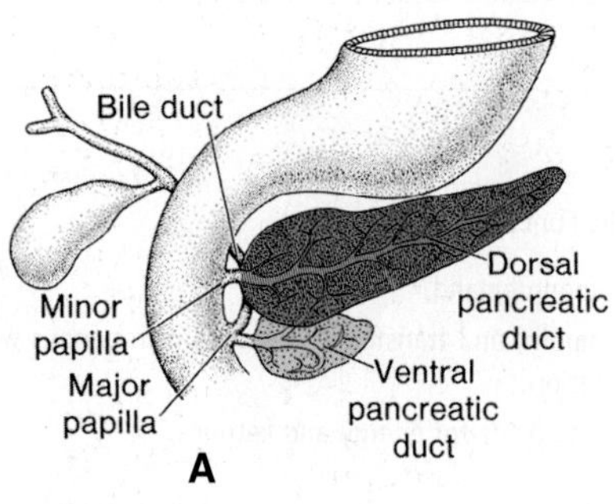

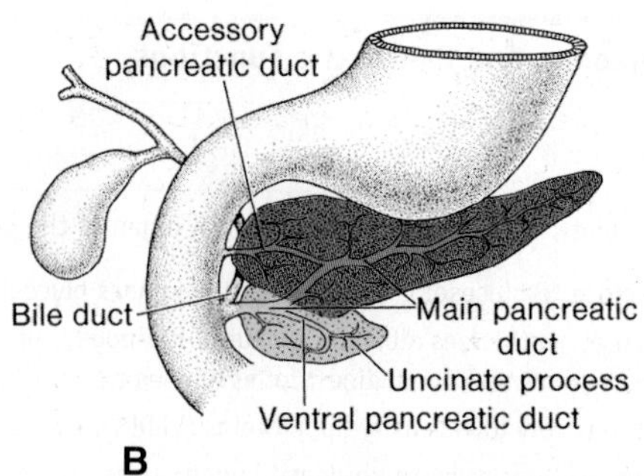

For More Information

- Abnormal Liver Function Test Algorithm
  http://www.uwgi.org/guidelines/ch_09/ch09txt.htm
- American Association for the Study of Liver Diseases
  http://www.aasld.org/
- American Liver Foundation
  http://www.liverfoundation.org/
- Centers for Disease Control and Prevention (CDC)—Fast Statistics
  http://www. cdc.gov/nchs/fastats/liverdis.htm
- National Digestive Diseases Information Clearinghouse
  http://digestive.niddk.nih.gov/

CITED REFERENCES

Giboney PT. Mildly elevated liver transaminase levels in the asymptomatic patient. *Am Fam Physician.* 1:1105, 2005.

Lesurtel M, et al. Role of serotonin in the hepato-gastroIntestinal tract: an old molecule for new perspectives. *Cell Mol Life Sci.* 65:940, 2008.

Leung PS, Chan YC. Role of oxidative stress in pancreatic inflammation. *Antioxid Redox Signal.* 11:135, 2009.

Lowenfels AB, et al. The epidemiology and impact of pancreatic diseases in the United States. *Curr Gastroenterol Rep.* 7:90, 2005.

LIVER DISORDERS

ALCOHOLIC LIVER DISEASE

NUTRITIONAL ACUITY RANKING: LEVEL 3

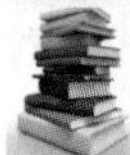

DEFINITIONS AND BACKGROUND

Alcohol is a hepatotoxin and is ulcerogenic, especially to the esophagus and other organs. Alcohol cannot be stored and is used preferentially over other energy fuels.

Alcoholic liver disease (ALD) is a major cause of illness and death. ALD affects about 2 million people in the United States. Signs and symptoms of alcoholism include restlessness, agitation, spider angiomas on the face or back or belly, insomnia, anorexia, weight loss, GI cramping, malnutrition, delirium tremens, and hand tremors. In men, altered hair distribution and gynecomastia may occur. Understanding alcohol addiction is key to treating ALD, since abstinence leads to improvement in all forms of alcoholic liver damage (Lucey, 2009). Section 4 addresses alcohol addiction. Table 8-2 lists stages and effects of alcoholism. Given the benefit of drug treatment, it is important to identify patients at risk of early mortality from alcoholic hepatitis using tools such as the Maddrey Discriminant Function, the Model of End-Stage Liver Disease score, and the Glasgow Alcoholic Hepatitis score (Maher, 2007).

Alcoholics may replace as much as one third of their daily energy requirements from alcohol. As a result, they are malnourished. Either they eat poorly or alcohol metabolism prevents them from properly absorbing, digesting, and using nutrients, particularly vitamin A (Plauth et al, 2006). Classic effects of malnutrition from alcoholism include Wernicke's encephalopathy, Korsakoff's psychosis, muscle wasting, weight loss, and liver disease.

Most tissues of the body contain enzymes capable of ethanol metabolism, but significant activity occurs only in

TABLE 8-2 Stages of Alcoholism-Related Effects

Stage	Condition	Effects
I.	Fatty liver (steatosis)	Reversible. Acetaldehyde promotes hepatic fat accumulation. Hepatomegaly, hypertriglyceridemia, hypoalbuminemia, cytochrome P-450 2E1 induction, free radical generation, lipid peroxidation, and increased transcription of proinflammatory mediators, including TNF-alpha, occur.
II.	Alcholic hepatitis	Fibrosis begins. Fever with tachycardia; liver enlargement is mild, and tenderness can occur.
III.	Cirrhosis	Not reversible. Diffuse necrosis and regeneration of fibrous tissue leading to loss of normal hepatic function.
IV.	Encephalopathy or Coma	May lead to death if not treated. Impaired mentation, altered neuromuscular function, and altered consciousness.

the liver and stomach (Lieber, 2005). Alcohol dehydrogenase is made with zinc. Alcohol decreases absorption of fats, fat-soluble vitamins, thiamin, folic acid, vitamin B_{12}, and zinc. Nicotine adenine dinucleotide (NADH) is significant in alcohol metabolism by reduction of pyruvate and promotion of steatosis.

Adequate nutrition is critical and should be provided by TF if necessary (Maher, 2007). A prompt decline in serum bilirubin within 1 week indicates a favorable response to therapy; nonresponders have a 6-month mortality rate of 50% or higher (Maher, 2007).

Plasma homocysteine levels are altered in actively drinking patients, causing brain atrophy and withdrawal seizures (Bleich et al, 2005). Methionine needs to be activated to S-adenosylmethionine (SAM); this metabolism is impaired in liver disease. Folate deficiency accentuates abnormal methionine metabolism, lipid oxidation, and liver injury (Halsted et al, 2002; Schalinske and Nieman, 2005). SAM, betaine, and folate decrease oxidative stress by upregulation of glutathione and interleukin-10 and downregulation of tumor necrosis factor-alpha, TNF-a (Purohit et al, 2008). No benefit has been found in randomized, placebo-controlled clinical trials of colchicine, S-adenosylmethionine (SAMe), or phosphatidylcholine (Lucey, 2009). Betaine may attenuate ALD by increasing synthesis of SAM and glutathione, decreasing homocysteine (tHcy) levels (Song et al, 2008). More research is indicated.

Alcohol-induced liver injury is an immunological response of the liver; neutrophils damage liver cells through cytotoxicity (Leevy and Elbeshbeshy, 2005). Men and women metabolize alcohol differently. It takes less time and lower doses of alcohol exposure to cause liver damage in females than in males. Community-dwelling heavy drinkers who are not in alcoholism treatment have dose-related gray matter volume losses (Cardenas et al, 2005).

Treatment strategies for ALD include lifestyle changes for abstinence from alcohol consumption. Nutrition therapy and medications are also important. Serious alcoholic hepatitis has a mortality record of up to 50%. If necessary liver transplantation may be life-saving.

ASSESSMENT, MONITORING, AND EVALUATION

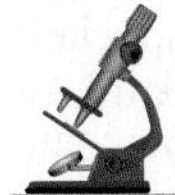

CLINICAL INDICATORS

Genetic Markers: The dopamine (DR2) receptor promotes effects of alcohol. People with a genetic deficit of beta-endorphin peptide are susceptible (Manzardo et al, 2005; Zalewska-Kaszubska and Czarnecka, 2005). The dopaminergic mesolimbic system activates the endogenous mu and delta opioid receptors; mu receptor polymorphisms may be associated with ethanol dependence (Job et al, 2007). Polymorphisms in cytochrome P450 2E1 (CYP2E1), the major microsomal ethanol metabolizing enzyme, can alter detoxification of alcohol by glutathione-S-transferases M1 (GSTM1) and gamma-aminobutyric acid receptor gamma2 (Khan et al, 2009).

Clinical/History

- Height
- Weight
- Body mass index (BMI)
- Usual body weight (UBW)
- Diet history
- Blood pressure (BP)
- Intake and output (I & O)
- Food intolerances, taste aversions
- Anorexia, nausea, vomiting, diarrhea
- Scurvy—ecchymoses, hemorrhagic gingivitis, perifollicular hemorrhages
- Leg edema, poor wound healing
- CT scan or ultrasound of abdomen
- Liver biopsy
- Ascites (mild, moderate, or severe)
- Fatigue
- CAGE test (Cut down, Annoyed, Guilty, Eye opener)
- Alcohol Use Disorders Identification Test (AUDIT)
- Dual-energy x-ray absorptiometry (DEXA) bone scan

Lab Work

- Glucose (increased or decreased)
- Glucose tolerance test (sensitive and reliable)
- AST (increased)
- ALT (normal or only mildly elevated)
- INR
- Bilirubin (often elevated)
- Serum ammonia (may be elevated)
- Blood urea nitrogen (BUN) (low?)
- Albumin or transthyretin (low?)
- C-reactive protein (CRP)
- Triglycerides (increased?)
- Cholesterol (increased or decreased)
- WBC count
- Serum B_{12} and folate
- Plasma homocysteine (high?)
- Na^+ (hyponatremia?)
- K^+
- Hemoglobin and hematocrit (decreased)
- Serum Fe, ferritin
- Transferrin
- Uric acid (UA, increased)
- Globulin
- Alk phos (mildly elevated)
- Mg^{++} (decreased)
- Ca^{++}
- Serum phosphorus (decreased)

INTERVENTION

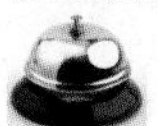

OBJECTIVES

- Remove alcohol to allow the disabled liver to function more effectively while protecting it from metabolic stress. Avoid alcohol in miscellaneous products, such as vinegar, sauces, and cough syrup.
- Improve health of liver so it can synthesize albumin and other serum proteins. Help liver tissue regenerate; replenish plasma proteins that are lost. Improve skeletal muscle synthesis.
- Prevent hypoglycemia from blocked gluconeogenesis. Correct metabolic syndrome, hyperglycemia, hypertension, or hypertriglyceridemia.
- Repair damage from fatty liver and diminished bile salt synthesis.
- Repair neural damage from malnutrition and malabsorption.

SAMPLE NUTRITION CARE PROCESS STEPS

Excessive Alcohol Intake

Assessment Data: Dietary intake records; low protein and energy intake for age/gender. Intake of one fifth of vodka per day to the exclusion of most meals.

Nutrition Diagnosis (PES): Excessive alcohol intake >25–30 g/d related to daily consumption above this level as evidenced by alcohol-induced liver injury, elevated LFTs and ascites.

Intervention:

Food and Nutrient Delivery: ND 1.1 General Healthful diet (avoid alcohol); ND 3.1.4 Modified food—increased calorie/protein intake.

Education: E 1.3 Survival Information. Educate about nutrient-dense foods and the role that alcohol plays in liver damage. E-1.1 Present concise and clear educational material with nutritional tips for patients with liver disease.

Counseling: C 2.5 Social support—avoid social outings with alcohol present.

Coordination of Care: RC 1.4 Referral to community agencies/programs. RC-1.3 Refer to social worker for alcohol rehabilitation. C-2.9 Relapse prevention by explaining the pros of following diet and medications as recommended, as the importance of maintain sober.

Monitoring and Evaluation: Track food intake through food diary or history. Coordinate care for rehabilitation program. Follow-up on intake of energy, protein and nutrients after omission of alcohol.

- Correct fluid and electrolyte imbalances, nutritional deficits such as iron deficiency anemia from chronic blood loss in varices, ulcers, and vomiting.
- Be honest and direct in approach. Gently confront conflicting information when stated by the patient.

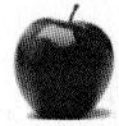

FOOD AND NUTRITION

- Avoid alcohol to allow the liver to begin heal (DiCecco and Francisco-Ziller, 2006).
- Malnourished alcoholics should consume a diet rich in carbohydrate and protein, preferentially via the oral or enteral route. Provide protein as 1.5 g/kg body weight if malnourished. Plan sufficient carbohydrates and fat to spare protein, but monitor for hyperglycemia or dyslipidemia.
- In hypertensive patients, a Dietary Approaches to Stop Hypertension (DASH) diet may be planned that provides a sufficient mixture of nutrients without excessive kilocalories. All fasting or very low–calorie diets should be avoided.
- Include a mix of fat from omega-3 (fish oils), omega-6 fatty acids, and medium-chain fatty acids.
- Micronutrient deficiencies require supplementation. Supplement the diet with B-complex vitamins, but supplemental vitamins A and D may not be well tolerated. Oral diet should provide adequate amounts of vitamins C, E, and K, phosphorus, potassium, selenium, magnesium, zinc, and calcium.
- Provide small frequent meals to prevent hypoglycemia, resulting from limited glycogen storage.
- Monitor iron intake to avoid excesses from diet or supplements, especially if there is the possibility of iron storage disease.
- Make meals appealing to stimulate the appetite.
- If TF is needed, avoid glutamine-enriched formulas which may increase ammonia levels.

Common Drugs Used and Potential Side Effects

- Corticosteroids have become the standard of care in patients with severe alcoholic hepatitis (Lucey, 2009). Methylprednisolone improves the ability to produce albumin and to normalize PT and bilirubin levels. Side effects may include negative nitrogen balance, hypocalemia, or hyperglycemia.
- Pharmacotherapy for alcoholism with naltrexone, acamprosate, topiramate, and baclofen is exciting (Lucey, 2009). Naltrexone is more effective in some individuals than in others (Rubio et al, 2005).
- Disulfiram (Antabuse) is given with patient's consent. It causes the patient to vomit after ingesting alcohol and can be dangerous.
- Beta-blockers (propranolol, nadolol) or octreotide (Sandostatin) may be used to reduce portal hypertension when varices occur.
- Insulin may be necessary; do not mix with alcohol. Alcohol intake may cause severe hypoglycemia in patients taking insulin (Pedersen-Bjergaard et al, 2005). Metformin should be avoided in patients with liver disease.

Herbs, Botanicals, and Supplements

- Antioxidants are increasingly used. Agents involved in methionine metabolism such as SAM and betaine have shown efficacy in liver disease. Milk thistle (*Silybum marianum*) may have some therapeutic effect as well. *Curcuma longa* (turmeric) and *Glycyrrhiza glabra* (licorice) are being evaluated. Tea polyphenols, especially green tea, may alleviate liver damage (Zhang et al, 2005).
- Herbs and botanical supplements should not be used without discussing with the physician. Chaparral is especially toxic to the liver and should be avoided; severe hepatitis or liver failure may result. Aloe vera should be avoided orally.

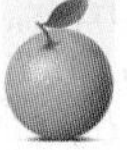

NUTRITION EDUCATION, COUNSELING, CARE MANAGEMENT

- Instruct patient on the sources of necessary nutrients in the diet and use of the prescribed multivitamins. Help patient in the planning and preparing of appetizing, nutrient-dense meals.
- Explain that alcohol is metabolized readily by the liver but cannot be used for muscular activity or energy production. Chemical addiction is a disease; self-help programs and follow-up can reduce dependency.
- General multivitamin–mineral supplementation may improve a poor appetite.

- Obesity, diabetes, and hyperinsulinemia play a role in the development of hepatic steatosis; weight loss remains a critical part of protecting the liver against damage.
- Identify sources of assistance for persons who need help with meal preparation or with access to meals.

Patient Education—Foodborne Illness

- If home TF is needed, teach appropriate sanitation and food-handling procedures.

For More Information

- Alcoholics Anonymous (AA) World Services http://www.alcoholics-anonymous.org/
- Alcoholic Hepatitis http://www.emedicine.com/med/topic101.htm
- International Society for Biomedical Research on Alcoholism http://www.isbra.com/
- National Council on Alcoholism and Drug Dependence http://www.ncadd.org/
- National Institute on Alcohol Abuse and Alcoholism (NIAAA) http://www.niaaa.nih.gov/
- International Research Society on Alcoholism http://www.rsoa.org/
- Substance Abuse and Mental Health Administration (DHHS) http://www.samhsa.gov/

ALCOHOLIC LIVER DISEASE—CITED REFERENCES

Bleich S, et al. Evidence of increased homocysteine levels in alcoholism: the Franconian Alcoholism Research Studies (FARS). *Alcohol Clin Exp Res.* 29:334, 2005.

Cardenas VA, et al. Chronic active heavy drinking and family history of problem drinking modulate regional brain tissue volumes. *Psychiatry Res.* 138: 115, 2005.

DiCecco SR, Francisco-Ziller N. Nutrition in alcoholic liver disease. *Nutr Clin Pract.* 21:245, 2006.

Halsted CH, et al. Folate deficiency, methionine metabolism, and alcoholic liver disease. *Alcohol.* 27:169, 2002.

Job MO, et al. Mu (mu) opioid receptor regulation of ethanol-induced dopamine response in the ventral striatum: evidence of genotype specific sexual dimorphic epistasis. *Biol Psychiatry.* 62:627, 2007.

Khan AJ, et al. Polymorphism in cytochrome P450 2E1 and interaction with other genetic risk factors and susceptibility to alcoholic liver cirrhosis. *Mutat Res.* 664:55, 2009.

Leevy CB, Elbeshbeshy HA. Immunology of alcoholic liver disease. *Clin Liver Dis.* 9:55, 2005.

Lieber CS. Metabolism of alcohol. *Clin Liver Dis.* 9:1, 2005.

Lucey MR. Management of alcoholic liver disease. *Clin Liver Dis.* 13:267, 2009.

Maher JJ. Alcoholic steatohepatitis: management and prognosis. *Curr Gastroenterol Rep.* 9:39, 2007.

Manzardo AM, et al. Developmental differences in childhood motor coordination predict adult alcohol dependence: proposed role for the cerebellum in alcoholism. *Alcohol Clin Exp Res.* 29:353, 2005.

Pedersen-Bjergaard U, et al. Psychoactive drugs, alcohol, and severe hypoglycemia in insulin-treated diabetes: analysis of 141 cases. *Am J Med.* 118: 307, 2005.

Plauth M, et al. ESPEN Guidelines on Enteral Nutrition: liver disease. *Clin Nutr.* 25:285, 2006.

Purohit V, et al. Role of S-adenosylmethionine, folate, and betaine in the treatment of alcoholic liver disease: summary of a symposium. *Am J Clin Nutr.* 86:14, 2008.

Rubio G, et al. Clinical predictors of response to naltrexone in alcoholic patients: who benefits most from treatment with naltrexone? *Alcohol.* 40: 227, 2005.

Schalinske KL, Nieman KM. Disruption of methyl group metabolism by ethanol. *Nutr Rev.* 63:387, 2005.

Song Z, et al. Inhibition of adiponectin production by homocysteine: a potential mechanism for alcoholic liver disease. *Hepatology.* 47:867, 2008.

Zalewska-Kaszubska J, Czarnecka E. Deficit in beta-endorphin peptide and tendency to alcohol abuse. *Peptides.* 26:701, 2005.

Zhang Y, et al. Effect of tea polyphenols on alcoholic liver injury. *Zhonghua Gan Zang Bing Za Zhi.* 13:125, 2005.

ASCITES AND CHYLOUS ASCITES

NUTRITIONAL ACUITY RANKING: LEVEL 2

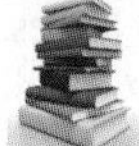

DEFINITIONS AND BACKGROUND

Ascites is defined as a distended abdomen due to pathological fluid in the peritoneal cavity. The development of ascites indicates a pathological imbalance between the production and resorption of intraperitoneal fluid; appearance and composition vary based on the underlying pathophysiology (Rochling and Zetterman, 2009). Ascites develops in decompensated cirrhosis, cardiac failure, or renal insufficiency. Portal hypertensive gastropathy (PHG) causes upper gastrointestinal bleeding in advanced cases. Liver transplantation may be the only way to improve survival in refractory ascites (Sandhu and Sanyal, 2005).

Although weight is not used for nutritional assessment here, it does help determine fluid balance. The goal of diuretic therapy in ascites is to promote weight loss of 1–3 kg/d. Nutrient depletion can occur if left untreated; fat, proteins, fat-soluble vitamins, and electrolytes may be lost. An oral diet devoid of long-chain triglycerides (LCTs) but that includes medium-chain triglycerides (MCTs) may be used in mild cases.

Management of ascites from decompensated liver disease focus on low-sodium diets and diuretics, supplemented by paracentesis or transvenous intrahepatic portosystemic shunts (Rochling and Zetterman, 2009). While paracentesis improves patient comfort and reduces intra-abdominal pressure and secondary renal dysfunction, it also carries risk for spontaneous bacterial peritonitis (SBP) or renal failure (Sargent, 2006). Bacterial contamination of ascites fluid leading to SBP is caused by bacterial translocation with subsequent bacteremia; proton pump inhibitors (PPIs) suppress gastric acid secretion, and possibly should be avoided in this population (Bajaj et al, 2009).

Chylous ascites is a rare form of ascites, resulting from increased hydrostatic pressure and lymphatic blockade. Accumulation of LCT-dense chyle occurs in the peritoneum. Chyle leaks are a rare complication following abdominal surgery, trauma, cancer, or fistula. Although the incidence of chyle leak post surgery is low (1–4%), this complication can present significant challenges (Smoke and Delegge, 2008). Any source of large fluid volume losses, lymph vessel obstruction, or leakage may cause chylous effusions in the peritoneal cavities. Most chylous effusions heal spontaneously. Early introduction of enteral feeding may encourage chyle leaks (Malik et al, 2007), whereas total parenteral nutrition along with somatostatin can relieve the symptoms rapidly (Huang et al, 2004).

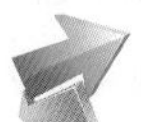

ASSESSMENT, MONITORING, AND EVALUATION

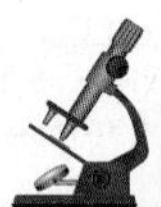

CLINICAL INDICATORS

Genetic Markers: No specific genetic causes are clear in cases of ascites.

Clinical/History	Lab Work	
Height	Serum ascites-albumin gradient (>1.1 g/dL = portal hypertension)	ALT
Weight	Alb (decreased)	AST
Dry weight or estimated dry weight	Transthyretin	H & H (high in hemochromatosis)
BMI	CRP	Serum Fe, ferritin
Diet history	Na^+, K^+	TIBC,% saturation
BP	Ca^{++}, Mg^{++}	Gluc
I & O	BUN, creatinine (Creat)	Chol
Temperature		Trig
Ascites, mild to severe		
Ultrasonography		

INTERVENTION

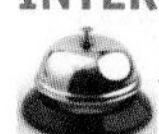

OBJECTIVES

- Reduce fluid retention, usually by diuretics. Mild ascites may present with fluid excess of 3–5 kg; moderate ascites may present with excess of 7–9 kg; and severe ascites may present with excess of 14–15 kg above usual weight.
- Prevent electrolyte imbalances.

SAMPLE NUTRITION CARE PROCESS STEPS

Excessive Sodium Intake-Ascites

Assessment Data: Dietary intake records.

Nutrition Diagnosis (PES): Excessive sodium intake related to presence of ascites and portal hypertension as evidenced by paracentesis of 7–8 kg over 24 hours.

Intervention: Food and Nutrient Delivery—manage sodium intake. Educate about sodium sources and requirements. Counsel about preferred foods that are high in sodium and ways to alter intake that are acceptable; how to shop, dine out, travel.

Monitoring and Evaluation: Track food intake through food diary. Follow-up on intake of sodium and alleviation of ascites.

- Prevent further pain, fatigue, loss of lean body mass (LBM), and anorexia.
- If possible, prevent hepatorenal syndrome, which can occur in patients with severe liver disease. If severe, it may require transplantation. Prepare for surgery, especially nutritionally (Hasse, 2006).
- Individualize diet as needs change.
- For **chylous ascites**, treat the underlying cause to decrease production of the chylous fluid. Malnutrition is a common result if left untreated; essential fatty acid deficiency must be avoided. Fluid and electrolyte replacement may be needed.

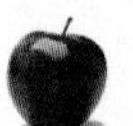

FOOD AND NUTRITION

- Energy needs are often as high as 1.5 times normal, and protein needs are often 1.5 g/kg of body weight (Hasse and Matarese, 2008). Smaller, more frequent meals are often better tolerated.
- If TF or central parenteral nutrition (CPN) is needed, use nutrient-dense formula but not glutamine-enriched formula; glutamine may increase ammonia production. While no high-quality data are available to prove that enteral nutrition is of benefit (Koretz, 2007), malnutrition should be addressed.
- Ensure that intake of vitamins and minerals is adequate. Water-soluble forms of vitamins may be needed; zinc and magnesium may be needed since levels are often low after diuretic therapy (Hasse and Matarese, 2008). Monitor for signs of malnutrition.
- Fluid restriction may be necessary (1–1.5 L/d), with two thirds with meals and one third for thirst/medicines.
- Restrict patient's intake of sodium to 2 g/d (Hasse and Matarese, 2008).
- Often, patients take spironolactone (Aldactone) or have renal insufficiency, which may increase potassium retention. Diet should be altered in potassium if serum levels so indicate. Other diuretics may cause potassium losses.
- For **chylous ascites**, a low-fat diet or enteral feeding is needed with MCTs as the preferred fat source; the addition of essential fatty acids (EFAs) will be needed. Adequate protein and calories are also needed since there may be significant losses. If oral diet fails, CPN may be needed (Assumpcao et al, 2008). Water-miscible forms of fat-soluble vitamins may be needed, along with extra fluid and electrolytes.

Common Drugs Used and Potential Side Effects

- Diuretics are the most important treatment (Rosner et al, 2006). Furosemide (Lasix) is not very effective. Check whether the specific drug retains or spares potassium; spironolactone spares potassium.
- Albumin replacement, while costly, may help to maintain oncotic pressure.
- Somatostatin analogs have been demonstrated to be effective (Huang et al, 2004).
- With bacterial peritonitis, antibiotic therapy is needed. Monitor for specific side effects. PPIs increase enteric bacterial colonization, overgrowth, and translocation (Campbell et al, 2008).

Herbs, Botanicals, and Supplements

- Herbs and botanical supplements should not be used without discussing with physician.
- Milk thistle may have some therapeutic effects in liver disease, but no controlled trials have shown efficacy for ascites at this time.

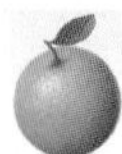

NUTRITION EDUCATION, COUNSELING, CARE MANAGEMENT

- Instruct patient concerning good sources of key nutrients to include and which nutrients to limit. Instruct patient to follow high-energy, high-protein diet to prevent wasting.
- Ensure that the patient follows a 2-g, low-sodium diet. Explain which foods have hidden sources of sodium, and share recipes if needed.
- For chylous ascites, treatment is generally managed through a hospital stay.

Patient Education—Foodborne Illness

- If home TF is needed, teach appropriate sanitation and food-handling procedures.

For More Information

- Ascites
  http://www.nlm.nih.gov/medlineplus/ency/article/000286.htm
- Chylous Ascites
  http://emedicine.medscape.com/article/185777-overview
- Medicine Net
  http://www.medicinenet.com/ascites/article.htm

ASCITES AND CHYLOUS ASCITES—CITED REFERENCES

Assumpcao L, et al. Incidence and management of chyle leaks following pancreatic resection: a high volume single-center institutional experience. *J Gastronintest Surg.* 12:1915, 2008.

Bajaj JS, et al. Association of proton pump inhibitor therapy with spontaneous bacterial peritonitis in cirrhotic patients with ascites. *Am J Gastroenterol.* 104:1130, 2009.

Campbell MS, et al. Association between proton pump inhibitor use and spontaneous bacterial peritonitis. *Dig Dis Sci.* 53:394, 2008.

Hasse J, Matarese L. Medical nutrition therapy for liver, biliary system, and exocrine pancreas disorders. In: Mahan L, Escott-Stump S, eds. *Krause's food nutrition and diet therapy.* 12th ed. St Louis: Elsevier, 2008.

Hasse JM. Examining the role of tube feeding after liver transplantation. *Nutr Clin Pract.* 21:299, 2006.

Huang Q, et al. Chylous ascites: treated with total parenteral nutrition and somatostatin. *World J Gastroenterol.* 10:2588, 2004.

Koretz RL. Do data support nutrition support? Part II. enteral artificial nutrition. *J Am Diet Assoc.* 107:1374, 2007.

Malik HZ, et al. Chyle leakage and early enteral feeding following pancreatico-duodenectomy: management options. *Dig Surg.* 24:418, 2007.

Rochling FA, Zetterman RK. Management of ascites. *Drugs.* 69:1739, 2009.

Rosner MH, et al. Management of cirrhotic ascites: physiological basis of diuretic action. *Eur J Intern Med.* 17:8, 2006.

Sandhu BS, Sanyal AJ. Management of ascites in cirrhosis. *Clin Liver Dis.* 9:715, 2005.

Sargent S. The management and nursing care of cirrhotic ascites. *Br J Nurs.* 15:212, 2006.

Smoke A, Delegge MH. Chyle leaks: consensus on management? *Nutr Clin Pract.* 23:529, 2008.

HEPATITIS

NUTRITIONAL ACUITY RANKING: LEVEL 2

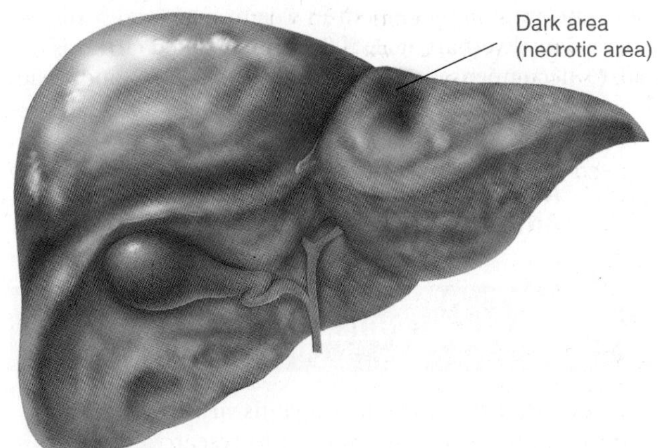

Asset provided by Anatomical Chart Co.

DEFINITIONS AND BACKGROUND

Hepatitis is defined as liver inflammation resulting from alcohol use, toxic materials (carbon tetrachloride), or viral infection (transmitted in food, liquids, or blood transfusions). There is also an autoimmune hepatitis and a NASH.

Acute viral hepatitis is a widespread inflammation of the liver and is caused by hepatitis viruses A, B, C, D, or E. Hepatitis causes nausea, fever, liver tenderness and enlargement, jaundice, pale stools, and anorexia. The first stage of viral hepatitis is preicteric/prodromal (with flu-like symptoms); the second stage is icteric (with jaundice, dark urine, and light stools). The third stage is posticteric/convalescent.

With chronic active hepatitis, inflamed liver cells continue for years, which is usually an autoimmune response. Metabolic diseases, such as Wilson's disease, hemochromatosis, and alpha-1 antitrypsin deficiency, and use of some drugs, such as methyldopa, nitrofurantoin, papaverine, dantrolene, clometacine, and ticrynafen, can cause chronic hepatitis (Hasse and Matarese, 2008). American Indian and Alaska Native (AI/AN) people suffer disproportionately from infectious diseases including **Hepatitis A virus** (**HAV**) and **Hepatitis B virus** (**HBV**); childhood immunizations have reduced these disease disparities (Singleton et al, 2009).

HAV, which is transmitted by fecal–oral route, comprises approximately 50% of hepatitis cases. **HBV** is considered a sexually transmitted disease; 20% of those affected develop

TABLE 8-3 **Hepatitis Symptoms, Transmission, and Treatment**

Type	Incubation	Symptoms	Transmission	Treatment
Hepatitis A Infectious HAV	30 days	Flu-like illness, jaundice, nausea, fatigue, abdominal pain, anorexia, diarrhea, fever	Ingestion of items contaminated with infected feces, drinking water or ice contaminated with raw sewage, eating fruits, vegetables, or uncooked food contaminated during handling. Risk factors: overseas travel, anal sex, IV drug use, living in poor sanitation.	Immunoglobulin 2–3 months before or 2 weeks after exposure. Vaccine is available.
Hepatitis B Serum HBV	Can survive 7 days outside of the body	Flu-like illness, jaundice, nausea, fatigue, vomiting, fever, often no symptoms	Contact with contaminated body fluids, exposure to sharp instruments that contain contaminated blood, human bites, blood transfusion before 1975. Risk factors: IV drug use, multiple sex partners, travel or work in developing countries, transfusion before 1975.	Interferon alfa and lamivudine. HBV immunoglobulin (HBIG) within 14 days of exposure. There are safe and effective vaccines. Ribavirin is under study.
Hepatitis C HCV	Average 7–9 weeks; can live 28 weeks	Often no symptoms until liver damage occurs, flu-like illness, fatigue, nausea headaches, abdominal pain	Blood-to-blood contact, especially IV drug use and shared needles. Exposure to items with contaminated blood, such as needles (tattoo, body piercing, acupuncture), razors, nail files, toothbrushes, scissors, tampons. Sexually transmitted disease with rashes or sores. Blood transfusions before July 1992. At risk: IV drug use, had a blood transfusion or organ transplantation before July 1992, snorts cocaine. Widespread—affects 4 million people. Silent. Leading cause of cirrhosis in the United States.	Interferon or combination drug treatments. Liver transplantation for end-stage. There are no vaccines. Treatment takes minimum of 1 year. Ribavirin is under study.
Hepatitis D HDV	Occurs only with HBV infection, cannot survive on own	Flu-like illness, jaundice, nausea, fatigue, vomiting, fever, often no symptoms	Sexual contact with HBV-infected person. Exposure to sharp instruments contaminated with HBV. At risk: IV drug use.	Interferon alpha for chronic cases. Vaccination against HBV provides protection against type D.
Hepatitis E HEV	2–9 weeks	Malaise, loss of appetite, abdominal pain, joint pain, fever	Fecal transmission, often through contaminated water. At risk: pregnant women, those who travel in developing countries.	No specific treatment.

some form of chronic liver disease. Table 8-3 provides symptoms and treatments for the many forms of hepatitis, including incomplete viral forms of **Hepatitis D and E**. Hepatitis E virus has been reported to result in chronic hepatitis in transplant patients.

Hepatitis C virus (HCV) is a complex and challenging medical condition. Nearly 20% of Americans test positive for HCV. Many persons with HCV develop chronic disease; 25% of cases lead to cirrhosis, liver cancer, or liver failure that requires transplantation. Recently, the gene marker that predicts response to HCV therapy has been identified; this is significant because about half of cases respond poorly to treatment. Regular coffee consumption is associated with lower rates of disease progression (Freedman et al, 2009) and may actually reduce onset of hepatocellular cancer (Inouye et al, 2005).

A deranged metabolic status and alcohol intake may trigger induction and progression of chronic HCV liver disease; variable intakes of carbohydrates, lipids, polyunsaturated fatty acids, iron, zinc, vitamin A, niacin, and alcohol are factors as are genotype, age, BMI, steatosis, and fibrosis (Loguercio et al, 2008). In the Hepatitis C Antiviral Long-Term Treatment Against Cirrhosis (HALT-C) trial, insulin resistance, histologic features of fatty liver disease, and weight change promoted poor outcomes; improvement in weight may modify disease progression (Everhart et al, 2009). HCV-related cirrhosis can lead to decompensation, end-stage liver failure, and death (Bruno et al, 2009).

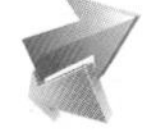

ASSESSMENT, MONITORING, AND EVALUATION

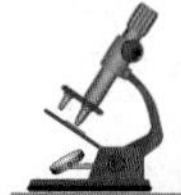

CLINICAL INDICATORS

Genetic Markers: How the hepatitis virus DNA evolves and changes is of great interest to researchers. Since the identification of the hepatitis viruses over the past decades, the understanding of host innate and adaptive immune responses has increased significantly (Rehermann, 2009). Drug-induced liver injury may stem from concomitant hepatic diseases, age, and poor health status; polymorphisms of CYP liver enzymes, phenotyping and genotyping studies may also be needed (Tarantino et al, 2009).

Clinical/History		
Height	Hepatitis B e antigen (*HBeAg*)	Absolute neutrophil count (ANC)
Weight	Hepatitis C Anti-body (HCV Ab, anti-HCV)	BUN
BMI	Hepatitis C viral load test (or PCR test)	Serum ammonia
I & O	Bilirubin (increased)	Lipase
Diet history	AST (increased)	Amylase (increased)
Right upper abdominal pain	ALT	PT or INR
Jaundice	Alk phos (increased)	Gluc
Temperature, fever	Chol	Transferrin (increased in acute stage)
Severe nausea, vomiting	Lactate dehydro-genase (LDH) (increased)	H & H, ferritin
Dark urine	Alb, transthyretin	WBC
Joint pain	Globulin	GGT
Lab Work	CRP	Na^+, K^+
IgM antibody for HAV		Ca^{++}, Mg^{++}
Hepatitis B surface antibody (*Anti-HBs or* core antibody (*Anti-HBc*)		

SAMPLE NUTRITION CARE PROCESS STEPS

Inadequate Bioactive Substance Intake

Assessment: Weight and diet history; abnormal liver tests. Intake <25% for past 3–4 weeks. Diet history reveals low intake of fruits, vegetables, whole grains, and coffee.

Nutrition Diagnosis (PES): Inadequate bioactive substance intake related to loss of appetite as evidenced by low intake of nutrient-dense foods and coffee.

Intervention: Food-Nutrient Delivery: high-protein, high-calorie diet in frequent small meals. Educate about the role of bioactive substances in protecting the liver; encourage use of coffee as tolerated.

Monitoring and Evaluation: Evaluate diet history and weight. Assess for improvement in appetite and intake of foods rich in bioactive substances.

INTERVENTION

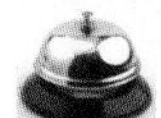

OBJECTIVES

- Promote liver regeneration and rest. Prevent further injury.
- Prevent or correct weight loss, which often results from poor appetite, nausea, and vomiting.
- Spare protein by providing a diet high in carbohydrates.
- Force fluids to prevent dehydration, unless contraindicated.
- Encourage intake of coffee and antioxidant foods.
- Prevent the spread to others by hand washing and safe hygiene practices.

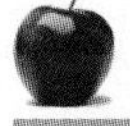

FOOD AND NUTRITION

- For patients with all forms of hepatitis, provide a complete and balanced diet. If nutritional support is necessary, consider TF. Nocturnal feedings may be beneficial.
- Use CPN only if necessary because of ileus or obstruction, and avoid products containing glutamine.
- Progress to a diet of small, frequent feedings of regular or soft foods.
- Diet should provide 30–35 kcal/kg body weight. Provide sufficient carbohydrate to replenish liver stores of glycogen; include 50–55% total energy as carbohydrate.
- Intake of protein should be 1–1.2 g/kg body weight for acute hepatitis. Well-nourished or chronic active hepatitis patients may need levels that just meet dietary reference intake (DRI).
- Fat intake should be moderate to liberal, depending on tolerance. Cut back if diarrhea or other signs of malabsorption occur.
- Supplement diet a multivitamin supplement with B-complex vitamins (especially thiamin, folate, and vitamin B_{12}), vitamin K (to normalize bleeding tendency), vitamin C, and zinc for anorexia and to improve encephalopathy. Monitor for excesses of iron and vitamin A, which may not be well tolerated in a supplemental form.
- Extra fluid should be encouraged, unless contraindicated. Encourage coffee intake (Freedman et al, 2009).

Common Drugs Used and Potential Side Effects

- A combined HAV and HBV vaccine, Twinrix, is available in many parts of the world. Hepatitis B vaccine is found singly as Engerix-B, Recombivax, or Cornvax. Because of vaccinations, the incidence of HAV and HBV has declined, especially among children.
- Two formulations of interferon (standard interferon (IFN) and pegylated IFN) can be used for sustained response to HBV and five nucleoside analogues (lamivudine, adefovir, entecavir, telbivudine, and tenofovir) for treatment-maintained response (Buster et al, 2008). Interferon (Intron-A) can lead to dry mouth, stomatitis, nausea, vomiting, and calcium depletion. The oral antiviral entecavir (Baraclude) is more effective than lamivudine (Dienstag et al, 2007) or adefovir (Leung et al, 2009).
- The gold standard for new patients with chronic HCV is the combination of pegylated interferon (Pegasys or PEG-Intron) and ribavirin (Copegus, Rebetol); individualizing dose and duration improves the sustained virologic response (Camma et al, 2005; Degertekin and Lok, 2009; McHutchison et al, 2009). There may be hemolytic side effects, depression, and weight or lipid changes. Etanercept as adjuvant therapy to interferon and ribavirin improves response and has decreased adverse effects (Zein et al, 2005).
- Steroids may cause sodium retention, nitrogen depletion, or hyperglycemia.

- Monitor for idiosyncratic drug-induced liver injury (DILI;) acute HCV may be present. DILI is caused by a single prescription medication in most cases and by multiple agents or dietary supplements in the remaining cases (Chalasani et al, 2008).

Herbs, Botanicals, and Supplements

- Chaparral and kava kava are especially toxic to the liver and should be avoided.
- Avoid excessive fat-soluble vitamin intake (vitamins A and D). Vitamin A toxicity is possible in compromised liver function; monitor all supplements carefully. Beta-carotene is much less toxic and may offer reasonable antioxidant protection.
- *Silybum marianum* (milk thistle) has been shown to have clinical applications in the treatment of toxic hepatitis and viral hepatitis via its antioxidant properties.
- Oregano, sage, peppermint, garden thyme, lemon balm, clove, allspice, and cinnamon as well as the Chinese medicinal herbs *Cinnamomi cortex* and *Scutellariae radix* contain very high concentrations of antioxidants. In a normal diet, intake of herbs contributes significantly to the total intake of plant antioxidants and can be an even better source of dietary antioxidants than other foods.
- Herbs and botanical supplements should not be used without discussing with the physician. Carrot, schisandra, dandelion, Indian almond, and licorice have been recommended but need research.

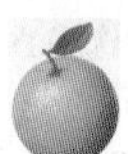

NUTRITION EDUCATION, COUNSELING, CARE MANAGEMENT

- Help patient make attractive, appetizing meals. Encourage frequent, small meals.
- Educate patient about how to increase calorie, protein, and vitamin intakes. Discuss pros and cons of supplemental products.
- Encourage coffee intake as well as intake of other antioxidant-rich foods.
- Ensure patient abstains from alcohol and drugs that are hepatotoxic. DILI may occur with antibiotics, acetominophen, CNS agents, herbal or dietary supplements.
- All children should receive Hepatitis B vaccinations.
- The NIH recommends that all immigrants be screened and treated for HBV when they move to the United States to prevent liver failure or hepatic carcinoma (NIH, 2008).
- In health care employment, follow standard precautions: handle needles and other sharps safely; report every needlestick on the job; get vaccinated against hepatitis B.
- Consider the risks of HCV before getting a tattoo or body piercing; infection is possible if the tools have someone else's blood on them, or if the artist or piercer does not follow practices such as washing hands and using disposable gloves.

Patient Education—Food Safety

- HAV is usually spread by putting something in the mouth that is contaminated by the stool of another person with hepatitis A. It is usually spread through household contact with an infected person, sharing utensils that are contaminated, eating or drinking contaminated food or water, touching a contaminated surface and then the mouth.
- Teach safe personal hygiene in regard to hand washing and use of disinfectants, especially when traveling overseas. Boil water or drink bottled water in areas where there is a risk for HAV contamination. Eat cooked foods and fruits that you can peel and avoid eating vegetables or fruits that could have been washed with contaminated water, such as lettuce. Avoid eating raw or steamed shellfish, such as oysters, that live in contaminated waters.
- Discuss other principles of food safety and personal hygiene. To protect against HCV, do not share items such as razors, toothbrushes, and other personal health items that might have had blood on them. Do not inject street drugs.

For More Information

- Centers for Disease Control and Prevention (CDC) Information http://www.cdc.gov/ncidod/diseases/hepatitis/
- Department of Veterans Affairs http://www.hepatitis.va.gov/vahep?page=basics-00-00
- Hepatitis Information Network http://www.hepnet.com/
- Hepatitis Information http://www.hepatitis.org
- Hepatitis B Foundation http://www.hepb.org/
- Hepatitis C Central http://www.hepatitis-central.com/
- Hepatitis Foundation International http://www.hepatitisfoundation.org/
- National HCV Prison Coalition http://www.hcvinprison.org/cms/index.php
- NIDDK—Hepatitis http://digestive.niddk.nih.gov/ddiseases/pubs/viralhepatitis/

HEPATITIS—CITED REFERENCES

Bruno S, et al. Predicting mortality risk in patients with compensated HCV-induced cirrhosis: a long-term prospective study. *Am J Gastroenterol.* 104:1147, 2009.

Buster EH, et al. Peginterferon for the treatment of chronic hepatitis B in the era of nucleos(t)ide analogues. *Best Pract Res Clin Gastroenterol.* 22: 1093, 2008.

Camma C, et al. Treatment of hepatitis C: critical appraisal of the evidence. *Expert Opin Pharmacother.* 6:399, 2005.

Chalasani N, et al. Causes, clinical features, and outcomes from a prospective study of drug-induced liver injury in the United States. *Gastroenterology.* 135:1924, 2008.

Degertekin B, Lok AS. Update on viral hepatitis: 2008. *Curr Opin Gastroenterol.* 25:180, 2009.

Dienstag JL, et al. Cross-study analysis of the relative efficacies of oral antiviral therapies for chronic hepatitis B infection in nucleoside-naive patients. *Clin Drug Investig.* 27:35, 2007.

Everhart JE, et al. Weight-related effects on disease progression in the hepatitis C antiviral long-term treatment against cirrhosis trial. *Gastroenterology.* 137:549, 2009.

Freedman ND, et al. Coffee intake is associated with lower rates of liver disease progression in chronic hepatitis C [published online ahead of print July 13, 2009]. *Hepatology.* 50:1360, 2009.

Hasse J, Matarese L. Medical nutrition therapy for liver, biliary system, and exocrine pancreas disorders. In: Mahan L, Escott-Stump S, eds. *Krause's food nutrition and diet therapy.* 12th ed. St Louis: Elsevier, 2008.

Inouye M, et al. Influence of coffee drinking on subsequent risk of hepatocellular carcinoma: a prospective study in Japan. *J Natl Cancer Inst.* 97:293, 2005.

Leung N, et al. Early hepatitis B virus DNA reduction in hepatitis B e antigen-positive patients with chronic hepatitis B: a randomized international study of entecavir versus adefovir. *Hepatology.* 49:72, 2009.

Loguercio C, et al. The impact of diet on liver fibrosis and on response to interferon therapy in patients with HCV-related chronic hepatitis. 103: 3159, 2008.
McHutchison JG, et al. Peginterferon alfa-2b or alfa-2a with ribavirin for treatment of hepatitis C infection. *N Engl J Med.* 361:580, 2009.
NIH. NIH consensus development statement on management of hepatitis B. *NIH Consensus Sci Statements.* 25:1, 2008.
Rehermann B. Hepatitis C virus versus innate and adaptive immune responses: a tale of coevolution and coexistence. *J Clin Invest.* 119:1745, 2009.
Singleton R, et al. Impact of immunizations on the disease burden of American Indian and Alaska native children. *Arch Pediatr Adolesc Med.* 163:446, 2009.
Tarantino G, et al. Drug-induced liver injury: is it somehow foreseeable? *World J Gastroenterol.* 15:2817, 2009.
Zein NN, et al. Etanercept as an adjuvant to interferon and ribavirin in treatment-naive patients with chronic hepatitis C virus infection: a phase 2 randomized, double-blind, placebo-controlled study. *J Hepatol.* 42:315, 2005.

HEPATIC CIRRHOSIS

NUTRITIONAL ACUITY RANKING: LEVEL 2–3

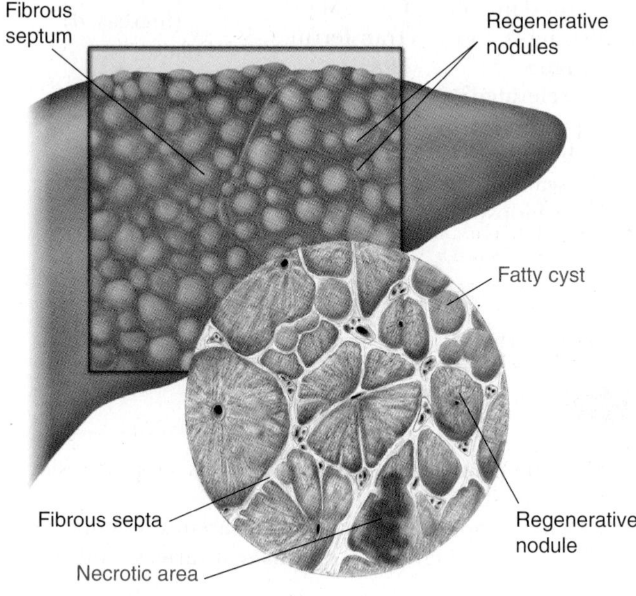

Asset provided by Anatomical Chart Co.

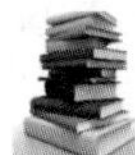

DEFINITIONS AND BACKGROUND

Cirrhosis is caused by chronic degeneration of the parenchymal liver cells and thickening of the surrounding tissue; the liver slowly deteriorates and malfunctions due to chronic injury. Alcoholism and hepatitis C are the most common causes; alcoholic cirrhosis is known as Laennec's cirrhosis. Cirrhosis may also result from biliary stenosis, hepatitis B-D, obesity with nonalcoholic fatty liver disease (NAFLD), autoimmune hepatitis, prolonged exposure to toxic chemicals, and inherited diseases such as glycogen storage disease, cystic fibrosis, alpha-1 antitrypsin deficiency, hemochromatosis, Wilson disease, or galactosemia.

Malnutrition plays a significant role in the pathogenesis of liver injury and should be carefully managed. Cirrhosis is a disease of accelerated use of alternative fuel (such as fat) since liver stores of glycogen tend to be depleted after an overnight fast. About 50% of energy kilocalories should be consumed from carbohydrate to minimize use of fat stores or protein for energy. Glucose intolerance, insulin resistance, and higher circulating glucagon may cause early satiety, hypophagia, and depleted nutrient stores. There is a high incidence of muscle wasting, weight loss, and malnutrition with cirrhosis. Table 8-4 list the related forms of malnutrition.

Exercise and protein-rich nutrition at the early stage of liver cirrhosis can help to maintain or increase muscular volume (Kotoh et al, 2005). Nutritionally depleted patients need extra attention. Both enteral and parenteral nutritional support can improve the general nutrition condition; EN has fewer complications (Zhang et al, 2005). Cirrhosis related to CPN may be rapidly reversible after isolated intestinal transplantation (Fiel et al, 2009).

Plasma aromatic amino acid (AAA) concentrations (phenylalanine, tyrosine, and tryptophan) tend to increase from rapid muscle proteolysis and decreased synthesis of proteins. Branched-chain amino acids (BCAAs) leucine, isoleucine, and valine are then imbalanced; the low BCAA to AAA ratio contributes to hepatic encephalopathy. When AAAs are high, BCAAs are more limited in cerebral uptake. A higher BCAA intake helps to improve cognitive status (Bianchi et al, 2005; Charlton, 2006). Long-term BCAA supplementation is associated with decreased frequency of hepatic failure and overall complication frequency, along with improved nutritional status (Charlton, 2006).

Severe cirrhosis may lead to decreased serum lipids. Omega-3 fatty acids in enteral supplementation completely protect the liver; IV sources provide only partial protection (Alwayn et al, 2005).

Liver damage from cirrhosis cannot be reversed, but treatment can stop or delay further progression and reduce complications. Participants who consume a diet high in protein are at a higher risk of hospitalization or death due to cirrhosis; those who report a diet high in carbohydrates are at a lower risk after adjusting for daily consumption of protein, carbohydrate, fat, tea or coffee, and alcohol, gender, race, age, educational attainment, U.S. geographical region, diabetes, and BMI ratio (Ioannou et al, 2009).

Treatment will depend on the cause of cirrhosis and any related complications. Serum ammonia levels may be high. Fermentable fiber or lactulose may be used for management of cirrhosis. Antibiotic therapy works to prevent infections, including SBP in cirrhosis (Saab et al, 2009).

Portal hypertension causes increased collateral flow, often with varices in parts of the GI tract. These veins become distended, may bleed, and cause pain. Esophageal varices are the most serious complication of cirrhosis. **Splenorenal shunting** with a trans-jugular intrahepatic portosystemic shunt

TABLE 8-4 Causes of Malnutrition in Cirrhosis

Decreased Oral Intake

- Anorexia
- Ascites
- Altered mental status or encephalopathy
- Delayed gastric emptying
- Early satiety
- Inadequate diet or strict limits on protein, fluid and salt
- Medications causing GI distress or taste changes
- Nausea
- Restrictive diets or NPO for several days

Maldigestion and Malabsorption

- Accelerated intestinal transit
- Accelerated protein breakdown
- Anemia from impaired GI and liver function
- Bacterial overgrowth
- Biliary flow changes
- Choline depletion and betaine
- Decreased hepatic production and storage of nutrients
- Decreased fat absorption
- Diuresis, paracentesis, and micronutrient losses
- Increased rate of gluconeogenesis
- Increased urinary and fecal losses
- Lactulose use
- Pancreatic insufficiency
- Villi damaged by alcohol
- Vomiting

Adapted from Caly WR, et al. Different degrees of malnutrition and immunological alterations according to the aetiology of cirrhosis: a prospective and sequential study. *Nutr J.* 2:10, 2003.
Stockslager JL, et al. *Nutrition made incredibly easy.* Baltimore: Lippincott Williams & Wilkins, 2003, p. 242.

(TIPS) is performed when the portal vein is obstructed. Portacaval blood flow is diverted from the liver by anastomosing the portal vein to the inferior vena cava. The shunt procedure is positive in most cases. Liver transplantation is needed when encephalopathy, ascites, or bleeding varices are uncontrollable.

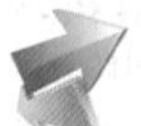

ASSESSMENT, MONITORING, AND EVALUATION

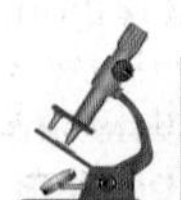

CLINICAL INDICATORS

Genetic Markers: Autoimmune hepatitis is caused by the body's immune system attacking liver cells and causing inflammation, damage, and cirrhosis; 70% of those with autoimmune hepatitis are female. A cirrhosis-risk score is being developed to assess host genetics and polymorphisms.

Clinical/History	Lab Work	
Height	MELD score for severity (INR for clotting, bilirubin, creatinine)	Alb, transthyretin (not valid in cirrhosis)
Weight	PT (prolonged); INR	ALT
BMI	BUN	AST (increased)
Weight loss?	Globulin	Bilirubin (increased)
I & O	Somatomedin C	Alk phos (increased)
Diet history	TP	WBC
Bowel changes	UA	Trig (increased)
Bleeding hemorrhoids	Gluc (increased or decreased)	Chol (low?)
Confusion	Na^+, K^+	LDH (increased)
Loss of libido	Ca^{++}, Mg^{++}	Copper, ceruloplasmin (increased)
Jaundice	Transferrin	Folate
Ascites	H & H (decreased)	GGT
Spider-like blood vessels on skin	Serum ammonia (elevated?)	
Itching		
Fatigue		
BP (elevated?)		
Easy bruising or bleeding		
CT scan		
Liver biopsy		

INTERVENTION

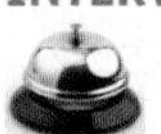

OBJECTIVES

- Slow the progression of scar tissue and support residual liver function.
- Provide supportive treatment for ascites, edema, muscle wasting, weight loss, esophageal varices, and portal hypertension.
- Monitor steatorrhea; offer suggestions for managing.
- Correct nutritional deficiencies, which are common. Tube feed if needed.

SAMPLE NUTRITION CARE PROCESS STEPS

Inadequate Oral Food and Beverage Intake

Assessment Data: Dietary intake records indicating poor appetite and intake of <50% at most meals; diagnosis of NASH; mild weight loss 5% in past 3 months; mild jaundice.

Nutrition Diagnosis (PES): Inadequate oral food and beverage related to anorexia as evidenced by intake only about 50% and weight loss of × lb in past 3 months (5% UBW).

Intervention: Food and Nutrient Delivery—offer smaller meals and snacks every few hours while awake; increase nutrient density and quality of foods chosen. Educate about the role of good nutrition in liver health and recovery. Assure no intake of alcohol.

Monitoring and Evaluation: Improvement in appetite, reduced nausea or side effects of liver disease. Gradual return of usual weight.

- Monitor closely for signs of hepatic encephalopathy such as drowsiness or confusion.
- Provide adequate glucose for brain metabolism but beware of glucose intolerance, especially with alcoholic cirrhosis.
- Prevent long-term bone disease, hyperkalemia or hypokalemia, hyponatremia, renal failure, and anemia. If hepatorenal failure occurs, hemodialysis may be necessary.
- Avoid hepatic insults from alcohol, drugs, vitamins and herbal products. Consult the physician first.

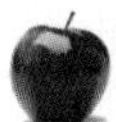

FOOD AND NUTRITION

- Increased energy is needed. Calculate energy at 50–75% above usual requirements if malabsorption is present or if repletion is needed. Use ideal or estimated dry weight.
- Diet should provide 1–1.5 g of high-quality protein/kg body weight with adequate carbohydrates to spare protein. Meat has a high level of AAAs; vegetable proteins or casein may be better tolerated.
- Fat is a preferred fuel in cirrhosis. Omega-3 fatty acids should be included (Alwayn et al, 2005). Malabsorption occurs from diminished lipase output; decrease LCTs in steatorrhea. Carefully monitor use of MCTs because they may cause diarrhea or acidosis.
- Supplement diet with B-complex vitamins, vitamins C and K, zinc, and magnesium through foods or supplements. Monitor need for vitamins A and D; do not use excesses in liver disease. Liquid form may be needed for patients with esophageal varices.
- TF can be used with cirrhosis or esophageal varices (Hasse and Matarese, 2008). PN is safe and improves mental state in patients with cirrhosis in whom enteral nutrition is insufficient or impossible (Plauth et al, 2009). Glutamine is not generally recommended in liver disease.
- Avoid alcoholic beverages.
- Control total carbohydrate intake with signs of hyperglycemia or with diabetes.
- Low sodium intake (2–4 g) is recommended with ascites.
- Decrease fluid if there is hyponatremia.
- Enhance nutrient density of food choices if malnourished.

Common Drugs Used and Potential Side Effects

- See Table 8-5.

Herbs, Botanicals, and Supplements

- People with liver disease must be particularly careful because the liver processes almost everything consumed. Herbs and botanical supplements should not be used without discussing with the physician. Some herbal tea preparations may be harmful (such as Comfrey tea) and should be avoided. Chaparral is an herbal product that may contribute to severe hepatitis or liver failure (Stickel et al, 2005). Mistletoe, kava kava, European barberry, and germander should also be avoided.
- Antioxidants, such as vitamin E and selenium, might help in treating cirrhosis. Supplements of vitamins A, C, E, selenium, methionine, and co-enzyme Q10 provide no specific benefit; fresh fruits, vegetables, and whole grains should be consumed instead.
- Betaine (10 g twice daily) reduces elevated homocysteine levels and might be helpful in treating alcohol-induced cirrhosis.
- Bupleurum (*Bupleurum chinese*) is a Chinese herb with anti-inflammatory properties that may lower risk of liver cancer in people with cirrhosis.
- Licorice root (*Glycyrrhiza glabra*) contains glycyrrhizin. Stronger neominophagen C (SNMC) is a Japanese preparation that contains 0.2% glycyrrhizin, 0.1% cysteine, and 2% glyceine that has anti-inflammatory or cytoprotective drug. Do not take licorice with high blood pressure, pregnancy, steroid use, digoxin (Lanoxin), diuretics, or anticoagulants (warfarin/Coumadin).
- Milk thistle (*S. marianum*) has been shown to have clinical applications in the treatment of cirrhosis through its antioxidative and anti-inflammatory effects. A total of 420 mg/d may protect the liver from damage caused by viruses, toxins, alcohol, and drugs such as acetaminophen, but milk thistle does not reduce mortality.
- SAM (*S*-adenosylmethionine 1200–1600 mg/d) may be effective in alcoholic cirrhosis. People with liver disease have low levels of SAMe, and glutathione. Avoid use with prescription antidepressants.
- Zinc deficiency has been implicated in the pathogenesis of liver diseases. Supplementation with zinc may have therapeutic benefits.

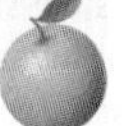

NUTRITION EDUCATION, COUNSELING, CARE MANAGEMENT

- Diet may be an important and potentially modifiable determinant of liver disease (Ioannou et al, 2009). Higher CHO and lower protein intake may be a reasonable goal.
- A better appetite at certain meals may be common; breakfast or another meal may be better tolerated. Some patients sleep late with a sleep reversal pattern.
- Discuss use of nutrient-dense foods and higher intakes of vegetable and dairy sources of protein.
- Dietary intake must be adjusted according to the changing status of the patient. Large meals increase portal pressure; recommend use of smaller meals throughout the day.
- Avoid skipping meals. Discuss proper menu planning.
- Avoid high doses of vitamins A and D, which may be toxic to the diseased liver. It is also not clear whether vitamin K supplementation is either safe or useful in cirrhosis. Vitamin E may be beneficial for its antioxidant properties; encourage dietary intake.

Patient Education—Foodborne Illness

- Avoid raw shellfish, which may contain *Vibrio vulnificus* which is dangerous to people with cirrhosis.

TABLE 8-5 Medications Used in Cirrhosis

Medication	Description
Antibiotics: tetracycline (Achromycin V), ampicillin (Polycillin), trimethoprim-sulfamethoxazole (Bactrim, Septra)	Antibiotics kill the bacteria that cause infections, a common complication of cirrhosis. Possible side effects include nausea and vomiting, poor appetite, diarrhea, sore mouth or tongue, and increased sensitivity to sunlight (tetracycline).
Antiviral medications: interferon-alpha (Alferon N, Roferon-A, Intron A), ribavirin (Virazole), lamivudine (Epivir, Epivir-HBV), baraclude (Entecavir)	These may be used if viral hepatitis B or C is the cause of cirrhosis. Treatment usually lasts for 4 months. Ribavirin is an oral antiviral agent that is given twice a day. Lamivudine is used to treat hepatitis B infection. Sometimes lamivudine is combined with interferon. Side effects may include severe GI pain, feeling of fullness, nausea, tingling, burning, numbness, or pain in the hands, arms, feet, or legs.
Anti-inflammatory medications (corticosteroids): prednisone, azathioprine (Imuran)	Corticosteroids reduce liver inflammation and prevent the progression of cirrhosis. High doses given long term are associated with an increase in serious side effects. Lower doses of prednisone may be used when combined with azathioprine. Possible side effects include: hypertension, glucose intolerance, and bone thinning.
Antihypertensives (beta-blockers): atenolol (Tenormin), metoprolol (Lopressor), nadolol (Corgard), propranolol (Inderal), timolol (Blocadren)	Beta-blockers are used to reduce venous blood pressure in the abdomen (portal hypertension) to reduce the risk of esophageal variceal bleeding and other complications. Possible side effects associated with beta-blocker use include: drowsiness, dizziness, cold sensitivity, and sleep disorders.
Diuretics: "Loop" diuretics: bumetanide (Bumex), furosemide (Lasix); thiazide diuretics: hydrochlorothiazide (HydroDIURIL, Esidrix), chlorothiazide (Diuril); potassium-sparing diuretics: amiloride (Midamor), triamterene (Dyrenium)	Diuretics are used to treat the buildup of excess fluid in the body that occurs with cirrhosis (as well as other diseases). These drugs act on the kidneys to increase urine output, which reduces the amount of fluid in the bloodstream. This can help to reduce portal vein hypertension and help alleviate some of the symptoms of cirrhosis, such as fluid accumulation in the abdomen and legs. Possible side effects associated with diuretic use include: loss of appetite, nausea and vomiting, dizziness, headache, lethargy, and altered blood potassium level.
Insulin	If insulin is needed, monitor carefully for hypoglycemic episodes.
Laxatives: beta-galactosidofructose (lactulose [Cephulac] and kristalose [Chronulac])	In cirrhosis, laxatives such as beta-galactosidofructose (lactulose) can help to absorb or bind toxins, such as ammonia, in the intestine and remove them from the body. Possible side effects associated with laxative use include: diarrhea, abdominal cramping, flatulence and bloating, dehydration, and weakness. Take with food or milk.
Metal Chelating Agents: penicillamine (Cuprimine, Depen), trientine (Syprine), deferoxamine (Desferal)	Metal chelating agents draw toxic metals from the bloodstream so that the body can excrete them. Chelating agents are used to rid the body of excess copper in Wilson's disease or excess iron in hemochromatosis. Both of these rare inherited diseases can produce liver damage resulting in cirrhosis. Possible side effects include: fever; joint pain; lesions on the face, neck, scalp, and/or trunk; rash, hives, or itching; swollen glands; sores or white spots on lips or in mouth; cyanosis; blurred vision; convulsions; wheezing or fast breathing; tachycardia; flushing of skin; nausea, vomiting or diarrhea; and blood in the urine.
Vitamin K: phytonadione (AquaMEPHYTON, Mephyton)	Bleeding abnormalities are common in cirrhosis. Vitamin K helps prevent excessive bleeding. Possible side effects include: flushing of the face and unusual taste.

- If home TF is needed, teach appropriate sanitation and food-handling procedures.

For More Information

- CDC—Cirrhosis
  http://www.cdc.gov/nchs/fastats/liverdis.htm
- Cirrhosis Diet
  http://digestive-system.emedtv.com/cirrhosis/cirrhosis-diet.html
- Hepatic Foundation International
  http://www.hepfi.org/
- Hep Net
  http://www.hepcnet.net/nutritionandcirhossis.html
- Medicine Net—Cirrhosis
  http://www.medicinenet.com/cirrhosis/article.htm
- Milk Thistle
  http://nccam.nih.gov/health/milkthistle/ataglance.htm
- National Institutes of Health—Cirrhosis
  http://www.nlm.nih.gov/medlineplus/cirrhosis.html
- University of Maryland
  http://www.umm.edu/altmed/articles/cirrhosis-000037.htm
- Veterans Administration
  http://www.hepatitis.va.gov/vahep?page=diet-03–00
- WebMD—Cirrhosis
  http://www.webmd.com/digestive-disorders/cirrhosis-liver

HEPATIC CIRRHOSIS—CITED REFERENCES

Alwayn IP, et al. Omega-3 fatty acid supplementation prevents hepatic steatosis in a murine model of nonalcoholic fatty liver disease. *Pediatr Res.* 57:445, 2005.

Bianchi G, et al. Update on branched-chain amino acid supplementation in liver diseases. *Curr Opin Gastroenterol.* 21:197, 2005.

Charlton M. Branched-chain amino acid enriched supplements as therapy for liver disease. *J Nutr.* 136:295S, 2006.

Fiel MI, et al. Rapid reversal of parenteral-nutrition-associated cirrhosis following isolated intestinal transplantation. *J Gastrointest Surg.* 13:1717, 2009.

Hasse J, Matarese L. Medical nutrition therapy for liver, biliary system, and exocrine pancreas disorders. In: Mahan L, Escott-Stump S, eds. *Krause's food nutrition and diet therapy.* 12th ed. St Louis: Elsevier, 2008.

Ioannou GN, et al. Association between dietary nutrient composition and the incidence of cirrhosis or liver cancer in the United States population. *Hepatology.* 50:175, 2009.

Kotoh K, et al. High relative fat-free mass is important for maintaining serum albumin levels in patients with compensated liver cirrhosis. *World J Gastroenterol.* 11:1356, 2005.

Plauth M, et al. ESPEN Guidelines on Parenteral Nutrition: hepatology. *Clin Nutr.* 28:436, 2009.

Saab S, et al. Oral antibiotic prophylaxis reduces spontaneous bacterial peritonitis occurrence and improves short-term survival in cirrhosis: a meta-analysis. *Am J Gastroenterol.* 104:993, 2009.

Stickel F, et al. Herbal hepatotoxicity. *J Hepatol.* 43:901, 2005.

Zhang K, et al. Early enteral and parenteral nutritional support in patients with cirrhotic portal hypertension after pericardial devascularization. *Hepatobiliary Pancreat Dis Int.* 4:55, 2005.

HEPATIC FAILURE, ENCEPHALOPATHY, AND COMA

NUTRITIONAL ACUITY RANKING: LEVEL 3–4

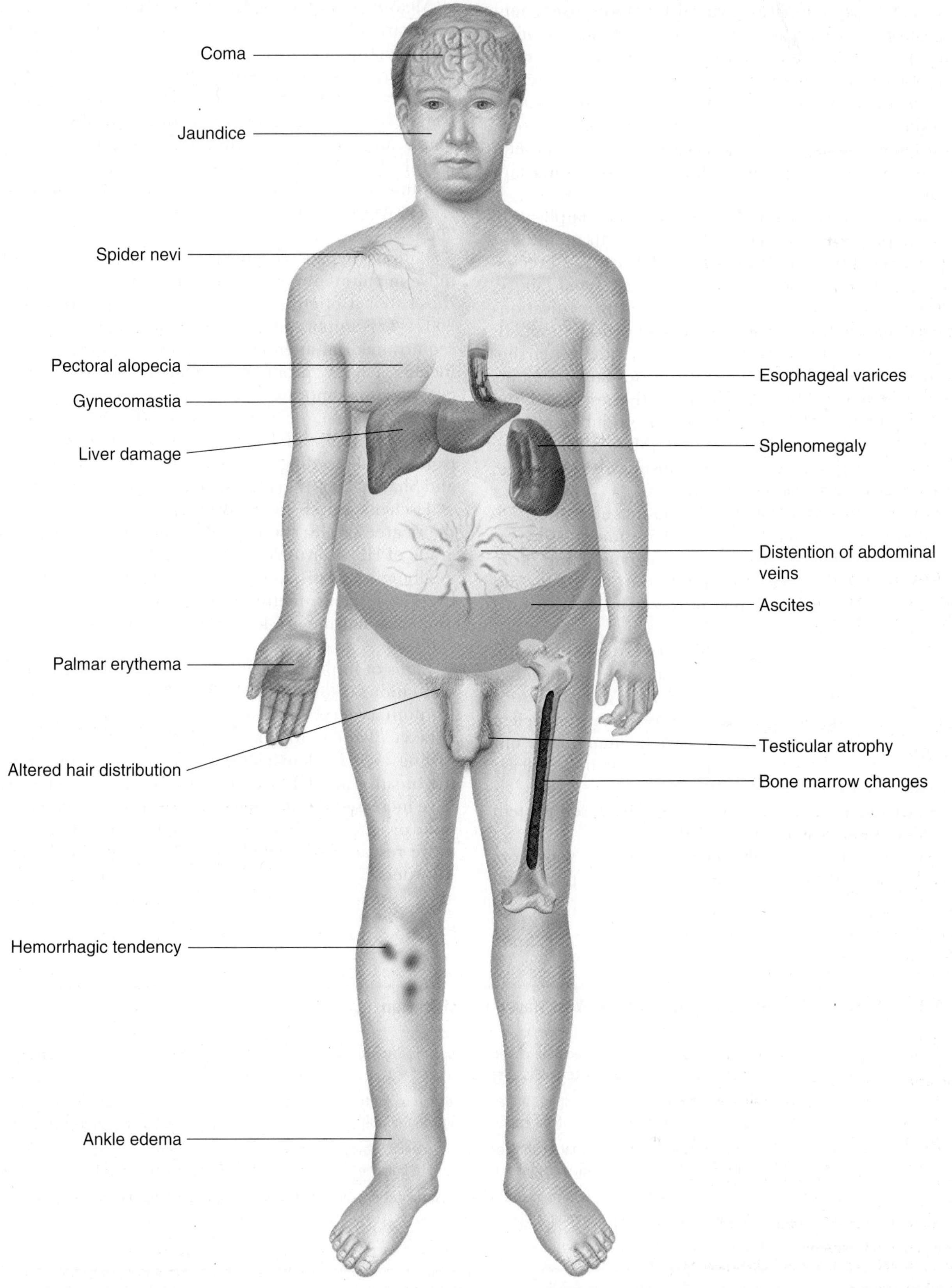

Asset provided by Anatomical Chart Co.

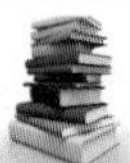

DEFINITIONS AND BACKGROUND

Hepatic failure is common in critical illnesses. Acetaminophen overdose is the leading cause of the acute form. Hallmarks include coagulopathy, usually an INR of 1.5 or more, and encephalopathy. Typical nutrition assessment measures may not reflect the severity of malnutrition because ascites can mask loss of LBM. Blood levels of lactate appear to be good markers for predicting which patients can be managed medically and which need a transplantation (MacQuillan et al, 2005). If hepatorenal syndrome occurs, hemodialysis may be needed; creatinine is not useful here but glomerular filtration rate (GFR) is an important measure.

Hepatic encephalopathy (HE) is a clinical complication caused by portosystemic venous shunting, with or without intrinsic liver disease (Munoz, 2008). HE can be precipitated by GI bleeding, abnormal electrolytes, renal failure, infection, diuretic therapy, use of sedatives or medications that affect the central nervous system, and constipation. HE is estimated to occur in 30–45% of patients with liver cirrhosis and in 10–50% of patients with portosystemic shunts (Eroglu and Byrne, 2009). Patients with HE present with the onset of mental status changes ranging from subtle psychologic abnormalities to profound coma (Munoz, 2008). See Table 8-6 for stages of HE. Acute forms may be reversible; chronic forms may worsen or lead to coma.

Brain glutamine, a byproduct of ammonia detoxification, is elevated in HE (Rama Rao et al, 2005). Causes of hyperammonemia include GI bleed, muscle catabolism, infection, dehydration, noncompliance with lactulose/neomycin, and constipation. The basis of neurotoxicity from ammonia, gamma-aminobutyric acid (GABA), or other agents is not clear. Astrocytes are the most abundant cell type in the brain; they buffer extracellular K(+), regulate neurotransmitter release, form the blood–brain barrier, release growth factors, and regulate the brain immune response (Gee and Keller, 2005). Acute exposure of the astrocytes to ammonia results in alkalinization, with calcium-dependent glutamate release and dysfunction (Rose et al, 2005).

Encephalopathy is usually not caused by altered protein in the diet (Shawcross and Jalan, 2005).

Protein restriction is only necessary in rare, refractory encephalopathy. Patients who have been given a portacaval shunt (TIPS) may benefit from mild protein restriction; nutritional status improves after the shunt.

Decreased dopamine and BCAAs occur in HE; increased AAAs and serotonin also occur. Nevertheless, the use of BCAA solutions is not fully supported by the literature.

Measuring nutritional status in HE can be a challenge. Subjective global assessment and other techniques are not very effective. Measuring handgrip strength may be useful in undernourished patients (Alvares da Silva and Reverbel da Silveira, 2005). Because oxidative stress is a possible trigger in the progression of chronic liver disease, antioxidants and omega-3 polyunsaturated fatty acids may be useful. In addition, because zinc improves taste and immune function, supplementation may improve neurological symptoms and nutrition (Grungrieff and Reinhold, 2005).

Minimal hepatic encephalopathy (MHE) is the mild cognitive impairment commonly seen in patients who have cirrhosis, but it often goes undiagnosed (Stewart and Smith, 2007). It is important to identify signs and symptoms that require medical attention. Commonly associated disorders include energy production deficiencies (hypoglycemia), coagulation abnormalities, immune system dysfunctions, cerebral edema, or **hepatic coma** (Cochran and Losek, 2009). Treatment of HE involves correction of sepsis, gastrointestinal bleeding, and electrolyte imbalance (Sundaram and Shaikh, 2009). Lactulose may be used.

Fischer's ratio between BCAAs and AAAs correlates with the degree of HE; the lower Fischer's ratio, the higher the grade of HE (Koivusalo et al, 2008). Some procedures, such as albumin dialysis, may be used; plasma levels of neuroactive amino acids, methionine, glutamine, glutamate, histidine, and taurine are lowered as a result (Koivusalo et al., 2008).

Signs of impending coma include irritability, change in mentation; disorientation to time and place; asterixis or involuntary jerky movements of the hands; constructional apraxia (inability to draw simple diagrams;) difficulty with writing; ascites, edema; fetor hepaticus (sweet, musty odor of the breath); and GI or esophageal bleeding. Coma patients have increased intracranial pressure and brain edema with a poor prognosis without liver transplantation. Clearly, much more research is needed to resolve these life-threatening disorders.

TABLE 8-6 Stages of Hepatic Encephalopathy—West Haven Classification

Grade 0	Minimal hepatic encephalopathy. Lack of detectable changes in personality or behavior. Minimal changes in memory, concentration, intellectual function, and coordination. Asterixis is absent.
Grade 1	Trivial lack of awareness. Shortened attention span. Impaired addition or subtraction. Hypersomnia, insomnia, or inversion of sleep pattern. Euphoria, depression, or irritability. Mild confusion. Slowing of ability to perform mental tasks. Asterixis can be detected.
Grade 2	Lethargy or apathy. Disorientation. Inappropriate behavior. Slurred speech. Obvious asterixis. Drowsiness, lethargy, gross deficits in ability to perform mental tasks, obvious personality changes, inappropriate behavior, and intermittent disorientation, usually regarding time.
Grade 3	Somnolent but can be aroused, unable to perform mental tasks, disorientation about time and place, marked confusion, amnesia, occasional fits of rage, present but incomprehensible speech.
Grade 4	Coma with or without response to painful stimuli.

Adapted from: Emedicine. Accessed September 5, 2009, at http://www.emedicine.com/med/topic3185.htm.

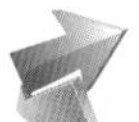

ASSESSMENT, MONITORING, AND EVALUATION

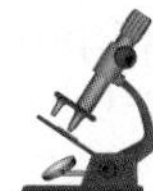

CLINICAL INDICATORS

Genetic Markers: HE is generally acquired.

Clinical/History

Height
Weight
Euvolemic (dry) weight
BMI
Diet history
I & O
BP
Muscle stiffness or rigidity
Changes in mentation or personality
Daytime sleepiness
Decreased self-care
Dysfunctional movements, agitation
Flapping tremor (positive Babinski reflex)
Jaundice
Ascites
Early satiety?
Musty odor of breath and urine
Electroencephalogram (EEG)
Handgrip strength
Acute Physiology and Chronic Health Evaluation (APACHE II) score

Lab Work

Serum lactate levels
BUN (decreased)
Creatinine (not valid?)
Bilirubin (increased)
Alk phos (increased)
AST (increased)
Tumor necrosis factor (elevated)
ALT, GGT
Ca^{++}, Mg^{++}
H & H (decreased)
Serum iron, ferritin
Na^{+}, K^{+}
Chol, Trig
UA
Ammonia
Alb (decreased)
Transthyretin
Nitrogen (N) balance
CRP
PT or INR
Transferrin
Gluc (decreased)
Actin-free Gc globulin (Af-Gc)
Plasma isoleucine, leucine, valine
Plasma tryptophan, phenylalanine, tyrosine
Fischer's ratio
Serum insulin, epinephrine
Thyroxine

INTERVENTION

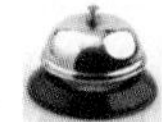

OBJECTIVES

- Treat specific causes and prevent multiple organ system failure. Stop any GI bleeding; offer life support if comatose.
- Provide nutrition support to promote regeneration of liver tissue. Support respiratory, neurological, GI, circulatory systems while the liver regenerates.
- Avoid skeletal muscle catabolism from inadequate oral intake, severely restricted diets or nothing by mouth (NPO) status.
- Decrease ammonia and toxin production. Normalize serum amino acid patterns.
- Avoid daytime or nocturnal fasting by using frequent meals and late evening snacks.
- Prevent hypokalemia, sepsis, starvation, and acute crises.

SAMPLE NUTRITION CARE PROCESS STEPS

Underweight and Altered Nutritional Lab Values

Assessment Data: Dietary intake records; temporal wasting; low weight and BMI of 17; loss of LBM in arms and legs; ascites; confusion and signs of impending coma. Altered LFTs and albumin 2.1 g/dL.

Nutrition Diagnoses (PES):

NC 3.1 Underweight related to decreased appetite prior to admission as evidenced by 90% DBW, BMI 17.

NC 2.2 Altered nutrition related lab value related to liver dysfunction as evidenced by elevated ALT, ALP, AST, NH3, albumin 2.7 g/dL.

Interventions:

Food and Nutrient Delivery: ND 1.2 Modify, distribution type or amount of food and nutrients within meals or specified time (recommend diet change to 2 g sodium, 60 g protein, and six small meals per day; focus on lower animal proteins)

Education: E 1.1 Purpose of nutrition education

Counseling: C 2.2 Goal setting(improve lab values with change)

Coordination of Care: RC 1.1 Team meeting

Monitoring and Evaluation: Track food intake (food diary or history); improvement in albumin or other lab values. Improvement in weight and BMI.

- Reduce circulating amines and lessen shunting of blood around the liver. Control hemorrhage and blood loss into the gut.
- Correct anemia, zinc, and other deficiencies such as magnesium, thiamin, and folate (see Table 8-7).
- Prevent progression to hepatic cancer and improve quality of life.

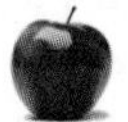

FOOD AND NUTRITION

Follow Practice Parameters of the American College of Gastroenterology (Blei and Cordoba, 2009):

- **Acute encephalopathy:** Withhold oral intake for 24–48 hours, and provide intravenous glucose until improvement is noted. Start TF if patient appears unable to eat after this period. Protein intake begins at a dose of 0.5 g/kg/d; progress to 1–1.5 g/kg/d.
- **Chronic encephalopathy:** Focus protein intake on dairy products and vegetable-based diets. Consider oral BCAAs for individuals intolerant of all protein.
- **Problematic encephalopathy:** Consider lactulose, neomycin, oral zinc, and surgical shunts.
- With coma, use TF with 0.5–0.6 g protein/kg body weight; advance to 1–1.5 g/kg euvolemic weight. Higher intake of BCAAs and glutamine-enriched products are not usually beneficial.
- Glucose is needed to reduce likelihood or presence of hypoglycemia. Start feeding slowly to prevent refeeding syndrome; then to progress to desired level of intake in the malnourished patient. It is prudent to start with

TABLE 8-7 Nutrient Relationships in Hepatic Failure and Hepatic Encephalopathy

Increased sodium and fluid	Edema; fluid retention
Decreased protein	Swollen belly (ascites) from decreased albumin production
Decreased protein and fat with malabsorption	Somnolence, euphoria, asterixis, coma
Decreased vitamin A	Increased respiratory infections
Decreased vitamins C and K	Hemorrhage; scurvy
Decreased magnesium, niacin, thiamin	Hallucinations, delirium, bei-beri, pellagra
Decreased B-complex vitamins, iron, and protein	Glossitis, anemias
Decreased thiamin	Amnesia, confabulation, Korsakoff's psychosis
Decreased niacin	Memory loss
Decreased folacin	Degeneration of spinal cord
Decreased vitamin K	Muscle weakness
Decreased magnesium	Marked anxiety, hyperirritability, confusion, seizures, tremor
Decreased zinc	Poor taste acuity, impaired wound healing

15–20 kcal/kg and progress as tolerated over several days.

- For the patient who is not comatose, diet should provide moderate-to-high levels of protein (Shawcross and Jalan, 2005). Protein restriction has been discontinued in most cases.
- Use enteral nutrition to correct protein–energy malnutrition. A calorie-dense product is desirable. A nasogastric tube placement may be better tolerated when there is ascites.
- To minimize muscle catabolism, diet should provide extra energy from carbohydrates and fats. Use 30 kcal/kg to maintain and 35 kcal/kg body weight to replete tissue; calculate needs using indirect calorimetry whenever possible. Fats should be 30–35% of kilocalories, using MCT if needed.
- When necessary, administer PN with 50% of energy as nonprotein kilocalories. Because PN does not use the gut, where bacteria may otherwise produce ammonia, parenteral protein is well tolerated and may be given as 1.0–1.5 g/kg. Parenteral solutions have risks of infection and metabolic complications.
- Ensure adequate intake of fluids and electrolytes as monitoring determines. Often, sodium is limited to aid diuresis. Restrict fluid only with dilutional hyponatremia (usually 1000–1500 mL).
- Vitamin–mineral supplements may be needed for niacin, thiamin, folate, phosphate, zinc, calcium, and magnesium.
- Monitor fat-soluble vitamin intake (vitamins A, D, E, and K) carefully and avoid excesses. Avoid copper and manganese at this time, and do not give iron supplements randomly.
- If oral diet is tolerated, use a bedtime snack to avoid hypoglycemia. Small meals and snacks throughout the day may increase intake; oral liquid supplements can be made readily available. Avoid severe restrictions of protein, sodium, fluid, fiber. Liquids are often better tolerated than bulky meals.

Common Drugs Used and Potential Side Effects

- Drug-induced ALF accounts for approximately 20% of ALF in children and a higher percentage of ALF in adults; the most common cause of drug-induced ALF in children is acetaminophen (Murray et al, 2008). N-acetylcysteine is effective in ALF caused by acetaminophen overdose, with better results related to how soon it is given (Khashab et al, 2007).
- For other treatments of HE, see Table 8-8.

Herbs, Botanicals, and Supplements

- Healthy enterocytes can degrade peptides and amino acids and use ammonia via glutamate, glutamine, citrulline, and urea synthesis (Bergen and Wu, 2009). Probiotic, CO_2-producing lactobacilli are useful for enhancing gut microbial metabolism in HE (Bergen and Wu, 2009; Bongaerts et al, 2005). Other treatments using prebiotics and probiotics are under study; see Table 8-9.
- Avoid high doses of vitamins A and D, which may be toxic to the diseased liver.
- Herbs and botanical supplements should not be used without discussing with physician. For example, chaparral use can lead to liver failure. Kava kava and many other products should also be avoided in this population. *Silybum marianum* (milk thistle) is not proven to have a therapeutic role in liver failure.

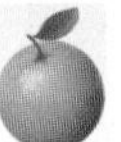

NUTRITION EDUCATION, COUNSELING, CARE MANAGEMENT

- Hospitalization is usually required; discuss symptoms that require immediate medical attention.
- Dietary intake must be adjusted according to the changing status of the patient. Large meals increase portal pressure; use smaller meals more frequently.
- Milk and eggs tend to produce less ammonia than meats or poultry.
- Discuss the importance of refraining from use of alcoholic beverages.
- A better appetite at certain meals may be common. Identify if breakfast or another meal is best tolerated. Some patients sleep late and have a sleep reversal pattern.
- Discuss proper menu planning. Avoid skipping meals.

Patient Education—Foodborne Illness

- If home TF is needed, teach appropriate sanitation and food-handling procedures.

TABLE 8-8 Medications Used for Hepatic Encephalopathy

Medication	Description
Antibiotics: Neomycin	Orally administered antibiotics kill some of the bacteria present within the intestines that produce the dangerous toxins. Be careful not to miss doses. Adverse side effects are common.
Rifaximin	Rifaximin is a nonabsorbed antibiotic with a broad spectrum of activity against aerobic and anaerobic Gram-positive and Gram-negative organisms. It has a better safety and tolerability profile than that of lactulose and possibly neomycin.
Cholestyramine or ursodeoxycholic acid	For itching.
Dietary supplements	Vitamin D and calcium may be needed if osteopenia occurs. Fat-soluble excesses should be avoided since the liver is damaged.
Laxatives: Lactulose (Chronulac, Duphalac, Cholac Syrup, Constulose)	Lactulose is a synthetic sugar used to treat constipation. It is broken down in the colon into products that pull water out from the body and into the colon to soften stools. It also removes ammonia. One or two bowel movements a day are needed. Take lactulose with juice. It may cause abdominal bloating or gas. Be careful not to miss doses, but avoid excesses which can cause diarrhea.
Zinc sulfate or acetate	RNA oxidation and an increase of free intracellular zinc is a consequence of astrocyte swelling and ROS/RNOS production. RNA oxidation may impair postsynaptic protein synthesis, which is critically involved in learning and memory consolidation. Zinc supplementation is recommended.
Medications to avoid	Certain medications can increase the brain's sensitivity to ammonia and other toxins and should not be taken: sedative drugs (Valium, Ativan, Xanax), pain medications (Darvocet, codeine, Vicodin, Percocet, Demerol), antinausea agents (Phenergan, Compazine), antihistamines (Benadryl)

TABLE 8-9 Prebiotics, Probiotics, and Healthy Foods Shopping List[a]

Grains	Beans and Peas (canned/dried)	Oils
Whole grain breads[b] (rye,[c] barley,[c] wheat,[c] oat,[b] buckwheat[b])	Beans:[b] black, pinto, garbanzo, kidney lima, soy, small red, small white, cannellini, Black eyed peas, exotics	Olive
Pasta,[b] whole grain[b]	Lentils:[b] black, red, brown, French	Canola or vegetable
Bulgur,[b] wheat berries[c]	Split peas (yellow, green)	Peanut
Polenta, cornmeal	Edamame (soy beans)	Sesame
Tortillas		Walnut
Flours,[b] whole grain (pastry)[b]		Exotic
Rice, brown		
Oats		
Wild rice		
Exotic grains (spelt, quinoa)		
Cereals, prepared whole grain		
Barley,[b] pearled[c]		
Baking	**Nuts and Seeds**	**Dairy and Cold Case**
Flour, whole grain	Almonds[b]	Pesto
Jam or jelly	Cashews	Salsa
Syrup	Coconuts, fresh	Yogurt[d]
Honey	Flaxseed[b]	Yogurt smoothies[d]
Sugar	Hazelnuts	Kefir[d]
Baking soda/powder	Macadamias	Cottage cheese[b] (check for live cultures or[d] prebiotic inulin)[b]
Tapioca	Peanuts	Skim Milk
Vanilla	Pecans	Acidophilus milk[d]
Yeast	Pine nuts	Cheese
Chocolate	Pistachios	Eggs
Corn Starch	Poppy seeds	Dips
Baking mixes	Pumpkin seeds	Spreads
Carob	Sesame seeds	Tofu[e]
	Sunflower seeds	Miso (soy paste)[e]
	Walnuts	
	Tahini (ground sesame seeds)	
	Nut butters from the above	

(continued)

TABLE 8-9 Prebiotics, Probiotics, and Healthy Foods Shopping List[a] *(continued)*

Beverages	Condiments	Meat, Poultry, Fish, Other
Coffee	Vinegar (apple cider, balsamic, red wine, malt)[e]	Chicken
Tea	Horseradish	Turkey
Chocolate or cocoa	Mustard	Beef
Beer[e]	Mayonnaise	Pork
Wine[e]	Catsup	Lamb
Soymilk	Worcestershire[e]	Fish
Nut milk	Soy sauce/Tamari[e]	Exotics: bison, ostrich, etc.
Rice milk	Chutney	Tofu[e]
Kombucha (tea/live cultures)[e]	Salsa	Tempeh (soy beans)[e]
	Chile oil or sauce	Seitan (wheat gluten)
	Wasabi	Natto (fermented beans)[e]
		Soy turkey, soy lunchmeat, etc.

Fermented/Pickled[e]	Snacks	Freezer Items	Deli
Pickled cucumbers	Popcorn	Vegetables	Bean salads
Olives	Dips made from beans, vegetables	Fruits	Grain salads
Pickled beets	Crackers with whole grain	Waffles	Vegetable salads
Kimchi (fermented cabbage)	Chips, whole grain		
Sauerkraut	Snack bars[b] (check ingredients for whole grains,[b] inulin,[b] probiotics[d])		

Vegetables		Fruits		Herbs and Spices
Artichokes[c]	Ginger root	Apples	Yacon[c]	Allspice
Asparagus[c]	Greens (spinach[c], chard, leafy greens etc.)	Apricots	Figs	Anise
Avocados	Horseradish	Asian pears	Gooseberries	Basil
Bamboo shoots	Jerusalem artichoke[c]	Bananas[c]	Grapefruit	Black Pepper
Beans, green or waxed	Jicama[c]	Berries (raspberry, blackberry, strawberry, gooseberry, elderberry, red currants, exotics)	Grapes	Caraway
Beans, lima (unshelled)	Kale	Cactus pears	Guava	Chili
Beets	Kohlrabi	Cherries	Jujubee	Cilantro
Bok choy	Leeks[c]	Coconut, fresh	Kiwi	Cinnamon
Broccoli	Lettuce, iceberg	Cranberries	Kumquat	Clove
Broccoli rabe	Lettuce, leaf	Currants	Lemon	Coriander
Brussel sprouts	Lettuce (dandelion greens[c], endive, watercress)	Dates	Lime	Cumin
Burdock[c]	Mushrooms	**Vegetables (continued)**	Mango	Dill
Cabbage (red, green, Chinese)	Okra	Rutabagas	Melon, musk	Fennel
Cauliflower	Onions[c]	Salsify[c]	Nectarines	Ginger
Carrots	Onions, dry[c]	Seaweed, edible	Oranges	Mace
Celery	Onions, green[c]	Shallots[c]	Papaya	Marjoram
Celery root	Palm hearts	Snow peas	Passion fruit	Mint
Chestnuts	Parsnips	Sprouts, bean, alfalfa, etc	Peaches	Nutmeg
Chicory[c]	Peas (unshelled)	Squash, summer varieties	Pears	Oregano
Corn (in husks)	Peppers, chili	Squash, winter varieties	Persimmon	Parsley
Cucumbers	Peppers, bell	Taro	Pineapple	Rosemary
Daikon radish	Potatoes	Tomatillo	Plantain	Sage
Dandelion greens[c]	Potatoes, sweet, yams	Tomatoes	Plums, pluot, plumcot	Savory
Eggplant	Pumpkin	Turnips	Pomegranate	Tarragon
Endive	Radishes	Watercress	Pommelo	Thyme
Fennel	Rhubarb		Raisins	Turmeric
Fiddleheads			Star fruit	Vanilla
Garlic[c]			Quince	
			Watermelon	

NOTE—read labels: Strain. What probiotic is inside? *Lactobacillus casei Shirota, Lactobacillus acidophilus, Bifidobacteriumlactis, Saccharomyces cereviase boullardii.* CFU (Colony Forming Units). How many live microorganisms are in each serving? When does it expire? Packaging should ensure an effective level of live bacteria through the "best by" or expiration date. Suggested serving size. How much do I take? Health benefits. What can this product do for me? Proper storage conditions. Where do I keep it to ensure maximum survival of the probiotic? Corporate contact information. Who makes this product? Where to do I go for more information?

From: International Scientific Association for Probiotics and Prebiotics, http://www.ISAPP.net.

Adapted from: Gut Insight © 2009 Gut Insight: probiotics and prebiotics for digestive health and well-being by Jo Ann Tatum Hattner, MPH, RD, with Susan Anderes, MLIS. San Francisco: Hattner Nutrition, 2009. Used with permission.

Other resources: U.S. Probiotics, http://www.usprobiotics.org/.

[a]Seventy percent of the body's immunity is in the gut. There are 300–1000 species of bacteria, 100 trillion in the gut (about 3 lb). Alcohol, smoking, stress, poor bowel hygiene, aging, intestinal infections, antibiotics, and a poor diet can affect intestinal microbiota. The normal levels of lactobacilli, bifidobacteria, and other "good bacteria" may be decreased. Imbalanced flora may lead to abnormal GI function, such as constipation, diarrhea, flares of inflammatory bowel disease or irritable bowel syndrome, other pancreatic or abdominal inflammations, allergic responses, and an impaired immune system. Choosing foods wisely can improve gut health.

[b]Prebiotic potentials.

[c]Prebiotic stars.*

[d]Probiotics.

[e]Fermented foods.

For More Information

- Hepatic Encephalopathy
  http://www.nlm.nih.gov/medlineplus/ency/article/000302.htm
- Medline
  http://www.nlm.nih.gov/medlineplus/ency/article/000302.htm

HEPATIC FAILURE, ENCEPHALOPATHY, AND COMA—CITED REFERENCES

Alvares da Silva MR, Reverbel da Silveira T. Comparison between handgrip strength, subjective global assessment, and prognostic nutritional index in assessing malnutrition and predicting clinical outcome in cirrhotic outpatients. *Nutrition.* 21:113, 2005.

Bergen WG, Wu G. Intestinal nitrogen recycling and utilization in health and disease. *J Nutr.* 139:821, 2009.

Blei AT, Cordoba J. Practice Guidelines: Hepatic Encephalopathy. Accessed October 9, 2009, at http://www.nature.com/ajg/journal/v96/n7/abs/ajg2001494a.html.

Bongaerts G, et al. Effect of antibiotics, prebiotics and probiotics in treatment for hepatic encephalopathy. *Med Hypotheses.* 64:64, 2005.

Cochran JB, Losek JD. Acute liver failure in children. *Pediatr Emerg Care.* 23:129, 2009.

Eroglu Y, Byrne WJ. Hepatic encephalopathy. *Emerg Med.* 27:401, 2009.

Gee JR, Keller JN. Astrocytes: regulation of brain homeostasis via apolipoprotein E. *Int J Biochem Cell Biol.* 37:1145, 2005.

Grungrieff K, Reinhold D. Liver cirrhosis and "liver" diabetes mellitus are linked by zinc deficiency. *Med Hypotheses.* 64:316, 2005.

Khashab M, et al. Epidemiology of acute liver failure. *Curr Gastroenterol Rep.* 9:66, 2007.

Koivusalo AM, et al. Albumin dialysis has a favorable effect on amino acid profile in hepatic encephalopathy. *Metab Brain Dis.* 23:387, 2008.

Macquillan GC, et al. Blood lactate but not serum phosphate levels can predict patient outcome in fulminant hepatic failure. *Liver Transpl.* 11:1073, 2005.

Munoz SJ. Hepatic encephalopathy. *Med Clin Am.* 92:795, 2008.

Murray KF, et al. Drug-related hepatotoxicity and acute liver failure. *J Pediatr Gastrointest Nutr.* 48:395, 2008.

Rama Rao KV, et al. Differential response of glutamine in cultured neurons and astrocytes. *J Neurosci Res.* 79:193, 2005.

Rose C, et al. Acute insult of ammonia leads to calcium-dependent glutamate release from cultured astrocytes: an effect of pH. *J Biol Chem.* 280:20937, 2005.

Shawcross D, Jalan R. Dispelling myths in the treatment of hepatic encephalopathy. *Lancet.* 365:431, 2005.

Stewart CA, Smith GE. Minimal hepatic encephalopathy. *Nat Clin Pract Gastroenterol Hepatol.* 4:677, 2007.

Sundaram V, Shaikh OS. Hepatic encephalopathy: pathophysiology and emerging therapies. *Med Clin N Am.* 93:819, 2009.

LIVER TRANSPLANTATION

NUTRITIONAL ACUITY RANKING: LEVEL 4

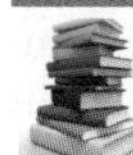

DEFINITIONS AND BACKGROUND

Liver transplantation (LT) is now a viable alternative for patients with end-stage hepatic failure due to cirrhosis, viral hepatitis, chronic active liver disease, alpha-1 antitrypsin deficiency, primary sclerosing cirrhosis, cholangiocarcinoma, hemochromatosis, autoimmune hepatitis, Budd–Chiari syndrome, hepatoma, primary biliary cirrhosis, or cystic fibrosis.

Nutritional depletion occurs in this population before surgery. Muscle wasting, cachexia, and decreased fat stores are common. Supportive care for all patients with ALF includes adequate enteral nutrition, aggressive screening and treatment of infection, prophylactic broad-spectrum antibiotics, and antifungal agents (Hay, 2004).

Patients are screened carefully for other underlying conditions; many will not be suitable for transplantation. Alcohol is a major contributor to cirrhosis and the need for transplantation. NASH, obesity, diabetes, and hyperinsulinism play a role in cirrhosis and the need for transplantation. Older age, higher BMI, diabetes and HTN are associated with poor outcomes (Malik et al, 2009).

Symptoms and signs leading to the need for transplantation include ascites, jaundice, edema, CNS dysfunction, and cachexia. In living donor liver transplantation (LDLT), a healthy, living person donates a portion of his or her liver to another person.

Preoperative and early postoperative nutrition may speed recovery, lessen time in the intensive care unit, and promote fewer infections. Subjective global assessment (SGA) is often useful because lab work varies so much in liver disease. SGA includes physical signs and symptoms, dietary changes and intolerances, medical/surgical history, GI symptoms and complaints, history of weight loss, and functional capacity. Transthyretin may be a reliable test when the inflammatory process resolves.

Patients with end-stage liver disease are prone to develop osteopenia and osteoporosis, and additional bone loss may occur with the use of immunosuppression agents after transplant. Bone loss occurs early after liver transplant and leads to postoperative fractures, especially with low bone mass. Calcium and vitamin D intake must be a priority.

In general, enteral nutrition is effective in maintaining nutritional status after transplantation. Nutritional supplementation after LT quickly restores protein synthesis. PN may be needed (Plauth et al, 2009). Patients with LT regain a normal life within months of surgery but have a lifetime of immunosuppressive treatment. Intravenous fish oil lipid emulsion may be useful.

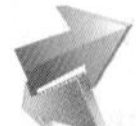

ASSESSMENT, MONITORING, AND EVALUATION

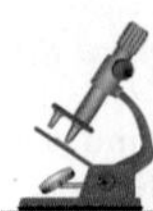

CLINICAL INDICATORS

Genetic Markers: Respiratory chain disorders may present with neonatal ALF, hepatic steatohepatitis, cholestasis, cirrhosis with chronic liver failure and the need for LT; molecular defects (mutations in nuclear genes such as SCO1, BCS1L, POLG, DGUOK, and MPV17 and the deletion or rearrangement of mitochondrial DNA) have been identified (Lee and Sokol, 2007). Methylmalonic acidemia with complete mutase deficiency (mut(0) type) is an inborn error of metabolism with high mortality and morbidity; LT may be a solution (Chen et al, 2009).

Clinical/History	Lab Work	
Height	Serum lactate levels	Serum Fe, ferritin
Weight—usual	BUN, Creat	Transferrin
Present weight	Alb, Transthyretin	BUN, creatinine
BMI	N balance	Chol, Trig
SGA with diet history	Na^+, K^+	Carotenoids
Cachexia?	CRP (elevated?)	AST, ALT
Edema	Alk phos	GGT
Nausea and vomiting	Bilirubin	Gluc
I & O	Amino acid profiles	PT or INR
BP	Serum ammonia	
Ascites?	Cerebrospinal fluid (CSF)	
Early satiety?	Ca^{++}, Mg^{++}	
Jaundice	H & H	
CNS dysfunction?		
DEXA		

SAMPLE NUTRITION CARE PROCESS STEPS

Inadequate Intake From Enteral Nutrition

Assessment Data: I & O records showing long periods without enteral infusion for testing, lab work and nursing shift changes. Dry weight beginning to drop below desired range.

Nutrition Diagnosis (PES): Inadequate intake of enteral nutrition (NI-2.3) related to infusion being held for >3 hours daily as evidenced by intake at 70% of expected protein and kilocalories.

Intervention: Food and Nutrient Delivery—recalculation of TF formula to provide appropriate protein and kilocalories over 21 versus 24 hours daily. Education of nursing staff about necessary change in the TF order; coordination of care.

Monitoring and Evaluation: Track intake of enteral infusion; identify if weight is stable and labs are normal. Determine if current intake meets estimated needs; continue therapy. Evaluate every other day until discharge.

INTERVENTION

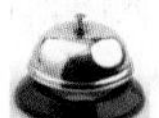

OBJECTIVES

Pretransplantation

- Correct malnutrition; lessen edema and ascites.
- Treat hyponatremia and electrolyte imbalances, depending on medications and renal function.
- Prevent or correct catabolic wasting of muscle mass from increased hormonal levels of insulin, glucagon, epinephrine, or cortisol.
- Provide nutritional support in an appropriate mode of feeding to provide a normalized nitrogen balance and other normalized laboratory values. Consider nausea, vomiting, anorexia, diarrhea.
- Correct fat malabsorption, with or without steatorrhea and diarrhea.
- Normalize blood glucose levels and prevent hypoglycemia; diabetes is common.
- Correct abnormal amino acid metabolism and neural accumulation of amino acids that are precursors for dopamine, serotonin, and norepinephrine. Normalize serum ammonia.

Posttransplantation

- Promote normalized protein synthesis in the liver for albumin, globulins, clotting factors. Monitoring nutritional parameters will not be a simple process; many usual measurements are not useful markers of nutritional decline (Shahid et al, 2005).
- Prevent or correct hyperglycemia, fasting hypoglycemia, and abnormal glucagon storage. Diabetes is a common complication from use of prednisone, cyclosporine, and tacrolimus.
- Prevent hypophosphatemia and refeeding syndrome.
- Support wound healing.
- Prevent infection and rejection, the most common complications. Portal venous complications have been well documented and can lead to graft failure (Woo et al, 2007).
- Manage long-term hypercholesterolemia, hypertension, obesity, osteopenia, or bone fractures.
- The role of probiotics in LT is unclear (Jenkins et al, 2005).

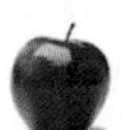

FOOD AND NUTRITION

Pretransplantation

- Energy should be 35–45 kcal/kg dry weight for malnourished patients and 30–35 kcal/kg dry weight to maintain weight (Hasse, 2005). Use sufficient carbohydrate and fat to spare protein and meet energy needs. Monitor closely for hyperglycemia.
- Protein needs will vary: 0.8–1.0 g/kg dry weight in compensated liver disease. Calculate 1.5–2.0 g/kg dry weight in decompensated liver disease and 0.6–1.0 g/kg dry weight for HE.
- Modify for fluid, sodium, potassium, and other electrolytes depending on lab values and renal status. Restrict

TABLE 8-10 Post–Liver or Pancreatic Transplant Nutrition Guidelines

Nutrient	LIVER Short-Term	LIVER Long-Term	Pancreas Short-Term	Pancreas Long-Term
Calories	20–30% above normal or measure through indirect calorimetry; increase for weight gain	Maintenance: 30–35 kcal/kg depending on activity level	20–30% above normal or measure through indirect calorimetry; increase for weight gain	Maintenance: 30–35 kcal/kg depending on activity level
Protein	1.3–2 g/kg/d	1 g/kg/d	1.3–2 g/kg/d	1 g/kg/d
Carbohydrate	50–70% of calories	50–70% of calories; restrict simple sugars	45–55% of kcals; use CHO counting	45–55% of kcals; use CHO counting
Fat	30% of calories; up to 50% with severe hyperglycemia	<30% of total calories; <10% saturated fats	25–35% of kcals, depending on lipid levels Up to 50% of calories with severe hyperglycemia	25–35% of total calories; <10% saturated fats
Calcium	800–1200 mg/d	1–1.5 g/d (consider the need for vitamin D supplements)	800–1200 mg/d	1000–1500 mg/d (consider the need for vitamin D supplements)
Sodium	2–4 g/d	3–4 g/d	2–4 g/d	3–4 g/d
Magnesium and phosphorus	Encourage intake of foods high in these nutrients	Encourage intake of foods high in these nutrients; supplement as needed	Encourage intake of foods high in these nutrients; supplement as needed	Encourage intake of foods high in these nutrients; supplement as needed
Potassium	Supplement or restrict based on serum levels	Supplement or restrict based on serum levels	Supplement or restrict based on serum levels	Supplement or restrict based on serum levels
Other vitamins and minerals	Multivitamin–mineral: supplement to DRI or RDA levels	Adequate vitamin D will be needed to prevent deficiency; multivitamin–mineral: supplement to DRI or RDA levels	Multivitamin–mineral: supplement to RDA levels	Multivitamin–mineral: supplement to RDA levels

Source: Hasse J, Matarese L. Medical nutrition therapy for liver, biliary system, and exocrine pancreas disorders. In: Mahan L, Escott-Stump S, eds. *Krause's food nutrition and diet therapy*. 12th ed. St Louis: Elsevier, 2008.

sodium to 2- to 4-g and limit fluid to 1000- to 1500-mL with edema.

- Use a low-volume TF if needed, diluting the concentration. Avoid glutamine-enriched solutions with elevated serum ammonia levels. Consider use of BCAA-enriched formulas.
- Vitamins and minerals should be given at levels that meet but not exceed recommended daily allowances. Fat malabsorption is common; use water-miscible forms of vitamins A, D, E, and K with steatorrhea. B-complex vitamins may be depleted. Stores of calcium, magnesium, potassium, phosphorus, manganese, copper, and zinc are often low and should be repleted.

Post-transplantation

- See Table 8-10.

Common Drugs Used and Potential Side Effects

- See Table 8-11.

Herbs, Botanicals, and Supplements

- Use of probiotics may be quite helpful in this population. A synbiotic composition in an enteral feeding, consisting of one lactic acid bacteria (LAB) and one fiber, greatly reduces incidence of postoperative bacterial infections (Rayes et al, 2005).
- Chaparral should be avoided after transplantation. Herbs and botanical supplements should not be used without discussing with physician. St. John's wort interferes with the metabolism of cyclosporine and should not be used.
- In one study, 50% of LT patients admitted to using vitamins after surgery, and 19% used herbal remedies combined with vitamins, mostly silymarin (Neff et al, 2004).

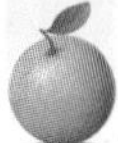

NUTRITION EDUCATION, COUNSELING, CARE MANAGEMENT

- Discuss the role of diet in wound healing, graft retention, and improvement in health status.
- Provide patient or family with recipes for no-added-salt and sugar-free foods as needed.
- Obesity can occur unless energy intake is controlled over the long term.
- Discuss sources of foods that contain calcium, magnesium, and other desirable nutrients. Individualize to patient preferences and needs.
- Discuss the need for alcohol rehabilitation, family counseling, or other available services. Ethanol (ETOH) abuse affects such key nutrients as niacin, folate, vitamin B_{12}, zinc, phosphorus, and magnesium.

TABLE 8-11 Medications Used after Liver Transplantation

Medication	Description
Analgesics	Analgesics are used to reduce pain. Long-term use may affect such nutrients as vitamin C and folacin; monitor carefully for each specific medication.
Azathioprine (Imuran)	Azathioprine may cause anorexia, leukopenia, thrombocytopenia, oral and esophageal sores, macrocytic anemia, pancreatitis, vomiting, diarrhea, and altered taste acuity. Folate supplementation and other dietary modifications (liquid or soft diet, use of oral supplements, and flavor enhancements) may be needed. The drug works by lowering the number of T cells; it is often prescribed along with prednisone for conventional immunosuppression.
Corticosteroids (prednisone or Solu-Cortef)	Corticosteroids such as prednisone and Solu-Cortef are used for immunosuppression. Side effects include increased catabolism of proteins, negative nitrogen balance, hyperphagia, ulcers, decreased glucose tolerance, sodium retention, fluid retention, and impaired calcium absorption and osteoporosis. Cushing's syndrome, obesity, muscle wasting, and increased gastric secretion may result. A higher protein intake and lower intake of carbohydrate and sodium may be needed.
Cyclosporine	Cyclosporine does not retain sodium as much as corticosteroids do. Intravenous doses are more effective than oral doses. Nausea, vomiting, and diarrhea are common side effects. Hyperlipidemia, hyperglycemia, and hyperkalemia may also occur; decrease fat intake as well as sodium and potassium if necessary. Magnesium may need to be replaced. The drug is also nephrotoxic; a controlled renal diet may be beneficial. Taking omega-3 fatty acids during cyclosporine therapy may reduce toxic side effects (such as high blood pressure and kidney damage) associated with this medication in transplantation patients. Avoid use with St. John's wort.
Diuretics	Diuretics such as furosemide (Lasix) may cause hypokalemia. Aldactone actually spares potassium; monitor drug changes closely. In general, avoid use with fenugreek, yohimbe, and ginkgo.
Immunosuppressants	Immunosuppressants such as muromonab (Orthoclone OKT3) and antithymocyte globulin (ATG) are less nephrotoxic than cyclosporine but can cause nausea, anorexia, diarrhea, and vomiting. Monitor carefully. Fever and stomatitis also may occur; alter diet as needed.
Insulin	Insulin may be necessary during periods of hyperglycemia. Monitor for hypoglycemic symptoms during use.
Mycophenolate mofetil	Diarrhea is common. Extra fluids will be needed.
Muromonab (Orthoclone OKT3)	This drug can lead to nausea, vomiting, diarrhea, and anorexia, and meal adjustments may be needed.
Tacrolimus (Prograf, FK506)	Tacrolimus suppresses T-cell immunity; it is 100 times more potent than cyclosporine, thus requiring smaller doses. Side effects include GI distress, nausea, vomiting, hyperkalemia, and hyperglycemia; adjust diet accordingly by reducing carbohydrate or elevating potassium intake.

- Maintain a good diet and physical activity to support bone density.

Patient Education—Foodborne Illness

- Careful food handling and hand washing are important to prevent introduction of foodborne pathogens to the transplantation individual who may be experiencing graft–host rejection.
- Prevent infections from foodborne illness; patients who have undergone transplantation may be prone to increased risk more than other individuals.

For More Information

- Medicine Net
  http://www.medicinenet.com/liver_transplant/article.htm
- National Institute of Diabetes and Digestive and Kidney Diseases (NIDDK)–Liver Transplant
  http://digestive.niddk.nih.gov/ddiseases/pubs/livertransplant/
- United Network for Organ Sharing
  http://www.unos.org/
- USC Liver Transplant Guide
  http://www.surgery.usc.edu/divisions/hep/patientguide/

LIVER TRANSPLANTATION—CITED REFERENCES

Chen PW, et al. Stabilization of blood methylmalonic acid level in methylmalonic acidemia after liver transplantation [published online ahead of print August 14, 2009]. *Pediatr Transplant.* 14:337, 2010.

Hay JE. Acute liver failure. *Curr Treat Options Gastroenterol.* 7:459, 2004.

Jenkins B, et al. Probiotics: a practical review of their role in specific clinical scenarios. *Nutr Clin Pract.* 20:262, 2005.

Lee WS, Sokol RJ. Mitochondrial hepatopathies: advances in genetics and pathogenesis. *Hepatology.* 45:1555, 2007.

Malik SM, et al. Outcome after liver transplantation for NASH cirrhosis. *Am J Transplant.* 9:782, 2009.

Neff GW, et al. Consumption of dietary supplements in a liver transplant population. *Liver Transpl.* 10:881, 2004.

Plauth M, et al. ESPEN Guidelines on Parenteral Nutrition: hepatology. *Clin Nutr.* 28:436, 2009.

Rayes N, et al. Supply of pre- and probiotics reduces bacterial infection rates after liver transplantation—a randomized, double-blind trial. *Am J Transplant.* 5:125, 2005.

Shahid M, et al. Nutritional markers in liver allograft recipients. *Transplantation.* 79:359, 2005.

Woo DH, et al. Management of portal venous complications after liver transplantation. *Tech Vasc Interv Radiol.* 10:233, 2007.

PANCREATIC DISORDERS

PANCREATITIS, ACUTE

NUTRITIONAL ACUITY RANKING: LEVEL 3–4

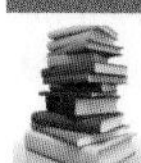

DEFINITIONS AND BACKGROUND

Acute pancreatitis is an inflammatory, clinical syndrome defined by a discrete episode of abdominal pain and elevations in serum enzyme levels (Gramlich and Taft, 2007). The exocrine pancreas secretes proteolytic, lipolytic, and amylolytic enzymes for nutrient digestion in the intestines. AP is initiated inside acinar cells by premature activation of digestive enzymes in the pancreas instead of the duodenum. Seventy-five percent to 85% of all pancreatic episodes are considered mild and self-limiting and do not require intervention with nutrition support (Gramlich and Taft, 2007). In the unfortunate 15–25% who need nutrition support, preventing multiple organ failure is important.

AP is common in men between the ages of 35 and 45 years, primarily from alcohol abuse or secondarily from gallstones (cholelithiasis). It is often difficult to differentiate between pancreatitis and acute cholecystitis; the correct diagnosis is important because treatments are very different. Other causes of AP include end-stage renal disease, lupus, biliary tract disease, abdominal trauma, certain dyslipidemias (especially triglycerides >1000 mg/dL), AIDS, and pancreatic cancer.

Symptoms of AP include sudden, severe abdominal pain, nausea, vomiting, and diarrhea. Complications include sepsis, acute renal failure, hypovolemia, circulatory shock, and pancreatic necrosis. Abdominal pain can be constant and disabling, causing some patients to become addicted to pain medications. About 25% of persons with AP go on to have chronic pancreatitis. Surgery for AP may include necrosectomy, pancreaticoduodenectomy, or sphincterotomy.

Oxygen free radical–mediated tissue damage is well established in the pathogenesis of AP. Cytokines involved in the systemic inflammatory response in AP include lipid mediators (prostanoids, thromboxanes, and leukotrienes) generated from arachidonic acid. Reactive oxygen species mediate inflammatory cytokine expression and apoptosis of pancreatic acinar cells (Parks et al, 2009). Omega-3 fatty acids DHA and alpha-linolenic acid (ALA), suppress the expression of inflammatory cytokines (IL-1beta, IL-6) and inhibit the activation of transcription factor activator protein-1 in cerulein-stimulated pancreatic acinar cells (Parks et al, 2009). Heat shock proteins (HSPs) that inhabit almost all subcellular locations and cellular membranes play a major role in the protection of cells against stressful and injury-inciting stimuli, including acinar cell injury in AP (Dudeja et al, 2009).

The role of the gut in maintaining immune system integrity is widely recognized. Therefore, nutrition support by the enteral route is preferred (Cao et al, 2008). Nasojejunal feeding tube and a low-molecular diet provide clear advantages compared to parenteral nutrition, such as fewer infectious complications, shorter length of hospital stay, lower cost, and less need for surgery (McClave et al, 2006; Meier and Beglinger, 2006; Petrov et al, 2008). Parenteral nutrition (PN) is used for short term when full nutritional requirements cannot be met enterally so that body composition is preserved (Chandrasegaram et al, 2005).

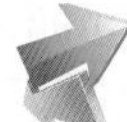

ASSESSMENT, MONITORING, AND EVALUATION

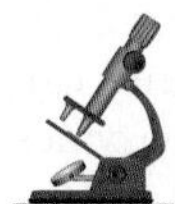

CLINICAL INDICATORS

Genetic Markers: Evaluation for a susceptible genotype is important (Balog et al, 2005). This is true for pancreatic carcinoma more than pancreatitis per se.

Clinical/History

- Height
- Weight
- BMI (obese?)
- Diet history
- BP (low)
- Rapid heart rate
- Left upper quadrant abdominal pain
- Nausea, vomiting
- Temperature
- Chvostek's sign
- Steatorrhea or oily stools
- Multiple Organ System Score (MOSS)
- CT scan showing interstitial pancreatic edema
- Magnetic resonance imaging (MRI)

Lab Work

- CRP (used to measure severity in AP)
- Procalcitonin (elevated?)
- Lipase (>110; more sensitive than amylase)
- Amylase (>250)
- K^+ (decreased)
- Na^+ (decreased)
- PT or INR
- Bilirubin (elevated)
- Ca^{++} (decreased)
- Gluc (increased, >200)
- Chol (total decreased)
- LDL cholesterol (elevated?)
- Trig (increased)
- Mg^{++} (decreased)
- LDH (>700)
- ALT (elevated)
- AST (>250)
- WBC (>10,000 cells/mm^3)
- Alb (low)
- Partial pressure of carbon dioxide (pCO_2) (increased)
- Partial pressure of oxygen (pO_2) (decreased)
- BUN
- H & H
- Serum folate
- Alk phos (increased)
- CT scan for necrosis
- Ultrasound
- Fecal fat study

SAMPLE NUTRITION CARE PROCESS STEPS

Impaired Nutrient Utilization

Assessment Data: Patient statement of not taking enzyme medication, reports of abdominal pain, diarrhea after eating, vomiting.

Nutrition Diagnosis (PES): Impaired nutrient utilization related to pancreatic enzyme deficiency as evidenced by abdominal pain and steatorrhea and report of medication noncompliance.

Intervention: Interventions would address the appropriate dose and frequency of medication intake.

Monitoring and Evaluation: Plan would include asking patient time of next clinic visit. Evaluate change in steatorrhea and improvement in enzyme medication compliance.

INTERVENTION

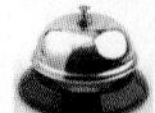

OBJECTIVES

- Reduce pain. Achieve pancreatic rest simultaneously with gut use.
- Use enteral nutrition to reduce the systemic inflammatory response syndrome (Gramlich and Taft, 2007). Failure to use the GI tract in AP may exacerbate disease severity (McClave et al, 2006).
- Avoid pancreatic irritants, especially alcohol and caffeine. Monitor for increased need for pancreatic enzymes with the use of TF.
- Avoid overfeeding.
- Correct fluid and electrolyte imbalances and malnutrition. Acid–base imbalance is common with nasogastric suctioning, fistula losses, renal failure, nausea, and vomiting.
- Reduce fever; prevent shock and hypovolemia, hypermetabolism, sepsis, and compression of the stomach or colon. Avoid cardiovascular, pulmonary, hematological, renal, neurological, or metabolic complications with organ failure. Extensive necrosis and infection are associated with the development of organ failure (Garg et al, 2005).
- Use CPN if abdominal pain is refractory. CPN use can promote positive nitrogen balance (Chandrasegaram et al, 2005).

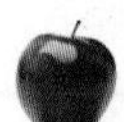

FOOD AND NUTRITION

- Postpyloric TF is often well tolerated (Niv et al, 2009). Products containing MCT are useful for TF, especially when there is steatorrhea. Omega-3 fatty acids are also helpful (Lasztity et al, 2005). Transition to jejunostomy can be considered when pain is refractory, using a standard formula and needle catheter jejunostomy.
- Progress to a diet given in six daily feedings used with pancreatic enzymes for all meals and snacks.
- Alcoholic beverages and nicotine are prohibited. Limit gastric stimulants, such as peppermint and black pepper, if not tolerated.
- Diet should include adequate amounts of vitamin C, B-complex vitamins, and folic acid for water-soluble vitamin needs. Vitamin B_{12} deficiency can occur because intrinsic factor is prevented from binding with vitamin B_{12}. Use fat-soluble vitamins in water-miscible form.
- Antioxidants including selenium may be needed (Musil et al, 2005). Adequate calcium, magnesium, and zinc supplementation should also be provided.

Common Drugs Used and Potential Side Effects

- Many drugs can trigger acute pancreatitis: furosemide (Lasix), azathioprine, dideoxyinosine, DDI (used for treating AIDS), 6-mercaptopurine, 6-MP (an immunosuppressant drug), angiotensin-converting enzyme (ACE) inhibitors, dapsone, acetaminophen, estrogens, methyldopa, nitrofurantoin, steroids, thiazides, cimetidine, erythromycin, salicylates, sulfonamides, and tetracyclines.
- The most common cause of death in AP patients is infection with enteric bacteria, but there is no convincing evidence for routine administration of prophylactic antibiotics (Wittau et al, 2008).
- See Table 8-12 for guidance on medications.

Herbs, Botanicals, and Supplements

- Antioxidants have protective properties that can be beneficial. See Table 8-13.
- Other herbs and botanical supplements should not be used without discussing with physician as many have hepatotoxic properties.
- Probiotics have had mixed results; they may actually promote higher mortality in patients with AP (Besselink et al, 2008).

TABLE 8-12 Medications Used in Pancreatitis

Medication	Description	Acute	Chronic
Antibiotics	Antibiotics may be needed to manage necrosis and systemic complications.	X	X
Bile salts	Bile salts or water-miscible forms of fat-soluble vitamins may be needed.	X	X
Diuretics	Diuretics such as acetazolamide (Diamox) may be needed to control fluid retention. Nausea, vomiting, and diarrhea may result.	X	X
H_2-receptor antagonists (cimetidine, ranitidine)	Cimetidine may deplete vitamin B_{12}, especially among the elderly. Histamine H_2-receptor antagonists or proton pump inhibitors can improve fat malabsorption and steatorrhea.	—	X
Insulin	Insulin may be necessary. Monitor for hypoglycemia during use.	X	X
Octreotide	Octreotide may have a beneficial role in the management of AP.	X	—
Opiates	Opiates may be prescribed for pain.	X	—
Painkillers	Pain control requires the use of morphine-like drugs (pethidine, morphine, and diamorphine), which have the risk of addiction, particularly if their use is not controlled.	—	X
Pancreatic enzymes	30,000 IU per meal may be needed to reduce steatorrhea to less than 20 g/d. Enteric coating is necessary to prevent destruction by enzymes. Take enteric-coated enzymes with cimetidine, food, or antacids. Capsules or tablets should be swallowed whole.	X	X

TABLE 8-13 Antioxidants and Sources[a]

Vitamins	Sources or Comments
• Vitamin A as beta carotene protects vegetables and fruits from solar radiation damage.	See beta-carotene (below). Supplements are not recommended for general use.
• Vitamin C (ascorbic acid) is a reducing agent.	Citrus fruits (oranges, sweet limes, grapefruit, tangerines), green peppers, broccoli, black currants, strawberries, blueberries, raw cabbage. Destroyed by long-term storage or cooking.
• Vitamin E (alpha-tocopherol) protects lipid membranes. It also protects glutathione peroxidase (GPX-4). Some tocotrienol isomers also have antioxidant properties.	Wheat germ, nuts, seeds, whole grains, green leafy vegetables, vegetable oil, fish oil. GPX4 is the only molecule that efficiently reduces lipid hydroperoxides within the cell membranes.
Vitamin Cofactors and Minerals	
• Coenzyme Q10	Ubiquinol is made in the body and is poorly absorbed from the gut
• Manganese	Part of the superoxide dismutase (SOD) enzyme in mitochondria
• Copper	Part of the superoxide dismutase (SOD) enzyme in the cytosol and extracellular fluid
• Zinc	Part of the superoxide dismutase (SOD) enzyme in the cytosol and extracellular fluid
• Iodide	Iodized salt and seafood
• Selenium and Glutathione	Liver contains a large amount as part of detoxification system. Glutathione is made from amino acids, but diet does not control its production. Acetylcysteine is a sulfur-containing amino acid that may increase glutathione levels.
Carotenoid Terpenoids	
• Alpha-carotene	Less active than beta-carotene
• Astaxanthin	Found naturally in red algae and animals higher in the marine food chain. It is a red pigment familiarly recognized in crustacean shells and salmon flesh/roe.
• Beta-carotene	Butternut squash, carrots, orange bell peppers, pumpkins, broccoli, cantaloupe, peaches, apricots and sweet potatoes
• Canthaxanthin	Edible mushrooms, crustaceans, fish such as carp.
• Lutein	Spinach, red peppers. Destroyed by long-term storage or cooking.
• Lycopene	Ripe red tomatoes, tomato sauces, watermelon
• Zeaxanthin	Yellow corn
Flavonoid Polyphenolics	
• Flavones:	Tea, coffee, soy, fruit, olive oil, red wine, chocolate, cinnamon, oregano
• Apigenin	Parsley, celery, dandelion. Potent inhibitor of CYP2C9, which metabolizes drugs.
• Luteolin	Celery, thyme, green pepper, chamomile tea
• Tangeritin	Tangerine and citrus peels. May help lower cholesterol or prevent Parkinson's disease.
• Flavonols:	The flavonols (kaempferol, quercetin, and myricetin) may reduce the risk of pancreatic cancer.
• Isorhamnetin	Quercetin 3-O-methyltransferase uses S-adenosyl methionine and quercetin to produce S-adenosylhomocysteine and isorhamnetin.
• Kaempferol	Tea, broccoli, grapefruit, brussel sprouts, applies
• Myricetin	Walnuts, grapes, berries, fruits, vegetables, herbs
• Proanthocyanidins, or condensed tannins	Sorghum bran, cocoa powder, and cinnamon are rich sources of procyanidins, found in many fruits and some vegetables
• Quercetin	Apples, onions, beans
• Rutin	Citrus rinds, buckwheat, asparagus, cranberries. Rutin as ferulic acid can help lower cholesterol levels.
• Flavanones:	
• Eriodictyol	From Yerba Santa plant; a glycoside found in rose hips
• Hesperetin	Found in citrus fruits. Metabolizes to hesperidin.
• Naringenin	Grapefruit and citrus fruits. Metabolizes from naringin. Lowers blood lipids, has anticancer activity, inhibits CYP3A4 and CUP1A2 enzymes.
• Flavanols and their polymers:	
• Catechin, gallocatechin and gallate esters	Strawberries, green and black teas
• Epicatechin, epigallocatechin	Cocoa, dark chocolate. Green tea. Improves blood flow.
• Theaflavin	Black tea
• Thearubigins	Formed during fermentation of tea leaves.
• Isoflavone phytoestrogens	Soy, peanuts, other members of the Fabaceae family
• Daidzein	Soybeans, tofu, textured vegetable protein
• Genistein	Soybeans, tofu, textured vegetable protein
• Glycitein	Soy food products

(continued)

TABLE 8-13 Antioxidants and Sources[a] *(continued)*

Vitamins	Sources or Comments
• Stilbenoids:	
• Resveratrol	Skins of dark-colored grapes, and concentrated in red wine
• Pterostilbene	Blueberries and grapes. Methoxylated analogue of resveratrol but not found in wine. May function like metformin to lower blood glucose; more research is needed.
• Anthocyanidins	
• Cyanidin	Grapes, bilberry, blackberry, blueberry, cherry, cranberry, elderberry, hawthorn, loganberry, acai berry and raspberry; apples, red cabbage, and plums.
• Delphinidin	Blue-red grapes, pomegranate, cranberries.
• Malvidin	Red wine
• Pelargonidin	Ripe raspberries, blueberries, blackberries, plums, cranberries, pomegranates.
• Peonidin	Raw cranberries; blueberries, plums, grapes, cherries. Not found in frozen fruits; raw only.
• Petunidin	Chokeberries, muscadine grapes
Phenolic Acids and Their Esters	
• Chicoric acid—a caffeic acid derivative	Found only in Echinacea purpurea.
• Chlorogenic acid—produced from esterification of caffeic acid.	High concentration in coffee (more concentrated in robusta than arabica beans), blueberries and tomatoes.
• Cinnamic acid and ferulic acid	Seeds of plants such as in brown rice, whole wheat and oats, as well as in coffee, apple, artichoke, peanut, orange and pineapple.
• Ellagic acid	Raspberry, strawberry. In ester form in red wine tannins.
• Ellagitannins—hydrolyzable tannin polymer	Formed when ellagic acid, a polyphenol monomer, esterifies and binds with the hydroxyl group of a polyol carbohydrate such as glucose
• Gallic acid	Found in gallnuts, sumac, witch hazel, tea leaves, oak bark, and many other plants
• Gallotannins—hydrolyzable tannin polymer	Formed when gallic acid, a polyphenol monomer, esterifies and binds with the hydroxyl group of a polyol carbohydrate such as glucose.
• Rosmarinic acid	High concentration in rosemary, oregano, lemon balm, sage, and marjoram.
• Salicylic acid	Found in most vegetables, fruits, and herbs; but most abundantly in the bark of willow trees (in aspirin).
Other Nonflavonoid Phenolics	
• Curcumin	Low bioavailability, because, much of it is excreted through glucuronidation. Chemopreventive.
• Eugenol	Oil of cloves. May be toxic if used in undiluted essential oils.
• Flavoglycosides	Gingko
• Flavonolignans—silymarin	Flavonolignans extracted from milk thistle.
• Xanthones—mangosteen and derivatives	Mangostin may only be found in inedible shell
Other Organic Antioxidants	
• Bilirubin, a breakdown product of blood	Possibly a significant antioxidant
• Cannabidiol, THC and synthetic cannabinoids	Cannabidiol is protective against glutamate neurotoxicity; a potent cerebral antioxidant.
• Citric acid	Lemons, limes, other citrus fruits. Part of citric acid cycle, so found in all living things.
• Lignan—antioxidant and phytoestrogen	Oats, flax seeds, pumpkin seeds, sesame seeds, rye, soybeans, broccoli, beans, and some berries.
• N-Acetylcysteine—water soluble	Augments glutathione reserves in the body to protect hepatocytes in the liver from acetaminophen toxicity. Precursor in the formation of the antioxidant glutathione in the body with antioxidant effects to reduce free radicals.
• Oxalic acid	Rhubarb, buckwheat, star fruit, black pepper, parsley, poppy seed, spinach, chard, beets, cocoa, chocolate, most nuts, berries, beans.
• Phytic acid (inositol, phytate)	Storage form of phosphorus in bran and seeds. Sesame seeds, pinto beans, Brazil nuts, peanuts, soybeans, linseed.
• R-α-Lipoic acid—fat and water soluble	Lipoic acid is found in almost all foods; slightly more in kidney, heart, liver, spinach, broccoli, and yeast extract.
• Uric acid	In humans, uric acid accounts for roughly half the antioxidant ability of plasma
Other Substances	
• Melatonin, a hormone	Easily crosses the blood-brain barrier. Once oxidized, it cannot be reduced to its former state.

[a]Antioxidants prevent or slow down oxidation where free radicals damage cells; they are often reducing agents. While supplements are available from many health food stores and nutraceutical companies, clinical trials have not found them to be useful and some may be harmful in elderly or vulnerable populations. See also, Table 1–23 and Table 2–2.

Sources:

1. Antioxidants. Accessed September 15, 2009, at http://en.wikipedia.org/wiki/List_of_antioxidants_in_food.
2. Nothlings U, et al. Flavonols and pancreatic cancer risk. *Am J Epid* 166:924, 2007.

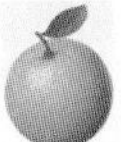

NUTRITION EDUCATION, COUNSELING, CARE MANAGEMENT

- Instruct patient to watch for signs and symptoms of diabetes, tetany, peritonitis, acute respiratory distress syndrome, and pleural effusion. These patients are best managed by a multidisciplinary team approach, especially in pediatrics (Stringer et al, 2005).
- Discuss omission of alcohol and gas-forming foods.
- Discuss tips for handling nausea and vomiting (e.g., dry meals, taking liquids a few hours before or after meals, use of ice chips, sipping beverages, asking physician about available antiemetics).
- If home enteral nutrition is needed, teach appropriate management methods.
- Teach use of a low-fat, high-protein, high-calorie oral diet when and if appropriate.
- Discuss the use of foods rich in antioxidants.

Patient Education—Foodborne Illness

- If home TF is needed, teach appropriate sanitation and food-handling procedures.

For More Information

- American Gastroenterological Association
  http://www.gastro.org/clinicalRes/brochures/pancreatitis.html
- Childhood Pancreatitis
  http://www.aafp.org/afp/990501ap/2507.html
- Medscape
  http://emedicine.medscape.com/article/775867-overview
- Merck—Pancreatitis
  http://www.merck.com/mmhe/sec09/ch124/ch124b.html

PANCREATITIS, ACUTE—CITED REFERENCES

Balog A, et al. Polymorphism of the TNF-alpha, HSP70–2, and CD14 genes increases susceptibility to severe acute pancreatitis. *Pancreas.* 30:46, 2005.

Besselink MG, et al. Probiotic prophylaxis in predicted severe acute pancreatitis: a randomised, double-blind, placebo-controlled trial. *Lancet.* 371:651, 2008.

Cao Y, et al. Meta-analysis of enteral nutrition versus total parenteral nutrition in patients with severe acute pancreatitis. *Ann Nutr Metab.* 53:268, 2008.

Chandrasegaram MD, et al, The impact of parenteral nutrition on the body composition of patients with acute pancreatitis. *J Parenter Enteral Nutr.* 29:65, 2005.

Dudeja V, et al. The role of heat shock proteins in gastrointestinal diseases. *Gut.* 58:1000, 2009.

Garg PK, et al. Association of extent and infection of pancreatic necrosis with organ failure and death in acute necrotizing pancreatitis. *Clin Gastroenterol Hepatol.* 3:159, 2005.

Gramlich L, TaftAK. Acute pancreatitis: practical considerations in nutrition support. *Curr Gastroenterol Rep.* 9:323, 2007.

Lasztity N, et al. Effect of enterally administered n-3 polyunsaturated fatty acids in acute pancreatitis—a prospective randomized clinical trial. *Clin Nutr.* 24:198, 2005.

McClave SA, et al. Nutrition support in acute pancreatitis: a systematic review of the literature. *J Parenter Enteral Nutr.* 30:143, 2006.

Meier RF, Beglinger C. Nutrition in pancreatic diseases. Nutrition in pancreatic diseases. *Best Pract Res Clin Gastroenterol.* 20:507, 2006.

Musil F, et al. Dynamics of antioxidants in patients with acute pancreatitis and in patients operated for colorectal cancer: a clinical study. *Nutrition.* 21:118, 2005.

Niv E, et al. Post-pyloric feeding. *World J Gastroenterol.* 15:1281, 2009.

Parks KS, et al. Inhibitory mechanism of omega-3 fatty acids in pancreatic inflammation and apoptosis. *Ann N Y Acad Sci.* 1171:421, 2009.

Petrov MS, et al. Enteral nutrition and the risk of mortality and infectious complications in patients with severe acute pancreatitis: a meta-analysis of randomized trials. *Arch Surg.* 143:1111, 2008.

Stringer MD, et al. Multidisciplinary management of surgical disorders of the pancreas in childhood. *J Pediatr Gastroenterol Nutr.* 40:363, 2005.

Wittau M, et al. The weak evidence base for antibiotic prophylaxis in severe acute pancreatitis. *Hepatogastroenterology.* 55:2233, 2008.

Xia Q, et al. Comparison of integrated Chinese and Western medicine with and without somatostatin supplement in the treatment of severe acute pancreatitis. *World J Gastroenterol.* 11:1073, 2005.

PANCREATITIS, CHRONIC

NUTRITIONAL ACUITY RANKING: LEVEL 3

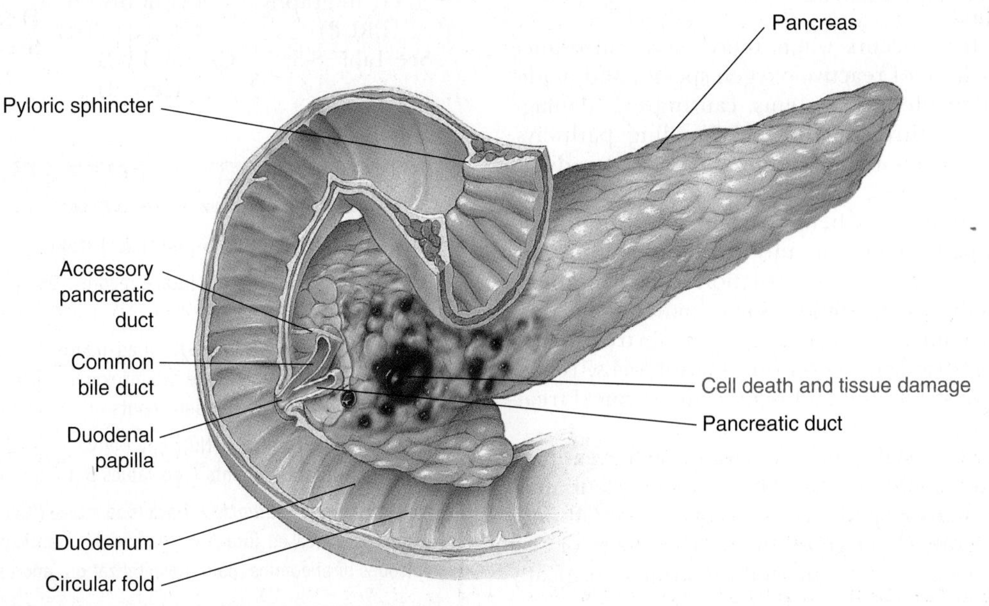

Asset provided by Anatomical Chart Co.

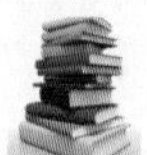

DEFINITIONS AND BACKGROUND

Chronic pancreatitis (CP) is an inflammatory disorder that results in permanent impairment of the pancreas. CP involves edema, fat necrosis, cellular exudate, fibrosis, and decreased enzymatic processes with abdominal pain, nausea, vomiting, and diarrhea. CP typically develops in people between the ages of 30 and 40, and can be caused by hereditary disorders of the pancreas, cystic fibrosis, hypercalcemia, excessive use of alcohol, hyperparathyroidism, hyperlipidemia, or lipase deficiency. The autoimmune forms of CP have been identified through elevated IgG4 levels. Approximately 5% of persons with acute pancreatitis go on to have CP.

Very heavy alcohol consumption and smoking are independent risks for CP (Yaday et al, 2009). Chronic alcohol abuse is the cause in 70% of adult cases, proportional to the dose and duration of alcohol consumption. The factors determining which alcoholic will develop alcoholic CP involve genetic and dietary factors or pancreatic injury from trauma, gallstones, and viruses. There is a gradual decrease in antioxidant enzyme expression in the pancreatic cells in CP and many patients will progress to having diabetes or pancreatic cancer.

Analysis of pancreatograms and textural changes of the parenchyma help diagnose CP (Kwon and Brugge, 2005). To avoid nutritional deterioration, screen early for fat malabsorption from decreased lipase levels. Steatorrhea occurs when fecal fat >7 g/dL is noted and over 90% of pancreatic enzyme secretion is lost. Weight loss is common, as is pain after intake of foods containing fat and protein. Jaundice, hypoalbuminemia, pancreatic pseudocysts or calcification, and splenic vein thrombosis may also occur.

Abstinence from alcohol, dietary modifications, use of oral supplements, and pancreatic enzyme supplementation will suffice in most patients (Meier et al, 2006). Enteral nutrition may be necessary for those in whom weight loss continues. Long-term use of a jejunostomy feeding may be needed (Stanga et al, 2005). PN is very seldom needed and is not as beneficial.

Oxidative stress occurs when there is an imbalance between generation of reactive oxygen species and inadequate antioxidant defense systems, causing cell damage either directly or through altering signaling pathways. Antioxidant supplementation relieves pain and reduces levels of oxidative stress (Bhardwaj et al, 2009; Verlaan et al, 2006). Patients may benefit from supplementation of vitamins A, C, E, selenium, and carotenoids. Episodes of inflammation and duct obstruction cause disabling pain (Gabbrielli et al, 2005). Some patients become dependent on pain medications. Supportive treatments, inhibition of gastric acid secretion, nerve blocks, reduction of oxidative stress, and endoscopic and surgical treatments are used.

Surgery, such distal pancreatectomy, achieves pain relief and better quality of life. The first successful autoislet cell transplants in patients who have severe CP were performed recently by surgeons at the University of Arizona Medical Center. This procedure avoids surgically caused diabetes.

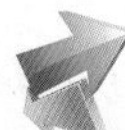

ASSESSMENT, MONITORING, AND EVALUATION

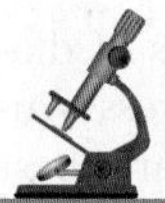

CLINICAL INDICATORS

Genetic Markers: Tropical calcific pancreatitis (TCP) is an idiopathic pancreatitis prevalent in Asia; trypsin inhibitor (SPINK1) N34S variant partially explains the genetic susceptibility (Sundaresan et al, 2009).

Clinical/History	Lab Work	
Height Weight BMI Diet history SGA evaluation Alcohol intake Smoking history Left upper quadrant abdominal pain Vomiting Anorexia, nausea Steatorrhea Temperature (fever?) I & O Chvostek's sign CT scan or MRI Endoscopic ultrasound Exploratory laparotomy Endoscopic retrograde cholangiopancreatography (ERCP) See Table 8-3 also	Bicarbonate levels (decreased; sensitivity 95) Secretin stimulation test IgG4 level, ESR, rheumatoid factor, ANA Thiobarbituric acid-reactive substances [TBARS] for oxidative stress Ferric-reducing ability of plasma [FRAP] for antioxidant status Fecal elastase (<200 μg/g) Sudan staining of feces Fecal fat test (24 hours on 100 g fat diet) CRP and WBC (elevated)	K^+, Na^+, Ca^{++} (decreased) Gluc (often increased) Lipase and Amylase (elevated?) Serum trypsinogen (low) Chol (LDL up, or total decreased) Trig (increased) Mg^{++} (decreased) LDH (>700) AST (>250) WBC (>200) Bilirubin and Alk phos (increased) pCO_2 (increased) and pO_2 (decreased) Alb, transthyretin BUN H & H Serum folate

SAMPLE NUTRITION CARE PROCESS STEPS

Inadequate Bioactive Substance Intake

Assessment Data: Dietary intake records, Dx of CP with frequent abdominal pain.

Nutrition Diagnosis (PES): Inadequate bioactive substance intake related to low intake of antioxidant-rich foods and beverages as evidenced by frequent bouts of abdominal pain with CP.

Intervention: Food and Nutrient Delivery—encourage intake of foods rich in antioxidants (see Tables 8-13 and 8-14).

Monitoring and Evaluation: Track food intake (food diary or history) to assess increased intake of foods rich in antioxidants and fewer episodes of abdominal pain, hospitalization, and use of analgesics.

TABLE 8-14 **Oxygen Radical Absorbance Capacity (ORAC) Rating of Foods**[a]

Food	USDA Data on Foods with High ORAC Scores				
	100 g Serving	Household Equivalent	Antioxidant capacity (TE) per 100 g	Other Common Unit	TE per Unit
Cinnamon, ground	100 g	14 Tbsp	264,543	1 Tbsp	19,110
Turmeric, ground	100 g	14 Tbsp	159,277	1 Tbsp	11,377
Sorghum, bran, black	100 g	1/3 cup	100,800	—	—
Cumin seed	100 g	14 Tbsp	76,800	1 Tbsp	5486
Parsley, dried flakes	100 g	4.7 cups	74,349	1/4 cup	3955
Basil, dried	100 g	4.7 cups	67,553	1/4 cup	3594
Curry powder	100 g	14 Tbsp	48,504	1 Tbsp	3465
Dutched chocolate powder	100 g	1 cup	40,200	1/4 cup	10,050
Sage, fresh	100 g	4.7 cups	32,004	1/4 cup	1702
Cloves, ground	100 g	14 Tbsp	31,446	1 Tbsp	2246
Mustard seed	100 g	8.75 Tbsp	29,257	1 Tbsp	3344
Pepper, black	100 g	14 Tsbp	27,618	1 Tbsp	1950
Marjoram	100 g	4.7 cups	27,297	1/4 cup	1452
Rice, brown	100 g	1/2 cup	24,287	—	—
Chili powder	100 g	14 Tbsp	23,636	1 Tbsp	1688
Dark chocolate candy	100 g	3.5 oz	21,800	1 oz	6229
Oregano powder, dried	100 g	4.7 cups	20,019	1/4 cup	1065
Semi-sweet chocolate morsels	100 g	1/2 cup	18,053	1/4 cup	9027
Pecans	100 g	7/8 cup	17,940	1/4 cup	5119
Paprika	100 g	14 Tbsp	17,919	1 Tbsp	1280
Tarragon, fresh	100 g	4.7 cups	15,542	1/4 cup	827
Ginger root, raw	100 g	1 cup	14,840	1/4 cup	3710
Elderberries, raw	100 g	1 cup	14,697	1/2 cup	7349
Peppermint, fresh	100 g	4.7 cups	13,978	1/4 cup	744
Oregano, fresh	100 g	4.7 cups	13,970	1/4 cup	743
Small Red Beans, dried	100 g	1/2 cup	13,727	—	—
Walnuts, English	100 g	7/8 cup	13,541	1/2 cup	3869
Wild blueberry	100 g	1 cup	13,427	1/2 cup	6713
Red kidney bean, dried	100 g	1/2 cup	13,259	—	—
Pinto beans	100 g	1/2 cup	11,864	—	—
Hazelnuts or filberts	100 g	3/4 cup	9645	—	—
Pears, dried	100 g	1/2 cup	9496	1/4 cup	4748
Blueberry, cultivated	100 g	1 cup	9019	1/2 cup	4510
Cranberry, whole	100 g	1 cup	8983	1/2 cup	4492
Pistachios	100 g	4 oz	7983	1 oz	1995
Artichoke hearts, cooked	100 g	1 cup	7904	1/2 cup	2635
Plums, black	100 g	1⅓ medium	7581	—	—
Prunes	100 g	1/2 cup	7291	—	—
Lentils, raw	100 g	1/2 cup	7282	—	—
Milk chocolate candy	100 g	3.5 oz	7203	1 oz	2058
Dried apples (to 40% moisture)	100 g	1/2 cup	6681	—	—
Garlic powder	100 g	14 Tbsp	6665	1 Tbsp	476
Chocolate syrup	100 g	1/3 cup	6330	—	—
Baby food, fruit, peaches	100 g	3.5 oz	6257	—	—
Raspberries	100 g	2/3 cup	6058	—	—

(continued)

TABLE 8-14 **Oxygen Radical Absorbance Capacity (ORAC) Rating of Foods[a] *(continued)***

	USDA Data on Foods with High ORAC Scores				
Food	**100 g Serving**	**Household Equivalent**	**Antioxidant capacity (TE) per 100 g**	**Other Common Unit**	**TE per Unit**
Strawberries	100 g	1 cup	5938	1/2 cup	2969
Red Delicious apple	100 g	1 apple	5900	—	—
Blackberry, cultivated	100 g	3/4 cup	5775	—	—
Soybean seeds, raw, mature	100 g	1/2 cup	5764	—	—
Onion powder	100 g	14 Tbsp	5735	1 Tbsp	410
Granny Smith apple	100 g	1 apple	5381	—	—
Garlic, raw	100 g	21 cloves	5436	1 clove	259
Cilantro (coriander leaves), raw	100 g	4.7 cups	5141		
Sweet cherries	100 g	10 cherries	4873	—	—
Baby food, fruit, apple and blueberry, Junior	100 g	3.5 oz	4822	—	—
Black plum	100 g	1 1/3 medium	4844	—	—
Russet potato	100 g	4 oz	4649	—	—
Almonds	100 g	3/4 cup	4454	1/4 cup	1485
Dill weed, fresh	100 g	4.7 cups	4392	1/2 cup	234
Black-eyed peas, cowpeas	100 g	1/2 cup	4343	—	—
Peaches, dried (40% moisture)	100 g	1/2 cup	4222	—	—
Black beans, dried	100 g	1/2 cup	4181	—	—
Plum	100 g	1 1/3 medium	4118	—	—
Gala apple	100 g	1 small	3903	—	—
Red table wine	100 g	3.5 oz	3873	—	—
Peanut butter, smooth, with salt	100 g	1/2 cup	3432	2 Tbsp	858
Currants, red, raw	100 g	2/3 cup	3387	1/3 cup	1694
Figs, dry	100 g	1/2 cup	3383	—	—
Peanuts, all types, raw	100 g	2/3 cup	3166	1/3 cup	1583
Raisins, seedless	100 g	2/3 cup	3037	1/3 cup	1519
Pear, raw	100 g	2/3 medium	2941	—	—
Blueberry juice	100 g	3.5 oz	2906	—	—
Lettuce, red leaf, raw	100 g	1 3/4 cup	2380	—	—
Concord grape juice	100 g	3.5 oz	2377	—	—
Cornflakes cereal, crumbs	100 g	1 cup	2359	1/2 cup	1180
Pomegranate juice	100 g	3.5 oz	2341	—	—
Oats, quick, plain, dry	100 g	1 1/4 cup	2308	—	—
Ready to eat cereal, granola with raisins	100 g	3.5 oz	2294	1 oz	655
Red cabbage, raw	100 g	7/8 cup	2252	1/2 cup	643
Ready to eat cereal, toasted oatmeal squares	100 g	3.5 oz	2143	1 oz	612
Sweet potato, baked in skin	100 g	2/3 medium	2115	—	—
Chives, raw	100 g	4.7 cups	2094	1/2 cup	111
Prune juice, canned	100 g	3.5 oz	2036	—	—
Cashew nuts	100 g	4 oz	1948	1 oz	487
Orange, raw, navel	100 g	1 average	1819	—	—
Red grape juice	100 g	3.5 oz	1788	—	—
Radishes, raw	100 g	11 radishes	1736	3 radishes	473
Macdamia nuts	100 g	3/4 cup	1695	1/2 cup	565

(continued)

TABLE 8-14 Oxygen Radical Absorbance Capacity (ORAC) Rating of Foods[a] *(continued)*

	USDA Data on Foods with High ORAC Scores				
Food	**100 g Serving**	**Household Equivalent**	**Antioxidant capacity (TE) per 100 g**	**Other Common Unit**	**TE per Unit**
Tangerines or mandarin oranges	100 g	1/3 cup	1620	—	—
Spinach, frozen	100 g	3/4 cup cooked	1515	—	—
Onions, red, raw	100 g	2/3 cup	1521	1/3 cup	761
Cranberry-grape juice	100 g	3.5 oz	1480	—	—
Butterhead lettuce, raw	100 g	1¾ cup	1423	—	—
Chocolate milk, fluid, commercial, low fat	100 g	3.5 oz	1263	8 oz	2887
Grapes, red, raw	100 g	2/3 cup	1260	—	—
Tea, brewed green	100 g	3.5 oz	1253	—	—
Lemon juice, raw	100 g	3.5 oz	1225	1 oz	350
Onions, yellow, raw	100 g	2/3 cup	1220	1/3 cup	610
Olive oil, extra virgin	100 g	7 Tbsp	1150	1 Tbsp	164
Onions, raw	100 g	2/3 cup	1034	1/3 cup	517
Sweet pepper, orange	100 g	2/3 cup	984	1/3 cup	492
Mangos, raw	100 g	1 cup	982	1/2 cup	491
Sweet pepper, yellow	100 g	2/3 cup	964	1/3 cup	482
Romaine lettuce raw	100 g	1¾ cup	963	—	—
Eggplant, raw	100 g	7/8 cup	933	1/2 cup	266
Sweet pepper, green	100 g	2/3 cup	923	1/3 cup	462
Kiwi fruit, raw	100 g	1 kiwi	882	1/2 kiwi	441
Cranberry juice blend, red	100 g	3.5 oz	865	—	—
Lime juice, raw	100 g	3.5 oz	823	1 oz	235
White table wine	100 g	3.5 oz	392	—	—

[a]Oxygen radical absorbance capacity (ORAC) is a method of measuring antioxidant capacities in biological samples. Values are expressed as the sum of the lipid soluble (e.g., carotenoid) and water-soluble (e.g., phenolic) antioxidant fractions (i.e., "total ORAC") reported as in micromoles Trolox equivalents (TE) per 100 g sample. Foods rich in antioxidants have an ORAC rating of 1000 per 100 g.

For household measurements:

- 100 g = 3.5 oz dry ingredients
- 3 tsp = 1 Tbsp.
- 48 tsp = 16 Tbsp = 1 cup.
- 1 Tbsp fresh herbs = ½ teaspoon, dried, crushed
- 1 oz = 4½ Tablespoons allspice, cinnamon, curry, paprika or dry mustard
  or 4 Tablespoons cloves or prepared mustard
  or 3½ Tablespoons nutmeg or pepper
  or 3 Tablespoons sage, cream of tartar or cornstarch
  or 2 Tablespoons salt or any liquid
- 1 pound = 2 cups liquid
  or 4 cups flour
  or 10 eggs without shells
  or 4 cups grated cabbage, cranberries, coffee or chopped celery
  or 3 cups corn meal
  or 2 cups uncooked rice
  or 2¾ cups raisins or dried currants

Sources:

Nutrient Data Laboratory, Agriculture Research Service, U.S. Department of Agriculture, Oxygen radical absorbance capacity (ORAC) of Selected Foods—2007. Accessed September 15, 2009, at http://www.ars.usda.gov/SP2UserFiles/Place/12354500/Data/ORAC/ORAC07.pdf.
Berry Health Fact Sheets. Accessed September 22, 2009, at http://berryhealth.fst.oregonstate.edu/health_healing/fact_sheets/index.htm.
Natural antioxidants. Accessed September 15, 2009, at http://naturalantioxidants.org/.

INTERVENTION

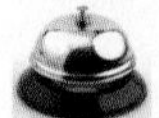

OBJECTIVES

- Decrease pain from oxidative stress. Abstain from alcohol and smoking.
- Correct fluid and electrolyte imbalances and malnutrition; avoid overfeeding. Acid–base imbalance is common with nasogastric suctioning, fistula losses, renal failure, nausea, and vomiting.
- Provide optimal nutrition support for weight gain as weight loss is common in the late course of CP (Stanga et al, 2005).
- Alleviate steatorrhea; decrease number of stools per day if there is diarrhea.
- Avoid or control complications (cardiovascular, pulmonary, hematological, renal, neurological, or metabolic); prevent multiple organ dysfunction.
- With diabetes, it may be better to have glucose elevated slightly (200 mg/dL) than to allow prolonged hypoglycemia to occur.
- If tube fed, monitor for abdominal pain or discomfort, and offer pain medication as needed. Administer pancreatic enzymes with meals or TF (Dominguez-Munoz et al, 2005; Stanga et al, 2005). CPN may be needed for resistant cases where pain does not subside.

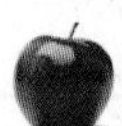

FOOD AND NUTRITION

- If tolerated, use a diet with low-to-moderate fat (0.7–1 g/kg) and high carbohydrates; calculate needs accordingly. Diet should be low in fiber with six small meals a day. Include adequate amounts of antioxidants (Tables 8-13 and 8-14), minerals (calcium, magnesium, selenium, and zinc), fat-soluble vitamins (A, D, E, and K) in water-miscible form, and water-soluble vitamins.
- High-energy, standard feeding by enteral pump is desirable for those who need it. Estimate needs at 35 kcals/kg, 1–1.5 g protein per kilogram. Jejunal feeding is more beneficial than gastric placement. Needle catheter jejunostomy may be used safely (Stanga et al, 2005), but not with ascites.
- Treat steatorrhea to minimize symptoms of the underlying disease and to promote weight retention or gain. MCTs and pancreatic replacement therapy combat maldigestion and malabsorption (Stanga et al, 2005). Monitor for hyperglycemia with a high-carbohydrate diet.
- When CPN is needed (in about 1% of cases), estimate needs according to similar parameters as for oral diet. The benefits of BCAAs and glutamine are not clear. If intravenous lipids are used, do not use more than 1.5 g/kg for adults. Provide no more than 5 mg/kg/min of glucose.
- Alcoholic beverages are absolutely prohibited.

Common Drugs Used and Potential Side Effects

- See Table 8-12 for guidance on medications.

Herbs, Botanicals, and Supplements

- Herbs and botanical supplements should not be used without discussing with physician.
- Antioxidant therapy with green tea polyphenols and gene therapy with superoxide dismutase can markedly attenuate disease (Dryden et al, 2005).
- The combination of pre- and probiotics (synbiotics) have mixed results in this population. In the acute form of pancreatitis, probiotic use may actually increase mortality (Besselink et al, 2008).

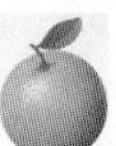

NUTRITION EDUCATION, COUNSELING, CARE MANAGEMENT

- Instruct patient to watch for signs and symptoms of diabetes, tetany, peritonitis, acute respiratory distress syndrome, and pleural effusion.
- Discuss omission of alcohol from the typical diet.
- Discuss tips for handling nausea and vomiting (e.g., dry meals, taking liquids a few hours before or after meals, use of ice chips, sipping beverages, asking physician about available antiemetics, etc.). Dietary counseling has been found to be as effective as dietary supplementation for managing CP (Singh et al, 2008). Gas-forming foods may need to be omitted. Teach high-calorie, high-protein, low-fat diet rich in antioxidant foods with a frequent small meal pattern.
- To prevent onset of pancreatic cancer, avoiding tobacco smoking.

Patient Education—Foodborne Illness

- If home TF is needed, teach appropriate sanitation and food-handling procedures.

For More Information

- Medline Plus
  http://www.nlm.nih.gov/medlineplus/ency/article/000221.htm
- Merck Manual—Chronic Pancreatitis
  http://www.merck.com/mmpe/sec02/ch015/ch015c.html#sec02-ch015-ch015c-901

PANCREATITIS, CHRONIC—CITED REFERENCES

Besselink MG, et al. Probiotic prophylaxis in predicted severe acute pancreatitis: a randomised, double-blind, placebo-controlled trial. *Lancet.* 371:651, 2008.

Bhardwaj P, et al. A randomized controlled trial of antioxidant supplementation for pain relief in patients with chronic pancreatitis. *Gastroenterology.* 136:149, 2009.

Dominguez-Munoz JE, et al. Effect of the administration schedule on the therapeutic efficacy of oral pancreatic enzyme supplements in patients with exocrine pancreatic insufficiency: a randomized, three-way crossover study. *Aliment Pharmacol Ther.* 21:993, 2005.

Gabbrielli A, et al. Efficacy of main pancreatic-duct endoscopic drainage in patients with chronic pancreatitis, continuous pain, and dilated duct. *Gastrointest Endosc.* 61:576, 2005.

Kwon RS, Brugge WR. New advances in pancreatic imaging. New advances in pancreatic imaging. *Curr Opin Gastroenterol.* 21:561, 2005.

Meier R, et al. ESPEN Guidelines on Enteral Nutrition: pancreas. *Clin Nutr.* 25:275, 2006.

Singh S, et al. Dietary counseling versus dietary supplements for malnutrition in chronic pancreatitis: a randomized controlled trial. *Clin Gastroenterol Hepatol.* 6:353, 2008.

Stanga Z, et al. Effect of jejunal long-term feeding on chronic pancreatitis. *J Parenter Enteral Nutr.* 29:12, 2005.

Sundaresan S, et al. Divergent roles of SPINK1 and PRSS2 variants in tropical calcific pancreatitis. *Pancreatology.* 9:145, 2009.

Verlaan M, et al. Assessment of oxidative stress in chronic pancreatitis patients. *World J Gastroenterol.* 12:5705, 2006.

Yaday D, et al. Alcohol consumption, cigarette smoking, and the risk of recurrent acute and chronic pancreatitis. *Arch Int Med.* 169:1035, 2009.

PANCREATIC INSUFFICIENCY

NUTRITIONAL ACUITY RANKING: LEVEL 2–3

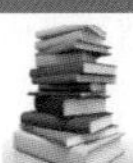

DEFINITIONS AND BACKGROUND

Pancreatic insufficiency is caused by the inability of the exocrine pancreas to secrete digestive enzymes such as lipase. Cystic fibrosis (CF), type 1 (autoimmune) diabetes, Shwachman-Diamond Syndrome (SDS), pancreatic cancer, or pancreatitis will often lead to pancreatic insufficiency. Other disorders of the gastrointestinal tract, such as celiac disease, inflammatory bowel disease, Zollinger–Ellison syndrome or gastric resection can either mimic or cause pancreatic exocrine Insufficiency (Keller et al, 2009).

Lipase is the key enzyme for breaking down triglycerides. Patients often have mild-to-moderate fat malabsorption. In CF, there may be recurrent problems with fatty acid abnormalities or pancreatitis (DeBoeck et al, 2005). Fecal elastase (FE) 1 levels indicate lipase activity; assessment should be used to verify pancreatic status (Cohen et al, 2005). A fecal fat or Steatocrit test may identify the problem.

Stool trypsin tests or low levels of trypsinogen are used to determine whether sufficient amounts of this pancreatic enzyme are reaching the intestines to metabolize proteins. Because the overt clinical symptoms of pancreatic exocrine insufficiency are steatorrhea and maldigestion (Keller et al, 2009), oral pancreatic enzyme supplements should be properly administered to ensure adequate gastric mixing with the food.

Nonendocrine pancreatic disease is a critical factor for development of diabetes; this "type 3c" affects over 8% of the general diabetic patient population (Hardt et al, 2008). There is a continuous interstitial matrix connection between the endocrine and exocrine pancreas; fibrosis and inflammation cause dysfunctional insulino-acinar-ductal-incretin gut hormone axis, resulting in pancreatic insufficiency and glucagon-like peptide deficiency and diabetes (Hayden et al, 2008).

The delivery of sufficient enzyme concentrations into the duodenal lumen simultaneously with meals can reduce nutrient malabsorption, improve the symptoms of steatorrhea, and in some cases alleviate pain (Ferrone et al, 2007). The best duodenal pH permits optimal efficacy of these extracts and the buffered, enteric-coated enzymes are most useful (Brady et al, 2006; Pezzilli, 2009).

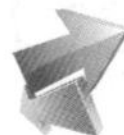

ASSESSMENT, MONITORING, AND EVALUATION

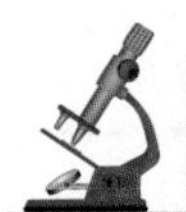

CLINICAL INDICATORS

Genetic Markers: Diagnosis of chronic pancreatic insufficiency is difficult in early stages; eventually, genetic testing may prove to be helpful. Hereditary pancreatitis involves a cationic trypsingen gene (PRSS1) gene, where treatment involves attempting to inactivate that gene before it causes pancreatic insufficiency. CF patients will have the CFTR gene that is associated with pancreatic insufficiency.

Clinical/History

Height
Weight
BMI
Weight loss?
Malabsorption
Steatorrhea
Diet history
I & O
Pale, bulky stools
Abdominal bloating
Stool weight
CT scan or MRI
ERCP

Lab Work

Amylase (increased)
Lipase
Trypsinogen
CRP
Serum carotene
FE 1
Ca^{++}, Mg^{++}
Trig, Chol
PT or INR
Bicarbonate
Gluc
Na^{+}, K^{+}
Alk phos
H & H

INTERVENTION

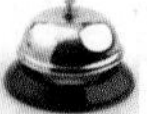

OBJECTIVES

- Maintain or achieve BMI >19.
- Correct fatty acid abnormalities, maldigestion, diarrhea, and steatorrhea. Prevent EFA deficiency.
- Provide adequate energy intake while lowering intake of fats.
- Provide fat-soluble vitamins A-D-E-K and zinc with malabsorption. Prevent overload of iron.
- Attenuate intestinal inflammation (Pezzilli, 2009). Prevent or manage type 2 diabetes.

SAMPLE NUTRITION CARE PROCESS STEPS

Malnutrition

Assessment Data: Dietary intake records; weight loss; steatorrhea; pale, bulky, foul stools.

Nutrition Diagnosis (PES): Malnutrition related to inability to digest nutrients as evidenced by steatorrhea and unintentional weight loss.

Intervention: Food and Nutrient Delivery—provide high kilocalories, high protein foods with low fat content. Include adequate pancreatic enzymes with every meal. Educate about the role of the pancreas in nutrient absorption. Counsel about ways to enjoy meals that are low fat while nutrient dense. Discuss the need for water-miscible forms of vitamins A, D E, and K if needed.

Monitoring and Evaluation: Track food intake (food diary or history). Evaluate for signs of malnutrition. Review lab test results. Monitor for improvement in weight, decrease in steatorrhea and pale, bulky stools.

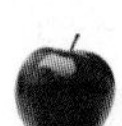

FOOD AND NUTRITION

- Encourage high-calorie, high-protein intake to maintain body weight. Dose pancreatic enzyme replacement adequately to minimize fat malabsorption.
- Use MCTs since they do not require lipase. They may be taken with simple sugars, jelly, jams and in mixed dishes.
- Increase use of omega-3 fatty acids from tuna, mackerel, salmon, and other fatty fish, as well as flaxseed. Probiotics may be considered.
- If diabetes is present, emphasize regular mealtimes and carbohydrate spacing to prevent hyperglycemia.
- Use tender meats and low-fiber fruits and vegetables.
- Alcoholic beverages are prohibited.
- Tube feed in severe cases of malnutrition. Night feeding may be a reasonable option.

Common Drugs Used and Potential Side Effects

- Pancreatic extract preparations contain pancreatin and pancrelipase; both contain principally amylase, protease, and lipase. Pancreatic enzymes (Cotazym, Creon) should be taken with food. Take enteric-coated tablets with cimetidine or antacids. Administration of lipase 25,000–40,000 units/meal is given by using pH-sensitive pancrelipase microspheres, along with dosage increases and compliance checks (Ferrone et al, 2007).
- Fat-soluble vitamins should be taken in water-miscible form, with the pancreatic enzymes.

Herbs, Botanicals, and Supplements

- New approaches may include the use of probiotics to reduce inflammation (Pezzilli, 2009).
- Lipase enzymes derived from microbial species show promise; plant-based enzymes, such as bromelain from pineapple, also serve as effective digestive aids in the breakdown of proteins (Roxas, 2008).
- Herbs and botanical supplements should not be used without discussing with physician.

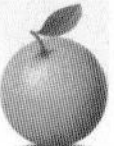

NUTRITION EDUCATION, COUNSELING, CARE MANAGEMENT

- Instruct patient in the role of the pancreas in digestion.
- Discuss how pancreatic enzymes should be taken with meals or afterward for best results.
- Discuss appropriate measures for recovery and control.
- Share menu planning tips for a high protein, low fat diet and how to include desired nutrients.

Patient Education—Foodborne Illness

- If home TF is needed, teach appropriate sanitation and food-handling procedures.

For More Information

- Cystic Fibrosis Foundation
  http://www.cff.org/
- Food and Drug Administration (FDA)
  http://www.fda.gov/cder/drug/infopage/pancreatic_drugs/default.htm
- Lab tests on line
  http://www.labtestsonline.org/understanding/conditions/pancreatic_insuf.html
- National Pancreas Foundation
  http://www.pancreasfoundation.org/
- Pancreas
  http://www.pancreas.org/
- Recipes, Low fat
  http://www.pancreasfoundation.org/live/recipes.shtml

PANCREATIC INSUFFICIENCY—CITED REFERENCES

Brady MS, et al. An enteric-coated high-buffered pancrelipase reduces steatorrhea in patients with cystic fibrosis: a prospective, randomized study. *J Am Diet Assoc.* 106:1181, 2006.

Cohen JR, et al. Fecal elastase: pancreatic status verification and influence on nutritional status in children with cystic fibrosis. *J Pediatr Gastroenterol Nutr.* 40:438, 2005.

DeBoeck K, et al. Pancreatitis among patients with cystic fibrosis: correlation with pancreatic status and genotype. *Pediatrics.* 115:e463, 2005.

Ferrone M, et al. Pancreatic enzyme pharmacotherapy. *Pharmacotherapy.* 27:910, 2007.

Hardt PD, et al. Is pancreatic diabetes (type 3c diabetes) underdiagnosed and misdiagnosed? *Diabetes Care.* 31:165S, 2008.

Hayden MR, et al. Attenuation of endocrine-exocrine pancreatic communication in type 2 diabetes: pancreatic extracellular matrix ultrastructural abnormalities. *J Cardiometab Syndr.* 3:234, 2008.

Keller J, et al. Tests of pancreatic exocrine function—clinical significance in pancreatic and non-pancreatic disorders. *Best Pract Res Clin Gastroenterol.* 23:r425, 2009.

Pezzilli R. Chronic pancreatitis: maldigestion, intestinal ecology and intestinal inflammation. *World J Gastroenterol.* 15:1673, 2009.

Roxas M. The role of enzyme supplementation in digestive disorders. *Altern Med Rev.* 13:307, 2008.

PANCREATIC TRANSPLANTATION

NUTRITIONAL ACUITY RANKING: LEVEL 4

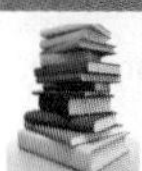

DEFINITIONS AND BACKGROUND

Pancreatic islet cell transplantation is a treatment alternative for patients with type 1 diabetes who experience hypoglycemic unawareness despite maximal care (Onaca et al, 2007). Islet transplant can restore pancreatic endocrine function, endogenous insulin secretion, and insulin independence in more than 80% of patients, and recover the metabolism of glucose, protein, and lipids (Bertuzzi et al, 2006). It helps to decrease nephropathy, early or mild retinopathy, and neuropathy.

Pancreas transplantation alone (PTA) involves transplanting a pancreas from a cadaver to a patient whose kidneys have not been damaged by diabetes. Simultaneous pancreas and kidney (SPK) transplantation involves kidney and pancreas being transplanted at the same time from a cadaver, often leading to freedom from both dialysis and insulin dependency. Pancreas after kidney (PAK) surgery is another option, as is islet cell or isolated beta-cell transplantation. Pancreatic islet cells are highly sensitive to hypoxia, which contributes to poor islet yield, inflammatory events, and cellular death during the early posttransplantation period (Lau et al, 2009). Pancreatic transplantation is major surgery, with risk of bleeding, infection, and reactions to anesthesia. Antirejection medicines, which have many side effects, have to be taken for a long time.

Whole pancreas transplantation is associated with a significant risk of surgical and postoperative complications (Meloche, 2007). Islet cell transplantation has fewer side effects but does not yield an ideal level of glucose control. Persistent graft function results in improved glucose control and avoidance of hypoglycemic events (Onaca et al, 2007). Improved control of glycated HbA1c, reduced risk of recurrent hypoglycemia and of diabetic complications are benefits of islet cell transplantation, irrespective of the status of insulin independence (Bertuzzi et al, 2006).

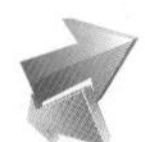

ASSESSMENT, MONITORING, AND EVALUATION

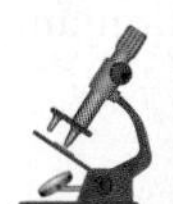

CLINICAL INDICATORS

Genetic Markers: Pancreatic transplantation is needed for type 1 diabetes, which has a genetic origin (American Diabetes Association, 2009).

Clinical/History

Height
Weight, dry
BMI
Diet history
Weight changes and goals
I & O
BP
Temperature

Lab Work

Gluc
BUN, Creat
H & H
Serum Fe
Serum amylase
Urinary amylase (only if bladder drained)
Na^+, K^+
Ca^{++}, Mg^{++}

SAMPLE NUTRITION CARE PROCESS STEPS

Inadequate Oral Food and Beverage Intake

Assessment Data: Dietary intake records pretransplantation indicate poor oral intake of both food and beverages; status posttransplant, 21 days on enteral nutrition; wishes to try some liquids and soft foods.

Nutrition Diagnosis (PES): Inadequate oral food and beverage related to inability to be fed orally posttransplant as evidenced by 14 days on EN and now asking to attempt oral intake.

Intervention: Food and Nutrient Delivery—offer one to two small items at mealtimes or every few hours while awake; gradually increase food intake as tolerated. Educate about the role of nutrition in liver health and recovery; discuss ways to progress orally and wean from enteral nutrition.

Monitoring and Evaluation: Improved oral appetite. No nausea or unplanned side effects after surgery Gradual return of usual weight and tolerance of oral intake closer to desired level.

INTERVENTION

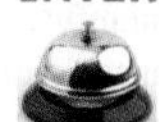

OBJECTIVES

- **Preoperatively:** Meet nutritional needs; improve visceral protein stores; maintain lean tissue. Nutritional management of candidates requires management of renal function, and treatment of obesity in advance as a BMI >27 kg/m^2 may delay wound healing.
- **Postoperatively:** Support graft survival. Promote wound healing. Improve or maintain nutritional status.
- **Long Term:** Weaned off CPN within the first year to achieve optimal nutritional status. Prevent weight gain. Prevent complications such as gastroparesis, hypertension, hyperlipidemia, hyperglycemia, and osteoporosis. Attain near-normal blood glucose control and normal hemoglobin A1c levels without risks of severe hypoglycemia (Meloche, 2007).

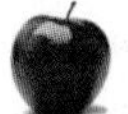

FOOD AND NUTRITION

- **Preoperatively:** Meet nutritional needs; improve visceral protein stores; maintain lean tissue.
- **Postoperatively:** Control carbohydrates if there is diabetes or hyperglycemia. Manage diet carefully to prevent hypoglycemia in patients who take insulin.

Common Drugs Used and Potential Side Effects

- See Table 8-15.

TABLE 8-15 Medications Used after Pancreatic Transplantation

Medication	Description
Analgesics	Analgesics are used to reduce pain. Long-term use may affect such nutrients as vitamin C and folacin; monitor carefully for each specific medication.
Azathioprine (Imuran)	Azathioprine may cause leukopenia, thrombocytopenia, oral and esophageal sores, macrocytic anemia, pancreatitis, vomiting, diarrhea, and other complex side effects. Folate supplementation and other dietary modifications (liquid or soft diet, use of oral supplements) may be needed. The drug works by lowering the number of T cells; it is often prescribed along with prednisone for conventional immunosuppression.
Corticosteroids (prednisone or Solu-Cortef)	Corticosteroids such as prednisone and Solu-Cortef are used for immunosuppression. Side effects include increased catabolism of proteins, negative nitrogen balance, hyperphagia, ulcers, decreased glucose tolerance, sodium retention, fluid retention, and impaired calcium absorption and osteoporosis. Cushing's syndrome, obesity, muscle wasting, and increased gastric secretion may result. A higher protein intake and lower intake of carbohydrate and sodium may be needed.
Cyclosporine	Cyclosporine does not retain sodium as much as corticosteroids do. Intravenous doses are more effective than oral doses. Nausea, vomiting, and diarrhea are common side effects. Hyperlipidemia, hyperglycemia, and hyperkalemia may also occur; decrease fat intake as well as sodium and potassium if necessary. Magnesium may need to be replaced. The drug is also nephrotoxic; a controlled renal diet may be beneficial. Taking omega-3 fatty acids during cyclosporine therapy may reduce toxic side effects (such as high blood pressure and kidney damage) associated with this medication in transplantation patients (Tsipas and Morphake, 2003). Avoid use with St. John's wort.
Diuretics	Diuretics such as furosemide (Lasix) may cause hypokalemia. Aldactone actually spares potassium; monitor drug changes closely. In general, avoid use with fenugreek, yohimbe, and ginkgo.
Immunosuppressants	Immunosuppressants such as muromonab (Orthoclone OKT3) and antithymocyte globulin (ATG) are less nephrotoxic than cyclosporine but can cause nausea, anorexia, diarrhea, and vomiting. Monitor carefully. Fever and stomatitis also may occur; alter diet as needed.
Insulin	Insulin may be necessary during periods of hyperglycemia. Monitor for hypoglycemic symptoms during use; teach patient self-management tips.
Pancreatic Enzymes	Pancreatic enzymes may be needed if pancreatitis occurs again after transplantation.
Tacrolimus (Prograf, FK506)	Tacrolimus suppresses T-cell immunity; it is 100 times more potent than cyclosporine, thus requiring smaller doses. Side effects include GI distress, nausea, vomiting, hyperkalemia, and hyperglycemia; adjust diet accordingly by controlling carbohydrate and enhancing potassium intake.

Herbs, Botanicals, and Supplements

- Herbs and botanical supplements should not be used without discussing with physician.
- St. John's wort interferes with the metabolism of cyclosporine and should not be used after transplantation.

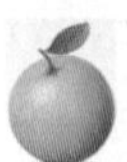

NUTRITION EDUCATION, COUNSELING, CARE MANAGEMENT

- Encourage activity to prevent excessive weight gain; 14–30 lb may be a common gain.
- Discuss surgical stress. Encourage positive protein balance to promote anabolism and wound healing.
- Over the long term, follow a low-cholesterol and low–saturated fatty acid dietary plan.
- Sudden abdominal pain, fever, and increased amylase and glucose can occur and are signs of pancreatitis even after transplantation. Report these warning signs immediately to the physician.
- Problems after transplantation include diabetic complications, bone loss, and failure of the pancreas graft. A multidisciplinary team is required to maximize long-term quality of life.

Patient Education—Foodborne Illness

- If home TF is needed, teach appropriate sanitation and food-handling procedures.

For More Information

- E-medicine
  http://emedicine.medscape.com/article/429408-overview
- Insulin
  http://www.insulin-free.org/
- Mayo Clinic—Pancreatic Transplant
  http://www.mayoclinic.com/health/pancreas-transplant/DA00047
- National Institute of Diabetes and Digestive and Kidney Diseases (NIDDK)
  http://diabetes.niddk.nih.gov/dm/pubs/pancreaticislet/
- NIH—Genetics of Diabetes
  http://www.ncbi.nlm.nih.gov/bookshelf/br.fcgi?book=diabetes&part=A987
- University of Minnesota—Diabetes Institute
  http://www.diabetes.umn.edu/diabinst/video/index.html
- USC Pancreatic Transplant Program
  http://www.pancreastransplant.org/

PANCREATIC TRANSPLANTATION—CITED REFERENCES

American Diabetes Association. Accessed September 19, 2009, at http://www.diabetes.org/diabetes-research/summaries/exploring-the-genetics-of-type1-diabetes.jsp.

Bertuzzi F, et al. Islet cell transplantation. *Curr Mol Med.* 6:369, 2006.

Lau J, et al. Oxygenation of islets and its role in transplantation [published online ahead of print September 9, 2009]. *Curr Opin Organ Transplant.* 14:688, 2009.

Meloche RM. Transplantation for the treatment of type 1 diabetes. *World J Gastroenterol.* 13:6347, 2007.

Onaca N, et al. Pancreatic islet cell transplantation: update and new developments. *Nutr Clin Pract.* 22:485, 2007.

ZOLLINGER–ELLISON SYNDROME

NUTRITIONAL ACUITY RANKING: LEVEL 3

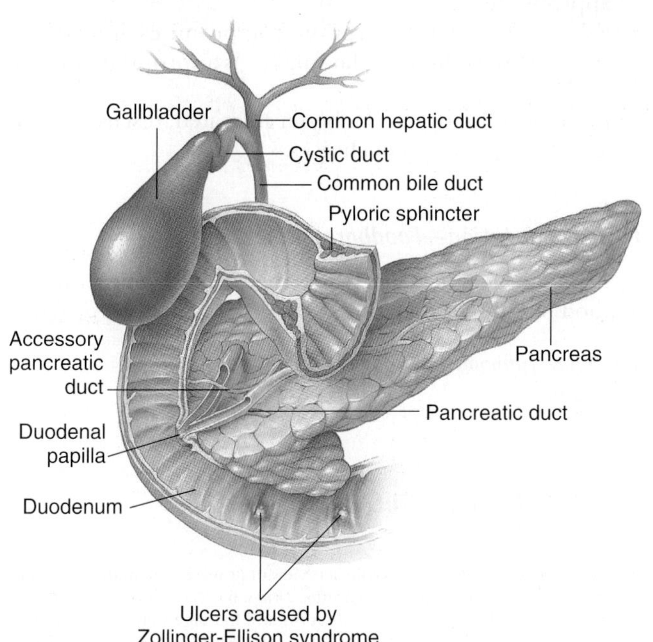

Asset provided by Anatomical Chart Co.

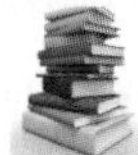

DEFINITIONS AND BACKGROUND

Zollinger–Ellison syndrome (ZES) is a severe disease with ulceratogenic tumor (gastrinoma) of the delta-cells of the pancreatic islets of Langerhans; the cells produce gastrin. Almost every patient with ZES has marked gastric acid hypersecretion and ulcerations in the esophagus, stomach, duodenum, and jejunum. It is more common among 30- to 50-year-old men. ZES occurs in less than 1% of all patients with duodenal ulcers.

Gastrinomas producing ZES are the most frequent symptomatic, malignant pancreatic endocrine tumors (Gibril and Jensen, 2005). They frequently are accompanied by secretory diarrhea. Interestingly, insulin production is often increased in the beta-cells. Of all cases, 60% occur in males; two thirds of cases are malignant. Widespread metastasis indicates a poor prognosis.

Gastric carcinoid tumors in patients with longstanding ZES may be symptomatic and aggressive and may metastasize to the liver; they require long-term medical treatment. Curing gastrinoma or appropriately inhibiting gastric acid hypersecretion in ZES patients prevents death and favors long-term survival (Quatrini et al, 2005).

Resection of localized gastrinomas often does not require extended surgical resection and is associated with excellent long-term outcomes (Mortellaro et al, 2009). Total gastrectomy is reserved for patients with extensive tumor involvement of the gastric wall or for patients with emergency bleeding.

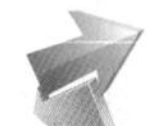

ASSESSMENT, MONITORING, AND EVALUATION

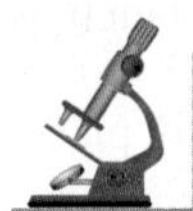

CLINICAL INDICATORS

Genetic Markers: The disease is more common in people who have an inherited condition called multiple endocrine neoplasia type 1 (MEN1). Evaluate for family history of hyperparathyroidism, nephrolithiasis, or gastrinoma.

Clinical/History		Lab Work
Height	Heartburn	N balance
Weight	Diarrhea or malabsorption	Na^+
BMI	BP	Ca^{++} (usually increased)
Weight loss?	Negative *H pylori* testing	Alb
Diet history	Upper GI endoscopy	H & H
I & O	Somatostatin receptor scintigraphy (SRS)	K^+ (decreased)
Burning abdominal pain	Gastrin radioimmunoassay	Mg^{++}
Nausea, vomiting	CT Scan	BUN
Severe esophageal reflux		Serum insulin
		Serum gastrin
		Trig, Chol
		Gluc

INTERVENTION

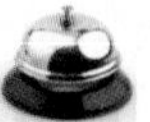

OBJECTIVES

- Relieve stomach acid to lessen ulcer symptoms, usually with medications. Surgery may be needed to remove tumors.

SAMPLE NUTRITION CARE PROCESS STEPS

Abnormal GI Function

Assessment Data: Dietary intake records, diarrhea, steatorrhea, weight loss, nausea and vomiting.

Nutrition Diagnosis (PES): Abnormal GI function related to excessive gastrin production as evidenced by gastrinoma with weight loss, nausea & vomiting, diarrhea and steatorrhea.

Intervention: Food and Nutrient Delivery—provide easily tolerated foods, low acid.

Monitoring and Evaluation: Track food intake (food diary or history).

- Overcome malabsorption and lessen diarrhea.
- Decrease problems with dysphagia and reflux.
- Prevent complications such as esophageal stricture or abdominal perforation.
- Manage or reduce cancer, which can occur in 25% of cases.

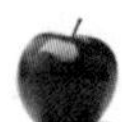

FOOD AND NUTRITION

- Modify fiber, seasonings, and textures as necessary. Decrease intake of acidic foods if not tolerated (such as citrus juices, tomato products).
- Alter feeding modality to TF such as jejunostomy placement as needed.

Common Drugs Used and Potential Side Effects

- PPIs are used for the treatment of acid-related disorders. Use of these medications can prevent the need for surgery (Hirschowitz et al, 2005). Take omeprazole (Prilosec), esomeprazole (Nexium), lansoprazole (Prevacid), or pantoprazole (Protonix) before meals. Iron and vitamin B_{12} levels may become depleted. Rabeprazole (Acifex) has been tested and has fewer side effects than some other PPIs (Baldwin and Keam, 2009).
- Chemotherapy may be needed if surgery to remove the tumors is not feasible. Streptozotocin (Zanosar), 5-fluorouracil (Adrucil) or doxorubicin (Doxil) may be used. Monitor for side effects.
- Octreotide or interferon may also be used.

Herbs, Botanicals, and Supplements

- Herbs and botanical supplements should not be used without discussing with physician.

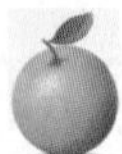

NUTRITION EDUCATION, COUNSELING, CARE MANAGEMENT

- Explain which modifications of fiber in the diet are appropriate.
- Explain how malabsorption compromises nutritional status. Discuss limiting fat intake, as appropriate for the patient.
- Lower acid foods may be better tolerated; discuss ways to adjust recipes or good choices.

Patient Education—Foodborne Illness

- If home TF is needed, teach appropriate sanitation and food-handling procedures.

For More Information

- **NIDDK**
  http://digestive.niddk.nih.gov/ddiseases/pubs/zollinger/

ZOLLINGER–ELLISON SYNDROME—CITED REFERENCES

Baldwin CM, Keam SJ. Rabeprazole: a review of its use in the management of gastric acid-related diseases in adults. *Drugs.* 69:1373, 2009.

Gibril F, Jensen JT. Advances in evaluation and management of gastrinoma in patients with Zollinger-Ellison syndrome. *Curr Gastroenterol Rep.* 7:114, 2005.

Hirschowitz BI, et al. Clinical outcome using lansoprazole in acid hypersecretors with and without Zollinger-Ellison syndrome: a 13-year prospective study. *Clin Gastroenterol Hepatol.* 3:39, 2005.

Mortellaro VE, et al. Long-term results of a selective surgical approach to management of Zollinger-Ellison syndrome in patients with MEN-1. *Am Surg.* 75:730, 2009.

Quatrini M, et al. Follow-up study of patients with Zollinger-Ellison syndrome in the period 1966–2002: effects of surgical and medical treatments on long-term survival. *J Clin Gastroenterol.* 39:376, 2005.

BILIARY DISORDERS

BILIARY CIRRHOSIS

NUTRITIONAL ACUITY RANKING: LEVEL 2

DEFINITIONS AND BACKGROUND

Biliary cirrhosis, also called cholangiolitic hepatitis or obstructive jaundice, occurs in two to five cases per 100,000 worldwide. Symptoms include pruritus, jaundice, and portal hypertension. Biliary atresia is the result of an inflammatory process that affects the intrahepatic and extrahepatic bile ducts, leading to fibrosis and obliteration of the biliary tract with development of biliary cirrhosis in infants (Tang et al, 2005).

Primary biliary cirrhosis (PBC) is characterized by progressive destruction of intrahepatic bile ducts; it primarily affects middle-aged women. Autoimmune factors may trigger the disease in genetically susceptible hosts; genetic susceptibility is a predisposing factor. Environmental factors (infection, chemicals, smoking) may also be relevant. Environmental xenobioticsmay aggravate genetic weaknesses in mechanisms of immune regulation, and subsequent immunopathology (Gershwin and Mackay, 2008). PBC that is associated with other autoimmune diseases such as Sjogren's syndrome, scleroderma, Raynaud's phenomenon, or CREST syndrome is regarded as an organ-specific autoimmune disease. Osteoporosis is prevalent in this population (Guanabens et al, 2005) and celiac disease is also commonly found (Duggan and Duggan, 2005).

Homocysteine has been proposed to be involved (Ebrahimkhani et al, 2005). In symptomatic patients, advanced age, elevated serum bilirubin levels, and decreased serum albumin levels lead to shortened survival. PBC slowly progresses and may lead to liver failure where transplantation is the only effective therapy.

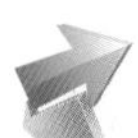

ASSESSMENT, MONITORING, AND EVALUATION

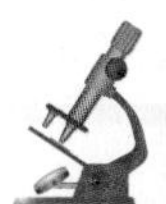

CLINICAL INDICATORS

Genetic Markers: There is a role for HLA to determine PBC susceptibility (Invernizzi et al, 2008). Vitamin D receptor polymorphisms are also being studied.

Clinical/History	Lab Work	
Height	Antimitochondrial antibodies (AMA)	Transferrin
Weight	Bilirubin (increased)	Tissue transglutaminase (for celiac disease)
BMI	Alk phos (increased)	Globulin
Diet history	ALT/AST	Gluc
Jaundice	Alb, transthyretin	Ca^{++}, Mg^{++}
Portal hypertension?	PT (decreased)	Na^{+}, K^{+}
Pruritus	Serum homocysteine	Chol (increased)
Xanthomas		Ceruloplasmin
Cholangiography		
Liver biopsy		

INTERVENTION

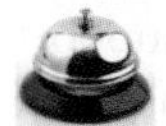

OBJECTIVES

- Correct diarrhea, steatorrhea, malnutrition, and osteomalacia. Prevention of bone density loss is important, as vitamin D deficiency is common.
- Limit or control symptoms. Prevent progression to end-stage liver disease when possible.
- Prevent or correct zinc and vitamin deficiencies.
- Manage related disorders (such as Sjögren's syndrome or celiac disease).

> **SAMPLE NUTRITION CARE PROCESS STEPS**
>
> **Altered Nutrition-Related Labs**
>
> ***Assessment Data:*** Dx biliary cirrhosis with presence of AMA, elevated bilirubin and alk phos.
>
> ***Nutrition Diagnosis (PES):*** Altered nutrition-related labs related to biliary cirrhosis with cholestasis as evidenced by AMA, elevated bilirubin and alk phos levels.
>
> ***Intervention:*** Food and nutrient delivery—use antioxidant-rich foods, supplement with fat-soluble vitamins.
>
> ***Monitoring and Evaluation:*** Track lab values.

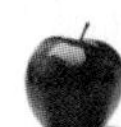

FOOD AND NUTRITION

- Increase vitamin D and calcium intake to protect against osteopenia. Vitamin K may also play an important role in protection of bone health and may be supplemented (Plaza and Lamson, 2005). Use water-miscible sources of vitamins A, D, E, and K with steatorrhea.
- Reduce cholesterol and saturated fats in hypercholesterolemia.
- Ensure adequate intake of zinc from diet.
- To lower elevated homocysteine levels, which seem to aggravate hepatic fibrogenesis, be sure the diet contains adequate amounts of folic acid and vitamins B_6 and B_{12} (Ebrahimkhani et al, 2005).
- If the patient also has celiac disease, omit gluten from the diet (e.g., wheat, rye, barley). Initiation of a gluten-free diet may help to resolve iron deficiency anemia, pruritus, and elevated serum liver biochemistries.
- Control carbohydrate intake with hyperglycemia.

Common Drugs Used and Potential Side Effects

- Prolonged administration of ursodeoxycholic acid (UDCA) in patients with PBC is associated with survival benefit and delay of LT. Ursodeoxycholic acid (UDCA) is the only currently known medication that can slow the disease progression. When UDCA is ineffective, cholestyramine is the treatment of choice; it decreases bile acids but can cause belching or constipation.
- Budesonide is a glucocorticoid that may help when given with UDCA to improve liver status (Rautiainen et al, 2005). Weight gain and increased appetite often result.
- Bezafibrate, a hypolipidemic drug, has been shown to benefit patients with PBC in some studies (Akbar et al, 2005).

Herbs, Botanicals, and Supplements

- Herbs and botanical supplements should not be used without discussing with physician.
- High doses of vitamin E (tocopherol) will elevate transaminases.

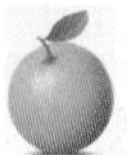

NUTRITION EDUCATION, COUNSELING, CARE MANAGEMENT

- Discuss the role of bile salts in fat and fat-soluble vitamin absorption. If supplements are used, water-miscible forms may be needed.
- Protection of bone mineral density will be important. Discuss the role of medications, calcium, and vitamin D on bone health (Plaza and Lamson, 2005).

Patient Education—Foodborne Illness

- If home TF is needed, teach appropriate sanitation and food-handling procedures.

For More Information

- Mayo Clinic—Primary Biliary Cirrhosis
  http://www.mayoclinic.com/health/primary-biliary-cirrhosis/DS00604
- Medicine Net
  http://www.medicinenet.com/primary_biliary_cirrhosis/article.htm

BILIARY CIRRHOSIS—CITED REFERENCES

Akbar SM, et al. Therapeutic efficacy of decreased nitrite production by bezafibrate in patients with primary biliary cirrhosis. *J Gastroenterol.* 40:157, 2005.

Duggan JM, Duggan AE. Systematic review: the liver in celiac disease. *Aliment Pharmacol Ther.* 21:515, 2005.

Ebrahimkhani MR, et al. Homocysteine alterations in experimental cholestasis and its subsequent cirrhosis. *Life Sci.* 76:2497, 2005.

Gershwin ME, Mackay IR. The causes of primary biliary cirrhosis: convenient and inconvenient truths. *Hepatology.* 47:737, 2008.

Guanabens N, et al. Severity of cholestasis and advanced histological stage but not menopausal status are the major risk factors for osteoporosis in primary biliary cirrhosis. *J Hepatol.* 42:573, 2005.

Invernizzi P, et al. Human leukocyte antigen polymorphisms in Italian primary biliary cirrhosis: a multicenter study of 664 patients and 1992 healthy controls. *Hepatology.* 48:1906, 2008.

Plaza SM, Lamson DW. Vitamin K2 in bone metabolism and osteoporosis. *Altern Med Rev.* 10:24, 2005.

Rautiainen H, et al. Budesonide combined with UDCA to improve liver histology in primary biliary cirrhosis: a three-year randomized trial. *Hepatology.* 41:747, 2005.

Tang ST, et al. Diagnosis and treatment of biliary atresia: a retrospective study. *Hepatobiliary Pancreat Dis Int.* 4:108, 2005.

CHOLESTASIS

NUTRITIONAL ACUITY RANKING: LEVEL 2–3

DEFINITIONS AND BACKGROUND

Cholestasis involves reduced bile flow in any liver disease with bilirubin over 2.0 mg/dL. Disturbance of the flow of bile leads to intracellular retention of biliary constituents. Hepatic causes of cholestasis include viral hepatitis, ALD, hemochromatosis, and autoimmune hepatitis. Biliary causes include primary sclerosing cholangitis (in which the intrahepatic and/or extrahepatic bile ducts undergo inflammation and fibrosis), choledocholithiasis, PBC, and biliary atresia. It can also occur with inflammatory bowel disease (Huang and Lichtenstein, 2005). Prolonged PN may be needed in the absence of GI tract stimulation.

Cholestasis interferes with excretion of the bile salts required for emulsification and absorption of dietary fat. Reduced bile secretion impairs micelle formation, which is needed for digestion of fat by pancreatic enzymes. Vitamin and mineral deficiencies and alterations are common, especially if cholestasis is significant. Zinc, magnesium, and calcium may be deficient because they are albumin-bound and the liver is not working properly. Deficiency of fat-soluble vitamins A, D, E, and K may occur. Of particular concern is vitamin E, which circulates in the blood almost exclusively attached to the lipoprotein fractions.

In chronic cholestasis with biliary obstruction, hyperlipidemia and accumulation of copper result, and manganese can accumulate in the brain; avoid overfeeding with copper or manganese. Hepatic copper overload in CPN patients occurs through chronic cholestasis in CPN-associated liver disease regardless of duration (Blaszyck et al, 2005).

Chronic CPN may induce fatty liver and inflammation, especially in patients with short bowel syndrome. Deficiency of choline in parenteral solutions has been proposed as the mechanism for liver disease. With CPN, cholestatic jaundice may occur from a lack of enteral nutrition and failure of biliary stimulation. In patients receiving home PN, prevalence of liver disease increases with duration.

Signs and symptoms of cholestasis can include glossitis from B-complex vitamin deficiency, protein and iron deficiency, hemorrhagic tendencies due to vitamin C or K inadequacy, and flatulence. Patients with steatorrhea may benefit from a low-fat diet or from use of MCTs. Intrahepatic cholestatic syndromes cause a decrease in bile flow with no overt bile duct obstruction; bile constituents accumulate in the liver and blood.

Ursodeoxycholic acid and adequate nutritional support are the usual treatments, with LT being performed in severe cases only (Huang and Lichtenstein, 2005). Depending on the cause (such as medication effects, postoperative jaundice, sepsis, CPN, or acalculous cholecystitis), treatment includes removal of offending drugs, supportive care, broad-spectrum antibiotic agents with drainage of infected fluids, CPN adjustment including cycling and limiting carbohydrates, and cholecystectomy.

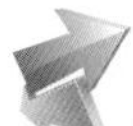

ASSESSMENT, MONITORING, AND EVALUATION

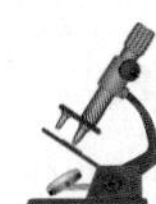

CLINICAL INDICATORS

Genetic Markers: Because ATP-binding cassette (ABC) transporters are important for normal bile secretion, hereditary and acquired ABC transporter defects play a central role in the pathogenesis of cholestasis (Trauner et al, 2007).

Clinical/History

- Height
- Weight
- BMI
- Diet history
- Ascites
- Edema
- I & O
- Jaundice
- Pale stools
- Fatty yellow deposits in skins
- Eas bleeding
- Small, spider-like blood vessels visible on skin
- Nausea
- Flatulence

Lab Work

- Chol, Trig (increased)
- PT (prolonged)
- AST, ALT (increased)
- Bilirubin (increased, >2 mg/dL)
- Somatomedin C
- Alk phos (increased)
- Gamma-glutamyl transpeptidase (very high)
- Serum carotene (increased or decreased)
- Bun, Creat
- H & H
- Serum Fe
- Alb, transthyretin
- Globulin
- Amylase, lipase
- Serum manganese
- Serum zinc
- Na^+, K^+
- Ca^{++}, Mg^{++}

INTERVENTION

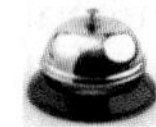

OBJECTIVES

- Promote return of normal liver function and bile flow.
- Treat fat malabsorption and deficiency of any additional nutrients.
- Correct steatorrhea, GI bleeding, and copper overloading when present.
- Prevent or correct for liver failure, osteomalacia, or osteoporosis.
- Correct nutrient excesses (e.g., manganese).
- Prepare for surgery when indicated.

SAMPLE NUTRITION CARE PROCESS STEPS

Excessive CPN Infusion

Assessment Data: Intake records indicating CPN solution exceeding estimated kilocalories requirements.

Nutrition Diagnosis (PES): Excessive CPN solution related to exceeding calculated needs as evidenced by cholestasis.

Intervention: Food and Nutrient Delivery—change CPN solution to meet and not exceed kilocalories needs.

Monitoring and Evaluation: Track CPN intake according to estimated needs; evaluate labs, weight, liver function.

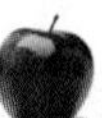

FOOD AND NUTRITION

- In chronic cases, 10–20% added kilocalories may be needed. Infants need more kilocalories, and adults tend to use CHO poorly. In acute stages, use IV glucose to prevent hypoglycemia and protein catabolism.
- In acute stages, infants will need 1.0–1.5 g/kg protein. Children, teens, and adults need 0.5–1.2 g protein/kg; highlight BCAAs sources. In chronic cases, use 3 g protein/d for infants and 1–1.5 g protein/kg in adults.
- Supplement with vitamins and minerals, especially fat-soluble vitamins. Vitamin D and calcium will be needed if osteopenia is present. Zinc and selenium may be needed.
- Small, frequent feedings and snacks may be better tolerated than large meals.
- Use enteral nutrition (where possible), if CPN has caused cholestasis. If CPN is required, early use of cyclic CPN may be useful. Avoid excesses of copper (Blaszyck et al, 2005) in the solutions.

Common Drugs Used and Potential Side Effects

- Ursodeoxycholic acid slows disease progression and should be used in relatively high doses as 20–30 mg/kg/d (Huang and Lichtenstein, 2005).
- Treat pruritus with bile acid–binding exchange resins such as cholestyramine or colestipol (Huang and Lichtenstein, 2005). Use with a low-fat diet and increase fluids and fiber. Constipation, nausea, or vomiting may be a side effect.
- Water-miscible forms of fat-soluble vitamins A, D, E, and K may be needed in cholestasis. Sample amounts of vitamin A may be given at 25,000–50,000 IU/d as Aquasol A; vitamin D may be given as 12,000–50,000 IU/d over a month; and vitamin E may be given as 10–25 IU/kg/d. Once nutrient stores are repleted and cholestasis is resolved, the supplementation can stop.
- Medications known to cause cholestasis include estrogens and anabolic steroids, chlorpromazine, erythromycin, and oxypenicillins.

Herbs, Botanicals, and Supplements

- Herbs and botanical supplements should not be used without discussing with physician. Cholestatic liver injury may occur from some herbal remedies, such as greater celandine, glycyrrhizin, chaparral.

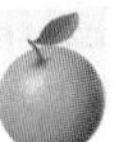

NUTRITION EDUCATION, COUNSELING, CARE MANAGEMENT

- Discuss the role of fat in normal metabolic processes; simplify explanation in correlation to absorption of fat-soluble vitamins and other nutrients affected by the liver.
- Discuss ways to increase satiety from the diet with appetizing recipes.
- Discuss use of over-the-counter (OTC) vitamin and mineral supplements, especially regarding possible toxicity if taken in large doses with liver disease.

- LT works best in a well-nourished patient. Promote good tolerance and intake.

Patient Education—Foodborne Illness

- If home TF is needed, teach appropriate sanitation and food-handling procedures.

For More Information

- Characteristics of Liver Disease
  http://www.umm.edu/liver/common.htm
- Merck Manual—Cholestasis
  http://www.merck.com/mmhe/sec10/ch135/ch135c.html

CHOLESTATIC LIVER DISEASE—CITED REFERENCES

Blaszyck H, et al. Hepatic copper in patients receiving long-term total parenteral nutrition. *J Clin Gastroenterol.* 39:318, 2005.

Huang CS, Lichtenstein DR. Treatment of biliary problems in inflammatory bowel disease. *Curr Treat Options Gastroenterol.* 8:117, 2005.

Trauner M, et al. MDR3 (ABCB4) defects: a paradigm for the genetics of adult cholestatic syndromes. *Semin Liver Dis.* 27:77, 2007.

GALLBLADDER DISEASE

NUTRITIONAL ACUITY RANKING: LEVEL 2

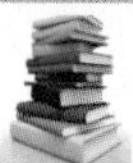

DEFINITIONS AND BACKGROUND

The **gallbladder**, located under the liver, collects and stores bile, which is made up of bile salts, electrolytes, bilirubin, cholesterol, and other fats. Bile helps the small intestine digest fats and remove waste products, especially through bilirubin. It passes from the liver's bile duct into the duodenum through the common bile duct. Bile contains 85–95% water; electrolytes (sodium, potassium, chloride, bicarbonate, calcium, magnesium); bile acids and bilirubin; lecithin, cholesterol and protein. Loss of bile can cause malabsorption and maldigestion of fat, electrolyte imbalances, and poor excretion of drugs or heavy metals.

Cholelithiasis is defined as the presence of gallstones. In developed countries, at least 10% of white adults harbor cholesterol gallstones, especially after age 65. Women have twice the risk (Shaffer, 2005). There is also prevalence among persons who have hepatitis C, diabetes, obesity, pregnancy, use of estrogens, insulin, oral contraceptives, cholestyramine (Bini and McGready, 2005; Ko et al, 2005). The western diet that is high in kilocalories, fat, and refined carbohydrate is also a factor. Being Hispanic or Native American predisposes to gallbladder disease, as does sickle cell anemia and some other genetic traits.

Gallstones are a hepatobiliary disorder due to biochemical imbalances in the gallbladder bile (Uppal et al, 2008). Some gallbladders can concentrate bile normally but cannot acidify it. The result is that calcium may be less soluble in bile and precipitates out. Increasing consumption of magnesium (Mg^{++}) appears to decrease the risk of symptomatic gallstones in men (Ko, 2008). Magnesium deficiency can cause dyslipidemia and insulin hypersecretion, which may facilitate gallstone formation (Tsai et al, 2008).

Gallstones contain primarily cholesterol, bilirubin, and calcium salts, formed into either cholesterol or pigment stones. Symptoms include steady pain in the upper abdomen that increases rapidly and lasts from 30 minutes to several hours, pain in the back between the shoulder blades or under the right shoulder, nausea, vomiting, abdominal bloating, intolerance for fatty foods, belching, and indigestion.

Gallstones also form if the gallbladder does not contract completely or often enough to empty bile; this can also occur after eating too little, after periods of starvation, or fasting. Rapid weight loss or crash dieting is to be avoided. Preventive measures include a controlled weight loss rate, reduction of the length of overnight fast, inclusion of a small amount of fat in the diet, and eating foods rich in magnesium (nuts, vegetable protein, beans, and soy).

Cholecystitis is inflammation of the gallbladder. Rather than a single clinical entity, cholecystitis is a class of related disease states with different causes, degrees of severity, clinical courses, and management strategies. Gallstones with low-grade inflammation, scarring, and thickening are common triggers. If the gallbladder is removed, fat absorption still occurs, but it is less efficient because bile is not as concentrated.

Endoscopic stent placement in the gallbladder is effective for patients with gallbladder disease who are poor surgical candidates (Conway et al, 2005). However, surgery is needed for most cases. There are over 700,000 cholecystectomies performed annually in the United States alone (Shaffer, 2005).

Laparoscopic cholecystectomy (LC) reduces the length of hospital stay and can be performed on patients who are morbidly obese (Simopoulos et al, 2005). Extracorporeal shock wave lithotripsy (ESWL) is also effective.

Gallbladder cancer is not common but is more prevalent in women who have had gallstones for many years. Jaundice, pain above the stomach, lumps in the abdomen, and fever should be addressed. Gallbladder cancer is usually associated with late diagnosis, unsatisfactory treatment, and poor prognosis.

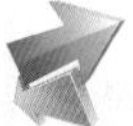

ASSESSMENT, MONITORING, AND EVALUATION

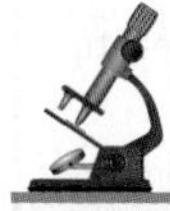

CLINICAL INDICATORS

Genetic Markers: Alagille syndrome is a genetic disorder with mutations in the JAG1 and NOTCH2 genes where there are too few bile ducts to function properly;

this occurs in one in 70,000 people. Activation of nuclear receptor liver X receptor (LXR) sensitizes mice to lithogenic diet-induced gallbladder cholesterol crystallization; studies are needed in humans (Uppal et al, 2008).

Clinical/History		Lab Work
Height	Magnetic resonance cholangiography (MRC)	Mg^{++} (low?)
Weight	Hepatobiliary iminodiacetic acid (HIDA) scan (cholescintigraphy)	Alk phos (ALP), elevated?
BMI	Endoscopic retrograde cholangiopancreatography (ERCP)	Bilirubin (increased)
Diet history	Cholecochoscopy	AST, ALT (elevated?)
Intolerance for fatty foods?		Amylase, Lipase (increased?)
WBC		Alb, transthyretin
Jaundice		Chol
Nausea, vomiting		Trig (elevated?)
I & O		H & H
Temperature		Na^+, K^+
CT scan or endoscopic ultrasound		Ca^{++}

INTERVENTION

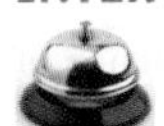

OBJECTIVES

- Lose excess weight, if needed but avoid fasting for rapid weight loss, which can lead to gallstones.
- Limit foods that cause pain or flatulence.
- For the patient with cholelithiasis, overcome fat malabsorption caused by obstruction and prevent stagnation in a sluggish gallbladder. Decreased bile secretion, bile stasis, bacteria, hormones, or fungi may be a problem; bacterial overgrowth alters bile acids so that they can no longer emulsify fats.
- Prevent biliary obstruction, cancer, or pancreatitis.
- Provide fat-soluble vitamins (ADEK) with signs of steatorrhea.
- Include a high magnesium food source daily.
- Ascorbic acid affects the catabolism of cholesterol to bile acids and the development of gallbladder disease; supplement the diet if needed.

SAMPLE NUTRITION CARE PROCESS STEPS

Excessive Fat Intake

Assessment Data: Dietary intake records indicating intake of fried foods at most every meal; dining at fast food restaurants six to seven times weekly; abdominal and back pain, nausea, vomiting for 3 days.

Nutrition Diagnosis (PES): Excessive fat intake related to extensive use of fried foods and fast food choices as evidenced by diet history and signs of cholecystitis.

Intervention: Food and Nutrient Delivery—offer lower fat meals; prep for surgery. Educate about the role of the gallbladder in fat metabolism. Counsel about postsurgical diet (low fat, frequent small meals perhaps better tolerated) and gradual return to a general diet that contains more nutrient-dense and lower fat options. Discuss the role of minerals such as magnesium in maintaining GB health.

Monitoring and Evaluation: Track food intake (food diary or history). Evaluate for resolution of abdominal pain, nausea and vomiting after surgery; tolerance for diet and use of foods that are more nutrient-dense and lower in fat.

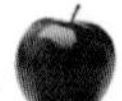

FOOD AND NUTRITION

- In **acute cholecystitis**, NPO or a low-fat diet may be needed. Progress to a diet with fewer condiments and gas-forming vegetables, which cause distention, increased peristalsis, and irritation.
- In **chronic cholecystitis**, use a fat/calorie-controlled diet to promote drainage of the gallbladder without excessive pain. Patient should consume adequate amounts of CHO, especially pectin, which binds excess bile acids.
- In **cholelithiasis**, encourage a diet that is high fiber, low in calories (as needed).
- Assure an adequate dietary intake of magnesium from nuts, bran, halibut, pollack, spinach, black or lima or white beans.
- Fat-soluble vitamins A-D-E-K may need to in water-miscible form.
- Increase dietary intake of sources of vitamin C such as citrus fruits and juices. Use supplemental forms if needed.

Common Drugs Used and Potential Side Effects

- Ursodiol (Actigall, Urso) is made from bile acid help dissolve small cholesterol gallstones over months or years. Take with food or milk. Ursodiol can lead to metallic taste, abdominal pain, mild diarrhea, or vomiting.
- The potent cholesterol absorption inhibitor ezetimibe reduces biliary cholesterol content and may be a promising strategy for preventing or treating cholesterol gallstones (Wang et al, 2008).
- Ursodeoxycholic acid decreases cholesterol saturation of bile and gallstone incidence during weight loss and may help to prevent gallstone formation. Orlistat is another option.
- Antibiotics may be used to counteract infection. Evaluate the need to take with food, milk or other liquids.
- If analgesics (Demerol, meperidine) are used to relieve pain, side effects such as nausea, vomiting, constipation, and GI distress can occur.
- Oral contraceptives and estrogens increase the risk of gallstones, especially after prolonged use. Orlistat has also been shown to cause gallstones for some patients. Thiazide diuretics have also been linked with gallstones (Leitzmann et al, 2005).

Herbs, Botanicals, and Supplements

- Herbal medicine such as turmeric and oregon grape may reduce gallbladder inflammation and relieve liver congestion.

- Herbs and botanical supplements should not be used without discussing with physician. Celandine, peppermint, couch grass, and goldenrod have been recommended for gallbladder disease, but no clinical trials have proven efficacy at this time.

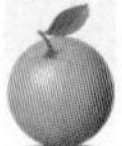

NUTRITION EDUCATION, COUNSELING, CARE MANAGEMENT

- After a cholecystectomy, fat intake should be limited for several months to allow the liver to compensate for the gallbladder's absence. Fats should be introduced gradually; excessive amounts at one meal should be avoided. Use more unrefined carbohydrates as well.
- If diarrhea persists after surgery, try using antidiarrheal medications, such as loperamide (Imodium) and a high-fiber diet for more bulk.
- Avoid fasting and rapid weight loss schemes.
- People who have had their gallbladders removed should have their cholesterol levels checked periodically. To prevent new gallstones from forming, maintain a healthy weight.

Patient Education—Foodborne Illness

- If home TF is needed, teach appropriate sanitation and food-handling procedures.

For More Information

- American College of Surgeons—Cholecystectomy
  http://www.facs.org/public_info/operation/cholesys.pdf
- Bile Duct Diseases
  http://www.nlm.nih.gov/medlineplus/bileductdiseases.html
- National Institute of Diabetes and Digestive and Kidney Diseases (NIDDK)—Gallstones
  http://digestive.niddk.nih.gov/ddiseases/pubs/gallstones/index.htm

GALLBLADDER DISEASE—CITED REFERENCES

Bini EJ, McGready J. Prevalence of gallbladder disease among persons with hepatitis C virus infection in the United States. *Hepatology.* 41:1029, 2005.

Conway JD, et al. Endoscopic stent insertion into the gallbladder for symptomatic gallbladder disease in patients with end-stage liver disease. *Gastrointest Endosc.* 61:32, 2005.

Ko CW, et al. Incidence, natural history, and risk factors for biliary sludge and stones during pregnancy. *Hepatology.* 41:359, 2005.

Ko CW. Magnesium: does a mineral prevent gallstones? *Am J Gastroenterol.* 103:383, 2008.

Leitzmann MF, et al. Thiazide diuretics and the risk of gallbladder disease requiring surgery in women. *Arch Intern Med.* 165:567, 2005.

Shaffer EA. Epidemiology and risk factors for gallstone disease: has the paradigm changed in the 21st century? *Curr Gastroenterol Rep.* 7:132, 2005.

Simopoulos C, et al. Laparoscopic cholecystectomy in obese patients. *Obes Surg.* 15:243, 2005.

Tsai CJ, et al. Long-term effect of magnesium consumption on the risk of symptomatic gallstone disease among men. *Am J Gastroenterol.* 103:375, 2008.

Uppal H, et al. Activation of liver X receptor sensitizes mice to gallbladder cholesterol crystallization. *Hepatology.* 47:1331, 2008.

Wang HH, et al. Effect of ezetimibe on the prevention and dissolution of cholesterol gallstones. *Gastroenterology.* 134:2101, 2008.

SECTION 9

Endocrine Disorders

CHIEF ASSESSMENT FACTORS

Warning Signs of Type 1 Diabetes

- Drowsiness, Lethargy, Blurred Vision
- Extreme Thirst
- Frequent Urination
- Fruity, Sweet, Wine-Like Odor on Breath
- Glucose or Ketones in Urine
- Heavy, Labored Breathing
- Increased Appetite
- Sudden Weight Loss
- Stupor, Unconsciousness

Risk Factors for Type 2 Diabetes

- Age ≥45 Years
- Ethnicity—African American, Hispanic American, Native American, Asian American, Pacific Islander
- Family History (Parents or Siblings with DM)
- Habitually Sedentary
- High-Density Lipoprotein Cholesterol Level ≤35 mg/dL and Triglyceride Level ≥250 mg/dL
- History of Gestational Diabetes Mellitus (GDM) or Women Delivering Babies Weighing >9 lb
- History of Impaired Fasting Glucose (IFG) or Impaired Glucose Tolerance (IGT)
- Hypertension (Blood Pressure ≥140/90 mm Hg)
- Obesity with Body Mass Index ≥25 kg/m^2
- Polycystic ovarian syndrome, other conditions associated with insulin resistance
- Vascular disease

Assessment in Diabetes

- Assessment for Mood Disorder
- Contraception; Reproductive and Sexual History
  - Current Treatment: Medications, Meal Plan, Results of Glucose Monitoring, Patients' Use of Data
  - Eating Patterns, Nutritional Status, and Weight History; Growth and Development in Children and Adolescents
    - Exercise History
    - Family History of Diabetes and Other Endocrine Disorders
    - Frequency, Severity, and Cause of Acute Complications Such as Ketoacidosis and Hypoglycemia

- History and Treatment of Other Conditions, Including Endocrine and Eating Disorders
- Infections: Skin, Foot, Dental, and Genitourinary Tract (Prior and Current)
- Laboratory Tests, Symptoms and Special Examination Results Related to the Diagnosis of Diabetes
- Lifestyle, Cultural, Psychosocial, Educational, and Economic Factors That Influence the Management of Diabetes
- Other Medications That May Affect Blood Glucose Levels
- Previous Treatment Programs (Nutrition and Diabetes Self-Management Education, Attitudes, and Health Beliefs)
- Prior HbA1c Records
- Risk Factors for Atherosclerosis: Smoking, Hypertension, Obesity, Dyslipidemia, and Family History
- Symptoms of Celiac Disease in Type 1 Diabetic Patients
- Symptoms and Treatment of Chronic Eye; Kidney; Nerve; Genitourinary (Including Sexual), Bladder, and Gastrointestinal Function; Heart; Peripheral Vascular; Foot; and Cerebrovascular Complications Associated with Diabetes
- Tobacco, Alcohol, and/or Controlled Substance Use

Assessment in Other Endocrine Conditions

- Adult Changes in Size of Head, Hands, Feet
- Altered Consciousness; Numbness, Tingling, or Paresthesia
- Anorexia, Nausea, Abdominal Pain, Malabsorption, Gastroparesis
- Bone Pain
- Decreased Libido, Erectile Dysfunction
- Diagnosis of Thyroid Disease or Other Endocrine Disorder
- Dysuria
- Goiter; Exophthalmos; Intolerance to Heat or Cold
- Headache, Seizures, Syncope
- Hormone Imbalances (Excess or Deficiency)
- Hormone Therapy: Anabolic Hormones—Growth Hormones, Androgens, Sex Hormones; Catabolic Hormones—Stress Hormones (Causing Gluconeogenesis from Protein) Such as Catecholamines (Epinephrine, Norepinephrine), Glucocorticoids (Cortisone, Cortisol), or Glucagon
- Hyperglycemia, Hypoglycemia
- Postural Hypotension, Weakness
- Pruritus, Dryness of Skin or Hair
- Shortness of Breath, Hoarseness
- Weight Changes

OVERVIEW OF DIABETES MELLITUS

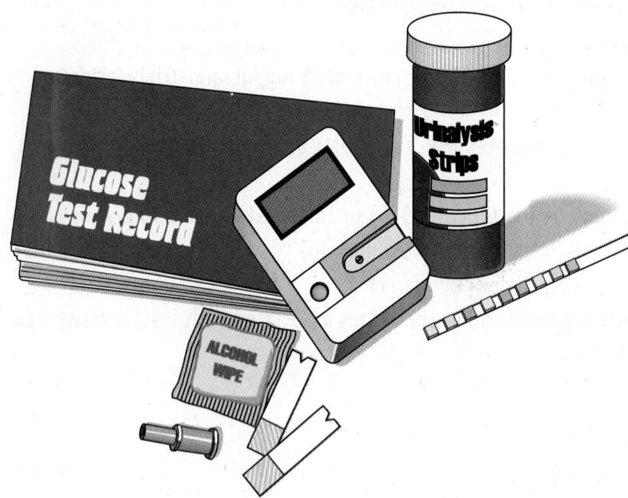

LifeART image copyright © 2010. Lippincott Williams & Wilkins.

Diabetes mellitus is a group of metabolic diseases characterized by hyperglycemia resulting from defects in insulin secretion, insulin action, or both. Hyperglycemia of diabetes is associated with long-term damage, dysfunction, and failure of various organs, especially the eyes, kidneys, nerves, heart, and blood vessels. Diabetes affects 24 million Americans; 54 million are estimated to have prediabetes, and over 200,000 individuals die each year of related complications (CDC, 2009; CMS, 2009).

Diabetes is divided into distinct types: type 1, type 2, gestational diabetes mellitus (GDM), and other types (see Table 9-1). Type 2 diabetes (T2DM), composing 90% of diabetes cases, is affected by both genetic and environmental factors. Types of diabetes affecting children and teens are listed in Table 9-2.

Adiposity-associated inflammation and insulin resistance are strongly implicated in the development of T2DM as well as the metabolic syndrome (Shah et al, 2008). Activation of nuclear transcription factor-B has been linked with a variety of inflammatory diseases, including diabetes. Antioxidant spices, herbs, and omega-3 fatty acids help to suppress inflammatory pathways.

Amino acids are also important; they support cell signaling, gene expression, and hormone synthesis. While physiological concentrations of amino acids and their metabolites (e.g., nitric oxide, polyamines, glutathione, taurine, thyroid hormones, and serotonin) are required, elevated levels of their products (e.g., ammonia, homocysteine, and asymmetric dimethylarginine) contribute to oxidative stress (Wu, 2009). Dietary supplementation with one or a mixture of arginine, cysteine, glutamine, leucine, proline, and tryptophan may be beneficial for ameliorating health problems including fetal growth restriction, neonatal morbidity and mortality, obesity, diabetes, cardiovascular disease (CVD), the metabolic syndrome, and infertility (Wu, 2009).

Medical nutrition therapy (MNT) replaced the term "diet therapy" years ago. There is no single "diabetic" or "ADA" diet. The recommended diet is an individualized nutrition prescription, based on assessment findings and treatment

TABLE 9-1 Etiologic Classification of Diabetes Mellitus

I. Type 1 diabetes (results from auto-immune beta-cell destruction, usually leading to absolute insulin deficiency).

II. Type 2 diabetes (results from a relative deficiency or insulin resistance).

III. Other specific types of diabetes due to other causes, for example, genetic defects in beta-cell function, genetic defects in insulin action, diseases of the exocrine pancreas (such as cystic fibrosis), or drug- or chemical-induced diabetes (such as in the treatment of AIDS or after organ transplantation).

   A. Genetic defects of beta-cell function: Maturity-onset diabetes of youth (MODY)
   B. Genetic defects in insulin action: Leprechaunism, Rabson–Mendenhall syndrome, Lipoatrophic diabetes
   C. Diseases of the exocrine pancreas: Pancreatitis, Trauma/pancreatectomy, Neoplasia, Cystic fibrosis, Hemochromatosis, Fibrocalculous pancreatopathy
   D. Endocrinopathies: Acromegaly, Cushing's syndrome, Glucagonoma, Pheochromocytoma, Hyperthyroidism, Somatostatinoma, Aldosteronoma
   E. Drug- or chemical-induced: Nicotinic acid, Glucocorticoids, Thyroid hormone, Beta-adrenergic agonists, Thiazides, Dilantin, Alpha-interferon
   F. Infections: Congenital rubella, Cytomegalovirus
   G. Other genetic syndromes sometimes associated with diabetes: Down's syndrome, Klinefelter's syndrome, Turner's syndrome, Friedreich's ataxia, Huntington's chorea, Myotonic dystrophy, Porphyria, Prader-Willi syndrome

IV. Gestational diabetes mellitus (GDM) is diabetes first diagnosed during pregnancy.

Adapted from American Diabetes Association. Diagnosis and classification of diabetes mellitus. Web site accessed September 20, 2009, at http://care.diabetesjournals.org/content/29/suppl_1/s43.full; American Diabetes Association. Standards of Medical Care in Diabetes–2009.

TABLE 9-2 Types of Diabetes in Children and Teens

Type 1 Diabetes (Immune-Mediated)

- Usually not obese; often recent weight loss.
- Short duration of symptoms (thirst and frequent urination).
- Presence of ketones at diagnosis, with about 35% presenting with ketoacidosis.
- Often a honeymoon period after blood sugars are in control during which the need for insulin diminishes for awhile. Low dose of long-acting insulin, such as glargine (Lantus), may prolong the honeymoon phase.
- Ultimate complete destruction of the insulin-producing cells needing exogenous insulin for survival.
- Ongoing risk of ketoacidosis.
- Only about 5% with a family history (in first- or second-degree relatives) of diabetes.

Type 2 Diabetes (Insulin-Resistant)

- Usually overweight at diagnosis; little or no weight loss.
- Usually have sugar in the urine but no ketones.
- As many as 30% will have some ketones in the urine at diagnosis.
- About 5% will have ketoacidosis at diagnosis.
- Often little or no thirst and minimal increased urination.
- Strong family history of diabetes.
- 45–80% have at least one parent with diabetes.
- Diabetes may span many generations of family members.
- 74–100% have a first- or second-degree relative with diabetes.
- Typically from African, Hispanic, Asian, or American Indian origin.
- Disorders likely to cause insulin resistance are common.
- About 90% of children with type 2 diabetes have dark shiny patches on the skin (acanthosis nigricans), which are most often found between the fingers and between the toes, on the back of the neck (dirty neck), and in axillary creases.
- Polycystic ovarian syndrome (PCOS).

Maturity-Onset Diabetes of the Young (MODY)

- Rare form of diabetes; several varieties exist.
- Early age of onset (ages 9–25 years) with autosomal dominant inheritability.
- Results from defects to insulin-producing cells caused by a genetic defect in the pancreatic beta-cell function.
- Symptoms run the gamut from mild elevation in blood sugar to a severe disturbance.
- MODY can occur in all ethnic groups.
- Gene abnormalities are rare and can only be identified through testing that is currently available only in research laboratories.
- Not usually obese.
- Environmental stressors, such as illness or puberty, may unmask the genetically limited insulin secretory reserve of patients with undiagnosed MODY.
- Unlike type 1 diabetes, MODY does not cause polyuria, thirst, or extreme hunger. The primary goal is euglycemia.
- Fasting insulin and C-peptide levels are usually normal or elevated slightly.

Sources: American Diabetes Association, Web site accessed September 20, 2009, at http://spectrum.diabetesjournals.org/content/18/4/249.full; Children with Diabetes Web site accessed September 20, 2009, at http://www.childrenwithdiabetes.com/clinic/mody.htm

goals. MNT considers usual eating habits and other lifestyle factors. Strategic patient counseling should identify benefits of the plan, self-efficacy, obstacles, and lifestyle changes the patient is willing to make; these interventions will help reach desired outcomes. Using open-ended discussion and counseling encourages the client to assess and determine a realistic self-management plan. MNT should be offered in phases, according to patient comprehension and readiness.

Screening for diabetes is outlined in Table 9-3. The nutrition care process include assessment, nutrition diagnosis, intervention, followed by monitoring and evaluation. Monitoring of blood glucose, medications, physical activity, education, behavior modification, and evaluation of cardiovascular and renal status are all relevant. In addition, prevention of complications is essential; see Table 9-4.

A diabetes educator is defined as a health professional who has mastered the core knowledge and skills, communication, counseling, and education. The credentials of certified diabetes educators (CDE) designate professionals who have at least 1000 hours of direct diabetes teaching and who have successfully completed an examination. An advanced credential has been developed for registered dietitians (RDs), nurses, and pharmacists who have advanced degrees and meet experiential requirements; this credential is known as BC-ADM.

TABLE 9-3 Evaluation for Diabetes

Screen for prediabetes and diabetes in high-risk, asymptomatic, undiagnosed adults and children. An oral glucose tolerance test (OGTT) may be considered in patients with impaired fasting glucose (IFG) to better define the risk of diabetes. Testing for diabetes should be considered in all individuals at age 45 years and above, particularly in those with a BMI of 25 kg/m^2, and if normal, testing should be repeated at 3-year intervals. The classic symptoms of diabetes include polyuria, polydipsia, and unexplained weight loss plus one of the following:

1. Symptoms of diabetes and a casual plasma glucose of 200 mg/dL. Casual is defined as any time of day without regard to time since last meal.
2. A fasting plasma glucose (FPG) test, a 2-hour OGTT (75-g glucose load), or both are appropriate. FPG ≥126 mg/dL. Fasting is defined as no caloric intake for at least 8 hours.
3. Two-hour plasma glucose of 200 mg/dL during an OGTT. The test should be performed using a glucose load containing the equivalent of 75 g anhydrous glucose dissolved in water.

American Diabetes Association. Standards of Medical Care in Diabetes–2009. Web site accessed September 22, 2009, at http://care.diabetesjournals.org/content/32/Supplement_1/S13.full

TABLE 9-4 Potential Complications of Diabetes

ACUTE	
Hyperglycemia	Symptoms include polyphagia, polydipsia, polyuria, dehydration, weight loss, weakness, muscle wasting, recurrent or persistent infections, hypovolemia, ketonemia, glycosuria, blurred or changed vision, fatigue, muscle cramps, and dry mouth. Blood glucose >250 mg/dL should be evaluated; monitor blood or urine ketones to check for diabetic ketoacidosis (DKA). Three forms of hyperglycemia may be noted in the hospitalized patient: (1) someone with a history of diagnosed diabetes; (2) previously unrecognized diabetes; (3) hospital-related fasting blood glucose of 126 mg/dL or random blood glucose of >200 mg/dL that reverts to normal after discharge.
DKA or nonketotic hyperosmolar state	The stress of illness, trauma, and/or surgery frequently aggravates glycemic control and may precipitate DKA or nonketotic hyperosmolar state. A vomiting illness accompanied by ketosis may indicate DKA, a life-threatening condition that requires immediate medical care to prevent complications and death (American Diabetes Association, 2009). Cerebral edema can occur. Early consultation with an endocrinologist is needed.
Hypoglycemia	Symptoms include shakiness, confusion, diplopia, irritability, hunger, weakness, headache, rapid and shallow breathing, numbness of mouth/lips/tongue, pulse normal or abnormal, convulsions, lack of coordination, dizziness, staggering gait, pallor, slurred speech, tingling, diaphoresis, nausea, sweating, tremors, and nightmares. Treat when blood glucose level is <70 mg/dL with 15 g of liquid or fat-free sources of glucose or carbohydrates (CHO); wait 15 minutes and retest, then treat with another 15 g of CHO if still <70 mg/dL. Evaluate blood glucose after 1 hour. Continue to monitor until next meal. Adding protein to carbohydrate does not affect the glycemic response and does not prevent subsequent hypoglycemia, but adding fat may retard and then prolong the acute glycemic response (American Diabetes Association, 2009). In rare, severe hypoglycemia (when the individual requires the assistance of another person and cannot be treated with oral carbohydrate), emergency glucagon kits may be used; these require a prescription and they can expire over time (American Diabetes Association, 2009).
Dawn phenomenon	The dawn phenomenon is the end result of a combination of natural body changes that occur during the sleep cycle. Between 3:00 a.m. and 8:00 a.m., the body naturally starts to increase the amounts of counter-regulatory hormones (growth hormone, cortisol, and catecholamines) which work against insulin's action to drop blood sugars. These cause a blood sugar levels to rise in the morning.
Somogyi effect	"Rebound hyperglycemia" leads to high blood sugar levels in the morning preceded by an episode of asymptomatic hypoglycemia. When blood sugar drops too low in the middle of the night, the body counters by releasing hormones to raise the sugar levels. Too much insulin earlier or not enough of a bedtime snack may be the problem.
Acute illness or infection	Any condition leading to deterioration in glycemic control necessitates more frequent monitoring of blood glucose and urine or blood ketones (American Diabetes Association, 2009). Aggressive glycemic management with insulin is needed with severe acute illness (American Diabetes Association, 2009). The risk for DKA is higher during this time; test blood glucose, drink adequate amounts of fluid, ingest CHO (50 g CHO every 3–4 hours) if blood glucose levels are low, and adjust medications to keep glucose in desired range and to prevent starvation ketosis. Marked hyperglycemia requires temporary adjustment of the treatment program and, if accompanied by ketosis, frequent interaction with the diabetes care team (American Diabetes Association, 2009). Hospitalization may be needed. In a pediatric case, cerebral edema may occur; referral to a pediatric endocrinologist is important.
Vaccines	Annually provide an influenza vaccine to all diabetic patients ≥6 months of age; provide at least one lifetime pneumococcal vaccine for adults with diabetes (American Diabetes Association, 2009). Persons who have diabetes tend to be at higher than normal risk for bacterial forms of pneumonia.
Critical illness	In critically ill patients, blood glucose levels should be kept as close to 110 mg/dL (6.1 μmol/L) as possible and generally <180 mg/dL (10 μmol/L); intravenous insulin is usually needed (American Diabetes Association, 2009). Scheduled prandial insulin doses should be given in relation to meals and should be adjusted according to point-of-care glucose levels; traditional sliding-scale insulin regimens may be ineffective and are not useful (American Diabetes Association, 2009).

(continued)

TABLE 9-4 Potential Complications of Diabetes *(continued)*

INTERMEDIATE	
Children with T1DM	Children's growth and development may be impaired with diabetes; adequate protein and energy must be provided. Children may be picky eaters. Blood glucose goals are less strict. Target range for normal blood glucose (90–130 mg/dL before eating for 13–19 year olds; 90–180 mg/dL for 6–12 year olds; and 100–180 mg/dL for 0–5 year olds) may be altered according to the health care provider's evaluation. Near-normalization of blood glucose levels is seldom attainable in children and adolescents after the honeymoon (remission) period (American Diabetes Association, 2009). The A1c goals also vary in children. Most children under 6 or 7 years of age have "hypoglycemic unawareness;" young children lack the cognitive capacity to recognize and respond to hypoglycemic symptoms (American Diabetes Association, 2009). Children with diabetes differ from adults in many ways, including insulin sensitivity related to sexual maturity, physical growth, ability to provide self-care, vulnerability to hypoglycemia, differing family dynamics, developmental stages, and physiological differences (American Diabetes Association, 2009). Work with the family and school to plan for emergencies such as low or high blood glucose levels.
Children with T2DM	Distinction between type 1 and type 2 diabetes in children can be difficult because autoantigens and ketosis may be present in a substantial number of patients (American Diabetes Association, 2009). Children with T2DM are usually overweight or obese and present with glycosuria with or without ketonuria, absent or mild polyuria and polydipsia, and little or no weight loss. Up to 33% have ketonuria at diagnosis; some may have ketoacidosis without any associated stress, illness, or infection.
Preconception	All women with diabetes and childbearing potential should be educated about the need for good glucose control before pregnancy, the need for family planning, and need for early treatment for diabetic retinopathy, nephropathy, neuropathy, and cardiovascular disease (American Diabetes Association, 2009). A1c levels should be normal or as close to normal as possible (<1% above the upper limits of normal) in an individual before conception is attempted (American Diabetes Association, 2009).
Pregnancy and diabetes	Infant mortality rates are approximately twice as high for babies born to women with uncontrolled diabetes compared with babies born to women without diabetes. To reduce the risk of fetal malformations and maternal or fetal complications, pregnant women and women planning to become pregnant require excellent blood glucose control. These women need to be seen frequently by a multidisciplinary team. Specialized laboratory and diagnostic tests may be needed. Women with diabetes must be trained in self-monitoring of blood glucose (SMBG). Nutrition recommendations for women with preexisting diabetes must be based on a thorough assessment. Monitoring blood glucose levels, blood or urine ketones, appetite, and weight gain is needed to develop an individualized nutrition prescription and to make adjustments to the meal plan. Plasma glucose should be maintained at 65–100 mg/dL before meals and in fasting; 110–135 mg/dL 1 hour after meals; and <120 mg/dL 2 hours after meals. Use an extra 300 kcal daily during the second and third trimester; 1 g/kg/d or an additional 25 g/d of protein; 175 g/d of CHO; 600 μg folic acid. Added iron and calcium may also be required.
Gestational diabetes	See the entry later in this chapter.
Lactation	Extra protein, calcium, and folic acid will be needed. Monitoring of blood glucose is recommended, but hypoglycemia should be avoided. Breastfeeding lowers blood glucose and may require women to eat a CHO-containing snack either before or during breastfeeding. Extra 330–400 kcal meets the needs of most lactating mothers.
Older adults	Unexplained weight loss should be viewed as a symptom of a problem. Diabetes is an important health condition for the aging population; at least 20% of patients over the age of 65 years have diabetes. These patients tend to have higher rates of premature death, functional disability, and coexisting illnesses such as hypertension, heart disease, and stroke than those without diabetes (American Diabetes Association, 2009). New-onset diabetes in adults over the age of 50 may signal underlying pancreatic cancer, which should be investigated. Strict diets in long-term care are not warranted and may lead to dehydration and malnutrition; specialized diabetic diets are not required, and a balanced diet with consistent timing of CHO is to be recommended. Modify medications, rather than diet, as needed. Lower hypertension gradually; implement the DASH diet whenever possible. A multivitamin-mineral supplement may be beneficial for this population.
CHRONIC	
A1c levels	Achieve and maintain normal blood glucose (BG) and lipids. Intensive therapy (IT) helps reduce onset or progression of vascular problems. Maintain hemoglobin A1c levels <7% (A1c level of 7 = BG 170). For evaluation, note that A1c of 5% = BG 100; 6% = BG 135; 7% = BG 170; 8% = BG 205; 9% = BG 240; 10% = BG 275; 11% = BG 310.
Microvascular	Retinopathy, ocular abnormalities, nephropathy, neuropathy (sensory or motor conditions, which may lead to ulceration or even limb amputation, orthostatic hypotension, intractable nausea and vomiting, and diabetic gastroenteropathy), diabetic cystopathy, and chronic diarrhea.

(continued)

TABLE 9-4 **Potential Complications of Diabetes *(continued)***

CHRONIC	
Retinopathy	Retinopathy from diabetes accounts for 12,000–24,000 cases of blindness each year. Optimal glycemic and blood pressure control can substantially reduce the risk and progression of diabetic retinopathy (American Diabetes Association, 2009). In the presence of proliferative diabetic retinopathy (PDR) or severe nonproliferative diabetic retinopathy (NPDR), vigorous aerobic or resistance exercise may be contraindicated because of the risk of triggering vitreous hemorrhage or retinal detachment (American Diabetes Association, 2009). Pregnancy in T1DM may aggravate retinopathy; laser photocoagulation surgery can minimize this risk (American Diabetes Association, 2009).
Microalbuminuria and nephropathy	Early signs of nephropathy include hyperfiltration, renal hypertrophy, and microalbuminuria (loss of 30–300 μg/mg creatinine in the urine). Protein losses at a rate of >300 μg/mg creatinine may indicate advancement toward chronic kidney disease (CKD). To reduce the risk and/or slow the progression of nephropathy, optimize glucose and blood pressure control (American Diabetes Association, 2009). Nephropathy is preceded by microalbuminuria for several years; onset of end-stage renal disease is about 5 years after onset of microalbuminuria. For diabetic nephropathy, liberalize CHO intake and control insulin levels accordingly. Controlled protein intake will slow down progression of nephropathy. Adults need <0.8–1 g protein/kg daily (American Diabetes Association, 2009). Protein restriction is of benefit in slowing the progression of albuminuria, glomerular filtration rate (GFR) decline, and occurrence of end-stage renal disease (ESRD). Protein restriction should be considered in patients whose nephropathy seems to be progressing despite optimal glucose and blood pressure control and use of angiotensin-converting enzyme (ACE) inhibitors and/or angiotensin receptor blockers (ARBs) (American Diabetes Association, 2009). Intensive diabetes management with the goal of achieving near normoglycemia has been shown to delay the onset of microalbuminuria (American Diabetes Association, 2009). Refer to a physician experienced in the care of diabetic renal disease when the estimated GFR has fallen to <60 mL/min or if difficulties occur in the management of hypertension or hyperkalemia (American Diabetes Association, 2009). ACE inhibitors are almost always prescribed to decrease progression. Phosphorus should be controlled at 8–12 mg/kg/d. Some people may need phosphate binders and calcium supplements.
End-stage renal disease	Diabetes is the leading cause of CKD, especially among blacks, Mexican Americans, and Native Americans. Diabetic nephropathy occurs in 20–40% of patients with diabetes and is the single leading cause of ESRD (American Diabetes Association, 2009). Creatinine and GFR should be assessed annually in this population. Microalbuminuria (30–299 mg/24 h) and macroalbuminuria (≥300 mg/24 h) should be carefully monitored (American Diabetes Association, 2009). While physical activity can acutely increase urinary protein excretion, there is no evidence that vigorous exercise increases the rate of progression of diabetic kidney disease (American Diabetes Association, 2009).
Autonomic neuropathy	About 70% of persons who have diabetes have some degree of neuropathy, including impaired sensation in the hands and feet, slowed digestion, or carpal tunnel syndrome. Autonomic neuropathy can decrease cardiac responsiveness to exercise, causing postural hypotension, impaired thermoregulation, impaired skin blood flow and sweating, impaired night vision, impaired thirst, risk of dehydration, and gastroparesis with unpredictable food delivery (American Diabetes Association, 2009). Neuropathy may be delayed with careful blood glucose management. Weight loss may be beneficial for obese persons.
Skin and joints	Decreased pain sensation in the extremities may increase risk of skin breakdown and infection and joint destruction; it may be best to encourage nonweight-bearing activities such as swimming, bicycling, or arm exercises (American Diabetes Association, 2009).
Genitourinary	Diabetic autonomic neuropathy is associated with recurrent genitourinary tract disturbances or bladder and/or sexual dysfunction.
Amputations	Lower extremity amputations are painful and disabling; prevention is desirable. Amputation and foot ulcers are the most common consequences of diabetic neuropathy and the major causes of morbidity and disability in people with diabetes (American Diabetes Association, 2009).
Cardiac neuropathy	Major clinical manifestations of cardiac neuropathy in diabetes include resting tachycardia, exercise intolerance, orthostatic hypotension, constipation, gastroparesis, erectile dysfunction, sudomotor dysfunction, impaired neurovascular function, "brittle diabetes," and hypoglycemic autonomic failure (American Diabetes Association, 2009). Evaluate cardiac status before starting an exercise program.
Gastrointestinal (GI) neuropathy	GI disturbances (esophageal enteropathy, gastroparesis, constipation, diarrhea, and fecal incontinence) are common, and any section of the GI tract may be affected. Gastroparesis should be suspected in individuals with erratic glucose control (American Diabetes Association, 2009).

(continued)

TABLE 9-4 Potential Complications of Diabetes *(continued)*

Macrovascular **Coronary artery disease and arterial vascular disease**	CVD is a major cause of mortality and also a major contributor to morbidity in diabetics. T2DM is an independent risk factor for macrovascular disease (American Diabetes Association, 2009). Other risk factors include insulin resistance, hyperglycemia, hyper tension, dyslipidemia, and smoking. Smoking is related to the premature development of microvascular complications of diabetes and may have a role in the development of T2DM (American Diabetes Association, 2009). Advise all patients not to smoke; include smoking cessation as a routine component of care (American Diabetes Association, 2009).
Dyslipidemia	Lifestyle modification focusing on the reduction of saturated fat and cholesterol intake, weight loss (if indicated), and increased physical activity has been shown to improve the lipid profile in patients with diabetes (American Diabetes Association, 2009). Guidelines promote low-density lipoprotein (LDL) cholesterol levels of <100 mg/dL as optimal for all patients and lowering of triglyceride levels when >150 mg/dL. Statins may be helpful. Elevate high-density lipoprotein (HDL) to levels >50 mg/dL. If HDL is <50 mg/dL and LDL is between 100 and 129 mg/dL, a fibric acid derivative or niacin might be used. Niacin raises HDL but can significantly increase blood glucose at high doses (American Diabetes Association, 2009). Use aspirin therapy (75–162 mg/d) as a secondary prevention strategy in those with diabetes with a history of CVD (American Diabetes Association, 2009). Tailor nutrition interventions according to each patient's age, type of diabetes, pharmacological treatment, lipid levels, and other medical conditions. Focus on the reduction of saturated fat, cholesterol, and trans fat intake (American Diabetes Association, 2009). Monitoring of homocysteine levels and related actions should be taken. Adequate insulin therapy often returns lipids to normal in T1DM. Elevated levels in T2DM require strict management; limit saturated fat to 7–10% of total calories. The rate of heart disease is about two to four times higher in adults who have diabetes; it is the leading cause of diabetes-related deaths. Since people with diabetes tend to have high triglyceride and low HDL levels, omega-3 fatty acids from DHA and EPA (fish and marine oils) can help.
Hypertension	Over 70% of adults with diabetes also have hypertension. Control of hypertension in diabetes has been linked to reduction in the progression of both microvascular and macrovascular disease. In T1DM, hypertension is often the result of underlying nephropathy, whereas in T2DM, it may be present as part of the metabolic syndrome (American Diabetes Association, 2009). Patients with systolic blood pressure ≥140 mm Hg or diastolic blood pressure ≥90 mm Hg should receive drug therapy in addition to lifestyle and behavioral therapy (American Diabetes Association, 2009). Blood pressure should be measured at every routine diabetes visit; patients with diabetes should be treated to reach a systolic blood pressure <130 mm Hg and a diastolic blood pressure <80 mm Hg (American Diabetes Association, 2009). In patients with T1DM with hypertension and any degree of albuminuria, ACE inhibitors have been shown to delay the progression of nephropathy. With T2DM, hypertension, and microalbuminuria, ACE inhibitors and ARBs have been shown to delay the progression to macroalbuminuria (American Diabetes Association, 2009). Modest weight loss is helpful. Prevent hypokalemia, which can blunt insulin release. Control glucose; limit alcohol and smoking; and add exercise. Use the DASH diet because it increases intake of calcium, magnesium, and potassium while lowering alcohol and excess weight.
Hypertension in pregnancy	Pregnancy-induced hypertension is two to four times more common in women with T1DM than in the general population. Screen for microalbuminemia as a strong predictor of pre-eclampsia. In pregnant patients with diabetes and chronic hypertension, blood pressure target goals are 110–129/65–79 mm Hg; avoid lower blood pressure because fetal growth may be impaired (American Diabetes Association, 2009). ACE inhibitors and ARBs are contraindicated during pregnancy (American Diabetes Association, 2009).
Stroke	Stroke risk is two to four times higher among persons with diabetes, and high blood pressure should be carefully controlled.
Catabolic illness	Catabolic illness (such as HIV infection, AIDS, or cancer) changes body compartments, with increased extracellular fluid and shrinkage of body fat and cell mass. Monitor unexplained weight losses carefully, especially 10% or more of usual weight. Standard tube feedings are usually well tolerated in persons with diabetes (50% CHO or lower); monitor fluid status, weight, plasma glucose and electrolytes, and acid–base balance. Overfeeding is to be avoided; start with 25–35 kcal/kg of body weight. Protein needs may be 1 g/kg up to 1.5 g/kg in stressed individuals, and pressure ulcers may require a higher level of protein and calories than normal for healing. Addition of insulin may be needed. Oral glucose-lowering medications need to be adjusted to achieve adequate control of glycemia.

Additional data from: American Diabetes Association, 2009; Centers for Disease Control and Prevention, 2009.

TABLE 9-5 Key Concepts in Diabetes Management

Glucose Control

- Improved glycemic control benefits people with either type 1 or type 2 diabetes.
- For every 1% reduction in results of A1c blood tests (e.g., from 8.0% to 7.0%), the risk of developing microvascular diabetic complications (eye, kidney, and nerve disease) drops by 40%.
- A1c is the primary target for glycemic control. More stringent glycemic goals (i.e., a usual A1c, <6%) may further reduce complications at the cost of increased risk of hypoglycemia. Less-intensive glycemic goals may be indicated in patients with severe or frequent hypoglycemia.
- Postprandial glucose may be targeted if A1c goals are not met despite reaching preprandial glucose goals.
- Goals should be individualized, and lower goals may be reasonable based on benefit-risk assessment.
- Certain populations (children, pregnant women, and elderly) require special considerations. See guidelines:

	Plasma Blood Glucose Goal			
Values by Age (years)	**Pre-prandial (mg/dL)**	**Bedtime/ Overnight**	**A1c**	**Rationale**
Toddlers and preschoolers age (0–6)	100–180	110–200	<8.5% (but >7.5%)	High risk and vulnerability to hypoglycemia
School age (7–12)	90–180	100–180	<8%	Risks of hypoglycemia and relatively low risk of complications prior to puberty
Adolescents and young adults (13–19)	90–130	90–150	<7%	Risk of severe hypoglycemia; developmental and psychological issues; a lower goal <7% is reasonable if achieved without excessive hypoglycemia
Adults (20+)	90–130		<7%	Peak post-prandial <180 mg/dL 1–2 hours after beginning of meal

Blood Pressure Control

- Goal: blood pressure <130/80 mm Hg.
- Restriction of sodium to 2400 mg/d assists in the control of hypertension.
- Blood pressure control can reduce cardiovascular disease (heart disease and stroke) by approximately 33–50% and can reduce microvascular disease (eye, kidney, and nerve disease) by approximately 33%.
- In general, for every 10-mm Hg reduction in systolic blood pressure, the risk for any complication related to diabetes is reduced by 12%.

Control of Blood Lipids

- Improved control of cholesterol or blood lipids (e.g., high-density lipoprotein [HDL], low-density lipoprotein [LDL], and triglycerides) can reduce cardiovascular complications by 20–50%.
- Goals: Total cholesterol minus HDL should be ≤130 mg/dL; LDL <100 mg/dL; Triglycerides<150 mg/dL; HDL<40 mg/dL in men, >50 mg/dL in women.

Preventive Care Practices for Eyes and Feet

- Detecting and treating diabetic eye disease with laser therapy can reduce the development of severe vision loss by an estimated 50–60%.
- Comprehensive foot care programs can reduce amputation rates by 45–85%.

Preventive Care for Kidneys (Prerenal Failure)

- Detecting and treating early diabetic kidney disease by lowering blood pressure can reduce the decline in kidney function by 30–70%. Angiotensin-converting enzyme (ACE) inhibitors and angiotensin receptor blockers (ARBs) are most effective in reducing the decline in kidney function.
- With protein intakes greater than 20% of energy intake, there is an association with increased albumin excretion rate.
- Once albuminuria is present, reduce protein to 0.8–1.0 g/kg/d with microalbuminuria and to 0.8 g/kg/d with macroalbuminuria. There may be a benefit to lowering phosphorus intake to 500–1000 mg/d.
- There is evidence for a benefit on renal function, glucose, lipids, and blood pressure from weight-maintaining diets.

Adapted from: National Diabetes Guidelines, Web site accessed September 20, 2009, at http://guidelines.gov/Compare/comparison.aspx?file=DIABETES_NUTRITION1.inc#t3general

Collaborative, multidisciplinary teams are best suited to provide such care for people with chronic conditions such as diabetes and to empower patients' performance of appropriate self-management (American Diabetes Association, 2009). MNT provided by RDs to patients with type 1 and T2DM has been shown to improve glycemic outcomes. Community-based education that incorporates Social Cognitive Theory and Stages of Change Theory, with three group sessions focused on meal planning with cooking demonstrations, is effective; the education successfully promotes use of herbs in place of salt, use of olive or canola oils, use of artificial sweeteners in baking, knowledge of diabetes and nutrition, and self-efficacy (Chapman-Novakofski and Karduck, 2005). Table 9-5 offers more tips for diabetes management.

It is also important to address culturally specific eating habits. For example, a recent study in South Dakota found that a diet patterned after the historical hunter–gatherer type diet (with the 25% of energy supplied from protein), provided better blood glucose control and lower the circulating insulin levels in Northern Plains Indians with T2DM. The same may be true for other high-risk groups.

For More Information

- American Association of Diabetes Educators
  http://www.aadenet.org/
- American Diabetes Association
  http://www.diabetes.org/
- American Diabetes Association Youth Zone
  http://www.diabetes.org/youthzone/youth-zone.jsp
- Calorie and Nutrient Information
  http://www.calorieking.com
- Canadian Diabetes Association
  http://www.diabetes.ca/
- Centers for Disease Control and Prevention (CDC) Diabetes Public Health Resources
  http://www.cdc.gov/diabetes/index.htm
- CDC Division of Diabetes
  http://www.cdc.gov/diabetes
- Centers for Medicare and Medicaid Services Diabetes Guidelines
  http://www.cms.hhs.gov/DiabetesScreening/
- Children with Diabetes
  http://www.childrenwithdiabetes.com
- Diabetes Care and Dietetic Practice Group
  http://www.dce.org/
- Diabetic Gourmet Magazine
  http://diabeticgourmet.com/dgarchiv2.shtml
- Diabetes Research Institute Foundation
  http://www.drinet.org/
- International Diabetes Federation
  http://www.idf.org
- Joslin Diabetes Center, Boston, MA
  http://www.joslin.org/
- Juvenile Diabetes Research Foundation International
  http://www.jdrf.org
- Low Literacy Information
  http://www.learningaboutdiabetes.com
- National Diabetes Education Program
  http://www.ndep.nih.gov/
- National Guideline Clearinghouse – Diabetes
  http://guidelines.gov/summary/summary.aspx?doc_id=12816&nbr=006618
- National Institute of Diabetes and Digestive and Kidney Diseases (NIDDK)
  http://www.diabetes.niddk.nih.gov/
- Park Nicollet–International Diabetes Center
  http://www.Parknicollet.com/diabetes
- School Guidelines
  http://www.ndep.nih.gov/diabetes/pubs/Youth_NDEPSchoolGuide.pdf
- Taking Control of Your Diabetes
  http://www.tcoyd.org

CITED REFERENCES

American Diabetes Association. Standards of Medical Care in Diabetes–2009. Web site accessed September 22, 2009, at http://care.diabetesjournals.org/content/32/Supplement_1/S13.full

CDC (Centers for Disease Control and Prevention). National diabetes fact sheet. Web site accessed September 21, 2009, at http://www.cdc.gov/diabetes/pubs/general.htm#impaired

Chapman-Novakofski K, Karduck J. Improvement in knowledge, social cognitive theory variables, and movement through stages of change after a community-based diabetes education program. *J Am Diet Assoc.* 105:1613, 2005.

CMS (Centers for Medicare and Medicaid Services). Diabetes Screening. Web site accessed September 20, 2009, at http://www.cms.hhs.gov/DiabetesScreening/

Shah A, et al. Adipose inflammation, insulin resistance, and cardiovascular disease. *JPEN J Parenter Enteral Nutr.* 32:638, 2008.

Wu G. Amino acids: metabolism, functions, and nutrition. *Amino Acids.* 37:1, 2009.

DIABETES MELLITUS, COMPLICATIONS, AND RELATED CONDITIONS

TYPE 1 DIABETES MELLITUS

NUTRITIONAL ACUITY RANKING: LEVEL 4

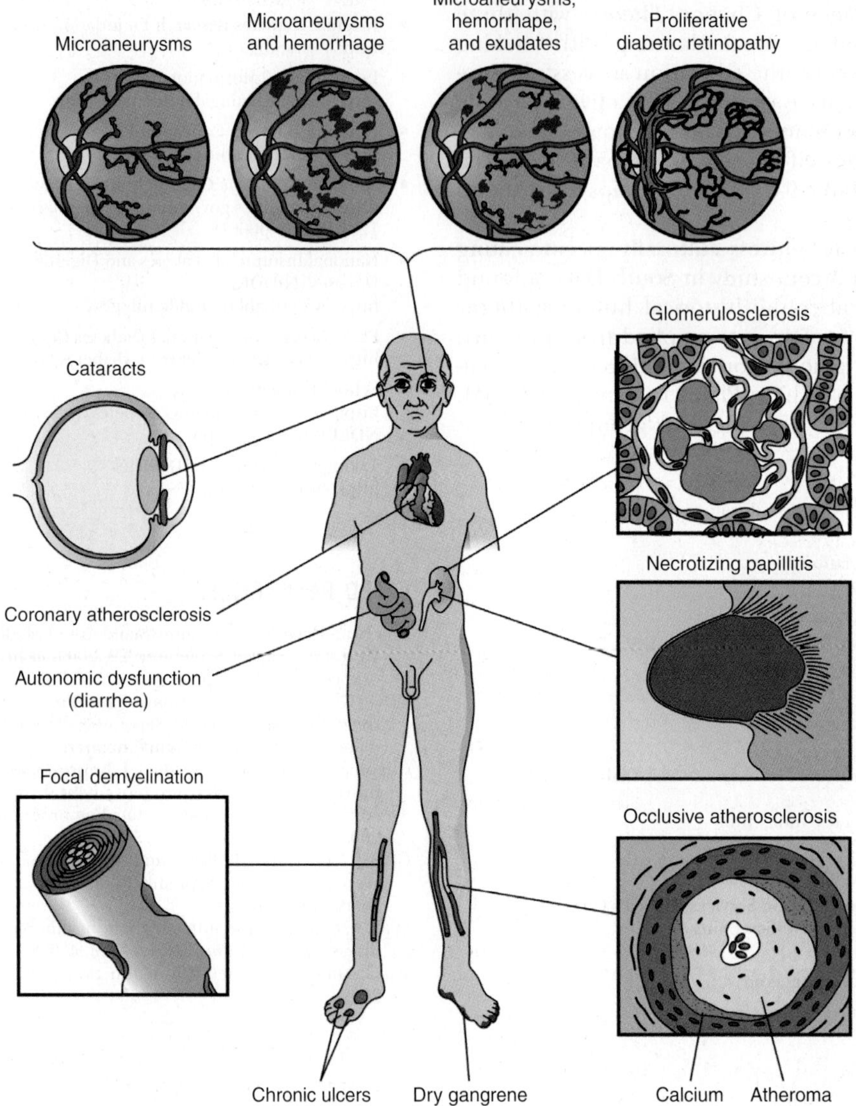

Adapted from: Raphael Rubin, David S. Strayer, *Rubin's Pathology: Clinicopathologic Foundations of Medicine,* 5th ed. Philadelphia: Lippincott Williams & Wilkins, 2008.

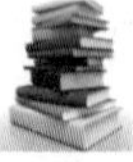

DEFINITIONS AND BACKGROUND

Type 1 diabetes mellitus (T1DM) is absolute insulin deficiency with total failure to produce insulin. Previously used terms include "type I," "insulin-dependent diabetes mellitus (IDDM)," "juvenile," "brittle," or "ketosis-prone" diabetes. T1DM involves autoimmune destruction of the pancreatic beta-cells (the islets of Langerhans). Onset often follows viral infection such as mumps. It usually starts in children or young adults, affecting 10% of cases of diabetes; beta-cell damage is often more severe in patients diagnosed before puberty.

Signs and symptoms of diabetes include polyuria (frequent urination, including frequent bedwetting in otherwise trained children), polydipsia (excessive thirst), polyphagia (extreme hunger), weakness, fatigue, irritability, and sudden weight loss. A fasting plasma glucose (FPG) test or an oral glucose tolerance test (OGTT) can be used. FPG is the preferred method; level of 126 mg/dL or higher is considered to be diabetes. With the OGTT, blood glucose is measured after fasting and 2 hours after drinking a glucose beverage; results between 140 and 199 mg/dL indicate prediabetes, and a level of 200 mg/dL represents diabetes. Hemoglobin A1c (HbA1c) test is not recommended for diagnosis; finger-prick tests are also not valid.

Serious complications begin earlier than previously thought. Glucose control really matters, as proven by the results of the Diabetes Control and Complications Trial (DCCT) and other trials. More than 65% of people with diabetes die from heart disease or stroke (American Diabetes Association, 2009). Diabetes is the chief cause of blindness, renal failure, and amputations and is a leading cause of birth defects.

Intensive therapy to achieve near-normal glucose levels results in lower onset and progression of complications. Caution is needed to prevent hypoglycemia, especially in the very young (<6-year old) and those with vision loss or kidney disease. Fasting blood glucose should be measured three to eight times daily when on a new insulin regimen; this may be tapered down when stable (American Dietetic Association, 2009).

Protein and nutrient metabolism are affected by insulin availability. The long-term effects of diets high in protein and low in carbohydrate (CHO) are unknown at this time. Vitamin and mineral intakes are being studied for their various impacts on blood glucose levels. In addition, it is important to note that antioxidant foods and spices may be helpful in lowering blood glucose levels.

Individuals using insulin should eat at consistent times synchronized with the time-action of the insulin preparation used, monitor their blood glucose levels, and determine their required insulin doses for the amount of food usually eaten. Intensified insulin therapy, including multiple daily injections, continuous subcutaneous insulin infusion with an insulin pump, and rapid-acting insulin, allows for more flexibility in the timing of meals and snacks, as well as in the amount of food eaten.

Medical costs for patients with diabetes account for a significant percentage of all health care costs. National Standards for Diabetes Self-Management have been written to support a team approach to patient care; they include the RD as an essential team member. Ongoing nutrition self-management education includes assessment, care plans, treatment goals, desired outcomes, and monitoring metabolic parameters such as blood glucose, lipids, A1c, and related lab values.

The use of evidence-based MNT can lead to effective lifestyle changes. Use of technology to track quarterly weight and lab values is an effective way to help patients with their self-management goals (Chima et al, 2005). Multidisciplinary team interventions are suggested to help improve patients' A1c levels and to reduce complications, hospital readmissions, and hospital stays. The American Dietetic Association recommends a specific number of MNT visits to promote the desired outcome (see Table 9-6).

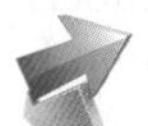

ASSESSMENT, MONITORING, AND EVALUATION

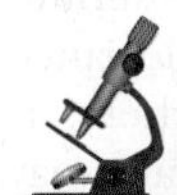

CLINICAL INDICATORS

Genetic Markers: The pathogenesis of most DM is multifactorial including both genetic and environmental factors. Interleukin, HLA-DR or HLA-DQ alleles, INS-23, and vitamin D receptor (VDR) gene polymorphisms may be associated with risk of developing T1DM. Much more research is needed to clarify how these present in various haplotypes or ethnic groups. Hormonal imbalance controls key proteins that regulate the folate-SAM-homocyteine pathways. Poor folate status has been associated with endothelial dysfunction in adolescents with type 1 diabetes (Wiltshire et al, 2008). The methylene-tetrahydrofolate reductase (MTHFR) A>C genotype may confer protection against early nephropathy with lower homocysteine (tHcy) levels, whereas MTHFR 677 TT genotypes may have earlier onset of retinopathy (Wiltshire et al, 2008).

Clinical/History	Lab Work	
Height	HbA1c (goal <7%)	High-density lipoprotein (HDL)
Weight	Fasting blood glucose (FBG) (goal 90–130 mg/dL)	Low-density lipoprotein (LDL)
Weight:height percentiles	OGTT results	Triglycerides (Trig)
Body mass index (BMI)	Urine glucose	Urinary ketones
Diet history	Blood urea nitrogen (BUN)	Na^+, K^+
Waist circumference	Creatinine (Creat)	Ca^{++}, Mg^{++}
Visual acuity	Microalbuminuria	Serum phosphorous (PO_4)
Blood pressure (BP)	C-reactive protein (CRP)	Thyroid-stimulating hormone (TSH)
Intake and output (I & O)	Total Cholesterol (Chol)	Serum D_3 level
Absence of menstruation?		
Increased hunger, thirst, urination		
Nausea, vomiting, abdominal pain		

INTERVENTION

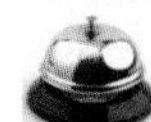

OBJECTIVES

- Individualize MNT as needed to achieve treatment goals, preferably provided by an RD familiar with the components of diabetes MNT (American Diabetes Association, 2009).

TABLE 9-6 Recommended Medical Nutrition Therapy Visits for Type 1 Diabetes

Encounter	Length of Contact	Time between Encounters
1	60–90 minutes	2–4 weeks
2, 3	30–45 minutes	2–4 weeks
4, 5	30–45 minutes	6–12 months
6, 7, 8	30–45 minutes	As indicated by clinical data and/or changes in medication

Adapted from: National Guideline Clearinghouse. Nutrition practice guidelines for type 1 and type 2 diabetes mellitus. Web site accessed September 20, 2009 at http://guidelines.gov/summary/summary.aspx?doc_id=12816&nbr=006618

SAMPLE NUTRITION CARE PROCESS STEPS

Altered Nutrition Labs-Type 1 Diabetes

Assessment Data: Blood glucose log and food history.

Nutrition Diagnosis (PES): Altered nutrition-related lab values related to wrong dose of insulin as evidenced by blood glucose readings consistently ≥250 mg/dL before lunch.

Intervention: Education and counseling to address appropriate timing of food and insulin dose; CHO counting.

Monitoring and Evaluation: Ask patient to fax blood glucose logs for next 3 days.

- Address the metabolic abnormalities of glucose, lipids, and BP (Kulkarni, 2006). Meet the specific needs of the patient; modify drug therapy to enhance outcomes and quality of life.
- Regularly evaluate food/nutrition history, physical exercise, activity patterns, excessive weight gain.
- Develop food/meal planning with client; share plan with medical team so an insulin regimen can be integrated into the client's usual lifestyle. In hospital settings, avoid use of restrictive diets.
- Promote lifestyle changes according to client readiness, educational, and skill level. Early referral for lifestyle changes and advice yields the most benefit (Kulkarni, 2006).
- Plan meal plan, exercise, and medication to achieve blood glucose and lipid goals. Minimize intake of trans fatty acids; saturated fat should be <7% of total calories (American Diabetes Association, 2009).
- Prevent early onset of complications by controlling glucose, lipids, and BP. If there are complications, delay or prevent consequences. The DCCT intensive therapy group had substantially lower complication rates; fewer than 1% became blind, required kidney replacement, or had an amputation because of diabetes (DCCT Research Group, 2009).
- Both the amount (grams) of carbohydrate as well as the type of carbohydrate in a food influence blood glucose level. Monitoring total grams of carbohydrate remains a key strategy in achieving glycemic control (American Diabetes Association, 2009).
- Teach individuals how to use carbohydrate counting and how to adjust insulin doses based on planned carbohydrate intake.
- Promote self-monitoring of blood glucose (SMBG) multiple times per day, and more often during illness.

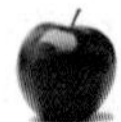

FOOD AND NUTRITION

- A meal plan based on the individual's usual food intake should be used as the basis for integrating insulin therapy into the usual eating and exercise patterns (American Diabetes Association, 2009).
- Choose a variety of heart-healthy foods, including an average of five servings of fruits and vegetables, six servings of grains (three whole grain), and two servings of low-fat dairy. Foods in the meat and fat groups do not directly affect blood glucose.
- Discourage meal skipping.
- Determine appropriate energy intake for age. Pregnant and growing individuals should receive more: sedentary, 25 kcal/kg; normal, 30 kcal/kg; undernourished or active, 45–50 kcal/kg. Reassess as activity or life stage changes.
- Monounsaturated fatty acids and carbohydrates combined should provide about 60–70% of daily energy intake; limit saturated fats to <10% of energy intake. Use a plan that includes CHO at 45–65% of total energy intake each day to prevent ketosis (American Diabetes Association, 2009).
- Apply carbohydrate counting, dietary guidelines, or MyPyramid food guidance principles. Focus on carbohydrates more than total energy or source of carbohydrate.
- Determine insulin to carbohydrate ratios for each individual. One CHO unit equals 15 g CHO (standard starch, fruit, sweet, or milk servings are based on 15 g CHO).
- Provide consistent carbohydrate with each meal and snack with set doses of insulin. Each of the following portions is one carbohydrate choice (15 g CHO):
  - Grains, breads, cereals: 1 oz bread (1 slice bread, 1/4 large bagel, 6″ tortilla); 1/2 cup cooked dried beans; 1/3 cup pasta or rice; 1 cup soup; 3/4 cup cold cereal; 1/2 cup cooked cereal.
  - Milk and yogurt: 1 cup milk; 2/3 cup unsweetened yogurt (6 oz) or sweetened with noncaloric sweetener.
  - Fruits: 1 small fresh fruit; 1/2 cup fruit; 1 cup melon or berries; 1/2 cup fruit juice; 1/4 cup dried fruit.
  - Sweets and snack foods: 3/4 oz snack food (pretzels, chips, 4–6 crackers); 1 oz sweet snack (two small sandwich cookies, five vanilla wafers); 1 tbsp sugar or honey; 1/2 cup ice cream.
  - Vegetables: 1/2 cup potato, peas, or corn; 3 cups raw vegetables; 1½ cups cooked vegetables; small portions of nonstarchy vegetables.
- Most women need about 3–4 carbohydrate choices (45–60 g CHO) at each meal; men generally need about 4–5 carbohydrate choices (60–75 g CHO) per meal. Active young women may need 2500 kcal, or about 75–90 g CHO/meal; an active young man who needs 3000 kcal/d may need 90–100 g CHO/meal. Use 1–2 carbohydrate choices (15–30 g CHO) for snacks; body size and activity level will determine the number of choices needed.
- Include plenty of fiber from rice, beans, vegetables, barley, oat bran, fruits, and vegetables. Recommendations for fiber intake for people with diabetes are similar to the recommendations for the general public (DRI: 14 g/1000 kcal) and diets containing 44–50 g of fiber daily truly improve glycemia (American Dietetic Association, 2009) Whole grains are good sources of vitamin E, fiber, and magnesium.
- To reduce the risk of nephropathy, protein intake should be limited to the recommended dietary allowance (American Diabetes Association, 2009). If there is microalbuminuria, a more controlled protein intake may be required.
- Cut down or eliminate fried and creamed foods. Include omega-3 fatty acids (as from salmon, mackerel, tuna, walnuts, and canola oil) to control blood lipids and reduce inflammatory processes. A high–monounsaturated fat diet seems to have a favorable effect on lipoproteins in diabetes.
- For minerals, assure adequacy of intake; routine supplementation is not advised. Replenish potassium and magnesium, if needed. Adequate calcium is important: 500 mg in 1–3 year olds, 800 mg in 4–8 year olds, 1300 mg

in 9–18 year olds, and 1000 mg in adults should be attained daily.

- Sodium intake should be limited to 2400 mg daily or less.
- Routine supplementation with antioxidant vitamins E and C and beta-carotene is not advised because of lack of evidence of efficacy (American Diabetes Association, 2009). Folate is important in women of childbearing ages; acquire 400 μg prepregnancy and 600 μg during pregnancy.
- Vitamin D has been found to play an important role in auto-immune disorders. Encourage intake of vitamin-D fortified foods, but also encourage adequate time in the sun.
- If foods containing sucrose are chosen, they should be substituted for other carbohydrate foods. Sucrose intakes of 10–35% of total energy intake do not affect on glycemic or lipid responses negatively when substituted for isocaloric amounts of starch (American Dietetic Association, 2009).
- If adults with diabetes choose to use alcohol, intake should be limited to 1 drink/d or less for adult women and 2 drinks/d or less for adult men. One drink is defined as 12 oz beer, 5 oz wine, or 1.5 oz distilled spirits (American Diabetes Association, 2009). To avoid hypoglycemia, alcohol should be consumed with a carbohydrate-containing food. Abstain in pregnancy, pancreatitis, advanced neuropathy, extremely elevated triglycerides, or a history of alcohol abuse.
- Nonnutritive sweeteners are safe when consumed within the acceptable daily intake levels established by the Food and Drug Administration (FDA) (American Diabetes Association, 2009). The FDA has approved use of several sweeteners; see Table 9-7.
- Adequate carbohydrate replacement during and after exercise is important to prevent hypoglycemia. Decrease rapid-acting insulin doses during the physical activity; 30–50% less is reasonable.
- In critical illness, blood glucose management is a challenge. Enteral feeding is generally preferred but specialty formulas are not usually required. Regular blood glucose monitoring and insulin replacement may be needed.
- If parenteral nutrition is needed, use strict blood glucose control. Hyperglycemia reflects illness severity and results in deleterious consequences. Plan 30% of nutrient intake as fat, 50% as CHO, and 15–20% as protein unless other disease states require alternative plans.

Common Drugs Used and Potential Side Effects

- Anti-CD3 mAbs may prolong beta cell function up to 2 years in patients with new onset Type 1 diabetes (T1DM) but studies are still ongoing (Herold et al, 2009).
- Insulin/diet correlation is essential. Persons with T1DM are usually dependent on insulin for life. The primary potential effect is hypoglycemia. Sources of insulin must be noted because they affect the peak times and duration of effect, and some affect the speed of absorption. Human insulin is produced synthetically from Escherichia coli or yeast with identical amino acid sequence to the human insulin. See Table 9-8 for insulin onset, peak, and duration times.
- Insulin pumps (continuous subcutaneous insulin infusion [CSII]) may be good to maintain glucose levels. If a pump is used, meal schedules are not as strict but should not be abused. With multiple daily insulin injections (MDI), test blood glucose before meals to determine insulin doses. Insulin pens available are convenient for insulin dosing. Insulin glargine (Lantus) is well tolerated in MDI regimens for pediatric patients with T1DM and may be more efficacious than NPH/Lente in those with elevated A1 c (White et al, 2009; Chase et al, 2008).
- Insulin analogs match postprandial blood glucose excursions better than traditional insulin. Bolus analogs are used for more rapid onset to cover meal CHO and to correct hyperglycemia. Basal agents release at a more constant rate to cover between-meal glucose needs or the body's basal insulin needs. Premixed insulins are discouraged except when patients are not able to be compliant with MDI. Adverse effects include the potential for hypoglycemia, especially when HbA1c is less than 7%. Analog insulins are less likely to lead to hypoglycemia, especially overnight hypoglycemia. Weight gain with use of insulin can be counteracted with attention to food intake and physical activity.

Herbs, Botanicals, and Supplements

- Herbs and botanical supplements should not be used without discussing with the physician. There is still insufficient evidence to draw definitive conclusions about the efficacy of beans, peanuts, onion, *Coccinia indica*, aloe vera, *Momordica charantia*, and bitter gourd.
- Adequate Vitamin D should be available, especially for bone health (Svoren et al, 2009).
- See Table 9-9 for guidance on specific herbs and supplements in diabetes. The American Diabetes Association also has a book on herbs and supplements for diabetes care, available from the Web site.

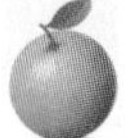

NUTRITION EDUCATION, COUNSELING, CARE MANAGEMENT

- The RD should assess food intake (focusing on carbohydrate), medication, metabolic control (glycemia, lipids, and BP), anthropometric measurements, and physical activity to serve as the basis for implementation of the nutrition prescription, goals, and intervention that are tailored for the individual (American Dietetic Association, 2009).
- Diabetes self-management education (DSME) is an essential element of diabetes care, and national standards have been based on evidence. DSME helps patients optimize metabolic control, prevent and manage complications, and maximize quality of life in a cost-effective manner (American Diabetes Association, 2009). Learning can lead to behavioral changes (healthy eating, being active, taking medications, monitoring glucose, problem-solving) which may then lead to desired clinical and health outcomes. Overall, improved health status includes better quality of life, fewer days lost from school or work, fewer complications and health care costs. Weekly problem-based, self-management support interventions can yield health benefits (Tang et al, 2005), as can even a single session with a dietitian (Gaetke et al, 2006).
- Teach patient about the importance of self-care, optimal functioning, the roles of carbohydrate intake and physical activity in maintaining metabolic control. Blood glucose testing is essential. Insulin injections must be given at planned, regular intervals for persons with T1DM.

TABLE 9-7 Sugar and Sweetener Summary

The percentage of calories from carbohydrate (CHO) in the diet for diabetes will vary; it is individualized based on eating habits and glucose and lipid goals.

Glycemic load (GL)	GL = glycemic index × available CHO amount	Although various starches do have different glycemic responses, first priority should be given to the total amount of CHO consumed rather than the source of the CHO. If the use of glycemic index (GI) is proposed as a method of meal planning, the RD should advise on the conflicting evidence of effectiveness of this strategy. Studies comparing high versus low GI diets report mixed effects on A1C.
Sweets	Sugar equivalents (teapoons)	Soft drink, 12 oz (10 tsp) Chocolate bar, 1.5 oz (5.5 tsp) Froot-loop cereal, 1 cup (3.5 tsp) Sweet pickle, 1 oz (2.25 tsp) Catsup, 1 Tbsp (1 tsp) Barbequed chips, 1 oz. (1/2 tsp) Unsweetened cereal, 1 cup (1/3 tsp)
Nutritive Sweeteners		
Sugar (sucrose)	Sucrose = 16 kcal/tsp (4 g CHO)	Sucrose is saccharose ($C_{12}H_{22}O_{11}$). Sucrose is a disaccharide; that is, it is made up of two monosaccharides—glucose and fructose. It is one of the sweetest of sugars. Sucrose-containing foods should be substituted for other carbohydrate foods. Sucrose intakes of 10–35% of total energy intake do not have a negative effect on glycemic or lipid responses when substituted for isocaloric amounts of starch.
Corn syrup, molasses, dextrose, glucose, and maltose	Corn sugar (called glucose, or dextrose), milk sugar (lactose), and malt sugar (maltose).	If sucrose is taken as a standard of 1, the sweetness of glucose is 0.5–0.6, that of lactose is 0.27, and that of maltose is 0.6 There is no evidence that foods sweetened with these sweeteners have any significant advantage or disadvantage over foods sweetened with sucrose in decreasing total calories or CHO content of the diet or in improving overall diabetes control.
Fructose and honey	Fructose: 11 kcal/tsp (3 g CHO); fruit sugar; 1.1–2 times as sweet as sucrose.	Fructose, found in fruits and honey, is the sweetest. Although dietary fructose produces a smaller rise in plasma glucose than equal amounts of sucrose and most starches, it is not to replace more than 20% of calories in adults because of its potential adverse effects on lipids, especially triglycerides. There is no reason to recommend that people with diabetes avoid consumption of fruits and vegetables, in which fructose occurs naturally. In children, fructose works well as a substitute in baked goods because their lipids are not yet a problem and fructose has little impact on blood glucose levels.
Sugar alcohols	Sugar alcohols: 2 kcal/g (50% of kilocalories of other nutritive sweeteners such as sucrose) Sorbitol: 50% as sweet as sucrose Xylitol: 16 kcal/tsp (4 g CHO)	Sugar alcohols produce a lower postprandial glucose response than sucrose or glucose and have lower available energy. With foods containing sugar alcohols, subtraction of one half of sugar alcohol grams from total CHO grams is appropriate, particularly when using the CHO counting method for meal planning. There is no evidence that the amounts of sugar alcohol likely to be consumed will result in significant reduction in energy intake or long-term improvement in glycemia. The use of sugar alcohols appears to be safe. Excessive amounts of polyols may have a laxative effect. The calories and CHO content from all nutritive sweeteners must be accounted for in the meal plan and have the potential to affect blood glucose levels.

(continued)

TABLE 9-7 Sugar and Sweetener Summary *(continued)*

Non-Nutritive Sweeteners		
Acesulfame potassium (Sunette®) **Alitame** **Aspartame (Equal®, NutraSweet®)** **Neotame** **Saccharin (Sweet 'N Low®)** **Sucralose (Splenda®)**	Acesulfame: 200 times sweeter than sugar; heat stable Alitame is made from amino acids, 2000 times sweeter than sugar. Still awaiting FDA approval. Aspartame: 180 times sweeter than sugar; 4 kcal/tsp; contains phenylalanine and cannot be used in PKU. Equally contains aspartame, dextrose, and maltodextrin. Neotame: 6000 times sweeter than sugar; heat stable Saccharin: 300–400 times sweeter than sugar; heat stable; leaves a slightly bitter aftertaste Sucralose: 600 times sweeter than sugar; heat stable	The Food and Drug Administration has approved five non-nutritive sweeteners for use in the United States. All have undergone rigorous scrutiny and have been shown to be safe when consumed by the public, including people with diabetes and women who are pregnant. If persons with diabetes choose to consume products containing U.S. Food and Drug Administration (FDA)-approved non-nutritive sweeteners, at levels that do not exceed the acceptable daily intakes (ADIs), the RD should advise that some of these products may contain energy and carbohydrate from other sources that needs to be accounted for. Research on non-nutritive sweeteners reports no effect on changes in glycemic response.

For more information: International Food Information Council, Web site accessed September 22, 2009, at http://www.ific.org/publications/factsheets/lcsfs.cfm; American Diabetes Association, 2009; National Diabetes Evidence-based guidelines, Web site accessed September 20, 2009, at http://guidelines.gov/summary/summary.aspx?doc_id=12816&nbr=006618

- Identify potential or real obstacles; discuss options for resisting temptations, dining away from home, feeling deprived, time pressures, food offers from others, competing priorities, handling social events, family or social support, and food intolerances.
- Encourage regular mealtimes and snacks. Children and teens in particular may need planned snacks.
- A nondiet approach to diabetes management encourages regular eating according to actual hunger and making gradual changes for healthier eating.
- Discuss visual assessment of portions. Practice with measuring cups, spoons, and scales.
- Teach patient how to read labels and how to identify carbohydrates in processed foods.
- Empowerment is important; help patients to gain mastery over their affairs and to effect change (Funnell et al, 2005). Discuss emotional eating, such as from boredom, anger, frustration, loneliness, and depression; alternative choices should be designed from the client perspective. Research reports sustained improvements in A1 c at 12 months and longer with long-term follow-up encounters with an RD (American Dietetic Association, 2009).
- Discuss the weight gain that occurs with intensive insulin therapy and improved glucose control.
- Low-carbohydrate diets are not recommended for the management of diabetes (American Diabetes Association, 2009).

TABLE 9-8 Insulin Onset, Peaks, and Duration[a]

Insulin Type	Begins Working	Peaks at	Ends Working in	Low Occurs at
Rapid, Bolus				
Humalog (Lispro)	15–20 minutes	30–90 minutes	3–4 hours	2–4 hours
Novolog (Aspart)	15–20 minutes	40–50 minutes	3–4 hours	2–4 hours
Short-Acting				
Regular (Novolin R, Humulin R)	30–60 minutes	80–120 minutes	4–6 hours	3–7 hours
Intermediate-Acting				
NPH	2–4 hours	6–10 hours	14–16 hours	6–12 hours
Lente	3–4 hours	6–12 hours	16–18 hours	7–14 hours
Ultralente	4–6 hours	10–16 hours	18–20 hours	12–24 hours
Long-Acting				
Lantus (Glargine)	2–3 hours	Almost no peak; flat action throughout duration	18–26 hours	4–24 hours

[a]Insulin can be used after 1 month if stored at cooler than 86°C and out of direct sunlight or heat. Unopened bottles of insulin should be stored in a refrigerator; do not freeze insulin. Syringes may be prefilled and stored in a refrigerator for up to 3 weeks. Roll the syringes before use to mix the insulin.

Adapted from: North Coast Medical Center, accessed September 22, 2009, at http://www.northcoastmed.com/insulin.htm; and Medscape, accessed September 22, 2009, at http://img.medscape.com/pi/emed/ckb/endocrinology/116364-138562-117853-118003.jpg

TABLE 9-9 Herbs and Supplements in Diabetes Management

Aloe vera	Studies in Japan found that the phytosterols in aloe vera might play a role in lowering blood glucose levels. Further research is needed.
Alpha lipoic acid (thitoic acid)	Alpha lipoic acid (thioctic acid) may have some potential benefits. It is found in the mitochondria and seems to have antioxidant properties that protect vitamin C, vitamin E, and glutathione. Natural sources include red meat, yeast, potatoes, and spinach. Supplementation may provide protection against cataracts, neuropathy in diabetes, cardiovascular disease; research is needed.
Antioxidants	Antioxidants from food should include good sources of beta carotene, vitamins C and E, selenium and zinc.
Bilberry	Bilberry contains anthocyanosides that counteract cellular damage to the retina. Mild drowsiness and skin rashes have been noted.
Biotin	Biotin shows preliminary evidence of being useful for controlling blood glucose.
Bitter melon (*Momordica charantia*)	Bitter melon has traditionally been used as a remedy for lowering blood glucose.
Chromium	Chromium enhances use of insulin. Skin allergies, renal toxicity, and altered iron and zinc absorption can occur. There are no proven benefits if a patient is not deficient (American Diabetes Association, 2009).
Cinnamon	Doses of 1, 3, or 6 g capsules of cinnamon daily lowered blood glucose levels in individuals with diabetes.
Essential oils	Essential oils from cinnamon, cumin, and oregano may enhance insulin sensitivity. Studies are ongoing.
Evening primrose oil	Evening primrose oil may prevent or limit neuropathy due to gamma linoleic acid, an essential fatty acid. It may cause headache and gastrointestinal distress.
Fenugreek	Fenugreek may lower glucose, triglyceride and cholesterol levels due to its psyllium content. Note that it is part of the peanut family and may cause allergic reactions. Do not take with monoamine oxidase (MAO) inhibitors; it has the potential for drug interactions with other medications as well.
Gamma linolenic acid	Evening primrose oil may be useful for preventing neuropathy in diabetes.
Garlic	Garlic may lower blood glucose levels if used in large amounts; more studies are needed.
Gingko biloba	Gingko biloba may help control neuropathy by maintaining integrity of blood vessels and reducing stickiness of blood and clotting. It has some antioxidant properties. Avoid taking with warfarin, aspirin, and other anticoagulant drugs. Headache and interactions with other drugs can occur.
Ginseng, American	Ginseng (American) may lower blood glucose levels. Avoid with warfarin, aspirin, MAO inhibitors, caffeine, antipsychotics, insulin, and oral hypoglycemics because of fluctuations in blood glucose levels, bleeding, platelet functioning, blood pressure and heart rate. Avoid taking with steroids. Headache, insomnia, nausea, or menstrual difficulties can occur. Take with a meal.
Guar gum	Guar gum is a fiber that normalizes the moisture content of the stool, absorbs excess liquid in diarrhea, softens the stool in constipation, and decreases the amount of cholesterol and glucose absorbed from the stomach and intestines.
Gymnema sylvestre	*Gymnema sylvestre* is a hypoglycemic herb. It is highly potent and should be used only under doctor's supervision because it may change insulin requirements.
Magnesium	Magnesium is needed for hundreds of biochemical reactions; it helps regulate blood sugar levels and blood pressure. Some studies suggest that low magnesium levels may worsen blood glucose control in type 2 diabetes. Magnesium supplementation may help with insulin resistance, but avoid high doses.
Turmeric	Turmeric, the rhizome of *Curcuma*, may decrease blood glucose levels.
Vanadum	Vanadium may lower glucose levels. It has been associated with cancer cell growth and can be toxic at therapeutic levels.
Vitamin B_6	Some studies suggest that an adequate intake of vitamin B_6 (pyrodoxine) can helo with both T1DM and T2DM,
Vitamin D	Supplementation of up to 2000 IU daily in infants were less likely to develop type 1 diabetes over the next 30 years in Finland. This vitamin has a strong, protective effect. Experts are now recommending supplementation at the upper end of the current recommendations (i.e., 1000 IU).
Zinc	Zinc is part of the production and storage of insulin in the body. Fresh oysters, ginger root, lamb, pecans, split peas, egg yolk, rye, beef liver, lima beans, almonds, walnuts, sardines, chicken, and buckwheat are sources from the diet. Zinc should not be used with immunosuppressants, tetracycline, ciprofloxacin, or levofloxacin because of potential antagonist effects.

- Discuss the risks for CVD and how to manage them (American Diabetes Association, 2009; American Dietetic Association, 2009).
- Eating disorders often occur in young women with diabetes; refer for psychotherapy if needed.
- A1 c is often unacceptably high in adolescents; there is a need to more fully assess and understand factors such as race/ethnicity, education, and socioeconomic status on treatment recommendations (Paris et al, 2009).
- For sick days: Patients may require more insulin when ill. Liquid diets should provide 200 g CHO in equally divided amounts at mealtime and snacks; liquids should not be sugar free.
- For surgery: Blood glucose should be in good control; perioperative hyperglycemia can be managed with doses of short-acting insulin. Correct abnormalities before surgery when possible.
- Discuss reasonable use of the glycemic index (see Table 9-10).

TABLE 9-10 Glycemic Index and Glycemic Load

Glycemic index (GI) is a measure of serum glucose response to a food relative to a reference food that contains equal amounts of carbohydrate. It does not refer directly to quantified food exchanges. Glycemic load = GI × available carbohydrate amount.

A mixed diet yields varying results on blood glucose levels. Choosing low-GI foods in place of conventional or high-GI foods has a small, clinically useful effect on medium-term glycemic control in patients with diabetes (Brand-Miller et al, 2003).

Carbohydrate Choices

Choose low-GI carbohydrates most often because they digest slower and will be less likely to elevate blood glucose. Each choice = 15 g of carbohydrate. Choose desired number of carbohydrate choices per meal or as needed by the individual. Children and teens, as well as young adults and athletes, will need much more per meal than sedentary adults.

Glycemic Index	Grain or Bean Choices	Fruit Choices	Vegetable Choices
Low (best choice)	Barley, 1/3 cup Beans (kidney, pinto, etc.), 1/2 cup cooked Lima beans, 2/3 cup Muesli, 1/4 cup Oat bran, 1/3 cup	Apple, orange, or pear Cherries, 12 Grapes, 17 Grapefruit, 1/2 Cantaloupe or berries (blueberries, raspberries, strawberries, etc.) = 1 cup	Corn, 1/2 cup Squash, acorn, 1 cup cooked Peas, green or lentils, 1/2 cup cooked 1½ cups cooked or 3 cups raw vegetables (asparagus, beets, broccoli, carrots, cucumbers, mushrooms, onions, peppers, tomatoes, zucchini, and others)
Medium (choose less often)	Baked beans, 1/4 cup Bran flakes, 1/2 cup Bread, 100% whole wheat, 1 slice English muffin, whole wheat, 1/2 Granola, low sugar, 1/4 cup Hamburger or hot dog bun, 1/2 Oatmeal, old fashioned, 1/2 cup Pasta, 1/3 cup cooked Raisin bran, 1/3 cup Rice, converted or wild, 1/3 cup cooked Special K, 3/4 cup Tortilla, 6″	Banana, 1 small Canned fruit, drained, 1/2 cup Dried fruit, 1/4 cup Watermelon, 1¼ cups Raisins, 2 tbsp Orange juice, 1/2 cup Apple juice, 1/2 cup Grape juice, 1/3 cup	Potato, small, "new," 1/2 cup Sweet potato, 1/2 cup cooked
High (choose rarely)	Bagel, large, 1/4 bagel Bread, white, 1 slice Cream of wheat, 1/2 cup cooked Cheerios, 3/4 cup Corn flakes, 3/4 cup Instant oatmeal, 1/2 cup cooked Pancake, 4″ Rice Krispies, 3/4 cup Rice, white, 1/3 cup cooked Shredded wheat, 1/3 cup Waffle, 4″		Potato, small russet, 3″ diameter Potato, mashed, 1/2 cup

(continued)

TABLE 9-10 Glycemic Index and Glycemic Load *(continued)*

Glycemic Index	Combination Foods	Sweets/Snacks	Milk/Yogurt/Milk Substitutes
Low	Soup, cream, low fat, 1 cup Chili, low fat, 1/2 cup	Ice cream, low fat, 1/2 cup Pudding, sugar free, 1/2 cup Chocolate candy, 15 kisses or 1-oz bar	Milk, skim or low fat (1%), 1 cup Yogurt, low fat, artificially sweetened, 1 cup
Medium	Burrito, bean, flour tortilla, 7″ long = 3 carb choices Pasta dish, 1/2 cup	Popcorn, microwave light, popped, 3 cups Cookie, 3″ across, 1 Muffin, small, 1/2	Soy milk, low fat or nonfat, 1 cup Yogurt, low fat, sweetened, with fruit, 1/3 cup
High	Pizza, thin crust, medium, 1 slice (= 2 carb choices) Pizza, thick crust, medium, 1 slice (= 3 carb choices)	Pretzel twists, mini, 15 pieces Brownie or cake, no frosting, 2″ square Doughnut, 3″, 1/2 doughnut Granola bar, 1 Potato or tortilla chips, 15 chips Syrup, 1 tbsp	

Source: Brand-Miller et al, 2003.

- Aim for 30 min/d of physical activity to burn a minimum of 1500 kcal/wk (see Table 9-11).

Patient Education—Foodborne Illness

- If home tube feeding is needed, teach appropriate sanitation and food-handling procedures.

For More Information

- American Dietetic Association: Type 1 Diabetes Evidence-Based Guidelines for Practice
  http://www.eatright.org/cps/rde/xchg/ada/hs.xsl/home_21231_ENU_HTML.htm
- American Diabetes Association–T1DM
  http://www.diabetes.org/type-1-diabetes.jsp
- Juvenile Diabetes Research Foundation
  http://www.jdrf.org/index.cfm?page_id=101982
- Mayo Clinic – T1DM
  http://www.mayoclinic.com/health/type-1-diabetes/DS00329

TABLE 9-11 American Diabetes Association General Guidelines for Regulating Exercise

Metabolic control before exercise	Avoid exercise if ketosis is present. Use caution if glucose levels are >300 mg/dL without ketosis. Ingest added carbohydrate if glucose levels are <100 mg/dL.
Blood glucose monitoring before and after exercise	Identify when changes in insulin or carbohydrate are necessary. Learn the glycemic response to different exercise conditions.
Food intake	Consume added carbohydrate, as needed, to avoid hypoglycemia. Carbohydrate-based foods should be readily available during and after exercise.

- Medline Plus
  http://www.nlm.nih.gov/medlineplus/ency/article/000305.htm

TYPE 1 DIABETES MELLITUS—CITED REFERENCES

American Diabetes Association. Diabetes: heart disease and stroke. Accessed September 22, 2009, at http://www.diabetes.org/diabetes-heart-disease-stroke.jsp

American Diabetes Association. Standards of Medical Care in Diabetes–2009. Web site accessed September 22, 2009, at http://care.diabetesjournals.org/content/32/Supplement_1/S13.full

American Dietetic Association. Evidence analysis library: Type 1 and Type 2 Diabetes. Web site accessed September 22, 2009, at https://www.adaevidencelibrary.com/topic.cfm?cat=3481

Chase HP, et al. Insulin glargine versus intermediate-acting insulin as the basal component of multiple daily injection regimens for adolescents with type 1 diabetes mellitus. *J Pediatr.* 153:547, 2008.

Chima CS, et al. Use of technology to track program outcomes in a diabetes self-management program. *J Am Diet Assoc.* 105:1933, 2005.

DCCT Research Group. Modern-day clinical course of type 1 diabetes mellitus after 30 years' duration: the diabetes control and complications trial/epidemiology of diabetes interventions and complications and Pittsburgh epidemiology of diabetes complications experience (1983–2005). *Arch Int Med.* 169:1307, 2009.

Funnell MM, et al. Implementing an empowerment-based diabetes self-management education program. *Diabetes Educ.* 31:53, 2005.

Gaetke LM, et al. A single nutrition counseling session with a registered dietitian improves short-term clinical outcomes for rural Kentucky patients with chronic disease. *J Am Diet Assoc.* 06:109, 2006.

Herold KC, et al. Treatment of patients with new onset Type 1 diabetes with a single course of anti-CD3 mAb Teplizumab preserves insulin production for up to 5 years. *Clin Immunol.* 132:166, 2009.

Kulkarni K. Diets do not fail: the success of medical nutrition therapy in patients with diabetes. *Endocr Pract.* 12:121S, 2006.

Paris CA, et al. Predictors of insulin regimens and impact on outcomes in youth with type 1 diabetes: the SEARCH for Diabetes in Youth study. *J Pediatr.* 155:183, 2009.

Svoren B, et al. Significant Vitamin D Deficiency in Youth with Type 1 Diabetes Mellitus. *J Pediatr.* 154:132, 2009.

Tang TS, et al. Developing a new generation of ongoing diabetes self-management support interventions: a preliminary report. *Diabetes Educ.* 31:91, 2005.

Williams KT, Schalinske KL. New insights into the regulation of methyl group and homocysteine metabolism. *J Nutr.* 137:311–314, 2007.

White NH, et al. Comparison of glycemic variability associated with insulin glargine and intermediate-acting insulin when used as the basal component of multiple daily injections for adolescents with type 1 diabetes. *Diabetes Care.* 32:387, 2009.

ISLET CELL TRANSPLANTATION

NUTRITIONAL ACUITY RANKING: LEVEL 4

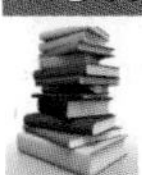

DEFINITIONS AND BACKGROUND

Some native pancreatic beta cell function persists even years after disease onset in most type 1 diabetic patients (Liu et al, 2009). However, the destruction of beta cells leads to permanent insulin dependence. Islet cell transplantation can lead to insulin independence with excellent metabolic control. Islet transplantation can require more than one donor pancreas to achieve insulin independence (Rickels et al, 2005). Transplants may be performed by a radiologist, who uses x rays and ultrasound to guide placement of a catheter through the upper abdomen and into the portal vein, where islets are slowly infused. If this is not feasible, a surgeon may perform the procedure under anesthesia.

The acute posttransplantation phase lasts up to 2 months; the chronic phase starts after 2 months. Drugs are needed to prevent rejection. Islet cell programs try to avoid using large doses of glucocorticoids. Most protocols are designed to use tacrolimus and sirolimus so that high-dose glucocorticoids would not have to be used.

During the acute period of care, there is the issue that patients are variably managed with insulin therapy to allow for recovery of the islets after they have been placed into their new and not totally adequate environment in the liver. Most centers treat patients for up to a month, and treating hypoglycemia during this time is a concern.

Long-term complications may include hyperlipidemia. In T1DM, the release of many hormones, not only from beta-cells, but also from adipocytes (adipokines) is altered (Stadler et al, 2009). After successful pancreas–kidney transplantation (PKTx), T1DM patients can revert to a nondiabetic metabolism, but altered adipokines are still present after PKTx; adipokines include visfatin, retinol-binding protein-4 (RBP-4), adiponectin, and high-molecular-weight (HMW) adiponectin (Stadler et al, 2009). More research in this area is needed.

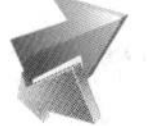

ASSESSMENT, MONITORING, AND EVALUATION

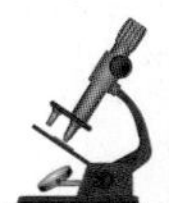

CLINICAL INDICATORS

Genetic Markers: Transplantation may occur for T1DM, where there is a genetic component.

Clinical/History

Height
Dry weight, present weight
BMI
Diet history
I & O
BP
Temperature

Lab Work

Albumin (Alb), transthyretin
HbA1c
Nitrogen (N) balance
Glomerular filtration rate (GFR)
Alkaline phosphatase (Alk phos)
Aspartate aminotransferase (AST)
Alanine aminotransferase (ALT)
Bilirubin
Na^+, K^+
Hemoglobin and hematocrit (H & H)
Serum Fe
Serum folacin
BUN, Creat
Ca^{++}, Mg^{++}
White blood cell (WBC) count
Total lymphocyte (TLC) count
Glucose (Gluc)
Chol, Trig
CRP

INTERVENTION

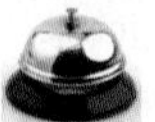

OBJECTIVES

- Meet the specific needs of the patient; modify drug therapy to enhance outcomes and quality of life.
- Prevent infection and promote healing.
- Monitor for abnormal electrolyte levels.
- Monitor CHO intolerance but make sure that diet provides enough CHO to spare proteins. Treatment goals should reflect those of the American Diabetes Association; adjust as new evidence suggests.
- Alleviate rejection episodes.
- Control infections, especially during the acute phase. Support protein intake to prevent additional infections.
- Force fluids unless contraindicated, as in retention. Match fluid output.
- Help patient adjust to a lifelong medical regimen during chronic phase. Improve survival rate by supporting immune response.
- Correct or manage complications that occur.
- Control weight gain in the first year after transplantation.

SAMPLE NUTRITION CARE PROCESS STEPS

Poor Nutrition Quality of Life

Assessment Data: Weight, labs, nutritional history prior to transplantation, statement of "not liking to eat any more because of the pain."

Nutrition Diagnosis (PES): Poor nutritional quality of life related to abdominal pain after meals as evidenced by weight changes, vacillating lab results and statements about not enjoying meals.

Intervention: Food and Nutrient Delivery—gradual weaning from nutritional support back to oral diet, using small portions of favorite foods. Education—how the transplant would eventually allow life without insulin shots and more normal meal experiences.

Monitoring and Evaluation: Tolerance after weaning from nutrition support to oral diet. Acceptance of several favorite foods, and trying new foods with assistance of family members.

TABLE 9-12 **Medications Used after Islet Cell Transplantation**

Medication	Description
Cyclosporine	Cyclosporine does not cause retention of sodium as much as corticosteroids do. Intravenous doses are more effective than oral doses. Nausea, vomiting, and diarrhea are common side effects. Hyperlipidemia, hyperglycemia, and hyperkalemia may also occur; decrease fat intake as well as sodium and potassium if necessary. Magnesium may need to be replaced. The drug is also nephrotoxic; a controlled renal diet may be beneficial. Take omega-3 fatty acids to reduce toxic side effects such as high blood pressure and kidney damage. Avoid St. John's wort.
Diuretics	Diuretics such as furosemide (Lasix) may cause hypokalemia. Aldactone actually spares potassium; monitor drug changes closely. In general, avoid use with fenugreek, yohimbe, and ginkgo.
Immunosuppressants	Immunosuppressants such as muromonab (Orthoclone OKT3) and antithymocyte globulin (ATG) are less nephrotoxic than cyclosporine but can cause nausea, anorexia, diarrhea, and vomiting. Monitor carefully. Fever and stomatitis also may occur; alter diet as needed.
Insulin	Insulin may be necessary during periods of hyperglycemia. Monitor for hypoglycemic symptoms during use; teach patient self-management tips.
Pancreatic enzymes	Pancreatic enzymes may be needed if pancreatitis occurs after transplantation.
Tacrolimus (Prograf, FK506)	Tacrolimus suppresses T-cell immunity; it is 100 times more potent than cyclosporine, thus requiring smaller doses. Side effects include gastrointestinal distress, nausea, vomiting, hyperkalemia, and hyperglycemia; adjust diet accordingly by controlling carbohydrate and enhancing potassium intake.
Tetranectin	Tetranectin binds plasminogen and may have a role in regulating pericellular proteolysis and in the survival of islets in the liver after islet transplantation.

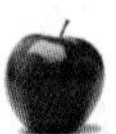

FOOD AND NUTRITION

- Progress solids as quickly as possibly postoperatively. Monitor fluid status, and adjust as needed.
- Daily intake of protein should be appropriate for age and sex; 1.5 g/kg while on steroids may be recommended. Energy needs should be calculated as 30–35 kcal/kg.
- Daily intake of sodium should be 2–4 g until the drug regimen is reduced. Adjust potassium levels as needed.
- Daily intake of calcium should be 1–1.5 times the daily requirements to offset poor absorption. Children especially need adequate calcium for growth. Daily intake of phosphorus should be equal to calcium intake.
- Supplement diet with vitamin D, magnesium, and thiamin as needed. Adequate vitamin intake will be essential to maintain immunity and to support wound healing.
- Control CHO intake with hyperglycemia (45–50% total kcal); encourage healthy food sources of carbohydrate. Transplantation patients are at risk of further glucose intolerance from multiple medications.
- Plan fats at 25–35% of total kilocalories (encourage monounsaturated fats and omega-3 fatty acids). Low saturated fats and cholesterol may be needed. A controlled fat intake is recommended for prevention and treatment of hyperlipidemia.
- Reduce gastric irritants as necessary if GI distress or reflux occurs.
- Monitor electrolytes carefully; hyperkalemia is common with cyclosporine or tacrolimus.
- Special diets may be discontinued when drug therapy is reduced to maintenance levels. Encourage exercise and a weight control plan thereafter.

Common Drugs Used and Potential Side Effects

- Thymoglobulin is an antibody preparation to prevent organ transplant rejection. The START trial is underway to determine whether Thymoglobulin treatment can halt the progression of newly diagnosed type 1 diabetes when given within 6 weeks of disease diagnosis.
- See Table 9-12 for other drugs used for the transplant.

Herbs, Botanicals, and Supplements

- Herbals should be discouraged after transplantation. Those who self-medicate with herbals are taking a chance that their use of a herb may interact with their immunosuppressive drugs and either cause higher or lower than desired drug levels of these agents.
- Chaparral is an herbal product that may cause severe hepatitis or liver failure. St. John's wort interferes with the metabolism of immunosuppressants and should not be used after transplantation.
- See Table 9-9 for guidance on more specific herbs and supplements.

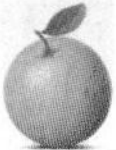

NUTRITION EDUCATION, COUNSELING, CARE MANAGEMENT

- Indicate which foods are sources of key nutrients such as protein in the diet. If patient does not like milk, discuss how other sources of calcium may be used in the diet.
- Alcohol should be avoided unless permitted by the doctor.
- Patients should know when to seek medical attention.
- Discuss problems with long-term obesity and hypercholesterolemia.
- Encourage moderation in diet; promote adequate exercise.

Patient Education—Foodborne Illness

- If home tube feeding is needed, teach appropriate sanitation and food-handling procedures.

For More Information

- American Diabetes Association–Islet Cell Transplantation http://www.diabetes.org/type-1-diabetes/islet-transplants.jsp
- Immune Tolerance Network (ITN) http://www.immunetolerance.org
- Insulin-Free http://www.insulin-free.org/
- NIDDK–Islet Cell Transplantation http://diabetes.niddk.nih.gov/dm/pubs/pancreaticislet/

PANCREAS OR ISLET CELL TRANSPLANTATION—CITED REFERENCES

Hermann M, et al. In the search of potential human islet stem cells: is tetranectin showing us the way? *Transplant Proc.* 37:1322, 2005.

Liu EH, et al. Pancreatic beta cell function persists in many patients with chronic type 1 diabetes, but is not dramatically improved by prolonged immunosuppression and euglycaemia from a beta cell allograft. *Diabetologia.* 52:1369, 2009.

Rickels MR, et al. Beta-cell function following human islet transplantation for type 1 diabetes. *Diabetes.* 54:100, 2005.

Stadler M, et al. Adipokines in type-1 diabetes after successful pancreas transplantation: Normal visfatin and retinol-binding-protein-4, but increased total adiponectin fasting concentrations. [published online ahead of print September 21, 2009] *Clin Endocrinol (Oxf).* 72:763, 2010.

METABOLIC SYNDROME

NUTRITIONAL ACUITY RANKING: LEVEL 3–4

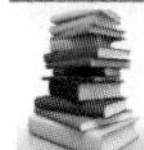

DEFINITIONS AND BACKGROUND

The metabolic syndrome (MetS; insulin resistance syndrome or syndrome X) has simultaneous clustering of low levels of HDL cholesterol, hyperglycemia, high waist circumference, hypertension, and elevated triglycerides. Any three of the following five criteria constitute diagnosis of MetS (Grundy et al, 2005):

- Elevated waist circumference: 40″ or 102 cm in men; 35″ or 88 cm in women.
- Elevated triglycerides (TG) ≥150 mg/dL or drug treatment for elevated TG.
- Reduced HDL cholesterol: <40 mg/dL in men and 50 mg/dL in women or drug treatment for low HDL cholesterol levels.
- Elevated BP: >130 mm Hg systolic BP or 85 mm Hg diastolic BP or drug treatment for hypertension.
- Elevated fasting glucose: >100 mg/dL or drug treatment for elevated glucose.

It is associated with CVD and often leads to T2DM. This condition affects some young people but usually affects persons aged 55 years and older. More than 64 million Americans have MetS, roughly one in four adults and 40% of adults aged 40 years and older.

Increased birthweight, excessive energy intake, physical inactivity, obesity, smoking, inflammation, and hypertension contribute to MetS. Individuals who are obese and insulin resistant are particularly prone to this syndrome. An "apple" shaped figure (high waist circumference) is riskier because fat cells located in the abdomen release fat into the blood more easily than fat cells found elsewhere.

Serum adiponectin levels are associated with insulin sensitivity; they are decreased in T2D and obesity. Genetic and environmental factors contribute to risk (Gable et al, 2006). The initial insult in adipose inflammation and insulin resistance is perpetuated through chemokine secretion, adipose retention of macrophages, and elaboration of pro-inflammatory adipocytokines (Shah et al, 2008). In women, depressive symptoms are associated with MetS, especially with elevated afternoon and evening cortisol (Muhtz et al, 2009). Clearly, more research is needed.

Management of MetS should focus on lifestyle modifications, especially reduced caloric intake and increased physical activity (Deedwania and Volkova, 2005). Phytochemicals, MUFA, antioxidant foods, spices such as turmeric, cumin, and cinnamon have anti-inflammatory effects. Intake of whole milk, yogurt, calcium, and magnesium protect against MetS whereas intake of cheese, low-fat milk, and phosphorus do not (Beydoun et al, 2008; McKeown et al, 2009). Mild-to-moderate alcohol consumption is acceptable but binges and early onset of drinking are not acceptable.

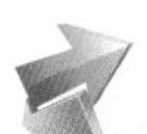

ASSESSMENT, MONITORING, AND EVALUATION

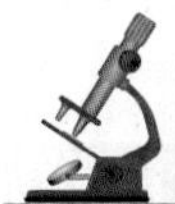

CLINICAL INDICATORS

Genetic Markers: Candidate genes associated with CVD represent potential risk factors for the MetS (Goulart et al, 2009). Chronic inflammation and IL1beta genetic variants may be a concern; genetic influences are more evident among subjects with low (n-3) PUFA intake (Shen et al, 2007).

Clinical/History		
Height	BMI	Waist circumference (35″ or 88 cm in women)
Weight	Diet history	BP (≥130/85 mm Hg)
Weight pattern history	Waist circumference (40″ or 102 cm in men)	
Central Obesity?		

Sleep apnea?	LDL Chol (high?)	High fibrinogen or plasminogen activator inhibitor [−1] in the blood?
Depression?	Trig (>150 mg/dL)	
Lab Work	Mg^{++}	
Gluc (>100 mg/dL)	Na^{+}, K^{+}	
HbA1 c	Serum insulin	Prothrombin time (PT)
HDL Chol (<40 mg/dL for men, <50 mg/dL for women)	Serum uric acid (elevated?)	International normalized ratio (INR)
	CRP (elevated)	

INTERVENTION

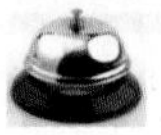

OBJECTIVES

- Reduce the inflammatory state and insulin resistance caused by excessive adipose tissue. Improve body weight; lessen abdominal obesity in particular. A realistic goal for weight reduction should be 7–10% over 6–12 months (Bestermann et al, 2005).
- Promote physical activity. Recommendations should include practical, regular, and moderated regimens of exercise, with a daily minimum of 30–60 minutes and equal balance between aerobic and strength training (Bestermann et al, 2005).
- Achieve and maintain cholesterol, blood glucose, and BP at levels indicated by the American Heart Association, as follows (Grundy et al, 2005):

For Atherogenic Dyslipidemia

- For elevated LDL cholesterol: Give priority to reduction of LDL cholesterol over other lipid parameters. Achieve LDL cholesterol goals based on patient's risk category. LDL cholesterol goals for different risk categories are:
  - High risk: seek 70–100 mg/dL
  - Moderately high risk: seek 100–130 mg/dL
  - Moderate risk: seek 130 mg/dL
  - Lower risk: 160 mg/dL is acceptable

SAMPLE NUTRITION CARE PROCESS STEPS

Inappropriate Intake of Types of CHO—Metabolic Syndrome

Assessment Data: Food intake records: high refined CHO and soft drink intake; high juice but minimal fruit intake; low dietary fiber intake.

Nutrition Diagnosis (PES): Inappropriate intake of types of CHO related to knowledge deficit about MetS as evidenced by FBS of 140 mg/dL and triglycerides of 300 mg/dL.

Intervention: Education about desirable CHO, whole grains, and fiber; shopping tips; dining out.

Monitoring and Evaluation: Improved labs in 3–6 months; dietary records showing improvement in intake of whole grains, whole fruits, and vegetables.

- If TG is >200 mg/dL, then goal for non-HDL cholesterol for each risk category is 30 mg/dL higher than for LDL cholesterol. If TG is >200 mg/dL after achieving LDL cholesterol goal, consider additional therapies to attain non-HDL cholesterol goal.
- If HDL cholesterol is <40 mg/dL in men or <50 mg/dL in women, raise HDL cholesterol to extent possible with standard therapies for atherogenic dyslipidemia. Either lifestyle therapy can be intensified or drug therapy can be used for raising HDL cholesterol levels, depending on patient's risk category.

For Elevated BP

- Reduce BP to at least achieve BP of >140/90 mm Hg (or <130/80 mm Hg if diabetes is present). Reduce BP further to extent possible through lifestyle changes.
- For BP >120/80 mm Hg: Initiate or maintain lifestyle modification via weight control, increased physical activity, alcohol moderation, sodium reduction, and emphasis on increased consumption of fresh fruits, vegetables, and low-fat dairy products in all patients with MetS.
- For BP >140/90 mm Hg (or >130/80 mm Hg if diabetes is present), add BP medication as needed to achieve goal BP.

For Elevated Glucose

- For IFG, delay progression to T2DM. Encourage weight reduction and increased physical activity.
- In diabetes, for hemoglobin A1 c at or above 7.0%, lifestyle therapy and pharmacotherapy, if necessary, should be used. Modify other risk factors and behaviors (e.g., abdominal obesity, physical inactivity, elevated BP, or lipid abnormalities).

For Prothrombotic State

- Reduce thrombotic and fibrinolytic risk factors. Low-dose aspirin therapy or prophylaxis is recommended.

For Proinflammatory State

- There are no specific therapies beyond lifestyle changes. The antioxidants and omega-3 fatty acids may be helpful.

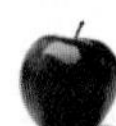

FOOD AND NUTRITION

- The general recommendations include low intake of saturated fats, trans fats, and cholesterol. Increase use of omega-3 PUFA intake (Shen et al, 2007) and MUFA (especially extra virgin olive oil).
- Plan a Mediterranean-type diet using more fiber and starches, especially whole grains, raw fruits, and vegetables. A plant-based diet may be useful (Barnard et al, 2005).
- The DASH diet contains 3–4 g sodium with good sources of potassium, calcium, and magnesium. Dairy products provide calcium, magnesium, and potassium.
- Monitor blood glucose levels. Carbohydrate restriction (CR) has been shown to improve dyslipidemias associated with MetS more than a low fat diet (Al-Sarraj et al, 2010).

- Encourage soy protein as a meat substitute several times a week; soy protein may help with weight reduction and dyslipidemia (Bestermann et al, 2005).
- Ensure adequate intake of folate, vitamins B_6, B_{12}, C, and E, preferably from food.
- Dark chocolate in small amounts regularly may help lower BP, improve cholesterol, and help with insulin sensitivity.
- Spread out the energy load by eating smaller meals.

Common Drugs Used and Potential Side Effects

- To lower lipids, a statin should be used initially unless contraindicated (Bestermann et al, 2005). Statins decrease biomarkers of inflammation and oxidative stress in a dose-related manner; atorvastatin 80 mg compared with a 10-mg dose is superior for decreasing oxidized LDL, hs-CRP, matrix metalloproteinase-9, and NF-kB activity (Singh et al, 2008).
- Glucose-lowering medications must be carefully prescribed and monitored. Metformin may be indicated (Orchard et al, 2005).
- BP medications may be prescribed; monitor for necessary restrictions of sodium and/or higher need for potassium. An ACE inhibitor or an angiotensin receptor blocker is usually the first medicine (Bestermann et al, 2005).
- Medications that diminish insulin resistance and directly alter lipoproteins are necessary; combination therapy is often required (Bestermann et al, 2005).
- If patients with MetS have elevated fibrinogen and other coagulation factors leading to prothrombotic state, aspirin is used (Deedwania and Volkova, 2005). Low-dose aspirin is not generally a problem; taken with a meal or light snack to prevent potential for GI bleeding.

Herbs, Botanicals, and Supplements

- Antioxidant supplements are not recommended, but intake of antioxidant-rich foods should be suggested (Czernichow et al, 2009). Thus far, trials with alpha tocopherol have been disappointing; further trials with gamma and alpha-tocopherols are warranted. Include phytochemicals, antioxidant foods, and spices such as turmeric, cumin, and cinnamon in the diet. See Tables 8-13 and 8-14.
- Chromium picolinate (CrPic) enhances insulin action by lowering plasma membrane (PM) cholesterol (Horvath et al, 2008). Coenzyme Q10 may have some merit, but further research is needed.
- High serum selenium concentrations have been associated with prevalence of higher FPG, LDL, TG, and glycosylated hemoglobin levels; further research is needed to determine its role in the development or the progression of MetS (Bleys et al, 2008).
- Other herbs and botanical supplements should not be used without discussing with physician. See Table 9-9 for guidance on more specific herbs and supplements.

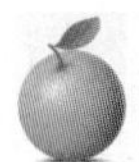

NUTRITION EDUCATION, COUNSELING, CARE MANAGEMENT

- Widespread screening is recommended to slow the growth of this syndrome. Prevention should start in childhood with healthy nutrition, daily physical activity, and annual measurement of weight, height, and BP beginning at 3 years of age (Bestermann, 2005).
- Discuss the role of nutrition (DASH or Mediterranean diet principles) in managing this syndrome. Obesity is a major contributor to the problem, so weight loss (even 10 lb) can help improve health status. A diet rich in antioxidants and DHA is beneficial. Finally, the 2005 Dietary Guidelines are consistent with lowering risk for MetS (Fogli-Cawley et al, 2007).
- Regular physical activity can help to lower elevated blood cholesterol levels and BP. Walking, or an exercise that is pleasant for the individual, is the one to select. Aerobic and strength training exercises are beneficial. Reduce sedentary activities, including television and computer time (Ford et al, 2005).
- Smoking cessation measures may be needed. Offer guidance on how not to gain weight after quitting.
- Limit consumption of alcoholic beverages, which can elevate triglycerides in large doses.

Patient Education—Foodborne Illness

- If home tube feeding is needed, teach appropriate sanitation and food-handling procedures.

For More Information

- American Diabetes Association–Metabolic Syndrome
  http://www.diabetes.org/diabetes-research/summaries/ekelund-metabolic.jsp
- American Heart Association
  http://www.americanheart.org/presenter.jhtml?identifier=534
- Mayo Clinic
  http://www.mayoclinic.com/health/metabolic%20syndrome/DS00522

METABOLIC SYNDROME—CITED REFERENCES

Al-Sarraj T, et al. Metabolic syndrome prevalence, dietary intake, and cardiovascular risk profile among overweight and obese adults 18–50 years old from the United Arab Emirates. *Metab Syndr Relat Disord.* 8:39, 2010.

Barnard ND, et al. The effects of a low-fat, plant-based dietary intervention on body weight, metabolism, and insulin sensitivity. *Am J Med.* 118:991, 2005.

Bestermann G, et al. Addressing the global cardiovascular risk of hypertension, dyslipidemia, diabetes mellitus, and the metabolic syndrome in the southeastern United States, part II: treatment recommendations for management of the global cardiovascular risk of hypertension, dyslipidemia, diabetes mellitus, and the metabolic syndrome. *Am J Med Sci.* 329:292, 2005.

Beydoun MA, et al. Ethnic differences in dairy and related nutrient consumption among US adults and their association with obesity, central obesity, and the metabolic syndrome. *Am J Clin Nutr.* 87:1914, 2008.

Bleys J, et al. Serum selenium and serum lipids in US adults. *Am J Clin Nutr.* 88:416, 2008.

Czernichow S, et al. Effects of long-term antioxidant supplementation and association of serum antioxidant concentrations with risk of metabolic syndrome in adults. *Am J Clin Nutr.* 90:329, 2009.

Deedwania PC, Volkova N. Current treatment options for the metabolic syndrome. *Curr Treat Options Cardiovasc Med.* 7:61, 2005.

Ellison RC, et al. Relation of the metabolic syndrome to calcified atherosclerotic plaque in the coronary arteries and aorta. *Am J Cardiol.* 95:1180, 2005.

Fogli-Cawley JJ, et al. The 2005 Dietary Guidelines for Americans and risk of the metabolic syndrome. *Am J Clin Nutr* 86:1193, 2007.

Ford ES, et al. Sedentary behavior, physical activity, and the metabolic syndrome among U.S. adults. *Obes Res.* 13:608, 2005.

Gable DR, et al. Adiponectin and its gene variants as risk factors for insulin resistance, the metabolic syndrome and cardiovascular disease. *Atherosclerosis.* 188:231, 2006.

Goulart AC, et al. Association of genetic variants with the metabolic syndrome in 20,806 white women: The Women's Health Genome Study. *Am Heart J.* 158:257, 2009.

Grundy S, et al. Diagnosis and management of the metabolic syndrome. *Circulation.* 112:105, 2005.

Horvath EM, et al. Antidiabetogenic effects of chromium mitigate hyperinsulinemia-induced cellular insulin resistance via correction of plasma membrane cholesterol imbalance. *Mol Endocrinol.* 22:937, 2008.

McKeown NM, et al. Dietary magnesium intake is related to metabolic syndrome in older Americans. *Eur J Nutr.* 47:210, 2009.

Orchard TJ, et al. The effect of metformin and intensive lifestyle intervention on the metabolic syndrome: the Diabetes Prevention Program randomized trial. *Ann Intern Med.* 142:611, 2005.

Shah A, et al. Adipose inflammation, insulin resistance, and cardiovascular disease. *JPEN J Parenter Enteral Nutr.* 32:638, 2008.

Shen J, et al. Interleukin1beta genetic polymorphisms interact with polyunsaturated fatty acids to modulate risk of the metabolic syndrome. *J Nutr.* 137:1846, 2007.

Singh U, et al. Comparison effect of atorvastatin (10 versus 80 mg) on biomarkers of inflammation and oxidative stress in subjects with metabolic syndrome. *Am J Cardiol.* 102:321, 2008.

Talpur N, et al. Effects of a novel formulation of essential oils on glucose-insulin metabolism in diabetic and hypertensive rats: a pilot study. *Diabetes Obes Metab.* 7:193, 2005.

PREDIABETES

NUTRITIONAL ACUITY RANKING: LEVEL 3–4

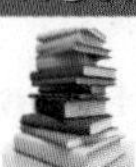

DEFINITIONS AND BACKGROUND

Prediabetes (impaired glucose tolerance, IGT) distinguishes those people who are at increased risk of developing diabetes. People with prediabetes have IFG or IGT, or both. More than 54 million Americans are affected with this combination of genes, obesity, and physical inactivity. People who have prediabetes may have a family history of heart disease and apple-shaped (intra-abdominal) obesity. Elevated triglycerides and low HDL cholesterol are risks for T2DM (Zacharova et al, 2005); adiposity-associated inflammation and insulin resistance are also implicated (Shah et al, 2008). NIH has also reported that smoking increases insulin resistance and prediabetes.

Under recent criteria, a normal blood glucose level is <100 mg/dL. Table 9-13 shows the tests and classification for IGT and IFG.

Most people with prediabetes go on to develop T2DM within 10 years unless they make lifestyle changes. Studies have evaluated various interventions among people with IGT and risks for developing diabetes. The Diabetes Prevention Program (DPP) was a large prevention study of people at high risk for diabetes (American Diabetes Association, 2006). Half of the participants had MetS at the beginning of the study; lifestyle intervention and metformin therapy reduced development of the syndrome in the remaining participants (Orchard et al, 2005). Lifestyle interventions include modest weight loss from a low-calorie, low-fat diet, and increased moderate-intensity physical activity (such as walking for 2½ hours each week).

People treated with an intensive lifestyle intervention reduce their risk of developing diabetes by half over 4 years, whereas people treated with metformin reduce their risk by only one third (American Diabetes Association, 2006). Metformin is most effective among younger, heavier people (those 25–40 years of age, 50–80 lb overweight) and less effective among older people and people with lower BMIs. In the STOP-NIDDM Trial, treatment of people with IGT with the drug acarbose reduced the risk of developing diabetes by 25% over 3 years.

The benefits of weight loss and physical activity strongly suggest that lifestyle modification should be the first choice to prevent or delay diabetes (American Diabetes Association, 2009). The dietitian plays an important role in nutrition education and counseling for these behavioral changes.

TABLE 9-13 Prediabetes Classifications and Tests

Condition/Classification	Test Used and Diagnostic Values
Impaired glucose tolerance (IGT)	• Oral Glucose Tolerance Test (OGTT), 75 g of glucose • 2-hour plasma glucose = 140–199 mg/dL
Impaired fasting glucose (IFG)	• Fasting plasma glucose (FPG) after 8-hour fast • Fasting plasma glucose = 100–125 mg/dL

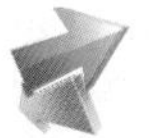

ASSESSMENT, MONITORING, AND EVALUATION

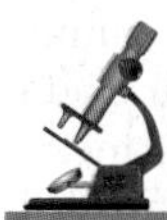

CLINICAL INDICATORS

Genetic Markers: Researchers are learning how to predict a person's odds of getting diabetes; Caucasians with type 1 diabetes have genes called HLA-DR3 or HLA-DR4 (American Diabetes Association, 2009). The HLA-DR7 gene may put African Americans at risk, and the HLA-DR9 gene may put Japanese at risk.

The MTHFR C>T polymorphism has a significant association with diabetic neuropathy in Caucasians and in persons with T2DM (Zintzaras et al, 2007). More rigorous studies are needed to define the role of genotypes in diabetes complications and management.

Clinical/History		
Height	Waist circumference	I & O
Weight	BMI	BP (>140/90?)
	Diet history	Smoker?
		PCOS?

Heart disease?	Fasting glucose after 8 hours (100–120 mg/dL?)	Alb, transthyretin
Hx gestational diabetes?	HbA1 c	Na^+, K^+
High risk ethnic background?	Chol, HDL and LDL profiles	H & H
Sedentary lifestyle?	Trig	Serum Fe
Family hx T2DM?	CRP	Serum folacin
		BUN, Creat
		Ca^{++}, Mg^{++}
		GFR

Lab Work

Gluc
OGTT with 2 hours post-prandial (140–199 mg/dL?)

> **SAMPLE NUTRITION CARE PROCESS STEPS**
>
> **Not Ready For Lifestyle Change**
>
> ***Assessment Data:*** Blood glucose log and food history; BMI 29 at age 48; family Hx diabetes (T2DM); previous counseling on lifestyle changes to prevent diabetes. Recent random blood glucose >140 mg/dL.
>
> ***Nutrition Diagnosis (PES):*** Not ready for lifestyle change related to potential for diabetes as evidenced by BMI 29, family history of diabetes, statement of "not being interested in many changes at this time."
>
> ***Intervention:*** Counseling about the importance of lifestyle changes to reduce likelihood of diabetes.
>
> ***Monitoring and Evaluation:*** Follow-up clinic visit indicating that client did make some lifestyle changes after considering the last counseling session; random blood glucose 100 mg/dL; weight loss of 5 lb in two months; increase in physical activity noted.

INTERVENTION

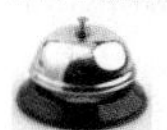

OBJECTIVES

- Increase the probability of reverting from IGT to normal glucose tolerance. Prevent further insulin resistance, hyperglycemia, or progression to diabetes.
- Modest weight loss (5–10% of body weight) and modest physical activity (30 minutes daily) are the recommended goals (American Diabetes Association, 2006). Walking can be encouraged for most people.
- Prevent or delay heart and kidney diseases, stroke, eye disease, and other undesirable conditions.
- Design a program that includes elements from the successful DPP trial:

Clearly defined weight loss and physical activity goals	A flexible maintenance program
Individual case managers or "lifestyle coaches"	Culturally appropriate materials and strategies
Intensive, ongoing intervention	Local and national network of training, feedback and clinical support
A core curriculum	Supervised exercise sessions at least twice weekly

Source: CDC, Web site accessed September 25, 2009, at http://www.cdc.gov/diabetes/faq/prediabetes.htm.

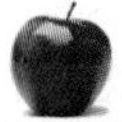

FOOD AND NUTRITION

- Control CHO intake (about 45–50% of total kilocalories) and limit excess added sugars. Encourage less processed carbohydrate and fiber food sources. Individualize according to lab work, BMI, and other risk reduction requirements.
- Maintain protein at about 20% of total energy.
- Plan fats at about 30–35% of total kcal (encourage monounsaturated fats and omega-3 fatty acids). Low saturated fats and cholesterol may be needed to prevent or treat hyperlipidemia.
- A moderate reduction in total energy intake is important. Modest weight loss of 5–7% of body weight may be recommended.
- Sufficient intake of minerals such as magnesium may be protective against diabetes. Include more almonds, whole wheat, cooked spinach, baked potatoes, and other magnesium-rich foods.
- Excesses of iron and selenium should be avoided; studies suggest that high intakes cause deposits in the internal organs, including the pancreas.
- Include adequate intake of fiber. A low fat vegan diet has been found to improve glycemia and elevated lipids (Barnard et al, 2009).
- Essential oils such as fenugreek, cinnamon, cumin, and oregano enhance insulin sensitivity (Talpur et al, 2005). Cinnamon may improve blood sugar and lipid levels (1/2 teaspoon daily).
- When a tube feeding is needed, there is insufficient evidence to support the use of specialty products as compared with standard products at this time.

Common Drugs Used and Potential Side Effects

- Acarbose treatment in IGT subjects decreases the risk of progression to diabetes by 36% (Delorme and Chiasson, 2005).
- Metformin reduces risk of developing diabetes, especially among younger, heavier people such as those 25–40 years of age who are 50–80 lb overweight (Herman et al, 2005). It is less effective among older people and people who were not as overweight.

Herbs, Botanicals, and Supplements

- Herbs and botanical supplements should not be used without discussing with physician. See Table 9-9 for tips.

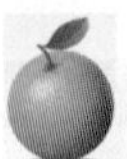

NUTRITION EDUCATION, COUNSELING, CARE MANAGEMENT

- Community Health Workers (CHW) may be trained for peer counseling when administered through a Diabetes Care Center (Katula et al, 2010). Lifestyle weight (LW) loss intervention has a goal of ≥7% weight loss achieved through increases in physical activity (180 min/wk) and decreases in caloric intake (approximately 1500 kcal/d) with CHW-led group-mediated cognitive behavioral meetings that occur weekly for 6 months and monthly thereafter for 18 months (Katula et al, 2010). Monthly small-group education sessions for a year are recommended by the CDC.
- Weight loss is a key goal (Davis et al, 2009; Norris et al, 2005). Discuss foods and meal patterns that will help to reduce risk factors for the individual client.
- Look AHEAD (Action for Health in Diabetes) trial participants (overweight adults diagnosed with diabetes) exceed recommended intake of fat, saturated fats, and sodium, which may contribute to increasing their risk of CVD and other chronic diseases (Vitolins et al, 2009). Therefore, it is important to address total fat intake (type of fat) and to suggest increasing intake of antioxidant-rich, high fiber foods. A vegan or vegetarian diet can be safely recommended (Barnard et al, 2009).
- Promote 8 oz or more of low fat milk, an ounce a day of nuts, filtered coffee, 1/2 teaspoon of cinnamon, and plenty of nonstarchy vegetables.
- Exercise seems to promote more reliable glycemic control compared with specific dietary protocols (Nield et al, 2007). Promote physical activity that matches client interest and ability. Discuss how to handle medication changes accordingly.

Patient Education—Foodborne Illness

- If home tube feeding is needed, teach appropriate sanitation and food-handling procedures.

For More Information

- American Diabetes Association–Prediabetes
  http://www.diabetes.org/diabetes-prevention/pre-diabetes.jsp
- CDC – Prediabetes
  http://www.cdc.gov/diabetes/faq/prediabetes.htm
- Mayo Clinic – Prediabetes
  http://www.mayoclinic.com/health/prediabetes/DS00624
- NIDDK–Prediabetes and Insulin Resistance
  http://diabetes.niddk.nih.gov/dm/pubs/insulinresistance/

PREDIABETES—CITED REFERENCES

American Diabetes Association. Genetics. Website accessed September 25, 2009, at http://www.diabetes.org/genetics.jsp.

Barnard ND, et al. A low-fat vegan diet and a conventional diabetes diet in the treatment of type 2 diabetes: a randomized, controlled, 74-wk clinical trial. *Am J Clin Nutr.* 89:1588S, 2009.

Davis N, et al. Nutritional strategies in type 2 diabetes mellitus. *Mt Sinai J Med.* 76:257, 2009.

Delorme S, Chiasson JL. Acarbose in the prevention of cardiovascular disease in subjects with impaired glucose tolerance and type 2 diabetes mellitus. *Curr Opin Pharmacol.* 5:184, 2005.

Herman WH, et al. Diabetes Prevention Program Research Group. The cost-effectiveness of lifestyle modification or metformin in preventing type 2 diabetes in adults with impaired glucose tolerance. *Ann Intern Med.* 142:323, 2005.

Katula JA, et al. Healthy Living Partnerships to Prevent Diabetes (HELP PD): Design and methods. [published online ahead of print September 13,2009] *Contemp Clin Trials.* 31:71, 2010.

Nield L, et al. Dietary advice for treatment of type 2 diabetes mellitus in adults. *Cochran Database Syst Rev.* 2007 Jul 18; (3):CD004097.

Norris SL, et al. Long-term effectiveness of weight loss interventions in adults with pre-diabetes. A review. *Am J Prev Med.* 28:126, 2005.

Orchard TJ, et al. The effect of metformin and intensive lifestyle intervention on the metabolic syndrome: the Diabetes Prevention Program randomized trial. *Ann Intern Med.* 142:61, 2005.

Shah A, et al. Adipose inflammation, insulin resistance, and cardiovascular disease. *JPEN J Parenter Enteral Nutr.* 32:638, 2008.

Talpur N, et al. Effects of a novel formulation of essential oils on glucose-insulin metabolism in diabetic and hypertensive rats: a pilot study. *Diabetes Obes Metab.* 7:193, 2005.

Vitolins MZ, et al. Action for Health in Diabetes (Look AHEAD) trial: baseline evaluation of selected nutrients and food group intake. *J Am Diet Assoc.* 109:1367, 2009.

Zacharova J, et al. The common polymorphisms (single nucleotide polymorphism [SNP] +45 and SNP +276) of the adiponectin gene predict the conversion from impaired glucose tolerance to type 2 diabetes: the STOP-NIDDM trial. *Diabetes.* 54:893, 2005.

TYPE 2 DIABETES IN ADULTS

NUTRITIONAL ACUITY RANKING: LEVEL 4

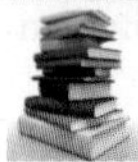

DEFINITIONS AND BACKGROUND

T2DM arises because of insulin resistance, when there is failure to use insulin properly combined with relative insulin deficiency. Increased and unrestrained hepatic glucose production as well as diminished glucose uptake and utilization results from insulin resistance occurring in the cells of the liver and other peripheral tissue, especially skeletal muscle. Previous names for T2DM include "non–insulin-dependent diabetes (NIDDM)," "adult-onset," "type II," "maturity-onset," and "ketosis-resistant" diabetes. T2DM accounts for 90% of all forms of diabetes. A significant percentage (about one third) of individuals who have T2DM are unaware of their diagnosis. Because T2DM is progressive, most patients will have already lost at least 50% of beta-cell function at the time of diagnosis.

The American Diabetes Association recommends diagnostic screening at 3-year intervals beginning at the age of 45, especially in individuals who have a BMI greater than 25 kg/m^2 (overweight). Risk factors include genetics, obesity, age, history of gestational diabetes, sedentary lifestyle, and smoking. Smoking cessation, decreasing BMI, and decreasing BP are major modifiable risk factors that are also major determinants of acquiring T2DM (Smith et al, 2005).

TABLE 9-14 Number of Medical Nutrition Therapy Visits Recommended for Type 2 Diabetes

Encounter Number	Length of Contact	Time between Encounters
1	60–90 minutes	2–4 weeks
2, 3	30–45 minutes	2–4 weeks
4, 5	30–45 minutes	6–12 months

From: National Guideline Clearinghouse. Nutrition practice guidelines for type 1 and type 2 diabetes mellitus. Accessed August 1, 2009, at http://guidelines.gov/summary/summary.aspx?doc_id=12816&nbr=006618&string=nutrition+AND+visits+AND+diabetes

For reducing BP, numerous clinical trials and experts support reduction of sodium intake; modest weight loss; increased physical activity; a low-fat diet that includes fruits, vegetables, and low-fat dairy products; and moderate alcohol intake. MNT from RDs in the treatment of T2DM improves glycemic outcomes with a decrease in A1 c of approximately 1–2%, depending on the duration of diabetes. Early referral for lifestyle changes and advice will yield the most benefit (Kulkarni, 2006).

The body's first defense against invading pathogens or tissue injury is the innate immune system; the cholinergic anti-inflammatory pathway is a neural mechanism that suppresses the innate inflammatory response such as excessive cytokine release in T2DM (Oke and Tracey, 2009). The use of antioxidant foods, spices and the Mediterranean diet has shown positive results as compared with a low fat diet (Esposito et al, 2009).

Patients should be educated about the progressive nature of diabetes and the importance of glycemic control with appropriate food choices and physical activity in conjunction with antidiabetes medication (Kulkarni, 2006). Maintain focus on lifestyle strategies that will improve blood glucose, BP, and lipids. Diabetes self-management training (DSMT), consisting of a 4-hour class, followed by individual dietitian consults and monthly support meetings can lower A1 c at a very low cost.

Weight management is especially helpful (Davis et al, 2009). Addition of a modest-cost, RD-led lifestyle case-management intervention to usual medical care does not increase health care costs and yields modest cost savings among obese patients with T2DM (Wolf et al, 2007). Weight loss significantly reduces diabetes costs; for every 1% weight lost, there is a 3.6% savings in total health costs and a 5.8% savings in diabetes care costs (Yu et al, 2007). The American Dietetic Association recommends four MNT visits initially, then one visit every 6–12 months Table 9-14). Referral to a dietitian within the first month after diagnosis is important.

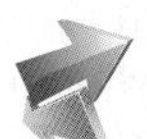

ASSESSMENT, MONITORING, AND EVALUATION

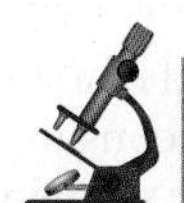

CLINICAL INDICATORS

Genetic Markers: T2DM has a stronger genetic basis than type 1, but depends more on environmental factors such as obesity and a western diet. From whole-genome studies, affected family members are studied; calpain 10 (CAPN10) and hepatocyte nuclear factor 4 alpha (HNF4A) have been identified.

Common genetic variation near melatonin receptor MTNR1B contributes to raised plasma glucose and increased risk of type-2 diabetes among Indian Asians and European whites (Chambers et al, 2009). Variants of the FTO (affectionately called the FATSO) gene are identified an obesity risk allele; this gene is associated with increased risk of TDM.

Clinical/History

- Height
- Weight
- BMI
- Obesity?
- Diet history
- Waist circumference
- BP (increased?)
- Blurred vision?
- Erectile dysfunction
- Fatigue
- Frequent, slow-healing infections
- Increased appetite, thirst, urination
- Numbness or burning sensation in feet, ankles, legs
- Signs of dehydration?
- Smoking history
- Electrocardiogram (ECG) before exercise program

Lab Work

- CRP
- FPG
- HbA1c
- Blood or urinary ketones
- Total Chol, LDL, HDL
- Trig (often increased)
- BUN, Creat
- Na^+, K^+
- ALT, AST
- Lactate dehydrogenase (LDH)
- Alk phos
- Ca^{++}, Mg^{++}
- Microalbuminuria
- Plasminogen activator inhibitor type 1
- Fasting insulin
- Fasting C-peptide levels

SAMPLE NUTRITION CARE PROCESS STEPS

Self-Monitoring Deficit In T2DM

Assessment Data: Blood glucose self-monitoring records, food diary worksheets and meal records, blood glucose levels (fasting, 2-hour postprandial and/or HbA1c levels).

Nutrition Diagnosis (PES): Self-monitoring knowledge deficit related to lack of understanding how to record food and beverage intake as evidenced by incomplete food records at last two clinic visits and lab of HbA1c = 8.5 mg/dL.

Intervention: Teaching patient and family member(s) about use of simple blood glucose self-monitoring records (recording of timing, amount, blood glucose levels) and meal records.

Monitoring and Evaluation: HbA1c levels (goal <7 mg/dL); other glucose labs, food diary and records, discussion about complications of using the records.

INTERVENTION

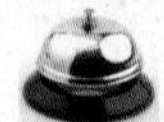

OBJECTIVES

- Provide persons with diabetes initial basic nutrition messages and schedule time for MNT with an RD who has expertise in diabetes management.
- Maintain as near-normal blood glucose levels as possible by balancing food intake with insulin (either endogenous or exogenous) or oral glucose-lowering medications and activity levels. Improvement with MNT, if successful, is usually seen within 6 weeks and up to a maximum of 6 months. Medication may be needed if blood glucose levels are not under control.
- Maintain glycosylated A1c levels <7%, preprandial capillary plasma glucose levels between 90 and 130 mg/dL, and peak postprandial capillary plasma glucose levels <180 mg/dL. The target goal range for the patient may vary by age and underlying disorders.
- Protect beta-cell function by controlling hyperglycemia. A1c tests should be done at least two times a year in patients who are meeting treatment goals and quarterly in patients whose therapy has changed or who are not meeting glycemic goals.
- Achieve optimal serum lipid levels to reduce the risk for macrovascular disease. Dyslipidemia is a central component of insulin resistance in all ethnic groups.
- Emphasis of MNT is on lifestyle strategies to reduce glycemia, dyslipidemia, and BP. Strategies should lead to reduced energy intake and increased energy expenditure through physical activity. The A to Z (Atkins to Zone Diet) weight loss diet analysis found that premenopausal overweight and obese women who followed the Atkins diet (lowest carbohydrate intake), lost more weight at 12 months than women assigned to follow the Zone diet (Gardner et al, 2007). Therefore, for some patients, a low-carbohydrate, high-protein, high-fat diet may be a feasible alternative recommendation for weight loss.
- Maintain or improve overall health. The Dietary Guidelines for Americans and the MyPyramid food guide illustrate healthy nutritional guidelines and can be used by people with diabetes.
- Encourage regular mealtimes. Maintain lifestyle changes through behavior modification, education, and problem-solving strategies.
- Address individual needs according to culture, ethnicity, and lifestyle, while respecting willingness to change. For older adults, meet nutritional and psychosocial needs. For pregnant or lactating women, provide adequate energy and nutrients for optimal outcomes. Encourage therapeutic lifestyle changes (TLC), considering client's readiness, skills, resources, and current needs.
- Achieve BP levels that reduce risk for vascular disease and renal function decline.
- Manage problems related to compulsive or binge eating. Patients often report deliberate omission of insulin or oral hypoglycemic agents (OHA) to lose weight.
- Manage children with T2DM or maturity-onset diabetes of youth (MODY) differently than children who have T1DM; see appropriate entries.
- Prevent and treat the acute and long-term complications of diabetes listed in Table 9-2.

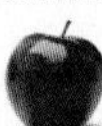

FOOD AND NUTRITION

- The dietitian should calculate CHO and fat requirements individually according to lipid and glucose levels. Assess dietary history, physical exercise, and activity patterns.
- Include foods containing CHO from whole grains, fruits, vegetables, and low-fat milk. A vegan diet is also an effective consideration (Barnard et al, 2009; Turner-McGrievy et al, 2008).
- Moderate weight loss in an obese patient (5–10% of starting weight) may reduce hyperglycemia, dyslipidemia, and hypertension. A moderate caloric restriction (250–500 calories less than average daily intake as calculated from a food history) and a nutritionally adequate meal plan should be recommended. Extremely low-calorie diets for adults should be performed only in a hospital setting.
- In morbidly obese patients, bariatric surgery may be the only effective treatment. There are risks from surgery and anesthesia, but the benefits often outweigh the risks.
- Space meals and spread nutrient intake, particularly carbohydrate, throughout the day.
- Eating breakfast has beneficial effects on fasting lipid and postprandial insulin sensitivity. Avoid meal skipping. Individualize meal plan according to patient preferences.
- Carbohydrate should be calculated between 45% and 65% of energy intake. Consistency is important.
- Protein should be calculated at 15–20% of daily energy intake with normal renal function and control at 0.8–1.0 g/kg with renal disease. Where weight loss is needed, use of a diet slightly higher in protein may help to enhance insulin sensitivity.
- Fat should be 25–35% of energy intake (7–10% of kcal saturated fats, 10% polyunsaturated fats, and 10–15% monounsaturated fats). Limit intake of cholesterol to <200–300 mg/d.
- Foods that benefit both the carbohydrate and lipid abnormalities should be consumed often. Recommendations are the same as for the general population concerning fiber: use more brown rice, beans, green leafy vegetables, oat bran, legumes, barley, produce with skins, apples, oranges, and other whole fruit and produce.
- As part of a healthy lifestyle and to manage hypertension, teach the principles of the DASH diet; <2400 mg/d of sodium is recommended.
- For most vitamins and minerals, ensure adequate dietary intakes. Higher levels of magnesium (Rumawas et al, 2006), chromium, and zinc are recommended. A multivitamin–mineral supplement may be used. Because altered vitamin D and calcium homeostasis may play a role in the development of T2DM, dual supplementation may prevent T2DM in high-risk populations (Tremblay and Gilbert, 2009; Pittas et al, 2007). Vitamin K as phylloquinone may also have a role in glucose management (Yoshida et al, 2008).
- Discuss usefulness of artificial sweeteners and food diaries.
- Discuss use of alcohol. Avoid hypoglycemia by consuming alcohol with food. Limit to 1 drink daily for women and two for men. Light-to-moderate amounts of alcohol do not increase triglyceride or BP levels. Indeed, moderate alcohol consumption has been associated with a decreased incidence of diabetes and heart disease; alcohol has been

reported to increase insulin sensitivity and raise HDL cholesterol levels. Alcoholic beverages should be considered an addition to the regular food/meal plan. If consumed daily, calories from alcohol are calculated into the total energy intake. Abstain from alcohol in pregnancy, pancreatitis, advanced neuropathy, severe hypertriglyceridemia, and a history of alcohol abuse.

Common Drugs Used and Potential Side Effects (see Table 9-15)

- T2DM is a progressive disease. Medications will need to be combined with lifestyle strategies. Insulin may be used in a combination with oral therapy or alone. If oral glucose-lowering medications do not achieve normoglycemia, combined oral therapies (drugs from two or more classes) can be initiated.
- If combination oral therapy does not work, insulin is needed. Insulin may also be needed for refractory hyperglycemia, diabetic ketoacidosis, stress, infection, or pregnancy.
- Multiple drug therapy is generally required to achieve BP targets. Angiotensin-converting enzyme (ACE) inhibitors, angiotensin receptor blockers (ARBs), beta-blockers, diuretics, and calcium channel blockers may all be helpful.
- Aspirin therapy (75–162 mg/d) is recommended to protect against cardiovascular events.
- Overwhelming evidence suggests that the renin-angiotensin system (RAS) plays an important role in the pathogenesis of DM and its associated cardiovascular risks; RAS blockers may delay or prevent the onset (Braga and Leiter, 2009).
- In individuals with diabetes over the age of 40 years and without overt CVD, statin therapy to achieve an LDL <100 mg/dL is recommended. For people with diabetes and overt CVD, an LDL cholesterol goal of <70 mg/dL is recommended. Lifestyle modifications focusing on reducing saturated fat and increasing physical activity are also important.
- Antipsychotic agents contribute to the development of the metabolic syndrome and increase the risk for T2DM and heart disease. Monitor their use carefully.

TABLE 9-15 Medications Used for Type 2 Diabetes

Combination therapy rather than monotherapy is typically used to achieve glucose control in patients who are not at glycemic goals.

Classification	Medication	Route	The Way it Works	Time and Dose	Comments
Sulfonylureas	Glimepiride (Amaryl) Glipizide (Glucotrol) Glipizide ER (Glucotrol XL) Glyburide (Diabeta, Micronase)	Oral	Increases insulin production. Long-acting.	One or two times a day	Never give to a patient who is fasting for any reason. Do not use with alcoholic beverages. May cause weight gain, nausea, diarrhea or heartburn. Check LFTs.
Biguanides	Glucophage (Metformin) Glucophage XR	Oral	Lowers glucose from digestion; inhibits glucose release from the liver. Sensitizer.	Two to three times a day, XR once a day	Take with food. May cause diarrhea, flatulence, abdominal pain. Do not use with inflammatory bowel disease. Enhances weight loss.
Alpha-Glucosidase Inhibitors	Miglitol (Glyset) Acrobose (Precose)	Oral	Slows digestion, slows glucose production. Starch blocker that delays intestinal glucose absorption.	Take before each meal; swallow with first bite of food.	GI intolerance can occur. Exercise enhances effectiveness.
Thiazolidinediones	Rosiglitazone (Avandia) Pioglitazone (Actos)	Oral	Lowers glucose production; increases tissue glucose utilization, mostly in muscle.	Once daily with or without food	Liver damage is possible. Can lead to weight gain or heart failure.
Meglitinides	Repaglinide (Prandin) Senaglinide (Starlix)	Oral	Increases insulin production; short-acting.	5–30 minutes before meals	Offers better control of postprandial hyperglycemia and is associated with a lower risk of delayed hypoglycemic episodes.
DPP-4 Inhibitors	Sitagliptin (Januvia)	Oral	Lowers glucose by blocking an enzyme	100 mg. Once a day	
Incretin Mimetics	Exenatide (Byetta)	Injectable	Helps the pancreas make insulin, slows digestion	10 μg. Inject within an hour of AM and PM meals	Acid or sour stomach, belching, diarrhea, dizziness, nervousness.
Anti-hyperglycemic	Amylin (Symlin)	Injectable	Controls postprandial blood glucose	15 μg. Inject before major meals	

Source: Diabetes Medications, NIDDK. Web site accessed September 22, 2009, at http://diabetes.niddk.nih.gov/dm/pubs/medicines_ez/.

- Medications such as steroids, beta-blockers, and diuretics may cause hyperglycemia in some patients. Supplements of Vitamin C may cause false-positive urinary glucose levels when given in large doses.
- Melatonin may have a role. Carriers of the risk genotype exhibit increased expression of MTNR1B in islet cells; these individuals may be more sensitive to the actions of melatonin, leading to impaired insulin secretion. Blocking the inhibition of insulin secretion by melatonin may be a novel therapeutic avenue for T2DM.
- Metformin improves insulin sensitivity in patients with IGT, but it does not reduce inflammatory biomarker levels (Pradhan et al, 2009).
- Xenical (fat blocker) may help cut heart risk in patients with T2DM. The obese diabetic patient who is poorly controlled may benefit from weight-reducing agents, such as sibutramine or orlistat.

Herbs, Botanicals, and Supplements

- Herbs and botanical supplements should not be used without discussing with physician. See Table 9-9 for more details.
- Vitamin D and calcium in combined supplementation may be beneficial in optimizing glucose metabolism (Pittas et al, 2007).

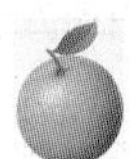

NUTRITION EDUCATION, COUNSELING, CARE MANAGEMENT

- Medical nutrition intervention in patients with diabetes should address the metabolic abnormalities of glucose, lipids, and BP (Kulkarni, 2006). To meet the specific needs of the patient, adapt drug therapy to enhance outcomes and quality of life.
- DSME is an essential element of diabetes care, and national standards have been based on evidence for its benefits. DSME helps patients optimize metabolic control, prevent and manage complications, and maximize quality of life in a cost-effective manner. Health care providers should refer newly diagnosed patients to a dietitian who should then regularly reassess patients over time for modification of medications and food intake patterns.
- Emphasize the importance of regular mealtimes, use of medications, self-care and optimal functioning with instructions on how to handle illness, stress, exercise, label reading, use of sucrose or fructose and sugar alcohols.
- Vegan diets increase intakes of carbohydrate, fiber, and several micronutrients even more than the American Diabetes Association recommended diet (Turner-McGrievy et al, 2008). It would be acceptable to promote a vegan lifestyle for diabetes management (Barnard et al, 2009).
- Some restaurants offer foods lower in cholesterol, fat, and sodium, and higher in fiber. All restaurants offer low calorie sweeteners in the blue, yellow, or pink packets, and diet drinks. Many offer reduced-calorie salad dressings, low-fat or fat-free milk, and salt substitutes. Choose salads, fish, vegetables, baked or broiled food, and whole-grain breads.
- Clinical trials using antihyperglycemic medications to improve glycemic control have not demonstrated the anticipated cardiovascular benefits in patients with T2DM (Jenkins et al, 2008).
- To improve glycemic control, assist with weight maintenance, and reduce risk of CVD, at least 150 min/wk of moderate-intensity aerobic physical activity (50–70% of maximum heart rate) is recommended or at least 90 min/wk of vigorous aerobic exercise (>70% of maximum heart rate). Activity should be distributed over at least 3 d/wk, with no more than 2 consecutive days without physical activity.
- While high-intensity exercise is beneficial, even in older adults, it should start gradually and increase to desired intensity and duration. Avoid high-intensity exercise and resistance training in persons with neuropathy, coronary heart disease, or retinopathy. In the absence of contraindications, people with T2DM should perform resistance exercise three times a week, targeting all major muscle groups and progressing to three sets of 8–10 repetitions.
- Decrease sedentary behaviors, especially prolonged TV or computer time.
- Identify potential or real obstacles. Discuss options for handling negative emotions, temptations, dining away from home, feeling deprived, time pressures, competing priorities, social events, family support, food refusal, and lack of support from friends.
- Regular consumption of breakfast, self-weighing, and infrequent intake of fast foods are strategies that work well (Raynor et al, 2008).
- Use culturally appropriate methods for teaching and guidance. For example, use of the Medicine Wheel in Plains Indians has shown more effective results than usual techniques (Kattelmann et al, 2009).
- Encourage group support, behavior modification, and nutritional counseling for overweight.
- Small changes lead to greater self-esteem. Sequential rather than simultaneous dietary changes work well for most people and can improve the sense of self-efficacy.
- A comprehensive lifestyle self-management program using the Mediterranean low–saturated fat diet, stress management training, exercise, group support, and smoking cessation can reduce cardiovascular risk factors.
- Dietitians have a distinct role in MNT versus DSME; but both education and counseling are more medically effective than either one alone (Daly et al, 2009).
- A low-literacy tool can be useful in teaching key changes for those who need it. The goal is to achieve a sense of control over self-management of the diabetes.
- Before any type of surgery, blood glucose should be maintained between 100 and 200 mg/dL. Perioperative hyperglycemia may be managed with doses of rapid-acting insulin. Correct abnormalities before surgery, when possible.
- In noncritically ill hospitalized patients, premeal blood glucose should be kept as close to 90–130 mg/dL as possible, with a postprandial blood glucose <180 mg/dL; use insulin when necessary.
- In critically ill hospitalized patients, blood glucose levels should be kept as close to 110 mg/dL as possible and generally <180 mg/dL. These patients will usually require intravenous insulin.

Patient Education—Foodborne Illness

- If home tube feeding is needed, teach appropriate sanitation and food-handling procedures.

For More Information

- American Diabetes Association
  http://www.diabetes.org/food-nutrition-lifestyle/nutrition.jsp
- American Diabetes Association–Medicare Policy and Benefits
  http://www.diabetes.org/for-health-professionals-and-scientists/recognition/dsmt-mntfaqs.jsp
- American Diabetes Association–Type 2 Diabetes
  http://www.diabetes.org/type-2-diabetes.jsp
- American Dietetic Association: Type 2 Diabetes Practice Guidelines
  http://www.eatright.org/cps/rde/xchg/ada/hs.xsl/index.html
- Annals of Internal Medicine – Mediterranean Diet Implications for Patients
  http://www.annals.org/cgi/summary_pdf/151/5/306.pdf
- Mayo Clinic – T2DM
  http://www.mayoclinic.com/health/type-2-diabetes/DS00585
- Web MD – T2DM
  http://diabetes.webmd.com/guide/type-2-diabetes

TYPE 2 DIABETES IN ADULTS—CITED REFERENCES

Barnard ND, et al. Vegetarian and vegan diets in type 2 diabetes management. *Nutr Rev.* 67:255, 2009.

Braga MG, Leiter LA. Role of renin-angiotensin system blockade in patients with diabetes mellitus. *Am J Cardiol.* 104:835, 2009.

Chambers JC, et al. Common genetic variation near melatonin receptor MTNR1B contributes to raised plasma glucose and increased risk of type-2 diabetes amongst Indian Asians and European whites. [published online ahead of print August 3,2009] *Diabetes.* 58:2703, 2009.

Daly A, et al. Diabetes white paper: Defining the delivery of nutrition services in Medicare medical nutrition therapy vs Medicare diabetes self-management training programs. *J Am Diet Assoc.* 109:528, 2009.

Davis N, et al. Nutritional strategies in type 2 diabetes mellitus. *Mt Sinai J Med.* 76:257, 2009.

Esposito K, et al. Effects of a Mediterranean-style diet on the need for antihyperglycemic drug therapy in patients with newly diagnosed type 2 diabetes: a randomized trial. *Ann Int Med.* 151:306, 2009.

Gardner CD, et al. Comparison of the Atkins, Zone, Ornish, and LEARN diets for change in weight and related risk factors among overweight premenopausal women: the A TO Z Weight Loss Study: a randomized trial. *JAMA*, 297:969, 2007.

Jenkins DJ, et al. Effect of a low-glycemic index or a high-cereal fiber diet on type 2 diabetes: a randomized trial. *JAMA.* 300:2742, 2008.

Kattelmann KK, et al. The medicine wheel nutrition intervention: a diabetes education study with the Cheyenne River Sioux Tribe. *J Am Diet Assoc.* 109:1532, 2009.

Kulkarni K. Diets do not fail: the success of medical nutrition therapy in patients with diabetes. *Endocr Pract.* 12:121S, 2006.

Oke SL, Tracey KJ. The inflammatory reflex and the role of complementary and alternative medical therapies. *Ann N Y Acad Sci.* 1172:172, 2009.

Pittas AG, et al. The role of vitamin D and calcium in type 2 diabetes. A systematic review and meta-analysis. *J Clin Endocrinol Metab.* 92:2017, 2007.

Pradhan AD, et al. Effects of initiating insulin and metformin on glycemic control and inflammatory biomarkers among patients with type 2 diabetes: the LANCET randomized trial. *JAMA.* 302:1186, 2009.

Raynor HA, et al. Weight loss strategies associated with BMI in overweight adults with type 2 diabetes at entry into the Look AHEAD (Action for Health in Diabetes) trial. *Diab Care.* 31:1299, 2008.

Rumawas ME, et al. Magnesium intake is related to improved insulin homeostasis in the Framingham offspring cohort. *J Am Coll Nutr.* 25:486, 2006.

Tremblay A, Gilbert JA. Milk products, insulin resistance syndrome and type 2 diabetes. *J Am Coll Nutr.* 28:91S, 2009.

Turner-McGrievy GM, et al. Changes in nutrient intake and dietary quality among participants with type 2 diabetes following a low-fat vegan diet or a conventional diabetes diet for 22 weeks. *J Am Diet Assoc.* 108:1636, 2008.

Wolf AM, et al. Effects of lifestyle intervention on health care costs: Improving Control with Activity and Nutrition (ICAN). *J Am Diet Assoc.* 107:1365, 2007.

Yoshida M, et al. Phylloquinone intake, insulin sensitivity, and glycemic status in men and women. *Am J Clin Nutr,* 88:210, 2008.

Yu AP, et al. Short-term economic impact of body weight change among patients with type 2 diabetes treated with antidiabetic agents: analysis using claims, laboratory, and medical record data. *Curr Med Res Opin.* 23:2157, 2007.

TYPE 2 DIABETES IN CHILDREN AND TEENS

NUTRITIONAL ACUITY RANKING: LEVEL 4

DEFINITIONS AND BACKGROUND

T2DM arises because of insulin resistance, when there is failure to use insulin properly combined with relative insulin deficiency. In children, obesity or puberty often unmasks T2DM in genetically susceptible individuals. For example, the emergence of T2DM presents a new challenge for pediatricians and other health care professionals; preventive efforts, early diagnosis, and collaborative care of the patient and family are essential.

Breastfeeding, reduced television and sedentary lifestyles, healthy eating principles, family-based approaches, and screening are all important in managing this epidemic. Screening should be available for children whose BMI is greater than the 85th percentile at puberty or at age 10 plus any two of the following risk factors: family history, increased risk by ethnicity, or signs of insulin resistance such as polycystic ovary syndrome (PCOS), hypertension, dyslipidemia, or acanthosis. Weight greater than 120% of ideal for height also warrants screening.

In addition to obesity, family history of T2DM, and absence of GAD-65 antibodies, children with new-onset T2DM may be distinguished from those with T1DM by a combination of biochemical parameters of C-peptide, IGFBP-1, CO(2), and urine ketones (Katz et al, 2007). However, one third of the children with T2DM may have at least one detectable beta-cell autoantibody, classified as latent autoimmune diabetes in youth.

Fasting blood glucose levels should be checked at least every 2 years in high-risk children. T2DM in childhood can lead to end-stage renal disease and mortality in middle age; long duration is more detrimental (Pavkov et al, 2006). There is an ongoing effort for diabetes prevention in trials specifically designed to address the adolescent population (Karam and McFarlane, 2009).

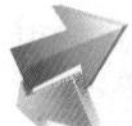

ASSESSMENT, MONITORING, AND EVALUATION

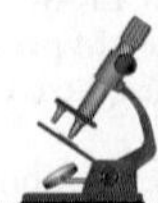

CLINICAL INDICATORS

Genetic Markers: The presence of multiple risk alleles amounts to a significant difference in children who have diabetes (Kelliny et al, 2009). Genetic variations for glucokinase (GCK), GCK regulatory protein (GCKR), islet-specific glucose 6 phosphatase catalytic subunit-related protein (G6PC2), and melatonin receptor type 1B (MTNR1B) are associated.

Clinical/History

- Height
- Weight
- BMI
- Diet history
- Waist circumference
- BP (often increased)
- Sleep-disordered breathing?

Lab Work

- FPG
- HbA1c
- C-peptide, IGFBP-1, CO(2)
- Beta-cell autoantibodies (anti-GAD, anti-IA-2, and anti-ICA)?
- Urine ketones
- CRP
- Urinary microalbuminuria
- Plasminogen activator inhibitor type 1
- Total Chol, LDL (high?)
- HDL (usually low)
- Trig (often increased)
- BUN, Creat
- Na^+, K^+
- ALT, AST
- LDH
- Alk phos
- Ca^{++}, Mg^{++}
- Alb

INTERVENTION

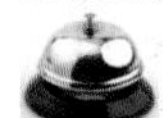

OBJECTIVES

- Maintain as near-normal blood glucose levels as possible by balancing food intake with insulin (either endogenous or exogenous) or oral glucose-lowering medications and activity levels.
- Try to maintain glycosylated A1c levels <7%. Target goal range for the patient may vary by age and underlying disorders: <6-year old, 7.5–8.5%; 6- to 12-year old, <8%; 13- to 9-year old, <7.5%. Preprandial capillary plasma glucose levels should be kept between 90 and 130 mg/dL.
- Protect beta-cell function by controlling hyperglycemia. A1c tests should be done at least twice a year in patients who are meeting treatment goals and quarterly in patients who are not meeting glycemic goals.
- Achieve optimal serum lipid levels to reduce the risk for macrovascular disease.
- Emphasis of MNT is on lifestyle strategies to reduce hyperglycemica, dyslipidemia, and hypertension.
- Prevent and treat acute complications, short-term illnesses, and exercise-related problems, the long-term complications of renal disease, autonomic neuropathy, hypertension, and CVD.
- Maintain BP levels that reduce risk for vascular disease. Elevated BP has a major impact on renal function.
- Improve overall health through optimal nutrition and physical activity. Dietary Guidelines for Americans and the MyPyramid food guidance system illustrate nutritional guidelines and can be used by young people with diabetes.
- Encourage regular mealtimes. Maintain lifestyle changes through behavior modification, education, and problem-solving strategies.
- Working with the whole family is important. Promote family and individualized psychosocial counseling to handle depression and emotions.
- Address individual needs according to culture, ethnicity, and lifestyle, while respecting willingness to change. Encourage TLC, considering the child's needs and family circumstances.
- Manage problems related to compulsive or binge eating. Patients often report deliberate omission of medication in order to lose weight.

SAMPLE NUTRITION CARE PROCESS STEPS

Altered Nutritional Labs – T2DM In Teenager

Assessment Data: Blood glucose self-monitoring records, food diary worksheets and meal records, hour HbA1c levels 9 mg/dL, BMI >85% for age. Family Hx T2DM (both parents). BP normal but LDL cholesterol slightly elevated

Nutrition Diagnosis (PES): Altered nutritional labs related to overweight, knowledge deficit about diabetes and self-monitoring difficulty as evidenced by HbA1c = 8.5 mg/dL and LDL chol >130 mg/dL and statement that "I don't really understand my diabetes very well."

Intervention: Teaching patient and family member(s) about use of simple blood glucose self-monitoring records (timing, blood glucose testing, role of HbA1c in evaluating past 3 months, meal records).

Monitoring and Evaluation: HbA1c levels <7 mg/dL. Other labs WNL; food diary and glucose records showing improvement in outcomes of lab testing.

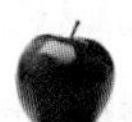

FOOD AND NUTRITION

- Calculate CHO and fat requirements individually according to age, serum lipid, and glucose levels. Assess dietary history, physical exercise, and activity patterns. Studies support the importance of carbohydrate from whole grains, fruits, vegetables, and low-fat milk.
- Moderate weight loss (5–10% of starting weight) may reduce hyperglycemia, dyslipidemia, and hypertension. A moderate restriction of 250–500 calories less than average daily intake (as calculated from a food history) and a nutritionally adequate meal plan are recommended.
- For teen boys over age 15, it may be useful to calculate caloric needs as 18 kcal/lb for usual activity and 16 kcal/lb if sedentary. Teen girls over age 15 have needs that are estimated the same as those for an adult.
- Extremely low-calorie diets are not recommended for children or teens. In morbidly obese children, gastric bypass surgery should be the last option as malnutrition is a permanent side effect.

- Spacing of meals (spreading carbohydrate throughout the day) and eating breakfast have beneficial effects on fasting lipid and postprandial insulin sensitivity.
- Meal skipping should be discouraged. Individualize meal plan according to patient preferences.
- Carbohydrate should be calculated as 45–65% of energy intake. Daily consistency is important.
- Protein should be calculated at 15–20% of daily energy intake with normal renal function; control at 0.8–1.0 g/kg with presence of renal disease.
- Fat should be 25–35% of energy intake, with 7–10% of kilocalories saturated fats, 10% polyunsaturated fats, and 10–15% monounsaturated fats. Limit intake of cholesterol to 200–300 mg/d.
- Recommendations for fiber include rice, beans, vegetables, oat bran, legumes, barley, produce with skins, apples, oranges, other produce. Include 19–38 g/d, larger amounts for older children and teens.
- As part of a healthy lifestyle and to manage hypertension, teach the principles of the DASH diet; 2400 mg/d of sodium is recommended.
- For vitamins and minerals, ensure that patient has adequate dietary intakes. Higher levels of magnesium, chromium, and potassium are recommended when serum levels are low. There is no need for supplements of any singular nutrient; a pediatric multivitamin–mineral supplement may be used.
- Include phytochemicals and antioxidants in the diet (see Table 8-14 in the pancreatic chapter).
- Discuss use of artificial sweeteners, food diaries, menu options at school, fast food choices that are lower in total fat, benefits and goals for physical activity, and the need for adequate fluid intake.

Common Drugs Used and Potential Side Effects (see Table 9-15 also)

- Oral agents may be used when blood glucose and other treatment goals are not met through diet and exercise alone. Glucophage should be the first oral agent used but not in children with known liver and kidney disease, low oxygen problems, or severe infections. Other oral agents such as a sulfonylurea or meglitinide can be added if control does not improve after 3–6 months. Thiazolidinediones probably should not be used in children.
- Insulin therapy should be started in children with severely elevated blood sugar levels or children with intense thirst and frequent urination. There are a wide variety of insulin regimens that can be used, anywhere from bedtime alone to multiple daily injections. Once blood sugars are under control, glucophage can be added while decreasing insulin dosage.
- Pharmacologic options for weight loss, including metformin, orlistat, and sibutramine have been studied (Miller and Silverstein, 2006). They should be used only under close medical supervision.

Herbs, Botanicals, and Supplements

- Herbs and botanical supplements should not be used in children and teens. There is insufficient evidence to draw definitive conclusions about the efficacy of individual herbs and supplements for diabetes, especially in children. However, inclusion of spices and seasonings in the diet would be acceptable.
- See Table 9-9 for guidance on more specific herbs and supplements that the client may be using.

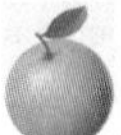

NUTRITION EDUCATION, COUNSELING, CARE MANAGEMENT

- Health care providers are encouraged to refer newly diagnosed patients to a dietitian. The dietitian should regularly reassess children and teens for overall growth and health status.
- Stress the importance of parental supervision and support.
- Children often benefit from attending diabetes camps for youth and support groups for family counseling. DSME is helpful for SMBG, medication use, physical activity goals, and meal planning.
- Emphasize the importance of regular mealtimes, proper use of medications, and balanced activity. Home blood glucose monitoring records and food/exercise records are important.
- Emphasize the importance of self-care and optimal functioning for illness, stress, dining out, exercise.
- Identify potential or real obstacles and discuss options for handling negative emotions, temptations, dining away from home, feeling deprived, time pressures, competing priorities, social events, family support, food refusal, and lack of support from friends.
- Explain food and nutrition labeling as well as how to manage sucrose, fructose, and sugar alcohols in the diet. Reduce sugar-sweetened beverage intake as much as possible.
- Encourage group support, behavior modification, and nutritional counseling for overweight. Small changes lead to greater self-esteem than continued failures. Sequential rather than simultaneous dietary changes work best and can improve self-efficacy.
- Reduce stress where possible. BMI and stress are independent determinants of TNF-alpha (an inflammatory cytokine) and adipocytokine among Latino children (Dixon et al, 2009).
- Suggest guidelines for physical activity: three to four times a week, exercise for 30–60 min/d. Aerobic exercise is protective against age-related increases in visceral adiposity (Kim and Lee, 2009).

Patient Education—Foodborne Illness

- If home tube feeding is needed, teach appropriate sanitation and food-handling procedures.

For More Information

- Centers for Disease Control and Prevention (CDC) Diabetes Projects
  http://www.cdc.gov/diabetes/projects/cda2.htm
- CDC Reference Documents
  http://www.cdc.gov/diabetes/projects/ref.htm
- Children with Diabetes
  http://www.childrenwithdiabetes.com/d_0n_d00.htm
- National Diabetes Education Program
  http://www.ndep.nih.gov/publications/PublicationDetail.aspx?PubId=154

TYPE 2 DIABETES IN CHILDREN AND TEENS—CITED REFERENCES

Dixon D, et al. Stress and body mass index each contributes independently to tumor necrosis factor-alpha production in prepubescent Latino children. *J Pediatr Nurs.* 24:378, 2009.

Karam JG, McFarlane SI. Prevention of type 2 DM: implications for adolescents and young adults. *Pediatr Endocrinol Rev.* 5:980S, 2009.

Katz LE, et al. Fasting c-peptide and insulin-like growth factor-binding protein-1 levels help to distinguish childhood type 1 and type 2 diabetes at diagnosis. *Pediatr Diabetes.* 8:53, 2007.

Kelliny C, et al. Common Genetic Determinants of Glucose Homeostasis in Healthy Children: The European Youth Heart Study (EYHS). [published online ahead of print September 9, 2009] *Diabetes.* 58:2939, 2009.

Kim Y, Lee S. Physical activity and abdominal obesity in youth. *Appl Physiol Nutr Metab.* 34:571, 2009.

Miller JL, Silverstein JH. The treatment of type 2 diabetes mellitus in youth: which therapies? *Treat Endocrinol.* 5:201, 2006.

Pavkov ME, et al. Effect of youth-onset type 2 diabetes mellitus on incidence of end-stage renal disease and mortality in young and middle-aged Pima Indians. *JAMA.* 296:421, 2006.

GESTATIONAL DIABETES

NUTRITIONAL ACUITY RANKING: LEVEL 4

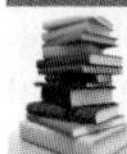

DEFINITIONS AND BACKGROUND

GDM involves glucose intolerance with first onset or recognition during pregnancy. It affects 14–25% of all pregnancies, increasing over the past decade (March of Dimes, 2009).

Pregnancy itself is a metabolic stress test. During the first half of pregnancy, transfer of maternal glucose to the fetus occurs; during the second half of pregnancy, placental hormones outweigh glucose transfer and insulin requirements typically double.

The placenta functions as a nutrient sensor, altering placental transport according to the maternal supply of nutrients. Placental transporters are regulated by hormones such as insulin. Insulin resistance occurs when gestational hormones such as human placental lactogen (HPL) interfere with insulin action. The accelerated fetal growth in women with diabetes is characterized by increased activity of placental and glucose transporters (Jansson and Powell, 2006). Cell signaling for insulin changes in GDM; women with diabetes or GDM may need one to two times more insulin than other pregnant women.

All pregnant women should be assessed for risk of GDM at the first prenatal visit; most women are screened between 24 and 28 weeks of gestation. One or more of the following factors identifies women at risk for GDM:

- Ethnicity: Hispanic American, African American, Asian, Pacific Islander, American Indian.
- Family history of diabetes in a first-degree relative (parents or siblings).
- Gestational diabetes or presence of a birth defect in a previous pregnancy.
- History of pregnancy-induced hypertension, urinary tract infections, or hydramnios (extra amniotic fluid).
- History of abnormal glucose tolerance.
- Older maternal age (>25-year old).
- Prepregnancy overweight or obesity; BMI >29.
- Previous birth of a large baby (>9 lb).
- Previous stillbirth or spontaneous miscarriage.

Hyperglycemia in pregnancy poses many complications and risks for the infant such as macrosomia, neural tube defects, hypocalcemia, hypomagnesemia, hyperbilirubinemia, birth trauma, prematurity, or neonatal hypoglycemia. Daily SMBG is important; fasting glucose levels should not exceed 105 mg/dL. Excellent blood glucose control with diet and, when necessary, insulin will result in improved perinatal outcome. HbA1c testing is not useful in GDM.

Women with a prior history of GDM and obesity are at significant high risk of developing MetS (Vohr and Boney, 2009). There is a higher risk of hypertension, pre-eclampsia, urinary tract infections, cesarean section, and future diabetes. About half of women who have GDM will proceed to have T2DM later, especially women who are hypertensive.

Nutrition recommendations should be based on a thorough nutrition assessment. Monitoring blood glucose levels, urine ketones, appetite, and weight gain guides the individualized nutrition prescription and meal plan. Adjustments should be made to the meal plan throughout pregnancy to ensure desired outcomes. See Table 9-16.

In women who have had bariatric surgery, close nutritional evaluation will be needed. Deficiencies in iron, vitamin A, vitamin B12, vitamin K, folate, and calcium can result in both maternal anemia and fetal complications, such as congenital abnormalities, IUGR and failure to thrive (Guelinckx et al, 2009).

Offspring of women with GDM are at increased risk for respiratory distress, macrosomia, jaundice, hypoglycemia, hyperinsulinemia, birth trauma, and developmental problems. Development of MetS in late adolescence and young adulthood is related to maternal glycemia in the third trimester, maternal obesity, neonatal macrosomia, and childhood obesity (Vohr and Boney, 2009).

Although treatment of mild GDM does not significantly reduce the frequency of stillbirth, perinatal death, or several neonatal complications, it does reduce the risks of fetal overgrowth, shoulder dystocia, cesarean delivery, and hypertensive disorders (Landon et al, 2009). Family planning, early screening for fetal abnormalities, compliance, glycemic and BP control during pregnancy, and improved neonatal care can make a difference.

After birth, rapid adaptation is necessary for infants to be able to maintain independent glucose homeostasis; this is compromised in infants who are small for gestational age (SGA), premature, or large for gestational age (Beardsall et al, 2008). Obesity, insulin resistance, and abnormal lipid metabolism bear ominous consequences for future generations (Vohr and Boney, 2009). For women who are offered treatment for mild GDM in addition to routine obstetric care,

TABLE 9-16 Glucose Testing for Gestational Diabetes Mellitus (GDM)

GDM often presents with hyperglycemia and glycosuria. Selective screening at 24–28 weeks of pregnancy is generally recommended, with a glucose challenge test and 1-hour assessment using either a 100-g or 75-g oral glucose load. Two or more of the venous plasma glucose concentrations must be met or exceeded for a positive diagnosis. The test should be done in the morning after an overnight fast.

American Diabetes Association criteria for GDM are noted below:

One-Step Approach

Perform a diagnostic oral glucose tolerance test (OGTT) without prior plasma or serum glucose screening. The one-step approach may be cost effective in high-risk patients or populations.

Two-Step Approach

Perform an initial screening by measuring the plasma or serum glucose concentration 1 hour after a 50-g oral glucose load (glucose challenge test [GCT]), and perform a diagnostic OGTT on the subset of women exceeding the glucose threshold value on the GCT. When the two-step approach is used, a glucose threshold value >140 mg/dL (>7.8 μmol/L) identifies approximately 80% of women with GDM, and the yield is further increased to 90% by using a cutoff of >130 mg/dL (>7.2 μmol/L).

Glucose Load	Glucose (mg/dL)
Glucose load, 100 g	
Fasting	95
1 hour	180
2 hours	155
3 hours	140

Sources: American Diabetes Association. Standards of Medical Care in Diabetes–2009.

additional charges are incurred but fewer babies experience serious perinatal complication or death (Moss et al, 2007). Nutritional intervention for GDM saves thousands of dollars per case. All women with GDM should receive nutritional counseling by an RD. MNT, initiated within 1 week of diagnosis and with a minimum of three nutrition visits, results in decreased hospital admissions and insulin use, improves likelihood of normal fetal and placental growth, and reduces risk of perinatal complications, especially when diagnosed and treated early (American Dietetic Association, 2009).

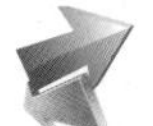

ASSESSMENT, MONITORING, AND EVALUATION

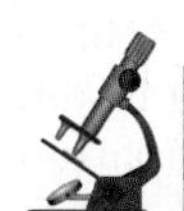

CLINICAL INDICATORS

Genetic Markers: GDM is associated with increased anti–human leukocyte antigen (HLA) class II antibodies in the maternal circulation (Steinborn, 2006). There may be some link between both autoimmune and nonautoimmune forms of diabetes and GDM.

Clinical/History

Height
Pregravid weight
Pregravid BMI
Pregravid waist circumference
Expected date of confinement (EDC)
No. of risk factors for GDM
Current weight
Goal weight
Weight gain pattern
Diet history
BP
Edema?
Periodontal disease?
Frequent urinary tract infections?
Ultrasonography for fetal growth

Lab Work

Ketones, fasting
H & H
Serum Gluc on awakening (95 mg/dL or lower)
1-hour postprandial glucose (not above 140 mg/dL)
2-hour postprandial glucose (not above 120 mg/dL)
Na^+, K^+
BUN
Creat (often elevated)
Alb, transthyretin
Microalbuminuria
Serum homocysteine levels
Ca^{++}, Mg^{++}
TSH (altered?)
OGTT
CRP

INTERVENTION

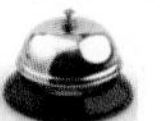

OBJECTIVES

- Prevent complications, perinatal morbidity, and mortality by normalizing the levels of glycemia and other metabolites (i.e., lipids and amino acids) to the levels of nondiabetic pregnant individuals.

SAMPLE NUTRITION CARE PROCESS STEPS

Inconsistent CHO Intake and Knowledge Deficit

Assessment Data: Blood glucose self-monitoring records, food diary worksheets and meal records, blood glucose levels (fasting, 2-hour postprandial).

Nutrition Diagnoses (PES):

(1) Inconsistent CHO intake (NI 5.8.4) related to lack of knowledge and confusion concerning gestational diabetic meal plan and CHO portion sizes as evidenced by postprandial blood sugars above and below desired ranges.

(2) Food and nutrition-related knowledge deficit (NB 1.1) related to gestational diabetic meal plan as evidenced by patient reported confusion and lack of confidence in meal planning and reported diet recall indicating inconsistent carbohydrate intake.

Interventions: E 2.2—review purpose of meal plan, CHO containing foods, portion sizes, CHO limits at meals/snacks. E 2.3, 2.5—provide advanced training in CHO counting, food label reading, menu planning, shopping tips.

Monitoring and Evaluation: Improvements in blood glucose levels; food diary and meal records showing more consistent intake of CHO throughout the day and before bedtime. Monitor at routine clinic visits for HgbA1c and weight gain. Assess need for further education/counseling; patient verbalizes better understanding of a meal plan and agrees to continue following plan.

- Optimize growth and development of the fetus. Desirable maternal weight gain will vary according to prepregnancy and current weight. Optimal weight gain is generally as follows: first trimester 0.5–1 kg (1–2 lb); second and third trimesters 0.2–0.5 kg/wk (0.5–1 lb/wk). Prevent weight loss.
- Obese women should control weight gain carefully. Excessive weight gain may be a forerunner of the MetS in offspring (Pirkola et al, 2008).
- Prevent infections and unexpected outcomes. Fetal glucose exposure and consequent fetal insulin secretion is normally tightly regulated by glucose delivery from the mother during pregnancy (Beardsall et al, 2008). The risk of spontaneous preterm birth increases with increasing levels of pregnancy glycemia.
- Control BP.
- Avoid incidents of starvation ketosis (where glucose is needed) and diabetic acidosis (where insulin and potassium are needed) by regular preprandial and postprandial SMBG. Ketosis is harmful to the baby.
- Use insulin when necessary, based on measures of maternal glycemia with or without assessment of fetal growth. Insulin therapy is recommended when nutrition intervention fails to maintain fasting whole-blood glucose at desired levels.
- Prevent hypoglycemic episodes, urinary tract infections, and candidiasis.
- Promote healthy lifestyle changes for the mother that will last long after delivery.
- Women with GDM should be encouraged to breastfeed.
- Physical activity, especially after meals, can help to maintain blood glucose control. Contraindications to exercise may include pregnancy-induced hypertension, intrauterine growth retardation, preterm labor or history of preterm labor, incompetent cervix/cervical cerclage, and persistent second or third trimester bleeding (American Dietetic Association, 2009).

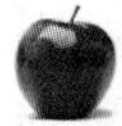

FOOD AND NUTRITION

- Use a carbohydrate-controlled meal plan with adequate intake to keep weight gain appropriate while preventing glycemic shifts or ketonuria; manage for age and weight goals. Provide adequate energy and nutrients to meet the needs maternal blood glucose goals that have been established. The typical diet may include 30–35 kcal/kg; 20% protein, 40–45% CHO, and 35–40% fat.
- Select CHO from whole grains, one fruit portion, or one milk portion at a time. Limit juices, sweets, or desserts. Sufficient CHO intake is needed, 175 g at minimum. Many women with GDM undereat out of fear of needing insulin; interval weight loss may indicate presence of fasting ketones. Insulin may be needed.
- While a low glycemic index diet may be beneficial for some outcomes for both mother and child, results are inconclusive at this time (Tieu et al, 2008).
- For obese women (BMI >30), a calorie limit ~25 kcal/kg actual weight per day has been shown to reduce hyperglycemia and plasma triglycerides with no increase in ketonuria. For many women, this translates to an energy intake around 1700–1800 kcal. Artificial sweeteners may be used, but not saccharin.
- Maintain an adequate intake of polyunsaturated fats; keep saturated fats to 10% of total fat or less.
- Most women require three meals and four to five snacks; snacks are eaten at least 2–3 hours between feedings and should contain carbohydrate.
- Smaller, more frequent meals and snacks will be beneficial because of insulin resistance. Work closely with a dietitian to establish the best pattern according to typical blood glucose levels. A snack before bedtime may be needed.
- DASH diet principles may be helpful if BP is elevated. Include regular use of antioxidant foods and spices such as cinnamon.
- Ensure intake of a prenatal vitamin–mineral supplement (especially containing 600 μg folic acid, 30–60 mg iron, vitamin C, and adequate calcium). Include adequate chromium intake from diet (as in yeast breads).
- Tube feeding may be useful in patients who cannot be fed orally or with hyperemesis. CHO-controlled products are not necessarily required; monitor closely.
- After delivery, a review of glucose tolerance and postpartum nutrition is suggested at 6–12 weeks.

Common Drugs Used and Potential Side Effects

- Investigators found no substantial maternal or neonatal outcome differences between use of glyburide or metformin compared with use of insulin in GDM (Nicholson et al, 2009). Insulin may be required to control blood glucose if diet and exercise do not help. Careful physician and self-monitoring is important. The insulin lispro is associated with fewer hypoglycemic events.
- Use prenatal vitamin–mineral supplements as prescribed. Avoid large doses of vitamin C, which may show false-positive urinary glucose levels; more than 200 mg/d is not needed.
- Low-dose estrogen–progesterone oral contraceptives may be used after GDM, if no medical contraindications exist. However, medications that worsen insulin resistance (e.g., glucocorticoids, nicotinic acid) should be avoided if possible.

Herbs, Botanicals, and Supplements

- In general, pregnant women should not take any herbs and botanical products. They should discuss concurrent or previous use with their physician.
- Supplements of 1,25-dihydroxyvitamin D_3 may influence glucose metabolism in GDM by increasing insulin sensitivity. More research is needed on postpartum requirements.
- Only limited evidence exists to support prenatal omega-3 supplementation; use caution for an unbalanced high DHA intake during the first two trimesters of pregnancy, that is, DHA without additional amino acid (AA) supplementation (Hadders-Algra, 2008).

- Conflicting results have been found for specific nutrients. Zinc and selenium seem to be protective, whereas chromium does not; more research is needed for micronutrient recommendations to be made (American Dietetic Association, 2009).

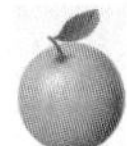

NUTRITION EDUCATION, COUNSELING, CARE MANAGEMENT

- The RD should monitor and evaluate blood glucose, weight, food intake, physical activity, and pharmacological therapy (if indicated) in women with GDM at each visit; MNT results in improved maternal and neonatal outcomes (American Dietetic Association, 2009).
- Communicate the importance of meal spacing, timing, adequacy, and consistency (i.e., patient should not skip meals). Instructions on what to eat and what to avoid will be important. Carrying a snack at all times is helpful (e.g., fruit, peanut butter, crackers). Follow current evidence-based guidelines.
- Regular aerobic exercise, such as walking, is beneficial. Exercise after meals may help to control blood sugar, but do not exercise until short of breath. Upper body exercises are also beneficial. Avoid exercises while lying on back as this decreases blood flow when the weight of the fetus presses on the main artery. Avoid exercises that increase the risk of falling.
- Encourage breastfeeding.
- Babies born to women who have GDM may have low levels of lipids such as arachidonic acid and docosahexaenoic acid (DHA); further studies are needed (Bitsanis, 2006).
- Encourage family planning to ensure optimal glucose regulation for all subsequent pregnancies. Women with a history of GDM are more likely to have recurrent diabetes if they are older, heavier and wait longer between pregnancies (e.g., 3 vs. 2 years) in many cases (Holmes et al, 2010). Recurrence of GDM is common, especially among non-Caucasian populations (Kim et al, 2007).
- Counsel regarding risk for T2DM. Any degree of abnormal glucose homeostasis during pregnancy independently predicts an increased risk of glucose intolerance and CVD postpartum (Retnakaran, 2009). Elevated FBG, OGTT 2-hour blood glucose, and OGTT glucose A1c are strong and consistent predictors of subsequent T2DM (Golden et al, 2009). Long-term lifestyle modifications, maintenance of normal body weight, and physical activity should be discussed.
- Discuss the potential impact of GDM on offspring, who are at increased risk of obesity, glucose intolerance, and diabetes in late adolescence or adulthood.

Patient Education—Foodborne Illness

- If home tube feeding is needed, teach appropriate sanitation and food-handling procedures.

For More Information

- American Diabetes Association
  http://www.diabetes.org/gestational-diabetes.jsp
- Baby Center – GDM
  http://www.babycenter.com/0_gestational-diabetes_2058.bc
- Diabetes and Pregnancy
  http://www.otispregnancy.org/pdf/diabetes
- NIDDK
  http://diabetes.niddk.nih.gov/dm/pubs/gestational/

GESTATIONAL DIABETES—CITED REFERENCES

American Dietetic Association. Evidence Analysis Library, Gestational Diabetes. Web site accessed October 9, 2009, at http://www.adaevidencelibrary.com/topic.cfm?cat=1399.

Bitsanis D, et al. Gestational diabetes mellitus enhances arachidonic and docosahexaenoic acids in placental phospholipids. *Lipids.* 41:341, 2006.

Golden SH, et al. Antepartum glucose tolerance test results as predictors of type 2 diabetes mellitus in women with a history of gestational diabetes mellitus: a systematic review. *Gend Med.* 6:109S, 2009.

Guelinckx I, et al. Reproductive outcome after bariatric surgery: a critical review. *Hum Reprod Update.* 15:189, 2009.

Hadders-Algra M. Prenatal long-chain polyunsaturated fatty acid status: the importance of a balanced intake of docosahexaenoic acid and arachidonic acid. *J Perinatal Med.* 36:101, 2008.

Holmes HJ, et al. Prediction of Diabetes Recurrence in Women with Class A1 (Diet-Treated) Gestational Diabetes. [published online ahead of print October 5, 2009] *Am J Perinatol.* 27(1):47, 2010.

Jansson T, Powell TL. IFPA 2005 Award in Placentology Lecture. Human placental transport in altered fetal growth: does the placenta function as a nutrient sensor?—a review. *Placenta.* 27:91S, 2006.

Kim C, et al. Recurrence of gestational diabetes mellitus: a systematic review. *Diabetes Care.* 30:1314, 2007.

Landon MB, et al. A multicenter, randomized trial of treatment for mild gestational diabetes. *N Engl J Med.* 361:1396, 2009.

March of Dimes. Gestational diabetes. Web site accessed October 8, 2009, at http://www.marchofdimes.com/pnhec/188_1025.asp.

Moss JR, et al. Costs and consequences of treatment for mild gestational diabetes mellitus—evaluation from the ACHOIS randomised trial. *BMC Pregnancy Childbirth.* 7:27, 2007.

Nicholson W, et al. Benefits and risks of oral diabetes agents compared with insulin in women with gestational diabetes: a systematic review. *Obstet Gynecol.* 113:193, 2009.

Pirkola J, et al. Maternal type 1 and gestational diabetes: postnatal differences in insulin secretion in offspring at preschool age. *Pediatr Diabetes.* 9:583, 2008.

Retnakaran R. Glucose tolerance status in pregnancy: a window to the future risk of diabetes and cardiovascular disease in young women. [published online ahead of print August 1, 2009] *Curr Diab Rev.* 5:239.

Steinborn A, et al. The presence of gestational diabetes is associated with increased detection of anti-HLA-class II antibodies in the maternal circulation. *Am J Reprod Immunol.* 56:124, 2006.

Tieu J, et al. Dietary advice in pregnancy for preventing gestational diabetes mellitus. *Cochrane Database Syst Rev.* 2008;16(2):CD006674.

Vohr BR, Boney CM. Gestational diabetes: the forerunner for the development of maternal and childhood obesity and metabolic syndrome? *J Matern Fetal Neonatal Med.* 21:149, 2009.

PRE-ECLAMPSIA AND PREGNANCY-INDUCED HYPERTENSION

NUTRITIONAL ACUITY RANKING: LEVEL 2

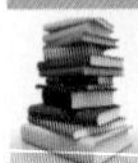

DEFINITIONS AND BACKGROUND

Pre-eclampsia is defined as the association of pregnancy-induced hypertension (PIH) and proteinuria of 300 mg/24 h or more after 20-weeks estation. It is more common in primigravidas and in patients with multiple gestation, T1DM, teenage mothers, family history of PIH, age over 40 years, or underlying vascular or renal disease. It affects 2–8% of pregnancies and is a severe complication, which may lead to fetal morbidity and mortality. Risks for the baby include poor growth and prematurity (Duley, 2009).

Pre-eclampsia can lead to problems in the liver, kidneys, brain, and the clotting system (Duley, 2009). Maternal morbidity includes placental abruption, HELLP syndrome (hemolysis, elevated liver enzymes, low platelets) or eclampsia; treatment consists of ending the pregnancy. Early sonogram is recommended; many women will have to have total bed rest. Severe pre-eclampsia that develops at <34 weeks of gestation is associated with high perinatal mortality and morbidity (Sibai and Barton, 2007). Women who are 37-week pregnant are induced immediately.

Criteria for **mild pre-eclampsia** include hypertension as defined at 140/90 to 159/109 mm Hg; proteinuria >300 mg/24 h; mild edema with weight gain >2 lb/wk or >6 lb/month; and urine output >500 mL/24 h. Signs and symptoms include increased BP, proteinuria, facial edema, pretibial pitting edema, irritability, nausea and vomiting, nervousness, headache, altered states of consciousness, epigastric pain, and oliguria.

Criteria for **severe pre-eclampsia** include: BP >160/110 mm Hg on two occasions with patient on bed rest; systolic BP rise >60 mm Hg over baseline; diastolic BP increase of >30 mm Hg over baseline; proteinuria >5 g/24 h or 3+ or 4+ on a urine dipstick; massive edema; and oliguria <400 mL/24 h. Symptoms include pulmonary edema, severe headaches, visual changes, right upper quadrant pain, elevated liver enzymes, and thrombocytopenia in addition to the symptoms listed for mild pre-eclampsia.

In **eclampsia,** a seizure occurs. Eclamptic seizures and symptoms of the HELLP syndrome occur. In severe cases, there may also be hepatic rupture, pulmonary edema, acute renal failure, placental abruption, elevated creatinine, intrauterine growth restriction, cerebral hemorrhage, cortical blindness, and retinal detachment. Maternal mortality rate is 8–36%.

Because plasma homocysteine is often increased, sufficient intakes of folic acid, vitamins B_{12} and B_6 are recommended (Mignini et al, 2005). Studies have also shown the effectiveness of magnesium in eclampsia and pre-eclampsia (Guerrera et al, 2009).

SAMPLE NUTRITION CARE PROCESS STEPS

Disordered Eating Pattern

Assessment Data: Food records, weight records. Diet hx reveals intake of one large meal daily, mostly canned soup and sandwiches; no fruits and few vegetables. BP 170/90 average; abnormal lung function tests (LFTs).

Nutrition Diagnosis (PES): Disordered eating pattern (NB 1.5) related to lack of knowledge concerning nutrition during pregnancy as evidenced by excessive prenatal weight gain, frequent meal skipping, increased BP, and diet lacking in vitamins and minerals and statement that "I can't eat more than once a day because it isn't good for the baby."

Intervention: ND 3.2.1—daily use of prenatal vitamin. Education and counseling about appropriate dietary intake and meal frequency during pregnancy; dangers of skipping meals; when to contact the doctor. E 1.2—priority modifications of diet include not skipping meals, ensure adequate calcium, folic acid, potassium and magnesium; control sodium intake. C 1.3—Health Belief Model of counseling used to motivate patient in making necessary dietary changes.

Monitoring and Evaluation: Weight and prenatal growth charts; improved intake. Lab reports and BP records showing improvement in all aspects. Check urine protein and presence of edema. Successful outcome for infant and mother, even if hospitalization is required.

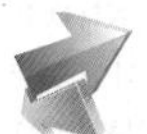

ASSESSMENT, MONITORING, AND EVALUATION

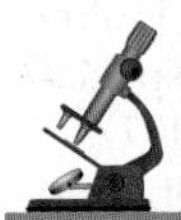

CLINICAL INDICATORS

Genetic Markers: Women with pre-eclampsia have higher levels of a peptide that increases BP in the pieces of tissue linking mother and fetus.

Clinical/History

Height
Pregravid weight
Pregravid BMI
Pregravid waist circumference
EDC
Current weight
Weight gain pattern
Diet history
Edema in lower extremities
BP (mild, ≥140/90 mm Hg; severe, >160/110 mm Hg)
Decreased urine output
Confusion, apprehension
Shortness of breath
Right upper quadrant abdominal pain
Dizziness
Visual changes (blurring, double vision)
Excessive nausea or vomiting
Severe headaches
Fever?
Blood in urine?

Lab Work

GFR
Alb, transthyretin (often low)

Proteinuria (>300 mg/d is mild; >500 mg/d is severe)	BUN	Liver function tests (AST, ALT, LDH)
H & H	Creat (may be elevated)	Microalbuminuria
Serum Fe	Homocysteine	
Chol, Trig (elevated?)	CRP	
Gluc	PT, INR	
Ca^{++}	HELLP syndrome (decreased platelets, abnormal liver function tests)	
Mg^{++}		
Na^{+}, K^{+}		
Uric acid (elevated)		

INTERVENTION

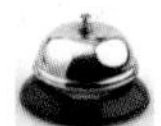

OBJECTIVES

- Reduce maternal and neonatal mortality and morbidity. In pregnant patients with diabetes and chronic hypertension, BP target goals of 110–129/65–79 mm Hg are suggested. Avoid lower BP because fetal growth may be impaired.
- Lessen edema when present. Correct any underlying malnutrition or micronutrient deficiencies.
- Monitor any sudden weight gains (1 kg/wk) that are unexplained by food intake.
- Prevent, if possible, chronic hypertension and MetS after delivery.

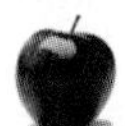

FOOD AND NUTRITION

- Maintain diet as ordered for age and pregnancy stage (generally 300 kcal more than prepregnancy diet). Use extra fruits and vegetables and less sucrose.
- Sources of magnesium include green leafy vegetables, nuts, legumes, and whole grains.
- Supplement with prenatal vitamins. Include folic acid, calcium, other B-complex vitamins, protein, selenium, and potassium from diet. The role of vitamins C and E does not benefit women at risk for pre-eclampsia (Villar et al, 2009). Antioxidant supplements are also not recommended (Rumbold et al, 2008).
- Sodium intake may need to be controlled to 2 g/d if edema is severe. Diuretics generally are not used.
- There may be some merit for including a sufficient intake of omega-3 fatty acids from salmon, tuna, walnuts, and flaxseed oil.

Common Drugs Used and Potential Side Effects

- The only interventions shown to prevent pre-eclampsia are antiplatelet agents, primarily low-dose aspirin, calcium supplementation and magnesium sulfate for eclamptic seizures (Duley, 2009). Avoid excessive magnesium from supplements if this medication is being used.
- Corticosteroids for lung maturity may be necessary.
- During pregnancy, typical diuretics and cardiac drugs are not used. ACE inhibitors and ARBs are contraindicated. Calcium pump inhibitors are often a first line choice.

Herbs, Botanicals, and Supplements

- Herbs and botanical supplements should not be used in pregnancy.
- Evening primrose has been suggested for this condition. Coenzyme Q10 and alpha-tocopherol are potent antioxidants.
- See Table 9-9 for guidance on more specific herbs and supplements that the client may have used.

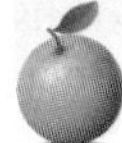

NUTRITION EDUCATION, COUNSELING, CARE MANAGEMENT

- Rest is essential during this time. Biofeedback, yoga, meditation, and other forms of stress reduction are often beneficial.
- Meal skipping should be avoided at all costs.
- Discuss adequate sources of calcium from the diet, especially if dairy products are not tolerated or preferred.
- Good sources of potassium and magnesium include nuts, fruits and vegetables. The DASH diet is an excellent diet to continue, even after pregnancy.

Patient Education—Foodborne Illness

- If home tube feeding is needed, teach appropriate sanitation and food-handling procedures.

For More Information

- Diabetes and Preeclampsia
  http://diabetes.healthcentersonline.com/womensdiabetes/preeclampsia.cfm
- Mayo Clinic
  http://www.mayoclinic.com/health/preeclampsia/DS00583
- Pregnancy and Preeclampsia
  http://familydoctor.org/064.xml

PRE-ECLAMPSIA AND PIH—CITED REFERENCES

Duley L. The global impact of pre-eclampsia and eclampsia. *Semin Perinatol.* 33:130, 2009.

Guerrera MP, et al. Therapeutic uses of magnesium. *Am Fam Physician.* 80:157, 2009.

Rumbold A, et al. Antioxidants for preventing pre-eclampsia. *Cochrane Database Syst Rev.* CD004227, 2008.

Sibai BM, Barton JR. Expectant management of severe preeclampsia remote from term: patient selection, treatment, and delivery indications. *Am J Obstet Gynecol.* 196:514, 2007.

Villar J, et al. World Health Organisation multicentre randomised trial of supplementation with vitamins C and E among pregnant women at high risk for pre-eclampsia in populations of low nutritional status from developing countries. *BJOG.* 116:8780, 2009.

DIABETIC GASTROPARESIS

NUTRITIONAL ACUITY RANKING: LEVEL 3–4

DEFINITIONS AND BACKGROUND

Gastroparesis occurs in approximately 50% of all cases of diabetes (Aring et al, 2005), with delayed gastric emptying (DGE) in the absence of mechanical obstruction. Diabetic gastroparesis is the result of ongoing damage to the nerves that are responsible for peristalsis and normal motility. Foods digest abnormally slowly or peristalsis is diminished so that it is difficult to match insulin action to digestion and absorption of the meals. If food stays in the stomach too long, infection is possible. Also, the food can harden into a solid lump; these bezoars may cause pain, nausea, and blockages in the digestive tract.

Hypoglycemia can occur if insulin is working and if food remains in the stomach too long. Later, insulin action is diminished and food finally digests, causing hyperglycemia. Problems occur more often in type 1 than in T2DM. Strict glycemic control is key.

A gastrostomy is rarely indicated, but a jejunostomy may be helpful in maintaining nutrition. Prokinetic agents are the best treatment option; see Section 7 for more details on management of gastroparesis. Gastric electrical stimulation may be used to send out brief, low-energy impulses to the stomach to decrease nausea and vomiting.

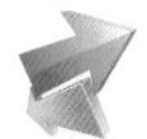

ASSESSMENT, MONITORING, AND EVALUATION

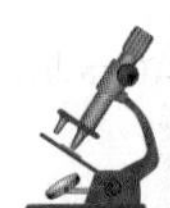

CLINICAL INDICATORS

Genetic Markers: T1DM has a genetic component, but gastroparesis would be individually acquired.

Clinical/History

- Height
- Weight
- BMI
- I & O
- Diet history
- Early satiety
- DGE
- Diarrhea or constipation
- Vomiting undigested food
- Nausea
- Reflux or heartburn
- Abdominal bloating or pain
- Upper endoscopy
- Barium x-ray
- Gastric emptying scintigraphy (GES)
- Gastric manometry

Lab Work

- HbA1c
- H & H
- Serum Fe
- Gastrin
- Gluc (fasting and 30 minutes after meals)
- Na^+, K^+
- Alb, transthyretin
- CRP
- Chol, Trig

SAMPLE NUTRITION CARE PROCESS STEPS

Abnormal GI Function

Assessment Data: Blood glucose self-monitoring records, nausea, gastroesophageal reflux (GERD) and reflux with meals, abdominal discomfort. Irregular FBG levels from day to day.

Nutrition Diagnosis (PES): Abnormal GI function related to gastroparesis as evidenced by nausea, GERD, and abdominal discomfort.

Intervention: Meal records and food diary listing symptoms and frequency of discomfort. Blood glucose self-monitoring records. Discussion about use of prokinetic agents.

Monitoring and Evaluation: Glucose records, food diary and records, discussion about GI symptoms.

INTERVENTION

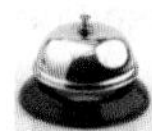

OBJECTIVES

- Correct the fluctuating blood glucose levels through careful food and insulin management, frequent blood glucose checks and monitoring records.
- For nausea and vomiting, restore volume and hydration and provide antiemetics generously.
- Relieve symptoms (pain, diarrhea, constipation) and maintain adequate nutritional status.
- Differentiate from ketoacidosis, which has similar symptoms of nausea and vomiting.
- Prevent infection or bezoar formation from accumulation of indigestible solids.

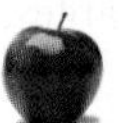

FOOD AND NUTRITION

- Monitor intake carefully; blood glucose fluctuations are common. Include 200–240 g CHO daily, spread throughout the day. Use two to three CHO servings per meal. Be consistent from day to day.
- Soft-to-liquid diet may be useful to prevent delay in gastric emptying. Six small meals may be better tolerated than large meals.
- Use a low-fat diet to improve digestion and to improve stomach emptying. Stay sitting after meals.
- Decrease overall fiber intake from meals or supplements. Oranges, broccoli, green beans, berries, figs, and fresh apples may be difficult to digest.
- For dry mouth, add extra fluids and moisten foods with broth or allowed sauces or gravies.
- If nausea occurs, cold foods and low-odor choices may be better tolerated.

- In severe problems, a percutaneous jejunostomy (PEJ) tube feeding may be indicated. It can be used temporarily if needed to correct malnutrition.

Common Drugs Used and Potential Side Effects

- Prokinetics such as metoclopramide (Reglan) may be given 30 minutes before meals to increase gastric contractions and to relax pyloric sphincter. Dry mouth, sleepiness, diarrhea or nausea can be side effects. Emitasol is a nasal spray form of this medication. Metoclopramide prophylaxis to reduce gastric volumes before elective surgery is unnecessary unless the patient has a prolonged history of poor blood glucose control (Jellish et al, 2005).
- Rapid-acting insulin should be injected with or after meals. Use SMBG to monitor delayed absorption and glucose changes. Insulin lispro (Humalog) is quite effective because it starts working shortly after injection. To control blood glucose, it may be necessary to take insulin more often, to take insulin after eating instead before, and to check blood glucose often after eating.
- If a liquid diet is used, more insulin may be needed. Insulin pumps may be beneficial because insulin delivery rates can be programmed to the patient's individual needs.
- Because there is a reciprocal relationship between gastric emptying and ambient glucose concentrations, newer diabetes therapies that decelerate the rate of gastric emptying may be a beneficial tool (Samsom et al, 2009).
- Antiemetics may be used for vomiting. Monitor for specific side effects. Zofran may cause constipation or headache.
- Erythromycin improves stomach emptying by increasing the contractions that move food through the stomach. Side effects are nausea, vomiting, diarrhea, and abdominal cramps.
- Dramamine (dimenhydrinate) is an antihistamine that helps prevent nausea and vomiting; slight-to-moderate drowsiness and thickening of bronchial secretions may occur.
- Motilium (domperidome) is used to manage the upper GI problems; side effects may include headache.

Herbs, Botanicals, and Supplements

- Herbs and botanical supplements should not be used without discussing with physician.
- See Table 9-9 for guidance on more specific herbs and supplements.

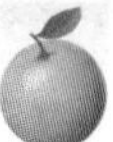

NUTRITION EDUCATION, COUNSELING, CARE MANAGEMENT

- Discuss delayed digestion and absorption of food.
- Discuss role of diet in maintaining weight and controlling discomfort. Emphasize nutrient-dense foods if intake has been poor. Blenderized foods or smoothies may be well tolerated.
- Bezoar formation may occur after eating oranges, coconuts, green beans, apples, figs, potato skins, Brussels sprouts, broccoli, sauerkraut, corn, sauerkraut, and other high-fiber foods.
- Discuss insulin management, as appropriate. Include information about SMBG and meal spacing. Advise the doctor if blood glucose levels are >200 mg/dL.

Patient Education—Foodborne Illness

- If home tube feeding is needed, teach appropriate sanitation and food-handling procedures.

For More Information

- American Diabetes Association
  http://www.diabetes.org/type-1-diabetes/Gastroparesis.jsp
- Ask the Dietitian
  http://www.dietitian.com/drugnutr.html
- Diabetic Gastroparesis
  http://digestive.niddk.nih.gov/ddiseases/pubs/gastroparesis/
- Gastroparesis and Dysmotilities Association (GPDA)
  http://www.digestivedistress.com/main/page.php?page_id=26

DIABETIC GASTROPARESIS—CITED REFERENCES

Jellish WS, et al. Effect of metoclopramide on gastric fluid volumes in diabetic patients who have fasted before elective surgery. *Anesthesiology.* 102:904, 2005.

Samsom M, et al. Diabetes mellitus and gastric emptying: questions and issues in clinical practice. *Diab Metab Res Rev.* 25:502, 2009.

van der Voort IR, et al. Gastric electrical stimulation results in improved metabolic control in diabetic patients suffering from gastroparesis. *Exp Clin Endocrinol Diabetes.* 113:38, 2005.

DIABETIC KETOACIDOSIS

NUTRITIONAL ACUITY RANKING: LEVEL 3–4

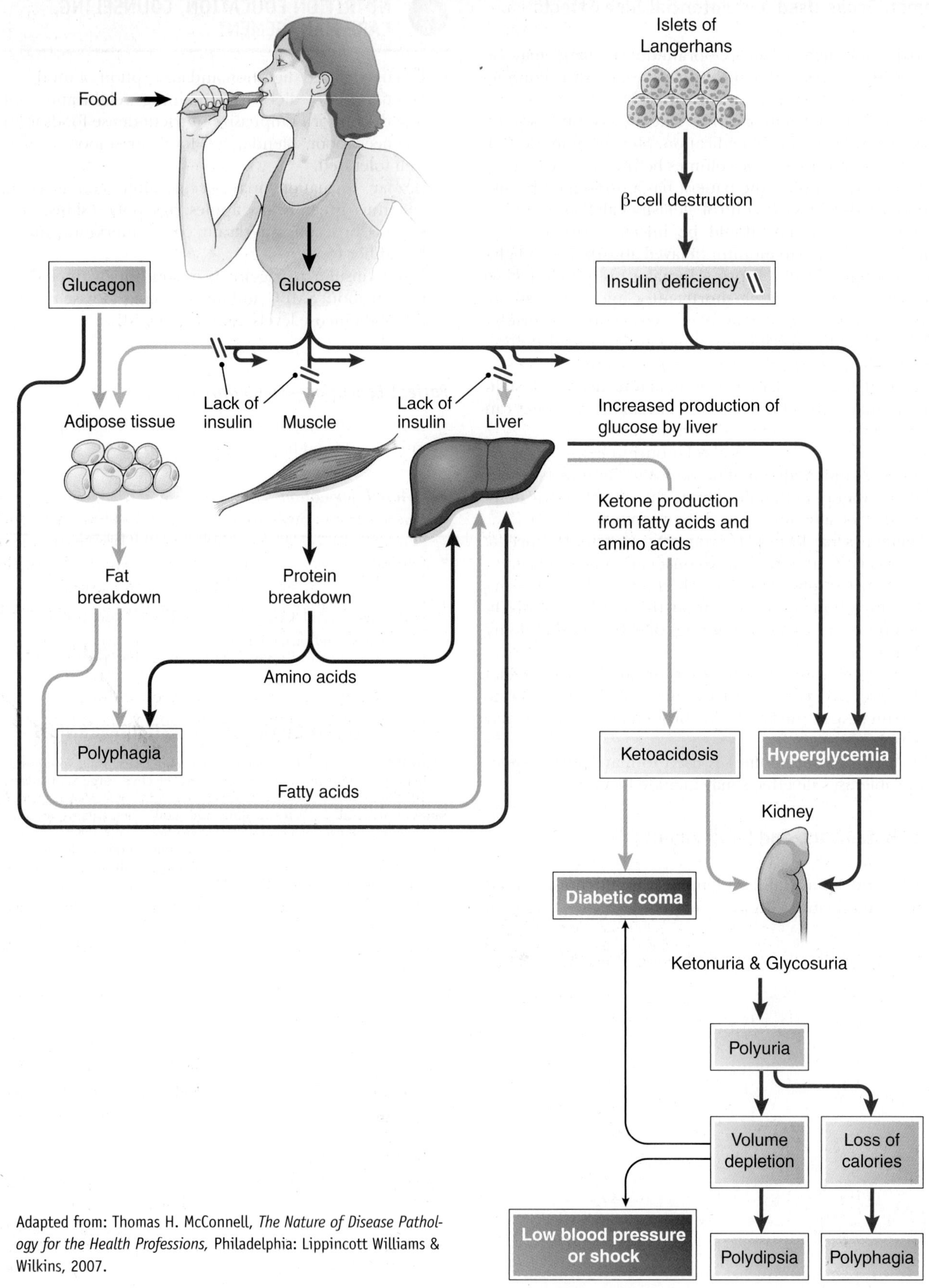

Adapted from: Thomas H. McConnell, *The Nature of Disease Pathology for the Health Professions*, Philadelphia: Lippincott Williams & Wilkins, 2007.

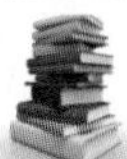

DEFINITIONS AND BACKGROUND

Ketones in the urine mean that the body is burning fat to get energy because glucose is not available. The lack of insulin leads to gluconeogenesis in the liver, then glucose spills into the urine and causes an osmotic diuresis with dehydration. Free fatty acids are released from the adipose tissue and converted into acidic ketones (acetoacetate and β-Hydroxybutyrate) by the liver.

Large amounts of ketones in the serum and urine can be dangerous. Diabetic ketoacidosis (DKA) is classic metabolic acidosis, a medical emergency that accounts for more than 100,000 hospital admissions yearly in the United States. A patient with a low serum potassium level should be assumed to have a potentially life-threatening crisis.

Causes of DKA include not getting enough insulin from missed injections; alkaline reserves depleted by too little insulin, flu or colds, fever, pregnancy, stress, trauma, or myocardial infarction; infection (leading cause); urinary tract infections and pneumonia. The triad of uncontrolled hyperglycemia, metabolic acidosis, and increased total body ketone concentration characterizes DKA. These metabolic derangements result from the combination of absolute or relative insulin deficiency and increased levels of the counterregulatory hormones of glucagon, catecholamines, cortisol, and growth hormone. Table 9-17 provides defining characteristics for DKA and hyperosmolar hyperglycemic state (HHS).

DKA is seen primarily in patients with T1DM; a few type 1 diabetic patients presenting with DKA on initial diagnosis. In children, DKA is a leading cause of hospitalization and is a cause of cerebral edema, which may lead to death if untreated. DKA can also occur in T2DM, usually from urinary tract infections, trauma, stress, pregnancy, surgery, or myocardial infarction. Inflammatory processes may play a role. Both DKA and its treatment produce varying degrees of immunological stress (Jerath et al, 2005). All individuals with DKA should be tested for hyperthyroidism (Potenza et al, 2009). Use of standardized written guidelines have merit.

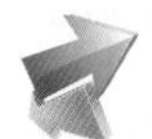

ASSESSMENT, MONITORING, AND EVALUATION

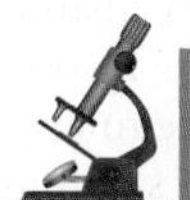

CLINICAL INDICATORS

Genetic Markers: There are no specific genes for DKA, but diabetes itself has a genetic component.

Clinical/History

Height
Weight
BMI
Diet history
Temperature
I & O
BP (often low)
Nausea and vomiting
Hot or dry and flushed skin
Diarrhea
Fruity breath
Intense thirst
Profound dehydration
Dim vision
Labored or rapid breathing (Kussmaul)
Pruritus
Polyuria
Cramping
Seizures or drowsiness

Lab Work

Mild: blood pH 7.25–7.30; bicarbonate 15–18 μmol/L; alert
Moderate: pH 7.00–7.25, bicarbonate 10–15, mild drowsiness
Severe: pH < 7.00, bicarbonate <10, stupor or coma
Gluc (>250 mg/dL)
HgbA1c
Beta-hydroxybutyrate levels
K^+ (low?)
Urinary glucose, ketones, osmolality
T3, T4, TSH levels
CRP
BUN (increased)
Creat
Na^+ (decreased)
Cl^- (decreased)
HbA1c
Amylase (increased)
WBC (elevated with infections)
pCO_2 (decreased)
pO_2
Uric acid (increased)
AST (decreased)
ALT, LDH, creatine kinase (CK) (increased)
Phosphate (often decreased)
Mg^{++} (often decreased)
Chol (increased), Trig
Ca^{++}

INTERVENTION

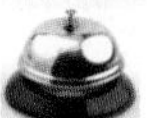

OBJECTIVES

- Correct the high blood glucose level by giving more insulin. Frequent blood glucose and ketone monitoring is necessary. Note that urine ketones lag behind serum ketones because it takes time to the empty the bladder, where they have accumulated and been stored.
- Replace fluids and electrolytes lost through excessive urination and vomiting.
- Promote return to wellness after poor health for several days.
- Evaluate precipitating factors such as surgery, trauma, urinary tract infection, pneumonia, or influenza.
- Monitor frequently to prevent recurrence of DKA.

TABLE 9-17 Diagnostic Criteria for Diabetic Ketoacidosis (DKA) and Hyperosmolar Hyperglycemic State (HHS)

	DKA			
Criteria	**Mild**	**Moderate**	**Severe**	**HHS**
Plasma glucose (mg/dL)	>250	>250	>250	>600
Arterial pH	7.25–7.30	7.00–7.24	<7.00	>7.30
Serum bicarbonate (mEq/L)	15–18	10–<15	<10	>15
Urine ketones	Positive	Positive	Positive	Small
Serum ketones	Positive	Positive	Positive	Small
Effective serum osmolality (mOsm/kg)	Variable	Variable	Variable	>320
Altered mental status	Alert	Alert/drowsy	Stupor/coma	Stupor/coma

Adapted with permission from Kitabchi AE, et al. Hyperglycemic crises in diabetes. *Diabetes Care.* 27:S95, 2004.

SAMPLE NUTRITION CARE PROCESS STEPS

Self Monitoring Deficit

Assessment Data: Admission to unit with DKA, random blood glucose levels >600, semi-comatose state, unable to eat orally.

Nutrition Diagnosis (PES): Self monitoring deficit (NB-1.4) related to blood glucose monitoring and diabetes management as evidenced by DKA, BG > 600, lethargy, nausea and vomiting past 2 days, and report by family that "he doesn't test his sugars as he should."

Intervention: Food and nutrient delivery with IVs and tube feeding until semicomatose state resolves and glucose levels are below 200 consistently. Educate patient when possible about the dangers of not monitoring BG levels. Teach methods for simplifying records, tracking lab results, and self-monitoring of glucose and activity levels to match insulin therapy.

Monitoring and Evaluation: Improved cognition and ability to resume an oral diet. Able to describe how to track glucose, lab results, physical activity, and insulin; defined own goals for reporting signs and symptoms to doctor when hyperglycemia persists. Able to state the signs of impending DKA and measures to take immediately.

- Prevent complications such as shock, arterial thrombosis, renal failure, or cerebral edema (CEDKA). CEDKA remains a significant problem with a high mortality rate (Lawrence et al, 2005). Young children are especially vulnerable and may slip into a coma.
- For chronically high fasting glucose levels, adjust evening intermediate- or long-acting insulin doses or timing.

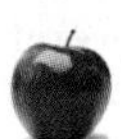

FOOD AND NUTRITION

- If patient is comatose, intravenous insulin, electrolytes, and fluids are used. A nasogastric tube may be placed to prevent aspiration during feeding. If patient is alert and oriented, offer plenty of fluids orally.
- As treatment progresses, a 5% glucose solution is usually given as glucosuria and hyperglycemia subside. If glucosuria and hyperglycemia do not decrease, try tea and salty broth. Later, fruit juices and liquids high in potassium may be given.
- Resolution of DKA leads to the ability to tolerate oral nutrition and fluids, normalization of blood acidity (pH>7.3), and absence of ketones in blood (<1 μmol/l). Once this has been achieved, insulin may be switched to the usual regimen.

Common Drugs Used and Potential Side Effects

- Insulin and fluid are usually given intravenously to decrease blood glucose by 50–75 mg/dL/h. Guidelines may recommend a bolus (initial large dose) of insulin of 0.1 unit of insulin/kg of body weight if potassium level is higher than 3.3. Regular and glulisine insulin are equally effective during the acute treatment of DKA; a basal bolus regimen with glargine and glulisine is safer than NPH and regular insulin after the resolution of DKA (Umpierrez et al, 2009).
- Dextrose in saline is given once plasma glucose decreases to avoid accidental hypoglycemia.
- Potassium, phosphate and magnesium levels may be low. Bicarbonate therapy is needed only rarely (Trachtenbarg, 2005).
- Intravenous antibiotic therapy will be needed where there is sepsis.
- Atypical antipsychotics, thiazide diuretics, and corticosteroids can lead to DKA if the patient is not carefully monitored.

Herbs, Botanicals, and Supplements

- Herbs and botanical supplements should not be used without discussing with physician.
- See Table 9-9 for guidance on more specific herbs and supplements.

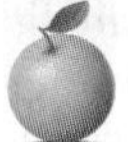

NUTRITION EDUCATION, COUNSELING, CARE MANAGEMENT

- Explain demand for more insulin during illness and infection. Use of a diabetes record may be useful if episodes of high blood glucose are frequent.
- Never exercise when there are ketones present.
- Because every episode of DKA implies breakdown in clinical communication, appropriate diabetes education should be reinforced. Education of patients and their social environment to promote frequent testing—especially during sick days—and to lower their glucose levels, as well as to recognize the early symptoms of hyperglycemia and DKA is of paramount importance in preventing the development of severe DKA (Weber et al, 2009).
- When strict control through insulin is administered, weight gain is common. Insulin omission and reduction, which are eating disorder symptoms unique to diabetes mellitus, are associated with an increased risk of DKA. Attention to this disorder is important in overall treatment planning and management.
- The biggest risk of insulin pump therapy is DKA since no long-acting insulin is used. Any interruption to insulin delivery or pump malfunctioning can cause DKA. To prevent this reaction, monitor blood glucose regularly. Insulin pump users also need to check often to see that insulin is still flowing through the tubing.

Patient Education—Foodborne Illness

- If home tube feeding is needed, teach appropriate sanitation and food-handling procedures.

For More Information

- American Diabetes Association
  http://www.diabetes.org/type-1-diabetes/ketoacidosis.jsp
- Merck manual – DKA
  http://www.merck.com/mmpe/sec12/ch158/ch158c.html
- NIDDK–Diabetic Ketoacidosis
  http://diabetes.niddk.nih.gov/DM/pubs/dictionary/K-O.htm

DIABETIC KETOACIDOSIS—CITED REFERENCES

Jerath RS, et al. Complement activation in diabetic ketoacidosis and its treatment. *Clin Immunol.* 116:11, 2005.

Lawrence SE, et al. Population-based study of incidence and risk factors for cerebral edema in pediatric diabetic ketoacidosis. *J Pediatr.* 146:688, 2005.

Potenza M, et al. Excess thyroid hormone and carbohydrate metabolism. *Endocrin Pract.* 15:254, 2009.

Trachtenbarg DE. Diabetic ketoacidosis. *Am Fam Physician.* 71:1705, 2005.

Umpierrez GE, et al. Insulin analogs versus human insulin in the treatment of patients with diabetic ketoacidosis: a randomized controlled trial. *Diabetes Care.* 32:1164, 2009.

Weber C, et al. Prevention of diabetic ketoacidosis and self-monitoring of ketone bodies: an overview. *Curr Med Res Opin.* 25:1197, 2009.

HYPEROSMOLAR HYPERGLYCEMIC STATE

NUTRITIONAL ACUITY RANKING: LEVEL 3–4

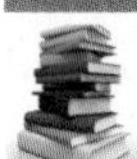

DEFINITIONS AND BACKGROUND

Diabetic HHS is a life-threatening emergency with marked elevation of blood glucose, hyperosmolarity, and minimal or no ketosis (Stoner, 2005). HHS is preventable if blood glucose is monitored regularly in order to correct elevating levels before problems occur. The condition occurs in patients older than age 70 years with T2DM and profound dehydration as precipitating factors. If recognized early, HHS can frequently be treated in the outpatient setting if the patient can take fluids. Table 9-18 provides diagnostic criteria. Sometimes DKA is the first time that diabetes is diagnosed.

Identification and treatment of the underlying and precipitating causes of HHS are absolutely essential. Predisposing factors for this syndrome include long-term uncontrolled hyperglycemia, pancreatic disease, infections or sepsis, stroke, surgery, extensive burns, renal or CVD, corticosteroid use, diuretics, excessive total parenteral nutrition (TPN), dialysis.

Underlying poor compliance with medications, infections, alcohol, or cocaine abuse are the most common causes. In children, corticosteroid use and gastroenteritis are common causes. The mortality rate is high at 10–20%. Areas of future research include prospective randomized studies to determine the pathophysiological mechanisms for the absence of ketosis in HHS and to investigate the reasons for elevated proinflammatory cytokines and cardiovascular risk factors (Kitabchi et al, 2008).

TABLE 9-18 Quick Sources of Glucose

4 oz grape, cranberry, or prune juice	19 g CHO
1 tbsp honey	17 g CHO
1/2 cup sweetened gelatin	17 g CHO
1 tbsp corn syrup, jam, jelly or glucose	15 g CHO
5 Lifesavers candies	15 g CHO
4 oz orange, apple, pineapple, grapefruit juice	12–15 g CHO
4 oz regular soft drink	13 g CHO
1 tbsp sugar, dissolved in water	13 g CHO
2 tablespoons raisins	10–15 g CHO
5–6 Lifesaver candies	10–15 g CHO
1 cup 2% or skim milk	12 g CHO
3–4 glucose tablets	4–5 g CHO each

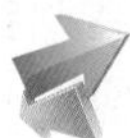

ASSESSMENT, MONITORING, AND EVALUATION

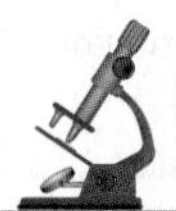

CLINICAL INDICATORS

Genetic Markers: HHS is acquired and not genetic, although T2DM has a genetic component. African Americans, Hispanics, and Native Americans have the highest rates.

Clinical/History

Height
Weight
BMI
Diet history
BP (hypotension?)
I & O
Profound dehydration (8–12 L)
Fever or hypothermia?
Excessive thirst and urination
Dry, parched mouth
Sunken eyes
Dry skin with no sweating
Weakness, lethargy
Leg cramps
Sleepiness or confusion
Rapid pulse and abnormal respirations
Convulsions, grand mal seizures, or coma

Lab Work

Gluc (>600 mg/dL)
Na^+, K^+
Bicarbonate >15 mEq/L
Serum osmolality (usually >320 mOsm)
pH levels greater than 7.30
Mild or absent ketonemia
Elevated serum urea nitrogen (BUN)-to-creatinine ratio
Alb
H & H
PO_4
Chol, Trig
CRP

INTERVENTION

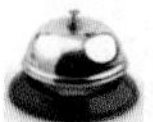

OBJECTIVES

- Correct dehydration, shock, and cardiac arrhythmias.
- Reduce elevated blood glucose levels with isotonic saline, then hypotonic saline along with insulin.
- Monitor fluid status and replace deficits, which may be 10–20% of total body weight. This may require up to 9 L in 48 hours (Stoner, 2005).

SAMPLE NUTRITION CARE PROCESS STEPS

Excessive Alcohol Intake

Assessment Data: Blood glucose self-monitoring records with FBG >650; recent heavy intake of alcohol; fever; profound dehydration and signs of HHS; admitted to Emergency Room from a wedding reception; lives with son and daughter-in-law.

Nutrition Diagnosis (PES): Excessive alcohol intake related to lack of understanding about the impact of alcohol on diabetes as evidenced by confusion, profound dehydration, FBG >650, and fever after intake of four alcoholic beverages within 3 hours at a wedding reception.

Intervention: Teaching patient and family members about dangers of large doses of alcohol mixed with diabetes medication, especially with aging. Counseling about how to include an occasional alcoholic beverage and ways to participate in social events without excessive intake.

Monitoring and Evaluation: Improved glucose labs, resolution of HHS, fever and dehydration.

- Prevent future crises by appropriate DSME and regular monitoring of blood glucose.
- Prevent acute renal failure, which could result from prolonged hypovolemia.

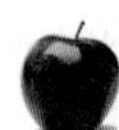

FOOD AND NUTRITION

- Offer fluid replacement, often 1 L/h until volume is restored; 9–12 L may be needed.
- Patient is likely to nothing by mouth (NPO) during a crisis or perhaps tube fed during a comatose state. As appropriate, intake may be progressed gradually to a balanced diet, controlling calories as needed.
- Correct electrolyte deficits. Potassium or magnesium may be needed.
- The reported sodium level should be corrected when the patient's glucose level is markedly elevated. In this circumstance, extracellular fluid (ECF) osmolality rises and exceeds that of intracellular fluid (ICF), since glucose penetrates cell membranes slowly in the absence of insulin, resulting in movement of water out of cells into the ECF (Merck Manual, 2009). Types of fluids administered will depend on the corrected serum sodium level, calculated using the following formula: measured sodium + [(serum glucose − 100)/100) × 1.6].
- A renal diet plan may be needed if renal failure is identified.

Common Drugs Used and Potential Side Effects

- Insulin is needed to normalize blood glucose levels. Infusions will be needed until full rehydration is complete. DKA and HHS are associated with elevation of proinflammatory cytokines; insulin therapy provides a strong anti-inflammatory effect (Stentz et al, 2004).
- Potassium replacements may be needed. Monitor carefully.
- Antibiotic therapy may be needed in cases of underlying infections.
- Drugs that may precipitate HHS include diuretics, beta blockers, clozapine, olanzapine, H2 blockers, cocaine, alcohol.

Herbs, Botanicals, and Supplements

- Herbs and botanical supplements should not be used without discussing with physician.
- See Table 9-9 for guidance on more specific herbs and supplements.

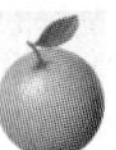

NUTRITION EDUCATION, COUNSELING, CARE MANAGEMENT

- Discuss, where possible, predisposing factors, how to avoid future incidents, and blood glucose monitoring.
- CHO-controlled diets may be beneficial if patient can comprehend. Family intervention may be required.
- Discuss possible neglect or abuse, if suspected.
- Continuous management of the fluid, electrolyte, and glucose disturbances is necessary until resolved.
- Provide diabetes teaching to prevent recurrence. Adjust insulin or oral hypoglycemic therapy on the basis of the insulin requirement once serum glucose level are stable.
- Coordinate home visits from nursing or dietitian if needed to evaluate the inadequate access to water.

Patient Education—Foodborne Illness

- If home tube feeding is needed, teach appropriate sanitation and food-handling procedures.

For More Information

- Diabetic Hyperosmolar Hyperglycemic State
  http://www.diabetes.org/type-2-diabetes/treatment-conditions/hhns.jsp
- E-medicine
  http://www.emedicine.com/emerg/topic264.htm

HYPEROSMOLAR HYPERGLYCEMIC STATE—CITED REFERENCES

Kitabchi AE, et al. Thirty years of personal experience in hyperglycemic crises: diabetic ketoacidosis and hyperglycemic hyperosmolar state. *J Clin Endocrinol Metab.* 93:1541, 2008.

Merck Manual. Hyperosmolar Hyperglycemic State. Web site accessed October 13, 2009, at http://www.merck.com/mmpe/sec12/ch158/ch158d.html.

Stentz FB, et al. Proinflammatory cytokines, markers of cardiovascular risks, oxidative stress, and lipid peroxidation in patients with hyperglycemic crises. *Diabetes.* 53:2079, 2004.

Stoner GD. Hyperosmolar hyperglycemic state. *Am Fam Physician.* 71:1723, 2005.

HYPOGLYCEMIA

NUTRITIONAL ACUITY RANKING: LEVEL 3

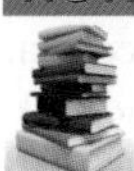

DEFINITIONS AND BACKGROUND

Hypoglycemia occurs primarily in patients with T1DM. Except in diabetic patients receiving insulin or sulfonylureas, hypoglycemia is a rare disorder. True low blood sugar (70 mg/100 dL or lower) releases hormones such as catecholamines, which produce hunger, trembling, headache, dizziness, weakness, and palpitations.

Sources of bodily glucose are from dietary intake, glycogenolysis, and gluconeogenesis. The metabolism of glucose involves oxidation and storage as glycogen or fat. The body makes great effort to supply glucose for the CNS and red blood cells. Glycogenolysis is stimulated by secretion of glucagon from the alpha-cells of the pancreas; this is impaired in patients with T1DM.

As different causes can stimulate hypoglycemia, treatments will differ accordingly. Skipped or insufficient meals, errors in insulin dosing, taking too much insulin, alcohol consumption, or extra physical exertion can lead to hypoglycemic episodes. Oxidative stress and zinc release contribute to neuronal death after hypoglycemia (Suh et al, 2008). Recurrent episodes of iatrogenic hypoglycemia induce a state of hypoglycemia unawareness and defective counterregulation, which defines hypoglycemia-associated autonomic failure (HAAF).

It is essential to manage these episodes carefully. A pro-oxidant state is promoted in certain brain regions during hypoglycemia and after glucose reperfusion, which results from the activation of several oxidative stress pathways; subsequent cell death occurs in particular brain regions including the cerebral cortex, the striatum, and the hippocampus (Haces et al, 2010).

Approaches to the prevention of hypoglycemia include glucose monitoring, patient education, meal planning, and medication adjustment. Adequate carbohydrate replacement during and after exercise seems to be an important measure to prevent hypoglycemia. Insulin dosage adjustment with a decrease from 20% to 30% is needed only for exercise duration over an hour (Grimm et al, 2004).

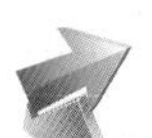

ASSESSMENT, MONITORING, AND EVALUATION

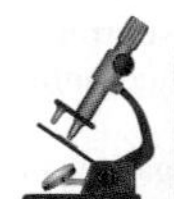

CLINICAL INDICATORS

Genetic Markers: A genetic deficiency in the p47(phox) subunit of NADPH oxidase may be relevant (Suh et al, 2008).

Clinical/History

Height
Weight
BMI
Diet history
I & O
Temperature
BP
Trembling
Headache
Dizziness, weakness
Palpitations
Seizures or coma
Blood glucose and insulin regimen records
Exercise history and habits
Hypoglycemia unawareness?
Type and duration of diabetes

Lab Work

Serum Gluc (≤70 mg/dL)
HbA1c
Serum insulin
Na^+, K^+
Alb
CRP
Chol, Trig
Ca^{++}
Mg^{++}
OGTT results using 1 g glucose/kg

INTERVENTION

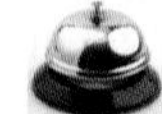

OBJECTIVES

- Normalize blood glucose levels. If the problem is recurrent, stabilize blood glucose levels through consistent mealtimes, CHO consistency, insulin dose adjustments, and blood glucose self-monitoring. For those individuals on insulin, appropriate insulin timing with food or use of CHO to insulin ratio are important factors to consider.
- Minimize length of time between meals.
- Prevent seizures and coma, with precipitating symptoms such as neuroglycopenia with confusion, light headaches, and aberrant behavior.
- Determine frequency, symptoms of hypoglycemia, activity levels for the individual.
- Delayed hypoglycemia after strenuous or prolonged exercise may occur up to 24 hours after exercise and is related to increased insulin sensitivity from exercise as well as

SAMPLE NUTRITION CARE PROCESS STEPS

Excessive Physical Activity

Assessment Data: Blood glucose self-monitoring records, food diary worksheets and meal records, blood glucose levels (fasting, 2-hour postprandial and/or HbA1c levels). Recent exercise program including aerobic dancing for >1 hour thrice weekly. Low blood glucose levels and signs/symptoms of hypoglycemia twice weekly.

Nutrition Diagnosis (PES): Excessive physical activity related to a new exercise regimen as evidenced by two bouts of blood glucose levels below 70 in past week.

Intervention: Education of patient, exercise partner, and family member(s) about blood glucose self-monitoring records (timing, blood glucose levels before and after exercise), insulin dosing, and activity records. Counseling about timing of FBG testing, insulin reductions, and close monitoring before and after dance sessions.

Monitoring and Evaluation: Glucose lab results within desirable range; no symptoms of hypoglycemia. Food diary and activity records showing effective self-management.

repletion of glycogen stores. Plan appropriately by increasing carbohydrate, decreasing insulin for periods of activity, and increasing frequency of blood glucose monitoring.

- Always recheck blood glucose 15–20 minutes after treatment to make sure that problem is resolved. Very low blood glucose levels (<50 g/dL) may take 30 g CHO or more to resolve, especially after exercise.

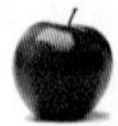

FOOD AND NUTRITION

- For insulin-induced hypoglycemia, use a normal diet with adequate CHO content. Consider a possible reduction of medication if the hypoglycemia is recurrent.
- Have patient ingest fruit juice when needed or use candy for an immediate corrective measure. If there are symptoms of hypoglycemia (blood glucose <70 g/dL), carry quick sources of glucose (see Table 9-18). Fat is not as effective as CHO in normalizing blood glucose.
- In most cases, mild hypoglycemia can be handled with use of readily available CHOs, including milk, fruit, and crackers. Balanced, regular mealtimes or frequent small snacks are also useful.
- For hypoglycemia at night that is caused by excessive insulin or insufficient dinner meal or evening snack, adjust evening and bedtime doses of insulin. A slightly larger dinner or snack containing CHO may be needed.

Common Drugs Used and Potential Side Effects

- Insulin and other glucose-lowering medications must be carefully prescribed and monitored. Careful use of sliding scales of insulin is the goal (Smith et al, 2005). Glycemic control to a lower glucose target range can be achieved using a computerized insulin dosing protocol with particular attention to timely measurement and adjustment of doses (Juneja et al, 2009).
- Glucose tablets have 4–5 g CHO per tablet. Patients should receive instructions regarding quantity, when to use, and when not to use. Most people will need three to four tablets to treat low blood glucose levels.
- If the individual passes out from hypoglycemia and uses insulin on a daily basis, it may be necessary to give a glucagon shot and call for emergency assistance. Glucagon can cause vomiting. Intravenous dextrose is administered by medical professionals.

Herbs, Botanicals, and Supplements

- Herbs and botanical supplements should not be used without discussing with physician. Clinical trials are lacking for this condition.
- See Table 9-9 for guidance on more specific herbs and supplements.

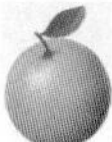

NUTRITION EDUCATION, COUNSELING, CARE MANAGEMENT

- Teach benefits of frequent blood glucose monitoring. Explain signs, symptoms, and treatment of hypoglycemia.
- Review appropriate timing of meals, snacks, and medications. Promote regular mealtimes, meal spacing, and planned exercise.
- Teach routine blood glucose before and after exercise. Discuss carrying a quick source of glucose.
- Encourage patients to obtain and carry diabetes identification.
- Discuss observations that require medical attention. Teach when to contact physician for medication adjustment.
- Discuss use of alcoholic beverages and potential effects. Excess alcohol increases the risk of hypoglycemia. Alcohol is processed in the liver to acetaldehyde at a time when the liver cannot do gluconeogenesis because nicotinamide adenine dinucleotide (NAD) is depleted. The biggest risk occurs when a patient drinks alcohol without carbohydrates being available, such as 4 hours or longer after the last meal. One drink takes 1–1.5 hours to process in the liver. Women should stick to one alcoholic beverage a day; men should limit their intake to two per day; both should consume a CHO with their drinks.
- In the elderly who are monitoring blood glucose levels closely, the benefits of intensive therapy in an effort to lower A1c must be weighed against the greater risk of unpredictable hypoglycemia (Alam et al, 2005).

Patient Education—Foodborne Illness

- If home tube feeding is needed, teach appropriate sanitation and food-handling procedures.

For More Information

- Mayo Clinic
  http://www.mayoclinic.com/health/hypoglycemia/DS00198
- NIDDK–Hypoglycemia in Diabetes
  http://diabetes.niddk.nih.gov/dm/pubs/hypoglycemia/

HYPOGLYCEMIA—CITED REFERENCES

Alam T, et al. What is the proper use of hemoglobin A1c monitoring in the elderly? *J Am Med Dir Assoc.* 6:200, 2005.

Grimm JJ, et al. A new table for prevention of hypoglycaemia during physical activity in type 1 diabetic patients. *Diabetes Metab.* 30:465, 2004.

Haces ML, et al. Selective vulnerability of brain regions to oxidative stress in a non-coma model of insulin-induced hypoglycemia. [published online ahead of print October 7, 2009] *Neuroscience.* 165:28, 2010.

Juneja R, et al. Computerized intensive insulin dosing can mitigate hypoglycemia and achieve tight glycemic control when glucose measurement is performed frequently and on time. *Crit Care.* 13:165, 2009.

Smith WD, et al. Causes of hyperglycemia and hypoglycemia in adult inpatients. *Am J Health Syst Pharm.* 62:714, 2005.

Suh SW, et al. Sequential release of nitric oxide, zinc, and superoxide in hypoglycemic neuronal death. *J Cereb Blood Flow Metab.* 28:1697, 2008.

HYPERINSULINISM AND SPONTANEOUS HYPOGLYCEMIA

NUTRITIONAL ACUITY RANKING: LEVEL 3–4

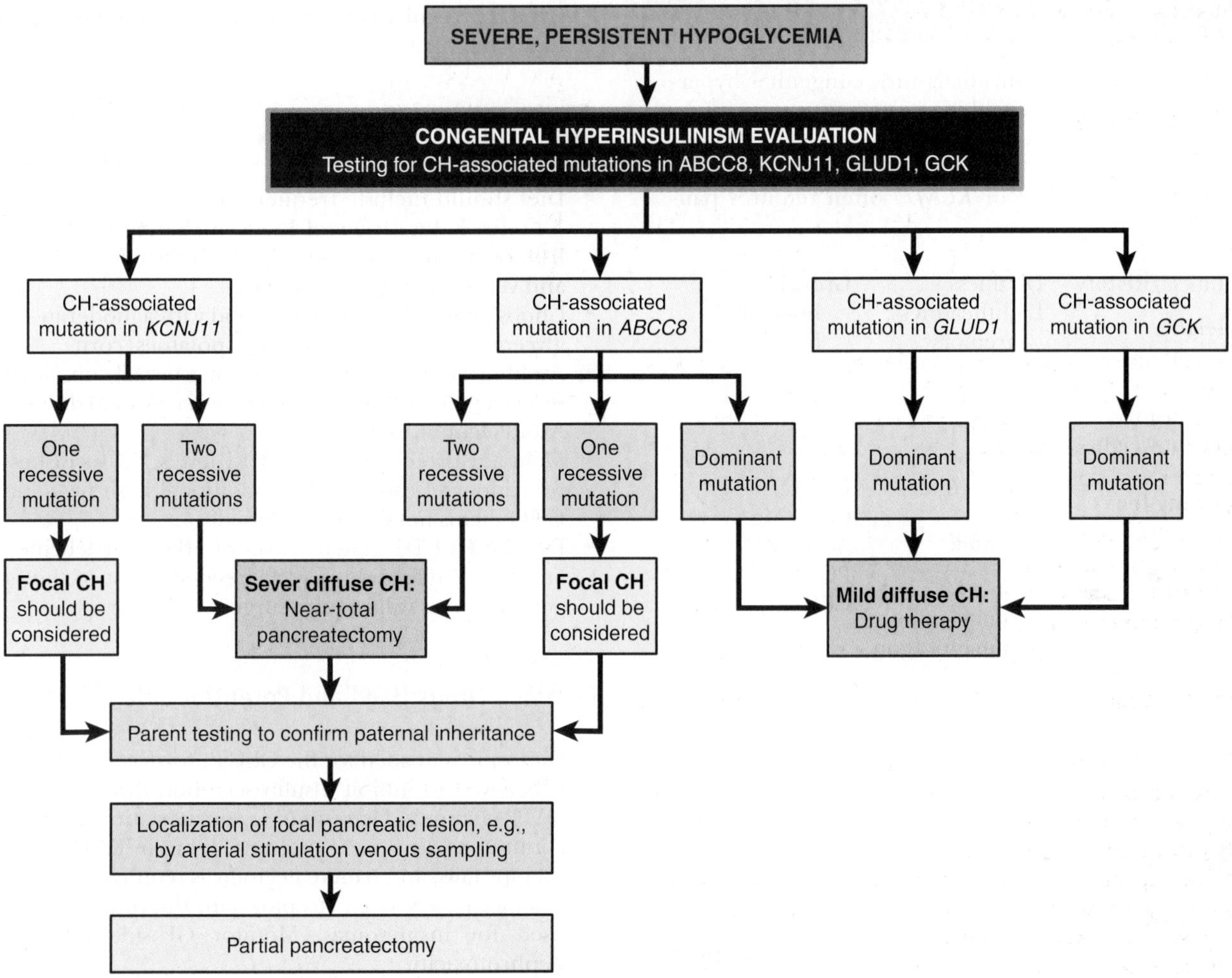

SEVERE, PERSISTENT HYPOGLYCEMIA

CONGENITAL HYPERINSULINISM EVALUATION
Testing for CH-associated mutations in ABCC8, KCNJ11, GLUD1, GCK

CH-associated mutation in *KCNJ11*

CH-associated mutation in *ABCC8*

CH-associated mutation in *GLUD1*

CH-associated mutation in *GCK*

One recessive mutation

Two recessive mutations

Two recessive mutations

One recessive mutation

Dominant mutation

Dominant mutation

Dominant mutation

Focal CH should be considered

Sever diffuse CH: Near-total pancreatectomy

Focal CH should be considered

Mild diffuse CH: Drug therapy

Parent testing to confirm paternal inheritance

Localization of focal pancreatic lesion, e.g., by arterial stimulation venous sampling

Partial pancreatectomy

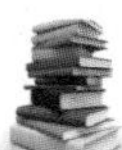

DEFINITIONS AND BACKGROUND

Hyperinsulinism consists of insulin levels above 3 μU/mL when glucose levels are below 50 mg/dL. Treatment depends on the cause and the severity of the hyperinsulinism. **Congenital hyperinsulinism (CH)** is familial hyperinsulism (FHI) with profound hypoglycemia because of excessive insulin secretion. CH can lead to developmental delay, mental retardation or death if untreated. CH occurs at an approximate frequency of 1/25,000 to 1/50,000 live births. New procedures spare healthy cells in the pancreas while allowing surgeons to remove abnormal tissue. **Spontaneous hypoglycemia** is an underlying symptom of some other diseases besides diabetes. Fasting and reactive hypoglycemias fall into the category of spontaneous forms. In **fasting hypoglycemia**, the body is not able to maintain adequate levels of sugar in the blood after a period without food in heavy drinkers who do not eat; people with islet cell tumors, viral hepatitis, cirrhosis, or liver cancer; and children with carbohydrate metabolic disorders. Hereditary fructose intolerance, galactosemia, leucine sensitivity can cause this type of hypoglycemia. **Reactive hypoglycemia** describes recurrent episodes of hypoglycemia occurring 2–4 hours after a high CHO or glucose load. Etiologies include alimentary hypoglycemia (dumping syndrome following gastric surgery); hypothyroidism or other hormonal disorders; *h. pylori*-induced gastritis; or occult diabetes with an exaggerated hyperglycemia during a glucose tolerance test. Symptoms include weakness and agitation 2–4 hours after meals, perspiration, nervousness, and mental confusion. Diet remains the main treatment, although alpha-glucosidase inhibitors and some other drugs may be helpful. Brain glycogen supports energy metabolism when glucose supply from the blood is inadequate and its levels rebound to levels higher than normal after a single episode of moderate hypoglycemia (Oz et al, 2009). Glutamate serves important intracellular signaling functions; glutamate dehydrogenase (GDH) catalyzes the oxidative deamination of glutamate to alpha-ketoglutarate in brain, liver, kidney, and the pancreatic islets (Stanley, 2009).

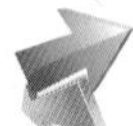

ASSESSMENT, MONITORING, AND EVALUATION

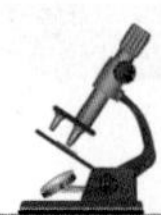

CLINICAL INDICATORS

Genetic Markers: Individuals with congenital hyperinsulinism (CH) should be tested for gene mutations. Mutations in *GLUD1, GCK,* or *HADHSC* are response to drug therapy, but CHI associated with mutations in *ABCC8* or *KCNJ11* often requires pancreatectomy.

Clinical/History
- Height
- Weight
- BMI
- Diet history
- Recent weight losses
- Craving for sweets
- BP
- Seizures, confusion
- Heart palpitation or fibrillation
- Dizziness
- Lightheadness, tremors
- Headache
- Flushing
- Irritability
- Numb or cold extremities

Lab Work
- Gluc
- Serum insulin
- Serum glucagon
- Growth hormone levels
- Chol
- Trig
- Na^+, K^+
- Trig
- HgA1c
- Ca^{++}, Mg^{++}
- Acetone
- PO_4
- CRP

INTERVENTION

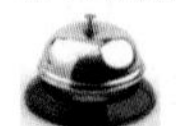

OBJECTIVES

- Reduce intake of concentrated CHO to a level that does not overstimulate the pancreas to secrete inappropriately large amounts of insulin, which may cause blood sugar to drop. Limit total intake of carbohydrate to 130 g/d to reduce the severity of symptoms.
- If required, ensure that patient loses weight gradually.
- Reduce counterregulatory hormone responses to excessive insulin.
- Exercise regularly and maintain consistency in meal times and daily routines.

SAMPLE NUTRITION CARE PROCESS STEPS

Excessive CHO Intake

Assessment Data: Recent bouts of low blood glucose, (<50 mg/gL) without Hx of diabetes or insulinoma. Dumping syndrome 2–3 hours after meals with weakness, perspiration, heart palpitations, headache, and craving for sweets. Diet history reveals CHO intake averaging 250 g/d, especially between meals and before bedtime.

Nutrition Diagnosis (PES): Excessive CHO intake related to high intake of sweets as evidenced by diet history.

Intervention: Food and nutrient delivery—tracking of CHO intake at meals and snacks. Education—sources of CHO from each food group. Counseling—ways to decrease hunger; food diary for episodes of hypoglycemia; signs and symptoms and when to call the doctor; glycemic index and glycemic load of foods.

Monitoring and Evaluation: Improvement through decreased episodes of hypoglycemia following meals and snacks with limitation of intake to 130–150 g daily.

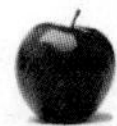

FOOD AND NUTRITION

- Diet should include frequent small meals, about every 3 hours. Eat a variety of foods, including meat, poultry, fish, or nonmeat sources of protein; whole grains; fruits and vegetables; dairy products.
- Choose high-fiber foods and food with a moderate-to-low glycemic load. Avoid white rice, potatoes, corn.
- Avoid or limit foods high in sugar, especially on an empty stomach; this includes sweetened beverages and dried fruits.
- Avoid alcohol, caffeine.
- Maintain protein intake at DRI levels; fat furnishes the remainder of calories. The traditional high protein, low CHO diet is not evidenced-based.
- For the GLUD1 genetic form of HI, a low leucine diet and use of diazoside may be needed. Most of the other genetic forms will require surgery or just drug use.

Common Drugs Used and Potential Side Effects

- Diazoside is needed for the GLUT1 form of HI. Diazoxide is believed to inhibit insulin secretion through opening KATP channels. Octreotide (a somatostatin analogue) or continuous dextrose is often used; but in KATP HI, drug therapy fails, and pancreatectomy is required.
- Chemotherapy (e.g., streptozocin, fluorouracil) may be used for insulinomas. Monitor GI side effects and nephrotoxicity.
- Alpha-glucosidase inhibitors may be where diabetes is identified.
- Monitor all medications for their potential hypoglycemic effects.

Herbs, Botanicals, and Supplements

- Products such as hemicelluose and pectin may help in dumping syndrome.
- Herbs and botanical supplements should not be used without discussing with physician.
- See Table 9-9 for guidance on more specific herbs and supplements.

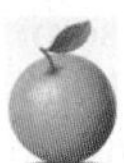

NUTRITION EDUCATION, COUNSELING, CARE MANAGEMENT

- Explain that alcohol blocks gluconeogenesis and should be avoided.
- Ensure that patient keeps snacks available such as cheese and crackers. More frequent feedings are needed.

- Avoid skipping meals; eat meals on time. Avoid any one meal that is unbalanced or especially high in carbohydrates.
- Control caffeine intake and use of other stimulants, which may aggravate condition.

Patient Education—Foodborne Illness

- If home tube feeding is needed, teach appropriate sanitation and food-handling procedures.

For More Information

- Congenital Hyperinsulinism
http://www.chop.edu/service/congenital-hyperinsulinism-center/home.html?id=47690
- Congenital Hyperinsulinism International
http://www.congenitalhi.org/
- NIDDK–Hypoglycemia (Nondiabetes)
http://diabetes.niddk.nih.gov/dm/pubs/hypoglycemia/#nodiabetes

HYPERINSULINISM AND SPONTANEOUS HYPOGLYCEMIA—CITED REFERENCES

Oz G, et al. Human brain glycogen metabolism during and after hypoglycemia. *Diabetes* 58:1978, 2009.
Stanley GA. Regulation of glutamate metabolism and insulin secretion by GDH in hypoglycemic children. *J Am Clin Nutr.* 90:862S, 2009.

Other Endocrine Disorders

Hormones can be separated into three categories: **amines**, these are simple molecules, **proteins and peptides**, which are made from chains of amino acids, and **steroids**, which are derived from cholesterol. **Glands** discharge hormones directly into the bloodstream, and they have feedback mechanisms that maintain a proper balance of hormones and prevent excess secretion. Endocrine disorders require varying levels of nutritional intervention. If medications are taken appropriately, many conditions can be readily managed. See Table 9-19.

TABLE 9-19 Other Endocrine Conditions

There are many other disorders of endocrine function besides those affecting the pancreas that require some level of nutritional intervention. Listed below are essential hormones and functions of the endocrine glands.

Gland	Hormones	Functions
Pancreas	Glucagon (from alpha-cells)	Alpha-cells in the pancreatic islets secrete the hormone glucagon in response to a low concentration of glucose in the blood.
	Insulin (from beta-cells)	Beta-cells in the pancreatic islets secrete insulin in response to high blood glucose concentrations. See diabetes section.
Gastric mucosa	Gastrin	Stimulates production of hydrochloric acid and the enzyme pepsin, used in digestive processes.
Small intestinal mucosa	Secretin	Stimulates the pancreas to produce bicarbonate-rich fluid to neutralize stomach acid.
	Cholecystokinin	Stimulates contraction of the gallbladder to release bile after a meal containing fat. Also stimulates the pancreas to secrete digestive enzymes.
Placenta	Human chorionic gonadotropin	Signals the mother's ovaries to secrete hormones to maintain the uterine lining during pregnancy.
Hypothalamus	Gonadotropin-releasing hormone (GnRH) and other releasing hormones	Hunger and thirst; emotional and sexual responses of the limbic system; heart rate and blood pressure; circadian cycles; body temperature; bladder function; moods. Hypothalamus links the nervous system by synthesizing and secreting neurohormones that stimulate release of hormones from the anterior pituitary gland.
Pituitary (anterior)	Adrenocorticotropic hormone (ACTH)	Reacts with receptor sites in the cortex of the adrenal gland to stimulate the secretion of cortical hormones, particularly cortisol.
	Human growth hormone (hGH or somatotropin hormone)	Growth of bones, muscles, and other organs by promoting protein synthesis; influences height.
	Thyroid-stimulating hormone (TSH or thyrotropin)	Causes thyroid to secrete thyroid hormone.
	Gonadotropins (follicle-stimulating hormone [FSH]; luteinizing hormone [LH])	React with gonads to regulate growth and function of these organs. In females, FSH stimulates egg production; in males, it stimulates sperm production. In females, LH causes ovulation; in males, it causes the testes to secrete testosterone.
	Prolactin (PRL)	Promotes development of glandular tissue in the female breast during pregnancy and stimulates milk production after the birth of the infant.
Pituitary (posterior)	Oxytocin (OT)	Causes contraction of the smooth muscle in the wall of the uterus. It also stimulates the ejection of milk from the lactating breast.
	Vasopressin (antidiuretic hormone [ADH])	ADH promotes the reabsorption of water by the kidney tubules; less water is lost as urine to conserve water for the body. Insufficient amounts of ADH cause excessive water loss in the urine.

(continued)

TABLE 9-19 Other Endocrine Conditions *(continued)*

Gland	Hormones	Functions
Pineal gland	Melatonin (5-methoxy-*N*-acetyl-tryptamine)	Reproductive development and daily sleep–wake cycles; skin blanching. Derived from tryptophan. Production is stimulated by darkness and inhibited by light. Beta-blockers decrease release of melatonin.
Adrenal cortex		Adrenal cortex has control of 28 hormones, all of which are steroids.
	Mineralocorticoids (such as aldosterone)	Aldosterone conserves sodium ions and water.
	Glucocorticoids (such as cortisol)	Cortisol increases blood glucose levels.
	Gonadocorticoids (sex hormones: androgens and estrogens)	Normal reproductive functioning.
Adrenal medulla	Epinephrine (adrenalin) and norepinephrine (noradrenalin)	These two hormones are secreted in response to stimulation by the sympathetic nerve, particularly during stressful situations. They cause faster heartbeat and increased blood glucose levels.
		A lack of hormones from the adrenal medulla produces no significant effects. Hypersecretion, usually from a tumor, causes prolonged or continual sympathetic responses.
Thyroid	Thyroid hormones: thyroxine (95%) and triiodothyronine (5%)	Growth and development, metabolism. Thyroid hormones need iodine.
	Calcitonin	Calcitonin is secreted by the parafollicular cells of the thyroid gland. This hormone opposes the action of the parathyroid glands by reducing the calcium level in the blood. If blood calcium becomes too high, calcitonin is secreted until calcium ion levels decrease to normal.
Thymus	Thymosin	Immunity; T cells; lymphocytes. Currently being studied for its possible role in AIDS and hepatitis.
Parathyroid glands	Parathyroid hormone (PTH)	Regulation of calcium and phosphorus; secreted in response to low blood calcium levels in order to increase those levels. PTH mobilizes calcium by increasing calcium resorption from bone and by raising calcium reabsorption in the proximal kidney tubule.
Gonads (testes and ovaries)	Androgens (testosterone)	Growth and development of the male reproductive structures; increased skeletal and muscular growth; enlargement of the larynx accompanied by voice changes; growth and distribution of body hair; increased male sexual drive.
	Estrogen and progesterone	Development of the breasts; distribution of fat evidenced in the hips, legs, and breasts; maturation of reproductive organs such as the uterus and vagina. Progesterone causes the uterine lining to thicken in preparation for pregnancy. Together, progesterone and estrogens are responsible for the changes that occur in the uterus during the female menstrual cycle.

Sources: Surveillance, Epidemiology, and End Results. Endocrine glands and their functions. Accessed July 1, 2005, at http://training.seer.cancer.gov/module_anatomy/unit6_3_endo_glnds.html and Cotterill S. The endocrine system (hormones). Accessed July 1, 2005, at http://www.cancerindex.org/medterm/medtm12.htm#function

For More Information on Other Endocrine Conditions

- American Association of Clinical Endocrinologists
  http://www.aace.com/
- American Medical Association
  http://www.ama-assn.org/ama/pub/category/7157.html
- Endocrine Society
  http://www.aace.com/
- The Hormone Foundation
  http://www.hormone.org/
- National Institutes of Health–Endocrine Disorders
  http://www.niddk.nih.gov/health/endo/endo.htm

Pituitary Gland

HYPOPITUITARISM

NUTRITIONAL ACUITY RANKING: LEVEL 1

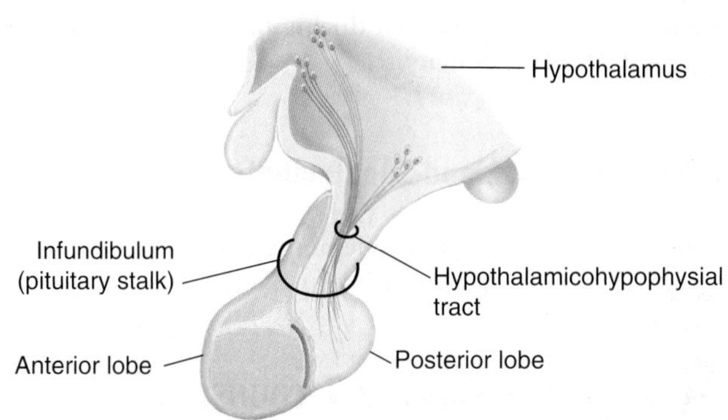

Asset provided by Anatomical Chart Co.

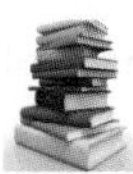

DEFINITIONS AND BACKGROUND

Hypopituitarism is an underactive pituitary gland. A deficiency in production of pituitary hormones may be caused by tumor, trauma, radiation to the brain, stroke or aneurysm, or surgery.

In hypopituitarism, there is a lack of one or more of these hormones and loss of function in the affected gland or organ. Table 9-20 lists symptoms of pituitary disorders. It may take years for an accurate diagnosis to be made. If all pituitary hormones are missing, this is panhypopituitarism; it is relatively rare.

Adrenocorticotropic hormone (ACTH) stimulates the adrenal gland to release cortisol to maintain BP and blood glucose levels. If ACTH is missing, depression, fatigue, low BP, nausea and diarrhea, dizziness, pale skin, weakness, and weight loss are signs and symptoms. A shortage of cortisol can be life threatening.

Arginine vasopression (AVP) was formerly known as antidiuretic hormone (ADH). AVP controls water loss by the kidneys. If AVP is deficient, severe thirst and excessive urination occur; diabetes insipidus may result. In rare instances, deficiency may occur after an event such as brain surgery.

TABLE 9-20 Symptoms of a Pituitary Disorder

Headaches	Short stature if during growth period
Depression	Cold intolerance
Mood/emotion swings	Weight loss
Abdominal pain, anorexia	Infertility in women
Loss of memory	Impotence in men
Loss of sleep	Cessation of or irregular menses
Sexual dysfunction	Lethargy, fatigue
Failure in lactation	Weakness
Low blood pressure	Loss of armpit, body, pubic or facial hair

Source: Pituitary Network Association. Available at http://www.pituitary.org/

Growth hormone (GH) regulates somatic growth, carbohydrate and lipid metabolism, and adipocyte functions. There is a complex interplay between GH and insulin signaling (Perrini et al, 2008). If GH is deficient in children, short stature (below 5 feet) can result. This condition causes 10% of all dwarfism. In adults, there is abnormal body composition, osteopenia, impaired quality of life, cardiac dysfunction, and an adverse lipid profile. Follicle-stimulating hormone (FSH) and Luteinizing hormone (LH) control sexual function and fertility in males and females. When gonadotropin (FSH, LH) deficiency occurs, men and women will lose interest in sex and can experience fatigue, weakness, loss of body hair, impotence in men, and loss of menstruation in women. Oxytocin stimulates the uterus to contract during labor and the breasts to release milk. Oxytocin mechanisms are necessary for successful pregnancies (Kubler et al, 2009). Pregnancy is uncommon when oxytocin levels are low.

Prolactin stimulates female breast development and milk production. Prolactin deficiency is rare but can stop milk production in women.

TSH stimulates the thyroid gland to release hormones that affect the body's metabolism. When TSH is deficient, this can lead to an underactive thyroid (hypothyroidism). Cold intolerance, constipation, weight gain, and pale and waxy or dry skin can occur.

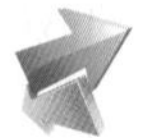

ASSESSMENT, MONITORING, AND EVALUATION

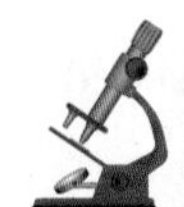

CLINICAL INDICATORS

Genetic Markers: Transcription factors have an impact on target genes; different phenotypes result when the gene encoding the relevant transcription factor is mutated. Many genes are involved.

Clinical/History	Lab Work	
Height	ACTH level	Protein-bound iodine (PBI) uptake (decreased?)
Weight	Cortisol	Glucose
BMI	Serum estradiol	Glucose tolerance test (GTT)
Diet history	Serum testosterone	Chol, Trig
BP	Serum IGF-1	Homocysteine
Brain scan	Thyroxine (T4) (decreased?)	CRP
Pituitary MRI	Triiodothyronine (T3)	Alb
Dual-energy x-ray absorptiometry (DEXA) scan	FSH, LH, TSH (decreased?)	Complete blood count (CBC)

Osmolarity	Serum Gluc	H & H, serum ferritin
Na^+, K^+	Uric acid	Transferrin
Ca^{++}, Mg^{++}		

INTERVENTION

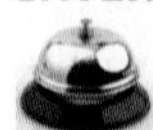

OBJECTIVES

- Replenish missing hormones.
- Prevent dehydration, hypoglycemia, and related problems.
- Improve lean muscle mass stores.
- Monitor serum levels of cholesterol and triglycerides; prevent vascular complications.

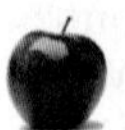

FOOD AND NUTRITION

- Dietary alterations may be needed, such as higher or lower energy intake, until hormone levels are normalized. A modified fat, cholesterol, and carbohydrate intake may be needed. Ensure sufficient intake of protein.
- Six small feedings may be better tolerated than larger meals.
- Increase fluids unless contraindicated.
- Ensure adequate intake of all vitamins and minerals. Calcium and vitamin D should be taken in sufficient amounts to prevent osteoporosis.

Common Drugs Used and Potential Side Effects

Hormone replacement therapy may include any of all of the following:

1. Corticosteroids (hydrocortisone [Cortef], cortisol) are often used and can alter glucose, calcium, and phosphate tolerance. Potassium and folacin must be increased; sodium must be decreased. Monitor for signs of hyperglycemia.
2. Thyroid preparations (levothyroxine) may be needed.
3. GH (somatotropin) requires no specific dietary interventions. It may help alleviate elevated triglycerides. Long-term GH replacement therapy in adults is safe for lifelong therapy in order to maintain the benefits.
4. Estrogen, progesterone, or testosterone replacement should be monitored for side effects related to heart disease and elevated lipids.
5. Cortisone may be needed during periods of stress or illness if ACTH is deficient.

Herbs, Botanicals, and Supplements

- Herbs and botanical supplements should not be used without discussing with physician.

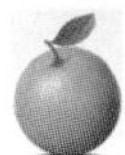

NUTRITION EDUCATION, COUNSELING, CARE MANAGEMENT

- Have patient avoid fasting and stress.
- Discuss the need to use small, frequent meals instead of large meals.
- Discuss the possibility of hyperglycemia and how to manage.
- Hormone replacement is usually permanent, so doctor visits will be needed to check for diabetes and signs of osteoporosis.

Patient Education—Foodborne Illness

- If home tube feeding is needed, teach appropriate sanitation and food-handling procedures.

For More Information

- Hormone Foundation–Pituitary Hormone
  http://www.hormone.org/public/pituitary.cfm
- Mayo Clinic
  http://www.mayoclinic.com/health/hypopituitarism/DS00479
- Medline Plus
  http://www.nlm.nih.gov/medlineplus/pituitarydisorders.html
- Pituitary Disorders Education and Support
  http://www.pituitarydisorder.net/
- The Pituitary Society
  http://www.pituitarysociety.org/

SAMPLE NUTRITION CARE PROCESS STEPS

Unsafe Food Handling

Assessment Data: On home tube feeding. Unsanitary habits noted during home visit.

Nutrition Diagnosis (PES): Unsafe food handling related to preparation and administration of tube feeding as evidenced by observations during home visit.

Intervention: Education on how to sanitize counters and maintain safe procedures while handling tubing and enteral product.

Monitoring and Evaluation: No signs of diarrhea or GI distress from contaminated TF.

HYPOPITUITARISM—CITED REFERENCES

Kubler K, et al. High-risk pregnancy management in women with hypopituitarism. *J Perinatol.* 29:89, 2009.

Perrini S, et al. Metabolic implications of growth hormone therapy. *J Endocrinol Invest.* 31:79, 2008.

Verhelst J, et al. Baseline characteristics and response to 2 years of growth hormone replacement of hypopituitary patients with growth hormone deficiency due to adult-onset craniopharyngioma in comparison to patients with non-functioning pituitary adenoma: data from KIMS. *J Clin Endocrinol Metab.* 90:4636, 2005.

PITUITARY GLAND (ANTERIOR)

ACROMEGALY

NUTRITIONAL ACUITY RANKING: LEVEL 1

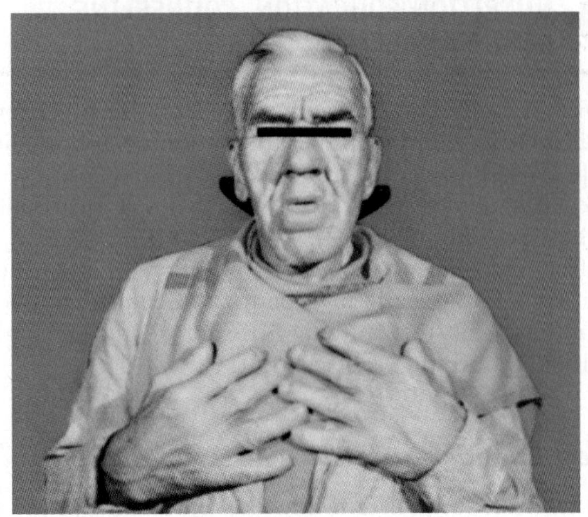

Adapted from: Weber J RN, EdD and Kelley J RN, PhD. *Health Assessment in Nursing*, 2nd ed. Philadelphia: Lippincott Williams & Wilkins, 2003.

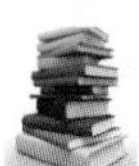

DEFINITIONS AND BACKGROUND

Acromegaly is a hormonal disorder caused by overproduction of human GH by the pituitary gland. Incidence is rare, with 50–70 cases per million in the U.S. population. Diagnosis is made common about a decade after oversecretion of GH begins. If GH-producing tumors occur in puberty, the condition is called gigantism. Genetics and nutrition impact the height of most children; unusual, continuing growth in stature beyond the twenties should be evaluated.

GH (somatotropin) affects the growth of almost all cells and tissues and has direct and indirect effects. Direct effects of excessive GH include hyperinsulinism, lipolysis, insulin resistance in peripheral tissues, ketogenesis, hyperglycemia, and sodium and water retention. In over 98% of cases, overproduction of GH is related to a benign pituitary tumor. In a few patients, acromegaly is caused by tumors of the pancreas, lungs, or adrenal glands. Symptoms and signs of acromegaly include enlarged extremities with disproportionate growth of nose, lips, brow, lower jaw, tongue, hands, and feet. Serious side effects include heart failure, colon polyps that become cancerous, and diabetes.

Elevated insulin-like growth factor I (IGF-I) also occurs in acromegaly, resulting in greater protein synthesis, amino acid transportation, muscle and bone growth, DNA and RNA synthesis, and cell proliferation. High levels of GH and increased IGF-1 levels (three to ten times above normal) may be used to diagnose acromegaly. Hormone-secreting pituitary tumors account for about 30% of all pituitary tumors (Patil et al, 2009). Surgical removal of the pituitary gland provides a 50–70% chance of cure (Vance and Laws, 2005). Acromegaly is complicated by an increased incidence of diabetes mellitus caused by impaired insulin sensitivity and reduced beta-cell function (Higham et al, 2009). Bone and cartilage growth may lead to arthritis. Acromegalic patients present with hypoadiponectinemia; studies suggest a link between adiponectin, visfatin, fat mass, and bone changes (Sucunza et al, 2009). Premature death may result if left untreated. Treatment may include surgical removal of the tumor, radiation therapy, or injection of a GH blocking drug. Somatostatin analogs have been key in medical therapy. Pegvisomant, a GH-receptor antagonist, competitively binds to the GH receptor, blocking IGF-I production and allowing for a better control of cardiac disorders and glucose metabolism (Vance and Lawes, 2005). Improved insulin sensitivity occurs after use from a reduction in overnight endogenous glucose production (Higham et al, 2009). Somatuline Depot (lanreotide) can be used for a long-term treatment in patients who have had an inadequate response to surgery and/or radiation.

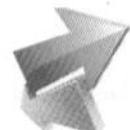

ASSESSMENT, MONITORING, AND EVALUATION

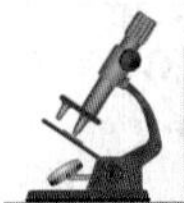

CLINICAL INDICATORS

Genetic Markers: Most pituitary tumors are from a genetic mutation that is acquired and not present from birth.

Clinical/History

Height
Weight
BMI
Weight changes
Diet history
BP (increased)
I & O
Increased coarse body hair
Coarse, leathery skin
Excessive diaphoresis and oily skin
Skin tags
Impaired vision
Osteoarthritis, carpal tunnel syndrome
Deepening voice
Headaches
Fluid retention

Lab Work

IGF-I levels (best marker)
GH (>5× higher than normal)
N balance
BUN
Serum Creat (increased)
Urine sugar
Gluc, HbA1c
GTT
Serum insulin
Ca^{++} (decreased)
Phosphorus (increased?)
Alb
Na^+, K^+
H & H

INTERVENTION

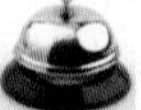

OBJECTIVES

- Control weight.
- Prevent or control diabetes, hypertension, or heart disease when present.
- Prevent osteoporosis with calcium balance, which is often negative.
- Monitor for complications such as colon polyps, which may lead to cancer.

SAMPLE NUTRITION CARE PROCESS STEPS

Involuntary Weight Gain

Assessment Data: Diagnosis of acromegaly with recent weight gain of 10 lb over 6 weeks; FBG 130 mg/dL.

Nutrition Diagnosis (PES): Involuntary weight gain (NC-3.4) related to excessive GH and IGF-1 levels as evidenced by 10 lb weight gain in 6 weeks.

Intervention: Education—importance of controlling CHO and energy intake to manage weight and prevent diabetes. Counseling—tips for identifying hidden CHO sources and controlling energy intake.

Monitoring and Evaluation: Weight stabilized; HgbA1c, FBS and other available lab results. No additional signs of hyperglycemia and no further weight gain.

- Achieve the goal for GH levels as 1–2 μg/L (Sheppard, 2005).

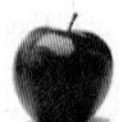

FOOD AND NUTRITION

- An CHO-controlled diet may be needed if diabetes is present.
- Extra fluid intake may be needed.
- Control sodium and fluid intake if there is heart failure.
- Offer sufficient intake of calcium and vitamin D; a multivitamin–mineral supplement may be useful.

Common Drugs Used and Potential Side Effects

- Bromocriptine (Parlodel) can be taken orally to reduce GH secretion. Side effects include gastrointestinal upset, nausea, vomiting, light-headedness when standing, and nasal congestion. Take with food.
- Octreotide (Sandostatin) injection is a synthetic form of somatostatin. Side effects include diarrhea, nausea, gallstones, and loose stools.
- Insulin may be needed if diabetes is also present. Be wary of excess doses; hypoglycemia is a dangerous side effect.
- Cardiac medications may be needed; monitor for specific side effects accordingly. Atorvastatin treatment is safe, well-tolerated, and effective (Mishra et al, 2005).
- Pegvisomant is used to normalize circulating levels of IGF-I, the principal mediator of GH action.
- Somatuline Depot delivers an injection subcutaneously instead of into the muscle; side effects include diarrhea, cholelithiasis, abdominal pain, nausea, injection site reactions, flatulence, arthralgia, and loose stools.

Herbs, Botanicals, and Supplements

- Herbs and botanical supplements should not be used without discussing with physician.

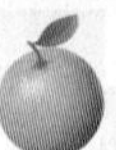

NUTRITION EDUCATION, COUNSELING, CARE MANAGEMENT

- Discuss body changes and altered self-image. Exercise can help to improve physical functioning and quality of life (Woodhouse et al, 2006).
- Teach patient about control of diabetes or heart failure, where present.
- After surgery, potential complications include cerebrospinal fluid leaks, meningitis, and damage to the surrounding normal pituitary tissue, requiring lifelong pituitary hormone replacement.

Patient Education—Foodborne Illness

- If home tube feeding is needed, teach appropriate sanitation and food-handling procedures.

For More Information

- Acromegaly
  http://www.acromegaly.org/
- NIDDK–Acromegaly
  http://www.niddk.nih.gov/health/endo/pubs/acro/acro.htm
- Pituitary Network Association
  http://www.pituitary.com/
- Skull Base Institute
  http://www.skullbaseinstitute.com/acromegaly_gigantism.htm
- Treatment Guidelines
  http://www.aace.com/pub/pdf/guidelines/AcromegalyGuidelines2004.pdf

ACROMEGALY—CITED REFERENCES

Higham CE, et al. Pegvisomant improves insulin sensitivity and reduces overnight free fatty acid concentrations in patients with acromegaly. *J Clin Endocrinol Metab.* 94:2459, 2009.

Mishra M, et al. The effect of atorvastatin on serum lipoproteins in acromegaly. *Clin Endocrinol.* 62:650, 2005.

Patil CG, et al. Non-surgical management of hormone-secreting pituitary tumors. *J Clin Neurosci.* 16:985, 2009.

Sheppard MC. GH and mortality in acromegaly. *J Endocrinol Invest.* 28:75S, 2005.

Sucunza N, et al. A link between bone mineral density and serum adiponectin and visfatin levels in acromegaly. *J Clin Endocrinol.* 94:3889, 2009.

Vance ML, Laws ER Jr. Role of medical therapy in the management of acromegaly. *Neurosurgery.* 56:877, 2005.

Woodhouse LJ, et al. The influence of growth hormone status on physical impairments, functional limitations, and health-related quality of life in adults. *Endocr Rev.* 27:287, 2006.

PITUITARY GLAND (ANTERIOR)

CUSHING'S SYNDROME

NUTRITIONAL ACUITY RANKING: LEVEL 1–2

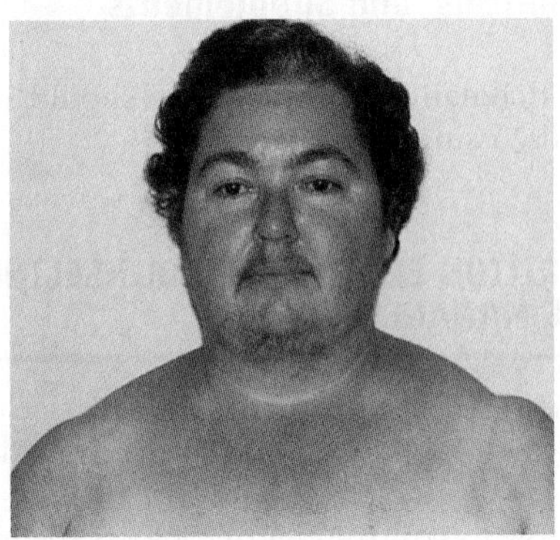

Adapted from: Rubin E. *Essential Pathology,* 3rd ed. Philadelphia: Lippincott Williams & Wilkins, 2000.

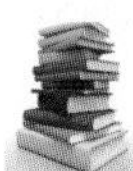

DEFINITIONS AND BACKGROUND

Cushing's syndrome (CS) is a disease caused by an excess of cortisol. It can be caused by extrinsic and excessive hormonal stimulation of the adrenal cortex by tumor of the anterior pituitary gland, adrenal hyperplasia, or exogenous cortisol use. Differential diagnosis is not simple. No existing test is accurate when used alone; focused imaging, including computed tomography (CT), magnetic resonance imaging (MRI), and nuclear imaging modalities can provide the diagnosis (Lindsay and Nieman, 2005).

Pituitary CS occurs after puberty with equal frequency in boys and girls. In adults, it has a greater frequency in women than men, with most diagnosed between ages 20 and 50 years. The total incidence is about 10–15 million people per year. It is a disorder characterized by virilism, upper body obesity with thin arms and legs, hyperglycemia, glucosuria, hypertension, red moon face, vertigo, emotional liability, buffalo hump, purple striae over obese areas, acne, female balding or hirsutism, blurry vision, and pitting ankle edema. In some cases, osteoporosis and severe depression are present.

Chronic cortisol hypersecretion causes central obesity, hypertension, insulin resistance, dyslipidemia, and prothrombotic state, manifestations of a MetS. There is a complex interaction between CS and inflammation; raised levels of IL-8 and OPG in CS patients, despite glucocorticoid excess, may represent an inflammatory and pro-atherogenic phenotype (Kristo et al, 2008). If left untreated, CS can be fatal. Diagnosis is not simple. Late-night salivary cortisol may be a useful test (Carroll et al, 2009). Treatments differ according to the cause: ACTH dependent (pituitary or ectopic) or independent (an adrenal tumor), or iatrogenic (from excessive steroid hormone use). If iatrogenic, depletion of steroid hormones will be needed. If pituitary, the gland may need to be removed. CS caused by ACTH production from solid tumors can result in life-threatening hypercortisolemia (Uecker and Janzow, 2005). Radiation, chemotherapy, or surgery may be needed. After surgical removal of the adrenal glands, most symptoms of CS disappear. Psychological impairment can persist despite successful treatment (Iacabone et al, 2005).

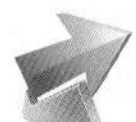

ASSESSMENT, MONITORING, AND EVALUATION

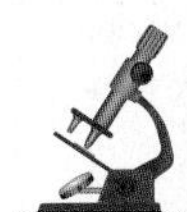

CLINICAL INDICATORS

Genetic Markers: Rarely, CS results from an inherited tendency to develop tumors of one or more endocrine glands. With multiple endocrine neoplasia type 1 (MEN1), hormone-secreting tumors of the parathyroid glands, pancreas, and pituitary develop and may lead to CS.

Clinical/History

Height
Weight
BMI
Diet history
BP (increased)
Edema
Buffalo hump
Moon face
Easy bruising, slow healing
Red or purple striae on skin
Weakened bones
Sore, aching joints in hip, back, shoulders
Excess facial hair in women
Decreased fertility in men
CT
MRI for tumors
DEXA scan

Lab Work

24-hour urinary free cortisol level (>50–100 μg/d)
Dexamethasone suppression test
Late-night salivary cortisol
Corticotropin-releasing hormone (CRH) stimulation test for ACTH levels (altered)
Urinary Gluc (increased)
Gluc (increased)
HbA1c
Ca^{++}, Mg^{++}
Urinary Ca^{+}
Lipid profile, Chol, Trig
K^{+} (decreased)
Na^{+} (increased)
Alb, N balance
CRP
pCO_2 (increased), pO_2
WBC, TLC (decreased)

INTERVENTION

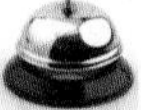

OBJECTIVES

- Control elevated blood glucose or lipids; manage diabetes and CVD.
- Promote weight loss if needed; decrease fat stores while increasing lean body mass.
- Control or lower BP.

SAMPLE NUTRITION CARE PROCESS STEPS

Excessive Sodium Intake

Assessment Data: Long-term corticosteroid use for lupus; dietary history reveals high intake of sodium from snack foods, canned soups and vegetables, luncheon meats; buffalo hump, slightly elevated glucose and lipids. BMI 27. BP averaging 190/80. Feet and hands edematous.

Nutrition Diagnosis (PES): Excessive sodium intake related to high intake of salted and processed foods as evidenced by diet history and requirement for corticosteroids.

Intervention: Education about a desirable lowering of sodium from dietary sources. Counseling about sources of well-flavored snack foods, use of more fruits and raw vegetables, use of varied spices and seasonings; choices in the supermarket, at restaurants, while traveling.

Monitoring and Evaluation: Evaluation of impact of lower sodium from diet on BP and edema. Improved intake of fruits, raw vegetables and nonprocessed meats. Improved quality of life.

- Prevent or control side effects of corticosteroid therapy: vertebral collapse, heart failure, bone demineralization, osteoporosis, and hypokalemia.

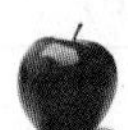

FOOD AND NUTRITION

- Restrict sodium if steroids are used.
- Use an energy-controlled diet, if needed. Calculate diet according to patient's desirable body weight.
- Control glucose levels when elevated; carbohydrate counting can be useful.
- Ensure adequate intake of calcium and potassium.
- Ensure adequate intake of protein if losses are excessive (e.g., 1 g protein/kg or more).
- Use an anti-inflammatory diet rich in omega-3 fatty acids, herbs, spices and antioxidant foods; see Tables 8-13 and 8-14.

Common Drugs Used and Potential Side Effects

- With glucocorticoid therapy, osteoporosis and hypercalciuria are common side effects. Withdrawal of these medications after autoimmune or cancer management may cause iatrogenic CS. Adrenal insufficiency or steroid withdrawal symptoms may occur (Hopkins and Leinung, 2005).
- Large doses of vitamin D may be necessary; do not use for extended periods without monitoring for toxicity.

Herbs, Botanicals, and Supplements

- Herbs and botanical supplements should not be used without discussing with physician.

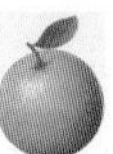

NUTRITION EDUCATION, COUNSELING, CARE MANAGEMENT

- Help patient control weight as needed.
- Explain which foods are good sources of calcium in the diet.
- Explain how to control elevated blood sugars and lipids through balanced dietary intake.
- Manage symptoms of MetS through dietary changes and exercise.

Patient Education—Foodborne Illness

- If home tube feeding is needed, teach appropriate sanitation and food-handling procedures.

For More Information

- Cushing's Support and Research Foundation
http://csrf.net/
- Hormone Foundation
http://www.hormone.org/Other/upload/cushings-syndrome-billingual-032309.pdf
- NIDDK–Cushing's Syndrome
http://www.niddk.nih.gov/health/endo/pubs/cushings/cushings.htm

CUSHING'S SYNDROME—CITED REFERENCES

Carroll T, et al. Late-night salivary cortisol for the diagnosis of Cushing syndrome: a meta-analysis. *Endocr Pract.* 15:335, 2009.

Hopkins RL, Leinung MC. Exogenous Cushing's syndrome and glucocorticoid withdrawal. *Endocrinol Metab Clin North Am.* 34:371, 2005.

Iacabone M, et al. Results and long-term follow-up after unilateral adrenalectomy for ACTH-independent hypercortisolism in a series of fifty patients. *J Endocrinol Invest.* 28:327, 2005.

Kristo C, et al. Biochemical markers for cardiovascular risk following treatment in endogenous Cushing's syndrome. *J Endocrinol Invest.* 31:400, 2008.

Lindsay JR, Nieman LK. Differential diagnosis and imaging in Cushing's syndrome. *Endocrinol Metab Clin North Am.* 34:403, 2005.

Uecker JM, Janzow MT. A case of Cushing syndrome secondary to ectopic adrenocorticotropic hormone producing carcinoid of the duodenum. *Am Surg.* 71:445, 2005.

PITUITARY GLAND (POSTERIOR)

DIABETES INSIPIDUS

NUTRITIONAL ACUITY RANKING: LEVEL 3

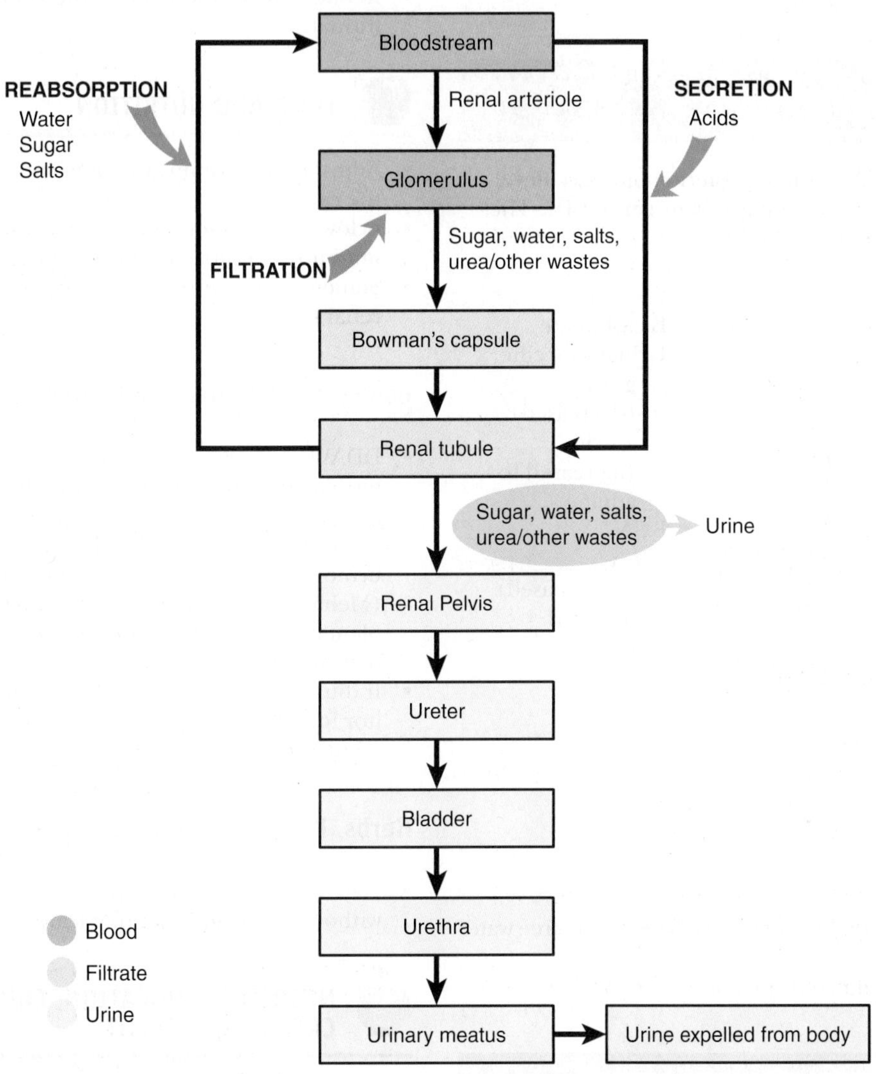

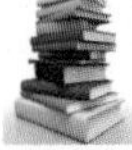

DEFINITIONS AND BACKGROUND

Diabetes insipidus (DI) can be caused by defects in the posterior pituitary gland or from an insufficient renal response to AVP, formerly ADH. Distinction is essential for effective treatment (Makaryus and MacFarlane, 2006). DI may be primary (congenital) or secondary (acquired after trauma, surgery, tumor, or infection). Both forms of DI are marked by excessive thirst, copious urination, and dry skin. There is potential for dehydration and weakness. Urine output may be 5–10 L/24 h.

Nephrogenic DI is characterized by the kidney's inability to respond to AVP. The multiple and complex functions of the renal tubule in regulating water, electrolyte, and mineral homeostasis make it prone to numerous genetic abnormalities (Chadra and Alon, 2009). Nephrogenic DI requires careful monitoring of body chemistry and adequate hydration.

Neurogenic (primary) DI is more common in males. Children with DI may be irritable or listless and may have problems with bedwetting, fever, vomiting, or diarrhea (Linshaw, 2007). Neurogenic DI responds to nasal administration of 1-deamino-8-D-arginine vasopressin (desmopressin acetate) (DDAVP), a vasopressin analogue.

Dipsogenic DI is a very rare forms of DI from a defect in the thirst mechanism in the hypothalmus.

Gestational DI (GDI) is also very rare. DI can complicate up to 1 in 30,000 pregnancies. If DI occurs with pre-eclampsia, the baby may have to be delivered early. DDAVP may be used (Ananthakrishnan, 2009).

Sometimes, the exact cause of DI is unknown. Patients undergoing surgery for pituitary tumors present with DI (Dumont et al, 2005). In acquired forms, the kidneys' ability to respond to AVP can be impaired by drugs such as lithium, or by chronic disorders including polycystic kidney disease, sickle cell disease, kidney failure, partial blockage of the ureters, and inherited genetic disorders.

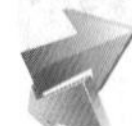

ASSESSMENT, MONITORING, AND EVALUATION

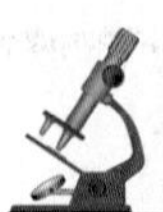

CLINICAL INDICATORS

Genetic Markers: Abnormal posterior pituitary development is found in genetic forms of central DI. The exact genes are being studied.

Clinical/History	Lab Work	
		Glucose
		Bicarbonate
Height	Arginine vasopressin (AVP) in serum, urine	Urinary specific gravity (decreased)
Weight	Urinary osmolality (may be <300 mOsm/kg)	Uric acid (increased in adults)
BMI	Fluid deprivation test (neurogenic vs. nephrogenic forms)	BUN
Diet history		Creat
BP		Na^+ (increased)
Excessive thirst and urination		K^+ (altered?)
I & O		Alb
Fever?		
Vomiting, diarrhea in children		
Brain MRI		

INTERVENTION

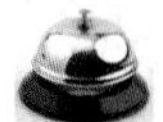

OBJECTIVES

- Reduce urine osmolality and increase electrolyte-free water excretion.
- Raise serum sodium concentration.
- Avoid fluid overload and rapid fluctuations in sodium concentration, especially in persons who cannot control their fluid intake themselves (Toumba and Stanhope, 2006).
- Check patient's weight three times weekly to determine fluid retention and effectiveness of drug therapy. At home, have weights recorded daily.
- Reduce excess workload for the kidney and prevent stone formation.

SAMPLE NUTRITION CARE PROCESS STEPS

Inadequate Fluid Intake

Assessment Data: Polyuria, polydipsia; preference for cold beverages or ice. Signs of poor skin turgor and dehydration; pale urine. Diagnosis of nephrogenic DI.

Nutrition Diagnosis (PES): Inadequate fluid intake related to losses from frequent urination and diagnosis of DI as evidenced by pale urine, urination 10 times daily and during the night.

Intervention: Education about the importance of taking prescribed medication and increasing fluid intake because of Dx of DI. Counseling about sources of fluid from beverages and foods; discussion of signs of dehydration and when to contact the physician.

Monitoring and Evaluation: Reports of improved hydration status. Consistent use of medication. No emergency visits to the doctor or emergency room. Improved quality of life.

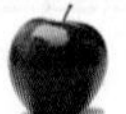

FOOD AND NUTRITION

- Adjust fluid, sodium, and potassium intakes according to the cause.
- A low-sodium diet and diuretics may also be needed to minimize workload of the kidney.
- Sometimes a controlled-protein diet is needed to protect renal function.

Common Drugs Used and Potential Side Effects

- DDAVP may cause abdominal pain, headaches, gastrointestinal distress, and weakness. It is administered parenterally, by pill, or by nasal spray. Patients should drink fluids or water only when thirsty, but be aware that a low urine volume is a risk factor for kidney stone formation (Mehandru and Goldfarb, 2005). Hyponatremic hypervolemia leading to seizures is a rare but potentially life-threatening side effect.
- If diuretics such as thiazides or amiloride are used, monitor for side effects. Potassium may be needed if a supplement is not used.

Herbs, Botanicals, and Supplements

- Herbs and botanical supplements should not be used without discussing with physician.

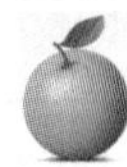

NUTRITION EDUCATION, COUNSELING, CARE MANAGEMENT

- Fluid adjustments will be made according to the type of DI. Caution patients not to limit fluid intake in an effort to lessen urine output.
- Cold or ice water may be preferred.
- Select low-calorie beverages to prevent excessive weight gain.
- Avoid stimulant/diuretic-type beverages (e.g., coffee, tea, alcohol).

Patient Education—Foodborne Illness

- If home tube feeding is needed, teach appropriate sanitation and food-handling procedures.

For More Information

- Diabetes Insipidus Foundation, Inc.
  http://diabetesinsipidus.com
- Nephrogenic Diabetes Insipidus Foundation
  http://www.ndif.org/

DIABETES INSIPIDUS—CITED REFERENCES

Ananthakrishnan S. Diabetes insipidus in pregnancy: etiology, evaluation, and management. *Endocr Pract.* 15:377, 2009.

Chadra V, Alon US. Hereditary renal tubular disorders. *Semin Nephrol.* 29:399, 2009.

Dumont AS, et al. Postoperative care following pituitary surgery. *J Intensive Care Med.* 20:127, 2005.

Linshaw M. Back to basics: congenital nephrogenic diabetes insipidus. *Pediatr Rev.* 28:372, 2007.

Makaryus AN, MacFarlane SI. Diabetes insipidus: diagnosis and treatment of a complex disease. *Cleve Clin J Med.* 73:65, 2006.

Mehandru S, Goldfarb DS. Nephrolithiasis complicating treatment of diabetes insipidus. *Urol Res.* 33:244, 2005.

Toumba M, Stanhope R. Morbidity and mortality associated with vasopressin analogue treatment. *J Pediatr Endocrinol Metab.* 19:197, 2006.

PITUITARY GLAND

SYNDROME OF INAPPROPRIATE ANTIDIURETIC HORMONE (SIADH)

NUTRITIONAL ACUITY RANKING: LEVEL 2

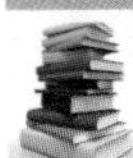

DEFINITIONS AND BACKGROUND

Syndrome of inappropriate antidiuretic hormone (SIADH) involves hyponatremia and hyperosmolarity of urine. Normal renal and adrenal functioning with abnormal elevation of plasma vasopressin occurs (inappropriate for serum osmolality). Hyponatremia and SIADH can occur among elderly long-term care patients with febrile illness (Arinzon et al, 2005). Other causes of SIADH are listed in Table 9-21.

Hyponatremia is usually the first symptom of SIADH. In severe hyponatremia, convulsions or coma can occur. Other signs and symptoms include irritability, lethargy, seizures, and confusion. SIADH or cerebral salt-wasting syndrome (CSWS) can occur after pituitary surgery; differential diagnosis can be difficult. SIADH syndrome often requires sodium replacement or use of loop diuretics.

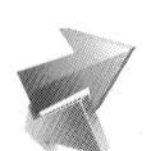

ASSESSMENT, MONITORING, AND EVALUATION

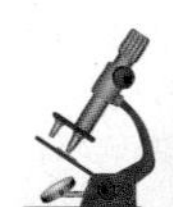

CLINICAL INDICATORS

Genetic Markers: SIADH is usually acquired and not genetic.

Clinical/History
- Height
- Current weight
- Edema-free weight
- BMI
- Diet history
- I & O
- Temperature
- Edema
- Irritability
- Lethargy, confusion
- Low urine volume

Lab Work
- Serum Na$^+$ <135 µmol/L
- Serum osmolality <280 mOsm/kg
- Serum AVP (elevated)
- Urine osmolality >500 µmol/kg
- Urinary Na$^+$ (elevated)
- BUN (low, <10 mg/dL)
- Creat
- K$^+$
- Ca^{++}, Mg^{++}
- Bicarbonate (normal)
- Uric acid (may be low)
- GFR (increased)

SAMPLE NUTRITION CARE PROCESS STEPS

Inadequate Sodium Intake

Assessment Data: Serum Na+ levels low at 110 mol/L; elevated urinary osmolality.

Nutrition Diagnosis (PES): Inadequate sodium intake related to salt wasting syndrome after pituitary surgery as evidenced by low serum Na+ (110) and high urinary mOsm.

Intervention: Food-nutrient delivery – Add extra salt to meals; send extra salt packet with delivered meals.

Monitoring and Evaluation: Normal serum Na+ and urinary osmolality at next lab visit.

TABLE 9-21 Causes of Syndrome of Inappropriate Antidiuretic Hormone

Acute leukemia
Brain abscess, stroke or meningitis
Drugs: chlorpropamide, cyclophosphamide, carbamazepine
Gillain-Barre syndrome
Head injury
Lung cancer (especially small-cell lung cancer)
Lymphoma
Olfactory neuroblastoma
Pancreatic cancer
Pituitary surgery
Pneumonia
Prostate cancer
Rocky Mountain spotted fever
Sarcoidosis
Temporal arteritis, polyarteritis nodosa

INTERVENTION

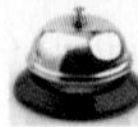

OBJECTIVES

- Treat the cause.
- Restrict water intake.
- Replace electrolytes as appropriate; usually intravenous saline is provided.
- Normalize hormone secretion through drug therapy.

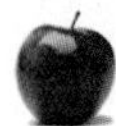

FOOD AND NUTRITION

- Restrict fluid intake, usually 1000–1200 mL/d.
- Alter dietary sodium and potassium, as deemed appropriate for the condition. This will vary by patient condition and medications used.
- When enteral feeding is needed, select a formula that is fluid restricted, such as those that are 2 kcal/mL. Monitor carefully for signs of dehydration. Check content of formula for sodium and potassium; select according to patient status and needs.

Common Drugs Used and Potential Side Effects

- Demeclocycline (Declomycin) may be used with side effects like those of tetracycline. Avoid taking with calcium or dairy products.
- Conivaptan is a new agent available for use to antagonize the effects of vasopressin, especially in heart failure patients (Schwarz and Sanghi, 2006).
- Hyponatremia as a result of SIADH is a relatively common serious side effect of the use of selective serotonin reuptake inhibitors (SSRIs) in (mostly elderly) adults (Vanhaesebrouk et al, 2005).

Herbs, Botanicals, and Supplements

- Herbs and botanical supplements should not be used without discussing with physician.

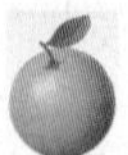

NUTRITION EDUCATION, COUNSELING, CARE MANAGEMENT

- Provide counseling regarding water and fluid restrictions as ordered.
- Discuss any underlying conditions that may have caused the syndrome; highlight needed dietary alterations.

Patient Education—Foodborne Illness

- If home tube feeding is needed, teach appropriate sanitation and food-handling procedures.

For More Information

- E-medicine
  http://www.emedicine.com/ped/topic2190.htm
- National Library of Medicine–Dilutional Hyponatremia
  http://www.nlm.nih.gov/medlineplus/ency/article/000394.htm

SIADH—CITED REFERENCES

Arinzon Z, et al. Water and sodium disturbances predict prognosis of acute disease in long term cared frail elderly. *Arch Gerontol Geriatr.* 40:317, 2005.

Casulari LA, et al. Differential diagnosis and treatment of hyponatremia following pituitary surgery. *J Neurosurg Sci.* 48:11, 2004.

Goh KP. Management of hyponatremia. *Am Fam Physician.* 69:2387, 2004.

Johnson AL, Criddle LM. Pass the salt: indications for and implications of using hypertonic saline. *Crit Care Nurse.* 24:36, 2004.

Schwarz ER, Sanghi P. Conivaptan: a selective vasopressin antagonist for the treatment of heart failure. *Expert Rev Cardiovasc Ther.* 4:17, 2006.

Vachharajani TJ, et al. Hyponatremia in critically ill patients. *J Intensive Care Med.* 18:3, 2003.

Vanhaesebrouk P, et al. Phototherapy-mediated syndrome of inappropriate secretion of antidiuretic hormone in an in utero selective serotonin reuptake inhibitor-exposed newborn infant. *Pediatrics.* 115:508, 2005.

OVARY

POLYCYSTIC OVARIAN DISEASE

NUTRITIONAL ACUITY RANKING: LEVEL 2

DEFINITIONS AND BACKGROUND

Polycystic ovarian disease (PCOD; or polycystic ovarian syndrome [PCOS]) is an endocrine disorder characterized by hyperandrogenism, bilaterally enlarged polycystic ovaries, and insulin resistance. This syndrome affects about 6–10% of women of childbearing age (Barbieri, 2000). There is a lack of consensus between endocrinologists and gynecologists in the definition, diagnosis, and treatment of PCOD (Cussons et al, 2005).

PCOD is currently considered as possibly the most frequent cause of female infertility; it is also closely associated with the MetS (Gleicher and Barad, 2006). Hyperandrogenism, insulin resistance, and acanthosis nigricans (HAIR-AN syndrome) cause presentation of the insulin-resistant syndrome PCOD (Barbieri, 2000). Insulin resistance and hyperandrogenism are caused by both genetic and environmental factors. Acanthosis nigricans is a dark, velvety patch of skin that indicates insulin resistance (Scalzo and McKittrick, 2000). Women of Caribbean-Hispanic or African American descent seem to be more prone to this condition.

Women with PCOD may have had a history of GDM. Many adolescents present with hirsutism and irregular menses. In PCOD, elevated LH to FSH ratio, hirsutism, acne, oily skin, male pattern baldness, menstrual irregularity, oligomenorrhea, and obesity can occur. Abnormally elevated levels of testosterone and LH disrupt the normal maturation process for ovulation. Immature cysts remain on the ovaries, giving the appearance of a "string of pearls."

Girls tested for anorexia nervosa (AN) may also have PCOD, with menstrual irregularities before weight loss and elevated LH and estrogen compared with individuals who have AN alone (Pinhas-Hamiel et al, 2006). In PCOD, biochemical abnormalities include hyperandrogenism, acyclic estrogen production, LH hypersecretion, decreased levels of steroid hormone–binding globulin (SHBG), and hyperinsulinemia (Mascitelli and Pezzetta, 2005). Infertility, hypertension, uterine cancer, diabetes, coronary heart disease, and endometrial carcinoma often follow (Legro, 2001).

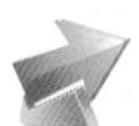

ASSESSMENT, MONITORING, AND EVALUATION

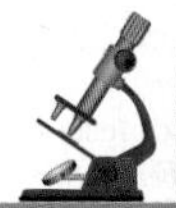

CLINICAL INDICATORS

Genetic Markers: Polymorphisms in the PPARGC1A, PPAR-delta and PPAR-gamma2 loci have been associated with PCOS.

Clinical/History

- Height
- Weight
- BMI
- Diet history
- Weight gain pattern
- History (Hx) of GDM
- Irregular menses
- Amenorrhea
- Hirsutism
- Infertility
- Acne
- Male pattern baldness
- Acanthosis nigricans (dark, velvety patches on skin)
- Vaginal ultrasound with enlarged ovaries
- Recurrent pregnancy loss?

Lab Work

- Glucose
- CRP
- Chol, Trig (elevated?)
- Homocysteine
- Fasting serum insulin (elevated)
- C-peptide levels for insulin secretion
- Serum estrogen
- Serum testosterone
- LH
- LH:FSH ratio (elevated)
- Plasminogen activator inhibitor-1 (PAI-1) (shows abnormal clotting)
- H & H
- Alb
- BUN, Creat
- ALT
- BP (elevated)

SAMPLE NUTRITION CARE PROCESS STEPS

Food-Drug Interaction

Assessment Data: Recent Dx of PCOD; wt at 110% of normal for height. Currently taking metformin but complaining of GI distress.

Nutrition Diagnosis (PES): Food-drug interaction related to metformin use as evidenced by GI distress and use of the medication on an empty stomach.

Intervention: Education about the need to eat before taking the prescription to evaliate if GI distress resolves.

Monitoring and Evaluation: Follow-up about GI distress or other side effects while taking metformin. Evaluation of timing for food and medication use.

INTERVENTION

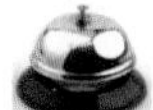

OBJECTIVES

- Lose weight or maintain a normal weight for height; obesity occurs in 50% of this population.
- Prevent heart problems, stroke, and heart attack. Improve lipid profile.
- Reduce serum androgens and improve menstrual regularity.
- Decrease risk for endometrial cancer.
- Alleviate glucose intolerance and insulin resistance.
- Improve anxiety, moods, and quality of life.

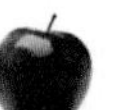

FOOD AND NUTRITION

- Offer a weight-control and exercise plan to meet weight goals. Loss of 5–10 lb may reduce symptoms.
- Lower elevated blood glucose and lipids. Eat five to six small meals per day.
- The DASH diet may be helpful to lower BP. Include low-fat dairy products and more fruits and vegetables.
- Avoid low-fat, high-CHO diets, which promote extra insulin secretion (McKittrick, 2002). A diet of 30–40% fat, 45–50% complex CHOs, and 15–20% protein may be useful.
- Include sufficient fiber (20–35 g/d).
- Include sources of omega-3 fatty acids (fish, walnuts, and flaxseed).
- Dietary or supplemental chromium should be included.

Common Drugs Used and Potential Side Effects

- Symptoms may be managed by antiandrogen medication (e.g., birth control pills, spironolactone, flutamide, or finasteride).
- Insulin-sensitizing drugs improve ovulation and hirsutism in PCOD (Azziz et al, 2001). Metformin (glucophage) allows for improved insulin sensitivity and reduced LH and testosterone. Metformin induces ovulation, has some marginal benefit in improving aspects of the MetS, improves objective measures of hirsutism, and seems to be effective in both obese and lean individuals (Lord and Wilkin, 2004). Do not use with heart failure, chronic obstructive pulmonary disease, or chronic kidney disease. Take with food; monitor for minor gastrointestinal side effects such as nausea, diarrhea, and flatulence. Hypoglycemia does not usually occur.
- Rosiglitazone (Avandia) and pioglitazone (Actos) pose minimal risk of hepatotoxicity compared with older medications.

Herbs, Botanicals, and Supplements

- Herbs and botanical supplements should not be used without discussing with physician.
- Chromium picolinate (1000 μg) may be useful as an insulin sensitizer in the treatment of PCOD (Lydic et al, 2006).

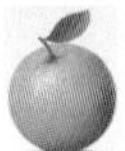

NUTRITION EDUCATION, COUNSELING, CARE MANAGEMENT

- Counsel about weight loss and nutrition. Regular mealtimes and snacks may help control cravings and overeating.
- Encourage regular exercise and reduced sedentary lifestyle.
- Explain relationship of insulin resistance and increased risk for T2DM.
- Medical treatments may be needed to support reproduction. Some women will need in vitro fertilization (IVF) treatments.

Patient Education—Foodborne Illness

- If home tube feeding is needed, teach appropriate sanitation and food handling procedures.

For More Information

- E-medicine: PCOS
  http://www.emedicine.com/med/topic2173.htm
- Polycystic Ovarian Syndrome Association, Inc.
  http://www.pcosupport.org

POLYCYSTIC OVARIAN DISEASE—CITED REFERENCES

Cussons AJ, et al. Polycystic ovarian syndrome: marked differences between endocrinologists and gynaecologists in diagnosis and management. *Clin Endocrinol.* 62:289, 2005.

Essah PA, Nestler JE. The metabolic syndrome in polycystic ovary syndrome. *J Endocrinol Invest.* 29:270, 2006.

Gleicher N, Barad D. An evolutionary concept of polycystic ovarian disease: does evolution favor reproductive success over survival? *Reprod Biomed Online.* 12:587, 2006.

Lydic ML, et al. Chromium picolinate improves insulin sensitivity in obese subjects with polycystic ovary syndrome. *Fertil Steril.* 86:243, 2006.

Mascitelli L, Pezzetta F. Polycystic ovary syndrome. *N Engl J Med.* 352:2756, 2005.

Pinhas-Hamiel O, et al. Clinical and laboratory characteristics of adolescents with both polycystic ovary disease and anorexia nervosa. *Fertil Steril.* 85:1849, 2006.

ADRENAL GLAND (CORTEX)

ADRENOCORTICAL INSUFFICIENCY AND ADDISON'S DISEASE

NUTRITIONAL ACUITY RANKING: LEVEL 1–2

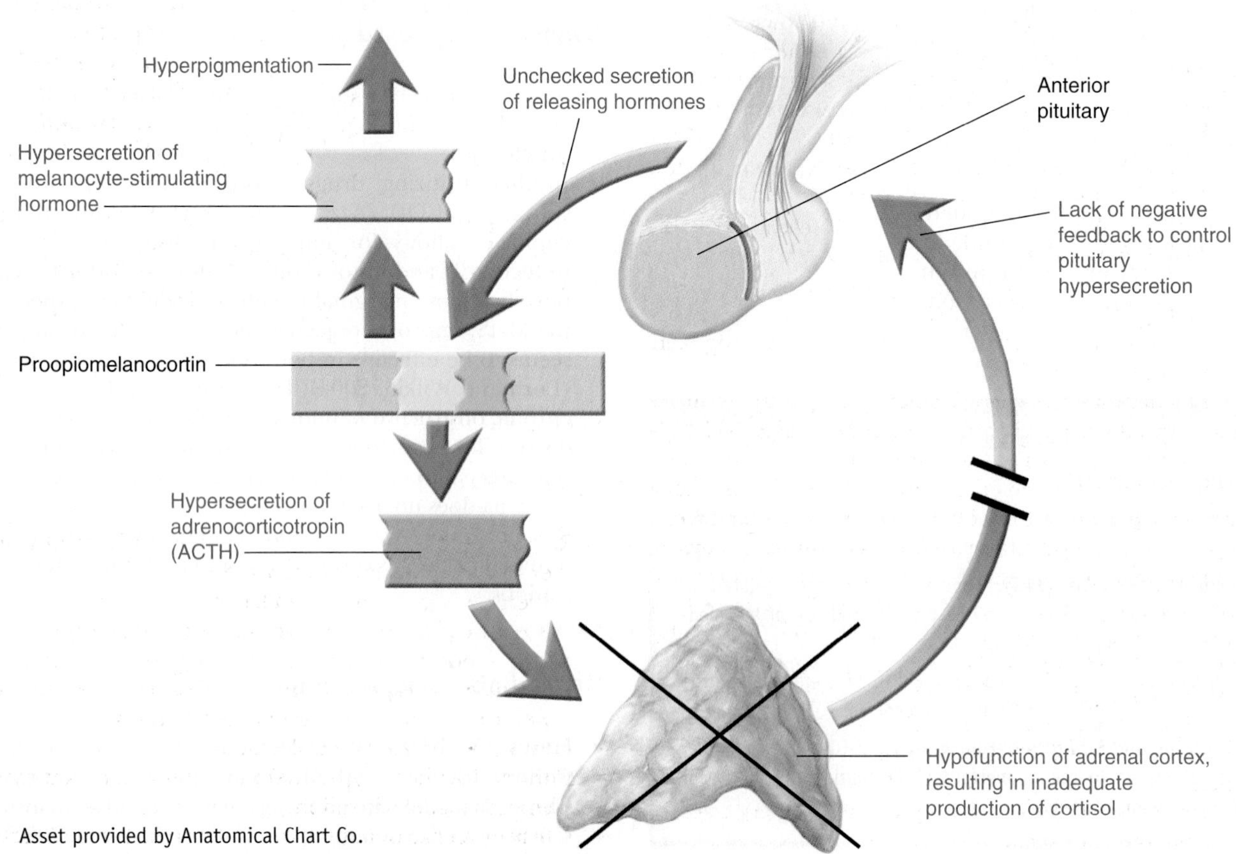

Asset provided by Anatomical Chart Co.

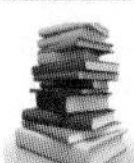

DEFINITIONS AND BACKGROUND

In adrenocortical insufficiency, the adrenal cortex atrophies with loss of hormones (aldosterone, cortisol, and androgens). Primary adrenal insufficiency in the pediatric population (0–18 years) is most commonly attributed to congenital adrenal hyperplasia, which occurs in about 1 in 15,000 births, followed by Addison's disease, with a likely autoimmune etiology (Perry et al, 2005). Secondary forms often result from tuberculosis, cancer, or surgery in which the adrenal glands are destroyed or damaged. Of patients with adrenocortical insufficiency, 33% also have diabetes. With T1DM, the expression of organ-specific autoantibodies is very high (Barker et al, 2005), and this suggests a need for careful screening in both of these conditions.

Cortisol, a glucocorticoid, affects almost every organ and tissue in the body. Cortisol helps the body respond to stress. Among other tasks, cortisol helps to maintain BP and cardiac functioning, the immune system's inflammatory response, the effects of insulin in breaking down sugar for energy through metabolism of macronutrients, and proper arousal and well-being.

Aldosterone functions to conserve sodium and excrete potassium. When aldosterone is no longer secreted, the following events occur: excretion of sodium takes place, and the body's store of water decreases, which leads to dehydration, hypotension, and decreased cardiac output. The heart becomes slower due to reduced workload. Increased serum potassium can lead to arrhythmias, arrest, and even death.

Primary adrenal insufficiency causes abdominal pain, vomiting, weakness, fatigue, weight loss, dehydration, nausea, diarrhea, hyperpigmented (tan or bronze) skin, hypotension, low serum sodium, high serum potassium, and low corticosteroid levels. It may be temporary or may become a chronic insufficiency. Salt cravings can occur.

Type I primary adrenal insufficiency (polyendocrine deficiency syndrome) occurs in children and exhibits underactive parathyroid glands, pernicious anemia, chronic *Candida* infections, chronic active hepatitis, and slow sexual development. Autoimmune thyroid diseases are often associated with T1DM and Addison's disease, characterizing the autoimmune polyendocrine syndrome. **Type II primary adrenal insufficiency (Schmidt's syndrome)** affects young adults and presents with underactive thyroid gland, slow sexual development, diabetes, vitiligo and changing skin pigmentation.

In **secondary adrenal insufficiency**, which is much more common than the primary form, there is a lack of ACTH. Production of cortisol drops but not production of aldosterone. A temporary form of secondary adrenal insufficiency may occur when a person who has been receiving a glucocorticoid hormone such as prednisone for a long time abruptly stops or interrupts taking the medication. Glucocorticoid hormones, which are often used to treat inflammatory illnesses such as rheumatoid arthritis, asthma, or ulcerative colitis, block the release of both CRH and ACTH. Normally, CRH instructs the pituitary gland to release ACTH. If CRH levels drop, the pituitary is not stimulated to release ACTH, and the adrenals then fail to secrete sufficient levels of cortisol. In secondary adrenal insufficiency, darkening of the skin does not occur, and GI symptoms are less common. Hypoglycemia, anxiety, nausea, and palpitations can occur.

Addison's disease is a strict insufficiency state of adrenal hormones, including cortisol and aldosterone. It affects about one in 100,000 people. Autoimmune Addison's disease is caused by autoreactivity toward the adrenal cortex; T cells seem to be involved. An Addisonian crisis can be precipitated by acute infection, trauma, surgery, or excessive body salt loss. Patients with adrenal insufficiency, although on treatment, have a poor quality of life and an increased mortality (Debono et al, 2009). A normal lifespan is possible if daily medications are taken as prescribed. Delayed and sustained release oral formulations of hydrocortisone will match the more natural circadian rhythms of the body. Adrenalectomy may require steroid replacement therapy, a 2-g sodium diet, and control of carbohydrate to prevent hyperglycemia. Possibly, the addition of dehydroepiandrosterone (DHEA) to the treatment plan may lead to improved well-being and sexual function (Hahner and Allolio, 2009).

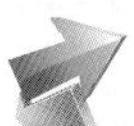

ASSESSMENT, MONITORING, AND EVALUATION

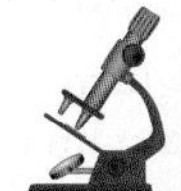

CLINICAL INDICATORS

Genetic Markers: Cytotoxic T lymphocyte antigen 4 (CTLA-4), protein tyrosine phosphatase nonreceptor type 22 (PTPN22), major histocompatibility complex class II transactivator (CIITA), and C-lectin type genes (CLEC16A) play a role in the primary form (Michels and Eisenbarth, 2009).

Clinical/History	Lab Work	
Height	Gluc	ACTH stimulation test
Weight	K^+ (increased)	BUN (increased)
BMI	N balance	Cortisol (decreased)
Diet history	Na^+ (decreased)	CRH stimulation test
BP (decreased)	Ca^{++} (increased)	Alb
I & O	Cl_2 (decreased)	Mg^{++} (increased)
Abdominal x-rays	WBC (decreased)	HbA1c
Skin changes	ACTH (increased)	

INTERVENTION

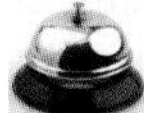

OBJECTIVES

- Relieve symptoms of hormone deficiency by taking synthetic hormones (but not to excess).
- Prevent hypoglycemia; avoid fasting.
- Prevent weight loss. Improve appetite and strength.
- Modify sodium according to drug therapy. Prevent hyponatremia, especially in warm weather when sodium losses from perspiration are higher than usual.
- Prevent dehydration and shock.
- Correct diarrhea, hyperkalemia, nausea, and improper medication administration.
- If hyperglycemia or diabetes occurs, insulin may be needed.

SAMPLE NUTRITION CARE PROCESS STEPS

Inadequate Sodium Intake

Assessment Data: Adrenal insufficiency with inadequate intake of medication replacement; recent labs showing elevated potassium and low serum sodium levels.

Nutrition Diagnosis (PES): Inadequate sodium intake related to insufficient medication for Addison's disease as evidenced by high serum potassium and low serum sodium and diet history revealing low sodium intake for the past week.

Intervention: Educate about the importance of taking sufficient medication to maintain normal electrolyte levels and when to add salt to the diet.

Monitoring and Evaluation: Review of serum electrolytes, quality of life, fewer episodes of Addisonian crisis, diet hx revealing controlled sodium intake as per medical advice.

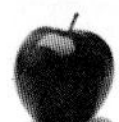

FOOD AND NUTRITION

- During an Addisonian crisis, low BP, low blood glucose, and high levels of potassium can be life threatening. Intravenous injections of hydrocortisone, saline, and dextrose are given by the medical team.
- Use a high-protein, moderate-carbohydrate diet. Snacks may be needed. Control carbohydrate amount and frequency according to blood glucose and HgbA1c levels.
- Ensure intake of sodium is adequate according to medications given. Monitor potassium levels and adjust diet if needed.
- Force fluids (2–3 L) when allowed.

Common Drugs Used and Potential Side Effects

- If aldosterone is missing, fludrocortisone (Florinef) is used as an oral, synthetic, sodium-retaining hormone. Be wary about overdosing, with potential side effects of hypertension and ankle edema. Postural hypotension can occur with a dose that is too low. Extra may be needed when exercising or in hot weather.
- Long-acting synthetic glucocorticoids, such as oral dexamethasone or prednisone, are given for replacement. Side effects can include loss of calcium, decreased bone density, or risk of osteoporosis. To decrease gastric irritation, take hormones with milk or an antacid.
- Signs of insufficient amounts of cortisol replacement include feeling weak and tired all the time, getting sick or vomiting, and anorexia. Weight loss can occur.

Herbs, Botanicals, and Supplements

- Herbs and botanical supplements should not be used without discussing with physician.

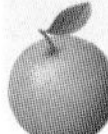

NUTRITION EDUCATION, COUNSELING, CARE MANAGEMENT

- Help patient individualize diet according to symptoms. During illness or injury, the body normally makes up to 10 times more cortisol than usual. Be prepared to avoid a crisis with a prompt treatment.
- Ensure patient does not skip meals. Instruct patient to carry cheese or cracker snack to prevent hypoglycemia.
- Discuss simple meal preparation to lessen fatigue.
- Discuss food sources of sodium and potassium according to the medical plan.
- Use of Medic-Alert identification is recommended. Patients with this condition may need to carry a syringe prefilled with dexamethasone.
- Pregnancy is possible, with carefully managed replacement medication. Evidence has accrued that fracture risk might be programmed during intrauterine life, mediated through pituitary-dependent endocrine systems such as insulin, growth hormone, and the HPA (hypothalamic-pituitary-adrenal) system (Cooper et al, 2009).

Patient Education—Foodborne Illness

- If home tube feeding is needed, teach appropriate sanitation and food-handling procedures.

For More Information

- Adrenal Gland Disorders
  http://www.nlm.nih.gov/medlineplus/adrenalglanddisorders.html
- JAMA – Patient Page for Adrenal Insufficiency
  http://jama.ama-assn.org/cgi/reprint/294/19/2528.pdf
- National Adrenal Diseases Foundation
  http://www.medhelp.org/nadf/
- National Institutes of Health
  http://www.cc.nih.gov/ccc/patient_education/pepubs/mngadrins.pdf

ADRENOCORTICAL INSUFFICIENCY AND ADDISON'S DISEASE—CITED REFERENCES

Barker JM, et al. Autoantibody "subspecificity" in type 1 diabetes: risk for organ-specific autoimmunity clusters in distinct groups. *Diabetes Care.* 28:850, 2005.

Cooper C, et al. Developmental origins of osteoporosis: the role of maternal nutrition. *Adv Exp Med Biol.* 646:31, 2009.

Debono M, et al. Novel strategies for hydrocortisone replacement. *Best Pract Res Clin Endocrinol Metab.* 23:221, 2009.

Hahner S, Allolio B. Therapeutic management of adrenal insufficiency. *Best Pract Res Clin Endocrinol Metab.* 23:167, 2009.

Michels AW, Eisenbarth GS. Autoimmune polyendocrine syndrome type 1 (APS-1) as a model for understanding autoimmune polyendocrine syndrome type 2 (APS-2). *J Intern Med.* 265:530, 2009.

Perry R, et al. Primary adrenal insufficiency in children: twenty years experience at the Sainte-Justine Hospital, Montreal. *J Clin Endocrinol Metab.* 90:3243, 2005.

ADRENAL GLAND (CORTEX)

HYPERALDOSTERONISM

NUTRITIONAL ACUITY RANKING: LEVEL 1–2

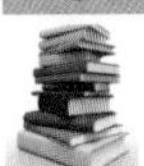

DEFINITIONS AND BACKGROUND

Hyperaldosteronism is an increased production of aldosterone by the adrenal cortex. Aldosterone controls water and electrolyte balance by acting on mineralocorticoid receptors in the kidney and in the vascular system (Oberleithner, 2005). Hyperaldosteronism causes endothelial dysfunction regardless of high BP. Patients may be quite vulnerable to cardiac events, including stroke (Milliez et al, 2005).

Primary aldosteronism (PA) is usually from an adenoma and involves hypertension, hypokalemia, and low plasma renin. Familial hyperaldosteronism type I (FH-I) represents about 1% of cases of primary hyperaldosteronism. It may be detected in asymptomatic individuals when screening the offspring of affected individuals, or patients may present in infancy with hypertension, weakness, and failure to thrive due to hypokalemia. It is inherited in an autosomal dominant manner.

Conn's syndrome is a benign tumor in one adrenal gland that can cause this condition. Urine 18-hydroxycortisol (18-OHF) measurements are used to detect Conn's syndrome with adrenal adenoma or glucocorticoid-suppressible hyperaldosteronism (Reynolds et al, 2005).

Secondary forms of aldosteronism may occur after cancer, heart failure, hyperplasia, malignant hypertension, pregnancy, estrogen use, or cirrhosis. Aldosteronism is a diagnosis that should be considered in refractory hypertension.

CT, MRI, and adrenal vein sampling (AVS) distinguish unilateral PA from the bilateral form; the unilateral form can be treated surgically, whereas bilateral PA is treated medically (Kempers et al, 2009).

SAMPLE NUTRITION CARE PROCESS STEPS

Excessive Sodium Intake

Assessment Data: Hypertension (190/95); diet hx indicating daily use of high sodium foods and salty snacks.

Nutrition Diagnosis (PES): Excessive sodium intake related to intake of high sodium foods and frequent salty snacks throughout the day as evidenced by dietary recall and food records estimated at about 8–9 g Na^+ daily.

Intervention: Food-nutrient delivery—limit dietary sources of sodium to 2–4 g sodium; monitor effects of medication. Educate about sources of sodium, potassium, and use of the DASH diet plan as appropriate. Counsel about ways to reduce sodium from foods and snacks; how to dine away from home; how to monitor for signs and symptoms requiring medical attention.

Monitoring and Evaluation: Lower BP; normal serum labs, especially potassium. Diet history indicating great improvement in sodium regulation. Able to verbalize use of the DASH diet principles.

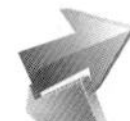

ASSESSMENT, MONITORING, AND EVALUATION

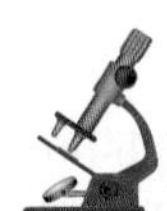

CLINICAL INDICATORS

Genetic Markers: Primary hyperaldosteronism may be the cause of essential hypertension in some people. Specific DNA mutations have emphasized the role of molecular genetics in this disorder (New et al, 2005).

Clinical/History

- Height
- Weight
- BMI
- Diet history
- I & O
- BP (high)
- Fatigue
- Headache
- Weakness, intermittent paralysis
- Numbness
- Abdominal CT scan for adrenal mass
- ECG with abnormalities from low K^+ levels

Lab Work

- Sodium load test (6 g common)
- Plasma renin (low)
- Plasma aldosterone (elevated)
- Urinary aldosterone (elevated)
- Aldosterone: renin ratio
- Urine sodium (altered)
- Urine 18-hydroxycortisol (18-OHF)
- Na^+ (altered)
- K^+ (low)
- Urine potassium (altered)
- Ca^{++}
- Mg^{++} (altered)
- pCO_2 (altered)
- H & H
- Serum Fe

INTERVENTION

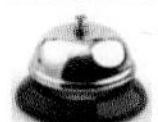

OBJECTIVES

- Hydrate adequately.
- Alter diet as needed (sodium, potassium).
- Correct hypokalemia and hypertension.
- Prepare for surgery if a tumor is involved. Laparoscopic adrenalectomy (LA) is quite successful, after which BP returns to normal. If a tumor is not involved, medical treatment will be for life.

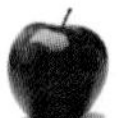

FOOD AND NUTRITION

- Provide adequate fluid intake (unless contraindicated for other reasons).
- A sodium-restricted diet may be needed. A high potassium intake and the DASH diet may be required, depending on the medical or surgical treatment used.
- Small, frequent feedings may be needed.

Common Drugs Used and Potential Side Effects

- Antihypertensives may be used; monitor side effects specifically for the medications prescribed. Aldosterone antagonists have been available for many decades; spironolactone may be used alone or with ACE inhibitors or ARBs.
- Eplerenone, a selective aldosterone antagonist, avoids the androgen and progesterone receptor–related adverse events that sometimes occur with spironolactone, such as breast tenderness, gynecomastia, sexual dysfunction, and menstrual irregularities (Pratt-Ubunama et al, 2005).
- Digitalis may be used. Avoid herbal teas, high-fiber intakes, and excessive amounts of vitamin D. Include adequate amounts of potassium. Take the drug 30 minutes before meals.

Herbs, Botanicals, and Supplements

- Herbs and botanical supplements should not be used without discussing with physician.
- Products containing natural licorice should be avoided in this condition.

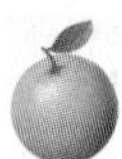

NUTRITION EDUCATION, COUNSELING, CARE MANAGEMENT

- Explain altered sodium and potassium requirements. Teach principles of the DASH diet.
- Have patient avoid fasting, skipping meals, and fad dieting.
- Provide recipe suggestions.
- Avoid consuming large amounts of real licorice, which can aggravate the condition.

Patient Education—Foodborne Illness

- If home tube feeding is needed, teach appropriate sanitation and food-handling procedures.

For More Information

- Medline
  http://www.nlm.nih.gov/medlineplus/ency/article/000330.htm
- Merck manual – Hyperaldosteronism
  http://www.merck.com/mmhe/sec13/ch164/ch164e.html
- National Adrenal Foundation – Hyperaldosteronism
  http://www.nadf.us/diseases/hyperaldosteronism.htm

HYPERALDOSTERONISM—CITED REFERENCES

Kempers MJ, et al. Systematic review: diagnostic procedures to differentiate unilateral from bilateral adrenal abnormality in primary aldosteronism. *Ann Intern Med.* 151:329, 2009.

Milliez P, et al. Evidence for an increased rate of cardiovascular events in patients with primary aldosteronism. *J Am Coll Cardiol.* 45:1243, 2005.

New MI, et al. Monogenic low renin hypertension. *Trends Endocrinol Metab.* 16:92, 2005.

Oberleithner H. Aldosterone makes human endothelium stiff and vulnerable. *Kidney Int.* 67:1680, 2005.

Pratt-Ubunama MN, et al. Aldosterone antagonism: an emerging strategy for effective blood pressure lowering. *Curr Hypertens Rep.* 7:186, 2005.

Reynolds RM, et al. The utility of three different methods for measuring urinary 18-hydroxycortisol in the differential diagnosis of suspected primary hyperaldosteronism. *Eur J Endocrinol.* 152:903, 2005.

ADRENAL GLAND (MEDULLA)

PHEOCHROMOCYTOMA

NUTRITIONAL ACUITY RANKING: LEVEL 1

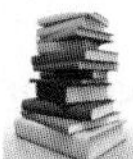

DEFINITIONS AND BACKGROUND

Pheochromocytoma (PHEO) is a rare tumor of the chromaffin cells most commonly arising from the adrenal medulla, resulting in increased secretion of epinephrine and norepinephrine. It is slightly more common in males. Hereditary PHEOs are typically intra-adrenal and bilateral, and patients typically present at a young age.

PHEO may occur as a single tumor or as multiple growths. Symptoms and signs include very high BP, headache, excessive diaphoresis, and palpitations. Less-common symptoms are anxiety, chest pain, fatigue, weight loss, abdominal pain, and nervousness. About 10% of these tumors are malignant and can spread. Persons who have difficult-to-treat hypertension, have onset before age 35 or after age 60, or are taking four or more BP medicines may need to be tested for PHEO.

BP often fluctuates up and down, daily testing is recommended. Diagnosis includes measurement of urinary catecholamines or their metabolites, vanillylmandelic acid and total metanephrines. The urinary metanephrines provide a highly sensitive clue to the presence of PHEO; see Table 9-22.

Treatment usually involves surgical removal of the tumor. Before surgery, alpha-adrenergic blockers may be used. After surgery, about one quarter of patients will still suffer from hypertension and require lifelong management.

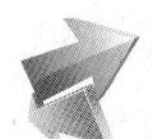

ASSESSMENT, MONITORING, AND EVALUATION

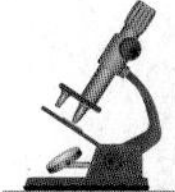

CLINICAL INDICATORS

Genetic Markers: PHEO may be transmitted as an autosomal dominant trait. At least five different gene mutations can cause PHEO. One type causes multiple endocrine neoplasia. Type IIB (MEN IIB) also leads to thyroid cancer and tumors of nerves in the lips, mouth, eyes and digestive tract. The NF1 neurofibromas may present with café-au-lait spots, an optic glioma, and PHEO.

Clinical/History

Height
Weight
BMI
Diet history
Increased appetite
BP (very elevated)
Orthostatic hypotension
Headache
Excessive diaphoresis, flushing
Intolerance of heat
Heart palpitations
Sleep disturbances
CT scan, MRI
Adrenal biopsy
Metaiodobenzylguanidine (MIBG) scanning

Lab Work (see Table 9-22)

Urinary epinephrine and norepinephrine (increased)
Urinary metabolites (vanillylmandelic acid and metanephrines)*
Gluc
Na^+, K^+
Alb
CRP
H & H
Glucagon test (positive)
T3, T4

*Testing may require dietary changes up to 3 days in advance.

INTERVENTION

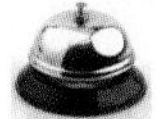

OBJECTIVES

- Prepare for surgery to remove tumor. Patients with preoperative endocrinopathies present a challenge because the "endocrine axis" is complex (Kohl and Schwartz, 2009). If the tumor cannot be removed, lifelong medication will be needed.

TABLE 9-22 Catecholamines

Catecholamine	Comments	Normal Urinary Value/24 h
Dopamine	A neurotransmitter (a chemical used to transmit impulses between nerve cells) found mainly in the brain. Metabolized by target tissues or by the liver to become inactive substances that appear in the urine—dopamine becomes homovanillic acid.	Dopamine 65–400 μg
Epinephrine	A brain neurotransmitter, but is also a major hormone secreted from the adrenal medulla in response to low blood glucose, exercise, and various forms of stress where the brain stimulates release of the hormone. Epinephrine causes a breakdown of glycogen to glucose in liver and muscle, the release of fatty acids from adipose tissue, vasodilation of small arteries within muscle tissue, and increases in the rate and strength of the heartbeat. In the urine: epinephrine becomes metanephrine and VMA.	Epinephrine 0.5–20 μg Metanephrine: 24–96 μg VMA: 2–7 mg*
Norepinephrine	The primary neurotransmitter in the sympathetic nervous system (controls the "fight or flight" reaction) and is also found in the brain. In the urine: norepinephrine becomes normetanephrine and vanillylmandelic acid (VMA).	Norepinephrine 15–80 μg Normetanephrine: 75–375 μg
Total		Total urine catecholamines: 14–110 μg

*For testing, a VMA-restricted diet may be required for lab results; omit chocolate, vanilla extract, and citrus.
Source: Medline Plus. Catecholamines–urine. Accessed September 22, 2009, at http://www.nlm.nih.gov/medlineplus/ency/article/003613.htm

SAMPLE NUTRITION CARE PROCESS STEPS

Excessive Intake of Bioactive Substances

Assessment Data: Hypertensive crisis following intake of caffeine and Chianti wine. Dx of PHEO; high levels of urinary epinephrine and norepinephrine, as well as vanillylmandelic acid and metanephrines. Diet history reveals recent intake of coffee, chocolate and Chianti wine at dinner meal, causing extreme heart palpitations and soaring BP.

Nutrition Diagnosis (PES): Excessive intake of bioactive substances (caffeine, tyramine) related to coffee, chocolate and Chianti wine as evidenced by very high BP and diet history.

Intervention: Education about foods to avoid, such as caffeine from food and beverages, tyramine-rich foods including beer, Chianti wine, processed meats, soy sauce, bananas, avocado.

Monitoring and Evaluation: No further hypertensive crises related to food and beverage intake.

- Stabilize BP before surgery. Avoid overstimulation from even slight exercise, cold stress, or emotional upsets.
- Correct nausea, vomiting, and anorexia.
- Manage long-term hypertension. A severe BP level is any reading above 180/110 mm Hg. Prevent hypertensive crises, which could cause sudden blindness, kidney failure, seizures, acute respiratory distress, arrthymias or stroke.
- Manage any complications such as heart attack or cardiomyopathy (Kassim et al, 2008).

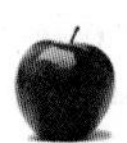

FOOD AND NUTRITION

- For urine testing, some doctors order a VMA diet where patient avoids bananas, caffeine from coffee or Pepsi/Coke, chocolate, tea, vanilla in foods, pineapple, alcoholic beverages, eggplant, plums, walnuts. While this was a common practice in the past, there is no strong evidence to support its use.
- Increase fluids but avoid caffeinated beverages. Avoid tyramine-rich foods, especially if taking MAO inhibitors.
- Six small feedings may be better tolerated than large meals.
- Increase protein and calories if patient is having surgery. Postoperatively, provide adequate vitamins and minerals for wound healing.
- Re-expansion of plasma volume may be accomplished by liberal salt or fluid intake with use of alpha-1 adrenergic receptor antagonists.
- In recurrent cases, long-term drug therapy will be needed. Monitor for specific dietary changes and side effects.

Common Drugs Used and Potential Side Effects

- Pharmacological treatment of catecholamine excess is mandatory.
- Phenoxybenzamine (or an alpha-1 adrenergic receptor antagonist such as prazosin) is needed to block alpha-adrenergic activity. Diuretics should not be used.
- Low doses of a beta-blocker such as propranolol are used to control BP and cardiac tachyarrhythmias but only after alpha blockade. Labetalol, an alpha- and beta-adrenergic blocker, has also been shown to be effective in the control of BP and symptoms of PHEO.
- Avoid decongestants, amphetamines, MAO inhibitors (Nardil, Parnate).
- High-dose MIBG may be used in the treatment of malignant PHEO but can have toxic side effects (Gonias et al, 2009).
- If diabetes occurs, insulin may be needed.

Herbs, Botanicals, and Supplements

- Herbs and botanical supplements should not be used without discussing with physician.

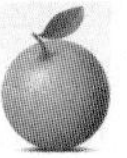

NUTRITION EDUCATION, COUNSELING, CARE MANAGEMENT

- Discuss avoidance of caffeinated foods and beverages (e.g., coffee, tea, and chocolate).
- Maintain a calm atmosphere for patient; prevent undue stress.
- Exercise should be limited until condition is under control.

Patient Education—Foodborne Illness

- If home tube feeding is needed, teach appropriate sanitation and food-handling procedures.

For More Information

- Endocrine Web
  http://www.endocrineweb.com/pheo.html
- Mayo Clinic
  http://www.mayoclinic.com/health/pheochromocytoma/DS00569
- Medline
  http://www.nlm.nih.gov/medlineplus/ency/article/000340.htm
- Merck Manual
  http://www.merck.com/mrkshared/mmanual/section2/chapter9/9d.jsp
- National Cancer Institute
  http://www.cancer.gov/cancerinfo/pdq/treatment/pheochromocytoma/patient
- National Library of Medicine
  http://www.nlm.nih.gov/medlineplus/pheochromocytoma.html
- Urology Health
  http://www.urologyhealth.org/adult/index.cfm?cat=04&topic=114

PHEOCHROMOCYTOMA—CITED REFERENCES

Gonias S, et al. Phase II study of high-dose [131I]metaiodobenzylguanidine therapy for patients with metastatic pheochromocytoma and paraganglioma. *J Clin Oncol.* 27:4162, 2009.

Kassim TA, et al. Catecholamine-induced cardiomyopathy. *Endocr Pract.* 14:1137, 2008.

Kohl BA, Schwartz S. Surgery in the patient with endocrine dysfunction. *Med Clin North Am.* 93:1031, 2009.

THYROID GLAND

HYPERTHYROIDISM

NUTRITIONAL ACUITY RANKING: LEVEL 1

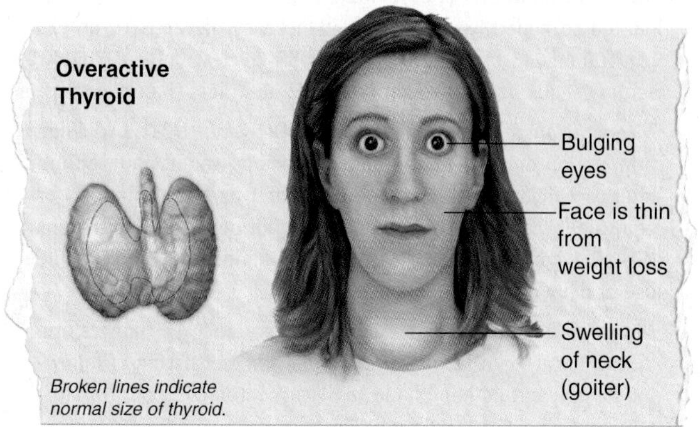

Asset provided by Anatomical Chart Co.

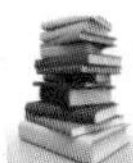

DEFINITIONS AND BACKGROUND

Hyperthyroidism results from oversecretion of the thyroid hormones, triiodothyronine (T3) or thyroxone (T4). These hormones affect every cell through controlling body temperature, heart rate, metabolism, and production of calcitonin. Thyroid hormone affects glucose homeostasis through increased hepatic glucose output, increased futile cycling of glucose degradation products between the skeletal muscle and the liver, decreased glycogen stores in the liver and skeletal muscle, altered oxidative and nonoxidative glucose metabolism, decreased active insulin output from the pancreas, and increased renal insulin clearance (Potenza et al, 2009). When the hypothalmus signals the pituitary gland to produce TSH, normally this is regulated to be just enough. See Table 9-23 for interpretation of lab results for thyroid disorders.

The autoimmune thyroid diseases (AITD), Graves' disease, and chronic lymphocytic thyroiditis (CLT) are among the most common endocrine diseases in childhood and adolescence (Brown, 2009). Usually in hyperthyroidism, the entire gland is overproducing thyroid hormone. Rarely, a single nodule is responsible for the excess hormone secretion. An elevated metabolic rate, tissue wasting, diaphoresis, tremor, tachycardia, goiter, heat intolerance, cold insensitivity, nervousness, increased appetite, exophthalmos, and loss of glycogen stores can occur. If left untreated, atrial fibrillation and osteoporosis can result.

Autoimmune thyroiditis (AITD) may start out temporary, then lead to hyperthyroidism. The most common causes include Hashimoto's thyroiditis, subacute granulomatous thyroiditis, or silent lymphocytic thyroiditis. The major environmental triggers of AITD include iodine, medications, infection, smoking, and possibly stress (Tomer and Huber, 2009). Specific digestive diseases (celiac disease or primary biliary cirrhosis) may be associated with autoimmune thyroid processes (Daher et al, 2009). Persons who have T1DM, mood disorders, psychosis, or Addison's disease also seem to be at higher risk.

Graves' disease (diffuse toxic goiter) is the most common form; **thyrotoxicosis** is more severe. Clinical thyrotoxicosis in Graves' disease patients is caused by thyrotropin receptor (TSHR)-stimulating autoantibodies (Schott et al, 2005). Most people who develop Graves' ophthalmopathy have one or more of the following symptoms: dry and itchy eyes, a staring or bug-eyed look (exophthalmos), sensitivity to light, excessive tearing, a feeling of pressure around the eyes, difficulty closing the eyes completely, and peripheral double vision. Thyrotoxicosis can alter carbohydrate metabolism in a type 2 diabetic patient to such an extent that DKA develops if untreated (Potenza et al, 2009).

Thyroid storm (thyroid crisis) is a potentially life-threatening condition that develops in a person with hyperthyroidism. The gland suddenly releases large amounts of thyroid hormone in a short period of time. Signs of thyroid storm include extreme irritability, high systolic BP, low diastolic BP, tachycardia, nausea, vomiting, diarrhea, high fever, confusion, and sleepiness. Shock, delirium, shortness of breath, fatigue, coma, heart failure, and death can result if not treated immediately. Emergency medical treatment is always needed.

If thyroidectomy is needed, antithyroid agents and iodine are often given 4–6 weeks before surgery to minimize the risk of thyroid crisis. With thyroidectomy, the patient may require a high-calorie, high-protein diet preoperatively. Evaluate needs postoperatively with the doctor's care plan.

TABLE 9-23 Thyroid Test Results

TSH	T4	T3	Interpretation
High	Normal	Normal	Mild (subclinical) hypothyroidism
High	Low	Low or normal	Hypothyroidism
Low	Normal	Normal	Mild (subclinical) hyperthyroidism
Low	High or normal	High or normal	Hyperthyroidism
Low	Low or normal	Low or normal	Nonthyroidal illness; rare pituitary (secondary) hypothyroidism

Source: Lab Tests On Line, web site accessed October 25, 2009, at http://www.labtestsonline.org/understanding/analytes/t3/test.html

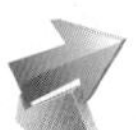

ASSESSMENT, MONITORING, AND EVALUATION

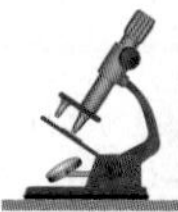

CLINICAL INDICATORS

Genetic Markers: In Graves' disease a specific combination of polymorphisms for thyroglobulin and HLA-DR markedly increases the odds ratio for developing disease

(Brown, 2009). Among the major AITD susceptibility genes that have been identified is the HLA-DR gene locus, as well as CTLA-4, CD40, PTPN22, thyroglobulin, and TSH receptor genes (Tomer and Huber, 2009).

Clinical/History		
Height	More frequent bowel movements	TSH (normal or low)
Weight	Fatigue, muscle weakness	Protein-bound iodine (PBI)
BMI	Changes in menstrual habits	Gluc (increased)
Rapid weight loss?	Protruding eyeballs?	Alb, transthyretin
Diet history	Excessive tearing from one or both eyes?	Ca^{++}
Temperature	Thyroid scan	Mg^{++} (decreased)
BP	Goiter (enlarged thyroid gland)	Na^+, K^+
I & O		H & H
Nervousness, anxiety	**Lab Work**	Serum ferritin
Tachycardia or palpitations	T3 (increased)	Chol, Trig (decreased)
Increased sensitivity to heat	T4 (increased)	BUN, Creat
Difficulty sleeping		N balance
Fine tremor of hands		Alk phos (increased)

INTERVENTION

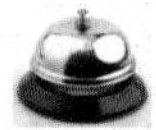

OBJECTIVES

- Achieve a euthyroid state to avoid the effects of triiodothyronine (T3) on the heart and cardiovascular system: decreased systemic vascular resistance and increased resting heart rate, left ventricular contractility, blood volume, and cardiac output (Dahl et al, 2008).
- Prevent or treat complications accompanying high metabolic rate, including bone demineralization. This seems to be a greater problem in older women than in adolescents (Poomthavorn et al, 2005).
- Replenish glycogen stores. Replace lost weight (usually 10–20 lb).
- Correct negative nitrogen balance.
- Replace fluid losses from diarrhea, diaphoresis, and increased respirations. However, exophthalmos, caused by increased accumulation of extracellular fluid in the eyes, may require fluid and salt restriction.
- Monitor or treat fat intolerance and steatorrhea.

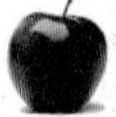

FOOD AND NUTRITION

- Use a high-calorie diet (start with 40 kcal/kg). The patient's caloric needs may be increased by 50–60% in this condition (or 10–30% in mild cases). Ensure adequate intake of carbohydrates.
- Provide protein in the range of 1–1.75 g/kg body weight.
- Fluid intake should be 3–4 L/d, unless contraindicated by renal or cardiac problems.
- Include 1 quart of milk or equivalent daily to supply adequate calcium, phosphorus, and vitamin D.
- Exclude caffeine and stimulants from diet because they aggravate excitability and nervousness.
- Supplement diet with vitamins A, C, and B-complex vitamins, especially thiamin, riboflavin, B_6, and B_{12}. A general multivitamin–mineral supplement may be beneficial; monitor for iodine content.
- Be aware of iodine in any supplements used. Chronic iodine intakes greater than 500 μg/L are associated with adverse effects (Zimmermann et al, 2005).
- Raw natural goitrogens (cabbage, Brussels sprouts, kale, cauliflower, soybeans, peanuts) should not be used with antithyroid medications because these substances increase side effects of the drugs. Cooking reduces this effect.

SAMPLE NUTRITION CARE PROCESS STEPS

Altered Nutrient Utilization

Assessment Data: Elevated T3 and T4, low TSH and serum calcium; BMI 18 with weight loss of 15 lb in 6 months. Dx hyperthyroidism.

Nutrition Diagnosis (PES): Altered nutrient utilization (NC-2.1) related to hyperthyroidism as evidenced by elevated T4 of 112 μg/100 mL; T3 of μg/100 mL; low TSH level at 0.10 μU/L; low serum calcium levels; weight loss of 15 lb in less than 6 months.

Interventions: Food and Nutrition Delivery: ND-1.3 provide information on high calorie diet to promote weight gain, ensure high carbohydrate intake, importance of 1 quart of milk daily or equivalent, caffeine to be avoided, be cautious of raw goitrogens ND-3.2.1 continue use of daily multivitamin. ND3.2.4 continue use of daily calcium supplement.

Nutrition Education: E-1.1 Discuss importance of high calorie diet (40 kcal/kg/d) to promote weight gain consisting of following healthy eating habits and to discuss interaction of raw natural goitrogens with antithyroid drugs.

Counseling: C-2.2 RD to work with patient to set goals of weight gain and taking antithyroid drug to be prescribed by MD.

Coordination of Care: RC-1.3 Collaboration with MD and referral to endocrinologist, to speak with MD about weight gain of 1–2 lb per week and drug–food interactions.

Monitoring and Evaluation: Prevent the thyroid from producing excess hormones with use of antithyroid drug, Tapazole. Follow a weight gain of 1–2 lb/wk till patient reaches normal body weight range of 125–130 lb. Daily use of multivitamin and calcium supplementation. Successful food recording in food diary. Patient can recite raw natural goitrogens to be avoid them in her diet. Patient eating frequent snacks. Patient successfully gained 1 lb in 2 weeks bringing her weigh to 116 lb, BMI now 19.3. Patient to visit endocrinologist in next week.

Common Drugs Used and Potential Side Effects

- The goal of drug therapy is to prevent the thyroid from producing excess hormones. Antithyroid drugs, also called thionamides, such as methimazole (Tapazole) and propylthiouracil (PTU), can cause nausea, vomiting, altered taste sensation, and gastrointestinal distress. They should be taken with food. Avoid use of natural goitrogens in raw form; cooked forms are not a problem.

- Thionamides represent the treatment of choice in pregnant women, during lactation, in children and adolescents, and in preparation for radioiodine therapy or thyroidectomy (Bartelena et al, 2005).
- Radioactive iodine may be used to damage or destroy some of the thyroid cells. It can cause a temporary burning sensation in the throat. Hydrochlorothiazide (HCTZ) may be used to improve radioiodine uptake in hyperthyroid patients; replace potassium.
- Some drugs can affect the thyroid glands. Amiodarone is a potent antiarrhythmic drug that also possesses beta-blocking properties; a 100-mg tablet contains an amount of iodine that is 250 times the recommended daily iodine requirement. Amiodarone-induced thyrotoxicosis is a difficult condition to diagnose and treat; monitor carefully (Basaria and Cooper, 2005).

Herbs, Botanicals, and Supplements

- Herbs and botanical supplements should not be used without discussing with physician. Bugleweed, verbena, lemon balm and kelp have been recommended; no clinical trials prove efficacy.
- Limit use of large quantities of iodine-rich seaweed such as kombu (*Laminaria japonica*).

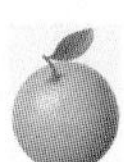

NUTRITION EDUCATION, COUNSELING, CARE MANAGEMENT

- Thyroid hormone affects adipokines and adipose tissue, predisposing the patient to ketosis (Potenza et al, 2009). Beware of hyperglycemia after carbohydrate-rich meals.
- Encourage quiet, pleasant mealtimes.
- Exclude use of alcohol, which may cause a hypoglycemic state.
- Frequent snacks may be needed. To avoid obesity, adjust patient's diet as condition corrects itself.

Patient Education—Foodborne Illness

- If home tube feeding is needed, teach appropriate sanitation and food-handling procedures.

For More Information

- American Thyroid Association
  http://www.thyroid.org/
- Endocrine Web–Hyperthyroidism
  http://www.endocrineweb.com/hyper1.html
- European Thyroid Society
  http://www.eurothyroid.com/
- Latin American Thyroid Society
  http://www.lats.org/
- National Graves Disease Foundation
  http://www.ngdf.org/
- University of Maryland Medical Center
  http://www.umm.edu/endocrin/hypert.htm

HYPERTHYROIDISM—CITED REFERENCES

Bartelena L, et al. An update on the pharmacological management of hyperthyroidism due to Graves' disease. *Expert Opin Pharmacother.* 6:851, 2005.

Basaria S, Cooper DS. Amiodarone and the thyroid. *Am J Med.* 118:706, 2005.

Brown RS. Autoimmune thyroid disease: unlocking a complex puzzle. *Curr Opin Pediatr.* 21:523, 2009.

Daher R, et al. Consequences of dysthyroidism on the digestive tract and viscera. *World J Gastroenterol.* 15:2834, 2009.

Dahl P, et al. Thyrotoxic cardiac disease. *Curr Heart Fail Rep.* 5:170, 2008.

Poomthavorn P, et al. Exogenous subclinical hyperthyroidism during adolescence: effect on peak bone mass. *J Pediatr Endocrinol Metab.* 18:463, 2005.

Potenza M, et al. Excess thyroid hormone and carbohydrate metabolism. *Endocrin Pract.* 15:254, 2009.

Schott M, et al. Thyrotropin receptor autoantibodies in Graves' disease. *Trends Endocrinol Metab.* 16:243, 2005.

Tomer Y, Huber A. The etiology of autoimmune thyroid disease: a story of genes and environment. *J Autoimmun.* 32:231, 2009.

Zimmermann MB, et al. High thyroid volume in children with excess dietary iodine intakes. *Am J Clin Nutr.* 81:840, 2005.

THYROID GLAND

HYPOTHYROIDISM

NUTRITIONAL ACUITY RANKING: LEVEL 1

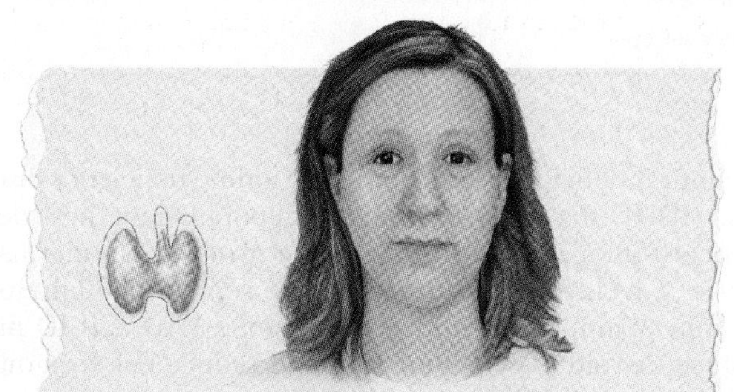

Asset provided by Anatomical Chart Co.

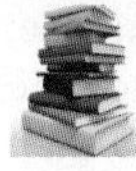

DEFINITIONS AND BACKGROUND

Hypothyroidism is caused by the underfunctioning of the thyroid gland. It can be classified as primary (thyroid failure), secondary (from pituitary TSH deficit), or tertiary (from hypothalamic deficiency of thyrotropin-releasing hormone) or result from peripheral resistance to the action of thyroid hormones. Primary hypothyroidism causes about 95% of all cases.

The most common cause of thyroid gland failure is **Hashimoto's thyroiditis**, which is inflammation caused by the patient's own antibodies (as in pernicious anemia, lupus, rheumatoid arthritis, diabetes, or chronic hepatitis). The second major cause of thyroid gland failure is from various medical treatments that affect the thyroid gland (e.g., surgery, chronic medication use).

Hypothyroidism affects up to 10% of adult women, usually middle-aged and older women. Women may experience menstrual irregularities or difficulty conceiving. Triiodothyronine (T3) and thyroxine (T4) are elevated during pregnancy and with oral contraceptive and estrogen use. Physicians must treat hypothyroidism to avoid long-term complications, such as depression, infertility, and CVD. Risk decreases if thyroid hormones are taken as directed.

Congenital hypothyroidism (CH) or cretinism is rare; incidence is one in 4000 births. Screening for this type of hypothyroidism is now common (Lanting et al, 2005). Treatment involves replacement of thyroid hormones and iodine. Cretinism can occur in areas where soil content of iodine is low.

Myxedema is a nonpitting edema that can occur in adults with hypothyroidism; hydrophilic mucopolysaccharide accumulates in the skin and muscles. In end-stage myxedema coma, untreated hypothyroidism leads to progressive weakness, stupor, hypothermia, hypoventilation, hypoglycemia, hyponatremia, water intoxication, shock, and even death. It occurs most often in older patients with underlying pulmonary and vascular disease. Signs and symptoms of hypothyroidism are listed in Table 9-24.

Thyroid autoimmunity is common and may contribute to miscarriages as well as to hypothyroidism. Infants are totally dependent on T4 from the mother during the first trimester for normal neurological development (Smallridge et al, 2005). Hypothyroidism from autoimmune disease or suboptimal iodine intake occurs in 2.5% of pregnant women; postpartum thyroid dysfunction (PPTD) occurs in 5–9% of women (Lazarus and Premawardhana, 2005). Because of the potential problems for mother and baby, screening, diagnosis, and treatment of thyroid problems among pregnant women is important.

Endemic goiter is an enlargement of the thyroid gland with swelling in front of the neck, resulting from iodine deficiency due to inadequate dietary intake or drug effects. Over 3 billion people in the world are on iodine supplementation programs. Optimal level of iodine intake to prevent thyroid disease is in a relatively narrow range around the recommended daily iodine intake of 150 μg.

Subclinical hypothyroidism (SCH) is mild thyroid failure and is diagnosed when peripheral thyroid hormone levels are within normal reference laboratory range but serum TSH levels are mildly elevated (Fatourechi, 2009). Iodine, iron, selenium, and zinc deficiencies can impair thyroid function. Iron deficiency impairs thyroid hormone synthesis by reducing activity of heme-dependent thyroid Peroxidase; iron supplementation may improve the efficacy of iodine supplementation. Anemia is a major manifestation in hypothyroidism not only because of impaired hemoglobin synthesis, but also because of iron deficiency from increased iron loss with menorrhagia, impaired intestinal absorption of iron, folate deficiency due to impaired intestinal absorption of folic acid, and pernicious anemia with vitamin B_{12} deficiency. Selenium deficiency and disturbed thyroid hormone status may develop in phenylketonuria, cystic fibrosis, as well as from poor nutrition in children, elderly people, or sick patients. In parts of the world where iodine and selenium are both deficient, dual supplementation may be advisable.

TABLE 9-24 Symptoms of Hypothyroidism By Life Stage

Infants
Constipation
Cyanosis
Developmental delay
Hoarse cry
Marked retardation of bone maturation
Persistent jaundice
Poor feeding
Respiratory difficulty
Somnolence
Umbilical hernia
Children
Evidence of mental retardation
Poor performance at school
Retarded growth
Stunting, short stature
Adults
Abnormal menstrual cycles
Brittle nails
Broad flat nose
Coarse features with protruding tongue
Coarse, dry hair
Cold intolerance
Dry, rough pale skin
Decreased libido
Delayed dentition
Difficulty losing weight
Easy fatigue
Hair loss
Hoarse, husky voice
Impaired mental development
Muscle cramps, frequent muscle aches
Puffy hands and face
Reduced conversion of carotene to vitamin A
Short stature
Weakness
Weight gain
Widely set eyes

Vitamin A deficiency (VAD) and the iodine deficiency disorders (IDD) affect >30% of the global population; these deficiencies often coexist in vulnerable groups (Zimmerman, 2007). Given alone, without iodine repletion, high-dose vitamin A supplementation in combined VAD and ID may reduce thyroid hyperstimulation and reduce risk for goiter (Zimmerman, 2007). More research on vitamin and mineral therapies will be beneficial.

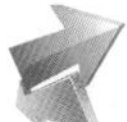

ASSESSMENT, MONITORING, AND EVALUATION

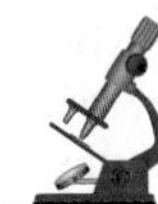

CLINICAL INDICATORS

Genetic Markers: Mutations in the DUOX2, PAX8, SLC5A5, TG, TPO, TSHB, and TSHR genes cause congenital hypothyroidism.

Clinical/History (see Table 9-24)

Height
Weight
BMI
Diet history
Temperature
BP
Goiter?
Thyroid scan

Lab Work

T4 (decreased)
T3 (decreased)
TSH (elevated)
Urinary iodine concentration (UIC)
Ca^{++}
Mg^{++} (increased)
H & H (decreased)
Serum ferritin
Chol, Trig (increased)
Gluc
Alk phos (decreased)
Serum copper (decreased)
Na^+ and K^+ (decreased)
Serum folic acid and vitamin B_{12} (low)
Creatine phosphokinase (CPK)
GFR (decreased?)
Thyrotropin
Somatomedin C (increased)
Uric acid (increased)
Carotenoids (increased)
Thyroglobulin (useful measure after introducing iodized salt)
Serum vitamin D_3

SAMPLE NUTRITION CARE PROCESS STEPS

Overweight (NC-3.3)

Assessment Data: Low serum levels of T4 and T3 with increased TSH. Unplanned weight gain of 30 lb in past 2 years. Recent Dx of hypothyroidism and initiation of synthroid. BMI 30.

Nutrition Diagnosis (PES): Overweight (NC-3.3) as related to excess food and nutrition related knowledge deficit and hypothyroidism as evidenced by reports of overconsumption of high fat/calorie dense food and beverages, BMI 30, waist circumference >40 inches, and a fat mass of 51.7%.

Interventions: Nutrition prescription (ND-1) of a weight control/exercise plan with promotion of a diet including 30–40% fat, 45–50% complex carbohydrates, and 15–20% protein with a goal of cutting out 250–500 calories a day resulting in a 0.5–1 lb weight loss each week. Recommend adequate intake of fluid and foods high in fiber. Support use of Synthroid 25 μg once daily. Initial/Brief nutrition education (E-1) to begin instruction on following a weight control/exercise plan with a diet including 30–40% fat, 45–50% complex carbohydrates, and 15–20% protein with a goal of cutting out 250–500 calories a day and provide basic nutrition related educational information on natural goitrogens, fiber, fluids, use of iodized salt, and physical activity.

Monitoring and Evaluation: Follow up in 1 month to repeat a TSH and free T4 to reassess thyroid function status; repeat TSH and free T4 and adjust dose of Synthroid accordingly. Evaluate progress in weight loss and healthy eating habits. Schedule a counseling session for in-depth nutrition related knowledge regarding weight loss as well as hypothyroidism.

INTERVENTION

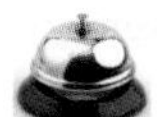

OBJECTIVES

- Control weight gain that results from a 15–40% slower metabolic rate, especially in the untreated patient. Measure weight frequently to detect fluid losses or retention.
- Correct underlying causes, such as inadequate intake of iodine or congenital deficiency. Hormone replacement will be given.
- Correct vitamin B_{12}, folic acid, or iron deficiency anemias when present.
- Because vitamin D_3 has implications in autoimmune disorders, assure an adequate diet and supplementary source as needed.
- Improve energy levels; reduce fatigue.
- Improve cardiac, neurological, and renal functioning.
- Screen for thyroid problems in pregnant or postpartum women; assure hormone replacement as needed.

FOOD AND NUTRITION

- Use an energy-controlled diet adjusted for age, sex, and height.
- A multivitamin–mineral supplement formula may be beneficial, especially to replace nutrients that have been poorly absorbed. Since T3 is an important hormone needed for vitamin A metabolism, serum levels may be low in this population. Include good sources of carotenoids such as lycopene.
- Ensure an adequate supply of antioxidant and fiber-rich foods as well as fluids.
- For pregnant women or children, make sure that adequate amounts of iodine are consumed.
- Natural goitrogens in cabbage, turnips, rapeseeds, peanuts, cassava, cauliflower, broccoli, and soybeans may block uptake of iodine by body cells; they are inactivated by heating and cooking.
- Achieve optimal iodine intakes from iodized salt (in the range of 150–250 μg/d for adults) to minimize thyroid dysfunction (Zimmerman, 2009). Zinc, copper, and tyrosine are needed.
- Ensure adequate iodine status during parenteral nutrition, particularly in preterm infants (Zimmerman, 2009).

Common Drugs Used and Potential Side Effects

- Thyroid hormones (liotrix, sodium levothyroxine, or Synthroid) are used. Use caution with use of soy protein products since they can decrease effectiveness of the hormones. Thyroid hormones elevate glucose and decrease cholesterol; monitor persons who have diabetes carefully. Monitor for weight changes and fluid shifts. If rapid weight loss, sweating, or other symptoms of hyperthyroidism occur, the doctor should be contacted for immediate follow-up.

- Lithium treatment for bipolar disorder has been associated with the development of goiter. Monitor patients closely.

Herbs, Botanicals, and Supplements

- Herbs and botanical supplements should not be used without discussing with physician.
- Avoid kelp tablets and "thyroid support" supplements. Gentian, walnut, mustard, radish, and St. John's wort have been recommended, but no clinical trials have proven efficacy.
- Curcumin and vitamins A, B_{12}, D_3, and E may be beneficial; longer human studies are needed.
- If large quantities of iodine-rich seaweed such as kombu (*Laminaria japonica*) are consumed, use should be monitored in patients who take thyroid replacement hormones.

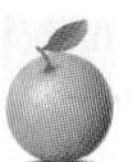

NUTRITION EDUCATION, COUNSELING, CARE MANAGEMENT

- Discuss goitrogens in cabbage and *Brassica* vegetables, turnips, rapeseeds, peanuts, cassava, and soybeans; they are inactivated by heating and cooking.
- Encourage use of iodized salt, as permitted. Avoid self-medication with iodine supplements.
- Encourage adequate fluid intake.
- Women who are considering pregnancy may want to be screened to rule out thyroid problems. If their iodine intake is low, or if they live in an area without use of iodized salt, they may need an iodine supplement prescribed from their physician. A normal urinary iodine level would be 150–249 μg/L.
- In many developing countries, children are at high risk of iodine deficiency, VAD, and iron deficiency anemia. Select the proper supplements.
- Because subclinical hypothyroidism is common in individuals who have chronic kidney disease, close monitoring of GFR is recommended (Chonchol et al, 2008).
- Exposure to large doses of metals such as lead, molybdenum, or arsenic may reduce thyroid function, with adverse effects on development, behavior, metabolism and reproduction (Meeker et al, 2009).

Patient Education—Foodborne Illness

- If home tube feeding is needed, teach appropriate sanitation and food-handling procedures.

For More Information

- American Thyroid Association
  http://www.thyroid.org/
- Endocrine Web
  http://www.endocrineweb.com/hypo1.html
- Mayo Clinic
  http://www.mayoclinic.com/health/hypothyroidism/DS00353/DSECTION=symptoms
- Synthroid Information
  http://www.synthroid.com/

HYPOTHYROIDISM—CITED REFERENCES

Chonchol M, et al. Prevalence of subclinical hypothyroidism in patients with chronic kidney disease. *Clin J Am Soc Nephrol.* 3:1296, 2008.

Fatourechi V. Subclinical hypothyroidism: an update for primary care physicians. *Mayo Clinic Proc.* 84:65, 2009.

Lanting CI, et al. Clinical effectiveness and cost-effectiveness of the use of the thyroxine/thyroxine-binding globulin ratio to detect congenital hypothyroidism of thyroidal and central origin in a neonatal screening program. *Pediatrics.* 116:168, 2005.

Lazarus JH, Premawardhana LD. Screening for thyroid disease in pregnancy. *J Clin Pathol.* 58:449, 2005.

Meeker JD, et al. Multiple metals predict prolactin and thyrotropin (TSH) levels in men. *Environ Res.* 109:869, 2009.

Smallridge RC, et al. Thyroid function inside and outside of pregnancy: what do we know and what don't we know? *Thyroid.* 15:54, 2005.

Zimmerman MB. Interactions of vitamin A and iodine deficiencies: effects on the pituitary-thyroid axis. *Int J Vitam Nutr Res.* 77:236, 2007.

Zimmerman MB. Iodine deficiency. *Endrocr Rev.* 30:376, 2009.

PARATHYROID GLANDS

The parathyroid glands have an overall regulatory role with action as a thermostat in the systemic calcium homeostasis to ensure tight regulation of serum calcium concentrations and appropriate skeletal mineralization. Parathyroid hormone (PTH) affects calcium, phosphorus, and vitamin D metabolism by removing calcium from bone to raise serum levels; it promotes hydroxylation of vitamin D to its active form. Calcitonin, in contrast to PTH, decreases serum calcium levels; it is secreted by the thyroid gland.

The body secretes PTH in response to hypocalcemia or hypomagnesemia; the hormone then stimulates osteoclasts to increase bone resorption. PTH also stimulates adenyl cyclase to increase renal tubular calcium resorption and phosphate excretion. PTH works with vitamin D to regulate total body calcium by activating conversion of 25-hydroxyvitamin D to 1,25-dihydroxyvitamin D, the active form that stimulates calcium and phosphate absorption from the GI tract. Calcitonin, in contrast to PTH, decreases serum calcium levels and is secreted by the thyroid gland.

Fibroblast growth factor-23 (FGF23) is a hormone that regulates mineral and vitamin D metabolism (Juppner, 2009). Research on the effects of various genes and hormones in bone homeostasis is on-going.

PARATHYROID GLANDS—CITED REFERENCE

Juppner H. Novel regulators of phosphate homeostasis and bone metabolism. *Ther Apher Dial.* 11:3S, 2007.

HYPOPARATHYROIDISM AND HYPOCALCEMIA

NUTRITIONAL ACUITY RANKING: LEVEL 2

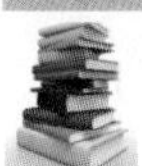

DEFINITIONS AND BACKGROUND

Hypoparathyroidism results from a deficiency of PTH from biologically ineffective hormones, damage or accidental removal of the glands, or impaired skeletal or renal response. In the hereditary form, parathyroid glands are either absent or not functioning properly; symptoms appear before age 10. Other causes include magnesium deficiency or neonatal immaturity. If untreated, hypoparathyroidism-retardation-dysmorphism (HRD) may result.

Cancellous bone in hypoparathyroidism is abnormal, suggesting that PTH is required to maintain normal trabecular structure (Rubin et al, 2010). Hypoparathyroidism with hypocalcemia is one of the most common results of damage to parathyroid glands during surgery; in fact, it may be diagnosed during a workup for hypocalcemia.

Vitamin D levels may also be deficient. Intraoperative PTH levels are used widely during parathyroidectomy as an indicator of parathyroid gland function; vitamin D supplementation after surgery may be given to anticipate decreased parathyroid gland function and to avoid symptomatic hypocalcemia (Quiros et al, 2005).

Hypoparathyroidism is a chronic condition that requires lifelong treatment with large doses of calcium and vitamin D supplements. Episodes of tetany are treated with calcium given intravenously to provide quick relief of symptoms. Controlled release of physiological concentrations of PTH can be achieved using a surgically implantable controlled-release delivery system (Anthony et al, 2005).

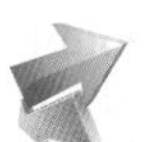

ASSESSMENT, MONITORING, AND EVALUATION

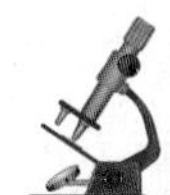

CLINICAL INDICATORS

Genetic Markers: There is a hypoparathyroidism-deafness-renal (HDR) dysplasia syndrome which is an autosomal dominant disorder caused by mutations of the GATA3 gene (Ali et al, 2007).

Clinical/History		Lab Work
Height	Seizures	PTH (low)
Weight	Muscle cramps and tetany	Ca^{++} (serum levels <2.5–3 mg/dL)
BMI	Tingling of the lips or fingers	Urinary Ca^{++} (altered)
Diet history	Hair loss, dry skin	Serum phosphorus (high)
Weakness, fatigue	Dental hypoplasia	Mg^{++} (may be low)
Hyperreflexia	Chronic cutaneous moniliasis	Na^{+}, K^{+}
Chvostek's sign positive (with tapping of facial muscles)	Abnormal heart rhythms on ECG	
Irritability or psychosis		

SAMPLE NUTRITION CARE PROCESS STEPS

Inadequate Mineral Intake

Assessment Data: Abnormal labs with low PTH, serum calcium 2.4 mg/dL, high serum phosphorus; positive for Chvostek's sign and tetany with muscle cramps and abnormal ECG. Diet history indicates no dairy intake for past several years. Medical diagnosis of hypoparathyroidism after thyroid surgery.

Nutrition Diagnosis (PES): Inadequate mineral (calcium) intake related to nutritional intake low in calcium and hypoparathyroidism as evidenced by low PTH, low serum calcium (2.4), high serum phosphorus, and signs of tetany.

Intervention: Food and nutrient delivery—provide foods rich in calcium (nondairy if necessary) and provide a calcium supplement calculated for body size and age. Educate about the role of calcium in alleviating signs of tetany and abnormal labs. Counsel about nondairy sources of calcium and tips for increasing intake throughout the day.

Monitoring and Evaluation: Resolution of low serum calcium and PTH, high phosphorus. No signs of tetany, muscle cramps, irritability. Improvement in dry skin or hair loss. Normal ECG.

INTERVENTION

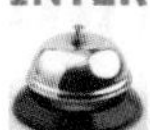

OBJECTIVES

- Normalize serum and urinary levels of calcium, phosphorus, and vitamin D.
- Prevent long-term complications such as cataracts, pernicious anemia, Parkinson's disease, and bone disease.
- Prevent mental retardation or malformed teeth in affected children.
- Decrease symptoms of tetany and improve overall health status.

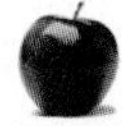

FOOD AND NUTRITION

- Use a high-calcium diet with dairy products, nuts, salmon, peanut butter, broccoli, and other green leafy vegetables. If tolerated, lactose should be included in the diet for better absorption of calcium.
- Oral supplements high in calcium should be used, such as calcium carbonate.
- Reduce excess use of meats, phytates (whole grains), and oxalic acid (spinach, chard, and rhubarb) if the diet contains large amounts.
- Intake of vitamin D and protein should be adequate, at least meeting recommended levels.

Common Drugs Used and Potential Side Effects

- Calcium lactate (8–12 g) may be used. Ergocalciferol (Calciferol) is a vitamin D analog that is used with calcium

supplements in this condition. Calcitriol (Rocaltrol) also may be useful.
- Diuretics sometimes are given to prevent too much calcium from being lost through the urine, which is a problem that can lead to kidney stones. Taking diuretics also reduces the amount of calcium and vitamin D supplements needed.
- Overuse of steroids may cause hypocalcemia.

Herbs, Botanicals, and Supplements

- Herbs and botanical supplements should not be used without discussing with physician.

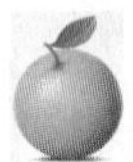

NUTRITION EDUCATION, COUNSELING, CARE MANAGEMENT

- Indicate which foods are good sources of calcium, phosphorus, and vitamin D.
- Indicate which foods are sources of phytates and avoided, if dietary intake is a concern.
- Discuss role of sunlight exposure in vitamin D formation and how it relates to individual needs.

Patient Education—Foodborne Illness

- If home tube feeding is needed, teach appropriate sanitation and food-handling procedures.

For More Information

- American Society for Bone and Mineral Research http://www.asbmr.org/
- Hypoparathyroidism Association http://www.hypoparathyroidism.org/
- Medline http://www.nlm.nih.gov/medlineplus/ency/article/000385.htm
- National Institutes of Health–Osteoporosis and Related Bone Diseases http://www.osteo.org/

HYPOPARATHYROIDISM AND HYPOCALCEMIA—CITED REFERENCES

Ali A, et al. Functional characterization of GATA3 mutations causing the hypoparathyroidism-deafness-renal (HDR) dysplasia syndrome: insight into mechanisms of DNA binding by the GATA3 transcription factor. *Hum Mol Genet.* 16:265, 2007.

Anthony T, et al. Development of a parathyroid hormone-controlled release system as a potential surgical treatment for hypoparathyroidism. *J Pediatr Surg.* 40:81, 2005.

Quiros RM, et al. Intraoperative parathyroid hormone levels in thyroid surgery are predictive of postoperative hypoparathyroidism and need for vitamin D supplementation. *Am J Surg.* 189:306, 2005.

Rubin MR, et al. Three dimensional cancellous bone structure in hypoparathyroidism. [published online ahead of print September 25, 2009] *Bone.* 46:190, 2010.

HYPERPARATHYROIDISM AND HYPERCALCEMIA

NUTRITIONAL ACUITY RANKING: LEVEL 2

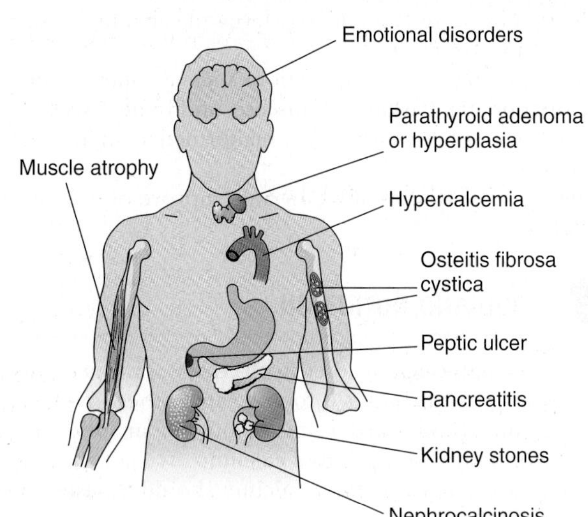

Adapted from: Raphael Rubin, David S. Strayer, *Rubin's Pathology: Clinicopathologic Foundations of Medicine,* 5th ed. Philadelphia: Lippincott Williams & Wilkins, 2008.

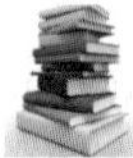

DEFINITIONS AND BACKGROUND

Primary hyperparathyroidism (pHPT) results from parathyroid adenoma in up to 80% of cases, hyperplasia of the parathyroid glands in 10–20% of cases, or cancer. Double parathyroid adenomas occur in 2–15% of pHPT cases (Abboud et al, 2005). pHPT has been associated with premature death in CVDs and should, therefore, be quickly managed (Nilsson et al, 2005).

Secondary hyperparathyroidism (sHPT) occurs in renal failure or even after renal transplantation. Calcitriol deficiency and phosphorus retention are involved in the pathogenesis. Parathyroid gland hyperplasia develops in azotemic patients, producing hypercalcemia and hyperphosphatemia. Secondary hyperparathyroidism in chronic kidney disease is stimulated by dietary phosphate loading and ameliorated by dietary phosphate restriction (Martin et al, 2005). The disorder is complex in that not enough phosphate is cleared from the body; phosphate is released from bone and Vitamin D is not produced. Thereafter, absorption of calcium in the gut is low and serum levels of calcium are lowered.

In children with renal failure, growth can be impaired. Postmenopausal women after Roux-en-Y gastric bypass may show evidence of secondary hyperparathyroidism with elevated bone resorption. There is an effect of early breast tumors on calcium homeostasis; subclinical hyperparathyroidism may increase the risk for breast cancer (Martin et al, 2010). Age-induced increased PTH plasma levels have been associated with cognitive decline and dementia. Increased PTH levels may become a biological marker of both dementia and osteoporosis (Braverman et al, 2009).

Parathyroidectomy can induce long-lasting improvement in regulation of BP, left ventricular diastolic function, and other signs of myocardial ischemia, with improved life expectancy (Nilsson et al, 2005). A minimally invasive procedure is available. After surgery, mild cognitive changes seem to improve, especially for depression and anxiety (Walker et al, 2009).

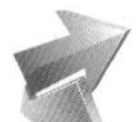

ASSESSMENT, MONITORING, AND EVALUATION

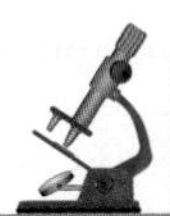

CLINICAL INDICATORS

Genetic Markers: Peroxisome proliferator-activated receptor gamma PPARgamma2 has a dominant role in controlling osteoblast differentiation and numerous gene–gene interactions suggests there is a "master" regulatory process (Shockley et al, 2009). Familial multiple endocrine neoplasia type 1 and familial tumoral calcinosis account for 2% of pHPT cases. In the second form, altered GALNT3 is usually present. More studies are needed on the effects of genes on calcium and bone homeostasis.

Clinical/History		
Height	Bone and joint pain	Urinary Ca^{++} (elevated)
Weight	Bone x-rays showing fractures or reabsorption	Serum phosphorus (high?)
BMI	X-rays, ultrasound, or Sestamibi scan of parathyroids	Calcium-phosphorus product (Ca × P)*
Diet history	**Lab Work**	Albumin-corrected calcium level (Ca corr)
BP	PTH (>60 pg/mL)	FGF23 assessment, as available
Weakness, fatigue	Serum Ca^{++} (>11 mg/dL)	Mg^{++}, Na^{+}, K^{+}
Constipation		Alb, BUN, Creatinine
Growth delay or rickets in children		H & H, serum ferritin
Anorexia, weight loss		Gluc
Increased thirst		
Dehydration		
Itchy skin		
Back pain		

*Calcium phosphate product (Ca× Pi) is a clinically relevant tool to estimate the cardiovascular risk of patients with renal failure.

INTERVENTION

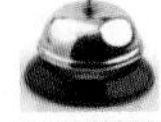

OBJECTIVES

- Lower elevated serum calcium and urinary calcium levels. Maintain calcium levels between 8.4 and 9.5 mg/dL.
- Normalize serum phosphate; keep phosphorus between 3.5 and 5.5 mg/dL and calcium × phosphorus product below 55 mg/dL.
- Alleviate constipation, anorexia, weight loss, and weakness.
- Avoid clinical consequences such as renal osteodystrophy, hyperphosphatemia, cardiovascular calcification, extraskeletal calcification, endocrine disturbances, neurobehavioral changes, compromised immune system, altered erythropoiesis, renal stones, and sleep disturbances.
- Prevent rickets and growth delay in children (Sabbagh et al, 2005).
- Prepare for surgery if parathyroidectomy is necessary.

SAMPLE NUTRITION CARE PROCESS STEPS

Excessive Mineral Intake

Assessment Data: Abnormal nutritional labs with PTH 65 pg/mL; serum Ca^{++} 12.5 mg/dL; urinary Ca^{++} levels elevated; elevated serum phosphorus; diagnosis of hyperparathyroidism related to early renal failure without dialysis. Signs of weakness and anorexia. Poor intake because of nausea. Unplanned weight loss of 2 lb recently.

Nutrition Diagnosis (PES): Excessive phosphorus intake related to inability of kidneys to metabolize vitamin D_3 in renal failure as evidenced by abnormal labs (PTH 65 pg/mL; serum Ca^{++} 12.5 mg/dL; urinary Ca^{++} levels elevated; serum phosphorus 6, anorexia and weight loss.

Intervention: Food-Nutrient Delivery—provide a low-phosphorus diet. Educate about foods to avoid and which to include (see Table 9-25). Counsel about dining away from home, packing a lunch, or other relevant guidelines, how to take Sevelamer and Sensipar according to doctor's orders.

Monitoring and Evaluation: Improvement in serum and urinary labs related to calcium, PTH and phosphorus. Resolution of symptoms including weight loss, nausea, anorexia. Able to state foods to avoid when PTH is elevated and when to contact the physician.

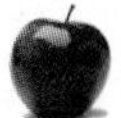

FOOD AND NUTRITION

- Use a low-calcium diet with fewer dairy products, nuts, salmon, peanut butter, and green leafy vegetables.
- Extra fluid is useful to correct or prevent dehydration, which can elevate serum calcium levels.
- Limit phosphorus-containing foods if hyperphosphatemia is present. See Table 9-25. Use alternatives such as nondairy creamer, sorbet, jams and jellies, white rice, noodles with margarine, cream cheese, whipped cream, popcorn, pretzels, gingerale or Kool-aid if extra calories are needed.
- Dietary protein 0.8 g/kg for a balanced intake of protein in adults.

Common Drugs Used and Potential Side Effects

- Vitamin D therapy sends a signal to the parathyroid gland to slow down the making of PTH. This helps to prevent many of the unwanted complications of hyperparathyroidism.

TABLE 9-25 Phosphorus Facts

Normal PO_4 levels in plasma: 2.5–4.5 mg/dL

Total body PO_4 content: 500–700 g (85% in bone)

Dietary Reference Intake: 700 mg

Typical U.S. dietary intake: 1200 mg

GI absorption—Mainly passive, through Na/Pi transporter; enhanced by vitamin D

Kidney is major regulator—mediated by brush border Na/Pi transporter; PTH increases excretion and Vitamin D decreases excretion

Phosphorus-Rich Foods

Dairy Products
- Milk
- Cheese
- Yogurt
- Ice cream
- Pudding and custard

Dried beans and lentils
- Kidney, lima, pinto
- Soy beans
- Split peas
- Black-eyed peas

Nuts and seeds
- Almonds
- Cashews
- Sunflower seeds
- Peanuts and Peanut Butter

Meats
- Liver
- Organ meats
- Sweetbreads
- Smelt, sardines, herring

Miscellaneous
- Beer
- Bran, bran flakes, wheat germ
- Chocolate
- Colas

- Treatment with active vitamin D from analogs can increase VDR expression, inhibit growth of parathyroid tumors, and reduce PTH levels (Akerstrom et al, 2005). Zemplar (paricalcitol) and Hectorol (doxercalciferol) are examples of vitamin D analogs. These products are especially useful for dialysis patients.
- Cinacalcet (Sensipar) has been approved to treat sHPT in renal patients and parathyroid cancer. It also appears to effectively treat pHPT. Cinacalcet normalizes serum calcium with only modest increases in PTH (Sajid-Crockett et al, 2008).
- Phosphate-binding agents that do not contain calcium offer therapeutic alternatives for managing renal osteodystrophy. Sevelamer (Renagel) lowers serum phosphorus and PTH levels without inducing hypercalcemia. Sevelamer binds drugs such as furosemide, cyclosporine, and tacrolimus, making them less effective. The timing of administration should allow several hours between these medicines. Standard protocols are recommended for use of phosphate binders.
- Once-yearly intramuscular cholecalciferol injections (600,000 IU) have been used to correct vitamin D deficiency; controlled trials are needed to determine the effect on PTH levels over time.
- Some antacids may contain high levels of calcium; monitor carefully.
- Bisphosphonates may be needed to decrease risks for osteoporosis.

Herbs, Botanicals, and Supplements

- Herbs and botanical supplements should not be used without discussing with physician.
- Conjugated linoleic acid (CLA) reduces prostaglandin E_2 synthesis, which is required for PTH release. More research is needed.

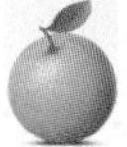

NUTRITION EDUCATION, COUNSELING, CARE MANAGEMENT

- Discuss foods that are sources of calcium, phosphorus, and vitamin D. Indicate food sources of phytates and oxalates, if intake is a concern.
- Discuss role of sunlight exposure in vitamin D formation and how it relates to individual needs.
- Drink plenty of liquids.
- In renal patients, focused counseling may help to clarify misunderstanding of simple dietary facts.
- The doctor should monitor Ca^{++} and P monthly and PTH quarterly after stabilization.
- Exercise and smoking cessation may be needed.

Patient Education—Foodborne Illness

- If home tube feeding is needed, teach appropriate sanitation and food-handling procedures.

For More Information

- American Society for Bone and Mineral Research http://www.asbmr.org/
- Endocrine Web http://www.endocrineweb.com/hyperpara.html
- National Institutes of Health–Osteoporosis and Related Bone Diseases http://www.osteo.org/
- NIDDK http://endocrine.niddk.nih.gov/pubs/hyper/hyper.htm

HYPERPARATHYROIDISM AND HYPERCALCEMIA—CITED REFERENCES

Abboud B, et al. Existence and anatomic distribution of double parathyroid adenoma. *Laryngoscope*. 115:1128, 2005.

Braverman ER, et al. Age-related increases in parathyroid hormone may be antecedent to both osteoporosis and dementia. *BMC Endocr Disord.* 9:21, 2009.

Martin DR, et al. Acute regulation of parathyroid hormone by dietary phosphate. *Am J Physiol Endocrinol Metab.* 289:E729, 2005.

Martin E, et al. Serum calcium levels are elevated among women with untreated postmenopausal breast cancer. [published online ahead of print October 24, 2009] *Cancer Causes Controls.* 21:251, 2010.

Nilsson IL, et al. Maintained normalization of cardiovascular dysfunction 5 years after parathyroidectomy in primary hyperparathyroidism. *Surgery.* 137:632, 2005.

Sabbagh Y, et al. Hypophosphatemia leads to rickets by impairing caspase-mediated apoptosis of hypertrophic chondrocytes. *Proc Natl Acad Sci U S A.* 102:9637, 2005.

Sajid-Crockett S, et al. Cinacalcet for the treatment of primary hyperparathyroidism. *Metabolism.* 57:517, 2008.

Shockley KR, et al. PPARgamma2 nuclear receptor controls multiple regulatory pathways of osteoblast differentiation from marrow mesenchymal stem cells. *J Cell Biochem.* 106:232, 2009.

Walker MD, et al. Neuropsychological features in primary hyperparathyroidism: a prospective study. *J Clin Endocrinol Metab.* 94:1951, 2009.

SECTION 10

Malnutrition—Obesity and Undernutrition

CHIEF ASSESSMENT FACTORS

- Anorexia, Nausea, Vomiting, Diarrhea—Frequency, Length of Time
- Blood Pressure, Either Elevated or Very Low Levels
- Body Mass Index (BMI) Using Height and Weight
- Frame Size—Small, Medium, Large
- Goal Weight and Current Percentage of Goal Weight
- Healthy Body Weight Range
- History of Usual Body Weight, Present Weight, Recent Weight Changes,% Usual Body Weight
- Laboratory Values—Glucose, Albumin/Transthyretin, Hemoglobin and Hematocrit (H & H), Lipids, C-Reactive Protein (CRP)
- Medical History—Disordered Eating; Cancer or Other Conditions or Disease States; Menstrual or Reproductive Problems in Women; Smoking and Alcohol Histories
- Physical Activity Level
- Sleep Apnea, Altered Lung Function; Sleep Disorder
- Triceps Skinfold (TSF) Measurements; Arm Muscle Circumference (AMC) Measurements—Comparing Individual Against Own Values Over Time
- Waist Circumference

TYPES OF MALNUTRITION

The malnourished state arises from a combination of inflammation and a disturbed nutrient balance in either undernutrition or overnutrition (Soeters and Schols, 2009). Malnutrition is defined by the American Society of Parenteral and Enteral Nutrition (ASPEN) as any derangement in the normal nutrition status.

Undernutrition may be *primary*—from insufficient intake—or *secondary*—from impaired utilization; see Table 10-1. Malnutrition originates not only from an imbalance of calories but also from psychological, economic, physical, and social factors. Health problems, alcoholism, depression, restricted diets, and mobility problems may play a part. Undernutrition contributes to half of the world's mortality in children, particularly in India and sub-Saharan Africa.

Nutrition Day, which originated in Europe, is now recognized in the United States. The intent is to identify the type and percentages of malnourished patients in hospitals and nursing homes in order to clarify their impact on health outcomes.

Overnutrition is caused by excessive calorie intake and/or inadequate activity; see Table 10-2. The thrifty genotype developed when food was scarce; now, an environment where food is plentiful contributes to the dilemma (Bouchard, 2007). The study of extreme human obesity caused by single gene defects has provided a glimpse into the long-term regulation of body weight through a disrupted hypothalamic leptin-melanocortin system and extremely heterogeneous factors (Ranadive and Vaisse, 2008).

In addition to the change in environment, thirst, hunger, and high calorie beverage intake have changed in the past few decades. The intake of energy-yielding beverages seems to be related to pleasure-oriented, hedonic factors rather than hunger or thirst (McKiernan et al, 2008). Pavlovian cues for rewards become endowed with incentive salience, guiding "wanting" to a learned reward (Tindell et al, 2009). Thus, the hedonic appetite has displaced genuine hunger in the current environment of plenty, perhaps in relation to conditioned stimuli. For example, salted food may be an addictive substance that stimulates the opiate and dopamine receptors in the brain's reward and pleasure center; both salted food and opiate withdrawal stimulate the appetite, increase calorie consumption, and augment the incidence of overeating, becoming overweight, and becoming obese (Cocores and Gold, 2009).

TABLE 10-1 Concerns with Undernutrition

- The lack of adequate macronutrients or selected micronutrients (zinc, selenium, iron, and the antioxidant vitamins) can lead to clinically significant immune deficiency (Cunningham-Rundles et al, 2005). Iron deficiency alters myelination, monoamine neurotransmitter synthesis, and hippocampal energy metabolism in the neonatal period (Georgleff, 2007). Zinc deficiency alters autonomic nervous system regulation and hippocampal and cerebellar development (Georgleff, 2007).
- Inflammation and oxidative stress fuel each other. Cachexia includes distinct metabolic changes that are the result of an acute-phase response (APR) mounted by the host, including increased muscle proteolysis, increased fat lipolysis, and increased hepatic production of acute-phase proteins such as C-reactive protein and fibrinogen (Gullett et al, 2009).
- Children who are undernourished may not reach their potential in many aspects of development. Stunting represents growth failure resulting from poor nutrition and health during the pre- and postnatal periods (Milman et al, 2005). Intrauterine and early neonatal life is a period during which environmental and nutritional influences may produce chronic and frequent infections, long-term effects, and disease risk in adulthood (Buckley et al, 2005).
- The effect of any nutrient deficiency or overabundance on brain development will be governed by the principle of timing, dose, and duration (Georgleff, 2007).
- Bourre (2006) reported on nutritional requirements for the brain. The use of glucose by nervous tissue requires thiamin. Vitamins B_6 and B_{12} are directly involved in the synthesis of some neurotransmitters. Supplementation with cobalamin improves cerebral and cognitive functions in the frontal lobe. Alpha-tocopherol is actively uptaken by the brain and is directly involved in the protection of nervous membranes. Vitamin K is also involved in nervous tissue biochemistry. Iron deficiency anemia is associated with apathy, depression, and fatigue. Iodine deficiency during pregnancy induces severe cerebral dysfunction, actually leading to cretinism.
- Long-chain polyunsaturated fatty acids are important for synaptogenesis, membrane function, and, potentially, myelination (Georgleff, 2007). The rise in autism, learning problems, cognitive decline with age, Alzheimer's, Parkinson's Disease, and the SIDS epidemic has a common link: dietary deficit in omega-3 brain-foods from fish and seafood (Saugstad, 2008).
- Undernutrition in adult women tends to be associated with high levels of undernutrition in children, reflecting overall food/nutrient insecurity (Nube, 2005). Prenatal exposure to famine can lead to low birth weight and cardiovascular disease in adulthood (Painter et al, 2005).
- A woman with a low body mass index (BMI) may have difficulty becoming pregnant; preconceptional undernutrition shortens gestation in those women who do become pregnant (Rayco-Solon et al, 2005).
- **Recent weight loss** appears to be the most important single indicator of nutritional status. Nutritional risk with muscle mass depletion increases lengths of stay in hospitals (Kyle et al, 2005). Undernutrition is associated with increased resting energy expenditure (REE; kcal/kg/d). Reduced respiratory quotient (RQ) and protein synthesis (g/kg/d) occur in patients with coexistent disease; refeeding normalizes this process (Winter et al, 2005).
- Involuntary weight loss can be categorized into one of three primary etiologies (Thomas, 2007): **Starvation** results in a loss of body fat and non-fat mass due to inadequate intake of protein and energy. **Sarcopenia** involves a reduction in muscle mass and strength occurring with normal aging, associated with a reduction in motor unit number and atrophy of muscle fibers; this leads to diminished strength and exercise capacity. **Cachexia** is severe wasting that accompanies disease states such as cancer or immunodeficiency disease.
- lnutrition in pediatric hospitals ranges from 15–30% of patients, with an impact on growth, morbidity, and mortality; nutrition-support interventions help (Agostoni et al, 2005).
- rson has a BMI below 18, there is an increased risk for nutrition-related complications such as infections, poor wound healing, and pressure ulcer ment.

(continued)

TABLE 10-1 Concerns with Undernutrition *(continued)*

- Approximately 25–50% of hospital patients have been found to be malnourished. Only 50% of malnourished patients are identified by the medical and nursing staff (Kruizenga et al, 2005).
- Over half of older adults have protein–energy malnutrition at admission or acquire nutritional deficits while hospitalized (Pepersack, 2005). Malnutrition may come from the "11 Ds": disease, drinking alcohol, drugs, deficits (sensory), desertion/isolation, dementia, delirium, depression, destitution, despair, and dysphagia. Cognitive function is particularly sensitive to glucose and insulin availability. Older individuals often have dementia, falls, mobility disorders, malnutrition, end-of-life issues, pressure ulcers, and urinary incontinence to consider.
- Nutritional screening and assessment must become routine. Subjective Global Assessment and the Mini Nutritional Assessment tools are used to detect patients who need preventive nutritional measures (Kyle et al, 2005). The short nutritional assessment questionnaire (SNAQ) is simple and may be used to screen for **appetite changes**—another important factor leading to undernutrition and its consequences (Wilson et al, 2005).
- Outcome monitoring and evaluation should include weight change, use of supplemental drinks and snacks between meals, use of tube feeding or parenteral nutrition, number of consultations by the hospital dietitian, and decreased length of hospital stay (Kruizenga et al, 2005).

REFERENCES

Agostoni C, et al. The need for nutrition support teams in pediatric units: a commentary by the ESPGHAN Committee on Nutrition. *J Pediatr Gastroenterol Nutr.* 41:8, 2005.
Bourre JM. Effects of nutrients (in food) on the structure and function of the nervous system: update on dietary requirements for brain. Part 1: micronutrients. *J Nutr Health Aging.* 10:377, 2006.
Buckley AJ, et al. Nutritional programming of adult disease. *Cell Tissue Res.* 322:73, 2005.
Cunningham-Rundles S, et al. Mechanisms of nutrient modulation of the immune response. *J Allergy Clin Immunol.* 115:1119, 2005.
Georgleff MK. Nutrition and the developing brain: nutrient priorities and measurement. *Am J Clin Nutr.* 85:214S, 2007.
Gullett N, et al. Cancer-induced cachexia: a guide for the oncologist. *J Soc Integr Oncol.* 7:155, 2009.
Kruizenga HM, et al. Effectiveness and cost-effectiveness of early screening and treatment of malnourished patients. *Am J Clin Nutr.* 82:1082, 2005.
Kyle UG, et al. Hospital length of stay and nutritional status. *Curr Opin Clin Nutr Metab Care.* 8:397, 2005.
Milman A, et al. Differential improvement among countries in child stunting is associated with long-term development and specific interventions. *J Nutr.* 135:1415, 2005.
Nube M. Relationships between undernutrition prevalence among children and adult women at national and subnational level. *Eur J Clin Nutr.* 59:1112, 2005.
Painter RC, et al. Prenatal exposure to the Dutch famine and disease in later life: an overview. *Reprod Toxicol.* 20:345, 2005.
Pepersack T. Outcomes of continuous process improvement of nutritional care program among geriatric units. *J Gerontol A Biol Sci Med Sci.* 60:787, 2005.
Rayco-Solon P, et al. Maternal preconceptional weight and gestational length. *Am J Obstet Gynecol.* 192:1133, 2005.
Saugstad LF. Infantile autism: a chronic psychosis since infancy due to synaptic pruning of the supplementary motor area. *Nutr Health.* 19:307, 2008.
Thomas DR. Loss of skeletal muscle mass in aging: examining the relationship of starvation, sarcopenia, and cachexia. *Clin Nutr.* 26:389, 2007.
Wilson MM, et al. Appetite assessment: simple appetite questionnaire predicts weight loss in community-dwelling adults and nursing home residents. *Am J Clin Nutr.* 82:1074, 2005.
Winter TA, et al. The effect of severe undernutrition and subsequent refeeding on whole-body metabolism and protein synthesis in human subjects. *JPEN J Parenter Enteral Nutr.* 29:221, 2005.

TABLE 10-2 Concerns with Overnutrition

- Obesity caused by excess nutrition or excess storage of fat relative to energy expenditure is a form of malnutrition that is increasingly seen in children (Cunningham-Rundles et al, 2005).
- Leptin is a cytokine-like immune regulator that has complex effects in both overnutrition and in the inflammatory response in malnutrition.
- BMI > 30 is the initial calculated measure used to determine obesity. If a person has too high a BMI, risks increase for high blood pressure, high blood cholesterol, diabetes, orthopedic problems, gallstones, gout, osteoarthritis, sleep apnea, and cancers of the breast, colon, gallbladder, and so on.
- Critical factors that may put a person at risk for obesity, as they accumulate and interact over an individual's life span, include rapid weight gain in infancy and childhood, early puberty, and excessive weight gain in pregnancy (Johnson et al, 2006).
- Obesity in women can lead to several health challenges. Epidemiological evidence shows that being overweight contributes to menstrual disorders, infertility, miscarriage, poor pregnancy outcome, impaired fetal well-being, and diabetes mellitus. Changes in sensitivity to insulin may occur. Pregnant women who are obese are more at risk for pregnancy-induced hypertension and preeclampsia.
- Weight management programs should include a strong component of nutrition education (Klohe-Lehman et al, 2006).
- Obesity in older adults is increasing in prevalence along with related macro- and micronutrient deficiencies (Flood and Carr, 2004).
- Individualized programs with the goal of achieving modest weight reduction in obese patients are likely to result in immediate (e.g., alleviation of arthritic pains and reduction of glucose intolerance) and possibly long-term (e.g., reduction in cardiovascular risk) healthcare benefits.
- Lifestyle modifications are best. Diets based on complex carbohydrates, fibers, red wine, fresh fruit and vegetables, and nonanimal fat may protect against age-related cognitive impairment and dementia (Flood and Carr, 2004).
- Permanent 100-kilocalorie reductions in daily intake among the overweight/obese would eliminate approximately 71.2 million cases of overweight/obesity; in the long term, this could increase national productivity by $45.7 billion annually, and more aggressive diet changes of 500 kilocalories would yield benefits of $133.3 billion (Dall et al, 2009).

REFERENCES

Cunningham-Rundles S, et al. Mechanisms of nutrient modulation of the immune response. *J Allergy Clin Immunol.* 115:1119, 2005.
Dall TM, et al. Predicted national productivity implications of calorie and sodium reductions in the American diet. *Am J Health Promot.* 23:423, 2009.
Flood KL, Carr DB. Nutrition in the elderly. *Curr Opin Gastroenterol.* 20:125, 2004.
Johnson DB, et al. Preventing obesity: a life cycle perspective. *J Am Diet Assoc.* 106:97, 2006.
Klohe-Lehman DM, et al. Nutrition knowledge is associated with greater weight loss in obese and overweight low-income mothers. *J Am Diet Assoc.* 106:65, 2006.

Food variety is another factor with a major influence on energy intake (Epstein et al, 2009). Obese individuals prefer and consume more highly palatable foods more frequently than do persons of normal weight. There are 10 neurophysiologic pathways involved in the selection of food, which include reflexive and uncontrollable neurohormonal responses to food images, cues, and smells; mirror neurons that cause people to imitate the eating behavior of others without awareness; and limited cognitive capacity to make informed decisions about food (Cohen, 2008).

A transition in patterns and food intake occurs for immigrants. Any intervention aimed at reducing obesity must consider ethnicity, income, and degree of acculturation (Chen 2009). The intake of both sweetened drinks and meat increases among individuals emigrating to the United States (Novotny et al, 2009). The use of low-energy dense food (fruits and vegetables) and routine healthy breakfast consumption can help to maintain or lose weight (Greenwood and Stanford, 2008).

Restaurant and fast food consumption, large portion sizes, and consumption of sugar-sweetened beverages are closely associated with weight gain. Fructose from both sucrose and high fructose corn syrup is a concern (Bray, 2009). Fructose acutely increases thermogenesis, triglycerides, and lipogenesis as well as blood pressure; this leads to changes in body weight, fat storage, and triglycerides and increases inflammatory markers (Bray, 2009).

Many tools are available to assess food habits and weight status. Body mass index (BMI) standards are used to determine weight status. BMI correlates well with body fat for most individuals. Table 10-3 provides important weight and BMI calculations and guidelines. Whenever possible, use body mass index (BMI) to estimate a desirable weight range for height. Table 10-4 provides resources and calculations for estimating one's ideal body weight range; the Hamwi method (1974) is listed but is not evidence-based. Table 10-5 provides the standard BMI tables for adults. Table 10-6 provides several short methods for calculating energy needs.

TABLE 10-3 Weight Calculations and Body Mass Index (BMI) Guidelines

Calculation of BMI: (Weight [lb] ÷ Height [in]^2) × 705

BMI more often correctly predicts risks for chronic disease or malnutrition than life insurance tables.

BMI Web sites: There are many Web sites that make it easy to calculate BMI, which may be downloaded to a hand-held device, such as http://www.cdc.gov/nccdphp/dnpa/bmi/calc-bmi.htm.

For both English and metric calculations: http://www.nhlbisupport.com/bmi/bminojs.htm.

Usual Body Weight and% Change:

Calculation of % usual body weight = (Actual Weight/Usual Weight) × 100.

Calculation of % weight change = (Usual Weight − Actual Weight/Usual Weight) × 100.

Waist measurements: Waist circumference correlates with intra-abdominal adipose tissue. It is the most practical anthropometric measurement for assessing a patient's abdominal fat content before and during weight loss treatment. Computed tomography (CT) and magnetic resonance imaging (MRI) are both more accurate but impractical for routine use. Upper body obesity is defined as a waist circumference of >40 inches for men and >35 inches for women; this is the "apple shape." If more weight is around the hips, this "pear shape" has lower metabolic risks. Waist-hip ratio is often more useful in special populations such as HIV-AIDS and in older adults.

Calculation of lean body mass: Body composition is often measured using dual-energy X-ray absorptiometry (DEXA) or electrical impedance absorptiometry (BIA). BIA may underestimate body fat percentage more than DEXA.

Ethnic-specific cut-off points: Compared to Caucasians, African-Americans of the same age, gender, waist circumference, weight, and height may have lower total and abdominal fat mass when measured with DEXA bone density scanning or computed tomography (CT).

Because muscle mass may be higher in blacks, ethnic-specific cutoffs for what values represent overweight and obesity are needed. Dr. Dagogo-Jack summarized these findings at the Endocrine Society's Annual Meeting in 2009. The determination of the health status of all individuals should be based on metabolic indicators of health rather than on BMI alone. Counselors should promote healthy lifestyles that include adequate amounts of physical activity and rest as well as a nutrient-dense diet.

BMI Clinical Guidelines

<18.5	Underweight
18.5–24.9	Normal
25–29.9	Overweight
≥30	Obese
≥40	Morbidly obese

http://www.nhlbi.nih.gov/guidelines/obesity/ob_home.htm.

BMIs for Pregnant Women

The amount of weight a woman should gain during her pregnancy depends on her prepregnant BMI. To avoid complications and long-term health risks, the woman wants to gain enough weight to have a healthy baby but not too much weight. For twins, ideal weight gain is about 35–45 pounds (National Academy of Sciences, http://books.nap.edu/books/0309041384/html/220.html#pagetop).

Prepregnant BMI	Weight Gain During Pregnancy (lb)
≤19.5	28–40
19.6–26	25–35
27–29	15–25
≥30	~13–15

(continued)

TABLE 10-3 Weight Calculations and Body Mass Index (BMI) Guidelines *(continued)*

BMIs for Children

Growth charts are used for children to watch the pattern of their growth. Charts cannot be used to diagnose obesity or malnutrition; if a child is over the 85th percentile or lower than the 5th percentile on the charts, the child should see a doctor. The curves on the growth chart show the pattern of growth. Growth charts for infants and children are calculated the same as for adults but interpreted differently based on BMI. Children are not just small adults; as they grow, their BMI will change. For example, it may be healthy for a 2-year-old child to have a BMI of 16.1 and for that same child to have a BMI of 15.5 at age 6 years and then a BMI of 20 at age 15 years. Children under the 5th percentile should be examined to see if they are normal but small children or if they have a problem that prevents normal growth rate. Growth charts can be found at http://www.cdc.gov/growthcharts. Tables adapted for use in WIC Clinics are at http://www.nal.usda.gov/wicworks/Learning_Center/WIC_growthcharts.html. A calculator for estimating requirements with physical activity levels can be found at http://www.mydr.com.au/tools/child-energy-calculator.

BMIs for Adolescents

An expert consensus panel suggests that a BMI of 95% for age and gender should define obesity. BMI charts are used for the specific age and sex of the adolescent. Being over the 95th percentile on this chart is "overweight," while 85th to 95th percentiles are "at risk of overweight." Most guidance for teens is similar to that for adults. BMI calculators for teens include http://kidshealth.org/teen/food_fitness/dieting/bmi.html or http://apps.nccd.cdc.gov/dnpabmi/Calculator.aspx.

Template for Calculating Total Energy Expenditure

An easy way to calculate daily EERs for adults includes a template based on physical activity level. The estimated energy requirement (EER) equations of the Institute of Medicine DRI Committee account for all factors and measurements to determine physical activity level and energy expended from daily physical activity.

$$\text{BEE} = 293 - 3.8 \times \text{age (years)} + 456.4 \times \text{height (meters)} + 10.12 \times \text{weight (kg)}$$

For women:

$$\text{BEE} = 247 - 2.67 \times \text{age (years)} + 401.5 \times \text{height (meters)} + 8.6 \times \text{weight (kg)}$$

$$\Delta\ \text{PAL} = (\text{METs} - 1) \times [(1.15/0.9) \times \text{Duration (minutes)}]/1440)$$

$$\text{BEE}/[0.0175 \times 1440 \times \text{weight (kg)}]$$

After the Δ PAL is calculated for each physical activity, the physical activity category (PAL: sedentary, low active, active, or very active) is determined based on the basal activity impact on energy expenditure (a factor of 1.1) and the sum of all activities (sum of Δ PAL). This factor accounts for TEF and postexercise increase in energy expenditure. The PAL is automatically calculated as PAL = 1.1 + sum of Δ PALi, where Δ PALi is the list of each reported activity impact on energy expenditure. The template is available in an Excel spreadsheet at http://www.ncbi.nlm.nih.gov/pmc/articles/PMC1784117/; accessed 11/7/09.

REFERENCE

Gerrior S, et al. An easy approach to calculating estimated energy requirements. *Prev Chronic Dis.* 3:129A, 2006.

BMI and Mortality

Both general adiposity and abdominal adiposity are associated with the risk of death and support the use of waist circumference or waist-to-hip ratio in addition to BMI in assessing the risk of death (Pischon et al, 2008). Lean men and women (BMI <18 kg/m^2) experience increased all-cause mortality compared with those with a BMI between 20 and 22 kg/m^2, particularly for cardiovascular and respiratory diseases.

It is important that public health messages regarding healthy eating are aimed at maintaining a healthy body weight rather than just "losing weight" (Thorogood, 2003). The following table indicates the lower ranges of BMI, below which mortality increases (Stevens, 2000).

Ages 20–29	BMI: Men 21.4; Women 19.5
Ages 30–39	BMI: Men 21.6; Women 23.4
Ages 40–49	BMI: Men 22.9; Women 23.2
Ages 50–59	BMI: Men 25.8; Women 25.2
Ages 60–69	BMI: Men 26.6; Women 27.3

REFERENCES

Pischon T, et al. General and abdominal adiposity and risk of death in Europe. *N Engl J Med.* 359:2105, 2008.

Stevens J. Impact of age on associations between weight and mortality. *Nutr Rev.* 58:129, 2000.

Thorogood M. Relation between body mass index and mortality in an unusually slim cohort. *J Epidemiol Community Health.* 57:130, 2003.

Using BMI for Older Adults

TEE and physical activity level (PAL, defined as the ratio of total to resting energy expenditure) decline progressively throughout adult life in both normal weight and overweight men and women (Roberts and Dallal, 2005). In normal weight individuals (defined as BMI 18.5–25) TEE falls by approximately 150 kilocalories per decade, and PAL falls from an average of 1.75 in the second decade of life to 1.28 in the ninth decade (Roberts and Dallal, 2005). Thermic effect of food does not appear to change.

Waist-to-hip ratio (WHR) rather than BMI appears to be a more appropriate yardstick for health risk among older adults over age 70 (Srikanthan et al, 2009).

REFERENCES

Roberts SB, Dallal AG. Energy requirements and aging. *Public Health Nutr.* 8:1028, 2005.

Srikanthan P, et al. Waist-hip-ratio as a predictor of all-cause mortality in high-functioning older adults. *Ann Epidemiol.* 19:724, 2009.

TABLE 10-4 Calculations of Ideal Body Weight Range

Estimated Ideal Body Weight (Hamwi Method)–Not a Validated Method

Medium-frame women: allow 100 lb for first 5 ft of height, plus 5 lb for each additional inch

Medium-frame men: allow 106 lb for first 5 ft of height plus 6 lb for each additional inch

Small/large frame: subtract/add 10%

REFERENCES

Hamwi GJ. Therapy: changing dietary concepts. In: Danowski TS, ed. *Diabetes mellitus: diagnosis and treatment.* New York: American Diabetes Federation, 1974:612–623.

Adjustment for Paraplegia or Quadriplegia

Paraplegic: ideal weight minus 5–10%

Quadriplegic: ideal weight minus 10–15%

REFERENCE

O'Brien RY. Spinal cord injury. In: Gines DJ, ed. *Nutrition management in rehabilitation.* Rockville, MD: Aspen Publishers, Inc., 1990:165.

Adjustment for Amputation

$Wt_E = Wt_O/1 - P$

Key: Wt_E = estimate of total body weight; Wt_O = observed body weight; P = proportion of total body weight represented by missing limb.

REFERENCE

Himes JH. New equation to estimate body mass index in amputees. *J Am Diet Assoc.* 95:646, 1995.

Adjustment for Obese Patients

Indirect calorimetry is the "gold standard" for determining energy requirements in the obese patient, or equations can be used, such as 21 kcal/kg actual weight. Formulas for adjusted body weight for obesity [(actual body weight − ideal body weight) × 0.25 + ideal body weight] have not been validated, and predictive equations for resting metabolic rates (RMR) have many flaws. The Harris-Benedict Equation (Harris and Benedict, 1919) may lead to overfeeding, particularly in older adults. Estimated energy needs should be based on RMR using indirect calorimetry; if RMR cannot be measured, then the Mifflin-St. Jeor equation using **actual** weight is the most accurate for estimating RMR for overweight and obese individuals.

Mifflin-St. Jeor Equation:

Men: $RMR = 9.99 \times \text{weight} + 6.25 \times \text{height} - 4.92 \times \text{age} + 5$

Women: $RMR = 9.99 \times \text{weight} + 6.25 \times \text{height} - 4.92 \times \text{age} - 161$

For the obese elderly (Frankenfield et al, 2009): Mifflin (0.71) + T_{max} (85) + Ve(64) − 3085 (ADA, Weight Management, 2009; Dobratz et al, 2007).

Adjustment for Critically Ill Patients

In critical illness, energy needs often fluctuate substantially. Nutrition delivery may be influenced by the risk of refeeding syndrome, hypocaloric feeding regimens, inadequate access, feeding intolerance, and feeding-delay for procedures (Walker and Heuberger, 2009). No equation accurately predicts REE in hospitalized patients. Only indirect calorimetry (IC) will provide accurate assessment of energy needs (Boullata et al, 2007).

When comparing popular equations (Harris-Benedict, Ireton-Jones, Penn State 1998 and 2003; Swinamer, 1990), prediction accuracy is rarely within 10% of the measured energy expenditure (Walker and Heuberger, 2009). Thirteen studies comparing RMR and the Harris-Benedict equation without adjustments report an underestimation of energy needs in the critically ill population, by as much as 1000 kilocalories or more (ADA, 2009).

Use of hand-held indirect calorimeters have significant advantages when metabolic carts are not available (Spears et al, 2009). Prediction of metabolic rate is imperfect and requires clinical judgment. The ADA evidence analysis library has described comparisons of these estimated calculations (ADA, 2009). The Penn State equation provides the most accurate assessment of metabolic rate in critically ill patients (79%) if indirect calorimetry is unavailable (Frankenfield et al, 2009). This equation follows: RMR = BMR (0.85) + V_E (33) + T_{max} (175) − 6433

REFERENCES

American Dietetic Association (ADA). Evidence analysis library. Critical illness project. Accessed November 7 2009 at http://www.adaevidencelibrary.com/evidence.cfm=evidence_summary_id=250444.

American Dietetic Association (ADA). Position Paper on Weight Management. *J Am Diet Assoc.* 100:330, 2009.

Boullata J, et al. Accurate determination of energy needs in hospitalized patients. *J Am Diet Assoc.* 107:393, 2007.

Dobratz JR, et al. Predicting energy expenditure in extremely obese women. *JPEN J Parenter Enteral Nutr.* 31:217, 2007.

Frankenfield DC, et al. Analysis of estimation methods for resting metabolic rate in critically ill adults. *JPEN J Parenter Enteral Nutr.* 33:27, 2009.

Harris J, Benedict F. *A biometric study of basal metabolism in man.* Washington, DC: Carnegie Institute of Washington, 1919.

Spears KE, et al. Hand-held indirect calorimeter offers advantages compared with prediction equations, in a group of overweight women, to determine resting energy expenditures and estimated total energy expenditures during research screening. *J Am Diet Assoc.* 109:836, 2009.

Walker RN, Heuberger RA. Predictive equations for energy needs for the critically ill. *Respir Care.* 54:509, 2009.

TABLE 10-5 Body Mass Index Table for Adults

Obese (>30) | Overweight (25-30) | Normal (18.5-25) | Underweight (<18.5)

HEIGHT in feet/inches and centimeters

WEIGHT lbs (kg)	4'8"	4'9"	4'10"	4'11"	5'0"	5'1"	5'2"	5'3"	5'4"	5'5"	5'6"	5'7"	5'8"	5'9"	5'10"	5'11"	6'0"	6'1"	6'2"	6'3"	6'4"	6'5"
	142cm		147	150	152	155	157	160	163	165	168	170	173	175	178	180	183	185	188	191	193	196
260 (117.9)	**58**	**56**	**54**	**53**	**51**	**49**	**48**	**46**	**45**	**43**	**42**	**41**	**40**	**38**	**37**	**36**	**35**	**34**	**33**	**32**	**32**	**31**
255 (115.7)	57	55	53	51	50	48	47	45	44	42	41	40	39	38	37	36	35	34	33	32	31	30
250 (113.4)	**56**	**54**	**52**	**50**	**49**	**47**	**46**	**44**	**43**	**42**	**40**	**39**	**38**	**37**	**36**	**35**	**34**	**33**	**32**	**31**	**30**	**30**
245 (111.1)	55	53	51	49	48	46	45	43	42	41	40	38	37	36	35	34	33	32	31	31	30	29
240 (108.9)	**54**	**52**	**50**	**48**	**47**	**45**	**44**	**43**	**41**	**40**	**39**	**38**	**36**	**35**	**34**	**33**	**33**	**32**	**31**	**30**	**29**	**28**
235 (106.6)	53	51	49	47	46	44	43	42	40	39	38	37	36	35	34	33	32	31	30	29	29	28
230 (104.3)	**52**	**50**	**48**	**46**	**45**	**43**	**42**	**41**	**39**	**38**	**37**	**36**	**35**	**34**	**33**	**32**	**31**	**30**	**30**	**29**	**28**	**27**
225 (102.1)	50	49	47	45	44	43	41	40	39	37	36	35	34	33	32	31	31	30	29	28	27	27
220 (99.8)	**49**	**48**	**46**	**44**	**43**	**42**	**40**	**39**	**38**	**37**	**36**	**34**	**33**	**32**	**32**	**31**	**30**	**29**	**28**	**27**	**27**	**26**
215 (97.5)	48	47	45	43	42	41	39	38	37	36	35	34	33	32	31	30	29	28	28	27	26	25
210 (95.3)	**47**	**45**	**44**	**42**	**41**	**40**	**38**	**37**	**36**	**35**	**34**	**33**	**32**	**31**	**30**	**29**	**28**	**28**	**27**	**26**	**26**	**25**
205 (93.0)	46	44	43	41	40	39	37	36	35	34	33	32	31	30	29	29	28	27	26	26	25	24
200 (90.7)	**45**	**43**	**42**	**40**	**39**	**38**	**37**	**35**	**34**	**33**	**32**	**31**	**30**	**30**	**29**	**28**	**27**	**26**	**26**	**25**	**24**	**24**
195 (88.5)	44	42	41	39	38	37	36	35	33	32	31	31	30	29	28	27	26	26	25	24	24	23
190 (86.2)	**43**	**41**	**40**	**38**	**37**	**36**	**35**	**34**	**33**	**32**	**31**	**30**	**29**	**28**	**27**	**26**	**26**	**25**	**24**	**24**	**23**	**23**
185 (83.9)	41	40	39	37	36	35	34	33	32	31	30	29	28	27	27	26	25	24	24	23	23	22
180 (81.6)	**40**	**39**	**38**	**36**	**35**	**34**	**33**	**32**	**31**	**30**	**29**	**28**	**27**	**27**	**26**	**25**	**24**	**24**	**23**	**22**	**22**	**21**
175 (79.4)	39	38	37	35	34	33	32	31	30	29	28	27	27	26	25	24	24	23	22	22	21	21
170 (77.1)	**38**	**37**	**36**	**34**	**33**	**32**	**31**	**30**	**29**	**28**	**27**	**27**	**26**	**25**	**24**	**24**	**23**	**22**	**22**	**21**	**21**	**20**
165 (74.8)	37	36	34	33	32	31	30	29	28	27	27	26	25	24	24	23	22	22	21	21	20	20
160 (72.6)	**36**	**35**	**33**	**32**	**31**	**30**	**29**	**28**	**27**	**27**	**26**	**25**	**24**	**24**	**23**	**22**	**22**	**21**	**21**	**20**	**19**	**19**
155 (70.3)	35	34	32	31	30	29	28	27	27	26	25	24	24	23	22	22	21	20	20	19	19	18
150 (68.0)	**34**	**32**	**31**	**30**	**29**	**28**	**27**	**27**	**26**	**25**	**24**	**23**	**23**	**22**	**22**	**21**	**20**	**20**	**19**	**19**	**18**	**18**
145 (65.8)	33	31	30	29	28	27	27	26	25	24	23	23	22	21	21	20	20	19	19	18	18	17
140 (63.5)	**31**	**30**	**29**	**28**	**27**	**26**	**26**	**25**	**24**	**23**	**23**	**22**	**21**	**21**	**20**	**20**	**19**	**18**	**18**	**17**	**17**	**17**
135 (61.2)	30	29	28	27	26	26	25	24	23	22	22	21	21	20	19	19	18	18	17	17	16	16
130 (59.0)	**29**	**28**	**27**	**26**	**25**	**25**	**24**	**23**	**22**	**22**	**21**	**20**	**20**	**19**	**19**	**18**	**18**	**17**	**17**	**16**	**16**	**15**
125 (56.7)	28	27	26	25	24	24	23	22	21	21	20	20	19	18	18	17	17	16	16	16	15	15
120 (54.4)	**27**	**26**	**25**	**24**	**23**	**23**	**22**	**21**	**21**	**20**	**19**	**19**	**18**	**18**	**17**	**17**	**16**	**16**	**15**	**15**	**15**	**14**
115 (52.2)	26	25	24	23	22	22	21	20	20	19	19	18	17	17	16	16	16	15	15	14	14	14
110 (49.9)	**25**	**24**	**23**	**22**	**21**	**21**	**20**	**19**	**19**	**18**	**18**	**17**	**17**	**16**	**16**	**15**	**15**	**15**	**14**	**14**	**13**	**13**
105 (47.6)	24	23	22	21	21	20	19	19	18	17	17	16	16	16	15	15	14	14	13	13	13	12
100 (45.4)	**22**	**22**	**21**	**20**	**20**	**19**	**18**	**18**	**17**	**17**	**16**	**16**	**15**	**15**	**14**	**14**	**14**	**13**	**13**	**12**	**12**	**12**
95 (43.1)	21	21	20	19	19	18	17	17	16	16	15	15	14	14	14	13	13	13	12	12	12	11
90 (40.8)	**20**	**19**	**19**	**18**	**18**	**17**	**16**	**16**	**15**	**15**	**15**	**14**	**14**	**13**	**13**	**13**	**12**	**12**	**12**	**11**	**11**	**11**
85 (38.6)	19	18	18	17	17	16	16	15	15	14	14	13	13	13	12	12	12	11	11	11	10	10
80 (36.3)	**18**	**17**	**17**	**16**	**16**	**15**	**15**	**14**	**14**	**13**	**13**	**13**	**12**	**12**	**11**	**11**	**11**	**11**	**10**	**10**	**10**	**9**

Note: BMI values rounded to the nearest whole number. BMI categories based on CDC (Centers for Disease Control and Prevention) criteria.

www.vertex42.com BMI = Weight[kg] / (Height[m] x Height[m]) = 703 x Weight[lb] / (Height[in] x Height[in])

For more information, see http://www.nhlbi.nih.gov/guidelines/obesity/bmi_tbl.htm.

TABLE 10-6 Short Methods for Calculating Energy Needs

Weight and Height Conversion Factors

1 kg	= 2.2 lb
1 lb	= 0.453 kg
1 ft	= 30.48 cm
1 in	= 2.54 cm
1 cm	= 0.39 in
1 m	= 39.37 in

Goal	Level of Activity or Illness: Low	Moderate	High
Lose weight	15 kcal/kg	20 kcal/kg	25 kcal/kg
Maintain weight	20 kcal/kg	25 kcal/kg	30 kcal/kg
Gain weight	25 kcal/kg	30 kcal/kg	35 kcal/kg

Energy Needs Based on Gender for Adults

Men, active women	15 kcal/lb body weight
Most women, sedentary men, and adults over 55 years	13 kcal/lb body weight
Sedentary women, obese adults	10 kcal/lb body weight
Pregnant women	
1st trimester	13–15 kcal/lb body weight
2nd and 3rd trimester	16–17 kcal/lb body weight
Lactating women	15–17 kcal/lb body weight

Energy Needs Based on Age for Children

There is a general decline in the calories needed per pound as a child gets older. These figures are not accurate for obese children.

0–12 months	55 kcal/lb body weight
1–10 years	45–36 kcal/lb body weight
11–15 years–young women	17 kcal/lb body weight
11–15 years–young men	30 kcal/lb body weight
16–20 years–young women	15 kcal/lb body weight
16–20 years–young men	**18 kcal/lb body weight**

REFERENCES

Bray G. Soft drink consumption and obesity: it is all about fructose [published online ahead of print Dec 2, 2009]. *Curr Opin Lipidol.*

Chen JL. Household income, maternal acculturation, maternal education level and health behaviors of Chinese-American children and mothers. *J Immigr Minor Health.* 11:198, 2009.

Cocores JA, Gold MS. The Salted Food Addiction Hypothesis may explain overeating and the obesity epidemic [published online ahead of print July 28, 2009]. *Med Hypotheses.*

Cohen DA. Neurophysiological pathways to obesity: Below awareness and beyond individual control. *Diabetes.* 57:1768, 2008.

Epstein LH, et al. What constitutes food variety? Stimulus specificity of food [published online ahead of print Sept 16, 2009]. *Appetite.*

Flagel SB, et al. Individual differences in the attribution of incentive salience to reward-related cues: Implications for addiction. *Neuropharmacology.* 56:139S, 2009.

Greenwood JL, Stanford JB. Preventing or improving obesity by addressing specific eating patterns. *J Am Board Fam Med.* 21:135, 2008.

McKiernan F, et al. Relationships between human thirst, hunger, drinking, and feeding. *Physiol Behav.* 94:700, 2008.

Novotny R, et al. US acculturation, food intake, and obesity among Asian-Pacific hotel workers. *J Am Diet Assoc.* 109:1712, 2009.

Ranadive SA, Vaisse C. Lessons from extreme human obesity: monogenic disorders. *Endocrinol Metab Clin North Am.* 37:733, 2008.

Soeters PB, Schols AM. Advances in understanding and assessing malnutrition. *Curr Opin Clin Nutr Metab Care.* 12:487, 2009.

Tindell AJ, et al. Dynamic computation of incentive salience: "wanting" what was never "liked". *J Neurosci.* 29:12220, 2009.

OVERNUTRITION

OVERWEIGHT AND OBESITY

NUTRITIONAL ACUITY RANKING: LEVEL 3–4

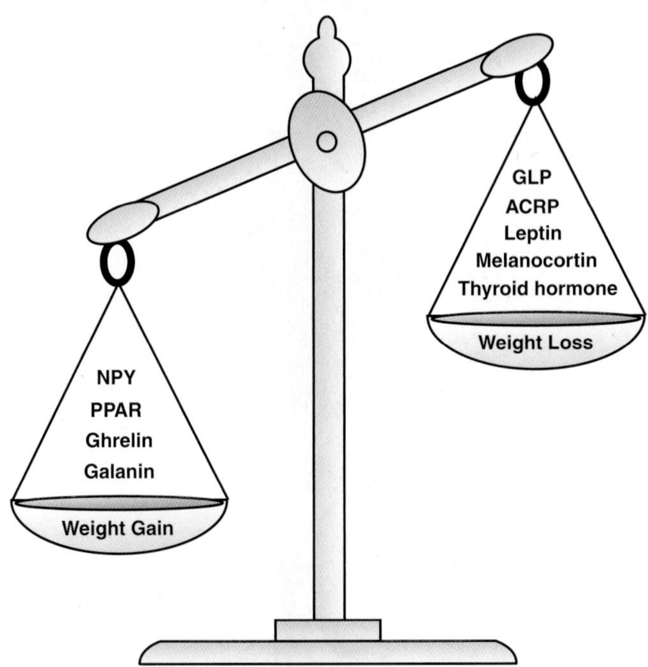

Adapted from: Raphael Rubin, David S. Strayer, *Rubin's Pathology: Clinicopathologic Foundations of Medicine,* 5th ed. Philadelphia: Lippincott Williams & Wilkins, 2008.

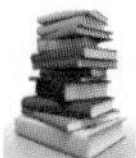

DEFINITIONS AND BACKGROUND

Overweight is defined as a BMI of 25–29; obesity is defined as a BMI of 30 or more. Obesity is a problem because the percentage of body fat is much greater than lean body mass. Micronutrients are often consumed at lower than desirable levels, while macronutrients are eaten in large amounts. Obesity has reached epidemic proportions in the United States, with 35.1% of adults being classified as obese (Catenacci et al, 2009). The World Health Organization (WHO) labels the increase in obesity and related syndromes as an epidemic in both industrialized countries and in developing countries (Misra and Khurana, 2008).

Obesity is a complex multifactorial chronic disease that develops from an interaction of genetic, social, behavioral, cultural, physiological, and metabolic factors (NHLBI, 2009; Thorleifsson et al, 2009). Genetics account for 30–40% of the variations in weight between individuals (Pi-Sunyer and Kris-Etherton, 2005). Indeed, weight and BMI are highly heritable (Thorleifsson et al, 2009). Environmental factors include low physical activity, energy intake, smoking cessation, overconsumption of high-fat foods.

The prevalence of overweight (BMI >25) and obesity (BMI >30) has steadily increased over the past decade. Approximately 34% of American adults are obese, and 14.6% of low-income, preschool-aged children are obese (CDC, 2009). Blacks have a 51% higher prevalence of obesity than whites, and Hispanics have a 21% higher obesity prevalence compared with whites (CDC, 2009). However, abdominal visceral adipose tissue (VAT) is significantly greater in white men and women; African American men and women have higher subcutaneous adipose tissue (SAT) than whites (Katzmarzyk et al, 2009). An increased understanding of race-based differences in adiposity in specific body depots helps to explain the differential health risks associated with obesity.

The current generation in the United States may have a shorter life expectancy than that of their parents if the obesity epidemic is not controlled (Catenacci et al, 2009). In Project EAT, researchers found that the use of low-calorie soft drinks was a marker for more general dietary behaviors and weight concerns; there was no association between sugar-sweetened beverage consumption, juice consumption, and adolescent weight gain over a 5-y period; and adolescents who consumed little or no white milk gained significantly more weight than their peers who consumed white milk (Vaneslow et al, 2009).

Recent evidence also shows a link between obesity and viral infections, particularly with human adenoviruses (Atkinson, 2007; Mitra and Clarke, 2009). The human distal gut harbors microbiota that provide important metabolic capabilities including the ability to extract energy from otherwise indigestible dietary polysaccharides (Turnbaugh et al, 2009). Metagenomic studies demonstrated that certain mixes of gut microbiota may protect or predispose the host to obesity by increasing dietary energy harvest, promoting fat deposition, and triggering systemic inflammation (Tsai and Coyle, 2009). Each person's gut microbial community varies in the specific bacterial lineages present, which may lead to differences in leanness or obesity (Turnbaugh et al, 2009).

Both overweight and obesity increase the risks of contracting chronic diseases, secondary symptoms, and impaired quality of life. Waist circumference, waist-hip ratio, and BMI may predict chronic disease and mortality. Hypertension is common in persons with central-type obesity, and women who have a BMI over 30 may have problems with fertility. Morbid obesity (BMI >40) is a strong predictor of premature death. When a patient reaches the overweight stage, he or she should be given guidance on how to avoid obesity (see Table 10-7 and figure).

Reimbursement for obesity counseling and management is a complicated issue. Not everyone loses weight easily or steadily, and there are indirect costs such as pain and suffering to consider. BMI can help predict those who may benefit from weight loss counseling, but there are no guarantees of success.

There are varied options for the management of overweight and obese patients including dietary approaches, altered physical activity patterns, behavior therapy techniques, pharmacotherapy, surgery, and combinations of these techniques. Studies have shown that small changes in weight and increases in physical activity can make significant improvements in health.

Starvation diets are not the solution. Orthostatic hypotension may complicate very low–calorie diets (VLCD) because of sodium depletion and depressed sympathetic nervous system activity. It is more desirable to calculate basal energy

TABLE 10-7 **Suggested Weights for Initiation of Weight Management Counseling**

Height (in)	Overweight in lb (BMI >25)	Obese in lb (BMI >30)
58	119	143
59	124	148
60	128	153
61	132	158
62	136	164
63	141	169
64	145	174
65	150	180
66	155	186
67	159	191
68	164	197
69	169	203
70	174	207
71	179	215
72	184	221
73	189	227
74	194	233
75	200	240
76	205	246

Derived from: National Heart, Lung, and Blood Institute. Body mass index table. Accessed August, 8, 2005 at http://www.nhlbi.nih.gov/guidelines/obesity/bmi_tbl.pdf.

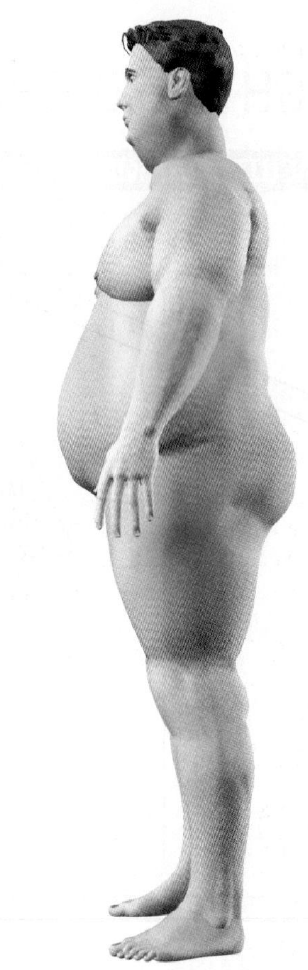

An obese male. LifeART image copyright © 2010 Lippincott Williams & Wilkins. All rights reserved.

requirements for the individual and to determine a reasonable energy intake accordingly. Evidence suggests that weight loss diets should include moderate carbohydrate (35–50% of energy), moderate fat (25–35% of energy), and protein as 25–35% of energy (Schoeller and Buchholz, 2005). Specifically, avoid consuming large portions of energy-dense foods or snacks, high-calorie beverages, and foods with empty calories (Pi-Sunyer and Kris-Etherton, 2005).

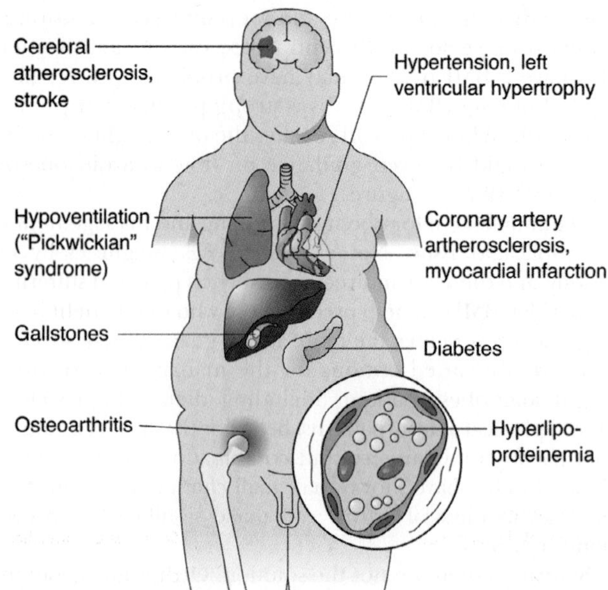

Consequences of Obesity. Adapted from: Raphael Rubin, David S. Strayer, *Rubin's Pathology: Clinicopathologic Foundations of Medicine,* 5th ed. Philadelphia: Lippincott Williams & Wilkins, 2008.

Energy-reduced, isocaloric very-low-carbohydrate, high-fat (VLCHF) diets and high-carbohydrate, low-fat (HCLF) diets produce similar weight loss results (Tay et al, 2008). However, the use of appropriate types of fat is important to protect the heart. Comparisons of the biological effect of popular diets such as Atkins, South Beach, and Ornish during weight maintenance periods show that the Atkins diet leads to the least favorable results in flow-mediated vasodilation (Miller et al, 2009). The HCLF diet has favorable effects on the blood lipid profile (Tay et al, 2008). To estimate the percentage of fat calories for a nutritional plan, review Table 10-8.

Hormones, genes, nutrients and the central nervous system converge to manage energy intake. Dysregulation in the system of fuel-sensing signals may underlie problems such as obesity and diabetes (Sandoval et al, 2008). Leptin is a mediator of long-term regulation of energy balance, suppressing food intake, and inducing weight loss. Leptin is produced within white adipose tissue, brown fat, the placenta, and in a fetal heart, bone, and cartilage. As the amount of fat stored in adipocytes rises, leptin is released into the blood and signals to the brain that the body has had enough to eat. Altered leptin receptor genes (LEPR) can lead to changes in BMI over time. Obesity markedly influences serum insulin, leptin, growth hormone (GH) secretion, and free fatty acid (FFA) levels. Most overweight people have altered levels of serum leptin.

TABLE 10-8 Calculation of Fat Grams

Divide desired body weight by 2. Examples:

120 lb/2 = 60 g	130 lb/2 = 65 g
140 lb/2 = 70 g	150 lb/2 = 75 g
160 lb/2 = 80 g	170 lb/2 = 85 g
180 lb/2 = 90 g	190 lb/2 = 95 g
200 lb/2 = 100 g	210 lb/2 = 105 g

Hormones and peptides such as melatonin, ghrelin, obestatin, and leptin perform dual functions in the pancreas by maintaining metabolic homeostasis; appetite-controlling neuropeptides such as ghrelin, orexin A, and neuropeptide Y regulate pancreatic secretions (Chandra and Liddle, 2009). Ghrelin acts quickly for meal initiation and is produced in the stomach.

Satiety signals from the pancreas and intestine include cholecystokinin, peptide YY, pancreatic polypeptide (PP), glucagon-like peptide 1 (GLP-1), oxyntomodulin (OXM), and amylin (Wren and Bloom, 2007). Cholecystokinin induces satiety by interacting through CCK-1 receptors located in the hindbrain; it also inhibits the expression of orexigenic peptides in the hypothalamus and prevents stimulation of specialized neurons by ghrelin (Chandra and Liddle, 2007). Ghrelin, peptide YY, and cholecystokinin are all influenced by macronutrient intake (Orr and Davy, 2005).

Elevated cholecystokinin levels decrease appetite and also reduce intestinal inflammation caused by parasites and bacterial toxins (Chandra and Liddle, 2007). Elevated inflammatory markers—such as tumor necrosis factor (TNF) alpha, soluble TNF receptor II (sTNF-RII), interleukin-6 (IL-6), and C-reactive protein (CRP)—are characteristically found in the serum in obese patients. Night eating syndrome (NES) is also affected by disordered neuroendocrine functioning; see Table 10-9.

It is important to discuss psychological well-being, particularly feelings about food and body image. The Power of Food Scale (PFS) assesses individual differences in appetitive responsiveness to rewarding properties of the food environment; it is a reliable and valid tool for assessing food cravings and binge eating (Lowe and Butryn, 2007). The PFS evaluates the appetite for palatable foods at three different levels of food proximity: food available, food present, and food tasted (Lowe et al, 2009). See Table 10-10 for the questions asked in the Power of Food Scale. Setting achievable goals will require individualized approaches (Nonas and Foster, 2009).

Self-esteem, body image, self-efficacy, locus of control, motivation, stress management, problem-solving and

TABLE 10-9 Night Eating Syndrome Description and Questionnaire

Night eating syndrome (NES) is a special condition that affects 1–1.5% of the general population, 6%–16% of patients in weight reduction programs, and 8%–42% of candidates for bariatric surgery (Stunkard et al, 2008). Viewed as a delay in the circadian rhythm of food intake, NES is defined by two core criteria: evening hyperphagia (ingestion of at least 25% of daily calories after supper) with awakenings and ingestions at least three times a week (Stunkard et al, 2008). Single PET scans have shown significant elevation of serotonin transporters in the midbrain of night eaters; this is from a genetic vulnerability transmitted as part of the established heritability triggered by stress (Lundgren et al, 2006). Because of elevations in serotonin transporter levels, sertraline (an SSRI) helps to alleviate impaired circadian rhythm and resulting NES (O'Reardon et al, 2006).

Night Eating Questionnaire

1. How hungry are you usually in the morning?
2. When do you usually eat for the first time?
3. Do you have cravings or urges to eat snacks after supper but before bedtime?
4. How much control do you have over your eating between supper and bedtime?
5. How much of your daily food intake do you consume after suppertime?
6. Are you currently feeling blue or down in the dumps?
7. When you are feeling blue, when is your mood lower?
8. How often do you have trouble getting to sleep?
9. Other than using the bathroom, how often do you get up in the middle of the night?
10. Do you have cravings or urges to eat snacks when you wake up at night?
11. Do you eat in order to get back to sleep when you awake at night?
12. When you get up in the middle of the night, how often do you snack?
13. If you snack in the middle of the night, how aware are you of your eating?
14. How much control do you have over your nighttime eating?

Allison KC, et al. The Night Eating Questionnaire (NEQ): psychometric properties of a measure of severity of the night eating syndrome. *Eat Behav.* 9:62, 2008. Accessed November 1, 2009 at http://www.med.upenn.edu/weight/nighteatingform.shtml.

REFERENCES

Lundgren JD, et al. Familial aggregation in the night eating syndrome. *Int J Eat Disord.* 39:516, 2006.
O'Reardon JP, et al. A randomized, placebo-controlled trial of sertraline in the treatment of night eating syndrome. *Am J Psychiatry.* 163:893, 2006.
Stunkard A, et al. Issues for DSM V: Night eating syndrome. *Am J Psychiatry.* 265:424, 2008.

TABLE 10-10 Power of Food Scale

Please indicate the extent to which you agree that the following items describe you. Use the following 1–5 scale for your responses:

1 don't agree at all
2 agree a little
3 agree somewhat
4 agree
5 strongly agree

1. I find myself thinking about food even when I'm not physically hungry.
2. When I'm in a situation where delicious foods are present, but I have to wait to eat them, it is very difficult for me to wait.
3. I get more pleasure from eating than I do from almost anything else.
4. I feel that food is to me like liquor is to an alcoholic.
5. If I see or smell a food I like, I get a powerful urge to have some.
6. When I'm around a fattening food I love, it's hard to stop myself from at least tasting it.
7. I often think about what foods I might eat later in the day.
8. It's scary to think of the power that food has over me.
9. When I taste a favorite food, I feel intense pleasure.
10. When I know a delicious food is available, I can't stop myself from thinking about having some.
11. I love the taste of certain foods so much that I can't avoid eating them even if they're bad for me.
12. When I see delicious foods in advertisements or commercials, it makes me want to eat.
13. I feel like food controls me rather than the other way around.
14. Just before I taste a favorite food, I feel intense anticipation.
15. When I eat delicious food, I focus a lot on how good it tastes.
16. Sometimes, when I'm doing everyday activities, I get an urge to eat "out of the blue" (for no apparent reason).
17. I think I enjoy eating a lot more than most other people.
18. Hearing someone describe a great meal makes me really want to have something to eat.
19. It seems like I have food on my mind a lot.
20. It's very important to me that the foods I eat are as delicious as possible.
21. Before I eat a favorite food, my mouth tends to flood with saliva.

Didie ER. The Power of Food Scale (PFS): development and theoretical evaluation of a self-report measure of the perceived influence of food. A thesis submitted to the faculty of Drexel University, June 2003. Accessed November 2, 2009 at http://dspace.library.drexel.edu/bitstream/1860/205/7/didie_thesis.pdf.

decision-making, and assertiveness are important considerations. Stress may cause those who are overweight to add more pounds (Block et al, 2009). Elevated cortisol or other hormone levels may be the trigger from stress.

Traditional weight management programs can be helpful. Sustained modest weight loss by obese adults can result in substantial health and economic benefits. Successful weight management to improve overall health for adults requires a lifelong commitment to healthy lifestyle behaviors emphasizing sustainable and enjoyable eating practices and daily physical activity (Seagle et al, 2007). The American Dietetic Association has recommended eight medical nutrition therapy visits for adult weight management. (See Figure on page 613)

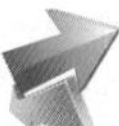

ASSESSMENT, MONITORING, AND EVALUATION

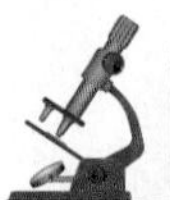

CLINICAL INDICATORS

Genetic Markers: Research into the genetics of obesity is extensive (Farooqi and O'Rahilly, 2007). The human Ob gene has been mapped to chromosome 7. The FTO (fat mass and obesity-associated) gene is found on chromosome 16. A genome-wide association (GWA) study has linked thousands of SNPs close to or in the FTO, melanocortin-4 receptor (MC4R,) brain-derived neurotrophic factor (BDNF), and SH2B adapter protein (SH2B1) genes (Thorleifsson et al, 2009). Other genes may play a role. The fatty-acid binding protein (FABP2) gene is associated with fat absorption and metabolism. The peroxisome proliferator-activated receptor gamma (PPARG) gene has a key role in the formation of fat cells. The adrenergic beta-2-receptor (ADRB2) gene mobilizes fat cells for energy, whereas the adrenergic beta-3-receptor (ADRB3) gene regulates the breakdown of fat from tissues in response to exercise. The glutamate decarboxylase 2 (GAD2) gene is released from pancreatic and brain cells. GAD2 codes for the GABA neurotransmitter, which regulates food intake. Clearly, these multiple hormones and genes suggest that future obesity treatment will require a genetic profile and individualized plan.

Clinical/History

Height
Weight
BMI
Desirable BMI
Weight changes
Percentage of excess weight
Percentage of body fat
Diet history
Blood pressure (BP)
Skinfold thickness
Waist circumference
Sleep apnea

Lab Work

CRP (elevated)
Ca^{++}, Mg^{++}
Na^+, K^+
Uric acid
Triiodothyronine (T3), thyroxine (T4)
Glucose (Gluc)
Cholesterol (Chol)
Triglycerides (Trig)
Hypoxemia
Plasma cortisol

INTERVENTION

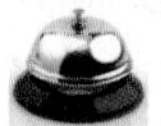

OBJECTIVES

The Clinical Guidelines on the Identification, Evaluation, and Treatment of Overweight and Obesity in Adults (NHLBI, 2009) suggest the following objectives:

1. Reduce body weight, maintain a lower body weight over the long term, and prevent further weight gain. It is better to maintain a moderate weight loss over a prolonged period than to regain from a marked weight loss. See Figure 10-6 for tips.

MAINTAINING A HEALTHY WEIGHT

Healthy Diet Plan

If you are concerned about your diet, no particular food plan is magical and no particular food must be either included or avoided. Your diet should consist of foods that you like or can learn to like, that are available to you, and that are within your means. The most effective diet programs for weight loss and maintenance are based on physical activity and reasonable serving sizes, with less frequent consumption of foods high in fat and refined sugars.

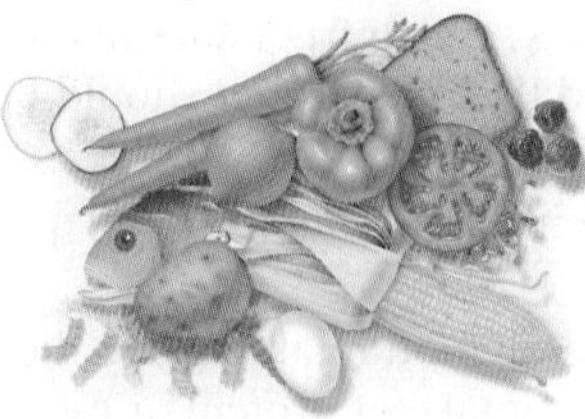

Physiological Hazards That Accompany Low-Carbohydrate Diets

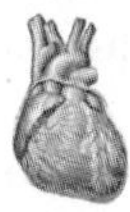

- **Heart Failure**
  Carbohydrates maintain sodium and fluid balance. A carbohydrate deficiency promotes loss of sodium and water, which can adversely affect blood pressure and cardiac function if not corrected.

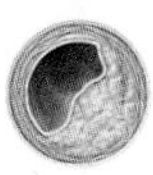

- **High Blood Cholesterol**
  Low-carbohydrate diets can raise blood cholesterol because in these diets, fruits, vegetables, breads, and cereals are replaced by meat and dairy products, which are rich in fat and protein. High fat and protein intakes, especially from meat and dairy products, raise LDL and total cholesterol.

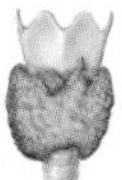

- **Metabolic Abnormalities**
  When carbohydrate intake is low, ketones are produced from fat to replace carbohydrates as a source of energy for the brain. Since ketones are acids, high levels can make the blood acidic, altering respiration and other metabolic processes that are sensitive to an increase or decrease in acidity.

The Risk in Low-Carbohydrate Diets

Low-carbohydrate diets, especially if undertaken without medical supervision, can be dangerous. Low-carbohydrate diets are designed to cause rapid weight loss by promoting an undesirably high concentration of ketone bodies (a byproduct of fat metabolism). The sales pitch is that you'll never feel hungry and that you'll lose weight faster than you would on any "ordinary diet". Both claims are true but the low-carb diets are true but misleading. Fast weight loss means loss of water and lean tissue, which are rapidly regained when people begin eating their usual diets again. The amount of body fat lost will be the same as with a conventional low- calorie diet. Fat loss is always equal to the difference between enegy consumed in food and energy expended in activity.

Overweight Problems

As the amount of body fat increases, especially around the abdomen, so does the risk of:

- Respiratory disease
- Obstructive sleep apnea
- Complications during surgery
- Gallbladder disease
- Stroke
- Non–insulin-dependent (type 2) diabetes
- Some forms of cancer, especially breast and colon
- Coronary heart disease
- Hypertension

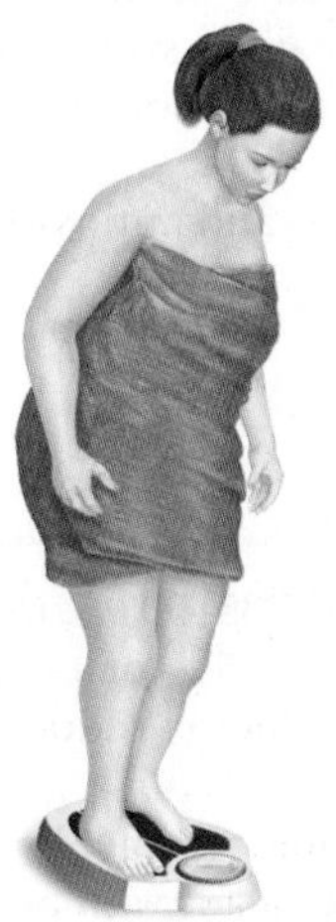

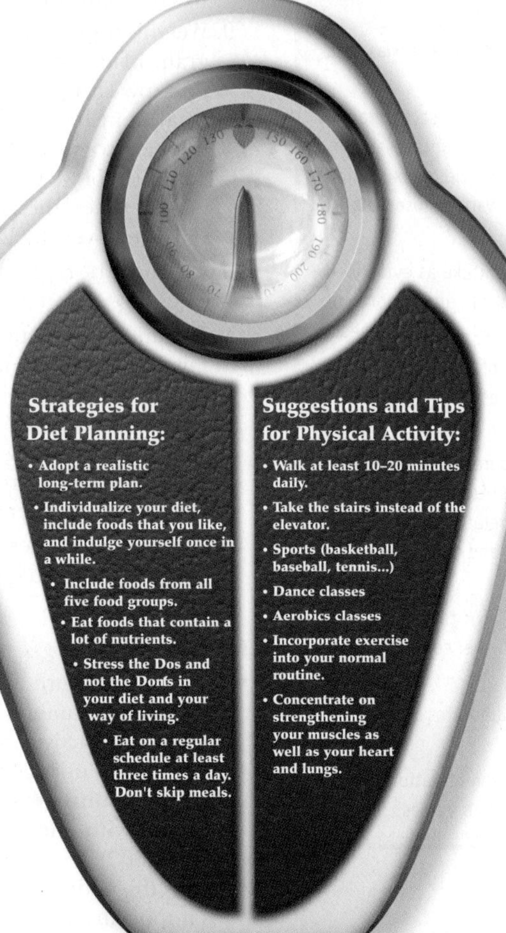

Strategies for Diet Planning:
• Adopt a realistic long-term plan.

• Include foods from all five food groups.

• Stress the Dos and not the Don'ts in your diet and your way of living.

• Walk at least 10–20 minutes daily.
• Take the stairs instead of the elevator.
• Sports (basketball, baseball, tennis...)
• Dance classes
• Aerobics classes
• Incorporate exercise into your normal routine.
• Concentrate on strengthening your muscles as well as your heart and lungs.

What Is Your Body Mass Index?

Your body mass index (BMI) is your weight in kilograms divided by the squae of your height in meters. It is used to indicate whether or not you are overweight or underweight.

How to Calculate Your Body Mass Index:

1. Convert your weight in pounds (lb) to kilograms (kg) by dividing your weight in pounds by 2.2 kg.
2. Convert your height in inches (in) to meters (m) by multiplying your height in inches by .0254 m.
3. Take your height in meters and square it by multiplying it by itself.
4. Divide your weight in kilograms by your height in meters squared (your calculated height fom step 3).

Example: Mark weighs 150 lb and is 5 ft, 10 in tall (70 in).

1. 150 lb ÷ by 2.2 kg = 68.18 kg
2. 70 in x .0254 m = 1.778 m
3. 1.778 m x 1.778 m = 3.161 m^2
4. 68.18 kg ÷ 3.161 m^2 = 21.56

Mark's BMI is 21.56

Acceptable Weight for Height Based on Body Mass Index

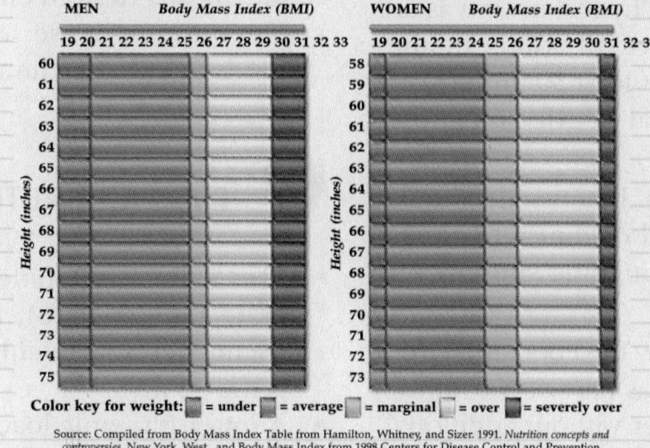

60 61 62 63 64 65 66 67 68 69 70 71 72 73 74 75

58 59 60 61 62 63 64 65 66 67 68 69 70 71 72 73

Color key for weight: = under = average = marginal = over = severely over

Source: Compiled from Body Mass Index Table from Hamilton, Whitney, and Sizer. 1991. *Nutrition concepts and controversies*. New York. West. and Body Mass Index from 1998 Centers for Disease Control and Prevention.

Excess Fat Distribution

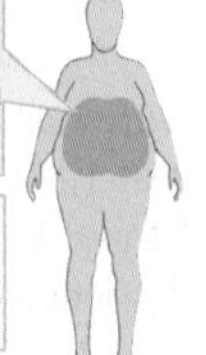

Apple Shaped Excess fat is distributed around the abdomen. Common in men, postmenopausal women, and with aging. Associated with increased risk of Type 2 diabetes.
Pear Shaped Excess fat is distributed around the hips and buttocks. Common in women. Associated with increased risk of osteoarthritis.

Understanding Calories

Calories are a standard measurement of heat energy. Technically, 1 calorie is 1 kilocalorie, which is the amount of heat required to raise the temperature of 1 kg. of water by 1° C.

A person's energy needs are determined by the amount of lean tissue or muscle and by the level of activity. A small, elderly, sedentary woman may need only about 1200 calories to meet her energy needs each day, whereas a tall, young, physically active man may need as many as 4000 calories daily.

How to Calculate Your Total Daily Energy (Calorie) Needs

1. Convert your weight from pounds (lb) to kilograms (kg) by dividing your weight in pounds by 2.2 lb/kg.
2. Multiply your weight in kilograms by 30 kcal/kg if you are a man and 25 kcal/kg if you are a woman.

Example

1. 150 lb– by 2.2 lb/kg = 68.18 kg
2. 68.18 kg x 30 kcal/kg = 2045 kcal

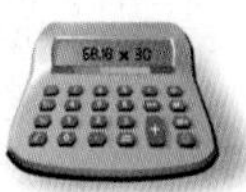

Result: A 150 lb man needs approximately 2045 kcal (calories) a day to maintain her weight.

Energy Demands of Activities

Activity	Body Weight (lb) 110	125	150	175	200
	CALORIES PER MINUTE				
Aerobics	6.8	7.8	9.3	10.9	12.4
Basketball (vigorous)	10.7	12.1	14.6	17.0	19.4
Bicycling					
13 miles per hour	5.0	5.6	6.8	7.9	9.0
Cross-country skiing					
8 miles per hour	11.4	13.0	15.6	18.2	20.8
Golf (carrying clubs)	5.0	5.6	6.8	7.9	9.0
Rowing (vigorous)	10.7	12.1	14.6	17.0	19.4
Running					
5 miles per hour	6.7	7.6	9.2	10.7	12.2
Soccer	10.7	2.1	14.6	17.0	19.4
Studying	1.2	1.4	1.7	1.9	2.2
Swimming					
20 yards per minute	3.5	4.0	4.8	5.6	6.4
Walking (brisk pace)					
3.5 miles per hour	3.9	4.4	5.2	6.1	7.0

Source: Compiled from Hamilton, Whitney, and Sizer. 1991. *Nutrition concepts and controversies*. New York. West.

Underweight Problems

When body weight decreases to 15–20% below desirable weight (BMI < 18.5), the amount of energy being consumed is not sufficient to support the function of vital organs. Lean tissue is being broken down and utilized for energy to make up the deficit. The results are:

- Low body temperature
- Abnormal electrical activity in the brain
- Altered blood lipids
- Dry skin
- Impaired immune response
- Loss of digestive function
- Abnormal hormone levels
- Malnutrition
- Anemia

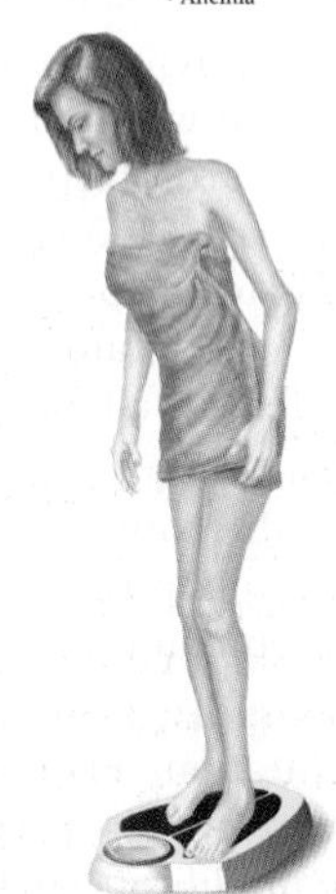

Asset provided by Anatomical Chart Co.

SAMPLE NUTRITION CARE PROCESS STEPS

Not Ready for Lifestyle Change

Assessment: Diet, weight, and physical activity histories and psychosocial issues.

Nutrition Diagnoses (PES): Not ready for diet/lifestyle change (NB 1.3) related to excessive oral food/beverage intake as evidenced by increased weight gain in spite of previous counseling sessions and statements such as, "I just don't want to lose weight; I can't see the point."

Overweight (NC-3.3) related to excess energy intake as evidenced by BMI >25, waist circumference >40 inches, and reports of overconsumption of high-fat/calorie-dense food and beverages.

Interventions: Nutrition prescription (ND-1) of 2200 kilocalories per day with approximately 25–30% of calories from fat and less than 10% of intake from saturated fat.

Initial/brief nutrition education (E-1) to address motivation to get to the next stage of change; reinforce instructions on following the diet plan; provide basic nutrition-related information; discuss the importance of physical activity and the benefits of weight loss.

Transtheoretical Model/Stages of Change (C-1.5): to help patient move from the precontemplation stage to the contemplation stage of change.

Collaboration (RC-1.3): MD and RD to collaborate on helping patient choose to lose weight.

Monitoring and Evaluation: Assess changes in motivation in one month. Evaluate for changes in weight, other lab values.

2. The initial goal of weight loss therapy should be to reduce body weight by approximately 10% from baseline. With success, further weight loss can be attempted if indicated through further assessment.
3. Weight loss should be about 1–2 lb/wk for a period of 6 months, with the subsequent strategy based on the amount of weight lost.
4. Promote use of low-calorie diets (LCDs). A diet that is individually planned to help create a deficit of 500–1000 kcal/d should be an integral part, aimed at achieving a weight loss of 1–2 lb/wk.
5. Increased physical activity is recommended since it produces some weight loss, decreases abdominal fat, and increases cardiorespiratory fitness. Physical activity is an integral part of weight maintenance. All adults should set a long-term goal to accumulate at least 30 minutes or more of moderate-intensity physical activity on most, and preferably all, days of the week.
6. Behavior therapy is a useful adjunct. Practitioners need to assess the patient's motivation and readiness to implement the plan; they must provide ongoing support for positive outcomes.
7. Weight-loss drugs that are approved by the Food and Drug Administration (FDA) may be used as part of a comprehensive weight-loss program but never without additional lifestyle modifications. Continual assessment of drug therapy for efficacy and safety is necessary.
8. Weight-loss surgery is an option for patients with morbid obesity (BMI ≥40 or ≥35 with comorbid conditions) when less invasive methods of weight loss have failed.
9. Weight-loss maintenance is enhanced by an ongoing program of dietary therapy, physical activity, and behavior therapy. Drug safety and efficacy beyond 1 year of total treatment has not been established. A weight maintenance program should be a priority after the initial 6 months of weight loss therapy; a high frequency of contacts between the patient and the practitioner should be provided over the long term.
10. All smokers, regardless of their weight status, should quit smoking.
11. In seniors, restrictions on overall food intake due to dieting could result in inadequate intake of protein or essential vitamins or minerals. Involuntary weight loss could be indicative of occult disease. Proper nutritional counseling and regular body weight monitoring in older persons is desirable. Weight reduction may improve cardiovascular risk factors in older and younger adults.
12. Tailor approaches to the needs of various patients or cultural/religious preferences.

Other Advice

- Reduce exposure and heighten awareness of the "obesogenic" environment, including calorie abundance, decreasing physical activity, and increasing automation.
- Maintain a normal or slightly higher protein intake to maintain nitrogen balance and to decrease perceived hunger with energy-restricted diets (Nickols-Richardson et al, 2005).
- Have the patient set his or her own goals. Self-monitoring is important for maintaining calorie, fat gram, and physical activity goals.
- Weigh weekly on the same scale with the same clothing at about the same time of day. After reaching a desired weight, daily weighing often helps maintain motivation for continuing effective lifestyle changes.
- Intake of foods with high water content reduces subsequent energy intake (Rolls et al, 2005). The DASH diet works well because it encourages intake of more fruits and vegetables.
- Avoid or correct disordered eating (e.g., abnormal eating, diet cheating, compulsive eating, addictive or manipulative habits, eating disorders, night eating syndrome). Healthy eating patterns, not constant evaluation of body fat, are the desired end behaviors.
- Use nutrient-dense, antimicrobial spices and antioxidant foods to enhance immunity.

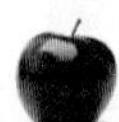

FOOD AND NUTRITION

- Plan a diet with moderate carbohydrate (35–50%), moderate fat (25–35%), and protein as 25–35% of energy (Schoeller and Buchholz, 2005). Total energy reduction is the goal.
- A lower glycemic load is helpful for some people. Foods that have a low glycemic index include salads with an oil and vinegar dressing, high-fat granola cereal, and most

fresh fruits and vegetables (Pittas et al, 2005). **Glycemic load = glycemic index × available carbohydrate amount.**

- Schedule 6–8 small meals at frequent intervals to prevent cheating and overeating.
- Breakfast should be emphasized (Song et al, 2005). Cereal consumption may play a role in helping to maintain a healthful BMI (Barton et al, 2005) and a high-fiber choice may curb appetite at lunch.
- Fiber-rich foods take longer to chew, are low in calories, and increase satiety. Encourage the consumption of 25–35 grams of fiber per day. For example, eating 4–6 walnuts before meals may curb appetite and intake. Oats and barley with their soluble fiber, beta-glucan, may also be particularly useful grains.
- The American Dietetic Association supports a "total diet approach," where the overall food pattern is more important than one food or meal (American Dietetic Association, 2007). If food is consumed in moderation with appropriate portion size and regular activity, a positive approach to food makes the client feel less anxious and guilty.
- Diet should provide adequate fluid intake to excrete metabolic wastes; use 30 cc/kg of body weight for an estimate.
- Decrease the overall salt intake if fluid retention is a concern. Use other spices and herbs.
- NHLBI guidelines recommend 35% kilocalories from fat, more from monounsaturated sources and less from saturated fats. Fat substitutes, when used in moderation, can be safely used to lower total energy intake. With elevated triglycerides, cut down on sugars and alcoholic beverages.
- For a modified fast, a meal replacement product for 1–2 meals per day can get the patient started. This method is not recommended for the long term unless sufficient fiber is also available.
- For obese patient in hospitals or critical care, estimating needs may be inaccurate. Indirect calorimetry is the gold standard. Most medical intensive care unit (ICU) patients require only 25 kcal/kg, with greater energy requirements needed in burn or trauma units.

Common Drugs Used and Potential Side Effects

- Some medications cause weight gain, particularly those affecting the neurological system. See Table 10-11.
- Phenylpropanolamine (PPA) produces dose-related, life-threatening cardiovascular and central nervous toxicity from adrenergic overstimulation. Because of these effects and the risk of hemorrhagic stroke, the FDA stopped the use of PPA in cold medicines and prescription diet aids.
- Pharmacotherapy alone is not sufficient for permanent weight loss. Behavior modification must be taught for long-term success. See Table 10-12 for approved weight management medications. Many products on the market are either not safe or not efficacious.

Herbs, Botanicals, and Supplements

- Herbs and botanical supplements should not be used without discussing it with a physician.
- Because supplements are often taken for stimulating weight loss, dietitians should check for information on efficacy and safety (Dwyer et al, 2005). Health providers must also disclose a real or perceived conflict of interest if they promote or sell supplements to their clients (American Dietetic Association, 2009).
- Bitter orange, chitosan, conjugated linolenic acid (CLA, calcium, and hydroxycitric acid have not shown efficacy (Dwyer et al, 2005).
- Chromium picolinate may improve glucose and lipid metabolism. There is little evidence for benefit in weight loss, but there are few adverse effects (Dwyer et al, 2005).
- Ephedra (ma huang) contains ephedrine and works as an anorexiant. The FDA removed it from the market because it elevates blood pressure and can cause significant problems.
- Garcinia is not effective; it has cytotoxic effects and is toxic in animals.
- Green tea contains polyphenols and catechins, which help to promote weight loss (Nagao et al, 2005).
- Melatonin may improve glucose control by restoring the vascular action of insulin; more studies are needed.
- Modulation of gut microbiota using probiotics or prebiotics will be possible in the future for obesity management (Tsai and Coyle, 2009). Antimicrobial spices such as oregano, thyme, cinnamon, bay leaf, palmarosa, clove bud, lemongrass, and allspice may be safely used.
- Stanols (Take Control) and sterols (Benecol) do not affect weight; they are safe when used as directed to lower elevated cholesterol levels.

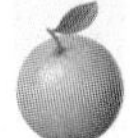

NUTRITION EDUCATION, COUNSELING, CARE MANAGEMENT

- A multidimensional program is best for weight management; it should include the formulation of reasonable goals, the prevention of unnecessary weight loss or gain, weight loss when necessary, prevention of relapse, and the acceptance of physique for "health at every size."
- Individualize according to psychosocial, behavioral, and biological factors. Obesity is a chronic condition that requires chronic care with varying levels of intensity (Nonas and Foster, 2009). Emphasize a balance of foods rather than any one food or meal (American Dietetic Association, 2007).
- Identify the mind–body connection. Teach the patient about physical hunger and how to identify true hunger from emotional "hunger." Practical advice and hunger rating scales are available.
- Low-energy diets tend to be higher in nutritional value if carefully planned using water-rich fruits, vegetables, cooked grains, and soups (Rolls et al, 2005). Noncalorie sweeteners and chewing sugarless gum are useful; chewing gum may help fight cravings for sweets and suppress the appetite.
- Develop reduced-calorie eating plans that meet personal food preferences and provide satisfying food portions (Rolls et al, 2005).
- Instruct the patient on how to plan menus and use recipes. Recipe modifications are useful for replacing fat in recipes (e.g., use applesauce or pear puree in muffins or sponge cake; prune or black bean puree in brownies or spice cake or chocolate cake; or white bean puree in cookies).

TABLE 10-11 Medications That Cause Weight Gain

Medications that affect the central nervous system can cause clinically relevant resting metabolic rate (RMR) effects (from 262–680 kcal/d) in all age groups (Dickerson and Roth-Yousey, 2005a). Sedation or analgesia may produce temporary reductions in RMR (Dickerson and Roth-Yousey, 2005a). Medications that may cause weight gain are listed here.

Medication	Description	Alternatives to Consider
Antianxiety Agents: benzodiazepine (alprazolam [Xanax], chlordiazepoxide [Librium])	Psychotropic drugs can cause weight gain.	
Antidepressants: Selective Serotonin Reuptake Inhibitors (SSRIs)—fluoxetine (Prozac), sertraline (Zoloft), paroxetine (Paxil), fluvoxamine (Luvox), Celexa	SSRIs cause weight loss at first and then weight gain within 6 months. Paxil causes the most weight change. Prozac is often used for patients with bulimia nervosa; it may cause hyperglycemia.	buproprion (Wellbutrin, Zyban)
Antidepressants: Tricyclics (TCAs)—amitriptyline (Elavil, Vanatrip), doxepin (Sinequan), imipramine (Tofranil), nefazodone (Serzone), nortriptyline (Aventyl; Pamelor), trimipramine (Surmontil), mirtazapine (Remeron)	General gains of 0.4–4.12 kg/month; minority of patients gain 15–20 kilograms in 2–6 months from slowed metabolism and increased carbohydrate cravings.	buproprion (Wellbutrin, Zyban)
Antidepressants: Monoamine Oxidase Inhibitors (MAOIs)—isocarboxazid [Marplan], phenelzine [Nardil], tranylcypromine [Parnate]	MAOIs cause more weight gain. Less profound than tricyclics; some gain with phenylzine.	MAOI selective reversible drugs (RIMAs), such as moclobemide (Aurorix, *Manerix*) or toloxatone (*Humoryl*) are not as weight-enhancing as other antidepressants.
Mood Stabilizers: lithium (Eskalith, Lithobid); Moban, Clozaril, Serlect, and Zeldox	Mood stabilizers made with lithium can cause weight gain in 11% to 65% of treated patients; up to 10 kilograms or more in 6 to 10 years.	
Antipsychotics: haloperidol [Haldol], perphenazine [Trilafon], thiothixene [Navane], thioridazine HCl (Mellaril], olanzapine [Zyprexa], risperidone [Risperdal]	Antipsychotics often cause weight gain.	ziprasidone (Geodon); quetiapine (Seroquel)
Anticonvulsants: valproic acid (Depakote/Depakene), gabapentin (Neurontin), carbamazepine (Tegretol)	These medications can increase appetite and insulin levels, and variable gains of up to 15 to 20 kilograms.	topiramate (Topamax), lamotrigine (Lamictal), zonisamide (Zonegran)
Antihistamines: diphenhydramine (Benadryl, Nytol)	Used for allergy management. If used to induce sleep, may mask sleep apnea.	Decongestants or inhalers
Cardiovascular Agents: beta-adrenergic blockers—Propranolol (Inderal), atenolol (Tenormin,) carvedilol, bisoprolol, metoprolol (Lopressor) alpha-adrenergic blockers—prazosin (Minipress), doxazosin (Cardura), terazosin (Hytrin)	These medications can reduce RMR by 4–12% over time (Dickerson and Roth-Yousey, 2005a).	ACE inhibitors such as enalapril (Vasotec) Angiotensin II Inhibitors such as candesartan (Atacand) Ca^{++} channel blockers such as amlodipine (Norvasc), verapamil (Calan, Isoptin), diltiazem (Cardizem)
Chemotherapy	Chemotherapy can decrease metabolic rate by 6–11% in patients with leukemia, breast cancer, and some solid tumors (Dickerson and Roth-Yousey, 2005b).	Treatment is short term.
Diabetes Agents: insulin (Humalog)	Weight gain of up to 8 kg with intensive treatment.	metformin (Glucophage; glucophage XR)
Diabetes Agents: thiazolidinediones	rosiglitazone (Avandia) pioglitazone Actos	acarbose (Precose) miglitol (Glyset)
Diabetes Agents: sulfonylureas	Glipizide (Glucotrol) may reduce RMR by 3.5% (Dickerson and Roth-Yousey, 2005b). Weight gain ≤5 kilograms over 3–12 months.	metformin (Glucophage; Glucophage XR); acarbose (Precose); miglitol (Glyset)
Steroid Hormones: corticosteroids	Hormones can cause weight gain if taken over a long time. cortisone, prednisolone, human growth hormone, somatotropin [Serostim]	NSAIDs if appropriate
Steroid Hormones: progestational agents; androgens	medroxyprogesterone acetate [Provera, Depo-Provera], oxymetholone [Anadrol-50], testosterone [Androderm, Testoderm])	—

REFERENCES

Blackburn G. Medications that cause weight gain. Accessed November 7, 2009 at http://medical.slim-fast.com/pdfs/medications_that_cause_weight_gain.pdf

Dickerson RN, Roth-Yousey L. Medication effects on metabolic rate: a systematic review (part 1). *J Am Diet Assoc.* 105:835, 2005a.

Dickerson RN, Roth-Yousey L. Medication effects on metabolic rate: a systematic review (part 2). *J Am Diet Assoc.* 105:835, 2005b.

DIABETES TREATMENTS (Up to 8 kilograms gained in an intensive 3-month treatment course)

TABLE 10-12 Medications Used for Weight Reduction in the United States

Diethylpropion (Tenuate)	Appetite suppressant. Dry mouth and GI upset can occur; short-term use is recommended. Average weight 4–6%, drug alone.
Orlistat (Xenical)	Decreases pancreatic lipase and decreases fat absorption. Soft stools and anal leakage may occur, particularly if a diet high in fat (>90 g) is consumed. Orlistat helps minimize weight regain after weight loss and appears to be well-tolerated for the long term. Fat-soluble vitamins may be required during chronic therapy because absorption may be decreased. Patients on orlistat should have a BMI over 27 with risk factors or a BMI over 30 without risk factors; the drug is not for everyone. Weight loss of 8% with behavioral approaches. Alli is an over-the-counter version, which contains a lower dose of orlistat; weight loss is slower.
Phentermine (Adipex, Ionamin)	Appetite suppressant; may cause excitability, gastrointestinal (GI) distress, and insomnia, as well as dry mouth. Average weight 4–6%, drug alone.
Sibutramine (Meridia)	Increases energy expenditure and satiety; it acts via the central nervous system (CNS) as a serotonergic and noradrenergic reuptake inhibitor. It can be used long term. Elevates plasma epinephrine, plasma glucose, and blood pressure. Weight loss of about 16% with behavioral approaches.

Adapted from: Nonas CA, Foster GD. *Managing obesity: a clinical guide*. 2nd ed. Chicago: American Dietetic Association, 2009.

- Steps to normalize eating include awareness training, changing thoughts and beliefs about food, handling issues of deprivation and guilt, and refocusing on areas other than food and weight. Self-efficacy is particularly important (Wamsteker et al, 2005). Correcting unrealistic weight goals is also an issue; it is better to correct them before treatment begins (Wamsteker et al, 2009).
- Provide guidance on how to eat at parties, events, and restaurants. Low-calorie snacking and the selection of low calorie food preparation methods are needed. Avoid buffets when possible.
- Teach portion control. Sometimes measuring and weighing foods can be useful. Table 10-13 provides a handy portion adjustment guide using everyday objects.
- Behavior therapy may be helpful in self-monitoring (food diaries, weights, activity). Teach stimulus control of cues, family intervention, slowing down while eating, and monitoring of intake while at parties and during work breaks.
- To delay automatic eating, drink a glass of water and wait 20 minutes. If the sensation persists, it is probably hunger. Make meals last 20 minutes or longer. Eat slowly; chew well.
- The best diet is "don't buy it" to reduce temptations later.
- The use of meal replacements for one meal a day can be beneficial for improving cholesterol levels, plasma glucose, and diastolic blood pressure.
- Avoid an energy level that is too low, which causes hypophagia and could lead to sudden death syndrome. Low energy intake (<1200 kilocalories for women or <1500 kilocalories for men) requires the use of a multivitamin supplement.
- Physical activity is integral to weight loss maintenance; see Table 10-14. Encourage moderate levels of physical activity for 30–60 minutes daily whenever possible. It is reasonable to encourage the expenditure of 1000 kcal/wk in some type of physical activity. Resistance training increases muscle mass; aerobic exercise should be directed at 70% of maximal oxygen consumption.
- Cultural emphasis on thinness may lead to unhealthy weight loss efforts. Instead, focus on enhancement of self-esteem.
- The real challenge involves keeping weight off after it has been lost. Teach the patient to splurge by plan and not by impulse. Special considerations are important in specific age groups.
- Pregnant mothers should follow established recommendations for diet, exercise, and weight gain during pregnancy. A weight gain of 15–25 pounds in an overweight or <15 pounds in an obese mother leads to better outcomes (Crane et al, 2009).
- New mothers should breastfeed, and then provide wholesome, nourishing foods with low energy density for their children (Melanson, 2009).
- Between pregnancies, women with a history of GDM who gain more than 10 pounds are at higher risk for C-section and adverse outcomes (Paramsothy et al, 2009).
- Parents of young children must help them to develop good eating habits early in life.
- In puberty, it is common for young women to begin gaining weight. Women should not assume that premenstrual fluid weight gain is permanent; this may vary from 2–5 pounds per month.
- Encourage adequate sleep; deprivation increases a hunger hormone that can trigger overeating. Table 10-15 discusses sleep apnea and Pickwickian syndrome; a sleep study may be needed.
- Smoking cessation can lead to weight gain; see Table 10-16.
- Multiple and relentless forms of marketing, poor foods promoted in schools, and a variety of other conditions undermine personal resources, individual responsibility, and parental authority for preventing obesity among children and teens (Brownell et al, 2009). The current environment tends to promote overeating and minimal activity, yet there are social stigmas against being overweight.
- Obesity is increasing across all socioeconomic groups and educational levels (Cohen, 2008). Overall, fat intake tends to be higher in poorer neighborhoods (Keita et al, 2009). Children who live with overweight or obese individuals are often unaware of their desirable body weight range.
- Reduced activity and metabolism are factors that should be addressed to manage weight changes among older adults.
- Permanent lifestyle changes are better than popular diets or trends. Avoid bizarre fad dieting, skipping meals, or

TABLE 10-13 Portion Adjustments Using Everyday Objects

Bread, Cereal, Rice, Pasta

1 cup potatoes, rice, or pasta = 1 tennis ball or 1 ice cream scoop or a fist
1 pancake = 1 compact disc (CD)
1/2 cup cooked rice = a cupcake wrapper full
1 piece cornbread = bar of soap
1 slice bread = audiocassette tape
2 oz of pretzels = 2 handfuls

Vegetables

1 cup green salad = 1 baseball or a fist
1 baked potato = a fist
1 cup of vegetables = a fist
1/2 cup tomato juice = small Styrofoam cup
1/2 cup broccoli = 1 scoop ice cream or one light bulb
1/2 cup serving = 6 asparagus spears, 7–8 baby carrots, or 1 ear of corn on the cob

Fruit

1/2 cup grapes (15) = a light bulb
1/2 cup fresh fruit = 7 cotton balls
1 medium size fruit = a tennis ball or a fist
1 cup cut-up fruit = a fist
1/2 cup raisins = 1 large egg

Milk, Yogurt, Cheese

$1\frac{1}{2}$ oz cheese = one 9-volt battery or 3 dominos
1 oz cheese = pair of dice or your thumb
1 cup ice cream = 1 large scoop the size of a baseball

Meat, Poultry, Fish, Dry Beans, Eggs, Nuts

2 tbsp peanut butter = ping pong ball
1 tsp peanut butter = fingertip
1 tbsp peanut butter = thumb tip
3 oz cooked meat, poultry, fish = your palm; a deck of cards
3 oz grilled or baked fish = a checkbook
3 oz cooked chicken = one chicken leg, thigh, or breast
1 oz of nuts = 1 handful
1 oz of cheese = your index finger

Fats, Oils

1 tsp butter or margarine = size of a stamp, the thickness of your finger or thumb tip
2 tbsp salad dressing = 1 ping pong ball

Adapted from: NIDDK Web site. Accessed November 7, 2009 at http://win.niddk.nih.gov/publications/just_enough.htm.

TABLE 10-14 Physical Activity Equivalents

According to the National Weight Control Registry, people who have lost weight and kept it off for 2 years or longer, limit their intake to about **1800 kilocalories daily** and **walk about 4 miles a day**. MET is a practical means of expressing the intensity and energy expenditure of physical activities.

Physical Activity	MET
Light Intensity Activities	<3
Sleeping	0.9
watching television	1.0
writing, desk work, typing	1.8
walking, less than 2.0 mph (3.2 km/h), level ground, strolling, very slow	2.0
Moderate Intensity Activities	3 to 6
bicycling, stationary, 50 watts, very light effort	3.0
sexual activity (position dependent)	3.3
calisthenics, home exercise, light or moderate effort, general	3.5
bicycling, <10 mph (16 km/h), leisure, to work or for pleasure	4.0
bicycling, stationary, 100 watts, light effort	5.5
Vigorous Intensity Activities	>6
jogging, general	7.0
calisthenics (e.g. pushups, sit-ups, pull-ups, jumping jacks), heavy, vigorous effort	8.0
running jogging, in place	8.0

Other beneficial activities that burn kilocalories include the following:

Warm Weather	Calories/hour	Cold Weather
Jogging 6 mph	450	Jumping rope
Hiking on steep hills	400	Indoor rappelling
Aerobics (low impact)	400	Snow shoveling, light
Rowing	400	Rowing machine
Swimming	400	Skiing cross-country
Tennis, singles	390	Racquetball
Cycling 10 mph	300	Stationary bike 10 mph
Golf with walking	300	Splitting logs
Gardening	280	Window cleaning
Mowing lawn	275	Mopping floors
Tennis, doubles	235	Indoor basketball
Badminton	250	Indoor volleyball
Walking 3 mph	**250**	**Mall walking**

Other good resources:
CDC: http://www.cdc.gov/physicalactivity/everyone/measuring/index.html.
Harvard School of Public Health: http://www.hsph.harvard.edu/nutritionsource/staying-active/.
Physical Activity Guide for Americans: http://www.health.gov/paguidelines/guidelines/summary.aspx.

TABLE 10-15 Weight Management for Sleep Apnea and Pickwickian Syndrome

Obstructive sleep apnea (OSA)	Short-duration (<1 minute), repetitive episodes of impaired breathing during sleep. It mostly occurs in obese individuals, which contributes to pharyngeal obstruction. OSA acutely impacts the cardiovascular system and can increase morbidity or mortality. Morbid obesity can be associated with excessive daytime sleepiness even in the absence of sleep apnea. See Section 5 for more details.
Pickwickian syndrome	The individual is obese and hypersomnolent with cor pulmonale, polycythemia, nocturnal enuresis, and personality changes. Even mild obesity can affect lung function, particularly in men. Weight loss is desirable.

emphasis on any one nutrient. A "no fad diet" approach encourages healthy eating patterns. Table 10-17 describes some weight loss programs, several popular diets, and available Web sites.

- Large permanent changes are required to keep weight off. Promote small changes in diet and physical activity to initially prevent further weight gain (Hill, 2009). America On the Move (AOM) is a national initiative that promotes an increase in walking by 2000 steps/d and reductions in energy intake by about 100 kcal/d; people seem to be able to make positive changes in response to these messages (Stroebele et al, 2009). Greater self-reported physical activity was the strongest correlate of weight loss in the Look-Ahead Trial, followed by treatment attendance and consumption of meal replacements (Wadden et al, 2009).
- Discourage weight cycling. Cyclers tends to have a larger body fat percentage, lower metabolic rates, and higher BMI than non-cyclers (Strychar et al, 2009).
- Group counseling or corporate wellness programs may be effective.
- Electronic feedback, one-on-one advice from a nutrition counselor, phone or mail follow-ups can also help to maintain positive momentum in weight loss or maintenance.
- Given that people have a limited ability to shape the food environment individually and have no ability to control automatic responses to unconscious food-related cues, society as a whole may need to regulate the environment through the number and types of food-related cues, portion sizes, food availability, and food advertising (Cohen, 2008).
- Overweight adults diagnosed with type 2 diabetes experience significant improvement in health-related quality of life (HRQOL) by enrolling in a weight management program that yields significant weight loss, improved physical fitness, and reduced physical symptoms (Williamson et al, 2009).

Patient Education—Food Safety

There are no specific food handling techniques that are unique to overweight or obesity.

TABLE 10-16 Smoking Cessation and Weight Gain

Nicotine addiction is a chronic, relapsing condition.

Smoking cessation lowers cardiovascular and cancer risks even when compensating for possible weight gain; cessation lengthens life by several years and is worth the effort.

Weight gain is common after cessation because of increased caloric consumption, changes in activity levels, and a decrease in the basal metabolic rate. Past smokers are more likely to be obese than current smokers.

Contemplation of and experimentation with smoking is often related to weight concerns among boys and girls. Women fear weight gain more than men.

Women who quit smoking typically gain 6–12 pounds in the first year after quitting.

Interventions that address weight control are recommended. Moderate to heavy smokers who attempt to quit may need to reduce intake by 100–200 kcal/d just to maintain weight.

Behavioral weight control counseling helps to slow the rate of weight gain. Fruit often helps relieve the craving for sweets.

Exercise often helps relieve the desire to smoke. Walking is a great stress reliever.

Sustained-release bupropion (bupropion SR) was the first non-nicotine pharmacological treatment approved for smoking cessation. Others are now available.

Teach good principles of weight management:

- Weight gain is a problem requiring lifelong, multidisciplinary management.
- Weight is regulated by a complex set of biologic/environmental factors, not by a lack of willpower.
- Modest weight loss has benefits.
- Work to alter fundamental thoughts and assumptions versus unrealistic expectations.
- Emphasize slow, steady loss, followed by maintenance.
- Focus on long-term outcomes/sustained changes.

For more tips, see http://www.smokefree.gov/pubs/FFree3.pdf.

TABLE 10-17 Diet Program Comparisons

Programs	Description	Web Address	Pro	Con
Diet Center	Personal counseling	http://www.dietcenter.com	Consider "Exclusively You" option	
eDiets.com	Online dieting	http://www.ediets.com	Bargain	Must be self-motivated
Jenny Craig	Personal counseling; at home	http://www.jennycraig.com	Well-structured	Expensive
LA Weight Loss	Personal counseling	http://www.laweightloss.com	Good exercise centers	Costly foods
NutriSystem	Online dieting	http://www.nutrisystem.com	Healthy choices; good structure	
Overeaters Anon	Group support	http://www.oa.org	Physical, emotional, spiritual support	
Registered Dietitian	Expert personal counseling	http://www.eatright.org	Most flexible; personalized concerns	
Take Off Pounds Sensibly	Group or online support	http://www.tops.org	Inexpensive	Not personalized
Weight Watchers	Group or online support	http://www.weightwatchers.com	Comprehensive and sound principles	

Popular diets such as Weight Watchers, Atkins, the Zone, and Ornish achieve weight loss and reductions in LDL cholesterol, CRP, and insulin as long as calories are reduced and adherence continues for up to a year (Dansinger et al, 2005). In another study of the popular diets, Gardner et al (2007) found that premenopausal overweight and obese women assigned to follow the low CHO Atkins diet lost more weight at 12 months than women assigned to follow the Zone diet and experienced comparable or more favorable metabolic effects than those assigned to the Zone, Ornish, or LEARN diets. In general, any diet or program that achieves macronutrient reduction should yield acceptable results.

Type of Diet	Total Calories	Fat grams (% calories)	Carb grams (% calories)	Protein grams (% calories)	Nutrition Adequacy
Typical American diet	2200	85 (35%)	275 (50%)	82.5 (15%)	Varies by food choice and nutrient density.
High fat Low-carbohydrate diet • Dr. Atkins Diet • Zone Diet • Sugar Busters • Protein Power	1414	96 (60%) Fat level range: 35–65%	35 (10%)	105 (30%)	Low in several nutrients: Vitamins A, B_6, D, E, thiamin, folate, calcium, magnesium, iron, zinc, potassium, and dietary fiber. This type of diet also contains excess amounts of total fat, saturated fat, and dietary cholesterol. Nutritional supplementation is highly recommended.
Moderate fat diet • USDA Food Guide Pyramid • DASH Diet • American Diabetes Association • Weight Watchers • Jenny Craig	1450	40 (25%) Fat level range: 21–34%	218 (60%)	54 (15%)	Usually a nutritionally balanced eating plan assuming the dieter eats a variety of foods from all food categories. Limiting any food categories can lead to deficiencies in certain nutrients particularly calcium, iron, and zinc. Weight watchers scores are the highest here for long-term adherence.
Low- and very low-fat diet • Volumetrics • Dean Ornish's Eat More, Weigh Less • New Pritikin Program	1450	20 (13%) Fat level varies: 10–20%	235–271 (70%)	54–72 (17%)	Deficient in zinc and vitamin B12 due to infrequent meat consumption. This type of diet can be inadequate in vitamin E—a nutrient found in oils, nuts, and other foods rich in fat. Volumetrics rates the highest in this group for helping people lose weight effectively.

REFERENCES AND RESOURCES

Dansinger ML, et al. Comparison of the Atkins, Ornish, Weight Watchers, and Zone diets for weight loss and heart disease risk reduction: a randomized trial. *JAMA.* 293:43, 2005.

Gardner CD, et al. Comparison of the Atkins, Zone, Ornish, and LEARN diets for change in weight and related risk factors among overweight premenopausal women: the A TO Z Weight Loss Study: a randomized trial. *JAMA.* 298:178, 2007.

Health.com. Accessed November 2, 2009 at http://www.health.com/health/diet-guide.

Morgan LM, et al. Comparison of the effects of four commercially available weight-loss programmes on lipid-based cardiovascular risk factors. *Public Health Nutr.* 12:799, 2009.

NIDDK. Accessed November 2, 2009 at http://win.niddk.nih.gov/publications/choosing.htm.

Northwestern University. Accessed November 2, 2009 at http://www.feinberg.northwestern.edu/nutrition/factsheets/fad-diets.html.

USDA. Accessed November 2, 2009 at http://www.ars.usda.gov/is/AR/archive/mar06/diet0306.htm.

WebMD. Accessed November 2, 2009 at http://www.webmd.com/diet/evaluate-latest-diets.

WIN Network. Diet Myths. Accessed November 2, 2009 at http://win.niddk.nih.gov/publications/myths.htm.

For More Information

- American Dietetic Association–Weight Management Protocol http://www.eatright.org/ada/files/wmnp.pdf
- California Adolescent Nutrition and Fitness Program http://www.canfit.org/
- Canadian Physical Activity Guide http://www.csep.ca/
- CDC, Genetics of Obesity http://www.cdc.gov/Features/Obesity/
- CDC, Healthy Weight Web site http://www.cdc.gov/healthyweight/
- CDC, Report of the Surgeon General on Physical Fitness http://www.cdc.gov/nccdphp/sgr/summ.htm
- Center for Weight and Eating Disorders http://www.med.upenn.edu/weight/foster.shtml
- DASH Diet in Weight Management http://www.nhlbi.nih.gov/hbp/prevent/h_weight/h_weight.htm
- Dietary Guidelines, Calories http://www.health.gov/dietaryguidelines/dga2005/healthieryou/html/chapter5.html
- Federal Trade Commission http://www.ftc.gov/bcp/edu/pubs/consumer/health/hea03.shtm
- Food Diary Format http://www.cdc.gov/healthyweight/pdf/Food_Diary_CDC.pdf
- Genome Studies of Obesity http://www.ncbi.nlm.nih.gov/disease/Obesity.html
- National Association to Advance Fat Acceptance (NAAFA) http://www.naafa.org/
- National Weight Control Registry http://www.nwcr.ws/
- NHLBI Obesity Education Initiative and Evidence Guidelines http://www.nhlbi.nih.gov/guidelines/obesity/ob_gdlns.htm
- Physical Activity Format http://www.cdc.gov/healthyweight/pdf/Physical_Activity_Diary_CDC.pdf
- Physical Activity Guidelines http://www.cdc.gov/physicalactivity/everyone/guidelines/index.html
- Shape Up America http://www.shapeup.org/
- Surgeon General http://www.surgeongeneral.gov/topics/obesity/
- Weight Watchers International http://www.weightwatchers.com/

OVERWEIGHT AND OBESITY—CITED REFERENCES

American Dietetic Association (ADA), Ethics Opinion. Weight loss products and medications. *J Am Diet Assoc.* 109:2109, 2009.

American Dietetic Association (ADA). Position of the American Dietetic Association: Weight management. *J Am Diet Assoc.* 109:330, 2009.

Atkinson RL. Viruses as an etiology of obesity. *Mayo Clin Proc.* 82:1192, 2007.

Barton BA, et al. The relationship of breakfast and cereal consumption to nutrient intake and body mass index: the National Heart, Lung, and Blood Institute Growth and Health Study. *J Am Diet Assoc.* 105:1383, 2005.

Block JP, et al. Psychosocial stress and change in weight among US adults. *Am J Epidemiol.* 170:181, 2009.

Bouchard C. The biological predisposition to obesity: beyond the thrifty genotype scenario. *Int J Obes.* 31:1337, 2007.

Brownell KD, et al. The need for bold action to prevent adolescent obesity. *J Adolesc Health.* 45:8S, 2009.

Catenacci VA, et al. The obesity epidemic. *Clin Chest Med.* 30:415, 2009.

Centers for Disease Control and Prevention (CDC). Obesity statistics. Accessed November 2, 2009 at http://www.cdc.gov/obesity/data/index.html.

Chandra R, Liddle RA. Cholecystokinin. *Curr Opin Endocrinol Diabetes Obes.* 14:63, 2007.

Chandra R, Liddle RA. Neural and hormonal regulation of pancreatic secretion. *Curr Opin Gastroenterol.* 25:441, 2009.

Cohen DA. Neurophysiological pathways to obesity: below awareness and beyond individual control. *Diabetes.* 57:1768, 2008.

Crane JM, et al. The effect of gestational weight gain by body mass index on maternal and neonatal outcomes. *J Obstet Gyneacol Can.* 31:28, 2009.

Dwyer JT, et al. Dietary supplements in weight reduction. *J Am Diet Assoc.* 105:S80, 2005.

Farooqi IS, O'Rahilly S. Genetic factors in human obesity. *Obes Rev.* 8:37, 2007.

Hill JO. Can a small-changes approach help address the obesity epidemic? A report of the Joint Task Force of the American Society for Nutrition, Institute of Food Technologists, and International Food Information Council. *Am J Clin Nutr.* 89:477, 2009.

Katzmarzyk PT, et al. Racial differences in abdominal depot-specific adiposity in white and African American adults [published online ahead of print Oct 14, 2009]. *Am J Clin Nutr.*

Lowe MR, et al. The Power of Food Scale. A new measure of the psychological influence of the food environment. *Appetite.* 53:114, 2009.

Lowe MR, Butryn ML. Hedonic hunger: a new dimension of appetite? *Physiol Behav.* 91:432, 2007.

Keita AD, et al. Neighborhood-level disadvantage is associated with reduced dietary quality in children. *J Am Diet Assoc.* 109:1612, 2009.

Melanson KJ. Dietary considerations for prevention and treatment of obesity in youth. *Am J Lifestyle Med.* 3:106, 2009.

Miller M, et al. Comparative effects of three popular diets on lipids, endothelial function, and C-reactive protein during weight maintenance. *J Am Diet Assoc.* 109:713, 2009.

Misra A, Khurana L. Obesity and the metabolic syndrome in developing countries. *J Clin Endocrinol Metab.* 93:9S, 2008.

Mitra AK, Clarke K. Viral obesity: fact or fiction? [published online ahead of print Oct 27, 2009] *Obes Rev.*

Nagao T, et al. Ingestion of a tea rich in catechins leads to a reduction in body fat and malondialdehyde-modified LDL in men. *Am J Clin Nutr.* 81:122, 2005.

National Heart, Lung, and Blood Institute (NHLBI). Clinical Guidelines on the Identification, Evaluation, and Treatment of Overweight and Obesity in Adults–Executive Summary. Accessed November 1, 2009 at http://www.nhlbi.nih.gov/guidelines/obesity/index.htm.

Nickols-Richardson SM, et al. Perceived hunger is lower and weight loss is greater in overweight premenopausal women consuming a low-carbohydrate/high-protein vs. high-carbohydrate/low-fat diet. *J Am Diet Assoc.* 105:1433, 2005.

Nonas CA, Foster GD. *Managing obesity: a clinical guide.* 2nd ed. Chicago: American Dietetic Association, 2009.

Orr J, Davy B. Dietary influences on peripheral hormones regulating energy intake: potential applications for weight management. *J Am Diet Assoc.* 105:1115, 2005.

Paramsothy P, et al. Interpregnancy weight gain and cesarean delivery risk in women with a history of gestational diabetes. *Obstet Gynecol.* 113:817, 2009.

Pi-Sunyer X, Kris-Etherton PM. Improving health outcomes: future directions in the field. *J Am Diet Assoc.* 105:14S, 2005.

Pittas AG, et al. A low-glycemic load diet facilitates greater weight loss in overweight adults with high insulin secretion but not in overweight adults with low insulin secretion in the CALERIE Trial. *Diabetes Care.* 28:2939, 2005.

Rolls BJ, et al. Changing the energy density of the diet as a strategy for weight management. *J Am Diet Assoc.* 105:98S, 2005.

Sandoval D, et al. The integrative role of CNS fuel-sensing mechanisms in energy balance and glucose regulation. *Annu Rev Physiol.* 70:513, 2008.

Schoeller DA, Buchholz AC. Energetics of obesity and weight control: does diet composition matter? *J Am Diet Assoc.* 105:24S, 2005.

Seagle HM, et al. Position of the American Dietetic Association: Total Diet Approach to Communicating Food and Nutrition Information. *J Am Diet Assoc.* 107:1224, 2007.

Song WO, et al. Is consumption of breakfast associated with body mass index in US adults? *J Am Diet Assoc.* 105:1373, 2005.

Stroebele N, et al. A small-changes approach reduces energy intake in free-living humans. *J Am Coll Nutr.* 28:63, 2009.

Strychar I, et al. Anthropometric, metabolic, psychosocial, and dietary characteristics of overweight/obese postmenopausal women with a history of weight cycling: a MONET (Montreal Ottawa New Emerging Team) study. *J Am Diet Assoc.* 109:718, 2009.

Tay J, et al. Metabolic effects of weight loss on a very-low-carbohydrate diet compared with an isocaloric high-carbohydrate diet in abdominally obese subjects. *J Am Coll Cardiol.* 51:59, 2008.

Tsai F, Coyle WJ. The microbiome and obesity: is obesity linked to our gut flora? *Curr Gastroenterol Rep.* 11:307, 2009.

Thorleifsson G, et al. Genome-wide association yields new sequence variants at seven loci that associate with measures of obesity. *Nat Genet.* 41:18, 2009.

Turnbaugh PJ, et al. A core gut microbiome in obese and lean twins. *Nature.* 457:480, 2009.

Vaneslow MS, et al. Adolescent beverage habits and changes in weight over time: findings from Project EAT. *Am J Clin Nutr.* 90:1489, 2009.

Wadden T, et al. One-year weight losses in the Look AHEAD study: factors associated with success. *Obesity.* 17:713, 2009.

Wamsteker EW, et al. Obesity-related beliefs predict weight loss after an 8-week low-calorie diet. *J Am Diet Assoc.* 105:441, 2005.

Wamsteker EW, et al. Unrealistic Weight-Loss Goals among Obese Patients Are Associated with Age and Causal Attributions. *J Am Diet Assoc.* 109:1903, 2009.

Williamson DA, et al. Impact of a weight management program on health-related quality of life in overweight adults with type 2 diabetes. *Arch Intern Med.* 169:163, 2009.

Wren AM, Bloom SR. Gut hormones and appetite control. *Gastroenterol.* 132:2116, 2007.

UNDERWEIGHT AND MALNUTRITION

UNDERWEIGHT AND UNINTENTIONAL WEIGHT LOSS

NUTRITIONAL ACUITY RANKING: LEVEL 3–4

Underweight Problems

When body weight decreases to 15–20% below desirable weight (BMI < 18.5), the amount of energy being consumed is not sufficient to support the function of vital organs. Lean tissue is being broken down and utilized for energy to make up the deficit. The results are:

- Low body temperature
- Abnormal electrical activity in the brain
- Altered blood lipids
- Dry skin
- Impaired immune response
- Loss of digestive function
- Abnormal hormone levels
- Malnutrition
- Anemia

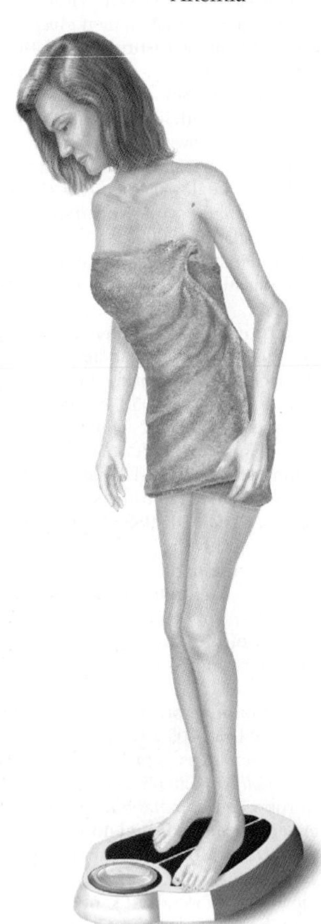

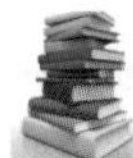

DEFINITIONS AND BACKGROUND

Underweight is defined as having a BMI below 18.5; approximately 8–9% of the population is underweight. Weight gain may be difficult for some healthy individuals because of a genetic tendency toward leanness, excessive activity, or routine eating patterns. Being underweight may or may not be associated with pathology. There are serious health risks associated with very low weight and with efforts to maintain an unrealistically lean body mass. Identification and treatment of disordered eating can be important for improving the health status of underweight individuals at any age. See Section 4 for eating disorder guidelines.

Body storage of glycogen is approximately 1100 kilocalories or about a 12- to 16-hour supply. Body storage of protein equals approximately 40,000 kilocalories of muscle tissue; the loss of 30–50% of lean body mass is incompatible with survival. Body fat is the remainder of calories in fuel storage; it varies depending on the weight of the individual compared with BMI tables for height and sex and by level of physical fitness.

Low BMI is a significant predictor of mortality among young as well as older hospitalized patients (Flegal et al, 2005; Sergi et al, 2005). A BMI value of 20 kg/m^2 seems to be a reliable threshold for defining underweight in older adults at high risk for short-term mortality (Sergi et al, 2005). The Women's Health Initiative Observational Study evaluated 40,657 women aged 65–79 years at baseline and measured frailty including muscle weakness, impaired walking, exhaustion, low physical activity, and unintended weight loss; hip fractures, activities of daily living disability, hospitalizations, and deaths were also tracked (Fugate Woods et al, 2005).

Underweight is often correlated with frailty and poor outcomes. Underweight is associated with significantly increased mortality from non-cancer, non-CVD causes (Flegal et al, 2007). Indeed, a low BMI tends to have the most risk for mortality (Heather et al, 2009).

The Ancel Keys studies (Keys et al, 1950) demonstrated that starvation results in food preoccupation, unusual eating habits, increased use of caffeine and tea, binge eating, depression, anxiety, social withdrawal, poor judgment, apathy, egocentrism, edema, sleep disturbances, hypothermia, gastrointestinal disturbances, and lowered basal metabolism. Death related to starvation is often from decreased respiratory muscle function and terminal pneumonia. In addition, patients who have chronic obstructive pulmonary disease (COPD) are more likely to have additional exacerbations when weight loss and poor intake occur (Hallin et al, 2006).

The most common cause of a person being underweight is inadequate access to food. While this problem is most significant in sub-Saharan Africa and south Asia, many Americans go to bed hungry every night. Financial resources, politics, geography, and economics play a role; food inadequacy may also relate to high prices and limited healthy choices at the local grocery store.

Unintentional weight loss with debility, cachexia, and loss of lean body mass suggests some undesirable condition or pathology, particularly among chronically ill or institutionalized individuals. Malnutrition in older adults is generally characterized by faulty or inadequate nutritional status, insufficient dietary intake, poor appetite, muscle wasting, and weight loss. Blunted responsiveness to neuropeptide Y (NPY)—a feeding stimulant—often occurs concurrently with age-related anorexia and hypophagia.

TABLE 10-18 Strengthening Tips

In healthy young people, 30% of body weight is muscle, 20% is adipose tissue, and 10% is bone; muscle accounts for 50% of lean body mass and 50% of total body nitrogen. By age 75, about half the body's muscle mass has disappeared: 15% of body weight is muscle, 40% is adipose tissue, and 8% is bone (Merck, 2009). Hospitalized or bedridden elderly people require early physical therapy and individualized exercise regimens (Merck, 2009). With restricted mobility, loss of muscle mass and strength (deconditioning) occurs, mostly in the antigravity muscles–those used to sit up, stand up, and pull up (Merck, 2009).

Up to 1.5%/d of muscle mass can be lost; for 1 day of absolute bed rest, up to 2 wks of reconditioning may be necessary to return to baseline function (Merck, 2009). Patients who can and will comply with a proper exercise program gain muscle protein mass, strength, and endurance and are often more capable of performing activities of daily living (NIA, 2009).

1. Start with a weight that can be lifted 5 times without too much effort.
2. When that is easy, rest a few minutes, and do it again (2 sets).
3. Increase to 3 sets.
4. Lift weight 10 times in each set.
5. Lift weight 15 times in each set.
6. Slowly increase weight and sets.

Sources:
Merck Manual of Geriatrics. Accessed November 7, 2009 at http://www.merck.com/mkgr/mmg/sec7/ch48/ch48d.jsp.
NIA. Exercise: a guide from the National Institute on Aging. Accessed November 7, 2009 at http://www.nia.nih.gov/HealthInformation/Publications/ExerciseGuide/chapter04a.htm.

Nutritional frailty includes sarcopenia with the loss of lean body mass, which leads to a failure to thrive and functional disability. Cytokines contribute to lipolysis, anorexia, muscle protein breakdown, and nitrogen loss. Patients with cardiac cachexia or chronic obstructive pulmonary disease (COPD) are often debilitated if they have lost weight rapidly. In older adults, micronutrient deficiency is a common result and should be addressed. Table 10-18 provides tips for helping debilitated persons to strengthen their muscles.

Carefully monitor for unintentional weight loss in adults following their admission into residential health care facilities. Red flags include early satiety, bloating, anorexia, dyspnea, fatigue, constipation, and dental problems.

Protocols must emphasize thorough assessment, interventions, frequent weighing and effective communications between all involved parties. Other populations who are at risk for weight loss and poor intake should be monitored (e.g., persons with chronic renal insufficiency, tuberculosis, HIV-AIDS, and cancer).

The American Dietetic Association Unintended Weight Loss (UWL) in Older Adults Evidence-Based Nutrition Practice Guideline was published in 2009. Qualified dietitians help to identify nutritional risk factors and recommend interventions based on the medical condition, needs, goals and desires of the individual. Studies support an association between increased mortality and underweight (BMI <20 kg/m^2 or current weight compared with usual or desired body weight) and/or unintended weight loss, such as 5% in 30 days (American Dietetic Association, 2009).

In long-term care, usual body weight is often more meaningful than comparison with an ideal body weight chart. Quality of life and resident-directed care plans ("I Care" plans) must be considered when designing interventions. The move from institutional to person-centered dining is a positive step in the right direction. The American Dietetic Association has recommended at least three MNT visits for adults who have had unintentional weight loss; it also has a Long-Term Care Toolkit for use during the nutrition care process with standardized language for that setting.

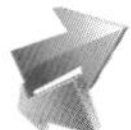

ASSESSMENT, MONITORING, AND EVALUATION

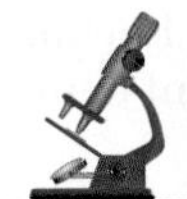

CLINICAL INDICATORS

Genetic Markers: Underweight may be part of a genetic disorder or inherited naturally.

Clinical/History

Height
Weight
Usual weight
Recent weight changes
BMI
Diet history
BP
Intake and output (I & O)
Dehydration?
DETERMINE checklist, MNA or other screening tool
Exercise tolerance
Parasitic infections?
Sarcopenia?
Xerostomia, mucositis?
Inflammatory bowel disease?
Cancer or HIV infection?
Loss of teeth or dental pain?
Nausea or frequent emesis?
Amenorrhea, anemia, hair loss?
Osteoporosis or fractures?
Stress, medication overuse?
Cognitive decline or depression?
Eating dependency?
Skinfold measurements (over time)

Lab Work

Hemoglobin and hematocrit (H & H)
Serum ferritin, if anemia is suspected
CRP (elevated?)
T3, T4, TSH
Albumin (Alb) below 3.5 g/dL
Transthyretin below 17 g/dL
Chol (may be low)
Trig
Fasting glucose
Blood urea nitrogen (BUN)
Creatinine (Creat)
Nitrogen (N) balance
Na^+, K^+
Alkaline phosphatase (Alk phos)
Ca^{++}, Mg^{++}

SAMPLE NUTRITION CARE PROCESS STEPS

Underweight

Assessment Data: Diet, weight, and physical activity histories. Medical history, frequent infections.

Nutrition Diagnosis (PES): Underweight related to a mismatch of energy intake and expenditure as evidenced by a 6-lb loss in 1 month without change in the usual oral intake.

Intervention: Address appropriate matching of energy intake and physical activity. Weight training may be beneficial. Counsel on food choices and ways to increase intake of energy-dense foods.

Monitoring and Evaluation: Ask patient to return in 2–4 weeks to assess weight. Review diet and activity logs, changes in BMI over time, fewer infections.

INTERVENTION

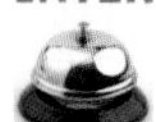

OBJECTIVES

- Increase body weight gradually if indicated. Encourage weight gain of approximately 1 lb weekly.
- Keep a food diary or log to determine changes that have been made and whether they are successful.
- Provide a 3-meal, 3-snack regimen as a baseline. Encourage increased consumption of calorie and nutrient-dense foods and beverages.
- In the case of recent acute illness or general chronic disease, provide diet as tolerated to improve nutritional status. Progress slowly; it may take several days to stimulate the patient's appetite.
- If confusion is present, dehydration may be a factor; evaluate carefully and rehydrate if appropriate.
- Try anabolic agents, exercise/physical activity, and cytokine inhibition.

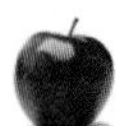

FOOD AND NUTRITION

- Calculate patient's goal weight: basal energy requirements plus kilocalories according to activity or stress factors. Each pound of fat requires 3500 kilocalories; therefore, diet should be increased by 500 kcal/d to promote a weight gain of 1 lb/wk.
- Use 15–20% protein, 60–70% CHO diet with frequent feedings, adequate micronutrients, and supplements as needed. Include healthy fats from avocado, nuts, fatty fish, olive, and canola oils.
- Plan meals and snacks according to appetite and preferences; encourage a small snack approximately every 2–3 hours. Patients who have cancer or other chronic illnesses may not want to eat large meals.
- Try serving the high calorie foods first if satiety is a problem; consume beverages between rather than with meals. Smaller, more frequent meals are recommended; avoid rushing mealtimes. Prepare items with fats, oils, extra sweets if feasible. Choose beverages with added calories such as a milkshake with chocolate syrup and peanut butter.
- Offer something to eat or drink every few hours, or keep snacks close at hand. If necessary, set an alarm to remember to eat something.
- With dyspnea, rest before meals and use bronchodilators in advance. Eat slowly and use pursed lip breathing between bites. Keep food and snacks within easy reach.
- For easy fatigue, rest before meals. Serve pre-prepared meals that are readily available. Use oral supplements between meals if intake is poor at mealtime.
- For constipation, a stool softener and adding extra fiber and fluid may be useful.
- For dental problems, change the food textures as needed (grind, chop, mash). Fix the problem with a dental appointment, or repair dentures if needed.
- For swallowing difficulty, work with the Speech and Language Pathologist (SLP) to identify appropriate solid and liquid consistencies.
- Provide enteral feeding if needed and appropriate. In some cases, feeding at night is well tolerated.

Common Drugs Used and Potential Side Effects

- Appetite may be stimulated through use of medications such as megestrol acetate, dronabinol, prednisone, or oxandrolone. Not everyone responds positively with an increased appetite and weight gain. Side effects vary and are most concerning with prednisone.
- Antidepressants may be warranted when a qualified professional has documented depression. Monitor for dry mouth and other side effects specific to ordered medication.

Herbs, Botanicals, and Supplements

- Herbs and botanical supplements should not be used without discussing with physician.

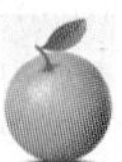

NUTRITION EDUCATION, COUNSELING, CARE MANAGEMENT

- When a registered dietitian, as part of the healthcare team, provides medical nutrition therapy (MNT) for older adults with unintentional weight loss, improved outcomes are seen for increased energy, protein and nutrient intakes, improved nutritional status, improved quality of life, and weight gain (American Dietetic Association, 2009).
- Help patient make meals in a simple manner, using attractive foods.
- Identify spices, seasonings, and other flavor enhancements that will stimulate the senses.
- The use of high-caloric density foods may be useful in programs where the patient refuses to eat or to take supplements. Adding them by "hiding" calories and extra protein in food may also be feasible (extra dry milk powder in soups, shakes, or mashed potatoes).
- Offer tips on weight gain such as eating a small snack every 2–3 hours. A high-calorie bedtime snack is often beneficial (for example, a milkshake or sandwich). If homemade items are not available, high calorie commercial supplements can be used.

- Dietary restraint and inadequate weight gain in pregnancy is not desirable. There are tools to assess restraint that may identify women at risk so that they can be counseled early in pregnancy (Mumford et al, 2008).
- Malnutrition often presents with loss, loneliness, dependency, and chronic illness, and it impacts morbidity, nutrition quality of life, and morbidity. Coordinate referrals such as home-delivered meals.
- Promote lean body mass development through strength training where appropriate. Increased physical activity appropriate for the clinical condition can help to improve appetite and intake in many cases. Exercise training has been successful for the treatment of wasting associated with sarcopenia, cancer, and some other conditions.
- Coordinate care with other health team members, as shown in this flow chart:

INTERDISCIPLINARY NUTRITION CARE PLAN
Involuntary Weight Loss

Client Name: ________ **#:** ________ **Initiated by:** ________ **Date:** ________

SCREENING
Nutrition Screen indicates Involuntary Weight Loss
Signed: ________ Date: ________

GOALS (Check any/all):
❑ Prevent nutritional decline/adverse events in ____ (goal time).
❑ Encourage improvement as evidenced by: wt gain/increased strength in ____ (goal time).
❑ Correct causes of involuntary weight loss where possible in ____ (goal time).

ASSESS ACUITY *(Check any/all)*
❑ Poor oral intake
❑ Complex diet order
❑ BMI <20 (high risk)
❑ Wt loss: >3 lb/wk or >5%/mo or >10%/6 mo
❑ Nausea/diarrhea/vomiting
❑ Infection (e.g., pneumonia, UTI, URI)
❑ Pressure ulcers, wounds
❑ Poor Strength
Signed: ________ Date: ________

None →

MODERATE RISK INTERVENTIONS *(Check any/all)*
❍ **Ways to Improve Nutrition** provided and reviewed
❍ **Food Record** provided and reviewed
❑ RD chart consult
❑ Weight monitoring q:_____
❑ BID/TID supplements
❑ **Other:**________
(See notes for documention.)
Signed: ________ Date: ________

KEY
❍ **Recommended intervention for best practice:**
- Patient Education Materials provided and assessed for comprehension

❑ **Optional intervention:**
- Nutrition support initiated (oral/enteral)
- Referrals
- Monitoring

1 or more ↓

HIGH-RISK INTERVENTIONS *(Check any/all)*
❍ **Ways to Improve Nutrition** provided and reviewed
❍ **Food Record** provided and reviewed
Obtain Dr. orders as needed:
❑ Weight monitoring q:_____
❑ RD referral for home visit(s)
❑ BID/TID supplements
❑ **Other:**________
(See notes for documention.)
Signed: ________ Date: ________

Next visit ↓

ASSESS RESPONSE *(Check any/all)*
❑ Further wt loss
❑ Wt gain < goal
❑ New onset infection
❑ Declining strength
❑ **Other:**________
(See notes for documention.)
Signed: ________ Date: ________

← 1 or more (to High-Risk Interventions); None →

OUTCOMES ACHIEVED
Document improved:
❑ Strength
❑ Weight
❑ **Other:**________
❑ Repeat Nutrition Screen in ____ days
(See notes for documention.)
Goals met
Signed: ________ Date: ________

Next visit ↓

ASSESS RESPONSE *(Check any/all)*
❑ Further wt loss
❑ Wt gain < goal
❑ New onset infection
❑ Declining strength
❑ **Other:**________
(See notes for documention.)
Signed: ________ Date: ________

None →

OUTCOMES ACHIEVED
Document improved:
❑ Strength
❑ Weight
❑ **Other:**________
❑ Repeat Nutrition Screen in ____ days
(See notes for documention.)
Goals met
Signed: ________ Date: ________

1 or more ↓

OUTCOMES NOT ACHIEVED
Reassess acuity/evaluate need for EN/PN (refer to Tube Feeding Nutrition Care Plan). Document on Nutrition Variance Tracking form.

Adapted with permission from www.RD411.com, Inc.

Patient Education—Food Safety

If enteral or parenteral nutrition is used, careful sanitation and handling techniques must be taught and used.

For More Information

- Health Line
  http://www.healthline.com/symptomsearch?addterm=Unintentional%20Weight%20Loss
- Unintentional Weight Loss
  http://www.nlm.nih.gov/medlineplus/ency/article/003107.htm
- Wrong Diagnosis
  http://www.wrongdiagnosis.com/u/underweight/symptoms.htm

UNDERWEIGHT AND UNINTENTIONAL WEIGHT LOSS—CITED REFERENCES

American Dietetic Association (ADA). Evidence analysis library: unintended weight loss. Accessed November 3, 2009 at http://www.adaevidencelibrary.com/topic.cfm?cat=3652.

Flegal KM, et al. Cause-specific excess deaths associated with underweight, overweight, and obesity. *JAMA*. 298:2028, 2007.

Flegal KM, et al. Excess deaths associated with underweight, overweight, and obesity. *JAMA*. 293:1861, 2005.

Fugate Woods N, et al. Frailty: emergence and consequences in women aged 65 and older in the Women's Health Initiative Observational Study. *J Am Geriat Soc*. 53:1321, 2005.

Hallin R, et al. Nutritional status, dietary energy intake and the risk of exacerbations in patients with chronic obstructive pulmonary disease (COPD). *Respir Med*. 100:561, 2006.

Heather M, et al. BMI and mortality: Results from a National Longitudinal Study of Canadian Adults. *Obesity*. 10:1038, 2009.

Keys A, et al. *The biology of human starvation*. Vol. 1. Minneapolis: University of Minnesota Press, 1950.

Mumford SL, et al. Dietary restraint and gestational weight gain. *J Am Diet Assoc*. 108:1646, 2008.

Sergi G, et al. An adequate threshold for body mass index to detect underweight condition in elderly persons: The Italian Longitudinal Study on Aging (ILSA). *J Gerontol A Biol Sci Med Sci*. 60:866, 2005.

UNDERNUTRITION AND PROTEIN-ENERGY MALNUTRITION

NUTRITIONAL ACUITY RANKING: LEVEL 3–4

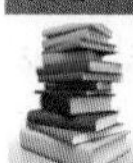

DEFINITIONS AND BACKGROUND

The undernourished category of malnutrition leads to the loss of body cell mass, which, together with inflammation, diminishes host response and quality of life (Soeters and Schols, 2009). Protein–energy malnutrition (PEM) decreases cardiac output, blood pressure, oxygen consumption, total lymphocyte count (TLC), number of T cells, and glomerular filtration rate (GFR). Undernutrition is associated with increased infection rates, emphysema and pneumonia, GI tract atrophy, intestinal bacterial overgrowth, hepatic mass losses, and anemia. In PEM, anemia is a result of ineffective erythropoiesis (Borelli et al, 2007).

Physical assessment and thorough clinical history are essential in determining the etiology of the PEM and appropriate interventions; see Table 10-19. Malnutrition may be assessed by estimating nutrient balance but, subsequently, to measure body composition (muscle mass), inflammatory activity (plasma albumin and C-reactive protein), and muscle endurance and force (Soeters and Schols, 2009).

Malnutrition is the leading cause of death among children in developing countries. Clinically, in children, PEM has three forms: dry (thin, desiccated), wet (edematous, swollen), or a combination; grading is mild, moderate, or severe. Grade is determined by calculating weight as a percentage of expected weight for length using international standards (normal 90–110%; mild 85–90%; moderate 75–85%; severe <75%). The dry form, **marasmus**, results from near starvation with a deficiency in protein and nonprotein nutrients. The wet form is called **kwashiorkor**—an African word meaning "first child–second child"—because the first child often develops malnutrition after the second child arrives and nutrient-poor foods replace breast milk. The combined form of malnutrition is called **marasmic kwashiorkor**; these children have some edema and more body fat than those with marasmus.

Nutrients and growth factors regulate brain development during fetal and early postnatal life. The rapidly developing brain is more vulnerable to nutrient insufficiency yet also demonstrates its greatest degree of plasticity (Georgleff, 2007). Chronic protein energy malnutrition (stunting) affects the ongoing development of higher cognitive processes during childhood and may also result in long lasting cognitive impairments (Kar et al, 2008). The nutrients that have greater effects on brain development than do others include protein, energy, certain fats, iron, zinc, copper, iodine, selenium, vitamin A, choline, and folate (Georgleff, 2007).

Adult malnutrition syndromes differ from those in underdeveloped countries; an understanding of the systemic inflammatory response should help guide assessment, diagnosis, and treatment (Jensen et al, 2009). In adult patients with acute illnesses, the prevalence of malnutrition is high, particularly related to age and metabolic stress (Martinez Olmos et al, 2005; Pirlich et al, 2006). Of patients admitted to hospitals, 35–55% are malnourished on admission and 25–30% more become malnourished during stay. Problems are common in gastrointestinal (GI) patients, particularly patients with inflammatory bowel disease (IBD); ventilator, radiation, or chemotherapy patients; burn and surgical patients; and patients with renal failure. Even with dialysis, renal patients are at high risk (Kopple, 2005), mostly from cardiovascular disease with markers of a malnutrition–inflammation complex syndrome (Colman et al, 2005).

Tissue catabolism usually begins with lowered plasma proteins, red blood cells, and leukocytes; later, wasting of organs, skeletal muscle, bone, skin, and subcutaneous tissue

TABLE 10-19 Complicating Effects of Chronic Malnutrition on Body Systems

Cardiac and Hematological System—Anemia; altered clotting time; decreased heart size; decreased amount of blood pumped; slow heart rate; decreased blood pressure; heart failure; decreased number of blood cells.

Digestive Tract—Frequent, chronic, or even fatal diarrhea; bacterial translocation in gut; low HCl production in stomach; progressive weight loss; gastrointestinal mucosal or villous atrophy with loss of immune function.

Endocrine System—Decreased body temperature (hypothermia); fluid accumulation in skin from lower subcutaneous fat and decreased albumin levels; vitamin and mineral deficiencies.

Immune System—Depressed cell-mediated immunity; increased infection, particularly gram-negative sepsis; impaired wound healing; more wound infections or disruption; impaired ability to fight infections; delayed response to cancer chemotherapy or radiation therapy.

Muscular System—Decreased activity; delayed physical rehabilitation; decreased muscle size and strength; delayed hospital discharge and ability to perform work.

Nervous System—Irritability, weakness, and apathy even if intellect remains intact.

Pulmonary System—Depressed ventilatory response to hypoxia; decreased lung capacity; slow breathing; pneumonia and eventually respiratory failure.

Quality of Life—Increased and prolonged use of hospitals, critical care units, and expensive drugs; excessive requirements of hospital support.

Renal System—Fluid, electrolyte, and acid–base malfunctioning; increased frequency of urinary tract infections; elevated blood urea nitrogen from muscle and tissue breakdown; decreased glomerular filtration rate.

Reproductive System—Decreased size of ovaries or testes; decreased libido; cessation of menstruation.

Skin and Skeleton—Pale, thin, dry inelastic skin; pressure ulcers; decreased subcutaneous fat; loss of bone density.

will occur. Chronic undernutrition of protein, calories, and micronutrients (particularly zinc) will compromise cytokine response and affect immune cell functioning. Nutrients act as antioxidants and as cofactors in cytokine regulation (Cunningham-Rundles et al, 2005). The central nervous system is the last system to be catabolized, and magnetic resonance imaging (MRI) scans taken of children who have moderate to severe malnutrition show cerebral atrophy (Odabas et al, 2005). Total starvation is fatal in 8–12 weeks.

Certain types of stress and surgery can lead to malnutrition; pancreatic surgery is one specific example (Schnelldorfer and Adams, 2005). Because malnutrition and involuntary weight loss are common problems in seniors, there is a significant increase in infection rate, a decrease in the rate of healing, and an increase in length of stay in older, malnourished burn patients when compared with those who are well nourished (Demling, 2005).

Common causes of malnutrition in the elderly involve decreased appetite, dependency on help for eating, impaired cognition and/or communication, poor positioning, frequent acute illnesses with GI losses, medications that decrease appetite or increase nutrient losses, polypharmacy, decreased thirst response, decreased ability to concentrate urine, intentional fluid restriction because of fear of incontinence or choking if dysphagic, psychosocial factors such as isolation and depression, monotony of diet, and higher nutrient density requirements, along with the demands of age, illness, and disease on the body (Harris and Fraser, 2004).

Poor nutritional state may be associated with an increase in postoperative complication rate; low serum albumin levels can be reflected by a higher rate of infectious complications as well as increased intensive care unit stays (Schnelldorfer and Adams, 2005). The Subjective Global Assessment (SGA) is a tool for nutritional screening that can be used on hospital admission. The SGA score, disease category, presence of malignancy, serum albumin level, percent triceps skinfold thickness, and percent arm muscle circumference are significant predictive parameters for hospital stay in patients with digestive diseases (Wakahara et al, 2007). SGA has also been found to be useful in chronic kidney disease, hemodialysis, and cardiac disorders as well as liver diseases and cancer.

It is important to use designated descriptions or codes for malnutrition in the medical record so that proper attention is given. Table 10-20 describes several types of undernutrition that are common in hospitals. Table 10-21 describes a malnutrition universal screening tool (MUST). The MUST tool has been developed to screen all adults, even if weight and/or height cannot be measured. This tool provides more complete information on malnutrition prevalence; MUST screening predicts clinical outcome in the hospitalized elderly where malnutrition is common in over half of the population (Stratton et al, 2006). Other tools are available in Appendix B.

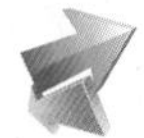

ASSESSMENT, MONITORING, AND EVALUATION

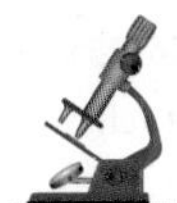

CLINICAL INDICATORS

Genetic Markers: While genetics are typically not responsible for malnutrition, some conditions make an individual prone to poor nutriture. Examples include inherited disorders such as cystic fibrosis, inflammatory bowel disease, and celiac disease. Recent studies have shown that vitamin D_3 and calcitriol impact over 1000 genes, and deficiency contributes to rickets, cancers, hypertension, stroke, heart attack, diabetes, bone fractures, multiple sclerosis, and periodontal disease (Edlich et al, 2010). Vitamin D up-regulates cathelicidin—a naturally occurring broad-spectrum antibiotic—and may even play a role in protecting against viral respiratory infections including the common cold and influenza (Cannell and Hollis, 2009).

Clinical/History	Lab Work	
Height, arm length, or knee length	CRP	Total iron-binding capacity (<250 mg/dL)
Stunting in a child	Alb, transthyretin (may be altered)	Urine acetone
Weight	Chol, Trig (decreased)	T3, T4
BMI	Serum Fe, ferritin	Ca^{++}, Mg^{++}
Recent weight; weight changes	Alk phos (decreased)	BUN (decreased)
Usual weight	Gluc	Creat
Desirable BMI	H & H	White blood cell count (decreased)
Diet history—poor appetite	Oxygen saturation levels	Na^+, K^+, Cl^-
I & O		Serum B_{12}, folate, B_6
BP		Serum D_3 [25(OH)D]*
Edema		
Muscle wasting		
Sarcopenia?		
Cachexia?		
TSF		
MAMC, MAC		

*Natural vitamin D levels in humans living in a sun-rich environment are between 40 and 70 ng/mL (Cannell and Hollis, 2009).

INTERVENTION

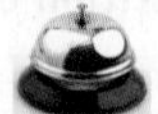

OBJECTIVES

- Provide adequate macronutrients and micronutrients. Work up to 100% of estimated needs over several days.
- Correct weight loss, weakness, infections, and poor wound healing. Improve signs of apathy and irritability.
- Reduce the costs of care. International studies suggest that disease-related malnutrition increases hospital costs by 30–70%; with this large cost of disease-related malnutrition, intervention can result in substantial absolute cost savings (Elia, 2009).
- Avoid hazards of refeeding (hypophosphatemia, low magnesium, and potassium). Fluid administration must be monitored carefully. Prevent sepsis, overfeeding, hyperglycemia, heart failure, or other organ failure by refeeding slowly.
- Allow normal growth of brain and prevent permanent IQ deficits in children.
- Correct malnutrition in patients who have dysphagia as it may contribute to further declines in the capacity for rehabilitation.
- Provide sufficient nutrients for gene expression.
- Prevent complications, which can include dehydration, electrolyte imbalances, infections, vitamin-mineral deficiencies, and other biochemical changes (Table 10-22).

TABLE 10-20 Indicators of Malnutrition

Category	Criteria for Nutrition Diagnosis of Malnutrition
Severe malnutrition	At least one of the following criteria must be met:
Protein-energy malnutrition	- BMI ≤16.0 - Weight loss of ≥26% of UBW within ≤6 months
Moderate malnutrition	At least one of the following criteria must be met:
Protein-energy malnutrition	- BMI 16.0–16.9 - Weight loss of 16–25% of UBW within ≤6 months
Mild malnutrition	At least one of the following criteria must be met:
Protein-energy malnutrition	- BMI 17–18.4 - Weight loss of 5–15% of UBW within ≤6 months - Weight loss of ≥5% of UBW within ≤1 month
Malnutrition, unspecified	Albumin must be below 3.4 and at least one of the following criteria must be met:
Disease/injury related malnutrition	- One indicator of malnutrition as described above - Peripheral edema or anasarca - Delayed wound healing - History of acute or chronic disease or trauma

Albumin should not be used as the sole indicator of visceral protein status in fluid imbalance, liver disease, post-operative states, infection, and nephrotic syndrome. Serum albumin levels drop when there is inflammation; when inflammation is corrected, levels may rise again regardless of nutritional intake. Albumin is a marker of severity of illness, not as a marker of protein nutriture.

Adapted from the Nutrition Support Committee, Emory Hospitals, Atlanta GA; 2008.

REFERENCE

American Dietetic Association (ADA). Unintentional weight loss and cachexia: medical nutrition therapy and nutrition care strategies from ADA Center for Professional Development. Accessed November 1, 2009 at http://www.eatright.org/cps/rde/xchg/ada/hs.xsl/nutrition_10448_ENU_HTML.htm.

TABLE 10-21 Malnutrition Universal Screening Tool (MUST)

MUST is a 5-step screening tool to identify adults who are malnourished, at risk of malnutrition (undernutrition), or obese. It includes management guidelines for care planning. It is used in hospitals, community care settings and other care settings and can be used by all care workers. It was established by the British Association for Enteral and Parenteral Nutrition (BASPEN). The guide contains the following:

- A flow chart showing 5 steps to use for screening and management
- BMI chart
- Weight loss tables
- Alternative measurements when BMI cannot be obtained by measuring weight and height

A more detailed MUST explanatory booklet should be used for procedures when weight and height cannot be measured and when screening with more interpretation is needed (e.g., those with fluid disturbances, plaster casts, amputations, or critical illness, or pregnant or lactating women).
The 5 MUST steps are as follows.

Step 1: Measure height and weight to get a BMI score using the chart provided.

If height cannot be measured: use recently documented or self-reported height (if reliable and realistic). If the subject does not know or is unable to report their height, use one of the alternative measurements to estimate height (ulna, knee height, or arm span).

If height and weight cannot be obtained: use mid upper arm circumference (MUAC) measurement to estimate BMI category.

If BMI cannot be determined: use subjective clinical impression—thin, acceptable weight, overweight. Obvious wasting (very thin) and obesity (very overweight) can also be noted.

BMI	Score
>20	☐ 0
18.5–20	☐ 1
<18.5	☐ 2
BMI score = ________	

Alternative procedures are available from the guide http://www.baspen.org.uk/the-must.htm.

Step 2: Note percentage of unplanned weight loss, and score using tables in the screening tool.

If recent weight loss cannot be calculated: use self-reported weight loss (if reliable and realistic).

Unplanned weight loss: clothes and/or jewelry have become loose fitting (weight loss); history of decreased food intake, reduced appetite or swallowing problems over 3–6 months; underlying disease or psychosocial/physical disabilities likely to cause weight loss.

Record presence of obesity. Control underlying conditions before treating obesity.

% of Unplanned weight loss in past 3–6 months	Score
<5%	= 0
5–10%	= 1
>10%	= 2
Weight loss score = __________	

Step 3: Establish the acute disease effect and score.

No nutritional intake or likelihood of no intake for more than 5 days = score 2.

Acute disease effect score = ________

Step 4: Add scores from steps 1, 2, and 3 to obtain the overall risk of malnutrition.

0 = Low Risk
1 = Medium Risk
≥2 = High Risk

(continued)

TABLE 10-21 Malnutrition Universal Screening Tool (MUST) *(continued)*

Step 5: Develop care plan and treat.
Observe and document dietary intake for 3 days if patient is in hospital or long-term care (LTC) facility.
If improved or adequate intake—little clinical concern. If no improvement—clinical concern; follow local policy. Repeat screening: Hospital, weekly; LTC facility, at least monthly; community, at least every 2–3 months.
Treat unless detrimental, no benefit is expected from nutritional support, or death is imminent:
Record need for special diets and follow local policy.
Record malnutrition risk category; as needed, refer to dietitian or nutritional support team or implement local policy.
Treat underlying condition and provide help and advice on food choices, eating, and drinking when necessary.
Improve and increase overall nutritional intake.
Monitor and review care plan: hospital, weekly; LTC facility, monthly; community, monthly.

SAMPLE NUTRITION CARE PROCESS STEPS

Malnutrition

Assessment Data: Diet, intake records, weight, medical history, frequency of infections, serum levels of vitamins such as vitamin A, lipids such as total cholesterol.

Nutrition Diagnoses (PES):

Malnutrition (NI-5.2) related to lack of appetite and poor food selection as evidenced by diet recall showing consumption of only 1200 kcal/d and 25 grams PRO, percent wt change of > 10% over the past 6 months, BMI of 18, serum cholesterol of 130, and albumin of 2.5 g/dL.

Involuntary weight loss (NC 3.2) related to inadequate dietary intake as evidenced by reported dietary recall and daily intake of 500–700 kilocalories was less than estimated needs.

Interventions:

Food and Nutrient Delivery: ND 1.3 Increase fiber and fluid intake

ND 1.2 High calorie, high protein diet

ND 5.7 Initiate meals on wheels

Education: E-1.2 Provide examples of high fiber, high protein foods, and high calcium foods

ND - 6.5 Develop regular schedule for taking iron supplements

Counseling: C-2.5 Discuss social support

C-2.4 Discuss fluid needs and how to practically incorporate them into daily meal plans

Coordination of Care: Contact psychologist to review ongoing depression and meds, make arrangements for dental clinics, refer to social worker for community and financial resources

Monitoring and Evaluation: Assess po intake of kilocalories, PRO, and fluid. Monitor weight and labs. Review intake and activity logs. Monitor for changes in BMI over time, fewer infections, and improved quality of life.

- Develop a targeted therapeutic approach to skeletal muscle loss and muscle strength in older persons (Thomas, 2007).
- Establish a nutritional plan according to patient prognosis (Table 10-23).

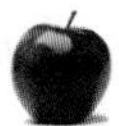

FOOD AND NUTRITION

- Monitor physical exam and clinical status to determine needed dietary changes.
- **Mild malnutrition:** Provide sufficient calories and protein, gradually increasing to meet needs. Diet should provide adequate carbohydrate (CHO) and caloric intake to spare protein and correct weight loss. Use tube feeding or CPN, if appropriate (see Section 17). Vitamin-mineral supplementation is recommended.
- **Severe malnutrition or cachexia:** Start treatment with intravenous glucose. Gradually add lactose-treated milk and soft, easily tolerated solids. Provide high-biologic value proteins with sufficient calories that are adequate to use nitrogen effectively. Avoid overfeeding (use 20–25 kcal/kg, progressing gradually to 35–40 kcal/kg). Add a vitamin–mineral supplement, particularly including thiamin. Provide enteral feeding, if needed; start with continuous versus intermittent or bolus feedings at a slow rate until serum electrolyte levels are stable.
- Practical suggestions for improving intake in debilitated patients include liberalizing previous diet restrictions where safe and appropriate, addressing impaired dentition and swallowing, addressing physical and cognitive deficits, encouraging family and friends to provide favorite foods, addressing poor consumption of specific foods, and providing appropriate nutrient supplements (Harris and Fraser, 2004).
- Oral nutritional supplements are feasible in nutritionally depleted patients, particularly between meals.

TABLE 10-22 Selected Biochemical Changes Observed in Severe Protein–Energy Malnutrition (PEM)

Body Composition	Energy Malnutrition	Protein Malnutrition/ Edema
Total body water	High	High
Extracellular water	High	Higher
Total body potassium	Low	Lower
Total body protein	Low	Low
Serum or plasma		
Transport proteins (transferrin, ceruloplasmin, retinol-, cortisol-, and thyroxine-binding proteins, beta-lipoproteins)[a]	Normal or low	Low
Enzymes such as amylase, alkaline phosphatase	Normal	Low
Transaminase	Normal or high	High
C-reactive protein	Varies by condition	Varies
Liver		
Glycogen	Normal or low	Normal or low
Urea cycle enzymes and other enzymes	Low	Lower
Amino acid synthesizing enzymes	High	Not as high

[a]Note. Inflammatory processes and their effects on hepatic protein metabolism (albumin, transferrin, and transthyretin) have been identified. Serum hepatic protein levels correlate with *severity* of illness but do not accurately measure effectiveness of nutritional repletion (Fuhrman et al, 2004). Evaluate their value cautiously.

REFERENCES

Fuhrman MP, et al. Hepatic proteins and nutrition assessment. *Am Diet Assoc.* 104:1258, 2004.

Torun B, Viteri F. Protein-energy malnutrition. In: Warren K, Mahmood A, eds. *Tropical and geographical medicine.* 2nd ed. New York: McGraw-Hill, 1990.

- Assure adequate intake of vitamin D_3 from sunlight exposure, diet, and supplements to support gene expression and health.

Common Drugs Used and Potential Side Effects

- Medications that are often used to increase intake by stimulating appetite include oxandrolone (Oxandrin), megestrol acetate (Megace), cyproheptadine HCl (Periactin), and dronabinol (Marinol).
- Experimental therapies for treating cachexia include nonsteroidal antiinflammatory drugs, tumor necrosis factor alpha antagonists, tetrahydrocannabinol, growth hormone, ghrelin, oxandrolone, and omega-3 fatty acids (Gullett et al, 2009). Comparing oxandrolone, strength training, and nutrition alone, strength training is most cost effective and improves quality of life more than nutrition alone or oxandrolone (Shevitz et al, 2005).

Herbs, Botanicals, and Supplements

- Herbs and botanical supplements should not be used without discussing it with the physician.

- Treatment of vitamin D deficiency in otherwise healthy patients with 2000–7000 IU vitamin D per day should be sufficient to maintain year-round 25(OH)D levels in the range of 40–70 ng/mL (Cannell and Hollis, 2009).

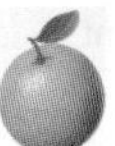

NUTRITION EDUCATION, COUNSELING, CARE MANAGEMENT

- Emphasize the importance of gradual refeeding.
- Discuss the complicating effects of malnutrition. Unless nutritional therapy is aggressive, infection and sepsis are major risks, and surgery becomes life threatening. PEM can increase fistula formation, reduce recovery and wound healing after surgery, and lead to pneumonia or poor drug tolerance.
- Allow patients to participate in feeding decisions. Set goals and help plan together with family.

Patient Education—Food Safety

Use of tube feeding or CPN at home warrants training to prevent foodborne illnesses. Handwashing, counter sanitation, and sterile techniques are important in handling these products and the administration kits.

TABLE 10-23 Poor Prognosis and Consequences of Not Feeding a Patient

Clinical manifestations of PEM relate to length of time, extent of nutritional deprivation, and prior health status. There are serious detrimental effects on every organ. "When maintained on a prolonged semi-starvation diet, otherwise healthy individuals experience a **loss of heart tissue** that parallels their loss of body mass. Respiratory rate, vital capacity, and minute volume of ventilation also decrease. These **changes in pulmonary function** are thought to result from reduced basal metabolic rate that accompanies starvation. In addition, **liver function declines, kidney filtration rates decline, and nearly every aspect of the immune system is compromised.** Defective ability to fight bacterial and viral infections occurs. Starvation therefore leads to **increased susceptibility to infection, delayed wound healing, reduced rate of drug metabolism, and impairment of both physical and cognitive function.** If starvation is prolonged, complications develop, **leading eventually to death**" (Sullivan, 1995).

Other consequences of not feeding an individual who *will not* or *cannot* eat orally in sufficient amounts include

- **Dehydration** with increased risk of urinary tract infections, fever, swollen tongue, sunken eyeballs, decreased urine output, constipation, nausea, vomiting, decreased blood pressure, mental confusion, and electrolyte disturbances.
- **Decreased awareness** of environment from decreased glucose availability for the brain.
- **Development of new or additional pressure ulcers** over bony prominences from lack of sufficient protein, calorie, vitamin, and mineral intakes and decreased body fat.
- **Decreased ability to participate in activities of daily living** (self-feeding, dressing, bathing, toileting).
- **Low body weight or rapid, involuntary weight loss,** which are highly predictive of illness and imminent death. The elderly are particularly unable to regain weight after a stress situation.

REFERENCE

Sullivan D. The role of nutrition in increased morbidity and mortality. *Clin Geriatr Med.* 11:663, 1995.

Poor prognosis may be seen in individuals with the following conditions who also have PEM:

Age <6 months

Cachexia from chronic renal failure

Clinical jaundice or elevated serum bilirubin level

Circulatory collapse: cold hands and feet, weak radial pulse, diminished consciousness

Deficit in weight for height >30% or in weight for age >40%

Dehydration and electrolyte disturbances, particularly hypokalemia and severe acidosis

Extensive exudative or exfoliative cutaneous lesions or deep pressure ulcers

Hypoglycemia

Hypothermia

Infections, particularly bronchopneumonia or measles

Petechiae or hemorrhagic tendencies (purpura is usually associated with septicemia or a viral infection)

Persistent tachycardia, signs of heart failure, or respiratory difficulty

Severe anemia with clinical signs of hypoxia

Stupor, coma, or other alterations in awareness

Cachexia is characterized by maladaptive responses such as anorexia, elevated basic metabolic rate, wasting of lean body tissue, and underutilization of fat tissue for energy. Inflammation secondary to cytokines is significant.

For More Information

- Abbott Health Nutrition Institute
  http://abbottnutritionhealthinstitute.org/
- Mayo Clinic
  http://www.mayoclinic.com/health/senior-health/HA00066
- Nestle Nutrition
  http://www.nestlenutrition.com/en
- Nutrition Day Worldwide
  http://www.nutritionday.org/
- World Health Organization
  http://www.wpro.who.int/health_topics/protein_energy/

MALNUTRITION—CITED REFERENCES

Borelli P, et al. Reduction of erythroid progenitors in protein-energy malnutrition. *Br J Nutr.* 97:307, 2007.

Cannell JJ, Hollis BW. Use of vitamin D in clinical practice. *Altern Med Rev.* 13:6, 2009.

Colman S, et al. The Nutritional and Inflammatory Evaluation in Dialysis Patients (NIED) study: overview of the NIED study and the role of dietitians. *J Ren Nutr.* 15:231, 2005.

Cunningham-Rundles S, et al. Mechanisms of nutrient modulation of the immune response. Mechanisms of nutrient modulation of the immune response. *J Allergy Clin Immunol.* 115:1119, 2005.

Demling RH. The incidence and impact of pre-existing protein energy malnutrition on outcome in the elderly burn patient population. *J Burn Care Rehabil.* 26:94, 2005.

Edlich RF, et al. Revolutionary advances in the diagnosis of vitamin d deficiency. *J Environ Pathol Toxicol Oncol.* 29:85, 2010.

Elia M. The economics of malnutrition. *Nestle Nutr Workshop Ser Clin Perform Programme.* 12:29, 2009.

Georgleff MK. Nutrition and the developing brain: nutrient priorities and measurement. *Am J Clin Nutr.* 85:214S, 2007.

Gullett N, et al. Cancer-induced cachexia: a guide for the oncologist. *J Soc Integr Oncol.* 7:155, 2009.

Harris CL, Fraser C. Malnutrition in the institutionalized elderly: the effects on wound healing. *Ostomy Wound Manage.* 50:54, 2004.

Jensen GL, et al. Malnutrition syndromes: a conundrum vs. continuum. *JPEN J Parenter Enteral Nutr.* 33:710, 2009.

Kar BR, et al. Cognitive development in children with chronic protein energy malnutrition. *Behav Brain Funct.* 4:31, 2008.
Kopple, JD. The phenomenon of altered risk factor patterns or reverse epidemiology in persons with advanced chronic kidney failure. *Am J Clin Nutr.* 81:1257, 2005.
Martinez Olmos MA, et al. Nutritional status study of inpatients in hospitals of Galicia. *Eur J Clin Nutr.* 59:938, 2005.
Odabas D, et al. Cranial MRI findings in children with protein energy malnutrition. *Int J Neurosci.* 115:829, 2005.
Pirlich M, et al. The German hospital malnutrition study. *Clin Nutr.* 25:563, 2006.
Schnelldorfer T, Adams DB. The effect of malnutrition on morbidity after surgery for chronic pancreatitis. *Am Surg.* 71:466, 2005.
Shevitz AH, et al. A comparison of the clinical and cost-effectiveness of 3 intervention strategies for AIDS wasting. *J Acquir Immune Defic Syndr.* 38:399, 2005.
Stratton R, et al. 'Malnutrition Universal Screening Tool' predicts mortality and length of hospital stay in acutely ill elderly. *Br J Nutr.* 95:325, 2006.
Thomas DR. Loss of skeletal muscle mass in aging: examining the relationship of starvation, sarcopenia, and cachexia. *Clin Nutr.* 26:389, 2007.
Wakahara T, et al. Nutritional screening with Subjective Global Assessment predicts hospital stay in patients with digestive diseases. *Nutrition.* 23:634, 2007.

REFEEDING SYNDROME

NUTRITIONAL ACUITY RANKING: LEVEL 4

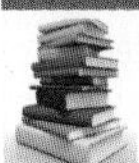

DEFINITIONS AND BACKGROUND

The effects of starvation are extensive and negatively affect the pituitary gland, thyroid gland, adrenal glands, gonads, and bones (Usdan et al, 2008). Refeeding syndrome (RFS) refers to these various metabolic abnormalities that may complicate carbohydrate and protein administration in undernourished patients, as in anorexia nervosa or head and neck cancer. Other conditions that can lead to refeeding syndrome can be found in Table 10-24.

During refeeding, insulin release is stimulated by the presence of carbohydrate and protein in the gut. Insulin plays a key role in the switch from using up body stores to using food; it stops the release of fat from stores and the production of glucose from protein. In refeeding, the increase in insulin lowers glucagon levels. With gluconeogenesis, glycogenolysis, and fatty acid mobilization, glucose is taken up rapidly into the cells. Phosphorus is driven inside the cells; the result is a dangerous hypophosphatemia. Adenosine triphosphate (ATP) levels drop, with major effects on the cardiac, pulmonary, CNS, hematological, and muscular systems. This process also stops sodium excretion and causes fluid retention in the first few days of refeeding or when caloric intake is increased.

TABLE 10-24 Conditions with High Risk for Refeeding Syndrome

Alcoholism
Anorexia nervosa
Chronic underfeeding
Hepatic failure
Malabsorption from GI damage or chronic use of phosphate binders such as aluminum-containing antacids or sucralfate
Morbid obesity with massive weight loss from fasting
Protein–energy malnutrition
Prolonged fasting
Prolonged parenteral nutrition
Respiratory alkalosis

The typical patient who experiences RFS has been malnourished for days to weeks and develops hypophosphatemia and, occasionally, hypokalemia and hypomagnesemia when administered a carbohydrate load in the form of glucose-concentrated fluids, total parenteral nutrition, tube feedings, or an oral diet (Marinella, 2009). Overwhelming cardiovascular and pulmonary manifestations can accompany refeeding with carbohydrate in chronically malnourished patients (Miller, 2008). Increases in heart rate, blood pressure, oxygen consumption, cardiac output, and an expansion of plasma volume are seen. The response is dependent on the amount of calories, protein, and sodium administered, and the malnourished heart can easily be given a metabolic demand that is too high for it to supply.

Stressed, critically ill patients may be at risk of refeeding following short periods of fasting (Miller, 2008). RFS usually occurs within 4 days of starting to feed again. The respiratory muscle, reduced in mass and ATP content by malnutrition, is unable to respond to the increased workload imposed by aggressive nutrition support. Excess carbon dioxide production and increased oxygen consumption can result from giving too much glucose and overfeeding. A person with malnutrition-induced respiratory muscle wasting can get short of breath and cannot sustain an increased ventilatory drive. Pulmonary edema may develop in some due to increased water load, and this may lead to respiratory failure. Clearly, RFS syndrome is a life-threatening, underdiagnosed but treatable condition (Gariballa, 2008).

Precipitous falls in electrolyte levels in persons with diabetes that occur due to intracellular shifts are a result of the anabolic effects of insulin doses (Parrish, 2009). This form of refeeding is common but not always recognized.

Problems with sodium derangements may lead to heart failure. When potassium shifts into cells, hypokalemia and arrhythmias can occur. When magnesium shifts intracellularly, tetany and seizures may be seen. Thiamin deficiency must be prevented during refeeding, because it is a cofactor in carbohydrate metabolism, important for both the heart and the brain. With thiamin deficiency, there can be signs such as mental confusion, ataxia, muscle weakness, edema, muscle wasting, tachycardia, and cardiomegaly. Wernicke's encephalopathy can be precipitated by carbohydrate feeding in thiamine-deficient patients.

The gut is also affected by malnutrition, where it begins to atrophy. Activity of the brush border enzymes and pancreatic enzyme secretion return to normal with refeeding, but it requires a period of readaptation to food to minimize GI complaints such as diarrhea, nausea, and vomiting.

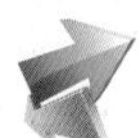

ASSESSMENT, MONITORING, AND EVALUATION

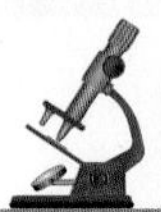

CLINICAL INDICATORS

Genetic Markers: Refeeding syndrome is not genetically derived.

Clinical/History

Height
Weight
BMI
Desirable BMI
Percentage of usual weight
History of weight changes
Diet history
I & O
Anorexia
Bone pain
Edema
Tachycardia
Temperature
Rhabdomyolysis
pCO_2, pO_2
Respiratory insufficiency or failure
Dizziness
Spontaneous diarrhea

Lab Work

Serum phos (low?)
Mg^{++} (low?)
K^+ (low?)
Gluc
Na^+
Chol, Trig
H & H
Serum Fe
Red blood cell dysfunction
Ca^{++}
BUN, Creat
Partial pressure of carbon dioxide (pCO_2)
Partial pressure of oxygen (pO_2)

INTERVENTION

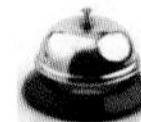

OBJECTIVES

- Correct starvation without overloading the system with nutrients of any type. Use less than full levels of calorie and fluid requirements. Weight gain is not a goal during the first week.
- Advance calories and volume with careful monitoring of cardiac and respiratory side effects.
- Increase nutrition support slowly while assuring adequate amounts of electrolytes. Check electrolytes 2–3 times daily until stable. Organ function and fluid balance also need to be monitored daily during the first week and less frequently after that time.
- Distinguish between constitutional thinness and malnutrition since the causes are different, as are risks for RFS.
- Monitor for neurological, hematological, and metabolic complications of hypokalemia, hypophosphatemia, and hyperglycemia. Prevent sudden death.

SAMPLE NUTRITION CARE PROCESS STEPS

Excessive Energy Intake—Refeeding Syndrome

Assessment Data: A 60-year old female with a 4-month history of poor dietary intake; connective tissue disease leading to myositis and dysphagia; respiratory failure needing mechanical ventilation. Low baseline electrolyte concentrations, including potassium, magnesium, calcium, and phosphate, and low serum albumin. Twelve hours after starting nasogastric tube feeding, she developed a cardiac arrest from which she was successfully resuscitated. Repeated attempts to wean her from the ventilator failed. BMI low at 16. Clinical nutrition team made the diagnosis of refeeding syndrome.

Nutrition Diagnosis: Excessive energy intake related to 4-month history of poor oral food and beverage intake as evidenced by diet history and respiratory failure with need for ventilator dependency.

Intervention: Food-nutrient delivery: high-protein, high-fat, low-carbohydrate diet, multivitamin and trace-element supplements, and electrolyte infusion. Education: role of proper pace of refeeding in someone who has been starving recently.

Monitoring and Evaluation: Monitor labs 2–3 times daily until labs improve (potassium, magnesium, calcium, and phosphate). Evaluate readiness for ventilator weaning after intake is managed and gradually increased over 14–21 days. Monitor for improvements in weight and BMI.

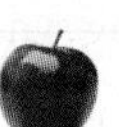

FOOD AND NUTRITION

Refeeding an Adult

- Avoid malnutrition—intervene early and use D5 (5% dextrose) with any saline infusion when patients are designated NPO or are on limited diets for procedures/surgery (Parrish, 2009).
- Start patients at 15–20 cal/kg for the first 3 days, but also start enteral nutrition or total parenteral nutrition at low infusion rates (Parrish, 2009). Feeding can be gradually increased and be up to desired levels by day 7.
- Protein should be started slowly (1.2 g/kg actual weight) and increased gradually to 1.5 g/kg to protect and restore some lean body mass.
- At first, restrict carbohydrate (CHO) intake to 150–200 g/d to prevent a rapid insulin surge. CHO in parenteral nutrition (PN) should be initiated at 2 mg/kg/min (about 150–200 mg/d). Provide insulin as needed to keep blood glucose within a normal range and to protect nutritional stores.
- Fat calories should make up the difference.
- Refeeding results in expansion of the extracellular space, and fluid must be given carefully during the first few days to weeks of refeeding. Weight gain greater than 1 kilogram in the first week is due to fluid retention. Fluid may need to be restricted to 800 to 1000 cc/d. Increases in blood pressure, heart rate, and respiratory rate may be early signs of fluid excess. Adjust when edema exists (e.g., fluid restriction according to I & O, tachycardia, peripheral edema).
- Rather than using boluses of potassium, phosphate, and magnesium via the enteral access, intravenous replacement can be slower and better tolerated (Parrish, 2009).

- Adjust electrolytes depending on laboratory values. Sodium must be given carefully to prevent overexpansion of the extracellular fluid. Additional phosphorus is required; 250–500 mg/d for up to 5–7 days may be needed to replenish. Potassium serum levels should be in the high normal range with 80 to 120 mEq/d needed.
- Magnesium and thiamin should also be given. Supplement with other vitamins and minerals as needed. Excesses are not required.

Refeeding a Child (Tips from the World Health Organization)

- Refeeding in a child should be through oral or tube feeding, not intravenous feedings. Use 100 kcal/kg actual weight; protein as 1–1.5 g/kg; 100–130 ml/g fluid daily. Breastfeeding may continue, but formula may be given first.
- Starter formula may be made with 300 milliliters of cow's milk, 100 grams of sugar, 20 milliliters of oil, 20 milliliters of electrolyte/mineral solution, and water to make 1000 milliliters. Feed the child every 2 hours at first, gradually decreasing to every 3 hours over the first week. If intake does not reach the 80 kcal/kg goal, then night tube feeding may be needed.
- Return of an appetite is often a first sign that the rehabilitative phase has begun; this may take a week. Continue a gradual increase to avoid heart failure. Increase each feed by 10 milliliters until some remains uneaten, usually around intakes of 200 ml/kg/d.
- After a gradual transition, give frequent feeds with unlimited amounts; 150–220 kcal/kg/d and 4–6 g/kg/d of protein are reasonable estimates. Catch-up formula can be made using 880 milliliters of milk, 75 grams of sugar, 20 milliliters of oil, 20 milliliters of electrolyte/mineral solution, and water to make 1000 milliliters.
- Sensory stimulation and emotional support is also a part of the therapy, so there is a need to provide tender loving care and a cheerful, stimulating environment. Structured play therapy for 15–30 minutes a day and physical activity as soon as the child is well enough are also important.
- The World Health Organization promotes healthy pregnancy in order to avoid chronic disease later in life (WHO, 2009). There is an association between low growth in the first year and an increased risk of CHD. Blood pressure has been found to be highest in those with retarded fetal growth and greater weight gain in infancy.
- Studies of children and health risk have found that the thinnest children, if they became obese as adults, have a greater risk of developing chronic diseases (WHO, 2009). With anorexia nervosa, short stature, osteoporosis, and infertility may be long-lasting complications (Usdan et al, 2008). Short stature may be associated with an increased risk of CHD, stroke, and even diabetes.

Common Drugs Used and Potential Side Effects

- Replacement of phosphorus, potassium, and magnesium may be needed if serum levels are depleted. ORS is responsible for saving the lives of millions of children worldwide; it is an inexpensive solution of sodium and glucose used to treat acute diarrhea.
- Monitor specific medications used and their side effects (e.g., gastrointestinal distress).
- Insulin is used to correct hyperglycemia levels. Monitor blood glucose levels as refeeding occurs.
- In clinical practice, it is not uncommon to give patients a 100-mg thiamine bolus daily for 3 days when they are at risk for refeeding syndrome (Francini-Pesenti, 2009; Parrish, 2009). Give the other B-complex and vitamins as well (Mehanna et al, 2009).
- Advances in leptin, ghrelin, and endocannabinoid systems may provide therapeutic breakthroughs. Ghrelin facilitates nutritional restoration and lowering serum leptin may be needed to avoid RFA (Stoving et al, 2009).

Herbs, Botanicals, and Supplements

- Herbs and botanical supplements should not be used without discussing it with the physician.

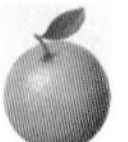

NUTRITION EDUCATION, COUNSELING, CARE MANAGEMENT

- Provide nutrition education to focus on adequate nutrient intake.
- Consider referral if food insecurity is a concern.
- Offer guidelines according to a discharge intervention plan for use at home or elsewhere. The physician may suggest long-term medication use or therapies.
- Encourage research in this area since evidence is lacking (Mehanna et al, 2009).

Patient Education—Food Safety

There are no specific food handling techniques that are unique to malnutrition. However, use of tube feeding or CPN at home warrants training to prevent infections.

For More Information

- Critical Care Tutorials
  http://www.ccmtutorials.com/
- Hypophosphatemia
  http://emedicine.medscape.com/article/767955-overview
- Refeeding Syndrome
  http://www.ccmtutorials.com/misc/phosphate/page_07.htm

REFEEDING SYNDROME—CITED REFERENCES

Francini-Pesenti F, et al. Wernicke's syndrome during parenteral feeding: not an unusual complication. *Nutrition.* 25:142, 2009.

Gariballa S. Refeeding syndrome: a potentially fatal condition but remains underdiagnosed and undertreated. *Nutrition.* 24:604, 2008.

Marinella MA. Refeeding syndrome: an important aspect of supportive oncology. *J Support Oncol.* 7:11, 2009.

Mehanna H, et al. Refeeding syndrome–awareness, prevention and management. *Head Neck Oncol.* 1:4, 2009.

Miller SJ. Death resulting from overzealous total parenteral nutrition: the refeeding syndrome revisited. *Nutr Clin Pract.* 23:166, 2008.

Parrish C. Peer viewpoint: the refeeding syndrome in 2009: prevention is the key to treatment. *J Support Oncol.* 7:21, 2009.

Stoving RK, et al. Leptin, ghrelin, and endocannabinoids: potential therapeutic targets in anorexia nervosa. *J Psychiatr Res.* 43:671, 2009.

Usdan LS, et al. The endocrinopathies of anorexia nervosa. *Endocr Pract.* 14:1055, 2008.

World Health Organization (WHO). Diet, nutrition and the prevention of chronic diseases. Accessed November 10, 2009 at http://www.who.int/hpr/NPH/docs/who_fao_expert_report.pdf.

SECTION 11

Musculo-Skeletal and Collagen Disorders

CHIEF ASSESSMENT FACTORS

- Actual Height, Measured Annually for Height Loss
- Arthritis—Warning Signs and Symptoms >2 Weeks: Early Morning Stiffness; Swelling in One or More Joints; Redness and Warmth in a Joint; Unexplained Weight Loss, Fever, or Weakness Combined with Joint Pain
- Bone Density Assessment
- Bone-Wasting Medications
- Contractures
- Easy Fatigue
- Edema
- Extremity Weakness
- Inflammation of Joints
- Movement Problems, Stiffness
- Pain in Muscles, Joints, Bones, Spine
- Psoriasis
- Unsteady Gait and Propensity to Fall
- Weight Loss, Anorexia, Depression, Insomnia
- Vitamin D_3 status (serum 25-OHD)

OVERVIEW—RHEUMATIC DISORDERS

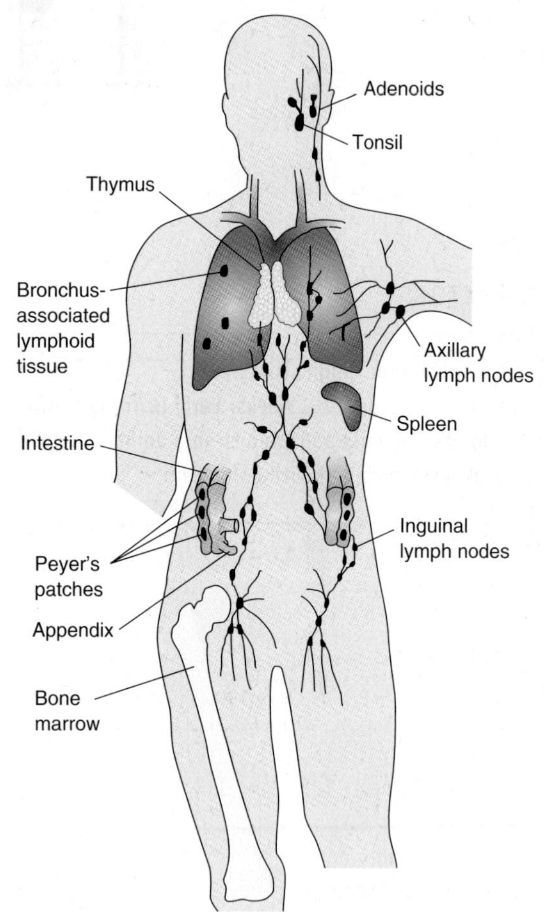

Adapted from: Porth CM. *Pathophysiology: Concepts of altered health states,* 5th ed. Philadelphia: Lippincott Williams & Wilkins, 1998.

TABLE 11-1 Autoimmune Rheumatic Disorders[a]

Blood and blood vessels	Lupus
	Polyarteritis nodosa
	Temporal arteritis and Polymyalgia rheumatica
Digestive tract and mouth	Scleroderma
	Sjögren's syndrome
Eyes	Sjögren's syndrome
	Uveitis
Heart	Ankylosing spondylitis
	Lupus
	Rheumatic fever
	Scleroderma
Joints	Ankylosing spondylitis
	Lupus
	Osteoarthritis
	Rheumatoid arthritis
Kidneys	Gout
	Lupus
Lungs	Lupus
	Rheumatoid arthritis
	Scleroderma
Muscles	Polymyositis
Nerves and brain	Lupus
Skin	Lupus
	Scleroderma

[a]When the immune system does not work right, the immune cells can mistake the body's own cells as invaders and attack them; these are called autoimmune diseases. In this table a sample list of body systems affected by autoimmune rheumatic disorders. Adapted from: National Institutes of Health (NIH). NIH Publication No. 02-4858. Available at http://www.niams.nih.gov/hi/topics/autoimmune/autoimmunity.htm.

Some rheumatic diseases involve connective tissues and others may be caused by autoimmune disorders, where the body attacks its own healthy cells and tissues. See Table 11-1. Rheumatic disorders include osteoarthritis (OA), rheumatoid arthritis (RA), juvenile RA, bursitis, tendonitis, infectious arthritis, spondyloarthropathies, polymyositis, psoriatic arthritis, systemic lupus erythematosus, scleroderma, polymyalgia rheumatica, polyarthritis nodosa, giant cell arteritis, gout, and fibromyalgia. Typically, treatment of these disorders includes a rheumatologist who specializes in the treatment of disorders that affect joints, soft tissue, bones and connective tissues.

Arthritis represents a group of more than 100 different rheumatic diseases that cause stiffness, pain, swelling in the joints, muscles, ligaments, tendons or bones. Over 15% (40 million) of Americans have some form of arthritis. *Spondylosis* is OA of the spine. *Infectious arthritis* is caused by bacterial invasion spread from nearby joints following chickenpox, rubella, or mumps. Autoimmune disorders, Crohn's disease, and psoriasis may cause *seronegative arthritis. Mixed connective tissue disease* shows features of RA, cutaneous systemic sclerosis, inflammatory myopathies and Raynaud's syndrome.

Mast cells and basophils are involved in several inflammatory and immune events and are known to produce a broad spectrum of cytokines (Rasheed et al, 2009). The activation of nuclear transcription factor-κB is linked with arthritis, osteoporosis, and psoriasis. The cytokine tumor necrosis factor alpha (TNFα) plays a key role in chronic inflammatory and rheumatic diseases.

Early recognition and treatment of these disorders are important. RA, juvenile idiopathic arthritis, the seronegative spondyloarthropathies, and lupus may have skeletal pathology (Walsh et al, 2005) and an inflammatory atherosclerosis. A multidisciplinary, multipronged approach is best. Physical and occupational therapies are beneficial for maintaining as much independence as possible in these conditions.

Most rheumatic conditions are managed by use of nonsteroidal anti-inflammatory drugs (NSAIDs) and TNFα antagonists. Etanercept, infliximab, and adalimumab significantly reduce symptoms and improve both functionality and quality of life (Braun et al, 2006; Nash and Florin, 2005). Fortunately, research is on-going for the autoimmune diseases. Gene profiling is helpful, especially in pediatrics (Jarvis, 2005). Osteoimmunology is a new branch of medical science, and anti-inflammatory therapies promise new treatments.

Role of Inflammation and Fatty Acids

Excessive and inappropriate inflammation contributes to acute and chronic human diseases. It is characterized by the production of inflammatory cytokines, arachidonic

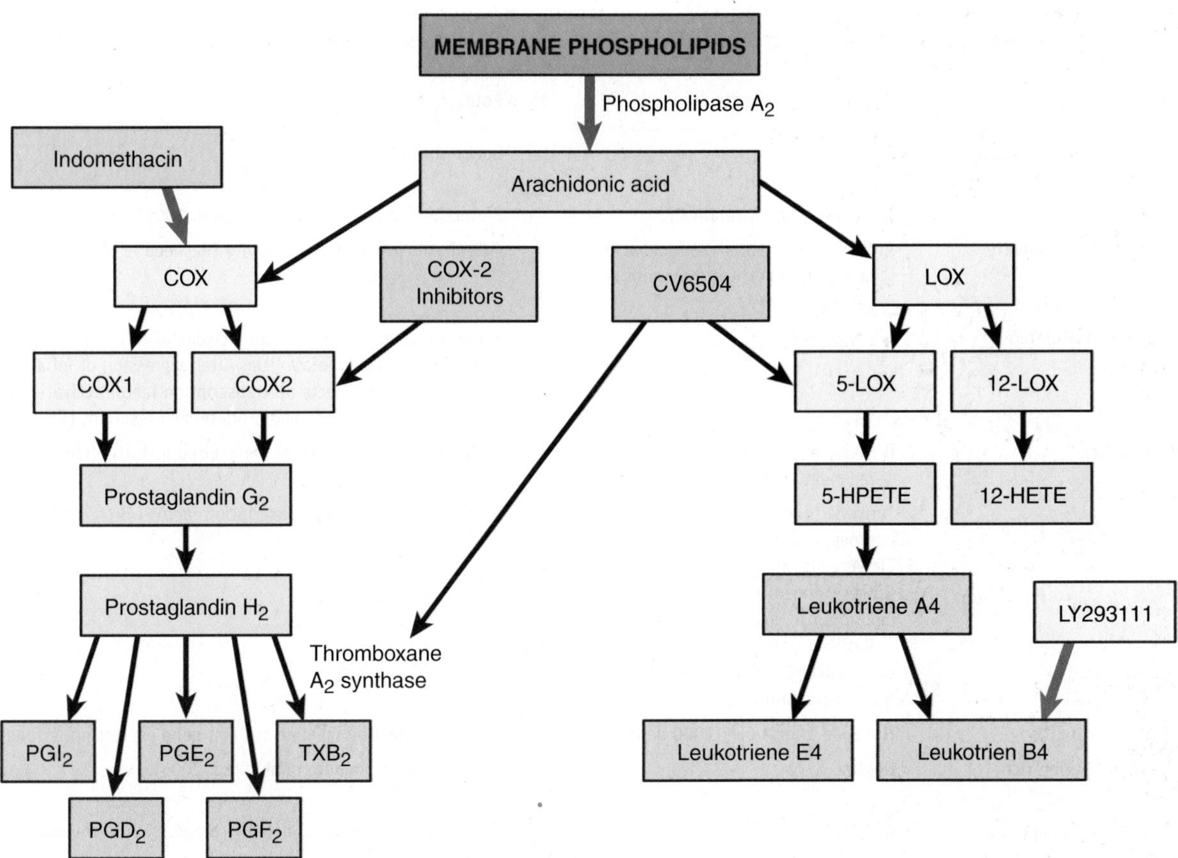

acid-derived eicosanoids (prostaglandins, thromboxanes, leukotrienes, and other oxidized derivatives), other inflammatory agents (e.g., reactive oxygen species), and adhesion molecules (Calder, 2006). Three major types of omega-3 fatty acids are ingested in foods: alpha linolenic acid (ALA), eicosapentaenoic acid (EPA), and docosahexaenoic acid (DHA). The body converts ALA to EPA and DHA, which are readily used by the body. Omega-3 fatty acids help reduce inflammation, while omega-6 fatty acids tend to promote inflammation. The precursor ALA does not appear to exert anti-inflammatory effects at achievable intakes (Calder, 2006).

A balance between omega-3 and omega-6 fatty acids in the diet is needed. The proper balance helps maintain and even improve health; one to four times more omega-6 fatty acids than omega-3 fatty acids is desirable, yet people who follow a Western diet consume a higher percentage of omega-6 fatty acids than they should.

Long-chain omega-3 polyunsaturated fatty acids (PUFAs) act by replacing arachidonic acid as an eicosanoid substrate, inhibiting arachidonic acid metabolism; by altering the expression of inflammatory genes through effects on transcription factor activation; and by leading to anti-inflammatory mediators known as resolvins (Calder, 2006).

Role of Phytochemicals and Total Diet

Phytochemicals known for their ability to protect tissue also appear to block the activity of an enzyme that triggers inflammation in joints. See Table 11-2.

Complementary and Alternative Medicine (CAM) Therapies

Controlled scientific studies of many patients can prove that a particular treatment is beneficial or that an apparent improvement is incidental. The important consideration is that treatment should do no harm.

Some studies have been done in alternative therapies, particularly diet in the treatment of arthritis, but none have shown any real long-term benefit. Patients often do benefit from complementary therapies, either because the treatment truly works or because of psychological (placebo) effects. While there is evidence of benefit for vitamin C, vitamin D, and nutraceuticals such as glucosamine, chondroitin, *S*-adenosylmethionine, ginger, and avocado/soybean unsaponifiables (McAlindon, 2006), specific diets and herbal or botanical products should only be used with medical consultation.

While the best nutrition-based strategy for promoting optimal health and reducing the risk of chronic disease is to wisely choose a wide variety of foods, additional nutrients from supplements can help some people meet their nutrition needs (American Dietetic Association, 2009). Physicians reported familiarity with acupuncture (80%), yoga (74%), and Tai-Chi (72%) yet almost all of their patients use CAM therapies (Mak et al, 2009). It is logical, then, that dietetics practitioners must keep up to date on the efficacy, safety, and the regulatory issues in order to provide the best advice.

TABLE 11-2 Phytochemicals and Dietary Factors Affecting Rheumatic Disorders

Component	Foods or Ingredients	Role
Cruciferous vegetables: broccoli, cauliflower, cabbage, bok choy	Sulforaphane	Boost phase 2 enzymes
Dairy products, low fat	To be identified; vitamin D?	Protective factors against gout (Choi, 2005).
Fruits: pomegranate, cranberry	Anthocyanins, tannins; ellagic acid; resverarol; quercetin; vitamins A, C; selenium	Potent anti-inflammatory activity (Rasheed et al, 2009).
Long-chain polyunsaturated fatty acids	EPA and DHA	Replace arachidonic acid as an eicosanoid substrate, inhibiting arachidonic acid metabolism. Alter expression of inflammatory genes through effects on transcription factor activation, leading to anti-inflammatory mediators termed resolvins (Calder, 2006).
Mediterranean diet	Resveratrol, olive oil, lower intake of red meat	Protects against severity of rheumatoid arthritis (Choi, 2005).
Spices	Turmeric (curcumin) Red pepper (capsaicin) Cloves (eugenol) Ginger (gingerol) Cumin, anise, and fennel (anethol) Basil, rosemary (ursolic acid) Garlic (diallyl sulfide, ajoene, *S*-allylmercaptocysteine)	Interrupts pathway for transcription factor-κB (Aggarwal and Shishodia, 2004).
Vitamin D	Hormone affects over 2000 genes	Needed for healthy immune system, gene expression, strong bones.
Total protein and purine-rich vegetables	Neutral	Do not tend to promote gout (Choi, 2005).
Vitamin E, beta-carotene, and retinol.	Neutral	Have NOT been shown to halt the progression of rheumatic disorders
Red meats, seafood, beer, and liquor	Undesirable	Tend to promote symptoms of gout, inflammatory polyarthritis, or rheumatoid arthritis (Choi, 2005).

Sources: Aggarwal BB, Shishodia S. Suppression of the nuclear factor-kappa B activation pathway by spice-derived phytochemicals: reasoning for seasoning. *Ann N Y Acad Sci.* 1030:434, 2004.

RHEUMATIC DISORDERS—CITED REFERENCES

Aggarwal BB, Shishodia S. Suppression of the nuclear factor-kappa B activation pathway by spice-derived phytochemicals: reasoning for seasoning. *Ann N Y Acad Sci.* 1030:434, 2004.

American Dietetic Association. Position of the American Dietetic Association: Nutrient supplementation. *J Am Diet Assoc.* 109;2073, 2009.

Braun J, et al. First update of the international ASAS consensus statement for the use of anti-TNF agents in patients with ankylosing spondylitis. *Ann Rheum Dis.* 65:316, 2006.

Calder PC. Omega-3 polyunsaturated fatty acids, inflammation, and inflammatory diseases. *Am J Clin Nutr.* 83:1505S, 2006.

Choi HK. Dietary risk factors for rheumatic diseases. *Curr Opin Rheumatol.* 17:141, 2005.

Jarvis JN. Gene expression profiling in pediatric rheumatic disease: what have we learned? What can we learn? *Curr Opin Rheumatol.* 17:606, 2005.

Mak JC, et al. Perceptions and attitudes of rehabilitation medicine physicians on complementary and alternative medicine in Australia. *Intern Med J.* 39:164, 2009.

McAlindon TE. Nutraceuticals: do they work and when should we use them? *Baillieres Best Pract Res Clin Rheumatol.* 20:99, 2006.

Nash PT, Florin TH. Tumour necrosis factor inhibitors. *Med J Aust.* 183:205, 2005.

Rasheed Z, et al. Polyphenol-rich pomegranate fruit extract (POMx) suppresses PMACI-induced expression of pro-inflammatory cytokines by inhibiting the activation of MAP Kinases and NF-kappaB in human KU812 cells. *J Inflamm (Lond).* 6:1, 2009.

Walsh NC, et al. Rheumatic diseases: the effects of inflammation on bone. *Immunol Rev.* 208:228, 2005.

OVERVIEW—BONE DISORDERS

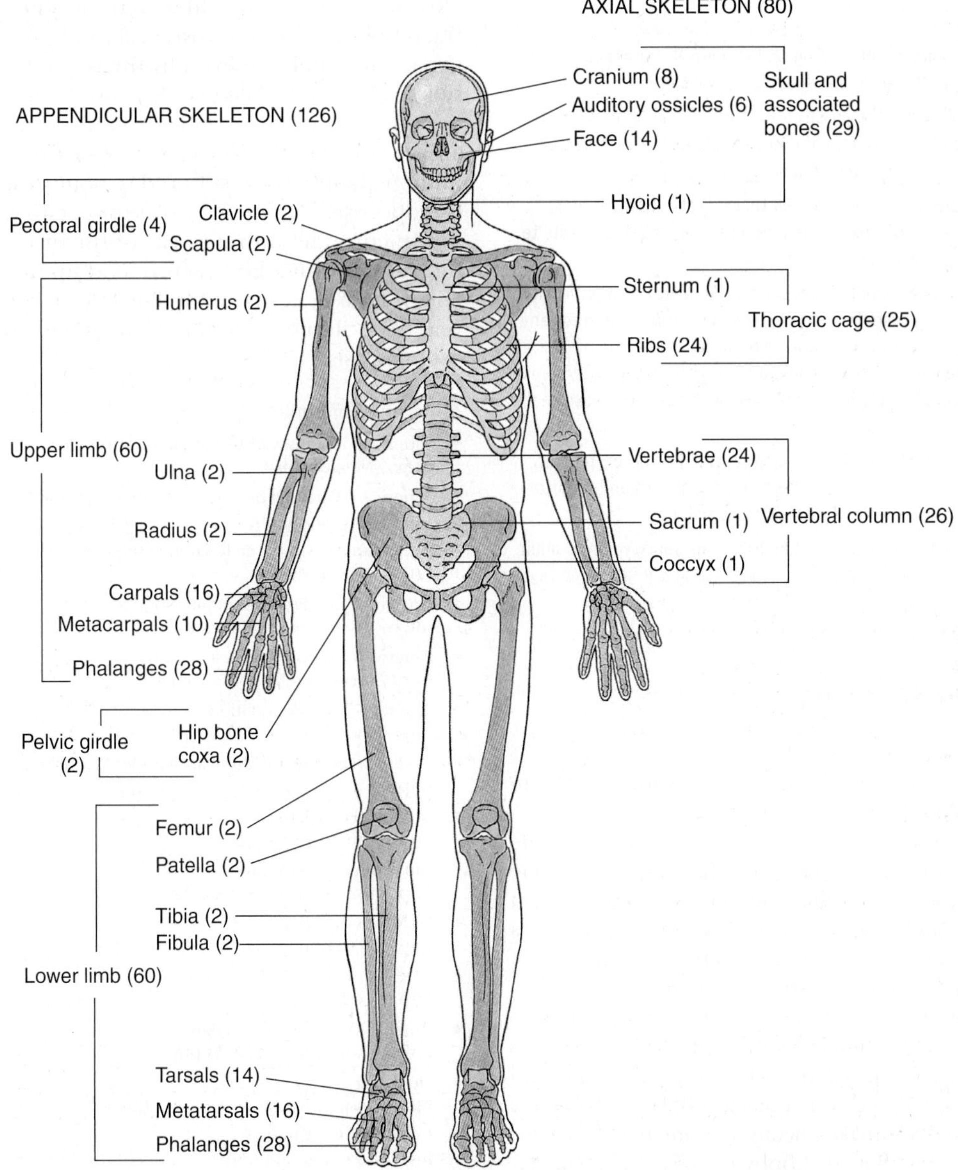

Adapted from: Moore KL, Agur AMR. *Essential Clinical Anatomy,* 2nd ed. Baltimore. Lippincott Williams & Wilkins

Bones are living, growing, and changing parts of the body. The human skeletal system consists of bones, cartilage, ligaments, and tendons and accounts for about 20% of the body weight. Osteoblasts are bone-forming cells, osteoclasts resorb or break down bone, and osteocytes are mature bone cells. The osteoblast is an endocrine cell type.

There is a reciprocal regulation of bone and energy metabolism by leptin and osteocalcin. Leptin inhibits insulin secretion by beta cells while osteocalcin favors it (Hinoi et al, 2009). Leptin deficiency leads to increased osteoblast activity and increased bone mass. Expression of the Esp gene, exclusive to osteoblasts, regulates glucose homeostasis and adiposity through controlling osteoblastic secretion of osteocalcin (Wolf, 2008). Osteocalcin deficiency leads to decreased insulin and adiponectin secretion, insulin resistance, higher serum glucose levels, and increased adiposity (Wolf, 2008). This recently understood concept has implications for diabetes and the metabolic syndrome.

There are 206 bones in the adult skeleton. The two types of bone tissue (compact and spongy) differ in density. Bone strength is derived from quantity (density and size) and quality (structure, consistency, and turnover). Bone mass is dependent upon individual genetic background. Adequate nutrient intake is needed from birth to achieve maximal bone mass and to prevent osteoporosis later in life.

The trace elements, calcium and phosphorus, are involved in skeletal growth. Parathyroid hormone (PTH) regulates calcium and bone homeostasis; it is expressed in the placenta, regulates the placental expression of genes involved in calcium and other solute transfer, and may directly stimulate placental calcium transfer (Simmonds et al, 2010).

Magnesium and fluoride are matrix constituents while zinc, copper and manganese are components of enzymatic systems involved in matrix turnover. A sufficient protein intake, along with adequate calcium, supports stronger

TABLE 11-3 Recommendations for Prevention of Osteoporosis

Get the recommended amounts of calcium and vitamin D_3 for age and sex; use supplements when diets are inadequate.

Maintain a healthy weight and be physically active 30+ minutes a day for adults and 60+ minutes a day for children, including weight-bearing activities to improve strength and balance.

Minimize the risk of falls by removing items that might cause tripping, improving lighting, and encouraging regular exercise and vision tests to improve balance and coordination.

Risks for patients of all ages should be evaluated by health care professionals. Obtain bone density tests for women over the age of 65 and for any man or woman who suffers even a minor fracture after the age of 50. "Red flags" for someone is at risk include a history of multiple fractures, those who take certain medications, and those who have a disease that can lead to bone loss.

A BMD test is used to detect osteoporosis before fractures occur, predict chances of future fractures, or determine rate of bone loss and monitor the effects of treatment. The DEXA scan is most common.

- Normal BMD: within 1 standard deviation (SD) of a "young normal" adult.
- Low bone mass (osteopenia): BMD is between 1 and 2.5 SD below that of a "young normal" adult.
- Osteoporosis: BMD is 2.5 SD or more below that of a "young normal" adult.

bone density; this fact contradicts past suggestions that high-protein diets deplete bone strength.

Changes in bone turnover markers may become accurate predictors of fracture risk. Assessing risk factors for low bone mass is important in monitoring the etiology of fracture in older individuals (Kelsey et al, 2006). In general, women's bone health has been studied more extensively than that of men. Studies on the predictors of fractures in men are needed, such as bone architecture, morphology, biochemical markers of bone turnover, and hormonal levels (Szulc et al, 2005).

Vitamins are important. Vitamin D_3 plays a role in calcium metabolism. Vitamins C and K are cofactors of key enzymes for skeletal metabolism. Another indicator of bone health is heart health. There are similar pathophysiological mechanisms underlying cardiovascular disease (such as dyslipidemia, oxidative stress, inflammation, hyperhomocysteinemia, hypertension, and diabetes) and low bone mineral density (BMD). Sufficient folic acid, vitamins B_6 and B_{12} can help improve bone health by lowering elevated homocysteine levels. Antioxidant nutrients, including vitamins A and C and selenium, play a role in bone health.

While calcium is widely recognized for bone health, other minerals are equally important. Iron promotes production of collagen in bone structure; 18 mg is most protective for women but balance is also critical as too much iron may throw off calcium balance. Finally, silicon in the form of choline-stabilized orthosilicic acid is the bioavailable form that enhances calcium and vitamin D_3 in bone health.

Omega-3 fatty acids such as EPA help increase levels of calcium in the body, deposit calcium in the bones, and improve bone strength. People who are deficient in EFAs EPA and gamma linolenic acid (GLA) are more prone to bone loss.

Former U.S. Surgeon General Richard H. Carmona (2005) warned in a landmark report that, by 2020, half of all American citizens older than 50 would be at risk for fractures from osteoporosis and low bone mass if immediate action is delayed by individuals at risk, doctors, health systems, or policymakers. At least 10 million Americans over the age of 50 have osteoporosis, another 34 million are at risk for developing osteoporosis, and roughly 1.5 million people have suffered a bone fracture related to osteoporosis. About 20% of senior citizens who suffer a hip fracture die within a year of fracture; another 20% of individuals with a hip fracture end up in a nursing home. Hip fractures account for 300,000 hospitalizations each year. See Table 11-3 for recommendations to prevent osteoporosis.

For More Information

- American Academy of Orthopaedic Surgeons
  http://www.aaos.org/
- American Academy of Physical Medicine and Rehabilitation
  http://www.aapmr.org
- American Autoimmune-Related Diseases Association (AARDA)
  http://www.aarda.org/
- American College of Rheumatology
  http://www.rheumatology.org/
- American Osteopathic Association
  http://www.do-online.osteotech.org/
- American Pain Foundation
  http://www.painfoundation.org/
- American Society for Bone and Mineral Research
  http://www.asbmr.org/
- Arthritis Foundation
  http://www.arthritis.org/
- Autoimmunity Resources
  http://www.aarda.org/links.php
- CAM Therapy Resources
  http://nccam.nih.gov/health/bydisease.htm
- CDC—Calcium for Bone Health
  http://www.cdc.gov/nutrition/everyone/basics/vitamins/calcium.html
- Clinical Trials Research Trials
  http://www.aarda.org/links.php
- Drug List
  http://www.rxlist.com/alternative.htm
- Journal of Immunology
  http://www.jimmunol.org/
- National Institute of Arthritis and Musculoskeletal and Skin Disorders
  http://www.niams.nih.gov/hi/index.htm
- Quack Watch for Unproven Remedies
  http://www.quackwatch.com/
- Rheumatic Diseases Internet Journal
  http://www.rheuma21st.com/

BONE DISORDERS—CITED REFERENCES

Hinoi E, et al. An osteoblast-dependent mechanism contributes to the leptin regulation of insulin secretion. *Ann N Y Acad Sci.* 1173:20S, 2009.

Kelsey JL, et al. Risk factors for fracture of the shafts of the tibia and fibula in older individuals. *Osteoporos Int.* 17:143, 2006.

Simmonds CS, et al. Parathyroid hormone regulates fetal-placental mineral homeostasis [published online ahead of print September 23, 2009]. *J Bone Miner Res.* 25:594, 2010.

Szulc P, et al. Bone mineral density predicts osteoporotic fractures in elderly men: the MINOS study. *Osteoporos Int.* 16:1184, 2005.

Wolf G. Energy regulation by the skeleton. *Nutr Rev.* 66:229, 2008.

ANKYLOSING SPONDYLITIS (SPINAL ARTHRITIS)

NUTRITIONAL ACUITY RANKING: LEVEL 1

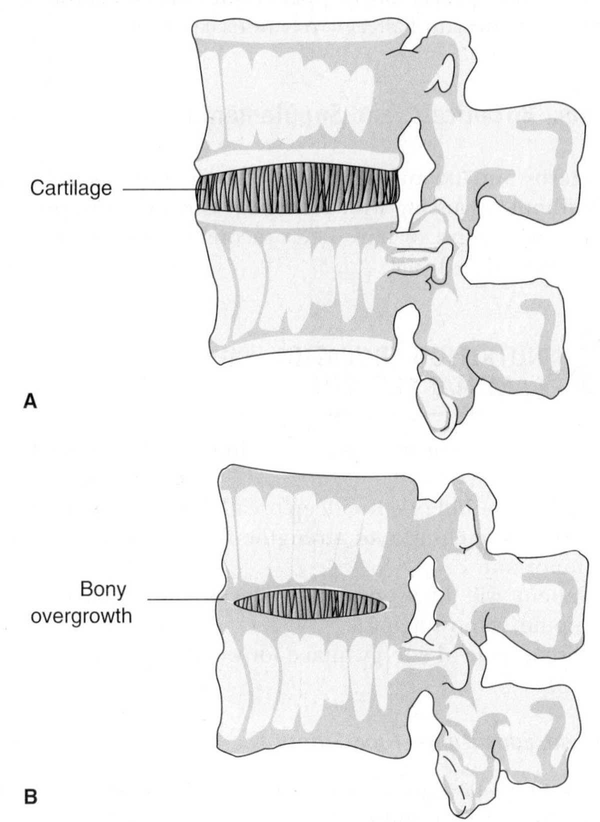

Carol Mattson Porth, *Pathophysiology Concepts of Altered Health States,* 7th ed. Philadelphia: Lippincott Williams & Wilkins, 2005.

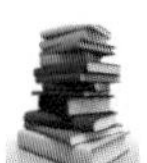

DEFINITIONS AND BACKGROUND

Among the 100 different rheumatic diseases that affect the joints and muscles is a group of five called **spondyloarthropathies**. These include ankylosing spondylitis, reactive arthritis (Reiter's syndrome), psoriatic arthritis or spondylitis, spondylitis of inflammatory bowel disease, and undifferentiated spondyloarthropathy. Spondylitis is inflammation of the joints linking the vertebrae (a fused spine is not uncommon). Spondylitis affects about 300,000 Americans and is more common in Caucasians than in African Americans. The condition is most common in men aged 16–35 years and may run in families.

In **ankylosing spondylitis**, inflammation of connective tissue recedes but leaves hardened and damaged joints that fuse together the bones of the spinal column. The sacroiliac joints generally are affected first. Symptoms and signs include chronic lower back pain, early morning stiffness in the lower back where the lower spine is joined to pelvis, vague chest pains, tender heels, weight loss, anemia, anorexia, slight fever, recurring iritis or reddened eyes, valvular heart disease. Pain may occasionally start in the knees and shoulders. There is a strong link between the bowel and the osteo-articular system, notably with the HLA-B27 gene where there are symptoms such as abnormal antigen presentation, the presence of autoantibodies against specific antigens shared by the colon and other extra-colonic tissues, increased intestinal permeability, osteoporosis and osteomalacia secondary to IBD (Rodriguez-Reyna et al, 2009).

Elevated tumor necrosis factor alpha (TNFα) is believed to be one of the causes of inflammation and bone destruction (Braun et al, 2006); therefore, anti-TNF therapy is effective (Barkham et al, 2005). Exercise to strengthen muscles that tend to cause pain on stooping or bending may be useful to relieve lower back pain. Attention to good posture will reduce some types of pain. Surgery may be needed to replace a joint or to relieve pain.

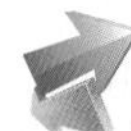

ASSESSMENT, MONITORING, AND EVALUATION

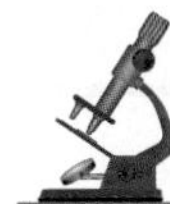

CLINICAL INDICATORS

Genetic Markers: Genetic marker HLA-B27 can be detected in these individuals.

Clinical/History

Height
Weight
Body mass index (BMI)
Weight changes
Anorexia
Fever?
Lower back pain
Pain in knees or shoulders
Iritis or reddened eyes
X-rays

Lab Work

HLA-B27 gene test (positive in 90%)
Erythrocyte sedimentation rate (ESR) (high)
C-reactive protein (CRP)
Ca^{++}, Mg^{++}
Na^{+}, K^{+}
Alkaline phosphatase (Alk phos)
Blood urea nitrogen (BUN)
Creatinine (Creat)
Phosphorus (P)
Hemoglobin and hematocrit (H & H)
Aspartate aminotransferase (AST)
Alanine aminotransferase (ALT)
Serum folate and B_{12}
Homocysteine levels
Vitamin D_3 status (serum 25-OHD)

INTERVENTION

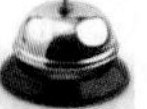

OBJECTIVES

- Reduce pain, inflammation, and disease activity; support improved functioning and ability to work or to maintain quality of life.
- Correct anorexia, nausea, poor intake or weight loss, anemia, or fever where present.

SAMPLE NUTRITION CARE PROCESS STEPS

Unintentional Weight Loss

Assessment: Loss of 15 lb this past 6 months, much pain and inflammation with ankylosing spondylitis, taking numerous medicines that cause GI distress and anorexia.

Nutrition Diagnosis (PES): *Unintentional weight loss* (NC-1.4) related to pain, inflammatory processes, and GI distress and evidenced by 15-lb unplanned weight loss in past 6 months.

Interventions:
Food and Nutrient Delivery: ND 1.2 Alter diet as tolerated. ND 32.3 and 32.4 Initiate vitamin and mineral supplementation.

Education: E-1.2 Discuss ways to increase energy and nutrient density in food choices.

Counseling: C 2.2 Agree to goal of consuming only nutrient-dense foods for the coming month until next visit. C-2.3 Keep a food diary for one month.

Monitoring and Evaluation: Review food diary after 1 month. Monitor weight for resolution of weight loss; goal is gain of 1–2 lb weekly.

- Improve ability to participate in physical activities of choice to maintain lean body mass.

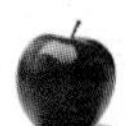

FOOD AND NUTRITION

- A normal diet is useful. Support gradual weight loss, if needed, to normalize weight. Some patients claim relief while using a vegetarian diet with less red meat.
- Preferred foods should be offered to stimulate appetite.
- Increase intake of foods rich in antioxidants such as vitamins E and C, selenium, and fish oils for rich sources of omega-3 fatty acids. Sufficient calcium and vitamin D are also important.
- Include phytochemicals derived from spices such as turmeric (curcumin); red pepper (capsaicin); cloves (eugenol); ginger (gingerol); cumin, anise, and fennel (anethol); basil and rosemary (ursolic acid); garlic (diallyl sulfide, *S*-allylmercaptocysteine, ajoene); and pomegranate (ellagic acid) (Aggarwal and Shishodia, 2004).

Common Drugs Used and Potential Side Effects

- Sulfasalazine, methotrexate, azathioprine, cyclosporine, leflunomide, and tumor necrosis factor-alpha blocking agents can be considered as first-line therapy but there are possible harmful effects on intestinal integrity, permeability, and even on gut inflammation (Rodriguez-Reyna et al, 2009).
- Etanercept (Enbrel), an anti-TNF therapy, may improve mobility and quality of life (Braun et al, 2006; Davis et al, 2005; Temel et al, 2005). Infliximab (Remicade), another monoclonal antibody, also targets TNFα and provides clinical improvement. Upper respiratory infections, psoriatic rashes, and allergic reactions can occur.

Herbs, Botanicals, and Supplements

- Herbs and botanical supplements should not be used without discussing with physician. Ginger, corn, pineapple, and pigweed have been recommended; no clinical trials prove efficacy.

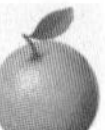

NUTRITION EDUCATION, COUNSELING, CARE MANAGEMENT

- Exercise is crucial, especially swimming, to relieve back pain.
- Patient should practice deep breathing exercises for pain relief. Stretching and strengthening exercises also are important.
- Patient will likely find that sleeping on a hard bed, supine, is most helpful.
- Discuss role of energy intake for weight control.

Patient Education—Food Safety

If enteral or parenteral nutrition is used, careful sanitation and handling techniques must be taught and used.

For More Information

- Ankylosing Spondylitis International Federation
http://www.asif.rheumanet.org/
- National Ankylosing Spondylitis Society (NASS)–United Kingdom
http://www.nass.co.uk/
- Spondylitis Association of America
http://www.spondylitis.org

ANKYLOSING SPONDYLITIS—CITED REFERENCES

Aggarwal BB, Shishodia S. Suppression of the nuclear factor-kappa B activation pathway by spice-derived phytochemicals: reasoning for seasoning. *Ann N Y Acad Sci.* 1030:434, 2004.

Barkham N, et al. The unmet need for anti-tumour necrosis factor (anti-TNF) therapy in ankylosing spondylitis. *Rheumatology (Oxford).* 44:1277, 2005.

Braun J, et al. First update of the International ASAS Consensus Statement for the use of anti-TNF agents in patients with ankylosing spondylitis. *Ann Rheum Dis.* 65:316, 2006.

Davis JC, et al. Reductions in health-related quality of life in patients with ankylosing spondylitis and improvements with etanercept therapy. *Arthritis Rheum.* 53:494, 2005.

Rodriguez-Reyna TS, et al. Rheumatic manifestations of inflammatory bowel disease. *World J Gastroenterol.* 15:5517, 2009.

Temel M, et al. A major subset of patients with ankylosing spondylitis followed up in tertiary clinical care require anti-tumour necrosis factor alpha biological treatments according to the current guidelines. *Ann Rheum Dis.* 64:1383, 2005.

GOUT

NUTRITIONAL ACUITY RANKING: LEVEL 2

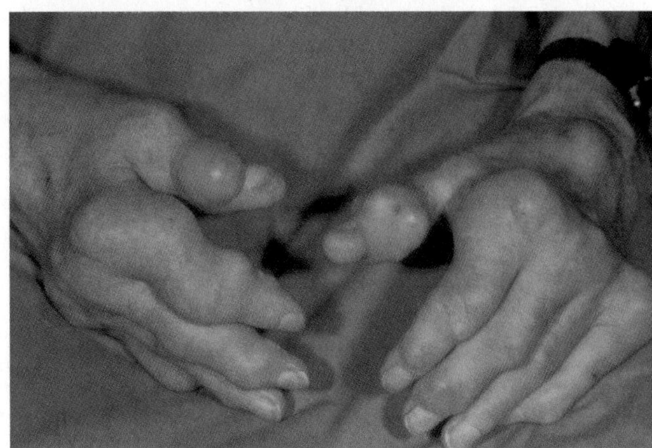

Adapted from: Rubin E MD and Farber JL MD. *Pathology,* 3rd ed. Philadelphia: Lippincott Williams & Wilkins, 1999.

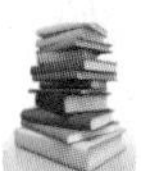

DEFINITIONS AND BACKGROUND

Uric acid is the end product of purine metabolism. Because humans have lost hepatic uricase activity, this leads to uniquely high serum uric acid concentrations when compared with other mammals. About 70% of daily urate disposal occurs via the kidneys; in 5–25% of the human population, impaired renal excretion leads to hyperuricemia.

Gout is a disorder of sudden and recurring attacks of painful arthritis with inflamed joints (usually the big toe, ankle, knees, and feet). Hyperuricemia promotes deposition of monosodium urate crystals in the joints and tendons. Gout affects more than 1% of adults in the United States and is the most common form of inflammatory arthritis among men (Saag and Choi, 2006). The disease tends to affect men between the ages of 30 and 50 years and is often hereditary.

Risks include genetic factors; high intake of seafood and red meats (Choi et al, 2005; Johnson et al, 2005) as well as beer and fructose (Doherty, 2009). Higher intakes of coffee, low-fat dairy products, and vitamin C are associated with lower risk (Doherty, 2009). See Table 11-4 for other etiologies of hyperuricemia. Gout prevalence increases in direct association with age, metabolic syndrome, hypertension, and use of thiazide diuretics (Saag and Choi, 2006). There is increased incidence in postmenopausal women, with polyarticular onset, hand involvement, and development of tophi (Ene-Stroescu and Gorbien, 2005). Tophi are hard lumps of urate crystals that are deposited under the skin around the joints and may be permanent.

Acute attacks may be triggered by surgery, sudden and severe illness, fasting, chemotherapy, or joint injury. Acute gout most commonly affects the first metatarsal joint of the foot, but other joints may also be involved. The joint swells, and skin turns warm, red, purplish, and shiny. Severe pain usually occurs, more so at night.

Gout progresses from asymptomatic hyperuricemia to acute gouty arthritis, intercritical gout (intervals between acute attacks), and finally to chronic tophaceous gout. Tophi may develop if the condition goes untreated. Although attacks of gout can subside in a few days, repeated attacks can cause permanent joint damage, and the disease often results in substantial disability and frequent medical care.

Treatment includes the pain-relieving NSAIDs and, for more serious outbreaks, corticosteroids. Most patients with gout eventually require long-term treatment with medications that lower blood uric acid levels. Patients with asymptomatic hyperuricemia should lower their urate levels by changes in diet or lifestyle.

TABLE 11-4 Acquired Causes of Hyperuricemia

Cause	Description
Increased urate production	
Nutritional	Excess ethanol or fructose intake
Hematological	Myeloproliferative and lymphoproliferative disorders, polycythemia
Drugs	Ethanol, cytotoxic drugs, vitamin B_{12} (treatment of pernicious anemia)
Miscellaneous	Obesity, psoriasis, hypertriglyceridemia
Decreased renal excretion of urate	
Drugs	Ethanol, cyclosporine (Sandimmune), thiazides, furosemide (Lasix) and other loop diuretics, ethambutol (Myambutol), pyrazinamide, aspirin(low-dose), levodopa (Larodopa), nicotinic acid (Nicolar)
Renal	Hypertension, polycystic kidney disease, chronic renal failure (any etiology)
Metabolic/endocrine	Dehydration, lactic acidosis, ketosis, hypothyroidism, hyperparathyroidism
Miscellaneous	Obesity, sarcoidosis, toxemia of pregnancy

Adapted from: Harris M, et al. Gout and hyperuricemia. *Am Fam Physician.* 59:925, 1999.

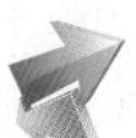

ASSESSMENT, MONITORING, AND EVALUATION

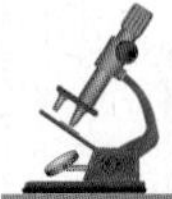

CLINICAL INDICATORS

Genetic Markers: About 10% of people with hyperuricemia develop gout. Genetic variants within the transporter gene, SLC2A9 (GLUT9), affect both fructose and uric acid transport. Other renal urate transporters have been identified, including URAT1.

Clinical/History

Height
Weight
BMI
Obesity
Swollen, painful big toe (podagra)
Arthritis
Urate crystals in urine
Use of thiazide diuretics?

Tophus, suspected or proven	Birefringent crystals in the synovial fluid	Ca^{++}, Mg^{++}
Asymmetrical swelling within a joint on X-ray	BUN (increased)	Na^{+}, K^{+}
Lab Work	Cholesterol (Chol)	Albumin (Alb)
CRP	Triglycerides (increased?)	Creat
Uric acid (increased)		Glucose (Gluc)
		AST, ALT
		Vitamin D_3 status (serum 25-OHD)

INTERVENTION

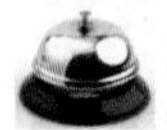

OBJECTIVES

- Lower bodily stores of uric acid crystal deposits to prevent the inflammatory processes and structural alterations. Increase excretion of urates and force fluid intake to prevent uric acid kidney stones.
- Data from NHANES III show a remarkably high prevalence of the metabolic syndrome among individuals with gout, along with an increased risk of myocardial infarction and cardiovascular mortality (Hak and Choi, 2008). Encourage lifestyle changes including reduction in energy intake, weight, alcohol intake, red meat intake.
- Promote gradual weight loss. In the obese, controlled weight management has the potential to lower serum urate (Schlesinger, 2005).
- Correct any existing dyslipidemia and prevent complications such as renal disease, hypertension, and stroke.

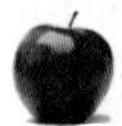

FOOD AND NUTRITION

- A low-fat, high-carbohydrate (CHO) diet increases excretion of urates. Vegetables such as peas, mushrooms, cauliflower, and spinach yield a protective effect (Choi, 2005).
- Develop a weight loss plan if needed.
- Avoid excessive intake of seafood such as anchovies, sardines, caviar, and herring. Reduce intake of beef, pork, duck, bacon, turkey, and ham.
- Ensure a high-fluid intake, especially water and skim milk. Nonfat milk, low-fat yogurt, dairy products, fruits such as cherries, and high intakes of vegetable protein may reduce serum urate (Schlesinger, 2005).
- Use of 4+ cups of coffee per day should be recommended (Choi and Curhan, 2007).
- Exclude alcoholic beverages (Schlesinger, 2005) and fructose or sugar-sweetened soft drinks (Choi et al, 2008).
- Use antioxidant-rich foods such as pomegranate, raspberries, and strawberries.

SAMPLE NUTRITION DIAGNOSES

Excessive Alcohol Intake

Assessment Data: Diet history and food records, medication history, alcohol and fluid intake.

Nutrition Diagnosis (PES): Excessive alcohol intake related to consuming large amounts of alcohol (36 oz whiskey daily) as evidenced by recent painful flare of gout with hyperuricemia.

Intervention: Food-nutrient delivery—Decrease alcohol intake (ND 3.3). Education: Discuss role of proteins, alcohol, diet, fluid intake, and medications in managing gout. Counseling: Motivational interviewing and goal setting with patient (C 2.1, 2.2) to implement recommended lifestyle modifications into daily plan.

Monitoring and Evaluation: Evaluation of alcohol intake records; improvement in symptoms of gout. Monitor need for additional education/counseling. Evaluate for decrease in uric acid levels and lower frequency of gouty attacks.

Common Drugs Used and Potential Side Effects

- Uricosuric drugs: Probenecid (Benemid) and sulfinpyrazone (Anturane) block renal absorption of urates. Serum uric acid levels should be kept below 360 μmol/L (6 mg/dL). Use adequate fluid.

  Anorexia, nausea, vomiting, and sore gums may result.
- The medication febuxostat (Uloric) shows promise.
- Xanthine oxidase inhibitors: Allopurinol (Aloprim) blocks uric acid formation. Adequate intake of fluid is needed. Mild gastrointestinal (GI) upset, taste changes, or diarrhea can occur; take after meals. Febuxostat is even more effective than allopurinol; side effects are transient (Schumacher, 2005).
- During more serious outbreaks, NSAIDs, colchicine (Colcrys), and corticosteroids (prednione) may be prescribed for short-term use.
- Medications that can increase uric acid levels include hydrochlorothiazide (a diuretic) and some transplantation medications (cyclosporine and tacrolimus). Monitor for signs of gout.

Herbs, Botanicals, and Supplements

- Herbs and botanical supplements should not be used without discussing with physician.
- Celery, avocado, turmeric, cat's claw, chiso, and devil's claw have been recommended; there are no clinical trials that prove efficacy.
- Vitamin C shows some effectiveness; 1000 mg may be beneficial in preventing gouty attacks (Gao et al, 2008).

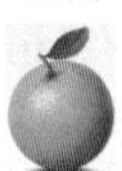

NUTRITION EDUCATION, COUNSELING, CARE MANAGEMENT

- The inflammatory response may be suppressed by omega-3 fatty acids from fish oils and from walnuts, flaxseed, and cherries. Use these foods several times a week.
- Alcohol, beef, sardines, anchovies, and pork may precipitate a gouty attack (Choi et al, 2005). Otherwise, there is little need for a traditional "low purine" diet (Hayman and Marcason, 2009).

- Weight loss may be helpful, but avoid fasting. Instruct patient to lose weight gradually.
- Discuss the importance of adequate fluid ingestion. Recommend coffee intake (Choi and Curhan, 2007). Avoid sugar-sweetened soft drinks and fructose, but diet soft drinks are acceptable (Choi et al, 2008; Hak and Choi, 2008).
- Aim to drink at least a half gallon of water and skim milk daily.

Patient Education—Food Safety

If enteral or parenteral nutrition is needed, sanitation and handwashing are essential.

For More Information

- American College of Rheumatology
  http://www.rheumatology.org/
- Arthritis–Gout
  http://www.arthritis.org/conditions/diseasecenter/gout.asp
- Diet for Gout
  http://www.gout.com/diet_gout/gout_friendly_foods.aspx
- Mayo Clinic—Gout
  http://www.mayoclinic.com/health/gout/DS00090/rss=1

GOUT—CITED REFERENCES

Choi HK. Dietary risk factors for rheumatic diseases. *Curr Opin Rheumatol.* 17:141, 2005.

Choi HK, et al. Intake of purine-rich foods, protein, and dairy products and relationship to serum levels of uric acid: the Third National Health and Nutrition Examination Survey. *Arthritis Rheum.* 52:283, 2005.

Choi HK, Curhan G. Coffee, tea, and caffeine consumption and serum uric acid level: the Third National Health and Nutrition Examination Survey. *Arthritis Rheum.* 57:816, 2007.

Choi JW, et al. Sugar-sweetened soft drinks, diet soft drinks, and serum uric acid level: the Third National Health and Nutrition Examination Survey. *Arthritis Rheum.* 59:1109, 2008.

Doherty M. New insights into the epidemiology of gout. *Rheumatology.* 48:2S, 2009.

Ene-Stroescu D, Gorbien MJ. Gouty arthritis. A primer on late-onset gout. *Geriatrics.* 60:24, 2005.

Gao X, et al. Vitamin C intake and serum uric acid concentration in men. *J Rheumatol.* 35:1853, 2008.

Hak AE, Choi HW. Lifestyle and gout. *Curr Opin Rheumatol.* 20:179, 2008.

Hayman S, Marcason W. Gout: is a purine-restricted diet still recommended? *J Am Diet Assoc.* 109:1652, 2009.

Johnson RJ, et al. Uric acid, evolution and primitive cultures. *Semin Nephrol.* 25:3, 2005.

Saag KG, Choi H. Epidemiology, risk factors, and lifestyle modifications for gout. *Arthritis Res Ther.* 8:2S, 2006.

Schlesinger N. Dietary factors and hyperuricaemia. *Curr Pharm Des.* 11:4133, 2005.

Schumacher HR Jr. Febuxostat: a non-purine, selective inhibitor of xanthine oxidase for the management of hyperuricaemia in patients with gout. *Expert Opin Invest Drugs.* 14:893, 2005.

IMMOBILIZATION

NUTRITIONAL ACUITY RANKING: LEVEL 2

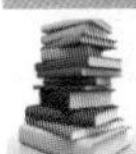

DEFINITIONS AND BACKGROUND

Extended periods of immobilization, for various reasons, may be nutritionally depleting. Patients with orthopedic injuries may lose 15–20 lb from stress, immobilization, trauma, and bed rest. Prolonged immobilization and nonuse of lower and upper limb muscles may cause atrophy. Nitrogen depletion can be extensive. A large nitrogen loss and high protein oxidation can be related to extensive injury and elevated energy expenditure.

Unloading of weight-bearing bones induced by immobilization has significant impacts on calcium and bone metabolism. Immobilization hypercalcemia involves nausea, vomiting, abdominal cramps, constipation, headache, and lethargy.

Persons with physical disabilities frequently are nonambulatory and have bone loss due to immobility. Prevention of osteoporosis and related fractures in this population includes calcium and vitamin D supplementation and risk-based screening. With careful attention to functional capacity enhancements, bone mass can be restored (Rittweger et al, 2005).

In older individuals, sarcopenia is the result of excessive loss of muscle mass and strength, loss of mobility, neuromuscular impairment, and balance failure. Falls and fractures can lead to immobilization, which induces more loss of muscle mass.

One final group at risk for the consequences of immobilization are those individuals who are in intensive care units (ICU) for a prolonged period. There is a need for physical therapy, as possible, to avoid a long recovery.

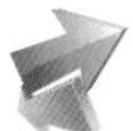

ASSESSMENT, MONITORING, AND EVALUATION

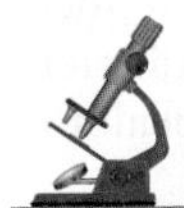

CLINICAL INDICATORS

Genetic Markers: Immobilization is usually from injury or other nongenetic causes, but may be a side effect of certain diseases with a genetic origin, such as spina bifida.

Clinical/History		Lab Work
Height or arm length/knee length	Dual-energy x-ray absorptiometry (DEXA)	H & H
Weight	Decreased range of motion?	Alb
BMI	Contractures; stiff joints?	Transthyretin, retinol-binding protein (RBP)
Weight changes	Blood clots	CRP
Triceps skinfold (TSF)	Pressure ulcers	Nitrogen (N) balance
Midarm muscle circumference (MAMC)	Constipation	Ca^{++} (increased?)
Midarm circumference (MAC)	Indigestion, anorexia?	Parathormone (PTH)
	Depression?	
	Change in quality of life?	

Urinary Ca^{++} (high?)	Alk phos	BUN, Creat
	Mg^{++}	Na^+, K^+
Vitamin D_3 status (serum 25-OHD)	Red blood cell (RBC) count	

INTERVENTION

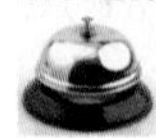

OBJECTIVES

- Correct negative nitrogen balance from increased losses (perhaps up to 2–3 g of nitrogen per day) to prevent pressure ulcers and infections. Moderate exercise is beneficial in altering the inflammatory milieu associated with immobility, and in improving muscle strength and physical function (Truong et al, 2009).
- Correct anorexia, indigestion, constipation.
- Prevent deossification and osteoporosis of bones. Prevent hypercalcemia from low serum levels of albumin, which normally binds calcium.
- Prevent kidney and bladder stones, urinary tract infections.
- Provide adequate fluid intake to aid excretion of nutrients.
- Prevent constipation, impactions, and obstruction.
- Prevent anemias that result from inadequate nitrogen balance.
- Prevent venous thrombosis (McManus et al, 2009).
- Improve or sustain a positive quality of life.

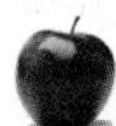

FOOD AND NUTRITION

- Diet should provide adequate intake of high–biological value proteins to correct nitrogen balance. An intake of 1.2 g protein/kg body weight is often recommended. Provide adequate energy to spare protein; use sufficient carbohydrates and fats, including 1–2% total kilocalories as essential fatty acids (EFAs).
- Encourage adequate intake of calcium since a high-protein diet raises the body's calcium requirements. Increased intake of phosphorus during the first few weeks may be useful.
- Diet should provide a high-fluid intake.
- Intake of vitamin C and zinc should be adequate to protect against skin breakdown.
- Diet should provide adequate amounts of fiber to prevent constipation. Avoid overuse of fiber in cases where there is impaction.

SAMPLE NUTRITION DIAGNOSES

Physical Inactivity

Assessment Data: Diet history, food records, medication history, fluid intake. New paraplegia following motorcycle accident.

Nutrition Diagnosis (PES): Physical inactivity (NB 2.1) related to paraplegia as evidenced by inability to walk voluntarily after motorcycle accident.

Intervention: Food-nutrient delivery—Offer food preferences to maintain desired intake; monitor calcium and protein intake in particular. Education: Discuss importance of physical therapy and nutrition in maintaining as much lean body mass as possible.

Monitoring and Evaluation: Evaluate ability to tolerate sufficient physical therapy to maintain adequate skin integrity, muscle mass, and urinary tract function; ability to achieve desirable nitrogen and calcium balance.

Common Drugs Used and Potential Side Effects

- Medications may be used to treat underlying conditions; they may have side effects that contribute to nutrient losses.
- Take pain medications as directed to maintain relief of pain, rather than only taking then when you feel very badly.
- Immobilization-induced hypercalcemia affects bone metabolism in Parkinson's disease; this inhibits secretion of PTH, which in turn suppresses 1,25-dihydroxyvitamin D production (Sato et al, 2005). These abnormalities may be corrected by the suppression of bone resorption with bisphosphonate; supplementations of calcium and vitamin D should be avoided in these patients (Sato et al, 2005).

Herbs, Botanicals, and Supplements

- Herbs and botanical supplements should not be used without discussing with physician.

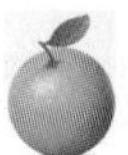

NUTRITION EDUCATION, COUNSELING, CARE MANAGEMENT

- Explain that calcium and nutrient intakes will have to be monitored for patients who will be tube fed or on a liquid diet for extended periods of time.
- Explain the need for adequate fiber and fluid (2–3 L) to prevent constipation, urinary tract infections, and so on. Early ambulation is the best treatment possible.
- Because prolonged bed rest in the ICU affects the development of ICU-acquired weakness, early mobility requires a reduction in heavy sedation and bed rest (Truong et al, 2009). Identify strengths and limitations, and alternate rest periods with activity. Do range of motion exercises every day.
- Monitor and report to a physician any symptoms such as pain and fatigue upon movement, new numbness in legs or arms, loss of motor strength, increased weakness, loss of bowel or bladder control, increased pain on movement.

Patient Education—Food Safety

If enteral or parenteral nutrition is needed, sanitation and handwashing are essential.

For More Information

- Family Care Research Program—Immobility and Movement
  http://www.cancercare.msu.edu/patients-caregivers/symptoms/immobility.htm
- Rehab Classworks
  http://www.rehabclassworks.com/mobility.htm

IMMOBILIZATION—CITED REFERENCES

McManus RA, et al. Thromboembolism. *Clin Evid (Online)*. 2009;pii: 0208.

Rittweger J, et al. Reconstruction of the anterior cruciate ligament with a patella-tendon-bone graft may lead to a permanent loss of bone mineral content due to decreased patellar tendon stiffness. *Med Hypotheses*. 64:1166, 2005.

Sato Y, et al. Abnormal bone and calcium metabolism in immobilized Parkinson's disease patients. *Mov Disord*. 20:1598, 2005.

Truong AD, et al. Bench-to-bedside review: mobilizing patients in the intensive care unit–from pathophysiology to clinical trials. *Crit Care*. 13:216, 2009.

LUPUS

NUTRITIONAL ACUITY RANKING: LEVEL 2

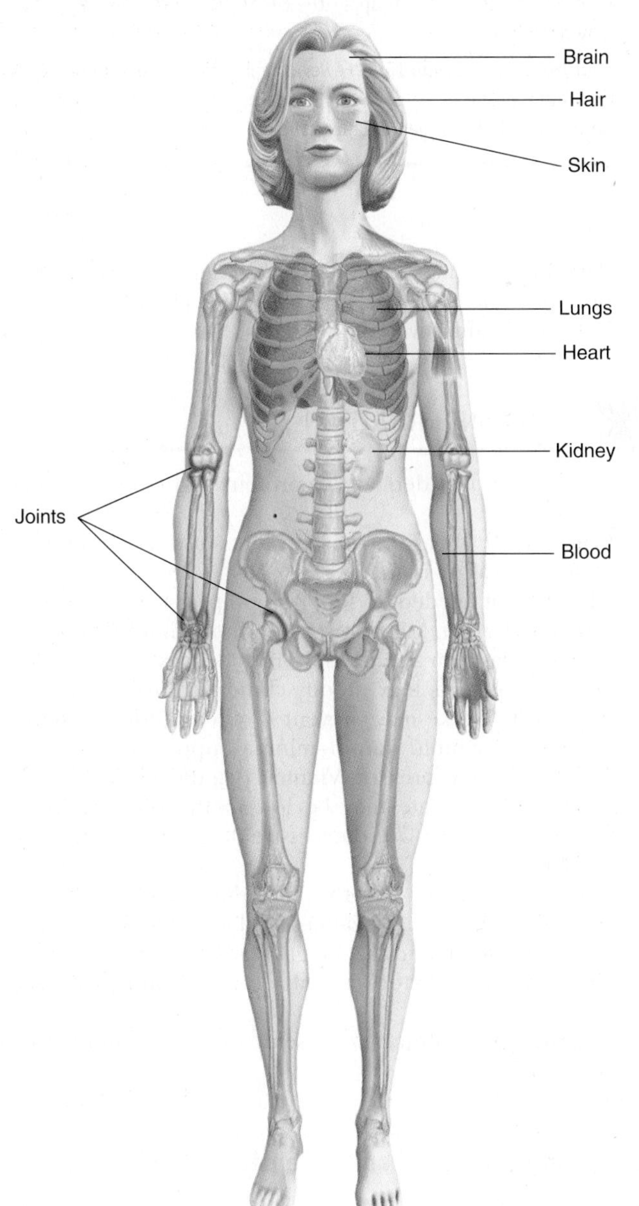

Asset provided by Anatomical Chart Co.

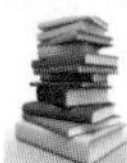

DEFINITIONS AND BACKGROUND

Lupus is an autoimmune disorder that involves areas of inflammation of the joints, tendons, other connective tissues, and skin. A pathologic CD4+T cell subset with impaired extracellular signal-regulated kinase (ERK) pathway signaling, DNA hypomethylation, and consequent aberrant gene expression contributes to disease pathogenesis (Gorelik and Richardson, 2010).

There are four types of lupus: neonatal, discoid, systemic, and drug induced. The systemic form (SLE) is the most common. One to two million people have lupus, especially Latino, African American, and Native American women, with onset in the late teens to thirties. For most people, lupus is a mild disease affecting only a few organs; for some, it may cause serious and even life-threatening problems. Because lupus has symptoms that mimic other disorders, careful diagnosis is important. Lupus may show symptoms similar to those of celiac disease.

Infections can bring on a lupus flare, increasing the risk of even more infections. Other environmental factors that may trigger the disease include antibiotics (especially sulfa and penicillin), other drugs, and exposure to phthalate in toys, plastics, and beauty products.

Active lupus contributes to coronary heart disease (CHD) risk (Haque et al, 2010). Premature cardiovascular disease in SLE patients is a consequence of inflammation. Type I interferons stimulate the cascade of atherosclerotic development, starting with endothelial damage and abnormal vascular repair (Von Feldt, 2008).

SLE is characterized by autoantibodies to nuclear antigens and immune complex deposition in organs such as the kidney (Gorelik and Richardson, 2010). Lupus nephritis is the term for this form of kidney disease that occurs. About a third of patients with lupus will develop it, requiring medical evaluation and nutritional management.

A cure for lupus is not yet possible, but treatments allow a more normal life. The use of methotrexate can reduce the dependency on steroids, which is desirable (Fortin et al, 2008). Antioxidant interventions have been studied extensively and show promise. Finally, supplementation with fish oil may reduce symptomatic disease activity.

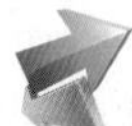

ASSESSMENT, MONITORING, AND EVALUATION

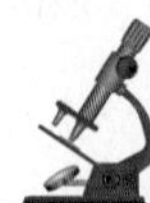

CLINICAL INDICATORS

Genetic Markers: Persons with close family members who have lupus have a 10 times greater frequency than the general population. Alleles in the TYK2 gene have been associated with SLE as well as multiple sclerosis.

Clinical/History

Height
Weight
BMI
BP
I & O
Fever over 100°F
Seizures and cognitive dysfunction
Butterfly rash across cheeks and nose
Skin rashes, red raised patches
Photosensitivity
Painless mouth or nose ulcers
Pale or purple fingers from cold or stress (Raynaud's syndrome)
Unusual hair loss
Pleuritis or pericarditis
Fatigue, prolonged
Achy joints (arthralgia)
Swollen and painful joints (nonerosive arthritis)
Protein or cellular casts in urine
Swollen ankles
Dry eyes
Easy bruising

Lab Work

LE prep
ESR or CRP (elevated?)
Complement protein test (C3, C4, CH50, CH100)
INR, abnormal blood clotting
Positive antinuclear antibody test (ANA)
Antibodies to double-stranded DNA
Serum copper (increased)
Total protein (decreased)
WBC (decreased)
Gluc (increased)
Low platelet count
H & H, serum ferritin (decreased)
Transferrin
Chol (increased)
BUN, Creat
Specific gravity, urine (decreased)
Alb, transthyretin
Transferrin
Ca^{++}, Mg^{++}
Na^{+}, K^{+}
Vitamin D_3 status (serum 25-OHD)

INTERVENTION

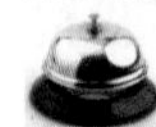

OBJECTIVES

- Counteract steroid therapy; replenish potassium and nutrient reserves.
- Reduce fever and replace nutrient losses and weight loss.
- Control disease manifestations.
- Manage cardiac effects. Accelerated atherosclerosis and premature CHD are recognized complications (Haque et al, 2010). Pericarditis is also common, with shortness of breath and chest pain.
- Rule out gluten intolerance.

> **SAMPLE NUTRITION CARE PROCESS STEPS**
>
> **Drug–Nutrient Interaction**
>
> ***Assessment Data:*** Weight and medical histories; medications; altered lab values for calcium, potassium. Complaints of swollen ankles and fluid retention.
>
> ***Nutrition Diagnosis (PES):*** Drug–nutrient interaction related to prolonged use of corticosteroids for lupus as evidenced by osteopenia, low serum calcium and potassium, negative nitrogen balance and sodium-fluid retention.
>
> ***Intervention:*** Food-nutrient delivery—Alter dietary intake to increase protein-rich foods, sources of potassium and calcium; decrease sodium intake. Education about the importance of managing specific nutrients while taking steroid medications (i.e., protein, calcium, potassium) and decreasing sodium-rich foods. Counseling about how to apply the DASH diet principles, which may be helpful.
>
> ***Monitoring and Evaluation:*** Fewer complaints of swollen ankles and fluid retention; improved lab values related to calcium, potassium, and nitrogen balance studies.

- Prevent or manage infections, such as urinary tract infections, shingles, respiratory infections such as colds, yeast infections, salmonella and herpes.

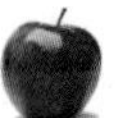

FOOD AND NUTRITION

- Diet should be adequate in protein and energy during fever.
- When renal disease is present, diet should be adjusted. Check lab values regularly.
- Alter diet, if needed, to lower blood pressure (BP) levels or excess weight. Mildly restrict sodium intake and monitor for potassium and phosphorus changes.
- Dietary nutrients may modify clinical course of disease. Vitamin C intake may prevent the occurrence of active disease; use a multivitamin–mineral supplement.
- Anemia is often present. Vitamin B_{12}, dietary fiber, iron, calcium, and folate may be low in the diets of lupus patients. However, avoid excessive doses of supplements; use DRI levels.
- Use a nutrient-rich diet that includes nuts, fish and fish oils, olive oil, fruits, vegetables, and whole grains that are rich in phytochemicals, omega-3 fatty acids, and antioxidants. Include phytochemicals derived from spices (see Table 11-2).
- If gluten intolerance is present, provide a gluten-free nutrition plan.

Common Drugs Used and Potential Side Effects

- Benlysta (belimumab), is a new drug developed specifically for people with systemic lupus. Many other drugs are in clinical trials.

- Steroid therapy may cause sodium retention, hyperglycemia, potassium and calcium depletion, and negative nitrogen balance. Side effects include weight gain, a round face, acne, easy bruising, fractures or osteoporosis, hypertension, cataracts, hyperglycemia or onset of diabetes, increased risk of infection, and stomach ulcers. Fish oil supplements may allow gradual reduction in use of steroids.
- Methotrexate (Rheumatrex) confers an advantage in participants with moderately active lupus by lowering daily prednisone dose and slightly decreasing lupus disease activity (Fortin et al 2008).
- Corticosteroid and cytotoxic drugs affect the immune system over time, making the individual prone to more infections. Immunosuppressive agents such as azathioprine (Imuran) and cyclophosphamide (Cytoxan) or methotrexate are used to control the overactive immune system but they have GI side effects.
- NSAIDs and acetaminophen may be useful.
- Sunscreens are needed to protect against the sun's harmful rays; there are no systemic side effects.
- Antimalarials, such as chloroquine (Aralen) or hydroxychloroquine (Plaquenil), may be used for skin and joint symptoms of lupus. Side effects are rare and consist of occasional diarrhea or rashes. Chloroquine can affect the eyes. Hydroxychloroquine may cause anorexia, nausea, abdominal cramps, and diarrhea.

Herbs, Botanicals, and Supplements

- Herbs and botanical supplements should not be used without discussing with physician.
- Coumestrol, a natural phytoestrogen, may relieve some symptoms.
- Use of indoles, conjugated linolenic acid (CLA), and vitamins C, E, and D may be beneficial.

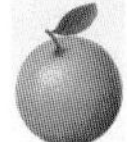

NUTRITION EDUCATION, COUNSELING, CARE MANAGEMENT

- Ensure patient has an adequate intake of fluids during febrile periods.
- Explain which foods are sources of sodium and potassium in the diet.
- Adequate rest is needed during flare-ups.
- Cortisone creams may be needed for persistent skin rashes. Sunblock should be used outdoors.
- Discuss how to manage diet for elevated blood glucose; insulin may be needed. Carbohydrate counting may be useful.
- Regular doctor visits and lab tests are important, especially blood and urine testing.
- Dietary strategies for the prevention of obesity, osteoporosis, and dyslipidemia deserve attention. Weight loss plans may be needed.

Patient Education—Food Safety

If enteral or parenteral nutrition is used, careful sanitation and handling techniques must be taught and used.

For More Information

- Lupus Alliance of America
  http://www.lupusalliance.org/
- Lupus Canada
  http://www.lupuscanada.org/
- Lupus Foundation of America
  http://www.lupus.org/
- Lupus Library
  http://www.lupusny.org/library.php
- Lupus Organizations
  http://www.lupusny.org/links.php#lupusorg
- SLE Foundation, Inc.
  http://www.lupusny.org/

LUPUS—CITED REFERENCES

Fortin PR, et al. Steroid-sparing effects of methotrexate in systemic lupus erythematosus: a double-blind, randomized, placebo-controlled trial. *Arthritis Rheum.* 59:1796, 2008.

Gorelik G, Richardson B. Key role of ERK pathway signaling in lupus [published online ahead of print December 7, 2009]. *Autoimmunity.* 37:322, 2010.

Haque S, et al. Risk Factors for Clinical Coronary Heart Disease in Systemic Lupus Erythematosus: The Lupus and Atherosclerosis Evaluation of Risk (LASER) Study [published online ahead of print December 1, 2009]. *J Rheumatol.* 37:322, 2010.

Tam LS, et al. Effects of vitamins C and E on oxidative stress markers and endothelial function in patients with systemic lupus erythematosus: a double blind, placebo controlled pilot study. *J Rheumatol.* 32:275, 2005.

Von Feldt JM. Premature atherosclerotic cardiovascular disease and systemic lupus erythematosus from bedside to bench. *Bull NYU Hosp Jt Dis.* 66:184, 2008.

MUSCULAR DYSTROPHY

NUTRITIONAL ACUITY RANKING: LEVEL 2

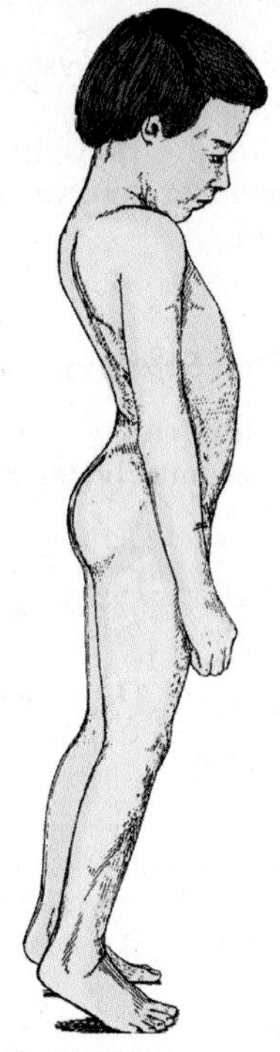

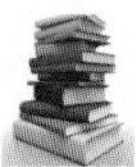

DEFINITIONS AND BACKGROUND

Actually a group of nine disorders, muscular dystrophy (MD) involves a hereditary condition with progressive degenerative changes in the muscle fibers, leading to weakness and atrophy. Most of the disorders are described in Table 11-5.

Muscular biopsy is required for the definitive diagnosis of the specific congenital type. BMI should be used with caution for the evaluation of the nutritional status of patients with Duchenne MD (DMD); assessment of the compartmental distribution of muscle and fat are more sensitive. Extremely elevated serum creatine kinase (CK) levels may indicate muscle disease. In the late stages, fat and connective tissue may replace muscle fibers.

Patients with MD may be prone to nutrient deficiency due to mobility limitations or oropharyngeal weakness (Motlagh et al, 2005). Micronutrient requirements are yet to be determined but, as a result of corticosteroid treatment, vitamin D and calcium should be supplemented (Davidson and Truby, 2009).

Many patients demonstrate inadequate nutrient intake of protein, energy, vitamins (especially E), and minerals (calcium, selenium, and magnesium), and significant correlations exist between measures of strength and copper and water-soluble vitamins (Motlagh et al, 2005).

Delayed growth, short stature, muscle wasting, and increased fat mass are characteristics that impact on nutritional status and energy requirements (Davidson and Truby, 2009). There may be loss of muscle mass, wasting, which may be hard to see because some types of MD cause a build-up of fat and connective tissue that makes the muscle appear larger (pseudohypertrophy).

Gene therapy, gene silencing, and cell therapy are potential therapies for MD patients. Some evidence exists supporting supplementation with creatine monohydrate to improve muscle strength (Davidson and Truby, 2009). Creatinine as a marker of renal function has limited value in DMD because of reduced muscle mass. There is potential value of cystatin C as a biomarker for monitoring renal function (Violett et al, 2009).

The prognosis of MD varies according to type and progression. Some cases may be mild and very slowly progressive, with a normal lifespan. Other cases may have more marked progression of muscle weakness, functional disability, and loss of ambulation. Life expectancy often depends on the degree of progression and late respiratory deficit. In DMD, death often occurs in the late teens or early twenties. Rehabilitation, orthopedic, respiratory, cardiovascular, gastroenterology, nutrition, pain issues, as well as general surgical and emergency-room considerations are essential to address (Bushby et al, 2010).

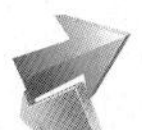

ASSESSMENT, MONITORING, AND EVALUATION

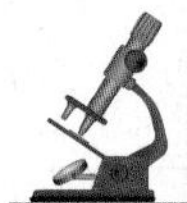

CLINICAL INDICATORS

Genetic Markers: Dystrophinopathies are due to a genetic defect of the protein dystrophin. Genetic counseling is advised when there is a family history of MD. Note that DMD can be detected by genetic studies performed during pregnancy.

Clinical/History

- Height
- Weight
- BMI (use only with other parameters)
- MAC, MAMC, TSF
- Muscle weakness
- Apparent lack of coordination
- Progressive crippling
- Scoliosis?
- Contractures of the muscles around the joints
- Clubfoot or clawhand?
- Hypotonia
- Loss of mobility
- Eyelid drooping (ptosis)
- Dysphagia?
- Drooling
- Chewing difficulty?
- Hand-to-mouth coordination
- Electromyography (EMG)
- Electrocardiography (ECG)
- DEXA

Lab Work

- Muscle biopsy
- Creatine phosphokinase (CPK), increased?
- Lactate dehydrogenase (LDH), increased
- Cystatin C
- Myoglobin-urine/serum
- Creat (often decreased)
- Aldolase, AST (altered)
- BUN
- N balance
- Alb, transthyretin
- CRP
- H & H, serum ferritin
- Serum P
- Gluc
- AST, ALT
- Ca^{++}, Mg^{++}
- Na^{+}, K^{+}
- Vitamin D_3 status (serum 25-OHD)

TABLE 11-5 Types of Muscular Dystrophy and Nutritional Implications

Type of MD	Comments	Nutritional Implications
Becker muscular dystrophy (BMD)	Very similar to DMD (see below), but onset is later (adolescence or adulthood). BMD patients live longer.	Weakness makes it difficult for self-feeding.
Congenital muscular dystrophy (CMD)	Caused by genetic mutations affecting some of the proteins necessary for muscles and some proteins related to the eyes and/or brain. Onset is at or near time of birth. Indicators include generalized muscle weakness with possible joint stiffness or looseness. Depending on the type, CMD may involve spinal curvature, respiratory insufficiency, mental retardation or learning disabilities, eye defects, and seizures.	Weakness makes it difficult for self-feeding.
Distal muscular dystrophy (DD)	DD is caused by a mutation in any of at least seven genes that affect proteins necessary to the function of muscles; it is usually passed on as an autosomal dominant or autosomal recessive trait. DD (Miyoshi form) first shows signs between ages 40 and 60 years, with weakness and muscle wasting of the hands, forearms, and lower legs; it progresses slowly.	Weakness and muscle wasting of the hands and forearms make self-feeding difficult.
Duchenne muscular dystrophy (DMD)	DMD primarily affects young boys, who inherit the disease through their mothers (X-linked recessive). Also called pseudohypertrophic. Caused by absence of dystrophin, a protein that helps keep muscle cells intact. DMD is the most severe form of dystrophinopathy. Aggressive forms appear in age 2–3, with frequent falls, difficulty in getting up from sitting or lying position. Generalized weakness and muscle wasting affect hip, thigh, shoulder, and trunk muscles first; large calf muscles. Weakness in lower leg muscles, resulting in difficulty running and jumping; waddling gait; mild mental retardation or scoliosis, in some cases. Survival is rare after the late twenties.	Facial muscles are involved; patient cannot suck, close lips, bite, chew, or swallow. DMD eventually affects all voluntary muscles, the heart, and lung muscles.
Emery-Dreyfus muscular dystrophy (EDMD)	EDMD is caused by gene mutations that produce emerin, lamin A, or lamin C, which are proteins in the membrane that surrounds the nucleus of each muscle cell. Onset in childhood, usually by age 10. Weakness and wasting of shoulder, upper arm, and shin muscles and joint deformities are common. Disease usually progresses slowly. Frequent cardiac complications are common, and a pacemaker may be needed.	Self-feeding becomes difficult.
Fascioscapulohumeral muscular dystrophy (FSHMD)	FSHMD (also called Landouzy-Dejerine) begins in childhood to early adulthood, with facial muscle weakness and weakness and wasting of the shoulders and upper arms. Caused by a missing piece of DNA on chromosome 4, it progresses slowly with some periods of rapid deterioration. Usually evident by age 20, it may span many decades. Inheritance is autosomal dominant, which means it can be passed on by either parent. It is considered to be the most common form.	Self-feeding becomes difficult; loss of skeletal muscle occurs. Abdominal muscles are affected.
Limb-girdle muscular dystrophy (LGMD)	LGMD is caused by a mutation in any of at least 15 different genes that affect proteins necessary for muscle function. LGMD has an onset in late childhood to middle age. Weakness and wasting affects shoulder and pelvic girdles first. Progression is slow, with cardiopulmonary complications often occurring in later stages of the disease. It is inherited as an autosomal recessive, autosomal dominant trait.	Self-feeding becomes difficult.
Myotonic dystrophy (MyD)	MyD (Steinert's disease) has onset anywhere from birth to middle age. Congenital myotonic form is more severe. Generalized weakness and muscle wasting affect the face, feet, hands, and neck first. Delayed relaxation of muscles after contraction. Progression is slow, sometimes spanning 50–60 years. Inheritance is autosomal dominant; there is a repeated section of DNA on either chromosome 19 or chromosome 3. Individuals with MyD have long faces and drooping eyelids; men have frontal baldness.	Progression is slow. Often complicated by diabetes. Prone to nutritional deficiencies from associated dysmotility of the entire GI. Handgrip is significantly lower; knee extension is higher compared to other dystrophies (Motlagh et al, 2005).
Oculopharyngeal muscular dystrophy (OPMD)	OPMD has onset in early adulthood to middle age. It affects muscles of eyelids (causing droopy eyelids) and throat. It progresses slowly, with swallowing problems common. Inheritance is autosomal dominant, and onset is usually in the fourth or fifth decade. The gene that is defective in OPMD is called the *poly(A) binding protein2* gene; extra amino acids in the protein made from the defective *PABP2* gene cause the protein to clump together in the muscle cell nuclei, interfering with cell function. OPMD can be diagnosed with a DNA test.	Swallowing difficulty is common. Tube feeding should be considered before wasting occurs.

From the Muscular Dystrophy Association, accessed November 16, 2009, at http://www.mdausa.org/publications/Quest/q65occup.html.

Type of CMD	Cause	Inheritance Pattern
Merosin-deficient CMD	Lack of merosin (laminin 2) or other defect leading to merosin deficiency	Chromosome 6 gene Other genes
Ullrich CMD	Abnormalities in collagen 6	Chromosome 2 or 21 genes, recessive or dominant
Bethlem myopathy	Abnormalities in collagen 6	Chromosome 2 or 21 genes, dominant
Integrin-deficient CMD	Lack of integrin alpha 7	Chromosome 12 gene, recessive
Fukuyama CMD (FCMD)	Lack of fukutin	Chromosome 9 gene, recessive
Muscle-eye-brain disease (MEB)	Lack of POMGnT1, fukutin or fukutin-related protein	Chromosome 1, 9, or 19 genes, recessive
Walker–Warburg syndrome (WWS)	Lack of POMT1, POMT2, fukutin or fukutin related protein	Chromosome 9, 14, or 19 genes, recessive
CMD with rigid spine syndrome	Lack of selenoprotein N1	Chromosome 1 gene, recessive

INTERVENTION

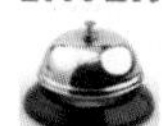

OBJECTIVES

- Encourage patient to lead a relatively active life; exercise programs can help prevent contractures.
- Prevent obesity, from inactivity; obesity complicates physical therapy.
- Encourage activities other than eating to prevent dependency on food as a source of pleasure.
- Malnutrition is a serious threat, especially with respiratory muscle weakness. Monitor nutritional intake and deficits on a regular basis. Prevent aspiration pneumonia or nasal regurgitation. Use a multidisciplinary approach, especially for feeding difficulties such as texture modification and supplemental feeding (Davidson and Truby, 2009).
- Avoid constipation because fecal impaction is frequent.
- Prevent osteoporosis and fractures, which can occur in this population.
- Manage long-term consequences, such as cardiomyopathy or respiratory failure.

SAMPLE NUTRITION CARE PROCESS STEPS

Abnormal GI Function—Constipation

Assessment Data: Weight and physical activity histories. Medical history, medications and lab values. Complaints of chronic constipation and GI discomfort. Diet hx showing low fiber and intake of <4 cups of fluid per day to avoid the need to urinate.

Nutrition Diagnosis (PES): Abnormal GI function related to constipation and physical inactivity as evidenced by infrequent evacuation, hard stools, and GI discomfort.

Intervention: Food and Nutrient Delivery—Increase fluid and fiber sources from tolerated foods such as whole grain cereals, fresh fruits, and vegetables. Educate about the desirable foods and fluid intake. Counsel about the importance of daily range of motion and physical exercises. Coordinate care with other disciplines according to needs, including PT, OT, nursing, medical team.

Monitoring and Evaluation: Alleviation of constipation. No further complaints of GI discomfort related to infrequent stooling pattern.

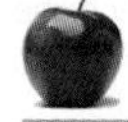

FOOD AND NUTRITION

- Work with the MyPyramid food guidance system as a basic guide. Check patient's BMI and adjust intake accordingly. Use a low-energy diet if necessary to control or lessen obesity. Some patients' requirements may be 30% lower than normal (Munn et al, 2005).
- Use foods that are easy to chew and swallow for DMD, such as pureed or blenderized foods. Tube feed only if necessary.
- Provide adequate fiber (prune juice, bran and other whole grains, fruits, and vegetables) if constipation becomes a problem.
- Ensure adequate intake of fluid to prevent fecal impaction, dehydration, and related effects.
- Adequate sodium chloride is important (Yoshida et al, 2006). Manage carefully if there are cardiac side effects or problems with BP.

Common Drugs Used and Potential Side Effects

- The myotonia (delayed relaxation of a muscle after a strong contraction) may be treated with medications such as phenytoin or quinine. Side effects can include folic acid depletion.

- Early introduction of steroids can exacerbate weight gain in a population already susceptible to obesity (Davidson and Truby, 2009).
- It may be useful to try beta$_2$-adrenergic agonists, which can increase muscle mass. Albuterol may be needed for some individuals prior to exercise and strength training.

Herbs, Botanicals, and Supplements

- Herbs and botanical supplements should not be used without discussing with physician.

Approximately 50% of children are on herbal preparations, 30% of adolescents take herbal medications, and 70% of adults use some aspect of complementary medicine (Buehler, 2007).

- Green tea extract may improve muscle health by reducing or delaying necrosis by an antioxidant mechanism (Dorchies et al, 2006).
- Traditional Chinese medicine has been advocated for treatment of types of MD, but studies are needed to identify active ingredients.
- Supplementation with creatine monohydrate may improve muscle strength (Davidson and Truby, 2009).

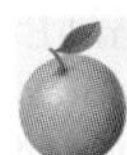

NUTRITION EDUCATION, COUNSELING, CARE MANAGEMENT

- Provide low-calorie snack tips for patients who are obese.
- Help patient modify food textures to meet needs.
- Discuss problems related to inactivity or weight gain.
- Discuss the importance of adequate fluid intake.
- Discuss methods to prevent aspiration and pneumonia.
- Comprehensive management strategies can improve function, quality of life, and longevity (Bushby et al, 2010). Work with the occupational therapist and other therapists to maintain optimal levels of function.

Patient Education—Food Safety

If enteral or parenteral nutrition is used, careful sanitation and handling techniques must be taught and used.

For More Information

- Facioscapulohumeral Dystrophy (FSHD) Society
  http://www.fshsociety.org
- Muscular Dystrophy Association (MDA)
  http://www.mdausa.org/
- Muscular Dystrophy Association of Canada
  http://www.mdac.ca/
- Muscular Dystrophy Family Foundation
  http://www.mdff.org/
- National Institute—MD
  http://www.ninds.nih.gov/health_and_medical/disorders/md.htm
- Neuromuscular Disorders in the MDA Foundation
  http://www.mdausa.org/disease/
- Parent Project for Muscular Dystrophy Research
  http://www.parentprojectmd.org
- Rare Muscular Dystrophy types
  http://www.mdausa.org/publications/fa-rareMD.html#dd

MUSCULAR DYSTROPHY—CITED REFERENCES

Buehler BA. Complementary and alternative medicine (CAM) in genetics. *Am J Med Genet A.* 143:2889, 2007.

Bushby K, et al. Diagnosis and management of Duchenne muscular dystrophy, part 2: implementation of multidisciplinary care [published online ahead of print November 27, 2009]. *Lancet Neurol.* 9:177, 2010.

Davidson ZE, Truby H. A review of nutrition in Duchenne muscular dystrophy. *J Hum Nutr Diet.* 22:383, 2009.

Dorchies OM, et al. Green tea extract and its major polyphenol (-)-epigallocatechin gallate improve muscle function in a mouse model for Duchenne muscular dystrophy. *Am J Physiol Cell Physiol.* 290:C616, 2006.

Motlagh B, et al. Nutritional inadequacy in adults with muscular dystrophy. *Muscle Nerve.* 31:713, 2005.

Munn MW. Estimate of daily calorie needs for a neuromuscular disease patient receiving noninvasive ventilation. *Am J Phys Med Rehabil.* 84:639, 2005.

Violett L, et al. Utility of cystatin C to monitor renal function in Duchenne muscular dystrophy. *Muscle Nerve.* 40:438, 2009.

Yoshida M, et al. Dietary NaCl supplementation prevents muscle necrosis in a mouse model of Duchenne muscular dystrophy. *Am J Physiol Regul Integr Comp Physiol.* 290:R449, 2006.

MYOFASCIAL PAIN SYNDROMES: FIBROMYALGIA AND POLYMYALGIA RHEUMATICA

NUTRITIONAL ACUITY RANKING: LEVEL 1–2

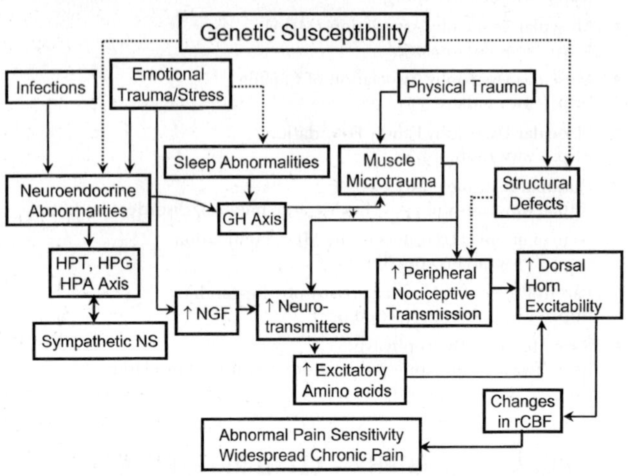

Adapted from: William J. Koopman, Larry W. Moreland, *Arthritis and Allied Conditions A Textbook of Rheumatology,* 15th ed. Philadelphia: Lippincott Williams & Wilkins, 2005.

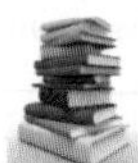

DEFINITIONS AND BACKGROUND

Myofascial pain syndromes are a group of disorders characterized by achy pain and stiffness in soft tissues, including muscles, tendons, and ligaments. In the United States, **fibromyalgia (FM)** is estimated to occur in 2% of adults (Mease, 2005). Diagnosis is difficult, and the etiology is not clear. Corticotropin-releasing hormone (CRH) and substance P (SP) are found in increased levels in the cerebral spinal fluid (CSF) of FM patients, and increased interleukin (IL)-6 and IL-8 are found in the serum where they release proinflammatory and neurosensitizing molecules (Lucas et al, 2006).

FM, or "fibrositis," is a central sensitivity syndrome with abnormalities in the peripheral, central, sympathetic nervous systems, and the hypothalomo–pituitary–adrenal axis stress response system (Mease, 2005). Etiology theories abound, including inadequate sleep, physical or psychological trauma, or exposure to viruses such as hepatitis B or C, or HIV infection. Serotonin and dopamine levels may be lower than normal. Insulin-like growth factor-1 (IGF-1) levels may also be low; they are a surrogate marker for low growth hormone secretion during stage 3 and 4 of sleep, when tissue repair occurs (Rosenzweig and Thomas, 2009).

FM causes widespread pain and stiffness either throughout the body or localized along the spine. Persistent symptoms may be disruptive but are not life threatening. Symptoms include sleep disturbance, depression, fatigue, headaches, irritable bowel syndrome, numbness in the hands and feet, and mood disorders. Acupuncture may offer relief (Martin et al, 2006).

Polymyalgia rheumatica (PMR) affects people over age 70 years, usually women. It causes aching, severe muscle stiffness, and pain. Symptoms start suddenly and may affect several areas in the neck, shoulders, hips, and/or thighs. It usually goes away with treatment but may reoccur. Symptoms include mild joint stiffness and swelling, face pain, anemia, extreme fatigue, unintentional weight loss, and anorexia. The cause of PMR is not known but may be related to aging. Diagnosis is difficult. Many people with PMR also have giant-cell arteritis with double vision, severe headaches, or vision loss. Low-dose corticosteroids may be needed for up to a year (Hernandez-Rodriguez et al, 2009).

Treatment of myofascial pain disorders may include exercise, medications such as glucocorticoids and NSAIDs, a healthy diet rich in antioxidants, and adequate rest. Massage and cognitive behavioral therapy (CBT) are helpful (Mease, 2005). After a warm-water swimming program, a significant decrease in IL-8, IFNgamma, and CRP has been noted (Ortega et al, 2009). Use of a phyochemical-rich diet results in a decrease in joint stiffness and pain as well as an improvement in self-reported quality of life. Plant foods are rich natural sources of antioxidants (quercetin, myristin, and kaempherol) in addition to fiber and other nutrients. A vegan diet often shows highly increased serum levels of beta- and alpha-carotenes, lycopene, lutein, and vitamins C and E.

Rapid-paced discovery is taking place in genetics, patient assessment, new therapeutic targets, and novel methods of treatment delivery (Williams and Clauw, 2009). The best multidisciplinary team includes a rheumatologist, physical therapist, exercise therapist, dietitian, and massage therapist (Lemstra and Olszynski, 2005).

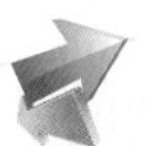

ASSESSMENT, MONITORING, AND EVALUATION

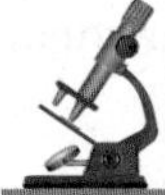

CLINICAL INDICATORS

Genetic Markers: A multigenic or genome-wide approach may be needed to alter individualized pain therapy according to the patient's genotype. For example, DRD2 polymorphisms decrease the functioning of the dopaminergic reward system; this could cause an individual to require more pain medicine. Research is ongoing to determine whether individuals with FM have the genetic tendency toward lower pain thresholds.

Clinical/History		
Height	Morning stiffness	FM-pain in shoulders, pelvis, and hips (pain in 11/18 trigger points)
Weight	Fatigue, sleep disturbances	Carpal tunnel syndrome (in PMR)
BMI	Fibromyalgia Impact Questionnaire (FIQ)	
Tender areas, back pain		
Headache		
Depression, mood disorders		

Lab Work	Trig, Chol	Alk phos
CRP or ESR (may be high)	Alb, transthyretin	Vitamin D_3 status (serum 25-OHD)
Plasma adreno-medullin (high in PMR)	BUN, Creat	
	Ca^{++}, Mg^{++}	
	Na^+, K^+	
	Gluc	

INTERVENTION

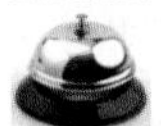

OBJECTIVES

- Relieve pain. Acupuncture, massage, cognitive-behavior therapy (CBT) and varied exercises may be recommended (Assefi et al, 2005; Rosenzweig and Thomas, 2009).
- Lose weight, if obese.
- Correct underlying problems such as hypertension.
- Support lifestyle changes, including stress reduction, relaxation techniques, and exercise.
- Prevent blindness in PMR when there is giant-cell arteritis.

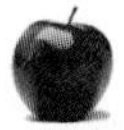

FOOD AND NUTRITION

- Use a balanced diet. The MyPyramid food guidance system is another useful tool for planning a healthy diet. Include phytochemicals; dietary quercetin should be encouraged (Lucas et al, 2006). Table 11-2 is also a useful reference.
- A vegan diet may be beneficial with berries, fruits, vegetables, roots, nuts, germinated seeds, and sprouts.
- A weight loss plan may be needed.

SAMPLE NUTRITION CARE PROCESS STEPS

Inadequate Intake of Bioactive Substances

Assessment Data: Weight and physical activity histories. Medical history, medications and lab values. Much pain; diagnosed FM. Diet hx and 3-day food record shows intake of <2 fruits and vegetables daily. No food allergies.

Nutrition Diagnosis (PES): Inadequate intake of bioactive substances related to low intake of fruits and vegetables as evidenced by diet history and intake records.

Intervention: Food and Nutrient Delivery—Provision of more spices, fruits, vegetables and juices. Education about the role of antioxidants, spices, and phytochemicals in reducing inflammation and the possibility of lessening pain symptoms. Counseling about menus, recipes and cooking tips for including more bioactive ingredients. Encourage intake of fish oils, walnuts, fatty fish such as salmon for omega-3 fatty acids.

Monitoring and Evaluation: Diet Hx showing improved intake of spices (such as turmeric, cumin, cinnamon), cocoa and coffee, fruits including berries and apples and pomegranates, vegetables such as broccoli and cabbage on a daily and weekly basis. Fewer complaints of overt pain.

- Increased intake of omega-3 fatty acids may help to reduce inflammation and relieve pain in some individuals. Increase intake of fatty fish, walnuts, and flaxseed.

Common Drugs Used and Potential Side Effects

- Medications that decrease pain and improve sleep may be prescribed. Low doses of tricyclic antidepressants (amitriptyline, Elavil; cyclobenzaprine, Flexeril) and the serotonin-3 receptor antagonist tropisetron may be helpful (Lucas et al, 2006; Rosenzweig and Thomas, 2009). Opioids, NSAIDs, sedatives, muscle relaxants, and antiepileptics have been used to treat FMS (Mease, 2005).
- Pregabalin (Lyrica) and duloxetine (Cymbalta) are used in FMS. Milnacipran (Savella) is a dual norepinephrine and serotonin reuptake inhibitor that has been shown to be safe (Arnold et al, 2009; Mease et al, 2009).
- Opioids are not recommended for FM (Rosenzweig and Thomas, 2009).
- For PMR, a trial of low-dose corticosteroids is given, usually in the form of 10–15 mg of prednisone (Deltasone, Orasone) per day. Side effects may include sleeplessness, weight gain, loss of nitrogen and calcium, cataracts, thinning of the skin, easy bruising. NSAIDS, such as ibuprofen (Advil, Motrin) and naproxen (Naprosyn, Aleve), are ineffective in the treatment of PMR.

Herbs, Botanicals, and Supplements

- Herbs and botanical supplements should not be used without discussing with physician. CAM is popular for musculoskeletal conditions. Some CAM modalities show significant promise, such as acupuncture (Martin et al, 2006). Excellent resources are available on the Internet from the National Center for Complementary and Alternative Medicine (http://nccam.nih.gov).
- Magnesium; sulfur compounds such as SAMe, dimethylsulfoxide (DMSO), taurine, glucosamine, and chondroitin sulfate; and reduced GSH may have clinical applications in the treatment of FMS; controlled trials are needed.

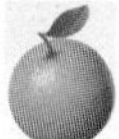

NUTRITION EDUCATION, COUNSELING, CARE MANAGEMENT

- Aerobic exercise, patient education and CBT are quite effective. Daily exercise will be important for strengthening weak muscles. Exercise adherence can help reduce the need for pain medications (Lemstra and Olszynski, 2005).
- Discuss weight management, as needed.
- Discuss the role of omega-3 fatty acids in reduction of inflammation.

Patient Education—Food Safety

If enteral or parenteral nutrition is used, careful sanitation and handling techniques must be taught and used.

For More Information

- American Fibromyalgia Syndrome Association, Inc.
  http://www.afsafund.org/
- Fibromyalgia Network
  http://www.fmnetnews.com/
- Mayo Clinic
  http://www.mayoclinic.com/health/myofascial-pain-syndrome/DS01042
- Myositis Association
  http://www.myositis.org/
- National Fibromyalgia Partnership, Inc.
  http://www.fmpartnership.org/FMPartnership.htm
- National Institute of Arthritis and Musculoskeletal and Skin Diseases
  http://www.niams.nih.gov/hi/topics/fibromyalgia/fibrofs.htm
- Polymyalgia Rheumatica
  http://www.rheumatology.org/public/factsheets/diseases_and_conditions/polymyalgiarheumatica.asp
- Polymyalgia Rheumatica and Giant Cell Arteritis
  http://www.niams.nih.gov/Health_Info/Polymyalgia/default.asp

MYOFASCIAL PAIN SYNDROMES—CITED REFERENCES

Assefi NP, et al. A randomized clinical trial of acupuncture compared with sham acupuncture in fibromyalgia. *Ann Intern Med.* 143:10, 2005.

Arnold LM, et al. Efficacy of duloxetine in patients with fibromyalgia: pooled analysis of 4 placebo-controlled clinical trials. *Prim Care Companion J Clin Psychiatry.* 11:237, 2009.

Hernandez-Rodriguez J, et al. Treatment of Polymyalgia Rheumatica. *Arch Intern Med.* 169:1839, 2009.

Lemstra M, Olszynski WP. The effectiveness of multidisciplinary rehabilitation in the treatment of fibromyalgia: a randomized controlled trial. *Clin J Pain.* 21:166, 2005.

Lucas HJ, et al. Fibromyalgia—new concepts of pathogenesis and treatment. *Int J Immunopathol Pharmacol.* 19:5, 2006.

Martin DP, et al. Improvement in fibromyalgia symptoms with acupuncture: results of a randomized controlled trial. *Mayo Clin Proc.* 81:749, 2006.

Mease P. Fibromyalgia syndrome: review of clinical presentation, pathogenesis, outcome measures, and treatment. *J Rheumatol.* 75:6S, 2005.

Mease PJ, et al. The efficacy and safety of milnacipran for treatment of fibromyalgia. a randomized, double-blind, placebo-controlled trial. *J Rheumatol.* 36:398, 2009.

Ortega E, et al. Exercise in fibromyalgia and related inflammatory disorders: known effects and unknown chances. *Exerc Immunol Rev.* 15:42, 2009.

Rosenzweig TM, Thomas TM. An update on fibromyalgia syndrome: the multimodal therapeutic approach. *Am J Lifestyle Med.* 10:226, 2009.

Williams DA, Clauw DJ. Understanding fibromyalgia: lessons from the broader pain research community. *J Pain.* 10:777, 2009.

OSTEOARTHRITIS AND DEGENERATIVE JOINT DISEASE

NUTRITIONAL ACUITY RANKING: LEVEL 1–2

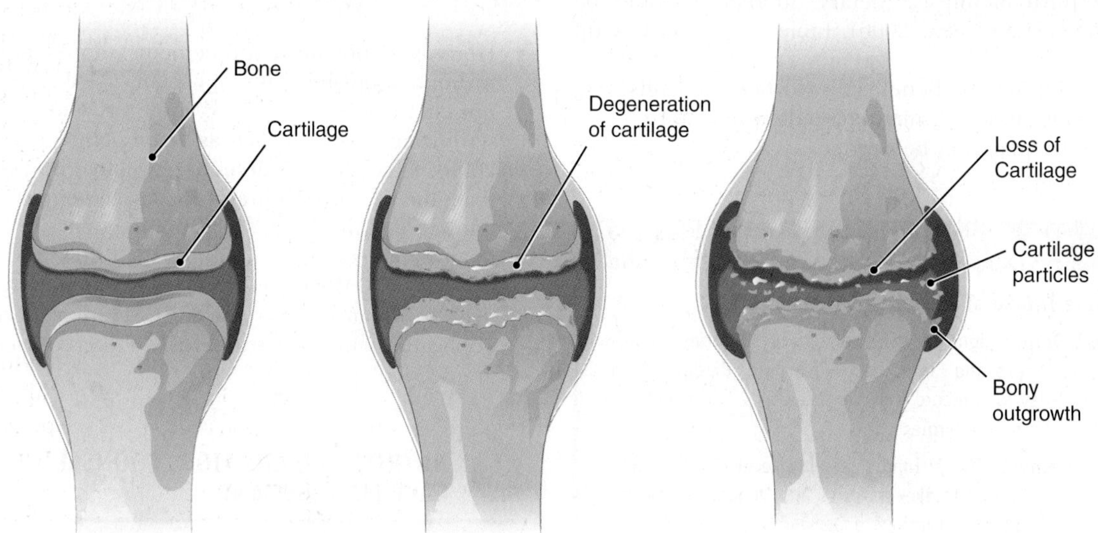

Adapted from: Cohen BJ. *Medical Terminology,* 4th ed. Philadelphia. Lippincott Williams & Wilkins 2003.

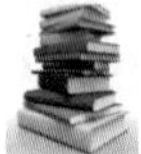

DEFINITIONS AND BACKGROUND

OA may be primary (in older individuals) or may follow an injury or disease involving the articular surfaces of synovial joints. The joint may lose its normal shape and bone spurs may grow on the edges of the joint. OA is a common health problem in populations over age 40 years, and it is a leading cause of pain and disability. OA mostly affects cartilage where the surface layer breaks down and wears away. The hands, knees, hips, and spine are most commonly affected.

Over 40 million Americans report that they have arthritis and many indicate that it limits their daily activities. High serum concentrations of tumor necrosis factor are associated with lower physical function and more pain, stiffness, and physical disability. Over a third of adults with arthritis experience limitations in their ability to work.

Treatments for OA combine nonpharmacological modalities, pharmacological agents, and surgical procedures. Exercise, weight control, rest, and relief from stress on joints, nondrug pain relief, and various types of complementary medical techniques may be useful. Continuous passive motion (CPM), massage, and heat treatments may be used. Surgery is reserved for those persons for whom other treatments have been unsuccessful.

Weight loss is a primary treatment for OA for individuals who are obese. Obesity is a significant risk factor for and contributor to increased morbidity and mortality from chronic diseases, including OA (Pi-Sunyer, 2009). Overweight causes strain on joints and should be managed early by health professionals (Gasbarrini and Piscaglia, 2005). An average weight loss of 5% in overweight and obese older patients brings an 18% gain in overall function (Messier et al, 2005), and a 10% weight loss improves function by 28% (Christensen et al, 2005).

While vitamins A, C, and E have major roles in modulating oxidative stress, immune responses, and cell differentiation, controlled trials found that these vitamins do not halt progression of OA (Choi, 2005). Vitamins D and K play a protective role (Bergink et al, 2009; Oka et al, 2009). Diets rich in omega-3 fatty acids may reduce joint stiffness and pain, increase grip strength, and enhance walking pace. Pomegranate fruit extracts can block interleukin-1β (IL-1β) enzymes that contribute to cartilage destruction and OA. Finally, cadgerin-11 is a protein that contributes to joint destruction and a related fabric has been developed for cartilage replacement.

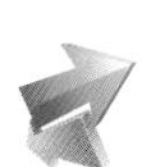

ASSESSMENT, MONITORING, AND EVALUATION

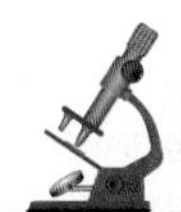

CLINICAL INDICATORS

Genetic Markers: OA is the breakdown and inflammation of joint cartilage, usually brought on by aging and repetitive joint usage. OA and cardiovascular disease share age and obesity as risk factors, but may also be linked by pathogenic mechanisms involving metabolic abnormalities and systemic inflammation (Puenpatom and Victor, 2009).

Clinical/History

Height
Weight
BMI
Obesity?
Pain, swelling of joints (arthralgia)
Synovial joint stiffness
Crunching sound of bone against bone
X-rays; DEXA
OA Index

Lab Work

Antistreptolysin titer (ASO)
Antirheumatoid factor
BUN, Creat
Sedimentation rate
CRP
Gluc
Alk phos
Uric acid
Ca^{++}, Mg^{++}
Na^{+}, K^{+}
Serum folate and B_{12}
Vitamin D_3 status (serum 25-OHD)

SAMPLE NUTRITION CARE PROCESS STEPS

Overweight

Assessment Data: Weight and physical activity histories; symptoms diary; medical history, medications, and lab values.

Nutrition Diagnosis (PES): Overweight with joint pain related to eating double portions at lunch and dinner meals as evidenced by diet history and BMI of 29.

Intervention: Food and Nutrient Delivery—Offer choices of lower fat and low energy foods and snacks. Educate about the role of excess weight and joint pain. Counsel and offer weight management tips, tips for dining out or snacking. Coordinate care with referral to physical therapy for exercises to reduce pain and stiffness in affected joints.

Monitoring and Evaluation: Weight changes, food intake records, symptoms diary.

INTERVENTION

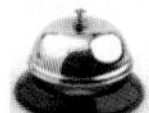

OBJECTIVES

- Control pain and improve joint function. If joint replacement is necessary, prepare for surgery accordingly.
- Maintain a normal body weight. If needed, weight loss may be beneficial to lessen pressure on weight-bearing joints.
- Maintain an active lifestyle as much as possible.
- Encourage patient (especially if older) to consume adequate amounts of vitamins D and K, protein and calcium from a healthy, nutrient-dense, antioxidant-rich diet.
- Maintain integrity of cartilage in affected joints. Omega-3 fatty acids may reduce the activity of enzymes that destroy cartilage. Include fish oils and certain plant seed oils that impact immune and inflammatory responses as precursors of eicosanoids.

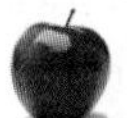

FOOD AND NUTRITION

- Use a calorie-controlled diet if obesity is present. Use of a meal replacement may help to promote weight loss.
- The inflammatory response may be suppressed by an increase in omega-3 fatty acids, as found in fatty fish (mackerel, herring, and salmon) and from walnuts and flaxseed. Use these foods several times a week.
- Calcium is found in dark green, leafy vegetables, such as kale and broccoli; canned sardines and salmon with bones; fortified orange juice; milk and dairy products, such as cheese and yogurt; fortified bread, tofu or soy milk.
- Vitamin C is needed for healthy collagen and cartilage. Good sources include citrus fruits, bell peppers, tomatoes, watermelon, strawberries, and kiwifruit.
- Low dietary vitamin D intake increases the risk of progression of knee OA, particularly in subjects with low baseline BMD (Bergink et al, 2009). Include vitamin D from sardines, herring, fish-liver oil; butter and cream; egg yolks; liver; fortified cow's milk and dairy

products, such as cheese and yogurt; and fortified cereals.

- Vitamin K may be found in leafy greens such as kale, Swiss chard, broccoli, spinach, raw parsley. It is also found in small amounts in olive, soybean or canola oils and in mayonnaise.
- Boron may help OA. Sources include apples, legumes, leafy vegetables, carrots, pears, grapes, and some drinking water.
- Include plenty of phytochemicals. Pomegranates and cranberries are especially protective because of the ellagic acid. See Table 11-2.

Common Drugs Used and Potential Side Effects

- Because of GI risks (including ulcer complications) and cardiovascular risks, including hypertension and thrombotic events associated with NSAIDs, acetaminophen is the first choice anti-inflammatory agent (Berenbaum, 2008). Table 11-6 gives more details on medicines used for OA. Evaluate risks as well as benefits for all drug therapies.

TABLE 11-6 Medications Commonly Used for Osteoarthritis

Medication	Comments	Side Effects
Anti-inflammatory drugs, nonsteroidal (NSAIDs)	Indomethacin (Indocin), aspirin piroxicam (Feldene), naproxen (Naprosyn), nabumetone (Relafen) and Ibuprofen (Advil, Motrin) may be recommended.	Nausea, GI distress, anorexia, flatulence, or vomiting can occur. Take with food. Prolonged use may cause GI bleeding or ulcers. Indomethacin may also cause renal failure, or diarrhea; naprosen may cause heartburn or increased risk of cardiovascular disease.
COX-2 Inhibitors	Cyclooxygenases are needed for the synthesis of prostaglandins. The COX-2 enzyme mediates inflammation and pain. Celecoxib (Celebrex) is the only FDA-approved drug at this time.	These agents may promote increased risk of heart attack and stroke. Rofecoxib (Vioxx) and valdecoxib (Bectra) were removed from the market in 2004 and 2005.
Misoprostol (Cytotec)	Misoprostol reduces stomach acid if NSAIDs are used.	Abdominal cramps may occur.
Frankincense (Boswellia frereana)	Interestingly, this herb may lessen arthritic pain. Epi-lupeol is the principal constituent of B. frereana. B. frereana prevents collagen degradation, and inhibits the production of pro-inflammatory mediators (Blain et al, 2010).	Fewer side effects than glucosamine and chondroitin.
Glucosamine sulfate and chondroitin	Glucosamine reduces cartilage damage and decreases pain associated with osteoarthritis. Taken with chondroitin, it may help relieve symptoms of osteoarthritis. Some pills do not contain sufficient levels to be effective; check brand with www.consumerlab.com to select the best choice.	Glucosamine can increase blood glucose levels andaggravate shellfish allergy because it is made from these shells. Chondroitin may alter blood clotting activity in a manner similar to that of aspirin.
Hyaluronic acid substitutes (viscosupplements)	These injections are designed to replace a normal component of the knee joint involved in joint lubrication and nutrition.	A series of injections are required. When used with methotrexate, the benefits may be greater (Homma et al, 2009).
Omega-3 fatty acids	Supplementation causes a decrease in both degradative and inflammatory aspects of chondrocyte metabolism.	May increase effects of blood-thinning drugs and herbs.
Steroids	Corticosteroids may cause sodium retention; calcium, nitrogen, and potassium depletion; truncal obesity; and hyperglycemia.	Corticosteroids may have a short-term effect in osteoarthritis (Bellamy et al, 2005). Injections are required.
Topical pain relievers (Zostrix, Icy Hot, Therapeutic Mineral Ice, Aspercreme, and Ben Gay)	Creams and rubs stimulate nerve endings to relieve pain; deplete the amount of neurotransmitter (substance P) that sends pain messages to the brain; and block prostaglandins that cause pain and inflammation.	No internal side effects.
Tramadol (Ultram)	Pain reliever that is prescribed when over-the-counter medications do not provide relief.	Potentially addictive.

REFERENCES

Arthritis drug guide, available at Web site accessed December 6, 2009, at http:// www.arthritis.org/conditions/DrugGuide/drug_index.asp.

Bellamy N, et al. Intraarticular corticosteroid for treatment of osteoarthritis of the knee. *Cochrane Database Syst Rev.* 2:CD005328, 2005.

Blain EJ, et al. Boswellia frereana (frankincense) suppresses cytokine-induced matrix metalloproteinase expression and production of pro-inflammatory molecules in articular cartilage [published online ahead of print November 26, 2009]. *Phytother Res*. 24:905, 2010.

Cranney A, et al. Effectiveness and safety of vitamin D in relation to bone health. *Evid Rep Technol Assess*. 158:1, 2007.

Homma A, et al. Novel hyaluronic acid-methotrexate conjugates for osteoarthritis treatment. *Bioorg Med Chem*. 17:4647, 2009.

National Institite of Arthritis and Musculoskeletal and Skin Disorders. Web site accessed December 13, 2009, at http://www.niams.nih.gov/Health_Info/Osteoarthritis/default.asp#4

TABLE 11-7 Side Effects of Herbs Commonly Used for Arthritis

Bromelain	May increase effects of blood-thinning drugs and tetracycline antibiotics.
Echinacea	Might counteract immunosuppressant drugs, such as glucocorticoids, taken for lupus and rheumatoid arthritis; might increase side effects of methotrexate.
Evening primrose oil	Can counteract the effects of anticonvulsant drugs.
Folic acid	Interferes with methotrexate.
Gamma linoleic acid (GLA)	May increase effects of blood-thinning drugs and herbs.
Garlic	Can increase effects of blood-thinning drugs and herbs
Ginger	Can increase nonsteroidal anti-inflammatory drug (NSAID) side effects and effects of blood-thinning drugs and herbs.
Ginkgo	May increase effects of blood-thinning drugs and herbs.
Ginseng	May increase effects of blood-thinning drugs, estrogens, and glucocorticoids; should not be used by those with diabetes; may interact with monoamine oxidase (MAO) inhibitors.
Kava	Can increase effects of alcohol, sedatives, and tranquilizers.
Magnesium	May interact with blood pressure medications.
***S*-adenosylmethionine (SAMe)**	SAMe may rebuild eroded joint cartilage. Enteric coating is needed because of gastrointestinal (GI) side effects.
Soy and avocado extracts	Antioxidant effects in reducing the symptoms of osteoarthritis; avoid excessive use in patients with hormonal cancers.
St. John's wort	May enhance effects of narcotics, alcohol, and antidepressants; increases risk of sunburn; interferes with iron absorption.
Valerian	May enhance effects of sedatives and tranquilizers.
Vitamin E	Gamma-tocopherol may worsen osteoarthritis; alpha-tocopherol is better.
Zinc	Can interfere with glucocorticoids and other immunosuppressive drugs.

Note: Herbs and botanical supplements should not be used without discussing with physician. Excerpted from The Arthritis Foundation's guide to alternative therapies, Web site accessed December 6, 2009, at http://www.arthritis.org.

Herbs, Botanicals, and Supplements

- Boswellia frereana (frankincense) suppresses cytokine-induced matrix metalloproteinase expression and production of pro-inflammatory molecules; studies are on-going (Blain et al, 2010).
- Glucosamine sulfate combined with omega-3 fatty acids may reduce OA symptoms, including morning stiffness and pain in hips and knees (Gruenwald et al, 2009). Undenatured type II collagen (UC-II) may be more effective in the treatment of OA than glucosamine and chondroitin (Crowley et al, 2009).
- Green tea's anti-inflammatory properties and ginger may aid in pain relief.
- Table 11-7 provides a description of some side effects of products often used for OA.

NUTRITION EDUCATION, COUNSELING, CARE MANAGEMENT

- Physical and occupational therapies, diet, and exercise play an extremely important role. Long-term exercise and dietary weight loss are most effective. Acupuncture may be used to relieve pain.
- Because OA allows muscles around the joints to become weak, exercise and stretching should be suggested to maintain flexibility. Repetitive, high-impact movements are not recommended whereas Tai Chi helps balance and protects bones. Exercises include a series for strengthening, aerobic, agility, and range of motion. Long-term weight training, walking programs, swimming, and flexibility exercises are helpful.
- Encourage patient to avoid fad diets for "arthritis cure." Ensure that the patient's diet is balanced and includes all nutrients. A weight-loss plan may be needed.
- To alleviate stress on the joints, pharmacological and behavioral techniques with self-monitoring, should be included (Berkel et al, 2005).
- Pain initiates and exacerbates sleep disturbance; therefore, improving the sleep of OA patients helps to reduce the pain (Vitello et al, 2009). Transcutaneous electrical nerve stimulation (TENS) directs mild electric pulses to nerve endings that lie beneath the skin in the painful area; it block messages to the brain and by modifies pain perception. CBT is also useful.
- Focus on abilities and strengths rather than on disabilities and weaknesses.

Patient Education—Food Safety

If enteral or parenteral nutrition is used, careful sanitation and handling techniques must be taught and used.

For More Information

- Arthritis Foundation
  http://arthritis.about.com/
- Arthritis Resource Center at Healingwell
  http://www.healingwell.com/arthritis
- NIAMS—Osteoarthritis
  http://www.niams.nih.gov/hi/topics/arthritis/oahandout.htm
- Johns Hopkins Arthritis Center
  http://www.hopkins-arthritis.som.jhmi.edu/

OSTEOARTHRITIS AND DEGENERATIVE JOINT DISEASE—CITED REFERENCES

Berenbaum F. New horizons and perspectives in the treatment of osteoarthritis. *Arthritis Res Ther.* 10:S1, 2008.

Bergink AP, et al. Vitamin D status, bone mineral density, and the development of radiographic osteoarthritis of the knee: The Rotterdam Study. *J Clin Rheumatol.* 15:230, 2009.

Berkel LA, et al. Behavioral interventions for obesity. *J Am Diet Assoc.* 105:35S, 2005.

Blain EJ, et al. Boswellia frereana (frankincense) suppresses cytokine-induced matrix metalloproteinase expression and production of pro-inflammatory molecules in articular cartilage [published online ahead of print November 26, 2009]. *Phytother Res.* 24:905, 2010.

Choi HK. Dietary risk factors for rheumatic diseases. *Curr Opin Rheumatol.* 17:141, 2005.

Christensen R, et al. Weight loss: the treatment of choice for knee osteoarthritis? A randomized trial. *Osteoarthritis Cartilage.* 13:20, 2005.

Crowley DC, et al. Safety and efficacy of undenatured type II collagen in the treatment of osteoarthritis of the knee: a clinical trial. *Int J Med Sci.* 6:312, 2009.

Gasbarrini A, Piscaglia AC. A natural diet versus modern Western diets? A new approach to prevent "well-being syndromes." *Dig Dis Sci.* 50:1, 2005.

Gruenwald J, et al. Effect of glucosamine sulfate with or without omega-3 fatty acids in patients with osteoarthritis [published online ahead of print September 4, 2009]. *Adv Ther.* 26:858, 2009.

Messier SP, et al. Weight loss reduces knee-joint loads in overweight and obese older adults with knee osteoarthritis. *Arthritis Rheum.* 52:2026, 2005.

Oka H, et al. Association of low dietary vitamin K intake with radiographic knee osteoarthritis in the Japanese elderly population: dietary survey in a population-based cohort of the ROAD study. *J Orthop Sci.* 14:687, 2009.

Pi-Sunyer X. The medical risks of obesity. *Postgrad Med.* 121:21, 2009.

Puenpatom RA, Victor TW. Increased prevalence of metabolic syndrome in individuals with osteoarthritis: an analysis of NHANES III data. *Postgrad Med.* 121:9, 2009.

Vitello MV, et al. Cognitive behavioral therapy for insomnia improves sleep and decreases pain in older adults with co-morbid insomnia and osteoarthritis. *J Clin Sleep Med.* 5:355, 2009.

OSTEOMYELITIS

NUTRITIONAL ACUITY RANKING: LEVEL 1–2

DEFINITIONS AND BACKGROUND

Acute osteomyelitis may be caused by localized infection of the long bones or injury to bone and surrounding soft tissue. *Staphylococcus aureus* is implicated in most patients with acute osteomyelitis; *S. epidermidis, S. aureus, Pseudomonas aeruginosa, Serratia marcescens,* and *Escherichia coli* may be found in the chronic form. When a bone is infected, the bone marrow swells and compresses against the rigid outer wall of bone, and blood vessels may be compressed or die; abscesses may form. Osteomyelitis and inflammatory arthritis affect many children (Pruthi and Thapa, 2009).

Some diseases predispose patients to osteomyelitis, including diabetes mellitus, sickle cell disease, acquired immunodeficiency virus (AIDS), intravenous drug abuse, alcoholism, chronic steroid use, immunosuppression, and chronic joint disease. Use of prosthetic orthopedic devices and recent orthopedic surgery or open fracture may also place a patient at risk for osteomyelitis. Patients with diabetes mellitus with poor glucose control may experience infections of the lower extremities, from superficial cellulitis to deep soft tissue infections and osteomyelitis. Because osteomyelitis is prevalent after diabetic foot ulcers, careful treatment is crucial to avoid amputation (Schinabeck and Johnson, 2005).

Prompt treatment is important. If not treated properly, the condition may become chronic with a poor prognosis. Treatment generally involves evaluation, staging, determination of etiology, antimicrobial therapy, and debridement or stabilization of bone. In children, serious musculoskeletal infections include osteomyelitis, septic arthritis, pyomyositis, and necrotizing fasciitis (Frank et al, 2005).

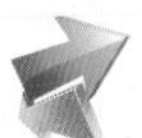

ASSESSMENT, MONITORING, AND EVALUATION

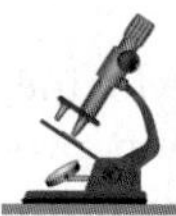

CLINICAL INDICATORS

Genetic Markers: Deficiency of the interleukin-1-receptor antagonist (DIRA) promotes neonatal osteomyelitis, an autosomal recessive autoinflammatory disease caused by mutations in IL1RN (Aksentijevich et al, 2009).

Clinical/History

Height
Weight
BMI
Intake and output (I & O)
BP
Bone pain
Sudden, acute pain in joints near the infection
Fever, chills
Tachycardia, diaphoresis
Nausea
Dehydration, electrolyte imbalance
Local swelling, redness
Contractures in affected extremities
Magnetic resonance imaging (MRI)
Bone densitometry or x-rays
Pressure ulcers or lesions with a sinus tract?

Lab Work

CRP and ESR (increased)
White blood cell (WBC) count (increased)
Gluc
Alb, transthyretin
BUN, Creat
Alk phos
AST, ALT
Ca^{++}, Mg^{++}
Na^{+}, K^{+}
Vitamin D_3 status (serum 25-OHD)

SAMPLE NUTRITION CARE PROCESS STEPS

Underweight

Assessment Data: Weight and physical activity histories. Medical history, medications, and lab values.

Nutrition Diagnosis (PES): Underweight related to poor nutrition quality of life and inadequate oral intake as evidenced by insufficient pain medicine before meals and BMI of 18.

Intervention: Food and nutrient delivery—offer nutrient and energy-dense favorite foods. Educate about the benefits of gaining weight to tolerate medical therapies more effectively, to gain energy, and to improve nutritional quality of life. Coordinate timing of medicines with meals to assure that pain medicine is given 20–30 minutes before meals.

Monitoring and Evaluation: Weight gain in 3–6 months; improved timing of meals with pain medicine to decrease anorexia at mealtime.

INTERVENTION

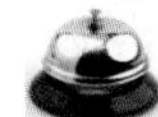

OBJECTIVES

- Characterize and treat the infection. Prevent further infection, dehydration, and other complications.
- Promote recovery and healing of any skin lesions or pressure ulcers.
- Correct defective blood flow to allow nutrients and oxygen to reach all tissues.
- Control serum glucose and alleviate hyperglycemia with insulin if needed.
- Correct anorexia, poor intake, weight loss, nausea and vomiting where present.

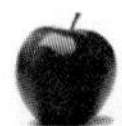

FOOD AND NUTRITION

- Encourage adequate fluid intake.
- Maintain a normal to high intake of calories, protein, zinc, vitamin A, and vitamin C in particular. A multivitamin–mineral supplement may be needed.
- With diabetes, control carbohydrate to promote more effective healing.

Common Drugs Used and Potential Side Effects

- For optimal results, antibiotic therapy must be started early, with antimicrobial agents administered parenterally for at least 4–6 weeks if needed. Vancomycin or amphotericin B may be used; monitor for side effects related to timing and meals.
- Analgesics may be used for pain. GI distress is a common side effect.

Herbs, Botanicals, and Supplements

- Herbs and botanical supplements should not be used without discussing with physician.
- It is reasonable to include phytochemical-rich foods each day. See Table 11-2.

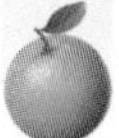

NUTRITION EDUCATION, COUNSELING, CARE MANAGEMENT

- Discuss role of nutrition in wound healing, immunity, and other conditions related to this disorder.
- Discuss signs that may indicate reversal of status or recovery, such as increased fever, elevated glucose levels, additional infections, more redness in affected areas.
- Promote use of nutrient-dense foods that are rich in antioxidants, phytochemicals, protein, zinc and vitamins.

Patient Education—Food Safety

- If enteral or parenteral nutrition is used, careful sanitation and handling techniques must be taught and used. Infection control is extremely important to avoid additional microbial contamination.

For More Information

- Cleveland Clinic—Osteomyelitis
  http://my.clevelandclinic.org/disorders/osteomyelitis/hic_osteomyelitis.aspx
- Mayo Clinic—Osteomyelitis
  http://www.mayoclinic.com/health/osteomyelitis/DS00759
- National Institutes of Health–Osteomyelitis
  http://www.nlm.nih.gov/medlineplus/ency/article/000437.htm

OSTEOMYELITIS—CITED REFERENCES

Aksentijevich I, et al. An autoinflammatory disease with deficiency of the interleukin-1-receptor antagonist. *N Engl J Med.* 360:2426, 2009.

Frank G, et al. Musculoskeletal infections in children. *Pediatr Clin North Am.* 52:1083, 2005.

Pruthi S, Thapa MM. Infectious and inflammatory disorders. *Radiol Clin North Am.* 47:911, 2009.

Schinabeck MK, Johnson JL. Osteomyelitis in diabetic foot ulcers. Prompt diagnosis can avert amputation. *Postgrad Med.* 118:11, 2005.

OSTEOMALACIA

NUTRITIONAL ACUITY RANKING: LEVEL 2

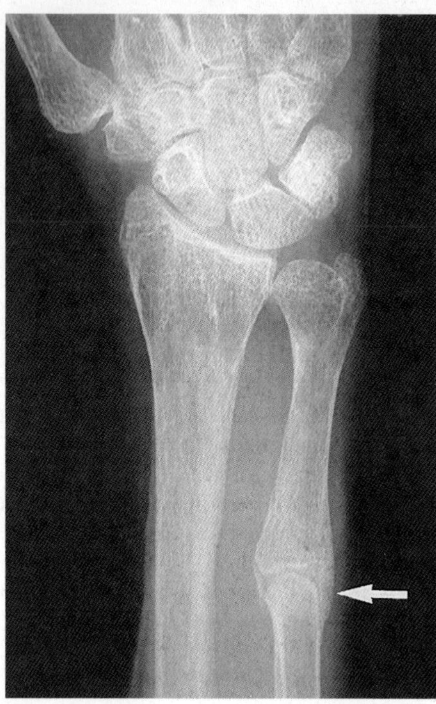

Adapted from: Yochum TR and Rowe LJ. *Yochum and Rowe's Essentials of Skeletal Radiology,* 3rd ed. Philadelphia: Lippincott Williams & Wilkins, 2004.

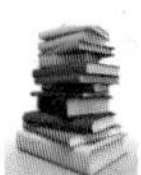

DEFINITIONS AND BACKGROUND

Osteomalacia, adult rickets, causes softening and demineralization of the bone from insufficient vitamin D. Osteomalacia may occur in conjunction with bone loss and hip fractures. It more commonly results from intestinal malabsorption as from Crohn's disease, colon resection, cystic fibrosis, celiac disease, or chronic use of anticonvulsants. It is also seen in kidney failure, liver disease, and some types of cancer. Severe vitamin D deficiency leads to secondary hyperparathyroidism, increased bone turnover and losses.

Derangements in serum phosphate level result in osteomalacia (Saito and Fukumoto, 2009). Matrix extracellular phosphoglycoprotein (MEPE) inhibits mineralization; altered expression is associated with oncogenic osteomalacia and hypophosphatemic rickets (Boskey et al, 2010). In addition, deficient actions of fibroblast growth factor, FGF23, result in hypophosphatemic osteomalacia; FGF23 works as a hormone (Saito and Fukumoto, 2009).

Osteomalacia often occurs in older people, in dark-skinned individuals who live in northern latitudes, and in those who have limited sunlight exposure. Vitamin D is produced in response to sun exposure, so the process works faster in pale individuals. Sun exposure of about 15 minutes without sunscreen a few times a week is needed. Darker skinned individuals may need to take supplements.

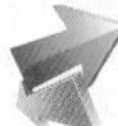

ASSESSMENT, MONITORING, AND EVALUATION

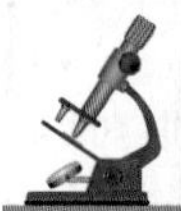

CLINICAL INDICATORS

Genetic Markers: The vitamin D receptor (VDR) is responsible for the expression of over 900 genes, or about 3% of the human genome.

Clinical/History	Lab Work	
Height	Serum P (decreased)	PTH
Weight	Serum Ca^{++} (decreased)	Mg^{++}
BMI	Urinary Ca^{++}	Na^+, K^+
Bone pain, aches	Vitamin D_3 (serum 25-OHD): normal >30 ng/mL; low between 15 and 30 ng/mL; very low at less than 15 ng/mL	Serum phos
Softened, deformed bones		Alk phos (increased)
Muscular weakness, listlessness		Alb, transthyretin
Numbness of arms, feet		CRP
Easy bone fractures		BUN, Creat
Bone densitometry, DEXA		
Bone biopsy		

SAMPLE NUTRITION CARE PROCESS STEPS

Inadequate Vitamin D Intake

Assessment Data: Weight, physical activity histories, medical history, medication use, lab values. Limited sunlight exposure; works indoors in a sedentary job. Complains of bone pain. Low serum vitamin D_3 at 17. Diet Hx shows limited to no intake from milk and milk products, dislike of fish, no use of multivitamin supplements.

Nutrition Diagnosis (PES): Inadequate vitamin D intake related to limited sunlight exposure, indoor job, and diet low in vitamin-D rich foods as evidenced by low serum vitamin D levels.

Intervention: Food-nutrient delivery—Encourage intake of more fortified dairy products, fish; use daily supplement containing the active form of vitamin D (cholecalciferol) in dose as prescribed by physician. Educate about the need to get sunlight exposure (20 minutes without sunscreen) several times weekly. Counsel about ways to use vitamin-D rich foods in menu planning and recipes that are acceptable to patient and/or family members.

Monitoring and Evaluation: Serum levels of 25-hydroxyvitamin D (25-OHD) at more desirable level after 2–3 months. Patient statement of acceptance of foods rich in vitamin D, such as cream soups and casseroles made with milk. No further signs of osteomalacia.

INTERVENTION

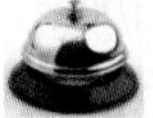

OBJECTIVES

- Provide correct amount of calcium, phosphorus, and vitamin D_3. Include other nutrients that support bone health; meet DRI levels. See Table 11-8.
- Prevent or reverse, if possible, bone density loss resulting from calcium loss in the bone matrix.
- Prevent heart disease and stroke, which may be consequences of severe vitamin D deficiency.

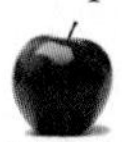

FOOD AND NUTRITION

- Diets should be high in calcium; adults will need 1200–1500 mg. If patient is lactose intolerant, try Lactaid or other forms of lactose-free milk, broccoli, greens, and other sources of calcium.
- Vitamin D is administered at high levels. Dietary sources include fish (particularly salmon, tuna, and mackerel) and fish liver oils. Small amounts are found in egg yolk and beef liver.
- Potassium, magnesium, vitamins C and K and other potentially important nutrients should be highlighted.

Common Drugs Used and Potential Side Effects

- Monitor treatment with calcium salts to prevent hypercalcemia; use with plenty of liquids. Avoid taking with iron supplements or bulk-forming laxatives. High-calcium diets may reduce zinc absorption and balance and may, therefore, increase zinc intake.

TABLE 11-8 Nutrients and Bone Health

Nutrient	Comments
Alcohol	Moderate drinking (1–2 glasses of wine daily) is associated with increased trochanteric bone mineral density (BMD), but higher intakes may be associated with lower BMD. Heavy alcohol consumption may be linked to tobacco use, poor dietary habits, and poor bone health.
B-complex vitamins	Folic acid and vitamins B_6 and B_{12} help to lower homocysteine when elevated.
Boron	Some role but not clearly defined.
Caffeine	Over 300 mg/d of caffeine can negatively impact the vitamin D receptor gene (*VDR*), and the Site Testing Osteoporosis Prevention and Intervention Trial (STOP-IT) found that greater amounts of caffeine affect BMD negatively (Rapuri et al, 2007). Limit intake to three cups of coffee daily and five servings of caffeinated soft drinks or tea; be sure to include adequate amounts of calcium.
Calcium and vitamin D	Dietary supplementation with calcium (1200 mg or more) and vitamin D (800–1000 IU) supports strong bone matrix, moderately reduces bone loss, and reduces the incidence of fractures. Vitamin D may actually be more important than calcium.
Copper	Copper is integral to the process of cross-linking of collagen and elastin molecules, and may have other roles in bone cells as well. Copper is found in meat, poultry, shellfish, organ meats; chocolate; nuts; cereal grains; dried legumes and dried fruits.
Dietary Fiber	A high intake of dietary fiber may interfere with calcium absorption; this may impact vegans, who consume 50 or more grams of fiber per day.
Iron	Iron is important for collagen maturation, and has other roles in osteoblasts and osteoclasts. Iron is found in organ meats, such as liver, kidney, heart; seafood; lean meat, poultry; dried beans; egg yolks; dried fruits; dark molasses; whole-grain and enriched breads or cereals.
Magnesium	Low intakes of magnesium contribute to bone loss. More than 50% of the total magnesium in the body is found in the bone, mostly in bone fluids. Magnesium is found in seeds, nuts; legumes; milled cereal grains; dark-green leafy vegetables such as spinach, broccoli, turnip greens, dark lettuces; milk.
Manganese	Manganese is necessary for the formation of bone matrix and is found in whole grains, nuts, legumes, tea, instant coffee, fruits, and vegetables.
Phosphorus	Meat, poultry, fish, eggs; cereals, grains; legumes; milk and dairy products, nuts.
Protein	70–100 g/d provides more bone building. Avoid larger doses, which can lead to excessive urinary calcium losses.
Silicon	There may be a role for silicon in stimulation of collagen synthesis and osteoblast differentiation. Intake of biologically active silicon, orthosilicic acid, enhances bone density and may help to preserve bone mass (Devine et al, 2005).
Sodium	Excesses can increase calcium excretion. Avoid using salt at the table, and limit total intake to 2400 mg/d.
Soy	Soy seems to be protective against fractures. Isoflavones increase bone density; use dietary sources.
Vitamin A	Too much retinal (not derived from the carotenoids found in plant sources) may contribute to hip fractures, especially in postmenopausal Caucasian women. Preformed vitamin A is found in liver, milk fat, fortified skim milk, eggs.
Vitamin C	Part of collagen, which supports healthy bone structure. Tissues saturate at 200 mg, therefore large doses are wasted.
Vitamin K	Supports osteocalcin for bone strength, reduces urinary calcium excretion, and modifies bone matrix proteins. A low intake of this fat-soluble vitamin increases the risk for bone fracture. Supplement with 120 μg if needed. Vitamin K is found in dark-green leafy vegetables, dairy products, meat, and eggs.
Zinc	The enzymes in osteoblasts require zinc in order to synthesize collagen. Zinc is found in animal products such as meat, fish, poultry; fortified and whole-grain cereals; milk and milk products; shellfish; liver. Zinc is also found in dry beans; nuts.

REFERENCES

Devine A, et al. Protein consumption is an important predictor of lower limb bone mass in elderly women. *Am J Clin Nutr.* 81:1423, 2005.

- Anticonvulsant therapy, tranquilizers, sedatives, muscle relaxants, and oral diabetic agents may deplete vitamin D. Phosphate binders with aluminum may precipitate osteomalacia; calcium carbonate may be useful, but do not take it with whole grains, bran, high-oxalate foods, or iron tablets.

Herbs, Botanicals, and Supplements

- Herbs and botanical supplements should not be used without discussing with physician.
- Many doctors believe that between 1000–2000 IU of vitamin D per day may be needed to maintain adequate serum levels of this hormone. The upper limit for vitamin D is 10,000 IU per day.

NUTRITION EDUCATION, COUNSELING, CARE MANAGEMENT

- Explain which foods are good sources of vitamin D. Encourage use of cholecalciferol (vitamin D_3) and not vitamin D_2.
- Encourage patient to spend time in the sun for skin synthesis of vitamin D; 15–20 minutes may be needed, after which use a sunscreen to avoid sunburn.
- A spoonful of cod liver oil contains about 1300 IU of vitamin D; an 8-oz glass of fortified milk contains about 100 IU.
- Vegetarians who avoid dairy products may be at risk for calcium and vitamin D depletion; discuss alternative sources from diet or from necessary supplementation.

Patient Education—Food Safety

If enteral or parenteral nutrition is used, careful sanitation and handling techniques must be taught and used.

For More Information

- Mayo Clinic—Osteomalacia
  http://www.mayoclinic.com/health/osteomalacia/DS00935
- Medline—Osteomalacia
  http://www.nlm.nih.gov/medlineplus/ency/article/000376.htm#Definition

OSTEOMALACIA—CITED REFERENCES

Boskey AL, et al. MEPE's Diverse Effects on Mineralization [published online ahead of print December 9, 2009]. *Calcif Tissue Int.* 86:42, 2010.

Rapuri PB, et al. Caffeine decreases vitamin D receptor protein expression and 1,25(OH)2D3 stimulated alkaline phosphatase activity in human osteoblast cells. *J Steroid Biochem Mol Biol.* 103:368, 2007.

Saito T, Fukumoto S. Fibroblast Growth Factor 23 (FGF23) and Disorders of Phosphate Metabolism. [published online ahead of print October 7, 2009] *Int J Pediatr Endocrinol.* 2009:496514.

OSTEOPENIA AND OSTEOPOROSIS

NUTRITIONAL ACUITY RANKING: LEVEL 2

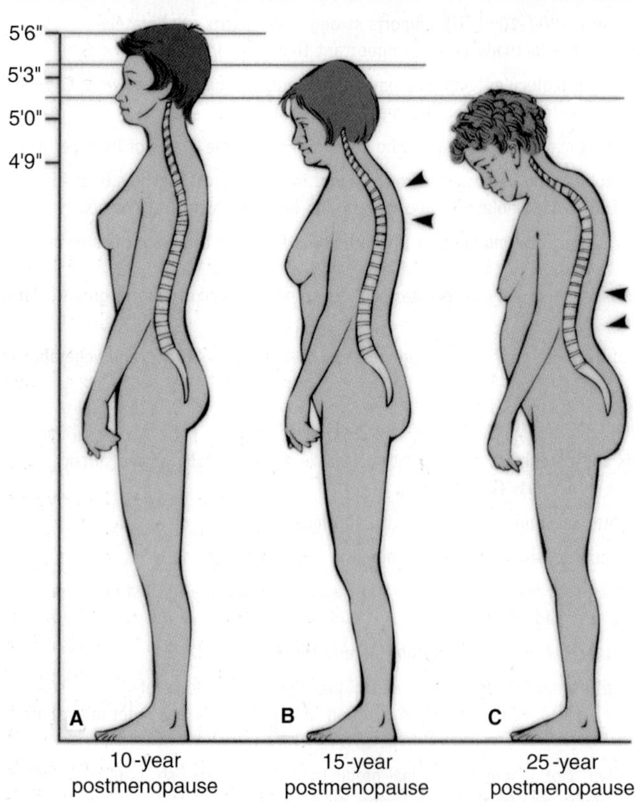

Adapted from: Smeltzer SC, Bare BG. *Textbook of Medical-Surgical Nursing,* 9th ed. Philadelphia: Lippincott Williams & Wilkins, 2000.

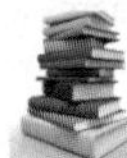

DEFINITIONS AND BACKGROUND

Osteopenia is a decrease in the amount of calcium and phosphorus in the bones. It is identified by a decrease in bone density, which is evident through a DEXA scan. It can occur in premature infants or in adults as a result of long-term inflammatory bowel disease, especially Crohn's disease, or from low BMI. Plasma 25-hydroxyvitamin D (25-OHD) is the most sensitive indicator of BMD and clinical vitamin D_3 status.

Osteoporosis is the most common bone disease in humans; it is characterized by low bone mass, structural deterioration, and decreased bone strength in an estimated 10 million Americans (NOF, 2009).

The aging population is highly affected. Seven percent of non-Hispanic white and Asian men aged 50 and older are estimated to have osteoporosis, and 35% are estimated to have low bone mass. Men are especially vulnerable when they have renal failure, smoke, or take medications on a regular basis, such as anticonvulsants, corticosteroids, or barbiturates.

The World Health Organization (2009) defines osteoporosis as a BMD value that is 2.5 standard deviations or more below the mean of a young adult of the same sex. The lower the BMD, the greater the fracture risk. Osteoporosis can be a silent disease until a fragility fracture occurs at the hip and proximal humerus, when significant physical disability can result.

TABLE 11-9 Risk Factors for Osteoporosis

Factors That Cannot Be Changed			
Advanced age	History of fracture in a first-degree relative		
Caucasians (e.g., Northern European and Asian)	Low body mass index (BMI) and low muscle mass		
Female gender	Personal history of fracture after age 50 years		
Family history of osteoporosis			
Factors That Might Be Altered			
Anorexia nervosa	Hypogonadism, as from low estrogen levels or anorexia nervosa		
Current smoking	Lifetime diet low in calcium (poor diet, excess fiber)		
Depression, past or current	Low testosterone levels in men		
Diabetes	Low vitamin D intake or sunlight exposure		
Estrogen deficiency (premature menopause, amenorrhea)	Sedentary lifestyle or extended bed rest (immobilization)		
Excessive use of alcohol	Use of chemotherapy, tamoxifen, glucocorticoids, lithium, and some anticonvulsants		
Homocysteine, elevated plasma levels	Total parenteral nutrition, long-term use		
Hypertension			
Conditions or Diseases That May Lead to Osteoporosis			
AIDS/HIV	Gastrectomy	Liver disease, severe	Primary biliary cirrhosis
Amyloidosis	Gaucher's disease	Lymphoma or leukemia	Rheumatoid arthritis
Ankylosing spondylitis	Hemochromatosis	Malabsorption syndromes	Spinal cord transection
Celiac disease	Hemophilia	Mastocytosis	Stroke
Chronic obstructive pulmonary disease	Hyperparathyroidism	Multiple myeloma	Thalassemia
Congenital porphyria	Hypophosphatasia	Multiple sclerosis	Thyrotoxicosis
Cushing's syndrome	Idiopathic scoliosis	Osteomalacia	Tropical sprue
Diabetes, type 1	**Inflammatory bowel disease**	Pernicious anemia	

Women can lose up to 20% of their bone mass in the 5–7 years following menopause; 50% of will experience an osteoporotic fracture at some point in time. About 20% of postmenopausal white women in the United States have osteoporosis and 1.5 million fractures occur annually, especially of the hip and spine. Falls are associated with a high risk of frailty fractures (Schwartz et al, 2005).

Spinal or vertebral fractures may lead to loss of height, severe back pain, and spinal deformities such as kyphosis or stooped posture. Hip fractures require hospitalization and major surgery; they impair the ability to walk and may cause disability or death. By 2050, the annual number of hip fractures is expected to triple (World Health Organization, 2009).

Awareness and management of risk factors is important for preventing osteoporosis and the related disability. Both genetic and lifestyle factors play a role. A family history of hip fracture carries a twofold increased risk of fracture among descendants; genetic factors play a major role in BMD and in osteoporosis risk (Ferrari, 2008). Yet BMD is just one of many contributors to bone strength and fracture risk reduction. Dairy, fruit, and vegetable intakes have emerged as an important modifiable protective factor for bone health (Tucker, 2009). Women may lose bone during lactation if their diets are low in calcium and other nutrients. Magnesium, potassium, vitamin C, vitamin K, several B vitamins, and carotenoids are important (Tucker, 2009); see Table 11-8.

In the skeleton, interleukin-1 protein causes an increase in the number and activity of osteoclastic cells—the cells that break down bone tissue. Depression and elevated plasma homocysteine levels are also associated with osteoporosis. See Table 11-9 for the full list of risk factors for osteoporosis.

Physical activity has different effects depending on its intensity, frequency, and duration, and the age at which it is started, with greater effects in adolescence and as a result of weight-bearing exercise. In addition, diet contributes significantly. Building strong bones during childhood and adolescence can be the best defense against developing osteoporosis later. By about age of 20, most women have acquired 98% of total bone mass. Acquisition of a high peak bone mass (reaching genetic potential) by 30 years of age helps reduce bone losses later in life.

Markers of bone turnover can be used to predict the rate of bone loss in post-menopausal women and can also be used to assess the risk of fractures (Eastell and Hannon, 2008). Markers of bone formation include serum bone alkaline phosphatase, total osteocalcin and the procollagen type I N-terminal propeptide assay (Eastell and Hannon, 2008).

Serotonin can serve as a marker for low bone mass. Circulating levels of the neurotransmitter serotonin are inversely associated with bone mass in women; this may have implications when using SSRIs. Bone formation is inhibited by serotonin in the gut. Inactivation of the leptin receptor in serotonergic neurons identifies a molecular basis for the common regulation of bone and energy metabolisms (Yadav et al, 2009). A drug that stops the gut from synthesizing serotonin may be able to reverse severe bone loss and prevent osteoporosis.

Measurements of the urinary excretion of N- and C-terminal cross-linked telopeptides and of serum C-terminal cross-linked telopeptides are sensitive and specific for bone resorption (Eastell and Hannon, 2008). These measures are as important as measurement of BMD.

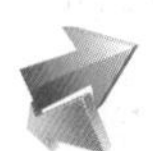

ASSESSMENT, MONITORING, AND EVALUATION

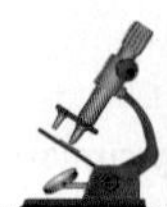

CLINICAL INDICATORS

Genetic Markers: Genes coding for the LDL-receptor related protein 5 (LRP5), estrogen receptor alpha (ESR1), and osteoprotegerin, OPG (TNFRSf11b) are known to pose a risk for osteoporosis (Ferrari, 2008). In a large-scale study, single nucleotide polymorphisms (SNPs) from nine gene loci (ESR1, LRP4, ITGA1, LRP5, SOST, SPP1, TNFRSF11A, TNFRSF11B, and TNFSF11) were associated with BMD, but not always in a predictable manner (Richards et al, 2009).

Clinical/History

Height
Weight
BMI
Back pain
BP
Bone densitometry, DEXA

Lab Work

Ca^{++}
Urinary Ca^{++} (24 hours)
Mg^{++}
Na^{+}, K^{+}
Vitamin D_3 status (serum 25-OHD)
Alb
CRP
PTH (useful in some patients)
Serum P (decreased with hyperparathyroidism)
TSH
Total testosterone in men
Serum homocysteine
Serum folate and vitamin B_{12}

INTERVENTION

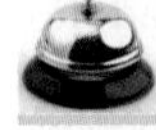

OBJECTIVES

- Preserve height, support independence, and improve functional status. Prevent fractures (Tussing and Chapman-Novakofski, 2005).

SAMPLE NUTRITION CARE PROCESS STEPS

Inadequate Vitamin Intake

Assessment Data: Food records, DEXA scan showing two deviations below normal. Weight and physical activity histories. Medical history, medications, and lab values.

Nutrition Diagnosis (PES): Inadequate intake of vitamin D (NI5.9.1.3) related to poor diet, no food sources, and no use of supplements as evidenced by very low BMD on DEXA.

Intervention: Food and Nutrient Delivery: ND 1.3—add calcium containing beverages and foods, vitamin-D rich foods, adequate protein. ND 3.2.3.3—Supplement use for Vitamin D.

Education: E 2.2—Educate patient concerning calcium and vitamin D food and beverage sources to meet needs along with supplement, sunlight exposure 10–30 min/d, protein needs, increased physical activity.

Counseling: Good sources of vitamin D from diet and supplements, meal planning and shopping tips, dining out guide, referral to Meals-on-Wheels or other social agencies as appropriate, appropriate role for sunshine exposure.

Monitoring and Evaluation: Improvements in dietary and supplemental intake of vitamin D as shown in food records, lab values. DEXA scan report showing no further decline, and a slight improvement in risk level. No fractures.

- Optimize bone health: choose a balanced diet rich in calcium and vitamin D; use weight-bearing and resistance-training exercises. Follow a healthy lifestyle with no smoking.
- Decrease precipitating factors, such as use of anticonvulsants or corticosteroids, lactase deficiency, low intake of fruits and vegetables and dairy, calcium malabsorption, sedentary lifestyle, and low BMI. Provide adequate time for evaluating improvement (6–9 months at least).
- Assure adequate intake of protein. Rather than having a negative effect on bone, protein intake appears to benefit bone status, particularly in older adults (Tucker, 2009).
- Intake of magnesium, potassium, fruit, and vegetables is positively associated with bone health and total bone mass.

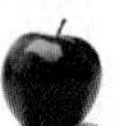

FOOD AND NUTRITION

- Advise all patients to consume adequate amounts of calcium ($\geq$1200 mg/d, including supplements if necessary) and vitamin D. Women after menopause or over age 65 years will need 1500 mg calcium daily. To fulfill the requirement, 1 quart of milk daily can be consumed. If fluid milk is not consumed, dry skim milk powder can be added to many foods. Aged cheeses and yogurt are sources as well.
- Calcium supplements can be used if dairy products are not tolerated; calcium absorption averages approximately 30–40% from most sources See Table 11-10. Space the supplements throughout the day; take no more than 500–600 mg two or more times daily with meals. Use with vitamin D and magnesium.
- For vitamin D, choose fortified milk, cod liver oil, egg yolks, and fatty fish. Supplements may be needed. Do not exceed 10,000 IU/d.

TABLE 11-10 Tips on Calcium Supplements[a]

Product	Source of Calcium (mg)	No. of Tablets/Day to Provide About 900–1000 mg Calcium Per Tablet
Caltrate 600	Carbonate (600 mg)	1.5
Os-Cal 500	Carbonate from oyster shell (500 mg)	2
Os-Cal 500 + Vitamin D	Carbonate from oyster shell (500 mg)	2
Posture (600 mg)	Phosphate (600 mg)	1.5
Posture–Vitamin D	Phosphate (600 mg)	1.5
Citracal	Citrate (200 mg)	5
Citracal + Vitamin D	Citrate (315 mg)	3
Citracal Liquitab	Citrate (500 mg)	2
Tums 500 mg	Carbonate from limestone (500 mg)	2
Tums E-X	Carbonate from limestone (300 mg)	3.5
Tums Ultra	Carbonate from shell (400 mg)	2.5
Calcet + Vitamin D	Carbonate, lactate, gluconate (300 mg)	3.5
Fosfree	Carbonate, gluconate, lactate (175 mg)	6

[a]Excesses of calcium supplements can cause hypercalcemia; monitor intakes carefully and take no more than 500–600 mg two or more times daily with meals. Avoid taking with iron supplements. Use extra water with supplements. Excess vitamin D can cause vitamin D calcinosis. Rates of calcium absorption vary, and dietary sources are the best absorbed; calcium maleate is also well absorbed. Elemental calcium varies in different supplements, as follows:

1. Calcium carbonate (Tums, Roxane, Os-Cal, Calciday, Oyst-Cal, Oystercal, Caltrate) contains 40%. Calcium carbonate temporarily decreases gastric acidity, which is needed for calcium absorption. Tricalcium phosphate provides 39%.
2. Calcium chloride contains 36%.
3. Bone meal or Dolomite contains 33% but should be avoided as it also contains lead.
4. Calcium acetate (Phos-Ex, PhosLo) contains 25%.
5. Calcium citrate (Citracal) contains 21%.
6. Calcium lactate contains 13%.
7. Calcium gluconate contains 9%.

Updated from: Shils M, et al, eds. *Modern nutrition in health and disease.* Baltimore: Lippincott Williams & Wilkins, 1999.

- Extra protein may be needed (Devine et al, 2005; Tucker, 2009).
- For sufficient intake of vitamin B_{12}, include dairy products, meat, poultry, fish, and fortified cereals.
- Isoflavones may also be beneficial; use two to three servings of soy foods daily.
- If patient is obese, use a nutrient-rich, calorie-controlled diet that provides adequate protein, vitamins, calcium, and other minerals. Adequate manganese, vitamins C and K, potassium, and magnesium should be consumed to meet at least the DRI levels. Include fruits and vegetables that contribute to bone health.
- Assure that folic acid and vitamins B_6 and B_{12} are adequate, especially if serum homocysteine levels are elevated.
- Sodium must be controlled. Keep sodium within desired limits while increasing potassium and magnesium.
- Beware of excesses of wheat bran because phytates may increase calcium excretion.
- Caffeine from coffee does not seem to be a problem if calcium (as from milk) is consumed in adequate amounts. However, cola drinks should be limited (Tucker, 2009).
- Moderate alcohol intake shows positive effects on bone, particularly in older women (Tucker, 2009).

Common Drugs Used and Potential Side Effects

- Adequate calcium is crucial; supplementation in bioavailable forms is necessary in individuals who do not achieve recommended intake from dietary sources (see Table 11-11). Side effects may include abdominal pain, anorexia, constipation, vomiting, nausea or dry mouth.
- Oral doses of vitamin D_3 in the range of 1800 to 4000 IU per day may be needed to take serum levels up to 75 to 110 nmol/L (Bischoff-Ferrari et al, 2010).
- Oral alendronic acid is the reference drug for menopausal women with osteopenia. It may be used with parathormone as well, but this has a 2-year limit (Black et al, 2005). See Table 11-12 for more guidance.
- The once monthly injections of risedronate (150 μg) are beneficial for those for which daily or weekly dosing is a challenge (Rackoff, 2009). Bone markers can be used to monitor the efficacy of antiresorptive therapy such as hormone-replacement therapy, raloxifene and bisphosphonates (Eastell and Hannon, 2008).
- SSRIs have been associated with lower BMD and increased rates of bone loss, as well as increased rates of fracture (Haney et al, 2010). Their use should be closely monitored.

Herbs, Botanicals, and Supplements

- Herbs and botanical supplements should not be used without discussing with physician.
- Cabbage, pigweed, dandelion, avocado, and parsley have been recommended, but have not shown efficacy.

TABLE 11-11 **Medications Commonly Used for Management of Osteoporosis**[a]

Medication Comments	Effects	Comments
Bisphosphonates: risedronate (Actonel); alendronate (Fosamax)	Effective agents for reducing vertebral and nonvertebral fracture risk. Alendronate is approved for the treatment of osteoporosis in men. Alendronate and risedronate are approved for use by men and women with glucocorticoid-induced osteoporosis. Zoledronic acid is under study. Bisphosphonates inhibit atherogenesis.	Risedronate may cause dysphagia, esophageal ulcer, and stomach ulcer. Take on an empty stomach 30 minutes before meals; sit upright. Take additional vitamin D and calcium. Headache, gastrointestinal (GI) distress, diarrhea, nausea, constipation, and rash may occur, although rarely. Alendronate may cause metallic taste, nausea, diarrhea, and decreased potassium and magnesium. Avoid in severe renal disease, pregnancy, or breastfeeding. Nausea, heartburn, irritation or pain of the esophagus, anorexia, vomiting, dysphagia, sensation of fullness, and constipation or diarrhea may occur.
Calcitonin-salmon (Miacalcin)	Bone loss is reduced, and bone mass increases, although not in the hip. A modest increase in bone mass occurs.	200 IU/d, the recommended regimen, reduces vertebral fracture risk by 33% in women with low bone mass. Calcitonin makes calcium more available to bones. It is given as an injection or nasal spray; it may cause allergic reactions and flushing of the face and hands, urinary frequency, anorexia, nausea, constipation, or skin rash.
Calcitriol (1,25-dihydroxyvitamin D)	Active form of vitamin D hormone that increases GI absorption of calcium from the gut, kidney reabsorption of calcium, stimulates bone resorption, decreases PTH production, and stimulates skeletal osteoblasts/osteoclasts. Larger doses than the DRI for vitamin D may be needed; 700–800 IU may be beneficial along with 500–1200 mg calcium (Cranney et al, 2007).	Anorexia, abdominal cramping, headache, lethargy, nausea, weight loss, and weakness may result from larger doses.
Ibandronate (Boniva)	Ibandronate is used to treat or prevent osteoporosis in women after menopause; it may increase bone mass by slowing loss of bone.	Should not be taken if hypocalcemia is a problem.
PTH (teriparatide; Forteo)	PTH is the only anabolic osteoporosis agent available for clinical use to lower vertebral fracture incidence by triggering formation of new bone.	Use only in ambulatory patients.
Raloxifene (Evista)	Significantly reduces vertebral fracture risk but not nonvertebral fracture risk.	Protects against thin, weak bones and fractures; also lowers serum cholesterol by 7% and low-density lipoprotein (LDL) by 11%. It may trigger menopausal symptoms, including hot flashes, but is less likely to have an estrogen-like increase in cancer risk.
Sodium fluoride	The slow-release form may increase bone formation and decrease the risk of fractures.	In patients with mild-to-moderate osteoporosis, long-term supplements with fluoride plus calcium result in lower rates of vertebral fracture than supplementation with calcium alone. Intake of fluoride in drinking water at 1 ppm does not appear to be associated with increased risk of hip fracture. Side effects may include abdominal pain, diarrhea, nausea, vomiting.
Statins	Statins, agents that reduce atherogenesis, stimulate bone formation.	Cardiovascular disease and low bone mineral density have some common etiologies.

[a]The FDA approves calcitonin, alendronate, raloxifene, and risedronate for the treatment of postmenopausal osteoporosis; alendronate, risedronate, and raloxifene are approved for the prevention of the disease. Current pharmacological options for osteoporosis prevention and/or treatment are bisphosphonates (alendronate and risedronate), calcitonin, estrogens and/or hormone therapy, parathyroid hormone (PTH 1–34), and raloxifene.
Source: National Osteoporosis Foundation Web site accessed December 14, 2009, at: http://www.nof.org/patientinfo/medications.htm.

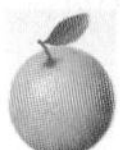

NUTRITION EDUCATION, COUNSELING, CARE MANAGEMENT

- Prevention is the best medicine. Encourage patient to stand upright, rather than sit or recline, as often as feasible. Measures to decrease fall frequency and to slow down the rapid life pace of healthy people with low bone mass should prevent some fractures (Kelsey et al, 2005).
- Change a sedentary lifestyle. Regular resistance and high-impact exercise, contributes to development of high peak bone mass and may reduce the risk of falls in older individuals (Moayyeri, 2008). Aerobic and strengthening exercises are helpful as well.
- Walking or running is beneficial. However, excessive weight-bearing exercise can cause amenorrhea in premenopausal women when a low-calorie diet is consumed.

TABLE 11-12 Features of Rheumatic Arthritis

Tender, warm, swollen joints
Symmetrical pattern of affected joints
Joint inflammation *often* affecting the wrist and finger joints closest to the hand
Joint inflammation *sometimes* affecting other joints, including the neck, shoulders, elbows, hips, knees, ankles, and feet
Fatigue, occasional fevers, a general sense of not feeling well
Pain and stiffness lasting for more than 30 minutes in the morning or after a long rest
Symptoms that last for many years
Variability of symptoms among people with the disease

Source: National Institute of Arthritis and Musculoskeletal and Skin Diseases. Available at http://www.niams.nih.gov/Health_Info/Rheumatic_Disease/default.asp#ra_14.

- An educational osteoporosis prevention program with hands-on activities can increase self-efficacy (Tussing and Chapman-Novakofski, 2005). Explain that calcium absorption declines with age and that adequate calcium and vitamin D are important throughout life. The overall benefit of healthful eating must be strongly emphasized. Consider calcium and vitamin D supplementation in the elderly.
- Describe importance of the use of milk, cheeses, yogurt, broccoli, kale and other greens, and soybeans. Provide recipes and shopping tips.
- Decrease the use of tobacco. Use only moderate amounts of alcohol.
- Caffeine poses a minimal risk unless it replaces calcium-containing beverages; BMD is not affected by caffeine if at least 1 glass of milk is consumed daily.
- Encourage adequate exposure to sunlight (10–30 min/d). Avoid sunburn and overexposure, with its risks of skin cancer.
- Remind all teenagers that osteoporosis is "kid stuff;" maintenance of weight-bearing activity is important during the growing years. Intake of carbonated beverages instead of milk is a big concern.
- Some mineral waters are excellent sources of calcium; bioavailability is good.
- Avoid long-term use of high doses of retinol from fortified foods or supplements.
- Persons with previous fractures are at risk and should be monitored carefully for osteoporosis. The National Osteoporosis Foundation supports an Awareness and Prevention Month in May of each year.
- When steroids are used, check on bone density changes; there is a high incidence of osteoporosis.
- Note that improvements in BMD may take up to 3 years to note improvement (Compston, 2009).

Patient Education—Food Safety

If enteral or parenteral nutrition is used, careful sanitation and handling techniques must be taught and used.

For More Information

- Clinical Guidelines–Osteoporosis
  http://www.nof.org/professionals/clinical.htm
- National Osteoporosis Foundation
  http://www.nof.org/
- Osteopenia
  http://www.nlm.nih.gov/medlineplus/ency/article/007231.htm

OSTEOPENIA AND OSTEOPOROSIS—CITED REFERENCES

Bischoff-Ferrari H, et al. Benefit-risk assessment of vitamin D supplementation [published online ahead of print December 3, 2009]. *Osteoporos Int.* 21:1121, 2010.

Black DM, et al. One year of alendronate after one year of parathyroid hormone (1–84) for osteoporosis. *N Engl J Med.* 353:555, 2005.

Compston J. Monitoring osteoporosis treatment. *Baillieres Best Pract Res Clin Rheumatol.* 23:781, 2009.

Eastell R, Hannon RA. Biomarkers of bone health and osteoporosis risk. *Proc Nutr Soc.* 67:157, 2008.

Ferrari S. Human genetics of osteoporosis. *Baillieres Best Pract Res Clin Endocrinol Metab.* 22:723, 2008.

Haney EM, et al. Effects of selective serotonin reuptake inhibitors on bone health in adults: time for recommendations about screening, prevention and management? *Bone.* 46:13, 2010.

Kelsey JL, et al. Reducing the risk for distal forearm fracture: preserve bone mass, slow down, and don't fall! *Osteoporos Int.* 16:681, 2005.

Moayyeri A. The association between physical activity and osteoporotic fractures: a review of the evidence and implications for future research. *Ann Epidemiol.* 18:827, 2008.

NOF. National Osteoporosis Foundation. Accessed December 14, 2009, at http://www.nof.org/osteoporosis/diseasefacts.htm.

Rackoff P. Efficacy and safety of risedronate 150 mg once a month in the treatment of postmenopausal osteoporosis. *Clin Interv Aging.* 4:207, 2009.

Richards JB, et al. Collaborative meta-analysis: associations of 150 candidate genes with osteoporosis and osteoporotic fracture. *Ann Intern Med.* 151: 528, 2009.

Schwartz AF, et al. Increased falling as a risk factor for fracture among older women: the study of osteoporotic fractures. *Am J Epidemiol.* 161:180, 2005.

Tucker KL. Osteoporosis prevention and nutrition. *Curr Osteoporos Rep.* 7:111, 2009.

Tussing L, Chapman-Novakofski K. Osteoporosis prevention education: behavior theories and calcium intake. *J Am Diet Assoc.* 105:92, 2005.

World Health Organization. Prevention and management of osteoporosis. Accessed December 14, 2009 at http://whqlibdoc.who.int/trs/WHO_TRS_921.pdf.

Yadav VK, et al. A serotonin-dependent mechanism explains the leptin regulation of bone mass, appetite, and energy expenditure. *Cell.* 138:976, 2009.

PAGET'S DISEASE (OSTEITIS DEFORMANS)

NUTRITIONAL ACUITY RANKING: LEVEL 1–2

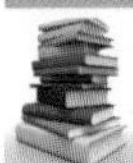

DEFINITIONS AND BACKGROUND

Paget's disease of the bone (PDB) is a disorder of skeletal remodeling, where areas on bone grow abnormally, enlarging and becoming soft. It is of unknown etiology, with excessive bone destruction and repairing. Of all persons older than 50 years of age, 3% have an isolated lesion; actual clinical disease is much less common. PDB is the second most common bone disease in the world. A systematic laboratory screening including serum alkaline phosphatase of an older subject complaining of bone pain, articular pain, or back pain is a strategy to improve the diagnosis of PDB (Varenna et al, 2009).

The disease tends to run in families. Genetic analysis indicates that 40% of patients with Paget's disease have an affected first-degree relative. Approximately 3 million Americans have the disease; it rarely occurs before age 40. Juvenile Paget's disease is very debilitating. Osteoclasts are larger than normal and increased in size (Deftos, 2005). Juvenile Paget's disease usually presents in infancy or childhood and results in progressive deformity, growth retardation, and deafness.

The disease is higher in frequency in people who are aged 65 or older. There is a slight male predominance. Prognosis is good in mild cases.

Sarcoma can also be found in this population (Mankin and Hornicek, 2005). There has been a decline in incidence of this complication but where it does occur, prognosis is still poor (Mangham et al, 2009).

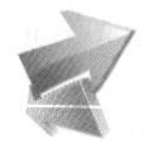

ASSESSMENT, MONITORING, AND EVALUATION

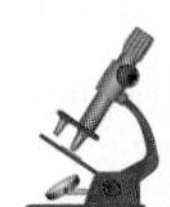

CLINICAL INDICATORS

Genetic Markers: There seem to be strong ties to European ancestry in Paget's disease, including Australia and New Zealand. A majority of cases harbor germline mutations in the SQSTM1, Sequestosome1 gene (Merchant et al, 2009).

Clinical/History

- Height
- Weight
- BMI
- Deep "bone pain"
- Joint pain, neck pain
- Skull enlargement
- Hearing loss
- Headaches
- Tickening of long bones
- Bowing of limbs
- Reduced height
- Spontaneous fractures
- X-rays (denser, expanded bones)
- Bone scans

Lab Work

- Alk phos (increased)
- Urinary Ca^{++} (altered)
- Vitamin D_3 status (serum 25-OHD)
- Uric acid (UA), elevated?
- PTH (abnormal)
- Ca^{++}, Mg^{++}
- Na^{+}, K^{+}
- Alb, transthyretin
- CRP
- Transferrin
- Serum P
- H & H
- Serum B_{12}
- Radiolabeled bisphosphonate

INTERVENTION

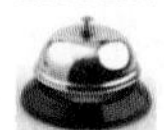

OBJECTIVES

- Prevent complications, especially related to the nervous system (e.g., fractures, spinal stenosis, paraplegia, cardiac failure, and deafness).
- Prevent side effects of drug therapy.
- Promote full recovery when possible.
- Differentiate from other conditions with bone lesions.
- Alleviate anemia and other complications.

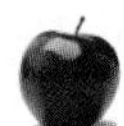

FOOD AND NUTRITION

- Adequate protein is important, with adequate calories to spare protein.
- Adequate levels of calcium and vitamins C and D may be needed.
- To correct anemia, monitor serum levels of iron and vitamin B_{12} to determine need for an altered diet.

Common Drugs Used and Potential Side Effects

- Drugs that inhibit bone resorption—bisphosphonates (etidronate, pamidronate, clodronate, or alendronate)—

SAMPLE NUTRITION CARE PROCESS STEPS

Abnormal Nutritional Labs

Assessment Data: Weight and physical activity histories. Medical history, medications, abnormal lab values for alk phos, uric acid, serum vitamin D_3, and PTH.

Nutrition Diagnosis (PES): Abnormal nutritional labs related to metabolic changes from Paget's disease as evidenced by increased alk phos, altered urinary calcium, abnormal PTH, elevated uric acid levels, diagnosis of anemia, and bone pain.

Intervention: Treatment with bisphosphonates to alter serum and urinary labs; careful monitoring for side effects affecting intake and appetite. Food-nutrient delivery—Correct iron-deficiency anemia from poor intake and disease process.

Monitoring and Evaluation: Improvement in serum lab values; resolution of anemia; decreased bone pain.

may be used to slow the progression. Bisphosphonates are pyrophosphate analogs that bind to bone at active sites of remodeling. The bisphosphonate zoledronic acid (Zometa), given in a single injection, yields a rapid and long-lasting improvement in bone health (Reid et al, 2005). The nitrogen-containing BPs pamidronate (Aredia) and zoledronic acid (Zometa) are capable of causing bisphosphonate-associated osteonecrosis of the jaw (Grewal and Fayans, 2008).

- Risedronate (Actonel) can cause dysphagia, esophageal ulcer, and stomach ulcer. Take on an empty stomach 30 minutes before meals; consume additional vitamin D and calcium. Headache, diarrhea, nausea, constipation, and rash may occur, although they are rare.
- Osteoprotegerin may be used in managing the juvenile form of Paget's disease (Cundy et al, 2005).
- Thyrocalcitonin or synthetic calcitonin may be used to decrease passage of calcium from bones to bloodstream. Methods of administration include a nasal spray. Monitor for nausea or vomiting.
- Analgesics may be needed for pain.

Herbs, Botanicals, and Supplements

- Herbs and botanical supplements should not be used without discussing with physician.
- Unusual bone diseases may be associated with use of Chinese herbs.

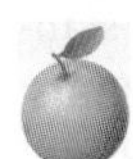

NUTRITION EDUCATION, COUNSELING, CARE MANAGEMENT

- Discuss appropriate dietary alterations for patient's condition, individualized for the current condition and status. Include good food sources of calcium, B-complex vitamins, iron, protein, and vitamin D. Monitor carefully, if supplements are used, in addition to dietary guidance.
- Discuss side effects for the specific drugs ordered.

Patient Education—Food Safety

If enteral or parenteral nutrition is used, careful sanitation and handling techniques must be taught and used.

For More Information

- National Association for the Relief of Paget's Disease http://www.paget.org.uk/
- National Institute of Arthritis and Musculoskeletal and Skin Diseases http://www.niams.nih.gov/bone/hi/paget/diagnosed.htm
- National Institutes of Health Osteoporosis and Related Bones Diseases http://www.niams.nih.gov/bone/
- Paget's Disease http://www.nlm.nih.gov/medlineplus/ency/article/000414.htm
- Paget Foundation http://www.paget.org/

PAGET'S DISEASE—CITED REFERENCES

Cundy T, et al. Recombinant osteoprotegerin for juvenile Paget's disease. *N Engl J Med.* 353:918, 2005.
Deftos LJ. Treatment of Paget's disease—taming the wild osteoclast. *N Engl J Med.* 353:872, 2005.
Grewal VS, Fayans EP. Bisphosphonate-associated osteonecrosis: a clinician's reference to patient management. *Todays FDA.* 20:38, 2008.
Mangham DC, et al. Sarcoma arising in Paget's disease of bone: declining incidence and increasing age at presentation. *Bone.* 44:431, 2009.
Mankin HJ, Hornicek FJ. Paget's sarcoma: a historical and outcome review. *Clin Orthop Relat Res.* 438:97, 2005.
Merchant A, et al. Somatic mutations in SQSTM1 detected in affected tissues from patients with sporadic Paget's disease of bone. *J Bone Miner Res.* 24:484, 2009.
Reid IR, et al. Comparison of a single infusion of zoledronic acid with risedronate for Paget's disease. *N Engl J Med.* 353:898, 2005.
Varenna M, et al. Demographic and clinical features related to a symptomatic onset of Paget's disease of bone [published online ahead of print December 1, 2009]. *J Rheumatol.* 37:155, 2010.

POLYARTERITIS NODOSA

NUTRITIONAL ACUITY RANKING: LEVEL 1–2

DEFINITIONS AND BACKGROUND

Polyarteritis nodosa (PAN) is characterized by necrotizing inflammation of medium- or small-sized arteries without glomerulonephritis or vasculitis in arterioles, capillaries, or venules (Colmegna and Maldonado-Cocco, 2005). Viral infections such as hepatitis B may trigger it.

In PAN, arteries become inflamed in several organs, causing damage in brain, heart, liver, GI tract, or renal tissues. Renal involvement develops and is accompanied by hypertension in half of patients. PAN also commonly involves the gut (abdominal angina, hemorrhage, perforation), heart (myocarditis, myocardial infarction), or eye (scleritis); rupture of renal or mesenteric microaneurysms can also occur. PAN is two to three times more common in men and usually develops between ages 40 and 50 years. Rarely, it occurs after a Hepatitis-B vaccination.

It is fatal if not treated. Treatment includes use of prednisone, plasmapheresis to remove immune complexes, and antiviral therapy (lamivudine) for the hepatitis B infection.

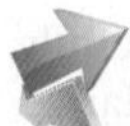

ASSESSMENT, MONITORING, AND EVALUATION

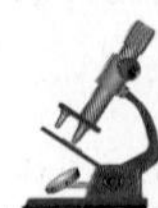

CLINICAL INDICATORS

Genetic Markers: Medium-sized artery vasculitides that occur in childhood manifest mostly as PAN, with high morbidity and mortality rates (Dillon et al, 2009). PAN is likely to have a genetic connection; MEFV is one gene under study.

Clinical/History		
Height	Myalgias, weakness	Hepatitis B antigen or antibody in serum
Weight	Neuropathy	Ca^{++}, Mg^{++}
BMI	Hematuria	Na^{+}, K^{+}
Weight loss >4 kg since onset of illness	Fatigue	Alb, transthyretin
Hematuria	Rash, nodules or Raynaud's disease	BUN, Creat (elevated but not from dehydration)
Edema	Biopsy of medium vessels	Transferrin
Chest pain	**Lab Work**	H & H
Tachycardia	ESR (elevated)	Vitamin D_3 status (serum 25-OHD)
Shortness of breath	CRP	
Fever?	Glucose	
Abdominal pain		
BP (elevated)		

INTERVENTION

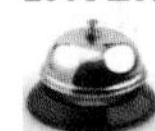

OBJECTIVES

- Treat as soon as possible to decrease heart and renal damage.
- Improve appetite and intake.
- Prevent weight loss.
- Increase calorie intake when there is fever.

SAMPLE NUTRITION CARE PROCESS STEPS

Inadequate Oral Food and Beverage Intake

Assessment Data: Weight and physical activity histories. Medical history, medications, and lab values.

Nutrition Diagnosis (PES): Inadequate oral food and beverage intake related to anorexia, fever and abdominal pain as evidenced by weight loss of 3 kg in 8 weeks.

Intervention: Food-Nutrient delivery—Offer preferred foods, enhanced with energy kilocalories from milk powder, fats, etc. Educate about how to manage nausea; suggest small, frequent meals throughout the day and liquids separate from meals. Coordinate care with nursing, medical teams if medications are needed.

Monitoring and Evaluation: Resolution of weight loss; no further losses. Improvement in nausea and abdominal pain.

- Reduce edema, anorexia, hypertension, and other effects of the disorder.

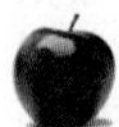

FOOD AND NUTRITION

- A high-energy intake may be beneficial in case of weight loss.
- A normal to high protein intake generally is required.
- Fluid or sodium intake may be limited with hypertension, kidney disease, or edema or with use of steroids.
- Include phytochemicals derived from spices such as turmeric (curcumin); red pepper (capsaicin); cloves (eugenol); ginger (gingerol); cumin, anise, and fennel (anethol); basil and rosemary (ursolic acid); garlic (diallyl sulfide, *S*-allylmercaptocysteine, and ajoene); and pomegranate (ellagic acid) (Aggarwal and Shishodia, 2004).

Common Drugs Used and Potential Side Effects

- Steroids such as prednisone may be used for 2 weeks. Side effects of long-term use include negative nitrogen and potassium balances; decreased calcium and zinc levels; CHO intolerance; and excessive sodium retention. With weight gain, a calorie-controlled diet may be useful.
- Pain relievers may be needed; monitor individually for side effects such as GI distress.
- Immunosuppressive cyclophosphamide may be used; long-term effects can reduce the ability to fight infections. Corticosteroids plus cyclophosphamide is the standard of care, in particular for patients with more severe disease, in whom this combination prolongs survival (Colmegna and Maldonado-Cocco, 2005).
- Infliximab may be used as an alternative agent for the treatment of patients with PAN refractory to conventional therapy (Al-Bishri et al, 2005).

Herbs, Botanicals, and Supplements

- Herbs and botanical supplements should not be used without discussing with physician.

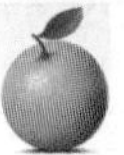

NUTRITION EDUCATION, COUNSELING, CARE MANAGEMENT

- Discuss alternate dietary guidelines as appropriate for medications and side effects of the disease.
- Discuss sources of nutrients as appropriate for the ordered diet. Provide guidance on enhancing nutrient and energy density from meals and snacks.
- With abdominal pain and GI bleeding, PAN occasionally is mistaken for inflammatory bowel disease. Be certain to see a trained specialist as needed.

Patient Education—Food Safety

If enteral or parenteral nutrition is used, careful sanitation and handling techniques must be taught and used.

For More Information

- Johns Hopkins Vasculitis Center
  http://vasculitis.med.jhu.edu/typesof/polyarteritis.html
- Polyarteritis Nodosa Foundation
  http://www.angelfire.com/pa3/autoimmunedisease/aifeindex.html
- Polyarteritis Nodosa
  http://www.emedicine.com/ped/topic1844.htm
- Vasculitis Foundation
  http://www.vasculitisfoundation.org/polyarteritisnodosa

POLYARTERITIS NODOSA—CITED REFERENCES

Aggarwal BB, Shishodia S. Suppression of the nuclear factor-kappa B activation pathway by spice-derived phytochemicals: reasoning for seasoning. *Ann N Y Acad Sci.* 1030:434, 2004.

Al-Bishri J, et al. Refractory polyarteritis nodosa successfully treated with infliximab. *J Rheumatol.* 32:1371, 2005.

Colmegna I, Maldonado-Cocco JA. Polyarteritis nodosa revisited. Polyarteritis nodosa revisited. *Curr Rheumatol Rep.* 7:288, 2005.

Dillon MJ, et al. Medium-size-vessel vasculitis [published online ahead of print November 28, 2009]. *Pediatr Nephrol.* 25:1641, 2010.

RHABDOMYOLYSIS

NURITIONAL ACUITY RANKING: LEVEL 3

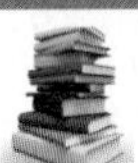

DEFINITIONS AND BACKGROUND

Rhabdomyolysis (RML) is a clinical and biochemical syndrome resulting from skeletal muscle injury with release of myoglobin into the plasma and breakdown of muscle fibers with release into the circulation. Some of these changes are toxic to the kidney, often resulting in kidney damage or acute renal failure. A disturbance in myocyte calcium homeostasis takes place.

RML may occur in infants, toddlers, and adolescents who have inherited enzyme deficiencies of carbohydrate or lipid metabolism, DMD, or malignant hyperthermia. RML may also occur from extensive muscle damage as from a crushing injury, major burn, electrical shock, toxins, bacterial infections, excessive exercise (Olpin, 2005), seizures, alcoholism, overdose of cocaine, or use of drugs such as cholesterol-reducing statins. The most common causes of RML in adults include crush injury, overexertion, alcohol abuse, use of certain medicines, and toxic substances. Postoperative RML in bariatric surgery occurs with prolonged muscle compression; potential consequences may lead to death (de Menezes Ettinger et al, 2005).

Muscle pain caused by RML may involve specific symptoms of groups of muscles or may be generalized throughout the body. Muscles in the calves and the lower back are commonly affected but each patient is different. Early complications of RML include severe hyperkalemia with cardiac arrhythmia and arrest. The most serious late complication is acute renal failure.

RML can be defined with CK values exceeding 10–25 times the upper limit of normal irrespective of renal function (Linares et al, 2009). Management of suspected drug-induced myopathy should include immediate discontinuation of the offending agent and supportive care (Mor et al, 2009).

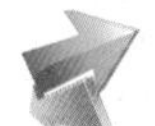

ASSESSMENT, MONITORING, AND EVALUATION

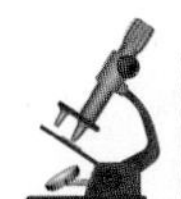

CLINICAL INDICATORS

Genetic Markers: RML may occur in infants, toddlers, and adolescents who have inherited enzyme deficiencies of carbohydrate or lipid metabolism or who have inherited myopathies. Elevated CK levels have been found with a high-density SNP genotype in a p.Trp3X allele; this mutation is associated with a mild Becker phenotype of MD (Flanigan et al, 2009).

Clinical/History

- Height
- Weight
- BMI
- Weight gain (unintentional)
- I & O
- Tea-colored urine
- Temperature
- BP (elevated)
- Exposure to toxic substances or chronic alcohol use
- Use of medications such as statins
- Muscle tenderness
- Weakness of the affected muscles
- Muscle stiffness or aching (myalgia)
- Seizures
- Joint pain
- Fatigue
- Abnormally dark colored urine from excretion of myoglobin

Lab Work

- Creatine phosphokinase (CPK) (very high)
- Serum myoglobin test (positive)
- Urinary casts or hemoglobin
- Ca^{++}, Mg^{++}
- Na^+
- K^+ (may be high from muscle breakdown)
- Alb, transthyretin
- CRP
- BUN
- Creat
- Transferrin
- H & H
- UA (elevated)
- Vitamin D_3 status (serum 25-OHD)

INTERVENTION

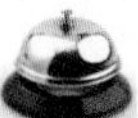

OBJECTIVES

- Preserve renal function.
- Eliminate myoglobin out of the kidneys with early and aggressive hydration. Medicines may also be needed to make the urine more alkaline.
- Treat kidney failure or hyperkalemia if needed.

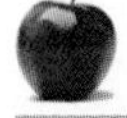

FOOD AND NUTRITION

- Hydration needs with muscle necrosis may approximate the massive fluid volume needs of a severely burned patient.

SAMPLE NUTRITION CARE PROCESS STEPS

Excessive Physical Activity

Assessment Data: Weight and physical activity histories. Medical history with diagnosis of RML.

Nutrition Diagnosis (PES): Excessive physical activity related to 2-hour workouts twice daily as evidenced by complaints of weakness, muscle stiffness and tenderness, and very high CPK levels.

Intervention: Education about a more desirable level of physical activity to lessen strain on muscles. Counseling about nutrition for athletics and maintenance of other healthy habits, including adequate rest and sleep. Physical activity logs.

Monitoring and Evaluation: Improvement in muscle stuffness and tenderness; CPK levels returning to a normal range. Physical activity logs showing workouts no longer than 30 minutes twice daily.

- Special dietary advice is required if there is renal disease or the need for dialysis.
- It is important to offer advice according to the medical condition that preceded RML. Avoidance of fasting, feeding with a high-carbohydrate and low-fat diet, and intravenous drip infusion soon after every onset of RML may be needed for children (Korematsu et al, 2009).

Common Drugs Used and Potential Side Effects

- Statins block the enzyme in the liver that is responsible for making cholesterol, hydroxy-methylglutaryl-coenzyme A reductase (HMG-CoA reductase).
- Despite the withdrawal of cerivastatin because of fatal RML, the risk of this complication with other statins is extremely low (Waters, 2005). Options for managing statin myopathy include statin switching, particularly to fluvastatin or low-dose rosuvastatin; nondaily dosing regimens; nonstatin alternatives, such as ezetimibe and bile acid-binding resins; and coenzyme Q10 supplementation (Joy and Hegele, 2009).
- Diuretic therapy may be needed if there is hypertension.
- If there is hyperkalemia, calcium chloride or calcium gluconate may be used.

Herbs, Botanicals, and Supplements

- Health care practitioners must take an active role in identifying patients who are using CAM and provide appropriate patient education (Gabardi et al, 2007). Herbs and botanical supplements should not be used without discussing with physician. There are 17 dietary supplements that have been associated with direct renal injury, CAM-induced immune-mediated nephrotoxicity, nephrolithiasis, RML with acute renal injury, and hepatorenal syndrome (Gabardi et al, 2007).
- Even brief exposure to atorvastatin causes a marked decrease in blood coenzyme Q10 concentration, with commonly reported adverse effects of exercise intolerance, myalgia, and myoglobinuria.

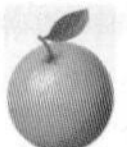

NUTRITION EDUCATION, COUNSELING, CARE MANAGEMENT

- Discuss alternate dietary guidelines as appropriate for medications and side effects of the disease.
- Discuss how to use diet and exercise to manage high serum cholesterol if this information has not been given before. Reinforce what the patient has been doing well.
- After damage to any muscles, extra fluid is needed to dilute urine and to eliminate myoglobin. Among soldiers, RML occurs in 25% of those who are injured (Carter et al, 2005).

Patient Education—Food Safety

If enteral or parenteral nutrition is used, careful sanitation and handling techniques must be taught and used.

For More Information

- E-medicine
  http://www.emedicine.com/emerg/topic508.htm
- Rhabdomyolysis
  http://www.nlm.nih.gov/medlineplus/ency/article/000473.htm

RHABDOMYOLYSIS—CITED REFERENCES

Carter R III, et al. Epidemiology of hospitalizations and deaths from heat illness in soldiers. *Med Sci Sports Exerc.* 37:1338, 2005.

de Menezes Ettinger JE, et al. Prevention of rhabdomyolysis in bariatric surgery. *Obes Surg.* 15:874, 2005.

Flanigan KM, et al. DMD Trp3X nonsense mutation associated with a founder effect in North American families with mild Becker muscular dystrophy. *Neuromuscul Disord.* 19:743, 2009.

Gabardi S, et al. A review of dietary supplement-induced renal dysfunction. *Clin J Am Soc Nephrol.* 2:757, 2007.

Joy TR, Hegele RA. Narrative review: statin-related myopathy. *Ann Intern Med.* 150:858, 2009.

Korematsu S, et al. Novel mutation of early, perinatal-onset, myopathic-type very-long-chain acyl-CoA dehydrogenase deficiency. *Pediatr Neurol.* 41:151, 2009.

Linares LA, et al. The modern spectrum of rhabdomyolysis: drug toxicity revealed by creatine kinase screening. *Curr Drug Saf.* 4:181, 2009.

Mor A, et al. Drug-induced myopathies. *Bull NYU Hosp Jt Dis.* 67:358, 2009.

Olpin SE. Fatty acid oxidation defects as a cause of neuromyopathic disease in infants and adults. *Clin Lab.* 51:289, 2005.

Waters DD. Safety of high-dose atorvastatin therapy. *Am J Cardiol.* 96:69, 2005.

RHEUMATOID ARTHRITIS

NUTRITIONAL ACUITY RANKING: LEVEL 1

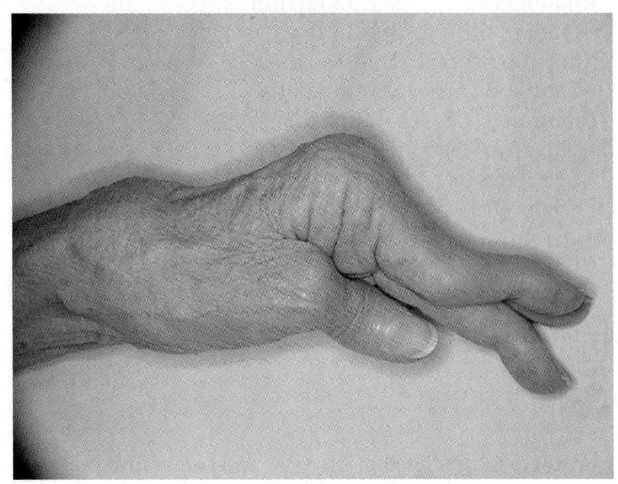

Adaprted from: Strickland JW, Graham TJ. *Master Techniques in Orthopeadic Surgery: The Hand*, 2nd ed. Philadelphia: Lippincott Williams & Wilkins, 2005.

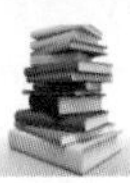

DEFINITIONS AND BACKGROUND

RA is a chronic polyarthritis mainly affecting the smaller peripheral joints and is accompanied by general ill health. Crippling deformities can occur. Of all cases, 75% are women. Most patients are between ages 20 and 40, and RA affects over 1.3 million Americans. To diagnose RA, symptoms must have been present for at least 6 weeks; see Table 11-12.

The cause of RA is increased inflammatory cytokine production, such as from mast cells, interleukin-6, tumor necrosis factor alpha (TNFα), and acute-phase proteins. Inflammation of synovial tissues is the dominant manifestation. Antibodies against IgG and collagen are noted. Hand involvement and knees or ankles/feet are involved in most. Table 11-13 provides a list of the variant forms of RA.

Some studies show an improvement in RA symptoms over the short term with a diet high in omega-3s or fish oil supplements. Omega-3 fatty acids reduce tenderness in joints, decrease morning stiffness, and reduce the amount

TABLE 11-13 Variant Forms of Rheumatic Arthritis (RA)

Condition	Background	Nutritional Implications
Juvenile RA (JRA)	JRA causes joint inflammation and stiffness for more than 6 weeks in a child 16 years of age or less. It is classified into three types, depending on symptoms, number of joints involved, and presence or absence of antibodies in the blood. Pauciarticular JRA is most common and affects mainly the knees. The polyarticular form affects 30% of children with JRA. Stills disease is the systemic form; it tests negative for the usual antibodies, may affect internal organs, may become chronic in adulthood and affects 20% of children with JRA. Both genetic factors and environmental factors, such as a virus, can trigger JRA. Because JRA often affects knees, limping can occur. Salicylates, gold salts, or glucocorticoids may be used.	Children suffering from JCA may have reduced serum levels of beta-carotene, retinol, and zinc.
Sjögren's syndrome	Dry eyes and dry mouth occur as a result of insufficient production of lacrimal and salivary secretions. Artificial tears and glucocorticoids may be needed. Sjögren's syndrome is relatively common and affects 4 million Americans, mostly women. It is most often related to RA, lupus, scleroderma, or polymyositis. Debilitating pain and fatigue can occur. Sensitivity to sunlight is common; sunscreen is helpful.	Plan meals and use artificial saliva for easier swallowing. Chewing sugar-free gum can stimulate saliva production if any is available. Gel-based saliva substitutes are useful. Sip water often, and avoid caffeinated drinks, which can be dehydrating. Drink water during meals to help with swallowing. Mouth infections are common; use good oral hygiene. With dry mouth or dysphagia, there is a risk for aspiration pneumonia. Weight loss and digestive problems are common.
Felty's syndrome	Felty's syndrome only affects about 1% of RA patients. This is a triad of RA, granulocytopenia, and splenomegaly. Painful, stiff, and swollen joints occur. Infections, leg ulcers, burning eyes, and anemia also can complicate the condition. Sometimes, splenectomy is indicated; drug therapy may be helpful to others.	Fever, weight loss, and brown pigmentation may occur. If immunosuppressive drugs are used, monitor for side effects.
Rheumatoid vasculitis	Rheumatoid vasculitis can be life threatening and usually occurs in patients with severe deforming arthritis and a high titer of rheumatoid factor. A majority have a strong human leukocyte antigen relationship. Vasculitic lesions include rheumatoid nodules, small nail fold infarcts, and purpura. Fatigue, weight loss, fever, organ ischemia, CNS infarctions, myocardial infarction, and peripheral neuropathy can occur.	Corticosteroids are the usual treatment. D-penicillamine and prednisone generally are used.

of medication needed; they also downregulate T-cell proliferation. People with RA who eat 4 oz of fish every day have less morning stiffness, swollen joints, and all-around pain. Fish oil and aspirin are blood thinners, and they should not be taken together for a long time.

Supplements of GLA, as from borage oil, may reduce generation of mediators of inflammation and attenuate symptoms but may cause potentially harmful increases in serum arachidonic acid unless EPA is also used. GLA increases prostaglandin E levels, which increase cyclic adenosine monophosphate (cAMP) levels which, in turn, suppress TNFα synthesis.

Epidemiological studies suggest that the antioxidant potential of dietary carotenoids may protect against the oxidative damage that can result in inflammation (Pattison et al, 2005). Proper antioxidant nutrients provide defense against increased oxidant stress. Supplementation of folate and vitamin B_{12} is needed in patients treated with methotrexate to reduce side effects and to offset elevated plasma homocysteine.

Complications of RA may include osteoporosis and chronic anemia. Calcium and vitamin D reduce the bone loss in patients who take steroids. An iron supplement may prevent anemia, and serum ferritin levels may be low. Patients benefit from a basic dietary supplement.

Higher intakes of meat and total protein and lower intakes of fruit, vegetables, and vitamin C are associated with an increased risk of RA (Choi, 2005). However, dietary factors such as fruit, coffee, long-chain fatty acids, olive oil, vitamins A, E, C, and D, zinc, selenium, and iron need to be studied over a longer time period (Pedersen et al, 2005).

Rheumatoid cachexia, loss of muscle mass and strength and increase in fat mass, is very common in patients with RA and persists even after joint inflammation improves (Roubenoff, 2009). Cardiovascular disease is a concern. Body composition studies are as important as BMI and other traditional assessment measures (Elkan et al, 2009).

ASSESSMENT, MONITORING, AND EVALUATION

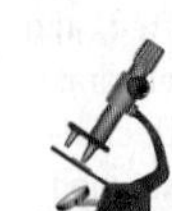

CLINICAL INDICATORS

Genetic Markers: B cell, cytokine and inflammation response, and antigen presentation pathways are associated with RA; this confirms the known biological mechanisms for auto-immunity (Ballard et al, 2009).

Clinical/History		Lab Work
Height	Pain and stiffness >30 minutes in the morning or after a long rest	RBC
Weight	Food allergies	CRP
BMI		LE prep
Temperature		Creat (may be decreased)

ESR (increases with inflammation)	Ceruloplasmin (may be increased)	Alb, transthyretin
ANA	H & H	Gluc
Rheumatoid factor (RF)	Serum ferritin	BUN
Antistreptococcal antibody titer	Serum B_{12}	Ca^{++}, Mg^{++}
Immunoglobulins (may be elevated in Sjögren's)	Transferrin	Na^{+}, K^{+}
	Serum folate, RBC folate	Vitamin D_3 status (serum 25-OHD)
	Serum copper	

INTERVENTION

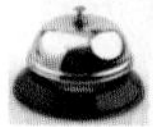

OBJECTIVES

- Preserve a high level of physical and social functioning to promote good quality of life; reduce the effects of pain and swelling.
- Maintain satisfactory nutritional status; malnutrition and loss of lean body mass are common in this condition. Monitor weight changes.
- Simplify meal preparation.
- Support the immune system. Consume foods rich in antioxidants, such as carotenoids (Pattison et al, 2005), vitamin E, selenium, and vitamin D. A vegetarian diet may have significant benefits.
- Promote adequate growth in children who have RA; stunting can occur from glucocorticoids.
- Promote return of fat-free body mass and improvement in muscle strength.
- Restrict sodium intake, if needed.

SAMPLE NUTRITION CARE PROCESS STEPS

Drug–Nutrient Interaction

Assessment Data: Weight and physical activity histories. Medical history, medications and lab values. DEXA scan results.

Nutrition Diagnosis (PES): Food-Medication interaction (NC-2.3) related to corticosteroid use secondary to diagnosis of RA as evidence by abnormal Ca^{++} level <8.4, DEXA scan at 80% of desirable range for age, perimenopausal status, low calcium and vitamin D intake from diet history.

Intervention: Food-Nutrient Delivery—include extra calcium-rich foods. Education about use of steroid therapy and its impact on nutritional status. Counseling about good sources of calcium and vitamin D from diet and supplements, meal planning and shopping tips, dining out guide, referral to Meals-on-Wheels or other social agencies as appropriate. Coordinate care with nursing and physician to administer calcium and vitamin D supplements at different time than corticosteroids to help increase absorption.

Monitoring and Evaluation: Improvements in dietary and supplemental intake of vitamin D and calcium as shown in food records, lab values, and DEXA scan report.

- Modify patient's diet if hyperlipidemia is present or if there is elevated homocysteine.
- Avoid or correct constipation.

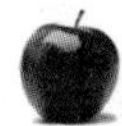

FOOD AND NUTRITION

- Use a high-protein and high-calorie diet if patient is malnourished. Cachexia is common (Marcora et al, 2005).
- A diet that lessens inflammation is useful; olive oil should be used often because it contains oleocanthal, a natural anti-inflammatory agent.
- Eating fatty fish, such as salmon, sardines, mackerel, herring, and tuna, two times per week is suggested. In addition to fatty fish, other good sources of omega-3s include flaxseed, walnuts, soy, canola oils. Try to acquire 3–6 g of omega-3 fatty acids per day for 4 months.
- An uncooked vegan diet may be useful, with berries, fruits, vegetables, roots, nuts, and seeds; see Table 11-2. There is improvement in RA when eating a lactovegetarian, vegan, or Mediterranean diet (Skoldstam et al, 2005).
- Adequate fluid, fiber, vitamins, and minerals are important. Use foods high in beta-carotene, lutein lycopene, selenium, vitamins C and E; choose nutrient-dense foods. Antioxidants such as beta-cryptoxanthin (as from one glass of freshly squeezed orange juice daily) can reduce the risk of developing RA (Pattison et al, 2005).
- Increase vitamin D intakes to decrease the incidence and severity of RA. Provide adequate intake of calcium, magnesium, B-complex vitamins, potassium, and zinc.
- Increase folic acid if methotrexate is used; enhance diet or encourage folic acid supplements.
- Provide meals that are easy to tolerate when the drugs being used cause gastric irritation. Avoid acidic or highly spiced foods if needed.
- With dysphagia, tube feed or use soft/thick, pureed foods as needed.
- Identify and eliminate any food allergens. Individualize the diet accordingly.

Common Drugs Used and Potential Side Effects

- With biologic therapies, such as TNF inhibitors, many patients with RA have seen significant improvement in symptoms, function, and quality of life (Barton et al, 2009). See Table 11-14.

TABLE 11-14 Medications Used in Rheumatoid Arthritis

Medications	Uses/Effects	Side Effects	Monitoring
Analgesics and nonsteroidal anti-inflammatory drugs (NSAIDs)	Analgesics relieve pain; NSAIDs relieve pain and reduce inflammation.	Upset stomach, peptic ulcer, bleeding, renal failure. Use of NSAIDs may increase rate of miscarriage for pregnant women.	For all traditional NSAIDs: avoid drinking alcohol or using blood thinners; avoid if there is sensitivity or allergy to aspirin or similar drugs, kidney or liver disease, heart disease, high blood pressure, asthma, or peptic ulcers.
Acetaminophen		Usually no side effects when taken as directed.	Not to be taken with alcohol or with other products containing acetaminophen. Not to be used for more than 10 days unless directed by a physician.
Aspirin: buffered, plain	Aspirin is used to reduce pain, swelling, and inflammation, allowing patients to move more easily and carry out normal activities. It is generally part of early and ongoing therapy.	Upset stomach; tendency to bruise easily; ulcers, pain, or discomfort; diarrhea; headache; heartburn or indigestion; nausea or vomiting.	Doctor monitoring is needed. Not used for children in whom Reye's syndrome is a risk, but otherwise useful in lessening inflammation.
Traditional NSAIDs: ibuprofen, ketoprofen, naproxen	NSAIDs help relieve pain within hours of administration in dosages available over the counter (available for all three medications). They relieve pain and inflammation in dosages available in prescription form (ibuprofen and ketoprofen). It may take several days to reduce inflammation.	For all traditional NSAIDs: abdominal or stomach cramps, pain, or discomfort; diarrhea; dizziness; drowsiness or light-headedness; headache; heartburn or indigestion; peptic ulcers; nausea or vomiting; possible kidney and liver damage (rare).	For all traditional NSAIDs: avoid drinking alcohol or using blood thinners; avoid if there is sensitivity or allergy to aspirin or similar drugs, kidney or liver disease, heart disease, high blood pressure, asthma, or peptic ulcers.
Cyclo-oxygenase (COX)-2 inhibitor NSAIDs: celecoxib, valdecoxib	COX-2 inhibitors, such as traditional NSAIDs, block COX-2, an enzyme in the body that stimulates an inflammatory response. Unlike traditional NSAIDs, however, they do not block the action of COX-1, an enzyme that protects the stomach lining. Vioxx was withdrawn by FDA.	Stomach irritation, ulceration, and bleeding may occur. Caution is advisable for patients with a history of bleeding or ulcers, decreased renal function, hepatic disease, hypertension, or asthma.	Doctor monitoring for possible allergic responses to valdecoxib and celecoxib is important.

(continued)

TABLE 11-14 Medications Used in Rheumatoid Arthritis *(continued)*

Medications	Uses/Effects	Side Effects	Monitoring
Corticosteroids	These are steroids given by mouth or injection. They are used to relieve inflammation and reduce swelling, redness, itching, and allergic reactions.	Increased appetite, indigestion, nervousness, or restlessness.	For all corticosteroids, advise the doctor if there is presence of the following: fungal infection, history of tuberculosis, underactive thyroid, herpes simplex of the eye, high blood pressure, osteoporosis, or stomach ulcer.
Methylprednisolone, prednisone	These steroids are available in a pill form or as an injection into a joint. Improvements are seen up to 24 hours after administration. There is potential for serious side effects, especially at high doses. They are used for severe flares or when the disease does not respond to NSAIDs and disease-modifying antirheumatic drugs.	Osteoporosis, mood changes, fragile skin, easy bruising, fluid retention, weight gain, muscle weakness, onset or worsening of diabetes, cataracts, increased risk of infection, and hypertension.	Doctor monitoring for continued effectiveness of medication and for side effects is needed.
Disease-modifying antirheumatic drugs (DMARDs)	These are common arthritis medications. They relieve painful, swollen joints and slow joint damage, and several DMARDs may be used over the disease course. They take a few weeks or months to have an effect and may produce significant improvements for many patients. Exactly how they work is still unknown.	Side effects vary with each medicine. DMARDs may increase risk of infection, hair loss, and kidney or liver damage.	Doctor monitoring allows the risk of toxicities to be weighed against the potential benefits of individual medications.
Azathioprine	This drug was first used in higher doses in cancer chemotherapy and organ transplantation. It is used in patients who have not responded to other drugs and in combination therapy.	Cough or hoarseness, fever or chills, loss of appetite, lower back or side pain, nausea or vomiting, painful or difficult urination, unusual tiredness or weakness.	Avoid with allopurinol or kidney or liver disease. May decrease immunity; contact doctor immediately with chills, fever, or a cough. Regular blood and liver function tests are needed.
Cyclosporine	This medication was first used in organ transplantation to prevent rejection. It is used in patients who have not responded to other drugs.	Bleeding, tender, or enlarged gums; high blood pressure; increase in hair growth; kidney problems; trembling and shaking of hands.	Avoid with sensitivity to castor oil (if receiving the drug by injection), liver or kidney disease, active infection, or high blood pressure. Using this drug may make you more susceptible to infection and certain cancers. Do not take live vaccines while on this drug. Avoid St. John's wort and echinacea.
Hydroxychloroquine	It may take several months to notice the benefits of this drug, which include reducing the signs and symptoms of rheumatoid arthritis.	Diarrhea, eye problems (rare), headache, loss of appetite, nausea or vomiting, and stomach cramps or pain.	Doctor monitoring is important, particularly with an allergy to any antimalarial drug or a retinal abnormality.
Gold sodium thiomalate (Ridaura)	This was one of the first DMARDs used to treat rheumatoid arthritis.	Redness or soreness of tongue; swelling or bleeding gums; skin rash or itching; ulcers or sores on lips, mouth, or throat; irritation on tongue. Monitor joint pain 1 or 2 days after injection.	Avoid with lupus, skin rash, kidney disease, or colitis. Periodic urine and blood tests are needed to check for side effects.
Leflunomide	This drug reduces signs and symptoms and slows structural damage to joints caused by arthritis.	Bloody or cloudy urine; congestion in chest; cough; diarrhea; difficult, burning, or painful urination or breathing; fever; hair loss; headache; heartburn; loss of appetite; nausea and/or vomiting; skin rash; stomach pain; sneezing; and sore throat.	Doctor must monitor for the following: active infection, liver disease, known immune deficiency, renal insufficiency, or underlying malignancy. Regular blood tests, including liver function tests, are needed. Leflunomide must not be taken during pregnancy; it may cause birth defects in humans.

(continued)

TABLE 11-14 **Medications Used in Rheumatoid Arthritis *(continued)***

Medications	Uses/Effects	Side Effects	Monitoring
Methotrexate (Rheumatrex)	This drug can be taken by mouth or by injection and results in rapid improvement (it usually takes 3–6 weeks to begin working). It is very effective, especially in combination with infliximab or etanercept. It produces more favorable long-term responses compared with DMARDs such as sulfasalazine, gold sodium thiomalate, hydroxychloroquine and may be used in pediatrics.	Abdominal discomfort, chest pain, chills, nausea, mouth sores, painful urination, sore throat, and unusual tiredness or weakness.	Doctor monitoring is important, particularly with an abnormal blood count, liver or lung disease, alcoholism, immune system deficiency, or active infection. Methotrexate must not be taken during pregnancy because it may cause birth defects in humans. Avoid Echinacea. Extra folic acid is needed.
Sulfasalazine	This drug suppresses the immune system.	Abdominal pain, aching joints, diarrhea, headache, sensitivity to sunlight, loss of appetite, nausea or vomiting, and skin rash.	Doctor monitoring is important, particularly with allergy to sulfa drugs or aspirin or with a kidney, liver, or blood disease.
Biological response modifiers	These drugs selectively block cytokines, which play a role in inflammation. Long-term efficacy and safety are uncertain.	Increased risk of infection, especially tuberculosis. Increased risk of pneumonia, and listeriosis (a foodborne illness caused by the bacterium *Listeria monocytogenes*).	Avoid eating undercooked foods (including unpasteurized cheeses, cold cuts, and hot dogs) to reduce listeriosis while taking biological response modifiers.
Tumor necrosis factor inhibitors: etanercept (Enbrel), golimumab (Simponi), infliximab (Remicade), and adalimumab (Humira)	Highly effective for treating patients with an inadequate response to DMARDs. Often prescribed in combination with methotrexate. Etanercept requires subcutaneous injections twice weekly. Infliximab is taken intravenously (IV) during a 2-hour procedure, along with methotrexate. Adalimumab requires injections every 2 weeks.	*Etanercept:* pain or burning in throat, redness, itching, pain, and/or swelling at injection site, runny or stuffy nose. *Infliximab:* abdominal pain, cough, dizziness, fainting, headache, muscle pain, runny nose, shortness of breath, sore throat, vomiting, wheezing. *Adalimumab:* redness, rash, swelling, itching, bruising, sinus infection, headache, nausea. *Golimumab:* respiratory infection, sore throat and nasal congestion.	Doctor monitoring is important, particularly with active infection, exposure to tuberculosis, or a central nervous system disorder. Evaluation for tuberculosis is necessary before treatment begins.
Interleukin-1 inhibitor: anakinra (Kineret)	This medication requires daily injections. Long-term efficacy and safety are uncertain.	Redness, swelling, bruising, or pain at the site of injection; headache; upset stomach; diarrhea; runny nose; and stomach pain.	Doctor monitoring is required.
Selective Costimulation Modulator: Abatacept	Abatacept is given intravenously in a 30-minute infusion. It may be given alone or with DMARDs.	Cough, dizziness, headache, infections, sore throat.	Doctor monitoring is needed.
CD20 Antibody: Rituximab	This medication is for people whose rheumatoid arthritis has not responded to other biologic agents. It is given by two IV infusions 2 weeks apart. It is given with methotrexate.	Abdominal pain, chills/shivering, fever, headache, infection, itching.	Doctor monitoring is needed.
Other medications	Pilocarpine hydrochloride (Salagen) and cevimeline (Evoxac).	Available to treat dry mouth associated with Sjögren's syndrome. They simulate the salivary glands.	

Adapted from: National Institutes of Health. Health topics. Accessed December 19, 2009 at http://www.niams.nih.gov/Health_Info/Rheumatic_Disease/default.asp#ra_16.

Herbs, Botanicals, and Supplements

- Herbs and botanical supplements should not be used without discussing with physician. Some people have tried acupuncture and other alternatives to traditional medicine, but it is important not to neglect regular health care or treatment of serious symptoms. Female patients tend to use alternative treatments for RA more than males; psychosocial intervention may be beneficial.
- With borage oil, concomitant NSAID use may undermine the effects. Borage oil is contraindicated in pregnancy given the teratogenic and labor-inducing effects of prostaglandin E agonists.
- St. John's wort and echinacea should not be used with cyclosporine or methotrexate.

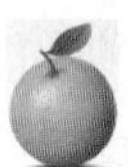

NUTRITION EDUCATION, COUNSELING, CARE MANAGEMENT

- Adoption of a Mediterranean diet confers health benefits in this population because of greater consumption of fruits and vegetables, lower consumption of animal products, and use of olive oil, which modulates immune function (Wahle et al, 2005). Inclusion of omega-3 fatty acids is also important (Berbert et al, 2005); herring, salmon, sardines, tuna, and mackerel are good dietary sources.
- No evidence exists to prove that foods from the nightshade family (potatoes, tomatoes, eggplant, and sweet and hot peppers) should be excluded.
- Encourage nutrient-dense foods. If intake is poor, a vitamin–mineral supplement may be needed. Dietary quinones, phenolics, vitamins, amino acids, isoprenoids, and other compounds in functional foods have become very popular (Losso and Bawadi, 2005).
- Instruct patient about simplified planning and preparation tips. Sandwiches, prepared meals, precut fruits and vegetables are easy to use. Cook double portions and freeze leftovers for another day.
- Discourage quackery and substitute sound health practices.
- Carbohydrate intolerance occurs because of chronic inflammation and use of steroids; planning must reflect individual needs.
- A support group may be helpful for coping.
- Physical therapy and exercise are beneficial for most patients. Strengthening exercises may help improve patient's ability to walk and may decrease joint pain and fatigue. Dynamic exercise is beneficial in RA (Hurkmans et al, 2009).
- Check on bone density; there is a high incidence of osteoporosis when steroids are used.

Patient Education—Food Safety

If enteral or parenteral nutrition is used, careful sanitation and handling techniques must be taught and used.

For More Information

- American Autoimmune Related Diseases Association
  http://www.aarda.org
- American College of Rheumatology
  http://www.rheumatology.org
- Arthritis Foundation
  http://www.arthritis.org
- Felty Syndrome
  http://rarediseases.about.com/od/rarediseasesf/a/121104.htm
- Information on Rheumatoid Arthritis
  http://www.niams.nih.gov/hi/topics/arthritis/rahandout.htm
- Juvenile Rheumatoid Arthritis
  http://www.niams.nih.gov/hi/topics/juvenile_arthritis/juvarthr.htm
- National Institute of Dental and Craniofacial Research–Sjögren's Syndrome
  http://www.nidcr.nih.gov/GrantsAndFunding/See_Funding_Opportunities_Sorted_By/ConceptClearance/CurrentCC/SjogrenSynd.htm
- National Sjögren's Syndrome Association
  http://www.sjogrenssyndrome.org/index.html
- Rheumatoid Vasculitis
  http://vasculitis.med.jhu.edu/typesof/rheumatoid.html
- Sjögren's Syndrome Foundation—Food Tips
  http://www.sjogrens.org/home/about-sjogrens-syndrome/living-with-sjogrens/diet-a-food-tips

RHEUMATOID ARTHRITIS—CITED REFERENCES

Ballard DH, et al. A pathway analysis applied to Genetic Analysis Workshop 16 genome-wide rheumatoid arthritis data. *BMC Proc.* 15;3:91, 2009.

Barton JL. Patient preferences and satisfaction in the treatment of rheumatoid arthritis with biologic therapy. *Patient Prefer Adherence.* 3: 335, 2009.

Berbert AA, et al. Supplementation of fish oil and olive oil in patients with rheumatoid arthritis. *Nutrition.* 21:131, 2005.

Choi HK. Dietary risk factors for rheumatic diseases. *Curr Opin Rheumatol.* 17:141, 2005.

Elkan AC, et al. Rheumatoid cachexia, central obesity and malnutrition in patients with low-active rheumatoid arthritis: feasibility of anthropometry, Mini Nutritional Assessment and body composition techniques. *Eur J Nutr.* 48:315, 2009.

Hurkmans E, et al. Dynamic exercise programs (aerobic capacity and/or muscle strength training) in patients with rheumatoid arthritis. *Cochrane Database Syst Rev.* 2009;(4):CD006853.

Losso JN, Bawadi HA. Hypoxia inducible factor pathways as targets for functional foods. *J Agric Food Chem.* 53:3751, 2005.

Marcora S, et al. Dietary treatment of rheumatoid cachexia with beta-hydroxy-beta-methylbutyrate, glutamine and arginine: a randomised controlled trial. *Clin Nutr.* 24:442, 2005.

Pattison DJ, et al. Dietary beta-cryptoxanthin and inflammatory polyarthritis: results from a population-based prospective study. *Am J Clin Nutr.* 82:451, 2005.

Pedersen M, et al. Diet and risk of rheumatoid arthritis in a prospective cohort. *J Rheumatol.* 32:1249, 2005.

Roubenoff R. Rheumatoid cachexia: a complication of rheumatoid arthritis moves into the 21st century. *Arthritis Res Ther.* 11:108, 2009.

Wahle KW, et al. Olive oil and modulation of cell signaling in disease prevention. *Lipids.* 39:1223, 2005.

RUPTURED DISC

NUTRITIONAL ACUITY RANKING: LEVEL 1

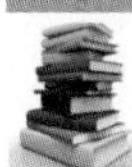

DEFINITIONS AND BACKGROUND

Determining the cause of back pain is complicated as it is often multifactorial; anatomical abnormalities are common in the spine and may not necessarily translate into clinical symptoms (Sheehan et al, 2010).

A slipped or ruptured disc is called a cervical radiculopathy, herniated intervertebral disc, lumbar radiculopathy, or prolapsed intervertebral disc. In this condition, slipping or prolapse of a cervical or lumbar disc occurs, with neck, shoulder, or low back pain accordingly. Degenerating changes in the disks begin around 30 years of age. Overweight and obesity increase the risk of low back pain and the need for medical attention (Shiri et al, 2010).

With **lumbar radiculopathy**, ambulation may be painful, and limping can occur. Muscular weakness, severe back pain that radiates to buttocks or legs and feet, pain that worsens with coughing or laughing, tingling or numbness in legs or feet, and muscle contractions or spasms may also result. With **cervical radiculopathy**, neck pain in back and sides is deep; pain may radiate to shoulders, upper arms, or forearms and worsens with coughing or laughing. Spasm of neck muscles and pain that worsens at night may occur.

A laminectomy surgically removes the lamina of a vertebra. Percutaneous automated discectomy (PAD) surgery can be performed in some cases; this surgery breaks up the disc and removes fragments. There is no convincing medical evidence to support routine use of lumbar fusion, but it may be useful in patients with associated spinal deformity, instability, or associated chronic low-back pain (Resnick et al, 2005). Surgery for radiculopathy with herniated lumbar disc and symptomatic spinal stenosis is associated with short-term benefits compared to nonsurgical therapy, though benefits diminish with long-term follow-up in some trials (Chou et al, 2009).

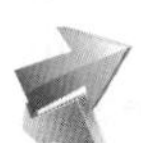

ASSESSMENT, MONITORING, AND EVALUATION

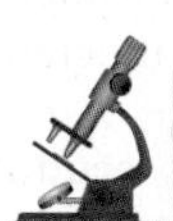

CLINICAL INDICATORS

Genetic Markers: This condition is acquired and not genetic.

Clinical/History

- Height
- Weight
- BMI
- I & O
- BP
- Constipation
- Edema
- MRI or computed tomography (CT) scan
- Myelography
- Discography
- Spinal or neck x-rays
- Nerve conduction velocity test

Lab Work

- H & H
- Ca^{++}, Mg^{++}
- Na^+, K^+
- Alb, transthyretin
- BUN, Creat
- Alk phos
- Gluc
- Vitamin D_3 status (serum 25-OHD)

SAMPLE NUTRITION CARE PROCESS STEPS

Abnormal GI Function

Assessment Data: Weight and physical activity histories. Medical history and medications.

Nutrition Diagnosis (PES): Abnormal GI function related to constipation and infrequent stooling pattern as evidenced by GI distress and evacuation every 3–4 days.

Intervention: Food-nutrient delivery—Assure intake of adequate fluid and fiber at all meals. Education—Discuss tips for alleviating constipation through use of specific foods rich in fiber (fruits, vegetables, whole grains, beans and legumes). Coordinate care—Work with nursing and physicians to determine if any medications that cause constipation can be changed, or if some type of laxative can be added.

Monitoring and Evaluation: Improvement in bowel habits; alleviation of constipation.

INTERVENTION

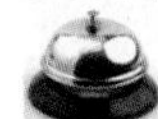

OBJECTIVES

- Maintain adequate rest and activity levels, as assigned by physician.
- Prevent weight gain from decreased activity.
- Encourage adequate hydration.
- Prevent constipation and straining.
- Assist with feeding, if patient is in traction.
- Relieve pain and promote healing.

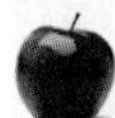

FOOD AND NUTRITION

- A regular diet generally is sufficient. For some, a strict energy-controlled diet may be beneficial to promote weight loss.
- Increased fluid and fiber intake can be helpful to reduce constipation. Fresh fruits and vegetables, dried beans, legumes, whole grains, bran, and other foods may be needed.

Common Drugs Used and Potential Side Effects

- Anti-inflammatory drugs may be used. NSAIDs are used for long-term pain control, but narcotics may be given if the pain does not respond. Nausea, GI distress, and anorexia may result. Follow directions regarding when to take (e.g., before or after meals).
- Analgesics may be helpful to relieve pain. Chronic use of aspirin may cause GI bleeding.
- Muscle relaxants may be ordered. GI distress or nausea can occur.

Herbs, Botanicals, and Supplements

- Herbs and botanical supplements should not be used without discussing with physician.

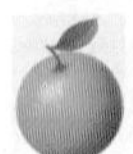

NUTRITION EDUCATION, COUNSELING, CARE MANAGEMENT

- Instruct patient regarding effective methods of relieving constipation.
- Discuss role of nutrition and exercise in health maintenance. Weight loss may be needed.
- After surgery, the role of nutrition in wound healing should be discussed.

Patient Education—Food Safety

If enteral or parenteral nutrition is used, careful sanitation and handling techniques must be taught and used.

For More Information

- Herniated Disk
  http://www.nlm.nih.gov/medlineplus/ency/article/000442.htm
- Lumbar Radiculopathy
  https://health.google.com/health/ref/Herniated+nucleus+pulposus

RUPTURED INTERVERTEBRAL DISC—CITED REFERENCES

Chou R, et al, Surgery for low back pain: a review of the evidence for an American Pain Society Clinical Practice Guideline. *Spine.* 34:1094, 2009.

Resnick DK, et al. Guidelines for the performance of fusion procedures for degenerative disease of the lumbar spine. Part 8: lumbar fusion for disc herniation and radiculopathy. *J Neurosurg Spine.* 2:673, 2005.

Sheehan NJ. Magnetic resonance imaging for low back pain: indications and limitations. *Ann Rheum Dis.* 69:7, 2010.

Shiri R, et al. The Association Between Obesity and Low Back Pain: A Meta-Analysis [published online ahead of print 2009]. *Am J Epidemiol.* 171:135, 2010.

SCLERODERMA (SYSTEMIC SCLEROSIS)

NUTRITIONAL ACUITY RANKING: LEVEL 1–2

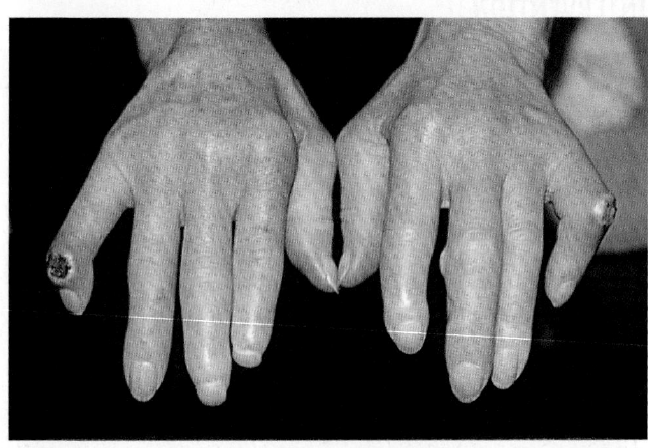

Adapted from: Goodheart HP, MD. *Goodheart's Photoguide of Common Skin Disorders,* 2nd ed. Philadelphia: Lippincott Williams & Wilkins, 2003.

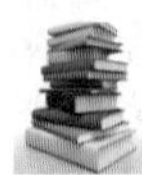

DEFINITIONS AND BACKGROUND

Scleroderma is a chronic disease characterized by fibrosis and autoantibodies. Approximately 2% of the population in Europe and North America suffers from disorders such as scleroderma (Chen and von Mikecz, 2005). Genetic, immunological, hormonal, and environmental factors are considered to be triggers (Molina and Shoenfeld, 2005).

The diffuse form affects a large area of the skin and several organs; it is also called **systemic sclerosis** (SSc). In SSc, pathological deposition of fibrous connective tissue in the skin and visceral organs occurs. Fibrosis involves an increase of hydroxylysine aldehyde collagen cross-linkages as well as an increase in inflammatory cytokines (Brinckmann et al, 2005). The GI tract is affected, and Raynaud's syndrome (ischemia of fingers) is common.

The limited form of scleroderma affects the skin and sometimes the lungs. The CREST syndrome (**limited cutaneous sclerosis**) is less severe than SSc and causes less internal organ damage. Calcium deposits, Raynaud's phenomenon, esophageal dysfunction, skin damage on fingers, and telangiectasia form the acronym for CREST.

As the disease progresses, large areas of the skin or just the fingers (sclerodactyly) may be affected. Skin on the face tightens and causes a mask-like appearance. Spider veins (telangiectasia) occur on the fingers, chest, face, lips, or tongue. Calcium deposits can occur on the fingers or other bony areas; sores or contractures may result from the scarring. Scarring of the esophagus may be especially detrimental, causing blockage or even cancer. Lungs can be affected, leading to shortness of breath with exercise.

Neurological involvement consists of epilepsy, central nervous system vasculitis, peripheral neuropathy, vascular malformations, headache, and neuroimaging abnormalities; ocular manifestations include uveitis, xerophthalmia, glaucoma, and papilledema (Zulian et al, 2005). SSc is characterized by vasculopathy, inflammation, vasospasm, microvascular involvement is common; an increased prevalence of distal peripheral artery disease in the digits has been found (Hetterna et al, 2008).

Scleroderma renal crisis (SRC) occurs in 5–10% of SSc patients, who may present with an abrupt onset of hypertension, acute renal failure, headaches, fevers, malaise, hypertensive retinopathy, encephalopathy, and pulmonary edema (Denton et al, 2009). Multiple organ system dysfunction may occur. Pulmonary hypertension, heart failure, and respiratory failure cause serious morbidity and mortality. There is no known cure, and SSc can be fatal.

There seems to be an increased prevalence of celiac disease in patients with scleroderma (Rosato et al, 2009). Both disorders require careful management. Current therapies for scleroderma target the immune system, with the goal of reducing inflammation, ischemic injury to the involved organs, and secondary tissue injury and fibrosis (Henness and Wigley, 2007).

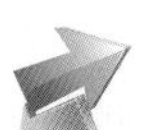

ASSESSMENT, MONITORING, AND EVALUATION

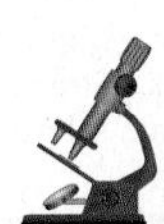

CLINICAL INDICATORS

Genetic Markers: Genetic factors contribute to disease susceptibility; transforming growth factor-ss is a cytokine that contributes to fibroblast activation, collagen overproduction, and pathological tissue fibrosis (Varga, 2008). T-cell polarization is implicated in the lung disease of SSc (Boin et al, 2008).

Clinical/History
- Height
- Weight
- BMI
- I & O
- Weight loss
- Fever?
- BP
- Thickening, swelling of the ends of the fingers
- Dysphagia
- Heartburn
- Fibrosis of salivary and lacrimal glands
- Abdominal pain, flatulence
- Nausea, vomiting
- Diarrhea, constipation
- Skinfold measurements

Lab Work
- ANA (high)
- RF (high)
- LDL Cholesterol (elevated)
- Trig (may be low)
- Anti-tTG antibody
- Serum folate
- H & H
- Serum B_{12}
- Gluc
- Prothrombin time (PT)
- Alb, transthyretin
- CRP
- GFR
- BUN, Creat
- Homocysteine
- Ca^{++}, Mg^{++}
- Na^{+}, K^{+}
- Alk phos
- Vitamin D_3 status (serum 25-OHD)
- Fecal fat test, hydrogen breath test for malabsorption

SAMPLE NUTRITION CARE PROCESS STEPS

Difficulty Swallowing

Assessment Data: Weight, medical history, medications. Low salivation and difficulty swallowing.

Nutrition Diagnosis (PES): Difficulty swallowing related to low saliva production as evidenced by fibrosis, inability to swallow solids.

Intervention: Food-Nutrient Delivery—Alteration in food choices to liquefy meals and make them easier to swallow. Educate about the use of saliva substitutes, more fluids, altered food choices as needed. Counseling about when to request changes, such as tube feeding.

Monitoring and Evaluation: Improvement in swallowing and tolerance for meals. No weight loss.

INTERVENTION

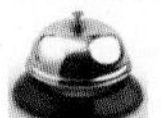

OBJECTIVES

- Prevent or correct protein-energy malnutrition and nutrient deficiencies.
- Correct xerostomia where present; decreased saliva, dysphagia, and difficulty in chewing will result.
- Monitor dysphagia with esophageal involvement; alter method of feeding as needed.
- Counteract vitamin B_{12} and fat maldigestion and absorption, which may be common.
- Monitor hypomotility and gastroparesis; alter fiber intake as appropriate. For many patients, nutritional support and relief of symptoms remain the primary management goals.
- Improve quality of life and reduce fatigue; allow return to work or maintenance of energy levels.

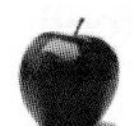

FOOD AND NUTRITION

- Diets high in energy (30–40 kcal/kg) and adequate to high in protein are often necessary. A soft diet with moistened foods and extra fluids is useful. Add fiber if constipation is a problem (such as adding crushed bran to hot cereal).
- Small, frequent feedings may be needed. Tube feed if patient is dysphagic or has obstruction.
- Use parenteral nutrition if GI tract is highly affected, with intractable diarrhea and severe malabsorption.
- If there is celiac sensitivity, omit gluten from the diet.
- Reduce lactose if intolerance occurs. Extra calcium may be needed if lactose is not tolerated orally.
- Give supplements of fat- and water-soluble vitamins.
- With hypertension and multiple organ system dysfunction, reduced sodium or fluid restriction may be needed.

Common Drugs Used and Potential Side Effects

- Topical or systemic corticosteroids, vitamin D analogs (calcitriol and calcipotriol), photochemotherapy, laser therapy, antimalarials, phenytoin, D-penicillamine, and colchicine all have varying degrees of success. Topical tacrolimus cream is an immunosuppressive antibiotic.
- Interstitial lung disease can be treated with cyclophosphamide, vascular disease of the lungs and digits with endothelin receptor antagonists, and general symptoms with phosphodiesterase inhibitor sildenafil or prostacyclins (Henness and Wigley, 2007).
- Early, aggressive treatment with angiotensin-converting enzyme inhibitors helps with a renal crisis (Denton et al, 2009).
- Anti-inflammatory agents, such as steroids, are often used in SSc. Monitor for nitrogen and calcium losses, altered electrolyte levels, and elevated glucose levels. Correct diet accordingly.
- Antihypertensives usually are needed; monitor BP results. Potassium supplements may or may not be required; determine need according to medication selected.
- Trental (pentoxifylline) is used for Raynaud's syndrome to improve circulation. Anorexia or GI distress may result.

Herbs, Botanicals, and Supplements

- Herbs and botanical supplements should not be used without discussing with physician.
- For Raynaud's disease, evening primrose, gingko, mustard, garlic, borage, and red pepper have been suggested, but there are no clinical trials that prove effectiveness.
- CAM is frequently used to treat stress-related disorders such as scleroderma; some merit can be noted (Hui et al, 2009).

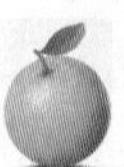

NUTRITION EDUCATION, COUNSELING, CARE MANAGEMENT

- Artificial saliva (Xero-Lube) or lemon glycerine may be useful.
- Chew sugarless gum.
- If eating orally, adequate chewing time will be required.
- Consume adequate fluids. Choose moist foods or foods with sauces/gravies.
- For heartburn, keep head elevated after meals; decrease or limit intake of chocolate, caffeine, fatty foods, alcohol, citrus, and tomatoes.
- Physical therapy and exercise may help maintain muscle strength but cannot totally prevent joints from locking into stiffened positions.

Patient Education—Food Safety

If enteral or parenteral nutrition is used, careful sanitation and handling techniques must be taught and used.

For More Information

- Scleroderma Foundation
  http://www.scleroderma.org/
- Scleroderma Research Foundation
  http://www.srfcure.org

SCLERODERMA—CITED REFERENCES

Boin F, et al. T cell polarization identifies distinct clinical phenotypes in scleroderma lung disease. *Arthritis Rheum.* 58:1165, 2008.

Brinckmann J, et al. Interleukin 4 and prolonged hypoxia induce a higher gene expression of lysyl hydroxylase 2 and an altered cross-link pattern: important pathogenetic steps in early and late stage of systemic scleroderma? *Matrix Biol.* 24:459, 2005.

Chen M, von Mikecz A. Xenobiotic-induced recruitment of autoantigens to nuclear proteasomes suggests a role for altered antigen processing in scleroderma. *Ann N Y Acad Sci.* 1051:382, 2005.

Denton CP, et al. Renal complications and scleroderma renal crisis. *Rheumatology* (Oxford). 48:32S, 2009.

Henness S, Wigley FM. Current drug therapy for scleroderma and secondary Raynaud's phenomenon: evidence-based review. *Curr Opin Rheumatol.* 19:611, 2007.

Hetterna ME, et al. Macrovascular disease and atherosclerosis in SSc. *Rheumatology* (Oxford). 47:578, 2008.

Hui KK, et al. Scleroderma, stress and CAM Utilization. *Evid Based Complement Alternat Med.* 6:503, 2009.

Molina V, Shoenfeld Y. Infection, vaccines and other environmental triggers of autoimmunity. *Autoimmunity.* 38:235, 2005.

Rosato E, et al. High incidence of celiac disease in patients with systemic sclerosis. *J Rheumatol.* 36:965, 2009.

Varga J. Systemic sclerosis: an update. *Bull NYU Hosp Jt Dis.* 66:198, 2008.

Zulian F, et al. Localized scleroderma in childhood is not just a skin disease. Localized scleroderma in childhood is not just a skin disease. *Arthritis Rheum.* 52:2873, 2005.

SECTION 12

Hematology: Anemias and Blood Disorders

CHIEF ASSESSMENT FACTORS

- Anorexia
- Beefy, Red Tongue or Magenta Tongue; Other Signs of Nutrient Deficiencies
- Blood Type
- Bruising
- Concurrent Asthma, Cancer, Cerebrovascular Disease, Hemorrhage, Myocardial Infarction, Renal Disease
- Dietary Habits: Use of Heme and Nonheme Iron, Vitamin and Mineral Deficiencies, Protein Intake, Vegan Lifestyle
- Exposure to Lead Paint, Other Toxins
- Family History of Allergies, Anemias, Cancer, Immune Disorders, and Leukemias
- Fatigue
- History of Alcohol and Nicotine Use
- Infections, Sepsis
- Lymphadenopathy
- Medication Use (Prescriptions, Over-the-Counter) and Use of Herbal or Botanical Medications
- Occupational or Environmental Exposure to Toxic Substances
- Previous Blood Disorder, Bleeding Tendencies, Blood Transfusion, or Exposure to Radiation
- Surgery, Especially Gastric, Hepatic, or Renal

GENERAL INFORMATION ABOUT ANEMIAS

Blood contains plasma and cells. Plasma is clear and yellow and makes up 55% of blood. It contains proteins, nutrients, hormones, and electrolytes. White cells, red blood cells (RBCs), and platelets make up the remaining 45% of blood. The white cells fight infection, platelets are necessary for blood clotting, and RBCs carry oxygen throughout the body. Hepcidin, the main iron regulatory hormone, is made primarily in hepatocytes in response to liver iron levels, inflammation, hypoxia, and anemia (Munoz et al, 2009). Erythropoietin is the hormone that stimulates RBC production. The erythrocyte life span is 120 days, after which the cells are destroyed by the spleen. Anemias are a set of hematological disorders with a reduced number of RBCs, reduced amount of hemoglobin (Hgb), or reduced number of volume-packed RBCs (hematocrit [Hct]). Excessive bleeding, decreased RBC production, and increased RBC destruction may lead to anemias. The main consequences of these disorders include hypoxia and decreased oxygen-carrying capacity. Overall, anemias affect over 3.4 million people in the United States. Chronic disease and iron deficiency are the most common causes. Other causes of anemias include peptic ulcers, inflammation, infection, cancers, gastritis, liver disease, renal disease, hypothyroidism, history of blood transfusions, blood coagulation disorders, and poor diet. Generally, Hgb, serum iron, TIBC or UIBC, and serum ferritin will establish iron status. In conditions due to blood cell production or cancers, other tests or procedures are needed to determine the cause for abnormal iron levels. These may include a complete blood count (CBC) with differential, zinc protoporphyrin (ZPP) immunological tests, hormone tests, reticulocyte count, C-reactive protein (CRP), sedimentation rate (SED rate), B_{12} or folate levels, genetic testing, tissue biopsy, MRI, ultrasound, bone marrow aspiration, blood smears, urine or fecal sampling, scopes (endoscope or colonoscopy), and tests associated with specific diseases or conditions that can have anemia or iron overload.

Anemias can be encountered with generalized or specific nutritional deficiencies (Table 12-1). The nutritional anemias are caused by deficits, but not all anemias require nutritional intervention. Use caution when evaluating single laboratory results; most anemias have a specific profile. For example, iron and copper participate in one-electron exchange reactions; the same property that makes them essential also generates free radicals that can be seriously deleterious to cells (Arredondo and Nunez, 2005). Table 12-2 provides some key definitions that are used to describe anemias.

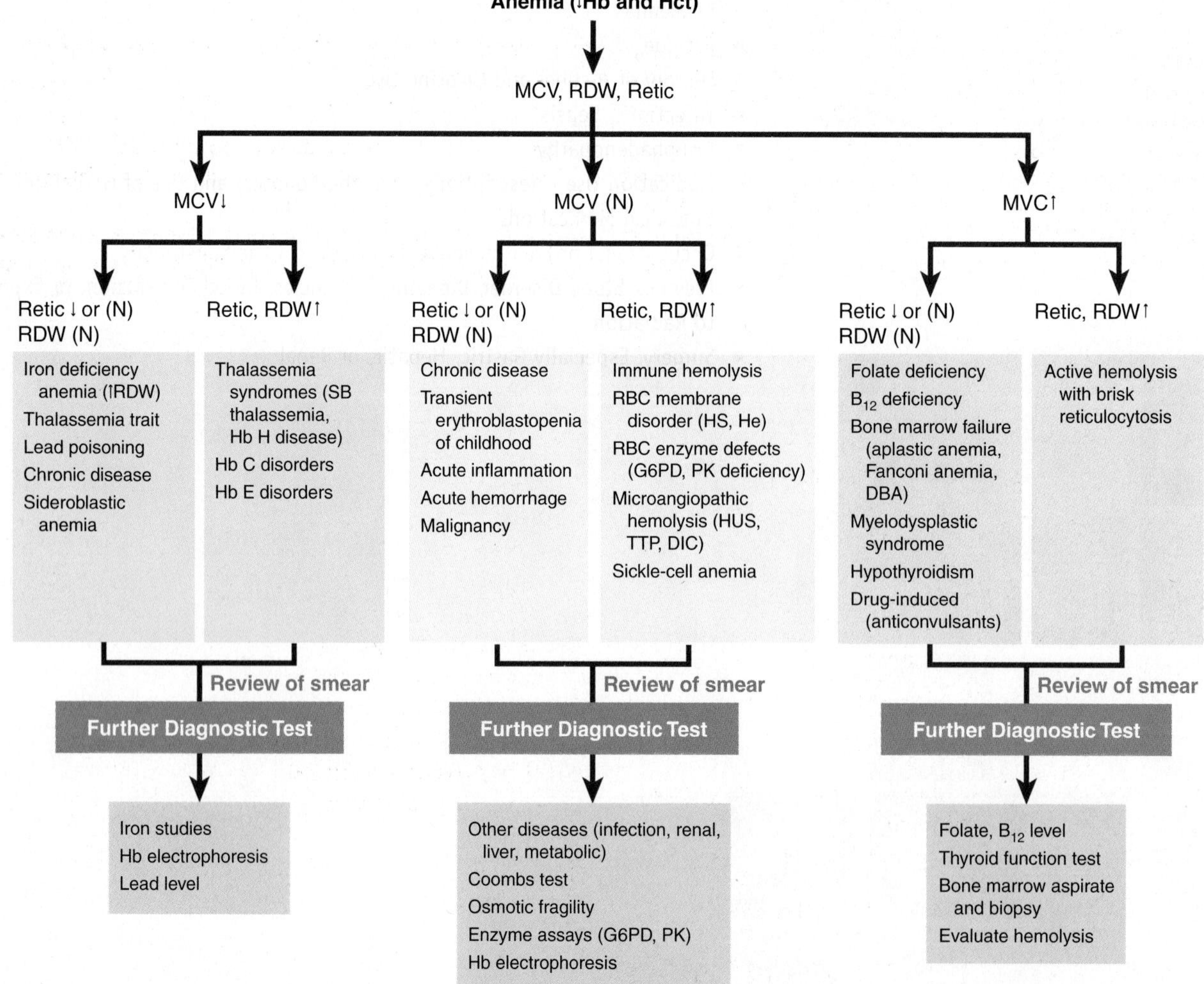

Red cell distribution width (RDW), a measure of heterogeneity in the size of circulating erythrocytes, is associated with some chronic diseases and predicts mortality.

TABLE 12-1 Nutritional Factors in Blood Formation

Protein
Iron
Vitamin C
Vitamin E
Folic acid
Vitamin B_6
Vitamin B_{12}
Vitamin K
Copper
Riboflavin (minute amounts)

Inadequate intakes of many nutrients are now known to contribute to several chronic diseases. Folic acid and vitamin B_{12} are among the key nutrients involved. Vitamin B_{12} deficiency, iron or folate deficiency, chronic gastrointestinal (GI) bleeding, and myelodysplastic syndrome are causes of anemia in the elderly. Anemias are more common in the hospitalized elderly than among those who live independently.

Iron is an essential micronutrient as it is required for adequate erythropoietic function, oxidative metabolism, and cellular immune responses (Munoz et al, 2009). Yet it is one of the most frequently lacking nutrients in both developing and developed countries. Iron-deficiency anemia (IDA) affects about 25% of infants worldwide. Adults, especially menstruating women, are also susceptible. Laboratory tests provide evidence of iron depletion in the body, or reflect iron-deficient red cell production; the appropriate combination of these laboratory tests help establish a correct diagnosis of ID status and anemia (Munoz et al, 2009). Table 12-3 lists some relevant tests and Table 12-4 lists common signs and symptoms of anemias.

Up to 10% of young women in developed countries are iron deficient. The problem is not easily resolved by adopting

TABLE 12-3 Iron Tests

Hemoglobin	Reflects the level of functional iron. Low levels can indicate iron-deficiency anemia or ACD. Hemoglobin values help determine if anemia is present and if a blood donation can be done
Serum ferritin	Measures the amount of iron in storage. One ferritin molecule can hold as many as 4500 iron atoms. Ferritin can be elevated when a person has an infection or inflammatory condition
Serum iron (Fe)	Free or unbound iron in serum. Ideal range is 40–180 µg/dL. Measurement is best done fasting because serum iron is sensitive to foods or supplements recently consumed, time of day, and menstruation
Transferrin	Iron-binding and transport protein that can bind to and transport two molecules of iron. Transferrin carries iron through the bloodstream to the bone marrow, the liver, and ferritin. Transferrin is no longer measured directly by most physicians, instead TIBC is used
TIBC	Demonstrates the iron-binding ability of transferrin. Serum iron divided by TIBC × 100% provides the transferrin-iron saturation percentage (Tsat%), which is also called iron saturation. Normally, Tsat% is 25–35%. Higher numbers are suggestive of iron loading. Lower numbers are suggestive of iron-deficiency anemia

From: Iron Overload Disease Association, http://www.irondisorders.org/Forms/irontests.pdf, accessed December 21, 2009.

TABLE 12-2 Definitions

Acute anemia	Precipitous drop in the RBC population due to hemolysis or acute hemorrhage
Anemia	Reduction in the number of circulating RBCs, the amount of hemoglobin, or the volume of packed RBCs (Hct)
Chronic anemia	Anemia that lasts 2 months or longer
Hypochromia	Blood condition in which there is a low level of hemoglobin and color
Hyperchromia	Blood that is excessively pigmented
Microcytic anemia	Usually caused by or resulting in iron deficiency; RBCs are small in size
Macrocytic anemia	Folic acid or vitamin B_{12} insufficiency; RBCs are larger than usual
Megaloblastic anemia	Anemias in which there are large, nucleated abnormal RBCs that are irregular in shape, from pernicious anemia or use of certain immunosuppressive or antitumor drugs
Normocytic anemias	Inhibition of marrow by infection or chronic disease; RBCs are of usual size
Normochromia	Blood with a normal color and level of hemoglobin

TABLE 12-4 General Signs and Symptoms of Anemia

- Anorexia
- Ascites
- Bowel irregularity
- Chest pain, palpitations
- Coldness of extremities
- Dizziness, especially postural
- Dyspnea, especially exercise intolerance
- Decreased libido or impotence
- Decreased urine output
- Difficulty sleeping or concentrating
- Fatigue, weakness, irritability
- Headache
- Mental status changes
- Pale conjunctiva
- Tachycardia
- Thirst
- Tinnitus
- Vertigo, syncope

Comparing Disorders of Iron

IRON PANEL TESTS	Serum Iron	Serum Ferritin	Transferrin Iron Saturation Percentage	Total Iron Binding Capacity (TIBC)	Transferrin	Hemoglobin
Hemochromatosis	↑	↑	↑	↓	↓	NORMAL
Iron Deficiency Anemia	↓	↓	↓	↑	↑	↓
Sideroblastic Anemia	↑	↑	↑	↓	↓	↓
Thalassemia	↑	↑	↑	↓	↓	↓
Porphyria Cutanea Tarda (PCT)	↑	↑	↑	↓	↓	NORMAL
Anemia of Chronic Disease (ACD)	↓	↑ OR NORMAL	↓	↓	↓	↓
African Siderosis (AS)	↑	↑	↑	↓	↓	NORMAL
Vitamin B_{12} Deficiency (pernicious anemia)	↑ OR NORMAL	↑ OR NORMAL	↑ OR NORMAL	↓ OR NORMAL	↓ OR NORMAL	↓

an iron-rich diet because absorption varies greatly. Although the absorption of dietary iron (1–2 mg/d) is regulated tightly, it is balanced with losses (Munoz et al, 2009). Dietary heme iron is important and more readily absorbed than nonheme iron derived from vegetables and grains. Most heme is absorbed in the proximal intestine.

Inherited Hgb disorders, such as sickle cell anemia and thalassemia, can be attributed to the effects of natural selection. In environments in which malaria was common, carriers were protected and survived to have more children.

For More Information

- National Anemia Action Center
  http://www.anemia.org/
- National Heart, Lung, and Blood Institute Information Center
  http://www.nhlbi.nih.gov/about/dbdr/

CITED REFERENCES

Arredondo M, Nunez MT. Iron and copper metabolism. *Mol Aspects Med.* 26:313, 2005.

Munoz M et al. An update on iron physiology. *World J Gastroenterol.* 15:4617, 2009.

ANEMIAS

ANEMIA OF CHRONIC DISEASE

NUTRITIONAL ACUITY RANKING: LEVEL 2

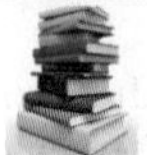

DEFINITIONS AND BACKGROUND

Anemia of chronic disease (ACD) is the condition of impaired iron utilization where functional iron (Hgb) is low, but tissue iron (such as in storage) is normal or high. ACD is known as anemia of inflammation (AI). Low Hgb, low total iron-binding capacity (TIBC), and low transferrin with elevated ferritin are identified. ACD is the second most common type of anemia after anemia of iron deficiency; it results in increased morbidity and mortality of the underlying disease (Agarwal and Prchl, 2009). ACD is seen in a wide range of chronic autoimmune, cancerous or leukemic, inflammatory, and infectious disease conditions. In rheumatoid arthritis, ACD and iron-deficiency anemia coexist, resulting from GI bleeding due to the use of many drugs. ACD is also found in approximately 50% of patients with lupus (Giannouli et al, 2006). In aging and heart failure, chronic anemia is common.

Hepcidin is the iron regulatory peptide that is synthesized in the liver to suppress iron absorption and utilization. Synthesis is suppressed by anemia, hypoxia, and erythropoiesis, and induced by inflammatory cytokines such as interleukin-6 (Matsumoto et al, 2009). ACD is characterized by macrophage iron retention induced by cytokines and hepcidin. Excess hepcidin causes proteolysis of the cellular iron exporter, ferroportin, trapping iron in macrophages, and iron-absorbing enterocytes (Ganz and Nemeth, 2009). Because circulating hepcidin levels affect iron traffic, its determination may aid to differentiate between ACD and iron-deficiency anemia to select an appropriate therapy (Theurl et al, 2009).

Hgb improvement is an independent predictor of quality of life improvement in anemic patients, yet supplementation with iron for those with ACD can be harmful and even result in death. Levels of erythropoietin are reduced in ACD. The genetically engineered form (epoetin) can correct anemia caused by cancer in about 50–60% of patients and may improve survival in HIV infection.

Epoetin can eliminate the need for transfusions but is very expensive.

Successful treatment of the underlying disease improves ACD, but if not possible, treatment with erythropoietic agents (ESAs), supplemented with iron if necessary, is helpful in many cases (Agarwal and Prchl, 2009). ESAs are safe and may forestall some of the target-organ damage (Nurko, 2006).

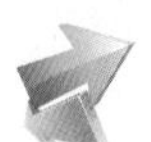

ASSESSMENT, MONITORING, AND EVALUATION

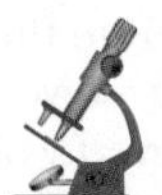

CLINICAL INDICATORS

Genetic Markers: Modifications of hepcidin gene expression suggest a key role for hepcidin in iron homeostasis. HAMP is the gene that encodes hepcidin.

Clinical/History
- Height
- Weight
- Body mass index (BMI)
- Diet history
- Intake and output (I & O)
- Blood pressure (BP)
- Fatigue and weakness
- Headache, irritability

Lab Work
- Complete blood count (CBC)
- RBC count
- Serum hepcidin level
- Total iron-binding capacity (TIBC) (low)
- Hgb and Hct (H & H) (high)
- Serum ferritin (high)
- Serum Fe
- Glucose (Gluc)
- Transferrin (low)
- Albumin (Alb)
- C-reactive protein (CRP)

SAMPLE NUTRITION CARE PROCESS STEPS

Abnormal Nutritional Laboratory Values

Assessment Data: Weight, BMI normal. Hgb is low at 10; ferritin is normal. GI bleeding and pain.

Nutrition Diagnoses (PES): Abnormal nutritional laboratory values related to chronic anemia and high doses of medications for lupus as evidenced by low Hgb, normal serum ferritin, and GI bleeding.

Interventions: Food-nutrient delivery—encourage nutrient-dense foods and frequent snacks; avoid fasting. Education about low-calorie, nutrient-dense foods and timing with medications. Counseling about timing of medications with food to reduce GI bleeding. Coordinate care with medical and nursing teams to review medications and determine which, if any, could be changed to reduce impact on GI tract.

Monitoring and Evaluation: No additional GI bleeding or distress. Resolution or improvement of anemia. Hgb closer to normal.

INTERVENTION

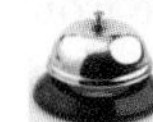

OBJECTIVES

- Prevent infections or sepsis.
- Reduce fever and excessive inflammation.
- Lessen bleeding tendencies and hemorrhages.
- Ensure adequate periods of rest. Simplify meal planning if needed.
- Prepare for bone marrow transplantation, if needed.
- Prevent further complications and decline in organ functioning.

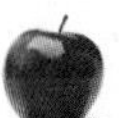

FOOD AND NUTRITION

- Provide a balanced diet that is easily prepared, with six small feedings.
- Provide extra fluid unless contraindicated.
- If steroids are used, limiting sodium intake may be needed.
- Correct iron overload where present.

Common Drugs Used and Potential Side Effects

- Genetically engineered erythropoietin (epoetin) is often used; given weekly, it can improve quality of life and levels of energy.
- Avoid iron supplements in this condition; they can be harmful and even result in death.
- Corticosteroids may be used. Watch side effects of chronic use such as elevated serum sodium levels, decreased potassium and calcium levels, and negative nitrogen balance. Hyperglycemia may occur; alter diet accordingly.
- Antibiotics may be required when infections are present. Monitor for GI distress and other effects.

Herbs, Botanicals, and Supplements

- Herbs and botanical supplements should not be used without discussing with the physician.
- Alpha tocopherol and *N*-acetylcysteine have been recommended, but more controlled studies are needed.

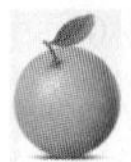

NUTRITION EDUCATION, COUNSELING, CARE MANAGEMENT

- Discuss needs of the patient, which are specific for signs, symptoms, and side effects of any medications.
- Discuss nutritious meal planning. If patient has diabetes, heart failure, or cirrhosis, counsel specifically for those issues.
- Correcting anemia in heart failure patients improves quality of life and exercise capacity in both men and women (Fox and Jorde, 2005). Once improvement is noted, activity levels can be increased.
- Counsel about reduction of iron overload if present. For example, iron-fortified cereals and oral supplements containing iron should be avoided. Increase grains, fruits, vegetables, cheese, and dairy foods; use fewer heme iron sources.
- Being female is often independently associated with lower Hgb, so assess using sex-specific laboratory values (Fox and Jorde, 2005).

Patient Education—Food Safety

If tube feeding or central parenteral nutrition (CPN) is needed, careful handwashing procedures should be followed.

For More Information

- Anemia of Chronic Disease
  http://www.emedicine.com/emerg/topic734.htm

ANEMIA OF CHRONIC DISEASE—CITED REFERENCES

Agarwal N, Prchl JT. Anemia of chronic disease (anemia of inflammation). *Acta Haematol.* 122:103, 2009.

Fox MT, Jorde UP. Anemia, chronic heart failure, and the impact of male vs. female gender. *Congest Heart Fail.* 11:129, 2005.

Ganz T, Nemeth E. Iron sequestration and anemia of inflammation. *Semin Hematol.* 46:387, 2009.

Giannouli S, et al. Anemia in systemic lupus erythematosus: from pathophysiology to clinical assessment. *Ann Rheum Dis.* 65:144, 2006.

Matsumoto M, et al. Iron regulatory hormone hepcidin decreases in chronic heart failure patients with anemia. *Circ J.* 2009 Dec 18. [Epub ahead of print]

Nurko S. Anemia in chronic kidney disease: causes, diagnosis, treatment. *Cleve Clin J Med.* 73:289, 2006.

Theurl I, et al. Regulation of iron homeostasis in anemia of chronic disease and iron deficiency anemia: diagnostic and therapeutic implications. *Blood.* 113:5277, 2009.

ANEMIAS IN NEONATES

NUTRITIONAL ACUITY RANKING: LEVEL 2

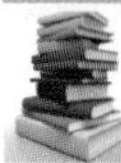

DEFINITIONS AND BACKGROUND

Anemia of prematurity (AOP) is a normocytic, normochromic anemia that presents with very low Hgb and low erythropoietin level. Inadequate RBC production may occur, and the average life span of these cells is about 35–50 days (compared with 120 days for adults). Three causes of AOP include inadequate RBC production, shortened RBC life span, or blood loss. AOP is very common among those born prematurely, where prevalence may be as high as 50% in those born before 32 weeks of gestation. It is also especially common in those born with weight below 1500 g (Haiden et al, 2006).

Hemolytic disease of the newborn (erythroblastosis fetalis) is a condition in which RBCs are broken down or destroyed more rapidly than normal, causing hyperbilirubinemia, anemia, or death; hemolytic disease of the newborn may occur in Rh-positive babies born to Rh-negative mothers (Merck Manual, 2009). Critically ill, extremely premature infants develop anemia because of intensive laboratory blood testing and undergo multiple RBC transfusions in the early weeks of life (Widness et al, 2005). Poor weight gain, apnea and tachypnea, lethargy, tachycardia, and pallor are symptoms.

Reducing anemia in infants may be a preventive measure to lower disease burden from infectious disease in this vulnerable population (Levy et al, 2005). Nutritional deficiencies of vitamin E, vitamin B_{12}, and folate exaggerate the degree of anemia. Vitamin E supplementation, however, when given to preterm infants, does not reduce the severity of this anemia. Administration of vitamin B_{12} and folate with erythropoietin and iron may enhance erythropoietin-induced erythropoiesis more than erythropoietin alone (Haiden et al, 2006).

When detected early in pregnancy, iron-deficiency anemia is associated with a greater risk of preterm delivery (Scholl, 2005). However, it is important not to overdo iron intake. High levels of Hgb, Hct, and ferritin are associated with an increased risk of fetal growth restriction, preterm delivery, and preeclampsia (Scholl, 2005).

Diamond-Blackfan anemia (DBA) (erythrogenesis imperfecta or congenital hypoplastic anemia) is a rare blood disorder characterized by deficiency of RBCs at birth. Other symptoms including slow growth, abnormal weakness, fatigue, pallor, characteristic facial abnormalities, protruding shoulder blades, abnormal shortening of the neck due to fusion of cervical vertebrae, hand deformities, and congenital heart defects. DBA may be inherited as either an autosomal dominant or recessive genetic trait, where the body's bone marrow produces little or no RBCs. A genetic error on chromosome

19 is associated with about 25% of cases, and there is a family history of the disorder in 10–20% of cases.

DBA affects approximately 600–700 million people worldwide but can be difficult to identify. The symptoms may also vary greatly, from very mild to severe and life threatening. DBA is usually diagnosed within the first 2 years of life, sometimes even at birth, on the basis of symptoms. The diagnosis of this anemia might not be recognized right away, however, because it is rare.

The first line of treatment for DBA is prednisone. About 70% of children with DBA will respond to this lifelong treatment, where the medication stimulates the production of more RBCs. If steroids do not work, the next treatment is blood transfusions. Regular blood transfusions will provide RBCs but can lead to iron overloading. Normally, the body uses iron when making new RBCs, but since the person with DBA is not making many cells, the iron builds up. The person then needs to take medication that takes the excess iron out of the body. The only cure available for DBA is bone marrow transplantation. Stem-cell transplantation with human leukocyte antigen (HLA)-matched stem cells has been used for DBA (Kuliev et al, 2005).

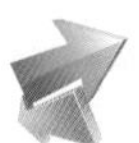

ASSESSMENT, MONITORING, AND EVALUATION

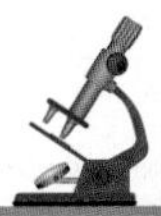

CLINICAL INDICATORS

Genetic Markers: Anemia in a newborn may be caused by a genetic condition such as congenital hypoplastic anemia. In DBA, a genetic alteration on chromosome 19 has been noted.

Clinical/History	Fatigue and pallor	Serum Fe and ferritin
Height	I & O	Gluc
Weight		Alb
BMI	**Lab Work**	CRP
Diet history		Serum folic acid and B_{12}
Slow growth in child (low height–weight percentiles)	CBC	K^+, Na^+
	RBC count	Calcium
	H & H (>2 standard deviations below mean for age)	
BP		
Weakness		

INTERVENTION

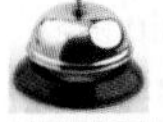

OBJECTIVES

- Provide improved oxygenation for tissues.
- Prevent infections or sepsis. Reduce fevers or excessive inflammation.
- Control hyperglycemia or other side effects of treatments.

> **SAMPLE NUTRITION CARE PROCESS STEPS**
>
> **Inadequate Vitamin-Mineral Intake**
>
> ***Assessment Data:*** Low birth weight (1450 g), poor suck. Lab work shows low Hgb and serum B_{12}; diagnosis of anemia. Pallor, listlessness, and tachycardia.
>
> ***Nutrition Diagnoses (PES):*** Inadequate vitamin and mineral intake related to poor suck and low birth weight as evidenced by lab work with low Hgb and serum B_{12}. Inadequate weight gain.
>
> ***Interventions:*** Nutrient delivery—specialized infant formula with added calories and administration of vitamin B_{12}, folate, erythropoietin and iron.
>
> ***Monitoring and Evaluation:*** Improvement in heart rate, growth, and pallor. Resolution of anemia.

- Prevent further complications.
- Support growth.

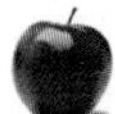

FOOD AND NUTRITION

- Provide an appropriate formula that is easily prepared, with small feedings given frequently.
- Provide extra fluid unless contraindicated.

Common Drugs Used and Potential Side Effects

- If corticosteroids are used, watch side effects of chronic use such as elevated serum sodium levels, decreased potassium and calcium levels, and negative nitrogen balance. Hyperglycemia may occur; alter diet accordingly. Besides diabetes, glaucoma, bone weakening, and high blood pressure can occur, and the medication may suddenly stop working for that person at any point in time.
- Antibiotics may be required when infections are present. Monitor for gastrointestinal distress and other side effects.

Herbs, Botanicals, and Supplements

- Herbs and botanical supplements should not be used without discussing with the physician.

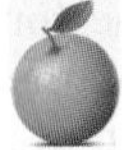

NUTRITION EDUCATION, COUNSELING, CARE MANAGEMENT

- Discuss needs of the patient, which are specific for signs and symptoms and for side effects of any medications.
- Discuss nutritious meal planning.
- If patient has diabetes, counsel specifically for nutritional management.
- Activity levels must be restricted to avoid accidents or falls that could promote bleeding.
- Referral to the Women, Infants, and Children (WIC) Program can be beneficial. WIC programs are helpful in

improving Hgb concentration among young children (Altucher et al, 2005). Age-specific values should be used to assess progress:

Age-Specific Values for Hemoglobin and Hematocrit

Age	Hb (g/dL)	Hct (%)
28-week gestation	14.5	45
32-week gestation	15	47
Term	16.5	51
1–3 days	18.5	56
2 weeks	16.6	53

Source: Merck Manual, http://www.merck.com/mmpe/print/sec19/ch273/ch273b.html, accessed December 22, 2009.

Patient Education—Food Safety

If tube feeding or CPN is needed, careful handwashing procedures should be followed.

For More Information

- Anemia of Prematurity
  http://www.emedicine.com/ped/topic2629.htm
- Diamond Blackfan Anemia
  http://www.diamondblackfan.org.uk/
- Perinatal Anemia
  http://www.merck.com/mmpe/sec19/ch273/ch273b.html

ANEMIAS IN NEONATES—CITED REFERENCES

Altucher K, et al. Predictors of improvement in hemoglobin concentration among toddlers enrolled in the Massachusetts WIC Program. *J Am Diet Assoc.* 105:716, 2005.

Haiden N, et al. A randomized, controlled trial of the effects of adding vitamin B12 and folate to erythropoietin for the treatment of anemia of prematurity. *Pediatrics.* 118:180, 2006.

Kuliev A, et al. Preimplantation genetics: improving access to stem cell therapy. *Ann N Y Acad Sci.* 1054:223, 2005.

Levy A, et al. Anemia as a risk factor for infectious diseases in infants and toddlers: results from a prospective study. *Eur J Epidemiol.* 20:277, 2005.

Merck Manual. Web site accessed December 22, 2009, http://www.merck.com/mmhe/sec23/ch264/ch264q.html

Scholl TO. Iron status during pregnancy: setting the stage for mother and infant. *Am J Clin Nutr.* 81:1218S, 2005.

Widness JA, et al. Reduction in red blood cell transfusions among preterm infants: results of a randomized trial with an in-line blood gas and chemistry monitor. *Pediatrics.* 115:1299, 2005.

ANEMIA OF RENAL DISEASES

NUTRITIONAL ACUITY RANKING: LEVEL 2

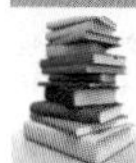

DEFINITIONS AND BACKGROUND

Anemia of renal disease occurs in both acute and chronic renal disease. This type of anemia is often normochromic, normocytic, and sometimes microcytic. When the kidneys become diseased, scar tissue forms and prevents the cells that make erythropoietin from functioning. The buildup of uremic toxins and decreased erythropoietin production adversely affects erythropoiesis. The accumulation of toxic metabolites, which are normally excreted by the kidneys, shortens the life span of circulating RBCs. Management is complicated by a vicious circle of cardiorenal anemia syndrome in which CKD, heart failure, and anemia exacerbate each other (Besarab et al, 2009).

There is an inverse relationship between blood urea nitrogen (BUN) levels and RBC life span, but there is also diminished renal production of erythropoietin. If no cause for anemia other than chronic kidney disease is detected on the basis of the workup and the serum creatinine is ≥2 mg/dL, anemia is most likely due to erythropoietin deficiency; measurement of serum erythropoietin levels is not needed.

Anemia usually starts during the third stage of renal disease, when glomerular filtration rate (GFR) is below 60 cc/minute but before dialysis has started. Short daily hemodialysis and daily home nocturnal hemodialysis can control blood pressure and manage anemia in this population (Pierratos, 2005). Correction of anemia appears to improve cardiac function and quality of life without a greater risk for adverse events (Besarab et al, 2009).

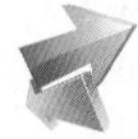

ASSESSMENT, MONITORING, AND EVALUATION

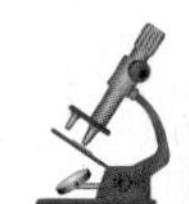

CLINICAL INDICATORS

Genetic Markers: In disorders such as type-2 diabetes, chronic kidney disease is common. Anemia may be present and cause fatigue and difficulty with daily activities such as climbing stairs.

Clinical/History

Height
Weight
BMI
Diet history
BP
I & O
Weakness
Fatigue and pallor
Dizziness
Difficulty concentrating
Shortness of breath

Lab Work

CBC and RBC count
Serum Fe
Hgb (may be <12 g/dL)
Hct (often <33%)
Serum ferritin: (100 absolute deficiency; overload >800 ng/dL
TIBC
[a]Transferrin saturation (serum iron × 100 ÷ TIBC) <20%?
[b]Reticulocyte hemoglobin content (CHr)
Serum soluble transferrin receptor (sTfR)—elevated?

Gluc	Test for occult blood	Creatinine (Creat)
Alb	Blood urea nitrogen (BUN)	
CRP		
Serum folic acid and B_{12}		

[a]The best indicator for iron availability for erythropoiesis.
[b]Half-life of reticulocytes is 1 day; it represents immediate availability of bone marrow iron.

INTERVENTION

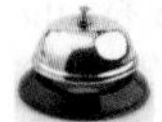

OBJECTIVES

- Prevent infections or sepsis. Reduce fever and excessive inflammation.
- Prevent further complications such as heart failure. Fluid may accumulate and build up in the lungs and liver.
- Support growth in children.
- Improve energy level and decrease fatigue, irritability, and infections.

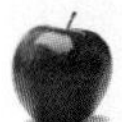

FOOD AND NUTRITION

- Provide a balanced diet that is easily prepared, with small feedings given frequently.
- Provide extra fluid unless contraindicated.
- Provide sufficient foods rich in iron and B-vitamins, as appropriate (depending on laboratory values, current status, predialysis, or dialysis).

Common Drugs Used and Potential Side Effects

- Iron therapy is effective in 30–50% of patients with CKD. A serum ferritin concentration of 100–500 ng/mL is the target during oral and IV iron therapy for predialysis and peritoneal dialysis patients. IV administration and a target serum ferritin concentration of 200–500 ng/mL is recommended for hemodialysis patients (Besarab et al, 2009; Grabe, 2007).
- Erythropoietin Stimulating Agents (ESAs) are given when Hgb falls below 10 g/dL. Epoetin (EPO) is used when oral iron therapy fails (Nurko, 2006). This can be given every week, or every 2 weeks, or monthly. The two formulations of EPO, epoetin alpha (ProCrit) and darbepoetin (Aranesp, DPO), are effective. Longer half-life of darbepoetin alpha permits administration on a once-monthly basis in patients with CKD and anemia (Grabe, 2007). A recent addition is methoxypolyethylene glycol-epoetin beta (Mircera) that has a longer half-life and can be given every 2 weeks.
- Iron deficiency and inflammation are possible causes of inadequate response to ESAs (Grabe, 2007). In the iron-replete patient with an inadequate response to epoetin, the following conditions should be evaluated and treated, if reversible: infection or inflammation (AIDS, lupus); chronic blood loss; aluminum toxicity; hemoglobinopathies (thalassemias, sickle cell anemia); folate or vitamin B_{12} deficiency; multiple myeloma; malnutrition; or hemolysis.
- Ferric gluconate maintains Hgb and allows lower epoetin doses in anemic hemodialysis patients with low TSAT and ferritin levels up to 1200 ng/mL (Kapoian et al, 2008).
- Parenteral iron is reserved for dialysis patients or those who are intolerant of oral iron. Iron dextran (In-FeD, Dexferrum), sodium ferric gluconate (Ferrlecit), and iron sucrose (Venofer) are available. Ferumoxytol is a new IV iron preparation for CKD (Schwenk, 2010). Iron dextran may cause serious allergic reactions.
- Vitamin C helps increase absorption. Dairy and antacids decrease absorption.
- Docusate helps alleviate constipation. Iron supplements can darken stools.

> **SAMPLE NUTRITION CARE PROCESS STEPS**
>
> **Inadequate Vitamin Intake**
>
> ***Assessment Data:*** CKD with low erythropoietin production; Hgb >12 and Hct >33% with EPO. Serum folic acid and vitamin B_{12} levels remain low. Physical signs of vitamin deficiency.
>
> ***Nutrition Diagnoses (PES):*** Inadequate vitamin intake related to poor oral intake as evidenced by diet history, recent anorexia, low serum levels of B_{12} and folate, and minimal use of prescribed water-soluble vitamins.
>
> ***Interventions:*** Food-Nutrient Delivery—In addition to EPO and iron, use vitamin B_{12} and folic acid supplements. Educate about the need to use the supplements daily and to retest lab work every 3–6 months. Counseling about good food sources of folic acid and vitamin B_{12}.
>
> ***Monitoring and Evaluation:*** Lab work showing normal B_{12} and folic acid levels. Fewer complaints of fatigue; no physical signs of vitamin deficiency.

Herbs, Botanicals, and Supplements

- Herbs and botanical supplements should not be used without discussing with the physician. Because the use of CAM is increasing among children and adults with chronic illnesses, efforts should be made to identify those therapies that are beneficial, harmless, and cheap for possible integration with conventional therapy (Oshikoya et al, 2008). Adverse side effects are possible.

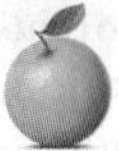

NUTRITION EDUCATION, COUNSELING, CARE MANAGEMENT

- Discuss needs of the patient that are specific for signs and symptoms and side effects of any medications.
- Discuss simplified, but nutritious, meal planning.
- If patient has diabetes, heart failure, or cirrhosis, counsel specifically for nutritional management.
- Activity levels must be restricted to avoid accidents or falls that could promote bleeding.

- People who take EPO shots should have regular tests to monitor their Hgb. If it climbs above 12 g/dL, their doctor should prescribe a lower dose of EPO.

Patient Education—Food Safety

If tube feeding or CPN is needed, careful handwashing procedures should be followed.

For More Information

- American Association of Kidney Patients http://www.aakp.org/aakp-library/Anemia-in-Chronic-Kidney-Disease/
- National Institute of Diabetes and Digestive and Kidney Diseases–Anemia http://kidney.niddk.nih.gov/kudiseases/pubs/anemia/
- National Kidney Foundation – Anemia http://www.kidney.org/Atoz/pdf/anemia.pdf

ANEMIA OF RENAL DISEASES—CITED REFERENCES

Besarab A, et al. Iron metabolism, iron deficiency, thrombocytosis, and the cardiorenal anemia syndrome. *Oncologist.* 14:22S, 2009.

Grabe DW. Update on clinical practice recommendations and new therapeutic modalities for treating anemia in patients with chronic kidney disease. *Am J Health Syst Pharm.* 64:8, 2007.

Kapoian T, et al. Ferric gluconate reduces epoetin requirements in hemodialysis patients with elevated ferritin. *J Am Soc Nephrol.* 19:372, 2008.

Nurko S. Anemia in chronic kidney disease: causes, diagnosis, treatment. *Cleve Clin J Med.* 73:289, 2006.

Oshikoya KA, et al. Use of complementary and alternative medicines for children with chronic health conditions in Lagos, Nigeria. *BMC Complement Altern Med.*8:66, 2008.

Pierratos A. New approaches to hemodialysis. *Annu Rev Med.* 55:179, 2005.

Schwenk MH. Ferumoxytol: a new intravenous iron preparation for the treatment of iron deficiency anemia in patients with chronic kidney disease. *Pharmacotherapy.* 30:70, 2010.

APLASTIC ANEMIA AND FANCONI'S ANEMIA

NUTRITIONAL ACUITY RANKING: LEVEL 1

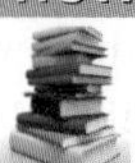

DEFINITIONS AND BACKGROUND

Aplastic anemia is a rare bone marrow disorder with normocytic, normochromic anemia in which normal marrow is replaced with fat. Aplastic anemia, myelodysplastic syndromes, and paroxysmal nocturnal hemoglobinuria (PNH) occur when the bone marrow stops making healthy blood-forming stem cells that produce RBCs, white blood cells, and platelets. Telomeres, repeat sequences at the ends of chromosomes, are protective chromosomal structures that shorten with every cell cycle; aplastic anemia is associated with inherited mutations in telomere repair or protection genes (Calado, 2009).

In about 50% of cases, the cause may be inherited or due to autoimmunity. In other cases, exposure to toxic agents (e.g., radiation, heavy metals, inorganic arsenic) or use of drugs (e.g., phenylbutazone, chloramphenicol, anticonvulsants) may be the cause. Use of interferon-gamma (IFN-γ) may be responsible for certain aspects of the pathology seen in bone marrow failure syndromes, including aplastic anemia (Zeng et al, 2006). Signs and symptoms are listed in Table 12-5.

Treatment includes blood transfusion, preventive antibiotics, careful handwashing, hormone therapy, immunosuppressive therapy, and medications to enhance bone marrow cell production. Severe aplastic anemia (SAA) is life threatening and can be treated with bone marrow transplantation, immunosuppressive therapy, and high-dose cyclophosphamide (Brodsky et al, 2009). Resolution of iron overload (such as serum ferritin >1000 ng/mL) should be addressed before transplant because it may lead to lethal infections (Storey et al, 2009).

Fanconi's anemia (FA) is a rare, genetic disorder characterized by multiple congenital anomalies, progressive bone marrow failure, and an increased prevalence of leukemia or liver cancer (Fagerlie and Bagby, 2006). FA is characterized by delayed bone marrow failure with progression to aplastic anemia. It may be apparent at birth or between ages 2 and 15 and is characterized by deficiency of all bone marrow elements including RBCs, white blood cells, and platelets (pancytopenia). FA is associated with cardiac, kidney, or skeletal abnormalities as well as vitiligo or patchy, brown discolorations (pigmentation changes) of the skin. There are

TABLE 12-5 Signs and Symptoms of Aplastic or Fanconi's Anemias
Blood in stool
Bronzing of skin (café au lait spots)
Dizziness
Headache, irritability
Hemorrhagic diathesis (gums, nose, GI tract, urinary tract, vagina)
Hemosiderosis with resulting cirrhosis, diabetes, heart failure
Increasing fatigue and weakness
Increasing or persistent infections
Irritability
Missing or horseshoe kidney (FA)
Missing or misshapen thumbs (FA)
Nausea
Oral thrush or lesions
Petechiae, ecchymosis
Scoliosis
Skeletal anomalies of spine, hips, ribs (FA)
Slow thought processes, headache
Small head, low birth weight (FA)
Tachycardia, tachypnea, dyspnea
Waxlike pallor

several different subtypes, each of which results from abnormal mutations of different genes. Prognosis is poor among those individuals with low blood counts. Treatment of FA involves transfusions, bone marrow transplantation, or gene therapy. FA patients do not tolerate radiation well and are prone to cancers, even after transplantation. Currently, life span is not long; many children do not survive to adulthood.

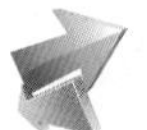

ASSESSMENT, MONITORING, AND EVALUATION

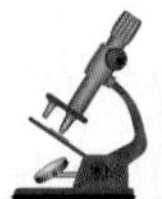

CLINICAL INDICATORS

Genetic Markers: In Caucasians, genetic variations in IFNG may be found. Mutations TERC and TERT genes are also seen in aplastic anemia. The FANCM or FNACJ gene mutations are responsible for some forms of Fanconi's anemia.

Clinical/History	Lab Work	
Height	RBC count (decreased)	White blood cell (WBC) count (<1500)
Weight	Prothombin time (PT)	Alb, transthyretin
BMI	Serum Fe	CRP
Diet history	Gluc	Alanine aminotransferase (ALT)
BP	Granulocytes (decreased)	Aspartate aminotransferase (AST)
GI problems	Transferrin	Bilirubin
See Table 12-5 also	H & H	
Bone marrow biopsy	Platelets (decreased)	
Ultrasound		
Hand x-ray or CT scan		

SAMPLE NUTRITION CARE PROCESS STEPS

Self-Feeding Difficulty

Assessment Data: Low BMI, medical hx with diagnosis of Fanconi's anemia, misshapen thumbs with difficulty holding utensils.

Nutrition Diagnoses (PES): Self-feeding difficulty (NB-2.6) related to hand deformity as evidenced by low BMI and difficulty consuming enough at mealtimes.

Interventions: Food-nutrient delivery—add extra kilocalories to foods and recipes, such as extra fats and carbohydrates. Include extra protein-rich foods as tolerated between meals. Serve finger foods and beverages that can be taken through a straw (milkshake, eggnog). Educate parents about changes in menus and foods for greater intake of nutrient and energy-dense foods. Counsel for ways to enhance self-feeding with use of adaptive feeding equipment.

Monitoring and Evaluation: Improvement in BMI over time and better intake from nutrient and energy-dense foods. Enhanced skills using adaptive feeding tools.

INTERVENTION

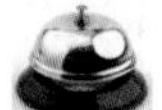

OBJECTIVES

- Prevent infections or sepsis. Reduce fevers.
- Reduce bleeding tendencies and hemorrhages.
- Ensure adequate periods of rest.
- Prepare for splenectomy or bone marrow transplantation.
- Prevent further complications, where possible, and decline in cardiovascular and hepatic functions.

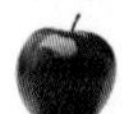

FOOD AND NUTRITION

- Replenish nutrient stores.
- Provide a balanced diet that is easily prepared, with six small feedings.
- Provide extra fluid unless contraindicated (35 cc/kg or more).
- If patient has mouth lesions, avoid excesses of hot or cold foods, spicy or acidic foods, or foods with rough textures.
- If steroids are used, limit sodium intake.

Common Drugs Used and Potential Side Effects

- Growth factors (erythropoietin, G-CSF, and GM-CSF) may help to improve blood counts.
  - Corticosteroids may be used. Side effects of chronic use include elevated serum glucose and sodium levels, decreased potassium and calcium levels, and negative nitrogen balance.
  - High-dose cyclophosphamide is highly effective therapy for SAA, but large randomized controlled trials are necessary to compare with either bone marrow transplantation or use of antithymocyte globulin and cyclosporine (Brodsky et al, 2009).
  - Antibiotics may be required for infections; monitor for GI distress and other side effects.
  - Aspirin should be avoided because it may aggravate blood losses. Other drugs that may aggravate the condition include chloramphenicol, phenylbutazone, sulfa drugs, and ibuprofen. Each of these has specific GI side effects that should be monitored (see index for more information).
  - A list of drugs that can cause acquired aplastic anemia is found at http://www.wrongdiagnosis.com/a/aplastic_anemia/medic.htm#medication_causes_list

Herbs, Botanicals, and Supplements

- Herbs and botanical supplements should not be used without discussing with the physician.

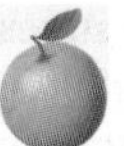

NUTRITION EDUCATION, COUNSELING, CARE MANAGEMENT

- Discuss needs of the patient, which are specific for signs and symptoms and for side effects of any medications.
- Discuss simplified, but nutritious, meal planning.

- If patient has diabetes, heart failure, or cirrhosis, counsel specifically to those issues for nutritional management.
- Activity levels must be restricted to avoid accidents or falls that could promote bleeding.
- Genetic counseling is advised for parents who wish to have more children.

Patient Education—Food Safety

If tube feeding or CPN is needed, careful handwashing procedures should be followed.

For More Information

- America's Blood Centers
  http://www.americasblood.org/
- Aplastic Anemia and MDS International Foundation, Inc.
  http://www.aplastic.org/
- Bloodline
  http://www.bloodline.net/
- Fanconi's Anemia
  http://www.fanconi.org/aboutfa/diagnosis.htm
- Medline—Fanconi's Syndrome
  http://www.nlm.nih.gov/medlineplus/ency/article/000334.htm
- Fanconi Canada
  http://www.fanconicanada.org

APLASTIC ANEMIA AND FANCONI'S ANEMIA—CITED REFERENCES

Brodsky RA, et al. High dose cyclophosphamide for severe aplastic anemia: long-term follow-up. *Blood.* 2009 Dec 16. [Epub ahead of print]

Calado RT. Telomeres and marrow failure. *Hematology Am Soc Hematol Educ Program.* 1:338, 2009.

Fagerlie SR, Bagby GC. Immune defects in Fanconi anemia. *Crit Rev Immunol.* 26:81, 2006.

Storey JA, et al. The transplant iron score as a predictor of stem cell transplant survival. *J Hematol Oncol.* 2:44, 2009.

Zeng W, et al. Interferon-gamma–induced gene expression in CD34 cells. Identification of pathologic cytokine-specific signature profiles. *Blood.* 107:167, 2006.

COPPER DEFICIENCY ANEMIA

NUTRITIONAL ACUITY RANKING: LEVEL 2

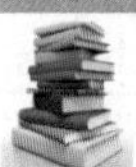

DEFINITIONS AND BACKGROUND

Copper has a role in the production of Hgb (the main component of RBCs), myelin (the substance that surrounds nerve fibers), elastin, collagen (a key component of bones and connective tissue), and melanin (a dark pigment that colors the hair and skin). It is required for the function of over 30 proteins, including superoxide dismutase, ceruloplasmin, lysyl oxidase, cytochrome c oxidase, tyrosinase, and dopamine beta-hydroxylase (Arredondo and Nunez, 2005).

One third of the total body pool of copper is found in skeletal muscle; one third is found in brain and liver; the final third is found in bone and other tissues. Copper is also found in trace amounts in all tissues in the body and is excreted primarily in the bile.

Copper is needed in minute amounts for the formation of Hgb. The metabolism of copper and iron are closely related. Systemic copper deficiency generates cellular iron deficiency, which results in diminished work capacity, reduced intellectual capacity, diminished growth, alterations in bone mineralization, and diminished immune response (Arredondo and Nunez, 2005). Copper deficiency also results in reduced activity of white blood cells and reduced thymus hormone production, thus resulting in increased infection rates.

Marginal deficits of this element can contribute to the development and progression of a number of disease states including cardiovascular disease and diabetes (Li et al, 2005; Urui-Adams and Keen, 2005). Homocysteine thiolactone accumulates when homocysteine is high; it inhibits lysyl oxidase, which depends on copper to catalyze cross-linking of collagen and elastin in arteries and bone. A copper deficiency should, therefore, be avoided. Betaine, copper, folate, pyridoxine, and vitamin B_{12} have proven to be beneficial in lowering serum homocysteine levels. Overall, supplementation with 3–6 mg of copper per day can improve copper status in otherwise healthy individuals; increased intake could reduce the risk of atherosclerosis by promoting improved fibrinolytic capacity (Bugel et al, 2005).

Copper, along with zinc and iron, is an essential metal for normal central nervous system development and function. Imbalances can result in neuronal death (apoptosis), which may contribute to Alzheimer's disease, Parkinson's disease, amyotrophic lateral sclerosis (ALS), and Huntington's disease. Imbalances can also result in neuron deaths in traumatic brain and spinal cord injury, stroke, and seizures (Levenson, 2005).

People with poor intake of protein or whose diets are very high in milk may become deficient in copper or iron. Infants fed on all cow's milk diet without copper supplements may develop copper deficiency. Acquired copper deficiency may be a delayed complication of gastric surgery.

Zinc supplementation (150 mg/d) or vitamin C (1500 mg or more) will reduce copper absorption and increase the potential for anemia. Other conditions that can lead to copper deficiency include burns, pancreatic or liver disease, kidney disease, diarrhea, and prematurity.

Bicytopenia (anemia and neutropenia) with normal platelet count is a feature of hematological disorders caused by copper deficiency; abnormalities improve within a few months after copper supplementation therapy (Nagano et al, 2005). Ceruloplasmin (Cp) is a copper-containing plasma protein with an important role in iron homeostasis; levels are low when copper intake is deficient.

Hospitalized patients should be evaluated carefully. Although enteral feedings contain adequate concentrations of trace elements, problems with bioavailability may occur, and patients receiving long-term enteral feeding should be monitored to avoid anemia and leukopenia (Ito et al, 2005; Oliver et al, 2005). Copper supplementation is essential in parenteral nutrition to prevent an adverse effect of deficiency; requirements in CPN amount to 0.3 mg/d in adults and 20 μg/kg body wt/d in infants or children (Shike, 2009). Nutritional deficiencies that can occur in otherwise asymptomatic normally growing children are often overlooked (Suskind, 2009). If present, they have a significant impact on the health of the child.

Another area for careful review is bariatric surgery. Serum copper levels should be monitored in patients with a neurologic syndrome, who have undergone gastric bypass surgery (Naismith et al, 2009; Griffith et al, 2009).

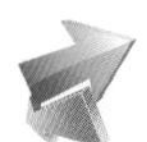

ASSESSMENT, MONITORING, AND EVALUATION

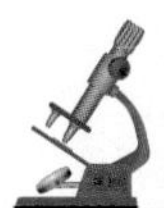

CLINICAL INDICATORS

Genetic Markers: Copper anemias are acquired.

Clinical/History
- Height
- Weight
- BMI
- Diet history
- BP
- See Table 12-6

Lab Work
- CBC
- Serum copper (low)
- Ceruloplasmin (low)
- H & H
- Serum Fe
- Serum ferritin (increased)
- Macrocytic, hypochromic anemia
- Platelets (normal)
- Erythropoietin levels (elevated)
- Serum zinc (Zn) (often elevated)
- Homocysteine
- Alb, transthyretin
- CRP
- Retinol-binding protein (RBP)

SAMPLE NUTRITION CARE PROCESS STEPS

Inadequate Mineral Intake

Assessment Data: Nutritional laboratories showing low-serum copper and Cp with high-serum zinc. Previous bariatric surgery (>1 year) with recent medical visit. Other laboratories are normal. Diet hx reveals low intake of copper from foods.

Nutrition Diagnoses (PES): Inadequate mineral intake of copper related to significant decrease in total food consumed each day for past year post-gastric bypass surgery as evidenced by low-serum Cu and Cp levels and regular use of Zn supplements.

Interventions: Education about ways to enhance copper from meals and snacks. Decrease use of single-Zn supplements and use a multivitamin-mineral supplement that contains copper.

Monitoring and Evaluation: Improved serum Cu and Cp levels after 3 months; better intake of copper-rich foods. Serum Zn within normal range.

TABLE 12-6 Symptoms of Copper Insufficiency and Anemia

Anorexia
Bone fractures
Cardiovascular disease, increased serum cholesterol levels
Diarrhea
Dermatitis or loss of pigmentation of skin, pallor
Edema
Fatigue
Growth retardation
Hair loss
Irregular heart rhythms
Labored respiration, decreased oxygen delivery
Nerve conduction problems
Neurological and immunological abnormalities in newborns if mothers are deficient (Urui-Adams and Keen, 2005).
Myeloneuropathy and myelopathy
Poor collagen formation, decreased wound healing
Reduced red blood cell function
Reduced thyroid function
Shortened red cell life span
Skeletal defects from bone demineralization
Skin sores
Weakness

INTERVENTION

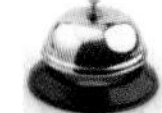

OBJECTIVES

- Correct copper deficiency and documented anemias.
- Instruct patient regarding good sources of protein, iron, and copper to prevent recurrences.
- Monitor use of zinc in supplements, diet, and enteral or parenteral sources to avoid overdosing and related copper depletion.

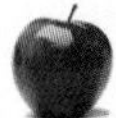

FOOD AND NUTRITION

- Good sources of copper include oysters, liver, nuts, dried legumes, and raisins. A typical diet provides about 2- to 3-mg copper/d, about half of which is absorbed. A supplement of 3- to 6-mg copper may be useful in adults.
- Protein should be at least 1 g/kg for adults; iron intake should be adequate for age and sex.
- Monitor use of multivitamin-mineral supplements to avoid large doses of zinc. Ascorbic acid can act as a pro-oxidant in the presence of metals such as iron or copper; large doses are not recommended.
- Monitor tube-fed patients to ensure that they are receiving sufficient amounts of copper (Ito et al, 2005; Oliver et al, 2005).

TABLE 12-7 Food Sources of Copper

Blackstrap molasses
Black pepper
Chicken
Chocolate (unsweetened or semisweet baker's chocolate and cocoa)
Enriched cereals (bran flakes, raisin bran, shredded wheat)
Fruits (such as cherries, dried fruits, bananas, grapes)
Legumes (such as soybeans, lentils, navy beans, and peanuts)
Nuts and nut butters (cashews, filberts, macadamia nuts, pecans, almonds, and pistachios)
Organ meats (beef liver, kidneys, and heart)
Potatoes
Seafood (oysters, squid, lobster, mussels, crab, and clams)
Seeds (pumpkin)
Tea
Vegetables (avocado, mushrooms, potatoes, sweet potatoes, tomatoes)
Whole grains

Common Drugs Used and Potential Side Effects

- Cupric sulfate is one brand of injectable copper supplement. Copper gluconate is given orally. Beware of excesses, which can be indicated by black or bloody vomit, bloody urine, diarrhea, heartburn, loss of appetite, lower back pain, metallic taste, nausea (severe or continuing), pain or burning while urinating, vomiting, yellow eyes or skin, dizziness or fainting, severe headache, or even coma.
- Do not refrigerate this supplement. Discard when outdated.
- Avoid taking copper supplements with nonsteroidal anti-inflammatory drugs (NSAIDs), birth control pills, allopurinol, estrogen hormones, or cimetidine.

Herbs, Botanicals, and Supplements

- Herbs and botanical supplements should not be used without discussing with the physician.

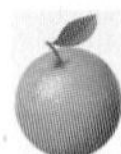

NUTRITION EDUCATION, COUNSELING, CARE MANAGEMENT

- Have patient avoid fad diets. Monitor vegetarian (nonheme iron) diets carefully.
- Zinc in large doses may deplete copper levels; discuss use of mineral supplements. (Rowan and Lewis, 2005).
- Patients at risk for copper deficiency should be counseled on how to avoid this condition. For example, patients with muscular dystrophy may not consume adequate amounts, and muscle strength can diminish as a result (Motlagh et al, 2005).
- Discuss foods that are good sources of protein, iron, and copper; see Table 12-7.
- Be aware that some denture creams contain a high amount of zinc that could be a concern (Spain et al, 2009).

Patient Education—Food Safety

If tube feeding or CPN is needed, careful handwashing procedures should be followed.

For More Information

- Merck Manual
  http://www.merck.com/mrkshared/mmanual/section1/chapter4/4j.jsp
- Northwestern University – Copper Fact Sheet
  http://www.feinberg.northwestern.edu/nutrition/factsheets/copper.html

COPPER DEFICIENCY ANEMIA—CITED REFERENCES

Arredondo M, Nunez MT. Iron and copper metabolism. *Mol Aspects Med.* 26:313, 2005.

Bugel S, et al. Effect of copper supplementation on indices of copper status and certain CVD risk markers in young healthy women. *Br J Nutr.* 94:231, 2005.

Griffith DP, et al. Acquired copper deficiency: a potentially serious and preventable complication following gastric bypass surgery. *Obesity (Silver Spring).* 17:827, 2009.

Ito Y, et al. Latent copper deficiency in patients receiving low-copper enteral nutrition for a prolonged period. *J Parenter Enteral Nutr.* 29:360, 2005.

Levenson CW. Trace metal regulation of neuronal apoptosis: from genes to behavior. *Physiol Behav.* 86:399, 2005.

Li Y, et al. Marginal dietary copper restriction induces cardiomyopathy in rats. *J Nutr.* 135:2130, 2005.

Motlagh B, et al. Nutritional inadequacy in adults with muscular dystrophy. *Muscle Nerve.* 31:713, 2005.

Nagano T, et al. Clinical features of hematological disorders caused by copper deficiency during long-term enteral nutrition. *Intern Med.* 44:554, 2005.

Naismith RT, et al. Acute and bilateral blindness due to optic neuropathy associated with copper deficiency. *Arch Neurol.* 66:1025, 2009.

Oliver A, et al. Trace element concentrations in patients on home enteral feeding: two cases of severe copper deficiency. *Ann Clin Biochem.* 42:136, 2005.

Rowin J, Lewis SL. Copper deficiency myeloneuropathy and pancytopenia secondary to overuse of zinc supplementation. *J Neurol Neurosurg Psychiatry.* 76:750, 2005.

Shike M. Copper in parenteral nutrition. *Gastroenterology.* 137:13S, 2009.

Spain RI, et al. When metals compete: a case of copper-deficiency myeloneuropathy and anemia. *Nat Clin Pract Neurol.* 5:106, 2009.

Suskind DL. Nutritional deficiencies during normal growth. *Pediatr Clin North Am.* 56:1035, 2009.

Urui-Adams JY, Keen CL. Copper, oxidative stress, and human health. *Mol Aspects Med.* 26:268, 2005.

FOLIC ACID DEFICIENCY ANEMIA

NUTRITIONAL ACUITY RANKING: LEVEL 2

Folic acid

Tetrahydrofolic acid

N^5, N^{10}-methylenetetrahydrofolic acid

Three steps for metabolism of dietary folic acid to the bioavailable form.

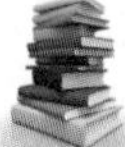

DEFINITIONS AND BACKGROUND

Folic acid is composed of a pterin ring connected to *p*-aminobenzoic acid (PABA). Humans do not generate folate because they cannot synthesize PABA. The amino acid histidine is metabolized to glutamic acid. Formiminoglutamic acid (FIGLU) is an intermediary in this reaction, and tetrahydrofolic acid is the coenzyme that converts it to glutamic acid. Under normal conditions, sufficient intake of dietary histidine can prevent anemia. When dietary intake of histidine is diminished or urinary excretion is greatly increased, anemia results. Folate deficiency depletes histidine through increased urinary excretion.

Folic acid is needed for the synthesis of DNA and maturation of RBCs. Deficiency of folate can lead to many clinical abnormalities, including macrocytic anemia, cardiovascular diseases, birth defects, and carcinogenesis (including colorectal cancer). Folic acid-deficiency anemia generally is caused by inadequate diet, intestinal malabsorption, alcoholism, or pregnancy (Table 12-8).

Folic acid deficiency yields a hyperchromic, macrocytic, megaloblastic anemia. Because similar hematological changes occur with vitamin B_{12} deficiency, it is important to check the serum levels of vitamin B_{12} along with folate tests. Folate is best measured by RBC folate because serum levels are misleading and reflect more recent intake.

Homocysteine elevation is a risk factor for vascular and thrombotic disease. Genetic and acquired influences have been evaluated. While neural tube defects result from maternal

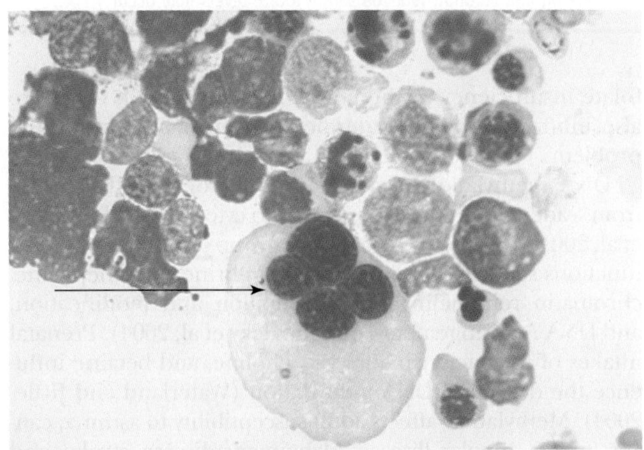

Folic acid anemic cells are hypochromic and macrocytic. Adapted from: *Anderson's Atlas of Hematology;* Anderson, Shauna C., PhD. Copyright 2003, Wolters Kluwer Health/Lippincott Williams & Wilkins.

TABLE 12-8 Conditions and Medications That Deplete Folic Acid

Aging
Alcoholism
Blind-loop syndrome
Burns
Cancers
Celiac disease
Crohn's disease
Dialysis
Elevated homocysteine levels
Hemolytic anemias
Hepatitis
Infection
Inflammatory diseases
Malabsorption
Megacolon
Pregnancy and lactation
Smoking
Stress
Surgery

Medications that interact with folic acid:

- Antiepileptic drugs (AED): phenytoin, carbamazepine, primidone, valproic acid, phenobarbital, and lamotrigine impair folate absorption and increase the metabolism of circulating folate
- Capecitabine: Folinic acid (5-formyltetrahydrofolate) may increase the toxicity of Capecitabine
- Dihydrofolate reductase inhibitors (DHFRI): DHFIs block the conversion of folic acid to its active forms, and lower plasma and red blood cell folate levels. DHFIs include aminopterin, methotrexate, sulfasalazine, pyrimethamine, triamterene, and trimethoprim. Administer leucovorin at the same time
- Nonsteroidal anti-inflammatory drugs (NSAIDs): NSAIDs inhibit some folate dependent enzymes. NSAIDs include ibuprofen, naproxen, indomethacin, and sulindac
- Cholestyramine, Colestipol, Cycloserine, Isotretinoin, oral contraceptives, Methylprednisolone, pancreatic enzymes, Pentamidine, Sulfasalazine either decrease folic acid absorption or increase excretion
- Smoking and alcohol: reduced serum folate levels may occur

folate insufficiency in the periconceptual period, there are also inborn errors of folate metabolism that aggravate the problem.

DNA methylation occurs by transfer of a methyl group from *S*-adenosylmethionine (SAM) to cytosine (Abdolmaleky et al, 2004). SAM serves as a methyl group donor in important functions such as changing norepinephrine to epinephrine, chromatin remodeling, RNA inhibition and modification, and DNA rearrangement (Abdolmaleky et al, 2004). Prenatal intakes of folic acid, vitamin B_{12}, choline, and betaine influence the degree of DNA methylation (Waterland and Jirtle, 2004). Methylation affects adult susceptibility to asthma, cancer, autism, bipolar disease, Alzheimer's disease, stroke, and schizophrenia.

Folate deficiency can result in congenital neural tube defects and megaloblastic anemia; inadequacy is associated with high blood levels of the amino acid homocysteine, which has been linked with the risk of arterial disease, dementia, and Alzheimer's disease (Malouf et al, 2008). Decreasing or low levels of folic acid may also be associated with depression in older adults.

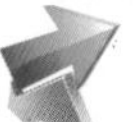

ASSESSMENT, MONITORING, AND EVALUATION

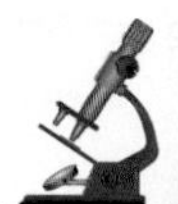

CLINICAL INDICATORS

Genetic Markers: Congenital folate malabsorption, methylenetetrahydrofolate reductase (MTHFR) deficiency, and formiminotransferase deficiency are genetic defects. MTHFR deficiency causes neurological problems even without megaloblastic anemia. MTHFR polymorphisms on chromosome 1 affect 10% of the world's population, especially Caucasians. Varied DNA methylation patterns influence the biological response to food components and vice versa (Milner, 2006).

Clinical/History

Height
Weight
BMI
Diet history
BP
I & O
Weight loss
Anorexia, malnutrition
Smooth and sore red tongue
Diarrhea
Fatigue, lethargy
Poor wound healing
Coldness of extremities
History of alcohol abuse?

Lab Work

RBC folate (<140 ng/mL) – best
Serum folate (<3 ng/mL)
MTHFR alleles?
Mild hyperhomocystinemia (15–25 mmol/L)
Moderate hyperhomocystinemia (26–50 mmol/L)
Low RBC H & H
CBC (macrocytic cells)
Transferrin
Serum B_{12}
Serum Fe (increased)
Mean cell volume (MCV)
Leukopenia, WBC
Urinary formiminoglutamic acid (FIGLU) after histidine load
Serologic testing for parietal cell and intrinsic factor (IF) antibodies (vs. Schilling test)

INTERVENTION

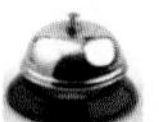

OBJECTIVES

- Increase folate in diet and supplemental folic acid to alleviate anemia.
- Improve diet to provide nutrients needed to make RBCs: folate and other B-complex vitamins, iron, and protein. Instruct patient to correct faulty diet habits if relevant.
- Check for malabsorption syndromes (celiac disease, blind-loop syndrome, congenital or acquired megacolon, Crohn's disease) and correct these as far as possible through use of medications and other treatments.
- Monitor serum folic acid status regularly.

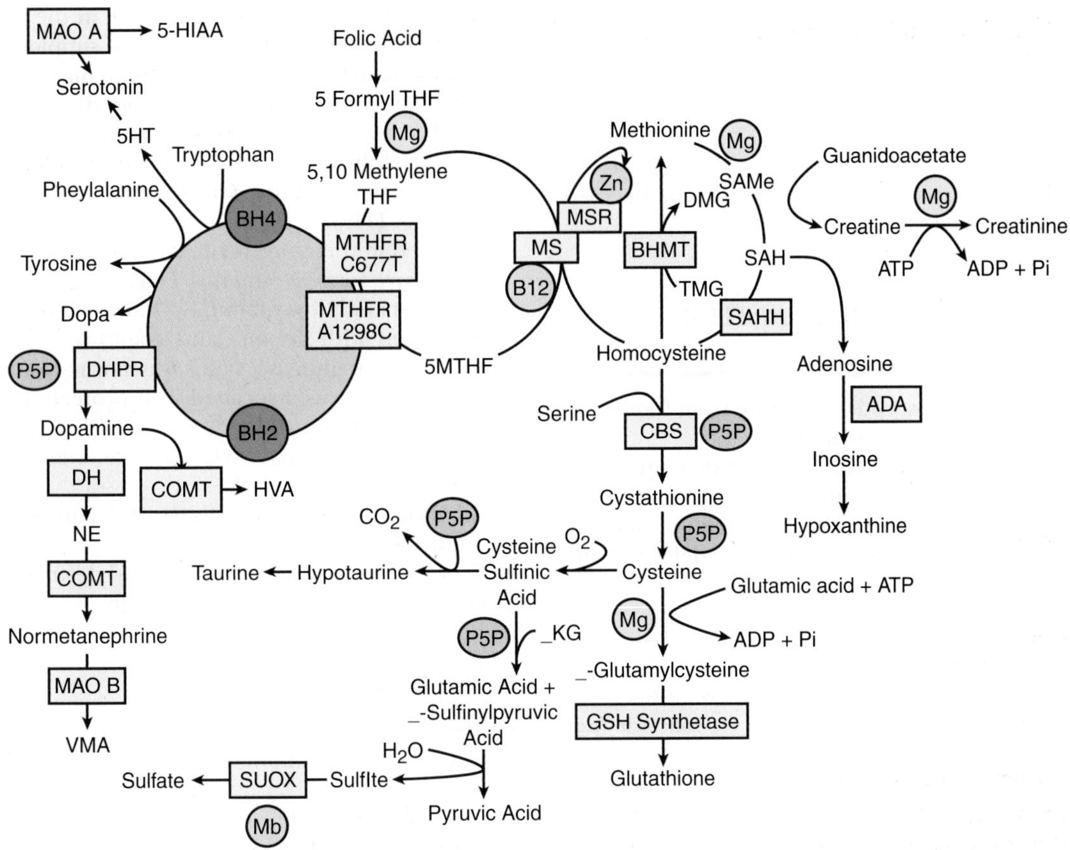

Folic acid-B_{12} pathway, showing the many substances that could be impacted by deficiency or genetic alterations.

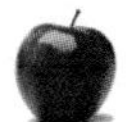

FOOD AND NUTRITION

- Provide a diet that is high in folate, protein, copper, iron, and vitamins C and B_{12}.

> **SAMPLE NUTRITION CARE PROCESS STEPS**
>
> **Inadequate Vitamin Intake and Food- and Nutrition–Related Knowledge Deficit**
>
> ***Assessment Data:*** Hx of MTHFR (C>T) allele and spina bifida in two infants. Diet Hx shows poor intake of folate from diet and no use of supplemental sources. Dislikes fruits and vegetables.
>
> ***Nutrition Diagnoses (PES):*** Inadequate vitamin intake of folate (NI 5.9.1.9) related to lack of folic acid food sources in daily diet as evidenced by headache, fatigue, decreased serum and RBC folate, and giving birth to two infants with spina bifida in the past 5 years. Food and nutrition-related knowledge deficit (NB 1.1) related to lack of prior exposure and interest in accurate nutrition-related information as evidenced by daily intake lacking sources of folate, especially from fruits and vegetables.
>
> ***Interventions:*** ND 3.2.1, 3.2.3.9—multivitamin/mineral supplement, folic acid supplement of additional 400 mcg/d. E 1.2—priority modifications to diet including addition of food sources rich in folic acid, basic information concerning food pyramid, and balanced meal planning.
>
> ***Monitoring and Evaluation:*** One month follow-up visit acceptance of supplements, dietary recall for daily use of folic acid sources, and efficacy of personal meal planning for meeting basic nutrition needs/food pyramid servings.

- Folic acid is distributed widely in green leafy vegetables, citrus fruits, and animal products. Ingestion of one fresh fruit or vegetable provides sufficient folic acid for most people. Other sources include fish, legumes (dried beans and peas), whole grains, leafy dark green vegetables, broccoli, citrus juices, berries, and meats.
- Food manufacturers in the United States have fortified grains with folic acid since 1998. These fortified foods include most enriched breads, flours, corn meal, rice, noodles, macaroni, and other grain products.
- Diets that provide bland, liquid, or soft foods may be needed for patients with a sore mouth; six to eight small meals may be helpful.

Common Drugs Used and Potential Side Effects

- Supplements of folic acid (Folvite) are better than diet alone to alleviate the anemia. Folate deficiency is generally treated with 800–1000 μg of folic acid daily. Leucovorin is an active reduced form.
- Be aware of the interdependence between vitamin B_{12} and folic acid, especially in older individuals. Vitamin B_{12} helps methylate folic acid so that it can travel into cells. The transport form is 5-methyltetrahydrofolate. Because B_{12} deficiency can produce anemia similar to folate deficiency, there is a risk that folate supplementation can delay the diagnosis of B_{12} deficiency, which can lead to irreversible neurological damage (Malouf, 2009).
- 5-methyltetrahydrofolate is an option for supplementation and fortification without masking the anemia of vitamin B_{12} deficiency (Pentieva et al, 2004). Metafolin is a

registered trademark of Merck; Deplin is one brand, containing 7.5 mg of L-methylfolate.

Herbs, Botanicals, and Supplements

- Herbs and botanical supplements should not be used without discussing with the physician.

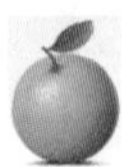

NUTRITION EDUCATION, COUNSELING, CARE MANAGEMENT

- Vitamin C promotes absorption of folate from foods. See Table 12-9 for a list of folate sources.
- Pregnant women should receive appropriate counseling; 30% may have a folate deficiency. Daily needs increase by approximately 200 μg over the adult requirements of 400 μg. Folate protects against neural tube defects in the first trimester.

TABLE 12-9 **Folic Acid Sources**

Source	Folic Acid (μg)
Breakfast cereals fortified with 100% of the DV	400
Beef liver, cooked, braised, 3 ounces	185
Black-eyed peas, immature, cooked, boiled, half cup	105
Spinach, frozen, cooked, boiled, half cup	100
Great Northern beans, boiled, half cup	90
Asparagus, cooked, four spears	85
Broccoli, cooked, half cup	84
Rice, white, long-grain, parboiled, enriched, cooked, half cup	65
Vegetarian baked beans, canned, one cup	60
Spinach, raw, one cup	60
Green peas, frozen, boiled, half cup	50
Broccoli, chopped, frozen, cooked, half cup	50
Egg noodles, cooked, enriched, half cup	50
Avocado, raw, all varieties, sliced, half cup sliced	45
Peanuts, all types, dry roasted, 1 ounce	40
Lettuce, Romaine, shredded, half cup	40
Wheat germ, crude, two tablespoons	40
Tomato Juice, canned, 6 ounces	35
Orange juice, chilled, includes concentrate, three-fourth cup	35

Derived from: NIH Fact Sheet, http://ods.od.nih.gov/factsheets/folate.asp, accessed December 27, 2009.

- Women who have a folic acid allele in the MTHFR gene may need to use a special brand of supplement, such as Neevo (pamlabs.com) during pregnancy.
- Large intakes of folic acid (>1 mg/d) can cure the anemia but may mask a correlated vitamin B_{12} anemia; monitor carefully. 5-methyl THFA enters cells via a diverse range of folate transporters where it may be demethylated to THFA, the active form. Because vitamin B_{12} is required in this conversion, its absence traps folic acid in its inactive form as 5-methyl THFA.
- In seniors with low vitamin B_{12} status, high-serum folate is associated with anemia and cognitive impairment but when not vitamin B_{12} status was normal; however, high-serum folate was associated with protection against cognitive impairment (Morris et al, 2009).
- Attractive meals may help appetite. Fad and restrictive diets should be avoided.
- Alcoholic beverages interfere with folate metabolism and absorption.
- Food folates are oxidized easily and destroyed by lengthy cooking; advise patients accordingly.

Patient Education—Food Safety

If tube feeding or CPN is needed, careful handwashing procedures should be followed.

For More Information

- E-medicine
  http://www.emedicine.com/med/topic802.htm
- Folic Acid Supplements
  http://ods.od.nih.gov/factsheets/folate.asp
- March of Dimes–Folic Acid Deficiency
  http://www.marchofdimes.com/professionals/19695_1151.asp

FOLIC ACID DEFICIENCY ANEMIA—CITED REFERENCES

Abdolmaleky AB, et al. Methylomics in psychiatry: modulation of gene-environment interactions may be through DNA methylation. *Am J Med Genet B Neuropsychiatr Genet.* 127:51, 2004.

Malouf R, et al. Folic acid with or without vitamin B12 for the prevention and treatment of healthy elderly and demented people. *Cochrane Database Syst Rev.* 4:CD004514, 2008.

Milner JA. Diet and cancer: facts and controversies. *Nutr Cancer.* 56:216, 2006.

Morris MS, et al. Folate and vitamin B-12 status in relation to anemia, macrocytosis, and cognitive impairment in older Americans in the age of folic acid fortification. *Am J Clin Nutr.* 85:193, 2007.

Ng TP, et al. Folate, vitamin B12, homocysteine, and depressive symptoms in a population sample of older Chinese adults. *J Am Geriatr Soc.* 57:871, 2009.

Pentieva K, et al. The short-term bioavailabilities of [6S]-5-methyltetrahydrofolate and folic acid are equivalent in men. *J Nutr.* 134:580, 2004.

Waterland RA, Jirtle RL. Early nutrition, epigenetic changes at transposons and imprinted genes, and enhanced susceptibility to adult chronic diseases. *Nutrition.* 20:63, 2004.

HEMOLYTIC ANEMIAS

NUTRITIONAL ACUITY RANKING: LEVELS 2–3

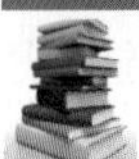

DEFINITIONS AND BACKGROUND

In **hemolytic anemia,** RBCs have an abnormal membrane, which results in hemolysis. RBCs are destroyed faster than they can be produced in bone marrow. In severe cases in infancy, encephalomalacia can result. The incidence of all types of hemolytic anemias is 4 in 100,000 persons in the United States. Treatment may involve splenectomy or steroid use. Most are not affected specifically by vitamin E.

Types of hemolytic anemias include Hgb-SC disease, hemolytic anemia due to glucose-6-phosphate dehydrogenase (G6PD) deficiency, hereditary elliptocytosis, hereditary spherocytosis, idiopathic autoimmune hemolytic anemia, nonimmune hemolytic anemia caused by chemical agents, and secondary immune hemolytic anemia. This text covers aplastic anemia, sickle cell anemia, and thalassemia. Table 12-10 describes some of these types of anemias.

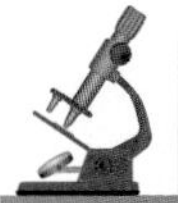

ASSESSMENT, MONITORING, AND EVALUATION

CLINICAL INDICATORS

Genetic Markers: Some types of hemolytic anemia have genetic links.

Clinical/History

Height
Weight
BMI
Diet history
Growth percentile
BP
Tachycardia
Shortness of breath
Dizziness
Edema
Pallor
Nosebleeds, bleeding gums
Dark urine
Jaundice, splenomegaly
Puffy eyelids
Weakness, confusion
Chills
Fatigue, intolerance for exercise
Heart murmur

Lab Work

RBC (low)
Hgb (low)
Reticulocyte count (increased)
Serum alpha-tocopherol levels
Hgb in urine
Hemosiderin in urine
TIBC
Bilirubin (elevated)
Transferrin
Gluc
AST (increased)
Blood test for G6PD
CRP

INTERVENTION

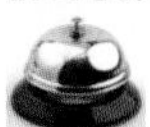

OBJECTIVES

- Prevent further complications.
- Correct anemia or deficits of nutrients, such as vitamin E.

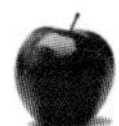

FOOD AND NUTRITION

- Provide diet as usual for age and sex.
- Avoid excesses of iron.
- Ensure adequate intake of vitamin E and zinc, which may become deficient. Good sources of vitamin E include wheat germ, almonds, sunflower seeds, sunflower or safflower oil, peanut butter, peanuts, corn oil, spinach, broccoli, and

TABLE 12-10 Types of Hemolytic Anemia

Type	Description
Acquired autoimmune hemolytic anemia	A rare autoimmune disorder characterized by the premature destruction of RBCs. Normally, RBCs have a life span of 120 days before the spleen removes them, but in this condition, RBCs are destroyed prematurely. Bone marrow production of new cells can no longer compensate. This anemia occurs in individuals who previously had a normal RBC system. Patients with autoimmune hemolytic anemia usually are associated with thrombosis
Familial hemolytic jaundice (spherocytic anemia)	A hereditary anemia in which RBCs are shaped like spheres rather than their normal, donut-like shape. Jaundice and anemia occur from destruction of the abnormal cells by the spleen. Surgical removal of the spleen usually is indicated. There is no permanent cure
Glucose-6-phosphate dehydrogenase (G6PD) deficiency anemia	This anemia is seen in about 10% of African-American males in the United States and is also common in persons from the Mediterranean area or Asia. The severity differs among different populations. In the most common form in the African-American population, the deficiency is mild, and the hemolysis affects primarily older RBCs. In Caucasians, G6PD deficiency tends to be more serious because even young red blood cells are affected. It affects millions of people worldwide, especially in malaria-prone areas
Hereditary nonspherocytic hemolytic anemia	A group of rare genetic blood disorders characterized by defective RBCs (erythrocytes) that are not abnormally "sphere shaped" (spherocytes). Membranes of RBCs, abnormal metabolism of a chemical contained in hemoglobin (porphyrin), and deficiencies in certain enzymes such as G6PD or pyruvate kinase are thought to be the cause of these disorders
Vitamin E-sensitive hemolytic anemia	This condition may occur in infants who receive polyunsaturated fatty acids (PUFAs) without adequate vitamin E. Children with cystic fibrosis should be screened for vitamin E-deficient hemolytic anemia

SAMPLE NUTRITION CARE PROCESS STEPS

Unintentional Weight Loss

Assessment Data: BMI 20, recent weight loss 10#. GI distress and pallor noted. Diagnosis of hemolytic anemia with splenectomy planned.

Nutrition Diagnoses (PES): Unintentional weight loss related to GI distress and loss of appetite as evidenced by recent weight loss of 10# in 6 weeks.

Interventions: Prepare for splenectomy; use nutrient-dense and energy-rich foods as tolerated, such as milkshakes or eggnogs with or between meals. Educate patient about ways to enhance food intake while not feeling well.

Monitoring and Evaluation: Postoperative evaluations; return of appetite and improved intake. No further weight loss; eventual weight regained.

soybean oil. Good sources of zinc include oysters, beef shank, crab, pork, chicken, lobster, baked beans, cashews, and yogurt.

Common Drugs Used and Potential Side Effects

- For hemolytic anemia that is sensitive to vitamin E deficiency, water-soluble vitamin E (alpha-tocopherol) is likely to be given daily. Avoid taking with an iron supplement, which could interfere with utilization.
- Persons with G6PD deficiency need to avoid exposing themselves to certain medicines such as aspirin (acetylsalicylic acid), certain antibiotics used to treat infections, fava beans, and mothballs.
- Medicines can improve autoimmune hemolytic anemia (AIHA). Where prednisone is used, monitor for side effects. Monoclonal antibody therapy such as rituximab is used in difficult cases; it appears to be a safe and effective option (Hoffman, 2009).

Herbs, Botanicals, and Supplements

- Herbs and botanical supplements should not be used without discussing with the physician.
- Flavonoid preparations, marketed for a variety of effects and generally safe, should be evaluated carefully because there have been reports of toxic flavonoid–drug interactions, hemolytic anemia, and other problems (Galati and O'Brien, 2004).

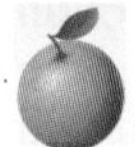

NUTRITION EDUCATION, COUNSELING, CARE MANAGEMENT

- For hemolytic anemia that is sensitive to vitamin E deficiency, discuss, in layman's terms, the role of vitamin E in lipid oxidation and utilization. Discuss sources of polyunsaturated fatty acids (PUFAs) and why excesses should be controlled. Discuss sources of vitamin E in the diet; natural sources are more bioavailable than synthetic sources.
- Discuss exercise tolerance and ability to eat sufficient amounts of food as related to fatigue.

Patient Education—Food Safety

If tube feeding or CPN is needed, careful handwashing procedures should be followed.

For More Information

- American Autoimmune Related Diseases Association, Inc.
  http://www.aarda.org
- Medline
  http://www.nlm.nih.gov/medlineplus/ency/article/000571.htm
- NIH – Hemolytic Anemias
  http://www.nhlbi.nih.gov/health/dci/Diseases/ha/ha_whatis.html

HEMOLYTIC ANEMIAS—CITED REFERENCES

Galati G and O'Brien PJ. Potential toxicity of flavonoids and other dietary phenolics: significance for their chemopreventive and anticancer properties. *ree Radic Biol Med.* 37:287, 2004.

Hoffman PC. Immune hemolytic anemia–selected topics. *Hematology Am Soc Hematol Educ Program.* 80–86, 2009.

IRON-DEFICIENCY ANEMIA

NUTRITIONAL ACUITY RANKING: LEVEL 2

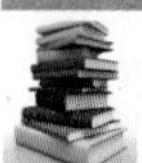

DEFINITIONS AND BACKGROUND

Hgb transports oxygen to the tissues and carbon dioxide back to the lungs where it is exhaled. Hgb levels are influenced by sex, age, altitude, and smoking. In the adult male and the elderly, iron deficiency is usually caused by chronic blood loss. In children and women, low intake of iron may be a problem. The nutrient most commonly deficient in the world is iron. Iron deficiency affects two billion people, mostly in developing countries (Lynch, 2005).

IDA results from inadequate intake, impaired erythropoiesis or absorption of iron, blood loss, or demands from closely repeated pregnancies (Table 12-11). Serious systemic consequences include impaired cognitive function, koilonychia, and impaired exercise tolerance. Hct is the measure of RBCs in a given volume of blood, packed by centrifuge. Transferrin is the carrier protein that picks up iron from the intestines.

Absorption of iron occurs in the ferrous form; storage is in the liver, spleen, and bone marrow. See Table 12-12 for

TABLE 12-11 Stages of Iron Deficiency

Stages of Iron Deficiency	Indicator	Diagnostic Range
Stage 1 Depletion of iron stores	Stainable bone marrow iron Total iron binding capacity Serum ferritin concentration	Absent >400 μg/dL <12 μg/L <20 μg/L + low Hb or Hct indicates iron deficiency
Stage 2 Early functional iron deficiency	Transferrin saturation Free erythrocyte protoporphyrin Serum transferrin receptor	<16% >70 μg/dL erythrocyte >8.5 mg/L
Stage 3 Iron deficiency anemia	Hemoglobin concentration Mean cell volume	<12 g/dL <80 fL

Adapted from: Dietary Reference Intakes for Vitamin A, Vitamin K, Arsenic, Boron, Chromium, Copper, Iodine, Iron, Manganese, Molybdenum, Nickel, Silicon, Vanadium, and Zinc (2002), Iron, p. 302 Food and Nutrition Board (FNB), Institute of Medicine (IOM).

content of iron in various body sources. Approximately 90% of the body's store of iron is reused. Diet replaces iron lost through sweat, feces, and urine. The duodenum (upper small intestine) is where iron is best absorbed. Damage or surgery of the duodenum can greatly inhibit total iron absorption, thus leading to greater risk of deficiency. Table 12-13 describes factors that can modify iron absorption.

IDA is the final stage of a long period of deprivation. Serum ferritin (storage form) is the most useful test to differentiate IDA from ACD. Iron deficiency is relatively common in toddlers, adolescent girls, and women of childbearing age. Ingestion of cow's milk causes occult intestinal blood loss in young infants. The Hgb content of reticulocytes (young RBCs) is a good indicator of iron deficiency and IDA in children. Risk of iron deficiency may be underestimated in high-risk populations.

Postpartum anemia is associated with breathlessness, tiredness, palpitations, and maternal infections, and blood transfusions and iron supplementation have been used in the treatment of IDA. Erythropoietin may be useful.

TABLE 12-12 Normal Iron Distribution in the Body

Forms	Men (mg iron/kg BW)	Women (mg iron/kg BW)
Storage—ferritin	9	4
Storage—hemosiderin	4	1
Transport protein: transferrin	<1	<1
Functional hemoglobin	31	31
Functional myoglobin	4	4
Enzymes	2	2
TOTAL	50	42

Based on data from: Insel P, Turner R, Ross D. *Nutrition*. Sudbury, MA: Jones & Bartlett Publishers, 2001.

TABLE 12-13 Factors That Modify Iron Absorption

Factor	Description
Physical state (bioavailability)	Heme > Fe^{2+} > Fe^{3+}
High gastric Ph	Hemigastrectomy, vagotomy, pernicious anemia, histamine H_2-receptor blockers, calcium-based antacids
Disruption of intestinal structure	Crohn's disease, celiac disease (nontropical sprue)
Inhibitors	Phylates, tannins, soil clay, laundry starch, iron overload
Competitors	Cobalt, lead, strontium
Facilitators	Ascorbate, citrate, amino acids, iron deficiency

From: Information Center for Sickle Cell and Thalassemic Disorders. Iron deficiency. Available at http://sickle.bwh.harvard.edu/fe-def.html.

Celiac disease may be present in children and is associated with IDA (Goel et al, 2005). In persistent IDA, screening for celiac disease (anti-tissue transglutaminase antibodies), autoimmune gastritis (gastric, anti-parietal, or anti-IF antibodies), and *Helicobacter pylori* (IgG antibodies and urease breath test) is recommended (Hershko and Ronson, 2009).

Because menstruation increases iron losses each month, women of childbearing age tend to become iron deficient. When there is not enough Hgb, free erythrocyte protoporphyrin (FEP) accumulates. Athletes are also at risk for iron deficiency. Recreational athletes should be screened for iron deficiency using serum ferritin, serum transferrin receptor, and Hgb (Sinclair and Hinton, 2005).

As many as 25% of children and 20% of those seen in mental health clinics have pica, which is characterized by persistent and compulsive cravings to eat nonfood items. Pica can occur in pregnant women, in autism, and in persons with brain injuries. Pica is seen in about half of patients with iron deficiency; it is a consequence of iron deficiency and is relieved by iron supplementation.

Exposure to lead also has a significant effect on Hgb and Hct levels. Serum levels above 50 mcg/dL are a problem. Lead poisoning reduces Hgb production, causes iron deficiency, and elevates FEP as the precursor.

Poor intake of vitamins A, B_{12}, C, and E, folic acid, and riboflavin is also linked to the development and control of IDA. Multiple micronutrient (MMN) supplementation during pregnancy reduces the risk of low birth weight, small-for-gestational age, and anemia; MMN supplementation improves CD4 counts and HIV-related morbidity and mortality in adults (Allen et al, 2009).

When Hgb levels are seriously low, the heart is particularly vulnerable. Anemia in heart failure patients is associated with reduced exercise tolerance, increased heart failure hospitalizations, and increased all-cause mortality (Stamos and Silver, 2009). Whole-blood transfusion or IV iron may be needed. Iron fortification of food is also a cost-effective method for reducing the prevalence of nutritional iron deficiency. In populations where young children are routinely fed cooked rice daily, fortifying it with iron helps improve iron status (Beinner et al, 2010).

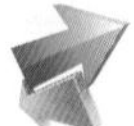

ASSESSMENT, MONITORING, AND EVALUATION

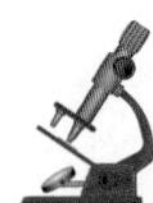

CLINICAL INDICATORS

Genetic Markers: Mutations in a type-II serine protease, matriptase-2/TMPRSS6, are associated with severe iron deficiency caused by inappropriately high levels of hepcidin expression; hemojuvelin is a cell surface protein that regulates hepcidin expression (Lee, 2009).

Clinical/History

- Weight
- BMI
- Diet history
- BP
- I & O
- Pallor
- Brittle, spoon-shaped fingernails (koilonychia)
- Stool examination for occult blood
- Impaired cognitive function
- Blue sclerae
- Impaired exercise tolerance
- Weakness, fatigue
- Vertigo
- Headache, irritability
- Heartburn
- Dysphagia
- Flatulence, vague abdominal pains
- Anorexia
- Diarrhea
- Glossitis, stomatitis
- Ankle edema
- Tingling in extremities
- Palpitations
- Alopecia

Lab Work

- Ferritin (decreased stores in liver, spleen, bone marrow; levels are <20 g/L)
- Serum iron (low)
- H & H (Hgb is more sensitive)
- Mean cell Hgb (MCH) (decreased)
- Mean cell Hct (MCHC) (decreased)
- CBC (every 3–6 months after initial)
- Transferrin (increased)
- MCV (<80)
- RBC (small, microcytic, hypochromic)
- WBC/differential (increased)
- TIBC (increased >350 μg/dL)
- Reticulocyte count
- Serum copper
- Cholesterol (Chol)
- Test for *H. pylori*

SAMPLE NUTRITION CARE PROCESS STEPS

Harmful Beliefs About Food

Assessment Data: Diet hx indicates pica during this pregnancy. Mom states that "the starch is good for my baby." Eats starch after each meal. Twenty-weeks pregnant; age 19. Low H & H.

Nutrition Diagnoses (PES): Harmful beliefs/attitudes (NB-1.2) about food or nutrition-related topics.

Interventions: Initial/Brief nutrition education (N.I.2.2) to provide basic nutrition-related educational about food and foods rich in iron; reasons to discontinue eating starch and to begin taking a prenatal vitamin. Counseling—work with client to set goals for a healthier pregnancy.

Monitoring and Evaluation: Improvement in H & H. Discontinuation of pica. Positive pregnancy outcome.

INTERVENTION

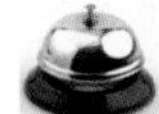

OBJECTIVES

- Alleviate cause of the anemia and associated anorexia.
- Provide adequate oral iron to replace losses or deficits, especially heme sources of protein (liver, beef, oysters, lamb, pork, ham, tuna, shellfish, fish, and poultry).
- Provide an acid medium to favor better absorption. Enhancers include gastric juice and ascorbic acid. Food sources of vitamin C should be included daily.
- Monitor and correct pica, including geophagia (clay eating), amylophagia (starch eating), ice eating, or any lead exposure.
- Avoid or correct constipation.
- Screen for IDA or sports anemia in athletes (Sinclair and Hinton, 2005).
- Reduce iron inhibitors, such as excessive fiber (as in whole grains), phytic acid (as in spinach, bran, legumes, and soy products), tannins in tea, and polyphenols in coffee or red wine. In many developing countries, cereal and legume-based diets contain low amounts of bioavailable iron, which may increase the risk of iron deficiency (Zimmermann et al, 2005).

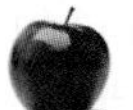

FOOD AND NUTRITION

- If IDA is related to inadequate iron in diet, usually adding three portions of lean red meat (heme iron sources) per week, along with all other essential vitamins and minerals, will correct the anemia. The average mixed diet contains approximately 6 mg of iron per 1000 kcal. Iron absorption increases as stores become depleted. Good sources of iron include liver, dried beans, egg yolks, kidney, lean beef, dark meat of chicken, salmon, tuna, dried fruits, enriched whole-grain cereals, molasses, and oysters.
- Heme iron is found readily in beef, pork, and lamb; consume with fruit or fruit juice. Heme iron is absorbed well, regardless of other foods in the diet.
- Nonheme iron absorption is greatly affected by other foods. Absorption of nonheme iron is best in the presence of foods rich in vitamin C or with heme-containing sources. Increase intake of vitamin C (oranges, grapefruit, tomatoes, broccoli, cabbage, baked potatoes, strawberries, cantaloupe, and green peppers), especially with an iron supplement.
- Detect pica and discuss with patient. Pica substance may displace other important foods, leading to nutrient malnutrition. The ingested substance may also be toxic.
- Tea, coffee, wheat brans, and soy products tend to inhibit absorption of nonheme iron. Monitor use carefully; avoid excesses.

Common Drugs Used and Potential Side Effects (Table 12-14)

- If anemia is caused by an increased demand for iron such as a growth spurt (toddlers, adolescents) or pregnancy, oral supplementation may be necessary: inorganic

TABLE 12-14 Medications to Correct Iron-Deficiency Anemia

Medication	Description
Ferrous salts (Feosol, Fer-In-Sol, Mol-Iron) or tablets (Feostat, Fergon, Feosol)	Prolonged-release ferrous sulfate (Slow Fe) improves iron absorption with fewer side effects than standard ferrous sulfate pills. Other forms include ferrous fumarate (Femiron, Feostat, Fumerin, Hemocyte, Ircon) and ferrous gluconate (Fergon, Ferralet, Simron). These may cause gastric irritation and constipation.
Enteric-coated or sustained-release iron	More expensive and often carry the iron past maximal absorption site in the upper intestine.
Heme iron (Proferrin Forte)	This is a medical food that contains heme iron plus folic acid. It is absorbed regardless of achlorhydria, and has fewer GI side effects than IV or ferrous iron sources. It can be taken with or without meals.
Parenteral or IV iron	Can be administered by injection or infusion. This therapy is reserved for cases of trauma where blood loss is life threatening and is not used for insufficiency due to inadequate dietary iron intake. Imferon can be given intramuscularly, if oral iron is not tolerated; pain and skin discoloration may result.

iron in ferrous form (50–200 mg/d for adults; 6 mg/kg for children) combined with increased consumption of heme-rich sources of iron. This is best absorbed on an empty stomach, but with food if there are GI side effects.

- Iron pills should be taken 2 hours before or after other medications. Iron can inhibit the effectiveness of thyroid medications, antibiotics, and some antidepressant drugs. Once ingested, it is imperative that the stomach contains acid to dissolve the iron salt; if taking antacids or H2 blockers such as cimetidine (Tagamet), the iron salt will not dissolve.
- The amount of elemental iron contained in iron pills will vary. A 325-mg supplement is probably made of ferrous fumarate or gluconate, with only 100 mg of elemental iron per pill.
- Heme iron supplements (such as Proferrin) can be taken with meals, unlike ionic iron preparations, which must be taken on an empty stomach between meals. However, individuals with allergies to beef, milk, or other dairy products should not be given Proferrin.
- It takes 4–30 days to note improvements after iron therapy, especially in Hgb levels. Hgb should rise 0.1–0.2 g/dL/day after the fifth day of treatment; then should rise 2.0 g/dL/week for 3 weeks. Iron therapy should be continued for at least 2 months after the Hgb has returned to normal to replenish the iron stores.
- Iron stores are replaced after 1–3 months of treatment. Increased supplementation in normal individuals can cause additional, unnecessary iron to go into storage, reflected by ferritin elevation.
- Aspirin or corticosteroids can cause GI bleeding or peptic ulceration. Vitamin C and nutrient levels may be decreased.
- Some medications, including antacids, can reduce iron absorption. Iron tablets may also reduce the effectiveness of other drugs, including the antibiotics tetracycline, penicillamine, and ciprofloxacin and the anti-Parkinson's drugs methyldopa, levodopa, and carbidopa. Wait 2 hours between doses of these drugs and iron supplements.

Herbs, Botanicals, and Supplements

- Herbs and botanical supplements should not be used without discussing with the physician.

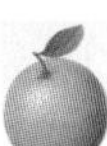

NUTRITION EDUCATION, COUNSELING, CARE MANAGEMENT

- Hgb is made from protein, iron, and copper. RBCs are made from vitamin B_{12}, folacin, and amino acids. Explain which foods are good sources of iron, protein, vitamin C, and related nutrients.
- Temporary changes in stool color (green or tarry and black) are common with supplements; this is not cause for alarm. To avoid side effects of supplements, take them with meals or milk; food iron has fewer side effects.
- Foods and substances that can interfere with the absorption of iron include calcium, tannins, which are found in coffee, tea, grapes, red wine, purple or red rice, and bran fiber or chocolate. Avoid excesses of oxalates, alkalis, and antacids; discuss sources. Iron supplementation is best taken 2 hours after consuming these substances.
- The average American diet contains 10–20 mg of iron daily, roughly 10% of which is absorbed. Avoid overdosing with iron supplements. The body can only synthesize 5–10 mg of Hgb per day, and excesses may work against the immune system.
- Local or systemic infections interfere with iron absorption and transport.
- In children under age 2, limit milk intake to no more than 500 mL/d for better iron status.
- Explain nonfood pica—clay, starch, plaster, paint chips—and the relationship with nutrition. In food pica in which singular foods are eaten instead of balanced meals, the foods chosen are often crunchy or brittle. Excessive consumption of lettuce, ice, celery, snack chips, and chocolate has been noted; after iron supplementation, cravings often subside.
- Iron deficiency may be partly induced by plant-based diets containing low levels of poorly bioavailable iron (Kesa and Oldewage-Theron, 2005). Young people who follow a vegan diet should have their iron status monitored closely.
- Use culturally appropriate nutrition counseling. In some cultures, boys may be fed iron-rich foods preferentially over girls; counseling should be designed to improve intake by girls (Shell-Duncan and McDade, 2005).

Patient Education—Food Safety

If tube feeding or CPN is needed, careful handwashing procedures should be followed.

For More Information

- E-medicine
  http://emedicine.medscape.com/article/202333-overview
- Iron Deficiency Anemia for Kids
  http://www.kidshealth.org/parent/medical/heart/ida.html
- Mayo Clinic
  http://www.mayoclinic.com/health/iron-deficiency-anemia/DS00323
- National Institutes of Health–Iron Deficiency Anemia
  http://www.nlm.nih.gov/medlineplus/ency/article/000584.htm
- University of Maryland
  http://www.umm.edu/blood/aneiron.htm

IRON DEFICIENCY ANEMIA—CITED REFERENCES

Allen LH, et al. Provision of multiple rather than two or fewer micronutrients more effectively improves growth and other outcomes in micronutrient-deficient children and adults. *J Nutr.* 139:1022, 2009.

Beinner MA, et al. Iron-fortified rice is as efficacious as supplemental iron drops in infants and young children. *J Nutr.* 140:49, 2010.

Goel NK, et al. Cardiomyopathy associated with celiac disease. *Mayo Clin Proc.* 80:674, 2005.

Hershko C, Ronson A. Iron deficiency, Helicobacter infection and gastritis. *Acta Haematol.* 122:97, 2009.

Kesa H, Oldewage-Theron W. Anthropometric indications and nutritional intake of women in the Vaal Triangle, South Africa. *Public Health.* 119:294, 2005.

Lee P. Role of matriptase-2 (TMPRSS6) in iron metabolism. *Acta Haematol.* 122:87, 2009.

Lynch SR. The impact of iron fortification on nutritional anaemia. *Best Pract Res Clin Haematol.* 18:333, 2005.

Shell-Duncan B, McDade T. Cultural and environmental barriers to adequate iron intake among northern Kenyan schoolchildren. *Food Nutr Bull.* 26:39, 2005.

Sinclair LM, Hinton PS. Prevalence of iron deficiency with and without anemia in recreationally active men and women. *J Am Diet Assoc.* 105:975, 2005.

Stamos TD, Silver MA. Management of anemia in heart failure. *Curr Opin Cardiol.* 2009 Dec 5. [Epub ahead of print]

Zimmermann MB, et al. Iron deficiency due to consumption of a habitual diet low in bioavailable iron: a longitudinal cohort study in Moroccan children. *Am J Clin Nutr.* 81:115, 2005.

MALARIA AND PARASITIC ANEMIAS

NUTRITIONAL ACUITY RANKING: LEVEL 1

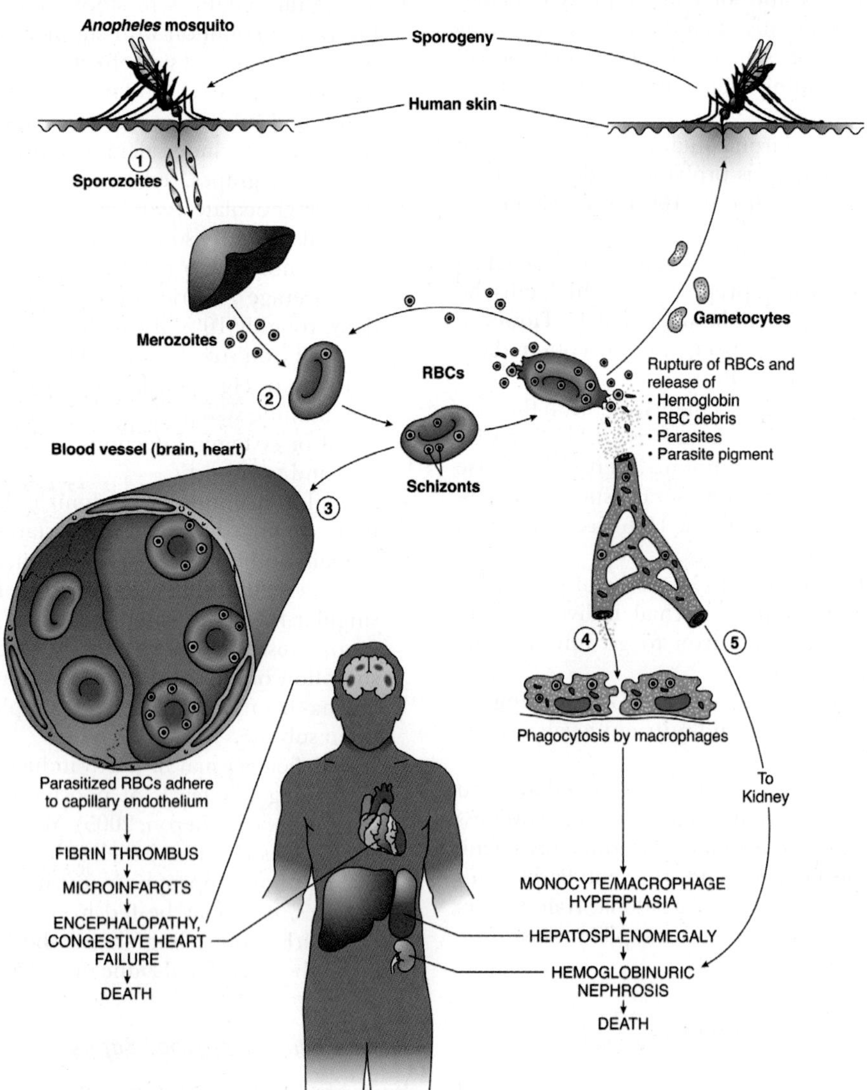

Adapted from: Rubin E MD and Farber JL MD. *Pathology,* 3rd ed. Philadelphia: Lippincott Williams & Wilkins, 1999.

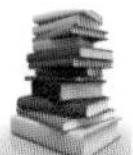

DEFINITIONS AND BACKGROUND

Gastrointestinal infestation by parasitic worms that feed on blood (hookworm) or on nutrients (tapeworm) may occur, especially in tropical or subtropical areas. Intestinal parasites that affect nutrition in particular include soil-transmitted helminths, *Giardia duodenalis*, *Entamoeba histolytica*, other parasites such as the coccidia, *Schistosoma* sp., and malarial parasites. Iron deficiency is found to be correlated with these parasites in tropical countries (Shell-Duncan and McDade, 2005).

The neglected infections of poverty are parasitic, bacterial, and viral infections that disproportionately affect impoverished populations in the United States; these include Chagas disease, cysticercosis, congenital cytomegalovirus (CMV), toxocariasis, toxoplasmosis, and trichomoniasis (CDC, 2009). Toxoplasmosis is considered to be the third leading cause of death attributed to foodborne illness in the United States (CDC, 2009).

Malaria is a bloodborne, parasitic infection transmitted by mosquitoes. It kills more than 1 million people annually, especially in Africa. Pregnant women, children, and immunocompromised individuals have the highest rates of morbidity and mortality (Schantz-Dunn and Nour, 2009). More than 1000 cases of malaria are reported to the Centers for Disease Control and Prevention each year in the United States. Travelers or immigrants present with fever, chills, nausea, vomiting, headache, abdominal pain, severe anemia, and acute renal failure (Vicas et al, 2005).

Risks for miscarriage, intrauterine demise, premature delivery, low birth-weight neonates, neonatal death, severe anemia, and maternal death are high among pregnant women with malaria (Schantz-Dunn and Nour, 2009). Between 150 and 300 children die each hour from malaria (Breman, 2009). For those who survive, neurologic impairment, anemia, hypoglycemia, and low birth weight imperil normal development and survival (Breman, 2009).

Malaria can be prevented with appropriate drugs, bednets treated with insecticide, and effective educational outreach. Resistance of *Plasmodium falciparum* to drugs and Anopheles mosquitoes to insecticides has stimulated discovery and development of artemisinin-based combination treatments (ACTs) and other drugs, long-lasting insecticide-treated bednets (with synthetic pyrethroids) and a search for nontoxic, long-lasting, affordable insecticides for indoor residual spraying (Breman, 2009). A malaria vaccine is under development (Greenwood, 2008).

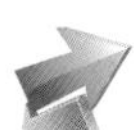

ASSESSMENT, MONITORING, AND EVALUATION

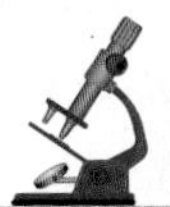

CLINICAL INDICATORS

Genetic Markers: Congenital CMV is passed from mother to infant during pregnancy.

Clinical/History

Height
Weight
BMI
Diet history
BP
I & O
Fatigue
Abdominal discomfort
Nausea, vomiting
Fever
Irritability
Pica?

Lab Work

Hgb (often <5 g/dL)
Hct
Serum Fe
Ferritin
Serum B_{12}
TIBC
Alb
Serum folic acid
CRP
Transferrin
Gluc
Serum Cu
Serum Zn

INTERVENTION

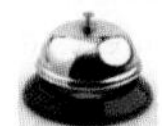

OBJECTIVES

- Correct anemia from blood losses; eliminate parasitic infestation.
- Prevent GI tract perforation or obstruction, when likely to exist.
- Improve nutritional status and appetite. Parasitic infections affect the intake of food, subsequent digestion and absorption, metabolism, and nutrient storage and cause subtle micronutrient deficiency, such as vitamin A deficiency.
- Prevent low birth weight and other adverse effects in pregnant or postpartum women and their infants.

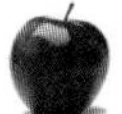

FOOD AND NUTRITION

- A diet high in protein, B-complex vitamins, and iron may be appropriate. Provide adequate energy to meet individual's needs for anabolism where needed.
- Foods rich in heme iron and vitamins C and A should be included in meals served or planned. Iron inhibitors should be excluded from diet as far as possible until recovery is complete.
- Include plenty of other nutrient-dense foods, such as good sources of zinc and other micronutrients (Table 12-15).

SAMPLE NUTRITION CARE PROCESS STEPS

Abnormal GI Function

Assessment Data: Weight loss, GI distress, Hgb <5, temperature averaging 101 degrees F. Dx of parasitic infection *Giardia* from drinking water at a campsite.

Nutrition Diagnoses (PES): Abnormal GI function related to parasitic infection of *Giardia* as evidenced by fever, low Hgb <5, GI distress, and weight loss.

Interventions: Food–Nutrient delivery—offer tolerated foods and beverages. Suggest use of a multivitamin-mineral supplement. Educate about risks of drinking potentially contaminated water from various sources.

Monitoring and Evaluation: Improvement in Hgb level; return of lost weight. Resolution of *Giardia*.

TABLE 12-15 **Micronutrient Deficiencies in Parasitic Anemias such as Malaria**

Micronutrient	Deficiency Effects
Vitamin A	Increased susceptibility to malarial anemia, altered iron metabolism, deficit of retinol for synthesis of acute phase reactants
Vitamin C	Impaired T-lymphocyte response, delayed cutaneous hypersensitivity, impaired complement function, reduced phagocytic function
Vitamin E	Impaired T-lymphocyte response, altered B-cell function and impaired humoral response, delayed cutaneous hypersensitivity, impaired cytokine function or production, reduced phagocytic function; deficiency can contribute to oxidant damage to erythrocytes, leading to hemolysis, but deficiency can make the parasite more vulnerable to oxidation generated with some antimalarial drugs
Riboflavin	Decreased iron absorption, increased erythrocyte fragility, depressed erythropoiesis; deficiency may protect against malaria by diminished parasite multiplication and growth
Folate	Impaired erythropoiesis; deficiency may protect against malaria through impaired parasite metabolism
Copper	Involvement in acute phase response to infection
Iron	Impaired erythropoiesis, decreased T-lymphocyte response, altered B-cell function and impaired humoral response, delayed cutaneous hypersensitivity, impaired cytokine function or production, reduced phagocytic function; deficiency and associated microcytosis may reduce malaria parasite multiplication. Avoid excesses.
Selenium	Unknown role
Zinc	Impaired immune function including decreased T-lymphocyte response, altered B-cell function and impaired humoral response, delayed cutaneous hypersensitivity, impaired cytokine function or production, reduced phagocytic function; can contribute to increased parasitemia

From: Nussenblatt V, Semba, RD. Micronutrient malnutrition and the pathogenesis of malarial anemia. *Acta Trop.* 82:321, 2002; and Scrimshaw NS, Sangiovanni JP. Synergism of nutrition, infection, and immunity: an overview. *Am J Clin Nutr.* 66:464S, 1997.

Common Drugs Used and Potential Side Effects

- Artemisinin combination therapy replaces ineffective chloroquine and sulphadoxine pyrimethamine for first-line treatment of malaria and for the provision of long-lasting, insecticide treated bednets (Greenwood, 2008).
- If needed, oral or parenteral iron may be given to correct anemia more rapidly. Beware of excessive use of oral supplements because of their potential side effects with iron overloading; monitor all sources (including iron-enriched foods).

Herbs, Botanicals, and Supplements

- Herbs and botanical supplements should not be used without discussing with the physician.

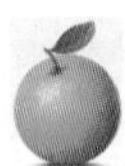

NUTRITION EDUCATION, COUNSELING, CARE MANAGEMENT

- Discuss ways to prevent further parasitic infestations, as with small children playing in soil. Pregnant women must be particularly careful, especially in developing countries where malaria, hookworm, and other parasites are common.
- Discuss ways to prepare foods high in necessary nutrients and methods to increase bioavailability (e.g., combining orange juice at breakfast with an iron-fortified cereal, etc.). In vulnerable populations, use fortified beverages to correct micronutrient deficiency.
- In areas of malaria transmission, anemia is apparent from the first few months of life, and there is a great need to target interventions at pregnant women and infants, which are the groups at highest risk. Food-fortification programs can be very beneficial.

Patient Education—Food Safety

- Avoid eating raw fish or meats.
- Washing vegetables thoroughly before eating them and cooking meat to recommended temperatures to avoid toxoplasmosis (CDC, 2009).
- If tube feeding or CPN is needed, careful handwashing procedures should be followed.
- To prevent the spread of CMV, do not share food, drinks, or eating utensils with young children. Wash hands with soap and water after touching diapers or saliva.

For More Information

- Parasites of the Intestinal Tract
  http://www.dpd.cdc.gov/dpdx/HTML/Para_Health.htm
- Parasitic Disorders
  http://www.oas.org/osde/publications/Unit/oea37e/ch10.htm
- World Health Organization–Malaria
  http://www.who.int/tdr/diseases/malaria/mim.htm

PARASITIC ANEMIA AND MALARIA—CITED REFERENCES

Breman JG. Eradicating malaria. *Sci Prog.* 92(Pt 1):1, 2009.

CDC. Web site accessed December 27,2009, at http://www.cdc.gov/ncidod/dpd/.

Greenwood B. Progress in malaria control in endemic areas. *Travel Med Infect Dis.* 6:173, 2008.

Schantz-Dunn J, Nour NM. Malaria and pregnancy: a global health perspective. *Rev Obstet Gynecol.* 2:186, 2009.

Shell-Duncan B, McDade T. Cultural and environmental barriers to adequate iron intake among northern Kenyan schoolchildren. *Food Nutr Bulletin.* 26:39, 2005.

Vicas AE, et al. Imported malaria at an inner-city hospital in the United States. *Am J Med Sci.* 329:6, 2005.

MEGALOBLASTIC ANEMIAS: PERNICIOUS OR VITAMIN B_{12} DEFICIENCY

NUTRITIONAL ACUITY RANKING: LEVEL 2

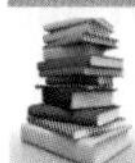

DEFINITIONS AND BACKGROUND

Megaloblastic anemias affect the nervous system if left untreated. Deficiency of folate and vitamin B_{12} changes in the concentrations of metabolites, such as methylmalonic acid and homocysteine.

Pernicious anemia (PA) is a macrocytic anemia caused by a vitamin B_{12} deficiency and intrinsic factor (IF). PA is thought to be an autoimmune disorder and is often found with other disorders such as thyroid or diabetes. The anti-parietal cell antibodies test measures the presence of antibodies against gastric parietal cells. Long-standing *Helicobacter pylori* infection probably plays a role with the irreversible destruction of the gastric body mucosa (Lahner and Annibale, 2009).

The three forms of PA are congenital PA, juvenile PA, and adult-onset PA. The forms are based on the age at onset and the precise nature of the defect causing impaired vitamin B_{12} utilization (e.g., absence of IF). PA affects 1–2% of older individuals. Defective RBC production occurs, caused by a lack of IF of the stomach. IF helps vitamin B_{12} produce RBCs. IF is present in gastric juice and binds to B_{12}. Once bound, IF changes and becomes less susceptible to digestion; this protects B_{12} and allows its absorption from gastric juice. When IF is not available, B_{12} cannot be properly absorbed. Vitamin B_{12} deficiency and achlorhydria have a detrimental effect on bone strength. Having PA increases the risk for hip fracture, even after treatment (Merryman et al, 2009).

Vitamin B_{12}-deficiency anemia may take 5–6 years to appear; this megaloblastic anemia is a reversible form of ineffective hematopoiesis. There may be almost 800,000 older adults in the United States who have undiagnosed and untreated vitamin B_{12} deficiency. It is often masked by high folate intakes. Hidden blood loss, gastric atrophy, and poor dietary intake should be addressed (Table 12-16).

The Schilling test is no longer used. Serologic testing for parietal cell and IF antibodies are used instead. With normal absorption, the ileum absorbs more vitamin B_{12} than the body needs and excretes excess into the urine. With impaired absorption, however, little or no vitamin B_{12} is excreted into the urine. Low serum levels cannot identify all cases of vitamin B_{12} deficiency; serum methylmalonic acid level may also be needed. Holotranscobalamin (holoTC), when compared with the other markers of vitamin B_{12} deficiency, shows promise for diagnosing early vitamin B_{12} deficiency (Hvas and Nexo, 2005).

Adequate selenium intake plays an important role in maintaining vitamin B_{12} adequacy. Glutathione forms a complex called glutathionylcobalamin, which could protect against diseases related to vitamin B_{12} depletion.

Areas of research include intermittent vitamin B_{12} supplement dosing and better measurements of the bioavailability of vitamin B_{12} from fermented vegetarian foods and algae. Vegetarians are at risk for vitamin B_{12} deficiency (Allen, 2008). Vitamin B_{12} anemia is corrected by the use of oral cyanocobalamin.

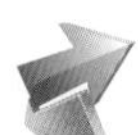

ASSESSMENT, MONITORING, AND EVALUATION

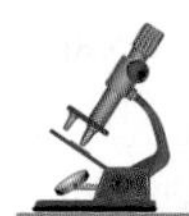

CLINICAL INDICATORS

Genetic Markers: Human leukocyte antigen-DR genotypes suggest a role for genetic susceptibility in PA (Lahner and Annibale, 2009). In congenital PA, IF is missing. Nearly all people with PA test positive for anti-parietal cell antibodies.

Clinical/History		
Height	Postural hypotension?	Diarrhea
Weight	Fatigue	Constipation
BMI	Flatulence, nausea, and vomiting	Anorexia
Diet history		Tachycardia, cardiomegaly
Weight loss?		Achlorhydria

TABLE 12-16 Risks and Causes of Pernicious Anemia or Vitamin B_{12}–Deficiency Anemia

Pernicious Anemia	Vitamin B_{12}–Deficiency Anemia
High risk:	High risk:
Family history of pernicious anemia; African, Scandinavian, or Northern European descent; autoimmune endocrine disorders	Vegans; elderly; persons with intestinal malabsorption or gastric atrophy or hypochlorhydria; stomach removal surgery; drug use (colchicine, neomycin); metabolic disorders (homocystinuria methylmalonic aciduria); breastfed infants of vitamin B_1–deficient mothers; poor diet in infancy or pregnancy
Causes:	Causes:
Autoimmune endocrine diseases such as type 1 diabetes, hypoparathyroidism, Addison's disease, hypopituitarism, testicular dysfunction, Graves' disease, chronic thyroiditis, myasthenia gravis, secondary amenorrhea, vitiligo, gastric surgery, anorexia nervosa, or bulimia nervosa	Poor intake of extrinsic factor (vitamin B_{12}). Chronic alcoholism. *Helicobacter pylori* infection with diminished production of intrinsic factor. Hidden blood loss. Fish tapeworm. Reduced intestinal absorption, as with celiac disease or Crohn's disease

Glossitis with beefy, red tongue	MCV, MCHC, MCH (increased)	TIBC
Lemon yellow or waxy skin	Macrocytic/nucleated cells	Urinary methylmalonic acid
Numbness or tingling in hands and feet	Reticulocyte count (low)	Serum folate
Impaired sense of smell	Hct (low)	Serum homocysteine (elevated?)
Lab Work	Lactate dehydrogenase (LDH) (increased)	Holotranscobalamin (holoTC)
Parietal cell and IF antibodies	CBC (altered platelets and WBC count)	Bilirubin
RBCs	Gastrin (increased)	Transferrin
Serum B_{12}		

INTERVENTION

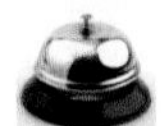

OBJECTIVES

- Alleviate the etiology of anemia, where possible.
- Provide foods that will not hurt a sore mouth. Glossitis decreases the desire to eat.
- Correct patient's anorexia.
- Prevent neurological defects if treatment is delayed or insufficient; depression, psychosis, and mania can appear.
- Where present, correct PA; prevent progression to gastric cancer. PA requires vitamin B_{12} injections.
- Prevent or correct hyperhomocysteinemia.

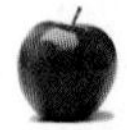

FOOD AND NUTRITION

- Diet should make liberal use of high biological value (HBV) proteins. Good sources of vitamin B_{12} include liver, other meats, fish, poultry, eggs, milk, cheese, yogurt, fortified products such as cereals, and soy milk. The daily average intake is 2–30 mg.
- Supplement diet with iron, vitamin C, folic acid and other B vitamins, copper, and selenium.
- If patient has a sore mouth, use a soft or liquid diet with fewer spicy or acidic foods.

SAMPLE NUTRITION CARE PROCESS STEPS

Abnormal Nutrition Laboratories

Assessment Data: PA with low serum vitamin B_{12}, Hgb, and Hct; elderly resident in long-term care facility.

Nutrition Diagnoses (PES): Altered nutrition-related laboratories related to resident's body inability to produce IF and to absorb cobalamin as evidence by abnormal vitamin B_{12} <200 pg/mL, Hgb <12 gm/dL, and Hct $<37\%$.

Interventions: Food and nutrient delivery—provide resident with foods/beverages with vitamin C such as orange juice, citrus fruits, and melon to be consumed at every meal to aid with iron absorption. Resident will eat two scrambled eggs at breakfast to increase vitamin B_{12}. Coordinate care with nursing and medical staff to administer vitamin B_{12} shots and support with adequate dietary intake.

Monitoring and Evaluation: Monitor monthly laboratories; goal vitamin B_{12} >200 pg/mL, Hgb >12, and Hct $>38\%$.

Common Drugs Used and Potential Side Effects

- Vitamin B_{12} deficiency is effectively treated with oral vitamin B_{12} supplementation. Crystamine or Rubramin PC is cyanocobalamin in drug form for vitamin B_{12} deficiency.
- For PA, vitamin B_{12} injections are given weekly until remission, after which six to eight injections yearly will suffice. For some, vitamin B_{12} supplements may be as effective as injections; high doses, such as 1000 μg, are needed daily for about 18 months.
- Trinsicon contains vitamin B_{12}, ferrous fumarate, vitamin C, folacin, and IF. It is less effective when taken with dairy products.
- Some medications that conflict with vitamin B_{12} absorption include chloramphenicol, proton pump inhibitors, histamine 2 inhibitors, and metformin.

Herbs, Botanicals, and Supplements

- Herbs and botanical supplements should not be used without discussing with the physician.

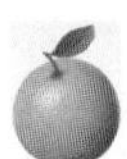

NUTRITION EDUCATION, COUNSELING, CARE MANAGEMENT

- True vegan diets do not contain vitamin B_{12}; it is found only in animal foods. Include eggs, meat, fish, shellfish, cheese, milk, milk products, or use B_{12} fortified soy products. Some fad diets may also be low in vitamins and protein; monitor intake carefully.
- PA develops after total gastrectomy unless vitamin B_{12} is administered. The problem may also occur in patients with partial gastrectomy or gastric bypass. Lifelong vitamin B_{12} replacement or injections are necessary.
- Avoid fatigue; plan simple meals and snacks.
- Megaloblastic B_{12} anemia may occur in elderly; careful food choices are essential.
- Breastfed infants of vitamin B_{12}–deficient mothers are at risk for severe developmental abnormalities, growth failure, and anemia. Counseling for lactating women is important.

Patient Education—Food Safety

If tube feeding or CPN is needed, careful handwashing procedures should be followed.

For More Information

- Medline–Pernicious Anemia
  http://www.nlm.nih.gov/medlineplus/ency/article/000569.htm
- Pernicious Anemia
  http://www.med.unc.edu/medicine/web/perniciousanemia.htm

- Vitamin B_{12} Deficiency Anemia
  http://www.nlm.nih.gov/medlineplus/ency/article/000574.htm

MEGALOBLASTIC ANEMIAS—CITED REFERENCES

Allen LH. Causes of vitamin B12 and folate deficiency. *Food Nutr Bull.* 29:20S, 2008.

Hvas AM, Nexo E. Holotranscobalamin—a first choice assay for diagnosing early vitamin B deficiency? *J Intern Med.* 257:289, 2005.

Lahner E, Annibale B. Pernicious anemia: new insights from a gastroenterological point of view. *World J Gastroenterol.* 15:5121, 2009.

Merryman NA, et al. Hip fracture risk in patients with a diagnosis of pernicious anemia. *Gastroenterology.* 2009 Dec 16. [Epub ahead of print]

SIDEROBLASTIC ANEMIA

NUTRITIONAL ACUITY RANKING: LEVEL 1

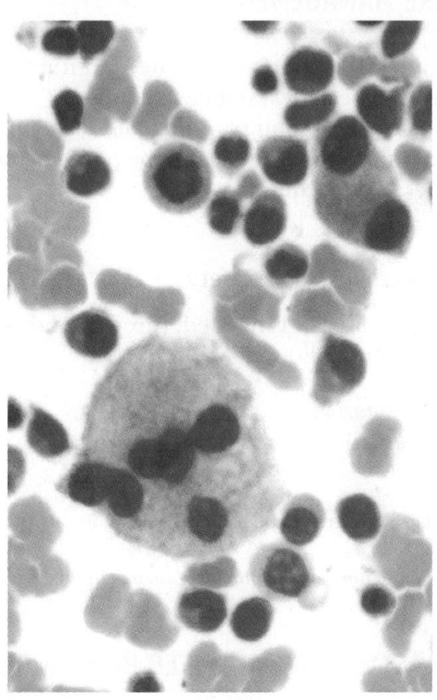

Adapted from: Raphael Rubin, David S. Strayer, *Rubin's Pathology: Clinicopathologic Foundations of Medicine,* 5th ed. Philadelphia: Lippincott Williams & Wilkins, 2008.

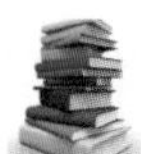

DEFINITIONS AND BACKGROUND

Sideroblastic anemias are a group of blood disorders characterized by an impaired ability of the bone marrow to produce normal RBCs. Inherited sideroblastic anemia comprises several rare anemias due to heterogeneous genetic lesions, all characterized by the presence of ringed sideroblasts in the bone marrow (Camaschella, 2009).

Abnormal RBCs called sideroblasts are found in the blood of people with these anemias. This anemia is a microcytic, hypochromic anemia similar to that caused by iron deficiency, except that serum iron is normal or elevated. The iron inside RBCs is inadequately used to make Hgb, despite adequate or increased amounts of iron. Therapy comprises application of antioxidants, vitamins, iron, bone marrow-stimulating factors, or substitution of cells (Finsterer, 2007).

The disease X-linked sideroblastic anemia with ataxia is due to a mutation in the protein transporter that is thought to transfer iron clusters from the mitochondrion to the cytoplasm (Napier et al, 2005). Another name for the congenital type of anemia is hereditary iron-loading anemia.

X-linked sideroblastic anemia (delta-aminolevulinate synthase deficiency) is vitamin B_6 responsive that responds to high pyridoxine doses (Clayton, 2006). Pyridoxal phosphate is the cofactor for over 100 enzyme-catalyzed reactions in the body. Vitamin B_6 is the main vitamin for processing amino acids and is also needed to make melatonin, serotonin, and dopamine.

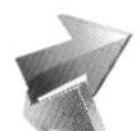

ASSESSMENT, MONITORING, AND EVALUATION

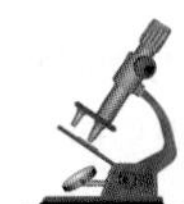

CLINICAL INDICATORS

Genetic Markers: Mutations in the mitochondrial carrier family gene SLC25A38 cause nonsyndromic autosomal recessive congenital sideroblastic anemia (Petkau, 2009). The enzyme directly relevant to sideroblastic anemia is ALAS-2 or ALAS-e on the X chromosome. However, most sideroblastic anemias are acquired.

Clinical/History
Height
Weight
BMI
Diet history
BP
I & O
Alcohol or drug toxicity?
Fatigue
Dizziness
Decreased tolerance for exercise

Lab Work
Serum B_6 levels
Hgb (low at 4–10 g/dL)
RBC
Transferrin saturation (often elevated)
Serum folic acid
Serum homocysteine
WBC
Serum Fe, ferritin
Serum Cu

INTERVENTION

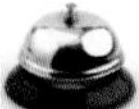

OBJECTIVES

- Identify causes and solutions.
- Remove any precipitating factors, such as specific drugs or alcohol use.
- Correct problems, such as suppression of bone marrow, iron loading, and anemia.

SAMPLE NUTRITION CARE PROCESS STEPS

Inadequate Vitamin Intake

Assessment Data: Diagnosis of sideroblastic anemia, pyridoxine-responsive. BMI normal. Complaints of fatigue and poor exercise tolerance. Diet indicates intake of B_6-rich foods to be infrequent. Lab work with high transferrin saturation, Hgb of 6, and low serum B_6 levels.

Nutrition Diagnoses (PES): Inadequate vitamin intake (B_6) related to X-linked genetic defect and low dietary intake as evidenced by diet and medical histories.

Interventions: Trial of 100- to 200-mg pyridoxine by mouth. Counseling about foods rich in vitamin B_6.

Monitoring and Evaluation: Improvement in symptoms (less fatigue and better exercise tolerance). Lab work showing improvement in serum B_6 and Hgb, and lower transferrin saturation levels.

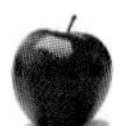

FOOD AND NUTRITION

- A diet high in vitamin B_6 may be beneficial with medication. Potatoes, bananas, raisin bran cereal, lentils, liver, turkey, and tuna are good sources of vitamin B_6.
- Protein and carbohydrate (CHO) intake should be adequate, and energy should also be adequate to spare protein. Folic acid and copper may also be needed.
- Alcohol intake should be severely limited.
- Balanced meals and snacks, as necessary, may be helpful.

Common Drugs Used and Potential Side Effects

- Vitamin B_6 may be ordered; age-dependent doses are specified. The National Academy of Sciences performed an analysis of vitamin B_6 studies. It is usually safe at intakes of up to 100 mg/d in adults, but neurological side effects can sometimes occur at or above that level. Vitamin B_6 toxicity damages sensory nerves, leading to numbness in the hands and feet as well as difficulty walking.
- Chloramphenicol may cause drug-induced bone marrow suppression, resulting in sideroblastic anemia. Isoniazid, busulfan, penicillamine, and cycloserine can cause abnormal vitamin B_6 metabolism. Monitor for gastrointestinal side effects.

Herbs, Botanicals, and Supplements

- Herbs and botanical supplements should not be used without discussing with the physician.

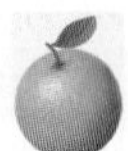

NUTRITION EDUCATION, COUNSELING, CARE MANAGEMENT

- Discuss adequate sources of all needed nutrients such as vitamin B_6, especially if deficiency caused the anemia.
- Discuss attractive menu planning and balancing of meals because appetite and intake may be poor chronically. Discuss snacks and frequency.

Patient Education—Food Safety

If tube feeding or CPN is needed, careful handwashing procedures should be followed.

For More Information

- Genetics Home Reference
  http://ghr.nlm.nih.gov/ghr/resource/health
- Harvard
  http://sickle.bwh.harvard.edu/sideroblastic.html
- Medline Plus: Anemia
  http://www.nlm.nih.gov/medlineplus/anemia.html

SIDEROBLASTIC ANEMIA—CITED REFERENCES

Camaschella C. Hereditary sideroblastic anemias: pathophysiology, diagnosis, and treatment. *Semin Hematol.* 46:371, 2009.

Clayton PT. B6-responsive disorders: a model of vitamin dependency. *J Inherit Metab Dis.* 29:317, 2006.

Finsterer J. Hematological manifestations of primary mitochondrial disorders. *Acta Haematol.* 118:88, 2007.

Napier I, et al. Iron trafficking in the mitochondrion: novel pathways revealed by disease. *Blood.* 105:1844, 2005.

Petkau TL. Same pathway, different gene: a second gene in the heme biosynthesis pathway causes inherited sideroblastic anemia. *Clin Genet.* 2009 Nov 11. [Epub ahead of print]

HEMOGLOBINOPATHIES

SICKLE CELL ANEMIA

NUTRITIONAL ACUITY RANKING: LEVEL 1

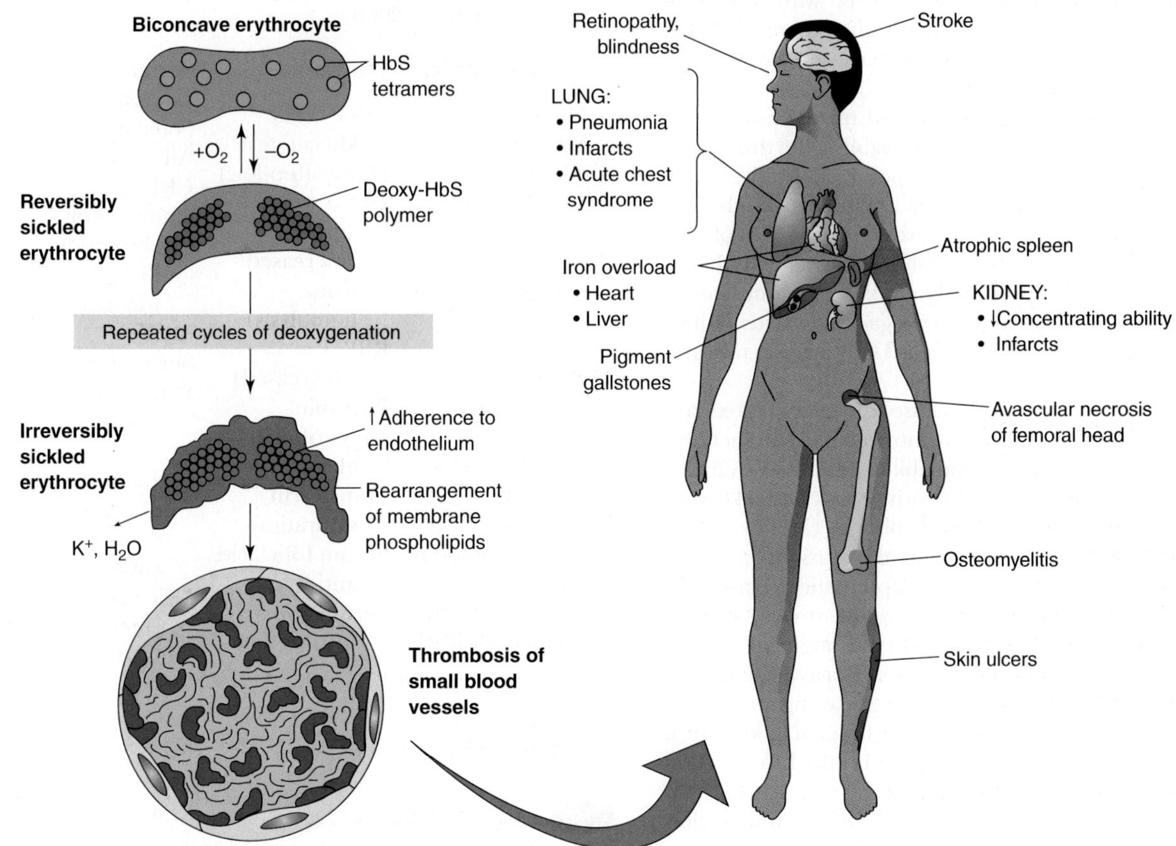

Adapted from: Raphael Rubin, David S. Strayer, *Rubin's Pathology: Clinicopathologic Foundations of Medicine,* 5th ed. Philadelphia: Lippincott Williams & Wilkins, 2008.

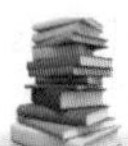

DEFINITIONS AND BACKGROUND

Sickle cell disease (SCD) is the most common genetic disorder of the blood. SCD involves anemia that is hereditary and hemolytic. Cells in SCD are crescent shaped and become rigid; they lodge themselves in the capillaries of the peripheral-blood system outside the heart. The sickling of RBCs occurs when partially or totally deoxygenated Hgb molecules distort their normal disk shape, producing stiff, sticky, sickle-shaped cells that obstruct small blood vessels; this causes vaso-occlusion as well as deprivation of oxygen to body tissues (Edwards et al, 2005). Everyone with SCD has chronic hemolytic anemia, vasculopathy, vaso-occlusive disease, acute and chronic organ damage, and shortened life span (Steinberg, 2008).

SCD has several forms including sickle cell anemia, sickle cell Hgb C disease, and sickle cell thalassemia disease. It is usually detected within the first year of life. Routine use of daily antibiotics until 5 years of age, immunization of children with pneumococcal vaccine, annual influenza vaccination after 6 months of age, and meningococcal vaccination after 2 years of age are important preventive measures (Mehta et al, 2006).

The largest population in the world with sickle cell anemia is in Africa. While this condition most commonly affects blacks of African descent, it is also found in people of Middle Eastern, East Indian, and Mediterranean origin. About 100,000 Americans have SCD (~1 in every 400–500 African–Americans). Carrier frequency varies, with high rates associated with zones of high malaria incidence. Carriers are often protected against malaria.

Patients with SCD are at risk for delayed growth and sexual maturation; acute and chronic pulmonary dysfunction; stroke; aseptic necrosis of the hip, shoulders, or both; sickle cell retinopathy; dermal ulcers; and severe chronic pain (Edwards et al, 2005). The homozygous state (SS) is associated with complications and a reduced life expectancy.

Chronic anemia, pallor, and jaundice result because sickled cells do not last as long as normal blood cells. Bone marrow functions at six times the normal rate. Because there are fewer cells, the blood is thinner or anemic. When RBCs are destroyed, bilirubin is released into the blood and turns the whites of the eyes to a shade of yellow.

Inadequate dietary intakes of folate are common, whereas vitamin B_{12} intakes are usually adequate. Low RBC folate levels may occur. Serum total homocysteine (tHcy) levels may be elevated in this population; greater intakes than normal of folate may be needed. Elevated tHcy levels contribute to thrombosis, a frequent event in this population. Children with sickle cell anemia have lower vitamin B_6 concentrations.

Infants and children who have SCD are at risk for nutritional deficiencies and loss of body mass during acute illness. Suboptimal vitamin A intake is common, with more frequent hospitalizations and poor growth. Low serum vitamin D status is highly prevalent in children with SCD; vitamin D status is associated with season and dietary intake. Prepubertal children with SCD may have zinc deficiency and may benefit from zinc supplementation.

There is an underlying defect in lipid metabolism associated with SCD, manifested during the fasting state; this abnormality in lipid homeostasis has the potential to alter RBC membrane fluidity and function in SCD patients (Buchowski et al, 2007). Individuals with SCD have reduced levels of EPA and DHA in red cells, platelets, and mononuclear cells due to peroxidation from compromised antioxidant competence (Ren et al, 2008). Because dietary omega-3 fatty acids reduce prothrombotic activity, include omega-3 fatty acids in diet and in supplemental form.

Cellular and tissue damage is caused by hypoxia, oxidant damage, inflammation, abnormal intracellular interactions, and reduced nitric oxide bioavailability (Steinberg, 2008). Young children with SCD are at a very high risk of stroke, with microvascular occlusion and painful episodes (Adams, 2007).

Aggressive antibiotic therapy and transfusions can save lives. Transfusion is indicated for symptomatic anemia and specifically to prevent stroke, during acute stroke, and for acute chest syndrome (Roseff, 2009). Although life saving, transfusion therapy has resulted in the majority of sickle cell anemia patients being at risk for iron overloading and hemosiderosis-induced organ damage (Vichinsky et al, 2005). Iron overload has become easier to manage with the introduction of an oral iron chelator (Adams, 2007).

Acute chest syndrome, triggered by infections and fat clots in the lungs, is the leading cause of death in sickle cell anemia. Treatment includes hydroxyurea therapy to decrease the frequency of painful episodes and hematopoietic cell transplantation (Mehta et al, 2006). Bone marrow transplantation requires a perfect match from a sibling. Because patients with SCD have problems with surgery, including prolonged bleeding, vitamin K should be given preoperatively (Raffini et al, 2006). Use of transcranial Doppler ultrasonography helps identify asymptomatic, at-risk children who should be considered for chronic blood transfusions (Mehta et al, 2006).

Studies of gene expression are bringing new solutions. Human progenitor cell (from bone marrow, peripheral blood stem cells, or umbilical blood) transplant can cure the disease and is used for patients with severe disease for whom conventional therapy may not be effective (Roseff, 2009).

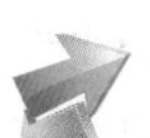

ASSESSMENT, MONITORING, AND EVALUATION

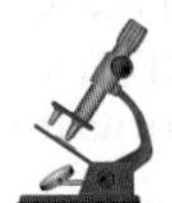

CLINICAL INDICATORS

Genetic Markers: Sickle cell anemia is an autosomal recessive disease caused by a mutation in the *hemoglobin beta gene* (*HBB*) found on chromosome 11p15.5. Genetic studies have identified regions on chromosome 6q23 and BCL11 A on chromosome 2p16 that account for 20–50% of the common variation in fetal Hgb levels in patients with sickle cell anemia (Thein et al, 2009). SNPs have also been found in KCNK6 (Sebastiani et al, 2009).

Clinical/History	Lab Work	
Height	CBC, WBC	Serum creatinine
Weight	Sickle cell test	N balance
BMI	Hgb (often low)	Alb
Diet history	Hct	CRP
BP	Serum Fe (increased from hemolysis)	Cholesterol
I & O	RBP (decreased)	Triglycerides (Trig) (decreased)
Chronic anemia, pallor	Bilirubin	MCV
Jaundice	tHcy (often elevated)	Serum ferritin
Bone pain	Transferrin saturation	Partial pressure of oxygen (pO_2)
Abdominal pain	Serum folic acid and B_{12}	Partial pressure of carbon dioxide (pCO_2)
Breathlessness	Serum and urinary zinc	Uric acid (increased)
Lower leg ulcers		PT and INR
Casts or blood in urine		
Excessive thirst		
CT scan or MRI		

INTERVENTION

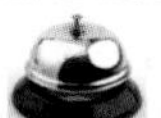

OBJECTIVES

- Supplement diet with missing nutrients. Correct any malnutrition.
- Reduce oxygen debt and hemolytic crises.
- Reduce painful cramps, liver dysfunction, cholelithiasis, jaundice, and hepatitis.
- Lessen likelihood of pressure ulcers, infections, and renal failure. Infections may include pneumonia, cholecystitis, osteomyelitis, or urinary tract infections.

SAMPLE NUTRITION CARE PROCESS STEPS

Involuntary Weight Loss

Assessment Data: Weight pattern, percent desirable body weight, diet history, problems with meal planning or shopping, financial challenges.

Nutrition Diagnosis (PES): Involuntary weight loss related to sick cell anemia with inadequate caloric intake as evidenced by 10% loss of usual body weight in the last 2 months.

Intervention: Nutrition counseling, encouraging energy-dense foods and favorites. Coordination of care with referral to social service agencies for help with meal preparation and delivery.

Monitoring and Evaluation: Weight records, improvements in appetite and intake.

TABLE 12-17 Equation to Predict Energy Needs in Adolescents with Sickle Cell Disease

Basal energy requirements are higher in adolescents with sickle cell anemia than in healthy control subjects (Buchowski et al, 2002)

Males: REE (kcal/d) = 1305 + 18.6 × weight (kg) − 55.7. hemoglobin (g/dL)

REE (kJ/d) = 5461 + 77.7 × weight (kg) − 233.2 × hemoglobin (g/dL)

Females: REE (kcal/d) = 1100 + 13.3 × weight (kg) − 30.2 × hemoglobin (g/dL)

REE (kJ/d) = 4603 + 55.6 × weight (kg) − 126.2 × hemoglobin (g/dL)

- Maintain adequate hydration.
- Promote normal growth and development, which tend to be stunted in children.
- Prevent chronic hypoxia, which can lead to lower intellectual performance.
- Improve quality of life and ability to participate in the activities of daily life.

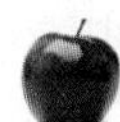

FOOD AND NUTRITION

- Include food sources of omega-3 fatty acids; vitamins D, C, A, B_{12}, and B_6; folic acid; and HBV proteins; ensure adequate zinc and riboflavin.
- Estimate fluid and energy needs; increase diet as needed (Table 12-17).
- A multivitamin–mineral supplement should be recommended; one without excess iron is important when transfusions are used. Avoid excesses of iron, including from tube feedings or parenteral nutrition.
- Energy deficits are common in this population. Nightly tube feeding can help to improve nutritional status. While supplementation with arginine has been suggested, more studies are needed.

Common Drugs Used and Potential Side Effects

- Pain medicines (such as ibuprofen) may be used. Monitor for all side effects and GI distress.
- Hydroxyurea therapy (Droxia, Hydrea) can be used to increase Hgb production.
- Rofecoxib is a cyclo-oxygenase-2 (COX-2) inhibitor approved for pain and has been tested in children with no adverse effects.
- Rituximab may be used to prevent delayed hemolytic transfusion reaction disorder in SCD.

Herbs, Botanicals, and Supplements

- Herbs and botanical supplements should not be used without discussing with the physician.
- A phytomedicine, Niprisan, may reduce episodes of SCD crisis associated with severe pain.

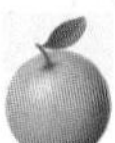

NUTRITION EDUCATION, COUNSELING, CARE MANAGEMENT

- Indicate which foods are good sources of folic acid, HBV proteins, zinc, riboflavin, and vitamins A, C, D, E, B_6, and B_{12}.
- Discuss ways for easy meal preparation because fatigue tends to be a problem.
- Quality of life is often decreased among adults with SCD, and health professionals should try to offer assistance that will help improve this quality (McClish et al, 2005).

Patient Education—Food Safety

If tube feeding or CPN is needed, careful handwashing procedures should be followed.

For More Information

- American Sickle Cell Association
  http://www.ascaa.org/
- National Institutes of Health (NIH)–Genes and Disease
  http://www.ncbi.nlm.nih.gov/disease/sickle.html
- NIH–Sickle Cell Anemia
  http://www.nlm.nih.gov/medlineplus/sicklecellanemia.html

SICKLE CELL ANEMIA—CITED REFERENCES

Adams RJ. Big strokes in small persons. *Arch Neurol.* 64:1567, 2007.

Buchowski MS, et al. Defects in postabsorptive plasma homeostasis of fatty acids in sickle cell disease. *JPEN J Parenter Enteral Nutr.* 31:263, 2007.

Edwards CL, et al. A brief review of the pathophysiology, associated pain, and psychosocial issues in sickle cell disease. *Int J Behav Med.* 12:171, 2005.

McClish DK, et al. Health related quality of life in sickle cell patients: the PiSCES project. *Health Qual Life Outcomes.* 3:50, 2005.

Mehta SR, et al. Opportunities to improve outcomes in sickle cell disease. *Am Fam Physician.* 74:303, 2006.

Raffini LJ, et al. Prolongation of the prothrombin time and activated partial thromboplastin time in children with sickle cell disease. *Pediatr Blood Cancer.* 47:589, 2006.

Ren H, et al. Patients with sickle cell disease have reduced blood antioxidant protection. *Int J Vitam Nutr Res.* 78:139, 2008.

Roseff SD. Sickle cell disease: a review. *Immunohematology.* 25:67, 2009.

Sebastiani P, et al. Genetic modifiers of the severity of sickle cell anemia identified through a genome-wide association study. *Am J Hematol.* 85:29, 2009.

Steinberg MH. Sickle cell anemia, the first molecular disease: overview of molecular etiology, pathophysiology, and therapeutic approaches. *Scientific World Journal.* 8:1295, 2008.

Thein SL, et al. Control of fetal hemoglobin: new insights emerging from genomics and clinical implications. *Hum Mol Genet.* 18:216, 2009.

Vichinsky E, et al. Comparison of organ dysfunction in transfused patients with SCD or beta thalassemia. *Am J Hematol.* 80:70, 2005.

THALASSEMIAS

NUTRITIONAL ACUITY RANKING: LEVEL 1

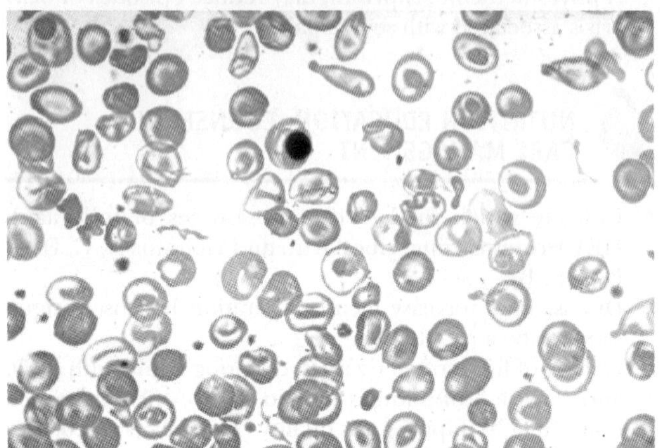

Adapted from: Raphael Rubin, David S. Strayer, *Rubin's Pathology: Clinicopathologic Foundations of Medicine*, 5th ed. Philadelphia: Lippincott Williams & Wilkins, 2008.

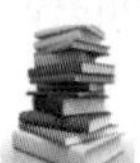

DEFINITIONS AND BACKGROUND

The thalassemias are inherited hematologic disorders caused by defects in the synthesis of one or more of the Hgb chains. Alpha thalassemia is caused by reduced or absent synthesis of alpha globin chains, and beta thalassemia is caused by reduced or absent synthesis of beta globin chains (Muncie and Campbell, 2009). Hemolysis and impaired erythropoiesis occur.

Collectively, the thalassemias are among the most common inherited disorders. Alpha-thalassemic syndromes have an increased frequency in African, American Indian, and Asian populations. Beta thalassemia is well recognized in persons of Greek and Italian descent; Cooley's or Mediterranean anemia is most severe. The beta thalassemias are more common and are a worldwide clinical problem due to an increasing immigrant population (Hahalis et al, 2005).

Silent carriers of alpha thalassemia and persons with alpha or beta thalassemia trait are asymptomatic and require no treatment. Alpha thalassemia intermedia (Hgb H disease) causes hemolytic anemia (Muncie and Campbell, 2009). The RBCs are fragile and contain abnormal Hgb.

Beta thalassemia major causes hemolytic anemia, poor growth, and skeletal abnormalities during infancy. Symptoms can begin as early as 3 months of age. In the first year or two of life and in the absence of transfusion, a child can demonstrate severe anemia and expansion of the facial and other bones. These children may be pale or jaundiced, have a poor appetite, fail to grow normally, and have an enlarged spleen, liver, or heart. The incidence of gallstones is unusually common in this population. Affected children will require regular lifelong blood transfusions (Hahalis et al, 2005).

Blood transfusions and increased gastrointestinal iron absorption result in iron overload and tissue damage. If splenomegaly occurs, a splenectomy may be needed. Excess iron accumulates, leading to liver, heart, and pituitary damage and failure of these organs. Cardiac complications caused by iron deposition, such as cardiomyopathy, are major causes of death (Hahalis et al, 2005). Chelation therapy may be needed.

Recent advances have been beneficial. Bone marrow transplants can be curative for some children with beta thalassemia major. Cord blood is the blood that remains in the umbilical cord and placenta following birth; it is a rich source of stem cells that reproduce into RBCs for the immune system. Stem cell transplantation offers opportunities for individuals with thalassemia to lead a more normal life.

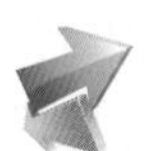

ASSESSMENT, MONITORING, AND EVALUATION

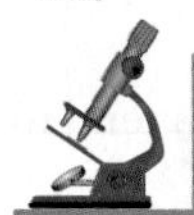

CLINICAL INDICATORS

Genetic Markers: In thalassemia, variations are caused by the severity of the genetic mutations. In thalassemia major or intermedia, reduction in the number of alpha globin genes can ameliorate the disease phenotype; conversely, excess alpha globin genes convert beta thalassemia trait to a clinical picture of thalassemia intermedia (Rund and Fucharoen, 2009). An increase in Hgb F level is variably associated with the presence of beta thalassemia trait. Levels relate to the presence of a polymorphism in the (G)gamma-158 (C>T) gene (Mosca et al, 2009).

Clinical/History

Height
Weight
BMI
Diet history
BP
Growth failure
Jaundice
I & O
Leg ulcers
Bone abnormalities
Enlarged spleen
Hypogonadism
Anemia
Jaundice

Lab Work

RBC, CBC
H & H (low?)
Quantitative Hgb A2 and Hgb F
Serum Fe (increased)
FEP
Transferrin iron saturation percentage (increased)
Serum lead
Transferrin (decreased)
Superconducting Quantum Interference Device (SQUID)
Serum ferritin (increased)
TIBC (decreased)
Thyroid-stimulating hormone (TSH)
Thyroxine (T4)
Alkaline phosphatase (Alk phos)
Gluc
Vitamin B_{12}
Serum zinc
Alb
CRP
Hypoparathyroidism

INTERVENTION

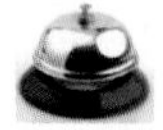

OBJECTIVES

- Offer temporary relief with blood transfusions; this will improve hematological status with oxygen availability.

SAMPLE NUTRITION CARE PROCESS STEPS

Unintentional Weight Loss

Assessment Data: Growth failure in 6-year old, weight loss of 3# in past 12 months. Poor oral intake and anorexia. Hx of thalassemia intermedia, diagnosed at age 2.

Nutrition Diagnoses (PES): Unintentional weight loss related to poor oral intake as evidenced by weight loss of 3# in past year and growth failure (previously 40th percentile, now at 25th percentile for age).

Interventions: Food–nutrient delivery: enhance meals and snacks with high-density foods such as milkshakes with dry milk powder and peanut butter added. Educate parents about ways to enhance energy and nutrient density in meals and snacks. Counsel about when to contact the physician (e.g., signs of jaundice, additional weight loss, or chronic anorexia).

Monitoring and Evaluation: Improved intake of energy-dense foods and beverages. Growth chart improving over past 3–6 months, closer to 40th percentile again.

Correct side effects of iron overloading from the necessary transfusions.

- Correct failure to thrive and GI problems.
- Prevent slow or stunted growth. Impaired growth is a problem in children.
- Reduce or correct infections. Promote healing of any ulcerations.
- Manage any hyperglycemia.

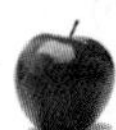

FOOD AND NUTRITION

- A diet high in quality protein, energy, B-complex vitamins (especially folic acid and vitamin B_{12}), and zinc will be beneficial. To prevent iron overloading, avoid use of multivitamin–mineral supplements that contain iron and vitamin C in large amounts.
- Provide adequate fluid intake.
- If hyperglycemia and diabetes are present, use carbohydrate counting and other accepted techniques for managing glucose levels.

Common Drugs Used and Potential Side Effects

- Iron-chelating therapy with deferoxamine in patients with thalassemia major has dramatically improved the prognosis of this disease (Taher et al, 2005). Side effects include allergic reactions, tinnitus, and erythematous rash. Overchelation may cause growth retardation and mineral deficiency.
- Oral iron-binding agents are capable of preventing dietary iron absorption from the diet; oral chelator deferiprone (Ferriprox) is one.

Herbs, Botanicals, and Supplements

- Herbs and botanical supplements should not be used without discussing with the physician.

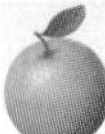

NUTRITION EDUCATION, COUNSELING, CARE MANAGEMENT

- Discuss ways to improve nutritional intake, when deficient.
- Discuss importance of diet in the maintenance of hematological health.
- Persons with thalassemia should be referred for preconception genetic counseling. Women with alpha thalassemia trait should consider chorionic villus sampling to diagnose infants with Hgb Bart's, which increases the risk of toxemia and postpartum bleeding (Muncie and Campbell, 2009).

Patient Education—Food Safety

If tube feeding or CPN is needed, careful handwashing procedures should be followed.

For More Information

- Cooley's Anemia Foundation
  www.thalassemia.org
- Cord Blood Information
  http://www.thalassemia.com/cord_blood.html
- Thalassemia International Federation
  http://www.thalassaemia.org.cy/

THALASSEMIA—CITED REFERENCES

Hahalis G, et al. Heart failure in beta-thalassemia syndromes: a decade of progress. *Am J Med.* 118:957, 2005.

Mosca A, et al. The relevance of hemoglobin F measurement in the diagnosis of thalassemias and related hemoglobinopathies. *Clin Biochem.* 42: 1797, 2009.

Muncie HL Jr, Campbell J. Alpha and beta thalassemia. *Am Fam Physician.* 80:339, 2009.

Rund D, Fucharoen S. Genetic modifiers in hemoglobinopathies. *Curr Mol Med.* 8:600, 2008.

Taher A, et al. Comparison between deferoxamine and deferiprone (L1) in iron-loaded thalassemia patients. *Eur J Haemetol.* 67:30, 2005.

OTHER BLOOD DISORDERS

BLEEDING DISORDERS: HEMORRHAGE AND HEMOPHILIA

NUTRITIONAL ACUITY RANKING: LEVEL 2

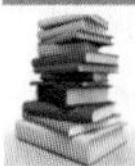

DEFINITIONS AND BACKGROUND

The circulatory system is a closed system, with low volume and high pressure. It provides efficient delivery of nutrients to all tissues. When there is volume loss, a large decrease in nutrient delivery occurs.

Hemorrhage is the excessive discharge of blood from a ruptured vessel. Bleeding (bright red in spurts from an artery; dark red and steady flow from a vein) can be external, internal, or into skin or other tissue. When massive, a hemorrhage can cause such symptoms as rapid, shallow breathing; cold, clammy skin; thirst; visual disturbances; and extreme weakness. Loss of more than 20% of blood volume causes hypotension and tachycardia; loss of more than 1 quart of blood may lead to shock. Peptic ulcer, hemophilia, spontaneous liver rupture, or stroke may lead to a hemorrhage. In some cases, surgery may be necessary. In chronic myelogenous leukemia (CML), a slowly progressive disease, platelets are increased in number and easy bleeding occurs.

To stop a hemorrhage, blood must clot properly. Blood clots when its fibrinogen is converted to fibrin by action of thrombin. Vitamin K works as a coenzyme that converts glutamic acid to gamma-carboxyglutamic acid; this helps to bind calcium and is required for the activation of the seven vitamin K–dependent clotting factors in the coagulation cascade (Table 12-18).

Hemophilia is an inherited bleeding disorder. Diagnosis may be early in life, or later after surgery or trauma. In severe cases, serious bleeding may occur without any cause. While internal bleeding may occur anywhere, bleeding into joints is common. Standard treatment involves replacing the missing clotting factor. In pregnant women who carry the trait, a C-section is often recommended. **Von Willebrand disease** is the most common hereditary bleeding disorder, where bleeding gums, abnormal menstrual bleeding, nose bleeds, and bruising are the symptoms. Desamino-8-arginine vasopressin (DDAVP) is given to raise the levels of von Willebrand factor, which reduces the bleeding tendency.

The immune response to coagulation factors VIII or IX with formation of inhibitory antibodies complicates the treatment of hemophilia; regulatory T cells (Treg) are an important component of the mechanism by which tolerance is maintained (Cao et al, 2009). New gene therapy and immune tolerance protocols are under study.

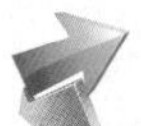

ASSESSMENT, MONITORING, AND EVALUATION

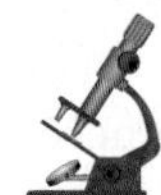

CLINICAL INDICATORS

Genetic Markers: Hemophilia A, which affects 80–90% of cases, shows a mutation in the FVIII gene. People with Hemophilia B have low or missing levels of clotting factor IX. Hemophilia affects mostly males, although women carry the trait.

Clinical/History		
Height	Temperature	Excessive or easy bleeding
Weight	I & O	Excessive bruising
BMI	Blood in urine or stool?	Nose bleeds
Diet history	Petechiae	Abnormal menstrual bleeding
BP	Hemophiliac arthropathy	
Pulse		

TABLE 12-18 Blood Clotting Factors That Involve Nutrition

The coagulation cascade involves a series of steps that stop bleeding through clot formation. Vitamin K–dependent coagulation factors are synthesized in the liver. Consequently, severe liver disease results in lower blood levels of vitamin K–dependent clotting factors and an increased risk of uncontrolled bleeding (hemorrhage). The following factors involve nutrition:

I. Fibrinogen
II. Prothrombin
III. Thromboplastin
IV. Calcium

In hemostatic (bleeding) disorders, it is important to evaluate for bleeding problems in the family history, history of heavy menses or easy bruising, and prior blood transfusions. Bleeding disorders include a number of conditions in which people tend to bleed longer. Clotting involves about 20 different plasma proteins (clotting factors). Normally, clotting factors form fibrin that stops bleeding. In bleeding disorders, the process does not occur normally

Some bleeding disorders are present at birth (hemophilia and von Willebrand's disease), or they can be acquired (such as vitamin K deficiency, severe liver disease, use of anticoagulant drugs or prolonged use of antibiotics, bone marrow problems, leukemia, pregnancy-associated eclampsia, or snake bite). In these disorders, vision loss can occur from bleeding into the eye, or anemia may result, or there may be neurological problems or even death. Gene therapy may one day be available to treat the bleeding disorders.

Lab Work

- Coagulation testing
- PT, International normalized ratio (INR)—prolonged?
- Activated partial thromboplastin time (aPTT)
- Thrombin time (thrombin added to plasma, and time to clot measured)
- Fibrinogen
- Platelet count (may be normal)
- Von Willebrand factor level (reduced?)
- Transferrin
- RBC
- Alb
- BUN
- CBC
- H & H
- Serum Fe
- Serum folic acid and B_{12}
- TIBC (increased)
- Creatinine
- CRP

INTERVENTION

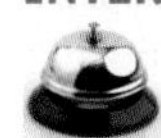

OBJECTIVES

- Medical management is designed to control bleeding, take care of the underlying cause of the bleeding, and replace lost blood. Transfusions may be needed. Less severe hemorrhages may require iron, vitamin B_{12}, and folic acid to help replace RBCs.
- Support erythropoiesis.
- Control intestinal impact of gastrointestinal bleeding, which can cause a protein overload.
- Prevent hypovolemic shock (low cardiac output, decreased blood pressure, and decreased urinary output) from uncontrolled bleeding.

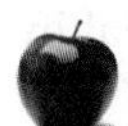

FOOD AND NUTRITION

- Ensure that diet is rich in proteins, iron, folic acid, vitamin B_{12}, and copper.
- Check need for vitamin K. Patients with intestinal or liver disease may become deficient. If medications to replace vitamin K are used, diet should provide a balance without excess. Monitor content of meals or enteral feedings and multivitamin supplements carefully to ensure that all RDAs are met without excesses (Table 12-19).

SAMPLE NUTRITION CARE PROCESS STEPS

Inadequate Vitamin Intake

Assessment Data: Bleeding disorder (Hemophilia A) with easy bruising and blood in urine and stool. Currently taking Alphanate; scheduled for dental surgery in 2 weeks. Serum vitamin K levels low. Diet hx shows little intake of any vitamin K–rich foods.

Nutrition Diagnoses (PES): Inadequate vitamin K intake related to hereditary bleeding disorder and minimal dietary intake as evidenced by low serum vitamin K levels, easy bruising and blood in urine and stool even while taking Alphanate.

Interventions: Food–nutrient delivery: identify foods that could be included and tolerated. Educate about the sources of vitamin K from diet. Counsel about multivitamin–mineral supplements that contain a desired dose of vitamin K (10–120 μg per dose).

Monitoring and Evaluation: Fewer episodes of blood in urine and stool; less easy bruising. Tolerance for multivitamin–mineral supplement and foods. Improved serum levels of vitamin K. No difficulty with dental surgery and excessive bleeding.

TABLE 12-19 Food Sources of Vitamin K

Food	Serving	Vitamin K (μg)
Kale, raw	One cup (chopped)	547
Broccoli, cooked	One cup (chopped)	420
Parsley, raw	One cup (chopped)	324
Swiss chard, raw	One cup (chopped)	299
Spinach, raw	One cup (chopped)	120
Leaf lettuce, raw	One cup (shredded)	118
Watercress, raw	One cup (chopped)	85
Soybean oil	One tbsp	26
Canola oil	One tbsp	20
Mayonnaise	One tbsp	12
Olive oil	One tbsp	7

Source: U.S. Department of Agriculture. USDA national nutrient database for standard reference, release 16. Available at http://www.nal.usda.gov/fnic/foodcomp/Data/SR16/wtrank/wt_rank.html.

Common Drugs Used and Potential Side Effects

- Avoid aspirin, NSAIDs, and other blood thinners. Oral anticoagulants, such as Warfarin, inhibit coagulation through antagonism of the action of vitamin K. Inadequate gamma-carboxylation of vitamin K–dependent proteins will inhibit clot formation. Patients taking these drugs are cautioned against consuming very large or highly variable quantities of vitamin K in their diets; they need a reasonably constant dietary intake.
- If vitamin K is needed, it is available in multivitamins and other supplements in doses that range from 10 to 120 μg per dose.
- Alphanate (antihemophilic factor) is approved to decrease bleeding in patients with bleeding diseases who must have surgery or other invasive procedures. People with hemophilia and their families can be taught to give factor VIII concentrates at home at the first signs of bleeding. XYNTHA is a new recombinant factor VIII product for both the control and prevention of bleeding episodes and surgical prophylaxis.
- FEIBA therapy, consisting of activated prothrombin complex concentrate (aPCC) and recombinant activated factor VII (rFVIIa), is effective and safe for reducing bleeding in hemophilia A (Valentino, 2009).

Herbs, Botanicals, and Supplements

- Herbs and botanical supplements should not be used without discussing with the physician.
- Potential adverse effects of high vitamin E intakes in humans, such as bleeding, are not clear (Hathcock et al, 2005).

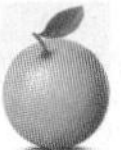

NUTRITION EDUCATION, COUNSELING, CARE MANAGEMENT

- Blood donors should be alerted to the need to replace daily iron intake by 0.7 mg for a year. Every pint is equivalent to 250 mg of iron lost.
- Discuss adequate dietary replacement for lost nutrients. A multivitamin–mineral supplement may be indicated.

Patient Education—Food Safety

If tube feeding or CPN is needed, careful handwashing procedures should be followed.

For More Information

- All About Bleeding
  http://www.allaboutbleeding.com/
- Anemia from Excessive Bleeding
  http://www.merck.com/mmhe/sec14/ch172/ch172b.html
- Blood Line
  http://www.bloodline.net/
- International Society on Thrombosis and Haemostasis
  http://www.isth.org/
- National Hemophilia Foundation
  http://www.hemophilia.org/about/programs.htm
- World Federation of Hemophilia
  http://www.wfh.org/2/docs/Publications/Diagnosis_and_Treatment/Gudelines_Mng_Hemophilia.pdf

HEMORRHAGE AND BLEEDING DISORDERS—CITED REFERENCES

Cao O, et al. Role of regulatory T cells in tolerance to coagulation factors. *J Thromb Haemost.* 7:88S, 2009.

Hathcock JN, et al. Vitamins E and C are safe across a broad range of intakes. *Am J Clin Nutr.* 81:736, 2005.

Valentino LA. Assessing the benefits of FEIBA prophylaxis in haemophilia patients with inhibitors. Haemophilia. 2009 Dec 16. [Epub ahead of print]

HEMOCHROMATOSIS AND IRON OVERLOAD

NUTRITIONAL ACUITY RANKING: LEVEL 2

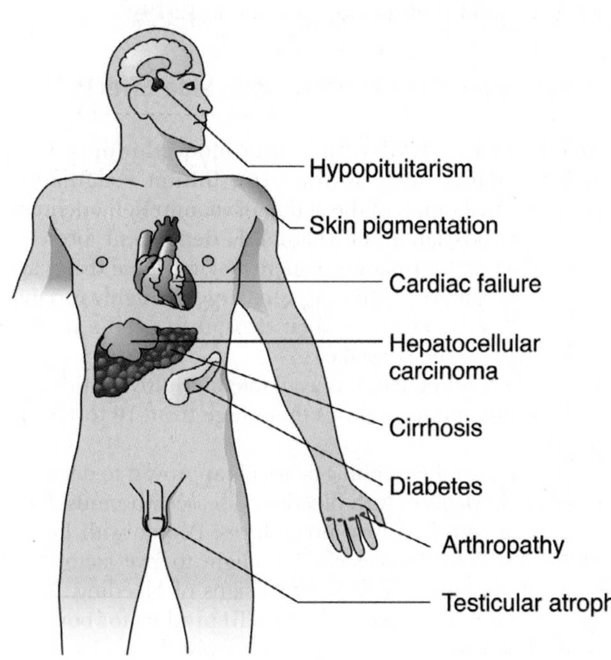

Adapted from: Rubin E MD and Farber JL MD. *Pathology*, 3rd ed. Philadelphia: Lippincott Williams & Wilkins, 1999.

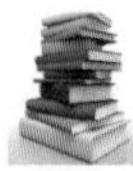

DEFINITIONS AND BACKGROUND

Hereditary hemochromatosis (HH) is one of the most common autosomal recessive disorders among Caucasians. One in 200–400 individuals of Northern European ancestry is at risk for hemochromatosis (Camaschella and Merlini, 2005). It is also common in Hispanics or people of Mediterranean descent and is 10 times more common in males than females. Irish Americans and African–Americans have double the usual frequency. Tragically, hemochromatosis remains underdiagnosed.

In hemochromatosis, iron stores are deposited in excess, often from excess intake or liver/pancreatic diseases, renal dialysis, or frequent and long-term transfusions. Healthy people may accumulate up to 1 g of iron, but people with this condition accumulate 15–30 g. Increased iron absorption leads to excessive accumulation of iron deposits within cells of the liver, heart, pituitary gland, pancreas, and other organs, gradually causing tissue damage.

Because hemochromatosis has many possible symptoms, it often goes undiagnosed. However, early detection is important and may prevent organ failure that can occur if it is left untreated. Long-term complications include liver cirrhosis, diabetes, cardiomyopathy, hypogonadism, arthropathy, skin pigmentation, and susceptibility to liver cancer (Camaschella and Merlini, 2005) (Table 12-20).

Iron overload patients may have diagnoses other than HH: non-alcoholic fatty liver disease (NAFLD), chronic hepatitis C, and chronic alcohol use are most common (Dever et al, 2009). Iron toxicity can also occur in aplastic anemia, chronic hemolytic anemia, porphyria cutanea tarda, sideroblastic anemia, thalassemias, diabetes, rheumatoid arthritis, or transfusional iron overload. Sometimes, individuals with Alzheimer's or Parkinson's disease may have heavy metal toxicities that contribute to an iron overload. Free iron is destructive to cells, and too much iron can be a carcinogen because cancer cells need it for their DNA synthesis. With chronic kidney disease, keep serum ferritin levels below 500 ng/dL.

Porphyrias are rare disorders caused by lack of the enzymes necessary for production of heme; this causes heme precursors, porphyrins, to accumulate in the bone marrow, liver, and bloodstream (MedlinePlus, 2009). The porphyrins may also

TABLE 12-20 Facts About Hemochromatosis

1. Undetected or untreated excess iron kills after inflicting injury to a variety of body organs. The physician's concern must be to detect any excess iron instead of establishing the diagnosis
2. Some literature suggests treatment when ferritin alone is elevated. Giving blood does no harm and, instead, is beneficial to health. About one fourth of patients have low hemoglobin; treatment is the same unless the anemia is so severe that blood transfusions are required. Severely anemic patients require iron removal by an iron chelator, Desferal
3. Iron overloading is preventable. When diagnosis is in doubt, the patient should begin a trial of weekly phlebotomies at the blood bank. Four to 6 weeks will usually provide the answer, and getting rid of a little excess iron will improve health
4. The patient should be taken to the blood bank upon the physician's order for weekly phlebotomies
5. A liver biopsy is not always necessary, and waiting can delay important treatment. DNA testing is not useful because it cannot detect all of the known mutations
6. When iron levels test low, the cause must be found. It is dangerous to medicate with iron without testing first and then finding the reason for any deficiency
7. Symptoms vary. Chronic fatigue, arthritis, anemia (iron-loading anemia is one symptom), and elevated liver enzymes must not be ignored. Hemoglobin level does not indicate iron status. A disorder of thyroid or any part of the body can be a symptom of iron overload
8. Excess iron lowers immunity. Many diseases (such as cancer, hepatitis, and AIDS) will show a poor outcome unless any excess iron is removed. Excess iron stored in the brain exacerbates severity in Alzheimer's, multiple sclerosis, Lou Gehrig's disease, Parkinson's disease, psychological problems, autism, and other diseases

Adapted from: Iron Overload Diseases Association, http://www.ironoverload.org/, accessed December 23, 2009.

be excreted in the urine or stool. Most porphyrias are hereditary, but attacks may also be triggered by drugs, alcohol, hormones, or infections.

Acute, hepatic porphyrias affect the nervous system. Symptoms include nerve damage with pain or paralysis, abdominal pain and liver damage, red or brown urine, anxiety and delirium, muscle pain or weakness, numbness or tingling, tachycardia, loss of deep tendon reflexes, low blood pressure, and electrolyte imbalances. Constipation or diarrhea may occur. A diet high in carbohydrate (55–60% of total kilocalories) and beta carotene may be beneficial (MedlinePlus, 2009).

Porphyria cutanea tarda (PCT) can occur without an inherited enzyme deficiency. The porphyrins accumulate in the liver and skin, causing photosensitivity, skin damage, and cirrhosis. Phlebotomy removes excess iron, and chloroquine or hydroxychloroquine removes the excess porphyrins from the liver (Anderson, 2007).

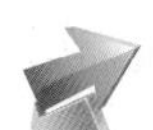

ASSESSMENT, MONITORING, AND EVALUATION

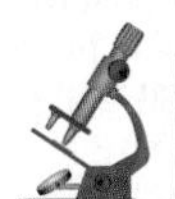

CLINICAL INDICATORS

Genetic Markers: HH is recessive, requiring the gene from two carrier parents. There are several types of genetic hemochromatosis: type I or classic (HHC); type II a, b, or juvenile (JHC); type III or transferrin receptor mutation; and type IV or ferroportin mutation. Iron overload can also occur in individuals with the HFE C2824 gene in 1 out of 200 people.

Clinical/History

Height
Weight
BMI
Diet history
BP
I & O
Bronzing of the skin
Profound fatigue (in HH)
Arthralgia (in HH)
Loss of body hair
Loss of libido
Lack of menstruation or early menopause
Abdominal pain
Chronic intermittent diarrhea
Irregular heartbeat
Cardiomegaly with congestive failure
Hepatomegaly
Enlarged spleen
Hypothyroidism
Depression
Liver biopsy
Bone marrow studies

Lab Work

Transferrin-Iron Saturation Percentage[a] (normal 25–35%)—best test
TIBC (normal, 12–45%)
Transferrin (increased)
Serum Cu (increased)
Alb
Serum Fe
Ferritin (increased >1000 ng/mL?)
Hgb (desirable = 10 g/dL)
Hct (desirable = 30–35%)
Gluc
Serum B_6
Serum B_{12}
Serum folic acid
Thyroid tests
Liver function tests
CRP

[a]Divide total serum iron by TIBC for percentage of tissue saturation (TS). Divide the serum iron level by TIBC for percentage of transferrin saturation.

INTERVENTION

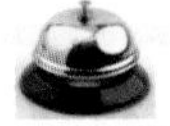

OBJECTIVES

- Remove excess iron from body (usually with phlebotomies of 500 mL weekly, performed by the physician over several months). Then therapy is repeated several times annually for rest of the life.
- Prevent liver cancer, heart attack, or stroke by unloading storage iron as fast as possible; keep serum ferritin at low normal range.
- If excess iron intake is a chronic problem, discontinue use in supplements and fortified foods (such as iron-fortified cereals). Read labels carefully.

SAMPLE NUTRITION CARE PROCESS STEPS

Excessive Mineral Intake

Assessment Data: Male with transferrin-iron saturation percentage (46%), ferritin (160 ng/mL), elevated H & H. Diagnosis of iron overloading. Diet hx reveals high intake of animal proteins and heme iron (about 20 g/day).

Nutrition Diagnoses (PES): Excessive iron intake related to diet high in animal proteins and heme iron as evidenced by transferrin-iron saturation percentage (46%), ferritin (160 ng/mL), elevated H & H.

Interventions: Food–nutrient delivery—encourage more vegetarian meals and fewer ounces of meats at mealtime. Educate about the role of heme iron intake in iron overloading disorders. Counsel and provide meal planning tips and portion guides for intake of meats.

Monitoring and Evaluation: Improvement in serum laboratories (transferrin-iron saturation percentage, ferritin, and H & H) with levels closer to normal. Diet hx reveals improved intake of 8–10 g/day.

- Teach principles of nutrition and menu planning to incorporate adequate intake of other nutrients that may be depleted with excessive phlebotomies (e.g., folate and other B-complex vitamins, protein).

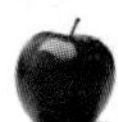

FOOD AND NUTRITION

- Provide a normal diet unless renal or hepatic function is altered. Do not consume foods or take supplements high in vitamin C. Read cereal labels and avoid those with 100% or more of the daily allowance for iron and vitamin C. A low-iron diet is not recommended.
- Ensure adequate protein and sufficient energy intake to meet estimated needs and activity levels.
- Avoid alcohol because of potential damage to a vulnerable liver.

Common Drugs Used and Potential Side Effects

- Avoid use of multivitamin supplements that contain iron and vitamin C because these can increase iron absorption.
- An iron chelator may be needed, such as deferoxamine (DFO). This is given intravenously 8–12 hours for up to five times in a week. It can be neurotoxic.

Herbs, Botanicals, and Supplements

- Herbs and botanical supplements should not be used without discussing with the physician.

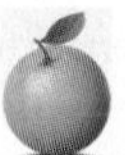

NUTRITION EDUCATION, COUNSELING, CARE MANAGEMENT

- All blood relatives of the patient must be evaluated and monitored yearly for iron overloading.
- Genetic testing of other family members is also recommended for those with inherited type.
- Discuss avoidance of alcohol and raw seafood. *Vibrio vulnificus* in some raw seafood kills people every year; many are those with undetected iron overload.
- Discuss nutrient sources as appropriate for the individual.

Patient Education—Food Safety

- If tube feeding or CPN is needed, careful handwashing procedures should be followed.
- Avoid eating raw seafood.

For More Information

- Iron Disorders Institute
  http://www.irondisorders.org
- Iron Facts
  http://ods.od.nih.gov/factsheets/iron.asp
- Iron Overload Diseases Association, Inc.
  http://www.ironoverload.org/
- Iron Tests
  http://www.irondisorders.org/Forms/irontests.pdf

HEMOCHROMATOSIS—CITED REFERENCES

Anderson K. The porphyrias. In: Goldman L, Ausiello D, eds. *Cecil Medicine.* 23rd ed. Philadelphia, Pa: Saunders Elsevier; 2007:229.

Camaschella C, Merlini R. Inherited hemochromatosis: from genetics to clinics. *Minerva Med.* 96:207, 2005.

Dever JB, et al. Phenotypic characteristics and diagnoses of patients referred to an iron overload clinic. *Dig Dis Sci.* 2009 Dec 24. [Epub ahead of print]

MedlinePlus. Porphyrias. Web site accessed December 28,2009, at http://www.nlm.nih.gov/medlineplus/ency/article/001208.htm.

POLYCYTHEMIA VERA

NUTRITIONAL ACUITY RANKING: LEVEL 1

DEFINITIONS AND BACKGROUND

Polycythemia vera (PV) is a chronic, progressive disease in which increased blood volume and increased erythrocyte production occur. Other names include erythremia, Osler–Vasquez disease, and polycythemia rubra vera. Hematological disorders like PV can result in elevated levels of cobalamin, which is released during hepatic cytolysis.

The cause of PV is unknown, and the disease is considered a hematological malignancy. The disease develops slowly and may progress to acute myelogenous leukemia. The average age at diagnosis is 50–60 years. Incidence is highest among those of Jewish ancestry, occurring in 2 of 100,000 of the population. Increased viscosity of the blood and number of platelets result in a high risk for clot formation and stroke, hemorrhage, or myocardial infarction.

Patients with PV frequently develop hyperhomocysteinemia due to discrete depletion of cobalamin or folate; vitamin therapy should be considered. With treatment, individuals with this condition may live for 15–20 years. Phlebotomy or medications may be used.

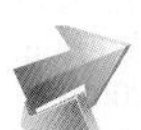

ASSESSMENT, MONITORING, AND EVALUATION

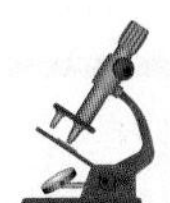

CLINICAL INDICATORS

Genetic Markers: The somatic V617 F mutation in the Janus kinase (JAK) 2 gene, which causes a valine to phenylalanine substitution at position 617, has recently been found in the majority of patients with PV (Meyer, 2009).

Clinical/History

- Height
- Weight
- BMI
- Diet history
- I & O
- BP (hypertension?)
- Belching, fullness
- Flatulence
- Peptic ulcer?
- Constipation
- Headache
- Vertigo
- Lassitude
- Tinnitus
- Pruritus after bathing
- Transient blurred vision, diplopia
- Dyspnea
- Chest pain
- Dusky reddish skin on face and hands
- Hemorrhagic tendency
- Seizures, confusion
- Splenomegaly
- Tinnitus
- Paresthesias
- Gout

Lab Work

- Hgb (>18 g/dL)
- Hct (>52% for men; >47% for women)
- Platelets (elevated)
- Leukocytes (elevated)
- Serum B_{12} (elevated)
- Erythropoietin (low)
- TIBC
- Erythrocyte sedimentation rate (ESR)
- Leukocyte Alk phos
- Serum ferritin
- Gluc
- RBC (7–12 million)
- Oxygen saturation >92%
- CRP
- Alb, transthyretin
- CRP
- Chol, Trig
- BUN, Creat
- Uric acid (elevated)
- Bone marrow biopsy

INTERVENTION

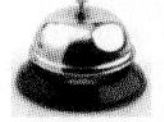

OBJECTIVES

- Prepare patient for phlebotomy by ensuring adequate nutrient stores.
- Prepare, as needed, for chemotherapy or radiation therapy, which may be provided.

SAMPLE NUTRITION CARE PROCESS STEPS

Abnormal GI Function

Assessment Data: BMI 20. Constipation, flatulence, history of gastric bleeding, and ulceration.

Nutrition Diagnoses (PES): Abnormal GI function related to discomfort and pain as evidenced by constipation, flatulence, GI ulceration, and bleeding.

Interventions: Food-nutrient delivery—use comfort foods and adequate CHO, fiber, and fluid intake; reduce acidic foods and items not well tolerated. Educate about good nutrition and inclusion of B-complex vitamins. Counsel about individualizing tolerance for medications with appropriate food, fluid, and snacks.

Monitoring and Evaluation: Daily use of prescribed medications. Improvement in GI function; resolution of constipation and flatulence. No additional GI bleeding.

- Correct or control condition.
- Manage any side effects such as heart failure, peptic ulcer disease, gastric bleeding, gout, leukemia, and seizures.

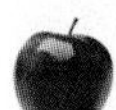

FOOD AND NUTRITION

- A high CHO diet with preferred foods and balanced meals should be offered. Monitor for the need for vitamin or mineral supplementation. Include foods rich in beta carotene.
- Extra fluids will be helpful (35–40 mL/kg, unless contraindicated, as with heart failure).
- Changes in dietary texture or content may be needed if radiation or chemotherapy alters nutrient or dietary needs.

Common Drugs Used and Potential Side Effects

- Myelosuppressive agents may be prescribed. Anagrelide hydrochloride (Agrylin) is an oral imidazoquinazoline agent that has been shown to reduce elevated platelet counts and the risk of thrombosis. Interferon alpha may be used in younger patients; pegylated interferon alpha-2a (PEG-IFN-alpha-2a) is beneficial (Quintas-Cardama et al, 2009).
- The antimetabolite hydroxyurea may be used. Side effects include anemia and skin ulcers.
- Chemotherapeutic agents (busulfan, chlorambucil, and cyclophosphamide) may cause nausea and vomiting or weight loss.
- Low-dose aspirin is sometimes used in patients with thrombotic or ischemic conditions. It can relieve some of the burning sensations in the feet and hands. Antihistamines can help reduce itching sensation.

Herbs, Botanicals, and Supplements

- Herbs and botanical supplements should not be used without discussing with the physician.

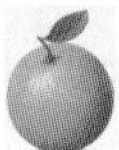

NUTRITION EDUCATION, COUNSELING, CARE MANAGEMENT

- Discuss need to maintain a healthy lifestyle and to eat adequate protein and calories because of the frequent phlebotomies, where completed.
- Discuss ways to make meals that are nutritious yet simple to prepare.
- Tepid oatmeal baths may help reduce pruritus.

Patient Education—Food Safety

If tube feeding or CPN is needed, careful handwashing procedures should be followed.

For More Information

- Mayo Clinic – PV
  http://www.mayoclinic.com/health/polycythemia-vera/DS00919
- Merck Manual–Blood Disorders
  http://www.merck.com/mmhe/sec14/ch178/ch178b.html
- Myeloproliferative Disorders
  http://www.acor.org/diseases/hematology/MPD/

POLYCYTHEMIA VERA—CITED REFERENCES

Meyer T. Activated STAT1 and STAT5 transcription factors in extramedullary hematopoietic tissue in a polycythemia vera patient carrying the JAK2 V617 F mutation. *Int J Hematol.* [Epub ahead of print]

Quintas-Cardama A, et al. Pegylated interferon alfa-2 a yields high rates of hematologic and molecular response in patients with advanced essential thrombocythemia and polycythemia vera. *J Clin Oncol.* 27:5418, 2009.

THROMBOCYTOPENIA

NUTRITIONAL ACUITY RANKING: LEVEL 1

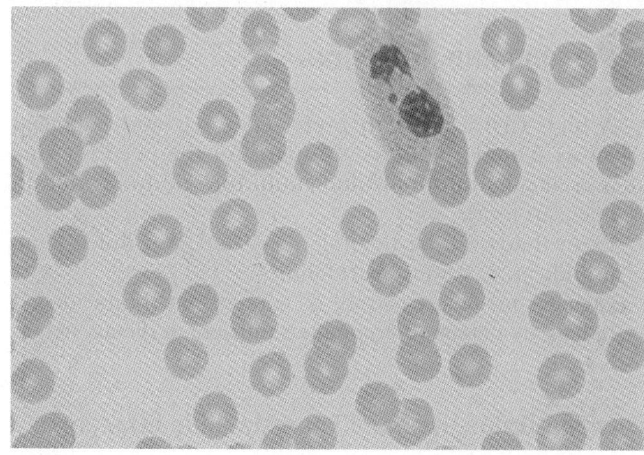

Adapted from: *Anderson's Atlas of Hematology;* Anderson, Shauna C., PhD. Copyright 2003, Wolters Kluwer Health/Lippincott Williams & Wilkins.

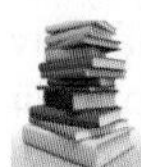

DEFINITIONS AND BACKGROUND

Thrombocytopenia purpura, a myeloproliferative disorder, is a blood disease affecting the clotting factor (platelets) of the blood, with an abnormally low platelet count and shorter than normal (10 days) platelet survival time. Thrombocytopenia is the most common cause of bleeding, usually from small capillaries. Women are more affected than men.

There are many reasons for the development of decreased marrow production or platelet destruction that causes thrombocytopenia, including some hereditary causes. These can sometimes be determined by examination of bone marrow. Idiopathic thrombocytopenic purpura (ITP) is caused by platelet destruction by antibodies. Thrombotic thrombocytopenic purpura (TTP) is manifested by vascular lesions.

Plasma exchange (plasmapheresis) is used to remove the abnormal antibody from the blood and replace the missing enzyme. Mortality of TTP has decreased from 90% to 10% (George, 2009); survival improved dramatically with plasma exchange treatments after the 1980s (Kremer-Hovinga et al, 2009). Unfortunately, adults with TTP of any etiology have a high risk for persistent minor cognitive abnormalities (George, 2009).

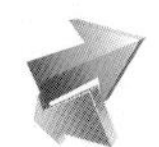

ASSESSMENT, MONITORING, AND EVALUATION

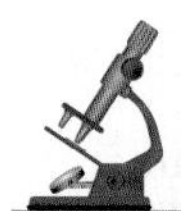

CLINICAL INDICATORS

Genetic Markers: Mutations in the ADAMTS13 gene cause the familial form of TPP. Alterations in the ADAMTS13 gene reduces instructions for the normal process of blood clotting.

Clinical/History

Height
Weight
BMI
Diet history
I & O
BP
Nosebleeds
Bleeding from other sites
Bruising
Pinpoint red spots on skin
Headache
Slurred speech
Numbness and weakness of extremities
Fever?
Pallor
Jaundice
Shortness of breath

Lab Work

CBC (low platelets)
H & H (decreased)
Alb, transthyretin
N balance
PT and PTT (normal)
Casts in urine
Proteinuria
CRP
Ca^{++}
Na^{+}, K^{+}

SAMPLE NUTRITION CARE PROCESS STEPS

Self-Feeding Difficulty

Assessment Data: BMI at lower end of normal, but some weight loss noted. Dx of TPP with numbness and weakness in hands and feet. Inability to feed self and remain independent; depression and easy frustration noted at mealtimes.

Nutrition Diagnoses (PES): Self-feeding difficulty related to numbness in hands as evidenced by inability to hold traditional utensils.

Interventions: Food–nutrient delivery—alter food choices to simplify options and offer more finger foods. Educate about use of adaptive feeding equipment that can be used for more independence. Counseling with tips on meal simplification.

Monitoring and Evaluation: Improved ability to feed self independently. No further weight loss. Less depression and frustration at mealtimes.

INTERVENTION

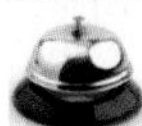

OBJECTIVES

- Avoid infections, especially upper respiratory infections and flu to prevent coughing, which increases intracranial pressure.
- Reduce bleeding tendency and complications, such as intracranial hemorrhage or GI bleeding (Goldman, 2007).
- Rest frequently.
- Prepare patient for splenectomy, if indicated. Ensure adequate nutrient stores.

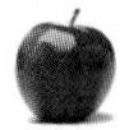

FOOD AND NUTRITION

- Maintain diet of preference. Use small, frequent feedings if patient has nausea or vomiting.
- Adequate folic acid will be needed.
- Increase fluids (e.g., 3 L/d) unless contraindicated.
- After splenectomy, patient will need adequate protein, energy, zinc, and vitamins A and C for wound healing. Vitamin K from the diet and supplements may need to be monitored.

Common Drugs Used and Potential Side Effects

- Most drugs are stopped because nearly any drug may aggravate the condition.
- Corticosteroids such as prednisone may be used to control bleeding. Side effects are numerous and may affect nutritional status (e.g., decreased serum calcium, potassium, and nitrogen; increased serum sodium; and glucose intolerance may occur).
- Myelosuppressive agents are often prescribed. Anagrelide hydrochloride (Agrylin) is an oral imidazoquinazoline agent that has been shown to reduce elevated platelet counts and the risk of thrombosis. Interferon alpha may be used.
- Rituximab seems to be a promising drug in the treatment of refractory autoimmune thrombocytopenia.

Herbs, Botanicals, and Supplements

- Herbs and botanical supplements should not be used without discussing with the physician.

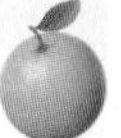

NUTRITION EDUCATION, COUNSELING, CARE MANAGEMENT

- Discuss altering nutrients as needed, depending on medications ordered and their use over time; surgery, if required; and ability to eat adequately.

Patient Education—Food Safety

If tube feeding or CPN is needed, careful handwashing procedures should be followed.

For More Information

- The ITP Society of the Children's Blood Foundation
  http://www.childrensbloodfoundation.org/
- Platelet Disorder Support Foundation
  http://www.pdsa.org/

THROMBOCYTOPENIA—CITED REFERENCES

George JN. The thrombotic thrombocytopenic purpura and hemolytic uremic syndromes: evaluation, management, and long-term outcomes experience of the Oklahoma TTP-HUS Registry, 1989–2007. *Kidney Int Suppl.* 112:52S, 2009.

Goldman L. *Ausiello D. Cecil Textbook of Medicine.* 23rd ed. Philadelphia, Pa: WB Saunders; 1291–1299, 2007.

Kremer-Hovinga JA, et al. Survival and relapse in patients with thrombotic thrombocytopenic purpura. *Blood.* 2009 Dec 23. [Epub ahead of print]

SECTION 13

Cancer

CHIEF ASSESSMENT FACTORS

American Cancer Society's Seven Warning Signs of Cancer

- Change in Bowel/Bladder Habits
- Indigestion or Dysphagia
- Nagging Cough or Hoarseness
- Obvious Change in Wart or Mole
- Sore That Does Not Heal
- Thickening or Lump in Breast or Elsewhere
- Unusual Bleeding or Discharge

Other Factors

- Anorexia or Chronic Nausea
- Changes in Food Intake, Usual Functional Capacity, Energy Levels
- Depression
- Diarrhea
- Dry Mouth
- Dysphagia, Esophagitis, Mouth Sores, Mucositis
- Edema or Ascites
- Fever of Unknown Origin (Hematological, Liver, Pancreatic, Brain, Kidney Cancers)
- History of Carcinogen Exposure, Tobacco Use, Excessive Alcohol Use
- Intolerance for Nauseating Odors
- Muscle Wasting
- Nutrient Intake and Immune Function
- Pain
- Participation in Complementary and Alternative Medicine Treatments
- Side Effects of Medications
- Vomiting
- Weight Changes—Unintended Weight Loss or BMI Less Than 22

TABLE 13-1 **Cancer Definitions**

Term	Definition
Adenocarcinoma	Cancer that starts in the glands.
Adenoma	Benign growth that may or may not transform into cancer.
Antiangiogenesis	Process of stopping a tumor from growing new blood vessels.
Antibodies	Proteins in the immune system; in cancer, antibodies are used to recognize specific cancer cell receptors and to act as smart bombs.
Basal cell carcinoma	Most common form of skin cancer, affecting 800,000 Americans each year. Chronic exposure to sunlight causes most basal cell carcinomas, which occur most frequently on exposed parts (e.g., face, ears, neck, scalp, shoulders, and back).
Biotherapy	Treatment to stimulate or restore the ability of the immune system to fight infection and disease and to lessen side effects that may be caused by some cancer treatments; also known as immunotherapy, biological therapy, or biological response modifier (BRM) therapy.
Cancer	Abnormal, uncontrolled growth of cells in a lump or mass that also destroys normal tissue. Oncogenes in a tumor cell may be identifying markers.
Carcinoma	Cancer involving epithelial tissue and coverings of internal and external surfaces; lungs, colon, breast, stomach, uterus, skin, and tongue cancers. 80–90% of all cancers.
Chemotherapy	Use of medications to kill malignant cells.
Curative Therapy	Permanent removal of the cancer from the body.
Endocrine system cancers	Adrenocortical carcinoma; gastrointestinal carcinoid tumor; pancreatic islet cell carcinoma; parathyroid cancer; pheochromocytoma; pituitary tumor; and thyroid cancer.
Epithelioma	Carcinoma consisting of many epithelial cells.
Gastrointestinal (GI) cancers	Anal cancer; bile duct cancer; colon cancer; esophageal cancer; gallbladder cancer; GI carcinoid tumor; liver cancers; pancreatic cancer; rectal cancer; small intestine cancer; stomach cancer.
Gynecological cancer	Female reproductive system: cervical cancer; endometrial cancer; gestational trophoblastic tumor; ovarian epithelial cancer; ovarian germ cell tumor; ovarian low malignant potential tumor; sarcoma; vaginal cancer; and vulvar cancer.
Hormonal therapy	Treatment by surgery or by shrinking or killing hormone-dependent cancers.
Leukemia	Cancer where bone marrow–produced abnormal white blood cells crowd out normal white blood cells, red blood cells, and platelets.
Lymphoma	AIDS-related lymphoma; cutaneous T-cell lymphoma; Hodgkin's lymphoma; mycosis fungoides; non-Hodgkin's lymphoma; primary central nervous system lymphoma; Sézary's syndrome; and Waldenstrom's macroglobulinemia.
Male reproductive cancers	Penile, testicular cancers, prostate cancers.
Meningiomas	Tumors affecting the meninges.
Mesothelioma	Rare cancer affecting the lining of the chest, heart, and abdominal cavity from exposure to asbestos.
Metastasis	Transfer of disease from one organ to another that is not directly connected to it; particularly the spread of carcinoma.
Monoclonal antibodies	Targeted therapy to locate and bind cancer cells. May be used alone or used to deliver drugs, toxins, or radioactive material directly to tumor cells.
Neuroma	A tumor composed of nerve cells, which may occur along any nerve.
Oat cell carcinoma	A rapidly spreading, highly fatal cancer of the bronchus.
Oncology	Scientific study of tumors.
Osteosarcoma	Most common bone cancer, which develops in new tissue in growing bones, affecting young people and more males.
Palliative therapy	Pain relief but not expected to cure the disease. Given to improve quality of life as much as possible.
Radiation	Treatment with high-energy rays to kill or damage cancer cells. May be external rays or internally placed radioactive material.
Sarcoma	Cancer arising from bone or connective tissue, which sometimes spreads into blood or lymphatic tissues.
Small cell carcinoma	Carcinoma that most commonly arises in the lung but can occur as a cancer in other body sites including the prostate, cervix, and head and neck; responsive to chemotherapy and radiation therapy.
Vaccine	To stimulate the immune system to mount a defense against cancer cells. Example – the cervical cancer vaccine.

Definitions: http://www.cancer.gov/dictionary/ and Types of cancers: http://www.cancer.gov/cancertopics/alphalist/a-d, accessed December 29, 2009.

For More General Information on Cancer: Table 13-1 provides a list of cancer definitions.

- AMC Cancer Research Center and Foundation
  http://www.amc.org/
- American Cancer Society
  http://www.cancer.org
- American Dietetic Association Oncology Nutrition Dietetic Practice Group
  http://www.oncologynutrition.org/
- American Institute for Cancer Research (AICR)
  http://www.aicr.org/
- Cancer Care
  http://www.cancercare.org/
- Cancer Screening Guidelines
  http://www.aafp.org/afp/20010315/1101.html
- Caring 4 Cancer
  http://www.caring4cancer.com/go/cancer/nutrition

- Eating Hints for Cancer Patients
  http://www.cancer.gov/cancertopics/eatinghints
- Genetics 101
  http://www.ornl.gov/sci/techresources/Human_Genome/project/info.shtml
- Harvard–Dana-Farber Cancer Institute
  http://www.dfci.harvard.edu/
- Harvard Center for Risk Analysis
  http://www.hcra.harvard.edu/#
- Hospice Net
  http://www.hospicenet.org/
- Human Carcinogens
  http://www.cancer.org/docroot/PED/ped_1_1.asp
- Journal of the National Cancer Institute
  http://jncicancerspectrum.oxfordjournals.org/
- Lance Armstrong Foundation
  http://www.laf.org
- National Cancer Institute
  http://www.nci.nih.gov/
- National Coalition for Cancer Survivorship
  http://www.canceradvocacy.org/
- National Institutes of Health Gene Testing
  http://www.genetests.org/
- National Toxicology Program
  http://ntp-server.niehs.nih.gov/index.cfm
- North American Cancer Registry
  http://www.naaccr.org/
- Oncology Association of Naturopathic Medicine
  http://www.oncanp.org/
- Oncology Nursing Society
  http://www.ons.org/
- Online Human Genome Resources
  http://www.genome.gov/10000464
- Vital Options
  http://www.vitaloptions.org/

CANCER PREVENTION AND RISK REDUCTION

Cancer results from dysregulated cell growth control and is caused by an interaction of dietary, genetic, and environmental risk factors. There are over 100 variations of cancer. Cancer has a strong genetic component, associated with initiation, promotion, and metastatic growth. The Human Genome Project has identified 30,000 human protein-coding genes. Individualized DNA methylation helps to control gene expression. Genotyping resources allow cancer prevention investigators to identify which genetic subsets of patients are likely to benefit most from chemoprevention and interventions. This emerging science of nutritional genomics is very promising (Kauwell, 2005).

Natural carcinogens include ultraviolet (UV) radiation, dyes, environmental chemicals from smoke or mines, viruses, nitrosamines, aflatoxins, and safrole. The most consistent carcinogen is tobacco. Approximately 30% of cancers also have a nutrition or dietary component (Williams and Hord, 2005). Functional food components greatly impact the incidence and treatment of cancer. In addition, food intake, aging, and immune function share a complex relationship; selenium, EPA, DHA, vitamin A, and sodium seem to be particularly important (Wardwell et al, 2008).

Nutritive and nonnutritive dietary constituents can either promote or hinder the development of cancer, individualized by genetic predisposition. Diets rich in carotenoids, antioxidative vitamins, phenolic compounds, terpenoids, steroids, indoles, and fibers reduce the risk of cancer and related chronic diseases (Aggarwal and Shishorida, 2004). Studies support the role of flavonoids, carotenoids, curcumin, ascorbic acid, and citrus liminoids (Patil et al, 2009). Polyphenols are the most abundant antioxidants in the average diet and are constituents of fruits, vegetables, cereals, dry legumes, chocolate, tea, coffee, and wine.

The strongest evidence linking specific foods to a decreased risk of certain cancers is related to the consumption of fruits, vegetables, and whole grains. Antioxidants protect against free radical damage, improving the resistance of cells to oxidative stress. In a study using HANES data, daily intakes of antioxidants from both diet and supplements averaged 208 milligrams of vitamin C, 20 milligrams of alpha-tocopherol, 223 retinol activity equivalents (RAE) of carotenes, 122 micrograms of selenium, and 210 milligrams of dietary flavonoids (Chun et al, 2009). Women, older adults, Caucasians, nonconsumers of alcohol, nonsmokers, and those with a higher income and exercise level than other tended to have better intakes (Chun et al, 2009). Key nutrients, chemoprotective phytochemicals, and functional food ingredients are listed in Table 13-2.

Promoting fruits, vegetables, and whole grains is the key message. Choose "better for you" foods, and make vegetables the central focus of the plate. Minimize meats, or use leaner cuts. Enhance the diet with nuts and whole grains (insoluble types to increase stool bulk and push bile out; soluble types for their cholesterol-lowering effect). A complete "anticancer" grocery list includes dark green, yellow, and orange fruits or vegetables; red grapes; cruciferous vegetables; orange juice; tomatoes; olive and canola oils; garlic; legumes; strong coffee; whole grains; soy; and other plant estrogens.

Dietary factors and physical inactivity contribute to approximately one-third of all cancers. Table 13-3 provides a list of important dietary factors. Excess body weight increases the risk of several cancers. There are five lifestyle habits to promote: maintain BMI <25, get 30 minutes of exercise, limit alcohol to—one to two drinks daily, do not smoke, and choose a healthy diet rich in phytochemicals.

Many cancer patients try CAM therapies; fish oil is the leading choice of adults. Yet the emphasis remains on food sources, not supplements or pills. The intake of whole foods and fortified, enriched, or enhanced foods has the most beneficial impact on health (American Dietetic Association, 2009).

TABLE 13-2 Phytochemicals, Functional Food Ingredients, and Cancer

Phytochemicals are functional foods or ingredients that occur naturally in fruits and vegetables and whole grains, often to protect against microorganisms. They are not "essential" nutrients, but some phytochemicals function as antioxidants to squelch free radicals.

Food	Functional Ingredient	Possible Roles in Reducing Cancer Risk
Apples (MALUS sp., Rosaceae)	Hydroxycinnamic acids, dihydrochalcones, catechins and oligomeric procyanidins	Also contain triterpenoids in apple peel and anthocyanins in red apples. Protect against skin, lung, breast, and colon cancer (Gerhauser, 2008).
Apples, black tea, grapefruit, onions, arugula	Quercetin, kaempferol, myricetin, isorhamnetin (flavonols)	Decreases ascorbate-dependent free radical oxidation; decreases inflammation and tumorigenesis. May be protective against colorectal cancer. Since apple skins retain pesticides, choose organic.
Beans and legumes, soybeans, whole grains, alfalfa, lentils, bean sprouts	Saponins: oleanic acid, hedagenin (terpenes)	Triterpene glycosides that neutralize enzymes in the intestine that may cause cancer; they boost immunity. Consume only moderate amounts of soy as part of a healthy plant-based diet.
Beef, lamb, yogurt, some cheeses and dairy products	Conjugated linoleic acid	Maintains immune function and normal body composition; some antitumor properties. Marinate meats in red wine or beer to cut heterocyclic amine exposure; do not burn meats.
Bell peppers, citrus fruits	Vitamin C	Protects against damage from free radicals.
Blueberries (particularly skins), blackberries, raspberries, strawberries, cherries, red grapes, red cabbage, eggplant, red onion, kidney beans, red beans, beets, black currants, elderberries, purple sweet potato skin, prunes	Anthocyanins (polyphenols/ flavonols)	Bolsters cellular antioxidant defenses particularly against UV radiation; maintain brain function and motor function; neutralize free radicals; have antimicrobial action.
Brazil nuts, lean meats, tuna, salmon, seafood	Selenium and Glutathione	Increases immune cell functioning, DNA methylation, and regulation of cytokine production. Protects from damage from free radicals. SELECT study found that a 200-milligram selenium supplement actually promotes prostate cancer.
Broccoli, broccoli sprouts, horseradish, cauliflower, cabbage, bok choy, Brussels sprouts, kale	Sulforaphane; thiols	Isothiocyanates (ITCs) protect the body from cancer by inducing detoxification enzymes such as quinone reductase. They increase periods of cancer latency and are effective agents against fungi such as *Aspergillus*. Protects against stomach and skin cancers. Lightly cooked broccoli has more; use a mix of raw and cooked vegetables.
Broccoli, peas, beans, and other vegetables; soybeans, clover, alfalfa	Coumestans (phytoestrogen)	High level of estrogenic activity that may reduce the risk for lung cancer. Estimated daily intake of coumestans is 0.6 micrograms; broccoli is the main source.
Cabbage, sauerkraut	Glucosinolate	May lower the risk of hormonal cancers
Carrots, American ginseng roots	Falcarinol, falcarindiol, panaxydol (polyacetylenes)	Inhibits cell proliferation in normal and cancer cells through synergism of bioactive polyacetylenes. More effective if whole and not chopped before cooking.
Carrots, sweet potatoes, pumpkin, butternut squash, cantaloupe, mangoes, apricots, peaches, papaya, watermelon	Beta-carotene (terpenes)	Beneficial effects on human cancer prevention; increases the activity of killer cells slightly; photoprotective; neutralize free radicals; serves as antioxidants. Avoid excesses of supplements as they act as pro-oxidants. Dietary fat is needed for proper absorption. Boil or steam to protect the antioxidants.
Cereals, legumes, nuts, sesame seeds, soybeans, brown rice, corn and wheat brans	Inositol	Found as phytic acid in plants. Used by all cells to relay outside messages to the cell nucleus. Aids in the metabolism of calcium and other minerals.
Cherry juice	Chlorogenic acid (phenolic acid)	Strong antioxidant properties.
Cinnamon, cocoa, apples, strawberries, purple grapes and wines, peanuts, cranberries	Proanthocyanidins	Decreases oxidative stress; supports urinary tract health.
Citrus fruits, lemon, cantaloupe, pomegranate, potato skins, wild leafy greens, celery stalks, lettuce, chili and sweet peppers, spinach, parsley, watermelon, whole grains, tomato sauce, red wines	Apigenin, luteolin (flavones)	Tumor growth inhibition and chemoprevention; may protect against skin cancer and ultraviolet damage. May protect women against ovarian cancer.
Citrus fruits, apples, pears		
Some vegetables	Caffeic acid, ferulic acid (flavanones)	Bolsters antioxidant defenses.

(continued)

TABLE 13-2 Phytochemicals, Functional Food Ingredients, and Cancer *(continued)*

Food	Functional Ingredient	Possible Roles in Reducing Cancer Risk
Corn, soy, wheat, wood oils	Plant stanols	Inhibits cholesterol absorption.
Cruciferous vegetables: Broccoli, cabbage, sauerkraut, Brussels sprouts, bok choy, arugula, Swiss chard, watercress, cauliflower, kale, kohlrabi, turnips, rutabaga	Indoles (indole-3-carbinol); glucosinolates (thiols)	Antimutagenics that may enhance detoxification of undesirable compounds. May contribute to a healthy immune system; downregulate estrogen and tumor formation. May yield a lower risk of breast, colon, prostate, and cervical cancers.
Cruciferous vegetables (*Brassica* family)	Jasmonates (thiols)	Plant signaling compounds that activate the coordinated gene expression in ascorbate and glutathione metabolic pathways. Important in defense responses to oxidative stress and biosynthesis of glucosinolate, a defense compound.
Dairy products	Vitamin D_3, calcium, sphingomyelin	May inhibit tumor cell growth and aid in cell death. Vitamin D_3 may protect against some skin cancers, but not melanoma. A level of 2000–4000 IU per day of vitamin D_3 is considered necessary for most adults. Sun exposure, diet, and supplements may be needed.
Flaxseed, rye, whole grains, berries, carrots, spinach, broccoli, tea, asparagus, linseeds; alcoholic beverages (red and white wines).	Lignans: matairesinol and secoisolariciresinol	Phytoestrogens attach to estrogen receptors and block real estrogen, lower cholesterol levels, and decrease cancer activity. Lignans may prevent prostate or lung cancer. Median intake of lignans is 578 micrograms (mainly from berries).
Garlic, onions	Allyl sulfides; selenium	Boosts levels of naturally occurring enzymes that may help maintain a healthy immune system. Garlic also contains arginine, oligosaccharides, sulfur and flavonoids. May be protective against cancers of the stomach, esophagus, colon, breast, and pancreas.
Ginkgo biloba	Ginkgolide A and B	Taken for 6 months or longer, may lower the risk of ovarian cancer. Involved in anti-inflammation processes.
Ginseng	Triterpene glycoside	Radioprotective capability, attributed to the ginsenosides, which are saponins with antioxidant properties. May increase lymphocyte production, stimulate natural killer cells and other immune activity; inhibit cancer cell growth; antioxidant.
Grapes, wine, raspberries, strawberries, tomatoes, citrus fruits, carrots, whole grains, nuts	Ellagic acid, Ferulic acid (phenolic acids)	May block the production of enzymes needed for cancer cells to reproduce. Protect against *Salmonella* and *Staphylococcus aureus* infections (particularly ellagitannins in raspberries).
Grape juices from green and black grapes	Gallic acid (phenolic acids)	Strong antioxidant properties
Green tea, oolong tea, black teas, dark chocolate, red wines, licorice root, cranberries and cranberry products	Catechins: epigallocatechin gallate (EGCG); glycyrrhizin; procyanidins/tannins (flavonols)	Decreases the growth of hydroquinone oxidase; decreases *COX-2* gene expression and cancer cell growth; and neutralizes free radicals. Tannins in green and black tea and strong coffee inhibit the proliferation of cancer cells in prostate, ovarian, breast, lung, and possibly other sites. Avoid excesses of caffeine, which dilute the effect of the tea.
Green tea extract, watermelon, prunes, raisins, plums, eggplant, grapes, berries, cherries, apples, cantaloupe	Polyphenols	May neutralize free radicals to help block damage to DNA. Superoxide anion radical (SOR) has scavenging activity; protects against oxidation of low-density lipoprotein and protects vision.
Green vegetables: Turnip, collard, and mustard; kale, spinach, broccoli. Green peas, kiwi, cilantro, parsley, lettuce. Corn; egg yolk.	Lutein and zeaxanthin (terpenes)	Antioxidants; anti-inflammatory; DNA repair. Good for healthy vision (protects against macular degeneration). Raw spinach is higher than cooked. Lutein may improve skin health and protect against skin cancer.
Leafy greens	Folic acid	Role in DNA synthesis, mitosis, and gene expression.
Legumes, whole grains, bananas, fish, chicken	Vitamin B_6	Supports a healthy immune system and increases lymphocyte numbers.
Licorice *Glycyrrhiza uralensis* and orange *Citrus* spp.	Coumarins; benzo-alpha-pyrones	Inhibits proteolysis and lipoxygenase; anti-inflammatory and antitumor effects.
Milk and dairy products, fish, liver	Vitamin A	Protects cells against free radical damage.
Nuts, nut butters, wheat germ, whole grains, oils, mayonnaise, creamy salad dressings, egg yolks, cereals, seeds	Vitamin E	Increases antibody production and B- and T-cell functioning; protects cells against free radical damage. SELECT study found that a 400 IU supplement actually promotes prostate cancer.
Oats	Avenanthramides; selenium	These polyphenols have strong antioxidant, anti-inflammatory properties (Meydani, 2009).

(continued)

TABLE 13-2 Phytochemicals, Functional Food Ingredients, and Cancer *(continued)*

Food	Functional Ingredient	Possible Roles in Reducing Cancer Risk
Oats, lima beans, navy beans, black beans, Brussels sprouts, ground psyllium seeds, peas, carrots, apples, barley, pectins, gums, mucilages	Soluble fiber	May lower cancer risk; helps lower cholesterol levels.
Olive and canola oils; tree nuts	MUFAs	Monounsaturated fats decrease tumorigenesis. Virgin olive oil phenols may reduce colorectal carcinogenesis.
Onions, garlic (particularly oil), leeks, chives, scallions, shallots	Allium and allicin (allyl sulfides, *S*-allylcysteine [SAC])	Organosulfurs decrease tumor cell growth; inhibit kinase activity; may protect the immune system, assist the liver in rendering carcinogens harmless, and reduce cholesterol production in the liver. Diallyl sulfide (DAS) inhibits the effects of PhIP that can cause DNA damage or transform substances into carcinogens.
Onions, garlic, leeks, shallots, inulin, Jerusalem artichokes, fructooligosaccharides (FOS); polydextrose in whole grains, some fruits, honey	Prebiotics	Support GI health and improve calcium absorption. Inulin may help protect against colon cancer.
Orange, grapefruit, lemon; cherries; citrus fruit peel	Limonoids/limonene (Terpenes); Naringenin, Hesperetin, Eriodictyol (flavanones)	Citrus glycosides decrease bacterial and fungal growth; decrease cancer cell growth by detoxifying enzymes in liver. Also cause cell apoptosis with certain types of cancers. Stimulate DNA repair with naringenin. Avoid grapefruit in estrogen+ breast cancer.
Oranges, grapefruit, lemons, tangerines, peaches, apricots, broccoli, tomatoes	Bioflavonoids, vitamin C	Minimizes damage to neutrophils; induces apoptosis; inhibits histamine
Pomegranate fruit and juice	Punicalagin (phenolic acid)	Potent antioxidant; protective against prostate cancer.
Red pepper, paprika	Capsaicin (8-methyl-*N*-vanillyl-6-nonenamide)	Red peppers of the genus *Capsicum*; it contains carotenoids that may be protective against cancer.
Salmon, mackerel, sardines	Coenzyme Q10 (ubiquinone) Omega-3 fatty acids	May reduce chemotherapy-related heart damage.
Seafood, canola oil, walnuts, flaxseed, marine and other fish oils	Omega-3 PUFAs	Reduce inflammation; may reduce cancer cachexia. Genetic variations affect response of COX-2 and its inflammatory impact on cancers such as prostate.
Soybean, corn and safflower oils	Omega-6 PUFAs	Keep omega-6 to omega-3 at a ratio of 5–10:1.
Soybeans (tofu, vegetable soy milk, soy nuts); legumes such as chick peas, beans, peas; nuts; grain products, coffee, tea; raisins and currants	Isoflavones: genistein, daidzein, biochanin A	Phytoestrogens attach to estrogen receptors and block real estrogen. Red clover and soy extracts contain isoflavones, with high affinity to estrogen receptor-alpha (ERα), estrogen receptor-beta (ERβ), progesterone receptor (PR), and androgen receptor (AR). Daily dose may be 40–50 milligrams of isoflavones (biochanin A, daidzein, formononetin, and genistein). Avoid excesses.
Spices: Cumin and turmeric, ginger, mint, rosemary, garlic, thyme, oregano, sage, basil, coriander, caraway, fennel, chili powder, black pepper, mint	Myricetin	Neutralizes free radicals, supports antioxidant defense system; preserves alpha-tocopherol, decreases inflammation; decreases ATPase; protects plasma DNA from radiation damage. May protect against prostate cancer.
Supplements, herbal	Astralgus, Echinacea, Silymarin	May increase macrophage activity and enhance immunity (interferon, killer cells, Interleukin-2). Silymarin protects the liver.
Sweet potatoes, carrots, turnips, spinach, papaya, tomato, red or green bell peppers, oranges	Retinoids; beta carotene	Important for cell growth, differentiation and death. May prevent some leukemias. Sweet potatoes are high in fiber, potassium, choline, vitamin C, magnesium, iron, and calcium as well.
Tomatoes and tomato products, ketchup, peppers; pink grapefruit; watermelon	Lycopene; vitamin C	Potent antioxidant; may reduce risk of prostate cancer. Tomato products must be cooked.
Vegetable oils, soy, peanuts, rice bran	Sterols: beta-sitosterol, campesterol, stigmasterol, squalene	Can reduce the risk of lung cancer and may reduce the tumor growth of other cancers. Sterols are found in vegetable oils. Sitosterol is the most studied.
Walnuts	Phytosterols, omega-3 fatty acid (ALA)	Antioxidant, anti-inflammatory properties that reduce tumor growth.
Wheat germ, lean beef, seafood, black-eyed peas	Zinc	Increases neutrophil function and killer cell numbers; decreases cytokines.
Whole grains, beans, seeds (soybeans, oats, barley, brown rice, whole wheat, flaxseed)	Phytates; insoluble fiber; vitamin E	Decreases oxidative damage to cells. Reduces the risk for breast or colon cancer.

(continued)

TABLE 13-2 Phytochemicals, Functional Food Ingredients, and Cancer *(continued)*

Food	Functional Ingredient	Possible Roles in Reducing Cancer Risk
Whole grains	Oligosaccharides; protease inhibitors	These increase short-chain fatty acid formation; decrease cholesterol and lower insulin levels; inhibit action of protein-splitting enzymes. May prevent cancer cell formation or decrease tumor size.
Wine, red grapes, grape juice, peanuts	Resveratrol; stilbenes (flavonoids)	Phytoalexin produced in plants in response to exposure to ultraviolet light or fungi. Decreases platelet activity, lowers cholesterol, suppresses proliferation of a variety of tumor cells.
Yogurt with *Lactobacilli, Bifidobacteria*; fermented milk such as Kefir.	Probiotic bacteria	Normalizes the intestinal microflora, blocks the invasion of potential pathogens in the gut, prevents colon cancer, modulates immune function, inhibits *H. pylori*, enhances calcium absorption; synthesizes niacin, folic acid, vitamin B_6, and biotin.

REFERENCES

American Cancer Society (ACS). Accessed December 31, 2009, at http://www.cancer/org

Gerhauser C. Cancer chemopreventive potential of apples, apple juice, and apple components. *Planta Med.* 74:1608, 2008.

International Food Information Council. Functional foods fact sheet: antioxidants Accessed December 30, 2009, at http://www.foodinsight.org/Resources/Detail.aspx?topic=Functional_Foods_Fact_Sheet_Antioxidants.

Linus Pauling Institute. Micronutrient information center. Accessed January 1, 2010, at http://lpi.oregonstate.edu/infocenter/index.html.

Medline Plus. Antioxidants. Accessed January 1, 2010, at http://www.nlm.nih.gov/medlineplus/antioxidants.html.

Meydani M. Potential health benefits of avenanthramides of oats. *Nutr Rev.* 67:731, 2009.

Seeram NP. Berry fruits for cancer prevention: current status and future prospects. *J Agric Food Chem.* 56:630, 2008.

USDA Phytochemical Database. Dr. Duke's Phytochemical and Ethnobotanical Databases. Accessed January 1, 2010, at http://www.ars-grin.gov/duke/index.html.

TABLE 13-3 Cancer Risk Factors by Site

Factors That are Known to Increase the Risk of Cancer

Cigarette Smoking and Tobacco Use

- Acute myelogenous leukemia (AML).
- Bladder cancer.
- Cervical cancer.
- Esophageal cancer.
- Kidney cancer.
- Lung cancer.
- Oral cavity cancer.
- Pancreatic cancer.
- Stomach cancer.

Infections

- Human papillomavirus (HPV) increases the risk for cancers of the cervix, penis, vagina, anus, and oropharynx.
- Hepatitis B and hepatitis C viruses increase the risk for liver cancer.
- Epstein-Barr virus increases the risk for Burkitt lymphoma.
- Helicobacter pylori increases the risk for gastric cancer.

Two vaccines to prevent infection by cancer-causing agents have already been developed and approved by the U.S. Food and Drug Administration (FDA). One is a vaccine to prevent infection with the hepatitis B virus. The other protects against infection with strains of human papillomavirus (HPV) that cause cervical cancer. Scientists continue to work on vaccines against infections that cause cancer.

Radiation

- Ultraviolet radiation from sunlight: This is the main cause of nonmelanoma skin cancers.
- Ionizing radiation from medical X-rays and radon gas in our homes: Scientists believe that ionizing radiation causes leukemia, thyroid cancer, and breast cancer in women. Ionizing radiation may also be linked to myeloma and cancers of the lung, stomach, colon, esophagus, bladder, and ovary.

Factors That May Affect the Risk of Cancer

Alcohol

- Oral cancer.
- Esophageal cancer.
- Breast cancer.
- Colorectal cancer (in men).
- Liver cancer
- Female colorectal cancer.

Diet

Foods may protect against cancer and other foods may increase the risk of cancer.

- Fruits and nonstarchy vegetables may protect against cancers of the mouth, esophagus, and stomach.
- Fruits may protect against lung cancer.
- Diet high in fat, protein, calories and red meat may increase risk of colorectal cancer, but studies have not confirmed this.
- It is not known if a diet low in fat and high in fruits, vegetables and fiber lowers the risk of colorectal cancer.

Physical Inactivity

- Colorectal cancer
- Postmenopausal breast cancer
- Endometrial cancer.

Obesity

- Postmenopausal breast cancer.
- Colorectal cancer.
- Endometrial cancer.
- Esophageal cancer.
- Kidney cancer.
- Pancreatic cancer.
- Gallbladder cancer

Adapted from: National Cancer Institute, http://www.cancer.gov/cancertopics/pdq/prevention/overview/Patient/page3, accessed December 29, 2009.

For More Information on Cancer Prevention

- Cancer Prevention and Control
  http://www.cdc.gov/cancer/
- Cancer Research and Prevention
  http://www.preventcancer.org/
- Complementary Treatments for Cancer
  http://nccam.nih.gov/health/cancer/
- Patient Advocate Foundation
  http://www.patientadvocate.org
- Wellness Community
  http://www.thewellnesscommunity.org/

REFERENCES

Aggarwal BB, Shishodia S. Suppression of the nuclear factor-kappaB activation pathway by spice-derived phytochemicals: reasoning for seasoning. *Ann N Y Acad Sci.* 1030:434, 2004.

American Dietetic Association. Position paper on functional foods. *J Am Diet Assoc.* 109:735, 2009.

Chun OK, et al. Estimation of antioxidant intakes from diet and supplements in U.S. adults [Published online ahead of print December 23, 2009]. *J Nutr.*

Kauwell GP. Emerging concepts in nutrigenomics: a preview of what is to come. *Nutr Clin Pract.* 20:75, 2005.

Patil BS, et al. Bioactive compounds: historical perspectives, opportunities, and challenges. *J Agric Food Chem.* 57:8142, 2009.

Wardwell L, et al. Nutrient intake and immune function of elderly subjects. *J Am Diet Assoc.* 108:2005, 2008.

Williams MT, Hord NG. The role of dietary factors in cancer prevention: beyond fruits and vegetables. *Nutr Clin Pract.* 20:451, 2005.

CANCER TREATMENT AND TIPS FOR LONG-TERM SURVIVAL

CANCER: TREATMENT GUIDELINES

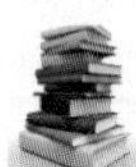

DEFINITIONS AND BACKGROUND

Cancer patients can be divided into three groups: those receiving standard or experimental therapy, those who have become unresponsive to these therapies, and those in remission who are at risk for recurrence or a second new cancer. Cancer cachexia—a wasting syndrome characterized by weight loss, anorexia, early satiety, progressive debilitation, and malnutrition—may lead to organ dysfunction and death (Mattox, 2005). Fatigue is the most common experience among cancer patients. Otherwise, each type of cancer has its own set of treatments and side effects.

TABLE 13-4 Use of Nutrition Support in Cancer Patients

ASPEN Cancer Guideline Updated (2009)

Nutrition support therapy should not be used **routinely** in patients undergoing major cancer operations. • Grade: A

Perioperative nutrition support therapy may be beneficial in moderately or severely malnourished patients if administered for 7–14 days preoperatively, but the potential benefits of nutrition support must be weighed against the potential risks of the nutrition support therapy itself and of delaying the operation. • Grade: A

Nutrition support therapy should not be used **routinely** as an adjunct to chemotherapy. • Grade: B

Nutrition support therapy should not be used **routinely** in patients undergoing head and neck, abdominal, or pelvic irradiation. • Grade: B

Nutrition support therapy is appropriate in patients receiving active anticancer treatment who are malnourished and who are anticipated to be unable to ingest and/or absorb adequate nutrients for a prolonged period of time. • Grade: B

The palliative use of nutrition support therapy in terminally ill cancer patients is rarely indicated. • Grade: B

Omega-3 fatty acid supplementation may help to stabilize weight in cancer patients on oral diets experiencing progressive, unintentional weight loss. • Grade: B

Indications for Enteral Feeding	Contraindications for Enteral Feeding
Inability to consume 50% of estimated needs orally for 1 week or longer—estimated or actual	Severe malabsorption that cannot be corrected with enteral nutrition
Functioning gastrointestinal (GI) tract with adequate capacity for nutrient absorption	Intestinal obstruction below feeding placement site
Patient willingness to use tube feeding method	Condition such as high-output fistula or high aspiration risk

Adapted from: ASPEN Guidelines. http://www.nutritioncare.org/wcontent.aspx?id=4054, accessed January 1, 2010.
Dixon SW. Nutrition care issues in the ambulatory (outpatient) head and neck cancer. *Support Line.* 27:3, 2005.

Weight loss and cachexia are common. Malnourished cancer patients commonly have high protein turnover and loss of nitrogen, significant loss of muscle mass, and impaired physical capacity. Tumor factors such as proteolysis-inducing factor (PIF), tumor necrosis factor (TNF), and lipid mobilizing factor (LMF) all tend to promote catabolism. Nutritional inadequacy mobilizes protein stores and, thus, causes a loss of lean body mass. Altered nutrient utilization causes glucose intolerance, insulin resistance, increased glucose turnover, lipolysis, hyperlipidemia, and increased protein turnover. Properly nourishing patients, particularly when malnourished, is essential therapy. The Subjective Global Assessment tool and scoring sheet is used for cancer patients. Indications for use of nutrition support are listed in Table 13-4. Parenteral nutrition (PN) should not be used to prolong life for patients at the end stages of disease but may be appropriate for patients with responsive cancers when enteral and oral feedings are poorly tolerated.

Many cancer therapies cause unpleasant side effects. Table 13-5 defines the types of side effects and treatments in cancer therapy. Patients who are unresponsive to standard or experimental therapies have few treatment options and usually experience poor quality of life for the remainder of their lives. An active nutritional protocol including high doses of multiple dietary antioxidants (vitamin C, alpha-tocopherol, and natural beta-carotene), when administered as an adjunct to other therapies, may increase tumor response and decrease toxicity. A maintenance nutritional protocol with lower doses of antioxidants, in addition to a modified diet and lifestyle, may reduce the risk of recurrence of the original tumor and development of a second cancer among survivors.

TABLE 13-5 Side Effects of Treatment and Common Problems of Cancer

Side Effect	Comments
Anemias	About half of the patients coming to cancer treatment are anemic. Use a balanced diet with high-quality proteins, B-complex vitamins, and vitamin C. Eat small meals every 2–3 hours. Heme sources of iron will increase iron bioavailability. Use beef, chicken, fortified grains, dried fruits such as prunes, nuts, and seeds, and blackstrap molasses. Avoid the long-term use of iron supplementation.
Anorexia	Medications, GI distress, altered sensory experiences often leads to cachexia. Treat symptoms, such as pain, constipation, and GI symptoms. Encourage small, frequent feedings. Consider pharmacological therapy with appetite-enhancing medications. Rinse mouth with baking soda or water before eating. Ginger ale or mint can mask metallic tastes; use plastic utensils if needed. Add flavorings to food, or suck on hard candy. Try chilled, frozen, sweet, or tart foods. Avoid unpleasant odors.
Aversion to foods or flavors	A lower threshold for urea causes aversion to meat; it "smells rotten." Substitute milk, cottage cheese, eggs, peanut butter, legumes, poultry, fish, and cheese. In addition, patient may have a decreased ability to taste salt and sugar. Add other seasonings, sauces, and more salt or sugar as desired by the patient; however, do not allow sweet foods to replace nourishing foods. Clear palate prior to meals by brushing teeth, gums, and oral cavity. Rinse with baking soda and salt water.
Cachexia	Cachexia is the clinical consequence of a chronic, systemic inflammatory response. Depletion of skeletal muscle and redistribution of the body's protein occur. Nutritional deprivation at diagnosis can lead to further depletion with treatments. Anorexia cachexia syndrome (ACS) is caused by numerous factors. Use small, frequent feedings and supplements. Teach ways to increase calories and protein. Fortify foods when possible. Relieve symptoms before meals whenever possible. Anabolic and anticatabolic agents, such as Megace and Oxandrin, may help. Use of omega-3 fatty acids (EPA and DHA) can disrupt the cachexia.
Chemotherapy	With all types (given daily, weekly, monthly for 1–2 months or even years), prompt attention to side effect management and appropriate use of supportive care (medications, nutrition, etc.) will be needed. Increase fluid intake for adequate hydration. After chemotherapy, cardiac, kidney, or pulmonary toxicity may occur. Some chemotherapy agents may cause infertility in both men and women. Nausea and vomiting can now be well controlled with Zofran (ondansetron), Kytril (granisetron), and Anzemet (dolasetron). Hemopoietic agents (e.g., Neupogen, Procrit, granulocyte colony-stimulation factor, granulocyte-macrophage colony-stimulating factor) may be needed if red blood cell production is too low; transfusions are a last resort. Avoid the risk of infection and cuts during chemotherapy. Monitor for nosebleeds, bruising, black or bloody stools, or reddish urine. Glutamine supplementation has been used with some success.
Cold food preference	Cold foods may be better accepted than hot foods. Use cold, clear fluids, carbonated beverages, ices, gelatin, watermelons, grapes and peeled cucumbers, cold meat platters, ice cream, and salted nuts. Serve supplements over ice between meals. Shakes, puddings, and custards are other alternatives.
Constipation	Establish an appropriate bowel program, including regular use of pharmacological agents. Add fiber and extra fluids to the diet. Milk is beneficial, if tolerated. Fresh or dried fruits, all vegetables, bran and a hot drink may help. Get adequate exercise, such as walking. Drink hot beverages, or use prunes or prune juice. Over-the-counter bulking agents may be useful in some cases. Avoid gas-forming foods in excess. Report any blood, vomiting, or no stool for 3+ days to the doctor.
Dental Caries	Avoid sweets and use sodium fluoride three times daily. Mouth care should be provided several times daily. Persons receiving irradiation to the head and neck area may benefit from use of fluoride trays and stannous fluoride.

(continued)

TABLE 13-5 Side Effects of Treatment and Common Problems of Cancer *(continued)*

Side Effect	Comments
Diarrhea	Evaluate all medications carefully. Assess hydration status and associated symptoms. Alter fiber in diet. Beware of lactose intolerance secondary to disease process, drug therapy, or abdominal or pelvic radiation therapy. Increase fluids that contain sodium and potassium; use of Gatorade or Pedialyte may be helpful. Use cool or room temperature foods. Avoid dairy products if lactose-intolerant. Consume small amounts of food throughout the day instead of three large meals. Decrease fatty, spicy, or acidic foods; caffeine; gas-forming vegetables; or carbonated beverages. Plain rice, potatoes, eggs, mild fish or skinless chicken may be well tolerated. Limit sorbitol and sugar substitutes. Oral glutamine may be useful.
Difficulty swallowing (dysphagia)	Modify diet consistency and follow swallowing techniques provided by speech pathologist. Use moist foods; add sauces or gravies. Semi-solid foods may be better tolerated than liquids, and pureed foods rather than regular items. Patient should sip fluids throughout meal. To prevent aspiration, try placing liquid under the tongue. Some patients find that tilting their heads back helps. Thickeners are available for liquids, if thin beverages are not tolerated well (as with choking, coughing with each swallow). Use of a straw may be beneficial. Spoons are easier to control than forks in the mouth. Avoid very hot or very cold foods. Chew sugarless gum or candy. Use artificial saliva if needed. Consider feeding tube if needed.
Dry mouth (xerostomia)	Surgical removal of salivary glands, atrophy of mucous membranes, or permanent damage from radiation to salivary glands may cause difficulty in eating and swallowing. Use salivary substitutes, lip balm, sugarless gum and candies, gravies, and sauces. Increase fluids and use softened, moist foods (custard, stews, and soups). Cut food into small pieces, or use pureed foods. Ice chips and popsicles also can help. Avoid salty foods. Tart foods, lemon drops, and lemonade may help to stimulate saliva production; avoid tart items if there are oral lesions. Sip on water or other fluids frequently throughout the day and with each bite of food. Synthetic saliva products such as Optimoist or MouthKote may help. Patients benefit from a thorough dental examination before treatment. Use fluoride trays, rinses, other measures. Avoid caffeine, alcohol and tobacco products. Salagen (pilocarpine) is approved to reduce radiation-related dry mouth.
Early Satiety	Rather than serving plain water, encourage a calorie-containing beverage. Take liquids between meals. Avoid fatty, greasy foods because they are more slowly digested and absorbed. Use small meals and frequent snacks between meals. Add protein and calories using extra butter, margarine, cheese, dry milk powder.
Edema	Fluid retention may require elevating the legs at rest, staying physically active (walking), and reducing salt intake overall. The doctor may prescribe a diuretic.
Fatigue	Fatigue is very common. Assess and treat causes such as anemia, infection, pain, neutropenia, depression, or medication side effects. Meals may be prepared in quantity when the patient is less tired. Use foods that require less chewing and provide frequent rest periods, particularly before meals. Exercise daily to build stamina. Maintain adequate sleep/nap patterns.
Graft-versus-host disease (GVHD), neutropenia	Fever, chills, sweating, coughing, shortness of breath, diarrhea. Avoid people with colds or flu. Wash hands frequently and use safe food handling procedures. Wash all produce carefully and cook thoroughly. Avoid raw eggs. Cook meats well.
Insulin resistance	Insulin resistance is common from the tumor itself, or may occur after pancreatic surgery. Control of CHO intake and oral agents may be indicated.
Loneliness, Emotional Changes	Social eating may improve food intake. Visitors should be encouraged to bring gifts of food, as appropriate. If anxiety occurs, discuss with healthcare provider.
Loss of lean body mass	Protein wasting and unintentional weight loss are common. Exercise is extremely helpful. Endurance activities can counteract loss of physical performance and improve lower and upper body strength. Patients who exercise also have less fatigue and depression. Taking hormones such as growth hormone, insulin-like growth factor (IGF-I), thyroid hormone, androgens, and cortisol makes a difference as well. Muscle protein synthesis can be increased accordingly.
Malabsorption	Elemental diets can only be used if patient has an intact duodenum and jejunum. Total parenteral nutrition should be used only in some cases, considering risk of infection. Tart beverages such as lemonade can be mixed with elemental products if they are to be taken orally.
Meal interruptions	Encourage a good breakfast and snacks to make up for interrupted meals. Keep kitchen well stocked. Meals-on-Wheels may be a useful way to serve meals to this population at home.
Mouth blindness (dysgeusia)	To alleviate disinterest and aversion to foods, emphasize the aroma and colors of foods. Foods that are served warm or hot have more flavor and aroma. Provide a variety of foods and use garnishes. Acidic foods (such as lemonade) may help stimulate patient's ability to taste foods. Use highly flavored foods and sauces. Try milk shakes that are coffee or mint flavored. Fresh vegetables, special breads, highly flavored snacks, olives and pickles may be well received.
Mouth or throat soreness or dry mouth (stomatitis, mucositis, esophagitis)	Swish mouth with lidocaine, mild saline, or sodium bicarbonate before meals. Changes in taste or enjoyment of foods may occur. Avoid acidic juices, salty foods or soups, dry toast, and coarse or grainy breads or cereals. Grind meats; use a "mechanical soft diet" as needed. Offer cold or tepid fluids frequently; use a straw if needed. Popsicles may help. Smaller meals are useful. Cut foods into small pieces; grind or puree if needed. Mix food with sauces or gravies to make it easier to swallow. Avoid smoking and use of alcohol. Oral glutamine has been used with some success. Avoid alcohol-based mouthwashes. Salagen (pilocarpine) reduces dry mouth and throat sprays or cough drops may be useful.

(continued)

TABLE 13-5 **Side Effects of Treatment and Common Problems of Cancer *(continued)***

Side Effect	Comments
Muscle wasting	Muscle weakness is frequently associated with tumor growth. Include adequate amounts of protein and amino acids in the diet or in enteral feeding, particularly arginine, glutamine and leucine. Depression, altered moods, immobility, and bed rest contribute to loss of muscle mass. Structured exercise, including resistance training and aerobic exercises, can improve muscle mass and strength. Increased physical activity improves emotional stability, self-confidence, and independence. Active patients have less fatigue, nausea, and insomnia; quality of life improves.
Nausea	Treated with slow, deep breathing, ice chips, or sips of ginger ale, tea, or candied dried ginger. Try a dry diet with liquids between meals. Eat small meals; rest upright afterward. Offer toast, yogurt, sherbet, popsicles, pretzels, angel food cake, canned fruit, baked chicken, lemonade, hot cereal such as oatmeal, clear liquids, or broth. Cut down on greasy, spicy, fried, fatty foods; foods with strong odors and excessive sweetness. Sit upright for meals and snacks; avoid tight clothing. If breakfast is the best meal, it can also be the largest of the day. Keep crackers or light snacks at hand; do not skip meals. Use antiemetics as directed by physician; underusage may aggravate the nausea. Drink plenty of water/liquids the day before and after chemotherapy.
Pain	Prevention is the key. Give pain medications with the first few bites of a meal or have the patient eat when pain is lowest. Encourage trying foods again after time lapse. Try biofeedback, acupuncture, massage, muscle relaxation techniques. Keep a pain journal and report any side effects to the doctor.
Radiation therapy	Radiotherapy may involve high-energy radiation from x-rays, cobalt-60, or radium. Brachytherapy provides internal, continuous local delivery of radiation to site of malignancy (concealed). Teletherapy provides external radiation to a localized area; 7000 rads usually causes damage, particularly to small intestine (radiation enteritis). Radiation therapy (daily for 2–8 weeks) can cause nausea or vomiting if administered to the brain or abdominal/pelvic fields. A light meal is encouraged before treatment. Diarrhea may occur in radiation enteritis; glutamine may be useful in supplements or in tube feeding (TF)/CPN. Formulas containing multiple antioxidants for biological protection against radiation damage in humans are needed. Use of oral glutamine has been used with some success. **In head and neck cancer: anorexia, dysgeusia, weight loss, odynophagia, dysphagia, difficulty chewing, xerostomia. In the thorax: nausea, esophagitis, vomiting. In abdominal, intestinal: lactose intolerance, diarrhea, distention, abdominal pain, nausea and vomiting; later–intestinal stenosis, edema, fluid and electrolyte loss, weight loss.
Radiation enteritis or colitis	About 50–80% of patients who have radiation to the pelvis end up with radiation enteritis; onset can occur up to years later. Symptoms include nausea, vomiting, mucoid diarrhea, abdominal pain, and bleeding; later, there may be colic, a decrease in stool caliber, and progressive obstipation with stricture and fibrosis. Serious injury to the intestinal epithelium and arterioles of the small or large intestines results in cell death, fibrosis, and obstruction. Radiation to the ileum is particularly devastating. If radiation must be given chronically, resection may be needed and the ability of the intestines to become hyperplastic and increase absorptive capacity is thus prevented. Of these persons, many will require home CPN.
Surgery, curative	Direct efforts at restoring nutritional health to pre-illness status. After GI surgery, effects include—Oropharynx: Difficulty with chewing and swallowing, dysgeusia, xerostomia. Esophagus: Heartburn, loss of normal swallowing, decreased motility, obstruction. Stomach: Dumping syndrome, delayed emptying, anemia, malabsorption. Small intestines: Lactose intolerance, bile acid depletion, steatorrhea, fat malabsorption, vitamin B_{12} deficiency and anemia, short-gut syndrome. Colon: Loss of electrolytes and water; diarrhea, constipation, gas, bloating.
Thick saliva	Thick, ropy saliva can produce more caries. Use less bread, milk, gelatin, and oily foods. Puree foods such as fruits and vegetables. Encourage the intake of plenty of fluids to decrease the viscosity of oral secretions. Encourage good oral intake and regular oral rinses.
Tooth loss	Loss of teeth makes the patient's mouth more sensitive to cold, heat, and sweets. Try serving foods at room temperature. Use ground, chopped, or pureed foods as needed until dental repair is possible.
Vomiting	Sip clear liquids every 10–15 minutes after vomiting episodes cease; keep head elevated. "Flat" carbonated beverages are useful. Call doctor if abdominal pains persist. Take antiemetic medications prior to meals. Use small feedings, avoid spicy or acidic foods and those with strong odor, use liquids between meals. Use low fat, light meals.
Weight loss	Calculate 40–45 kcal/kg for repletion. Add fats to foods, dry milk to mashed potatoes and shakes, and extra sugar to coffee and cereals. Use small, frequent feedings and the patient's favorite foods. Add cream sauces, extra meat or cheeses in casseroles, and gravies. Encourage patients to be as physically active as possible, particularly using long muscles to promote lean body mass.

Derived from: National Cancer Institute, http://www.cancer.gov/cancertopics/pdq/supportivecare/nutrition/Patient, accessed January 5, 2010.

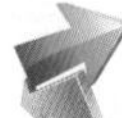

ASSESSMENT, MONITORING, AND EVALUATION

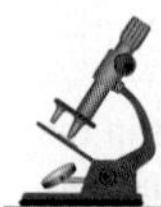

CLINICAL INDICATORS

Genetic Markers: HMGB1 protein—a danger signaling protein—can act as a proinflammatory and proangiogenic mediator when actively secreted by macrophages or passively released from necrotic cells; this plays an important role in the pathogenesis of cancer (Winter et al, 2009). Other genetics information for cancer can be found at http://www.cancer.gov/cancertopics/genetics-terms-alphalist/a-e.

Sample Clinical/History

- Height
- Weight
- Weight changes
- Body mass index (BMI)
- Diet history
- Input and output (I & O)
- Pain?
- Limited use of affected area
- Fatigue
- Warmth in a local area?
- Fever, temperature
- Cough
- X-ray
- Dual-energy x-ray absorptiometry (DEXA) scan
- Computed tomography (CT) scan or magnetic resonance imaging (MRI)

Lab Work

- Glucose (Gluc)
- Hemoglobin and hematocrit (H&H)
- Serum Fe, ferritin
- Serum folate, B_{12}, B_6
- Serum homocysteine
- Ca^{++}, Mg^{++}
- Na^+, K^+
- Albumin (Alb)
- C-reactive protein (CRP)
- Total lymphocyte count (TLC) (varies)

SAMPLE NUTRITION CARE PROCESS STEPS

Knowledge Deficit

Assessment: Medications, lab values, current use of herbs and botanical products.

Nutrition Diagnosis (PES): Knowledge deficit as evidenced by patients requesting information regarding the proper use of herbs and botanicals for cancer treatment.

Intervention: Education about herbs and botanical products in cancer; resources and Web sites; label reading. Counseling with responses to specific questions according to type of cancer, prevention versus treatment, side effects.

Monitoring and Evaluation: No reports of adverse side effects with herbs and botanicals, medications, or foods (such as allergic reactions).

INTERVENTION

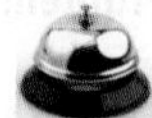

OVERALL OBJECTIVES IN CANCER TREATMENT

- Coordinate total care plan with doctor, nurse, patient, family, caregivers, and other team members.
- Review each case individually and honor patient's wishes regarding more aggressive intervention.
- Prevent or minimize weight changes. Some patients are hypometabolic; others are hypermetabolic by 10–30% above normal rates. Greatest losses occur from protein stores and body fat.
- Use indirect calorimetry to determine energy requirements; Resting Metabolic Rate (RMR) or Resting Energy Expenditure (REE) is measured after 30 minutes of recumbent rest, preferably fasting but not necessarily early in the morning, with as little physical activity as possible before the measurement (American Dietetic Association, 2010).
- Diminish toxicity of treatments and improve quality of life. Good nutritional status early on is a good prognostic indicator.
- Correct cachexia from weakness, anorexia, redistribution of host nutrients, and nutritional depletion.
- Prevent depletion of humoral and cellular immunity from malnutrition. Improved nutritional status may allow neoplastic cells to become more susceptible to medical treatment.
- An improved nutritional status reduces side effects, promotes better rehabilitation, and improves quality of life while perhaps increasing survival rates. Malnutrition can potentiate the toxicity of antineoplastic agents.
- Prevent infection or sepsis, further morbidity, or death.
- Control complications such as anemia or multiple organ dysfunction.
- Preserve body mass through structured exercise programs and specialized nutritional supplementation.
- Control gastrointestinal symptoms, which are more common with weight loss greater than 10%.
- Work with the interdisciplinary team using a sample algorithm (courtesy of RD411.com). (See Algorithm on page 743)

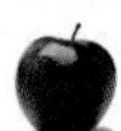

FOOD AND NUTRITION

- Determine cancer-specific energy and protein requirements (American Dietetic Association, 2010).
- If indirect calorimetry is not available, calculate energy as 30 kcal/kg body weight to maintain and 35–45 kcal/kg body weight to replete lost stores or if the patient is febrile, septic, or very active.
- In general, the intake of protein should be high (1–1.5 g/kg body weight to maintain; 1.5–2 g/kg body weight to replete lean body mass) to protect from muscle wasting, malnutrition, cachexia, and treatments.
- Provide appropriate and adequate, but not excessive, micronutrient supplementation. Avoid excesses of iron, but correct anemias when diagnosed. There is no evidence for use of vitamin E or arginine prior to radiation

INTERDISCIPLINARY NUTRITION CARE PLAN
Cancer

Client Name: ____________ **#:** ________ **Initiated by:** ________ **Date:** ________

SCREEN
Nutrition Screen diagnosis: Cancer
Signed: ____________ Date: ______

GOALS (Check any/all):

❑ Maintain or improve nutritional status in_____ (goal time).

❑ Prevent hospitalization due to dehydration/poor nutrional intake in _____ (goal time).

❑ Prevent or alleviate nutrition-related complications of cancer or cancer therapy in _____ (goal time).

❑ Avoid delay of cancer therapy due to poor nutrition in _____ (goal time).

ASSESS *(Check any/all)*
❑ **Receiving chemotherapy/radiation therapy**
❑ **Weight loss: _____lb/wk**
❑ **Receiving enteral or parenteral nutrition or complex diet order**
❑ **Dehydration**
Nutrition Impact Symptoms*
- ❑ Problems chewing/swallowing
- ❑ Mouth pain/dryness
- ❑ Nausea/vomiting
- ❑ Diarrhea/constipation
- ❑ Fatigue
- ❑ Anorexia
- ❑ Altered taste perception

Signed: ____________ Date: ______

None →

MODERATE RISK INTERVENTIONS
(Check any/all)
❑ **Build Up Your Diet** provided and explained
❑ **Food Record** provided and explained
❑ **Fluid intake** encouraged
Obtain Dr. orders as needed:
- ❑ RD chart consult
- ❑ Monitor weight q:_____
- ❑ BID/TID supplements

❑ **Other:** ____________
(See notes for documention.)

Signed: ____________ Date: ______

1 or more ↓

HIGH-RISK INTERVENTIONS *(Check any/all)*
❑ **Build Up Your Diet** provided and explained
❑ **Food Record** provided and explained
❑ **Fluid intake stressed**
Obtain Dr. orders as needed:
- ❑ RD referral for home visit(s)
- ❑ Monitor weight q:_____
- ❑ Monitor I & O q: _____
- ❑ BID/TID supplements

❑ **Other:** ____________
(See notes for documention.)

Signed: ____________ Date: ______

Next visit ↓

ASSESS RESPONSE *(Check any/all)*
❑ Further weight loss
❑ Exhibiting Nutrition Impact Symptoms*
❑ Dehydration
❑ **Other:** ____________
(See notes for documention.)

Signed: ____________ Date: ______

← 1 or more | None →

OUTCOMES ACHIEVED
❑ Weight stabilized or improved
❑ Hydration status maintained or improved
❑ Cancer therapy initiated without delay
❑ **Other:** ____________
(See notes for documention.)
❑ Repeat Nutrition Risk Screen in _____ days

Signed: ____________ Date: ______

Next visit ↓

ASSESS RESPONSE *(Check any/all)*
❑ Further weight loss
❑ Continued dehydration
❑ Exhibiting Nutrition Impact Symptoms*
❑ **Other:** ____________
(See notes for documention.)

Signed: ____________ Date: ______

None →

OUTCOMES ACHIEVED
❑ Weight stabilized or improved
❑ Hydration status maintained or improved
❑ Cancer therapy initiated without delay
❑ **Other:** ____________
(See notes for documention.)
❑ Repeat Nutrition Risk Screen in _____ days

Signed: ____________ Date: ______

1 or more ↓

OUTCOMES NOT ACHIEVED
Reassess/evaluate need for EN/PN (refer to Tube Feeding Nutrition Care Plan). Document on Nutrition Variance Tracking form.

or chemotherapy (American Dietetic Association, 2010). Use foods that are high in phytochemicals and antioxidants.
- Use adequate fluid for hydration.
- Schedule larger meals earlier in the day. If needed, schedule five to six small meals daily, with tube feeding or intravenous feeding. If the gut works, use it.
- Parenteral nutrition (PN) is not likely to benefit advanced cancer patients who are unresponsive to treatment and should be used with caution in current or potentially septic patients because of the risks (American Dietetic Association, 2010). Use CPN if enteral nutrition is contraindicated and if the patient is at low risk for infection.
- After surgery or abdominal radiation, glutamine may be useful to protect from enteropathy, lower morbidity, augment tumor cell kill, and boost natural killer (NK) cell activity.

Common Drugs Used and Potential Side Effects

- Drugs used will be matched to the specific type of cancer. Tables 13-6 and 13-7 list drugs and some common side effects.
- See the NCI list available at http://www.cancer.gov/drugdictionary/.

Herbs, Botanicals, and Supplements

- Answer questions about the use of herbs and botanicals in cancer treatment plans. Use of complementary and alternative medicine (CAM) therapy is common in the cancer population.
- Some products are harmless, but some may lead to serious problems. Table 13-8 describes herbs that are commonly used and some general comments.

TABLE 13-6 Cancer Drugs and Chemotherapy Agents

There are many chemotherapy drugs available. With chemotherapy, patients may suffer severe side effects such as nausea, hair loss, infection, and injury to the GI tract. Serotonin antagonists such as Anzemet (dolasetron), if administered at the same time as chemotherapy, can prevent nausea and vomiting, but abdominal pain, headache, and constipation may occur. Biologic therapies such as interferon and interleukin may cause flu-like symptoms and myalgias, shortness of breath, or edema. Monoclonal antibodies such as Herceptin and Rituxan are also used to treat cancer and may cause chills, fever, lethargy and muscle aches. With antineoplastic agents, side effects include nausea, anorexia, stomatitis, diarrhea, taste alterations, some vomiting, and possibly sloughing of colonic mucosa (see Table 13-7 also).

Drug	Description
Alkylating agents: cyclophosphamide, fluorouracil	These drugs kill cancer cells by stopping their growth or by making it hard for cancer cells to repair damage. Nausea, vomiting, hyperuricemia.
Antiangiogenic agent: humanized monoclonal antibody bevacizumab (Avastin)	Tumors require nutrients and oxygen in order to grow; angiogenesis provides access to these nutrients.
Antimetabolites: flucytosine	This is a DNA substrate analog that leads to incorrect DNA synthesis affecting the cancer cells. Nausea, vomiting, diarrhea, and stomatitis can occur.
Antiemetics: granisetron or ondansetron; medical cannabis, Marinol; domperidone, promethazine (Phenergan); metoclopramide (Reglan)	May be useful for anorexia/cachexia syndrome. Also used to relieve nausea and vomiting after chemotherapy. Headache may result. Other side effects include nausea, diarrhea, increased gastric emptying, or drowsiness.
Aspirin and anti-inflammatory agents	May prevent some types of cancer, including colon cancer. The use of herbal nonsteroidal anti-inflammatory drugs (NSAIDs) may be recommended with these medications to enhance effectiveness.
Irinotecan (Camptosar)	For the treatment of stage 1–4 breast, lung, prostate, colon, skin, and most other metastatic or nonmetastatic forms of cancer.
Corticosteroids: prednisone	Hyperglycemia, sodium and fluid retention, weight gain, and calcium losses can occur.
Folate antagonist: methotrexate	Use of folate preparations can alter drug response. Folate, lactose, vitamin B_{12}, and fat are less well absorbed. Mouth sores are common.
Immunotherapy: interleukin-2 and interferon	Lymphokine is administered to decrease tumor growth. Nausea, vomiting, abdominal pain, fatigue, and anorexia can result. In addition, low levels of folate and vitamins A and B_6 may result.
Monoclonal antibodies (MAbs): cetuximab, Campath-1 H, rituximab (Rituxan), and Bexxar	These drugs correct the abnormal enzyme that causes cancerous cells to grow out of control. These attack only abnormal elements of cells ("kinder and gentler" cancer therapies). Cetuximab specifically binds to the epidermal growth factor receptor with high affinity.
Vinca alkaloids: vincristine, vinblastine	Nausea and vomiting can occur.

Derived from: American Cancer Society, http://www.cancer.org/docroot/CDG/cdg_0.asp, accessed January 3, 2010.
Chemotherapy Drugs http://www.chemocare.com/BIO/.
National Cancer Institute http://www.cancer.gov/DRUGDICTIONARY/.
Oncology Channel http://www.oncologychannel.com/chemotherapy/medsideeffects.shtml.

TABLE 13-7 **Antineoplastic Agents: Generic and Brand Names**

Generic	Brand	Generic	Brand
Altretamine	Hexalen	Interferon-α2 a	Roferon-A
Asparaginase	Elspar	Interferon-α2b	Intron-A
Bevacizumab	Avastin	Interferon-αn3	Alferon-N
BCG	TheraCys, TICE BCG	Irinotecan	Camptosar
Bleomycin sulfate	Blenoxane	Leucovorin calcium	Wellcovorin
Busulfan	Myleran	Leuprolide	Lupron, Lupron-Depot
Carboplatin	Paraplatin	Levamisole	Ergamisol
Carmustine	BiCNU	Lomustine	CeeNU
Chlorambucil	Leukeran	Megestrol	Megace
Cisplatin (*cis*-platinum, *cis*-diammine-dichloroplatinum)	Platinol, Platinol-AQ	Melphalan, L-phenylalanine mustard, L-sarcolysin	Alkeran (R)
Cladribine, 2-chlorodeoxyadenosine	Leustatin	Melphalan hydrochloride	IV Alkeran
Cyclophosphamide	Cytoxan, Neosar	Mercaptopurine	Purinethol Tablets
Cytarabine, cytosine arabinoside	Cytosar-U	Mesna	Mesnex
Dacarbazine, imidazole carboxamide	DTIC-DME	Mechlorethamine, nitrogen mustard	Mustargen
Dactinomycin	Cosmegen	Methylprednisolone	Solumedrol, Medrol
Daunorubicin, daunomycin	Cerubidine	Methotrexate, amethopterin	Trexall
Dexamethasone	Decadron, Tobradex	Mitomycin	Mutamycin
Doxorubicin	Adriamycin	Mitoxantrone	Novantrone
Erlotinib	Tarceva	Paclitaxel	Taxol
Etoposide (epipodophyllotoxin)	VePesid	Plicamycin, mithramycin	Mithracin
Floxuridine	FUDR	Prednisone	Deltasone
Fludarabine	Fludara	Procarbazine	Matulane
Fluorouracil	Fluorouracil Injection	Streptozocin, streptozotocin	Zanosar
Fluoxymesterone	Halotestin	Tamoxifen	Nolvadex
Flutamide	Eulexin	6-Thioguanine	Tabloid
Goserelin	Zoladex	Thiotepa, triethylene thiophosphoramide	Thiotepa
Hydroxyurea	Hydrea	Vinblastine	Velban
Idarubicin HCL	Idamycin	Vincristine	Oncovin
Ifosfamide	IFEX	Vinorelbine tartrate	Navelbine Injection
Interferon-alfa	Roferon-A, Intron-A		

Source: Medicine Online. Antineoplastic agents generic abbreviations, http://www.medicineonline.com/reference/Health/Conditions_and_Diseases/Cancer, accessed January 3, 2010.

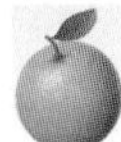

NUTRITION EDUCATION, COUNSELING, CARE MANAGEMENT

- Educate family about special patient needs (Dixon, 2005).
- There is evidence that cancer survivors who adopt a healthy lifestyle reap physical and emotional benefits. See Table 13-9 for more guidance and patient education tips.

Patient Education—Food Safety for Cancer Patients

- Clean: Wash hands and surfaces often.
- Separate: Don't cross-contaminate. Keep raw meat and poultry apart from cooked foods.
- Cook: Use a food thermometer to be sure meat and poultry are safely cooked.
- Chill: Refrigerate or freeze food promptly.
- Avoid:
  - Hot dogs, luncheon, and deli meats unless they are reheated until steaming hot.
  - Refrigerated plate, meat spreads from a meat counter, smoked seafood, and raw or undercooked seafood.
  - Raw (unpasteurized) milk and foods that contain unpasteurized milk.
  - Soft cheeses such as Feta, queso blanco, queso fresco, Brie, Camembert cheeses, blue-veined cheeses, and Panela unless it is labeled as made with pasteurized milk.
  - Salads made in the store such as ham salad, chicken salad, egg salad, tuna salad, or seafood salad.
  - Soft-boiled or "over-easy" eggs, as the yolks are not fully cooked.

TABLE 13-8 Herbs, Dietary Supplements, and Cancer

Most patients diagnosed with cancer explore complementary and alternative medicine (CAM), particularly herbal medicine. Dietetics professionals must evaluate the risks and benefits of the use of herbs and botanical products in various cancers; indicate whether **"guidance" or "promotion"** is being offered. Alternative therapies should be reviewed in the light of potential harm. Herbs should be appropriately labeled to alert consumers to potential interactions when used with drugs, and consultation with a general practitioner is recommended.

Ashwagandha (Withania somnifera)	Used for cancer treatment, diabetes, epilepsy, fatigue, gastrointestinal (GI) disorders, pain, rheumatoid arthritis (RA), skin infections, and stress.	Should not be used in pregnant women because it is an abortifacient.
Astragalus	Stimulates interferon and positively impacts the immune system. Possibly reduces the effectiveness of chemotherapy. Strong immune booster.	A type of legume used for years in Chinese medicine. No convincing evidence in cancer.
Black cohosh (Remifemin)	May relieve the symptoms of menopause. No known side effects with chemotherapy. Source of vitamin A and pantothenic acid. Drug interactions: may increase the toxicity of doxorubicin and docetaxel.	Used to lower hot flashes, which can be a challenge for breast cancer patients.
Bromelain	Bromelain (from pineapple extract) positively impacts the immune system. Improved tumor boundaries.	Studies have not demonstrated evidence in cancer therapy.
Cat's claw	May have some effect on the immune system, but more comprehensive studies are needed. Antioxidant.	Contains alkaloids.
Chamomile	No proven efficacy in cancer. May promote sedation or allergic reactions.	
Chili powder	Capsaicin may actually have tumor-promoting effects; chili powder has been implicated in several GI cancers, but the results are conflicting.	In Mexico, higher use of chili powder is related to more stomach cancer.
Chinese herbal medicine	Chinese herbal medicine uses a variety of herbs, in different combinations, to restore balance to the body.	See Astragalus, Ginkgo, Ginseng, Green tea, and Siberian ginseng.
Chinese PC-SPES	Contains chrysanthemum, isatis, licorice, Panax ginseng, saw palmetto, skullcap; Rabdosia rubescens is the most potent ingredient. PC-SPES contains flavonoids, alkaloids, polysaccharides, amino acids, and trace minerals such as selenium, calcium, magnesium, zinc, and copper.	Antiestrogenic effects.
Cloves	Contains eugenol, which reduces lipid peroxidation and reduces cancer cell proliferation.	
Dehydroepiandrosterone (DHEA)	DHEA is a steroid hormone produced by the adrenal gland and converted into estrogen and testosterone.	It is normally found in humans, plants, and animals. DHEA extracted from a wild yam plant is available as a dietary supplement.
Echinacea	No evidence of usefulness in reducing incidence or symptoms of cancer.	May reduce colds or flu for some people.
Eleuthero (Siberian ginseng)	May boost energy. More studies are needed.	
Essiac	Mixture of four herbs: burdock root (Arctium lappa), sheep sorrel (Rumex acetosella), slippery elm bark (Ulmus rubra), and Indian rhubarb root (Rheum officinale) to make a tea. Watercress (Nasturtium officinale R. Br.), blessed thistle (Cnicus benedictus L.), red clover (Trifolium pratense L.), and kelp (Laminaria digitata [Hudson] Lamx.) have been added to a product sold as Flor Essence.	Potent antioxidant and DNA-protective activity. Possibly estrogenic, antioxidant, anti-inflammatory, antimicrobial, and anticarcinogenic.
Evening primrose oil or gamma linolenic acid (GLA)	Proposed to reduce the effects of cancer treatments. GLA is an omega-6 unsaturated fatty acid made in the human body from other essential fatty acids. The main supplemental sources of GLA are oils of the seeds of evening primrose, borage, and black currant plants.	GLA is found in human breast milk. Claimed to slow cancer cell growth. Increases effectiveness of chemotherapy; boosts efficiency of tamoxifen; antioxidant; boosts immune system.
Falcarinol	A cancer-fighting substance found only in carrots.	Human studies are needed.
Flaxseed	Flaxseed supplements along with low-fat diets may be useful in men with early-stage prostate cancer.	Controlled clinical studies are needed.

(continued)

TABLE 13-8 Herbs, Dietary Supplements, and Cancer *(continued)*

Garlic	Seems to have reduced gastric and prostate cancers. Sulfur compounds tend to be the most chemoprotective. Useful in treatment as well as prevention. Garlic appears to induce cytochrome P-450 3A4 and may enhance metabolism of many medications such as cyclosporine and saquinavir. Antimicrobial properties are helpful.	Supplements are not as effective as real garlic for allicin and S-allylcysteine activity. Garlic poultices may cause burns in infants. Used as spice and to treat hyperlipidemia, hypertension, atherosclerosis, cancer, and infections, but sustained response has not been found. Mixed effects regarding reduction of blood glucose levels, blood pressure, or cardiovascular diseases. Garlic should not be used in patients on anticoagulants and patients with platelet dysfunction.
Ginger (6-gingerol)	May help to reduce the side effects of cancer treatments as an antiemetic, anti-inflammatory agent. Effective in preventing nausea and vomiting in some patients. It is a relatively safe herb, but patients taking blood thinners or about to undergo surgery should avoid ginger supplements. Interaction with many drugs including antacids, anticoagulants and antiplatelets, antidiabetics, antihypertensives, H_2 blockers, proton pump inhibitors (PPI), and barbiturates.	Ginger may be effective in treating chemotherapy-induced nausea and vomiting.
Ginkgo biloba (maidenhair tree)	Antioxidant and anti-inflammatory effects; role in cancer is being studied (see Table 13-2). Stimulates blood circulation and helps improve memory.	Ginkgo causes bleeding when combined with warfarin or aspirin (acetylsalicylic acid), raises blood pressure when combined with a thiazide diuretic, and causes coma when combined with trazodone. Lowers the threshold for seizures in seizure-prone individuals.
Ginseng, Asian (Panax ginseng)	The dried roots of the plants are used in some traditional medicines to treat a variety of conditions, including cancer. Rh2 is a ginsenoside extracted from ginseng that has effects on cell proliferation, induction of apoptosis, and stimulation of natural killer cells and other immune activity.	Asian ginseng may prevent some cancers. Proposed to give strength and stamina. Interactions with monoamine oxidase (MAO) inhibitors.
Ginseng, American (Panax quinquefolius)	A plant with similar (but not exactly the same) properties, is grown mainly in the United States.	Used for health maintenance, strength, stamina, and immunostimulation. Contraindicated in patients with hypertension and in premenopausal women.
Glucarate (calcium glucarate)	Proponents claim that glucarate may reduce the risk of colon, lung, liver, skin, prostate, and other cancers by increasing the body's ability to eliminate cancer-causing toxins that come from diet and the environment. May help the body remove excess estrogen and other hormones that promote these diseases.	Glucarate is found in many fruits and vegetables including apples, grapefruit, broccoli, Brussels sprouts, and bean sprouts. It also occurs naturally in the body in very small amounts.
Green tea (Camellia sinesis)	Contains polyphenols and may slow the delivery of nutrients to cancer cells by inhibiting the formation of new blood vessels (angiogenesis). Recent research has focused on green tea for the prevention of breast, prostate, skin, esophagus, stomach, colon, pancreas, lung, and bladder cancers.	The use of skin products that contain green tea may be somewhat protective against skin cancers. Epigallocatechin gallate (EGCG). EGCG may cause cancer cells to die and may stop new blood vessels from forming, thereby cutting off the supply of blood to cancer cells. Do not use with pregnant or lactating mothers. Use with caution with many drugs particularly anticoagulants.
Isatis root (Ban lan gen, Radix isatidis baphicacanthi, Isatis tinctoria, Isatis indigotica)	Used for common cold, sore throat, mumps, respiratory ailments, and malignant tumors. Leaves are used in one of the herbal formulas to treat prostate cancer. No adverse reactions known.	This herb is also used to treat chronic myelogenous leukemia. Studies also indicate that this plant has antiviral and immunostimulatory effects.
Licorice	Licorice root is an ingredient in many traditional Chinese herbal remedies. More research is needed to find out whether licorice extract has any role in cancer prevention or treatment.	May cause serious side effects, including hypertension or muscle weakness or paralysis.

(continued)

TABLE 13-8 Herbs, Dietary Supplements, and Cancer *(continued)*

Lipoic acid (alpha lipoic acid)	Lipoic acid plays an important role in metabolism. Recent research has shown that it is beneficial in treating nerve damage in diabetics. It may be helpful for other conditions as well. There is currently no evidence that lipoic acid prevents the development or spread of cancer.	Lipoic acid is an antioxidant found in certain foods including red meat, spinach, broccoli, potatoes, yams, carrots, beets, and yeast. It is also made in small amounts in the human body. Its possible role as a form of complementary therapy to reduce the side effects of radiation therapy or chemotherapy is still unclear.
Lyprinol (green-lipped mussel)	This is a fatty acid complex extracted from Perna canaliculus—a green-lipped mussel (shellfish) native to New Zealand. It contains omega-3 fatty acids. Lyprinol is promoted as a dietary supplement with anti-inflammatory properties to work against leukotrienes.	It is available in capsule form as a dietary supplement.
Macrobiotic diet	The standard macrobiotic diet today consists of 50–60% organically grown whole grains, 20–25% locally and organically grown fruits and vegetables, and 5–10% soups made with vegetables, seaweed, grains, beans, and miso (a fermented soy product). Early versions of the diet included no animal products at all.	Potatoes, tomatoes, eggplant, peppers, asparagus, spinach, beets, zucchini, and avocados are excluded. The diet also advises against eating bananas, pineapples, and other tropical fruits. The use of dairy products, eggs, coffee, sugar, stimulant and aromatic herbs, red meat, poultry, and processed foods is discouraged.
Melatonin	May aid in the effectiveness of chemotherapy and in improving survival in numerous types of cancer. Melatonin inhibits tumorigenesis with the suppression of tumor linoleic acid (LA) uptake and its metabolism. Melatonin may also stimulate natural killer cells, which attack tumors. Inhibits cachexia.	Circadian rhythm may be enhanced with use of melatonin; this may help to alleviate fatigue associated with cancer.
Milk thistle (Silymarin)	Antioxidant for treating liver diseases such as cirrhosis or chronic hepatitis. May help with cancer prevention; human studies are needed.	It contains flavonolignans; perhaps has a role in decreasing skin or prostate cancer.
Mistletoe (Iscador)	Lectin-rich mistletoe extract should be further evaluated.	There may be toxic side effects.
Mulberry	Anthocyanins in mulberry have an anticancer effect.	More research is needed.
Mustard seed (Brassica campestris)	Mustard seeds enhance the antioxidant defense system and provide protection against the toxic effects of carcinogens.	May protect against stomach and uterine cancers.
Oleandrin, odoroside (Nerium odorum)	Raw leaves are toxic. May cause apoptosis in various cancer cell lines.	Side effects include nausea, vomiting and diarrhea, tachycardia, and arrhythmia.
Noni juice (Morinda citrifolia)	An immunomodulatory polysaccharide-rich substance from the fruit juice is rich in potassium.	Common in Polynesian diets. High sugar content.
Pokeweed (Poke salad)	Pokeweed antiviral protein has anti-tumor effects in mice and laboratory studies. Clinical trials have not yet been done.	All parts of the mature plant contain chemically active substances such as phytolaccine, formic acid, tannin, and resin acid; all are mildly poisonous when eaten.
Probiotics	Evidence suggests the following beneficial effects: normalization of the intestinal microflora, the ability to block the invasion of potential pathogens in the gut, prevention of colon cancer, modulation of immune function, inhibition of H. pylori.	Regular use of yogurt and other natural functional foods may be useful for cancer patients. Daily intake of Bifidobacterium lactis enhances natural immune function.
Pycnogenol; pine bark extract (Pinus pinaster)	Pycnogenol is the name of a group of bioflavonoids with proanthocyanidins taken from a number of natural sources, such as grape seeds.	The maritime pine tree contains naturally occurring proanthocyanidins.
Quercetin	Quercetin is promoted to help prevent or treat different types of cancer.	See Table 13-2.
Reishi mushroom (Ganoderma lucidum)	The medicinal mushroom Reishi has been widely used to treat cancer, diabetes, and neurasthenia in many Asian countries. Used for fatigue, high cholesterol, HIV and AIDS, hypertension, immunostimulation, inflammation, strength and stamina, and viral infections.	Can interfere with immunosuppressants and chemotherapeutic drugs. Adverse reactions may include dry throat and nose, GI upset, itchiness, nausea, and vomiting.
Rosemary and marjoram (ursolic acid)	Terpenoids in these spices provide anticancer effects.	Triterpenoid compound that occurs naturally in a large variety of vegetarian foods, medicinal herbs, and plants.

(continued)

TABLE 13-8 Herbs, Dietary Supplements, and Cancer *(continued)*

Saffron (Crocus sativus)	This spice contains glutathione and crocetin, which decreases tumor growth and protects platelets from aggregation.	Being studied for effects on depression and Parkinson's disease also.
Saw palmetto (Serenoa repens)	Permixon, a phytotherapeutic agent derived from the saw palmetto plant, is a lipid/sterol extract; mixed research results.	Often used to prevent prostate cancer; no side effects noted.
Shark cartilage	It seems to have a role in inhibiting angiogenesis. Frequently recommended to cancer patients by family members.	No evidence that it plays a role in cancer. Prolonged use can have adverse side effects.
Shark oil	Alkylglycerols, found in shark liver oil, may fight cancer by killing tumor cells indirectly and activating the immune system by stimulating macrophages.	Depending on the supplement, it may be rich in omega-3 fatty acids and vitamin A.
Shiitake mushrooms	Contains lentin, which stimulates T-cell and natural killer cell production; antitumor, cholesterol-lowering, and virus-inhibiting effects.	Additional research is needed.
Skullcap (Scutellaria barbata)	It seems to play a role in the reduction of aflatoxin toxicity. Contains flavanone compounds such as scutellarein, scutellarin, carthamidin, and isocarthamidin.	Do not take orally.
Soy isoflavones	Role in cancer prevention is not clear. Exact dosage and effects on specific genes are not currently known. The best advice is to encourage usual dietary use and not to change drastically. Reduces menopausal symptoms.	Soy should not be used in estrogen-dependent breast cancer or with endometrial cancer. Avoid with use of tamoxifen.
Spirulina; blue-green algae (Spirulina spp)	Adverse effects are uncommon unless contaminated. Used to treat cancers, viral infections, weight loss, oral leukoplakia, increased cholesterol.	If contaminated, it is hepato-, nephro-, and neurotoxic.
St. John's wort (Hypericum perforatum)	Not effective against acute depression. Avoid with all types of chemotherapy; cyclosporine, midazolam, tacrolimus, amitriptyline, digoxin, indinavir, warfarin, and theophylline.	It accelerates the effects of tamoxifen and must be used cautiously. May cause breakthrough bleeding and unplanned pregnancy when used with oral contraceptives. Avoid with selective serotonin reuptake inhibitors and in pregnancy or lactation.
Turkey tail mushroom (Coriolus versicolor; Yunzhi)	A mushroom used in traditional Asian herbal remedies. Polysaccharide K (PSK) and polysaccharide peptide (PSP), are being studied as possible complementary cancer treatments.	
Turmeric (Curcuma longa)	Turmeric and other phenols have an anticancer effect. Additional research is needed about the efficacy of turmeric as a cancer treatment).	Warn breast cancer patients on cyclophosphamide to restrict the intake because it inhibits the antitumor action of these chemotherapeutic agents.
Valerian	Used to promote natural sleep; 2–4 weeks of use is needed. People who are going to have surgery should not use valerian or should taper down slowly, starting several weeks before surgery.	Avoid taking with alcohol, certain antihistamines, muscle relaxants, mental health drugs, sedatives, antiseizure drugs, or narcotics. Talk with their doctors or pharmacists about possible drug interactions before taking valerian.
Wheatgrass	Few scientific studies in humans to support claims made for wheatgrass.	Proponents suggest that wheatgrass strengthens the immune system.
White Birch (betulinic acid)	Potential role in treating melanoma and certain brain cancers; clinical trials are needed.	Birch bark, buds, and leaves are used as folk medicines but have not been studied to find out if they are safe or effective.
HARMFUL	**Avoid oral use:** Aconite (bushi, monkshood) aloe vera arnica (wolfbane, mountain tobacco) aveloz (pencil cactus) belladonna (deadly nightshade) blue cohosh (squaw root) boragebroom (broom tops, Irish broom) calamus (sweet root/flag) cesium chloride chaparral (creosote bush; Larrea tridentate)	May have serious side effects.

(continued)

TABLE 13-8 Herbs, Dietary Supplements, and Cancer *(continued)*

HARMFUL	**Avoid oral use:** coltsfoot comfrey (bruisewort; Symphytuen officinale) Convallaria (lily of the valley) DiBella (DMB) ephedra (ma huang) germander germanium horse chestnut Hoxsey herbal treatment jimson weed jin bu huan Kava (Piper methysticum) Kombucha tea krebiozin (creatine) laetrile (amygdalin)–cyanide toxicity licorice (Glycyrrhiza glabra) liferoot (golden senecio, ragwort) lobelia (Indian or wild tobacco) mandrake oleander Pau d'Arco (Taebuia) pennyroyal periwinkle poke root sassafras sea cucumber tea tree oil wormwood (madder, mug or Ming wort, Artemisia) yohimbe

This table was developed with assistance of Dr. Vijay Erankl and Valerie Kogut, MS, RD. See also:
American Cancer Society. Herbs, vitamins, and minerals.
http://www.cancer.org/docroot/ETO/ETO_5_2_5.asp?sitearea=&level=.
National Center for Complementary and Alternative Medicine
http://nccam.nih.gov/health/decisions/.

TABLE 13-9 General Patient Education Tips

For **cancer treatment**, start "where the patient is." Instruct patient to use unscientific treatments with caution. Discuss these issues with compassion and an understanding of patient's perspective. Patients want *faith* in their health provider, *hope* for coping and for strength, and *respect* for their wishes.

For **cancer survivors**, optimal attention to physical activity and nutrition should continue. Because there are different phases of cancer survivorship, from active treatment to advanced disease, existing evidence must be reviewed and informed decisions made regarding dietary choices. Obese and overweight patients can pursue modest weight loss provided that close monitoring occurs. Healthy food intake, low in energy density but high in nutrient and phytochemical content, is the goal. This translates into 5–9 fruits and vegetables, more fish, and plenty of whole grains. Teach good sources of folate, vitamin A, calcium and iron; highlight antioxidant foods rich in selenium, vitamins C and E, and beta-carotene. Excellent resources are available from the cancer survivor Web site at http://www.cancerrd.com/ and from the American Institute for Cancer Research Web site http://www.aicr.org/site/PageServer?pagename=reduce_diet_recipes_test_kitchen.

For **family member counseling**, teach that nutrition is fundamental in the molecular basis of cancer. Tailor interventions according to nutritional status, genotype, current health status, and nutritional requirements of the individual. Changes in diet, lifestyle and behaviors may be required.

For **terminal, palliative care**, emotional support and comfort may be the best treatment. The counselor should be aware of the stages of death and dying to identify where the patient is: (a) denial, (b) anger, (c) bargaining, (d) depression and loss, or (e) acceptance.

The patient must be included in all decisions. If not competent, follow the living will or advanced medical directives to follow. A court-appointed legal guardian may be needed. Evaluate the benefits and burdens of the illness on the patient, as well as any court or family decisions. Forego heroic measures, including tube feeding and CPN, if so chosen. Otherwise, maintain measures and re-evaluate at a later date. Hydration is the priority when "palliative care" orders are written.

For More Information

- Cancer Information
  http://www.cancerguide.org/std_books.html
- Cancer Treatments
  http://www.cancer.org/docroot/MBC/MBC_6.asp
- Clinical Trials
  http://www.cancer.gov/clinical_trials/
- Food Safety for Cancer Patients
  http://www.seattlecca.org/food-safety-guidelines.cfm
  http://www.fsis.usda.gov/
- Medicine Online
  http://www.meds.com/
- OncoLink: University of Pennsylvania Cancer Center
  http://oncolink.upenn.edu/
- Supportive Treatments
  http://www.cancer.gov/cancerinfo/pdq/supportivecare/
- Texas Cancer Data Center
  http://www.texascancer.info/
- Treatment Decisions
  http://www.cancer.org/docroot/ETO/eto_1_1a.asp

CANCER: TREATMENT GUIDELINES—CITED REFERENCES

American Dietetic Association (ADA). Evidence analysis library–Oncology. Accessed October 5, 2010, at http://www.adaevidencelibrary.com/topic.cfm?cat=1058.

Dixon SW. Nutrition care issues in the ambulatory (outpatient) head and neck cancer. *Support Line.* 27:3, 2005.

Mattox TW. Treatment of unintentional weight loss in patients with cancer. *Nutr Clin Pract.* 20:400, 2005.

Winter N, et al. Elevated levels of HMGB1 in cancerous and inflammatory effusions. *Anticancer Res.* 29:5013, 2009.

BONE CANCER AND OSTEOSARCOMA

NUTRITIONAL ACUITY RANKING: LEVEL 3

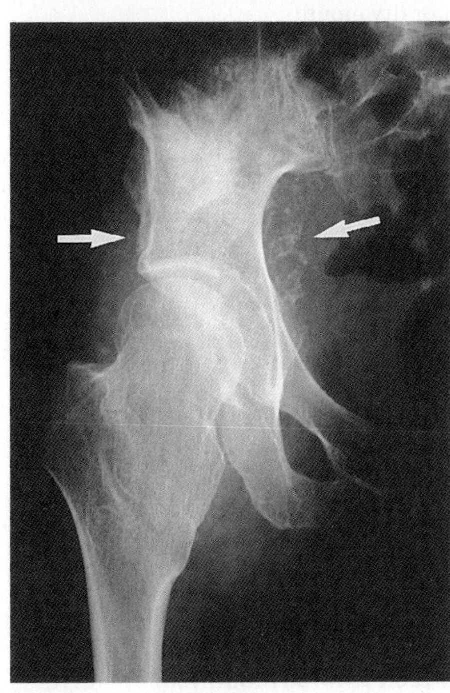

Adapted from: Yochum TR and Rowe LJ. *Yochum and Rowe's Essentials of Skeletal Radiology,* 3rd ed. Philadelphia: Lippincott Williams & Wilkins, 2004.

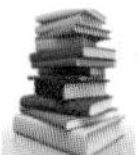

DEFINITIONS AND BACKGROUND

Bone is a fertile ground for cancer cells to flourish (Clines and Guise, 2005). Bone cancers include osteosarcomas, chondrosarcomas, and the Ewing family of tumors. The correct diagnosis depends on an evaluation of clinical, radiologic, pathologic, and genetic features (Li and Siegel, 2010).

Osteosarcoma involves a rapidly growing malignant bone tumor of unknown origin, occurring most often in the long bones of young people. It is most common in males between 10 and 25 years of age.

People who have had previous high doses of radiotherapy to a bone or Paget's disease have an increased risk of developing bone cancer. This type of cancer often spreads to the lung. When metastases from other organs occur, it is considered a secondary bone cancer. Patients with metastasis to the spine may present with pain, neurological deficit, or both. Optimal treatment should include consideration of the patient's neurological status, general health, age, quality of life, and the anatomical extent of the disease (Ecker et al, 2005).

Staging on bone cancer is as follows: stage 1 – low grade, no spread; stage 2 – high grade but not spread; stage 3 – bone cancer of any grade that has spread beyond the bone in which it started to other organs in the body, such as the lungs. In recurrent bone cancer, the cancer has returned after initial treatment.

The most common treatment for bone cancer pain is radiation. Radiation decreases bone cancer pain by direct effects on tumor cells (Goblirsch et al, 2005). Chemotherapy may also be needed; sore mouth or anemia may result. Surgery is reserved for neurological compromise, radiation failure, or spinal instability (Ecker et al, 2005). When possible, limb-sparing surgery is effective. Occasionally, amputation is necessary when the cancer has spread from the bone into the surrounding blood vessels.

Quality of life in this population is affected by depression, socialization problems, and physical limitations (Rustoen et al, 2005). Bisphosphonates are the standard of care for preventing skeletal morbidity and treating hypercalcemia of malignancy in patients with bone metastases; zoledronic acid may be given intravenously at the rate of 4 milligrams monthly (Gnant, 2009).

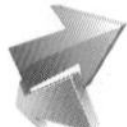

ASSESSMENT, MONITORING, AND EVALUATION

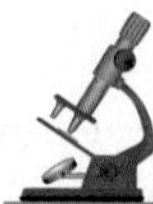

CLINICAL INDICATORS

Genetic Markers: Bone morphogenetic proteins (BMPs) may impact tumorigenesis and promote tumor spread (Thawani et al, 2009).

Specific Clinical/ History		
Height	Fever and cough	Na^+, K^+
Weight	Bone scan	Albumin (Alb)
BMI	CT scan	C-reactive protein (CRP)
Weight loss	**Lab Work**	Total lymphocyte count (TLC) (varies)
Leg, shin, shoulder pain?	H&H	Alanine aminotransferase (ALT) (increased)
Limited use of the extremity	Alkaline phosphatase (Alk phos) (increased)	
Fatigue	Glucose (Gluc)	
Warmth in a local area	Ca^{++}	
	Mg^{++}	

INTERVENTION

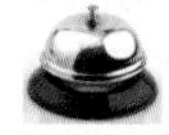

OBJECTIVES

- Prevent dehydration; correct fever.
- Relieve pain; prolong and improve quality of life.
- Correct side effects, such as sore mouth or anemia.
- Counteract effects of surgery (perhaps limb amputation), radiation therapy, or chemotherapy.
- Meet needs related to growth or elevated metabolic rate in children.

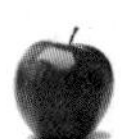

FOOD AND NUTRITION

- A balanced diet (high in energy and protein) will be needed.
- Extra fluids are used, unless contraindicated.
- Supplement with nutrients that are low in the patient's dietary intake. A diet rich in zinc, vitamins A and C, and other key nutrients will help with wound healing after surgery. A multivitamin–mineral supplement may be suggested.
- Small, frequent feedings may be better tolerated than large meals.

Common Drugs Used and Potential Side Effects

- Bisphosphonates may be used to restrict the action of the osteoclasts, help reduce the breakdown of the bone, reduce the risk of fracture and hypercalcemia, and reduce bone pain.
- Cisplatin, carboplatin (Paraplatin), cyclophosphamide (Cytoxan), doxorubicin (Adriamycin), high-dose methotrexate with leucovorin, ifosfamide (Ifex) may be used.
- Dry mouth, anemia, stomatitis, nausea, esophagitis, or vomiting may occur.

Herbs, Botanicals, and Supplements (see Table 13-8)

- Herbs and botanical supplements should not be used without discussing it with the physician.

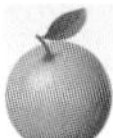

NUTRITION EDUCATION, COUNSELING, CARE MANAGEMENT

- Discuss ways to make meals more attractive and appetizing.
- Discuss with the patient and family how to adjust diet for therapies given.
- Encourage the patient to address depression or other issues that affect quality of life.
- Offer suggestions according to side effects such as sore mouth or dry mouth.

Patient Education—Food Safety

- Educate the patient about food safety issues. Discuss safe food handling and preparation, keeping foods at proper temperatures, the use of sterile water, and reheating foods properly.

For More Information

- American Cancer Society – Bone Cancer
  http://www.cancer.org/docroot/CRI/CRI_2_3x.asp?dt=2
- Bone Cancer Information
  http://www.cancerbacup.org.uk/Cancertype/Bone
- Bone Tumor
  http://www.bonetumor.org/
- Clinical Guidelines for Bone Cancer
  http://www.nccn.org/professionals/physician_gls/PDF/bone.pdf
- Medicine Net – Bone Cancer
  http://www.medicinenet.com/bone_cancer/article.htm

BONE CANCER AND OSTEOSARCOMA—CITED REFERENCES

Clines GA, Guise TA. Hypercalcaemia of malignancy and basic research on mechanisms responsible for osteolytic and osteoblastic metastasis to bone. *Endocr Relat Cancer.* 12:549, 2005.

Ecker RD, et al. Diagnosis and treatment of vertebral column metastases. *Mayo Clin Proc.* 80:1177, 2005.

Gnant M. Bisphosphonates in the prevention of disease recurrence: current results and ongoing trials. *Curr Cancer Drug Targets.* 9:824, 2009.

Goblirsch M, et al. Radiation treatment decreases bone cancer pain through direct effect on tumor cells. *Radiat Res.* 164:400, 2005.

Li S, Siegel GP. Small cell tumors of bone. *Adv Anat Pathol.* 17:1, 2010.

Rustoen T, et al. Predictors of quality of life in oncology outpatients with pain from bone metastasis. *J Pain Symptom Manage.* 30:234, 2005.

Thawani JP, et al. Bone morphogenetic proteins and cancer: review of the literature [Published online ahead of print Dec 29, 2009]. *Neurosurgery.*

BONE MARROW OR HEMATOPOIETIC STEM-CELL TRANSPLANTATION

NUTRITIONAL ACUITY RANKING: LEVEL 4

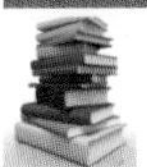

DEFINITIONS AND BACKGROUND

Hematopoietic stem cells are cells from which all blood cells evolve. Since bone marrow contains the greatest concentration of blood stem cells, most transplantations, historically, have been bone marrow transplantations. However, with the administration of an artificial growth factor called granulocyte colony-stimulating factor (G-CSF), stem cells are stimulated to grow and leave marrow and can be collected from the bloodstream by apheresis.

The terms "hematopoietic stem-cell transplantation" and "peripheral-blood stem-cell transplantation" are used when referring to bone marrow transplantation. Peripheral-blood stem-cell transplantations are being used with increased frequency because it is much less invasive. Traditional bone marrow harvest requires the use of general anesthesia.

Treatment consists of a preparative regimen that includes high-dose chemotherapy and may also include total-body irradiation. An infusion of autologous (the patient's own), syngeneic (from an identical twin), or allogeneic (from a histocompatible related or unrelated donor) marrow follows.

Hematological malignancies, including leukemias, lymphomas, multiple myeloma, and aplastic anemia, are the main indications for stem-cell transplantation. Nonhematological malignancies, such as testicular cancer and some autoimmune conditions, are also indications for stem-cell transplantation. Stem-cell transplantations are performed in both adult and pediatric populations. Stem-cell transplantations in patients with matched siblings versus unrelated donors have been associated with significantly better long-term survival (Talano et al, 2006).

After transplantation, the patient is often neutropenic, and nutritional status may decline rapidly. Children undergoing bone marrow transplantation may have suboptimal nutritional status; body mass index (BMI) is not an accurate indicator in these cases (White et al, 2005). Hospitalized transplantation patients resume oral intake sooner than ambulatory patients.

Treatment is aggressive and has many side effects. Early side effects are basically the same as those of any other type of high-dose chemotherapy and are caused by damage to bone marrow and other rapidly reproducing tissues of the body. Hepatic veno-occlusive disease (VOD) occurs after high doses of chemotherapy in preparation for bone marrow transplantation. Rapid weight gain, elevated bilirubin, right upper quadrant (RUQ) pain, ascites, jaundice, and hepatomegaly can occur.

Long-term side effects could include radiation damage to the lungs with shortness of breath, graft-versus-host disease (GVHD), damage to the ovaries causing infertility and loss of menstrual periods, damage to the thyroid gland causing problems with metabolism, cataracts, bone damage, and growth changes in children. GVHD causes erythroderma, jaundice, abdominal pain, emaciation, pneumonitis, infections, and gastrointestinal tract problems. Hemolytic uremic syndrome (HUS) is an uncommon but potentially life-threatening complication of stem-cell transplantation.

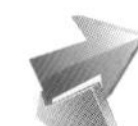

ASSESSMENT, MONITORING, AND EVALUATION

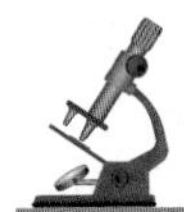

CLINICAL INDICATORS

Genetic Markers: Umbilical cord blood may be used in children born after a genetic diagnosis for human leucocyte antigen (HLA) matching for donation to a sick sibling.

Specific Clinical/History

- Height
- Weight
- BMI
- Weight changes
- Diet history
- I & O
- Temperature
- Ascites, jaundice
- Frequent infections
- Hepatomegaly?
- RUQ pain?
- Rectal biopsy for GVHD[a]

Lab Work

- H & H
- Bilirubin
- Gluc
- Mg^{++}, Ca^{++}
- Complete blood count (CBC)
- Absolute neutrophil count (ANC) to evaluate engrafting
- Na^{+}, K^{+}
- Alb, transthyretin
- Viral hepatitis screening
- CRP
- Serum phosphorus (low from cyclosporine A)
- Uric acid
- Cholesterol (Chol)
- Triglycerides (Trig)
- TLC (varied reliability)
- Ferritin
- Transferrin
- Blood urea nitrogen (BUN)
- Creatinine (Creat)

[a]Severe colonic crypt loss predicts severe clinical GI-GvHD that is more likely to be refractory to steroid treatment and have high mortality (Melson et al, 2007).

INTERVENTION

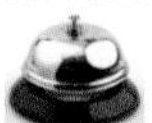

OBJECTIVES

Pretransplantation

- Replace the malignant or defective hematopoietic system for the production and development of blood cells.
- Provide adequate nutrient stores (glucose, calories, vitamins, minerals, and protein). Supplementation with EPA

SAMPLE NUTRITION CARE PROCESS STEPS

Decreased Oral Food–Beverages Intake

Assessment Data: Analysis of oral intake compared to requirements from nursing flow sheet; patient states pain while eating; physical examination of the oral cavity.

Nutrition Diagnosis (PES): NI-2.1 oral intake related to pain and mucositis as evidenced by the refusal of food at mealtimes.

Intervention: Diet modification for consistency. Education about foods that may be better tolerated. Counseling about taking pain medicines ahead of meals.

Monitoring and Evaluation: Follow-up in 24 hours to evaluate improvement and changes in oral intake.

fish oil improves energy intake and may reduce complications and inflammatory markers when compared with usual care (Elia et al, 2006).

- Assure adequate hydration.

Posttransplantation

- Restore normal hematopoiesis and immunological function.
- Individualize needs; promote engraftment of marrow.
- Prevent or manage gastrointestinal Graft-Versus-Host Disease (GI-GvHD). Rejection occurs less often in well-nourished patients.
- Prevent infections, viral hepatitis, mucositis, gastroenteritis, and pneumocystosis.
- Reduce nausea, vomiting, diarrhea, appetite loss and fatigue, which can seriously affect nutritional status (Iversen et al, 2009).
- Improve weight status; promote anabolism. Most patients are in the hospital for 4–6 weeks.
- Correct early satiety, anorexia, stomatitis, xerostomia, and depression—all of which reduce total intake.
- Provide nutrition support due to hypermetabolism and side effects of treatments. Promote positive nitrogen balance when possible.
- Correct hyperglycemia from metabolic stress, insulin resistance, and medication side effects.
- Monitor closely for renal insufficiency and necessary changes for diet.
- Prevent or prepare for long-term complications such as hyperphagia and obesity, insulin resistance and diabetes, hyperlipidemia, hypertension, and osteoporosis.
- Maximize quality of life. Health-related quality of life (HRQoL) is reduced before, during, and after intensive therapy (Iversen et al, 2009).

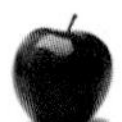

FOOD AND NUTRITION

- Protective isolation may be needed. A low-bacteria (neutropenic) diet may be useful for several months before and after transplantation. A neutropenic diet guide is found in Table 13-10.
- CPN may be needed to initiate recovery after transplantation or with severe intestinal GVHD. Where possible, the use of intravenous fluids and oral diet should be considered as a preference to parenteral nutrition; however, with severe gastrointestinal failure, even with a trial of enteral feeding, use PN (Murray and Pindoria, 2009). A naso-jejunal (NJ) feeding is associated with less vomiting and aspiration. The use of glutamine to decrease oral mucositis or diarrhea among patients receiving autologous or allogeneic HCT is not necessary (American Dietetic Association, 2010).
- Use indirect calorimetry to determine energy requirements where possible (American Dietetic Association, 2010). Provide 30–35 kcal/kg for the first month; increase for weight gain, infection, GVHD, or neutropenia.
- Protein intake should be 1.5–2 g/kg of weight; increase during corticosteroid therapy.
- Fat intake should be 25–30% of total kilocalories to prevent fatty acid deficiency and to support blood glucose control (American Dietetic Association, 2010). Monitor for hyperlipidemia. An olive oil-based lipid emulsion compared with a MCT/LCT emulsion can be well tolerated; maintain essential fatty acids, and support a favorable plasma lipid profile (Hartman et al, 2009).

TABLE 13-10 Neutropenic Diet Guidelines

To reduce the introduction of pathogenic organisms into the gastrointestinal tract of immunocompromised patients, food safety practices and dietary changes are in order. The following are practices that may be helpful to patients after bone marrow transplantation (for 3 months or until immunosuppressive therapies are complete):

- Ensure careful hand washing.
- Keep foods at a safe temperature to prevent food infection.
- Microwave hot foods immediately before service.
- Avoid foods that fall into the following categories:
- All moldy or outdated food products
- Deli cheeses and foods
- Hot dogs, bacon, sausage, luncheon meats
- Miso and tempeh products
- Pickled fish, cold smoked salmon, and lox
- Powdered infant formula
- Raw and unpasteurized milk and dairy products
- Raw brewer's yeast
- Raw honey
- Raw or undercooked meats, fish, shellfish, poultry, eggs, game meats
- Raw vegetable sprouts
- Salad dressings made with raw eggs
- Soft or mold-containing cheese (Brie, feta, blue)
- Stir fried vegetables or fruits
- Tofu
- Unboiled well water (it should be boiled at least one minute)
- Unpasteurized beer or fruit juices
- Unrefrigerated cheese-based salad dressings
- Unwashed fruits or vegetables
- Yogurt and other dairy products with active cultures

Adapted from: Oncology Nutrition Practice Group. *The clinical guide to oncology nutrition*. 2nd ed. Chicago, IL: American Dietetic Association, 2006.

- If there is hyperglycemia, keep carbohydrate intake at a steady amount each day.
- Sterile water may be used for hydration and renal health. Maintain 1 mL/Kg intake.
- A multivitamin–mineral supplement may be useful. Assure adequate intake of vitamin D and calcium with long-term steroid use. Potassium and magnesium can be depleted by some medications; monitor carefully. Avoid iron in supplements if transfusions have been frequent; iron overload may occur.
- Patient may need a low-lactose, low-fiber, low-fat diet. Progress, as tolerated, to normal diet.
- As patient recovers and no longer requires a protective setting, the use of live-culture pasteurized yogurt may be beneficial to increase bowel flora. *Lactobacillus acidophilus* therapy can also be helpful.

Common Drugs Used and Potential Side Effects

- See Table 13-11.

Herbs, Botanicals, and Supplements (see Table 13-8)

- Herbs and botanical supplements should not be used without discussing it with the physician.
- St. John's wort and echinacea should not be taken with cyclosporine, because they alter drug functioning.

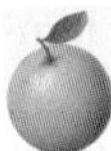

NUTRITION EDUCATION, COUNSELING, CARE MANAGEMENT

- The neutropenic, low-bacteria diet protocol should be made available, as appropriate.
- Help the patient and family to manage signs of gastrointestinal GVHD; this usually includes anorexia, nausea, vomiting, watery diarrhea, abdominal pain, and GI bleeding (Xu et al, 2008).
- Small, frequent meals of bland, cold consistency may be well-tolerated.
- Discuss any necessary nutritional support methods and procedures to be used at home or in discharge planning.

TABLE 13-11 Drugs Commonly Used in Bone Marrow or Stem-Cell Transplantation

Conditioning chemotherapy or irradiation is given immediately before the transplant to suppress immune reactions.

Drug	Comments
Analgesics, antihistamines, and antidepressants	Monitor for specific side effects.
Antibiotics	Amphotericin may be used to fight infections. Nausea, stomach pain, or vomiting may occur.
Antivirals	Acyclovir may be given prophylactically to resolve oral ulcers. Headaches, gastrointestinal(GI) distress, or diarrhea may occur.
Bisphosphonates	These may be needed if there is osteopenia or osteoporosis.
Chemotherapy	Busulfan (to destroy marrow stem cells) and cyclophosphamide (Cytoxan) are given to prevent rejection of the transplant. They can cause nausea, vomiting, diarrhea, and anorexia. Methotrexate, fludarabine, carmustine, and cyclophosphamide may cause anorexia, mucositis, and esophagitis; some also cause diarrhea. Gleevec interferes with an abnormal enzyme that sends signals to the nucleus of a cancer cell. Nausea, extensive diarrhea, and vomiting are potential side effects. Useful for leukemia or advanced stomach cancer.
Immunosuppressive therapy (graft-versus-host disease [GVHD] prophylaxis)	GVHD prophylaxis consists of T-cell depletion (antibody T10B9 or OKT3 and complement) with posttransplantation cyclosporine (Talano et al, 2006). Antithymocyte globulin may cause vomiting, nausea, diarrhea, and stomatitis. Azathioprine may cause vomiting, nausea, diarrhea, mucosal ulceration, esophagitis, and steatorrhea. Beclomethasone can lead to thrush, nausea, and xerostomia. Corticosteroids cause sodium and fluid retention, weight gain, hyperglycemia, skeletal muscle wasting, growth retardation in children, peptic ulceration, and elevated triglycerides. Cyclosporine (Sandimmune) may cause nausea and vomiting, skin rashes, hemorrhagic cystitis, and altered potassium metabolism. Methotrexate causes nausea and vomiting, mucositis, esophagitis, diarrhea, renal and liver changes, decreased absorption of vitamin B_{12}, fat, and D-xylose, and taste changes. Monoclonal antibodies cause nausea and vomiting. Sirolimus elevates triglycerides. Tacrolimus can be nephrotoxic or cause hyperglycemia, hyperkalemia, or hypomagnesemia. Ursodeoxycholic acid can cause nausea and vomiting, diarrhea, and GI distress.
Filgrastim (Neupogen)	Neutropenia secondary to immune suppression may be managed with Neupogen and a low-bacteria diet.
Insulin	May be needed if there is hyperglycemia.
Oral hygiene	Clotrimazole (Mycelex) may cause nausea or vomiting; it is used for oral hygiene and prevention of oral candidiasis.
Total-body irradiation (TBI)	Side effects vary for each individual, but anorexia, diarrhea, and mucositis or esophagitis are common.

Transition from CPN and PN to enteral nutrition or oral diet will be helpful.
- Physical therapy may be helpful to maintain strength and to regain mobility.

Patient Education—Food Safety

- Educate about food safety issues. Discuss safe food handling and preparation, keeping foods at proper temperatures, the use of sterile water, and reheating foods properly.
- The neutropenic, low-bacteria diet includes the careful use of raw fruits and vegetables, milk, and shellfish—all of which may be contaminated easily with bacteria. These diets are often used in bone marrow transplantation units.

For More Information

- Bone Marrow Support Group
  http://www.bmtsupport.ie/
- Medline Plus – BMT
  http://www.nlm.nih.gov/medlineplus/ency/article/003009.htm
- National Bone Marrow Transplant Link
  http://www.nbmtlink.org/
- National Cancer Institute – BMT
  http://www.cancer.gov/cancertopics/factsheet/Therapy/bone-marrow-transplant

BONE MARROW AND HEMATOPOIETIC STEM-CELL TRANSPLANTATION—CITED REFERENCES

American Dietetic Association (ADA). Evidence analysis library: Oncology. Accessed January 3, 2010, at http://www.eatright.org.

Elia M, et al. Enteral (oral or tube administration) nutritional support and eicosapentaenoic acid in patients with cancer: a systematic review. *Int J Oncol.* 28:5, 2006.

Hartman C, et al. Olive oil-based intravenous lipid emulsion in pediatric patients undergoing bone marrow transplantation: a short-term prospective controlled trial. *Clin Nutr.* 28:631, 2009.

Iversen PO, et al. Reduced nutritional status among multiple myeloma patients during treatment with high-dose chemotherapy and autologous stem cell support [Published online ahead of print Dec 29, 2009]. *Clin Nutr.* Melson J, et al. Crypt loss is a marker of clinical severity of acute gastrointestinal graft-versus-host disease. *Am J Hematol.* 82:881, 2007.

Murray SM, Pindoria S. Nutrition support for bone marrow transplant patients. *Cochrane Database Syst Rev.* 1:CD002920, 2009.

Talano JM, et al. Alternative donor bone marrow transplant for children with Philadelphia chromosome ALL. *Bone Marrow Transplant.* 37:135, 2006.

White M, et al. Nutritional status and energy expenditure in children pre-bone-marrow-transplant. *Bone Marrow Transplant.* 35:775, 2005.

Xu CF, et al. Endoscopic diagnosis of gastrointestinal graft-versus-host disease. *World J Gastroenterol.* 14:2262, 2008.

BRAIN TUMOR

NUTRITIONAL ACUITY RANKING: LEVEL 3

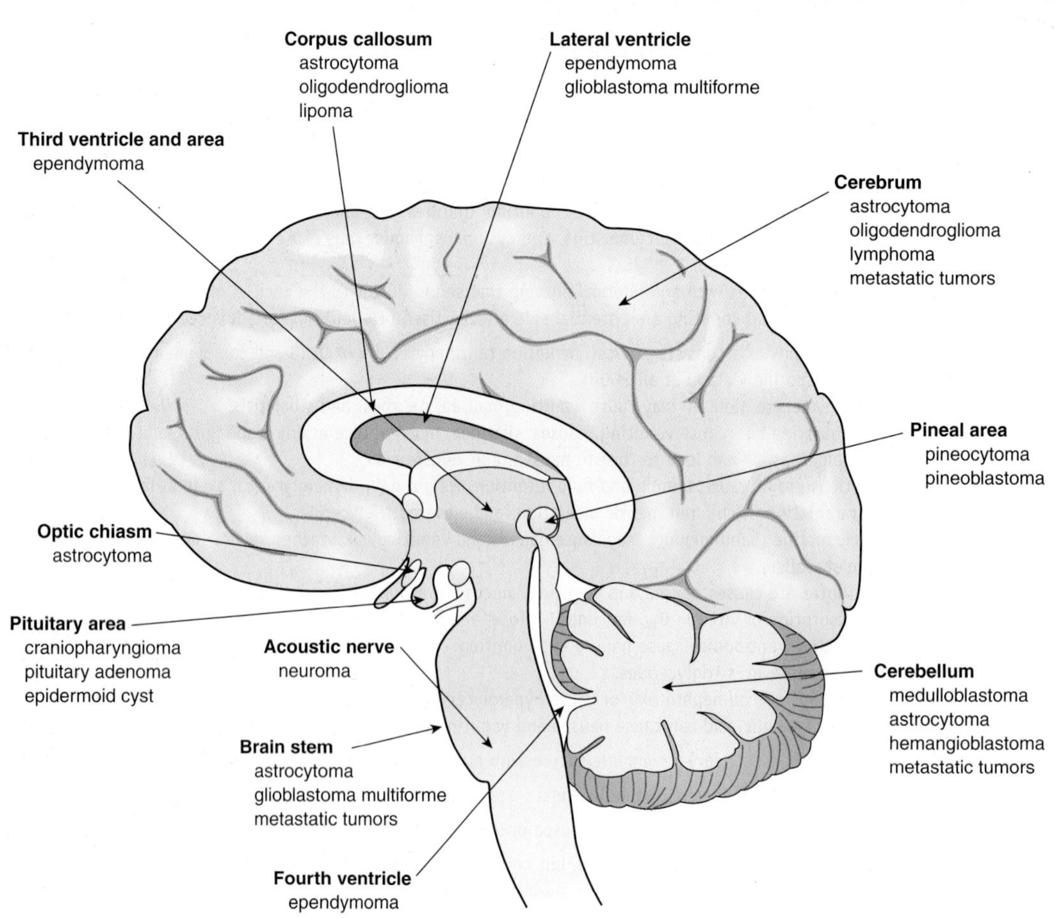

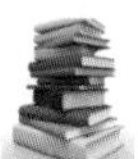

DEFINITIONS AND BACKGROUND

Tumors are either primary or secondary when they are found in the brain. Primary brain tumors start their growth in the brain and can be benign or malignant. They can occur in children, particularly girls between the ages of 5 and 9. Approximately 17,000 Americans each year are diagnosed with a primary brain tumor. Secondary brain tumors are more common, with about 90,000 cases diagnosed each year. These tumors result from cancer that has metastasized to the brain from the lung, breast, melanoma, kidney, or other part of the body.

Brain tumors destroy or damage brain cells by producing inflammation, compressing other parts of the brain as the tumor grows, and causing swelling and pressure inside the skull. Headache is the most common symptom. Brain tumor headaches are usually worse upon awakening and do not respond to the usual headache medicines. Depression, fatigue, and memory and personality changes may complicate care (Stewart-Amidei, 2005). Table 13-12 describes types of brain tumors and cells of origin.

The nerve cells (neurons) carry signals, and the cells that support them are called glial cells. There are a number of different types of glial cells, all with different names and functions, and they outnumber the neurons by a ratio of 10:1. A glioma is a tumor of neurological origin; it constitutes over 50% of all brain tumors.

Glioblastoma multiforme (GBM) is the most frequent and devastating primary malignant brain tumor in adults. Surgery followed by standard radiotherapy with temozolomide chemotherapy is the standard of care, but the prognosis remains poor with survival in the range of 12–15 months (Minniti et al, 2009). While fruit, vegetables, and carotenoids do not increase the risk of glioma (Holick et al, 2007), adequate GLA and DHA fatty acids, lycopene, beta carotene, and other antioxidants are under study. There is also no evidence that the intake of meat, nitrate, nitrite, or nitrosamines is related to the risk of glioma (Michaud et al, 2009).

Meningiomas are also common and may be classified as benign, atypical, or malignant. While surgical excision is curative for most patients, up to 20% recur (Lee et al, 2009).

Because malignant brain tumors are largely dependent on glycolysis for energy, normal neurons and glia readily transition to ketone bodies (beta-hydroxybutyrate) for energy when glucose levels are reduced (Seyfried and Mukherjee, 2005). Increased melanocortin activity and reduced neuropeptide Y function lead to catabolism with reduced energy intake, increased energy expenditure, increased muscle proteolysis, and adipose tissue loss (Laviano et al, 2008).

Nutritional status and weight decline early in treatment (Ward et al, 2009). Anorexia, early satiety, changes in taste/smell, and nausea are frequently reported. Ghrelin has anti-inflammatory properties that may help to alleviate cachexia and improve weight gain; ghrelin receptor agonists show promise (DeBoer 2008).

Some brain tumors can be treated successfully with surgery, radiation therapy, and chemotherapy. Emerging technologies allow physicians to target and treat brain tumors more precisely. Antiangiogenesis approaches have the potential to be particularly effective in the treatment of glioblastoma tumors (Anderson et al, 2008). Convection-enhanced delivery (CED) has emerged as a leading investigational delivery technique for the treatment of brain tumors (Bidros et al, 2010).

TABLE 13-12 Types of Brain Tumors

Type of Tumor	Location, Cell Origin, or Function
CNS Lymphoma	Affects the body's immune system, which defends against infection and foreign substances.
Craniopharyngiomas	Located around the pituitary gland.
Germinomas	Germ cell tumors.
Gliomas	Originate in the glial supporting tissues. Types include astrocytoma; brain stem glioma; oligodendroglioma that affects myelin production; ependymoma affects the ventricles that aid in the circulation of cerebrospinal fluid.
Meningioma	The meninges cover and protect the brain and spinal cord.
Medulloblastoma	These cells normally do not remain in the body after birth; primitive neuroectodermal tumors (PNET).
Neuroblastoma	Originate in the brain.
Pineal gland tumors	Pineocytoma or pineoblastoma are around the pineal gland.
Schwannoma	Affects the myelin that protects the acoustic nerve for hearing; acoustic neuromas are in this category.

Source: National Cancer Institute, http://www.cancer.gov/cancertopics/alphalist/a-d, accessed January 5, 2010.

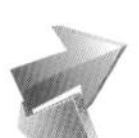

ASSESSMENT, MONITORING, AND EVALUATION

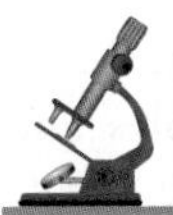

CLINICAL INDICATORS

Genetic Markers: Five "classes" of meningiomas have been detected by gene expression analysis where chromosomes 22q, 6q, and 14q are involved (Lee et al, 2009). Genomic deletion of chromosomes 6, 21, and 22 represents new targets for further research (Lassman et al, 2005).

Specific Clinical/History

- Height
- Weight
- BMI
- Weight changes
- Diet history
- BP (hypertension?)
- Inability to follow commands
- Aphasia
- Cerebral edema, headaches
- Vertigo
- Altered consciousness or convulsions
- Mental or personality changes
- Unequal pupil response
- Hemianopsia, blurred or decreased vision
- Ptosis
- Altered gait or immobility
- Dysphagia
- Vomiting (with or without nausea)
- Tinnitus

	Lab Work	
Loss of sense of smell	Gluc (elevated)	TLC, white blood cell count (WBC) (altered)
CT scan	Cerebrospinal fluid (CSF)—elevated protein levels	WBC in CSF (normal or increased)
Diffusion MRI	Alb, transthyretin	Transferrin
Skull x-ray	CRP	ALT (elevated)
Electroencephalogram (EEG)		NA^+, K^+
Lumbar puncture		Serum folate

INTERVENTION

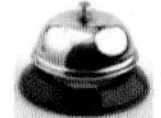

OBJECTIVES

- Provide adequate energy (30 kcal/kg or more if needed).
- Provide adequate protein for surgery: 1.2–1.5 g/kg body weight; for radiation: 1.0–1.2 g/kg body weight. Adjust for renal/hepatic dysfunction; obesity; skin breakdown or wound healing.
- Avoid constipation and straining.
- Prevent lower respiratory infections; coughing can increase intracranial pressure.
- Counteract side effects of therapy (e.g., radiation, surgery).
- Monitor carefully for elevated blood glucose levels, which may occur with corticosteroids that are used to control brain edema.
- Prevent complications such as the loss of ability to interact, care for self, or permanent neurological losses.

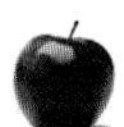

FOOD AND NUTRITION

- Maintain diet, as ordered. Include extra fluid, unless contraindicated.
- If oral diet is possible, include fish, fruits, vegetables, and adequate fiber. Include green tea, food sources of beta carotene, and fish oil to enhance neuroprotection.
- Alter texture and liquids, if necessary, for dysphagia. If necessary, tube feed or offer CPN.
- Limit sodium to 4–6 g/d to correct cerebral edema.

SAMPLE NUTRITION CARE PROCESS STEPS

Swallowing Difficulty

Assessment Data: Weight loss of 10# in 6 weeks; cognitive changes; brain tumor. Mealtime observation shows choking on thin liquids and inability to swallow solids.

Nutrition Diagnosis (PES): NC-1.1 Swallowing difficulty related to neurological changes as evidenced by inability to consume solids, choking on thin liquids, and 10# weight loss in 6 weeks.

Intervention: Enteral nutrition support with gastrostomy. Educate the patient and family about the benefits of tube feeding.

Monitoring and Evaluation: Recovery of lost weight; tolerance for chemotherapy and radiation treatments.

- Offer meal setup and assistance with eating, altered liquid/food textures, and/or enteral tube feedings for patients with cognitive deficits, swallowing difficulties, or limited function of upper extremity.

Common Drugs Used and Potential Side Effects

- Seizures are best managed with antiepileptic drug therapy (Stewart-Amidei, 2005). Levetiracetam (Keppra), an anticonvulsant, reduces seizures in malignant brain tumors and may help improve chemotherapy outcomes. Monitor for decreased serum folic acid levels and other nutrients.
- The use of procarbazine (an antineoplastic) may warrant the restriction of tyramine-containing foods that are secondary to its monoamine oxidase (MAO) inhibitor–like action.
- Nonsteroidal anti-inflammatory agents may help to reduce inflammation (Byrne, 2005).
- Steroid therapy may be used. Decrease sodium and increase potassium if appropriate. Negative nitrogen balance or hyperglycemia may result. Maintain near-normal blood glucose levels if possible.
- Osmotic diuretics may be needed for edema. Antacids or antihistamines may be needed for stress ulcers.
- Temozolomide (Temodar) was approved for brain cancer and GBM in particular.

Herbs, Botanicals, and Supplements (see Table 13-8)

- Herbs and botanical supplements should not be used without discussing it with the physician.

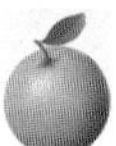

NUTRITION EDUCATION, COUNSELING, CARE MANAGEMENT

- The importance of regular and attractive meals should be stressed to help appetite if fair or poor. Keep in mind that sense of smell may have declined recently.
- Discuss the importance of a balanced diet with good sources of protein at meals.
- Early discussion about end-of-life issues is necessary because the disease can impair the patient's decision-making ability (Stewart-Amidei, 2005).
- A multidisciplinary approach using physical, occupational, and speech therapies is essential to maximize neurological function and activities of daily living.

Patient Education—Food Safety

- Educate the patient about food safety issues. Discuss safe food handling and preparation, keeping foods at proper temperatures, the use of sterile water, and reheating foods properly.

For More Information

- Brain Tumor Clinical Trials: Musella Foundation
  http://www.virtualtrials.com/musella.cfm

- Interactive Tour of the Brain
  http://www.braintumor.org/TourBrain/index.html
- National Brain Tumor Foundation
  http://www.braintumor.org/
- OncoLink—Brain Cancer
  http://www.oncolink.org/types/article.cfm?c=2&s=4&ss=25&id=9534

BRAIN TUMOR—CITED REFERENCES

Anderson JC, et al. New molecular targets in angiogenic vessels of glioblastoma tumours. *Expert Rev Mol Med.* 10:e23, 2008.

Bidros DS, et al. Future of convection-enhanced delivery in the treatment of brain tumors. *Future Oncol.* 6:117, 2010.

Byrne TN. Cognitive sequelae of brain tumor treatment. *Curr Opin Neurol.* 18:662, 2005.

DeBoer MD. Emergence of ghrelin as a treatment for cachexia syndromes. *Nutrition.* 24:806, 2008.

de Meijia EG, et al. Bioactive components of tea: cancer, inflammation and behavior. *Brain Behav Immun.* 23:721, 2009.

Holick CN, et al. Prospective study of intake of fruit, vegetables, and carotenoids and the risk of adult glioma. *Am J Clin Nutr.* 85:877, 2007.

Lassman AB, et al. Molecular study of malignant gliomas treated with epidermal growth factor receptor inhibitors: tissue analysis from North American brain tumor consortium trials. *Clin Cancer Res.* 11:7841, 2005.

Laviano A, et al. NPY and brain monoamines in the pathogenesis of cancer anorexia. *Nutrition.* 4:802, 2008.

Lee Y, et al. Genomic landscape of meningiomas [Published online ahead of print November 20, 2009]. *Brain Pathol.*

Michaud DS, et al. Prospective study of meat intake and dietary nitrates, nitrites, and nitrosamines and risk of adult glioma. *Am J Clin Nutr.* 90:570, 2009.

Minniti G, et al. Chemotherapy for glioblastoma: current treatment and future perspectives for cytotoxic and targeted agents. *Anticancer Res.* 29:5171, 2009.

Seyfried TN, Mukherjee P. Targeting energy metabolism in brain cancer: review and hypothesis. *Nutr Metab (London).* 2:30, 2005.

Stewart-Amidei C. Managing symptoms and side effects during brain tumor illness. *Expert Rev Neurother.* 5:71S, 2005.

Ward E. et al. Nutritional problems in children treated for medulloblastoma: implications for enteral nutrition support. *Pediatr Blood Cancer.* 53:570, 2009.

COLORECTAL CANCER

NUTRITIONAL ACUITY RANKING: LEVEL 3–4

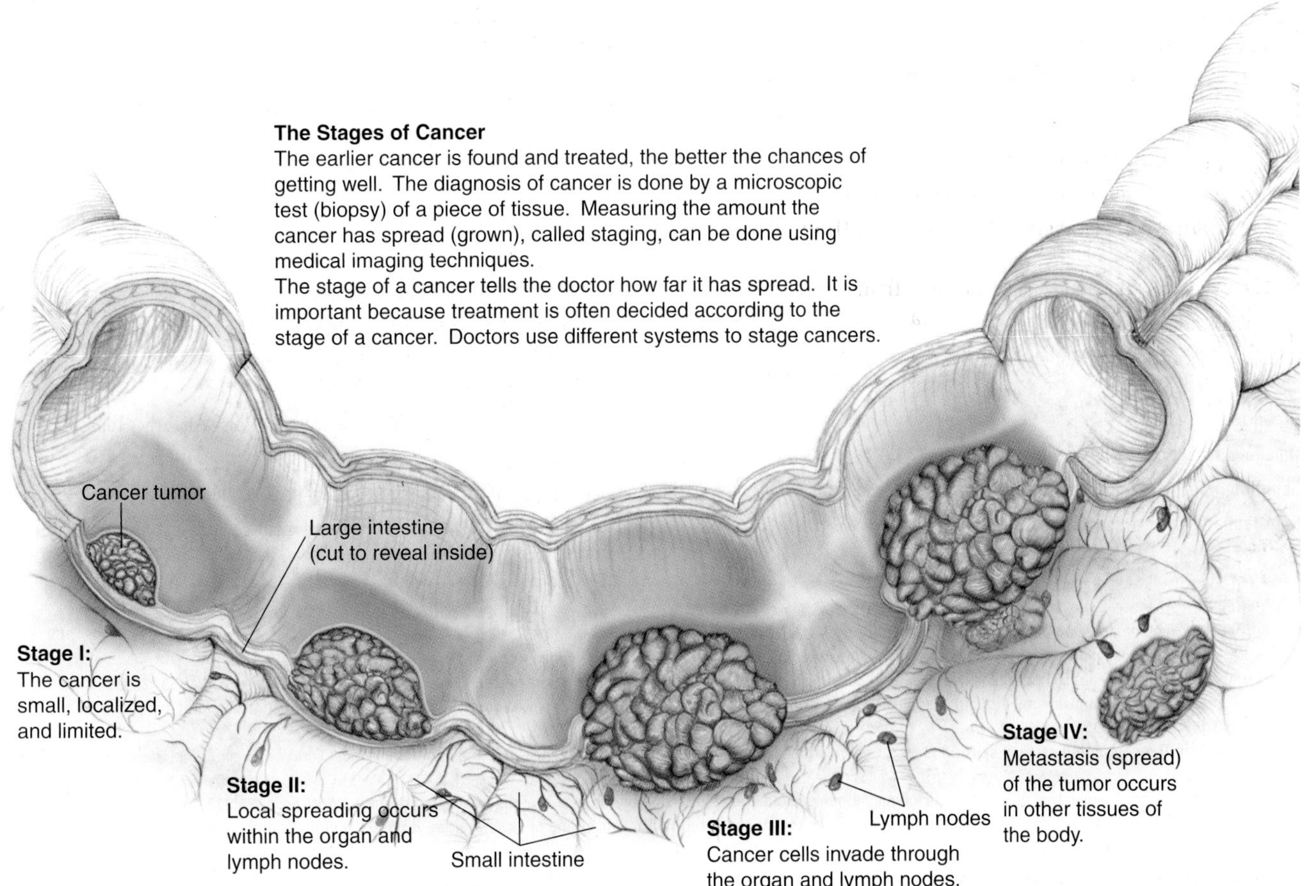
The Stages of Cancer
The earlier cancer is found and treated, the better the chances of getting well. The diagnosis of cancer is done by a microscopic test (biopsy) of a piece of tissue. Measuring the amount the cancer has spread (grown), called staging, can be done using medical imaging techniques.
The stage of a cancer tells the doctor how far it has spread. It is important because treatment is often decided according to the stage of a cancer. Doctors use different systems to stage cancers.
Cancer tumor
Large intestine (cut to reveal inside)
Stage I: The cancer is small, localized, and limited.
Stage II: Local spreading occurs within the organ and lymph nodes.
Small intestine
Stage III: Cancer cells invade through the organ and lymph nodes.
Lymph nodes
Stage IV: Metastasis (spread) of the tumor occurs in other tissues of the body.

Asset provided by Anatomical Chart Co.

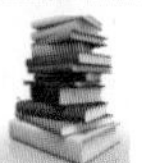

DEFINITIONS AND BACKGROUND

Colorectal cancer (CRC) is the third most common type of cancer in the United States, but the second leading cause of cancer deaths. Family history of colorectal cancer is a risk factor in 25% of cases. Hereditary nonpolyposis colorectal cancer (HNPCC, or Lynch syndrome) is one inherited form.

High risk for CRC exists among patients with ulcerative colitis and Crohn's disease after 8 or more years of duration. The incidence of colorectal cancer rises significantly after age 50 and doubles with each successive decade. Cyclooxygenase-2 (COX-2) and its proinflammatory metabolite, prostaglandin E_2 (PGE2), enhance colon cancer progression (Castellone et al, 2005).

Obesity is a risk factor (Fuemmeller et al, 2009). Bile acid deoxycholic acid (DCA) promotes the hyperproliferation of colonic epithelial cells and the risk of colon cancer (Zeng et al, 2009). Table 13-13 lists other factors that either promote or prevent CRC.

The adenomatous polyp is the precursor of most colorectal cancers. In Stage 0 CRC, early cancer is on the innermost layer of the intestine; in Stage 1, it is in the inner layers of the colon; in Stage 2, cancer has spread through the muscle wall of the colon. In Stage 3, the cancer has spread to the lymph nodes and in Stage 4, it has spread to other organs and is usually incurable.

Biomarkers may become a way to find or treat CRC. The 8-OH-dG in colorectal crypts is a biomarker of risk from oxidative DNA damage (Fedirko et al, 2010). Ibuprofen-type drugs, IL6 polymorphisms (rs1800796), and dietary alpha-tocopherol and lycopene significantly decrease the effects of TP53 mutations; beta-carotene and ibuprofen lower the risk of KRAS2 tumors (Slattery et al 2009). The interactions between genes, inflammation, and diet have been elucidated.

Fecal occult blood test and flexible sigmoidoscopy are used for diagnosis. Either standard colonoscopy (optical) or computed tomography (CT) colonoscopy may be used, but the CT (virtual) colonoscopy is not available at all facilities. In **cancer of the small intestine**, malignancy generally is found in the lower duodenum and lower ileum, with a high rate of mortality and few early symptoms; it presents in only 5% of cases. **Rectal cancer** is more common in men than in women and often occurs after middle age, with bleeding, pain, and irregular bowel habits.

In the **colon**, slow-growing malignancies are usually found in the cecum, lower ascending colon, and sigmoid colon. Few early symptoms are found, but the prognosis is optimistic. The right side of the colon (ascending) absorbs fluids and salts; cancer spreads upward here and obstruction is rare. The left side of the colon (the descending colon) stores feces; cancer here tends to encircle the bowel and cause obstructions. If surgery is required, maintaining the ileocecal valve is crucial.

TABLE 13-13 Risks and Protective Factors for Colorectal Cancer

Protective Factors	Risk Factors
Alpha-tocopherol and beta carotene (Slattery et al, 2009)	
Aspirin or nonsteroidal anti-inflammatory drugs (Kaur Saini et al, 2009; Slattery et al, 2009)	Age >50
Calcium and vitamin D_3 (Fedirko et al, 2010; Jenab et al, 2009)	Alcohol intake, excessive (Emmons et al, 2005)
Folic acid (Ulrich, 2005)	Chronic inflammatory and inflammatory cytokines (Bowen et al, 2009)
Lutein and lycopene (Slattery et al, 2009)	Family history of familial adenomatous polyposis (FAP) or hereditary non-polyposis colon cancer (HNPCC)
Green tea	Medical history of colon polyps, inflammatory bowel disease, other types of cancer
Omega-3 fatty acids	Overweight and obesity
Selenium; methylselenol is a critical metabolite (Zeng et al, 2009)	Smoking, particularly at an early age (Botteri et al, 2008; McCleary et al, 2010)
Sulforaphane (broccoli, cruciferous vegetables)	Western-style diet, high in red meat and fat; low in vegetables, folic acid, calcium and vitamin D (Emmons et al, 2005)

REFERENCES

Botteri E, et al. Smoking and colorectal cancer: a meta-analysis. *JAMA*. 300:2765, 2008.

Bowen KA, et al. PTEN loss induces epithelial-mesenchymal transition in human colon cancer cells. *Anticancer Res*. 29:4439, 2009.

Emmons KM, et al. Project PREVENT: a randomized trial to reduce multiple behavioral risk factors for colon cancer. *Cancer Epidemiol Biomarkers Prev*. 14:1453, 2005.

Fedirko V, et al. Effects of supplemental vitamin D and calcium on oxidative DNA damage marker in normal colorectal mucosa: a randomized clinical trial. *Cancer Epidemiol Biomarkers Prev*. 19:280, 2010.

Jenab M. Vitamin D receptor and calcium sensing receptor polymorphisms and the risk of colorectal cancer in European populations. *Cancer Epidemiol Biomarkers Prev*. 18:2485, 2009.

Kaur Saini M, et al. Chemopreventive response of diclofenac, a non-steroidal anti-inflammatory drug in experimental carcinogenesis. *Nutr Hosp*. 24:717, 2009.

McCleary NJ, et al. Impact of smoking on patients with stage III colon cancer: results from Cancer and Leukemia Group B 89803 [Published online ahead of print Jan 5, 2010]. *Cancer*.

Ulrich CM, et al. Polymorphisms in the reduced folate carrier, thymidylate synthase, or methionine synthase and risk of colon cancer. *Cancer Epidemiol Biomarkers Prev*. 14:2509, 2005.

Zeng H, et al. Deoxycholic acid and selenium metabolite methylselenol exert common and distinct effects on cell cycle, apoptosis, and MAP kinase pathway in HCT116 human colon cancer cells. *Nutr Cancer* 62:85, 2010.

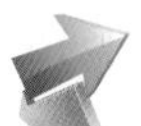

ASSESSMENT, MONITORING, AND EVALUATION

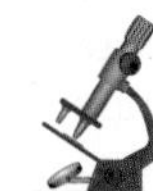

CLINICAL INDICATORS

Genetic Markers: Both cellular factors and genetic changes enhance tumor invasion. Vitamin D receptor (VDR) genes regulate the epithelial changes that initiate tumor cells; the BB genotype of the VDR polymorphism is associated with a reduced risk of colon cancer (Jenab et al, 2009). Chemokine receptor CCR5 expression and increased CD8(+) T-cell infiltration may be found (Zimmermann et al, 2010). While folate status may be linked with CRC because of its role in DNA synthesis, the C>T MTHFR polymorphism decreases risk by 15–18% (Levine et al, 2010). Finally, phosphatase and tensin homolog deleted on chromosome 10 (PTEN) is associated with late stage CRC (Bowen et al, 2009).

Specific Clinical/History

Height
Weight
BMI
Obesity?
Unintentional weight loss?
Diet history
Rectal bleeding, pain
Irregular bowel habits
Alternating diarrhea and constipation
Abdominal distention, bloating
Thin, pencil stools
Weakness
Anorexia
Dehydration, electrolyte imbalances
Intestinal obstruction, bowel abscess
Fistula
Proctoscopy
Colonoscopy
Digital rectal examination

Lab Work

CEA level (CEA 125)
8-OH-dG in colorectal crypts
Colon lavage cytology
Serum folate, B_{12}
Serum homocysteine
MTHFR genotyping
Fecal occult blood test (FOBT)
H & H (decreased)
Serum Fe
Transferrin
Na^+
K^+ (often decreased)
Chol, Trig
TLC (varies)
WBC, ESR (increased)
Alb, transthyretin
CRP
Mg^{++}, Ca^{++}
Serum zinc

INTERVENTION

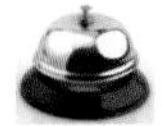

OBJECTIVES

- Decrease residue, particularly with obstruction, until fiber is better tolerated.
- Prevent rapid weight loss; correct anemia. Maintain hydration.
- Counteract side effects of therapies: chemotherapy, resection, or radiation. Nutrition counseling improves patient outcomes in radiotherapy (Ravasko et al, 2005).
- Provide nutrients in a tolerable form—oral, parenteral, or enteral.
- Include sufficient total amounts of folate and vitamin B_6 since disrupted DNA synthesis affects carcinogenesis (Sharp et al, 2008).
- Provide sufficient vitamin D_3 (Grant, 2009).
- Prevent or ameliorate starvation diarrhea.
- Protect against recurrence by dietary changes indicated in Table 13-13.

SAMPLE NUTRITION CARE PROCESS STEPS

Abnormal Gi Function

Assessment Data: Recent weight loss (10# in 2 months). Diarrhea and constipation; hx of dark, thin stools and blood. Dx of colon cancer.

Nutrition Diagnosis (PES): Abnormal GI function related to alternating diarrhea and constipation as evidenced by dark stools, and constipation 3× weekly on average followed by bloody diarrhea.

Intervention: Food-nutrient delivery—oral nutritional supplement between meals; mild fiber supplement as tolerated. Educate the patient about dietary changes that can be beneficial. Provide counseling about possible nutritional procedures (i.e., colostomy) after surgical resection.

Monitoring and Evaluation: No further weight loss before surgery. Tolerance for fiber in diet and from supplement. Adequate preparation for surgery, followed with appropriate changes in feeding method and counseling after colostomy.

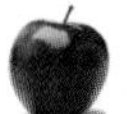

FOOD AND NUTRITION

- CPN or TF may be needed for an extended period of time; include glutamine.
- Administer parenteral fluids with adequate electrolytes, vitamins C and K, and selenium (if used over a long time). Monitor vitamin D, calcium, iron, zinc, and fat intakes for adequacy.
- With ileal resection, vitamin B_{12} deficiency can occur, and bile salts may be lost in diarrhea. Hyperoxaluria and renal oxalate stones can be a problem. With massive bowel resection, malabsorption, malnutrition, metabolic acidosis, and gastric hypersecretion may result.
- With ileostomy and colostomy, salt and sodium/water balance are problems. Ostomy diets may be needed (see ileostomy and colostomy entries in Section 7). Increase energy and ensure adequate protein.
- Decrease fiber until tolerated. Eventually, increase whole grains including rye bread, cereals, fruits, and vegetables.
- Consume less alcohol and more folic acid from spinach, broccoli, asparagus, avocado, orange juice, dried beans, and fortified cereals (Kim, 2007).
- Eat less red meat; use more poultry, fish, tofu, and beans as protein sources.
- Discuss the inclusion of other protective foods, such as calcium-rich foods; lutein and lycopene (tomato products, watermelon, spinach, kale, greens, broccoli, romaine lettuce, and pink grapefruit); cumin; cereal, bean, vegetable, and fruit fiber; flavonoids (apples, onions, green tea, and chamomile tea); cruciferous vegetables; coffee; omega-3

fatty acids from fish and walnuts; selenium foods such as Brazil nuts; and unsaturated fats such as flaxseed, salmon, and canola and olive oils.

- A multivitamin supplement is beneficial, particularly for folic acid and vitamins B_6 and D_3.
- Monitor carefully for lactose intolerance. Use lactase enzyme products when indicated.
- Physical activity should be encouraged as much as possible.

Common Drugs Used and Potential Side Effects

- Chemotherapy may be used for 6–8 months, particularly with stage 3 colon cancer. Monitor for side effects because these agents may further impact bowel function.
- The multidrug combination of oxaliplatin, fluorouracil, and leucovorin is standard treatment for metastatic colorectal carcinoma (Caraglia et al, 2005). Fluorouracil plus levamisole, methotrexate, mitomycin, lomustine, and vincristine may lead to diarrhea, nausea, vomiting, low WBC, and mouth sores.
- Bevacizumab (Avastin) use leads to a significant decrease in colon cancer deaths. Cetuximab (Erbitux), when added to chemotherapy, will shrink tumors and delay progression.
- COX-2 inhibitors may be helpful because 50% of polyps and 85% of colonic tumors in humans overexpress COX-2 (Samoha and Arber, 2005). The nonsteroidal anti-inflammatory drug, Diclofenac, is a preferential COX-2 inhibitor, which can be an effective chemopreventive agent in colon cancer (Kaur et al, 2009).
- Regular low doses of aspirin may reduce prostaglandin production; GI bleeding can result.

Herbs, Botanicals, and Supplements (see Table 13-8)

- Herbs and botanical supplements should not be used without discussing it with the physician.
- Folate vitamers (tetrahydrofolate, 5,10-methylenetetrahydrofolate) should be studied further for their roles in CRC (Sharp et al, 2008).
- With methotrexate (Rheumatrex), avoid echinacea; it may damage the liver.
- A vitamin D_3 supplement, such as 1100 IU daily, seems to be of benefit (Grant, 2009).
- Low-dose fish oil supplementation may be useful to reduce inflammation.
- Sea cucumber extract contains Frondanol A5—a glycolipid extract with potential chemopreventive properties (Janakiram et al, 2009).
- Sour orange (cirtus aurantium) has protective liminoid properties (Perez et al, 2009).

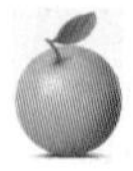

NUTRITION EDUCATION, COUNSELING, CARE MANAGEMENT

- At first, limit foods that may cause gas, such as corn, broccoli, cauliflower, beans, cabbage, melon, and carbonated beverages. Provide instruction on hydration and the use of fiber to help with bowel management, particularly for rectal cancer patients.
- Family members (offspring and other first-degree relatives) should have a digital examination annually at 40 years of age, stool tests for blood after 50 years of age, and sigmoidoscopy or colonoscopy after age 50 every 3–5 years.
- Medical advice may include regular use of aspirin or nonsteroidal anti-inflammatory drugs (NSAIDs).
- Discuss an appropriate dietary regimen for any specific problems. Weekly Medical Nutrition Therapy (MNT) that includes an individualized nutrition prescription and counseling improves calorie and protein intake, nutrition status, quality of life (QOL), and reduces symptoms of anorexia, nausea, vomiting and diarrhea (American Dietetic Association, 2010).
- Encourage family participation in all levels of care.
- Discuss how to prevent future polyps. High compliance with a low-fat, high-fiber diet is associated with a reduced risk of adenoma recurrence (Sansbury et al, 2009). Omit trans-fatty acids as much as possible (Vinikoor et al, 2009). A high intake of flavonols, which are at greater concentrations in beans, onions, apples, and tea, is also associated with decreased risk (Bobe et al, 2008).
- Suggest an intake of berries, chocolate, coffee, soy foods, folate from foods and supplements, lutein and carotenoids from fruits or vegetables, and whole grains such as rye.
- Encourage dairy products for calcium, vitamin D, and lactose content. If necessary, use lactase enzymes.
- Encourage physical activity when feasible.
- Surveillance following curative treatment generally includes history and physical exams every 6 months for 5 years, then every 3 months for 2 years, and then every 6 months for 3–5 years (Sunga et al, 2005).

Patient Education—Food Safety

- Educate the patient about food safety issues. Discuss safe food handling and preparation, keeping foods at proper temperatures, the use of sterile water, and reheating foods properly.

For More Information

- Colon Cancer Page
  http://jama.ama-assn.org/cgi/reprint/300/23/2816.pdf
- Medline Information–Colorectal Cancer
  http://www.nlm.nih.gov/medlineplus/colorectalcancer.html
- National Colorectal Cancer Action Campaign
  http://www.cdc.gov/cancer/screenforlife/

COLORECTAL CANCER—CITED REFERENCES

American Dietetic Association (ADA). Evidence analysis library: Oncology. Accessed January 8, 2010, at http://www.adaevidencelibrary.com/topic.cfm?cat=3250.

Bobe G, et al. Dietary flavonoids and colorectal adenoma recurrence in the Polyp Prevention Trial. *Cancer Epidemiol Biomarkers Prev.* 17:1344, 2008.

Bowen KA, et al. PTEN loss induces epithelial–mesenchymal transition in human colon cancer cells. *Anticancer Res.* 29:4439, 2009.

Caraglia MD, et al. Chemotherapy regimen GOLF induces apoptosis in colon cancer cells through multi-chaperone complex inactivation and increased Raf-1 ubiquitin-dependent degradation. *Cancer Biol Ther.* 4:1159, 2005.

Castellone MD, et al. Prostaglandin E2 promotes colon cancer cell growth through a novel Gs-axin-beta-catenin signaling axis. *Science.* 310:1504, 2005.

Fedirko V, et al. Effects of supplemental vitamin D and calcium on oxidative DNA damage marker in normal colorectal mucosa: a randomized clinical trial. *Cancer Epidemiol Biomarkers Prev.* 19:280, 2010.

Fuemmeller ER, et al. Weight, dietary behavior, and physical activity in childhood and adolescence: implications for adult cancer risk. *Obes Facts.* 2:179, 2009.

Grant WB. A critical review of Vitamin D and cancer: a report of the IARC Working Group. *Dermatoendocrinol.* 1:25, 2009.

Janakiram NB, et al. Chemopreventive effects of Frondanol A5, a Cucumaria frondosa extract, against rat colon carcinogenesis and inhibition of human colon cancer cell growth. *Cancer Prev Res (Phila Pa).* 3:82, 2010.

Jenab M. Vitamin D receptor and calcium sensing receptor polymorphisms and the risk of colorectal cancer in European populations. *Cancer Epidemiol Biomarkers Prev.* 18:2485, 2009.

Kaur Saini M, et al. Chemopreventive response of diclofenac, a non-steroidal anti-inflammatory drug in experimental carcinogenesis. *Nutr Hosp.* 24:717, 2009.

Kim DH. The interactive effect of methyl-group diet and polymorphism of methylenetetrahydrofolate reductase on the risk of colorectal cancer. *Mutat Res.* 622:14, 2007.

Levine AJ, et al. Genetic variability in the MTHFR gene and colorectal cancer risk using the colorectal cancer family registry. *Cancer Epidemiol Biomarkers Prev.* 19:89, 2010.

Perez JL, et al. Limonin methoxylation influences the induction of glutathione S-transferase and quinone reductase. *J Agric Food Chem.* 57:5279, 2009.

Ravasko P, et al. Dietary counseling improves patient outcomes: a prospective, randomized, controlled trial in colorectal cancer patients undergoing radiotherapy. *J Clin Oncology.* 23:1431, 2005.

Samoha S, Arber N. Cyclooxygenase-2 inhibition prevents colorectal cancer: from the bench to the bed side. *Oncology.* 69:33S, 2005.

Sansbury LB, et al. The effect of strict adherence to a high-fiber, high-fruit and -vegetable, and low-fat eating pattern on adenoma recurrence. *Am J Epidemiol.* 170:576, 2009.

Sharp L, et al. Polymorphisms in the methylenetetrahydrofolate reductase (MTHFR) gene, intakes of folate and related B vitamins and colorectal cancer: a case-control study in a population with relatively low folate intake. *Br J Nutr.* 99:379, 2008.

Slattery ML, et al. Tumor markers and rectal cancer: support for an inflammation-related pathway. *Int J Cancer.* 125:1698, 2009.

Sunga AY, et al. Care of cancer survivors. *Am Fam Physician.* 71:699, 2005.

Vinikoor LC, et al. Trans-fatty acid consumption and its association with distal colorectal cancer in the North Carolina colon cancer study II [Published online ahead of print October 20, 2009]. *Cancer Causes Control.*

Zeng H, et al. Deoxycholic acid and selenium metabolite methylselenol exert common and distinct effects on cell cycle, apoptosis, and MAP kinase pathway in HCT116 human colon cancer cells. *Nutr Cancer.* 62:85, 2010.

Zimmermann T, et al. Low expression of chemokine receptor CCR5 in human colorectal cancer correlates with lymphatic dissemination and reduced CD8(+) T-cell infiltration [Published online ahead of print Jan 7, 2010]. *Int J Colorectal Dis.*

ESOPHAGEAL, HEAD AND NECK, AND THYROID CANCERS

NUTRITIONAL ACUITY RANKING: LEVEL 3–4

Mouth and Throat Cancer

Cancer-causing chemicals from tobacco products increase the risk of cancer of the lip, cheek, tongue, and larynx (voice box). The removal of these cancers can be disfiguring and can result in loss of the larynx.

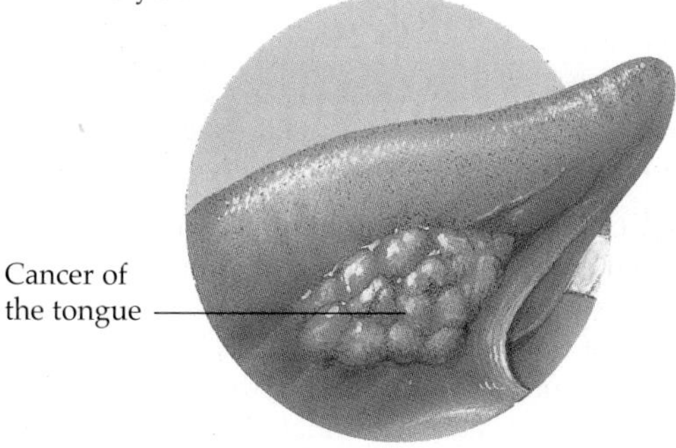

Asset provided by Anatomical Chart Co.

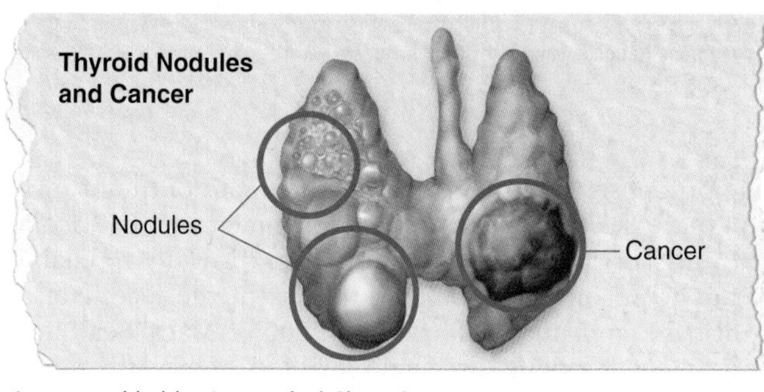

Asset provided by Anatomical Chart Co.

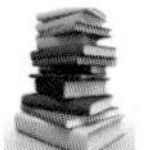

DEFINITIONS AND BACKGROUND

Head and neck cancers affect esophageal, hypopharyngeal, laryngeal, lip and oral cavity, nasopharyngeal, oropharyngeal, paranasal sinus and nasal cavity, parathyroid, or salivary glands. Annually, approximately 38,000 people in the United States are diagnosed with a head or neck cancer; the highest overall incidence rate is in black males. Tobacco is linked with 85% of these cancers; alcohol is another risk. Obesity is a factor in many cases (Steffen et al, 2009). See Table 13-14 for more details.

Damage from acid reflux may contribute to esophageal cancer. Folate and homocysteine derangements are common. A diet rich in fruits, vegetables, selenium, zinc, and folate is associated with a reduced risk of head and neck cancer (Falciglia et al, 2005; Kane, 2005; Steevens et al, 2010).

Head and neck squamous cell carcinoma (HNSCC) is an aggressive cancer with low survival rates in advanced stages.

TABLE 13-14 **Key Factors in Types of Head and Neck Cancer**

Site	Comments
Oral cavity	Caused by sun exposure (lip); possibly human papillomavirus (HPV) infection; paan (betel quid) used by Southeast Asians; intake of mate, a tea-like beverage habitually consumed by South Americans. May present with gingival swelling, pain, bleeding, and loosening teeth. The disorder is rare in persons younger than age 40. Risk of metastasis is great; only about half of these individuals will live longer than 5 years.
Nasopharynx	More common in Chinese ancestry. Caused by Epstein-Barr virus infection; occupational exposure to wood dust; and consumption of certain preservatives or salted foods. Signs include unilateral obstruction, epistaxis, pain, otological changes, and nasal obstruction.
Oropharynx	Caused by poor oral hygiene; HPV infection and the use of mouthwash that has a high alcohol content are possible, but not proven, risk factors. There may be a dull ache, dysphagia, referred otalgia, and trismus.
Paranasal sinuses and nasal cavity	Caused by industrial exposures, such as wood or nickel dust inhalation. Tobacco and alcohol use play less of a role in this type of cancer.
Hypopharynx	Plummer-Vinson syndrome is a rare disorder that results from iron and other nutritional deficiencies with severe anemia. Dysphagia results as webs of tissue grow across the upper part of the esophagus.
Larynx	Caused by exposure to airborne particles of asbestos, particularly in the workplace. Voice changes, dysphagia, odynophagia, and dyspnea occur.
Parotid and salivary glands	Caused by radiation to the head and neck. This exposure can come from diagnostic X-rays or from radiation therapy for noncancerous conditions or cancer. Unilateral symptoms and impaired jaw mobility can occur. The parotid gland is the largest salivary gland. Cancer here is rare. Surgery is often curative.
Esophageal cancer	Develops in the middle or lower third of the esophagus. It is one of the more common types of head and neck cancer. It presents as adenocarcinoma or squamous cell cases that require surgical resection. This condition is more common in persons older than 50 years of age, particularly males. Barrett's esophagus (BE) is a premalignant condition associated with esophageal cancer; cyclooxygenase-2 (COX-2) is overexpressed. Aspirin and other nonsteroidal anti-inflammatory drugs may help prevent esophageal cancer. Stage 0 is very early and affects only the first layer of cells; in Stage V, the cancer has metastasized.
Thyroid cancer	A lump on the side of the neck, hoarseness, and dysphagia can be signs. Thyroidectomy may be used, or radioactive iodine (RDI) can be used to destroy cancerous cells that remain after surgery. A low-iodine diet may be needed about 2 weeks before the RDI treatment.

Derived from: National Cancer Institute, http://www.cancer.gov/cancertopics/factsheet/sites-types/head-and-neck, accessed January 9, 2010.

The prognosis for cure worsens as the depth of tumor invasion increases. Surgery is possible for some cases. Cervicofacial and cervicothoracic rotation flaps provide a reliable means to reconstruct complex defects of the face, lateral skull base, and neck (Moore et al, 2005). Many head and neck cancer patients are malnourished before treatment begins, and those who are treated with radiotherapy are at an increased risk of malnutrition due to the severe side effects (Moore et al, 2005; Wood, 2005). Radiation therapy side effects may include odynophagia, dysphagia, mucositis, esophagitis, xerostomia (with occasional osteoradionecrosis), dental caries, weight loss, taste changes, and decreased appetite. Prophylactic placement of a gastrostomy feeding tube is useful.

Thyroid cancer affects approximately 26,000 people in the United States. Thyroid-stimulating hormone (TSH) from the pituitary causes the thyroid gland to produce thyroid hormones and to release thyroglobulin. Papillary tumors are the most common type; they arise as an irregular, solid, or cystic mass from otherwise normal thyroid tissue. Distant metastasis is uncommon, but lung and bone are the most common sites. Tumors that invade or extend beyond the thyroid capsule have a worse prognosis. Often, the thyroid gland is surgically removed as a cure. Thyroxine medicine (Synthroid, Levoxyl, and Unithroid) is needed to keep TSH levels low.

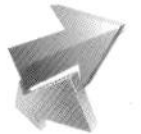

ASSESSMENT, MONITORING, AND EVALUATION

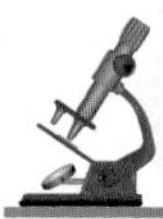

CLINICAL INDICATORS

Genetic Markers: An epigenome-wide screen has revealed a set of genes that are commonly methylated and downregulated in head and neck cancers (SEPT9, SLC5A8, FUSSEL18, EBF3, and IRX1). All five interact with components of the TGF-beta pathway; their silencing results in a coordinated decrease in apoptosis, increased proliferation, and decreased differentiation (Bennett et al, 2009).

Specific Clinical/History

Height
Weight
BMI
Obesity?
Unplanned weight loss
Diet history
BP
I & O
Dehydration?
Temperature
Dysphagia, painful swallowing
Substernal pain or feeling of fullness
Regurgitation of undigested food
Malaise
Malnutrition
Anemia

Regurgitation after eating	Taste changes, decreased appetite	CRP
Hiccups, foul breath	Loosening teeth	Transferrin
Aspiration	Oral biopsy	H & H
Increased salivation	Esophageal webs with achalasia?	ALT (increased)
Hoarseness and coughing	Palpable mass	Gluc
Gingival swelling, pain, bleeding, or hyperplasia	Barium swallow	Serum zinc (low?)
Nonhealing ulcerative oral lesions	Endoscopy	Triiodothyronine (T3)
Mucositis, esophagitis	Nasopharyngoscopy	Thyroxine (T4)
Xerostomia	Direct laryngoscopy, esophagoscopy	Thyroid-stimulating hormone (TSH)
Dental caries	Biopsy	Ca^{++}, Mg^{++}
	Lab Work	Na^{+}, K^{+}
	Alb, transthyretin	Alb, transthyretin
		Chol
		Bicarbonate

INTERVENTION

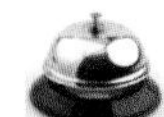

OBJECTIVES

- Prepare for treatments such as surgery, radiation, or chemotherapy. The dietitian should provide a pretreatment evaluation and weekly visits for 6 weeks during chemoradiation treatment to reduce weight loss, unplanned hospitalization, length of stay, and tolerance for full treatment (American Dietetic Association, 2010).
- Prevent malnutrition, further weight loss, cachexia, and aspiration. Weight loss, caused by acute mucositis and dysphagia, is common during concurrent chemotherapy and irradiation (chemoradiotherapy) of head and neck cancer (Lin et al, 2005).
- Because nutrition support for patients with head and neck cancer is associated with a significant increase in total energy ingestion, placing gastrostomy tubes prophylactically prevents disruption to treatment plans (Moore et al, 2005; Wood, 2005).
- Meet nutritional needs with tube feeding, as needed. Progress to goal with minimal signs and symptoms of intolerance (nausea, fullness). Transition to full or partial oral intake when feasible.
- If resection is needed, fat malabsorption, reflux, dumping syndrome, increased mediastinal pressure, and increased food transit time may be side effects.
- Hydrate adequately; encourage fluids between meals and limit fluid intake at meals to improve intake of other foods.
- Promote adequate wound healing, positive nitrogen balance, and retention of lean body mass.
- Prevent or correct anemia, sepsis, abscesses.
- Monitor for dysphagia, difficulty chewing, mucositis, xerostomia, fibrosis, and dental caries after treatments. Assure adequate mouth care.
- Omit alcoholic beverages and abstain from tobacco, including chewing snuff.
- In patients with advanced cancer: reduce symptoms, preserve organ function, and improve quality of life as much as possible. Provide palliative care if needed.

SAMPLE NUTRITION CARE PROCESS STEPS

Involuntary Weight Loss

Assessment: Recurrent squamous cell carcinoma of the larynx; s/p emergency tracheostomy, radiation and chemotherapy. NPO due to swallowing difficulty; on GT bolus feeding. Elevated BUN & creatinine levels. On oxycodone for pain.

***Nutrition Diagnosis (PES)*:** Involuntary weight loss (NC-3.2) related to decreased oral intake and dysphagia as evidenced by weight loss of 21% in 17 months.

Interventions: Nutrient delivery—ND 2.41 enteral feeding tube; ND 3.21 multivitamin supplement.

Education: Discuss home tube feeding that is appropriate for the patient's condition.

Counseling: C-2.2 goal setting: minimize weight loss, maintain adequate hydration, prevent aspiration, and improve quality of life.

Coordination of Nutrition Care: RC-1.1 Interdisciplinary team meeting with nursing, speech therapy, social worker, and recreational therapy.

Monitor and Evaluation: Monitor for weight improvement. No GI problems or enteral nutrition intolerance. Improvement in renal lab values. Reassess nutritional needs via GT. Reassess with speech evaluation for possible transition to full or partial oral intake when feasible.

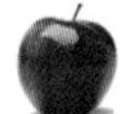

FOOD AND NUTRITION

- Adjust diet individually to meet the patient's needs. Nutrition support enhances desirable outcomes (Odelli et al, 2005). After radiation: xerostomia, ulceration, bleeding, and pain may result; after chemotherapy, nausea, vomiting, weakness, and fatigue may occur (Dixon, 2005).
- Be careful not to create refeeding syndrome, which is potentially fatal. Progress slowly in patients who have been malnourished for a week or longer. Begin with 10 kcal/kg per day and increase slowly; use thiamin and other B-complex vitamins in a supplement (Mehanna et al, 2009).
- Eventually, provide a diet high in energy and protein with bland or pureed foods as required: 30–35 kcal/kg; 1.0–1.5 g protein/kg.
- A dysphagia diet (thick pureed foods, decrease in thin liquids) may be needed. Tolerance will vary for hot and cold foods and drinks; monitor and alter intake accordingly.
- Patients are often fed with gastrostomy or jejunostomy feedings. Cellular and morphological changes follow a period of malnutrition; enteral feeding is an important strategy for maintaining gut integrity and function (Sica et al, 2005). Use enteral feeding formulas that are high in omega-3 fatty acids (Aiko et al, 2005) and arginine (De Luis et al, 2009).
- Increase fluid intake as tolerated; dehydration is common.

- Increase intake of vitamins D_3, A and C; zinc; and other nutrients that may be low. Otherwise, a multivitamin–mineral supplement is indicated if oral intake is not possible.
- If esophagectomy has been performed, gastric stasis or dumping syndrome may occur. The use of needle catheter jejunostomy (NCJ) is safe, with an extremely low rate of complications over a prolonged period at low costs (Sica et al, 2005).
- If an oral diet is possible, omit irritants such as black pepper and chili powder and dilute acidic fruits or juices such as orange, grapefruit, and tomato.
- Use protective foods to prevent recurrence; use beans, vegetables, fish, foods rich in zinc and lycopene, whole grains, citrus fruits, and vitamin C–rich foods.
- Polyphenols show great promise; EGCG in green tea is particularly beneficial (Baumeister et al, 2009).
- With thyroid cancer, a low-iodine diet may be needed prior to surgery or treatment.
- In advanced cases, offer palliative care. Hydration and comfort are the focus.

Common Drugs Used and Potential Side Effects

- Aspirin can lower esophageal cancer risk by 90% by reducing prostaglandin production. Some doctors will prescribe a low daily dose to prevent recurrence.
- Chemotherapy with cisplatin may be used, along with radiation therapy. Cisplatin can cause nausea, vomiting, altered taste, changes in renal function, and diarrhea. Weight loss during cisplatin-containing chemoradiotherapy is associated with reduced kidney function; findings highlight the importance of intensive supportive measures of nutrition and hydration beyond standard measures, and these steps should be started before 10% weight loss occurs (Lin et al, 2005).
- Bleomycin and methotrexate can lead to nausea, vomiting, anorexia, or stomatitis.
- Steroids may be used to reduce inflammation; hyperglycemia, sodium retention, potassium depletion, and negative nitrogen balance can result.
- Pilocarpine may be used as a saliva substitute for xerostomia.

Herbs, Botanicals, and Supplements (see Table 13-8)

- Herbs and botanical supplements should not be used without discussing it with the physician.
- Avoid the use of echinacea with cyclosporine or methotrexate (Rheumatrex) because of potential damage to the liver. Avoid St. John's wort also.
- Curcumin is a powerful inhibitor of COX-2 expression (Khafif et al, 2009).
- L-carnitine is sometimes used to decrease toxicity from agents such as bleomycin.
- Zinc supplementation helps in managing mucositis after radiation.

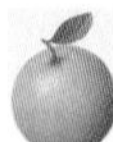

NUTRITION EDUCATION, COUNSELING, CARE MANAGEMENT

- Discuss a diet rationale that is appropriate for the patient's condition. If the patient can eat orally, encourage him or her to chew slowly.
- If jejunostomy feeding is required after esophagastric surgery, teach the patient/family/caretaker how to prepare feedings and how to produce the item in a clean environment.
- During radiation therapy/surgical recovery, patients with gastrostomy tubes should be encouraged to practice swallowing exercises, as prescribed by the speech pathologist, to maintain swallowing function and reduce the risk of fibrosis. Encourage help from speech therapy.
- Hypothyroid status can cause dysphagia; counsel accordingly.
- If oral diet is possible, discuss the use of protective foods.
- Relaxation therapy or biofeedback can be beneficial.
- Radiation-induced fibrosis (RIF) is caused by reduced blood supply months or years later. Rinse with vitamin E solutions and use 1000 IU tocopherol with pentoxifylline to decrease mucositis (Chiao and Lee, 2005; Haddad et al, 2005). Use small frequent feedings and oral supplements.

Patient Education—Food Safety

- Educate the patient about food safety issues. Discuss safe food handling and preparation, keeping foods at proper temperatures, the use of sterile water, and reheating foods properly.
- For home tube feeding or CPN, teach the principles of safe handling and administration. Discuss the signs of infection or intolerance and when to contact the health team.

For More Information

- CancerLinks USA–Esophageal Cancer
  http://www.cancerlinksusa.com/esophagus/wynk/
- Liquid Diets
  http://www.cancer.gov/cancertopics/eatinghints/page7
- Low Iodine Cookbook
  http://www.thyca.org/Cookbook.pdf
- Medline–Esophageal Cancer
  http://www.nlm.nih.gov/medlineplus/esophagealcancer.html
- National Cancer Institute–Esophageal Cancer – Nutrition
  http://www.cancer.gov/cancertopics/wyntk/esophagus/page12
- National Institutes of Health Cancer Information
  http://www.nidr.nih.gov/Spectrum/NIDCR3/3menu.htm
- Thyroid Cancer Survivors' Association
  http://www.thyca.org/
- Thyroid Cancer – Mayo Clinic
  http://www.mayoclinic.com/health/thyroid-cancer/DS00492

ESOPHAGEAL, HEAD AND NECK, AND THYROID CANCERS—CITED REFERENCES

Aiko S, et al. The effects of immediate enteral feeding with a formula containing high levels of omega-3 fatty acids in patients after surgery for esophageal cancer. *J Parent Enter Nutr.* 29:141, 2005.

American Dietetic Association (ADA). Evidence analysis library: Oncology. Accessed January 9, 2010, at http://www.adaevidencelibrary.com/.

Baumeister P, et al. Epigallocatechin-3-gallate reduces DNA damage induced by benzo[a]pyrene diol epoxide and cigarette smoke condensate in human mucosa tissue cultures. *Eur J Cancer Prev.* 18:230, 2009.

Bennett KL, et al. Disruption of transforming growth factor-beta signaling by five frequently methylated genes leads to head and neck squamous cell carcinoma pathogenesis. *Cancer Res.* 69:9301, 2009.

Chiao TB, Lee AJ. Role of pentoxifylline and vitamin E in attenuation of radiation-induced fibrosis. *Ann Pharmacother.* 39:516, 2005.

DeLuis DA, et al. High dose of arginine enhanced enteral nutrition in postsurgical head and neck cancer patients. A randomized clinical trial. *Eur Rev Med Pharmacol Sci.* 13:279, 2009.

Dixon SW. Nutrition care issues in the ambulatory (outpatient) head and neck cancer. *Support Line.* 27:3, 2005.

Falciglia GA, et al. A clinical-based intervention improves diet in patients with head and neck cancer at risk for second primary cancer. *J Am Diet Assoc.* 105:1609, 2005.

Haddad P, et al. Pentoxifylline and vitamin E combination for superficial radiation-induced fibrosis: a phase II clinical trial. *Radiother Oncol.* 77:324, 2005.

Kane MA. The role of folates in squamous cell carcinoma of the head and neck. *Cancer Detect Prev.* 29:46, 2005.

Khafif A, et al. Curcumin: a potential radio-enhancer in head and neck cancer. *Laryngoscope.* 119:2019, 2009.

Lin A, et al. Metabolic abnormalities associated with weight loss during chemoirradiation of head-and-neck cancer. *Int J Radiat Oncol Biol Phys.* 63:1413, 2005.

Mehanna H, et al. Refeeding syndrome – awareness, prevention and management. *Head Neck Oncol.* 1:4, 2009.

Mercuri A, et al. The effect of an intensive nutritional program on daily setup variations and radiotherapy planning margins of head and neck cancer patients. *J Med Imaging Radiat Oncol.* 53:500, 2009.

Moore BA, et al. Cervicofacial and cervicothoracic rotation flaps in head and neck reconstruction. *Head Neck.* 27:1092, 2005.

Odelli C, et al. Nutrition support improves patient outcomes, treatment tolerance and admission characteristics in oesophageal cancer. *Clin Oncol.* 17:639, 2005.

Sica GS, et al. Needle catheter jejunostomy at esophagectomy for cancer. *J Surg Oncol.* 91:276, 2005.

Steevens J, et al. Selenium status and the risk of esophageal and gastric cancer subtypes: the Netherlands cohort study [Published online ahead of print Jan 6, 2010]. *Gastroenterology.*

Steffen A, et al. Anthropometry and esophageal cancer risk in the European prospective investigation into cancer and nutrition. *Cancer Epidemiol Biomarkers Prev.* 18:2079, 2009.

Wood K. Audit of nutritional guidelines for head and neck cancer patients undergoing radiotherapy. *J Hum Nutr Diet.* 18:343, 2005.

GASTRIC CANCER

NUTRITIONAL ACUITY RANKING: LEVEL 3–4

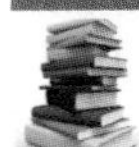

DEFINITIONS AND BACKGROUND

Gastric cancer (GC) is a carcinoma that most commonly occurs in the pyloric segment and along the lesser curvature. Cancer that begins in the glandular cells is an adenoma; this type is over 90% of gastric cancers. If the cancer starts in the immune system, it is a lymphoma; if it starts in the hormonal system, it is called carcinoid syndrome. Another very rare form starts in the nervous system and is called a gastrointestinal stromal tumor (GIST). Diffuse forms have a poor prognosis.

In GC, early definitive signs are rare. GC may follow long-term pernicious anemia, Ménétrier's disease, or chronic gastritis. It is generally found in males aged 50–70 years and among smokers. While frequency is low in the United States, it is high in Japan and China. Gastric carcinoma is the second leading cause of cancer-related deaths in the world, accounting for more than 700,000 deaths each year (Hatakeyama, 2009).

Helicobacter pylori infection plays a role. Chemokine production and antiapoptosis are mediated by *H. pylori* and may drive lymphocytes to malignancy. Infection with cagA-positive *H. pylori* plays an essential role; this protein is delivered into gastric epithelial cells via the bacterial secretion system where it contributes to the transformation of gastric epithelial cells (Hatakeyama, 2009). See Table 13-15 for other risk factors.

A recent study shows a protective role for riboflavin and vitamin B_6 (Eussen et al, 2010). Physical activity and eating a diet high in fruits, vegetables, beta-carotene, and vitamin C may also decrease the risk for GC (Kim et al, 2005; Vigen et al, 2006). Greater adherence to a Mediterranean dietary pattern is associated with a significant reduction in the risk of incident GC (Buckland et al, 2009).

Surgery is the most common treatment. Very small, stage 1 cancers that are limited to the inside lining of the stomach may be removed using endoscopy. In a subtotal gastrectomy, only the affected stomach portion is removed. In stages 3 or 4, it may be necessary to remove the entire stomach and connect the esophagus to the small intestine. Laparoscopic surgery is less invasive and recovery is faster.

Neoadjuvant radiation may be used before surgery to shrink a stomach tumor, or it can also be used after surgery to kill any remaining cancer cells. Radiation therapy may cause diarrhea, nausea, or vomiting. Chemotherapy may also be used along with radiation therapy or for advanced cancers that cannot be treated through surgery.

TABLE 13-15 Risks for Gastric Cancer

Risks for Gastric Cancer
Advanced age
Chronic atrophic gastritis, pernicious anemia, gastric polyps
Diet high in red meat
Diet high in salt, salted foods, smoked and preserved foods
Diet low in vitamin E or selenium
Eating foods contaminated with aflatoxin fungus
Ethnicity—young white and Hispanic males; African-Americans from poor socioeconomic backgrounds
Family history of gastric cancer, Ménétrier's disease, intestinal metaplasia
H. pylori gastric infection
Low use of fruits and vegetables
Male gender
Smoking

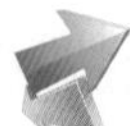

ASSESSMENT, MONITORING, AND EVALUATION

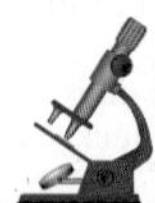

CLINICAL INDICATORS

Genetic Markers: Genetic predisposition is a risk factor in gastric cancer. Aberrant methylation of several genes is noted; some have a poor prognosis. E-cadherin is involved with diffuse forms; and SNP analysis (including IL1B) may elucidate the role of inflammation and stem cells in premalignant lesions (Milne et al, 2009).

Specific Clinical/History

- Height
- Weight
- BMI
- Weight loss?
- Diet history
- I & O
- Dehydration?
- BP
- Feeling of fullness
- Indigestion, belching
- Dysphagia
- Anorexia
- Anemia, pallor
- Vertigo
- Nausea or vomiting
- Melena
- MRI or CT scan
- Barium swallow
- Endoscopy

Lab Work

- *H. pylori*
- Low serum pepsinogen I/II ratio
- Alb, transthyretin
- CRP
- Ca^{++}, Mg^{++}
- Na^{+}, K^{+}
- Gluc
- H & H
- Transferrin
- ALT (increased)
- Melena, occult blood
- Serum folic acid, B_{12}

SAMPLE NUTRITION CARE PROCESS STEPS

Inadequate Mineral Intake

Assessment Data: Diagnosis of gastric cancer, stage 1; several small polyps found on endoscopy. BMI normal, no sign of *H. pylori*. Lives in region known to have low levels of selenium in the soil (coastal Carolinas). Diet history indicates no intake of selenium-rich foods or multivitamin-mineral supplementation. Some nausea and melena noted.

Nutrition Diagnosis (PES): Inadequate selenium intake related to poor diet and supplementation as evidenced by diet history and residence in area known to have selenium-poor soil.

Intervention: Food-Nutrient Delivery—Provide foods high in selenium; encourage the use of a daily multivitamin supplement that contains the daily value for selenium. Educate—teach the patient and family about food sources of selenium. Counseling—provide tips on other cancer preventive factors. Coordinate care with the medical team after the surgical removal of the gastric polyps.

Monitoring and Evaluation: Successful minor surgery. Improvement in intake of selenium from food and daily supplement; better intake of other protective factors. Able to maintain BMI within desirable range. No further melena or nausea.

INTERVENTION

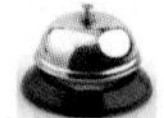

OBJECTIVES

- Prevent or reverse weight loss and further malnutrition.
- Encourage fluids.
- Counteract side effects of chemotherapy, radiation, or gastrectomy. If gastrectomy is performed, dumping syndrome or hypochlorhydria may result.
- Promote wound healing. Replete visceral proteins as stress level decreases.
- Correct protein-losing enteropathy.
- Prevent cancer recurrence by including protective foods.
- Improve quality of life.

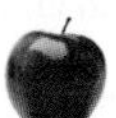

FOOD AND NUTRITION

- Parenteral therapy may be used, particularly before surgery.
- If oral diet is possible, include protective foods such as *Allium* in garlic (raw or lightly cooked), carotenoids and lycopene (Ito et al, 2005), fish, fruits, nonherbal tea, indoles and sulforaphane from cruciferous vegetables, and quercetin from apples and yellow onions. Vitamin B_6 and riboflavin should be included (Eussenn et al, 2010) as should selenium and vitamin E (Qiao et al, 2009).
- After resection, patients are often volume-sensitive and need small meals and snacks with fluids between meals. When oral intake is allowed, try light meals that are nutrient-dense, high-protein/high-energy. Drink 35 mL/kg of fluid or more, unless contraindicated.
- After gastrectomy, manage dumping syndrome, where undigested food enters the small intestine too quickly. Small, frequent feedings may be better tolerated. Concentrated carbohydrates, alcohol, and carbonated beverages should be severely limited or omitted. See entry in Section 7 also.
- Jejunostomy feeding may be needed at the time of a resection. Monitor tolerance carefully.
- Be sure that dietary intake and supplementation includes selenium, zinc, vitamin C, and other key nutrients for wound healing and correction of anemia. Take supplements with food.

Common Drugs Used and Potential Side Effects

- Antibiotic therapy is needed to eradicate *H. pylori* bacteria where present.
- Cytotoxic drugs such as mitomycin C may cause fever, nausea, vomiting, anorexia, and stomatitis.
- With fluorouracil (FU), anorexia and nausea are common. Sore mouth, taste changes, and vomiting also may result. Added thiamin is recommended, and leucovorin is often used with FU.
- In a rare form of gastrointestinal stromal tumor (GIST), imatinib (Gleevec) is useful; it interferes with an abnormal enzyme that sends signals to the nucleus of a cancer cell. Nausea and vomiting are potential side effects. Imatinib shrinks tumors by more than half with minimal side effects (Heinrich and Corless, 2005).

- Sunitinib (Sutent) is useful in stomach cancer when imatinib is not effective.

Herbs, Botanicals, and Supplements (see Table 13-8)

- Herbs and botanical supplements should not be used without discussing it with the physician.
- Treatment with a combination of 50 micrograms of selenium, 30 milligrams of vitamin E, and 15 milligrams of beta-carotene leads to decreased mortality from gastric cancer (Qiao et al, 2009).

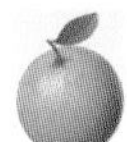

NUTRITION EDUCATION, COUNSELING, CARE MANAGEMENT

- Feeding tubes such as jejunostomy may be useful in the home setting.
- If eating orally, instruct patient on postgastrectomy diet. Encourage patient to chew slowly and well.
- Discuss protective foods and phytochemicals.
- If the stomach was resected, vitamin B_{12} anemia is likely to occur within several years; monitor carefully. Injections will likely be needed for life.

Patient Education—Food Safety

- Educate the patient about food safety issues. Discuss safe food handling and preparation, keeping foods at proper temperatures, the use of sterile water, and reheating foods properly.
- With tube feeding, discuss the safe handling of formula and tubing.

For More Information

- *H. pylori* and Cancer Fact Sheet
  http://www.cancer.gov/cancertopics/factsheet/risk/h-pylori-cancer
- Memorial Sloan-Kettering Cancer Center
  http://www.mskcc.org/mskcc/html/1467.cfm
- National Cancer Institute–Gastric Cancer
  http://www.cancer.gov/cancerinfo/pdq/treatment/gastric/healthprofessional
- OncoLink–Gastric Cancer
  http://cancer.med.upenn.edu/types/

GASTRIC CANCER—CITED REFERENCES

Buckland G, et al. Adherence to a Mediterranean diet and risk of gastric adenocarcinoma within the European Prospective Investigation into Cancer and Nutrition (EPIC) cohort study [Published online ahead of print Dec, 2010]. *Am J Clin Nutr.*

Eussen SJ, et al. Vitamins B_2 and B_6 and genetic polymorphisms related to one-carbon metabolism as risk factors for gastric adenocarcinoma in the European prospective investigation into cancer and nutrition. *Cancer Epidemiol Biomarkers Prev.* 19:28, 2010.

Hatakeyama M. Helicobacter pylori and gastric carcinogenesis. *J Gastroenterol.* 44:239, 2009.

Heinrich MC, Corless CL. Gastric GI stromal tumors (GISTs): the role of surgery in the era of targeted therapy. *J Surg Oncol.* 90:195, 2005.

Ito H, et al. Polyphenol levels in human urine after intake of six different polyphenol-rich beverages. *Br J Nutr.* 94:500, 2005.

Kim HJ, et al. Effect of nutrient intake and *Helicobacter pylori* infection on gastric cancer in Korea: a case-control study. *Nutr Cancer.* 52:138, 2005.

Milne AN, et al. Nature meets nurture: molecular genetics of gastric cancer. *Hum Genet.* 126:615, 2009.

Qiao YL, et al. Total and cancer mortality after supplementation with vitamins and minerals: follow-up of the Linxian General Population Nutrition Intervention Trial. *J Natl Cancer Inst.* 101:507, 2009.

Vigen C, et al. Occupational physical activity and risk of adenocarcinomas of the esophagus and stomach. *Int J Cancer.* 118:1004, 2006.

LIVER CANCER

NUTRITIONAL ACUITY RANKING: LEVEL 3–4

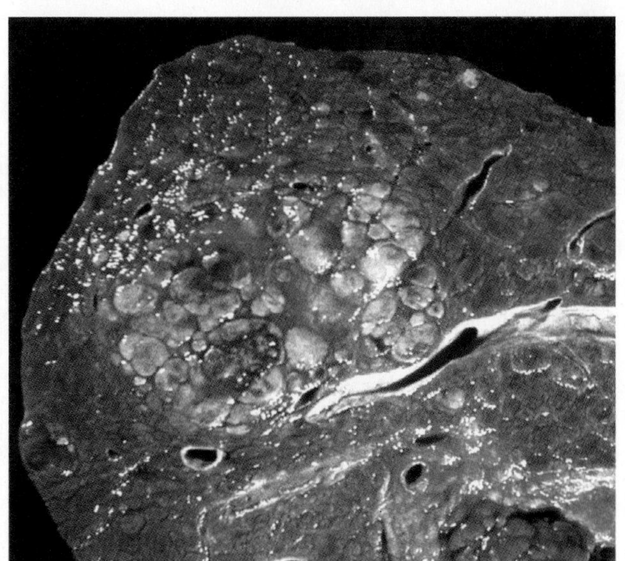

Adapted from: Rubin E MD and Farber JL MD. *Pathology,* 3rd ed. Philadelphia: Lippincott Williams & Wilkins, 1999.

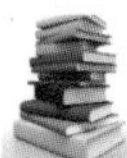

DEFINITIONS AND BACKGROUND

Liver cancer (hepatocellular carcinoma, HCC) is the fifth most common cancer and is one of the leading causes of cancer death worldwide (Yam et al, 2010). Primary hepatic tumors are common with alcohol abuse, aflatoxin ingestion, chronic hepatitis, or low weight at birth (see Table 13-16). HCC may develop after years of chronic inflammation and persistent mucosal or epithelial cell colonization by hepatitis B or C viruses. Malignant hepatic tumors are common due to metastatic lesions from other organs. HCC accounts for almost half a million cancer deaths a year, and the incidence is escalating in the Western world and in developing countries. HCC progresses in a stepwise manner, mostly regulated by gene expression; untreated liver cancer may rapidly lead to death within a year.

Early identification of malnutrition status is required for proper intervention. In one study, over 60% of hospitalized patients were malnourished; the prevalence was higher in

TABLE 13-16 Risk Factors for Liver Cancer

Aflatoxins (Voight, 2005)
Anabolic steroids
Arsenic in drinking water
Cirrhosis from alcohol abuse or hemochromatosis (Kuper et al, 2001)
Male gender
Liver disease: hepatitis B virus (HBV) and hepatitis C virus (HCV)
Obesity
Oral contraceptive use (higher dose estrogen)
Tobacco use
Vinyl chloride and thorium dioxide (Voight, 2005)

male patients with long hospital stays, readmitted patients, and patients who had liver cancer (Wie et al, 2009).

Surgical resection is sometimes possible in some cases; laparoscopic procedures are becoming more common. Laser-induced thermotherapy for the treatment of liver metastases may be an option. In some cases, liver transplantation may be possible.

Chemotherapy may be administered. Where radiation is used, radioactive substances are sent into the artery that leads directly to the liver. Computed tomography–guided focal liver irradiation combined with chemotherapy delivered via the hepatic artery may extend the lives of patients with unresectable cancer.

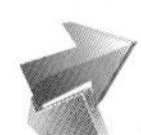

ASSESSMENT, MONITORING, AND EVALUATION

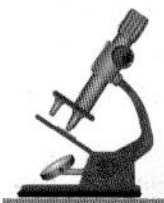

CLINICAL INDICATORS

Genetic Markers: HCC is strongly linked to increases in allelic losses, chromosomal changes, gene mutations, epigenetic alterations, and alterations in molecular cellular pathways (Yam et al, 2010).

Specific Clinical/History

Height
Weight
BMI
Progressive weight loss
I & O, dehydration
Anorexia, weakness
Nausea and/or vomiting
Increased flatulence
Steatorrhea, diarrhea
Abdominal fullness
Low-grade fever
Anemia, malnutrition
Portal hypertension
Dyspnea
Jaundice, ascites
Hepatic coma?
Melena
Hepatomegaly
Temperature (fever?)
Alcohol abuse?
Pesticide exposure?
CT or MRI

Lab Work

Alpha-fetoprotein (AFP)
Prothrombin time (PT) (prolonged)
H & H
Transferrin
Aspartate aminotransferase (AST) – altered?
ALT (abnormal)
Sedimentation rate (ESR), increased?
Ca^{++}, Mg^{++}
Na^{+}, K^{+}
Ammonia
Alb (decreased), transthyretin
CRP
Gluc (decreased)
Alk phos
TLC (varies)

INTERVENTION

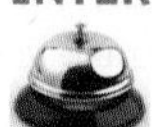

OBJECTIVES

- Reduce fluid retention and ascites.
- Correct serum protein levels and improve hepatic production capacity.
- Prevent further nausea and vomiting, weight loss, anorexia, and malnutrition.
- Counteract side effects of therapy (e.g., surgery, chemotherapy, radiation).
- Improve overall nutritional and hematologic status.
- Maintain adequate hydration.
- Improve prognosis and prolong life as long as possible. Improve quality of life.

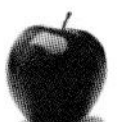

FOOD AND NUTRITION

- Tube feed if oral diet is not feasible; patients with hepatic cancer usually have significant fluid balance/overload/retention problems. Avoid CPN.
- Progress, if and when tolerated, to high-protein diet with sufficient carbohydrate intake. Managing weight will be important to prolong life; a carefully planned weight loss diet is needed in those patients who are obese.
- If hepatic coma occurs, decrease protein and supplement with amino acids (see hepatic encephalopathy in Section 8). Branched-chain amino acids may be beneficial (Togo et al, 2005).

SAMPLE NUTRITION CARE PROCESS STEPS

Poor Nutritional Quality of Life

Assessment Data: Liver cancer patient, weight loss of 5# in the past 2 weeks. Anorexia, nausea, and vomiting while on chemotherapy. Very fatigued.

Nutrition Diagnosis (PES): Poor nutritional quality of life related to chemotherapy treatments as evidenced by fatigue, anorexia, nausea, and vomiting.

Intervention: Food and nutrient delivery—offer preferred foods and beverages. Educate the patient about ways to enhance nutrient and energy density in smaller, more frequent meals. Counsel about ways to manage nausea and vomiting during chemotherapy weeks.

Monitoring and Evaluation: Improvement in intake. Tolerance of chemotherapy. No further weight loss. Improved nutritional quality of life.

- Reduce sodium if ascites and edema are significant; extra protein may be needed if albumin is also low. Monitor serum levels of other electrolytes to determine if other restrictions are needed.
- Supplemental vitamins may be beneficial. Monitor serum levels of vitamins A, D, and K because of poor hepatic clearance.
- With surgery, monitor nutritional intake for adequate wound healing and recovery.
- Encourage small meals and snacks as tolerated throughout the day.
- Decreased calcium absorption may occur after surgery. Calcium supplementation is needed, particularly in postmenopausal women.

Common Drugs Used and Potential Side Effects

- Antiemetics may be used for vomiting.
- Diuretics are used commonly; monitor side effects carefully.
- Chemotherapy may include cisplatin, interferon, doxorubicin, and fluorouracil.

Herbs, Botanicals, and Supplements (see Table 13-8)

- Herbs and botanical supplements should not be used without discussing it with the physician.
- Use of prebiotics (inulin and oligosaccharides) and silymarin may be protective.
- Polyphenols, mainly flavonoids and tannins, prevent oxidative stress-induced injury (Soory, 2009). Resveratrol has anti-inflammatory action through hepatic cyclooxygenase (COX-2) inhibition (Luther et al, 2009).
- Vitamin D_3 can be used to treat HCC, but hypercalcemia limits its use; a lower dose is possible if fish oil is given at the same time (Chiang et al, 2009).

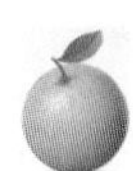

NUTRITION EDUCATION, COUNSELING, CARE MANAGEMENT

- Hepatic cancer from hepatitis C virus infection warrants maintaining a lean weight to prolong life.
- Teach the patient about the signs of deficiency of vitamins K and C, such as bleeding gums and easy bruising.
- Discuss signs of hepatic coma that require dietary alterations.
- Encourage hepatitis B virus vaccination and offer information.
- Provide education related to diet (regular, six small feedings) or jejunostomy tube feeding.
- Community-based programs to discourage and deal with excessive alcohol intake, to promote tobacco smoking awareness, and to avoid exposure to aflatoxin and other food toxins and measures taken to reduce the pandemic of obesity and diabetes are vital for lowering the incidence of HCC from nonviral liver disease (Fan et al, 2009).

Patient Education—Food Safety

- Educate the patient about food safety issues. Discuss safe food handling and preparation, keeping foods at proper temperatures, the use of sterile water, and reheating foods properly.
- Offer tips for managing jejunostomy tube feeding safely at home under sanitary preparation and storage methods.

For More Information

- American Liver Foundation
  http://www.liverfoundation.org/
- Liver Cancer in Children
  http://www.childrenshospital.org/az/Site1015/mainpageS1015P0.html
- Medline–Liver Cancer
  http://www.nlm.nih.gov/medlineplus/livercancer.html

HEPATIC CANCER—CITED REFERENCES

Chiang KC, et al. Fish oil enhances the antiproliferative effect of 1alpha, 25-dihydroxyvitamin D_3 on liver cancer cells. *Anticancer Res.* 29:3591, 2009.

Fan JG, et al. Prevention of hepatocellular carcinoma in nonviral-related liver diseases. *J Gastroenterol Hepatol.* 24:712, 2009.

Luther DJ, et al. Chemopreventive doses of resveratrol do not produce cardiotoxicity in a rodent model of hepatocellular carcinoma [Published online ahead of print Oct 8, 2009]. *Invest New Drugs.*

Soory M. Relevance of nutritional antioxidants in metabolic syndrome, ageing and cancer: potential for therapeutic targeting. *Infect Disord Drug Targets.* 9:400, 2009.

Togo S, et al. Usefulness of granular BCAA after hepatectomy for liver cancer complicated with liver cirrhosis. *Nutrition.* 21:480, 2005.

Wie GA, et al. Prevalence and risk factors of malnutrition among cancer patients according to tumor location and stage in the National Cancer Center in Korea [Published online ahead of print Aug 7, 2009]. *Nutrition.*

Yam JW, et al. Molecular and functional genetics of hepatocellular carcinoma. *Front Biosci (Schol Ed).* 2:117, 2010.

KIDNEY, BLADDER, AND URINARY TRACT CANCERS

NUTRITIONAL ACUITY RANKING: LEVEL 3

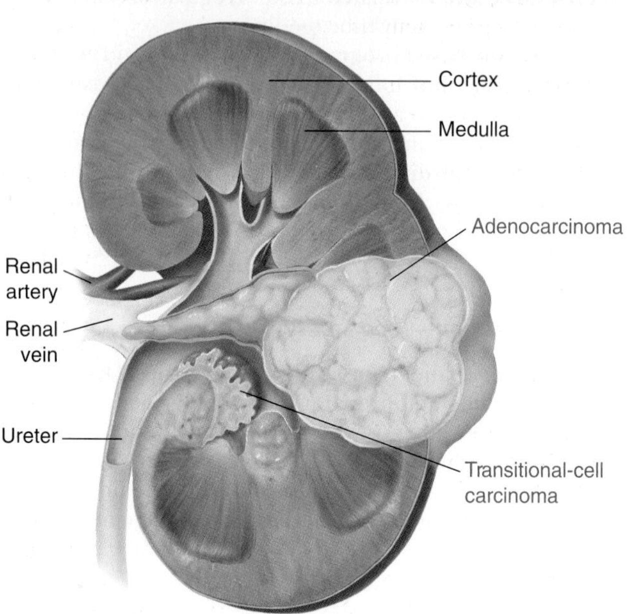

Asset provided by Anatomical Chart Co.

DEFINITIONS AND BACKGROUND

Urinary tract cancers affect more than 50,000 Americans each year. Men are more prone to this type of cancer than women. Surgery is usually required; prognosis with early intervention is good. Survival has improved. Fruit, extra fluids, vitamin C, retinol, daily multivitamin supplements, and green and nonherbal tea tend to be protective. It is likely that vitamin D_3 plays a role as well (Grant, 2009).

Renal cell cancer (RCC) accounts for approximately 2% of cancers worldwide. It is most common in persons over 45 years of age, particularly among blacks. Blood in the urine and an increased frequency of urination are the most common symptoms. Smoking, long-term dialysis, occupational exposure to dyes, rubber, and leather products are risk factors. Hypertension increases the risk of RCC in both sexes, while effective blood pressure control may lower the risk (Weikert et al, 2008). Finally, obesity contributes to morbidity and mortality in renal cancer (Anderson and Caswell, 2009). Total consumption of fruits, vegetables, fat, red meat, processed meat, poultry, and seafood are not associated with the risk of RCC (Lee et al, 2008; Weikert et al, 2006). RCC can often be cured if it is diagnosed and treated when still localized to the kidney. Fortunately, the majority of patients are diagnosed at that time. Surgical resection or nephrectomy may be needed.

Wilms' tumor (nephroblastoma or embryoma of the kidney) is a highly malignant tumor occurring almost exclusively in children younger than 6 years of age. It is more common in girls than in boys, and in African-American children. Symptoms and signs include weight loss, anorexia, enlarged kidney, hypertension, fever, anemia, and abdominal pain. A cure may be possible if metastasis has not occurred before nephrectomy. There is now an overall survival rate of 85%, and treatment-related morbidity has been reduced by chemotherapy (Gommersall et al, 2005). Metastasis to lungs, liver, and brain can occur.

Bladder cancer can be caused by factors such as smoking, exposure to chemicals at work (such as hair dyes, textiles, and paint), old age, chronic bladder infections, and infectious parasites. Well water should be tested for arsenic. Bladder cancer is more common in Caucasians. It can often be cured in the early stages using surgery, radiation, chemotherapy, or immunotherapy. If dual nephrectomy is needed, as in a stage 5 tumor, permanent dialysis may be required until a transplant is possible.

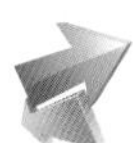

ASSESSMENT, MONITORING, AND EVALUATION

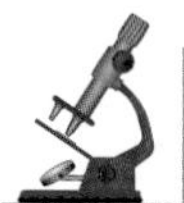

CLINICAL INDICATORS

Genetic Markers: Mutation of the VHL gene is associated with the development of RCC and the overexpression of the angiogenesis pathway (George and Bukowski, 2009). Some cases of Wilms' tumor are related to defects in either Wilms' tumor 1 (WT1) or Wilms' tumor 2 (WT2) or to several other genes.

Specific Clinical/History

- Height
- Weight
- Weight changes
- BMI (obesity?)
- Growth percentile in child
- Diet history
- BP (increased)
- I & O; dehydration?
- Hematuria
- Anorexia
- Enlarged kidney?
- Fever?
- Abdominal or lower back pain
- Smoking history
- Painful urination
- Frequent urinary tract infections
- Incontinence
- Abdominal CT scan
- Cystoscopy
- X-ray (intravenous pyelogram)
- Bone scan for metastasis
- Urine cytology

Lab Work

- Urinalysis
- Ca^{++}, Mg^{++}
- Na^{+}, K^{+}
- Alb, transthyretin
- CRP
- BUN
- Creat
- Gluc
- H & H (low?)
- Serum Fe, ferritin
- Transferrin
- Liver function tests
- ALT

SAMPLE NUTRITION CARE PROCESS STEPS

Unintentional Weight Loss

Assessment Data: BMI 20, down from the usual BMI of 24. Poor appetite, stomatitis. Taking temsirolimus for renal cancer.

Nutrition Diagnosis (PES): Unintentional weight loss related to anorexia and stomatitis as evidenced by a BMI of 20 when the usual is 24.

Intervention: Food-Nutrient Delivery—Suggest small, frequent meals of low-acid, mild foods and beverages. Educate the patient about foods that are more easily tolerated with stomatitis. Counsel about the long-term efforts to regain lost weight to tolerate cancer therapies; surgery is a possibility.

Monitoring and Evaluation: No further weight loss; tolerating medication and treatments while managing side effects.

INTERVENTION

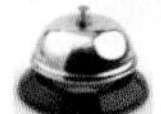

OBJECTIVES

- If needed, prepare patient for surgery and for postsurgical wound healing.
- Control the side effects of radiotherapy and chemotherapy.
- Promote normal growth and development, as far as possible, in children and teens.
- Control hypertension; correct anemia, which is common.
- Maintain adequate hydration.
- Minimize unplanned weight loss.
- Promote adequate bowel function.

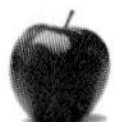

FOOD AND NUTRITION

- Provide adequate energy and protein according to age and to compensate for weight loss. In obese adults, weight loss regimens are not recommended until several months after surgery.
- Restrict excessive sodium with hypertension. Provide sufficient potassium, calcium, and magnesium; supplement if necessary.
- Monitor protein tolerance and adjust according to lab values, blood pressure, edema, and other signs of renal failure.
- Ensure adequate fluid intake, particularly water.
- Follow the Mediterranean or DASH diets, which encourage plenty of fruits and vegetables that are rich in antioxidants. Include fish that contains omega-3 fatty acids.

Common Drugs Used and Potential Side Effects

- Rapamycin (mTOR) controls translation of key proteins during cancer cell proliferation; temsirolimus is the first mTOR inhibitor approved for the treatment of advanced RCC (Hudes et al, 2009). Side effects may include hyperglycemia, hyperlipidemia, stomatitis, rash, or even pneumonitis.
- Interferon and interleukin-2 may also be used in advanced kidney cancer. Interferon often causes patients to have flu-like symptoms, and nausea and vomiting are common; interleukin-2 can cause nausea and vomiting or fluid retention. Sunitinib (Sutent) is useful in advanced kidney cancer where chemotherapy has not been effective.
- Zoledronic acid is a bisphosphonate that is approved for preventing fractures after bone metastasis from renal cancer.
- For **bladder cancer,** chemotherapy often involves carboplatin, fluorouracil, cisplatin, cyclophosphamide, methotrexate, or vinblastine. Many side effects are common, including nausea, anorexia, diarrhea, or vomiting. The use of gemcitabine and cisplatin is as useful as older treatments.
- **Wilms' tumor** requires perioperative vincristine and dactinomycin, with or without doxorubicin or radiotherapy (Gommersall et al, 2005).

Herbs, Botanicals, and Supplements (see Table 13-8)

- Herbs and botanical supplements should not be used without discussing it with the physician. Herbal preparations are subject to contamination with metals such as mercury or may contain potassium—all of which can be harmful to the kidney.
- Some studies promote the use of green tea for prevention, but others have not identified its efficacy.

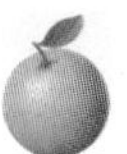

NUTRITION EDUCATION, COUNSELING, CARE MANAGEMENT

- Discuss the side effects that the patient is experiencing in light of the therapies used (e.g., radiation therapy, chemotherapy, or surgery).
- Discuss normal growth and/or desirable weight for the patient. Obesity is a concern.
- Highlight meals that are attractive so that the patient eats as well as possible. Cut down on fried meats and fats.
- Discuss how to manage anemia through appropriate medications or dietary measures.
- There is no risk for bladder or renal cancers from the use of artificial sweeteners.

Patient Education—Food Safety

- Educate the patient about food safety issues. Discuss safe food handling and preparation, keeping foods at proper temperatures, the use of sterile water, and reheating foods properly.
- In some countries, schistosomiasis infestation is a risk. Monitor for water and food safety.

For More Information

- Bladder Cancer
  http://www.mayoclinic.com/health/bladder-cancer/DS00177
- Kidney Cancer Association
  http://www.kidneycancerassociation.org/

- Medine – Bladder Cancer
  http://www.nlm.nih.gov/medlineplus/ency/article/000486.htm
- Medline–Kidney Cancer
  http://www.nlm.nih.gov/medlineplus/kidneycancer.html
- National Kidney Foundation – Council on Renal Nutrition
  http://www.kidney.org/professionals/CRN/
- Wilms' Tumor – Mayo Clinic
  http://www.mayoclinic.com/health/wilms-tumor/DS00436

KIDNEY, BLADDER, AND URINARY TRACT CANCERS—CITED REFERENCES

Anderson AS, Caswell S. Obesity management–an opportunity for cancer prevention. *Surgeon.* 7:282, 2009.

George S, Bukowski RM. Role of everolimus in the treatment of renal cell carcinoma. *Ther Clin Risk Manag.* 5:699, 2009.

Gommersall LM, et al. Current challenges in Wilms' tumor management. *Nat Clin Pract Oncol.* 2:298, 2005.

Grant WB. How strong is the evidence that solar ultraviolet B and vitamin D reduce the risk of cancer? An examination using Hill's criteria for causality. *Dermatoendocrinol.* 1:17, 2009.

Hudes GR, et al. Clinical trial experience with temsirolimus in patients with advanced renal cell carcinoma. *Semin Oncol.* 36:26S3, 2009.

Lee JE, et al. Fat, protein, and meat consumption and renal cell cancer risk: a pooled analysis of 13 prospective studies. *J Natl Cancer Inst.* 100:1695, 2008.

Weikert S, et al. Blood pressure and risk of renal cell carcinoma in the European prospective investigation into cancer and nutrition. *Am J Epidemiol.* 167:438, 2008.

Weikert S, et al. Fruits and vegetables and renal cell carcinoma: findings from the European prospective investigation into cancer and nutrition (EPIC). *Int J Cancer.* 118:3133, 2006.

LUNG CANCER

NUTRITIONAL ACUITY RANKING: LEVEL 3–4

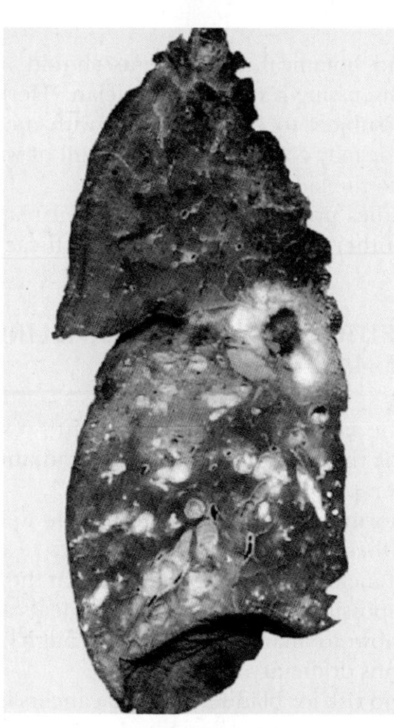

Bronchiolar carcinoma infiltrating growth

Adapted from: Moore KL, PhD, FRSM, FIAC & Dalley AF II, PhD. *Clinical Oriented Anatomy,* 4th ed. Baltimore, Lippincott Williams & Wilkins 1999.

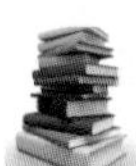

DEFINITIONS AND BACKGROUND

Lung (bronchial) cancer begins in the lungs and is the most common type of cancer in the Western world. There are two main types of lung cancer: non–small-cell lung cancer and small-cell lung cancer. **Non–small-cell lung cancer (NSCLC)** has three major subtypes: adenocarcinoma (40% of cases), squamous carcinoma (30–35% of cases, slow growing, and formerly called epidermoid carcinoma), and large-cell carcinoma (affecting 5–15% of cases). NSCLC is the leading cause of cancer-related death in the United States (Budde and Hanna, 2005).

Small-cell lung cancer (SCLC) is a more aggressive type of lung cancer that comprises 15% of all lung cancer diagnoses. It is highly correlated to smoking. SCLCs grow quickly but tend to respond to specific chemotherapy protocols. Oat cell cancer is a highly fatal form of SCLC; aggressive chemotherapy is needed.

In 85% of cases, smoking causes lung cancer. Heavy tobacco or marijuana smokers are 25 times more susceptible to lung cancer. Other causes include exposure to industrial chemicals, radon, and passive smoke. Smoking is associated with lower levels of vitamin C. The best protection against lung cancer is the avoidance of airborne carcinogens and increased consumption of fruits and vegetables (Cranganu and Camporeale, 2009).

Foods rich in flavonoids may protect against certain types of lung cancer. Onions and apples have quercetin. Vitamin E food sources (gamma-tocopherol) are protective; supplemental alpha-tocopherol is not. Resveratrol may be beneficial, but excess alcohol is not (Barnardi et al, 2010). Antioxidant sources seems to be an important issue.

The focus should be on food; supplemental beta-carotene is a concern (Roswall et al, 2010) whereas dietary beta-carotene is protective against lung cancer. Cryptoxanthin, alpha-carotene, and ascorbic acid need to be investigated further as potentially protective factors (Comstock et al, 2008). Isothiocyanates from cruciferous vegetables are anticarcinogenic. Because the glutathione S transferase M1 (GSTM1) gene promotes urinary isothiocyanate excretion, the reduced lung cancer risk with higher isothiocyanate intake may be slightly stronger among individuals with a deletion of GSTM1 and GSTT1 (Carpenter et al, 2009; Lam et al, 2009). Novel interventions to prevent lung cancer should be developed based on the ability of diet and dietary supplements to affect reprogramming of the epigenome (Stidley et al, 2010).

Lung cancer's 5-year survival rate is only 15%, which is worse than many other types of cancer. Cancer cells of the lung often spread to the brain, bone, liver, and skin. Radiation and chemotherapy are needed, but surgery after standard chemotherapy and radiation can be an option for some patients. Medical nutrition therapy is often required for the nutrition-related side effects of cancer treatment, which include anorexia, nausea and vomiting, and esophagitis (Cranganu and Camporeale, 2009).

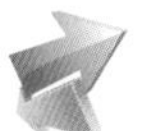

ASSESSMENT, MONITORING, AND EVALUATION

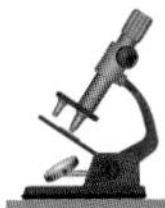

CLINICAL INDICATORS

Genetic Markers: Eight genes are commonly silenced in lung cancer and are associated with risk. Smoke-induced methylation may reduce HtrA3 expression, which is one concern (Beleford et al, 2010). Promoter methylation factors are controlled with the use of leafy green vegetables, folate, and the use of multivitamins (Stidley et al, 2010). Epidermal growth factor receptor (EGFR) mutations in tumors are prognostic markers in patients with early stage lung cancer. Tumor microRNAs may help to predict SCLC patients who are resistant to chemotherapy.

Specific Clinical/History

- Height
- Weight
- BMI
- Diet history
- I & O
- Weight loss?
- Fever of unknown cause
- Persistent cough
- Bloody sputum
- Chest pain
- Recurring pneumonia or bronchitis
- Fatigue
- Hoarseness
- Shortness of breath
- Swelling of neck or face
- Bronchoscopy
- Biopsy
- MRI, CT scan
- Thoracentesis
- Chest x-ray
- Sputum cytology

Lab Work

- Partial pressure of carbon dioxide (pCO_2)
- Partial pressure of oxygen (pO_2)
- CEA
- Alb, transthyretin
- Gluc
- CRP
- Ca^{++}, Mg^{++}
- Na^{+}, K^{+}
- ALT (increased)

INTERVENTION

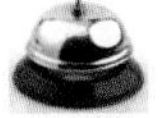

OBJECTIVES

- Patient must stop smoking, avoid passive smoke, or discontinue exposure to radon or other contributors.
- Prepare patient for therapy (e.g., surgery, radiation, or chemotherapy).
- Meet energy needs, which are often elevated as much as 30% above normal. The use of indirect calorimetry to measure REE is more accurate than estimation (American Dietetic Association, 2010).

SAMPLE NUTRITION CARE PROCESS STEPS

Inadequate Intake From Parenteral Infusion

Assessment Data: Inability to eat due to esophagitis over the past 1–2 days. Patient has been receiving chemotherapy treatment for lung cancer. Patient is only on PPN. Patient's weight has been stable at home; lung cancer is a recent diagnosis yet quite advanced. Labs: WBC 1.8, slightly below normal for Na, phosphorus, magnesium, Hgb and Hct.

Nutrition Diagnosis (PES):

1- Inadequate intake from parenteral infusion (NI 2.3) related to limitations of peripheral access as evidenced by the inability to meet energy requirements through PPN.

2- Inadequate oral food intake (NI 2.1) related to esophagitis as evidenced by the inability to swallow and decreased food intake over the past 2–3 days.

Interventions: Food and Nutrient Delivery: ND 4.2 Insert enteral nutrition feeding tube; NPO until PEG is surgically placed. ND 2.2 Modify rate, concentration, composition, or schedule. Once the PEG was placed, Jevity 1.5 was started 8 hours later at a rate of 35 ml/h. This was increased as tolerated by 10 milliliters every 8 hours until the goal rate of 65 ml/hr was reached.

Education: Discuss appropriate feeding using a PEG tube; safe handling; signs of intolerance.

Counseling: Adequate intake of tube feeding and how to adjust when oral intake is possible.

Coordination of Care: RC 1.3 Collaboration/referral to other providers; patient to have home health; instruct patient on tube feeding at home.

Monitoring and Evaluation: Patient tolerating goal rate of 65 ml/hr; discharged from hospital. Follow patient weight, tolerance, and intake status in 1 week. Evaluate for progress back to oral diet if esophagitis subsides.

- Maximize intake through side-effects management. Cachexia, infections, atelectasis, syndrome of inappropriate antidiuretic hormone (SIADH), esophagitis, weight loss, and anorexia may occur.
- Minimum weight loss.
- Maximize pulmonary health and improve quality of life. Increase disease-free time.

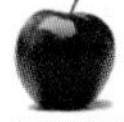

FOOD AND NUTRITION

- Increase the intake of protein, CHO, energy, and fluids.
- Tube feedings are highly recommended if weight loss, decreased appetite, dehydration, or electrolyte imbalance occurs.
- Alter diet as appropriate for side effects (see general cancer entry). Adequate vitamin-mineral intake should come from diet as much as possible. Providing medical nutrition therapy may help to improve protein and calorie intake, which may prevent weight loss and improve quality of life (American Dietetic Association).
- Small, frequent meals may be beneficial.

- If oral diet is possible, promote a protective diet. Include citrus fruits, vegetables, sesame seeds and pecans (for gamma-tocopherol), quercetin (apples and onions) and other flavonoids, selenium, lycopene, carotenoids, and natural estrogens (such as soy foods). Use curcumin as seasoning if tolerated.
- Include phytosterols from sunflower seeds, pistachio nuts, sesame seeds, and wheat germ (Phillips et al, 2005).
- Include more omega-3 fatty acids from fish, shellfish, flaxseed, and walnuts.
- Include resveratrol from red grapes and juice, berries, peanuts, or red wine if tolerated.

Common Drugs Used and Potential Side Effects

- Cytotoxic drugs are often used. Vincristine can cause severe constipation.
- With methotrexate, nausea and vomiting are common; doxorubicin (Adriamycin) causes stomatitis, anorexia, hair loss, and diarrhea. Coadministration of methotrexate with intravenous glucose may alleviate some of the toxic gastrointestinal (GI) effects.
- Cyclophosphamide (Cytoxan) and other combinations of therapy may cause anorexia, stomatitis, nausea, or vomiting.
- Toxicity is far less than with docetaxel if vitamin B_{12} and folate supplements are used (Budde and Hanna, 2005).
- Tarceva modestly improves survival in NSCLC patients.
- With immunotherapy, bacillus Calmette-Guérin (BCG) vaccine is often used.

Herbs, Botanicals, and Supplements (see Table 13-8)

- The use of complementary and alternative medicine by lung cancer patients is prevalent. Clinicians should investigate to avoid any potential side effects and interactions with conventional therapies (Cranganu and Camporeale, 2009). Herbs and botanical supplements should not be used without discussing with the physician.
- Five promising herbs have been identified in Chinese herbal medicine (CHM) that, when used in conjunction with chemotherapy, may improve quality of life in NSCLC (Chen et al, 2009).
- Luteolin, 3′,4′,5,7-tetrahydroxyflavone, exists in many types of plants and in Chinese medicinal herbs; it functions as an antioxidant with anticancer properties (Lin et al, 2009). Luteolin is found in carrots, celery, olive oil, oregano, peppers, peppermint, rosemary, and thyme.
- Avoid beta-carotene supplements. Diet is more protective.
- Clinical trials using dietary garlic, selenium, N-acetylcysteine, vitamins B_6 and C are needed.

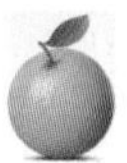

NUTRITION EDUCATION, COUNSELING, CARE MANAGEMENT

- Discuss alternate methods of intake if oral is not feasible.
- A diet high in antioxidant-rich foods such as fruits, vegetables, and spices is protective and a prudent preventive strategy (Roswall et al, 2010).
- Discuss the side effects of drugs being used.
- Dietary acrylamide affects carcinogenesis but not through genetic alterations (Hogervorst et al, 2009). Researchers are reviewing its role from heat-treated foods.
- Self-reported smoking consistently explains approximately 50% of the inequalities in lung cancer risk due to differences in education (Menvielle et al, 2009). Smokers who quit will allow their lung tissues to repair much of the damage.
- Smokers who cannot quit should use a brand of cigarettes with lower nicotine and low tar. Avoid smoking prior to or with meals; smoking may decrease appetite.
- Chewing tobacco or snuff is also carcinogenic and should be stopped.
- Offer tube feeding or nutritional build-up education as appropriate.

Patient Education—Food Safety

- Educate the patient about food safety issues. Discuss safe food handling and preparation, keeping foods at proper temperatures, the use of sterile water, and reheating foods properly.
- If tube feeding is needed, safe preparation, handling, storage, and administration will be important.

For More Information

- Alliance for Lung Cancer
  http://www.alcase.org/
- Cancer Net–Lung Cancer
  http://cancernet.nci.nih.gov/cancertopics/wyntk/lung/page1
- Focus on Lung Cancer
  http://www.lungcancer.org/
- Lung Cancer Information Library
  http://www.meds.com/lung/lunginfo.html
- Lung Cancer Online
  http://www.lungcanceronline.org/
- National Cancer Institute – Small Cell Cancer
  http://www.nci.nih.gov/cancerinfo/pdq/treatment/small-cell-lung/patient

LUNG CANCER—CITED REFERENCES

American Dietetic Association (ADA). Evidence analysis library: Oncology. Accessed January 14, 2010, at http://www.adaevidencelibrary.com/topic.cfm?cat=3250.

Bagnardi V, et al. Alcohol consumption and lung cancer risk in the Environment and Genetics in Lung Cancer Etiology (EAGLE) study. *Am J Epidemiol.* 171:36, 2010.

Budde LS, Hanna NH. Antimetabolites in the management of non-small cell lung cancer. *Curr Treat Options Oncol.* 6:83, 2005.

Carpenter CL, et al. Dietary isothiocyanates, glutathione S-transferase M1 (GSTM1), and lung cancer risk in African Americans and Caucasians from Los Angeles County, California. *Nutr Cancer.* 61:492, 2009.

Chen S, et al. Oral Chinese herbal medicine (CHM) as an adjuvant treatment during chemotherapy for non-small cell lung cancer: A systematic review [Published online ahead of print Dec 16, 2009]. *Lung Cancer.*

Comstock GW, et al. The risk of developing lung cancer associated with antioxidants in the blood: ascorbic acids, carotenoids, alpha-tocopherol, selenium, and total peroxyl radical absorbing capacity. *Am J Epidemiol.* 168:831, 2008.

Cranganu A, Camporeale J. Nutrition aspects of lung cancer. *Nutr Clin Pract.* 24:688, 2009.

Hogervorst JG, et al. Lung cancer risk in relation to dietary acrylamide intake. *J Natl Cancer Inst.* 101:651, 2009.

Lam TK, et al. Cruciferous vegetable consumption and lung cancer risk: a systematic review. *Cancer Epidemiol Biomarkers.* 18:184, 2009.

Lin Y, et al. Luteolin, a flavonoid with potential for cancer prevention and therapy. *Curr Cancer Drug Targets.* 8:634, 2008.
Menvielle G, et al. The role of smoking and diet in explaining educational inequalities in lung cancer incidence. *J Natl Cancer Inst.* 101:321, 2009.
Phillips KM, et al. Phytosterol composition of nuts and seeds commonly consumed in the United States. *J Agric Food Chem.* 53:9436, 2005.
Roswall N, et al. Source-specific effects of micronutrients in lung cancer prevention [Published online ahead of print Jan , 2010]. *Lung Cancer.*
Stidley CA, et al. Multivitamins, folate, and green vegetables protect against gene promoter methylation in the aerodigestive tract of smokers. *Cancer Res.* 70:568, 2010.

PANCREATIC CANCER

NUTRITIONAL ACUITY RANKING: LEVEL 3–4

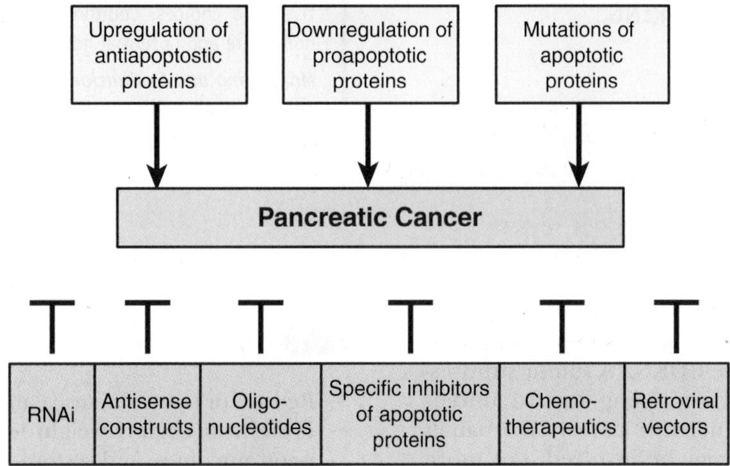

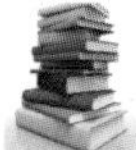

DEFINITIONS AND BACKGROUND

Pancreatic cancer is the fourth most common cause of death from cancer in men and the fifth for women, primarily occurring between 65 and 79 years of age. Development of pancreas cancer progresses over many years before symptoms appear, and many people with pancreatic cancer die within 6 months of diagnosis. Nearly all pancreatic cancers are primary pancreatic adenocarcinomas.

About 50–70% of patients have cancer in the head of the pancreas, and 50% have cancer in the body and tail. Patients who have cancer in the head of the pancreas often present with cholangitis, nausea, anorexia, weight loss, new-onset diabetes, light-colored stools, dark urine, steatorrhea, jaundice, and pruritus. Those who have cancer in the body or tail of the pancreas present with vague abdominal pain, dyspepsia, nausea, intermittent diarrhea, unexpected diabetes, and constant back pain. When there are spontaneous blood clots in the portal blood vessels, this may be associated with pancreatic cancer; this thrombophlebitis is called Trousseau sign.

Risks for pancreatic cancer increase with age. It is slightly more common in men, in smokers, in African-Americans, and in people who are obese. Almost a third of the cases of pancreatic cancer are due to cigarette smoking. Persons with a history of pancreatitis are also at risk; type 2 diabetes is not a true risk factor. Diets high in red meat or low in fruits and vegetables may also be linked to pancreatic cancer. Doses of alcohol greater than 30 grams per day contribute to only a modest increase for this type of cancer.

Exercise, such as walking 4 hours or more weekly, may protect against this cancer. Good folate, B_{12}, and pyridoxine status also helps (Schernhammer et al, 2007), as does an increased intake of citrus fruits (Bae et al, 2009). Lifestyle choices are the most preventive steps; cut down on smoking, alcohol and poor food choices (Whitcomb and Greer, 2009).

Nutrition intervention together with chemotherapy improves outcomes in these patients. An increased risk has been found for dietary intakes of saturated and polyunsaturated fat (Thiebault et al, 2009; Zhang et al, 2009). A diet high in omega-3 fatty acids may mitigate pancreatic precancer by inhibition of cellular proliferation through induction of cell cycle arrest and apoptosis (Strouch et al, 2009). DHA may be the primary fatty acid that is beneficial. However, the use of supplemental omega-3 fatty acids is not recommended (American Dietetic Association, 2010).

Malignancy in the pancreas has a high mortality rate from a lack of early symptoms, symptoms that mimic other conditions, and rapid metastasis to other organs. Medical treatment consists of radiation, chemotherapy, immunotherapy, or vaccine therapy. When the tumor has spread (metastasized) to other organs such as the liver, chemotherapy alone is usually used. The standard chemotherapy drug is gemcitabine, which can help some patients.

Unfortunately, only about 20% of patients with pancreatic cancer have a form that can be resected. **Whipple's procedure** (pancreaticoduodenectomy) involves many operations. The entire duodenum is usually removed, and the pancreas, gallbladder, and spleen may also be removed. It has many nutritional implications (Petzel, 2005; Tang et al, 2005). After surgery, the diet can be liberalized after 10–14 days, adding one new food at a time and using supplements when appetite is poor.

Survival rates have improved; approximately 30% will live for 3 years after diagnosis and treatment. But the 5-year survival rate is low; 95% of the people diagnosed with it will not be alive 5 years later.

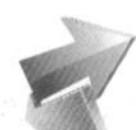

ASSESSMENT, MONITORING, AND EVALUATION

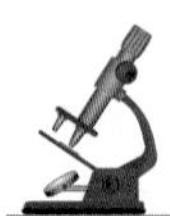

CLINICAL INDICATORS

Genetic Markers: Five to ten percent of cases are related to family history, such as mutations in BRCA2 or PALB2 genes, Lynch syndrome, Peutz-Jeghers syndrome, familial atypical mole-malignant melanoma (FAMMM), familial adenomatous polyposis, or mutations in the CDKN2 A tumor suppressor gene. Much research is going toward understanding the genes in pancreatic cancer (Hruban et al, 2008). Folate genes may be involved, but more studies are needed.

Specific Clinical/History

Height
Weight
BMI
Rapid weight loss
Midepigastric pain
Temperature
BP
Jaundice, pruritus
Dark urine?
Biliary obstruction?
Pancreatic insufficiency (indigestion, cramping, bloating)
Belching
Steatorrhea or loose stools
Anorexia
Nausea and vomiting
Thrombophlebitis (Trousseau sign).
Fatigue
Ascites
Angiography
Abdominal CT scan or MRI
Endoscopic ultrasound
Fine-needle biopsy
Endoscopic retrograde cholangiopancreatography (ERCP)

Lab Work

Ca 19–9 (>37 U/mL)
Elevated microRNAs (miR-155, miR196a)
Alk phos (increased)
Bilirubin (increased)
PT (increased)
Gluc (increased)
Serum lipase (increased)
Secretin
PSCA levels
Serum amylase (increased)
ALT, AST (increased)
Transferrin
Serum insulin
TLC (varies)
Serum B_{12}, folic acid
Homocysteine levels
Cholecystokinin
Alb
CRP
Chol, Trig
H & H
Ca^{++}, Mg^{++}
Na^{+}, K^{+}

SAMPLE NUTRITION CARE PROCESS STEPS

Undesirable Food Choices

Assessment Data: BMI 20, recent weight loss of 2#. Diet history reveals high red meat and saturated intake, low use of fruits and vegetables. Dx pancreatic cancer in past month.

Nutrition Diagnosis (PES): Undesirable food choices related to nutrient density and cancer diagnosis as evidenced by diet history showing high intake of red meats and low intake of fruits and vegetables.

Intervention: Food-nutrient delivery—offer acceptable fruit and vegetable choices and juices. Educate the patient and family about the role of diet in cancer. Counsel about tips for managing symptoms, weight changes, and anorexia while including protective food choices. Coordinate care with the medical team for home care and potential hospice care.

Monitoring and Evaluation: No further weight loss; good tolerance for small meals that are nutrient-dense but not high in fat.

INTERVENTION

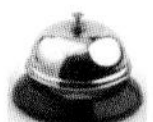

OBJECTIVES

- Reduce or control nausea and vomiting.
- Prevent or correct weight loss, which is associated with poor outcomes, and restore lean body mass.
- Control side effects of therapies and the disease such as diabetes, anemia, pancreatic fistula, wound infection, bile leak, cholangitis, dumping syndrome, weight loss, and lactose intolerance (Petzel, 2005).
- Provide foods or supplements that include all necessary nutrients to prolong health. Augment nutritional intake; correct anemia. Include protective foods.
- Monitor for depression; encourage the use of antidepressants if needed to help with appetite.
- Manage problems such as pancreatic cancer–related diabetes and vitamin B_{12} malabsorption.
- Parenteral nutrition (PN) is indicated mainly for perioperative use in patients with known malnutrition preoperatively. Postoperatively, tube feeding is the nutrition support method of choice.
- Wean off tube feeding with increasing oral intake and resolving gastroparesis, usually 4–6 weeks postoperatively.

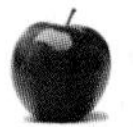

FOOD AND NUTRITION

- **For pancreatic insufficiency:** Medium-chain triglycerides (MCT), fat-soluble vitamins (water-miscible form), and essential fatty acids (EFAs) should be included. Calcium, selenium, zinc, and iron may become deficient unless supplemented.
- After Whipple's procedure, if pain is severe, tube feeding should be attempted before CPN. If possible, feed after bowel sounds return. Pancreatic enzyme replacement will be needed. Use a low-lactose, low-fat diet (40–60 g) and omit fried foods, nuts, and seeds.

- Small meals are best tolerated—six to eight feedings may be better tolerated than three large meals. Delayed gastric emptying is common, so avoidance of simple sugars and hot liquids may also be needed.
- Increased energy and protein intake should be provided to restore lost weight, unless the patient is hyperglycemic or has extensive liver impairment. Carbohydrate control may be needed to manage diabetes.
- Include protective foods, particularly tomato products for lycopene, other vegetables, and citrus fruits (Bae et al, 2009; Nkondjock et al, 2005). Onions, garlic, beans, orange and yellow vegetables, spinach, broccoli, kale, and raw vegetables are particularly protective.

Common Drugs Used and Potential Side Effects

- Chemotherapy may include gemcitabine.
- Pancreatic enzymes (pancrelipase and pancreatin) are given. Enteric coating aids in maintaining the integrity of enzymes until they reach the small intestine. If a pork allergy is present, there may be a reaction to these enzymes; a pork-free product is PAN-2400. As much as 20,000–30,000 units of lipase may be needed per meal; 10,000 units may be needed with snacks. They must be swallowed whole and not chewed.
- Insulin may be needed if the patient is hyperglycemic. In islet cell tumors, hypoglycemia may occur instead. Monitor with meal timing.
- Acid-reducing medications (such as proton-pump inhibitors or H_2 blockers) are usually needed.
- Vitamin B_{12} supplements may be required with total pancreatectomy, particularly with steatorrhea.
- Water-miscible fat-soluble vitamins A, D, E, and K will be needed until intake of pancreatic enzymes is sufficient. Brands may include Vitamax, Source CF, and ADEKs.
- Antiemetics, diuretics, and analgesics may be needed. Monitor side effects according to medications prescribed.
- Calcium carbonate twice daily may be useful to help bulk stools that are loose. Antidiarrheal medications (e.g., Lomotil, opiates, or Imodium) may be needed if loose stools are persistent. Guar gum and psyllium can be used to add soluble fiber.
- Targeted drug therapy blocks chemicals that signal cancer cells to grow and divide. Erlotinib (Tarceva) is usually combined with chemotherapy for advanced pancreatic cancer.
- A pancreatic cancer vaccine is under study.

Herbs, Botanicals, and Supplements (see Table 13-8)

- Herbs and botanical supplements should not be used without discussing it with the physician.
- There are potential drug-nutrient interactions (e.g., anticoagulant and anti-hypertensive medications/herbal supplements) with the use of EPA fish oil supplements; they are not recommended for pancreatic cancer (American Dietetic Association, 2010).

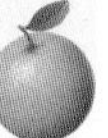

NUTRITION EDUCATION, COUNSELING, CARE MANAGEMENT

- Discuss specific dietary recommendations appropriate for the patient's condition and therapies.
- Discuss the use of pancreatic enzymes.
- Provide education for diet and jejunostomy feeding.
- With pancreatectomy, a diabetic diet may be absolutely essential. Discuss the rationale with the patient.
- Explain how diet affects malabsorption in regard to fat, protein, vitamins, and minerals.
- Research does not support the theory that high intakes of sugar or sugar-sweetened beverages cause this cancer.
- Lactase enzymes may be helpful if lactose intolerance persists.
- Family members may need genetic counseling. The fundamental problem underlying pancreatic cancer is altered genetics (Whitcomb and Greer, 2009).

Patient Education—Food Safety

- Educate the patient about food safety issues. Discuss safe food handling and preparation, keeping foods at proper temperatures, the use of sterile water, and reheating foods properly.

For More Information

- JAMA Patient Page – Pancreatic Cancer
  http://jama.ama-assn.org/cgi/reprint/297/3/330.pdf
- Johns Hopkins–Pancreatic Cancer Home Page
  http://www.path.jhu.edu/pancreas
- Lustgarten Foundation for Pancreatic Cancer Research
  http://www.lustgartenfoundation.org/
- Mayo Clinic – Pancreatic Cancer
  http://www.mayoclinic.com/health/pancreatic-cancer/DS00357
- Medline–Pancreatic Cancer
  http://www.nlm.nih.gov/medlineplus/pancreaticcancer.html
- National Pancreas Foundation
  http://www.pancreasfoundation.org/
- Pancreatic Cancer Action Network
  http://www.pancan.org/

PANCREATIC CANCER—CITED REFERENCES

American Dietetic Association (ADA). Evidence analysis library: Oncology. Accessed January 14, 2010, at http://www.adaevidencelibrary.com/topic.cfm?cat=3250.

Bae JM, et al. Citrus fruit intake and pancreatic cancer risk: a quantitative systematic review. *Pancreas.* 38:168, 2009.

Hruban RH, et al. Emerging molecular biology of pancreatic cancer. *Gastrointest Cancer Res.* 2:10S, 2008.

Nkondjock A, et al. Dietary intake of lycopene is associated with reduced pancreatic cancer risk. *J Nutr.* 135:592, 2005.

Petzel M. Nutrition support of the patient with pancreatic cancer. *Nutr Support.* 27:11, 2005.

Schernhammer E, et al. Plasma folate, vitamin B_6, vitamin B_{12}, and homocysteine and pancreatic cancer risk in four large cohorts. *Cancer Res.* 67:5553, 2007.

Strouch MJ, et al. A high omega-3 fatty acid diet mitigates murine pancreatic precancer development [Published online ahead of print May 15, 2009]. *J Surg Res.*

Tang CN, et al. Endo-laparoscopic approach in the management of obstructive jaundice and malignant gastric outflow obstruction. *Hepatogastroenterology.* 52:128, 2005.

Thiebault AC, et al. Dietary fatty acids and pancreatic cancer in the NIH-AARP diet and health study. *J Natl Cancer Inst.* 101:1001, 2009.

Whitcomb D, Greer J. Germ-line mutations, pancreatic inflammation, and pancreatic cancer. *Clin Gastroenterol Hepatol.* 7:S29, 2009.

Zhang J, et al. Physical activity, diet, and pancreatic cancer: a population-based, case-control study in Minnesota. *Nutr Cancer.* 61:457, 2009.

SKIN CANCERS

NUTRITIONAL ACUITY RANKING: 1–2

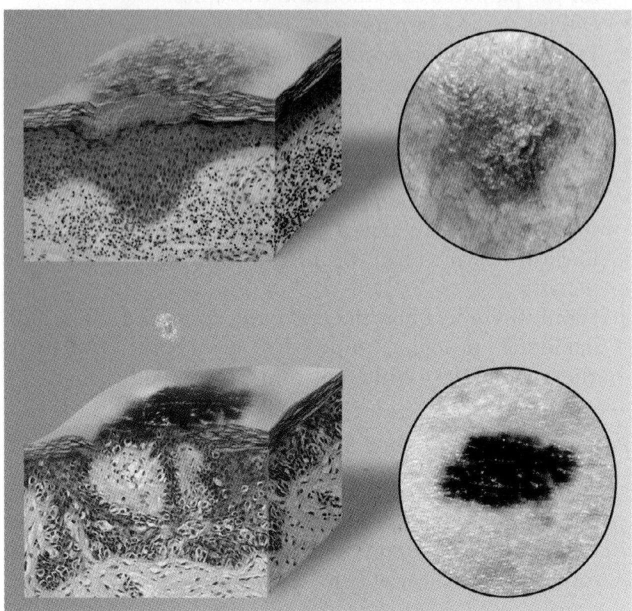

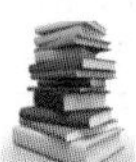

DEFINITIONS AND BACKGROUND

Skin cancer is the most common cancer in the United States, and the incidence is increasing. Vitamin D is made in the skin upon exposure to solar radiation; regular use of a tanning bed that emits vitamin D–producing ultraviolet (UV) radiation is associated with higher 25-hydroxyvitamin D concentrations, which may benefit the skeleton but not necessarily the skin. UVB–induced skin damage places individuals more at risk for basal cell and squamous cell carcinomas than for malignant melanoma.

Risk factors for skin cancer include certain types or a large number of moles; excessive exposure to sun and ultraviolet light with susceptible vitamin D receptor genes; family or personal history of skin cancer; freckles; light skin color, hair color, or eye color; and sunburns early in life. Since carcinogenesis and photoaging are multistep processes, tumor development may be halted at several points. The intake of flavonols may be protective (McNaughton et al, 2005).

Deficiency of the prohormone calcidiol (25OH vitamin D_3) seems to be associated with cancer, but not calcitriol (Tuohimaa, 2008). Daily brief exposure of a substantial area of the skin to ultraviolet light, climate allowing, provides adults with a safe, physiologic amount of vitamin D, equivalent to an oral intake of approximately 10,000 IU vitamin D_3 per day; the plasma 25-hydroxyvitamin D (25(OH)D) concentration potentially reaches 88 ng/mL (Vieth, 2009). The occupational sun exposure rate is positively correlated with a lower risk of overall organ mortality. Adequate vitamin D_3 is protective; benefits of sunlight may outweigh some risks (Krause et al, 2006).

Skin cancer and photoaging are the result of excessive ultraviolet radiation exposure. UVB (280–315 nm) in natural sunlight is associated with skin cancer through keratinocyte proliferation and cell cycle progression (Han and He, 2009). Excessive UVB light exposure in childhood promotes the development of melanomas (Wolpowitz and Gilchrest, 2006).

Basal cell cancer (BCC) starts as small, shiny, firm nodules that enlarge slowly, bleed and scab, then heal, and finally repeat the cycle. These are the most common type of skin cancer. Basal cell tumors should be removed to avoid destruction to other tissues. Most basal cell carcinomas occur on parts of the body that are excessively exposed to the sun—particularly the face, ears, neck, scalp, shoulders, or back. Rarely, these tumors come from exposure to arsenic or radiation, open sores that will not heal, chronic inflammatory skin conditions, and complications of burns, scars, infections, vaccinations, or tattoos.

Squamous cell carcinoma (SCC) originates in the middle layer of the epidermis and may develop on sun-damaged skin or even in the mouth lining or tongue. This type begins as a reddened area with a scaly, crusted surface that does not heal. A precursor is often an actinic keratosis (solar keratosis) that appears on the bald scalp, face, ears, lips, backs of the hands and forearms, shoulders, neck, or any other areas of the body that are frequently exposed to the sun. SCC may have the appearance of a wart and eventually becomes an open sore. Removal is important before it can spread. Leukoplakia anywhere in the mouth may be an early sign. SCC is more common in men than in women and is most likely to occur after age 50. In addition, people who use tanning beds are twice as likely to get SCC.

Melanoma, the deadliest type of skin cancer, originates in the melanocytes and tends to spread rapidly. Biopsy is essential. It is the most common cancer for women aged 25–29 years and the second most common cancer for women aged 30–34 years. Most melanomas are black or brown, but some may even be skin-colored, pink, red, blue, or white. Early warning signs of melanoma have been identified by the acronym "ABCDE" (A stands for Asymmetry, B stands for Border, C for Color, D for Diameter, and E for Evolving or changing was recently added). Individuals who have had breast cancer are at risk for melanoma and vice versa. Disfiguring surgery is no longer necessary to remove a melanoma. Mohs micrographic surgery is available.

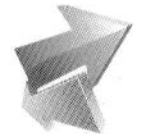

ASSESSMENT, MONITORING, AND EVALUATION

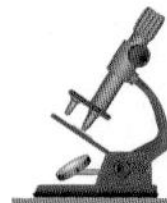

CLINICAL INDICATORS

Genetic Markers: The melanocortin 1 receptor (MC1R) is a highly polymorphic G protein-coupled receptor; MC1R alleles have been associated with a red hair/fair skin phenotype, increased incidence of skin cancer, and altered sensitivity to ultraviolet (UV) radiation (Smith et al, 2007). Specific alleles of the gene that codes for the melanocortin 1 receptor are also predictive of skin cancer risk, independent of skin type and hair color (Lynde and Sapra, 2010).

Specific Clinical/ History	Changes in skin or mole	H & H
Height	Itching, bleeding of mole	Serum ferritin
Weight	Nausea and vomiting	Transferrin
Weight changes	Anorexia	Ca^{++}, Mg^{++}
BMI		Na^{+}, K^{+}
Diet history	**Lab Work**	Serum 25(OH)D
Light-colored hair, skin, eyes	Alb	
	CRP	

INTERVENTION

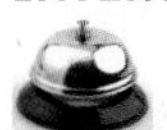

OBJECTIVES

- Maintain appropriate weight for height.
- General healthy dietary guidelines should be followed.
- Prevent or correct nutritional deficiencies and improve patient tolerance of treatment.
- Minimize potential treatment side effects.
- Optimize immune function to increase effectiveness of therapy.
- Enhance quality of life.
- Ensure appropriate healing of surgical sites, if applicable.

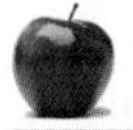

FOOD AND NUTRITION

- Eat a variety of foods, particularly fruits and vegetables and whole grains such as oats. Use flavonols such as apples, tea, and coffee.

> **SAMPLE NUTRITION CARE PROCESS STEPS**
>
> **Inadequate Bioactive Substance Intake**
>
> ***Assessment Data:*** Diagnosis of skin cancer. Hx of tanning bed use for psoriasis. Diet history indicates low intake of fruits and vegetables. Patient has been following a macrobiotic diet to lose weight for 6 months, eating mostly rice.
>
> ***Nutrition Diagnosis (PES):*** Inadequate bioactive substance intake related to low consumption of fruits and vegetables as evidenced by diet history.
>
> ***Intervention:*** Food-nutrient delivery—Provide a nutrient-dense diet that includes flavonols and anti-inflammatory foods. Educate the patient about the role of bioactive substances in reducing future skin cancer risks. Counsel about returning to a balanced diet with plenty of phytochemicals.
>
> ***Monitoring and Evaluation:*** Improved diet with balanced intake of nutrients and phytochemicals.

- A high-fat diet may influence the UV-induced inflammatory responses in the skin (Meeran et al, 2009). Choose a diet that is moderate in fat while controlled in saturated fat and cholesterol. Include good sources of omega-3 fatty acids regularly (i.e., salmon, tuna, mackerel, herring, and sardines).
- Use sugars, salt, and alcoholic beverages in moderation.
- If anemic, a diet that meets at least DRI requirements for blood-forming nutrients will be needed.
- Weight gain caused by fluid retention is commonly seen in patients receiving biological therapy (immunotherapy). Use a diet with 2–4 grams of sodium or fluid restriction if needed.
- Provide adequate amounts of vitamin D_3 and dietary beta carotene. Consumption of 40 IU/d of vitamin D(3) raises plasma 25(OH)D by approximately 0.4 ng/mL (Vieth, 2009).

Common Drugs Used and Potential Side Effects

- Aldara skin cream reduces basal cell lesions without surgery.
- Interferon-α2b (Intron-A) is used in adult patients who have surgically treated melanoma considered at high risk of recurrence. This immunotherapy (biologic therapy) makes use of chemicals that occur naturally in the body.
- Immunomodulating agent histamine dihydrochloride (Maxamine), when used in combination with interleukin-2 (IL-2), improves survival for stage 4 malignant melanoma patients.

Herbs, Botanicals, and Supplements (see Table 13-8)

- Herbs and botanical supplements should not be used without discussing it with the physician.
- Evidence from clinical trials shows that a prolonged intake of 10,000 IU/d of vitamin D(3) poses no risk of adverse effects for adults (Vieth, 2009).

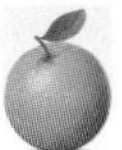

NUTRITION EDUCATION, COUNSELING, CARE MANAGEMENT

- Discuss the rationale for spacing meals throughout the day to avoid fatigue.
- Offer recipes and meal plans that provide the nutrients required to improve status and immunological competence.
- Patients undergoing treatment should be allowed flexibility in their food selections, while focusing on high-energy, high-quality protein, and phytochemical-rich choices whenever possible.
- Offer recipes and menu options for individual planning.
- Use sunscreen with sun protective factor (SPF) 15 or higher and both UVA and UVB protection; apply sunscreen after about 10–15 minutes in the sun.
- Biofeedback and stress management techniques may be useful.
- Dietary protection is provided by carotenoids, tocopherols, ascorbate, flavonoids, or omega-3 fatty acids.

Patient Education—Food Safety

- Educate the patient about food safety issues. Discuss safe food handling and preparation, keeping foods at proper temperatures, the use of sterile water, and reheating foods properly.

For More Information

- CDC – Skin Cancer
  http://www.cdc.gov/cancer/skin/basic_info/
- Melanoma Research Foundation
  http://www.melanoma.org/
- Mohs Micrograhic Surgery
  http://www.mohscollege.org/about/
- Web MD
  http://www.webmd.com/melanoma-skin-cancer/melanoma-guide/skin-cancer-melanoma-surgery

SKIN CANCERS—CITED REFERENCES

Benlloch M, et al. Bcl-2 and MnSOD antisense oligodeoxynucleotides and a glutamine-enriched diet facilitate elimination of highly resistant B16 melanoma cells by TNF-alpha and chemotherapy. *J Biol Chem.* 281:69, 2006.

Bergomi M, et al. Trace elements and melanoma. *J Trace Elem Med Biol.* 19:69, 2005.

Han W, He YY. Requirement for metalloproteinase-dependent ERK and AKT activation in UVB-induced G1-S cell cycle progression of human keratinocytes. *Photochem Photobiol.* 85:997, 2009.

Krause R, et al. UV radiation and cancer prevention: What is the evidence? *Anticancer Res.* 26:2723, 2006.

Lynde CW, Sapra S. Predictive testing of the melanocortin 1 receptor for skin cancer and photoaging. *Skin Therapy Lett.* 15:5, 2010.

McNaughton SA, et al. Role of dietary factors in the development of basal cell cancer and squamous cell cancer of the skin. *Cancer Epidemiol Biomarkers Prev.* 14:1596, 2005.

Meeran SM, et al. High-fat diet exacerbates inflammation and cell survival signals in the skin of ultraviolet B-irradiated C57BL/6 mice. *Toxicol Appl Pharmacol.* 241:303, 2009.

Smith G, et al. Melanocortin 1 receptor (MC1R) genotype influences erythemal sensitivity to psoralen-ultraviolet A photochemotherapy. *Br J Dermatol.* 157:1230, 2007.

Tuohimaa P. Vitamin D, aging, and cancer. *Nutr Rev.* 66:S147, 2008.

Vieth R. Vitamin D and cancer mini-symposium: the risk of additional vitamin D. *Ann Epidemiol.* 19:441, 2009.

Wolpowitz D, Gilchrest BA. The vitamin D questions: how much do you need and how should you get it? *J Am Acad Dermatol.* 54:301, 2006.

Woolcott CG, et al. Plasma 25-hydroxyvitamin D levels and the risk of colorectal cancer: the multiethnic cohort study. *Cancer Epidemiol Biomarkers Prev.* 19:130, 2010.

HORMONAL CANCERS

BREAST CANCER

NUTRITIONAL ACUITY RANKING: LEVEL 2–3

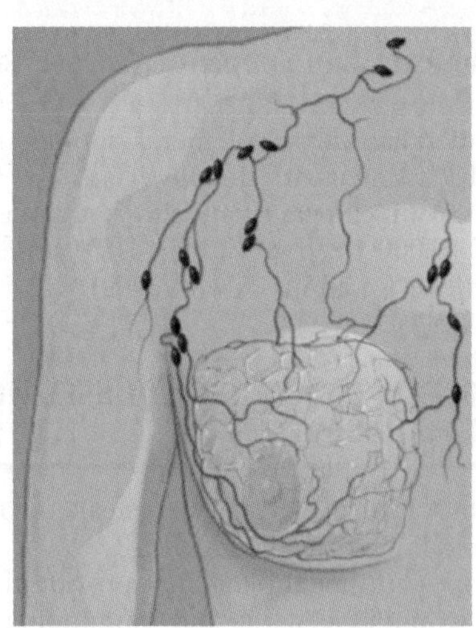

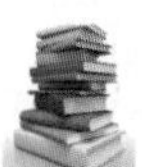

DEFINITIONS AND BACKGROUND

Breast (mammary) carcinoma is the second most common cancer in women, with over 200,000 cases diagnosed annually in the United States. It affects one in eight women. Having routine breast screenings for cancer is important. When a woman has specific family history patterns that put her at risk for gene mutations, her primary care physician should suggest DNA testing, but only about 2% of women have this level of risk. Age >30, health history related to fertility, ovarian function, and estrogen exposure play a role in the onset of breast cancer. Exposure to diets that produce high levels of estrogen seems to be most important in utero and after menopause; high estrogen levels during reproductive years seems to be protective. A longer duration of breastfeeding may be associated with a reduced risk. Breast cancer in men is less common and is generally preceded by gynecomastia.

Some breast cancer cells have a high proportion of estrogen and/or progesterone receptors in the nucleus. Those women who are ER/PR positive might benefit from hormonal therapy with tamoxifen or aromatase inhibiters; these drugs block hormone receptors in the cancer cell. Protein phosphatase 2A (PP2A) is a major cellular phosphatase that plays key regulatory roles in growth, differentiation, and apoptosis; its role in the suppression of breast cancer is being studied (Dupont et al, 2009).

Breast cancer may be related to oxidative stress. Receptor CXCR1 (IL-8) is a protein produced during chronic inflammation and tissue injury; it may play a role in breast cancer. Recent studies show that the intake of anthocyanins and ellagic acid can prevent cancer cells from developing (Stoner et al, 2009). Berries and pomegranates are particularly protective.

Being physically active is also protective, whereas obesity and Western dietary patterns increase cancer risk. Weight gain in the years preceding the onset of puberty is a promoter; increased fat cell adiposity increases estrogen availability at this time (Michels et al, 2006). Overweight breast cancer survivors commonly have metabolic syndrome (MetS) and elevated CRP (Thomson et al, 2009). Weight reduction is a reasonable goal.

TABLE 13-17 Staging of Breast Cancer

Stage 0	In situ—Cancer cells are present in either the lining of a breast lobule or a duct, but they have not spread to the surrounding fatty tissue.
Stage 1	Rarely metastasizing/noninvasive (<2 cm or 1 inch in diameter)—Cancer has spread from the lobules or ducts to nearby tissue in the breast; cancer has not spread to the lymph nodes.
Stage 2	Rarely metastasizing/invasive—The tumor can range from 2 cm to <5 cm in diameter (approximately 1–2 inches); sometimes, cancer may have spread to the lymph nodes.
Stage 3	Moderately metastasizing/invasive (≥2 inches)—Cancer cells have grown extensively into axillary (underarm) lymph nodes.
Stage 4	Highly metastasizing/invasive into other parts of the body, such as bone, liver, lung, or brain.

Eating soy foods yields greater benefits than taking isoflavone supplements (Li et al, 2005). Early exposure in childhood or early adolescence to phytoestrogens may be protective (Duffy et al, 2007).

Alcohol intake is a problem if folic acid intake is low; 600 micrograms of folic acid is protective. High intake of well-done meat and high exposure to meat carcinogens, particularly HCAs, may increase the risk of breast cancer (Zheng and Lee, 2009).

Breast cancer can be treated very effectively, particularly when it is diagnosed in the early stages. Staging of breast cancer is described in Table 13-17. Tumors are frequently found in the upper/outer quadrant of the breast (45%) and nipple area (25%), with 30% identified in other breast areas. In the early stages, a single nontender, firm, or hard mass with poorly defined margins may exist. Later, skin or nipple retraction, axillary lymphadenopathy, breast enlargement, redness, mild edema, and pain may occur. In the late stages, ulceration, moderate edema, and metastases to bone, liver, or brain are common.

Four standard types of therapy are used to treat breast cancer: surgery for the removal of cancerous tissue and, sometimes, other tissue; radiation therapy; chemotherapy; and hormonal therapy. New therapies are being researched through clinical trials.

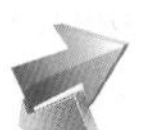

ASSESSMENT, MONITORING, AND EVALUATION

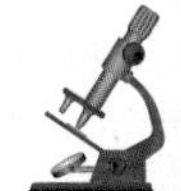

CLINICAL INDICATORS

Genetic Markers: Mutations in the *BRCA1* gene (on chromosome 17) result in an elevated risk of breast cancer and ovarian cancer (Kroiss et al, 2005). The *HER2* (Her2/neu, c-erb-2 or erb-2) gene produces a protein that acts as a receptor on the surface of all cells; some cancer cells have more receptors than normal, and they receive more messages to grow and divide. The C677 T polymorphism of the folic acid (*MTHFR*) genotype increases the risk of postmenopausal breast cancer, particularly with low intakes of folate and vitamin B_6 (Maruti et al, 2009).

Specific Clinical/History

Height
Weight
BMI
Weight changes
Diet history
Anorexia, nausea
Breast self-examination—masses
Calcifications
Biopsy
Skin or nipple retraction
Axillary lymphadenopathy
Breast enlargement
Redness, mild edema, pain
Ulceration, moderate edema
I & O
Temperature

Lab Work

Estrogen receptors (positive or negative)
Serum estrogen
Carcinoembryonic antigen (CEA)
Prolactin
Serum carotenoid levels
Mg^{++}, Ca^{++}
H & H
Gluc
Alk phos
Erythrocyte sed rate (ESR) to evaluate metastasis
Complete blood cell count (CBC)
Chol, Trig
Alb, transthyretin
CRP
Mammography

INTERVENTION

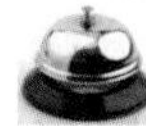

OBJECTIVES

- Control side effects of therapy and treatments (e.g., local or extensive mastectomy, chemotherapy, external-beam radiation therapy, brachytherapy).
- Promote intake of phytochemicals and protective foods to reduce inflammation.
- Promote good nutritional status to reduce future incidents and recurrence. Encourage regular breast self-examinations, physical activity, and other healthy behavior changes.
- Maintain or attain appropriate weight for height. Obese patients should lose weight before treatment; be careful not to lose lean body mass (LBM).
- Increase the likelihood of survival, wellness, and improved quality of life.
- For mastectomy patients, promote wound healing and prevent infection.

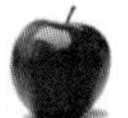

FOOD AND NUTRITION

- Because most studies have found that exercise, weight reduction, low-fat diet, and reduced alcohol intake are associated with a decreased risk of breast cancer, a diet with controlled total energy and fat is helpful (Cummings et al, 2009). While the Western style of diet should be discouraged (Adebamowo et al, 2005), meat, eggs and low-fat dairy foods can be used in moderation (Pala et al, 2009). Use fewer processed meats and less red meat, particularly if well-done (Zheng and Lee, 2009).

SAMPLE NUTRITION CARE PROCESS STEPS

Poor Nutrition Quality of Life

Assessment Data: Status post partial mastectomy; dysphagia and cachexia noted. Poor appetite and BMI dropped to 18.5 from 24 over the past 6 months.

Nutrition Diagnosis (PES): Poor nutrition, quality of life (NB-2.5) related to dysphagia, depression, and cachexia as evidenced by appetite <50% and BMI of 18.5.

Nutrition Intervention:

Food and Nutrient Delivery: ND 1.3 specific food/beverage: Puree, nectar, thick liquids and thinned soft foods. ND 3.1.1 commercial beverage supplement: 1 can 2× daily. ND 3.2.1: MVI.

Counseling:

C-2.2 Goal setting: Minimize weight loss, maintain adequate weight loss, monitor for signs and symptoms of aspiration, improve quality of life with exercise, and improve intake of phytochemical and nutrient-dense foods and tea.

Coordination of Nutrition Care:

RC 1.1 Interdisciplinary team meeting with nursing, social worker, recreational therapy, physical therapy, speech therapy.

Monitoring and Evaluation: No signs of aspiration, nausea, vomiting, speech evaluation follow-up, promote wound healing and prevent infection; reassess nutrition and quality of life.

- Promote use of the Mediterranean diet (Cottet et al, 2009; Masala et al, 2006). Olive/sunflower/canola oils, grape juice, red wine, and cheese are beneficial. Calorie restriction and use of omega-3 fatty acids decrease inflammation (Jolly, 2005).
- High fiber diets reduce hormone production and decrease cancer risk (Gaskins et al, 2009). At least 5–9 fruits and vegetables (Ahn et al, 2005; Rock et al, 2005) and 6 grain foods daily should be encouraged. The fruits and vegetables should include sources of alpha- and beta-carotene, zeaxanthin, and lycopene. Berries, pomegranate, garlic, and spices such as curcumin should be used often. Use cruciferous vegetables often (Warin et al, 2009).
- Sources of choline and betaine should be included (Xu et al, 2009). Choline is found in beef liver, wheat germ, and eggs. Betaine is found in beets.
- Alcohol may promote estrogen receptor–positive tumors (Suzuki et al, 2005). Red wine and resveratrol may be acceptable; limit to one drink per day.
- While some women are estrogen-sensitive (Fang et al, 2005; Li et al, 2005), overall, soy-enhanced diets are significantly associated with a decreased risk of death and recurrence (Shu et al, 2009; Steiner et al, 2008). This may be due to a new phytochemical found in soy called glyceollin I (Zimmermann et al, 2010). An isoflavone-rich diet might include wild leafy greens (as in the Greek diet), celery stalks, shredded lettuce, sweet peppers, raw spinach, fresh lemon, and sprigs of fresh parsley.
- A general supplement also may be safely recommended for folic acid (Zhang et al, 2005), calcium, vitamin D, vitamin A, vitamin C, and vitamin E as alpha-tocopherol.

Common Drugs Used and Potential Side Effects

- For patients who are **estrogen receptor positive**, hormonal therapy may be a breast cancer promoter; oral contraceptive use should be monitored or discontinued. Estrogen replacement (to prevent osteoporosis) increases risk levels.
- Antiestrogen therapy with tamoxifen (Noraldex) may be prescribed to treat estrogen-dependent breast cancer or be used in women at high risk. Nausea, vomiting, and hot flashes are common side effects. Avoid high doses of soy when using tamoxifen.
- For patients who are **estrogen receptor negative**, hormonal therapy actually may be recommended (e.g., progesterone and androgen therapy). Megestrol acetate (a hormonal antineoplastic drug and a synthetic derivative of progesterone) may reverse anorexia and weight loss.
- Chemotherapy may be used. Cyclophosphamide (Cytoxan) requires extra fluid intake. Doxorubicin, fluorouracil, and methotrexate are also commonly used; many gastrointestinal (GI) side effects are noted. Taste alterations are common for beef, chicken, and coffee. Anastrozole (Arimidex) can cause anorexia, weight changes, nausea, vomiting, dry mouth, constipation, and diarrhea. Gemcitabine (Gemzar) in combination with paclitaxel is used with metastatic breast cancer after failure of other chemotherapy.
- Trastuzumab (Herceptin) helps with early-stage HER2 breast cancer as an adjunct to chemotherapy to decrease recurrence.
- Repertaxin, originally developed to prevent organ transplant rejection, blocks receptor CXCR1 and kills breast cancer stem cells. It is under study in humans.

Herbs, Botanicals, and Supplements (see Table 13-8)

- Herbs and botanical supplements should not be used without discussing it with the physician. Women with a history of breast cancer may seek out "natural" phytoestrogens in the belief that they are safe or perhaps even protective against recurrence, but studies do not support a protective role (Duffy et al, 2007). The following herbal/botanical supplements should be avoided by patients with breast cancer because of their phytoestrogen content: Ginseng, Gingko biloba, Licorice root, Black cohosh, Wild yam root, DHEA.
- Grape seed extract, berry powder, and pomegranate products are beneficial (Kim, 2005; Stoner, 2009). Dietary sources of omega-3 fatty acids, vitamin C, vitamin E, beta-carotene, selenium, and coenzyme Q10 may be of particular value.
- With the use of methotrexate (Rheumatrex), avoid echinacea because of potential damage to the liver.

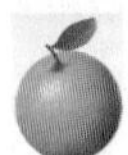

NUTRITION EDUCATION, COUNSELING, CARE MANAGEMENT

- Breast cancer detection projects are available throughout the United States; check with local chapters of the National Cancer Institute (NCI) and the American Cancer Society (ACS). Early detection of new tumors is crucial because lower stage tumors are much easier to control.

- Attain or maintain healthy body weight. Low total energy or lower fat dietary patterns may also be helpful (Elias et al, 2005). Reduce intake of sweets and high-glycemic index foods (Tavani et al, 2006). Eat a diet high in whole grains, fruits, and vegetables (Ahn et al, 2005).
- Discuss ways to make meals more appetizing, particularly if appetite is poor.
- Use of moderate amounts of soy may be encouraged. Increase use of cruciferous vegetables (Warin et al, 2009).
- Exercise and consumption of tea are important preventive factors to reduce depression among breast cancer survivors (Chen et al, 2010). Yoga and hypnosis may also be beneficial.
- Daughters of women with breast cancer should have a first mammogram before 40 years of age as a baseline and annually every 1–2 years thereafter. Lumps and changes should be reported immediately to a physician.
- Limit alcoholic beverages to one drink per day (Suzuki et al, 2005) and avoid high intakes of well-done meats and processed meats (Zheng and Lee, 2009).
- Calcium and vitamin D_3 supplementation may be indicated for patients who are menopausal or postmenopausal as they are at increased risk for developing osteoporosis.

Patient Education—Food Safety

- Educate the patient about food safety issues. Discuss safe food handling and preparation, keeping foods at proper temperatures, the use of sterile water, and reheating foods properly.

For More Information

- Breast Cancer
  http://www.breastcancer.org/
- Cornell University
  http://envirocancer.cornell.edu/factsheet/diet/fs49.BCRisk.cfm
- National Alliance of Breast Cancer Organizations
  http://www.nabco.org/
- National Breast Cancer Coalition
  http://www.stopbreastcancer.org/
- Sisters Network
  http://www.sistersnetworkinc.org/
- Y-Me National Breast Cancer Organization
  http://www.y-me.org/

BREAST CANCER—CITED REFERENCES

Adebamowo CA, et al. Dietary patterns and the risk of breast cancer. *Ann Epidemiol.* 15:789, 2005.

Ahn J, et al. Associations between breast cancer risk and the catalase genotype, fruit and vegetable consumption, and supplement use. *Am J Epidemiol.* 162:943, 2005.

Chen X. Exercise, Tea Consumption, and Depression Among Breast Cancer Survivors [Published online ahead of print Jan 4, 2010]. *J Clin Oncol.*

Cottet v, et al. Postmenopausal breast cancer risk and dietary patterns in the E3 N-EPIC prospective cohort study. *Am J Epidemiol.* 170(10):1257, 2009.

Cummings SR, et al. Prevention of breast cancer in postmenopausal women: approaches to estimating and reducing risk. *J Natl Cancer Inst.* 101:384, 2009.

Duffy C, et al. Implications of phytoestrogen intake for breast cancer. *CA Cancer J Clin.* 57:260, 2007.

Dupont WD, et al. Protein phosphatase 2 A subunit gene haplotypes and proliferative breast disease modify breast cancer risk [Published online ahead of print Nov 4, 2010]. *Cancer.*

Elias SG, et al. The 1944–1945 Dutch famine and subsequent overall cancer incidence. *Cancer Epidemiol Biomarkers Prev.* 14:1981, 2005.

Fang CY, et al. Correlates of soy food consumption in women at increased risk for breast cancer. *J Am Diet Assoc.* 105:1552, 2005.

Gaskins AJ, et al. Effect of daily fiber intake on reproductive function: the BioCycle Study. *Am J Clin Nutr.* 90:1061, 2009.

Jolly CA. Diet manipulation and prevention of aging, cancer and autoimmune disease. *Curr Opin Clin Nutr Metab Care.* 8:382, 2005.

Kim H. New nutrition, proteomics, and how both can enhance studies in cancer prevention and therapy. *J Nutr.* 135:2715, 2005.

Kroiss R, et al. Younger birth cohort correlates with higher breast and ovarian cancer risk in European BRCA1 mutation carriers. *Hum Mutat.* 26:583, 2005.

Li Y, et al. Inactivation of nuclear factor kappaB by soy isoflavone genistein contributes to increased apoptosis induced by chemotherapeutic agents in human cancer cells. *Cancer Res.* 65:6934, 2005.

Maruti SS, et al. MTHFR C677 T and postmenopausal breast cancer risk by intakes of one-carbon metabolism nutrients: a nested case-control study. *Breast Cancer Res.* 11:91, 2009.

Masala G, et al. Dietary and lifestyle determinants of mammographic breast density. A longitudinal study in a Mediterranean population. *Int J Cancer.* 118:1782, 2006.

McCann SE, et al. Dietary lignan intakes in relation to survival among women with breast cancer: the Western New York Exposures and Breast Cancer (WEB) Study [Published online ahead of print Dec 22, 2010]. *Breast Cancer Res Treat.*

Michels KB, et al. Preschool diet and adult risk of breast cancer. *Int J Cancer.* 118:749, 2006.

Pala V, et al. Meat, eggs, dairy products, and risk of breast cancer in the European Prospective Investigation into Cancer and Nutrition (EPIC) cohort. *Am J Clin Nutr.* 90:602, 2009.

Rock CL, et al. Plasma carotenoids and recurrence-free survival in women with a history of breast cancer. *J Clin Oncol.* 23:6631, 2005.

Shu XO, et al. Soy food intake and breast cancer survival. *JAMA.* 302:2437, 2009.

Steiner C, et al. Isoflavones and the prevention of breast and prostate cancer: new perspectives opened by nutrigenomics. *Br J Nutr.* 99:78S, 2008.

Stoner GD. Foodstuffs for preventing cancer: the preclinical and clinical development of berries. *Cancer Prev Res (Phila Pa).* 2:187, 2009.

Suzuki R, et al. Alcohol and postmenopausal breast cancer risk defined by estrogen and progesterone receptor status: a prospective cohort study. *J Natl Cancer Inst.* 97:1601, 2005.

Tavani A, et al. Consumption of sweet foods and breast cancer risk in Italy. *Ann Oncol.* 17:341, 2006.

Thomson CD, et al. Metabolic syndrome and elevated C-reactive protein in breast cancer survivors on adjuvant hormone therapy. *J Womens Health (Larchmt).* 18:2041, 2009.

Warin R, et al. Prevention of mammary carcinogenesis in MMTV-neu mice by cruciferous vegetable constituent benzyl isothiocyanate. *Cancer Res.* 69:9473, 2009.

Xu X, et al. High intakes of choline and betaine reduce breast cancer mortality in a population-based study. *FASEB J.* 23:4022, 2009.

Zhang SM, et al. Folate intake and risk of breast cancer characterized by hormone receptor status. *Cancer Epidemiol Biomarkers Prev.* 14:2004, 2005.

Zheng W, Lee SA. Well-done meat intake, heterocyclic amine exposure, and cancer risk. *Nutr Cancer.* 61:437, 2009.

Zimmermann MC, et al. Glyceollin I, a novel antiestrogenic phytoalexin isolated from activated soy. *J Pharmacol Exp Ther.* 332:35, 2010.

CHORIOCARCINOMA

NUTRITIONAL ACUITY RANKING: LEVEL 3

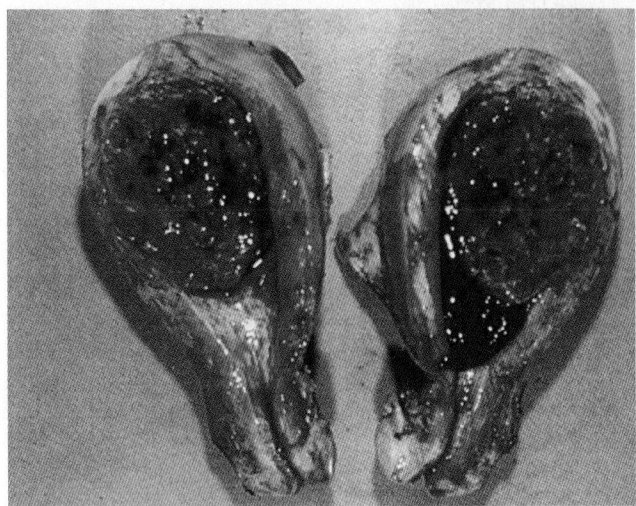

Adapted from: Michael S. Baggish, Rafael F. Valle, Hubert Guedj, *Hysteroscopy: Visual Perspectives of Uterine Anatomy, Physiology and Pathology*. Philadelphia: Lippincott Williams & Wilkins, 2007.

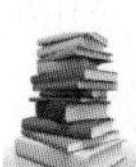

DEFINITIONS AND BACKGROUND

Choriocarcinoma involves a highly malignant neoplasm of the placenta with a secretion of human chorionic gonadotropin (hCG). It may develop in women after a molar pregnancy (where the fetus does not develop but a tumor develops instead), a miscarriage, or a full-term delivery.

Gestational choriocarcinoma occurs in approximately 1 in 20,000–40,000 pregnancies (Alvarez et al, 2005). It is more common among Asian women. Alternative names include chorioblastoma, trophoblastic tumor, chorioepithelioma, gestational trophoblastic disease, and gestational trophoblastic neoplasia. Rarely, a hydatidiform mole grows as a mass inside the uterus at the beginning of a pregnancy. When choriocarcinoma occurs in males, it presents as a testicular neoplasm, with skin hyperpigmentation (from excess beta hCG cross-reacting with the alpha MSH receptor), gynecomastia, and weight loss.

Diet affects the development of this type of cancer, because the placenta has such a large role in nutrient availability (Briese et al, 2005). Placental trophoblasts and immunomodulatory molecules are under investigation (Petroff et al, 2005). Phytoestrogens (PEs) induce biologic responses by mimicking or modulating the action or production of endogenous hormones; isoflavonoids and coumestrol increase progesterone receptor protein expression and decrease ERalpha expression (Taxvig et al, 2010).

Fatty acid synthase (FASN) is a tumor-associated marker found in all choriocarcinomas (Ueda et al, 2009). After the initial diagnosis, a careful examination is done to rule out metastasis. It can be fatal if there is metastasis to the kidney.

Gestational choriocarcinoma is responsive to chemotherapy; surgical excision or D & C is reserved for acute emergencies (Alvarez et al, 2005). A hysterectomy is rarely indicated but may be used for some women under age 40.

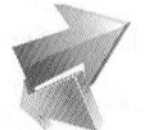

ASSESSMENT, MONITORING, AND EVALUATION

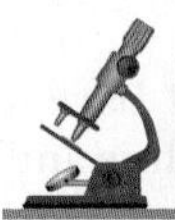

CLINICAL INDICATORS

Genetic Markers: Trophoblast factors are activated by hypoxia; interleukin (IL)-6, CD126, CD130, vascular endothelial growth factor (VEGF), and hypoxia inducible factor-1alpha (HIF-1alpha) are silenced in JEG-3 choriocarcinoma cells (Dubinsky et al, 2010).

Specific Clinical/ History	Cough, hemoptysis	Alb, transthyretin
Height	Chest pain	CRP
Weight	Headache	Transferrin
BMI	Chest X-ray	Gluc
Weight loss?		H & H
Diet history	**Lab Work**	Serum Fe, ferritin
Nausea, vomiting	Human chorionic gonadotropin β-hCG levels	Mg^{++}, Ca^{++}
I & O	Elevated TSH	Na^{+}, K^{+}
BP; hypertension?		ALT (increased)
Vaginal bleeding		Kidney function tests

SAMPLE NUTRITION CARE PROCESS STEPS

Inadequate Bioactive Substance Intake

Assessment Data: Pregnancy 6 months ago; still breastfeeding but showing high levels of β-hCG. Diagnosis of choriocarcinoma. BMI 25. No other unusual medical history. Diet history completed.

Nutrition Diagnosis (PES): Inadequate bioactive substance intake related to phytoestrogens as evidenced by food frequency records showing no intake of soy or other isoflavonoids.

Intervention: Food-nutrient delivery—Offer recipes and tips for ways to increase the intake of isoflavonoids from soy, legumes, spinach, and Brussels sprouts. Educate the patient about the role of bioactive substances in isoflavonoids in the prevention of relevant forms of cancer. Coordinate care with the medical team for the methotrexate treatment.

Monitoring and Evaluation: No undesirable outcomes (e.g., no renal metastasis); methotrexate treatment successful.

INTERVENTION

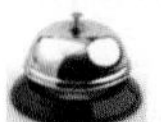

OBJECTIVES

- Maintain appropriate weight for height. Correct weight loss and cachexia.
- Increase intake of isoflavonoids and other bioactive substances.
- Correct side effects of chemotherapy if used.
- Treat and correct all other side effects of therapy and disease state.
- Prepare patient for surgery, if necessary.

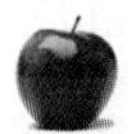

FOOD AND NUTRITION

- Modify diet to patient preferences. Include isoflavonoids and coumestrol from soy products, legumes, spinach, and Brussels sprouts.
- Increase liquids as needed.
- Provide adequate protein, B-complex vitamins, iron, calories, and other nutrients for wound healing, as appropriate. Use RDA and DRI levels as a guide.
- Alter the texture of the diet if the patient is fatigued at mealtimes or if stomatitis occurs after chemotherapy.

Common Drugs Used and Potential Side Effects

- Methotrexate or actinomycin D may be used; nausea and vomiting are common side effects. Administer with glucose to reduce toxicity.
- Combined EMACO therapy (etoposide, methotrexate, actinomycin D, cyclosphosphamide, and oncovin) may be used with high-risk disease; thinning hair or GI distress can occur.
- A new FASN inhibitor, C93, is being developed to initiate apoptosis in these cells (Ueda et al, 2009).

Herbs, Botanicals, and Supplements (see Table 13-8)

- Herbs and botanical supplements should not be used without discussing it with the physician.
- Phytoestrogens from isoflavonoids may prove to be quite effective in the treatment of this cancer.

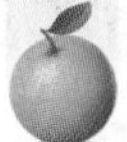

NUTRITION EDUCATION, COUNSELING, CARE MANAGEMENT

- Nausea or vomiting may require small, frequent feedings and control of fluid intake at mealtimes.
- With the high hCG levels, menstrual periods stop; periods start again when the levels are normal again. Delay pregnancy for 6 months or longer after treatment. With chemotherapy, periods will stop temporarily, and there may be early menopause.

Patient Education—Food Safety

- Educate the patient about food safety issues. Discuss safe food handling and preparation, keeping foods at proper temperatures, the use of sterile water, and reheating foods properly.

For More Information

- Cancer Help – UK
  http://www.cancerhelp.org.uk/type/GTT/choriocarcinoma/about/index.htm
- Family Practice Notebook–Choriocarcinoma
  http://www.fpnotebook.com/OB65.htm
- Medline–Choriocarcinoma
  http://www.nlm.nih.gov/medlineplus/ency/article/001496.htm

CHORIOCARCINOMA—CITED REFERENCES

Alvarez NR, et al. Metastatic choriocarcinoma to the pancreas. *Am Surg.* 71:330, 2005.

Briese J, et al. Osteopontin expression in gestational trophoblastic diseases: correlation with expression of the adhesion molecule, CEACAM1. *Int J Gynecol Pathol.* 24:271, 2005.

Dubinsky V, et al. Role of regulatory and angiogenic cytokines in invasion of trophoblastic cells [Published online ahead of print Dec 29, 2009]. *Am J Reprod Immunol.* 63:193, 2010.

Petroff MG, et al. The immunomodulatory proteins B7-DC, B7-H2, and B7-H3 are differentially expressed across gestation in the human placenta. *Am J Pathol.* 167:465, 2005.

Taxvig C, et al. Effects of nutrition relevant mixtures of phytoestrogens on steroidogenesis, aromatase, estrogen, and androgen activity. *Nutr Cancer.* 62:122, 2010.

Ueda SM, et al. Trophoblastic neoplasms express fatty acid synthase, which may be a therapeutic target via its inhibitor C93. *Am J Pathol.* 175:2618, 2009.

PROSTATE CANCER

NUTRITIONAL ACUITY RANKING: LEVEL 2

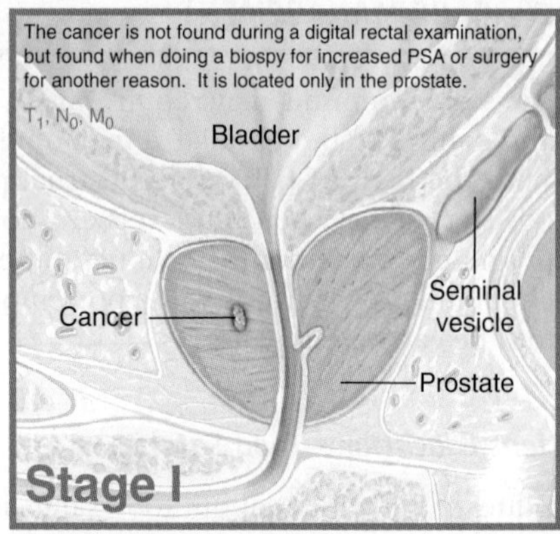

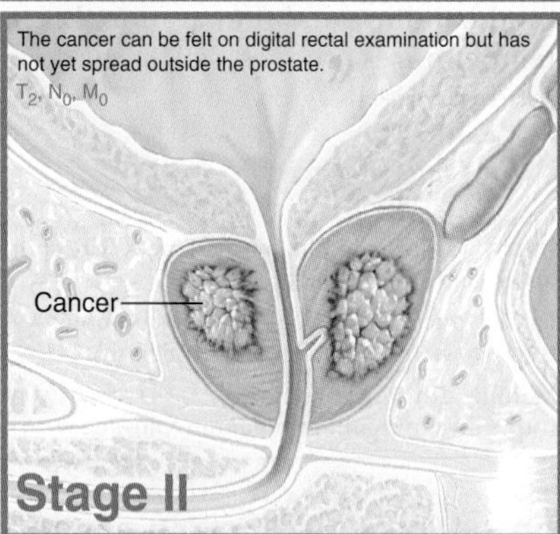

The cancer can be felt on digital rectal examination but has not yet spread outside the prostate.
T_2, N_0, M_0
Cancer
Stage II

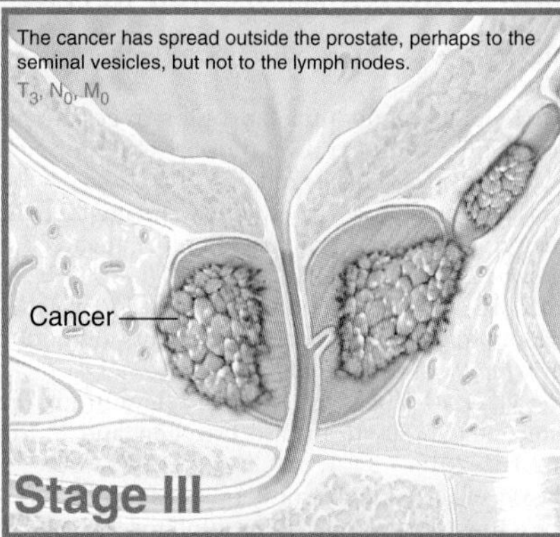

The cancer has spread outside the prostate, perhaps to the seminal vesicles, but not to the lymph nodes.
T_3, N_0, M_0
Cancer
Stage III

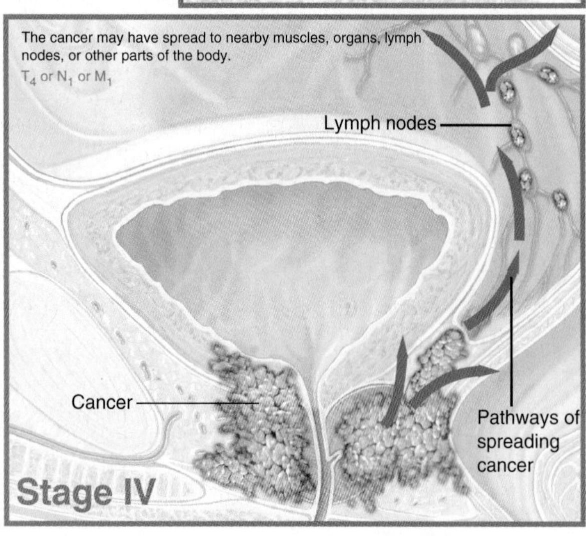

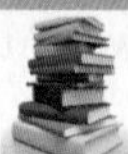

The cancer may have spread to nearby muscles, organs, lymph nodes, or other parts of the body.
T_4 or N_1 or M_1

Pathways of spreading cancer

DEFINITIONS AND BACKGROUND

Prostate cancer is third to lung and colon cancer as the cause of cancer-related deaths in American men (Colli and Amling, 2009). Prevalence is high in northwestern Europe and the United States, highest among African-American males worldwide. Men also at great risk are those with abdominal obesity, those with family history of the disease, and those whose diets are low in fiber and high in saturated fats or red meats. High serum cholesterol levels may be linked with the progression of prostate cancer (Freedman and Aronson, 2009).

An effective chemoprevention strategy for prostate cancer serves as a model for chemoprevention of other adult malignancies (Canby-Hagino and Thompson, 2005). Diets rich in specific vitamins, grains, fish, fruits, and vegetables may be associated with lower cancer rates (Chan et al, 2005; Lamb and Zhang, 2005). Chemoprotective factors are listed in Table 13-18.

Surgical intervention, radiation, and hormonal therapy are used. Radiation therapy may cause temporary changes in bowel habits (such as increased frequency, increased flatulence, and bowel cramping). Brachytherapy is internal radiation therapy in which small radioactive pellets are inserted or implanted into the prostate gland.

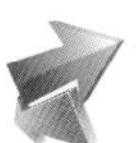

ASSESSMENT, MONITORING, AND EVALUATION

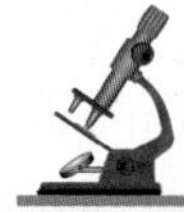

CLINICAL INDICATORS

Genetic Markers: Overexpression of the *AMACR* gene is associated with prostate cancer risk (Xu et al, 2005). Strict nutritional interventions can change gene expression (Ornish et al, 2008). Secondary analyses of two randomized, controlled phase III trials have demonstrated that selenium and vitamin E could reduce prostate cancer incidence through cell type- and zone-specific tissue effects (Tsavachidou et al, 2009).

Clinical/History

Height
Weight
BMI
Weight changes
Diet history
I & O
Urine testing (infections, enlarged prostate)
Urinary dribbling, frequency, pain, burning
Persistent pain (pelvis, lower back, upper thighs)
BP
Transrectal ultrasound
Doppler scan
Digital rectal examination
Bone scan, chest x-ray
CT scan, MRI

Lab Work

Prostate-specific antigen (PSA) (>2.5 ng/mL is a concern)

Alb, transthyretin	BUN, Creat	H & H
	Serum vitamin D	Ca^{++}, Mg^{++}
CRP	Transferrin	Na^{+}, K^{+}

INTERVENTION

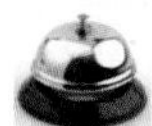

OBJECTIVES

- Prepare patient for surgery, radiation, medications, chemotherapy, or hormone therapy.
- Prevent or correct side effects such as nausea, vomiting, and diarrhea.
- Prevent or correct weight loss.

TABLE 13-18 Preventive Dietary Factors for Prostate Cancer

Allium vegetables (garlic, scallions, onions, chives, and leeks)
Apigenin
Cruciferous vegetables (Chan et al, 2005)
Curcumin
Epigallocatechin gallate (EGCG)
Grains, nuts, cereals
Grape seed extract
Green tea (Trottier et al, 2010)
Herbs and herbal supplements (saw palmetto)
Lignans
Lower fat diet
Lycopene, other carotenoids (Trottier et al, 2010)
Omega-3 fatty acids, EPA and DHA (Chan et al, 2005)
Physical activity and exercise (Jian et al, 2005; Zeegers et al, 2005)
Polyphenols (Chan et al, 2005)
Pomegranate (Trottier et al, 2010)
Quercetin
Resveratrol
Selenium (Chan et al, 2005; Trottier et al, 2010)
Soy genistein and isoflavones (Chan et al, 2005; Trottier et al, 2010)
Statins, 5-alpha-reductase inhibitors, and NSAIDs
Vegan diet
Vitamin D_3 (Schwartz, 2005; Tokar and Webber, 2005; Trottier et al, 2010)
Vitamin E as gamma-tocopherol in walnuts, pecans, sesame seed, corn and sesame oils (Chan et al, 2005; Trottier et al, 2010)

REFERENCES

Jian L, et al. Moderate physical activity and prostate cancer risk: a case-control study in China. *Eur J Epidemiol.* 20:155, 2005.

Schwartz, GG. Vitamin D and the epidemiology of prostate cancer. *Semin Dial.* 18:276, 2005.

Tokar EJ, Webber MM. Cholecalciferol (vitamin D_3) inhibits growth and invasion by up-regulating nuclear receptors and 25-hydroxylase (CYP27A1) in human prostate cancer cells. *Clin Exp Metastasis.* 22:275, 2005.

Trottier G, et al. Nutraceuticals and prostate cancer prevention: a current review. *Nat Rev Urol.* 7:21, 2010.

Zeegers MP, et al. Physical activity and the risk of prostate cancer in the Netherlands cohort study, results after 9.3 years of follow-up. *Cancer Epidemiol Biomarkers Prev.* 14:1490, 2005.

SAMPLE NUTRITION CARE PROCESS STEPS

Increased Energy Needs

Assessment Data: 90-year-old male resident in a long-term care facility; diagnosed with prostate cancer 1 year ago. Gradual weight loss, recently 5# in past month. Intake records show 25–50% at mealtime in the past month; previously 50–75% at all meals and taking oral supplements between meals.

Nutrition Diagnosis (PES): NC-3.2 Increased energy needs related to the inflammatory process and diagnosis of prostate cancer as evidenced by the insidious weight loss over six months.

Intervention:

Food and Nutrient Delivery—Provide fortified foods such as super oatmeal and potatoes because of increased energy needs; MVI with minerals to ensure adequate nutrients are available. Coordinate care—Continue high calorie supplements between meals and with medication passes by nursing.

Monitoring and Evaluation: No further weight loss. Improved intake of kilocalories as noted on 3-day calorie count.

- Promote intake of protective foods and phytochemicals. Support intensive nutrition and lifestyle intervention to change gene expression, where appropriate (Ornish et al, 2008).
- Maintain or achieve a healthy body weight.

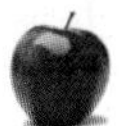

FOOD AND NUTRITION

- Provide adequate calories and protein; avoid excesses.
- It may be beneficial to have some weight loss prior to surgery using a low-fat, low glycemic index diet (Schenk et al 2009).
- After surgery, a multiple vitamin—mineral supplement may be indicated to promote wound healing.
- Monitor the need for lower sodium if corticosteroids are prescribed.
- Increase the use of fruits and vegetables, particularly green and yellow-orange, and sources of folic acid. Tomato products, pizza sauce, strawberries, and salsa provide lycopene. Pomegranate juice may reduce the likelihood of recurrence (Malik et al, 2005).
- Increase the use of isoflavonoids (Haddad et al, 2006; Steiner et al, 2008). Choose beans, soybeans, lentils, tofu, tempeh, soy nuts, soymilk, and dried fruit often.
- Low-fat, vegan, and high-fiber diets may be indicated (Dewell et al, 2008; Van Patten et al, 2008).
- Increased use of omega-3 fatty acids has been shown to be useful; include salmon, sardines, tuna, mackerel, and herring in the diet.
- Vitamin D_3 is needed; drink fortified milk, get a modest exposure to the sun, and take a vitamin pill that contains cholecalciferol.

Common Drugs Used and Potential Side Effects

- Aspirin improves survival after prostate cancer. NSAIDs and statins may also be beneficial.

TABLE 13-19 Antioxidant Color Link

Colors	Examples of Fruits-Vegetables	Antioxidants
Red	Grapes, red wine	Resveratrol
Red/Pink	Tomatoes, pink grapefruits, watermelon	lycopene
Red/Purple	Pomegranates, grapes, plums, berries	Anthocyanins
Orange	Carrots, mangoes, apricots, cantaloupes, pumpkin, sweet potato	Alpha and beta carotenes
Orange/Yellow	Oranges, peaches, papaya, nectarines	Beta-cryptoxanthin
Yellow/Green	Spinach, collard, yellow corn, green peas, avocado, honeydew melon	Lutein and zeaxanthin
Green	Broccoli, Brussels sprouts, cabbage, bok choy, kale	Sulforaphane, isothiocyanates, indoles
Whit/Green	Garlic, onions, asparagus, leeks, shallots, chives	Allyl sulfides

Source: Prostate Cancer Foundation, http://www.prostatecancerfoundation.org/atf/cf/%7B705B3273-F2EF-4EF6-A653-E15C5D8BB6B1%7D/Nutrition_Guide.pdf, accessed January 15, 2010.

- Chemotherapy drugs have varying side effects; monitor closely. Fatigue, nausea and vomiting, mouth sores, hair loss, and a low white blood cell count are common.
- The Prostate Cancer Prevention Trial (PCPT) identified the benefits of reducing prostate cancer risk with the use of 5alpha-reductase inhibitors (Crawford et al, 2009). Finasteride lowers prostate cancer risk and can be available to men who are at high risk (Kaplan et al, 2009).
- Hormonal therapy may be used as the treatment of choice (Bracarda et al, 2005). Luteinizing hormone–releasing hormone (LH-RH) agonists can decrease the amount of testosterone produced by a man's testicles as effectively as surgical removal. Lupron Depot (leuprolide acetate for depot suspension), an LH-RH agonist, is used in the palliative treatment of advanced prostate cancer.

Herbs, Botanicals, and Supplements (see Table 13-8)

- Complementary and alternative medicine (CAM) includes the use of vitamin and mineral supplements, herbs, antioxidants, saw palmetto, selenium, vitamin E, and lycopene (Chan, Elkin et al, 2005). Herbs and botanical supplements should not be used without discussing it with the physician.
- Saw palmetto has some efficacy. Avoid taking it with estrogens, testosterone, anabolic steroids, oral contraceptives, or finasteride because the herb and drugs function in similar ways and additive effects are possible.
- Phytoestrogens found in common herbal products are effective inhibitors of prostate tumor cell growth through different mechanisms; these include quercetin, genistein, epigallocatechin gallate (EGCG), curcumin, apigenin, resveratrol, and isoflavones in soy and red clover.
- Pygeum and nettle are being studied at this time.

NUTRITION EDUCATION, COUNSELING, CARE MANAGEMENT

- Discuss the side effects of therapy and the long-term plans for recovery.
- Maintain adequate hydration.
- Discuss lifestyle and dietary changes. This may include lowering the intake of red meats and saturated fats, increasing fruits and vegetables and tomato products, increasing fiber and whole grains, and consuming vitamin D–fortified milk.
- Chemopreventive agents include 5-alpha-reductase inhibitors; statins; NSAIDs; selenium; vitamins E and D; lycopene; allium vegetables (garlic, scallions, onions, chives, and leeks); soy/isoflavones; pomegranate and green tea polyphenols (Colli and Amling, 2009; Trottier et al, 2010; Van Patten et al, 2008). Table 13-19 provides a color chart to remember the antioxidant foods.
- Lifestyle changes tend to correlate with quality of life after prostate cancer treatments (Sheriff et al, 2005). Diet and exercise changes are important.
- Offer menu plans for sufficient intake of protective nutrients. Lycopene can be found in foods such as tomatoes, watermelon, guava, and red grapefruit. Include pomegranates, soy, fish, and more vegan or plant-based choices.
- Help to maintain a positive, optimistic outlook to yield favorable results (Kronenwetter et al, 2005).

Patient Education—Food Safety

- Educate the patient about food safety issues. Discuss safe food handling and preparation, keeping foods at proper temperatures, the use of sterile water, and reheating foods properly.

For More Information

- Association for the Cure of Prostate Cancer
  http://www.capcure.org/
- Medline
  http://www.nlm.nih.gov/medlineplus/prostatecancer.html
- Minorities and Underserved Populations
  http://www.ustoo.org/Minority_Program.asp
- Prostate Cancer Research Institute
  http://www.prostate-cancer.org/
- Prostate Cancer Support Group
  http://www.ustoo.com/

PROSTATE CANCER—CITED REFERENCES

Bracarda S, et al. Cancer of the prostate. *Crit Rev Oncol Hematol.* 56:379, 2005.

Canby-Hagino ED, Thompson IM. Mechanisms of disease: prostate cancer—a model for cancer chemoprevention in clinical practice. *Nat Clin Pract Oncol.* 2:255, 2005.

Chan JM, et al. Role of diet in prostate cancer development and progression. *J Clin Oncol.* 23:8152, 2005.
Colli JL, Amling CL. Chemoprevention of prostate cancer: what can be recommended to patients? *Curr Urol Rep.* 10:165, 2009.
Crawford ED, et al. Reduction in the risk of prostate cancer: future directions after the prostate cancer prevention trial [Published online ahead of print Dec 24, 2009]. *Urology.*
Dewell A, et al. A very-low-fat vegan diet increases intake of protective dietary factors and decreases intake of pathogenic dietary factors. *J Am Diet Assoc.* 108:347, 2008.
Freedland SJ, Aronson W J. Dietary intervention strategies to modulate prostate cancer risk and prognosis. *Curr Opin Urol.* 19:263, 2009.
Haddad AQ, et al. Novel antiproliferative flavonoids induce cell cycle arrest in human prostate cancer cell lines. *Prostate Cancer Prostatic Dis.* 9:68, 2006.
Kaplan SA, et al. PCPT: Evidence that finasteride reduces risk of most frequently detected intermediate- and high-grade (Gleason score 6 and 7) cancer. *Urology.* 73:935, 2009.
Kronenwetter C, et al. A qualitative analysis of interviews of men with early stage prostate cancer: the prostate cancer lifestyle trial. *Cancer Nurs.* 28:99, 2005.
Lamb DJ, Zhang L. Challenges in prostate cancer research: animal models for nutritional studies of chemoprevention and disease progression. *J Nutr.* 135:3009S, 2005.
Malik A, et al. Pomegranate fruit juice for chemoprevention and chemotherapy of prostate cancer. *Proc Natl Acad Sci USA.* 102:14813, 2005.
Ornish D, et al. Changes in prostate gene expression in men undergoing an intensive nutrition and lifestyle intervention. *Proc Natl Acad Sci U S A.* 105:8369, 2008.
Schenk JM, et al. A dietary intervention to elicit rapid and complex dietary changes for studies investigating the effects of diet on tissues collected during invasive surgical procedures. *J Am Diet Assoc.* 109:459, 2009.
Sheriff SK, et al. Lifestyle correlates of health perception and treatment satisfaction in a clinical cohort of men with prostate cancer. *Clin Prostate Cancer.* 3:239, 2005.
Steiner C, et al. Isoflavones and the prevention of breast and prostate cancer: new perspectives opened by nutrigenomics. *Br J Nutr.* 99:78S, 2008.
Trottier G, et al. Nutraceuticals and prostate cancer prevention: a current review. *Nat Rev Urol.* 7:21, 2010.
Tsavachidou D, et al. Selenium and vitamin E: cell type- and intervention-specific tissue effects in prostate cancer. *J Natl Cancer Inst.* 101:306, 2009.
Van Patten CL, et al. Diet and dietary supplement intervention trials for the prevention of prostate cancer recurrence: a review of the randomized controlled trial evidence. *J Urol.* 180:2314, 2008.

Hematological Cancers

LEUKEMIAS

NUTRITIONAL ACUITY RANKING: LEVEL 3–4

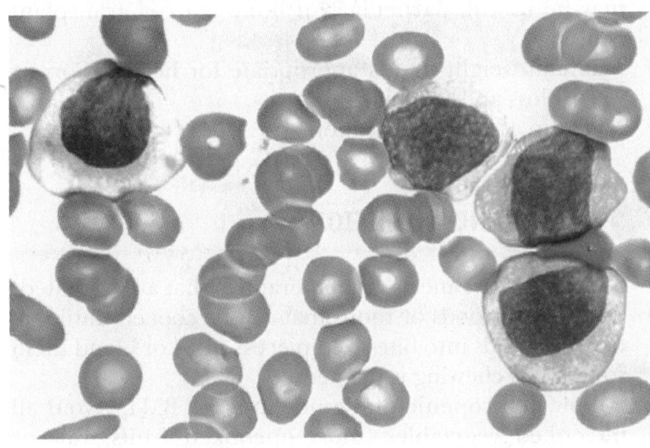

Adapted from: McClatchey KD M.D., D.D.S. *Clinical Laboratory Medicine,* 2nd ed. Philadelphia: Lippincott Williams & Wilkins, 2002.

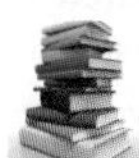

DEFINITIONS AND BACKGROUND

Leukemia involves the uncontrolled proliferation of leukocytes and their precursors in blood-forming organs, with infiltration into other organs (Table 13-20). The blood has a grayish-white appearance. Leukemia incidence is highest among whites and lowest among American Indians/Alaskan natives and Asian and Pacific Islander populations. Acute leukemia progresses rapidly, with an accumulation of immature, functionless cells in the marrow and blood. Then, the marrow stops producing enough normal red cells, white cells and platelets and anemia develops. Chronic leukemias progress more slowly.

Leukemia is the most common childhood cancer. Because chromosomal abnormalities are present at birth in children who later develop leukemia, nutrition during pregnancy affects their risk. Insulin-like growth factor I (IGF-I) is associated with high birth weight and an increased risk of childhood leukemia (Tower and Spector, 2007). Both insulin and IGF-I act to promote cell proliferation and to inhibit apoptosis (Fair and Montgomery, 2009). Obesity is a well-known problem in children with ALL; it may be the result of an excess in energy intake, reduced energy expenditure, or both (Jansen et al, 2009).

Dietary exposures to cured/smoked meat or fish, nitrites, and nitrosamines are associated with leukemia in children and adolescents (Liu et al, 2009). It may be prudent for women to consume a diet rich in vegetables, fruit, iron, soybean curd, and protein (particularly fish and seafood) prior to and during pregnancy to reduce the ALL risk in their children (Kwan et al, 2009; Liu et al, 2009; Petridou et al, 2005).

Phytochemicals, such as grape extract, apigenin, quercetin, kaempferol, and myricetin, are protective against cancer cell survival (Chen et al, 2005). Red wine polyphenolic extract may inhibit leukemia cell growth (Sharif et al, 2010). In adults with AML, individuals who smoke, do not drink coffee, and eat more meat have a higher risk (Ma et al, 2009).

The primary treatment of leukemias currently involves chemotherapy to kill attacking abnormal blood cells. Bone marrow transplantation may be feasible in some cases. Table 13-21 lists various types of leukemias, relevant signs and symptoms, and treatments.

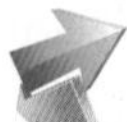

ASSESSMENT, MONITORING, AND EVALUATION

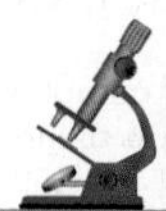

CLINICAL INDICATORS

Genetic Markers: FLT3 is a receptor tyrosine kinase that plays an important role in hematopoietic stem cell proliferation, differentiation and survival; alterations have a role in leukemia. BCR-ABL cancer gene is another gene of importance in leukemias. Persons with Down syndrome, Fanconi's anemia, and other genetic disorders have a high risk of leukemia. Lack of maternal folate causes DNA hypomethylation and increased DNA strand breaks; *MTHFR* gene polymorphisms have been associated with adult and childhood ALL (Smith et al, 2005; Tower and Spector, 2007). Chronic lymphocytic leukemia (CLL) is a malignancy of B cells of unknown etiology; deletions of the chromosomal region 13q14 are commonly associated with CLL (Klein et al, 2010).

Specific Clinical/ History

- Height
- Weight
- BMI
- Weight changes (slight weight loss?)
- Diet history
- BP
- Fever (over 101°F?)
- Frequent infections
- Malaise, irritability
- Pallor
- Hemorrhage
- Petechiae, ecchymosis, purpura
- Palpitations
- Shortness of breath
- Bone or joint pain
- Cough, sternal tenderness
- Splenomegaly, hepatomegaly
- Hemorrhages, nosebleeds
- Headache
- Anorexia
- Nausea and vomiting
- Mouth ulcers
- Bleeding
- Enlarged lymph nodes?
- Night sweats?
- Lumbar puncture

Lab Work[a]

- WBC (increased)
- Ferritin (increased)
- Platelets
- Lactate dehydrogenase (LDH) (elevated)
- Zinc (decreased)
- Uric acid (increased)
- Immunocytochemistry
- Cytogenetics (FISH test)
- Molecular genetic studies
- Alb, transthyretin
- CRP
- Serum copper (increased)
- Gluc
- H & H, Serum Fe, Ferritin
- Transferrin
- PT or International Normalized Ratio (INR)
- Na^+, K^+
- Ca^{++}, Mg^{++}

[a]A useful Web site describing lab tests is available at http://www.leukemia-lymphoma.org/attachments/National/br_1216925469.pdf.

INTERVENTION

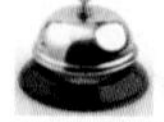

OBJECTIVES

- Prevent hemorrhage and infections.
- Promote recovery and stabilization before bone marrow transplantation, if performed.

SAMPLE NUTRITION CARE PROCESS STEPS

Intake of Unsafe Foods

Assessment Data: Status post bone marrow transplant for ALL in a 14-year old male. Now at the emergency room, complaining of gastric pain and vomiting after eating items at a restaurant salad bar. BMI normal for age. Labs all within normal limits.

Nutrition Diagnosis (PES): Intake of unsafe foods related to raw vegetables and salad items at public restaurant following BMT procedure, as evidenced by gastric pain and vomiting.

Intervention: Education about the benefits of the low bacteria (neutropenic) diet for a few months longer until the immune system and tolerance improves. Counseling about the use of cooked fruits and vegetables and avoidance of salad bars until tolerance is better.

Monitoring and Evaluation: No further episodes of vomiting and GI pain with the use of the neutropenic diet. Good acceptance of the restrictions until immunity improves.

- Correct anorexia and nausea or vomiting.
- Prevent complications and further morbidity, such as veno-occlusive disease (VOD).
- Alter diet according to medications and therapies such as chemotherapy. A low-bacteria (neutropenic) diet may be useful, particularly if bone marrow transplant is used.
- Maintain weight that is appropriate for height. Correct weight loss and cachexia.
- Maintain adequate hydration.

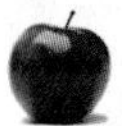

FOOD AND NUTRITION

- Serve attractive meals at temperatures that are tolerated.
- Choose soft foods or foods that can be cooked until tender. Cut foods into bite-sized pieces; grind or blend them so that less chewing is needed.
- Follow neutropenic diet guidelines for BMT. Avoid all uncooked vegetables, most uncooked fruits, raw or rare-cooked meat, fish. All eggs should be thoroughly cooked. Avoid salad bars and deli counters. Buy vacuum-packed luncheon meats rather than freshly sliced meats. Eat or drink only pasteurized milk, yogurt, cheese, or other dairy products. Avoid soft mold-ripened and blue-veined cheeses including Brie, Camembert, Roquefort, Stilton, Gorgonzola, and Blue. At home, use tap water or bottled water; avoid well water or boil it for one minute before using.
- Small meals may be better tolerated than large ones. In some cases, cold or iced foods may be preferred.
- A high-protein, high-energy, high-vitamin/mineral intake should be offered. Tube feeding in these patients is often useful, but intolerance due to treatment side effects may be an obstacle.
- Extra fluids will be important during febrile states or with the use of interferon, but avoid overload. Sip water and

TABLE 13-20 **Various Forms of Leukemia**

Form	Description
Acute Leukemias	Sx: easy fatigue, malaise, irritability, fever, pallor, petechiae, bruising, purpura, hemorrhage, palpitations, shortness of breath, slight weight loss, bone or joint pain, painless lumps in underarm or stomach, cough, sternal tenderness, splenomegaly, hepatomegaly, anemia, hemorrhages or nosebleeds, headache, nausea, vomiting, and mouth ulcers.
Acute lymphocytic leukemia (ALL)	ALL affects bone marrow and lymph nodes. It progresses rapidly and mainly affects children; it accounts for 50% of all childhood leukemias. Control of bone marrow and systemic disease is the goal. Treatment may include monthly lumbar punctures. ALL often spreads to the coverings of the brain and spinal cord; patients may receive chemotherapy into spinal fluid, or radiation therapy to the head. Bone marrow transplantation (BMT) treatment or peripheral-blood stem-cell transplant (PBSCT) may lead to bloody diarrhea, fever, and other symptoms of graft-versus-host disease (GVHD).
Acute myelogenous leukemia (AML)	AML starts in the bone marrow but moves into the blood and to the lymph nodes, liver, spleen, central nervous system, and testes. AML consists of proliferation of myeloblasts, which are immature polynuclear leukocytes. AML is more common in adult males but also accounts for just under half of cases of childhood leukemia. Average onset of AML is the sixth decade. Smoking, obesity, chronic workplace exposure to benzene, large doses of irradiation have been established as causes. Treatments vary according to the age of the patient and according to the specific subtype. The goal is to control bone marrow, CNS, and systemic disease.
Chronic Leukemias	Sx: anemia, increased infections, bleeding, enlarged lymph nodes (in lymphatic form), night sweats, fever, weight loss, and anorexia.
Chronic lymphocytic leukemia (CLL)	CLL involves a crowding out of normal leukocytes in lymph glands, interfering with the body's ability to produce other blood cells. CLL is more common in people older than 50 years of age and in males. It is twice as common as CML. Treatment depends upon the stage and symptoms of the individual patient. Low-grade disease does not benefit from treatment. With complications or more advanced disease, treatment may be needed. Hairy cell leukemia is a subtype of CLL.
Chronic myelogenous leukemia (CML)	CML affects mostly adults and is very rare in children. The standard of care for newly diagnosed patients is oral administration of imatinib (Gleevec), which has few side effects and makes CML a chronic, manageable condition.
T-cell prolymphocytic leukemia	Has similar overproduction of white blood cells in the bone marrow; less common than the other types. Difficult to treat and does not respond well to chemotherapy drugs. Alemtuzumab (Campath) is a monoclonal antibody that attacks white blood cells with some success.

other clear liquids such as broth, ginger ale, or lemonade frequently.
- Vitamins A and D may be beneficial (Trump et al, 2005) but avoid excesses above the UL levels.
- Include protective foods such as isoflavones in soy and flavonoids in grapes, coffee, tea, nuts, seeds, fruits, and vegetables.

Common Drugs Used and Potential Side Effects

- See Tables 13-22.
- Methadone kills leukemia cells while not affecting the normal ones; it activates the mitochondrial pathway, which activated specific enzymes within the cancer cell, causing pre-programmed death. This is a great breakthrough in leukemia research.

TABLE 13-21 **Medications for Acute Leukemias**

Induction: The first phase destroys as many cancer cells as quickly as possible to bring about a remission.

Consolidation: The goal is to get rid of leukemia cells where they reside.

Maintenance: After the number of leukemia cells has been reduced by the first two phases of treatment, lower doses of chemotherapy drugs are given over 2 years.

CEP-701 (lestaurtinib) inhibits the receptor tyrosine kinase FLT3 in AML patients

Chemotherapy often includes methotrexate, 5-azacitidine, cytarabine, thioguanine, and daunorubicin, which may cause stomatitis, nausea, or vomiting. Coadministration of these agents with glucose and adequate fluid is needed. When methotrexate is used, neurotoxicity is a concern; use low-dose folinic acid rescue (Leucovorin).

Gemtuzumab ozogamicin (Mylotarg) may be added. Granulocyte colony-stimulating factors (Neupogen, Leukine) may improve response to chemotherapy. This intensive therapy, which usually takes place in the hospital, typically lasts 1 week.

L-asparaginase (Elspar) may be used; hepatitis or pancreatitis may result; watch carefully.

Pegaspargase (Oncaspar) can cause nausea, vomiting, anorexia, and glucose changes.

Interferon may be used.

Prednisone may be used, with side effects related to steroids with chronic use. Alter diet and intake accordingly to manage hyperglycemia, hypokalemia, and nitrogen losses.

TABLE 13-22 Medications for Chronic Leukemias

Chemotherapeutic agents may be used with varying side effects. Chlorambucil (Leukeran) and busulfan are common; nausea, severe fatigue, flu-like symptoms, low-grade temperature, vomiting, glossitis, and cheilosis may occur. Avoid hot, spicy, or acidic foods, if not tolerated.

Pegaspargase (Oncaspar) can cause nausea, vomiting, anorexia, and glucose changes.

Imatinib (Gleevec), for CML, interferes with an abnormal enzyme that sends signals to the nucleus of a cancer cell. Nausea and vomiting are potential side effects. Dasatinib (Sprycel) and nilotinib (Tasigna) block the BCR-ABL cancer gene, but each works in a different way than Gleevec. Sprycel and Tasigna are approved for certain CML patients who are resistant or intolerant to prior therapy including Gleevec. All three drugs are given orally.

For CLL: Multiple treatments include purine analogs, monoclonal antibodies, and stem-cell transplantation.

Antifungals, antivirals, or antibiotic drugs may be used; side effects vary.

Herbs, Botanicals, and Supplements (see Table 13-8)

- Herbs and botanical supplements should not be used without discussing it with the physician.
- For CML, bioflavonoids, vitamin A, Retin-A, vitamin D_3, vitamin E, vitamin B_{12}, indirubin (found in herbs including *Indigofera tinctoria* and *Isatis tinctoria*), and *Curcuma longa* have shown promise (Matsui, 2005).
- Omega-3 fatty acid supplements may increase the blood-thinning effects of aspirin or warfarin.
- St. John's wort reduces the effectiveness of imatinib, which is used to treat CML and Philadelphia-positive ALL.

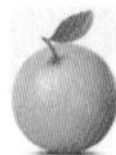

NUTRITION EDUCATION, COUNSELING, CARE MANAGEMENT

- A well-balanced diet is essential; discuss ways to improve or increase intake.
- Tumor lysis syndrome is a side effect caused by the rapid breakdown of leukemia cells. When these cells die, they release substances into the bloodstream that can affect the kidneys, heart, and nervous system. Giving patient extra fluids or certain drugs that help rid the body of these toxins can prevent this problem.
- Offer guidelines to transition from CPN or PN to enteral nutrition and oral intake.
- Discuss guidance for graft-versus-host disease (acute vs. chronic symptoms).
- Discuss alternative ways to make meals more attractive and appealing.
- Instruct patient on nutrition repletion if appropriate. For extra calories, blend cooked foods or soups with high-calorie liquids such as gravy, milk, cream or broth instead of water.

Patient Education—Food Safety

- People who are being treated for leukemia have weakened immune systems and increased risk for food-borne illness.
- Keep hands, counters, dishes, cutting boards, and utensils clean. Change sponges and dishtowels often.
- Keep foods at proper temperatures, reheating foods properly.
- Wash fruits and vegetables thoroughly.
- Use separate dishes, cutting boards, and utensils for preparing raw meat, fish, or poultry.
- Thaw frozen items in the microwave or refrigerator, not on the kitchen counter.
- Use a food thermometer to make sure that meat is fully cooked.
- Read the expiration dates on food products. Look for signs of food spoilage; if in doubt, throw it out.

For More Information

- Leukemia and Lymphoma Society
  http://www.leukemia-lymphoma.org
- People Living With Cancer
  http://www.plwc.org
- Partnership for Food Safety Education (PFSE)
  http://www.fightbac.org
- University of Virginia Health System
  http://www.healthsystem.virginia.edu/internet/hematology/hessidb/leukemias.cfm

LEUKEMIAS—CITED REFERENCES

Chen D, et al. Dietary flavonoids as proteasome inhibitors and apoptosis inducers in human leukemia cells. *Biochem Pharmacol.* 69:1421, 2005.

Fair AM, Montgomery K. Energy balance, physical activity, and cancer risk. *Methods Mol Biol.* 472:57, 2009.

Jansen H, et al. Acute lymphoblastic leukemia and obesity: increased energy intake or decreased physical activity? *Support Care Cancer.* 17:103, 2009.

Klein U, et al. The DLEU2/miR-15 a/16–1 cluster controls B cell proliferation and its deletion leads to chronic lymphocytic leukemia [Published online ahead of print Jan 6, 2010]. *Cancer Cell.*

Kwan ML, et al. Maternal diet and risk of childhood acute lymphoblastic leukemia. *Public Health Rep.* 124:503, 2009.

Liu CY, et al. Cured meat, vegetables, and bean-curd foods in relation to childhood acute leukemia risk: a population based case-control study. *BMC Cancer.* 9:15, 2009.

Ma X, et al. Diet, lifestyle, and acute myeloid leukemia in the NIH-AARP Cohort [Published online ahead of print Dec 30, 2009]. *Am J Epidemiol.*

Matsui J, et al. Dietary bioflavonoids induce apoptosis in human leukemia cells. *Leuk Res.* 29:573, 2005.

Petridou E, et al. Maternal diet and acute lymphoblastic leukemia in young children. *Cancer Epidemiol Biomarkers Prev.* 14:1935, 2005.

Sharif T, et al. Red wine polyphenols cause growth inhibition and apoptosis in acute lymphoblastic leukaemia cells by inducing a redox-sensitive up-regulation of p73 and down-regulation of UHRF1 [Published online ahead of print Jan 12, 2010]. *Eur J Cancer.*

Smith MT, et al. Molecular biomarkers for the study of childhood leukemia. *Toxicol Appl Pharmacol.* 206:237, 2005.

Tower RL, Spector LG. The epidemiology of childhood leukemia with a focus on birth weight and diet. *Crit Rev Clin Lab Sci.* 44:203, 2007.

Trump DL, et al. Anti-tumor activity of calcitriol: pre-clinical and clinical studies. *J Steroid Biochem Mol Biol.* 90:519, 2005.

LYMPHOMAS

NUTRITIONAL ACUITY RANKING: LEVEL 3

DEFINITIONS AND BACKGROUND

Chronic antigenic stimulation leads to lymphoid malignancy (Anderson et al, 2009). There are two types: **Hodgkin's lymphoma (HL)** and non-Hodgkin's lymphoma (NHL), which is far more common. In HL, patients present with enlarged lymph nodes that are firm and rubbery, severe pruritus, jaundice, night sweats, fatigue and malaise, weight loss, slight fever, alcohol-induced pain, cough, dyspnea, and chest pain. It presents most commonly in males between the ages of 15 and 34 or after age 60 in persons who have lupus, Epstein-Barr virus (mononucleosis) or HIV infection. Abnormal B cells, called Reed-Sternberg cells, develop and enlarge. The treatment of HL involves radiation and chemotherapy. Stage 1 is limited to one body part; stage 2 involves two or more areas on the same side of the diaphragm; stage 3 involves lymph nodes above and below the diaphragm; and stage 4 involves lymph nodes and other areas such as the lungs, marrow, and liver. Patients who present with weight loss initially have a worse prognosis than those without weight loss. The 5-year survival rate for Hodgkin's disease is 84%; it is one of the more curable forms of cancer. Unfortunately, survivors may have a stroke later in life, and young women who receive high-dose radiation for Hodgkin's disease are more at risk for breast cancer. **Non-Hodgkin's lymphoma (NHL)** is a malignant tumor of lymphoid tissue, resulting from an invasion of the lymph nodes and other tissues by lymphocytes. NHL is relatively common among individuals whose immune system is suppressed. Rheumatoid arthritis, Sjögren syndrome, T-cell lymphoma with hemolytic anemia, psoriasis, discoid lupus erythematosus, and celiac disease are associated with an increased risk of NHL (Anderson et al, 2009). *H. pylori* is associated with the development of lymphoma in the stomach wall. Burkitt's lymphoma is most common in children, young adult males, and patients with AIDS; it originates from a B lymphocyte and requires chemotherapy. This lymphoma is associated with a prior infection with the Epstein-Barr virus.

Exposure to certain chemicals (such as nitrates) in herbicides and pesticides promotes risk. Enteropathy-associated T-cell lymphoma (EATL) is a rare form of high-grade, T-cell NHL of the upper small intestine that is specifically associated with celiac disease (Catassi et al, 2005). Capsule endoscopy is used to evaluate this celiac disease–associated enteropathy (Joyce et al, 2005). Strict adherence to the gluten-free diet protects against NHL, particularly if started early (Hervonen et al, 2005).

Symptoms and signs of NHL include difficulty breathing, swelling of face, thickened or dark, itchy skin areas, increased incidence of bacterial infections, night sweats, weight loss, fever, anemia, and pleural effusion. It is possible, as well, to develop chylous ascites or chyloperitoneum. By the time of NHL diagnosis, it is often widely spread. It may spread to the cervix, uterus, and vagina in women. Radiation is a common treatment for the early stages. A cure is less likely for those over age 60.

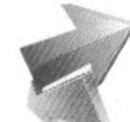

ASSESSMENT, MONITORING, AND EVALUATION

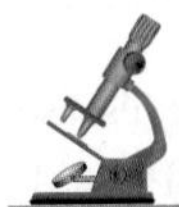

CLINICAL INDICATORS

Genetic Markers: HL and NHL have several gene mutations. The presence of the Reed-Sternberg cell in HL is an expression of the CD30 antigen. In NHL, t(14;18)(q32;q21) chromosomal translocations occur in the BCL2 gene.

Specific Clinical/History

- Height
- Weight
- BMI
- Weight loss?
- Diet history
- Enlarged, rubbery lymph nodes
- Painless adenopathy
- Pruritus, severe
- Jaundice
- Night sweats
- Fatigue and malaise
- Slight fever, temperature
- Alcohol-induced pain
- Cough, dyspnea, and chest pain
- Diarrhea
- I & O
- Lymphangiogram
- X-ray or CT scan
- Bone marrow biopsy

Lab Work

- Ceruloplasmin (increased)
- Reed-Sternberg cells (more than one nucleus)
- ESR
- Uric acid (increased)
- PT (increased)
- Gluc
- CRP
- Serum Cu (increased)
- H & H
- Bilirubin (increased)
- Alk phos (often increased)
- Ferritin (increased)
- ALT (increased)
- Serum lipids—Chol, Trig
- Ca^{++}, Mg^{++}
- Na^{+}, K^{+}

SAMPLE NUTRITION CARE PROCESS STEPS

Obesity

Assessment Data: BMI 42, new diagnosis of NHL. Diet hx indicates low intake of whole grains and vegetables and high intake of sugary, refined foods and beverages.

Nutrition Diagnosis (PES): Obesity related to poor food choices as evidenced by BMI 42 and preference for sugary, refined foods.

Intervention: Food-Nutrient Delivery—Promote the use of low energy foods and beverages. Educate the patient about the risks of obesity in cancer promotion. Counsel about ways to safely lose weight, with the focus on a healthy body weight and nutrient density.

Monitoring and Evaluation: Reasonable amount of weight lost, slowly and without loss of lean body mass but with tolerance for chemotherapy treatments. Improved BMI.

INTERVENTION

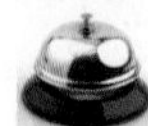

OBJECTIVES

- Prevent or correct weight loss, fever, malaise, and infections such as candidiasis.
- Correct dysphagia, nausea and vomiting, and anorexia.
- Control protein-losing enteropathy, chylous ascites, and other side effects.
- Control enteropathy in patients who also have celiac disease.
- Modify diet according to the side effects of therapy (e.g., radiation or chemotherapy).
- If obese, a gradual weight loss plan may be indicated.

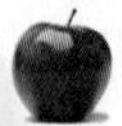

FOOD AND NUTRITION

- Increase protein and fluids. Balance energy intake to meet the needs of treatments without causing weight gain.
- Six small feedings are generally better tolerated than three large meals. Alter diet according to symptoms.
- Bland, low acidic foods may be better accepted for a while.
- With celiac disease, the gluten-free diet is required.
- With hyperglycemia, control carbohydrates and overall energy intake.
- Support the use of a protective diet with folate and B vitamins, vegetables, and legumes. Include vitamin D_3, particularly from sunlight (Grant, 2009; Kelly et al, 2009).

Common Drugs Used and Potential Side Effects

HL

- Chemotherapy is often given in combination. The regimen MOPP, which includes mechlorethamine (nitrogen mustard), vincristine (Oncovin), procarbazine, and prednisone may cause nausea, vomiting, diarrhea, weakness, constipation, and mouth sores. The regimen ChlVPP, which includes chlorambucil, vinblastine, procarbazine, and prednisone, may cause similar side effects. After chemotherapy, young women may have amenorrhea.
- Corticosteroids can aggravate the electrolyte status and will decrease the calcium, potassium, and nitrogen balance over time. Hyperglycemia may also occur; monitor blood glucose levels.

NHL

- Chemotherapy is often given as a regimen called CHOP, which includes cyclophosphamide, doxorubicin, vincristine (Oncovin), and prednisone. CHOP may cause nausea, vomiting, anorexia, diarrhea, and other gastrointestinal (GI) side effects. Single agents may also be used. Methotrexate causes GI pain, mouth ulcers, nausea, and folic acid depletion.

Herbs, Botanicals, and Supplements (see Table 13-8)

- Herbs and botanical supplements should not be used without discussing it with the physician.
- Lymphoma survivors tend to use CAM therapies more than the general population (Habermann et al, 2009). Chiropractic, massage, and use of St. John's wort and shark cartilage have been noted.
- Acupuncture, coenzyme Q10, and polysaccharide K are under study.

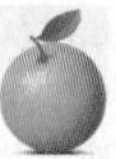

NUTRITION EDUCATION, COUNSELING, CARE MANAGEMENT

- Discuss methods of improving appetite by the use of attractive meals.
- Encourage rest periods before and after meals to reduce fatigue.
- Encourage a diet that is protective with plenty of vegetables and legumes.
- Vitamin D_3 may protect against both types of lymphomas (Grant, 2009; Kelly et al, 2009).

Patient Education—Food Safety

- Educate the patient about food safety issues. Discuss safe food handling and preparation, keeping foods at proper temperatures, the use of sterile water, and reheating foods properly.

For More Information

- Cancer Information Network
  http://www.ontumor.com/
- Leukemia and Lymphoma Society
  http://www.leukemia-lymphoma.org/all_page?item_id=7030
- Lymphoma Information Network
  http://www.lymphomainfo.net/lymphoma.html
- National Cancer Institute–Hodgkin's Lymphoma
  http://www.cancer.gov/cancerinfo/types/hodgkinslymphoma
- National Library of Medicine
  http://www.nlm.nih.gov/medlineplus/hodgkinsdisease.html
- Non-Hodgkin's Lymphoma
  http://www.nlm.nih.gov/medlineplus/ency/article/000581.htm
- Wellness After Treatment
  http://www.cancer.gov/cancertopics/life-after-treatment/page4

LYMPHOMAS—CITED REFERENCES

Anderson LA, et al. Population-based study of autoimmune conditions and the risk of specific lymphoid malignancies. *Int J Cancer.* 125:398, 2009.

Catassi C, et al. Association of celiac disease and intestinal lymphomas and other cancers. *Gastroenterology.* 128:S79, 2005.

Grant WB. How strong is the evidence that solar ultraviolet B and vitamin D reduce the risk of cancer? An examination using Hill's criteria for causality. *Dermatoendocrinol.* 1:17, 2009.

Habermann TM, et al. Complementary and alternative medicine use among long-term lymphoma survivors: a pilot study. *Am J Hematol.* 84:795, 2009.

Hervonen K, et al. Lymphoma in patients with dermatitis herpetiformis and their first-degree relatives. *Br J Dermatol.* 152:82, 2005.

Joyce AM, et al. Capsule endoscopy findings in celiac disease associated enteropathy-type intestinal T-cell lymphoma. *Endoscopy.* 37:594, 2005.

Kelly JL. et al. Vitamin D and non-Hodgkin lymphoma risk in adults: a review. *Cancer Invest.* 27:942, 2009.

Yee KW, O'Brien SM. Chronic lymphocytic leukemia: diagnosis and treatment. *Mayo Clin Proc.* 81:1105, 2006.

MYELOMA

NUTRITIONAL ACUITY RANKING: LEVEL 3

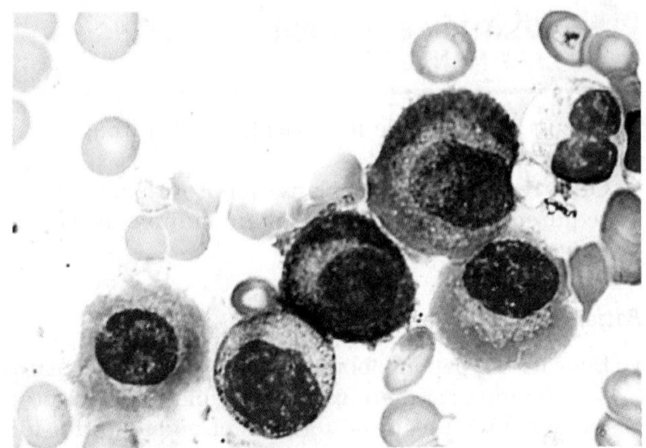

Adapted from: Raphael Rubin, David S. Strayer, *Rubin's Pathology: Clinicopathologic Foundations of Medicine,* 5th ed. Philadelphia: Lippincott Williams & Wilkins, 2008.

DEFINITIONS AND BACKGROUND

Myeloma is the second most common blood cancer. Multiple myeloma (MM) is a malignant cancer in which plasma cells proliferate, invade bone marrow, and produce abnormal immunoglobulin. Different types of myeloma are classified by the type of immunoglobulin produced by the abnormal cells. The condition is rare, affecting only 4/100,000 persons and representing only 1% of all cancers. Males are affected more often than females, and the disorder usually strikes after age 50. African-Americans are twice as likely to acquire MM as Caucasians, Hispanics, or Asians.

Obesity promotes this type of cancer. MM affects several areas of bone marrow. If significant bone lesions, renal failure, or hypercalcemia occur, chemotherapy or transplantation is recommended. Stem-cell transplantation or radiation therapy may be administered (Iversen, 2009).

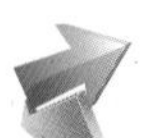

ASSESSMENT, MONITORING, AND EVALUATION

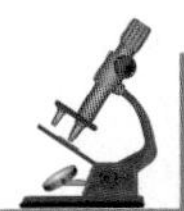

CLINICAL INDICATORS

Genetic Markers: The premalignant condition of monoclonal gammopathy of undetermined significance (MGUS) precedes all cases of MM (Jagannath, 2010).

Specific Clinical/History

- Height
- Weight
- BMI
- Weight loss?
- Shortened stature?
- I & O
- BP
- Bone pain
- Pathological fractures
- Nausea and vomiting
- Anorexia
- History of bleeding
- Fatigue, weakness, apathy
- Sudden confusion
- Renal disorders
- Bleeding tendency (particularly gums)
- Frequent urinary tract infections
- Pneumonia?
- Skeletal survey

Lab Work

- Ca^{++} (increased)
- Mg^{++}
- Na^+, K^+
- Total protein
- Parathormone (PTH) (increased)
- TLC (varies)
- Hypercalciuria
- Alb (often increased)
- CRP
- Transferrin
- H & H
- Proteinuria (Bence Jones proteins)
- Sedimentation rate (increased)
- Uric acid (increased)
- RBP
- ALT (increased)

INTERVENTION

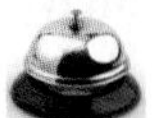

OBJECTIVES

- Avoid fasting. Space meals and snacks adequately.
- Counteract episodes of fatigue and weakness.
- Manage pain effectively.
- Counteract side effects of antineoplastic therapy, steroid therapy, and radiotherapy.
- Avoid infections and febrile states.
- Prevent spontaneous fractures, as far as possible.
- Correct anorexia, nausea and vomiting, and weight loss.

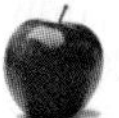

FOOD AND NUTRITION

- Provide diet as usual, with six small feedings rather than large meals.
- A higher protein intake may be useful to counteract losses.
- Provide adequate energy to meet requirements of weight control, preventing unnecessary losses.

SAMPLE NUTRITION CARE PROCESS STEPS

Inadequate Oral Food and Beverage Intake

Assessment Data: Mucositis following chemotherapy for the treatment of multiple myeloma. Unable to chew and swallow comfortably because of inflamed oral tissues.

Nutrition Diagnosis (PES): Inadequate oral food and beverage intake (NI-2.1) related to sore mouth as evidenced by mucositis after chemotherapy and difficulty finding tolerated foods and beverages.

Intervention: Food-nutrient delivery—offer soft, ground, or pureed foods that are low in acid and spices. Educate the patient about the use of a soft, easily tolerated diet that has nutrient-density. Counsel with tips for gradually increasing the oral diet as mucositis subsides.

Monitoring and Evaluation: Resolution of mucositis with an improvement in oral intake.

- Avoid dehydration by including adequate fluid intake (e.g., 3 L daily). This is important.
- Ensure sufficient intake of omega-3 fatty acids, vitamins, minerals, and phytochemicals, particularly from fruits and vegetables.

Common Drugs Used and Potential Side Effects

- Arsenic trioxide (Trisenox), carmustine (BiCU, BCNU), cyclophosphamide (Cytoxan), doxorubicin (Adriamycin, Rubex), idarubicin (Idamycin), interferon-alpha (Roferon-A, Intron-A), lenalidomide (Revlimid), pamidronate (Aredia), vincristine (Oncovin), or zoledronic acid (Zometa) may be given as chemotherapy, often with several in a mixture. Melphalan (Alkeran) or nitrosoureas may also be used; monitor for anorexia, anemia, nausea, vomiting, and stomatitis.
- Bisphosphonates may be used to prevent bone fractures.
- Pamidronate may be used. Ensure adequate fluid intake but not excess. Avoid use with calcium and vitamin D supplements. Extra phosphorus may be needed. Nausea, vomiting, gastrointestinal bleeding or distress, and constipation can occur.
- Prednisone, if used chronically, can increase nitrogen losses and potassium and magnesium depletion and can cause hyperglycemia and sodium retention.
- Lenalidomide delays disease progression in late-stage multiple myeloma. It also helps to reduce the need for blood transfusions.
- The immunomodulatory agents thalidomide and lenalidomide and the proteasome inhibitor bortezomib are now routine components of MM therapy (Jagannath, 2010). However, all patients with MM eventually relapse; efforts to identify novel synergistic combinations and agents are ongoing (Jagannath, 2010).
- Bortezomib (Velcade), a proteasome inhibitor, delays disease progression and extends survival.

Herbs, Botanicals, and Supplements (see Table 13-8)

- Herbs and botanical supplements should not be used without discussing it with the physician.

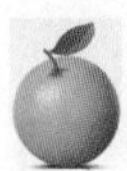

NUTRITION EDUCATION, COUNSELING, CARE MANAGEMENT

- Discuss the rationale for spacing meals throughout the day to avoid fatigue.
- Offer recipes and meal plans that provide the nutrients required to improve status and immunological competence.

Patient Education—Food Safety

- Educate the patient about food safety issues. Discuss safe food handling and preparation, keeping foods at proper temperatures, the use of sterile water, and reheating foods properly.

For More Information

- Cleveland Clinic–Multiple Myeloma Programs
  http://www.clevelandclinic.org/myeloma/
- International Myeloma Foundation
  http://www.myeloma.org/
- Mayo Clinic Myeloma
  http://www.mayoclinic.com/health/multiple-myeloma/DS00415
- Multiple Myeloma Foundation
  http://www.multiplemyeloma.org/
- National Library of Medicine
  http://www.nlm.nih.gov/medlineplus/multiplemyeloma.html

MYELOMA—CITED REFERENCES

Iversen PO, et al. Reduced nutritional status among multiple myeloma patients during treatment with high-dose chemotherapy and autologous stem cell support [Published online ahead of print Dec 29, 2009]. *Clin Nutr.*

Jagannath S, et al. The current status and future of multiple myeloma in the clinic. *Clin Lymphoma Myeloma.* 10:1E, 2010.

Pan SL, et al. Association of obesity and cancer risk in Canada. *Am J Epidemiol.* 159:259, 2004.

SECTION 14

Surgical Disorders

CHIEF ASSESSMENT FACTORS

Presurgical Status

- Anemia, Blood Loss
- Appetite Changes
- Blood Pressure, Abnormal
- Electrolyte Status
- History of Illness—Acute or Chronic (Such as Diabetes, Cerebrovascular Disease, Coronary Heart Disease)
- Hydration Status
- Infections
- Nausea, Vomiting
- Obesity and Anesthesia Risk
- Recent Starvation or Prolonged Malnutrition
- Recent Weight Changes, Especially Unintentional Loss
- Respiratory Function, Oxygen Saturation
- Serum Albumin, Transferrin, Retinol-Binding Protein, and C-Reactive Protein (CRP) (Inflammation)
- Surgical Procedure with Gastrointestinal (GI) Impact

Postsurgical Status

- Abnormal GI Function (diarrhea, constipation, obstruction)
- Altered Labs Such as Glucose, CRP, Electrolytes
- Breathing Rate
- Fever
- Impaired Skin Integrity, Wound Dehiscence
- Infection or Sepsis
- Nausea, Vomiting
- Pain, Sleep Disturbance
- Paralytic Ileus, Abdominal Distention
- Pneumonia or Lung Collapse
- Respiratory Function, Oxygen Saturation
- Urinary Tract Infection

GENERAL SURGICAL GUIDELINES

SURGERY

NUTRITIONAL ACUITY RANKING: LEVEL 2

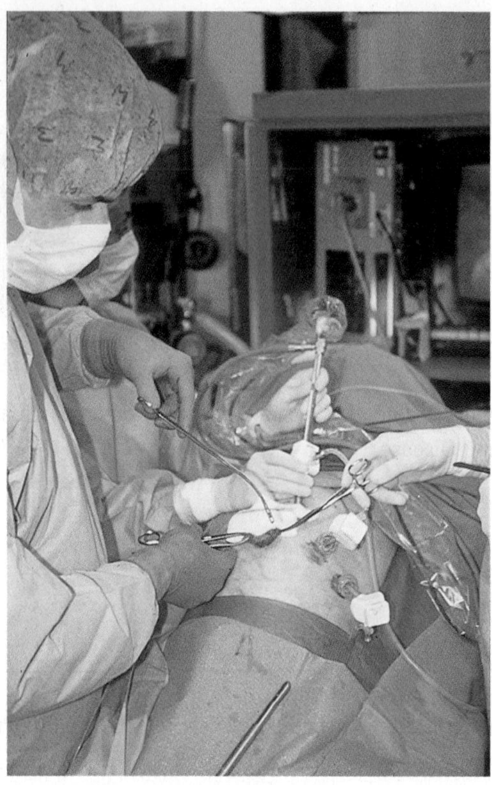

Adapted from: Smeltzer SC, Bare BG. *Textbook of Medical-Surgical Nursing*, 9th ed. Philadelphia: Lippincott Williams & Wilkins, 2000.

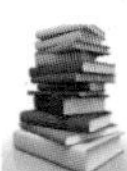

DEFINITIONS AND BACKGROUND

Nutritional risk from surgery is related to the extent of surgery, prior nutritional state of the patient, and the effect of surgery on the patient's ability to digest and absorb nutrients. Weight loss is one of the most important assessment tools to predict surgical risk as related to nutritional status. Techniques to assess body composition help to quantify weight loss and clarify the impact of malnutrition on postsurgical status.

Surgery is the term used for treatments that involve cutting or stitching tissue, laser surgery, and robotic surgical procedures. Major surgery involves opening a major body cavity, such as the abdomen (laparotomy) or the skull in a craniotomy. "General anesthesia," a surgical team, and a hospital stay are required. Minor surgery may be done in an outpatient or emergency room setting, often with minimal anesthetic treatment. Surgeries with high risk include hip replacement, open heart surgery, and prostatectomy. Patients who are at high surgical risk include those with heart or renal failure, those who have had a recent heart attack, those who are severely malnourished, and those with chronic lung or liver diseases.

After surgery or injury with extensive tissue damage, plasma cortisol generally increases rapidly and fat breaks down rapidly to fatty acids and glycerol. The metabolic response to surgical or accidental injury leads to breakdown of skeletal muscle protein and the transfer of amino acids to visceral organs and the wound. At the wound site, substrate serves to enhance host defenses and support vital organ function and wound repair. Increased excretion of nitrogen and sodium retention occur, but these are reversed in approximately 5–7 days or as late as 12–14 days in elderly individuals and after severe burns. Increased excretion of potassium occurs but begins to reverse itself 1–2 days after surgery.

Malnutrition is prevalent among surgical patients and is associated with higher surgical complication rates and mortality (Figure 14-1). Some causes of poor nutritional status are related to the underlying disease, socioeconomic factors, age, and length of hospitalization. If medical teams overlook malnutrition, patients are at risk for malnutrition and complications. Use of tools such as the Subjective Global Assessment identifies malnutrition in many patients.

Elective surgery involves minimal increases in nitrogen loss and a 10–15% increase in energy requirements. Major surgery involves greater intensity and duration that will increase catabolic effects. Prevention of hypoxia in surgical wounds is especially important and preventable; fluid and temperature management are key factors. Table 14-1 defines the average length of time and stages of catabolic response after surgery, followed by anabolism.

The presence of cancer, infection, age more than 60 years, upper gastrointestinal (GI) disease, and longer length of hospital stay all negatively influence nutritional status. Nutritional status plays an important role in determining outcome after many types of operations. Enteral immunonutrition is an important consideration preoperatively as well, if time permits. Early postoperative enteral nutrition with a formula supplemented with arginine, omega-3 fatty acids, and RNA increases hydroxyproline synthesis and improves surgical wound healing in patients undergoing gastric surgery (Farreras et al, 2005).

Fever causes increased nutritional needs; for every 1°F increase, there is an increased energy requirement of 7–8% and the need for extra fluid. Optimal wound healing requires integration of responses to inflammatory mediators, growth factors, cytokines, and mechanical forces (Falanga, 2005). Extra protein is needed for wounds, burns, and hemorrhage; major wounds and burns can cause a loss of greater than 50 g of protein per day. With hemorrhage

TABLE 14-1 Postsurgical Phases in Nutrition

3–7 days	Marked catabolic response
2–5 weeks	Turning point and anabolic phase at which spontaneous improvement begins
>6 weeks	Fat gain phase; vigorous nutritional support could promote excessive fat stores

or major blood loss, or even when much blood is drawn for laboratory tests, loss of iron and plasma protein may be significant; loss of 1 L of blood equals a loss of 500 mg of iron and 50 g of plasma protein.

C-reactive protein (CRP) is a risk factor for cardiovascular outcomes and mortality in the general population; it predicts all-cause mortality (Winklmayer et al, 2005). Preoperative serum albumin concentration may predict surgical outcomes such as sepsis, renal failure, and major infections. Early identification of high-risk patients undergoing major surgery allows aggressive management. After surgery, the presence of systemic inflammatory response syndrome is a predictor of later sepsis (Mokart et al, 2005). Other patient risk factors predictive of postoperative morbidity include anesthesia and complexity of the operation.

A complete, balanced diet is recommended after surgery. A clear liquid diet has about 600 kcal/d and D5W solutions have only 170 kcal/L. Early postoperative oral feeding has been demonstrated to be safe (Lucha et al, 2005). Enhanced rate of recovery can be achieved by enhancing the metabolic status of the patient before (e.g., carbohydrate and fluid loading), during (e.g., epidural anesthesia), and after (e.g., early oral feeding) surgery (Fearon and Luff, 2003).

Healing of wounds involves blood cells, tissues, cytokines, growth factors, and metabolic demand for nutrients. Vitamin A is required for epithelial and bone formation, cellular differentiation, and immune function. Vitamin C is necessary for collagen formation, for proper immune function, and as a tissue antioxidant. Adequate protein is absolutely essential for proper wound healing.

Tissue levels of the amino acids arginine and glutamine (GLN) influence wound repair and immune function. GLN depletion in skeletal muscle is an outstanding metabolic marker related to acute skeletal muscle wasting (Roth and Oehler, 2010.) Energy-saving signals may be switched on to protect organs in a mode similar to hibernation; this may explain the low energy expenditure in septic patients (Roth and Oehler, 2010.) Its use in various enteral or parenteral products is accepted in many facilities.

Patients who receive enteral immunonutrition with multiple nutrients before and after major GI surgery often have lower treatment costs. Arginine is helpful in wound healing after trauma (Wilmore, 2004; Wittman et al, 2005). Major surgery, skeletal trauma, prolonged immobilization, and soft tissue damage are followed by increased calcium loss. Vitamin C may be destroyed by extensive inflammation in postoperative conditions. Table 14-2 indicates the extent of body reserves of nutrients. Higher nutrient reserves are advantageous in most surgeries.

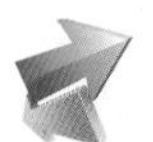

ASSESSMENT, MONITORING, AND EVALUATION

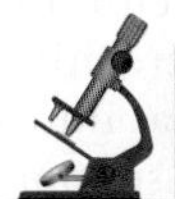

CLINICAL INDICATORS

Genetic Markers: Surgery may be needed to repair a genetic condition, such as a congenital heart disorder.

Clinical/History

Height
Weight
Body mass index (BMI)
Weight changes
Diet history
Blood pressure (BP)
Intake and output (I & O)
Nausea, vomiting
Constipation
Anorexia
Urinary tract infection
Skin integrity; pressure ulcers
History of dehydration or slow wound healing
Transfusions

Lab Work

Glucose (Gluc)
C-reactive protein (CRP)
Platelet count
Albumin (Alb), transthyretin
Blood urea nitrogen (BUN)
Creatinine (Creat)
Na^+
K^+
Ca^{++}
Mg^{++}
Phosphorus (P)
Urinary electrolytes
Serum osmolality (Osm)
N balance
Transferrin
Prothrombin time (PT) or international normalized ratio (INR)
Hemoglobin and hematocrit (H & H)
Serum Fe
Vitamin B_{12}

INTERVENTION

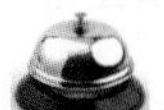

OBJECTIVES

Preoperative

- Maintain or enhance reserves. Many patients admitted to hospitals are malnourished; therefore, proper presurgical assessment and nourishment should be emphasized.

TABLE 14-2 Time Required to Deplete Body Nutrient Reserves in Well-Nourished Individuals

Nutrient	Time
Amino acids	Several hours
Carbohydrate	13 hours
Sodium	2–3 days
Water	4 days
Zinc	5 days
Fat	20–40 days
Thiamin	30–60 days
Vitamin C	60–120 days
Niacin	60–180 days
Riboflavin	60–180 days
Vitamin A	90–365 days
Iron	125 days (women); 750 days (men)
Iodine	1000 days
Calcium	2500 days

From: Guthrie H. *Introductory nutrition.* 7th ed. St Louis: Times Mirror/Mosby College Publishers, 1989.

SAMPLE NUTRITION CARE PROCESS STEPS

Involuntary Weight Loss

Assessment Data (sources of info): Food records, input and output reports, medication history, assessment of depression.

Nutrition Diagnosis (PES): NC-3.2 Involuntary weight loss related to depression and poor intake after above-knee (AK) amputation as evidenced by weight loss of >6% in past 2 weeks and statement that "I just don't feel like eating any more."

Intervention: Food-Nutrient Delivery—Offer nutrient and energy-dense foods until appetite improves. Counsel about desired food and beverage intake for wound healing. Coordinate care—Discuss status of depression and medications or counseling with health care team.

Monitoring and Evaluation: Improved food intake as per I & O records. Better weight status and rate of wound healing. Improvement in symptoms of depression with medication.

TABLE 14-3 Measuring Energy Expenditure in Critical Illness

Measuring energy expenditure via indirect calorimetry (IC) is the most accurate method of determining needs. For short-term use, predictive equations such as the Ireton-Jones calculation for nutrition support are recommended.

Ireton-Jones Equations for Estimated Energy Expenditure (EEE) (Ireton-Jones and Jones, 1998)

1. Spontaneously Breathing Patient: EEE = 629 − 11(A) + 25(W) − 609(O)
2. Ventilator-Dependent Patient: EEE = 1784 − 11(A) + 5(W) + 244(G) + 239(T) + 804(B)

Key: A = age in years; W = weight in kg; O = obesity (>130% ideal body weight); G = gender (female = 0, male = 1); T = diagnosis of trauma (absent = 0, present = 1); B = diagnosis of burn (absent = 0, present = 1).

Some facilities use glucose and potassium intravenous loading in nondiabetic, nonrespiratory patients for surgical preparation.

- Identify risks for cardiac events after surgery, which are common and costly (Maddox, 2005).
- Prepare patients who are morbidly obese. Fatty tissues are not resistant to infections, hard to suture, and prone to dehiscence. A large amount of anesthesia is needed in the morbidly obese patients, and it is difficult to awaken them. Controlled weight loss should be instituted before surgery whenever possible.
- Elevated serum glucose on admission is an accurate predictor of postoperative infection, length of stay, and mortality (Bochicchio et al, 2005). Reducing hyperglycemia is important.

Postoperative

- Replete nutrient stores, such as protein and iron from hemorrhage or other blood losses. Replace important vitamins and minerals (vitamin C, 100–200% recommended amounts; vitamin K, zinc, and vitamin A).
- Correct imbalances in fluid, sodium, potassium, and other electrolytes.
- Promote wound healing. The surgical wound has priority only for the first 5–10 days. Wound tensile strength peaks at 40–50 days.
- Use enhanced immunonutrition where needed to provide sufficient amounts of protein and energy to preserve muscle function; stimulate and protect enterocytes while limiting bacterial translocation; keep liver function as normal as possible; and prevent or compensate for disturbances in the immune response. Arginine triggers anabolic hormones (e.g., insulin, growth hormone) and speeds wound healing (Zaloga et al, 2004). Arginine is important for growth, wound healing, cardiovascular function, immune function, inflammatory responses, energy metabolism, urea cycle function, and other metabolic processes (Zaloga et al, 2004). While somewhat controversial, it may be helpful to select an immune-enhanced tube feeding (TF) product for GI surgeries.
- Attend to special needs such as fever, trauma, pregnancy, and growth in infants and children.
- Prevent infection and sepsis, which can occur in more than 10% of surgical cases.
- Prevent aspiration, a leading cause of pneumonia and the most serious complication of enteral TF. Traditional clinical monitors of glucose oxidase strips and blue food coloring (BFC) should never be used; evaluation of gastric residual volumes is recommended.
- Minimize weight loss, which is not obligatory.
- Prevent or correct sarcopenia and protein—energy malnutrition (PEM). Table 14-3 describes the use of estimated energy requirement calculations when indirect calorimetry is not available. With complete bed rest, young adults lose about 1% of their muscle per day; seniors lose up to 5% per day because of lower levels of growth hormone, which maintains muscle tissue. Sitting up in bed, moving, standing, and exercising as soon as possible and safe is good for surgical patients.
- Manage pain, blood clots, and other complications. Constipation or difficulty urinating may also occur, especially with opioids and anticholinergic drugs, inactivity, and not eating.

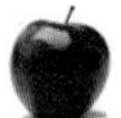

FOOD AND NUTRITION

Preoperative

- Because malnutrition is a recognized risk factor for perioperative morbidity, the Nutrition Risk Screening 2002 score should be used to identify patients at nutritional risk who may benefit from nutritional support therapy; it has been officially adopted by the European Society of Parenteral and Enteral Nutrition (Schiesser et al, 2008.)

- Use a high-protein/high-energy diet, a TF, or parenteral nutrition, if needed. Enteral nutrition is effective, poses lower risks than parenteral nutrition, reduces infection rates, and shortens hospital length of stay of critically ill patients (Grimble, 2005).
- If patient is obese, use a low-energy diet that includes carbohydrates adequate for glycogen stores and protein to protect lean body mass. Elevated serum glucose on admission is an accurate predictor of postoperative infection, length of stay, and mortality (Bochicchio et al, 2005).
- Ensure that intakes of zinc and vitamins C and K are adequate.
- Bowel cleansing regimens commonly require adherence to liquid diets for 24–48 hours before examination, which often leads to poor compliance. Offering patients a regular breakfast and a low-residue lunch before bowel cleansing with sodium phosphate oral solution may be better tolerated.
- Gradually restrict diet to clear liquids and then nothing by mouth (NPO).

Postoperative

- Immediately after surgery, use intravenous glucose, insulin, or electrolytes as needed (Bossingham et al, 2005). As treatment progresses, advance diet as tolerated to a combination of liquid and solid items.
- A complete, balanced mix of nutrients is best. Excessive vitamin and mineral supplements do not increase rate of healing. In fact, because zinc and iron are bacterial nutrients, excesses may be detrimental.
- If oral feeding is not possible, use enteral nutrition. Initiate TF within 12–18 hours for less sepsis and fewer complications. The gut can generally tolerate early feedings, even in patients with pancreatitis (Gabor et al, 2005; Lucha et al, 2005; Marek and Zaloga, 2004). Early postoperative feeding is generally safe, effective, and cost-effective (Braga and Gianotti, 2005).
- When necessary, because of prolonged GI compromise or short bowel syndrome, use central parenteral nutrition (CPN). Use caution with intravenous lipids due to proinflammatory omega-6 fatty acids. Omega-3 fatty acids are acceptable and not inflammatory. The adaptive role of the small intestine after surgery is described in Table 14-4.
- For elective GI surgery, specialized immunonutrition does not have to be routine (Klek et al, 2008.) Enteral nutrition is preferred over parenteral nutrition when the GI tract is functional (Zaloga, 2006). GLN-enhanced products are useful, especially in malnourished patients; they improve antioxidant levels (Grimble, 2005; Luo et al, 2008). If PN is needed, glutamine-supplemented parenteral nutrition (GLN-PN) significantly decreases infections in surgical intensive care patients after cardiac, vascular, and colonic surgery (Estivarez et al, 2008.)
- With oral diet, offer increased fluid and include sources of protein, zinc, and vitamins C and A for wound healing. Use 25–45 kcal/kg and 1–1.5 g protein/kg; this varies depending on extent of surgical intervention and degree of catabolism. Losses of 5–15 g of nitrogen daily may occur.
- An analysis of clinical studies using enteral formulas with supplemental arginine suggests overall benefits (Zaloga et al, 2004). Arginine is found in shrimp, lean ground beef, pumpkin seeds, garbanzo beans, cottage cheese, peanuts, and soymilk.
- Hyperglycemia is associated with poor wound healing, increased susceptibility to infection, and other complications. While perioperative hyperglycemia has been associated with increased surgical site infections, there is insufficient evidence to support strict versus conventional glycemic control (Kao et al, 2009.)
- Electrolyte imbalances are common after surgery; see Table 14-5.
- Fluid imbalances are also common. Monitor for changes in urine output or concentration. Check labs such as BUN, albumin, sodium, and glucose. Check for

TABLE 14-4 The Small Intestine After Surgery

- The small intestine has a large adaptive capacity, with resection of small segments generally not causing nutritional problems.
- If the terminal ileum is removed, vitamin B_{12} and bile salts will not be reabsorbed.
- Diarrhea can be massive if the ileocecal valve is removed with the terminal ileum, with great electrolyte losses and hypovolemia.
- Cholestyramine may be needed to bind bile salts.
- Fat malabsorption with steatorrhea and inadequate vitamin A, D, E, and K absorption may also occur. Medium-chain triglycerides (MCT) and water-miscible supplements may be necessary.
- Hyperoxaluria and renal stones may occur. Calcium supplements, altered polyunsaturated fatty acid (PUFA) intake, and aluminum hydroxide binders may be needed.

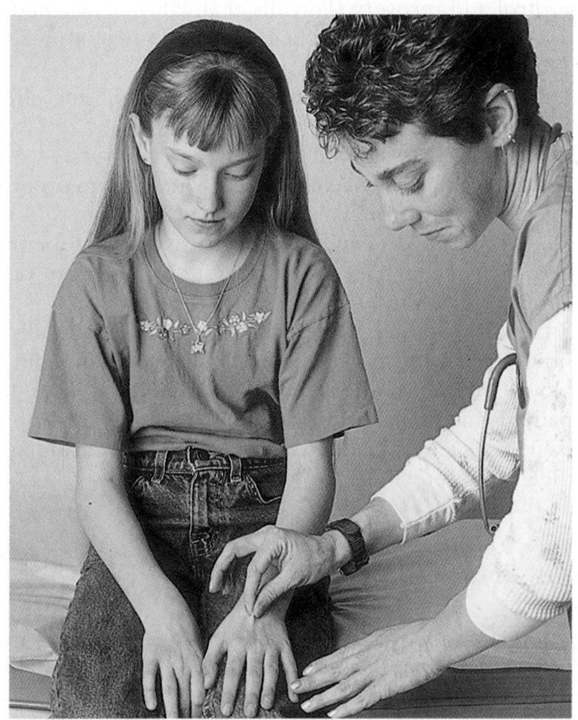

Adapted from: Nettina, Sandra M., MSN, RN, CS, ANP, *The Lippincott Manual of Nursing Practice*, 7th ed. Lippincott Williams & Wilkins, 2001.

fever. Calculate fluid needs; evaluate using I & O records. Be sure that medications are given with 4 oz of fluid and that sufficient fluid is served with and between meals.

- Intravenous therapy will likely be used to give fluids directly into a vein. IVs can be intermittent or continuous. Risks of IV therapy may include infiltration, fluid overload, electrolyte imbalances, phlebitis, or infection. It is important to calculate the content of IV fluids when they contain glucose, as indicated in this example:

Solution	Name	Na^+ (mmol/L)	Cl^- (mmol/L)	K^+ (mmol/L)	Ca^{2+} (mmol/L)	Glucose (mg/dL)
D5W	*5% dextrose*	0	0	0	0	5000
2/3D & 1/3 S	3.3% dextrose/0.3% saline	51	51	0	0	3333
Normal saline	0.9% NaCl	154	154	0	0	0
Ringer's lactate	Lactated Ringer	130	109	4	3	0

Follow an interdisciplinary protocol for managing dehydration, as shown on the following page.

Common Drugs and Anesthesia Used with Surgery and Potential Side Effects

- Anesthesia delays peristalsis; eat ice chips or sip carbonated beverages until nausea subsides.
- Analgesics should provide effective pain relief. Epidural analgesia in GI surgery yields shorter duration of postoperative ileus, attenuation of the stress response, fewer pulmonary complications, and improved postoperative pain control and recovery (Fotiadis et al, 2004). Pain medications should be taken sufficiently in advance of meals to allow a pleasant, pain-free mealtime.
- Antibiotics may be needed; monitor specific side effects for selected medication.
- Insulin may be needed if hyperglycemia persists.
- Laxatives may deplete electrolytes. When able to progress, use a higher fiber intake and plenty of liquids.
- Metoclopramide (Reglan) may help with postoperative ileus (Chan et al, 2005). Dry mouth or nausea can result after prolonged use.
- Vitamin K can help with clotting. There are generally no side effects with this injection. Warfarin (Coumadin), a blood thinner used to prevent emboli, requires that patients maintain steady intake of vitamin K foods (cabbage, kale, and spinach) to control levels. Heparin has no dietary consequences.

Herbs, Botanicals, and Supplements

- Interactions between herbs, anesthesia, and surgery must be noted. For surgical patients, herbs can affect sedation, pain control, bleeding, heart function, metabolism, immunity, and recovery. As many as one third of presurgical patients take herbal medications, and many of those patients fail to disclose herbal use during preoperative assessment, even when prompted. Table 14-6 describes these potential interactions.
- Antioxidant foods are protective. Consume plenty of tea and foods listed in Table 13-2. Coenzyme Q10 may help to lower angiogenesis markers and lipid levels; studies are ongoing.

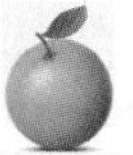

NUTRITION EDUCATION, COUNSELING, CARE MANAGEMENT

- Immobilization of the patient can produce unwanted side effects. Have patient drink plenty of fluids and ambulate as soon as possible.
- Patients tend to lose 0.5 lb daily early in postoperative period. Weight gain during this time suggests fluid excess.
- Eat and drink slowly to prevent gas formation from swallowed air.
- Discuss the role of surgery as "planned trauma," allowing adequate time for return to homeostasis. Discuss wound healing priority, tensile strength, and role of nutrients (zinc, vitamin C, vitamin A, and amino acids). Note that poor nutrient intake can decrease anabolism, delaying scar formation. B-complex vitamins are also beneficial. While zinc deficiency impairs wound healing, supplementation in people who are not deficient does not accelerate wound healing and an excess can interfere with immune system function and copper absorption.
- During the rehabilitative anabolic stage (3 months to 1 year postoperatively), energy intake should be adequate but not excessive.
- With amputation, determine the percentage of body mass lost and decrease estimated energy needs accordingly; see Table 14-7.
- Table 14-8 lists other types of surgeries and their specific nutritional impact.

Patient Education—Food Safety

Surgical patients may be vulnerable to foodborne illness; safe food handling and handwashing are essential.

INTERDISCIPLINARY NUTRITION CARE PLAN
Dehydration

Client Name: ______________________ **#:** __________ **Initiated by:** __________ **Date:** __________

SCREEN
Nutrition Screen diagnosis: Dehydration
Signed: ______________ Date: ________

↓

ASSESS *(Check any/all)*
Hydration status
❑ Fluid intake ≤ fluid output
❑ Diuretics' multiple medications
❑ Ostomy*
❑ Increased environmental temperature/ no air conditioning/low humidity
Biochemistries
❑ ↑BUN ❑ ↑Serum sodium
Complex diet order
❑ High-protein, high-calorie diet
❑ Fluid restriction
Infection/Wounds
❑ Fever ❑ Pneumonia, UTI, URI
❑ Pressure ulcers, wounds
Poor Oral Intake Symptoms
❑ Anorexia ❑ Nausea/vomiting*
❑ Poor appetite ❑ Diarrhea*

Signed: ______________ Date: ________

None → MODERATE RISK INTERVENTIONS
1 or more ↓ HIGH-RISK INTERVENTIONS

GOALS (Check any/all):

❑ Assure intake of minimum daily water need of _____ mL in _____(goal time). (Calculate using **Daily Water Need for Adults**.)

❑ Maintain or improve hydration status as indicated by weight gain, fluid intake greater than or equal to output and normalization of biochemistries in ____ (goal time).

❑ Prevent dehydration-related adverse events in ____ (goal time).

❑ Reduce or eliminate dehydration risk factors in _____ (goal time).

MODERATE RISK INTERVENTIONS
(Check any/all)
Getting the Fluid You Need provided and explained
Food Record provided and explained
Obtain Dr. orders as needed:
❑ RD chart consult
❑ Monitor weight q:_____
❑ **Other:**____________________
(See notes for documention.)

Signed: ______________ Date: ________

Next visit ↓

ASSESS RESPONSE *(Check any/all)*
❑ Weight loss
❑ Fluid intake less than fluid output
❑ Onset of new infection
❑ Dehydration
❑ Exhibiting Poor Oral Intake symptoms
❑ **Other:**____________________
(See notes for documention.)

Signed: ______________ Date: ________

None → OUTCOMES ACHIEVED
1 or more ← HIGH-RISK INTERVENTIONS

OUTCOMES ACHIEVED
❑ Hydration status maintained or improved
❑ Weight maintained or improved
❑ Nutrition status maintained or improved
❑ **Other:**____________________
(See notes for documention.)
❑ Repeat Nutrition Risk Screen in ____ days

Signed: ______________ Date: ________

HIGH-RISK INTERVENTIONS *(Check any/all)*
❑ **Getting the Fluid You Need** provided and explained
❑ **Food Record** provided and explained
❑ Assure intake of a 2qt (2L) of appropriate fluids/day
Obtain Dr. orders as needed:
❑ RD referral for home visit(s)
❑ Monitor weight q:_____
❑ Monitor I & O q: _____
❑ Oral rehydration fluid if diarrhea, vomiting, ostomy are present
❑ **Other:**____________________
(See notes for documention.)

Signed: ______________ Date: ________

Next visit ↓

ASSESS RESPONSE *(Check any/all)*
❑ Further weight loss
❑ Fluid intake less than fluid output
❑ Onset of new infection
❑ Dehydration
❑ Exhibiting Fewer Oral Intake symptoms
❑ **Other:**____________________
(See notes for documention.)

Signed: ______________ Date: ________

None → OUTCOMES ACHIEVED
1 or more ↓ OUTCOMES NOT ACHIEVED

OUTCOMES ACHIEVED
❑ Hydration status maintained or improved
❑ Weight maintained or improved
❑ Nutrition status maintained or improved
❑ **Other:**____________________
(See notes for documention.)
❑ Repeat Nutrition Risk Screen in ____ days

Signed: ______________ Date: ________

OUTCOMES NOT ACHIEVED
Notify physician. Reassess/evaluate need for EN/PN (refer to Tube Feeding Nutrition Care Plan). Document on Nutrition Variance Tracking form.

* Requires replacement of water and electrolytes.

TABLE 14-5 Managing Electrolyte Imbalances

Three variables regulate pH in blood plasma: carbon dioxide, electrolyte concentrations, and total weak acid concentrations.

Acid–base balance is when blood pH is out of the normal range (7.35–7.45). An excess of acid leads to acidosis (pH < 7.35) and an excess of base leads to alkalosis (pH > 7.45). Imbalance is classified according to the source: respiratory or metabolic.

There are four basic conditions: metabolic acidosis, respiratory acidosis, metabolic alkalosis, and respiratory alkalosis.

Dietitians typically address electrolyte imbalances, which involve calcium, potassium, magnesium, and sodium and are discussed here.

Normal Range	Causes of Elevation	Causes of Decline
Sodium (Na): 135–145 mEq/L	**Hypernatremia:** Excessive loss of water through GI system, lungs, or skin; fluid restriction, certain diuretics, hypertonic IV solutions, tube feeding; hypothalamic lesions, hyperaldosteronism, corticosteroid use, Cushing's syndrome, diabetes insipidus	**Hyponatremia:** Congestive heart failure, cirrhosis, nephrosis, excess fluid intake, syndrome of inappropriate antidiuretic hormone secretion (dilutional hyponatremia); sodium depletion, loss of body fluids without replacement, diuretic therapy, laxatives, nasogastric suctioning, hypoaldosteronism, cerebral salt-wasting disease
Potassium (K): 3.5–5.0 mEq/L	**Hyperkalemia:** Aldosterone deficiency, sodium depletion, acidosis, trauma, hemolysis of red blood cells, potassium-sparing diuretics	**Hypokalemia:** Lack of dietary intake of potassium, vomiting, nasogastric suctioning, potassium-depleting diuretics, aldosteronism, salt-wasting kidney disease, major GI surgery, diuretic therapy with inadequate potassium replacement
Calcium (Ca): 8.5–10.5 mg/dL	**Hypercalcemia:** Excessive vitamin D, immobility, hyperparathyroidism, potassium-sparing diuretics, ACE inhibitors, malignancy of bone or blood	**Hypocalcemia:** Hypoparathyroidism, malabsorption, insufficient or inactivated vitamin D or inadequate intake of calcium, hypoalbuminemia, diuretic therapy, diarrhea, acute pancreatitis, bone cancer, gastric surgery
Magnesium (Mg): 1.5–2.5 mg/dL	**Hypermagnesemia:** Excessive use of magnesium-containing antacids and laxatives, untreated diabetic ketoacidosis, excessive magnesium infusions	**Hypomagnesemia:** Malabsorption related to GI disease, excessive loss of GI fluids, acute alcoholism/cirrhosis, diuretic therapy, hyper- or hypothyroidism, pancreatitis, preeclampsia, nasogastric suctioning, fistula drainage

Kee J, et al. *Fluids and electrolytes with clinical applications: a programmed approach*. 7th ed. Clifton Park, NY: Delmar Learning, 2004.

Signs and Symptoms	Comments and Nutritional Concerns
HYPONATREMIA Lethargy, anorexia, nausea, vomiting, cramping, muscular twitching, confusion, fingerprinting over the breastbone, seizures, and coma. Hyponatremia is associated with increased morbidity and mortality.	Distinguish between the different types of hyponatremia and their treatments. Contracted extracellular fluid volume may occur; a hypertonic or isotonic saline solution is given (perhaps salty broth). Avoid giving large water flushes with isotonic tube feeding. Fluid restriction and low-sodium diet with diuretics may cause hyponatremia. D5W used in excess can cause hyponatremia with water intoxication.
HYPERNATREMIA Thirst, dry and sticky mucous membranes, fever, dry and swollen tongue, disorientation, and seizures. Flushing, fever, loss of sweating, dry tongue and mucous membranes, tachycardia, hallucinations, or coma.	High-protein tube feedings without adequate water flushes, excessive diaphoresis, diabetes insipidus, or watery diarrhea may cause problems. Correct dehydration. Monitor thirst, the first sign of water loss. High doses of steroids, solutions that contain NaCl, other sodium additives, and sodium-containing analgesics should be managed or omitted. Determine patient's fluid needs (generally 30 mL/kg or 1 mL/kcal given in enteral or total parenteral infusions. Adjust according to the renal or cardiovascular status, especially in seniors. Patients with dysphagia may have difficulty obtaining enough fluid; monitor closely.
HYPOKALEMIA Severe muscle weakness, electrocardiogram (ECG) changes and arrhythmias, lethargy, hypotension, shallow breathing, fatigue, anorexia, constipation, confusion, and impaired carbohydrate (CHO) tolerance. Chloride depletion usually accompanies hypokalemia; alkalosis is also common.	Replace potassium (generally done with intravenous or oral KCl, except in renal tubular acidosis). Kaochlor, Kay-Ciel, K-Lor, K-Lyte, K Tab, Klotrix, Micro-K, K-Dur, Klor-Con, Ten-K, and Slow-K are all sources of potassium. Some products are slow release. Diarrhea, nausea, or vomiting may occur; take with meals. A potassium-rich diet may also be needed. Monitor serum levels and adjust accordingly. Be sure fluid intake is adequate.

(continued)

TABLE 14-5 **Managing Electrolyte Imbalances *(continued)***

Signs and Symptoms	Comments and Nutritional Concerns
HYPERKALEMIA Weakness, anxiety, altered ECGs (with >7 mEq/L, a fatal arrhythmia can occur), flaccid muscle paralysis, or even respiratory arrest, if severe.	Immediate treatment is needed to prevent arrhythmias, bradycardia, heart block, and respiratory arrest. If all else fails, dialysis may be needed. Intravenous feedings are likely to be used (glucose, insulin, bicarbonate) to shift potassium intracellularly. Sodium or calcium may also be needed as physical antagonists; infusions will be given until serum potassium is corrected. Monitor closely. Avoid high-potassium foods and K^+ in salt substitutes. Kayexalate may be needed and should be given with sorbitol to prevent constipation; take separately from calcium or antacids. Read labels of oral supplements to be sure total K^+ is calculated.
HYPOCALCEMIA Tetany, seizures, and cardiac arrest. In the long term, bone demineralization with bone pain and compression fractures may result.	Correct symptomatic condition (usually calcium gluconate intravenously). Supplement with vitamin D_3 as needed. When able to eat orally, provide a high-calcium intake; dry milk can be added to foods. Avoid excesses of caffeine, oxalate, fiber, and aluminum-containing antacids. Calcium carbonate (as in Tums) provides 40% elemental calcium. Drink extra water. Avoid use of iron supplements at the same time. Beware of bone meal and dolomite because of their toxic metal content.
HYPERCALCEMIA Drowsiness, lethargy, stupor, muscle weakness, decreased reflexes, nausea and vomiting, anorexia, constipation, ileus, polyuria, renal stones, azotemia, nocturia, hypertension, bradycardia, pruritus, and eye abnormalities.	Correct underlying condition with rehydration (usually with normal saline) and hemodilution. Correct nausea, vomiting, constipation, and other side effects. Avoid excesses of milk, vitamins A or D, calcium supplements and antacids, and lactose. Potassium and magnesium may also be depleted; monitor carefully. Extra caffeine, oxalates, fiber, and phytates can help to decrease calcium absorption and can help excretion. Sometimes furosemide or prednisone is used to excrete calcium also. Intravenous etidronate (Didronel) may be used; nausea and vomiting could occur.
HYPOMAGNESEMIA Anxiety, hyperirritability, confusion, hallucinations, seizures, tremor, hyperreflexia, tetany, tachycardia, hypertension, arrhythmias, vasomotor changes, profuse sweating, muscle weakness, grimaces of facial muscles, and refractory hypocalcemia.	Correct low serum magnesium levels to prevent sudden death. Discuss long-term measures to prevent further episodes. Long-term use of magnesium-free CPN can be one aggravating source of the problem. Monitor intake from all sources (oral, TF, CPN.) Milk of magnesia (MOM) can be used for liquid form of magnesium hydroxide; nausea, cramps, or diarrhea may result. Normal renal function is needed for use of magnesium sulfate; diarrhea can occur. Chocolate, nuts, fruits and green vegetables, beans, potatoes, wheat, and corn are considered good sources.
HYPERMAGNESEMIA Lethargy, hyporeflexia, and respiratory depression. Bradycardia, myocardial infarction, and respiratory failure may be fatal.	Reduce or eliminate sources of exogenous magnesium from diet, supplements, CPN solutions, and medications until resolved. Calcium-containing medications may be given to help with excretion of excessive magnesium. Avoid megadoses of multivitamin–mineral supplements.
HYPOPHOSPHATEMIA Anorexia, weakness, bone pain, dizziness, and waddling gait may be observed. In severe cases, elevated creatine phosphokinase (CPK) levels are seen, with rhabdomyolysis superimposed on myopathy. Hypophosphatemia may result in sudden death, rhabdomyolysis, red cell dysfunction, and respiratory insufficiency. Heart failure can result if phosphorus is not administered. Low serum phosphorus levels will result in lowered 2,3-diphosphoglyceric acid (2,3-DPG), which facilitates oxyhemoglobin dissociation and leads to tissue hypoxia and low partial pressure of oxygen.	Phosphorus is a major component of bone and is one of the most abundant constituents of all metabolic processes and tissues; 85% is found in the skeleton. Only about 12% is bound to proteins; a typical laboratory assessment is of elemental phosphorus, with some values for HPO_4 and $NaHPO_4$ as well. Prevent further complications. Use appropriate measures according to the cause; for example, low-phosphorus diet with high calcium and adequate vitamin D will be needed in renal osteodystrophy. Note that 50–60% of dietary phosphorus is absorbed, and more is absorbed in depleted persons. If potassium phosphate (K-Phos) is used as an acidifier, it may cause nausea, vomiting, or diarrhea.
HYPERPHOSPHATEMIA Phosphorus levels tend to be higher in children and to rise in women after menopause.	Provide appropriate levels of phosphorus according to age and serum status. Monitor glucose and phosphorus intake, especially from enteral or parenteral nutrition. Monitor dietary intake of milk, meat, and other foods high in phosphorus. Observe serum levels regularly, especially in renal patients. Antacids containing aluminum will prevent phosphorus absorption in intestinal lumen. Calcium acetate is useful in dialysis patients.

Resources:
FreeMD, http://www.freemd.com/electrolyte-imbalance/, accessed January 19, 2010.
Medline Plus, http://www.nlm.nih.gov/medlineplus/fluidandelectrolytebalance.html, accessed January 19, 2010.
Merck Manual, http://www.merck.com/pubs/mmanual_ha/sec3/ch18/ch18d.html, accessed January 19, 2010.

TABLE 14-6 Herbal Medications and Recommendations for Discontinued Use before Surgery

Most commonly used herbs and antidepressant medications have potentially deleterious effects on the patient during surgery, ranging from increased risk of bleeding to fatal interactions (Chin et al, 2009.) The top four used by the general public are Echinacea, garlic, ginseng, and ginger (Heller et al, 2006.)

Herb	Relevant Effects	Perioperative Concerns	Recommendations
Echinacea	Boosts immunity	Allergic reactions, impairs immune system, especially for transplantation patients	Discontinue as far in advance as possible.
Ephedra (ma huang)	Increases heart rate and increases blood pressure	Risk of heart attack, arrhythmias, stroke, kidney stones, interaction with other drugs	Discontinue 24 hours before surgery.
Garlic	Prevents clotting	Risk of bleeding, especially when combined with other drugs that inhibit clotting	Discontinue at least 7 days before surgery.
Ginkgo	Prevents clotting	Risk of bleeding, especially when combined with other drugs that inhibit clotting	Discontinue at least 36 hours before surgery.
Ginseng	Lowers blood glucose, inhibits clotting	Increases risk of bleeding; interferes with warfarin (an anticlotting drug)	Discontinue at least 7 days before surgery.
Kava	Sedates, decreases anxiety	May increase sedative effects of anesthesia	Discontinue 24 hours before surgery.
St. John's wort	Inhibits reuptake of neurotransmitters	Alters metabolisms of other drugs	Discontinue at least 5 days before surgery.
Valerian	Sedates	Could increase effects of sedatives. Long-term use could increase amount of anesthesia needed.	If possible, taper dose weeks before surgery. Withdrawal symptoms resemble diazepam (Valium) addiction.

Sources:
Ang-Lee M, et al. Herbal medicines and perioperative care. *JAMA*. 286:208, 2001.
Chin SH, et al. Perioperative management of antidepressants and herbal medications in elective plastic surgery. *Plast Reconstr Surg*. 123:377, 2009.
Heller J, et al. Top-10 list of herbal and supplemental medicines used by cosmetic patients: what the plastic surgeon needs to know. *Plast Reconstr Surg*. 117:436, 2006.
Yuan CS, et al. Brief communication: American ginseng reduces warfarin's effect in healthy patients: a randomized, controlled Trial. *Ann Intern Med*. 141:23, 2004.

TABLE 14-7 Percentage of Body Weight in Amputees

Body weight is a good indicator of a person's size and is widely used in assessments. Body mass index (BMI) values in subjects with limb amputation are not useful unless lost weight of the limbs is not considered in the calculation. To reduce the underestimation of nutritional status in persons with limb amputation, estimation of body weight is necessary so that BMI can be reliably estimated for persons with limb amputation. Estimated body weight after amputation uses the following formula:

Estimated Ideal Body Weight (IBW) = (100 − % amputation)/100 × IBW for original height.

Body Part and % Loss from Amputation
Below knee 6.5%
Bilateral below knee (BK) 13%
Bilateral above knee (AK) 16%
BK + AK 14.5%
Foot 1.5%
Both feet 3%
Hand 0.7%
Both hands 1.4%
Forearm and hand 3%
Both forearms/hands 6%
Entire arm 5%
Both entire arms 10%
Entire leg 16%
Both entire legs 32%

Adapted from: Osterkamp LK. Current perspective on assessment of human body proportions of relevance to amputees. *J Am Diet Assoc*. 95:215, 1995.
Amputee BMI calculator, http://touchcalc.com/calculators/bmi_amputation, accessed January 20, 2010.

TABLE 14-8 Surgeries, Level of Nutritional Acuity, and Nutritional Recommendations

Background	Specific Objectives	Food and Nutrition Recommendations
Amputation, Level 2 Amputations may result from poorly controlled diabetes, trauma, peripheral artery disease, congenital deformity, chronic infections, gangrene, or tumors such as osteosarcoma.	Postoperative: Determine percentage of body weight of amputated area and calculate changes from preoperative to postoperative status in height, weight, and body mass index (BMI). Provide adequate protein, calories, zinc, vitamins C, K, and A for healing. Low albumin levels, serum carotene, zinc, and vitamin C are commonly found.	Postoperative: Use a high-protein/high-energy diet for healing. Supplement diet with vitamins and minerals, especially zinc, vitamins A, C, and K, and arginine. Use tube feeding (TF) if necessary; consider use of an immune-enhanced product. For hand or arm amputations, consider adaptive feeding equipment with Occupational therapy (OT) specialists.
	Long Term: Provide a low-calorie diet, if needed. For patients who lose too much weight, a higher energy diet should be used. Otherwise, immobilized patients tend to gain weight and will need weight control measures.	Long Term: Discuss how to control or increase calories in diet for energy use. Patients with an AK amputation who walk with or without prosthesis use 25% more energy than a nondisabled person who walks at the same speed; these patients have difficulty maintaining weight.
Appendectomy, Level 1 Appendectomy generally is an uncomplicated procedure with minimal recovery time. A low-fiber diet may contribute to appendicitis.	Preoperative: White blood cell count and erythrocyte sedimentation rate may be increased.	Postoperative: Use a balanced diet with adequate amounts of zinc and vitamins C, K, and A.
	Postoperative: Reduce fever. Lower risks of infection or sepsis, peritonitis, or abscess formation.	Long-Term: After recovery, include more fruits, vegetables, and whole grain for fiber.
Cesarean delivery (C-section), Level 1 C-section is performed for numerous reasons, including HIV infection, maternal diabetes, or edema-proteinuria-hypertensive (EPH) gestosis.	Postoperative: Manage nausea, which is common after anesthesia. Replenish stores of nutrients from blood and fluid losses. Reduce likelihood of complications such as hemorrhage, infection, fever, drainage, cystitis, anemia, or pneumonia after the operation.	Postoperative: Nothing by mouth (NPO) with intravenous or clear liquids and ice chips will be given until nausea subsides. Progress to usual diet, with increased fiber and fluid to soften stools. Promote wound healing with protein and energy; include iron, vitamins C and A, and zinc in diet or supplemental form.
Coronary Artery Bypass Graft (CABG), Level 3 Open heart procedures require use of a cardiopulmonary machine for extracorporeal circulation. Narrowed or blocked arteries are bypassed; the vein usually comes from the leg. Blood can then flow directly into the heart muscle. CABG usually takes 4–5 hours.	Preoperative: Monitor serum levels of electrolytes, albumin, and glucose. Provide the diet as prescribed (may be sodium, energy, or fluid restricted). Provide ample amounts of glycogen for stores. Use nutrition support, if needed, for malnourished cardiac patients.	Postoperative: Control fluid intake by measuring previous day's output plus 500 mL for insensible losses. Provide adequate protein, kilocalories, and micronutrients for wound healing. Use TF or CPN if severely malnourished. Replete slowly and keep head of bed elevated 30° to prevent worsening of heart failure. Low-sodium, high-calorie, low-volume TF products may be useful.
Heart valve replacement involves replacing the damaged valve with a mechanical prosthesis (St. Jude valve) or biological tissue valve. This may be done with robotic techniques, which are less invasive than open heart procedures.	Postoperative: Promote wound healing and restore normal fluid and electrolyte balance. Promote weight control. Wean from ventilator support when possible. Prevent hyperglycemia, coma, sepsis, renal failure, cardiac tamponade, wound dehiscence, and atelectasis. Maintain comfort and educate regarding follow-up.	
	Long Term: Avoid excessive weight gain, which can further aggravate heart condition. Teach appropriate measures for changes in daily diet to prevent further problems while wound is healing. Discuss need to alter lifestyle (diet, exercise, and stress) to prevent additional problems; many patients have atherogenic effects even after heart surgery. Control carbohydrates in patients with diabetes or hypertriglyceridemia.	Long-Term: Modify diet to control sodium and potassium intake, lessen edema, and improve blood pressure. Diuretics and digoxin may deplete potassium; anorexia, nausea, and diarrhea may occur. Beta-blockers, ace inhibitors, and other cardiac drugs may require use of low-sodium, low-calorie diets. Hypoalbuminemia can cause digoxin toxicity. National Cholesterol Education Program guidelines may be used if serum cholesterol remains high.

(continued)

TABLE 14-8 **Surgeries, Level of Nutritional Acuity, and Nutritional Recommendations *(continued)***

Background	Specific Objectives	Food and Nutrition Recommendations
Craniotomy, Level 2 Craniotomy involves removing and replacing the bone of the skull to provide access to intracranial structures, usually for a brain tumor.	Postoperative: Prevent aspiration. Prevent or correct dysphagia, constipation, urinary tract infection (UTI), nausea and vomiting, and diabetes insipidus. Normalize electrolyte levels. Prevent blood clots using anticoagulant therapy. If anticonvulsants are used, prevent folic acid depletion. Prevent or manage nausea, vomiting, facial or extremity paralysis, wound drainage, hyperthermia, dysphagia, diabetes insipidus, and syndrome of inappropriate antidiuretic hormone (SIADH). Monitor consciousness, gag reflex, results of examinations such as ECG and cerebrospinal fluid (CSF) levels.	Postoperative: NPO is needed until nausea and vomiting subside. Progress from liquids to soft diet as tolerated. Patient should be fed while lying on his/her side or with his/her head elevated 30° to prevent aspiration. Check swallowing reflex. Assist with feeding if needed, and TF may be required. Adequate fiber may be beneficial. If steroids are used, reduce sodium intake to 4–6 g/d (or less). Long-Term: Discuss importance of diet in correcting any malnutrition or anemia. As needed, teach family about a diet for dysphagia (e.g., thick, pureed foods with reduced thin liquids). When oral intake is possible, suggest slow chewing and eating. Aphasia occurs in some patients, making it hard to communicate their needs.
Hip Replacement, Level 2 A total hip replacement (arthroplasty) is the formation of an artificial hip joint. Prostheses are either cemented in place or uncemented. The procedure is performed for severe degenerative joint disease, rheumatoid arthritis, or congenital deformities.	Preoperative: Enhance nutritional intake in preparation for surgery. Postoperative: Replenish stores. Prevent side effects of immobilization (renal calculi, pressure ulcers, and UTIs). Promote adequate wound healing. Regain maximum mobility. Use small, frequent meals if nausea is a problem. Long-Term: Promote early ambulation, when possible, to promote healing and increase strength.	Preoperative: Nutritional status before arthroplasty is a good predictor of surgical outcomes after surgery; albumin levels >3.4 often predict a better outcome. Postoperative: Use a high-protein/high-energy diet. Supplement diet with zinc and vitamins A, C, and K. Determine whether blood loss can cause anemia; provide sufficient iron and protein in cooperation with medical team. Long-Term: If weight loss is needed, provide a balanced, low-energy diet after wound healing is completed. Include calcium and phosphorus.
Hysterectomy, abdominal, Level 1 Abdominal hysterectomy is the surgical removal of the uterus through an abdominal incision. This approach is used if the uterus is enlarged or if an oophorectomy (ovary removal) and salpingectomy (removal of the fallopian tubes) are also performed.	Postoperative: Promote wound healing and rapid recovery. Replete nutrient reserves and glycogen stores. Replace protein, iron, and vitamin K if blood loss was extensive. Prevent complications such as UTIs, incisional infections, fever, nausea, vomiting, or diverticular colovaginal fistula. Long-Term: Support gradual return to normal activity; exercise improves nutrient repletion and tissue repair.	Postoperative: Use a high-protein/high-calorie diet. Ensure that adequate fiber and fluid are provided to alleviate constipation. Provide a diet with adequate iron, zinc, and vitamins K, C, and A. Long-Term: Emphasize the importance of a good diet for wound healing.
Pancreatic Surgery, Level 3 This may include total pancreatectomy with or without islet cell autotransplantation for chronic pancreatitis and cancer; subtotal or pancreatoduodenectomy (Whipple's procedure) for islet cell tumors.	Preoperative: Monitor for history of ethanol (ETOH) abuse with resulting malnutrition and malabsorption; replete if possible. Postoperative: Prevent or correct sepsis, which is a common complication. Encourage nourishing and well-balanced meals; control CHO if diabetes occurs or is present. Determine pancreatic function according to type and extent of resection and underlying disorder. Whipple's procedure results in dumping syndrome, diarrhea, dyspepsia, ulceration at gastroenterostomy site, and extensive weight loss unless a pylorus-saving technique is used. Long-Term: Monitor impact of medications and replacement enzymes or hormones that are ordered. Alter fat source with malabsorption or steatorrhea. Offer resources for control of diabetes or for alcohol addiction, as needed.	Preoperative: Use enteral nutrition or CPN to prepare patient for a major operation. Postoperative: Enteral nutrition, CPN, or oral intake may progress as tolerated. Enteral nutrition has better outcomes if the tube is placed in the jejunum. Standard treatment following major pancreatic surgery includes the administration of pancreatic enzymes and inhibition of acid secretion by proton pump inhibitors; monitor effects on vitamin B_{12} status. Long-Term: A carbohydrate-controlled diet may be needed, along with small, frequent feedings. Most patients develop diabetes that may require insulin; hypoglycemia is the most difficult problem to manage.

(continued)

TABLE 14-8 Surgeries, Level of Nutritional Acuity, and Nutritional Recommendations *(continued)*

Background	Specific Objectives	Food and Nutrition Recommendations
Parathyroidectomy, Level 1 Surgical removal of the parathyroid glands	Preoperative: Prepare patient for surgery. Postoperative: Manage hypoparathyroidism (with tingling, tetany, hoarseness, and seizures.) Long-Term: Vitamin D, calcium, and chemotherapy are often required. A low-phosphorus diet with aluminum hydroxide (Amphojel) may be needed; constipation is one side effect.	Postoperative: IV or TF may be needed. Avoid CPN because of high risk for sepsis in the neck area. Provide extra fluids. Long-Term: A high-calcium/low-phosphorus diet may be necessary. Monitor carefully. Counsel about follow-up measures and potential medication interactions.
Pelvic Exenteration, Level 1 This surgery involves removal of all female reproductive organs and adjacent tissues (i.e., radical hysterectomy, pelvic node dissection, cystectomy and formation of an ileal conduit, vaginectomy, and rectal resection with colostomy). Cancer is usually the reason.	Preoperative: A low-residue or elemental diet may be needed, regressing to clear liquids, NPO. Vitamin K may be needed 24–48 hours before the procedure. Postoperative: Colonic stasis occurs after major abdominal surgery and persists for approximately 3 days. Prevent hemorrhage, infection, urinary or GI problems, shock, fever, anemia, and sepsis. Long-Term: Promote wound healing and recovery. Provide colostomy teaching if needed.	Postoperative: Parenteral fluids with electrolytes may be needed (3–4 L/d unless contraindicated). CPN or TF may also be appropriate. If nausea is an extensive problem, give fluids between meals. Long-Term: Progress, as tolerated, to a high-protein/high-calorie intake with snacks (eggnog, custard, oral supplements). Adequate iron, zinc, and vitamins A and C help with wound-healing process.
Spinal Surgery, Level 2 This surgery generally is performed to relieve pressure on spinal nerves or cord due to herniated discs, trauma, displaced fractures, osteoporosis, or incomplete vertebral dislocation from rheumatoid arthritis. Laminectomy, discectomy, or spinal fusion may be performed.	Preoperative: Nutrients may be needed for adequate stores (e.g., glucose, protein, vitamins A, C, and K, and zinc). Postoperative: Correct nausea and vomiting if a problem. Prevent calculi, UTIs, and pressure ulcers. Fluid and fiber will be important, but prevent overhydration. Long-Term: Avoid weight gain.	Postoperative: Parenteral fluids may be given as ordered. A balanced diet, when patient is ready, with control of total energy intake to prevent excessive weight gain, may be used. If patient has been malnourished, a gradual increase in calories may be beneficial. Adequate hydration will be necessary unless contraindicated. Long-Term: Increase fiber intake if constipation is a problem; prune juice, crushed bran, and other items may be used. If tolerated, extra fruits and raw vegetables may be used.
Tonsillectomy/Adenoidectomy, Level 1 These tissues are considered to be part of the protective immune system; removal is for severe and chronic ear, throat, and sinus infections.	Preoperative: Supply adequate nourishment for glycogen stores. Long-Term: Help patient select nonirritating foods for use at home. Avoid hot, spicy foods, raw vegetables, toast and crackers, citrus juices, and other related foods until full recovery.	Postoperative: Give cold liquids (sherbet, ginger ale, nectars, and gelatin). Do not use red gelatin as it may mask blood if there is any vomiting. Use extra fluid intake; large swallows are less painful than many small ones. Avoid milk products only if patient cannot tolerate them. On day 2 or 3, use soft, smooth foods (pudding, strained cereals, soft-cooked eggs). Progress to regular diet when tolerated. Long-Term: Use supplements of vitamin C if patient cannot tolerate juices. Evaluate zinc intake and encourage dietary sources when possible.

For More Information

- American Academy of Physical Medicine and Rehabilitation
  http://www.aapmr.org/
- Amputees
  http://www.nlm.nih.gov/medlineplus/amputees.html
- Amputee Resource Foundation of America
  http://www.amputeeresource.org/
- National Library of Medicine—Surgery
  http://www.nlm.nih.gov/medlineplus/surgery.html
- Refeeding Syndrome
  http://www.ccmtutorials.com/misc/phosphate/page_07.htm

SURGERY—CITED REFERENCES

Bochicchio GV, et al. Admission preoperative glucose is predictive of morbidity and mortality in trauma patients who require immediate operative intervention. *Am Surg.* 71:171, 2005.

Bossingham MJ, et al. Water balance, hydration status, and fat-free mass hydration in younger and older adults. *Am J Clin Nutr.* 81:1342, 2005.

Braga M, Gianotti L. Preoperative immunonutrition: cost-benefit analysis. *JPEN J Parenter Enteral Nutr.* 29:S57, 2005.

Chan DC, et al. Preventing prolonged post-operative ileus in gastric cancer patients undergoing gastrectomy and intra-peritoneal chemotherapy. *World J Gastroenterol.* 11:4776, 2005.

Estivarez CF, et al. Efficacy of parenteral nutrition supplemented with glutamine dipeptide to decrease hospital infections in critically ill surgical patients. *JPEN J Parenter Enteral Nutr.* 32:389, 2008.
Falanga V. Wound healing and its impairment in the diabetic foot. *Lancet.* 366:1736, 2005.
Farreras N, et al. Effect of early postoperative enteral immunonutrition on wound healing in patients undergoing surgery for gastric cancer. *Clin Nutr.* 24:55, 2005.
Fearon KC, Luff R. The nutritional management of surgical patients: enhanced recovery after surgery. *Proc Nutr Soc.* 62:807, 2003.
Fotiadis RJ, et al. Epidural analgesia in gastrointestinal surgery. *Br J Surg.* 91:828, 2004.
Gabor S, et al. Early enteral feeding compared with parenteral nutrition after oesophageal or oesophagogastric resection and reconstruction. *Br J Nutr.* 93:509, 2005.
Grimble RF. Immunonutrition. *Curr Opin Gastroenterol.* 21:216, 2005.
Kao LS, et al. Peri-operative glycaemic control regimens for preventing surgical site infections in adults. *Cochrane Database Syst Rev.* (3):CD006806, 2009.
Klek S, et al. The impact of immunostimulating nutrition on infectious complications after upper gastrointestinal surgery: a prospective, randomized, clinical trial. *Ann Surg.* 248:212, 2008.
Lucha PA Jr, et al. The economic impact of early enteral feeding in gastrointestinal surgery: a prospective survey of 51 consecutive patients. *Am Surg.* 71:187, 2005.
Luo M, et al. Depletion of plasma antioxidants in surgical intensive care unit patients requiring parenteral feeding: effects of parenteral nutrition with or without alanyl-glutamine dipeptide supplementation. *Nutrition.* 24:37, 2008.
Maddox TM. Preoperative cardiovascular evaluation for noncardiac surgery. *Mt Sinai J Med.* 72:185, 2005.
Marek PE, Zaloga GP. Meta-analysis of parenteral nutrition versus enteral nutrition in patients with acute pancreatitis. *BMJ.* 328:1407, 2004.
Mokart D, et al. Predictive perioperative factors for developing severe sepsis after major surgery. *Br J Anaesth.* 95:776, 2005.
Roth E, Oehler R. Hypothesis: Muscular glutamine deficiency in sepsis-A necessary step for a hibernation-like state? [published online ahead of print January 11, 2010]. *Nutrition.* 26:571, 2010.
Schiesser M, et al. Assessment of a novel screening score for nutritional risk in predicting complications in gastro-intestinal surgery. *Clin Nutr.* 27:565, 2008.
Wilmore D. Enteral and parenteral arginine supplementation to improve medical outcomes in hospitalized patients. *J Nutr.* 134:2863S, 2004.
Winkelmayer WC, et al. C-reactive protein and body mass index independently predict mortality in kidney transplant recipients. *Am J Transplant.* 4:1178, 2005.
Wittman F, et al. L-arginine improves wound healing after trauma-hemorrhage by increasing collagen synthesis. *J Trauma.* 59:162, 2005.
Zaloga GP. Parenteral nutrition in adult inpatients with functioning gastrointestinal tracts: assessment of outcomes. *Lancet.* 367:1101, 2006.
Zaloga GP, et al. Arginine: mediator or modulator of sepsis? *Nutr Clin Pract.* 19:201, 2004.

GASTROINTESTINAL SURGERIES

BARIATRIC SURGERY AND GASTRIC BYPASS

NUTRITIONAL ACUITY RANKING: LEVEL 3

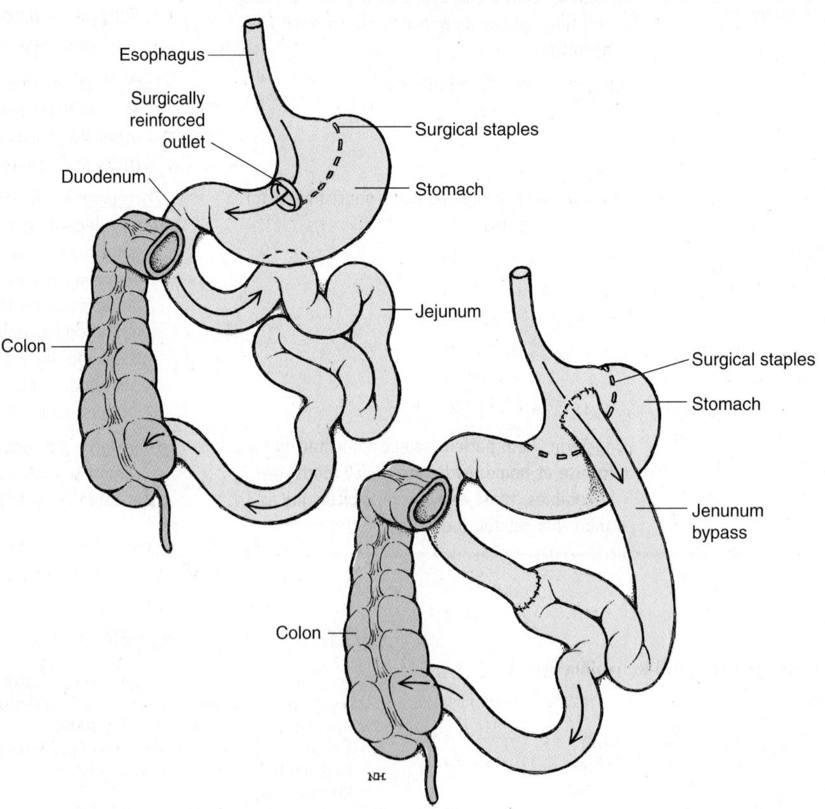

The gastric bypass procedure has replaced the jejunal bypass, which had many undesirable nutritional consequences. Adapted from: Neil O. Hardy. Wesport, CT. *Stedman's Medical Dictionary,* 27th ed. Baltimore: Lippincott Williams & Wilkins, 2000, p. 1249.

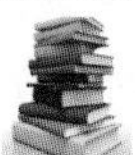

DEFINITIONS AND BACKGROUND

More than 10 million Americans are severely obese. Bariatric surgery is a viable option for the treatment, resulting in long-term weight loss and improved health risk factors. Bariatric surgery is expensive, \$20,000 and \$25,000, but is an effective weapon against the consequences of morbid obesity. Candidates should be 100 lb or more over ideal weight range, have a BMI greater than 40, or a BMI greater than 35 in addition to serious medical comorbidities. Obesity surgery is superior to medical intervention in this population (Leslie et al, 2007.) Results show lower incidence rates of diabetes, hypertriglyceridemia, and hyperuricemia. In fact, bariatric surgery should be considered for adults who have type 2 diabetes and a BMI greater than 35 kg/m^2, especially if the diabetes is difficult to control with lifestyle and pharmacologic therapy (American Diabetes Association, 2009.)

Bariatric surgery may be implemented in carefully selected, older, severely obese adolescents (Jen et al, 2010). However, surgical treatment should be considered only when adolescents have tried for at least 6 months to lose weight and have not been successful, have a BMI greater than 40, have reached their adult height (usually 13 or older for girls and 15 or older for boys), **and** have serious weight-related health problems such as T2DM, heart disease, or sleep apnea (NIDDK, 2010). Teens should be referred only to specialized adolescent bariatric centers.

Gastric bypass (GBP) achieves permanent and significant weight loss. The **Roux-en-Y gastric bypass (RYGB)** induces long-term remission of type 2DM, returning impaired glucose tolerance to euglycemia in a matter of days (Pories and Albrecht, 2001). Exclusion of food and alteration in signals from the antrum, duodenum, and proximal jejunum to the pancreatic islet cells improve glucose tolerance. While altered gut and pancreatic hormone secretion may resolve insulin resistance after RYGB, the independent effects of weight loss and hormonal secretion on peripheral glucose disposal are observed only after substantial weight loss (Campos et al, 2010.)

GBP procedures reduce capacity to 40–60 mL and induce physiological and neuroendocrine changes that affect the weight regulatory centers in the brain. Major adverse events include anastomosis leakage, pneumonia, pulmonary embolism, band slippage, and band erosion (Picot et al, 2009.) **Laparoscopic Roux-en-Y gastric bypass (LRYGB)** has fewer side effects, but anastomotic leak is one of them.

Biliopancreatic diversion with duodenal switch reduces the stomach to 20%, like a thin sleeve. The duodenal switch (valve) remains along with a limited portion of the duodenum; the intestine is connected to the duodenum near the stomach (biliopancreatic diversion). This weight loss leads to more malnutrition and vitamin deficiencies and requires close monitoring.

Lap-band adjustable gastric banding uses an inflatable band to divide the stomach into two parts by wrapping a band around the upper part and tightening it like a belt. Lap-band adjustable gastric banding is simple, has a lower complication rate, and can be adjusted or removed if necessary.

Most patients lose more than 60% of their excess weight after bariatric surgery. GBP and laparoscopic isolated sleeve gastrectomy are more effective for weight loss than vertical banded gastroplasty and adjustable gastric banding; more research is needed (Picot et al, 2009.) Because gallstones are common after the surgery, cholecystectomy may be done at the same time as the bariatric procedure.

Bariatric surgery appears to be a clinically effective and cost-effective intervention for moderately to severely obese people compared with nonsurgical interventions (Picot et al, 2009.) Expected long-term outcomes include improvement or resolution of diabetes, metabolic syndrome, coronary artery disease, dyslipidemia, gastroesophageal reflux disease, sleep apnea, hypertension, osteoarthritis, and cardiovascular mortality (Jhaveri et al, 2009; Madan et al, 2006; Torquati et al, 2005.)

Deficiencies in protein, iron, vitamin B_{12}, folate, calcium, fat-soluble vitamins (A, D, E, and K), and other micronutrients are common and become clinically significant if not recognized and treated with supplements (Carlin et al, 2006.) Copper deficiency, for example, has been noted in this population with cardiovascular and neurological changes (Tan et al, 2006).

Rhabdomyolysis is a risk from extended immobilization. It is accompanied by pain in the region of the referred muscle group, increase in creatine phosphokinase levels, myoglobinuria, severe renal failure, multiorgan system failure, and death if not treated in time (Filis et al, 2005). Another rare complication is hyperfunction of the pancreatic beta cells (nesidioblastosis) which can lead to life-threatening hypoglycemia (Service et al, 2005). Weight regain after RYGB occurs in approximately 20% of patients and constitutes another serious complication; failure to sustain elevated plasma PYY concentrations occurs (Meguid et al, 2008.)

Quality assurance produces better outcomes (Rendon and Pories, 2005). A multidisciplinary clinical pathway, preprinted orders, discharge home instruction sheet, and daily guidelines are important aspects of treatment. As long as obesity and the popularity of bariatric surgery continue, medical practitioners must be aware of preexisting nutritional deficiencies and treat any nutritional deficiencies that may arise or worsen following surgery (Xanthakos, 2009.) Monitoring and follow-up with a dietitian should be standard procedure. Tips are available in Table 14-9.

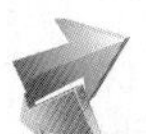

ASSESSMENT, MONITORING, AND EVALUATION

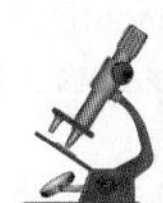

CLINICAL INDICATORS

Genetic Markers: The usual reason for GBP is morbid obesity, some of which may be genetically related, but it is believed that environment plays a greater role.

Clinical/History

- Height
- Weight
- Postoperative weight
- BMI (pre-/post-surgery)
- Diet history
- Waist-hip ratio (WHR)
- Waist circumference
- Vomiting
- I & O
- BP
- Sleep apnea
- Endoscopy

Lab Work

- Gluc
- Hemoglobin A1c
- CRP

TABLE 14-9 Tips for Diet after Gastric Bypass

Diet Order	Timing	Beverage and Food Choices
Clear Liquids (*no more than 1/2 cup total*)	1–2 days after surgery	Water, unsweetened drinks, sugar-free gelatin or popsicles, and clear broths. Diluted (pulp-free) juices (1 part juice to 10 parts water.) Decaffeinated tea. NO CARBONATED BEVERAGES. Sip at least 48–64 oz of liquid (especially water) each day. Take a prescribed multivitamin every day.
Full Liquids (*gradually increase to no more than 3/4 cup total*)	Days 3–21	*Items listed above, plus:* Use nonfat acidophilus milk, sugar-free Carnation Instant Breakfast drink, plain soymilk, low-fat cream soups made with skim milk for protein in this stage. May also add cream of wheat or rice cereal; sugar-free yogurt or pudding; unsweetened applesauce or strained infant fruits; sugar-free powdered drinks or iced tea. Sip at least 48–64 oz of liquid (especially water) each day. Take a prescribed multivitamin every day.
Pureed (*gradually increase to no more than 1 cup total*)	3–6 weeks after surgery	*Items listed above, plus:* Low-fat cottage cheese, eggs, tofu, baby food chicken or turkey for protein in this stage. May also add hummus, regular unflavored oatmeal, baby food or toddler fruits and vegetables, blended fruit smoothies, chicken or vegetable broth. Sip at least 48–64 oz of liquid (especially water) each day. Take a prescribed multivitamin every day.
Regular (*small meals and snacks with no more than 1 cup total; 2 oz total meat*)	6 weeks on	*Items listed above, plus:* Low-fat foods (<5 g fat per serving) such as plain rice, well-cooked pasta. Avoid concentrated sweets and sugar (>10 g sugar per serving). For protein, use lean chicken or deboned fish and most tender meats except for tough meats like beef or pork. Allow 30–45 minutes for each meal. Take small bites, and chew food until fairly liquefied before swallowing. Sip at least 48–64 oz of liquid (especially water) each day. Take a prescribed multivitamin every day.

Interleukin-6	Serum Fe	Alkaline phosphatase
Na^+, K^+	Serum B_{12}	
Ca^{++}, Mg^{++}	Serum folic acid	Cholesterol
Alb, transthyretin	Serum vitamin D	Triglycerides
H & H	Serum copper	

SAMPLE NUTRITION CARE PROCESS STEPS

Inadequate Vitamin Intake

Assessment Data: Medication history. Intake records after GBP surgery indicating no animal protein sources. Not taking prescribed vitamin-mineral supplement. BMI >50 before surgery; 6-month postoperation, BMI 48. Low serum B12 level. Recent complaints of tingling and numbness in extremities.

Nutrition Diagnosis (PES): NI-5.9.11 Inadequate vitamin B_{12} intake related to inadequate intake and not taking vitamin supplement as evidenced by diet history, low serum B_{12} level, and symptoms of neurological changes (tingling in hands and feet.)

Intervention: Food-nutrient delivery—Encourage use of milk products as tolerated throughout the day. Educate—Discuss the importance of vitamin B_{12} from supplemental intake when dietary intake is poor. Counsel about acceptable sources of B_{12} while on the highly restricted GBP diet. Coordinate care with medical team and family members to emphasize improving the diet.

Monitoring and Evaluation: Pill count for prescribed vitamin supplements. Improvement in neurological symptoms; normalized vitamin B_{12} lab values within 1–2 months of therapy.

INTERVENTION

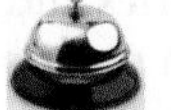

OBJECTIVES

Preoperative

- Provide adequate glycogen stores and vitamins C and K for surgical procedure. Consider enteral immunonutrition.
- Patients with diabetes should be under fairly good glucose control or at least stable.

Postoperative

- Promote wound healing and restoration of depleted glycogen in the liver.
- Prevent side effects during weight loss. The weight loss results of GBP surgery average 10 lb per month and stabilize between 18 and 24 months after surgery. Most patients will never achieve an ideal body weight, but they will be closer to a healthy body weight.
- Prevent complications such as alkaline reflux gastritis, esophagitis, perforation, gastric dilation, stomal obstruction, peptic ulcer, staple line disruption, and excessive vomiting.
- Monitor and manage rare conditions such as rhabdomyolysis, nesidioblastosis, bowel obstruction, and acute renal failure (Capella et al, 2006; Sharma et al, 2006.)
- At 4–6 weeks postoperatively, patients often report that foods taste sweet and will modify intake accordingly. Aversions to meat may occur. Pica may be found in some patients who also have iron deficiency anemia (Kushner and Shanta Retelny, 2005).
- Have patient eat and sip liquids slowly to prevent vomiting; take meat and toast in small bites.

- Prevent neurological, hematological, and cardiovascular side effects of thiamin, vitamin B_{12} deficiency, and other nutrients that may be inadequate (Bloomberg et al, 2005).

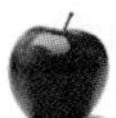

FOOD AND NUTRITION

Preoperative

- Use a balanced diet with adequate energy, protein, vitamins, and minerals. Enteral immunonutrition may be useful.
- Diet should regress from liquids to NPO.

Postoperative

- Over several days, progress from clear to full liquids. Enteral feeding with a high-protein intake may be useful to promote healing. Provide at least 1000 kcal/d with 1.5–2.0 g protein/kg.
- Until weight loss is achieved, add semisolid or pureed foods in small amounts. Initial gastric capacity is 30–60 mL; progression is up to 250 mL. Three meals and two snacks are better tolerated than three meals.
- Include 60–80 g of protein per day when possible. High-protein, low-fat foods such as milk, eggs, yogurt, boneless fish, and skinless poultry are important for maintaining adequate lean body mass while losing weight.
- Carbohydrate should be less than 30 g total per meal. A minimum of 130 g of carbohydrate per day should be included to meet Dietary Reference Intakes (DRIs).
- Patients will vomit if they eat too rapidly, drink fluids right after eating, lie down after eating, or overeat. Recommend chewing slowly and consuming liquids 30 minutes before or after meals.
- Dumping syndrome may also occur. Avoid alcoholic beverages, soft drinks, high-fat food such as fried foods and pastries, and high-carbohydrate foods such as cookies, cake, and candies.
- Ensure adequate fluid intake to prevent dehydration. Use at least 40 mL/Kg of noncaffeinated/noncaloric fluid daily, especially water.
- Meet micronutrient requirements, such as a daily liquid multivitamin–mineral supplement and a monthly vitamin B_{12} injection (Johnson et al, 2005). Monitor for iron and calcium deficiencies. Progress to a chewable supplement that meets 100% of the DRIs.
- Avoid obstructive foods, such as popcorn, celery, nuts, seeds, and membranes of citrus fruits.

Common Drugs Used and Potential Side Effects

- Drugs used will be for the specific condition and side effects of surgery.
- Combining RYGB with pharmacologic stimulation of PYY secretion may increase long-term success of surgical weight reduction in morbidly obese adults (Meguid et al, 2008.)

Herbs, Botanicals, and Supplements

- Answer questions about the use of herbs and botanicals; stop them before surgery.

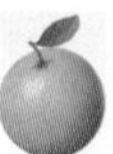

NUTRITION EDUCATION, COUNSELING, CARE MANAGEMENT

- **Preoperative evaluations** include: all weight loss attempts and outcomes; usual eating patterns and nutritional intake evaluations; frequency of eating away from home; cooking and shopping habits; reasons and motives for surgery; knowledge about protein, vitamins, and minerals; awareness of signs of dehydration; and food allergies and intolerances. Keeping a food diary and sharing it with the dietitian is important. Continuous nutrition monitoring can prevent poor outcomes if the patient and the dietitian work together.
- **Postoperative education** includes: use of high-protein supplemental beverages, especially for wound healing. Thinned baby food, low-fat and sugar-free milk shakes, thinned hot cereals, blenderized soups, vegetable juices, and sugar-free instant breakfast drinks are useful.
- Patients require close monitoring, with special regard to the rapidity of weight loss and vigilant screening for signs and symptoms of subclinical and clinical nutritional deficiencies (Bloomberg et al, 2005.)
- Discuss appropriate quantities and qualities of foods that will be consumed; overeating may stretch the stoma or cause dumping syndrome. Have patient take small bites and sip liquids slowly to prevent vomiting.
- Help patient progress to normalized diet with 120–200 mL per meal. Increase awareness of the eating and satiety process.
- A multivitamin–mineral preparation is definitely needed. Vitamin B_{12}, folacin, iron, potassium, copper, and vitamins A and D are special risks for deficiency. Nutritional deficiencies may become apparent, including PEM (Shuster and Vasquez, 2005).
- Discuss methods for blenderizing foods and recipes.
- Avoid fasting, as it may cause hypoglycemia.
- Promote adequate sleep, exercise, and other lifestyle measures that support a sense of well-being.
- Discuss how to manage dumping syndrome by avoiding simple sugars.
- Most patients lose a significant amount of weight and maintain their weight loss for long term, thereby having an improved quality of life. Unfortunately, between 5% and 30% of patients lose little weight or are unable to maintain their weight loss postoperatively (Puzziferri, 2005). Encourage exercise to help with weight loss and self-esteem.

Patient Education—Food Safety

Surgical patients may be vulnerable to foodborne illness; safe food handling and handwashing are essential.

For More Information

- American Society for Metabolic & Bariatric Surgery
  http://www.asbs.org/
- Cleveland Clinic
  http://cms.clevelandclinic.org/bariatricsurgery/
- Consumer Guide to Bariatric Surgery
  http://www.yourbariatricsurgeryguide.com/intro/
- Gastric Bypass
  http://www.nlm.nih.gov/medlineplus/ency/article/007199.htm

- Longitudinal Assessment of Bariatric Surgery (LABS)
http://www.niddklabs.org
- Mayo Clinic
http://www.mayoclinic.com/health/gastric-bypass/HQ01465
- Presurgical Psychological Assessment
http://www.asbs.org/html/pdf/PsychPreSurgicalAssessment.pdf
- Weight-Control Information Network
http://win.niddk.nih.gov/

GASTRIC BYPASS—CITED REFERENCES

American Diabetes Association. Standards of Medical Care in Diabetes 2009. *Diabetes Care.* 32:25S, 2009.

Bloomberg RD, et al. Nutritional deficiencies following bariatric surgery: what have we learned? *Obes Surg.* 15:145, 2005.

Campos GM, et al. Improvement in peripheral glucose uptake after gastric bypass surgery is observed only after substantial weight loss has occurred and correlates with the magnitude of weight lost. *J Gastrointest Surg.* 14:15, 2010.

Capella RF, et al. Bowel obstruction after open and laparoscopic gastric bypass surgery for morbid obesity. *J Am Coll Surg.* 203:328, 2006.

Carlin AM, et al. Prevalence of vitamin D depletion among morbidly obese patients seeking gastric bypass surgery. *Surg Obes Relat Dis.* 2:98, 2006.

Filis D, et al. Rhabdomyolysis following laparoscopic gastric bypass. *Obes Surg.* 15:1496, 2005.

Jen HC, et al. Trends and outcomes of adolescent bariatric surgery in California, 2005–2007. *Pediatrics.* 126:746, 2010.

Jhaveri RR, et al. Cardiac remodeling after substantial weight loss: a prospective cardiac magnetic resonance study after bariatric surgery. *Surg Obes Relat Dis.* 5:648, 2009.

Johnson JM, et al. Effects of gastric bypass procedures on bone mineral density, calcium, parathyroid hormone, and vitamin D. *J Gastrointest Surg.* 9:1106, 2005.

Kushner RF, Shanta Retelny V. Emergence of pica (ingestion of non-food substances) accompanying iron deficiency anemia after gastric bypass surgery. *Obes Surg.* 15:1491, 2005.

Leslie D, et al. Bariatric surgery primer for the internist: keys to the surgical consultation. *Med Clin North Am.* 91:353, 2007.

Madan AK, et al. Metabolic syndrome: yet another co-morbidity gastric bypass helps cure. *Surg Obes Relat Dis.* 2:48, 2006.

Meguid MM, et al. Weight regain after Roux-en-Y: a significant 20% complication related to PYY. *Nutrition.* 24:832, 2008.

NIDDK. Web site accessed January 22, 2010 at http://win.niddk.nih.gov/publications/gastric.htm#adolescent.

Picot J, et al. The clinical effectiveness and cost-effectiveness of bariatric (weight loss) surgery for obesity: a systematic review and economic evaluation. *Health Technol Assess.* 13:1, 2009.

Pories W, Albrecht R. Etiology of type II diabetes mellitus: role of the foregut. *World J Surg.* 25:527, 2001.

Puzziferri N. Psychologic issues in bariatric surgery—the surgeon's perspective. *Surg Clin North Am.* 85:741, 2005.

Rendon SE, Pories WJ. Quality assurance in bariatric surgery. *Surg Clin North Am.* 85:757, 2005.

Service GJ, et al. Hyperinsulinemic hypoglycemia with nesidioblastosis after gastric-bypass surgery. *N Engl J Med.* 353:249, 2005.

Sharma SK, et al. Acute changes in renal function after laparoscopic gastric surgery for morbid obesity. *Surg Obes Relat Dis.* 2:389, 2006.

Shuster MH, Vasquez JA. Nutritional concerns related to Roux-en-Y gastric bypass: what every clinician needs to know. *Crit Care Nurs Q.* 28:227, 2005.

Tan JC, et al. Severe ataxia, myelopathy, and peripheral neuropathy due to acquired copper deficiency in a patient with history of gastrectomy. *JPEN J Parenter Enteral Nutr.* 30:446, 2006.

Torquati A, et al. Is Roux-en-Y gastric bypass surgery the most effective treatment for type 2 diabetes mellitus in morbidly obese patients? *J Gastrointest Surg.* 9:1112, 2005.

Xanthakos SA. Nutritional deficiencies in obesity and after bariatric surgery. *Pediatr Clin North Am.* 56:1105, 2009.

BOWEL SURGERY

NUTRITIONAL ACUITY RANKING: LEVEL 3

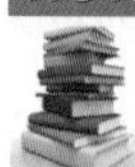

DEFINITIONS AND BACKGROUND

Small bowel surgery may be needed for inflammatory bowel disease, intestinal blockage, precancerous polyps, cancer, necrotizing enterocolitis, and other problems. Emergency surgical procedures in patients with inflammatory bowel disease are rare but can have a high morbidity unless carefully managed. Patients with short bowel syndrome (SBS) may have a higher than average prevalence of small intestinal bacterial overgrowth and may be at risk for septicemia due to bacterial translocation while on PN (Walzer and Buchman, 2010.) Failure to provide enteral nutrients creates a physiologic profile that exacerbates oxidative stress and increases the systemic inflammatory response syndrome (McClave and Heyland, 2009.)

After small bowel surgery, SBS occurs. Earlier feeding may reduce the risk of postsurgical complications after gastrointestinal (GI) surgery (Andersen et al, 2006.) When possible, early enteral feeding should be attempted (Lewis et al, 2009.). Residual small bowel length remains an important predictor of duration of the need for PN.

Most people with SBS experience spontaneous small bowel adaptation over time, when they can be weaned from PN. There are some individuals who cannot be weaned and are potential candidates for techniques to promote intestinal adaptation. Small bowel transplantation has become the treatment of choice for patients with chronic intestinal failure, whose illness cannot be managed with medications or who cannot be maintained on home parenteral nutrition. Rejection, bacterial translocation, and sepsis rates are high.

Colectomy removes part or all of the colon. A colostomy or ileostomy creates an opening on the abdomen (stoma) for the drainage of feces; it may be permanent or temporary. Patients who have an ileostomy lose a considerable amount of fluid that contains sodium and potassium. Fat and vitamin B_{12} absorption is reduced. See section 7 for more details on nutritional management.

Patients who have had a **hemorrhoidectomy** usually tolerate a low-residue diet to delay defecation and allow healing at operative site. After patient is healed, it is important to have patient return to a high-fiber diet to prevent constipation.

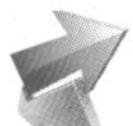

ASSESSMENT, MONITORING, AND EVALUATION

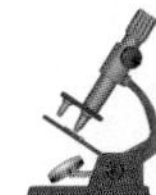

CLINICAL INDICATORS

Clinical/History

Height
Weight
Body mass index (BMI)
Weight changes
Diet history
Blood pressure (BP)
Intake and output (I & O)
Nausea, vomiting, anorexia
Constipation
Infection or pressure ulcers
History of dehydration?

Lab Work

Gluc
CRP
Platelet count
Alb, transthyretin
BUN, Creat
Na^+, K^+
Ca^{++}, Mg^{++}
Serum Osm
N balance
PT, INR
H & H
Serum Fe, ferritin
Vitamin B_{12}

INTERVENTION

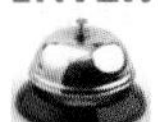

OBJECTIVES

Preoperative

- Replenish depleted reserves by using special immune-enhanced formulas. Uninterrupted enteral nutrition (before, during, and after surgery) is popular in practice to achieve energy intake goals.
- Mechanical bowel preparation before surgery offers no major benefits.

Postoperative

- Restore enteral autonomy (Weseman and Gilroy, 2005).
- Early enteral feeding is generally recommended; this downregulates systemic immune responses, reduces oxidative stress, and improves patient outcome (McClave and Heyland, 2009.)
- Slowly progress back to a normal diet. Progress from clear liquids to soft—solid diet and avoid dairy products if there is lactose intolerance. Modify diet, as needed, for part of bowel that was affected.
- Correct inadequate digestion or absorption of fluid, electrolytes, and nutrients (Matarese et al, 2005).
- Prevent complications, such as peritonitis or ileus. Chewing gum can prevent ileus in some patients.
- Coordinate efforts with a transplantation team to restore nutritional autonomy to transplantation recipients (Weseman and Gilroy, 2005). Successful transplantation recipients can resume unrestricted oral diet eventually.
- Fight surgical infections by adding probiotics to enteral nutrition (EN) improve the immune status of the colon.

SAMPLE NUTRITION CARE PROCESS STEPS

Inadequate Fluid Intake

Assessment Data: Food records, input and output reports showing poor fluid intake, medication history, assessment of depression following bowel surgery for cancer. Showing signs of dehydration.

Nutrition Diagnosis (PES): Inadequate fluid intake related to semiconscious state after bowel surgery and decreased oral intake as evidenced by I & O records showing only 800 mL intake for the past 3 days. Poor skin turgor, sunken eyeballs.

Intervention: Food-Nutrient Delivery—Add extra fluids to meal trays; encourage nursing to provide at least 4–5 oz with each medication given. Educate family and nursing staff about desired fluid intake; ensure that I & O records are kept accurately. Counsel about the dangers of dehydration. Coordinate care with medical team to increase fluid intake.

Monitoring and Evaluation: Improved fluid intake as per I & O records; achieving 35 mL/Kg fluid goal.

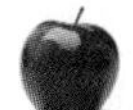

FOOD AND NUTRITION

Preoperative

- Regress from soft diet to full liquids and then clear liquids.
- If needed, use a hydrolyzed formula or jejunostomy.

Postoperative

- Enteral nutrition is a primary therapy. Growth hormone, GLN, short-chain fatty acids, and fermentable fiber sources are useful. Intestinal rehabilitation regimens provide specialized oral diets, soluble fiber, oral rehydration solutions, and tropic factors to enhance absorption (Matarese et al, 2005).
- Probiotics may be beneficial (Floch et al, 2006).
- Slowly progress from a low-residue diet to a normal diet. Suggest that patient eat slowly and chew foods well. Excesses of fiber should be avoided. Probiotics may be included (Jenkins et al, 2005).
- Focus on adequate fluids; needs are usually greater than normal.
- Long-term nutritional support may be needed; CPN may be required for a short time.

Common Drugs Used and Potential Side Effects

- Drugs used will be for the specific condition and side effects of surgery. New medications to reduce rejection in transplant patients are under study.

Herbs, Botanicals, and Supplements

- Answer questions about the use of herbs and botanicals; stop them before surgery.
- Patients may benefit from prebiotics and probiotics to decrease sepsis. Use with caution.

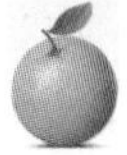

NUTRITION EDUCATION, COUNSELING, CARE MANAGEMENT

- Evaluate and discuss preoperative weight loss, eating problems and fears, nutritional intake evaluations, frequency of eating away from home, and cooking and shopping habits. Discuss changes that will be needed after the specific bowel surgery. See section 7 for ileostomy and colostomy guidance.

Patient Education—Food Safety

Surgical patients may be vulnerable to foodborne illness; safe food handling and handwashing are essential.

For More Information

- The American College of Gastroenterology
  http://www.acg.gi.org
- Atlas of Gastrointestinal Endoscopy
  http://www.endoatlas.com/atlas_1.html
- Bowel Sounds
  http://www.nlm.nih.gov/medlineplus/ency/article/003137.htm
- Ileostomy, Colostomy, and Other Surgery
  http://digestive.niddk.nih.gov/ddiseases/pubs/ileostomy/index.htm
- Ostomy
  http://www.cpmc.org/learning/documents/crm-ostomysurg-ws.html
- Small Bowel Resection
  http://www.nlm.nih.gov/medlineplus/ency/article/002943.htm
- Society for American Gastroenterological and Endoscopic Surgeons
  http://www.sages.org/
- Society for Surgery of the Gastrointestinal Tract
  http://www.ssat.com/

BOWEL SURGERY—CITED REFERENCES

Andersen AK, et al. Early enteral nutrition within 24 h of colorectal surgery versus later commencement of feeding for postoperative complications. *Cochrane Database Syst Rev.* (4):CD004080, 2006.

Floch MH, et al. Recommendations for probiotic use. *J Clin Gastroenterol.* 40:275, 2006.

Jenkins B, et al. Probiotics: a practical review of their role in specific clinical scenarios. *Nutr Clin Pract.* 20:262, 2005.

Lewis SJ, et al. Early enteral nutrition within 24 h of intestinal surgery versus later commencement of feeding: a systematic review and meta-analysis. *J Gastrointest Surg.* 13:569, 2009.

Matarese LE, et al. Short bowel syndrome: clinical guidelines for nutrition management. *Nutr Clin Pract.* 20:493, 2005.

McClave SA, Heyland DK. The physiologic response and associated clinical benefits from provision of early enteral nutrition. *Nutr Clin Pract.* 24:305, 2009.

Walzer N, Buchman AL. Development of Crohn's disease in patients with intestinal failure: A role for bacteria? [published online ahead of print January 5, 2010]. *J Clin Gastroenterol.* 44:361, 2010.

Weseman RA, Gilroy R. Nutrition management of small bowel transplant patients. *Nutr Clin Pract.* 20:509, 2005.

S E C T I O N 15

AIDS and Immunology, Burns, Sepsis and Trauma

CHIEF ASSESSMENT FACTORS

- Accidents or Trauma
- Altered Breathing
- Altered White Blood Cell (WBC) Count and Differential
- Anemia
- Anorexia, Malnutrition
- Culture Results, Specimens
- Environmental Sanitation and Level of Personal Hygiene
- Fever, Chills
- Fluid Status, Edema
- Infection, Sepsis (Heat, Pain, Redness, Swelling, or Drainage in Any Area)
- Indicators of Immunity (T Cells, Other Lymphocytes)
- Medications, Prescription and Over-the-Counter
- Metabolic Rate (Indirect Calorimetry or Estimated)
- Multiple Organ Dysfunction Syndrome (MODS)
- Nutritional Status for Zinc, Iron, Selenium; Vitamins A, C, E; Albumin, CRP
- Presence of Chronic Diseases
- Pulse Rate
- Recent Illness or Surgery
- Urinary Changes (Frequency, Urgency, Burning)

OVERVIEW OF NUTRITION AND IMMUNOCOMPETENCE

The interdependency between the disciplines of nutrition and immunology has been recognized for many decades. Fetal and early infant programming of thymic function suggests that early environments have long-term implications for immunocompetence and adult disease risk. Nutrition and physical growth affect immunocompetence and morbidity from infections.

Common diseases such as atopy and allergy, autoimmunity, chronic infections, and sepsis are characterized by a dysregulation of the pro- versus anti-inflammatory and T helper (Th) 1 versus Th2 cytokine balance. Proinflammatory cytokines promote atherosclerosis, major depression, visceral-type obesity, metabolic syndrome, and sleep disturbances (Elenkov et al, 2005).

Studies regarding the role of nutrients on gene expression and cytokine production have established the importance of maintaining a balanced immune system throughout life. Lack of adequate macronutrients or selected micronutrients, especially zinc, selenium, iron, and the antioxidant vitamins, can lead to clinically significant immune deficiency and infections, especially in children (Cunningham-Rundles et al, 2005). Reduced number of lymphocytes causes loss of host defense in zinc deficiency. In turn, infections aggravate micronutrient deficiencies by reducing nutrient intake, increasing losses, and altering metabolic pathways (Wintergerst et al, 2007). See Table 15-1 and Table 15-2.

Large variations in immunity relate to genetics, age, gender, smoking habits, exercise habits, alcohol consumption, diet, stage in the female menstrual cycle, stress, history of infections, vaccinations and early life exposures. Sound nutritional practices, stress management, good hygiene and sanitation, adequate rest and sleep, and maintaining healthy physical activity can enhance immunocompetence and reduce risks of infection in any population. Even in older adults, improved nutrition can decrease risks for infection. Nutritional supplementation may reduce this risk and reverse some of the immune dysfunction associated with advanced age. The role of calorie restriction and zinc on immunity, aging, autoimmunity, and malignancy has been studied extensively; adding omega-3 fatty acids (fish oil) is also beneficial (Fernandes, 2008).

Hospital admission screening that best identifies patients who are at risk for malnutrition-related complications include presence of a wound, poor oral intake or evident malnutrition, low serum albumin or hemoglobin values, and low total lymphocyte count (TLC) (Brugler et al, 2005). The ability of admission information to accurately reflect malnutrition-related complication risk is crucial to early initiation of restorative medical nutritional therapy (Brugler et al, 2005). New approaches exploring the link through nutrigenomics, proteomics, and metabolomics may provide insight into controlling age-related diseases by following a balanced diet intake (Fernandes, 2008). Table 15-3 provides a list of key nutrients for immunocompetence. Table 15-4 provides important factors to consider in critical illness. Table 15-5 lists nutritional implications in some specific conditions, and Table 15-6 lists virulence increased by iron supplementation.

TABLE 15-1 How the Immune System Works

The immune system is designed to provide protection from invading organisms, including bacteria and viruses, tumor cells, dirt, pollen, and other foreign material. Normally, barriers from the skin and linings of the lungs and gastrointestinal (GI) and reproductive tracts protect the underlying tissues from the outside environment. Whenever there is a breakdown in the protective lining, germs and other irritants can enter the body. The immune system is designed to conquer these foreign molecules by engulfing them or by destroying them with enzymes or other detoxifying means. In addition to fighting off these foreign invaders, the immune system has evolved to destroy abnormal cells (such as tumor cells) but occasionally reacts against the body's own normal tissues (autoimmunity).
Innate and Acquired Immunity
The two principal types of immune response, innate and adaptive (acquired) immunity, are distinguished from one another by both their speed and specificity. The innate immune system, present from birth, involves nonspecific responses that are the first line of defense against common infectious agents, including bacteria and viruses. This system is generally able to recognize foreign organisms but is unable to distinguish between particular invaders. Thus, an innate response does not require stimulation by sophisticated cell-to-cell interactions to remove bacteria or other foreign material and degrade it. The more specific adaptive (acquired) immune system must be triggered by a specific virus, bacterium, or other foreign material, which stimulates lymphocytes to produce antibodies that can combat the foreign substance. At the next exposure, the preformed antibodies will allow the person to respond with an even stronger, more specific response known as *immunological memory*.
Cells of the Immune System
The immune system consists of white blood cells (WBCs, leukocytes), which are produced in the bone marrow and mature there or in the thymus and other lymphoid organs. Leukocytes circulate in the blood along with oxygen-carrying red blood cells. Under normal conditions, leukocytes leave the circulation and migrate into organs where germs can appear, including the skin, lungs, intestine, and reproductive tract. There, they can wait for infectious agents, or they can migrate back through the circulation to other organs.

(continued)

TABLE 15-1 How the Immune System Works *(continued)*

There are three major types of leukocytes. *Neutrophils* are the most plentiful and are the first line of defense; they contain an arsenal of preformed enzymes that are capable of destroying bacteria. In addition, they are phagocytic, and they engulf viruses, bacteria, or other foreign material, protecting the host from further damage. Neutrophils are very short-lived, often destroyed during the fight. *Monocytes* are leukocytes that migrate to tissues and mature into macrophages. Macrophages are phagocytic and can remove foreign material and parts of dead cells from the tissues. They contain enzymes that can destroy infectious material but live longer than neutrophils and do not tend to self-destruct as easily. The tissue macrophage in the liver is called the Kupffer cell. *Lymphocytes* are selective, specialized WBCs that combat specific infectious agents.

The two types of lymphocytes are B cells and T cells. *B cells* are responsible for humoral immunity in the body fluids (classically known as the humors); they release specialized, soluble protein antibodies into the blood and other body fluids. The antibodies recognize and bind to the surface of foreign substances (i.e., pathogens), immobilizing them and further labeling them as foreign so that they can be more readily taken up by phagocytic cells. *T cells*, in contrast, act directly on other cells rather than manufacturing antibodies. Because of this direct interaction with other cells, T cells are responsible for cellular immunity. They can be further divided into *helper T cells*, which recognize foreign invaders and stimulate immune responses from other cells, and *cytotoxic T cells*, which destroy infected cells. Some of these cells are extremely long-lived "memory cells," capable of remembering certain features on the foreign molecules so that, if the organism encounters that foreign molecule in the future, it can quickly stimulate a response.

Communication Between Immune Cells: Cytokines

One form of communication between immune cells is *direct cell-to-cell contact*, which can occur either as a loose, transient association or as a tighter, long-lasting encounter. Either way, cells must make physical contact with one another. In the second form of contact, cells release small proteins called *cytokines*, which bind to specific receptors on the surface of target cells.

Cytokines interact only with the appropriate target cell and not with surrounding cells. Although many of the effects of cytokines are local, they have been called the hormones of the immune system because they are transported by the circulating blood. Cytokines can affect the same cell that produced them, a neighboring cell, or a cell far away. They stimulate or dampen cell proliferation (replication), production of other cytokines, killing of damaged cells or tumor cells (cytotoxicity), and cell migration (chemotaxis). The latter response is controlled by a subset, chemokines. Just as there are cells that can stimulate or inhibit immune response, cytokines can regulate a variety of cell functions either positively or negatively. *Interleukin-6* is an important cytokine. Excessive production of proinflammatory cytokines or their production in the wrong biological context may lead to chronic inflammation and negative health consequences.

Gut Immunity

An extremely important function of the GI tract is its ability to regulate the flow of macromolecules between the environment and the host through a barrier mechanism. The GI immune response maintains critical pathways in the body. Gut-associated lymphoid tissue (GALT) is the dominant location for initiation of mucosal immune response and is dependent on fats, amino acids, and micronutrients. A healthy GI mucosal immune system provides barriers against systemic access for food antigens and microbes. Changes in the GALT immune response may contribute to intestinal dysfunction and susceptibility to postinjury gut-derived sepsis. Together with GALT and the neuroendocrine network, the intestinal epithelial barrier controls the equilibrium between tolerance and immunity to non–self-antigens (Fasano and Shea-Donohue, 2005). Because genetic and mucosal immunity strongly influence the composition and function of enteric bacteria, strategies are needed to correct dysfunctional microbiota in genetically susceptible individuals and to correct dysbiosis in many inflammatory disorders (Hansen et al, 2010).

REFERENCE

Fasano A, Shea-Donohue T. Mechanisms of disease: the role of intestinal barrier function in the pathogenesis of gastrointestinal autoimmune diseases. *Nat Clin Pract Gastroenterol Hepatol.* 2:416, 2005.
Hansen J, et al. The role of mucosal immunity and host genetics in defining intestinal commensal bacteria. *Curr Opin Gastroenterol.* 26:564, 2010.

TABLE 15-2 Immunocompetence and Immunity Concerns

Almost all nutrients in the diet play a crucial role in maintaining an optimal immune response. Thus, deficient and excessive intakes can have negative consequences on immune status and susceptibility to a variety of pathogens. In addition, botanical and herbal products can be a concern. While Echinacea is used to reduce symptoms of the "common cold" or flu, there is a risk of hepatotoxicity, exacerbation of allergies or asthma, and even anaphylactic reactions. Garlic is also used to relieve cough, colds, and rhinitis but gastrointestinal disturbances, allergic reactions, or hypoglycemia can occur. Other agents, including angelica, German chamomile flower, ephedra, ginkgo, grape seed extract, licorice root, St. John's wort, kava-kava rhizome, peppermint, stinging nettle, and ginseng, may also have undesirable side effects (see Section 2).

Nutrition and dietary patterns have been shown to have direct impact on health of the population and of selected patient groups, related to a reduction of oxidative damage from free radical production (Berger, 2005). Insufficient intake of micronutrients occurs in people with eating disorders, in smokers (both active and passive), in individuals with chronic alcohol abuse, in patients who are immunocompromised or malnourished, during pregnancy and lactation, and in the elderly (Wintergerst et al, 2007; Happel and Nelson, 2005). Concerns are listed here.

Infants	Undernutrition in critical periods of gestation and neonatal maturation and during weaning impairs the development of a normal immune system. There is a high prevalence of micronutrient deficiencies and infectious diseases in infants in developing countries. Breastfed infants have lower morbidity and mortality due to diarrhea than those fed formula; human milk oligosaccharides protect against pathogens (Newburg et al, 2005).

(continued)

TABLE 15-2 Immunocompetence and Immunity Concerns *(continued)*

Young children	Risks and adverse functional and health outcomes may be associated with deficient and excessive intakes and nutrition status of iron, iodine, zinc, vitamins A and D, folate, vitamin B_{12}, and riboflavin in children. Altered growth and development, mental and neuromotor performance, immunocompetence, physical working capacity, and morbidity can result. Vitamin C and zinc may reduce the incidence and improve the outcome of pneumonia, malaria, and diarrhea infections, especially in developing countries (Wintergerst et al, 2005).
Older adults	Adults 65 years and older comprise the fastest-growing segment of the U.S. population. Older adults experience greater morbidity and mortality due to infection than do young adults (High et al, 2005). Nutritional factors can modify susceptibility to disease and promote healthy aging. Interleukin-6 (IL-6), a cytokine, is tightly controlled by hormonal feedback (estrogen, testosterone) that is lost in the aging process. Elevated IL-6 levels progressively increase and may promote tumorigenesis, osteoporosis, neurodegenerative diseases, and sarcopenia. Zinc is important for immune efficiency (innate and adaptive), antioxidant activity (superoxide dismutase), and cell differentiation (Mocchegiani et al, 2007). Use of a daily multivitamin/mineral supplement that contains 100% of the Dietary Reference Intakes (DRIs) may be encouraged.
Upper respiratory infections	The role of large doses of vitamin C to reduce duration or severity of cold symptoms has been inconclusive. Vitamin E supplementation may reduce the incidence of respiratory infections among the elderly. Echinacea or ginseng may also be modestly protective (Predy et al, 2005).
Immunocompromised persons (cancer, AIDS, tuberculosis)	Supplementation of vitamin C improves antimicrobial and natural killer cell activities, lymphocyte proliferation, chemotaxis, and delayed-type hypersensitivity (Wintergerst et al, 2005). Glutamine, arginine, fatty acids, and vitamin E provide some additional benefits for immunocompromised persons or patients who suffer from various infections but avoid excesses of arginine in septic patients. Chronic undernutrition and infection further weaken the immune response. Assessment of immunocompetence by available methods can identify individuals who are most in need of appropriate nutritional support to enhance host defense to infectious pathogens
Undernutrition	Iron and vitamin A deficiencies and protein–energy malnutrition are highly prevalent worldwide. Vitamin A and zinc play important roles in protecting individuals from severity in illnesses such as diarrhea and HIV infection. Zinc undernutrition or deficiency impairs cellular phagocytosis, natural killer cell activity, and the generation of oxidative burst (Wintergerst et al, 2005).
Overnutrition	Obesity caused by excess nutrition or excess storage of fats relative to energy expenditure is a form of malnutrition. Leptin is a cytokine-like immune regulator that has complex effects in both overnutrition and in the inflammatory response in malnutrition.
Surgical patients	Preoperative oral intake of immunonutrition containing omega-3 fatty acids, arginine, and nucleotides at home may prevent the risks of hospitalization and may lead to immunomodulating effects, which can improve nutritional status (see Section 14). Postsurgical or septic patients given branched-chain amino acids intravenously show improved immunity and improved outcomes (Calder, 2006).
Trauma	Sepsis and multiple organ failure have mortality rates of up to 80%. Vitamin C concentrations in the plasma and leukocytes rapidly decline during infections and stress (Wintergerst et al, 2005).

REFERENCES

Berger MM. Can oxidative damage be treated nutritionally? *Clin Nutr.* 24:172, 2005.
Calder PC. Branched-chain amino acids and immunity. *J Nutr.* 136:288S, 2006.
Happel KI, Nelson S. Alcohol, immunosuppression, and the lung. *Proc Am Thorac Soc.* 2:428, 2005.
High KP, et al. A new paradigm for clinical investigation of infectious syndromes in older adults: assessment of functional status as a risk factor and outcome measure. *Clin Infect Dis.* 40:114, 2005.
Mocchegiani E, et al. Zinc, metallothioneins, and longevity—effect of zinc supplementation: zincage study. *Ann N Y Acad Sci.* 1119:129, 2007.
Newburg DS, et al. Human milk glycans protect infants against enteric pathogens. *Annu Rev Nutr.* 25:37, 2005.
Predy GN, et al. Efficacy of an extract of North American ginseng containing poly-furanosyl-pyranosyl-saccharides for preventing upper respiratory tract infections: a randomized controlled trial. *CMAJ.* 173:1043, 2005.
Wintergerst ES, et al. Immune-enhancing role of vitamin C and zinc and effect on clinical conditions. *Ann Nutr Metab.* 50:85, 2005.
Wintergerst ES, et al. Contribution of selected vitamins and trace elements to immune function. *Ann Nutr Metab.* 51:301, 2007.

TABLE 15-3 Nutritional and Host Factors in Immunity

Nutrient status is an important factor contributing to immune competence; undernutrition impairs the immune system, suppressing immune functions that are fundamental to host protection. Both macronutrients and micronutrients are essential. Protein is very important. Branched-chain amino acids (BCAAs) and other essential amino acids support synthesis of protein, RNA, and DNA in lymphocytes to respond to pathogens. Arginine and glutamine support a healthy gut and healing processes, but excesses are to be avoided. To prevent protein use for energy, sufficient carbohydrate intake is needed. Fats, especially omega-3 fatty acids, provide needed calories and support the immune system.

Vitamin A deficiency impairs both innate and adaptive immune responses to infection. Carotenoids such as beta-carotene, lycopene, and zeaxanthin protect the immune system. As a precursor of NAD+, the substrate for DNA repair, niacin contributes to genomic stability (Moccegiani et al, 2008). Antioxidant vitamins C and E counteract damage caused by reactive oxygen species and modulate immune cell function (Wintergerst et al, 2007). Excesses of vitamin E must be avoided as they can also be immunosuppressive. Vitamin D_3 regulates the differentiation, growth, and function of monocytes, dendritic cells, and T and B lymphocytes (Equils et al, 2006). Vitamins B_6, folate, B_{12}, C, and E support the Th1 cytokine-mediated immune response with sufficient production of proinflammatory cytokines (Wintergerst et al, 2007). Protection against macular degeneration has been noted with prescriptions that contain omega-3 fatty acids, lutein and zeaxanthin, vitamins C, E, beta-carotene, zinc and copper (Krishnadev et al, 2010).

Minerals and other substances also play an important role. Chromium can enhance the ability of white blood cells to respond to infection. Iron, as lactoferrin, deprives invading cells of their defense systems. Manganese can enhance natural killer cells and macrophage activity; CoQ10 is thought to do the same. Selenium deficiency may allow viruses to mutate into more dangerous pathogens. Selenium, copper, and zinc modulate immune cell function; they, along with iron, help to produce proinflammatory cytokines (Wintergerst et al, 2007). A summary of important factors is listed here.

Infectious Disease Determinants

- Environmental sanitation
- Microorganismic virulence
- Host immunity, including nutritional status
- Personal hygiene

Host-Resistance Factors

- Cell-mediated T cells
- Complement system
- Immunoglobulins, antibodies (B cells)
- Monocytes and dendritic cells
- Mucus and cilia on epithelial surfaces
- Oligosaccharides and other prebiotics
- Phagocytes (leukocytes, macrophages)
- Physical barriers (skin, mucous membranes)
- Probiotic bacteria

Immune System

- Bone marrow (B cells)
- GALT
- Luster patches in bronchioles
- Lymph nodes
- Peyer patches in gut
- Spleen
- Thymus gland (T cells)
- Tonsils

Nutrients of Immunocompetence

- **Macronutrients**
  - Arginine and glutamine
  - Dietary nucleotides (RNA)
  - Essential amino acids (especially BCAAs)
  - Linoleic acid (essential fatty acid)
  - Omega-3 fatty acids
- **Micronutrient Vitamins**
  - Vitamin A; carotenoids
  - Iron
  - Magnesium and CoQ10
  - Manganese
- Folic acid, vitamin B_6, vitamin B_{12}
- Niacin
- Vitamin C
- Vitamin D
- Vitamin E
- **Micronutrient Minerals**
  - Chromium
  - Copper
  - Selenium
  - Zinc

Immunonutrition

- To provide immunonutrition, enteral feeding can be supplemented with arginine, glutamine, omega-3 polyunsaturated fatty acids (PUFAs), and nucleotides.
- Immunonutrition is a less invasive alternative to immunotherapy to lessen chronic inflammation.
- Excessive intravenous lipid can be deleterious due to the proinflammatory effects of omega-6 fatty acids. Omega-3 fatty acids are anti-inflammatory and, combined with medium-chain triglycerides and olive oil, they are more desirable (Grimble, 2005).
- Antioxidants, plant fibers, and live lactic acid bacteria are also important to boost the immune system and reduce inflammation (Bengmark, 2005).

(continued)

TABLE 15-3 Nutritional and Host Factors in Immunity *(continued)*

Nutrient–Nutrient Interactions, Excesses, and Immunocompetence

- Under most circumstances the systemic inflammatory response is beneficial to the host, improving the eventual outcome of injury or infection.
- Chronic, excessive inflammation may lead to cardiac, hepatic, and mitochondrial dysfunction.
- Excessive counterinflammation leads to immune depression; excesses of iron, zinc, vitamin E, and PUFA interfere with immunity, especially if given intravenously or intramuscularly.
- Excess calcium interferes with leukocyte function by displacing magnesium.
- Long-term parenteral nutrition reduces immune functions (Bengmark, 2005). Parenteral iron and zinc are to be used with great caution; central parenteral nutrition is contraindicated in septic patients.
- Associations for "zinc plus selenium and niacin" have a role in healthy immunity, especially in the aging process (Moccegiani et al, 2008).

REFERENCES

Bengmark S. Bio-ecological control of acute pancreatitis: the role of enteral nutrition, pro and synbiotics. *Curr Opin Clin Nutr Metab Care.* 8:557, 2005.

Grimble RF. Immunonutrition. *Curr Opin Gastroenterol.* 21:216, 2005.

Krishnadev N, et al. Nutritional supplements for age-related macular degeneration. *Curr Opin Ophthalmol.* 21:184, 2010.

Moccegiani E, et al. Zinc, metallothioneins and longevity: interrelationships with niacin and selenium. *Curr Pharm Des.* 14:2719, 2008.

Wintergerst ES, et al. Contribution of selected vitamins and trace elements to immune function. *Ann Nutr Metab.* 51:301, 2007.

TABLE 15-4 Factors of Importance in Critical Care

Metabolic complications can occur from overfeeding critically ill patients. In general, current practice is to underfeed slightly rather than to overfeed: 20–25 kcal/kg actual body weight ABW is recommended; use 30% fat.

Indirect calorimetry (IC) remains the best method of determining a patient's energy needs. IC decreases complications from overfeeding and saves costs by reducing length of stay. Use a combination of prediction equations, clinical judgment, and monitoring of the appropriateness of the nutrition prescription.

- Harris–Benedict equation: using ABW or IBW in the calculation tends to underestimate energy needs (Campbell et al, 2005).
- Ireton–Jones formula: tends to overestimate the energy needs of mechanically ventilated patients (Campbell et al, 2005).

Maintain protein at approximately 1.5 g/kg. In critical illness, glutamine levels are much higher in the duodenal mucosa than during starvation; glutamine supplementation may be beneficial (De-Souza and Greene, 2005).

Arginine is a conditionally essential amino acid. It is a substrate for protein synthesis but can also be metabolized to various compounds, including nitric oxide, ornithine, and creatine phosphate, that are important for growth, wound healing, cardiovascular function, immune function, inflammatory responses, energy metabolism, urea cycle function, and other metabolic processes. Arginine supplementation improves outcomes with sepsis, wounds, ischemia-reperfusion injury, and burns.

The use of specific nutrients to modify immune, inflammatory, and metabolic processes offers the possibility for reducing morbidity following major surgery (Heys et al, 2005). Trace elements and antioxidant nutrients, especially selenium, are important for use in critical care and may reduce mortality (Heyland et al, 2005). Vitamin E levels tend to be low and may be supplemented accordingly. Use of omega-3 fatty acids is also important.

In general, enteral nutrition poses fewer risks than parenteral nutrition. Calories and protein that are delivered early by the enteral route have a significant effect on outcome in patients in critical care units; specific nutrients may also be needed to replace acute deficiencies brought on by specific injury or disease states (Wischmeyer and Heyland, 2010).

Control of hyperglycemia is very important to lessen infection and sepsis (Butler et al, 2005).

REFERENCES

Butler SO, et al. Relationship between hyperglycemia and infection in critically ill patients. *Pharmacotherapy.* 25:963, 2005.

Campbell CG, et al. Predicted vs measured energy expenditure in critically ill, underweight patients. *Nutr Clin Pract.* 20:276, 2005.

De-Souza DA, Greene LJ. Intestinal permeability and systemic infections in critically ill patients: effect of glutamine. *Crit Care Med.* 33:1125, 2005.

Heyland DK, et al. Antioxidant nutrients: a systematic review of trace elements and vitamins in the critically ill patient. *Intensive Care Med.* 31:327, 2005.

Heys SD, et al. Nutrition and the surgical patient: triumphs and challenges. *Surgeon.* 3:139, 2005.

Wischmeyer PE, Heyland DK. The future of critical care nutrition therapy. *Crit Care Clin.* 26:433, 2010.

TABLE 15-5 Infections and Febrile Conditions and Nutritional Implications

Emergence of new infectious diseases and old diseases with new properties may affect the whole world; severe acute respiratory syndrome and avian flu are examples.

Condition, Nutritional Acuity, Background	Nutritional Implications
Bacterial endocarditis, Level 3 Bacterial endocarditis is an infection (often *Streptococcus*) of the membrane lining the heart chambers, often occurring after rheumatic fever. It accounts for 2% of all cases of organic heart disease. Symptoms and signs include fever, chills, joint pain, lassitude, anorexia, weight loss, and malaise.	Restore patient's nutritional status to normal. Replenish electrolytes and fluids. Reduce edema, if present. Prevent heart failure, infections, anemia, embolism, and nephritis. Penicillin, erythromycin, and other antibiotics may be used; monitor for timing of meals and drugs. Use a high-energy and high-protein diet. If patient's appetite is poor, encourage intake of favorite foods. Ensure adequate intake of fluids, vitamins, and minerals, especially vitamins A and C. Antibiotic prophylaxis is generally needed before dental work.
Candidiasis, Level 2 *Candida albicans* is normally found in the mouth, feces, and vagina. Greater colonization occurs in debilitated persons in whom thrush or vaginitis or cutaneous lesions are common. Susceptible individuals are those with leukemias, those who are immunosuppressed or on long-term central parenteral nutrition, and those who are obese or have diabetes.	Prevent or treat systemic infections. Prevent endocarditis, emboli, splenomegaly, and other complications. Correct underlying conditions when possible. Ensure a diet high in quality proteins, fluid, and calories. Use regular meals and small, frequent snacks; avoid skipping meals or fasting. Increase vitamin and mineral intake from tolerated fruits and vegetables, especially for vitamins A and C. Nystatin or amphotericin B may be used; diarrhea, nausea, and stomach pain may occur. Synthetic antimicrobial peptides are under development for use in oral candidiasis.
***Clostridium difficile*-infection, Level 3** The common name is *Clostridium difficile*-associated disease (CDAD;) it is hard to treat. Suppression of gastric acid with proton pump inhibitor drugs such as Prilosec (omeprazole) or Nexium (esomeprazole) is associated with a 2–3 times increase in community-acquired CDAD. *C. difficile* causes one fourth of nosocomial antibiotic-associated diarrheas. The incidence is rising, with more colectomy and mortality.	Repeat antibiotics are indicated, either metronidazole or vancomycin. Tapering the dose after a 10-day course decreases the incidence of recurrences compared with abruptly stopping antibiotics. Long-term use of metronidazole may cause neurotoxicity. Vancomycin followed by rifaximin or immune therapy are treatments under study. Probiotics such as *Saccharomyces boulardii* may decrease recurrences when combined with high-dose vancomycin.
Chronic fatigue and immune dysfunction syndrome (CFIDS), Level 1 CFIDS is a serious health concern affecting more than 800,000 Americans of all ages, races, socioeconomic groups, and genders. CFIDS involves severe exhaustion, weakness, headaches, sore throat, tender lymph nodes, unrefreshing sleep, fever, muscle aches, inability to concentrate, and depression. Symptoms tend to mimic lupus or even cancer. Testing for viral load is helpful. There may be a link to Hodgkin disease or multiple sclerosis; patients may have neurally mediated hypotension.	Improve immunological status and prevent malnutrition. Lessen severity of symptoms. Avoid infections and stress to prevent recurrent attacks, where possible. Discourage use of high fat diets. Provide adequate protein (0.8–1 g/kg) and 35 kcal/kg. Include adequate vitamins, minerals, and antioxidant foods. Extra salt or fluids may be needed for hypotension. Fludrocortisone promotes sodium retention. Use analgesics for aches and pain. A multidisciplinary approach is beneficial. Traditional Chinese medicine has shown some merit in reducing sleeplessness and fatigue.
Encephalitis and Reye syndrome, Level 2 Encephalitis involves an inflammation of brain cells, usually by a virus such as measles, mumps, mononucleosis, or herpes simplex. If caused by the tsetse fly, it is known as *African sleeping sickness*. **Reye syndrome** is a disease of the brain and liver, affecting mostly children and teenagers after viral illness. Symptoms include headache, lethargy, nightmares, heavy vomiting; stupor and fatty liver; coma, double vision; hypoglycemia; multiple organ failure, or even death.	Ease symptoms. Allow natural defense system to work. Assist breathing with respirator if necessary. Control any pernicious vomiting. Tube feed if patient is comatose. A ketogenic diet may help when there are seizures. Otherwise, use a high-protein, high-calorie diet with a multivitamin–mineral supplement and extra fluids. If steroid therapy is used, monitor glucose, potassium, and nitrogen levels carefully; reduce sodium in foods if there is edema. Aspirin should be avoided.
Fever, Level 2 Fever is considered to be elevated body temperature >37.5–38.3°C (100–101°F). Fever (pyrexia) may be caused by acute (pneumonia, measles, flu, or chicken pox) or chronic causes (tuberculosis, hepatitis, or malaria). Disturbed thermoregulation is controlled by the hypothalamus. Prostaglandin E2 (PE2) is released from the arachidonic acid pathway and can help increase leukocyte, phagocyte, T cell and interferon activity. **Hyperpyrexia** is considered to be 41.5°C (106.7°F). **Fever of unknown origin (FUO)** involves illness for more than 3 weeks with a temperature higher than 101°F. Approximately 40% of FUO is from infections, 20% from cancer, 15% from connective tissue disease, and 25% from undetermined causes.	Meet increased nutrient needs caused by patient's hypermetabolic state, especially energy requirements. Each 1°F elevation causes a 7% increase in metabolic rate. Replace nitrogen losses. Replenish carbohydrate since liver stores last only 18–24 hours. Normalize electrolyte status, replace losses from perspiration, and facilitate toxin elimination through increased urine output. Prevent dehydration but avoid water intoxication. Treat anorexia, nausea, or vomiting. Adults need 30–40 kcal/kg/day; infants and children need additional calories as well. Monitor weight changes closely. Adults need 1.5–2 g protein/kg if temperature is high and chronic. If fever is acute, patient may prefer liquids. With longer duration, thiamin and vitamins A and C may be depleted, and a supplement may be used. Parenteral zinc or iron supplementation may significantly increase temperature in patients with recent injury or infection; avoid until fever improves. As treatment progresses, a diet with small, frequent feedings can be used. Offer preferred foods according to appetite, such as puddings, shakes, and soups.

(continued)

TABLE 15-5 Infections and Febrile Conditions and Nutritional Implications *(continued)*

Condition, Nutritional Acuity, Background	Nutritional Implications
	Take antipyretics/aspirin with food or milk and avoid alcoholic beverages. Take erythromycin with a full glass of water on an empty stomach to avoid sore mouth, nausea, or diarrhea. Penicillins should not be taken with acidic food or fluids such as fruit juice; so use adequate protein. Take tetracycline on an empty stomach with a full glass of water; avoid milk and dairy products for 2 hours before or after taking tetracycline. Avoid use in pregnancy and in children.
Herpes simplex, Level 1 Herpes simplex involves a viral infection of skin or mucous membranes (herpes simplex I for oral lesions, whereas herpes simplex II usually involves genital/anal area) with vesicular eruptions of repeated frequency. Oral lesions ("cold sores" or "fever blisters") are latent in the nerve cell ganglia of the trigeminal nerve and are triggered by stress. This virus is similar to the chicken pox virus. Testing includes polymerase chain reaction, herpes simplex virus test, and swollen lymph nodes. Herpetic outbreaks are common in HIV-positive and other immunocompromised patients.	Reduce inflammation and duration. Lessen recurrences and virulence. Reduce stress, febrile states, or further complications such as encephalitis or aseptic meningitis. Highlight relaxation and stress reduction techniques. Use high-quality protein and adequate calories. Increase intakes of vitamins A and C. Discuss relationship of nutrition to immune status. Take prescribed medication at first sign of an outbreak. Acyclovir (Zovirax), famciclovir (Famvir), and antiviral agents such as Valtrex are available; nausea, vomiting, or headaches may occur. If interferon is used, gastrointestinal (GI) distress, stomatitis, nausea and vomiting, abdominal pain, and diarrhea may be side effects. A herpes vaccine is being tested.
Herpes zoster (shingles), Level 1 Herpes zoster is an acute viral infection with vesicles, usually confined to a specific nerve tract, and neuralgic pain in the area of the affected nerve. It is a reactivation of the *Varicella* virus (chicken pox); severity correlates with age. Symptoms include pain along the affected nerve tract, fever, malaise, anorexia, and enlarged lymph nodes. Bacterial infection of the lesions, poor nutritional status, and risk of dehydration may occur if rehabilitation requires a long period. There is a comprehensive, sensitive assay that detects simultaneous HSV-1, HSV-2, varicella-zoster virus, human cytomegalovirus, and Epstein–Barr virus (EBV). The Zostavax vaccine is effective.	Facial nerves may be affected; alter diet as needed. Prevent further systemic infection; reduce fever. Correct or prevent malnutrition, constipation, and encephalitis. Hydrate adequately. Prevent or correct unplanned weight loss. Prevent or reduce severity of postherpetic neuralgia, which is a very painful complication. A balanced diet with frequent, small feedings may be needed. Increased fiber may be useful to correct constipation. Adequate vitamins E and B_{12} have been suggested for postherpetic neuralgia. Use adequate vitamins A and C. Acyclovir or famciclovir may shorten the duration and decrease pain. Monitor for GI distress, nausea and vomiting, or diarrhea. Valacyclovir is effective at facilitating healing lesions, reducing pain and postherpetic neuralgia. Narcotics and analgesics are needed to reduce pain. Capsaicin cream from hot peppers has proven to be useful for pain relief. Injecting lidocaine and prednisone directly into spinal column for pain relief of postshingles neuralgia has been tested. Oral prednisone may be used; alter sodium intake and monitor for glucose intolerance.
Infection, Levels 1–2 Infection results from successful invasion, establishment, and growth of microorganisms in a host. Responses involve general and antigen-specific immunological defense systems. In infectious processes, vitamin A is excreted in large amounts from the urine. Correct iron-deficiency anemia, but do not use excesses as microbes depend on iron for growth and proliferation. Iron is mostly protein bound as transferrin. Avoid parenteral or intravenous iron and zinc until fever is resolved.	Provide adequate nourishment to counteract hypermetabolic state. Support body's host defense system. Prevent or correct dehydration, hypoglycemia, complications, and anorexia. Replace nutrient losses (potassium, nitrogen, magnesium, phosphorus, and sulfur). Discuss role of nutrients in maintaining skin and mucous membrane integrity and preventing bacterial invasion and subsequent infections. Use a high-protein, high-calorie diet, rich in vitamins, minerals, and fluids. Needs increase up to 20% in mild infection, 20–40% in moderate, or 40–60% in septic conditions. Administration of antibiotics with or without food is specific to the type of drug used. Avoid caffeine, sodas, and fruit juices when taking penicillins. For tetracycline, avoid milk and dairy products 2 hours before and after taking drug. With amoxicillin (Augmentin), diarrhea, nausea, and vomiting may occur. Cephalosporins (e.g., Ceclor, Cephalexin, Duricef) may cause diarrhea, nausea and vomiting, sore mouth, hypokalemia, and vitamin K deficiency. Griseofulvin for fungal infections should be taken with a high-fat meal; dry mouth, nausea, and diarrhea are common effects. Ketoconazole (Nizoral) is used in fungal infections and should be taken with an acidic liquid such as orange juice; avoid taking ketoconazole within 2 hours of use of calcium or magnesium. Metronidazole (Flagyl) may cause nausea and vomiting, diarrhea, and anorexia; avoid alcoholic beverages.
Influenza (flu) and the common cold, Level 1 The common cold and influenza are the most common syndromes of infection in human beings. Influenza virus is transmitted by respiratory route, generally in the fall and winter months. Incubation is 1–4 days, with abrupt onset. Signs and symptoms include chills, fever for 3–5 days, malaise lasting 2–3 weeks, muscular aching, substernal soreness, nasal stuffiness, sore throat, some nausea, nonproductive cough, and headache. Annual vaccinations are suggested for high-risk populations, including elderly individuals and those individuals with pulmonary diseases. Low humidity, cold weather, or psychological stress may increase susceptibility. Adequate rest and hydration are essential. Discuss infection control.	Reduce fever and relieve symptoms. Chicken soup is actually useful by providing potassium and sodium, as well as fluid; it increases mucus flow. Prevent complications such as Reye syndrome, secondary bacterial infections (especially pneumonia), otitis media, and bronchitis. Promote bed rest, adequate hydration, and calorie intake. Replace fluid and electrolyte losses. Increase fluids from salty broths, juices, and other fluids. A high-energy and protein intake should be encouraged. Small meals and snacks may be better tolerated than three large meals. Adequate vitamins A and C, sodium, and potassium should be considered. Adequate zinc and low zinc status may be a risk factor for pneumonia in the elderly Barnett et al, 2010). Antibiotics may be needed if secondary bacterial infections occur; monitor for proper timing of administration with food and beverages. Amantadine or rimantadine may be helpful, especially in type A flu. Nausea, dry mouth, and constipation may occur. Avoid use of aspirin in children.

(continued)

TABLE 15-5 Infections and Febrile Conditions and Nutritional Implications *(continued)*

Condition, Nutritional Acuity, Background	Nutritional Implications
Meningitis, Level 1 Infection of the meninges causes inflammatory reactions, usually in the pia mater or arachnoid membranes. The condition may be viral or bacterial. Bacterial forms are more likely to be fatal if left untreated. Bacterial forms include *Listeria monocytogenes, Neisseria meningitidis, Haemophilus influenzae,* or *Streptococcus pneumoniae.* Meningitis can be caused by lung or ear infections or by a skull fracture. Symptoms and signs include headache, neck rigidity, fever, tachycardia, tachypnea, nausea and/or vomiting, disorientation, diplopia, altered consciousness, photophobia, petechial rash, irritability, malaise, seizure activity, and dehydration. Spinal tap or lumbar puncture is needed to assess cerebrospinal fluid. Meningitis could lead to septic shock, respiratory failure, or death. It most commonly affects children aged 1 month–2 years. Chronic meningitis can affect people with cancer or HIV/AIDS.	Prevent or correct weight loss. Force fluids but do not overhydrate, especially if there is cerebral edema. Prevent or correct constipation, fever, and other symptoms. Maintain intravenous feedings as appropriate; prevent overhydration. Progress diet, as possible, to high-calorie, high-protein intake. Unless contraindicated, provide 2–3 L of fluid. Adequate fiber will be beneficial to correct or prevent constipation. Gradually return to normal caloric intake for age. Ensure adequate intake of vitamins A and C from fruits, juices, and vegetables. In the long term, control obesity. Antibiotics (penicillin, ampicillin, and cephalosporin) may be used in bacterial forms or to prevent complications in viral forms; nausea, vomiting, and diarrhea can result. If corticosteroids are used, side effects may include nitrogen and calcium losses and sodium retention.
Mononucleosis, Level 1 Infectious mononucleosis is an acute disease caused by EBV; it causes gland swellings in the neck and elsewhere ("glandular fever"). It causes fatigue, malaise, headache, chills, and other symptoms such as sore throat, fever, abdominal pain, jaundice, stiff neck, chest pain, breathing difficulty, cough, and hepatitis. Incubation is 5–15 days. It is most common in those between ages 10 and 35 years. Lab work may include evaluation of increased cerebrospinal fluid pressure, EBV titer, uric acid, and liver enzymes. It is also useful to evaluate a serum agglutination test.	Use a high-protein, high-calorie diet. Use liquids when swallowing solid foods is difficult. Use small, frequent feedings to improve overall nutritional quality and quantity. Ensure adequate intakes of vitamins A and C, especially from fruits and vegetables. Modify food textures when swallowing is difficult. Emphasize importance of exercise in restoring lean body mass. Restore fluid balance. Replenish glucose stores. Spare protein. Restore lost weight. Reduce fever. Prevent complications such as myocarditis, hepatitis, and encephalitis. Acyclovir (Zovirax) may be useful in initial infection, preventing typical persistence; nausea, anorexia, and vomiting may occur. Other antibiotics may be needed for related infections.
Pelvic inflammatory disease (PID), Level 1 PID involves inflammation of the pelvic cavity, affecting the fallopian tubes (salpingitis) and ovaries (oophoritis) with acute pelvic and abdominal pain, low back pain, fever, purulent vaginal discharge, nausea and vomiting, urinary tract infection (UTI), diarrhea, maceration of the vulva, and leukocytosis. Long-term sequelae may include tubal infertility or chronic pelvic pain.	Promote good nutritional status to maintain weight and immunity. Increase hydration as tolerated. Lessen diarrhea, nausea, and vomiting. If nausea or vomiting is extensive, discuss need for small meals and consumption of fluids separately from meals. Provide diet as tolerated with small, frequent feedings until nausea and vomiting subside. Alter fiber and fluid, as needed. Increase energy and protein if needed to improve patient's nutritional status. Ensure adequate intake of all vitamins and minerals, especially vitamins A and C. Antibiotics may be used; quinolones, cephalosporins, metronidazole, and doxycycline may be prescribed. Analgesics are generally used to reduce pain; chronic use may cause GI distress.
Poliomyelitis, Level 1 A highly contagious enterovirus, poliomyelitis attacks the motor neurons of the brain stem and spinal cord; it may or may not cause paralysis. Polio is transmitted by personal contact, by eating contaminated food, or by drinking contaminated fluids. Polio is rare in areas where the vaccine is available, but there are risks in areas where the vaccine is not administered to all members of the population. Extra immunization may be needed for persons traveling to tropical areas. Symptoms and signs include headache, sore throat, fever, and neck and back pain. For breathing problems, a ventilator may be needed. Postpolio syndrome produces neuromuscular symptoms 25–30 years after attack; serious swallowing difficulties can ensue. Beware of possible choking or aspiration in the bulbar type of paralysis; patient may be unable to swallow. Provide adequate nourishment. Correct electrolyte imbalances.	For patient with acute paralysis, use a high-protein, high-calorie diet in liquid form. Use intravenous feeding and tube feeding when needed. Use vitamin supplements with 1–2 times the DRI; extra calcium and potassium may be needed to replace losses. As the treatment progresses, diet may be changed from a liquid to a solid diet as tolerated. A dysphagia diet may be useful, with varying levels of thickened liquids to enhance swallowing. Wean to oral diet as intake increases. Frequent high nutrient-density snacks are recommended. Instruct patient regarding how to puree or blend foods as needed, including how to add thickeners to liquids. Discuss appropriate recipes for high-energy and high-protein foods. Prevent complications of prolonged immobilization: renal stones, pressure ulcers, and negative N balance. Current antiviral drugs do not work; polio has no cure.

(continued)

TABLE 15-5 Infections and Febrile Conditions and Nutritional Implications *(continued)*

Condition, Nutritional Acuity, Background	Nutritional Implications
Rheumatic fever, Level 1 Rheumatic fever is an inflammatory condition affecting the connective tissues that causes joint pain, swelling, fever, rash, jerky movements (Sydenham chorea), facial grimacing, and carditis. It usually ensues 3 weeks after streptococcal infection. Lab work includes testing for serum antibodies to streptococci; albumin, transthyretin, and cholesterol may be decreased; erythrocyte sedimentation rate and white blood cell (WBC) level may be increased. Heart inflammation usually disappears but may cause permanent damage to the valves (especially the mitral valve), with a resulting heart murmur. Long-term effects are called rheumatic heart disease.	Use a full-liquid diet for acute rheumatic fever. As treatment progresses, gradually change diet, first to a soft diet, then to a regular diet. Restrict sodium intake if edema is present or if steroids are used. Increase intake of vitamin C, protein, and calories. Include adequate vitamin A as well. Reduce inflammation in joints and heart. Decrease physical activity and encourage rest while heart is inflamed. Recover lost weight. Reduce fluid retention, if present. Cure the infection and prevent its recurrence. Prevent complications such as bacterial endocarditis, atrial fibrillation, and heart failure. Explain increased need for calories and protein. Adequate rest, exercise, and nutrition are essential to prevent recurrence. Explain increased need for calories and protein. Adequate rest, exercise, and nutrition are essential to prevent recurrence. Restrict sodium if prednisone or adrenocorticotropic hormone is given for severe heart inflammation. Side effects include depletion of nitrogen, calcium, potassium, and hyperglycemia. Antibiotics are used. Monitor for specific side effects such as GI distress. Penicillin may be needed for 10 days. Lifelong use of antibiotics before surgery and dental work protects against bacterial invasion of heart valves. Aspirin or nonsteroidal anti-inflammatory drugs may be used to reduce joint pain and inflammation.
***Staphylococcus aureus* and methicillin-resistant *Staphylococcus aureus* (MRSA) infection, Level 1** *Staphylococcus aureus* is a gram-positive bacterium that developed resistance to the penicillin-derivative methicillin. MRSA emerged as a bacterium that became less susceptible to the actions of methicillin and thus developed the ability to colonize and cause life-threatening infections. *S. aureus* and MRSA population estimates are in the millions of persons.	MRSA colonization should be contained by infection control measures and not treated. Hand-washing technique is very important. The most potent anti-MRSA drug at the present time is daptomycin, especially to treat endocarditis.
Toxic shock syndrome (TSS), Level 1 TSS is an acute bacterial infection caused by *S. aureus* and most often is associated with prolonged use of tampons during menses. Symptoms include sudden onset of high fever, severe headache, red eyes, myalgia, vomiting, watery diarrhea, red rash on palms and soles (with desquamation), decreased circulation to fingers and toes, disorientation, peripheral edema, pulmonary edema, respiratory distress syndrome, and sudden hypotension progressing to shock. Anemia, kidney, liver, and muscle damage; septic shock; respiratory distress can occur. Monitor labs for increased levels of WBC, blood urea nitrogen, creatinine, bilirubin, liver enzymes, and creatine phosphokinase. Platelets may be decreased.	Increase fluid intake to 3 L daily, unless contraindicated. Discuss need for adequate fluid intake and small meals, especially with vomiting or nausea. Control diarrhea and vomiting. Improve well-being. Stabilize hydration and electrolyte balance. Prevent renal, heart, and lung problems and other complications. Antibiotics are required. Monitor for GI side effects. Determine how to administer specific drugs (such as with food, water, or milk).
Typhoid (enteric) fever, Level 2 Enteric fever includes typhoid and paratyphoid fever. It is a systemic infection caused by *Salmonella enterica,* and it is most common among travelers. This infectious fever is spread by contamination of food, water, or milk with *S. typhi* or *paratyphi*, which can come from sewage, flies, or faulty personal hygiene. The problem practically has been eradicated in areas of proper sanitary practices. Most infections are found in people who are in contact with carriers who have persistent gallbladder or UTIs. Incubation is 5–14 days. Symptoms include malaise, headache, cough, sore throat, "pea soup" diarrhea, constipation, rose spots, and splenomegaly. Lab work includes stool and urine for Widal test.	Reduce fever and prevent irritation. Replace nutrient losses from diarrhea. Replace tissue losses. Prevent complications such as intestinal hemorrhage or shock and pulmonary or cardiac side effects. Gradually add pectin and other fiber. Especially, include good dietary sources of vitamins A and C. Explain which foods are high-protein, high-calorie sources. Discuss how to prevent future reinfection. For patients with acute fever, use a diet of high-protein, high-calorie liquids. A low-residue diet may be needed temporarily. As treatment progresses, gradually add soft, bland foods. Try small, frequent feedings. First-line therapy is ceftriaxone, and fluoroquinolones can also be given. Monitor for GI distress. Preventive measures include educating travelers about hygiene precautions and vaccinations.

REFERENCE

Barnett JB, et al. Low zinc status: a new risk factor for pneumonia in the elderly? *Nutr Rev*. 68:30, 2010.

TABLE 15-6 Virulence Increased by Iron

To successfully sustain an infection, nearly all bacteria, fungi, and protozoa require a continuous supply of host iron. Iron is a cofactor in oxidation-reduction reactions. Iron deficiency has opposing effects on infectious disease risk, decreasing susceptibility by restricting iron availability to pathogens, and increasing susceptibility by compromising cellular immunocompetence (Wander et al, 2009). Studies suggest that moderate iron deficiency protects against acute infection and may represent a nutritional adaptation to endemic infectious disease stress (Wander et al, 2009). Zinc and manganese may also play a role in host defense mechanisms.

Acid-fast and gram-positive bacteria	*Bacillus, Clostridium, Listeria, Mycobacterium, Staphylococcus, Streptococcus*
Fungi	*Candida, Cryptococcus, Histoplasma, Mucor, Pneumocystis, Rhizopus*
Gram-negative bacteria	*Campylobacter, Chlamydia, Escherichia, Klebsiella, Legionella, Proteus, Pseudomonas, Salmonella, Shigella, Vibrio, Yersinia*
Protozoa	*Entamoeba, Leishmania, Plasmodium, Toxoplasma, Trypanosoma*

REFERENCES

Robien M. Iron and microbial infection. *Support Line.* 22:23, 2000.
Wander K, et al. Evaluation of iron deficiency as a nutritional adaptation to infectious disease: an evolutionary medicine perspective. *Am J Hum Biol.* 21:172, 2009.

CITED REFERENCES

Brugler L, et al. A simplified nutrition screen for hospitalized patients using readily available laboratory and patient information. *Nutrition.* 21:650, 2005.
Cunningham-Rundles S, et al. Mechanisms of nutrient modulation of the immune response. *J Allergy Clin Immunol.* 115:1119, 2005.
Elenkov IJ, et al. Cytokine dysregulation, inflammation and well-being. *Neuroimmunomodulation.* 12:255, 2005.
Fernandes G. Progress in nutritional immunology. *Immunol Res.* 40:244, 2008.
Wintergerst ES, et al. Contribution of selected vitamins and trace elements to immune function. *Ann Nutr Metab.* 51:301, 2007.

AIDS AND HIV INFECTION

NUTRITIONAL ACUITY RANKING: LEVEL 4

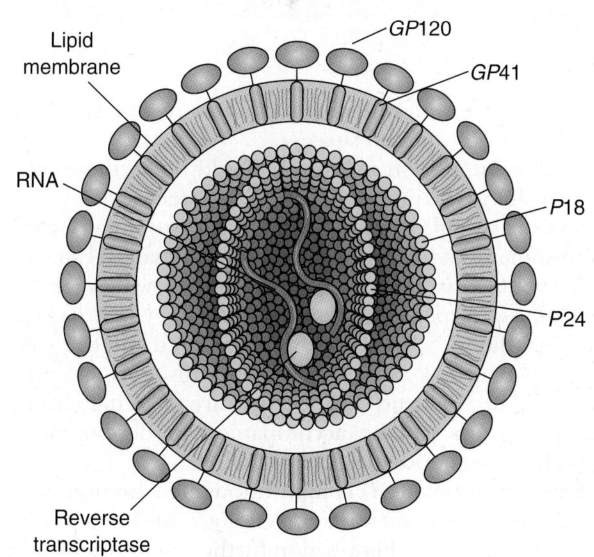

Adapted from: Porth CM. *Pathophysiology: Concepts of altered health states,* 5th ed. Philadelphia: Lippincott Williams & Wilkins, 1998.

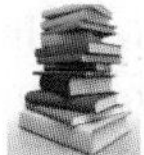

DEFINITIONS AND BACKGROUND

The human immunodeficiency virus (HIV) infects T cells (CD4+) and macrophages. Levels of CD41 (helper) and CD81 (nonhelper) subsets of T cells are used to evaluate immunological competency. After levels have been identified, staging is identified to plan therapeutic interventions; see Table 15-7. Many people will develop acquired immunodeficiency syndrome (AIDS) after a decade, following an opportunistic infection or a decline in the immune system. Prognosis for AIDS ranges from 1 year, if not treated with antiretroviral therapy (ART), to 5 years, if treated.

HIV is not easily transmitted except by exchange of bodily fluids during sexual contact, by receipt of infected blood through a blood transfusion, by sharing contaminated needles with intravenous drug injection, or from an HIV-infected mother to neonate (children represent 15–20% of the affected population). Persons at high risk include homosexual and bisexual males, hemophiliacs, intravenous drug addicts, heterosexuals with multiple partners, and infants of HIV-positive mothers. Breastfeeding by HIV-infected mothers can result in HIV transmission to the infant, especially with mastitis. In some developing countries, the relative risk of HIV transmission may be less significant than malnutrition for the infant; risks and benefits must be weighed individually.

HIV infection involves multiple organs. It targets the immune system and impairs the ability to mount an adequate immune response. Malnutrition and its complications further impair the body; HIV often depletes nutritional status (Sztam et al, 2010). Immune reconstitution inflammatory syndrome develops in a substantial percentage of HIV-infected patients who have an underlying opportunistic infection and receive ART (Danaher et al, 2010). AIDS-related malignancies are another major complication.

TABLE 15-7 **WHO Clinical Staging of HIV/AIDS for Adults and Adolescents**

Clinical stage 1—Asymptomatic	Clinical stage 4—Clinical signs
Acute retroviral syndrome	Chronic herpes simplex infection (orolabial, genital, or anorectal >1 month)
Persistent generalized lymphadenopathy	Central nervous system toxoplasmosis
Clinical stage 2	Esophageal candidiasis
Angular cheilitis	Extrapulmonary TB
Fungal nail infections of fingers	HIV encephalopathy
Herpes zoster	HIV wasting syndrome
Moderate unexplained weight loss (<10% of body weight)	Kaposi sarcoma
Papular pruritic eruptions	Pneumocystis pneumonia
Recurrent oral ulcerations	Recurrent severe or radiological bacterial pneumonia
Recurrent respiratory infections (sinusitis, bronchitis, otitis media, pharyngitis)	**Diagnostic testing needed for:**
Seborrheic dermatitis	Candida of trachea, bronchi or lungs
Clinical stage 3—Clinical signs	Cryptosporidiosis
Acute necrotizing ulcerative stomatitis, gingivitis, or periodontitis	Cytomegalovirus infection (retinitis or of an organ other than liver, spleen, or lymph nodes)
Oral candidiasis	Disseminated mycosis (e.g., histoplasmosis, coccidiomycosis, penicilliosis)
Oral hairy leukoplakia	Disseminated non-tuberculous mycobacteria infection
Pulmonary tuberculosis (TB) diagnosed in last 2 years	Extrapulmonary cryptococcosis including meningitis
Severe infections (e.g., pneumonia, empyema, pyomyositis, bone/joint infection, meningitis, bacteremia)	Invasive cervical carcinoma
Severe weight loss (>10% of body weight)	Isosporiasis
Unexplained chronic diarrhea >1 month	Lymphoma (cerebral or B-cell non-Hodgkin)
Unexplained persistent fever >1 month	Progressive multifocal leukoencephalopathy
Diagnostic test needed for: anemia (<8 g/dL), neutropenia (<500/mm^3), or thrombocytopenia (<50,000/mm^3) > 1 month	Recurrent non-typhoidal salmonella septicemia
	Visceral herpes simplex infection
	Visceral leishmaniasis

Kaposi sarcoma and Hodgkin and non-Hodgkin lymphomas are the most common malignancies (Wood and Harrington, 2005).

HIV infections are considered pandemic, and AIDS has killed more than 25 million people, especially in the sub-Sahara. Worldwide, hepatitis B virus affects 370 million people, hepatitis C virus (HCV) affects 130 million, and HIV affects 40 million (Alter, 2006). Fortunately, ART has reduced mother-to-child transmission rates.

HIV infection requires lifelong, vigilant polypharmacy. Nutrition directly impacts immune-cell triggering and indirectly impacts DNA and protein synthesis in HIV progression. Decline in body cell mass and deficiencies in vitamins and minerals occur; some clinicians recommend a series of antioxidant supplements to augment cellular immunity. Because of the crucial role that nutrition plays throughout the course of HIV, medical nutrition therapy (MNT) is an integral part of disease management.

During starvation, there is generally a loss of adipose tissue with maintenance of lean body mass (LBM); in HIV/AIDS, there is loss of LBM (wasting) while maintaining body fat. *Wasting syndrome* is defined by the World Health Organization as the involuntary loss of at least 10% of body weight and is a common AIDS-defining diagnosis. Weight loss is an independent prognostic indicator of outcomes, including mortality. Weight loss, fatigue, anorexia, diarrhea, and low-grade fevers may occur. As long as an infection remains untreated, nutritional support regimens will meet needs with only limited success.

Body composition measures should be accurate, ideally taken prior to the initiation of ART. Bioelectrical impedance analysis is useful, whereas skinfold measurements tend to overestimate fat-free mass and underestimate fat mass. Fat redistribution is part of a syndrome known as *peripheral lipodystrophy* in patients receiving ART; they lose facial and extremity fat with redeposition into visceral and truncal adiposity. Abnormal fatty deposits are disfiguring and are found in the neck and dorsocervical area ("buffalo hump"). These changes can be accompanied by development of hyperlipidemia or diabetes.

Gastrointestinal (GI) complications are common. Weight loss is often multifactorial in etiology, and reduced oral intake is common. Malnutrition further compromises those who have tuberculosis (TB) or persistent diarrhea (Wanke, 2005). Nutritional supplements, dietary counseling, and use of specific nutrients such as vitamin D_3, are critically important (Villamor, 2006).

While central parenteral nutrition (CPN) is often indicated with HIV patients experiencing severe GI dysfunction, there is a concern over infection with the use of central venous catheters in patients with advanced HIV/AIDS. Medication interactions, coinfection with other infections and diseases, wasting, lipodystrophy, and other issues make individualized nutrition care plans extremely important

TABLE 15-8 Guidelines for Nutrition Therapy in HIV Management

I. High risk (see RD within 1 week)
   A. Poorly controlled diabetes mellitus
   B. Pregnancy (mother's nutrition; infant: artificial infant formula)
   C. Poor growth, lack of weight gain, or failure to thrive in pediatric patients
   D. 110% unintentional weight loss over 4–6 months
   E. 15% unintentional weight loss within 4 weeks or in conjunction with the following:
      1. Chronic oral (or esophageal) thrush
      2. Dental problems
      3. Dysphagia
      4. Chronic nausea or vomiting
      5. Chronic diarrhea
      6. Central nervous system (CNS) disease
      7. Intercurrent illness or active opportunistic infection
   F. Severe dysphagia
   G. Enteral or parenteral feedings
   H. Two or more medical comorbidities, or dialysis
   I. Complicated food–drug–nutrient interactions
   J. Severely dysfunctional psychosocial situation (especially in children)

II. Moderate risk (see RD within 1 month)
   A. Obesity
   B. Evidence for body fat redistribution
   C. Elevated cholesterol (1200 mg/dL) or triglycerides (1250 mg/dL) levels, or cholesterol level <100 mg/dL
   D. Osteoporosis
   E. Diabetes mellitus, controlled or new diagnosis
   F. Hypertension
   G. Evidence for hypervitaminoses or excessive supplement intake
   H. Inappropriate use of diet pills, laxatives, or other over-the-counter medications
   I. Substance abuse in the recovery phase
   J. Possible food—drug–nutrient interactions
   K. Food allergies and intolerance
   L. Single medical comorbidity
   M. Oral thrush
   N. Dental problems
   O. Chronic nausea or vomiting
   P. Chronic diarrhea
   Q. CNS disease resulting in a decrease in functional capacity
   R. Chronic pain other than oral/gastrointestinal tract source
   S. Eating disorder
   T. Evidence for sedentary lifestyle or excessive exercise regimen
   U. Unstable psychosocial situation (especially in children)

III. Low risk (see RD as needed)
   A. Stable weight
   B. Appropriate weight gain, growth, and weight-for-height in pediatric patients
   C. Adequate and balanced diet
   D. Normal levels of cholesterol, triglycerides, albumin, and glucose
   E. Stable HIV disease (with no active intercurrent infections)
   F. Regular exercise regimen
   G. Normal hepatic and renal function
   H. Psychosocial issues stable (especially in children)

Source: Hayes C et al. Integrating nutrition therapy into medical management of human immunodeficiency virus. Web site accessed February 5, 2010, at http://www.aidsetc.org/aidsetc?page=etres-display&resource=etres-175.

(American Dietetic Association, 2010). Although the incidence of most AIDS-defining opportunistic infections, including HIV wasting syndrome, has dramatically decreased since the introduction of ART, weight loss and wasting are still common in HIV-infected persons who use injected drugs; live below the federal poverty level; have a lower CD4 cell count or higher HIV viral load; or have diarrhea, nausea, or fever (Tang et al, 2005).

Work on an HIV vaccine is important. The International AIDS Vaccine Initiative has established a consortium to elucidate mechanisms of protection from such a vaccine (Koff et al, 2006). In addition, a new, inactivated mycobacterial vaccine may significantly reduce TB cases among HIV-positive individuals.

MNT for HIV/AIDS patients can reduce illness, hospital stays, and related medical costs. MNT helps the patient have an improved quality of life along with better CD4 counts and weight gain (American Dietetic Association, 2010). See Table 15-8 for guidelines on risk levels. The American Dietetic Association has recommended three MNT visits per year for adults with stage 1 HIV/AIDS; three to six visits per year for adults with stage 2 or 3 HIV/AIDS; and a minimum of five visits per year for children or adolescents with HIV/AIDS. Through the Ryan White Comprehensive AIDS Resources Emergency (CARE) Act, treatment is available even when other funds have been depleted.

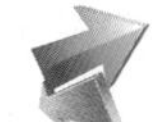

ASSESSMENT, MONITORING, AND EVALUATION

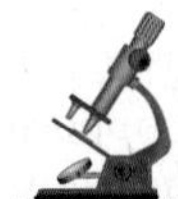

CLINICAL INDICATORS

Genetic Markers: HIV-1 has a minimal genome of only nine genes, which encode 15 proteins; the virus depends on the human host for every aspect of its life cycle (Balakrishnan et al, 2009). Polymorphisms cause the 15% of variation in viral load between individuals during the asymptomatic phase of infection. Alleles of the HLA-B5701 gene and the HLA-C gene are affected.

Clinical/History

Height
Pre-illness weight
Current weight
Waist to hip ratio
Body mass index (BMI)
Skinfolds; fat-free mass (low?)
Blood pressure (BP)
Intake and output (I & O)
Weight changes
Swollen lymph nodes
Rash
Sore throat, headache
Night sweats
Dyspnea on exertion, rales, or rhonchi
Nausea, vomiting
Anorexia
Temperature (fever, chills)
Dysphagia, chewing problems
Stomatitis
Diarrhea
Cyanosis, pneumonia
Frequent viral or herpes infections
Opportunistic infections (in AIDS)
Stool tests for malabsorption
Biopsies (lymph nodes, skin lesions)
Dual-energy x-ray absorptiometry scan
Bioelectrical impedance analysis

Lab Work

Complete blood count with differential
Platelets
Cholesterol (Chol)
Triglycerides (Trig) (increased)
Glucose (Gluc)
CD4 lymphocytes (active AIDS, <200 T cells)
CD8 lymphocytes
TLC
Viral load
Polymerase chain reaction for herpes virus
P24 antigen
Albumin (Alb) or transthyretin (decreased)
C-reactive protein (CRP)
Prealbumin:CRP ratio
Aspartate aminotransferase (AST)
Alanine aminotransferase (ALT)
Bilirubin
Prothrombin time (PT), international normalized ratio
Hemoglobin and hematocrit (H & H) (decreased?)
Ferritin (increased?)
Creatine (Creat), blood urea nitrogen (BUN)
Transferrin
Lactose test
Serum B_{12} and folate (decreased?)
Schilling test
Serum vitamin A
Serum testosterone

INTERVENTION

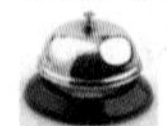

OBJECTIVES

- Improve nutrition-related immunity to prevent opportunistic infections, such as oral candidiasis; cirrhosis or hepatocellular carcinoma from chronic infection with hepatitis B or C; and other conditions such as immune reconstitution inflammatory syndrome.
- Enhance response to therapy through continuous counseling, nutritional alterations, and drug effectiveness monitoring. Follow guidelines according to levels of risk (see Table 15-8).
- Use 3-day food records rather than food frequencies (American Dietetic Association, 2010).

SAMPLE NUTRITION CARE PROCESS STEPS

Increased Nutrient Needs

Assessment Data: Three-day food records. Input and output, weight loss, and medication records. Diagnosis of AIDS 3 years ago. Complaints of GI distress after meals.

Nutrition Diagnosis (PES): NI 5.1 Increased nutrient needs related to unintentional weight loss of 21% in 5 months as evidenced by weight only 80% of desirable BMI range.

Interventions:

Food-Nutrient Delivery.

ND 1.3 Specific foods (yogurt) 2 times daily.

ND 3.1.1 Commercial beverage 3 times daily.

Education:

E 1.1 Purpose of nutrition education: to explain importance of adequate nutrient intake and compliance with all medical/nutritional/emotional care.

Counseling:

C2.2 Goal setting—Gain 1–1/2 lb per week until ideal body weight (IBW) range is reached.

Coordination of Care:

RC 1.1 Team meeting—Discuss interventions with interdisciplinary team.

Monitoring and Evaluation: Weight records, fewer reports of GI distress and symptoms. Greatly improved intake on 3-day food records.

- Maintain body weight at 95–100% of usual body weight levels. LBM is especially affected; increased resting energy expenditure occurs (American Dietetic Association, 2010).
- Prevent weight loss from fever, poor intake with oral pain, infection, nausea, diarrhea, malabsorption, swallowing difficulties, effects of medications, inflammation, viral load, and lipodystrophy, and vomiting; offer early nutritional intervention (American Dietetic Association, 2010).
- Reduce mealtime fatigue to encourage better intake. Avoid unnecessary distractions and stresses.
- Lower the temperature when febrile.
- Manage altered GI function including diarrhea, malabsorption, vomiting, and HIV-induced enteropathy.
- If necessary, use CPN to prevent further weight loss and potential malnutrition. CPN will stop weight loss, but it will not prevent further immunodeficiency.
- Keep body well hydrated. Fluids are critical to prevent kidney stones and other complications.
- Support depleted levels of nutrients such as linoleic acid, selenium, and vitamin B_{12}.
- Counteract problems such as dysphagia, mouth pain, taste alterations (dysgeusia), or difficulty chewing. Alleviate nutritional effect of fatigue, anemia, anorexia, depression, and dyspnea. Optimize nutritional status.
- Maintain fat intake at prudent levels (30–35% total kcal) to maintain or achieve normal lipid levels.
- Alter dietary regimen if there is renal or hepatic impairment.
- Maintain honest discussions regarding use of alternative therapies such as herbs, special diets, and megavitamin therapy.

- Encourage physical activity, which has been shown to improve cardiopulmonary fitness and to reduce symptoms of depression (American Dietetic Association, 2010).
- Comply with food and water safety guidelines.

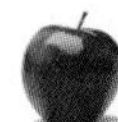

FOOD AND NUTRITION

- Maintain diet as appropriate for patient's condition; use a high-energy/high-protein diet with adequate nutritional supplements. Weight gain or maintenance is possible in patients with HIV infection and early stages of AIDS by use of oral liquid supplements.
- From 2–2.5 g protein/kg and 35–45 kcal/kg are needed. Fever and infection may further elevate need for these nutrients. Increase energy intake in cases of infection, fever, and pneumonia. Use indirect calorimetry when available; estimates are often incorrect (Frankenfield et al, 2005).
- Keep the body well hydrated. Estimate 35–40 cc/kg unless there is a reason to restrict fluids.
- Use TF, especially gastrostomy, if warranted. Low-lactose/low-fat TF products may need to be fed continuously to reduce gastroenteritis or reflux. CPN may be necessary if weight loss exceeds 20% of usual body weight.
- Increase use of omega-3 fatty acids and decrease saturated fat intake. There may be advantages to using a medium-chain triglyceride formula in the presence of AIDS-associated malabsorption (American Dietetic Association, 2010).
- Small, frequent feedings (6–9 times daily) are usually better tolerated but may be difficult to achieve given complex medication regimens.
- A general multivitamin–mineral supplement should be recommended, not to exceed 100% of the recommended dietary allowances (RDAs). Low serum micronutrient levels are common and have been associated with immune impairment, HIV disease progression, or mortality (Mehta and Fawzi, 2007). Use of vitamin A and beta-carotene may reduce some of the gut permeability and lessen watery diarrhea (American Dietetic Association, 2010). Vitamin K deficiency is common with antibiotic use.
- Use nutrient-dense snacks, such as pudding, if tolerated, nonacidic juices for sore mouth, ices made with tolerated juices, and sandwiches made with cold meat salads. Add protein powders and glucose polymers, if desired. Use oral supplements when needed.
- With bouts of diarrhea, use small meals and avoid extremes in temperatures; room temperature is often best. Avoid excesses of caffeine, alcohol, and fried and high-fat foods. Use soft cooked chicken, turkey, fish, and lean beef. Replace electrolytes with foods such as broth soups or Gatorade for sodium, potassium, magnesium, and chloride.
- If lactose intolerant, avoid milk and use a low-lactose diet.
- Sucrose and gluten may not be tolerated. Individualize as needed.
- Children present unique nutritional needs, further compounded by HIV infection; see Section 3.

Common Drugs Used and Potential Side Effects (see Table 15-9)

- Antiretroviral regimens are complicated and difficult. Because nonalcoholic fatty liver disease is a prominent feature induced by ART, hepatitis A and B virus vaccinations and close monitoring of liver parameters are suggested (Kahraman et al, 2006). Malabsorption can occur if antiretroviral agents are taken improperly with regard to meals or if they are taken with certain other drugs or herbal remedies. Suboptimal use of antiretrovirals because of noncompliance or malabsorption can result in viral resistance.
- Recombinant human growth hormone and growth hormone–releasing hormone are options for reducing visceral adipose tissue and coronary heart disease (Cofrancesco et al, 2009).

Herbs, Botanicals, and Supplements

- Ethical dilemmas may be presented by CAM use. HIV-infected patients often seek complementary therapies due to unsatisfactory side effects, high cost, nonavailability, or adverse effects of conventional medicines (Liu et al, 2005).
- CAM use is nearly 100% in the HIV-infected population, with half reporting daily use of a dietary supplement (especially vitamin C, vitamin E, and soy) as an adjunct to other treatments (Milan et al, 2008). However, there may be risks for herb–drug and herb–nutrient interactions. Many herbals may also interact with prophylactic medicines, such as antibiotics.
- Herbs and botanical supplements should not be used without discussing with the physician. Older, college-educated, or insured patients are more likely to disclose their CAM use to health care providers, and there is a need to find ways to discuss CAM between more patients and their providers (Liu et al, 2009).
- Licorice, capsaicin, astragalus, and burdock are not confirmed; large, rigorous trials are needed (Liu et al, 2005).
- Rosemary and marjoram have pentacyclic triterpenoic acids with anti-inflammatory, hepatoprotective, gastroprotective, antiulcer, anti-HIV, cardiovascular, hypolipidemic, antiatherosclerotic, and immunoregulatory effects. There would be no harm in seasoning foods with these herbs.
- Echinacea is not recommended as an antiviral agent. Do not use with warfarin or immunosuppressants.
- Garlic and St. John's wort may make saquinavir or indinavir less effective.

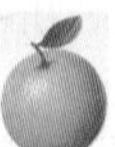

NUTRITION EDUCATION, COUNSELING, CARE MANAGEMENT

- Discuss the role of nutrition in infection and immunity; patients should also decrease the use of drugs and cigarettes because of their effects on overall health status and immunocompetence. They should avoid sharing razors, toothbrushes, tweezers, nail clippers or piercing jewelry with others.

TABLE 15-9 Medications Used for HIV Infections and AIDS

Class and Purpose	Generic Name	Brand and Other Names	Nutritional Implications and Comments
Nucleoside reverse transcriptase inhibitors (NRTIs)—*faulty versions of building blocks that HIV needs to make more copies of itself; when HIV uses an NRTI instead of a normal building block, reproduction of the virus is stalled*			Can cause severe bone marrow depletion and anemia, altered taste, constipation, nausea, indigestion, or vomiting. Adequate folate and vitamin B_{12} may prevent toxicity. NRTIs can cause lactic acidosis, hypersensitivity reactions, neuropathies, pancreatitis, anemia, and neutropenia.
	Abacavir	Ziagen, ABC	Diarrhea may be a side effect. Malaise, fever, rash, and liver inflammation can occur.
	Abacavir, lamivudine	Epzicom	Diarrhea may be a side effect. Malaise, fever, rash, and liver inflammation can occur.
	Abacavir, lamivudine, zidovudine	Trizivir	Diarrhea may be a side effect. Malaise, fever, rash, and liver inflammation can occur.
	Adefovir	Hepsera, ADV, Preveon	Often used in chronic hepatitis B virus treatments. Has nephrotoxic potential. Nausea, diarrhea, and vomiting can occur.
	Aptivus	Tipranavir	For the adjunctive treatment of HIV-1 infections.
	Didanosine	Videx, ddI Videx EC	May cause liver toxicity in low-weight patients. Neuropathy and pancreatitis may result.
	Emtricitabine	Emtriva, FTC, Coviracil	Well tolerated. Anorexia and fatigue are side effects.
	Emtricitabine, tenofovir DF	Truvada	May cause diarrhea, nausea, and vomiting. Take with food.
	Lamivudine	Epivir, 3TC	May cause nausea and vomiting, pancreatitis, and depression. Avoid alcohol. Take without regard for meals.
	Lamivudine, zidovudine	Combivir	Headache, liver inflammation, and fatigue can occur. Take with meals.
	Stavudine	Zerit, d4 T	Severe anemia may occur. Avoid alcohol.
	Tenofovir DF	Viread, TDF	Gastrointestinal (GI) distress, hypophosphatemia, acute renal failure.
	Zalcitabine	Hivid, ddC	Can cause oral ulcers, nausea, vomiting, dry mouth, and neuropathy. Take on empty stomach. Avoid taking with antacids.
	Zidovudine	Retrovir, AZT, ZDV	Can cause severe bone marrow depletion and anemia, altered taste, constipation, nausea, indigestion, or vomiting. It works better in sequence with acyclovir. Adequate folate and vitamin B_{12} may prevent toxicity. Take with food.
Nonnucleoside reverse transcriptase inhibitors (NNRTIs)—*bind to and disable reverse transcriptase, a protein that HIV needs to make more copies of itself*			Nausea, vomiting, and diarrhea are common side effects. Liver inflammation may occur; avoid alcohol and St. John's wort. NNRTIs can cause rashes and hepatotoxicity.
	Delavirdine	Rescriptor, DLV	Monitor for abnormal liver enzymes. Headaches are common.
	Efavirenz, emtricitabine, and tenofovir DF	Atripla	Hyperlipidemia can occur. Contains two NRTIs and one NNRTI.
	Nevirapine	Viramune, NVP	Take with food or on an empty stomach; fever, headache, hepatitis, general fatigue, mouth sores, and rash can occur.
Protease inhibitors (PI)—*disable protease, a protein that HIV needs to make more copies of itself*			Associated with hyperlipidemia, hyperglycemia, GI symptoms, and body fat distribution abnormalities. Disguising their taste is important; add a small amount to cold foods such as ice cream, shakes, and fruit ices; thick sweet foods such as honey, jellies, and frozen juice; or small amounts of peanut butter, pudding, applesauce, or yogurt.
	Atazanavir	Reyataz	May cause a tendency to bleed. Take with food.
	Darunavir	Prezista	May cause GI distress.
	Fosamprenavir	Lexiva, FPV	May cause a tendency to bleed. Take without regard for meals.

(continued)

TABLE 15-9 Medications Used for HIV Infections and AIDS *(continued)*

Class and Purpose	Generic Name	Brand and Other Names	Nutritional Implications and Comments
	Indinavir	Crixivan, IDV	Best absorbed on an empty stomach or with a light, nonfat snack and increased fluids (but not skim milk, coffee, or tea), even juice if calories are needed. Nausea and vomiting, change in taste, and diarrhea can occur.
	Lopinavir/ ritonavir	Kaletra, LPV/r	Elevated lipid levels and GI distress may occur. Take with food. Abnormal mouth sensations are noted. Hyperglycemia can occur.
	Nelfinavir	Viracept, NFV	Take with food; flatulence, loose stools, or diarrhea can occur. Hyperglycemia may result.
	Ritonavir	Norvir, RTV	Take with a high-energy, high-fat meal. Side effects include weakness, diarrhea, nausea and vomiting, loss of appetite, abdominal pain, abnormal mouth sensations of burning or prickling, dyslipidemia, and coronary events.
	Saquinavir	Invirase	Best absorbed after a high-energy, high-fat meal; contains some lactose; may cause GI distress, diarrhea, or nausea.
	Tipranavir	Aptivus	May cause GI distress.
Entry inhibitors: **Integrase inhibitors**—*stop HIV from inserting its own genetic code into the cell by slowing integrase, the chemical HIV needs to unlock the CD4 command center.*	**Raltegravir**	Isentress	
Entry inhibitors: **Fusion inhibitors**—*prevent HIV entry into cells.*	**Enfuvirtide**	Fuzeon, T-20	Pneumonia has been one side effect. Take without regard for meals. Nausea, diarrhea, fatigue, and pancreatitis are possible side effects.
	Maraviroc	Selzentry	May cause GI distress.
Antineoplastic agents—*for Kaposi sarcoma*	**Adriamycin, bleomycin, vincristine**		Numerous side effects include nausea and vomiting, diarrhea, anorexia, stomatitis, and weight loss.
	Doxorubicin		Administer with riboflavin to decrease toxicity. Dry mouth, esophagitis, stomatitis, nausea, and vomiting are common.
Other medications—*to manage other side effects of HIV.*	**Acyclovir**	Zovirax	May cause headache, nausea, anorexia, sore throat, fatigue, altered taste, and diarrhea.
	Antidepressants	Zoloft, Wellbutrin, others	May be useful before interferon therapy if there is a history of depression.
	Antifungals	Amphotericin-B, clotrimazole, flucytosine, ketoconazole	May cause nausea and vomiting, diarrhea, weight loss, metallic taste, and GI distress.
	Antioxidants	Multivitamin–mineral supplement that meets 100% DRI levels	Antioxidant supplementation may decrease markers of oxidative stress. Selenium may enhance immune function by modulating cytokine production.
	Cidofovir	Vistide	A cytosine nucleotide analog for treatment of cytomegalovirus (CMV), herpes simplex, papilloma, and pox viruses.
	Corticosteroids	Prednisone, others	Sodium retention and potassium, calcium, and vitamin C depletion can occur; protein malnutrition can occur with extended use. Glucose intolerance also may result.
	Foscarnet	Foscavir	Used for CMV retinitis (used intravenously only) and may cause anorexia, nausea and vomiting, abdominal pain, and diarrhea.
	Ganciclovir	Cytovene	Approved for use with CMV. May cause diarrhea, fever, neuropathy, elevated blood urea nitrogen and creatinine levels, and hypoglycemia.

(continued)

TABLE 15-9 Medications Used for HIV Infections and AIDS *(continued)*

Class and Purpose	Generic Name	Brand and Other Names	Nutritional Implications and Comments
	Pancreatic enzymes	Various	May be used with malabsorption.
	Peginterferon-α plus ribavirin		Standard for hepatitis C virus/HIV coinfection. Flu-like symptoms, fatigue, weight loss, and depressive mood changes are frequent.
	Topical microbicides	Many microbicides are in development. Alkyl sulfate microbicides, such as sodium dodecyl sulfate agents	Proposed to break the chain of transmission by providing chemical, biological, and physical barriers to infection by blocking or inactivating pathogens at the mucosal surface.
	Trimethoprim–sulfamethoxazole	Bactrim, Septra	Used for *Pneumocystis carinii* pneumonia for 1 month; may cause hepatitis, azotemia, anorexia, stomatitis, and thrombocytopenia. Monitor carefully. Folate may be needed.
	Valganciclovir	Valcyte	Approved for CMV.
Appetite stimulants and anabolic steroids—*to improve appetite and intake*			Appetite stimulants and anabolic steroids lead to significant increase in body weight and fat-free mass.
	Dronabinol	Marijuana derivative	Takes 4–6 weeks to show effects; somnolence and impaired memory can occur.
	Megestrol acetate	Megace	Useful for stimulating appetite.
	Anabolic steroids: oxandrolone, nandrolone decanoate	Oxandrin	Synthetic testosterone (anabolic steroid) that promotes weight gain, linear growth in children, and increased muscle mass. Hepatic changes or tumors have been reported. Elevation of low-density lipoprotein can occur with prolonged use; this may have cardiovascular effects. Nutritional status and the quality of life can improve.

For more information, see the FDA Web site. Accessed February 6, 2010, at http://www.fda.gov/ForConsumers/ByAudience/ForWomen/FreePublications/ucm118597.htm#nucleo

- Patients and caregivers should report all weight loss, anorexia, and fever to doctor. Even a 5% weight loss in 6 months markedly increases the risk of death (Tang et al, 2005).
- Diet must be altered whenever necessary. Evaluation of nutrition assessment parameters on a regular basis requires a comprehensive process. Continuing contact with a dietitian is essential regarding alternative feeding methods, changes in medications, need for home-delivered meals, simplified menu planning, and treatment of GI side effects.
- Aversion to meat may be countered by use of cold protein foods such as cottage cheese, yogurt, skim milk, and cheeses.
- Education should address any decline in self-care abilities, as well as alternative therapies and consequences.
- Address the consequences of protease-inhibiting therapy, such as hyperlipidemia. Studies show that managing fat, alcohol, and fiber intakes and increasing exercise can be very beneficial (American Dietetic Association, 2010).
- Resistance and strengthening exercises should be maintained. Twenty minutes three times weekly is quite effective (American Dietetic Association, 2010; Cade et al, 2007).
- New mothers who are HIV positive will want to use formula or milk from a surrogate mother instead of breastfeeding.
- In the short term, nutrition counseling and oral supplements can achieve a substantial increase in energy intake. Importance of maintaining a balanced, nutritious diet should be addressed. Dietary patterns in HIV-positive individuals may be reflected in changes in BMI, CD4 counts, and viral load (Hendricks et al, 2008). Rest periods before and after meals are suggested.
- Patients are living longer because of ART therapy, and they may be susceptible to other age-related diseases (Gerrior and Neff, 2005). They should receive appropriate nutrition counseling to meet their individual needs. A new standard of care is also needed where malnourished patients may easily access nutritional therapies within HIV treatment (Sztam et al, 2010).
- Patients should be screened and treated for depression (Kacanek et al, 2010).
- Use of stress management and coping mechanisms will be important to maintain nutritional health (Tromble-Hoke et al, 2005). Massage therapy may also be beneficial.
- In home care, continuing education should be offered to caregivers to prevent transmission of the disease and to reduce other infections.

Patient Education—Food Safety

- Educate about food safety issues. Studies show that education helps to reduce the instances of foodborne illness in this vulnerable population (American Dietetic Association, 2010).
- Reducing infections is very important. Meticulous hand washing is essential because immune-compromised individuals are more susceptible to foodborne illness. Preparation and home delivery methods must also be scrupulously clean (American Dietetic Association, 2010).
- Tips include the following:
  - Separate raw meats from other raw foods such as fruits and vegetables.
  - Avoid cross-contamination from raw meats by storing and preparing raw meat so it does not come in contact with fruits, vegetables, and uncooked foods.
  - Use separate cutting boards and cooking utensils so that juices from raw meats are not allowed to contact uncooked foods.
  - Keep hot foods hot (>140°F) and cold foods cold (<40°F). Limit the amount of time that food is left at room temperature to prevent germs from growing in it.
  - Wash all fruits and vegetables with warm water and a soft bristle brush.
  - Thaw frozen meat or poultry in a refrigerator or under cold running water, not at room temperature.
  - Avoid raw fish or shellfish, unpasteurized juices or milk, and uncooked eggs (and dishes containing uncooked eggs).
- Exceptional hand-washing techniques should be used by all caregivers and by patient. Safe food-handling techniques are imperative to reduce exposure to *Cryptosporidia*, *Giardia*, and *Salmonella*.

For More Information

- AEGIS (AIDS Education Global Information System)
  http://www.aegis.com/
- AIDS Clinical Guidelines
  http://aidsinfo.nih.gov/Guidelines/
- AIDS Info
  http://www.aidsinfo.nih.gov
- American Foundation for AIDS Research
  http://www.amfar.org/
- Body: An AIDS and HIV Information Resource
  http://www.thebody.com/
- HIV InSite
  http://hivinsite.ucsf.edu/InSite
- International AIDS Vaccine Initiative
  http://www.iavi.org
- National AIDS Information Clearinghouse (NAIC)
  http://www.cdcnpin.org/

AIDS AND HIV INFECTION—CITED REFERENCES

Alter MJ. Epidemiology of viral hepatitis and HIV co-infection: epidemiology of viral hepatitis and HIV co-infection. *J Hepatol.* 44:S6, 2006.

American Dietetic Association. Evidence Analysis Library: HIV infection. Web site accessed February 5, 2010 at http://www.adaevidencelibrary.com/topic.cfm?cat=1404.

Balakrishnan S, et al. Alternative paths in HIV-1 targeted human signal transduction pathways. *BMC Genomics.* 10:30S, 2009.

Cade WT, et al. Blunted lipolysis and fatty acid oxidation during moderate exercise in HIV-infected subjects taking HAART. *Am J Physiol Endocrinol Metab.* 292:E812, 2007.

Cofrancesco J Jr, et al. Treatment options for HIV-associated central fat accumulation. *AIDS Patient Care STDS.* 23:5, 2009.

Danaher RJ, et al. inflammatory syndrome? HIV protease inhibitors alter innate immune response signaling to double-stranded RNA in oral epithelial cells: implications for immune reconstitution. *AIDS.* 24:2587, 2010.

Frankenfield D, et al. Comparison of predictive equations for resting metabolic rate in healthy nonobese and obese adults: a systematic review. *J Am Diet Assoc.* 105:775, 2005.

Gerrior JL, Neff LM. Nutrition assessment in HIV infection. *Nutr Clin Care.* 8:6, 2005.

Hendricks KM, et al. Dietary patterns and health and nutrition outcomes in men living with HIV infection. *Am J Clin Nutr.* 88:1584, 2008.

Kacanek D, et al. Incident depression symptoms are associated with poorer HAART adherence: a longitudinal analysis from the nutrition for healthy living study. *J Acquir Immune Defic Syndr.* 53:266, 2010.

Kahraman A, et al. Non-alcoholic fatty liver disease in HIV-positive patients predisposes for acute-on-chronic liver failure: two cases. *Eur J Gastroenterol Hepatol.* 18:101, 2006.

Koff WC, et al. HIV vaccine design: insights from live attenuated SIV vaccines. *Nat Immunol.* 7:19, 2006.

Liu C, et al. Disclosure of complementary and alternative medicine use to health care providers among HIV-infected women. *AIDS Patient Care STDS.* 23:965, 2009.

Liu JP, et al. Herbal medicines for treating HIV infection and AIDS. *Cochrane Database Syst Rev.* 3:CD003937, 2005.

Mehta S and Fawzi W. Effects of vitamins, including vitamin A, on HIV/AIDS patients. *Vitam Horm.* 75:355, 2007.

Milan FB, et al. Use of complementary and alternative medicine in inner-city persons with or at risk for HIV infection. *AIDS Patient Care STDS.* 22:811, 2008.

Sztam KA, et al. Macronutrient supplementation and food prices in HIV treatment. *J Nutr.* 140:213S, 2010.

Tang AM, et al. Increasing risk of 5% or greater unintentional weight loss in a cohort of HIV-infected patients, 1995 to 2003. *J Acquir Immune Defic Syndr.* 40:70, 2005.

Tromble-Hoke SM, et al. Severe stress events and use of stress-management behaviors are associated with nutrition-related parameters in men with HIV/AIDS. *J Am Diet Assoc.* 105:1541, 2005.

Villamor E. A potential role for vitamin D on HIV infection? *Nutr Rev.* 64:226, 2006.

Wanke C. Nutrition and HIV in the international setting. *Nutr Clin Care.* 8:44, 2005.

Wood C, Harrington W Jr. AIDS and associated malignancies. *Cell Res.* 15:947, 2005.

BURNS (THERMAL INJURY)

NUTRITIONAL ACUITY RANKING: LEVEL 3 (MINOR), LEVEL 4 (MAJOR BURNS)

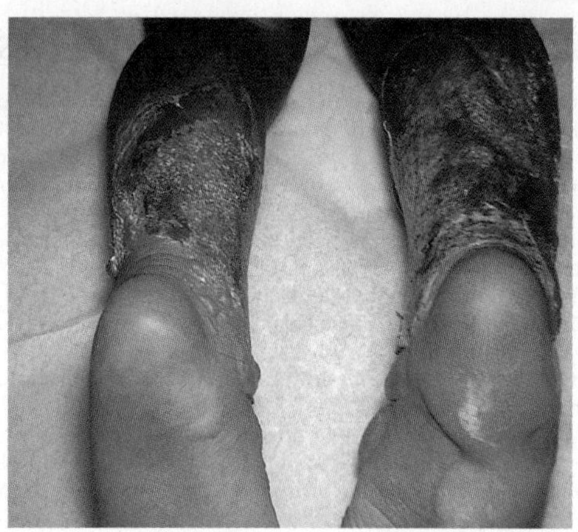

Adapted from: Fleisher GR, MD, Ludwig S, MD, Baskin MN, MD. *Atlas of Pediatric Emergency Medicine.* Philadelphia: Lippincott Williams & Wilkins, 2004.

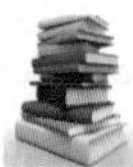

DEFINITIONS AND BACKGROUND

Electrical, thermal, chemical, or radioactive agents can cause burns. Burns are the third leading cause of accidental death in the United States; 35% of burn victims are children. Unfortunately, a significant proportion of critically ill children admitted to pediatric intensive care units (ICUs)present with nutritional deficiencies; younger age, burn injury, and need for mechanical ventilation support are some factors that are associated with worse nutritional deficiencies (Mehta and Duggan, 2009).

With a first-degree burn, simple redness of epidermis occurs. In a second-degree burn, redness and blistering occur. In a third-degree burn, skin and tissue destruction occurs. The hypermetabolic response to burn injury is mediated by hugely increased levels of circulating catecholamines, prostaglandins, glucagon, and cortisol. This response causes profound skeletal muscle catabolism, immune deficiency, peripheral lipolysis, reduced bone mineralization, reduced linear growth, increased energy expenditure, and marked increase in metabolic rate. Local cytokines are released from inflammatory cells, attracting more to the affected area. Interleukin (IL)-1, IL-6, and tumor necrosis factor (TNF) are involved. Fever, evaporative losses, and infections may occur. Determination of total body surface area (TBSA) burned is often documented in the medical record by using charts such as the Lund-Browder chart, shown in Figure 15-3 (http://www.rch.org.au/clinicalguide/cpg.cfm?doc_id=5158).

Before the modern era of early enteral nutrition therapy, significant weight loss led to impaired wound healing, infectious morbidity, and increased mortality (Lee et al, 2005). Loss of 1 g of nitrogen equals a 30 g loss of LBM. Therefore, nitrogen balance becomes a matter of life and death in a major burn victim. Survival depends on medical treatment and early, effective nutritional support. Weight loss of up to 10% is acceptable; 40–50% shows great catabolism and hypermetabolism. Systemic inflammation, acute lung injury, and multiple organ failure (MOF) are common causes of mortality (Magnotti and Deitch, 2005).

Early institution of enteral feeding can attenuate the stress response, abate hypermetabolism, and improve patient outcome (Lee et al, 2005). Adding high doses of ascorbic acid (25 mg/mL) to resuscitation fluid during the first 24 hours after severe burns significantly reduces edema and severity of respiratory dysfunction.

Thermal injury produces a profound hypermetabolic and hypercatabolic stress response characterized by increased endogenous glucose production via gluconeogenesis and glycogenolysis, lipolysis, and proteolysis (Jeschke, 2009; Jeschke et al, 2005). Severity of thermal injury and presence of systemic infection increase risk for developing ischemic bowel disease. If the GI tract becomes nonfunctional, parenteral support may be needed.

Estimating the percentage of total body burned is important because total burn thickness affects metabolic rate more than body surface area. A 25–30% TBSA burn leads to systemic edema and catabolic responses. A 90% TBSA burn is usually fatal; 60% or more in an older person is also usually fatal. The Harris–Benedict equation (with or without activity and stress factors), the Mifflin–St. Jeor equation, the 1997 Ireton–Jones equation, and the Fick equation should not be considered for use in resting energy expenditure (REE) determination, as these equations do not have adequate prediction accuracy (American Dietetic Association, 2010). If a

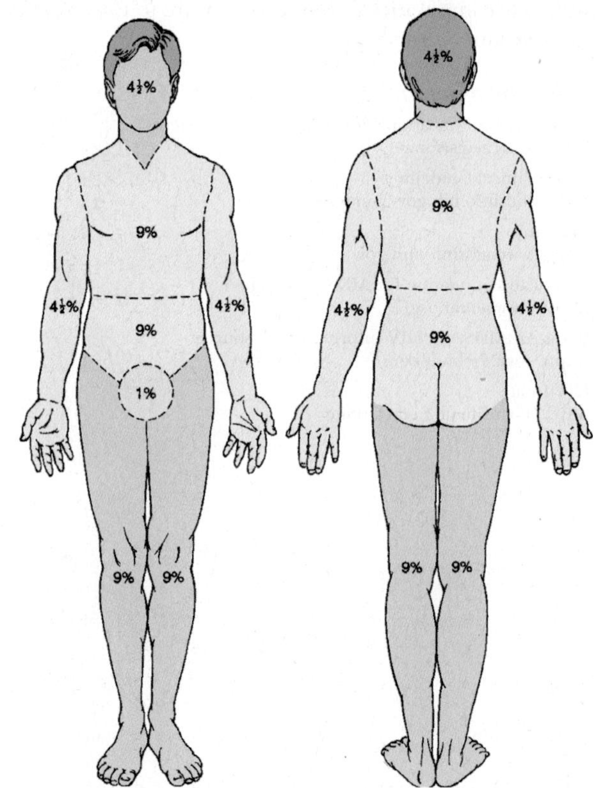

Figure 3. LifeART image copyright © 2010 Lippincott Williams & Wilkins. All rights reserved.

metabolic cart is not available, the following Penn State equation may be used for nonobese patients, where V is ventilation per minute (American Dietetic Association, 2010):

$$\text{PENN STATE EQUATION RMR} = \text{BMR}\ (0.85) + V_E\ (33) + T_{max(175)} - 6433.$$

The liver, with its metabolic, inflammatory, immune, and acute phase functions, plays a pivotal role in patient survival and recovery by modulating multiple pathways (Jeschke, 2009). Healing takes place in three stages: establishment of the epithelial barrier, scar tissue formation (dermal replacement), and contraction (shrinkage). Eschars cut off blood supply to an extremity or may impair breathing; they are often cut open in a surgical escharotomy. Bleeding occurs, but because the burn causing the eschar has destroyed the nerve endings in the skin, there is little pain. Hepatic acute phase proteins are strong predictors for postburn survival (Jeschke, 2009).

The burn patient is best cared for in a dedicated burn center where resuscitation and monitoring focus is on the pathophysiology of burns, inhalation injury, and edema management (Latenser, 2009). Most dietitians working in burn centers report having advanced training or education (Graves et al, 2009).

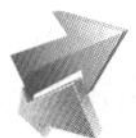

ASSESSMENT, MONITORING, AND EVALUATION

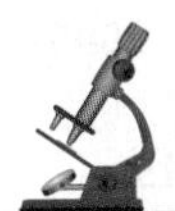

CLINICAL INDICATORS

Genetic Markers: Burns are an injury and not genetic in origin.

Clinical/History

Height
Preburn weight
Weight changes
Daily weight (beware of heavy exudate, edema)
BMI
Diet history
Measured energy expenditure (MEE)
Percentage body burned
Burn classification (first, second, third degree)
Edema
I & O
BP
Temperature
Urine acetone, sugars
Ability to chew
Ability to swallow
Hypovolemic shock = tachycardia, low BP, decreased urinary output

Lab Work

Alb
Prealbumin: CRP ratio
CRP
Transthyretin (decreased)
BUN, Creat
H & H
Gluc (increased)
AST (increased)
Na^+ (decreased)
Chloride
K^+
Total urinary N (TUN)
Ca^{++}, Mg^{++}
Partial pressure of carbon dioxide (pCO_2)
Partial pressure of oxygen (pO_2)
Transferrin
Chol, Trig
WBC, TLC
Serum catecholamines (increased)
Ceruloplasmin
Alkaline phosphatase (Alk phos)
N balance

SAMPLE NUTRITION CARE PROCESS STEPS

Unintentional Weight Loss

Assessment Data: Analysis of preferences, dislikes, and allergies; intake compared with measured or estimated requirements; confirmation of severity and extent of burn from medical record; recorded weights.

Nutrition Diagnosis (PES): NC-3.2 Unintentional weight loss related to inadequate intake after burns of 45% of upper extremities as evidenced by weight loss of 10 lb in past 14 days.

Intervention: Food-Nutrient Delivery—If needs cannot be met by oral route due to extent and severity of burn, patient will need nutrition therapy or feeding assistance. Eliminate distractions at mealtime and avoid lab work and painful procedures before meals. Educate family and nursing staff about not using empty-calorie foods or beverages and offering nutrient-dense beverages, especially with medication passes. Counsel about long-term nutritional implications, as appropriate.

Monitoring and Evaluation: Monitor and evaluate weights. Determine whether nutritional needs are being met. Anticipate 2–3 months total for optimal recovery time.

INTERVENTION

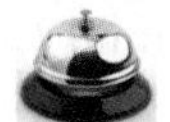

OBJECTIVES

- Restore fluid and electrolyte balance to prevent hypovolemic shock and to stabilize body temperature. Fluid resuscitation during the first 24–48 hours after injury remains a significant challenge (White and Renz, 2008).
- Prevent renal insufficiency or failure from decreased plasma volume, cardiac output, and excessive pigment overload from necrosis, toxins, or hemolysis. Exudate losses may be as high as 20–25% of total daily nitrogen losses.
- Promote wound healing and graft retention while minimizing loss of LBM (Lee et al, 2005). Close wound surface with grafts to reduce the likelihood of organ failure. Grafts may be autograft (own body) or from cultured keratinocytes.
- Provide early operative intervention and wound closure, metabolic interventions, early enteral nutrition, and intensive glucose control (Latenser, 2009).
- Anabolic steroid, glutamine, and glucose protocols (≤120 mg/dL) are widely used (Graves et al, 2009).
- Avoid weight losses greater than 10% of preburn weight. Minimize catabolism of protein tissues to avoid consequences of impaired immunity, decreased wound healing, decreased vigor and muscle strength, retarded synthesis of blood proteins and hemoglobin, and increased rates of infection.
- Use indirect calorimetry where possible. Patients require only small adjustment for physical activity levels; bedridden patients may need only 1.0–1.2 times the determined REE. Patients who are also malnourished benefit from a gradual increase in intake of 1.1–1.3 times the REE.
- Achieve positive nitrogen balance and minimize losses. Albumin therapy may be considered for the management

of ascites and volume resuscitation (Mendez et al, 2005). In children, growth must continue.
- Prevent ischemic gut, sepsis, and organ failure (Magnotti and Deitch, 2005). Prevent hypothermia and other complications.
- Reduce evaporative water losses, especially with occlusive wound dressings.
- Correct syndrome of inappropriate antidiuretic hormone, hypertonic dehydration, or overhydration.
- Relieve pain and alleviate problems such as postburn pruritus, deep venous thrombosis, peptic ulceration, or pressure ulcers.
- Manage psychosocial problems such as acute stress syndrome, depression, and posttraumatic stress syndrome, and reduce their effect on intake.
- Avoid overfeeding and minimize the negative consequences of hyperglycemia.
- Restore skin's protection to reduce infection. Sepsis is a major cause of mortality, often occurring 2–3 weeks after injury.

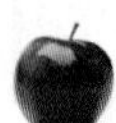

FOOD AND NUTRITION

- Immediately use intravenous fluids to replace deficits; prevent gastric distention and paralytic ileus. Prevent overhydration (Kattelmann et al, 2006). Add vitamin C (25 mg/mL) to promote healing.
- If hemodynamically stable with a functional GI tract, then EN is recommended over parenteral nutrition (PN) to lower sepsis and complication rates (American Dietetic Association, 2010; Chan and Chan, 2009). Start within a few hours to decrease the hypermetabolic response to injury (Magnotti and Dietch, 2005).
- A duodenal placement, especially in the early postburn phase, is superior to gastric feeding. Use specialty immunoenhanced products with peptides and glutamine to preserve gut function (De-Souza and Greene, 2005). Provide the feeding at a 45-degree angle, where possible, to reduce risks for pneumonia and aspiration; do not use blue dye to test for aspiration (American Dietetic Association, 2010).
- Protein intake should be from 2–3 times the RDA or 1.5–3 g/kg body weight; adjust for children. Add modular protein supplements as needed, especially glutamine. Leucine-supplemented nutrition is also very promising (De Bandt and Cynober, 2005).
- Use 20% protein, 50–60% carbohydrates (CHOs), and 20–30% fat (2–4% essential fatty acids and slight increase in omega-3 fatty acids). CHO may be given at rate of 5 mg/kg/min. Intravenous lipids can be given at 4 g/kg maximum in pediatric population.
- Gradually progress to oral diet when possible; use a high-calorie, high-protein diet with 5–6 small meals and snacks. Add CHO additives as needed. Suitable snacks may include peanut butter cookies, brownies, cake, shakes, pasteurized eggs in milkshakes or eggnog, protein in broths, and dextrins added to coffee. (See tips for adding protein and calories to the diet in Section 5).
- Supplemental glutamine granules with oral feeding or TF can abate glutamine depletion, promote protein synthesis, inhibit protein decomposition, improve wound healing, and reduce hospital stay (Peng et al, 2005).
- Provide adequate fluid intake: encourage intake of fruit juices (cranberry, grapefruit, prune, or orange juice) for adequate supplies of potassium. Water losses may be 10–12 times normal during first few weeks.
- Supplement diet with 5–10 times the RDA of vitamin C; 2 times the RDA of zinc sulfate; and 2–3 times the RDA of B-complex vitamins. Two times the RDA for vitamins A and D may be useful at first. Vitamins K and B_{12} may need to be given weekly; check serum levels as needed.
- For children, vitamins should be given at twice the RDA until recovery.
- Provide adequate copper (for collagen cross-linkage). Arginine (up to 2% of kilocalories) and carnitine also may be beneficial. Phosphorus should be added intravenously as potassium phosphate, enterally, or orally as Neutra-Phos.
- Essential fatty acids are included to reduce inflammation and promote wound healing. Omega-3 fatty acids help to promote a healthy balance of proteins in the body and to reduce inflammation.
- Administration of high-calorie total enteral nutrition in any highly septic phase should be avoided. Avoid large doses of linoleic acid, iron, and zinc, which can depress immunocompetence.
- Do not discontinue nutritional support because of watery diarrhea; this type of diarrhea is likely to occur for reasons other than CHO intolerance (Thakkar et al, 2005).

Common Drugs Used and Potential Side Effects

- See Table 15-10.

Herbs, Botanicals, and Supplements

- Herbs and botanical supplements should not be used without discussing with physician.
- Large amount of vitamin C supplements may be considered in severe burns because of increased requirements resulting from oxidative stress and wound healing; a 3-g dose/day may be needed to restore normal plasma ascorbate concentrations (Berger, 2009).
- Calendula may be used topically as an ointment or a tea. Gotu kola and bee resin (propolis) may also be useful. Aloe vera has some merit but should never be taken orally.
- Probiotic supplements containing *Lactobacillus acidophilus* can help restore GI and immune health.
- Vitamin E helps to promote healing; it may also be recommended for topical use. However, avoid excessive doses before any surgery.

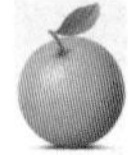

NUTRITION EDUCATION, COUNSELING, CARE MANAGEMENT

- Considering possible consequences of long-term immobilization (renal calculi, pneumonia, contractures, and pressure ulcers), increase activity as pain tolerance allows. Discuss importance of the balance between appetite, nutritional intake, and physical activity.

TABLE 15-10 Pharmacotherapy for Burns

Antimicrobial control, analgesia, sedation, and anxiety management are required for burn management. Given acutely and during rehabilitation, supportive therapy uses growth hormone, insulin and related proteins, oxandrolone, and propranolol.

Medication	Description
Anabolic steroids	Oral oxandrolone 0.1 mg/kg twice daily increases protein synthesis, lean body mass accretion, and muscle strength; improves serum visceral protein concentrations; promotes weight gain; and increases bone mineral content (Miller and Btaiche, 2008). Close monitoring of liver transaminase levels should be undertaken.
Analgesics	Pain medications may have some effect on gastrointestinal (GI) function and appetite.
Antacids	Used to prevent Curling ulcer. Cimetidine is also useful.
Antibiotic ointments	Early burn wound excision and complete coverage with autograft will reduce septic complications. Bacitracin may be used for first-degree burns, but other ointments (silver sulfadiazine, silver nitrate, mafenide, or povidone-iodine) may also be used. If Silvadene is used, nutrients may be leached out (i.e., sodium, copper, potassium, magnesium, calcium, and B-complex vitamins).
Antibiotics, oral	Oxacillin, mezlocillin, and gentamicin are used to treat infection.
Growth hormone	Growth hormones may be used to decrease the catabolic effect of burns.
Insulin	Used for stress-induced hyperglycemia.
Interferon-gamma or -alpha-2b	Used to decrease keloid formation. Dry mouth, stomatitis, nausea and vomiting, diarrhea, and abdominal pain may result.
Pain medicine	Prescription medications (acetaminophen with codeine, morphine, or meperidine) are used for severe burns.
Promotility agents (metoclopramide)	If the patient has gastroparesis or repeated high gastric residuals, a promotility agent may help increase GI transit and improve feeding tolerance.

From Miller JT, Btaiche IF. Oxandrolone in pediatric patients with severe thermal burn injury. *Ann Pharmacother.* 42:1310, 2008.

- Review the fact that fat is high in energy while low in volume. Fat is helpful in normalizing elimination; however, excesses may negatively affect immunocompetence.
- Explain that adequate intake of fiber is important.
- The family's attitude toward patient's dietary intake should be firm but understanding. A daily nutrient intake record may be a good way to track goals and to assess total intake. Discuss problems to monitor and report, such as fever or wound drainage.
- Offer a written care plan for home use.

Patient Education—Food Safety

- Educate about food safety, reducing risk of infection, and meticulous hand washing.
- Reinforce kitchen fire safety issues. Clean cooking surfaces to prevent food and grease buildup. Turn pan handles inward to avoid hot food spills. Avoid wearing loose clothing while cooking. Stay in the kitchen while cooking.
- Burn patients are more susceptible to minor illnesses, including foodborne illness. Tips include the following:
  - Separate raw meats from other raw foods such as fruits and vegetables.
  - Avoid cross-contamination from raw meats by storing and preparing raw meat so it does not come in contact with fruits, vegetables, and uncooked foods.
  - Use separate cutting boards and cooking utensils so that juices from raw meats are not allowed to contact uncooked foods.
  - Keep hot foods hot (>140°F) and cold foods cold (<40°F). Limit the amount of time that food is left at room temperature to prevent germs from growing in it.
  - Wash all fruits and vegetables with warm water and a soft bristle brush.
  - Thaw frozen meat or poultry in a refrigerator or under cold running water, not at room temperature
  - Avoid raw fish, shellfish, unpasteurized juices, and uncooked eggs (and dishes containing uncooked eggs).

For More Information

- American Burn Association
  http://www.ameriburn.org/
- Burn Care Foundation
  http://www.burnsurvivor.com/index.html
- Burn Prevention
  http://kidshealth.org/parent/firstaid_safe/sheets/burns_sheet.html
- Centers for Disease Control and Prevention (CDC) Emergency Treatment of Burns
  http://www.bt.cdc.gov/masscasualties/burns.asp
- Fire Safety
  http://www.nlm.nih.gov/medlineplus/firesafety.html
- Mayo Clinic
  http://www.mayoclinic.com/health/first-aid-burns/FA00022
- NIH—Burns
  http://www.nigms.nih.gov/Publications/Factsheet_Burns.htm
- National Library of Medicine—Burns
  http://www.nlm.nih.gov/medlineplus/burns.html

BURNS—CITED REFERENCES

American Dietetic Association. Evidence Analysis Library: critical illness. Web site accessed February 7, 2010 at http://www.adaevidencelibrary.com/topic.cfm?cat=2809.

Berger MM. Vitamin C requirements in parenteral nutrition. *Gastroenterology.* 137:70S, 2009.

Chan MM, Chan GM. Nutritional therapy for burns in children and adults. *Nutrition.* 25:261, 2009.

De Bandt JP, Cynober L. Therapeutic use of branched-chain amino acids in burn, trauma, and sepsis. *J Nutr.* 136:308S, 2006.

De-Souza DA, Greene LJ. Intestinal permeability and systemic infections in critically ill patients: effect of glutamine. *Crit Care Med.* 33:1125, 2005.

Graves C, et al. Actual burn nutrition care practices: an update. *J Burn Care Res.* 30:77, 2009.

Jeschke MG. The hepatic response to thermal injury: is the liver important for postburn outcomes? *Mol Med.* 15:337, 2009.

Jeschke MG, et al. Endogenous anabolic hormones and hypermetabolism: effect of trauma and gender differences. *Ann Surg.* 241:759, 2005.

Kattelmann K, et al. Preliminary evidence for a medical nutrition therapy protocol: enteral feedings for critically ill patients. *J Am Diet Assoc.* 106:226, 2006.

Latenser BA. Critical care of the burn patient: the first 48 hours. *Crit Care Med.* 37:2819, 2009.

Lee JO, et al. Nutrition support strategies for severely burned patients. *Nutr Clin Pract.* 20:325, 2005.

Magnotti LJ, Deitch EA. Burns, bacterial translocation, gut barrier function, and failure. *J Burn Care Rehabil.* 26:383, 2005.

Mehta NM, Duggan CP. Nutritional deficiencies during critical illness. *Pediatr Clin North Am.* 56:1143, 2009.

Mendez CM, et al. Albumin therapy in clinical practice. *Nutr Clin Pract.* 20:314, 2005.

Peng X, et al. Clinical and protein metabolic efficacy of glutamine granules-supplemented enteral nutrition in severely burned patients. *Burns.* 31:342, 2005.

Thakkar K, et al. Diarrhea in severely burned children. *JPEN J Parenter Enteral Nutr.* 29:8, 2005.

White CE, Renz EM. Advances in surgical care: management of severe burn injury. *Crit Care Med.* 36:318S, 2008.

FRACTURES

NUTRITIONAL ACUITY RANKING: LEVEL 2

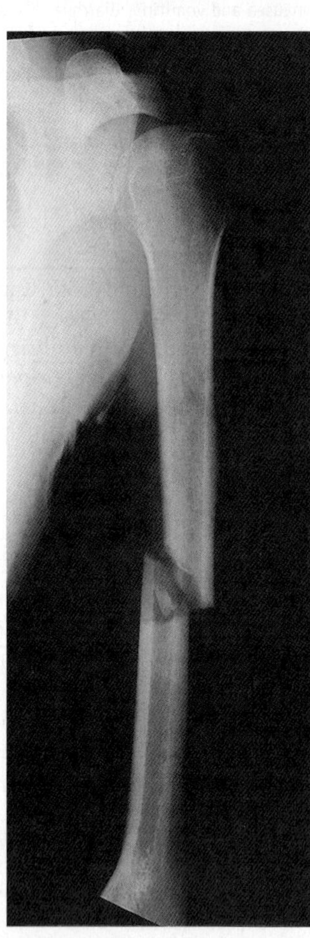

Adapted from: Koval KJ, MD and Zuckerman, JD, MD. *Atlas of Orthopaedic Surgery: A Multimeidal Reference.* Philadelphia: Lippincott Williams & Wilkins, 2004.

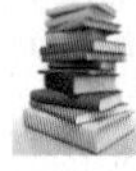

DEFINITIONS AND BACKGROUND

Stress fractures occur from prolonged stress on normal bones. Here, broken bones result from a physical force greater than stress that cannot be withstood. They are common in athletes, especially gymnasts, runners, and basketball or tennis players. *Simple (closed) fractures* involve bones that do not protrude. A *compound (open) fracture* allows bone to protrude. A *long-bone fracture* generally is an emergency and may be complicated by shock, wound infection, bleeding, or inadequate hydration; traction is used for internal immobilization. The most commonly broken bones are the collarbone (clavicle) and the bones of the wrist. In persons older than 75 years, the hip is more commonly broken.

A *complete fracture* has separated bone fragments complete, whereas they are still partially joined in an *incomplete fracture.* In *comminuted fractures,* the bones are split into multiple pieces. Orthopedic surgeons have elaborate nomenclature for the type of fracture, its location, and its geometric shape (transverse, oblique, spiral, and so on). After a break, edema of surrounding tissue causes discomfort, and muscle spasms occur to hold the bone in place.

Healing occurs in stages, starting with the *inflammation phase*; a blood clot (fracture hematoma) between the bone fragments, followed by new blood vessels with phagocytosis to remove dead tissue. Fibroblasts can then produce collagen fibers and new tissue. The second, *reparative stage* begins approximately 2 weeks after the fracture. In this stage, proteins produced by the osteoblasts and chondroblasts form new bone matrix (soft callus) from calcium hydroxyapatite crystals. This healing shows on a radiograph after approximately 4–6 weeks. The soft callus hardens forms into a hard callus over a 6- to 12-week period. In the third, *remodeling phase,* mature lamellar bone replaces the woven bone in the period of 3–18 months after the injury. Both osteoblasts and osteoclasts are involved.

Good nutrition is essential during all phases of healing. With multiple fractures, metabolic rate may increase by 20% or more for several weeks. Aggressive refeeding can decrease morbidity and mortality in malnourished patients (Bonjour, 2005).

Compression fractures involve weakened bones breaking from osteoporosis or from bone cancer. Incidence increases after 60 years of age, especially in women. Osteoporosis is responsible for more than 1.5 million fractures annually, including more than 300,000 hip fractures; 700,000 vertebral fractures; 250,000 wrist fractures; and 300,000 fractures at other sites. Bone resorption markers at levels above the upper limit of the premenopausal range are associated with an increased risk of hip, vertebral, and nonvertebral fracture; the most sensitive markers include serum osteocalcin, bone-specific alkaline phosphatase, the N-terminal propeptide of type I collagen for bone formation, and the cross-linked C- (CTX) and N- (NTX) telopeptides of type I collagen for bone resorption (Garnero, 2008).

A *broken hip* includes fractures of the femur head (intracapsular), femur neck (extracapsular), and greater Hesser trochanter. Osteoporotic fractures lower one's quality of life. Up to 50% of women and 20% of men at the age of 50 years may have a fragility fracture in their remaining lifetimes (Earl et al, 2010). The most common risk factors for osteoporotic fracture are advanced age, low bone mineral density, and previous fracture as an adult (NAMS, 2010). Women with one hip fracture are at a fourfold greater risk of having a second one.

Maternal nutrition may have critical and far-reaching persistent consequences for offspring health; reduced maternal fat stores and low levels of circulating 25-hydroxyvitamin D in pregnancy are associated with reduced bone mass in the offspring (Earl et al, 2010). Low birth-weight and poor childhood growth are also linked to risk of hip fracture later in life (Cooper et al, 2006). Clearly, optimizing nutrition throughout life is protective. Deficiency in dietary proteins causes marked deterioration in bone mass, microarchitecture, and strength (Bonjour, 2005). Vitamin A in amounts greater than 5000 IU/day may increase the risk of hip fractures; intake should be limited to 100% RDA levels.

After hip fracture, aligning the bone through an open "reduction" with internal fixation (ORIF) may be necessary. In spinal fracture, vertebroplasty involves inserting glue (methylmethacrylate) into the center of the collapsed spinal vertebra to stabilize and strengthen the crushed bone. Here, adequate nutrition must be provided to heal and to reduce infectious processes. Sometimes the medical team uses electrical bone growth stimulation or osteostimulation to support bone recovery. Once healed, it is important to return to some level of physical activity if possible.

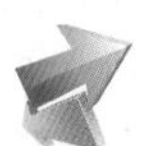

ASSESSMENT, MONITORING, AND EVALUATION

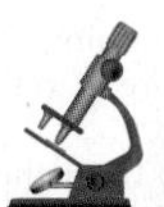

CLINICAL INDICATORS

Genetic Markers: Bone density and family history can predict fracture risk (Cosman, 2005). Many genes are implicated. BMD candidate genes, ADAMTS18 (ADAM metallopeptidase with thrombospondin type 1 motif, 18) and TGFBR3 (transforming growth factor, beta receptor III) seem to predict bone density and risk for skeletal fracture (Xiong et al, 2009).

Clinical/History	Lab Work	
Height	Serum Ca^{++}	Prealbumin: CRP ratio
Weight (may need chair scales)	Urinary Ca^{++}	CRP
Weight changes	Mg^{++}	Gluc
BMI	BUN, Creat	WBC, TLC
Diet history	H & H	Total iron-binding capacity (TIBC)
I & O	Serum Fe	Alk phos (increased)
BP	N balance	Na^+, K^+
Temperature	Alb, transthyretin	

INTERVENTION

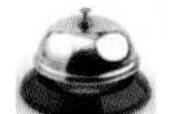

OBJECTIVES

- Support formation of bone matrix. Complete union may take 4–8 months.
- Supply adequate nutrition for collagen formation and calcium deposition.
- Prevent side effects of long-term immobilization, such as renal calculi, pressure ulcers, urinary tract infections, embolus, contractures, and neurovascular dysfunction.
- Use fluoridated water. Monitor bottled waters and well water, which are often not fluoridated.
- For long-bone fracture, meet energy needs, which are increased by 20–25%. Keep nearby joints as active as possible and prevent complications such as pressure ulcers, renal calculi, and effects from spinal anesthesia.

SAMPLE NUTRITION CARE PROCESS STEPS

Inadequate Oral Food and Beverage Intake

Assessment Data: Diet history and intake records showing intake of <50% at most meals following hip fracture and ORIF. Weights not available at that time. Medications include morphine and heparin. Patient shows signs of depression and anorexia.

Nutrition Diagnosis (PES): NI-2.1 Inadequate oral food and beverage intake related to anorexia and depression as evidenced by food records showing <50% oral intake at most meals for past 5 days.

Intervention: Food-Nutrient Delivery—Consider use of tube feeding if oral intake continues to be low. Offer liquid nutritional supplements between meals to enhance protein and calorie intake. Educate patient and family about the importance of nutrition for healing. Counsel about ways to increase nutrient density without increasing the total amount of food consumed. Coordinate care with medical team for gradual increments of physical activity, which should help with depression and anorexia; review medications and determine whether morphine can be decreased to lessen sleepiness during the day.

Monitoring and Evaluation: Improved oral intake for total protein and calories. Gradual improvement in cognition and the ability to participate in physical activity. Decline in signs of depression.

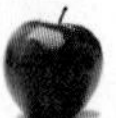

FOOD AND NUTRITION

- Use a high-protein, high-energy diet; needs may increase as much as 20–25%.
- Use adequate levels of calcium, phosphorus, and vitamins D, C, and K. Encourage these nutrients to be taken in diet; if a supplement is used, avoid levels >100% RDA for vitamin A.
- Although the main source of dietary calcium is dairy products, calcium contained in mineral water is highly bioavailable and can provide another valuable source.
- Supply zinc for wound healing after surgical procedures.
- Prevent or correct fever, pneumonia, and possible embolism.
- Ensure adequate fluid intake to excrete calcium excesses.

Common Drugs Used and Potential Side Effects

- Pharmacological therapy can reduce the risk of fractures, but many patients take their medication incorrectly, stop it prematurely, or have malabsorption (Hamdy et al, 2010).
- Bisphosphonates (alendronate, risedronate, and ibandronate), selective estrogen-receptor modulators (raloxifene), parathyroid hormone, estrogens, and calcitonin may be necessary (NAMS, 2010). Parathyroid hormone (teriparatide) is an anabolic agent that stimulates new bone formation, repairs architectural defects, and improves bone density.
- Some drugs, such thiazolidinedione, anticonvulsants, and opioids, significantly reduce bone mineral density. Selective serotonin reuptake inhibitors may also have an undesirable effect on bone health; their use should be carefully monitored (Haney et al, 2010).
- Pain medications such as morphine or meperidine (Demerol) may cause vomiting, nausea, and constipation. When analgesics are needed, monitor for GI distress or bleeding.

Herbs, Botanicals, and Supplements

- Herbs and botanical supplements should not be used without discussing with the physician.
- Creatine supplementation, with and without resistance training, has the potential to influence bone biology; however, the longer-term effects of creatine supplementation are not known (Candow and Chilibeck, 2010).

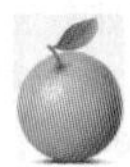

NUTRITION EDUCATION, COUNSELING, CARE MANAGEMENT

- Emphasize nutrition, especially adequate calcium, vitamin D, protein, and vitamin K (Earl et al, 2010).
- Encourage activity and the use of physical therapy after the healing has progressed. Use of oral supplements with resistance training can be very beneficial (Miller et al, 2006).
- Refer to appropriate agencies, such as home health, Visiting Nurses Association, or Meals-on-Wheels, as needed.
- All women should have a bone density test by the age of 65 years or at the time of early menopause.
- Discourage smoking. Smoking cigarettes hinders the healing of bones by decreasing collagen production and oxygen availability.
- Prevention focuses first on measures such as a balanced diet, adequate calcium and vitamin D intake, adequate exercise, smoking cessation, avoidance of excessive alcohol intake, and fall prevention (NAMS, 2010). Encourage frequent fish consumption, especially in winter, for vitamin D (Nakamura, 2006).

Patient Education—Food Safety

- Educate about basic food safety and hand washing.

For More Information

- American College of Physicians—Guidelines for Reducing Fractures
  http://www.annals.org/content/149/6/404.full
- Fracture Healing
  http://www.betterbones.com/bonefracture/speedhealing.aspx
- NIH—Medline
  http://www.nlm.nih.gov/medlineplus/ency/article/000001.htm
- Orthopedic Trauma Association
  http://www.hwbf.org/ota/bfc/
- Penn State University—Hershey Medical Center
  http://www.hmc.psu.edu/healthinfo/b/bonefracture.htm
- Web MD
  http://www.webmd.com/a-to-z-guides/understanding-fractures-basic-information
- WHO On-Line Risk Assessment Tool: FRAX
  http://www.shef.ac.uk/FRAX/

FRACTURES—CITED REFERENCES

Bonjour JP. Dietary protein: an essential nutrient for bone health. *J Am Coll Nutr.* 24:526S, 2005.

Candow DG, Chilibeck PD. Potential of creatine supplementation for improving aging bone health. *J Nutr Health Aging.* 14:149, 2010.

Cooper C, et al. Review: developmental origins of osteoporotic fracture. *Osteoporos Int.* 17:337, 2006.

Cosman S. The prevention and treatment of osteoporosis: a review. *Med Gen Med.* 7:73, 2005.

Earl S, et al. Session 2: other diseases: dietary management of osteoporosis throughout the life course. *Proc Nutr Soc.* 69:25, 2010.

Garnero P. Biomarkers for osteoporosis management: utility in diagnosis, fracture risk prediction and therapy monitoring. *Mol Diagn Ther.* 12:157, 2008.

Hamdy RC, et al. Algorithm for the management of osteoporosis. *South Med J.* 103:1009, 2010.

Haney EM, et al. Effects of selective serotonin reuptake inhibitors on bone health in adults: time for recommendations about screening, prevention and management? *Bone.* 46:13, 2010.

Miller MD, et al. Nutritional supplementation and resistance training in nutritionally at risk older adults following lower limb fracture: a randomized controlled trial. *Clin Rehabil.* 20:311, 2006.

Nakamura K. Vitamin D insufficiency in Japanese populations: from the viewpoint of the prevention of osteoporosis. *J Bone Miner Metab.* 24:1, 2006.

NAMS. Management of osteoporosis in postmenopausal women: 2010 position statement of The North American Menopause Society. *Menopause.* 17:25, 2010.

Xiong DH, et al. Genome-wide association and follow-up replication studies identified ADAMTS18 and TGFBR3 as bone mass candidate genes in different ethnic groups. *Am J Hum Genet.* 84:388, 2009.

INTESTINAL PARASITE INFECTIONS

NUTRITIONAL ACUITY RANKING: LEVEL 1

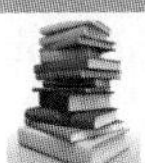

DEFINITIONS AND BACKGROUND

Intestinal parasite infections cause significant morbidity and mortality. These infections, especially from helminths and untreated water, represent major health problems that increase iron-deficiency anemia in developing countries (Alaofe et al, 2008). Protein–energy malnutrition causes immune deficiency, especially in developing countries. Newborns are especially vulnerable, where morbidity is often secondary to intestinal parasites (Steer, 2005). In addition, transmission of parasites is common in refugee or displacement camps. *Cryptosporidium parvum, Giardia lamblia, Entamoeba histolytica, Ascaris lumbricoides,* hookworm infection, *Schistosoma haematobium, S. mansoni* and *Strongyloides stercoralis* are important intestinal parasites that are common among children, the immunocompromised, and displaced populations (Gbakima et al, 2007). Infections caused by *Enterobius vermicularis, G. lamblia, Ancylostoma duodenale, Necator americanus,* and *E. histolytica* occur in the United States (see Table 15-11).

Mucin-secreting intestinal goblet cells are an important component of the innate defense system (Hasnain et al, 2010). Parasites modulate GI immunity, possibly by inhibiting migration of CD8α to the draining lymph nodes while increasing IL-6, TNF-α, and, in particular, IL-10 (Balic et al, 2009). Activation of the mucosal immune system of the GI tract results in altered intestinal physiology, which changes in intestinal motility and mucus production (Kahn and Collins, 2004). The protective immune response that develops following infection with intestinal parasites is characterized by increased numbers of $CD4^+$ T cells, granulocytes, and macrophages (Patel et al, 2009).

Toxoplasmosis is considered to be the third leading cause of death attributed to foodborne illness in the United States. More than 60 million men, women, and children in the United States carry the *Toxoplasma* parasite, but very few have symptoms because their healthy immune system usually keeps the parasite from causing illness. Washing vegetables thoroughly before eating them and cooking meat to the recommended temperatures are just a few ways to reduce risk of toxoplasmosis.

TABLE 15-11 Intestinal Parasites and Treatments

Parasite	Description and Treatment
Ancylostoma duodenale, Necator americanus (hookworms)	Cause blood loss, anemia, pica, and wasting. Finding eggs in the feces is diagnostic. Treatments include albendazole, mebendazole, pyrantel pamoate, iron supplementation, and blood transfusion. Preventive measures include wearing shoes and treating sewage.
Ascariasis (intestinal roundworms)	Common in warm or humid climates or when personal hygiene is inadequate. Adult worms live in the small intestine, with eggs that pass out in human feces. These eggs become infective within 2–3 weeks. When ingested by humans through fecally contaminated food or water, the eggs hatch and penetrate the intestines. Eventually, they reach the heart. Larvae mature within 2–3 months, and adult worms may live for 1 year or more. Hemorrhage can occur in lung tissue and cause pneumonitis. Vague abdominal discomfort can occur with small intestine involvement. Malnutrition can cause an imbalance in T-cell subpopulations that may lead to a defective T-cell maturation, thereby increasing susceptibility to parasitic infection (Di Pentima, 2009).
Enterobius vermicularis (pinworm)	Causes irritation and sleep disturbances. Diagnosis can be made using the "cellophane tape test." Treatment includes mebendazole and household sanitation.
Giardia	*Giardia intestinalis* is one of the most common intestinal parasites in the world, and it contributes to diarrhea, nutritional deficiencies, stunting, and cognitive impairment in children in developing regions (CDC, 2010). It causes nausea, vomiting, malabsorption, diarrhea, and weight loss. Stool ova and parasite studies are diagnostic. Treatment includes metronidazole. Sewage treatment, proper hand washing, and consumption of bottled water can be preventive.
Entamoeba histolytica	Can cause intestinal ulcerations, bloody diarrhea, weight loss, fever, gastrointestinal obstruction, and peritonitis. Amebas can cause abscesses in the liver that may rupture into the pleural space, peritoneum, or pericardium. Stool and serological assays, biopsy, barium studies, and liver imaging have diagnostic merit. Therapy includes luminal and tissue amebicides to attack both life-cycle stages. Metronidazole, chloroquine, and aspiration are treatments for liver abscess. Careful sanitation and use of peeled foods and bottled water are preventive.
Trichinella spiralis	*T. spiralis* is a roundworm that causes an acute infection (trichinosis) and is usually acquired by eating encysted larvae in raw or undercooked pork. Larvae mature and mate in the small intestine; larvae reaching striated muscle will encyst and live for years. Usual incubation is 5–15 days. The disorder has a 4% prevalence in the United States. Symptoms and signs include swelling of the upper eyelids, bleeding under the nails, skin rash, diarrhea, abdominal cramps, and malaise; later, low-grade fever, edema, sweating, dyspnea, cough, and muscle pain occur. In nonstriated muscle tissues such as the heart, brain, kidney, or lung, death can follow in 4–6 weeks, if untreated. Most symptoms disappear by the third month.

REFERENCES

CDC. Centers for Disease Control. Website accessed 10/16/10 at http://www.cdc.gov/ncidod/dpd/parasites/giardiasis/factsht_giardia.htm.

Di Pentima C. Burden of non-sexually transmitted infections on adolescent growth and development in the developing world. *Adolesc Med State Art Rev.* 20:930, 2009.

Risks are more significant for individuals with AIDS and for pregnant women. Most intestinal protozoan infections can cause acute or chronic diarrhea in healthy individuals but may result in intractable, life-threatening illness in patients with immunosuppressive diseases such as AIDS (Escobedo et al, 2009). Vaccines or immunotherapies may be developed to treat these pathogens.

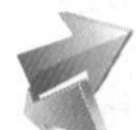

ASSESSMENT, MONITORING, AND EVALUATION

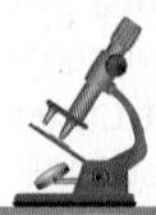

CLINICAL INDICATORS

Genetic Markers: The T-helper (Th) 2–type immune response causes infection-induced intestinal muscle hypercontractility and goblet cell hyperplasia (Kahn and Collins, 2004). The genetics of this form of immunity are under study.

Clinical/History

- Height
- Weight
- BMI
- Diet history
- Temperature
- I & O
- BP

Lab Work

- Stool examination
- Positive skin and serological tests for eosinophilia and leukocytosis
- Trichinosis—biopsy of skeletal muscle after fourth week (for larvae or cysts)
- Alb, transthyretin
- Prealbumin:CRP ratio
- CRP
- H & H
- Serum Fe, ferritin
- Transferrin
- TIBC
- Na^+, K^+, Cl^-
- Ca^{++}, Mg^{++}
- TLC, WBC
- Gluc

SAMPLE NUTRITION CARE PROCESS STEPS

Altered GI Function

Assessment Data: Diet history and intake records showing normal intake of all macronutrients. History of (Hx) explosive diarrhea for the past month. Tested positive for *G. lamblia* after a camping trip where patient drank untreated water from a stream. Other family members tested negative.

Nutrition Diagnosis (PES): NC-1.4 Altered GI function related to infection with *Giardia* as evidenced by explosive diarrhea for the past month and no changes in usual dietary intake.

Intervention: Food-Nutrient Delivery—discuss options for decreasing fiber and tolerating medications while under treatment for *Giardia.* Educate patient and family about the importance of drinking only treated water while camping. Counsel about monitoring tolerance for fiber-rich foods when infection has resolved. Coordinate care with medical team for pharmacotherapy and any nutritional side effects.

Monitoring and Evaluation: Resolution of *Giardia* infection and diarrheal disease. No undesirable side effects from medications.

INTERVENTION

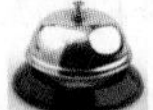

OBJECTIVES

- Differentiate symptoms and correctly identify condition as rapidly as possible; treat as needed.
- Treat infections and diarrhea.
- Prevent or correct malnutrition; prevent stunting and allow growth in children.
- Prevent blockage, inflammation, volvulus, and bowel perforation.
- Correct any complications such as anemia, pneumonia, and cardiac failure.
- Teach ways to prevent further infections.

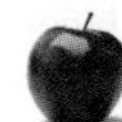

FOOD AND NUTRITION

- Provide balanced intake of all macronutrients. Protein intake, especially lysine, is important. Adequate, but not excessive, iron and zinc are also useful.
- Encourage adequate intake of food sources of vitamins A and C, especially from fruits, juices, and vegetables. Vitamin E and selenium may be especially protective (Smith et al, 2005). Supplements with retinol may be used in some cases.
- Ensure an adequate fluid intake, especially with diarrheal losses. Replace electrolytes with broths and juices.
- With poor appetite, offer small, frequent meals and snacks to correct malnutrition or weight loss that is undesirable.
- Ensure safe food handling at all meals.

Common Drugs Used and Potential Side Effects

- The albendazole–praziquantel combined regimen is a useful single-dose therapy for **giardiasis** in children.
- Pyrantel pamoate (Povan) may be used for **ascariasis**. Rarely, vomiting or diarrhea may occur.
- For **trichinosis**, mebendazole or thiabendazole may be used. GI distress is a common side effect. Aspirin or analgesics may be needed for muscular pain.
- Corticosteroids such as prednisone are often used temporarily to reduce inflammation of the heart or brain.

Herbs, Botanicals, and Supplements

- Herbs and botanical supplements should not be used without discussing with the physician. Chincona, elecampane, golden seal, ipecac, and papaya are not proven through clinical trials.

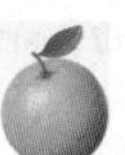

NUTRITION EDUCATION, COUNSELING, CARE MANAGEMENT

- Discuss the importance of personal hygiene in maintaining a sanitary environment and in preventing reinfestation.
- Children who play outside should always wash their hands before eating meals or snacks. Diarrhea caused by

parasites such as *Cryptosporidium* may be severe in malnourished or immunodeficient children; recovery is achieved only after sufficient nutritional repletion.

- Protozoa intestinal infection is still frequent in some marginalized populations; improvement in sanitation might decrease the prevalence of these diseases (Korkes et al, 2009). A mass campaign to educate about the role of sanitation in reducing intestinal parasite infection is recommended (Mehraj et al, 2008).

Patient Education—Food Safety

- Educate about food safety issues. Reducing new infection is very important. Meticulous hand washing is essential.
- Many of these parasites can be transmitted by food, water, soil, or person-to-person contact. Occasionally, helminthic roundworms, tapeworms, and flukes are transmitted in foods such as undercooked fish, crabs, and mollusks; undercooked meat; raw aquatic plants such as watercress; raw vegetables that have been contaminated by human or animal feces; and foods contaminated by food service workers with poor hygiene or working in unsanitary facilities.

For More Information

- CDC—An Ounce of Prevention
http://www.cdc.gov/ounceofprevention/
- Index of Parasitic Diseases
http://www.cdc.gov/ncidod/dpd/parasites/index.htm
- National Center for Emerging and Zoonotic Infectious Diseases
http://www.cdc.gov/ncezid/index.html

INTESTINAL PARASITES—CITED REFERENCES

Alaofe H, et al. Intestinal parasitic infections in adolescent girls from two boarding schools in southern Benin. *Trans R Soc Trop Med Hyg.* 102:653, 2008.

Balic A, et al. Dynamics of CD11 c(+) dendritic cell subsets in lymph nodes draining the site of intestinal nematode infection. *Immunol Lett.* 127:68, 2009.

Escobedo AA, et al. Treatment of intestinal protozoan infections in children. *Arch Dis Child.* 94:478, 2009.

Gbakima AA, et al. Intestinal protozoa and intestinal helminthic infections in displacement camps in Sierra Leone. *Afr J Med Med Sci.* 36:1, 2007.

Hasnain SZ, et al. Mucin gene deficiency in mice impairs host resistance to an enteric parasitic infection. *Gastroenterology.* 138:1763, 2010.

Kahn WI, Collins SM. Immune-mediated alteration in gut physiology and its role in host defence in nematode infection. *Parasite Immunol.* 26:319, 2004.

Korkes F, et al. Relationship between intestinal parasitic infection in children and soil contamination in an urban slum. *J Trop Pediatr.* 55:42, 2009.

Mehraj V, et al. Prevalence and factors associated with intestinal parasitic infection among children in an urban slum of Karachi. *PLoS One.* 3:e3680, 2008.

Patel N, et al. Characterisation of effector mechanisms at the host:parasite interface during the immune response to tissue-dwelling intestinal nematode parasites. *Int J Parasitol.* 39:13, 2009.

Smith A, et al. Deficiencies in selenium and/or vitamin E lower the resistance of mice to *Heligmosomoides polygyrus* infections. *J Nutr.* 135:830, 2005.

Steer P. The epidemiology of preterm labor—a global perspective. *J Perinat Med.* 33:273, 2005.

MULTIPLE ORGAN DYSFUNCTION SYNDROME

NUTRITIONAL ACUITY RANKING: LEVEL 4

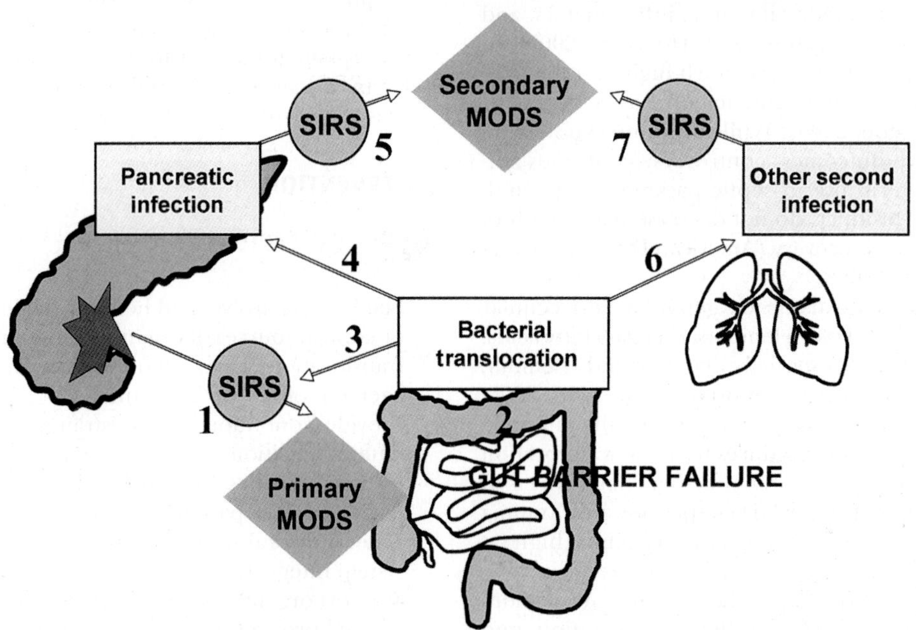

Adapted from: Sherwood L. Gorbach, John G. Bartlett, et al. *Infectious Diseases.* Philadelphia: Lippincott Williams & Wilkins, 2004.

DEFINITIONS AND BACKGROUND

Multiple organ dysfunction syndrome (MODS) involves two or more systems in failure at the same time (e.g., renal, hepatic, cardiac, or respiratory). The condition is also called MOF.

Etiology may be from sepsis (gram-positive/negative bacteria, fungal or viral,) shock, hemorrhage, allergy, burns, or trauma. Conditions leading to MOF may also include unnecessary deep sedation, excessive blood glucose levels, prolonged immobilization, or corticosteroid use (de Jonge et al, 2009).

Cytokines are direct mediators. MODS is triggered by TNF-α and by a cytokine cascade with IL-6 and other ILs, platelets, endothelial cells, and leukocytes. Lactate level is often used as a prognostic indicator of problems with tissue perfusion. High baseline serum cortisol level is also a marker of severity and poor prognosis. Cortisol levels <20 g/dL in a highly stressed patient (with respiratory failure, hypotension) may diagnose adrenal insufficiency, which should be treated (Marik et al, 2005). Early aggressive resuscitation of critically ill patients limits or prevents progression to MODS.

Gut injury and impaired gut barrier function have a high impact on the development of MODS. Mucosal lesions and increased intestinal permeability cause translocation of bacteria and endotoxins and initiate a local or systemic inflammatory response syndrome (SIRS). There are sequential metabolic changes following induction of SIRS, with an elevation in REE from 4–21 days and loss of LBM. Some experts suggest use of the phrase "nutrition therapy" versus "nutrition support" to strengthen the role in attenuating this metabolic response, preventing oxidative stress, and modifying the immune response with the use of appropriate lipids, glutamine, arginine, and antioxidants. Indeed, the quality of nutrition therapy is more important than the quantity.

Specific nutrients to modify immune, inflammatory, and metabolic processes have been helpful (Heys et al, 2005). In critical illness, glutamine levels are much higher in the duodenal mucosa; glutamine supplementation may be beneficial (De-Souza and Greene, 2005). While arginine supplementation may improve outcomes, controversy continues surrounding its long-term use in septic patients. In general, immune-enhanced products do not decrease ICU length of stay or improve rates of recovery (American Dietetic Association, 2010).

Maintaining adequate tissue oxygenation and cellular nutrition are priorities. Trace elements, omega-3 fatty acids, and antioxidant nutrients, especially vitamin E and selenium, are important and may reduce mortality (Grimble, 2005; Heyland et al, 2005). Enteral nutrition provides the intestinal mucosa with nutrients, which reduces bacterial translocation and septic complications. There may be beneficial effects of immune-enhancing diets for MODS, especially after trauma or surgery. However, overall mortality remains high at 30–100%, especially if multiple organs are involved.

The treatment of MODS is complex. Treatment includes correction of ischemia through fluid resuscitation and mechanical ventilation; antibiotics; and stabilization of water, electrolyte, and acid–base imbalance. Stress hyperglycemia promotes the proinflammatory response, whereas insulin has the opposite effect; therefore, tight glycemic control is important.

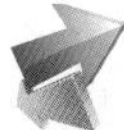

ASSESSMENT, MONITORING, AND EVALUATION

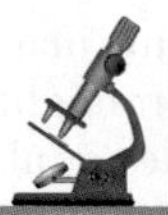

CLINICAL INDICATORS

Genetic Markers: The development of techniques for measuring the expression level of all of a person's genes may make it possible to develop an injury scoring system based on the degree of gene activation related to having more infections and organ failure (Warren et al, 2009).

Clinical/History	Lab Work	
Height	Serum procalcitonin (PCT)	Lactic acid (elevated?)
Weight	BUN (often elevated)	Serum pH <7.35 (acidosis)
BMI	Creat (often elevated)	Alanine, pyruvate (retention?)
Dry weight	ALT, AST (elevated)	Serum cortisol
Weight changes	Alb, transthyretin	pCO_2, pO_2
Edema, ascites	Albumin:CRP ratio	Chol, Trig
Diet history	CRP	Glomerular filtration rate
Temperature	Na^+, K^+	TLC, WBC
I & O	Ca^{++}, Mg^{++}	H & H
BP	Cl^-	Serum Fe
Acute Physiology and Chronic Health Evaluation (APACHE)	Creatine kinase (CK)	TIBC
Injury Severity Score (ISS)	Phosphorus	Serum phosphorous
Ultrasonography	Gluc—serum, urine	Serum folate
Echocardiography	Serum insulin	Serum zinc
Electroencephalogram (EEG)		

INTERVENTION

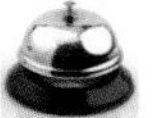

OBJECTIVES

- Stabilize electrolyte and hemodynamic balances. Remove or control sources of organ dysfunction, such as bacterial translocation. Early identification and aggressive management of MODS is essential.
- Provide continuous administration of at least minimal enteral nutrition to prevent gut mucosa atrophy.
- In patients with a functional GI tract, enteral nutrition is preferred over parenteral nutrition (Casaer et al, 2008). Enteral or oral nutrition preserves the gut and immune system integrity.
- Support organs with appropriate substrate. "Immunonutrition" provides formulas supplemented with arginine, omega-3 fatty acids, ribonucleic acids, and glutamine; however, there is no clear evidence that these products promote faster recovery (American Dietetic Association, 2010).
- Control hyperglycemia to decrease infection and sepsis.

SAMPLE NUTRITION CARE PROCESS STEPS

Excessive Infusion of Parenteral Nutrition

Assessment Data: Patient in ICU for 3 days, on CPN with order changed Day 2 to provide CHO and lipid in excess of estimated requirements. Indirect calorimetry identifies needs as 1400 kcal/day; patient receiving 1800 kcal/day. Admitted with acute pancreatitis; now showing signs of heart and liver failure. Glucose >200 mg/dL; fever with temperature of 102° F.

Nutrition Diagnosis (PES): Excessive infusion of parenteral nutrition related to current CPN order as evidenced by solution providing 1800 kcal/day with CHO and lipid exceeding daily requirements.

Intervention: Food-Nutrient Delivery—Decrease CPN order to 1400 kcal/day; lipid calculated at 30% total calories and CHO calculated as 50% total kilocalories. Patient may benefit from jejunostomy instead of CPN because of MODS.

Coordinate care with medical team—discuss importance of not overfeeding CPN solution. Discuss merits of using jejunostomy feeding instead of parenteral feeding.

Monitoring and Evaluation: CPN order discontinued. Jejunostomy tube placed; new feeding order that meets needs of 1400 kcal and 50% CHO, 30% fat, and 20% protein with extra fluid. Glucose monitoring and use of insulin to bring levels back below 120 mg/dL. Patient tolerating jejunostomy. Fever gradually subsiding. Signs of improvement in MODS.

- Promote prompt and immediate responses to all changing parameters. Until organ dysfunction resolves, monitor weight, relevant laboratory parameters, and nutrient intake.
- Consider short- and long-term consequences of all actions (e.g., treatments must incorporate a consensus of opinions about which therapy precedes another).
- Manage complications such as anemia, gastric reflux, or delayed bowel motility.
- Promote wound healing if surgery is required. Prevent additional sepsis.
- Promote recovery and improved well-being.

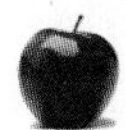

FOOD AND NUTRITION

- If there is gastric reflux or delayed bowel motility, a nasoduodenal or jejunal feeding tube or feeding jejunostomy is required. Ensure that the formula is appropriate.
- The recommended energy intake is 20–30 kcal/kg/day with a protein intake of 1.2–1.5 g/kg/day (Casaer et al, 2008). Evaluate organ function and provide a correctly calculated feeding and product for patient's diagnosis and condition.
- Immunoenhanced or glutamine-enriched products used to preserve gut integrity do not necessarily speed rates of recovery or reduce time in ICUs (American Dietetic Association, 2010).
- Review current vitamin and mineral intakes; adjust according to changing needs. Antioxidants may play a role in supporting recovery.
- Avoid excesses of iron, zinc, polyunsaturated fatty acids (PUFAs), and linoleic acid—especially parenterally—because of their effects on the immune system.
- When possible, return to oral feeding to acquire the benefits of phytochemicals from whole foods.
- Patients requiring ventilator support may need a higher lipid content in their feeding, even with cardiac failure.

Common Drugs Used and Potential Side Effects

- Hypertonic saline solution is commonly used.
- Anti-inflammatory treatment is vital for intervention in severe infectious disease.
- All medications should be reviewed for potential drug–nutrient incompatibility and stability with formulas. Try to avoid inclusion of medications with EN products because of drug–nutrient interactions and because drugs may then be less available to the patient.
- Drug metabolism with the liver cytochrome P-450 (CYP450) system can result in drug toxicities, reduced pharmacological effect, and adverse drug reactions. Foods such as grapefruit, alcoholic beverages, teas, and herbs may inhibit or induce the activity of CYP3A4 (Flanagan, 2005).
- Review all vitamin and mineral supplements and enteral products to determine whether the potential of hypervitaminosis and mineral toxicities exists.
- Insulin may be required because of the hyperglycemia that occurs with stress.
- With continuous seizures, lorazepam or anticonvulsants may be needed. Weight and appetite changes are common if used long term.

Herbs, Botanicals, and Supplements

- Herbs and botanical supplements should not be used without discussing with the physician. Herbs often possess the ability to inhibit or induce the activity of CYP3A4.
- Chinese herbs for reducing inflammatory reaction are being studied.

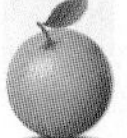

NUTRITION EDUCATION, COUNSELING, CARE MANAGEMENT

- When possible, discuss implications of MODS in relation to nutritional support. Include a realistic assessment of potential for recovery and use of EN in the home setting, as discussed with the physician.
- Family should be included in discussions about nutritional support measures that are taken. As appropriate, prepare patient and family for home nutritional needs and total parenteral nutrition/EN/oral diet requirements.
- Alleviate fears associated with eating or nutritional support therapies.
- Discuss any signs or problems that should require professional intervention.

Patient Education—Food Safety

- Educate about food safety issues. Reducing more infection is very important.

- Meticulous hand washing is essential because immunocompromised individuals are more susceptible to minor illnesses, including foodborne illness.

For More Information

- eMedicine—MODS
  http://emedicine.medscape.com/article/169640-overview
- Merck—Shock
  http://www.merck.com/mmpe/sec06/ch067/ch067b.html

MULTIPLE ORGAN DYSFUNCTION SYNDROME—CITED REFERENCES

American Dietetic Association. Evidence Analysis Library: critical illness. Web site accessed February 11, 2010 at http://www.adaevidencelibrary.com/topic.cfm?cat=2809.

Casaer MP, et al. Bench-to-bedside review: metabolism and nutrition. *Crit Care.* 12:222, 2008.

de Jonge B, et al. Intensive care unit-acquired weakness: risk factors and prevention. *Crit Care Med.* 37:309S, 2009.

De-Souza DA, Greene LJ. Intestinal permeability and systemic infections in critically ill patients: effect of glutamine. *Crit Care Med.* 33:1125, 2005.

Flanagan D. Understanding the grapefruit-drug interaction. *Gen Dent.* 53:282, 2005.

Grimble RF. Immunonutrition. *Curr Opin Gastroenterol.* 21:216, 2005.

Heyland DK, et al. Antioxidant nutrients: a systematic review of trace elements and vitamins in the critically ill patient. *Intensive Care Med.* 31:327, 2005.

Heys SD, et al. Nutrition and the surgical patient: triumphs and challenges. *Surgeon.* 3:139, 2005.

Marik PE, et al. The hepatoadrenal syndrome: a common yet unrecognized clinical condition. *Crit Care Med.* 33:1254, 2005.

Warren HS, et al. A genomic score prognostic of outcome in trauma patients. *Mol Med.* 15:220, 2009.

SEPSIS AND SYSTEMIC INFLAMMATORY RESPONSE SYNDROME

NUTRITIONAL ACUITY RANKING: LEVEL 4

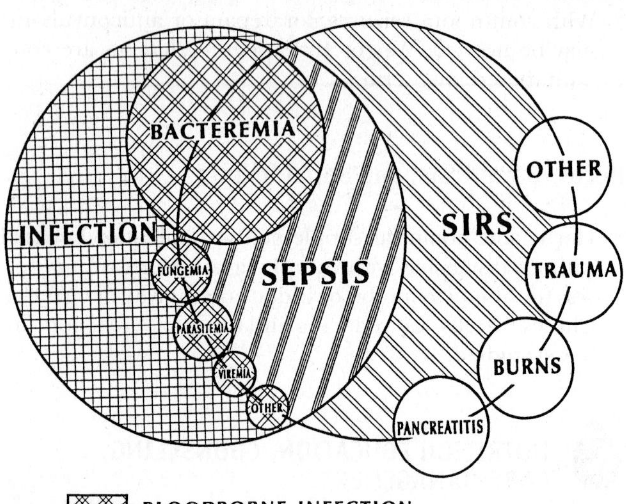

Adapted from: Sherwood L. Gorbach, John G. Bartlett, et al. *Infectious Diseases.* Philadelphia: Lippincott Williams & Wilkins, 2004.

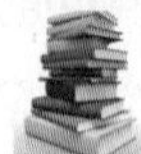

DEFINITIONS AND BACKGROUND

Sepsis involves a SIRS, with infection that has spread to other areas from its original site. Similar to the stress response, the inflammatory reaction is crucial for survival and is meant to be tailored to the stimulus and time (Elenkov et al, 2005). Sepsis may be a complication of vascular access devices or intravenous catheters and may be bacterial or fungal in origin. The most common sources of infection are lung and abdominal infections (Russell, 2008). The stages of sepsis are listed in Table 15-12.

Natural killer cells are a crucial component of the innate immune response to various viruses, fungi, parasites, and bacteria (Fauci et al, 2005). Systemic inflammation stimulates an acute-phase reaction and the stress response, mediated by the hypothalamic–pituitary–adrenal axis and the sympathetic nervous system (Elenkov et al, 2005). GI tract dysmotility increases permeability of intestinal mucosa and bacterial translocation, contributing to sepsis and MODS (Ukleja, 2010). Synergistic effects of TNF-α, IL-1β, other cytokines, and nitric oxide are also implicated. In SIRS, reduced TNF production occurs; this is immunosuppression rather than an excessive inflammatory response (Cavaillon et al, 2005).

In sepsis, activated phagocytes release leukocytic endogenous mediators; hepatic uptake of amino acids and increased prostaglandin synthesis occur. Hormonal responses include increases in adrenocorticotropic hormone (ACTH), aldosterone, and catecholamines (with increased gluconeogenesis, glycolysis, proteolysis, and lipolysis). Decreased triiodothyronine (T3) cause tissue degradation and mobilized triglycerides.

Host defense peptides modulate inflammation (Bowdish and Hancock, 2005). While albumin, transthyretin, and transferrin have a transport role in the body, acute-phase proteins (CRP, α-acid glycoprotein, and α-trypsin) help with host defense. These parameters drop in sepsis independent of nutritional status; monitor all protein levels as markers of inflammation in this population.

Vitamin D_3 plays a role in immune activation of endothelial cells during gram-negative bacterial infections (Equils et al, 2006). It may enhance the innate immune response by induction of cathelicidin (LL-37), an endogenous antimicrobial peptide produced by macrophages and neutrophils (Jeng et al, 2009).

Enteral feeding is preferred over parenteral feeding, where catheter infection is a risk. A key issue in providing nutrition to critically ill patients is intolerance of enteral feeding as a result of impaired GI motility (Ukleja, 2010). Overfeeding sometimes increases sepsis.

TABLE 15-12 Stages of Sepsis

Definitions of the various stages of sepsis can be summarized as follows:

- Infection is a microbial phenomenon in which an inflammatory response to the presence of microorganisms or the invasion of normally sterile host tissue by these organisms is characteristic.
- Bacteremia is the presence of viable bacteria in the blood.
- Systemic inflammatory response syndrome (SIRS) may follow a variety of clinical insults, including infection, pancreatitis, ischemia, multiple trauma, tissue injury, hemorrhagic shock, or immune-mediated organ injury.
- Sepsis is a systemic response to infection. This is identical to SIRS, except that it must result from infection.
- Septic shock is sepsis with hypotension (systolic blood pressure <90 mm Hg or a reduction of 40 mm Hg from baseline) despite adequate fluid resuscitation. Concomitant organ dysfunction or perfusion abnormalities (e.g., lactic acidosis, oliguria, coma) are present in the absence of other known causes.
- Multiple organ dysfunction syndrome (MODS) is the presence of altered organ function in a patient who is acutely ill such that homeostasis cannot be maintained without intervention. Primary MODS is the direct result of a well-defined insult in which organ dysfunction occurs early and can be directly attributable to the insult itself. Secondary MODS develops as a consequence of a host response and is identified within the context of SIRS. The inflammatory response of the body to toxins and other components of microorganisms causes the clinical manifestations of sepsis.

Sepsis syndrome is recognized clinically by the presence of two or more of the following:

- Temperature >38°C or <36°C
- Heart rate >90 beats/min
- Respiratory rate >20 breaths/min or partial pressure of carbon dioxide in arterial gas <32 mm Hg
- White blood cell count >12,000 cells/μL, <4000 cells/μL, or >10% band forms

Adapted from: American College of Chest Physicians/Society of Critical Care Medicine Consensus Panel guidelines. Web site accessed February 11, 2010 at http://chestjournal.chestpubs.org/content/101/6/1644.abstract.

Management of septic shock requires an ABCDEF approach: Airway, Breathing, Circulation, Drugs, Evaluate, and Fix the source of sepsis (Russell, 2008). Improvements in the management of sepsis and MODS have resulted from improvements in critical care practices (Sullivan et al, 2005). Yet, the incidence of septic shock is increasing; mortality ranges from 30% to 70% (Russell, 2008). Severe sepsis leading to shock is still a common cause of death in critically ill patients.

Sepsis may involve the bloodstream from gram-negative or gram-positive bacteria. Diseases caused by group A *Streptococcus* include acute rheumatic fever, rheumatic heart disease, poststreptococcal glomerulonephritis, and invasive infections. Pathogenic *Escherichia coli* causes infections such as urinary tract infection and meningitis, which are prevalent (Kim et al, 2005). *Yersinia enterocolitis* can cause bacteremia or abdominal abscess, especially in states of iron overload. Neonatal sepsis is a major cause of death, especially in low birth-weight infants. In addition, while sepsis during pregnancy is uncommon, it is potentially fatal (Fernandez-Perez et al, 2005). In the elderly, poor immune response and poor functional status may be indicators of sepsis (Gavazzi et al, 2005).

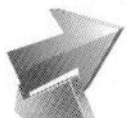

ASSESSMENT, MONITORING, AND EVALUATION

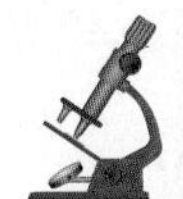

CLINICAL INDICATORS

Genetic Markers: The genetics involved with various inflammatory responses to sepsis are being studied. A variety of polymorphisms may play a role in sepsis.

Clinical/History

- Height
- Weight
- BMI
- Diet history
- I & O
- BP (hypotension?)
- Fever, chills
- Fatigue, malaise
- Decreased urine output
- Skin rash?
- Mild confusion
- Catabolism of lean body mass
- Tachycardia

Lab Work

- Elevated WBC
- Alb, transthyretin
- Albumin: CRP ratio
- CRP
- Chol (decreased)
- pO_2, pCO_2
- Gluc (altered)
- Decreased glucose tolerance?
- Glucagon (increased)
- Serum insulin
- Plasma 25(OH)D—low?
- Plasma lactate
- Transferrin
- Trig (increased)
- AST (increased)
- BUN, Creat
- Urinary urea nitrogen
- Na^+, K^+
- Ca^{++}, Mg^{++}
- Cl^-
- H & H
- Serum Fe
- N balance
- T3 (decreased)
- 5-Hydroxyindole acetic acid (5-HIAA) (increased)
- Phosphate (decreased)
- Osmolality

INTERVENTION

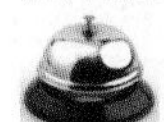

OBJECTIVES

- Prevent septic shock with increased cardiac output, tachycardia, low blood pressure, decreased renal output, and warm flushed skin. Support medical, goal-directed resuscitation of the septic patient and use of broad-spectrum antibiotic therapy within 1 hour of diagnosis of septic shock (Dellenger et al, 2008).
- Support the body's antimicrobial defense system and keep the environment as germ free as possible to prevent MODS. Use strict guidelines and protocols for insertion, care, and maintenance of any catheters and feeding tubes.
- Meet increased energy needs. Mild infection elevates resting energy expenditure between 15% and 40%; sepsis increases it by 40–70% and doubles nitrogen losses. Use indirect calorimetry whenever possible, and do not overfeed.

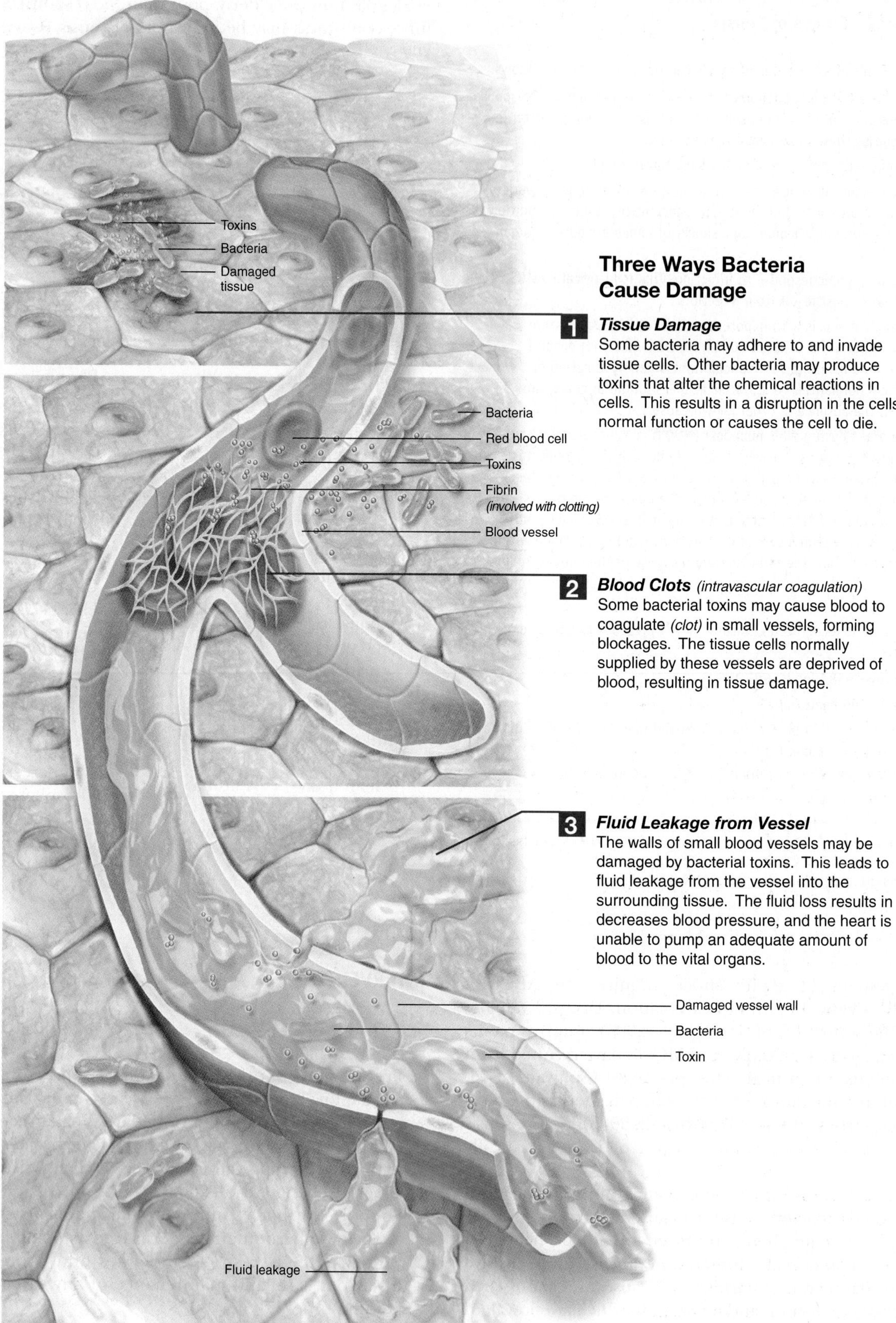

Toxins
Bacteria
Damaged tissue
Three Ways Bacteria Cause Damage
1 Tissue Damage
Some bacteria may adhere to and invade tissue cells. Other bacteria may produce toxins that alter the chemical reactions in cells. This results in a disruption in the cells' normal function or causes the cell to die.
Bacteria
Red blood cell
Toxins
Fibrin (involved with clotting)
Blood vessel
2 Blood Clots (intravascular coagulation)
Some bacterial toxins may cause blood to coagulate (clot) in small vessels, forming blockages. The tissue cells normally supplied by these vessels are deprived of blood, resulting in tissue damage.
3 Fluid Leakage from Vessel
The walls of small blood vessels may be damaged by bacterial toxins. This leads to fluid leakage from the vessel into the surrounding tissue. The fluid loss results in decreases blood pressure, and the heart is unable to pump an adequate amount of blood to the vital organs.
Damaged vessel wall
Bacteria
Toxin
Fluid leakage

Asset provided by Anatomical Chart Co.

SAMPLE NUTRITION CARE PROCESS STEPS

Increased Nutrient Needs

Assessment Data: Nursing home resident with urosepsis; fever with temperature 101°F; albumin 2.4 g/dL; requires feeding assistance; hip replacement surgery 1 month ago.

Nutrition Diagnosis (PES): NI 5.1 Increased nutrient needs for protein related to urosepsis and recent surgery as evidenced by albumin 2.4 g/dL and intake <50% of dairy-meat items at meals.

Intervention

Food-Nutrient Delivery—ND 3.1.1 Commercial high-protein beverage

Education E 2.1 Adding protein powder, 30 mL BID for increased protein

Counseling C2.2 Goal setting—meet protein needs daily (1.5 g/kg)

Coordination of Care RC 1.1 Team meeting—nursing to focus on better intake of dairy and meat items on trays.

Monitoring and Evaluation: Improved oral intake of protein sources from dairy products, meat group choices, and protein powder; 75–100% at meals. Meeting daily protein needs of 1.5 g/kg. Resolution of urosepsis. Wound healing continues.

- Promote tissue repair and wound healing. Protein turnover is often 30–50% higher than normal.
- Treat nausea, vomiting, and anorexia.
- Prevent or treat metabolic derangements such as hyperglycemia, glycosuria, hyperosmolar/nonketotic coma, electrolyte abnormalities (e.g., decreased potassium, decreased phosphate, elevated chloride), osmotic diarrhea, and fluid overload. Glycemic control, targeting a blood glucose <150 mg/dL after initial stabilization (Dellenger et al, 2008).
- Correct anemia, which prevents tissue oxygenation. Target a hemoglobin level of 7–9 g/dL (Dellenger et al, 2008). Prevent or manage stress ulcers and upper GI bleeding.

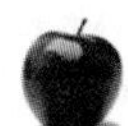

FOOD AND NUTRITION

- Protein should be provided in levels of 1.5–2.0 g/kg daily. Branched-chain amino acids (BCAAs) are useful for energy because they do not need to be metabolized to glucose.
- Provide calories at 30–35 kcal/kg. Monitor daily actual intake.
- Enteral nutrition should be initiated within 48 hours of injury or admission and average intake actually delivered within the first week should be **at least** 60–70% of total estimated energy requirements as determined by patient assessment (American Dietetic Association, 2010).
- When patient can eat, soft diet and liquids of high nutrient and energy value are beneficial.
- Vitamins A, C, D, K, thiamin, and folic acid may become depleted with infection. Urinary excretion of phosphorus, potassium, magnesium, zinc, and chromium also occur; monitor for signs of malnutrition. Replace in feedings or diet as appropriate.
- Include omega-3 fatty acids (Babcock et al, 2005). Inclusion of fish oil in parenteral nutrition provided to septic ICU patients increases plasma eicosapentaenoic acid, modifies inflammatory cytokine concentrations, improves gas exchange, and shortens the length of hospital stay (Barbosa et al, 2010).
- Monitor fluid requirements and intake carefully to excrete wastes properly.
- If tube feeding is needed, there are no benefits for using immune-enhancing formulas (American Dietetic Association, 2010).

Common Drugs Used and Potential Side Effects

- Antibiotics are used for bacterial sepsis; monitor for side effects and GI distress.
- Activated protein C, a vitamin K–dependent serine protease, is an anticoagulant that is also cytoprotective and has anti-inflammatory role for use in septic shock (Russell, 2008).
- Antiseptic-impregnated catheters, such as those with minocycline–rifampicin or chlorhexidine/silver sulfadiazine, may be needed to reduce catheter-related sepsis.
- Insulin may be needed for hyperglycemia; glucose control is important.
- Iron and zinc are bacterial nutrients; omit them in CPN solutions in septic patients.
- Prevent upper GI bleeding by using H2 blockers or proton pump inhibitors (Dellenger et al, 2008).
- Steroids may be used. Greater nitrogen depletion and hyperglycemia, sodium retention, and potassium losses can occur. Monitor carefully. Corticosteroid therapy induces potentially detrimental hyperglycemia in septic shock (COIITSS Study Investigators, 2010).

Herbs, Botanicals, and Supplements

- Herbs and botanical supplements should not be used without discussing with physician.
- Optimal vitamin D is important for innate immunity in the setting of sepsis (Jeng et al, 2009).
- Fish oil may play an important role in reducing the hospital length of stay in septic patients (Barbosa et al, 2010).

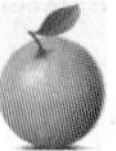

NUTRITION EDUCATION, COUNSELING, CARE MANAGEMENT

- Use of aseptic techniques for feedings and meals will be essential.
- Need for a well-managed convalescence and gradual refeeding process will be needed to support patient's resistance and immunity. Terminate the cycle of infection, malnutrition, reinfection, and further protein–energy malnutrition.

Patient Education—Food Safety

- Educate about food safety issues. Reducing infections is very important.

- Meticulous hand washing is essential; immunocompromised individuals are more susceptible to minor illnesses, including foodborne illness.

For More Information

- JAMA—Sepsis Page
http://jama.ama-assn.org/cgi/reprint/301/23/2516.pdf
- MEDLINE—Sepsis
http://www.nlm.nih.gov/medlineplus/ency/article/000666.htm

SEPSIS AND SYSTEMIC INFLAMMATORY RESPONSE—CITED REFERENCES

American Dietetic Association. Evidence Analysis Library: critical illness. Web site accessed February 11, 2010 at http://www.adaevidencelibrary.com/topic.cfm?cat=2809.

Babcock TA, et al. Experimental studies defining omega-3 fatty acid antiinflammatory mechanisms and abrogation of tumor-related syndromes. *Nutr Clin Pract.* 20:62, 2005.

Barbosa VM, et al. Effects of a fish oil containing lipid emulsion on plasma phospholipid fatty acids, inflammatory markers, and clinical outcomes in septic patients: a randomized, controlled clinical trial [published online ahead of print January 19, 2010]. *Crit Care.* 14:R5, 2010.

Bowdish DM, Hancock RE. Anti-endotoxin properties of cationic host defence peptides and proteins. *J Endotoxin Res.* 11:230, 2005.

Cavaillon JM, et al. Reprogramming of circulatory cells in sepsis and SIRS. *J Endotoxin Res.* 11:311, 2005.

COIITSS Study Investigators. Corticosteroid treatment and intensive insulin therapy for septic shock in adults: a randomized controlled trial. *JAMA.* 303:341, 2010.

Dellenger RP, et al. Surviving Sepsis Campaign: international guidelines for management of severe sepsis and septic shock: 2008. *Crit Care Med.* 36:296, 2008.

Elenkov IJ, et al. Cytokine dysregulation, inflammation and well-being. *Neuroimmunomodulation.* 12:255, 2005.

Equils O, et al. 1,25-Dihydroxyvitamin D inhibits lipopolysaccharide-induced immune activation in human endothelial cells. *Clin Exp Immunol.* 143:58, 2006.

Fauci AS, et al. NK cells in HIV infection: paradigm for protection or targets for ambush. *Nat Rev Immunol.* 5:835, 2005.

Fernandez-Perez ER, et al. Sepsis during pregnancy. *Crit Care Med.* 33:286S, 2005.

Gavazzi G, et al. Nosocomial bacteremia in very old patients: predictors of mortality. *Aging Clin Exp Res.* 17:337, 2005.

Jeng L, et al. Alterations in vitamin D status and anti-microbial peptide levels in patients in the intensive care unit with sepsis. *J Transl Med.* 7:28, 2009.

Kim BY, et al. Invasion processes of pathogenic *Escherichia coli*. *Int J Med Microbiol.* 295:463, 2005.

Russell JA. The current management of septic shock. *Minerva Med.* 99:431, 2008.

Sullivan KJ, et al. Critical care of the pediatric hematopoietic stem cell recipient in 2005. *Pediatr Transplant.* 9:12S, 2005.

Ukleja A. Altered GI motility in critically ill patients: current understanding of pathophysiology, clinical impact, and diagnostic approach. *Nutr Clin Pract.* 25:16, 2010.

TRAUMA

NUTRITIONAL ACUITY RANKING: LEVEL 3

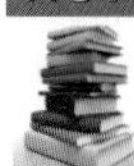

DEFINITIONS AND BACKGROUND

Physical trauma is caused by major injury or accidents; 50% are from traffic accidents. Trauma is the third leading cause of death and the number one killer of people younger than 45 years (Compton and Rhee, 2005). Multiple traumas involve at least two injuries. Long-bone fractures, pelvic or vertebral fractures, and damage to body cavities (head, thorax, or abdomen) generally are involved. The first assessment by emergency medical technicians involves airway, breathing, and circulation (A-B-C), followed by disability and exposure (D-E). For a neurological disability evaluation, clinicians use the Glasgow Coma Scale (GCS) to determine the level of consciousness; see Table 15-13.

Metabolic changes may include increased oxygen consumption and energy expenditure; increased secretion of ACTH, cortisol, epinephrine, norepinephrine, insulin, and growth hormone; and decreased total T3 levels (Jakob and Stanga, 2010). Reperfusion injury, a potential life-threatening disorder, is an acute inflammatory response after periods of ischemia resulting from trauma (Zhang et al, 2006). The heart and brain are the organs most affected.

The first 60 minutes, or the "golden hour" after trauma, may involve early deaths from severe brain or spinal cord injuries. Days later, death may occur from subdural or epidural hematoma. Late deaths may occur after several weeks. Therefore, nutritional support is an integral part of the management of trauma victims. Skeletal muscle is a major protein source for catabolism; BCAAs are cannibalized (Laviano et al, 2005). Nitrogen excretion increases after injury, peaks after 7 days, and eventually stabilizes. Insulin has been shown to increase synthesis and decrease degradation of skeletal muscle protein when amino acids are provided intravenously. Malnutrition caused by hypercatabolism and hypermetabolism parallels the severity of illness (Wooley et al, 2005).

Trauma is best managed by emergency department or critical care teams. Most countries have adopted measures known as Advanced Trauma Life Support (ATLS). In this process, teams address the most life-threatening issues first.

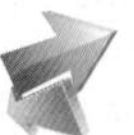

ASSESSMENT, MONITORING, AND EVALUATION

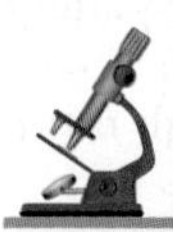

CLINICAL INDICATORS

Genetic Markers: Trauma is not genetic in origin, but individuals respond to trauma while using their innate and acquired immune systems accordingly.

Clinical/History

Height
Weight before trauma
Weight after trauma
Percentage weight change
Resting energy expenditure (indirect calorimetry)
BMI
Diet history
Temperature
I & O
BP
ISS
GCS
Respiratory rate
Arteriography
Radiographs, computed tomography

Lab Work

Alb, transthyretin (monitor fluid levels)
Albumin:CRP ratio
CRP
Na^+, K^+
Ca^{++}, Mg^{++}
Cl^-
H & H
Serum Fe
TLC
WBC
Serum lactate
Chol, Trig
Phosphorus
BUN, Creat
Gluc (increased?)
Creatine phosphokinase (increased)
pCO_2, pO_2
Bilirubin, AST (increased)
Serum amino acids
N balance

SAMPLE NUTRITION CARE PROCESS STEPS

Inadequate Oral Food and Beverage Intake

Assessment Data: Car accident victim; closed head injury and comatose. Indirect calorimetry measures REE at 1800 kcal.

Nutrition Diagnosis (PES): Inadequate oral food and beverage intake related to inability to eat orally as evidenced by comatose state and ventilator dependency.

Intervention: Food-Nutrient Delivery—Initiate enteral tube feeding at slow rate, gradually increasing to meet needs of 1800 kcal/24 hours. Avoid overfeeding and monitor hydration status carefully. Coordinate care with medical team to follow progress.

Monitoring and Evaluation: Tube feeding tolerance: glucose, BUN, other lab values; hydration without excess.

INTERVENTION

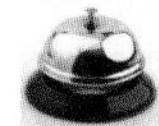

OBJECTIVES

- Assess and monitor extent of injury and resulting problems. Restore hemodynamic and metabolic functions and acid–base and fluid balance.
- Prevent infection, respiratory failure, shock, sepsis, and reperfusion injury.
- Determine GI function; provide nutrients in the most effective mode. Use the gut if possible. Enteral nutrition is more efficacious and poses lower risks than parenteral nutrition; it reduces infection rates and shortens hospital length of stay (American Dietetic Association, 2010).
- Decrease nitrogen losses; promote nitrogen balance. Glutamine and arginine may be indicated.
- Meet elevated energy requirements (up by 20–45%). Spare proteins and LBM.
- Prevent overfeeding with respiratory distress from increased carbon dioxide production.
- Determine and monitor fluid requirements and balance. Do not overhydrate; persistent positive fluid balance in older surgical patients prolongs mechanical ventilation (Epstein and Peerless, 2006).
- Promote healing and rapid recovery.

TABLE 15-13 Glasgow Coma Scale (GCS)

The GCS is a neurological scale for recording the conscious state of a person, for initial and subsequent assessments. A patient is assessed against the criteria of the scale, and the resulting points give patient a score between 3 (indicating deep unconsciousness) and either 14 (original scale) or 15 (the more widely used modified or revised scale). The scale comprises three tests: eye, verbal, and motor responses. The three values are considered separately, as well as their sum. The lowest possible GCS score (the sum) is 3 (deep coma or death), whereas the highest score is 15 (fully awake person). The lower the score, the worse the prognosis.

Key: Severe, with GCS ≤ 8
Moderate, GCS 9–2
Minor, GCS ≥ 13

Glasgow Coma Scale

	1	2	3	4	5	6
Eyes	Does not open eyes	Opens eyes in response to painful stimuli	Opens eyes in response to voice	Opens eyes spontaneously	N/A	N/A
Verbal	Makes no sounds	Incomprehensible sounds	Utters inappropriate words	Confused, disoriented	Oriented, converses normally	N/A
Motor	Makes no movements	Extension to painful stimuli (decerebrate response)	Abnormal flexion to painful stimuli (decorticate response)	Flexion/withdrawal to painful stimuli	Localizes painful stimuli	Obeys commands

From Teasdale G, Jennett B. Assessment of coma and impaired consciousness. A practical scale. *Lancet.* 2:81, 1974.

- Treat ileus, fistula, glucose abnormalities, and other complications such as venous thromboembolism (VTE). VTE causes major morbidity in adults after trauma and occurs in up to 50% of patients without prophylaxis (Hanson et al, 2010).
- Promote rehabilitation.
- Correct anorexia and depression; improve the quality of life.

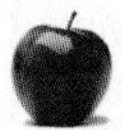

FOOD AND NUTRITION

- **Day 1: Immediately**—Intravenous feedings are given for fluid resuscitation for approximately 24 hours until stable. Life support measures and careful monitoring are required.
- **Days 2–5: Transition Phase**—Assess changing status. Implement nutrition by the most effective means, dictated by injury location and extent. Controversy exists regarding the optimal nutrition regimen; therefore, individualize for each patient (Thompson and Fuhrman, 2005). When goals are not achieved enterally, early PN use may be associated with a greater risk of nosocomial infection and worse clinical outcomes (Sena et al, 2008). Initiation of enteral feedings within 24–48 hours of injury or admission to ICU generally reduces infectious complications (Kattelmann et al, 2006). Feed patients in the semirecumbent rather than supine position to reduce aspiration pneumonia and formula reflux (Kattelmann et al, 2006). Provide adequate energy and nutrients: 35–45 kcal/kg and 1.5–2 g protein/kg. Advance feeding rate over several days; gastrostomy may be useful in head/neck trauma. Actual delivery of 14–18 kcal/kg/day or 60–70% of goal is associated with improved outcomes, whereas greater intake may not be beneficial (Kattelmann et al, 2006). Blue food coloring should not be used to detect aspiration with enteral feedings (American Dietetic Association, 2010).
- **Days 5–10: Adaptive Phase**—Use products with glutamine, arginine, and high percentage of BCAAs; include lipids. Osmolarity should be monitored to be close to 300 mOsm. In general, 25 kcal/kg/d is an acceptable and achievable target intake, but patients with trauma may require almost twice as much energy during the acute phase of their illness. Provide 1.5–2 g protein/kg. CHOs should be given as 5 mg/kg/min. A diet providing 50% CHO, 15% protein, and 35% fat should be adequate. A slight increase in vitamin–mineral intake should be addressed, with vitamins A, B-complex, and C in particular. Avoid large doses of iron and zinc.
- **Day 11 Onward: Rehabilitative Phase**—Patient can be weaned to oral diet, if possible, and off the ventilator support. Liquid to regular diets are usually tolerated at this time.

Common Drugs Used and Potential Side Effects

- Albumin therapy is considered for trauma, hypovolemia, shock, hypoalbuminemia, and volume resuscitation (Mendez et al, 2005).
- Analgesics may have an effect on nutritional status. Evaluate individually. Lidocaine can be used to alleviate neuropathic pain.
- Antibiotics generally are used to reduce bacterial infection. Monitor for GI distress and side effects.
- Barbiturates, used for closed head injury, will decrease metabolic rate.
- Intensive insulin therapy and the use of a continuous glucose sensor may be used for hyperglycemia (Mraovic, 2009).
- Promotility agents may reduce gastric residual volume in tube-fed patients (Kattelmann et al, 2006).

Herbs, Botanicals, and Supplements

- Herbs and botanical supplements should not be used without discussing with the physician.
- Capsaicin and resveratrol have been used for some patients to decrease inflammation after trauma.

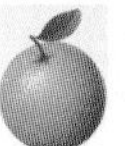

NUTRITION EDUCATION, COUNSELING, CARE MANAGEMENT

- Need for specific nutrients should be discussed, according to the mode tolerated.
- Rehabilitation should progress according to individual requirements and injury sites, side effects, and complications.

Patient Education—Food Safety

- Educate about food safety issues. Reducing infections is very important. Meticulous hand washing is essential because immunocompromised individuals are more susceptible to minor illnesses, including foodborne illness.

For More Information

- Medscape—Trauma
  http://emedicine.medscape.com/trauma
- Trauma
  http://www.trauma.org/

TRAUMA—CITED REFERENCES

American Dietetic Association. Evidence Analysis Library: critical illness. Web site accessed February 13, 2010 at http://www.adaevidencelibrary.com/topic.cfm?cat=2809.

Compton C, Rhee R. Peripheral vascular trauma. *Perspect Vasc Surg Endovasc Ther.* 17:297, 2005.

Epstein CD, Peerless JR. Weaning readiness and fluid balance in older critically ill surgical patients. *Am J Crit Care.* 15:54, 2006.

Hanson SJ, et al. Incidence and risk factors for venous thromboembolism in critically ill children after trauma. *J Trauma.* 68:52, 2010.

Jakob SM, Stanga Z. Perioperative metabolic changes in patients undergoing cardiac surgery. *Nutrition.* 26:349, 2010.

Kattelmann KK, et al. Preliminary evidence for a medical nutrition therapy protocol: enteral feedings for critically ill patients. *J Am Diet Assoc.* 106:1226, 2006.

Laviano A, et al. Branched-chain amino acids: the best compromise to achieve anabolism? *Curr Opin Clin Nutr Metab Care.* 8:408, 2005.

Mendez CM, et al. Albumin therapy in clinical practice. *Nutr Clin Pract.* 20:314, 2005.

Mraovic B. Analysis: continuous glucose monitoring during intensive insulin therapy. *J Diabetes Sci Technol.* 3:960, 2009.

Sena MJ, et al. Early supplemental parenteral nutrition is associated with increased infectious complications in critically ill trauma patients. *J Am Coll Surg.* 207:459, 2008.

Thompson C, Fuhrman MP. Nutrients and wound healing: still searching for the magic bullet. *Nutr Clin Pract.* 20:331, 2005.

Wooley JA, et al. Metabolic and nutritional aspects of acute renal failure in critically ill patients requiring continuous renal replacement therapy. *Nutr Clin Pract.* 20:176, 2005.

Zhang M, et al. Identification of the target self-antigens in reperfusion injury. *J Exp Med.* 203:141, 2006.

SECTION 16

Renal Disorders

CHIEF ASSESSMENT FACTORS

Ten Symptoms of Kidney Disease

- Changes in urination
- Confusion
- Feeling dizzy
- Headache
- High blood pressure
- Loss of appetite or change in taste
- Nausea or vomiting
- Severe itching not related to a bite or rash
- Shortness of breath
- Swelling of face, hands, and/or feet

Other Factors

- Altered Lipid and Amino Acid Levels
- Abnormal Blood Urea Nitrogen (BUN):Creatinine Ratio
- Anorexia
- Bone Pain, Altered Height, or Lean Body Mass
- Burning or Difficulty During Urination
- Changes in Glomerular Filtration Rate (GFR)
- Chronic Inflammation
- Flank Pain
- Frequent Weight Shifts
- Ghrelin and Obestatin Ratios
- Insomnia
- Itching, Dry Skin
- Leg Cramps
- More Frequent Urination and Nocturia
- Pain in Small of Back Just Below Ribs, Not Aggravated by Movement
- Passage of Bloody-Appearing Urine (Hematuria)
- Presence or History of Urinary Tract Infections or Stones
  - Proteinuria, Microalbuminuria
  - Protein–Energy Malnutrition or Wasting
  - Puffiness Around Eyes
  - Serum Creatinine 1.7 mg/dL
    - Unbalanced Calcium:Phosphorus Ratios
    - Uremia
    - Weakness, Pallor, Anemia

OVERVIEW OF RENAL NUTRITION

According to the National Institute of Diabetes and Digestive and Kidney Diseases, more than 16% of adults 20 years and older (23 million people) have evidence of chronic kidney disease (CKD), with moderately or severely reduced glomerular filtration rate (GFR) (NIDDK, 2010). The Kidney Disease Outcomes Quality Initiative (KDOQI) classifies CKD on the basis of the level of kidney function. Simple blood tests, as follows, can be done to determine renal status but are not always ordered (Aase, 2010):

- Reduction of kidney function—eGFR < 60 mL/min/1.73 m^2 and/or
- Evidence of kidney damage/persistent albuminuria—≥30 mg of urine albumin per gram of urine creatinine (UACR)
- Kidney failure eGFR < 15 mL/min/1.73 m^2

The kidney plays an important role in blood pressure management through the renin–angiotensin system and identifies the damage from inflammation following scarlet fever, flu, or tonsillitis. Table 16-1 gives a brief background about the kidneys.

A registered dietitian (RD) with renal experience should be a central and integral part of the management of both pediatric and adult patients (NKF, 2010). In pediatrics, the evaluation of growth as well as physical, developmental, educational, and social needs is essential. Table 16-2 lists terms and abbreviations commonly used in renal disorder management.

Renal patients need a detailed nutritional assessment by dietitians (Chauveau, 2009). Subjective Global Assessment (SGA) is used and includes weight change over the past 6 months, dietary intake, gastrointestinal (GI) symptoms, visual assessment of subcutaneous tissue and muscle mass. While weight change is assessed by evaluating weights during the past 6 months, edema might obscure a greater amount of weight loss. Dietary intake is evaluated by using a comparison of the patient's usual or recommended intakes to current intake. Duration and frequency of GI symptoms (e.g., nausea, vomiting, and diarrhea) are also assessed. The interviewer rates a 7-point scale with higher scores if the patient has little or no weight loss, a better dietary intake, better appetite, and the absence of GI symptoms. See Appendix B for the SGA questionnaire.

Nutritional interventions and specifically supplemented diets have many advantages in terms of managing the progression of renal failure, better metabolic and endocrine control, and decreased proteinuria (Chauveau, 2009). Because anorexia and weight loss are associated with wasting, morbidity, and mortality, dietitians must be aware of the impact of hormones, such as the orexigenic ghrelin and the anorexigenic obestatin, on intake (Mafra et al, 2010). In addition, the role of inflammation must be understood. Inflammation causes increased levels of cytokines (interleukin [IL]-6 and tumor necrosis factor [TNF]-α) and acute-phase proteins (C-reactive protein [CRP] and serum amyloid A); loss of muscle mass; changes in plasma composition; decreases in serum albumin, transthyretin, and transferrin; altered lipoprotein structure and function to favor atherogenesis. Knowing that fish oils may decrease the loss of renal function by affecting eicosanoid and cytokine production, altering renal dynamics, and decreasing inflammation is important for all dietitians to understand.

Renal replacement therapy (RRT) includes dialysis and renal transplantation. RRT is designed to normalize the volume and composition of the body fluids and to remove uremic toxins. But because renal disease is often related to diabetes and hypertension, a multidisciplinary approach is warranted.

Not everyone with CKD needs a strict hemodialysis (HD) diet. Appropriate, individualized use of one- and two-page information sheets on sodium, phosphorous, potassium,

TABLE 16-1 Human Kidney Functions

Waste excretion: Kidneys remove the waste products of metabolism (urea, uric acid, creatinine).

Acid–base balance: Kidneys regulate pH by eliminating excess hydrogen ion concentration and controlling composition of the blood. Blood plasma pH is maintained by the kidney at a neutral pH of 7.4. Urine is either acidic (pH 5) or alkaline (pH 8). Potassium and phosphate require renal control as well.

Blood pressure control: Sodium ions are controlled in a homeostatic process involving aldosterone, which increases sodium ion absorption in the distal convoluted tubules. When blood pressure is too low, *renin* is secreted by cells of the distal convoluted tubule. Renin acts on the blood protein, *angiotensinogen*, converting it to *angiotensin I*. Angiotensin I is then converted by the angiotensin-converting enzyme in the lung capillaries to *angiotensin II*, which stimulates the secretion of *aldosterone* by the adrenal cortex. Aldosterone stimulates increased reabsorption of sodium ions from the kidney tubules, which causes an increase in the volume of water that is reabsorbed from the tubule. This increase in water reabsorption increases the volume of blood, which ultimately raises the blood pressure.

Plasma volume and osmolality: Any rise or drop in blood osmotic pressure due to a lack or excess of water is detected by the *hypothalamus*, which notifies the *pituitary gland* via negative feedback. A lack of water causes the *posterior pituitary gland* to secrete *antidiuretic hormone*, which results in water reabsorption and an increase in urine concentration. Tissue fluid concentration thus returns to normal. Body fluid is two thirds extracellular and one third intracellular.

Hormone secretion: *Erythropoietin* is secreted for red blood cell production; deficiency is common in chronic renal anemia. *Urodilatin* is a natriuretic peptide that mediates natriuresis. *Vitamin D_3* is converted from an inactive form (D2) for calcium:phosphorus homeostasis; the final stage of conversion of vitamin D to its active form, 1,25-dihydroxyvitamin D occurs in the proximal tubule.

Carnitine synthesis: Carnitine carries fatty acids from cytoplasm to mitochondria for heart and skeletal muscle fuel. Lysine, methionine, vitamin C, iron, vitamin B_6, and niacin are needed to produce carnitine.

Glucose homeostasis: The kidney plays a role in gluconeogenesis and glucose counterregulation.

Prostaglandin E_2: It is a major renal cyclooxygenase metabolite of arachidonic acid that impacts renal hemodynamics and salt and water excretion.

TABLE 16-2 Renal Abbreviations

Abbreviation	Description	Abbreviation	Description
a1-AG	a1-Acid Glycoprotein	IPAA	Intraperitoneal Amino Acids
aBWef	Adjusted Edema-Free Body Weight	Kt/V_{urea}	A measure of dialysis; K is the dialyzing membrane clearance, t is the time of dialysis delivered in minutes, and V_{urea} is the volume of distribution of urea
AMA	Arm Muscle Area	MAC	Midarm Circumference
APD	Automated Peritoneal Dialysis	MAMA	Midarm Muscle Area
BIA	Bioelectrical Impedance Analysis	MAMC	Midarm Muscle Circumference
BUN	Blood Urea Nitrogen	MD	Maintenance Dialysis
CANUSA	Canada/United States Peritoneal Dialysis Study	MHD	Maintenance Hemodialysis
CAPD	Continuous Ambulatory Peritoneal Dialysis	NHANES	National Health and Nutrition Evaluation Survey
CCPD	Continuous Cyclic Peritoneal Dialysis	nPCR	Protein Catabolic Rate normalized to body weight
CoA	Coenzyme A	nPNA	Protein Equivalent of Total Nitrogen Appearance normalized to body weight
CPD	Chronic Peritoneal Dialysis	PCR	Protein Catabolic Rate
CPN	Central Parenteral Nutrition	PNA	Protein Equivalent of Total Nitrogen Appearance
CrCl	Urinary Creatinine Clearance	PTH	Parathyroid Hormone
CRF	Chronic Renal Failure (GFR < 20 mL/min)	RTA	Renal Tubular Acidosis
CRI	Chronic Renal Insufficiency (GFR less than normal but >20 mL/min)	SBW	Standard Body Weight
CRP	C-Reactive Protein	SDS	Standard Deviation Score
CVVHD	Continuous Venovenous Hemofiltration with Hemodialysis	SGA	Subjective Global Assessment
DXA	Dual Energy X-Ray Absorptiometry	SUN	Serum Urea Nitrogen
ESRD	End-Stage Renal Disease	TBW	Total Body Water
GFR	Glomerular Filtration Rate	TNA	Total Nitrogen Appearance
HD	Hemodialysis	TSF	Triceps Skinfold
IDWG	Interdialytic Weight Gain	UBW	Usual Body Weight
IDPN	Intradialytic Parenteral Nutrition	UNA	Urea Nitrogen Appearance
IGF-I	Insulin-Like Growth Factor-I		

and protein will enable dietitians to advise their clients more effectively than using complex documents (Aase, 2010).

Ideally, dietitians who work with renal patients are certified renal dietetic specialists ("CS-R" credential), which requires experience and a successful examination score. However, because there is a gap between the dialysis unit (where renal dietitians practice) and the doctor's office (where gradual changes in CKD may not be detected), all dietitians must be comfortable with the basics of renal intervention (Aase, 2010).

While **diabetic renal disease** (diabetic nephropathy) is the leading cause of end-stage renal failure, the process cannot be reversed by glycemic control but by control of blood pressure and protein restriction. Therefore, specific nutrition care is needed for all renal patients—whether before starting dialysis, while on dialysis, or after a kidney transplant. Early dietary intervention is most critical to reduce sodium intake, control blood pressure, manage diabetes, and reduce excessive protein intake in early stages of CKD (Aase, 2010).

Standards of professional performance and standards of practice for dietitians in nephrology care set the expectations for renal practice (Brommage et al, 2009; Joint Standards Task Force, 2009). In addition, the American Dietetic Association evidence analysis library provides regular updates on research in the field. Medicare CKD–related medical nutrition therapy (MNT) reimbursement requires use of these evidence-based guidelines (EBGs) and currently begins at approximately stage 3 (GFR between 13 and 50 mL/min/1.73 m^2).

The National Kidney Disease Education Program (NKDEP) has developed multiple tools, tear-off sheets, and guidelines that can be used (see Web site http://nkdep.nih.gov/professionals/index.htm). There are clever lists of "kidney-friendly" foods, supermarket tips, and other simplified ways to enhance patient understanding. Once NKDEP brings primary care clinicians up to speed, referrals to RDs and rates of reimbursement for qualified CKD-related MNT should increase (Aase, 2010). Go to the Medicare MNT reimbursement Web site for more details at http://www.cms.hhs.gov/MedicalNutritionTherapy/01_Overview.asp#TopOfPage.

For More Information

- American Association of Kidney Patients
  http://www.aakp.org/
- American Kidney Fund
  http://www.kidneyfund.org/

- American Society of Pediatric Nephrology http://www.aspneph.com/
- Cyber Nephrology http://www.cybernephrology.org/
- Dialysis and Transplantation http://www.eneph.com/
- European Dialysis and Transplant Association http://www.era-edta.org/
- Home Dialysis http://www.homedialysis.org/
- International Society of Nephrology http://www.isn-online.org/
- International Society for Peritoneal Dialysis http://www.ispd.org/
- Kidney Disease: Improving Global Outcomes http://www.kdigo.org/
- Kidney Options Diet and Nutrition http://www.kidneyoptions.com/dietnutrition.html
- Kidney School http://www.kidneyschool.org/
- NKF http://www.kidney.org/
- NKF Handouts http://www.kidney.org/atoz/atozTopic_Brochures.cfm
- National Kidney and Urologic Diseases Information Clearinghouse http://kidney.niddk.nih.gov/
- Nephron Information Center http://www.nephron.com/
- Northwest Kidney Centers http://www.nwkidney.org/
- Renal Physicians Association http://www.renalmd.org/
- Renal World http://www.renalworld.com/
- UNC Kidney Center—Links http://www.unckidneycenter.org/about/links.html
- Vitamin D and Vitamin D Receptors in Kidney Disease http://www.kidney.org/professionals/tools/pdf/Vit_D_ReceptorsTool.pdf

REFERENCES

Aase S. Kidney friendly: what the National Kidney Disease Education Program strategic plan means for dietetic practice. *J Am Diet Assoc.* 110:346, 2010.

Brommage D, et al. American Dietetic Association and the National Kidney Foundation standards of practice and standards of professional performance for registered dietitians (generalist, specialty, and advanced) in nephrology care. *J Am Diet Assoc.* 109:1617, 2009.

Chauveau P. Nutritional intervention in chronic kidney disease. *J Ren Nutr.* 19:1S, 2009.

Joint Standards Task. American Dietetic Association and the National Kidney Foundation Standards of Practice and Standards of Professional Performance for Registered Dietitians (generalist, specialty, and advanced) in nephrology care. *J Am Diet Assoc.* 109:1617, 2009.

Mafra D, et al. Endocrine role of stomach in appetite regulation in chronic kidney disease: about ghrelin and obestatin. *J Ren Nutr.* 20:68, 2010.

NIDDK. National Institute of Diabetes and Digestive and Kidney Diseases. Web site accessed February 15, 2010, at http://kidney.niddk.nih.gov/kudiseases/pubs/kustats/index.htm.

National Kidney Foundation (NKF). Web site accessed February 20, 2010, at http://www.kidney.org/Professionals/kdoqi/.

COLLAGEN-IV NEPHROPATHIES: ALPORT SYNDROME AND THIN GLOMERULAR BASEMENT MEMBRANE NEPHROPATHY

NUTRITIONAL ACUITY RANKING: LEVEL 2–3

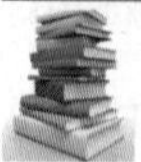

DEFINITIONS AND BACKGROUND

Alport syndrome (ATS) is a progressive inherited (usually X-linked) nephritis. ATS is characterized by irregular thinning, thickening, and splitting of the renal glomerular basement membrane. It is often associated with hearing loss and ocular symptoms (Longo et al, 2006). Both ATS and **thin glomerular basement membrane nephropathy (TBMN)** are genetically heterogeneous conditions with initial presentation that usually involves hematuria (Haas, 2009). In ATS, kidney function is lost, with eventual progression to end-stage renal disease (ESRD) between adolescence and age 30 years (Tan et al, 2010). Mutational analysis of the affected genes will be a valuable adjunct to the treatment options, avoiding the need for transplantation and dialysis (Thorner, 2007).

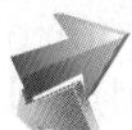

ASSESSMENT, MONITORING, AND EVALUATION

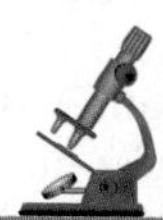

CLINICAL INDICATORS

Genetic Markers: Both ATS and TBMN can be considered as genetic diseases of the glomerular basement membrane (GBM) involving the alpha3/alpha4/alpha5 network of type IV collagen (Thorner, 2007).

Clinical/History

Height
Weight
Body mass index (BMI)
Diet history
Input and output (I & O)

- Edema-free adjusted body weight (aBWef)
- Edema, ankles and feet
- Abnormal urine color
- Hypertension?
- Hearing loss before age 30? (males)
- Cataracts?
- Microscopic hematuria?
- Temperature
- Renal biopsy, genetic testing

Lab Work

- Blood urea nitrogen (BUN)
- Creatinine (Creat)
- Chloride (Cl_2)
- GFR
- Creatine clearance (CrCl)
- Cholesterol (Chol)—increased?
- Albumin (Alb), transthyretin
- CRP
- Na^+, K^+
- Phosphorus
- Aspartate aminotransferase (AST)
- Ca^{++}
- Proteinuria
- Hemoglobin and hematocrit (H & H)
- Serum Fe, ferritin
- Total iron-binding capacity (TIBC), percentage saturation
- Parathormone (PTH)
- Serum Cu (decreased?)

INTERVENTION

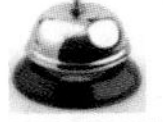

OBJECTIVES

- Reduce renal workload. Improve or control excretion of waste products such as urea and sodium.
- Manage edema resulting from sodium and fluid retention.
- Prevent uremia from nitrogen retention.
- Adjust electrolyte intakes (sodium, potassium, and chloride) if needed.
- Prevent systemic complications, where possible, and protein catabolism, as from poor intake.

SAMPLE NUTRITION CARE PROCESS STEPS

Excessive Sodium Intake

Assessment: Dx of ATS at age 11, now 20 and away from home at college. Recent admission to hospital with edema and hypertension, despite use of a diuretic each day. Diet history indicates frequent use of canned soups and a bag of chips with a sandwich at lunch every day. Normally uses a lower sodium breakfast and dinner.

Nutrition Diagnosis (PES): NI-5.10.7 Excessive sodium intake related to the use of canned soups, chips, and sandwich for lunch every day as evidenced by recent severe edema and hypertension.

Interventions:

Food-Nutrient Delivery: Low-sodium diet plan for lunch; alternatives identified that are easy to pack and take to college or campus.

Education: Review the requirements for the low sodium diet; has had previous teaching two times by a RD back in hometown.

Counseling: Supportive counseling about food choices that are lower in sodium.

Coordination of Care: Work with medical team to determine whether diuretic is indicated.

Monitoring and Evaluation: Improvement in edema and blood pressure. No further problems following the low sodium diet; change in lunch choices well received.

- Manage hypertension.
- Recommend genetic counseling for those with ATS. A family history and a renal biopsy may be needed (Thorner, 2007).

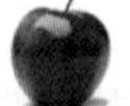

FOOD AND NUTRITION

- Determine fluid intake (measured output plus 500 mL insensible losses).
- Restrict sodium intake to 2–3 g if patient has hypertension or edema.
- In the case of renal failure, protein intake should be low, as 0.6–0.8 g/kg of adjusted edema-free BW. Use 50% high biological value proteins to ensure positive nitrogen balance. If needed, follow dialysis guidelines.
- Check need for vitamin A, which may be low.
- Decrease elevated phosphorus levels with a low-phosphate diet (5–10 mg/kg/d) as needed.
- Provide adequate energy intake (35 kcal/kg BW).
- Use fish oils to reduce inflammation.

Common Drugs Used and Potential Side Effects

- Antihypertensive, antibiotic, and immunosuppressive medications are commonly used. Monitor for specific side effects, especially with long-term use.

Herbs, Botanicals, and Supplements

- Herbs and botanical supplements should not be used without discussing with the physician.
- Discuss the varied sources of fish oil supplements and how much to take.

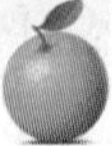

NUTRITION EDUCATION, COUNSELING, CARE MANAGEMENT

- Ensure dietary measures are appropriate for patient's current status.
- Discuss ways to include more omega-3 fatty acids and fish in diet.

Patient Education—Food Safety

- Foodborne illness can occur when there is contamination of food at any point during the preparation process. Because renal patients are at high risk for foodborne illness, follow the four-step guidelines established by the U.S. Department of Agriculture: clean, separate, cook, and chill.
- Details are available at the Kidney Foundation Web site at http://www.kidney.org/atoz/content/foodsafety.cfm.

For More Information

- Alport Syndrome Foundation
  https://www.alportsyndrome.org/
- Hearing Loss
  http://www.entnet.org/

ALPORT SYNDROME AND NEPHRITIS—CITED REFERENCES

Haas M. Alport syndrome and thin glomerular basement membrane nephropathy: a practical approach to diagnosis. *Arch Pathol Lab Med.* 133:224, 2009.

Longo I, et al. Autosomal recessive Alport syndrome: an in-depth clinical and molecular analysis of five families. *Nephrol Dial Transplant.* 21:665, 2006.

Tan R, et al. Alport retinopathy results from "severe" COL4A5 mutations and predicts early renal failure. *Clin J Am Soc Nephrol.* 5:34, 2010.

Thorner PS. Alport syndrome and thin basement membrane nephropathy. *Nephron Clin Pract.* 106:82, 2007.

CHRONIC KIDNEY DISEASE AND RENAL FAILURE

NUTRITIONAL ACUITY RANKING: LEVEL 4

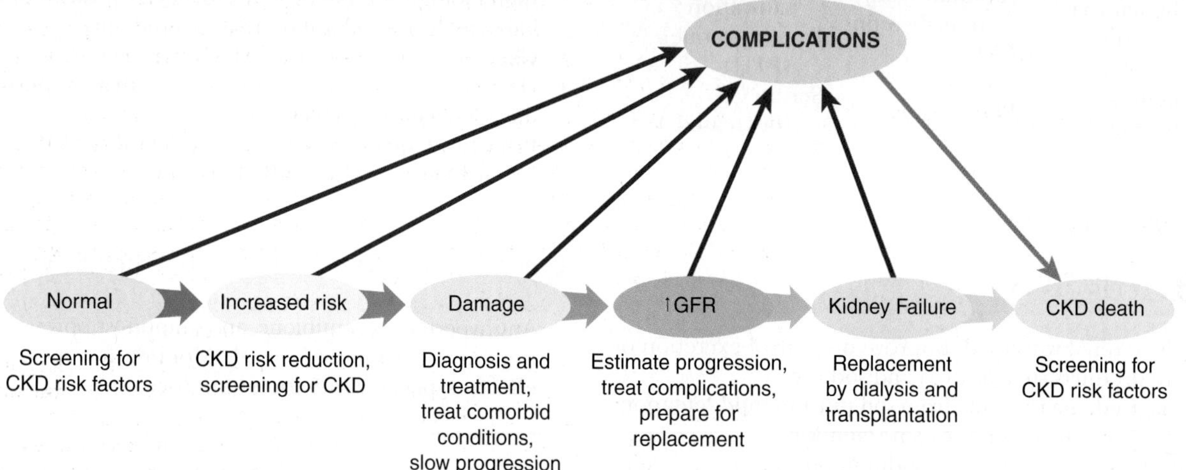

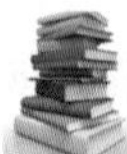

DEFINITIONS AND BACKGROUND

CKD is characterized by the inability of kidney function to return to normal after acute kidney failure or progressive renal decline from disease. Excess urea and nitrogenous wastes accumulate in the bloodstream (azotemia). CKD causes permanent reduction in function, eventually leading to end-stage ESRD. Early stages of CKD are defined by GFR and urinary albumin:creatinine ratio (Castro and Coresh, 2009). Table 16-3 describes the five stages of CKD.

Approximately 23 million Americans have some degree of CKD. Fifty percent of individuals with CKD have diabetes; hypertension is the second highest risk factor. Other risk factors include cardiovascular disease, family history of CKD, use of certain medications, and age >60 years. Undiagnosed CKD is especially common in people who have diabetes. The Pima Indians of Arizona have the world's highest incidence of type 2 diabetes and ESRD. Incorporating estimated GFR into screening for CKD would identify individuals earlier and enable early effective treatment (Middleton et al, 2006).

Depending on the form of disease, renal function may be lost in a matter of days or weeks, or may deteriorate slowly and gradually over the course of decades. Potentially modifiable risk factors in CKD include proteinuria, hypertension, dyslipidemia, anemia, oxidative stress, infections, depression, hyperglycemia, bone disease, and obesity. A low-protein diet (LPD) and low phosphorus intake may retard the progression of kidney disease and should be used in the renal population (Kent, 2005). Studies have shown that LPDs can reduce patient morbidity, preserve renal function, relieve uremic symptoms, improve nutritional status, postpone the start of dialysis for 6 months, and entail substantial cost-savings (Eyre et al, 2008).

Acute renal failure (ARF) involves abrupt decline in renal function with waste retention. ARF occurs when the kidneys fail to function because of circulatory, glomerular, or tubular deficiency resulting from an abrupt cause. ARF is caused by diabetes or hypertension in most cases. Other causes include glomerulonephritis (GN), polycystic kidney disease (PKD), and other causes (burns, severe crush injuries, transfusions, antibiotics, nephrotoxicity from drugs such as tacrolimus or cyclosporine, surgery or anesthesia, cardiac transplantation, shock, or sepsis). In children, ARF has been caused by hemolytic uremic syndrome from a specific strain of *Escherichia coli* (0157:H7) that is associated with undercooked ground beef. ARF occurs also in approximately 5% of surgical or trauma cases; frequently, this is reversible. Intermittent HD and continuous RRT are equally beneficial for patients with ARF (Pannu et al, 2008). In ARF, the patient gradually improves, although some loss of function may be permanent. If toxic accumulation occurs, ARF may be fatal. The phases of ARF include the following:

- Prodromal phase—varies in duration depending on cause—urine output may be normal
- Oliguric (average 10–14 days)—output typically between 50 and 400 mL/d
- Postoliguric phase (average 10 days)—urine output gradually returns to normal
- Recovery (from 1 month or up to 1 year).

TABLE 16-3 Stages, Symptoms, and Preventive Measures for Chronic Kidney Disease (CKD)

Stage	Glomerular Filtration Rate (GFR)	Symptoms and Preventive Measures
Stage 1	≥90 mL/min/1.73 m^2	Kidney damage with normal or increased GFR occurs. Blood flow through the kidney increases (hyperfiltration), and the kidneys are larger than usual. A person with stage 1 CKD usually has no symptoms. Regular testing for protein in the urine and serum creatinine can show whether the kidney damage is progressing. Living a healthy lifestyle can help slow the progression of kidney disease.
Stage 2	60–89 mL/min/1.73 m^2	A person with stage 2 CKD has kidney damage with a mild decrease in GFR. Filtration rate remains elevated or nearly normal. Glomeruli show signs of damage. Blood pressure is usually normal. Albuminuria is <30 mg/d. If people find out they have stage 2 CKD, it is usually because they were being tested for diabetes or high blood pressure.
Stage 3	30–59 mL/min/1.73 m^2	A person with stage 3 CKD has kidney damage with a moderate decrease in the GFR. Microalbuminuria becomes constant. Losses increase to 30–300 mg/d. This can occur after about 7 years of having diabetes. As kidney function declines, uremia occurs. Complications such as high blood pressure, anemia, and early bone disease may occur. Consult a nephrologist to perform specific lab tests. Limit protein from diet to 0.8 g/kg.
Stage 4	15–29 mL/min/1.73 m^2	A person with stage 4 CKD has advanced kidney damage with a severe decrease in the GFR. Nephropathy occurs with passage of large amounts of protein in the urine (>300 mg/d); blood pressure continues to rise. Creatinine rises >1.1–1.3 mg/dL and waste products build up (uremia). New symptoms include nausea, taste changes, uremic breath, anorexia, difficulty concentrating, and numbness in fingers and toes. Visits to the nephrologist every 3 months will be needed to test for creatinine, hemoglobin, calcium, and phosphorus levels and for management of hypertension and diabetes. An arteriovenous (AV) fistula and AV graft are created surgically and need a few months or so to mature before dialysis is needed. By doing everything possible to help prolong kidney function and overall health, the goal is to put off dialysis or transplantation for as long as possible. Limit protein to 0.8 g/kg.
Stage 5	<15 mL/min/1.73 m^2	A person with stage 5 CKD has end-stage renal disease where kidney failure occurs. The kidneys have lost all their ability to do their job effectively. Renal replacement therapy (RRT) is initiated with dialysis or renal transplantation. Dialysis is started when renal Kt/V (urea) falls below 2.0/wk or when kidney function is 15% or less. New symptoms that can occur in stage 5 CKD include anorexia, nausea or vomiting, headaches, fatigue, anuria, swelling around eyes and ankles, muscle cramps, tingling in hands or feet, and changing skin color and pigmentation.

REFERENCES

National Kidney Foundation. Clinical practice guidelines for nutrition in chronic renal failure. Accessed February 15, 2010, at http://www.kidney.org/professionals/kdoqi/guidelines.

Nephron Online. Web site accessed February 16, 2010, at http://www.nephronline.org/management/ckd.html

Chronic renal failure (CRF) is the slow, gradual loss of kidney function. Causes include lupus, ATS, chronic hypertension, prolonged urinary obstruction, nephrotic syndrome, PKD, cystinosis, or diabetes. Diabetic nephropathy may be delayed by tightly controlling blood glucose levels and using angiotensin-converting enzyme (ACE) inhibitors.

Some forms of CRF can be controlled or slowed down but never cured. Partial loss of renal function means that some of the patient's nephrons have been scarred and cannot be repaired. In patients with progressive CRF who consume uncontrolled diets, progressive declines in spontaneous protein and energy intake, serum proteins, cholesterol, total creatinine excretion, and anthropometric values are evident below a CrCl of approximately 25 mL/min. Mortality increases greatly with serum albumin levels below 3.5 g/dL and low cholesterol level (<150–180 mg/dL).

Chronic inflammation predicts mortality in the CKD population; IL-6 is a significantly better predictor of mortality than CRP, albumin, or TNF-α (Barreto et al, 2010).

Most CKD patients also have elevated serum total homocysteine (tHcy) and low selenium levels. Suggest a multivitamin supplement that contains 800 μg folic acid, adequate vitamins B_6 and B_{12} and selenium if needed. Glutathione peroxidase helps prevent generation of free radicals and decreases the risk of oxidative damage to tissues, including the kidney and its vascular supply.

The African American Study of Kidney Disease and Hypertension (AASK) supports tight blood pressure control (<130/80 mm Hg) in CKD. Adherence to practices known to be of clinical benefit not only improves patient outcomes but also reduces costs of care. A multidisciplinary effort is needed.

ESRD is stage 5 CKD. Care involves early detection of progressive renal disease, interventions to retard its progression, prevention of uremic complications, control of related conditions, adequate preparation for RRT, and timely initiation of dialysis. Higher blood pressure and lower income are associated with a higher incidence of ESRD in both white and African American men. Mortality is remarkably high in ESRD, usually from cardiovascular disease (Shen et al, 2006). Decreasing complications may reduce death rates.

Wasting and protein–energy malnutrition (PEM) are complications of ESRD. Cachexia from anorexia, acidosis, and inflammation can lead to the **Malnutrition-Inflammation Complex Syndrome**. The decline in nutritional status may be caused by disturbances in protein and energy metabolism, hormonal derangement, and spontaneous reductions in dietary energy and protein intake. Factors that can worsen PEM include poor dentition, infections or sepsis,

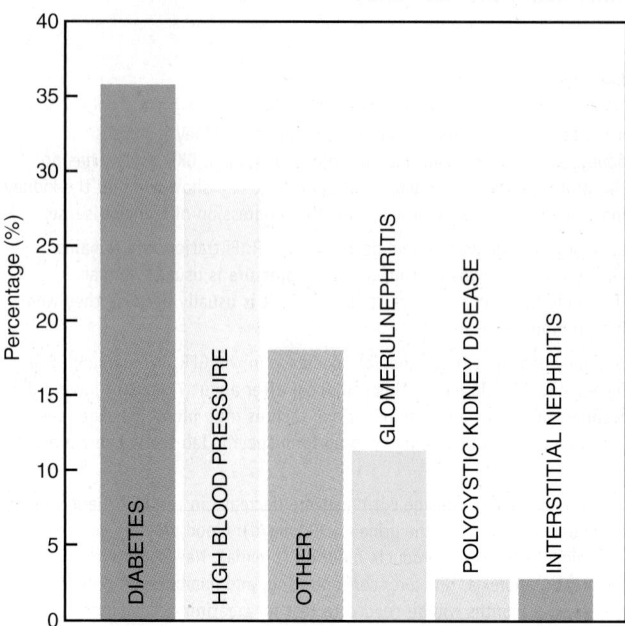

multiple medications, and pain. Worsening of PEM over time is associated with a greater risk for cardiovascular death form the **cardiorenal syndrome.**

Other CKD complications that should be managed include metabolic acidosis due to reduced acid (hydrogen ion) excretion, anemia due to impaired erythropoiesis and low iron stores, hyperkalemia, and dyslipidemia. In addition, secondary hyperparathyroidism (HPT) and **bone and mineral metabolism disorder** may start as early as stage 2 or 3 CKD, and dietitians must monitor vitamin D and calcium levels and restrict dietary phosphorous intake (Aase, 2010). Vitamin D receptor activation improves endothelial function in CKD, and this area of research is very promising (Wu-Wong et al, 2010).

The Kidney Early Evaluation Program (KEEP) is a free screening program designed to detect CKD early, promote follow-up evaluation with clinicians, and ultimately improve outcomes (Vassolotti et al, 2010). The program screens individuals with diabetes, hypertension, or those with a first-degree relative with diabetes, hypertension, and/or kidney disease. African Americans, Native Americans, Hispanics, and Asians/Pacific Islanders have a 3 times higher risk for CKD and anemia (McFarlane et al, 2008; Vassolotti et al, 2010). Such health disparities must be addressed (NKF, 2009).

Management of CKD is costly, yet adverse effects can be prevented. Early nutritional intervention may delay or prevent rapid progression of many complications. KDOQI guidelines recommend that patients on dialysis achieve an albumin level of 3.7 g/dL. SGA scores and other nutritional indicators, such as BMI, handgrip strength for measures of muscle mass, waist circumference, serum albumin level, and serum creatinine level are a good place to start; see Table 16-4. All patients with diabetes and CKD should receive nutritional interventions (NKF, 2007).

Current EBGs should always be followed. The NKF-KDOQI guidelines address strategies for diabetes, hypertension, dyslipidemia, bone disease, anemia, and heart disease in CKD patients. Guidelines are also available for managing CKD in children.

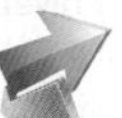

ASSESSMENT, MONITORING, AND EVALUATION

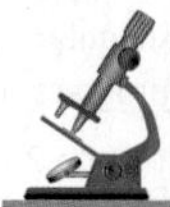

CLINICAL INDICATORS

Genetic Markers: Potential markers of CKD include asymmetric dimethylarginine, factors involved in calcium–phosphate metabolism, adrenomedullin, A-type natriuretic peptide, N-terminal pro-brain natriuretic peptide, liver-type fatty acid–binding protein, kidney injury molecule 1, neutrophil gelatinase-associated lipocalin, apolipoprotein A-IV, adiponectin, and genetic polymorphisms (Kronenberg, 2009). Apolipoprotein E polymorphisms are relevant, with e2 allele conferring risk and e4 providing protection; these associations differ between ethnic groups (Chu et al, 2009).

Clinical/History

- Height
- Weight
- aBWef
- Pitting edema in hands and legs
- BMI
- Waist circumference
- Waist:hip ratio
- Diet history
- BP (increased)
- I & O
- Severe headaches
- Dyspnea
- Failing vision
- Poor appetite
- Nausea, vomiting
- Abdominal pain
- Mouth ulcers, hiccups
- Bone and joint pain
- Fatigue
- Pale skin
- Uremic convulsions
- Pericarditis
- Skin changes and pigmentation
- Body composition (SGA score)
- Electrocardiogram
- Renal sonography
- Renal biopsy
- Dual-energy x-ray absorptiometry (DEXA) scan

Lab Work

- Urine flow:
  - Normal, 1–1.5 L/d
  - Nonoliguria, >500 mL/d
  - Oliguria, <500 mL/d
  - Anuria, <100 mL/d
  - Polyuria, 3 L/d
- Azotemia (excess urea and nitrogen in blood)
- Urine albumin:creatinine ratio
- Alb (goal, >4.0 g/dL)
- Transferrin saturation (goal, >20%)
- CRP
- IL-6
- BUN
- Creat
- BUN:creatinine ratio
- GFR (if <10–15 mL/min, consider dialysis)
- Glucose (goal, <140–160 mg/dL random)
- Hemoglobin A1c (HbA1c) (goal, <7%)
- Na^+
- K^+ (goal, 3.5–5.5 mEq/L)
- Ca^{++} (goal, 8.5–10.2 mg/dL)
- Phosphorus (increased?)
- Uric acid (increased?)
- Mg^{++} (increased?)
- Serum bicarbonate
- PTH
- Hemoglobin (goal, 12 g/L for men; 11 g/L for women)

TABLE 16-4 Protein–Energy Malnutrition (PEM) in Renal Patients

Etiology	Comments
Blood loss	Loss of blood may be due to gastrointestinal bleeding, frequent blood sampling, and blood sequestered in the hemodialyzer and tubing.
Dialysis	The process promotes wasting by removing such nutrients as amino acids, peptides, protein, glucose, water-soluble vitamins, and other bioactive compounds, and may promote protein catabolism, due to bioincompatibility.
Endocrine changes	Endocrine disorders of uremia include resistance to the actions of insulin and IGF-I, hyperglucagonemia, and hyperparathyroidism.
Inadequate food intake	Poor intake is secondary to anorexia caused by the uremic state; altered taste sensation; intercurrent illness; emotional distress or illness; impaired ability to procure, prepare, or mechanically ingest foods; and unpalatable prescribed diets.
Inflammation and the catabolic response	Chronic inflammation from cardiovascular disease, diabetes mellitus, and other illnesses may produce anorexia, hypercatabolism, and malnutrition. Diminished appetite relates to high concentrations of proinflammatory cytokines. Inflammatory cytokines, such as tumor necrosis factor-α and interleukin-6, are associated with protein synthesis and catabolism in the body, and they downregulate albumin synthesis. Serum albumin is altered by systemic inflammation; a low serum albumin concentration is strongly associated with mortality in CKD.
Other issues	Sleep disturbances, pain, erectile dysfunction, patient dissatisfaction with care, depression, symptom burden, and perception of intrusiveness of illness may all lead to poor quality of life, resulting in poor appetite and intake. Suggest psychotherapy, anti-depressants, or other treatments.
Oxidative stress	PEM and low body mass index may be associated with increased oxidative stress and impaired endothelium-dependent vasodilation with reduced bioavailability of nitric oxide. Elevated C-reactive protein is a risk factor for mortality in chronic kidney disease (Menon et al, 2005).
Toxins	There may be accumulation of endogenously formed uremic toxins or the ingestion of exogenous toxins.
Wasting	Wasting may be due to anorexia, nausea, emesis, uremia, inflammation, infections, diabetes, underdialysis, or dental problems. Supplementation with branched-chain amino acids spares lean body mass during weight loss, promotes wound healing, may decrease muscle wasting with aging, and may have beneficial effects in renal disease (Tom and Nair, 2006).
Assessments	**Comments**
Lab values—BUN: creatinine ratio	BUN:creatinine ratio is altered by catabolic stress, low urine volume, and muscle mass changes.
Lab values—creatinine	Creatinine is a waste product that comes from muscle activity. When kidneys are working well, they remove creatinine from the blood. As kidney function slows, blood levels of creatinine rise. Serum creatinine concentration reflects muscle mass, somatic protein stores, and dietary protein intake. Because it predicts outcome in CKD, it may be a useful marker of nutritional status or loss of muscle mass in CKD. However, creatinine levels are affected by inflammation, age, sex, race, residual kidney function, variation in creatinine metabolism, and dialysis. The assessment of dietary intake is more commonly used to assess protein status.
Lab values—creatinine index	The creatinine index is directly related to the normalized protein equivalent of total nitrogen appearance (nPNA) and independent of the dialysis dose. A low or declining creatinine index correlates with mortality independently of the cause of death. People with catabolic diseases may have larger and faster declines in the creatinine index before death.
Lab values—glomerular filtration rate (GFR)	GFR is a good measure of kidney function. A math formula using the person's age, race, gender, and serum creatinine is used to calculate the GFR.
Lab values—nitrogen balance	Because the nitrogen content of protein is relatively constant at 16%, the protein equivalent of total nitrogen appearance (PNA) can be estimated by multiplying total nitrogen appearance (TNA) by 6.25 (PNA is mathematically identical to the protein catabolic rate or PCR). In the clinically stable patient, PNA can be used to estimate protein intake. However, PNA approximates protein intake only when the patient is in nitrogen equilibrium (steady-state). In the catabolic patient, PNA will exceed protein intake to the extent that there is net degradation and metabolism of endogenous protein pools to form urea.
Lab values—serum cholesterol	Low serum cholesterol is an indicator of chronically inadequate protein–energy intake. It may be an indicator for mortality in maintenance hemodialysis patients.
Lab values—transthyretin (prealbumin)	Transthyretin is a good index of liver protein synthesis, but it is reabsorbed and metabolized by the proximal tubule; serum levels rise as kidney function declines. Transthyretin levels correlate strongly with serum albumin.

(continued)

TABLE 16-4 Protein–Energy Malnutrition (PEM) in Renal Patients *(continued)*

Assessment Frequency	Suggested Evaluation for PEM Status
Monthly assessments	Predialysis or stabilized serum albumin
	Percentage of usual postdialysis (MHD) or postdrain (CPD) body weight
	In hemodialysis: nPNA
Every 3–4 months	In peritoneal dialysis: nPNA
Every 4 months	Percentage of standard (NHANES II) body weight
Every 6 months	Subjective global assessment
	Dietary interview and/or diary
As needed to confirm or extend the data obtained earlier	Predialysis or stabilized serum prealbumin
	Skinfold thickness
	Midarm muscle area, circumference, or diameter
	Dual-energy x-ray absorptiometry
If low, to identify the need for more rigorous examination	Low predialysis or stabilized serum creatinine level (<10 mg/dL)
	Low or declining creatinine index
	Low predialysis or stabilized serum urea nitrogen level
	Low predialysis or declining serum cholesterol level (150–180 mg/dL)

Developed using:

- KDOQI Guidelines. Web site accessed February 23, 2010, at http://www.kidney.org/Professionals/kdoqi/guidelines_updates/doqi_nut.html.
- Menon V, et al. C-reactive protein and albumin as predictors of all-cause and cardiovascular mortality in chronic kidney disease. *Kidney Int.* 68:766, 2005.
- Tom A, Nair KS. Assessment of branched-chain amino acid status and potential for biomarkers. *J Nutr.* 136:324S, 2006.

Serum Fe, serum ferritin	Serum 23-hydroxyvitamin D (goal, >30 ng/mL)	Serum chloride
Mean cell volume (MCV)	pH	Chol (goal, >160–<200 mg/dL)
Red blood cell (RBC) folate (≥200 ng/mL)	CO_2 (goal, 24–32 mEq/L)	Triglycerides (goal, <150 mg/dL)

SAMPLE NUTRITION CARE PROCESS STEPS

Inadequate Enteral Nutrition Infusion

Assessment Data: Dietary recall and I & O records, nursing flow sheets. Renal lab values: K+ 6.0 mEq/L, BUN 60 mg/dL, serum creat 1.5 mg/dL. On tube feeding with fluid restriction.

Nutrition Diagnosis (PES): NI-2.3 Inadequate intake from enteral nutrition (EN) infusion related to volume restriction as evidenced by recorded infusion of 900 mL of enteral formula over the past 24 hours providing only 70% of estimated energy and protein needs.

Interventions:

Food-Nutrient Delivery: Increase tube feeding by concentrating formula and increasing protein.

Coordinate Care: Work with the medical team to monitor for tolerance and lab changes.

Monitoring and Evaluation: Monitor by I & O intake to monitor change in enteral formula administration, output, and serum creatinine levels.

INTERVENTION

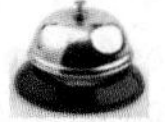

OBJECTIVES

- Postpone dialysis as long as possible. Work with high-risk conditions, such as diabetes or when urine albumin:creatinine ratio is abnormal (>30). Start working with other patients when serum creatinine is >1.5 mg/dL (women) or >2.0 mg/dL (men) to limit further renal impairment and reduce kidney workload. Patients should see a renal team, including a dietitian.
- Maintain or improve nutritional status. Protect lean body mass, minimize tissue catabolism. Consume adequate calories to spare protein.
- Keep protein intake at 0.6–0.75 g/kg/d to postpone dialysis (Eyre et al, 2008). Provide amino acids in proportion to protein status; attempt to keep serum albumin level of 4.0 g/dL.
- Control uremic symptoms and reduce complications from accumulation of nitrogenous waste. Evaluate the BUN: creatinine ratio; typically, a 10:1 ratio is desirable (urinary creatinine doubles when renal function is <50%).
- Treat hypertension aggressively. Limit dietary sodium, use moderate alcohol intake, obtain regular exercise, lose weight in those with a BMI >25, and reduce saturated fats. Blood pressure goal is <130 mm Hg systolic and <80 mm Hg diastolic for all CKD patients.
- Keep blood glucose under control with HbA1c ≤ 7%. Control carbohydrate (CHO) intake if needed.
- Include a variety of grains, especially whole grains, fresh fruits, and vegetables. Limit intake of refined and processed foods high in sugar and sodium.

- Choose low saturated fat, low cholesterol, and moderate total fat foods to normalize lipid profiles.
- Restore and maintain electrolyte balance; correct acidosis. Individualize potassium and phosphorus plans if blood levels are high.
- Consume the dietary recommended intake (DRI) for vitamins and minerals; preventing osteodystrophy.
- Have regular checkups and take medicines as prescribed. Exercise regularly, stop smoking, and eat a healthy diet.
- Aim for a healthy weight and include physical activity each day; obesity causes a decline in kidney function.
- Treat anemia, defined as a hematocrit <36% in women and <39% in men.
- Maintain growth in children with adequate calories, vitamins, and minerals.
- Correct other physiological changes such as constipation, diarrhea, blurred vision, pruritus, ecchymosis, pallor, crackles in the lungs, loss of muscle tone, and tingling of lips or fingertips.

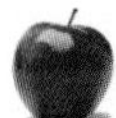

FOOD AND NUTRITION

- Consume adequate calories. Nondialyzed patients younger than 60 years with advanced CKD (GFR <25 mL/min) need 35 kcal/kg/d; those older than 60 years need 30–35 kcal/kg.
- CHO should be 50–60% of total calories per day (Burrowes, 2008). CHO intolerance is common; fructose, galactose, or sorbitol may be better tolerated than sucrose.
- With diabetes or heart disease, limit total fat to 30% or less of total calories per day; saturated fat less than 10% of the total calories; 200 mg cholesterol per day (Burrowes, 2008).
- In stages 1, 2, or 3 of CKD, limit protein to 12–15% of calories per day. Use 0.8 g to 1.0 g protein/kg BW from high-quality protein sources.
- In stage 4 CKD, reduce protein to 10% of calories per day. For nondialyzed patients with GFR <25 mL/min, use 0.6 g protein/kg/d, 50% from high–biological value sources. Amino acid analogs (CHO skeleton of amino acids minus the amino group) may also be used.

TABLE 16-5 Spices and Condiment Substitutes for Salt

Allspice	Dry mustard	Paprika
Bay leaf	Garlic, fresh or powder	Rosemary
Black pepper	Ginger	Scallions
Caraway seeds	Green bell pepper	Shallots
Celery seed	Lemons and limes	Sugar substitute
Chili powder	Mint	Sweet basil
Chives	Mrs. Dash	Tabasco sauce
Cinnamon	Nutmeg	Thyme
Cloves	Onions	Turmeric or cumin
Curry powder	Oregano	Vanilla extract
Dill	Pan spray, nonstick	Vinegar

- Limit sodium to 2.3 g/d for those with diabetes, high blood pressure, or fluid retention. Limit intake of processed foods high in sodium. Use less salt at the table and fewer high-sodium ingredients. See Table 16-5 for seasoning ideas instead of salt.
- Phosphorus and potassium are modified on the basis of the stage of CKD (Burrowes, 2008):
  Phosphorus: stages 1–2: 1.7 g/d; stages 3–4: 0.8–1.0 g/d
  Potassium: stages 1–2: less than 4 g/d; stages 3–4: 2.4 g/d

See Table 16-6 for tips on managing these potassium and phosphorus in the diet. Limit use of salt substitutes. Liberalize K+ when there is diarrhea or vomiting.

- Limit elemental calcium to <2000 mg, including that from phosphorus binders, as needed. Initiate vitamin D therapy if PTH is high, calcium is <9.5 mg/dL, or phosphorous is <4.6 mg/dL.
- Fluid intake should be output plus 500–1000 mL for insensible losses. Monitor regularly.
- Avoid over-the-counter dietary supplements unless approved by the nephrologist. Supplement with the DRI for the water-soluble vitamin B complex, and limit vitamin C to 100 mg/d from supplemental sources. Vitamin A and iron may not be desirable, levels can build up as kidney function declines.
- EN significantly increases serum albumin concentrations and improves total dietary intake (Stratton et al, 2005). Renal-specific enteral products may be needed; monitor content according to lab data. Because EN can help infants and children overcome malnutrition and promote catch-up growth, noctural feedings may be useful. If central parenteral nutrition (CPN) is needed, avoid excesses of micronutrients.
- Work with the interdisciplinary team, as shown on page 871.

Common Drugs Used and Potential Side Effects

- See Table 16-7.

Herbs, Botanicals, and Supplements

- Herbs and botanical supplements should not be used without discussing with the physician. Some products may actually contribute to renal failure, such as aristolochic acid, found in Mu Tong or Fangchi in Taiwanese prescription medicines (Lai et al, 2010).
- Probiotic dietary supplements are being designed to metabolize nitrogenous waste that has diffused from the bloodstream into the bowel.

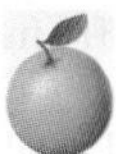

NUTRITION EDUCATION, COUNSELING, CARE MANAGEMENT

- Counseling interventions should include aggressive blood pressure control, reduction of dietary protein to

TABLE 16-6 Tips for Managing Potassium and Phosphorous in the Diet

Most high-potassium foods come from plants (fruits and vegetables). High-phosphorus foods are mainly from animals (meats, poultry, fish, eggs, cheese, dairy foods), but dried beans and peas also tend to be high in phosphorus. Foods that are high in both potassium and phosphorus are dairy foods, nuts, seeds, chocolate, and whole grain foods.

Category	Tips and Alternatives for Lowering Potassium (K+)
Beverages	Drink ice water with sliced lemon and cucumber, instead of drinking tomato or vegetable juices.
Cooking	Cook with onion, bell peppers, mushrooms, or garlic, instead of tomatoes, tomato or chili sauces.
Desserts and snacks	Choose vanilla- or lemon-flavored desserts, instead of chocolate desserts. A plain donut is acceptable. Choose unsalted popcorn or pretzels, rice cakes, jelly beans, red licorice, or hard candies. Avoid products made with molasses and nuts.
Fruit	Choose apples, berries, canned peaches, canned pears, dried cranberries, fruit cocktail, grapes, pineapple, and plums. Avoid bananas, oranges, cantaloupe, honeydew, dried fruits, mango, or kiwi.
Fruit juice	Drink apple, cranberry, pineapple, or grape juice, instead of orange or prune juice.
Potatoes	Leach potatoes by cooking in water first to lower the potassium content. Prepare mashed potatoes or hash browns from leached potatoes instead of eating a baked potato, sweet potatoes, yams, or French fries.
Pumpkin or squash	Use summer squashes such as crookneck or zucchini, instead of pumpkin or winter squashes (acorn, banana, hubbard).
Seasonings	Season with pepper, lemon, or low-sodium herb and spice blends, instead of salt substitutes or seeds.
Vegetables	Choose green beans, wax beans, carrots, cabbage, cauliflower, or snow peas, instead of spinach, dried beans or peas.
Vegetables for dips, salads	Prepare salads and vegetable appetizers with cucumber, cauliflower, eggplant, lettuce and sweet peppers. Avoid avocado and artichokes.
High K+ and High Phosphorus	**Alternatives for a Lower K+/Phosphorus Diet**
Cheese	Vegan rella cheese, low-fat cottage cheese, sprinkle of parmesan cheese; very small amounts of extra sharp cheeses for the maximum flavor
Chocolate	Desserts made with lemon or apple, white cake, rice-crispy treats
Cream soup	Broth-based soups made with pureed vegetables or make soups with Mocha Mix® nondairy creamer, Rich's Coffee Rich®, or Dairy Delicious® milk
Dried beans and peas	Green beans, wax beans
Ice cream	Mocha Mix® frozen dessert, sorbet, sherbet, popsicles
Milk	Dairy Delicious® milk, Mocha Mix® nondairy creamer, Coffeemate®, Rich's Coffee Rich®, Rice Dream® original, unenriched rice beverage
Nuts	Low-salt snack foods including pretzels, tortilla chips, popcorn, crackers, Sun Chips®
Peanut butter	Low-fat cream cheese, jam, or fruit spread

Derived from: Davita Dialysis Centers, http://www.davita.com/diet-and-nutrition/c/diet-basics, accessed February 22, 2010.

recommended levels, weight loss, and control of hyperlipidemia. Referral to a qualified dietitian is important.

- For diabetic kidney disease (DKD), provide tips on controlling CHOs from the diet. The NKF recommends intense measures to manage hyperglycemia, hypertension, and dyslipidemia (NKF, 2007). Maintain HbA1c <7.0% regardless of the stage of CKD. Keep high blood pressure controlled (<130/80 mm Hg); low-density lipoprotein (LDL) cholesterol <100 mg/dL; dietary protein intake at 0.8 g/kg BW per day. Avoid high-protein diets with 20% of calories from protein.
- As eGFR declines, renal metabolism of insulin and oral medication is reduced, potentially causing hypoglycemia; cranberry juice cocktail, grape, apple juice, or glucose tablets may be helpful (Aase, 2010).
- Teach the Dietary Approaches to Stop Hypertension (DASH) diet that emphasizes sources of protein other than red meat for hypertension, diabetes, and CKD stages 1–2 (NKF, 2007).
- Discuss reading food labels, measuring portions, reading restaurant menus, planning box lunch foods, and dining away from home.
- LPDs are safe when properly planned. They reduce the accumulation of metabolic products and can suppress progressive loss of kidney function (Mitch, 2005). Have patient consume the designated proteins throughout the day. Low-protein wheat starch, hard candy, and jelly can be used to increase calories.
- Foods with sharp, distinct flavors may be needed. Lack of interest in red meats is common, and taste changes can occur.

INTERDISCIPLINARY NUTRITION CARE PLAN
End-Stage Renal Disease (Hemodialysis)

Client Name: ________________ **#:** ________ **Initiated by:** ________ **Date:** ________

SCREENING
Nutrition Screen diagnosis: End-Stage Renal Disease (or dialysis)
Signed: ____________ Date: ______

GOALS (Check any/all):

❑ Maintain or improve nutritional status in ____ (goal time).

❑ Improve serum albumin in ____ (goal time).

❑ Maintain or improve adherence to renal diet in ____ (goal time).

Weight ❑ maintained, or ❑ loss/ ❑ gain of ____ lb in ____ (goal time).

ASSESS *(Check any/all)*
Blood chemistries
❑ Serum albumin
❑ Serum transferrin, iron, or ferritin
❑ Total iron-binding capacity (TIBC)
❑ Serum ferritin
❑ Hematocrit, hemoglobin
❑ RBC indices, reticulocyte count
❑ BUN, creatinine
❑ Potassium/phospohorus, calcium
❑ Glucose
❑ Other: ____________
Weight/BMI
❑ Weight loss >3 lb/wk or > 5%/mo or >10%/6 mo
❑ Weight gain >2 lb/d (fluid weight gain)
❑ BMI <20 (High Risk)
Poor Oral Intake Symptoms
❑ Complex diet order
❑ Nausea/vomiting
❑ Poor appetite/early satiety
❑ Problems chewing/swallowing
❑ Depression/anxiety
❑ GI distress
Signed: ____________ Date: ______

None →

MODERATE-RISK INTERVENTIONS
(Check any/all)
❑ **Hemodialysis and Your Renal Diet** provided and explained
Obtain Dr. orders as needed:
❑ RD chart consult
❑ Social Services chart consult
❑ Monitor blood chemistry
❑ Monitor weight q:_____
❑ Medication adjustments
❑ BID/TID supplement or sole source
❑ **Other:** ____________
(See notes for documention.)
Signed: ____________ Date: ______

Next visit ↓

ASSESS RESPONSE *(Check any/all)*
❑ Abnormal blood chemistries
❑ Exhibiting Poor Oral Intake Symptoms
❑ Weight change not appropriate per goal
❑ Declining strength
❑ **Other:** ____________
(See notes for documention.)
Signed: ____________ Date: ______

None →

OUTCOMES ACHIEVED
❑ Weight maintained or improved
❑ Adherence to renal diet
❑ Normal blood chemistries
❑ **Other:** ____________
(See notes for documention.)
❑ Repeat Nutrition Screen in ____ days
Signed: ____________ Date: ______

← 1 or more

1 or more ↓

HIGH-RISK INTERVENTIONS *(Check any/all)*
❑ **Hemodialysis and Your Renal Diet** provided and reviewed
Obtain Dr. orders as needed:
❑ RD referral for home visit(s)
❑ Social Services referral for home visit(s)
❑ Labs: ____________
❑ Monitor weight q:_____
❑ Medication adjustments
❑ BID/TID supplement or sole source
❑ **Other:** ____________
(See notes for documention.)
Signed: ____________ Date: ______

Next visit ↓

ASSESS RESPONSE *(Check any/all)*
❑ Abnormal blood chemistries
❑ Continued Poor Oral Intake Symptoms
❑ Weight change not appropriate per goal
❑ Declining strength
❑ **Other:** ____________
(See notes for documention.)
Signed: ____________ Date: ______

None →

OUTCOMES ACHIEVED
❑ Weight maintained or improved
❑ Adherence to renal diet
❑ Normal blood chemistries
❑ **Other:** ____________
❑ Repeat Nutrition Screen in ____ days
(See notes for documention.)
Signed: ____________ Date: ______

1 or more ↓

OUTCOMES NOT ACHIEVED
Reassess acuity/evaluate need for further nutrition support. Document on Nutrition Variance Tracking form.

Adapted with permission from www.RD411.com, Inc.

TABLE 16-7 Drugs Used in Chronic Kidney Disease (CKD) and Dialysis Patients

Medication	Comments
Angiotensin-converting enzyme (ACE) inhibitor or angiotensin receptor blocker	First-line pharmacological intervention should be an ACE inhibitor or angiotensin receptor blocker in those with >200 mg protein/g creatinine on a urine sample.
Antidepressants	Depression is common in this population. Antidepressant treatment may be needed to improve appetite and intake.
Carnitine	Carnitine is formed from lysine and methionine, requiring adequate vitamin C, niacin, iron, and vitamin B_6. Red meat and dairy products are typical dietary sources. Because the kidneys cannot make it, carnitine supplements are sometimes recommended.
Cinacalcet	**Cinacalcet (Sensipar)** has been approved to treat secondary hyperparathyroidism.
	Cinacalcet can be used to lower PTH despite elevations in calcium and/or phosphorus. Parathyroidectomy may be needed to lower PTH when pharmacologic intervention fails.
Growth hormone	Pharmacological doses of recombinant human growth hormone constitute an effective anabolic therapy.
Insulin	Insulin may be needed to control blood glucose levels. It is an anabolic hormone and can protect lean body mass for some patients.
Iron supplements and epoetin	**Recombinant human erythropoietin (rHuEPO)** is used to treat anemia; an iron supplement will be necessary. Be careful not to overload with excesses, and do not take supplements at the same time as calcium.
	Retacrit (epoetin zeta) is being evaluated for intravenous administration.
Lipid-lowering medications	Lipoprotein metabolism is often impaired in CKD. Patients with low-density lipoprotein ≥100 mg/dL should be treated with diet and a statin.
Phosphate binders	Phosphate binders offer options for phosphorus reduction; newer binders are available that will not increase serum calcium. Nausea or vomiting may occur.
	Aluminum-containing binders are effective but can accumulate in tissues or may lead to bone disease, encephalopathy, or anemia.
	Calcium-containing binders (gluconate, carbonate, or lactate) may increase calcium intake, which may be otherwise inadequate if milk is limited. They are widely used but can lead to hypercalcemia or calcification.
	Lanthanum carbonate (Fosrenol) has good potency and minimal absorption; long-term studies on tolerability needed. Does not cause hypercalcemia.
	Magnesium carbonate can lead to hypermagnesemia, but long-term studies are lacking. It has the potential to minimize calcium load.
	Sevelamer (Renagel) causes less vascular calcification than calcium binders; it also reduces triglycerides and LDL cholesterol. It is costly and tolerability is variable.
Vitamin supplement	Renal multivitamins (such as Diatx) may be useful in providing B-complex vitamins (especially folic acid, B_6, and B_{12}) for hyperhomocysteinemia and CKD.
Vitamin D	In CKD, the patient's kidney is unable to convert vitamin D to its active form; osteodystrophy can result. Take the supplements with extra water if possible because constipation may be a problem.
	Calcitriol (Calcijex®, Rocaltrol®) is the active vitamin D form that increases calcium and phosphorus absorption; it loses effectiveness with high serum P. The active form should not be taken if calcium or phosphorus levels are too high; it can increase phosphorus deposits in soft tissues such as arteries, lungs, eyes, and skin.
	Vitamin D analogs lower parathyroid hormone and increase bone mineralization but may raise calcium and phosphorus. **Paricalcitol (Zemplar®) and Doxercalciferol (Hectorol®)** are active vitamin D analogs that are less calcemic.

- Check for weights daily. Offer tips for maintaining fluid balance and managing thirst; see Table 16-8.
- Discuss dietary sources of vitamin D (see Appendix A).
- Manage high levels of phosphorus by dietary changes and prescribed medicines.
- Teach the patient how to monitor for signs of hyperkalemia, including nausea, weakness, numbness, tingling, slow pulse, or irregular heartbeat.
- Exercising regularly, maintaining a healthy weight, and not smoking prolong kidney health. Patients should talk to their doctors about an exercise plan.

Patient Education—Food Safety

- Foodborne illness can occur when there is contamination of food at any point during the preparation process.

TABLE 16-8 Tips for Managing Thirst and Fluid Restrictions

Fluid Equivalents	Sample Fluid Content
30 mL = 1 fluid oz = 2 tablespoons	1 whole popsicle = 90 mL
240 mL = 8 fluid oz = 1 cup	4 oz soup = 120 mL
2 cups = 1 lb fluid weight	6 oz juice = 180 mL
2.2 lb = 1 kg fluid weight	8 oz beverage = 240 mL
1 kg fluid weight = 4 cups liquid	12 oz soda = 360 mL
	16 oz milkshake = 480 ml

Tips for Managing Thirst

Control high blood glucose; thirst is a side effect of hyperglycemia.

Limit foods that contain hidden or large amounts of fluid (popsicles, soup, gravy, watermelon, and ice cream).

Reduce intake of salty and spicy foods.

Rinse often with mouthwash or suck on a lemon to decrease dry mouth.

Sipping beverages will make them last longer.

Stay cool in warm weather; drink cool instead of warm beverages.

Take medicines with applesauce instead of beverages.

Using ice instead of beverages may seem more satisfying; freeze the allotted amount of beverages (such as fruit juice) and track intake accordingly.

Derived from: Davita Dialysis Centers, http://www.davita.com/diet-and-nutrition/diet-basics/a/477, accessed February 22, 2010.

- To prevent contamination from *E. coli* bacteria (0157:H7) that is associated with undercooked meats, cook until juices run clear (155°F for ground meat or hamburger).
- Because renal patients are at high risk for foodborne illness, follow the four-step guidelines established by the U.S. Department of Agriculture: clean, separate, cook, and chill. See the Kidney Foundation Web site at http://www.kidney.org/atoz/content/foodsafety.cfm.

For More Information

- End-Stage Renal Disease Clinical Performance Measures (CPMs) Project http://www.cms.hhs.gov/CPMProject/
- ESRD Quality Initiative http://www.cms.hhs.gov/ESRDQualityImproveInit/downloads/ESRDOverview.pdf
- KDOQI Guidelines for Managing Diabetes and CKD http://www.ajkd.org/article/S0272–6386(06)01843–9/fulltext
- MEDLINE—ESRD http://www.nlm.nih.gov/medlineplus/ency/article/000500.htm
- NKF—CKD http://www.kidney.org/kidneydisease/ckd/index.cfm
- NKF-KDOQI Guidelines http://www.ajkd.org/content/kdoqiguidelines
- NKF-KDOQI Guidelines for Pediatrics http://www.kidney.org/professionals/KDOQI/guidelines_updates/pdf/CPGPedNutr2008.pdf

CHRONIC KIDNEY DISEASE AND RENAL FAILURE—CITED REFERENCES

Aase S. Kidney friendly: what the National Kidney Disease Education Program strategic plan means for dietetic practice. *J Am Diet Assoc.* 110:346, 2010.

Barretto DV, et al. Plasma interleukin-6 is independently associated with mortality in both hemodialysis and pre-dialysis patients with chronic kidney disease. *Kidney Int.* 77:550, 2010.

Burrowes JD. New recommendations for the management of diabetic kidney disease. *Nutr Today.* 43:65, 2008.

Castro AF, Coresh J. CKD surveillance using laboratory data from the population-based National Health and Nutrition Examination Survey (NHANES). *Am J Kidney Dis.* 53:46S, 2009.

Chu AY, et al. Association of APOE polymorphism with chronic kidney disease in a nationally representative sample: a Third National Health and Nutrition Examination Survey (NHANES III) Genetic Study. *BMC Med Genet.* 10:108, 2009.

Eyre S, et al. Positive effects of protein restriction in patients with chronic kidney disease. *J Ren Nutr.* 18:269, 2008.

Kent PS. Integrating clinical nutrition practice guidelines in chronic kidney disease. *Nutr Clin Pract.* 20:213, 2005.

Kronenberg F. Emerging risk factors and markers of chronic kidney disease progression. *Nat Rev Nephrol.* 5:677, 2009.

Lai MN, et al. Risks of kidney failure associated with consumption of herbal products containing Mu Tong or Fangchi: a population-based case-control study. *Am J Kidney Dis.* 55:507, 2010.

McFarlane SI, et al. Prevalence and associations of anemia of CKD: Kidney Early Evaluation Program (KEEP) and National Health and Nutrition Examination Survey (NHANES) 1999–2004. *Am J Kidney Dis.* 51:46S, 2008.

Menon V, et al. Effect of a very low-protein diet on outcomes: long-term follow-up of the Modification of Diet in Renal Disease (MDRD) Study. *Am J Kidney Dis.* 53:208, 2009.

Middleton RJ, et al. The unrecognized prevalence of chronic kidney disease in diabetes. *Nephrol Dial Transplant.* 21:88, 2006.

Mitch WE. Beneficial responses to modified diets in treating patients with chronic kidney disease. *Kidney Int Suppl.* 94:S133, 2005.

National Kidney Foundation. KDOQI clinical practice guidelines and clinical practice recommendations for diabetes and chronic kidney disease. *Am J Kidney Dis.* 49:1S, 2007.

National Kidney Foundation. *National Kidney Disease Education Program. Reducing disparities, improving care: a summary report.* Bethesda, MD: NIH Publication No. 09-7381. Reprinted August 2009.

Pannu N, et al. Renal replacement therapy in patients with acute renal failure: a systematic review. *JAMA.* 299:793, 2008.

Shen Y, et al. Should we quantify insulin resistance in patients with renal disease? *Nephrology.* 10:599, 2006.

Stratton RJ, et al. Multinutrient oral supplements and tube feeding in maintenance dialysis: a systematic review and meta-analysis. *Am J Kidney Dis.* 46:387, 2005.

Vassolotti JA, et al. Kidney early evaluation program: a community-based screening approach to address disparities in chronic kidney disease. *Semin Nephrol.* 30:66, 2010.

Wu-Wong JR, et al. Vitamin D receptor activation mitigates the impact of uremia on endothelial function in the 5/6 nephrectomized rats. *Int J Endocrinol.* 2010:625852, 2010.

DIALYSIS

NUTRITIONAL ACUITY RANKING: LEVEL 4

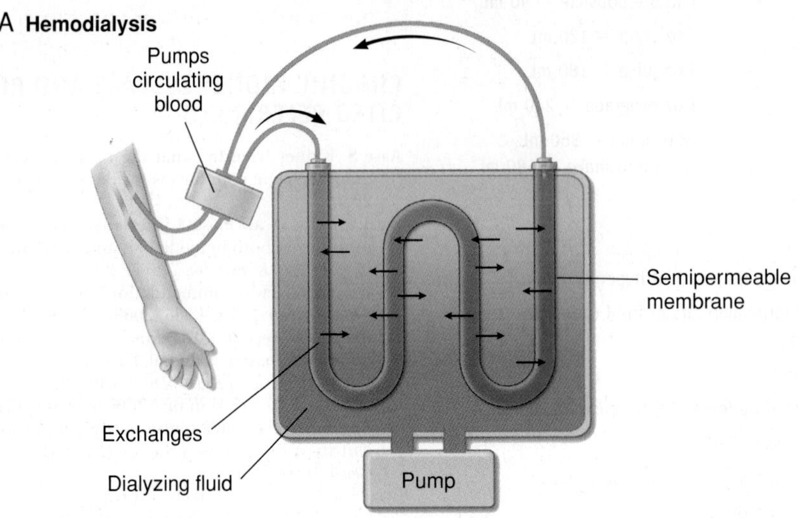

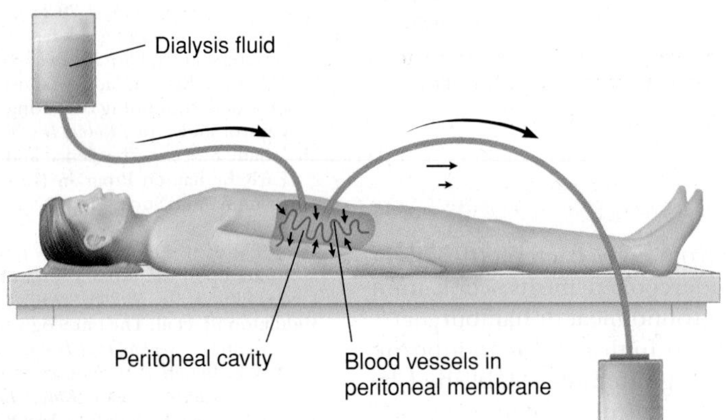

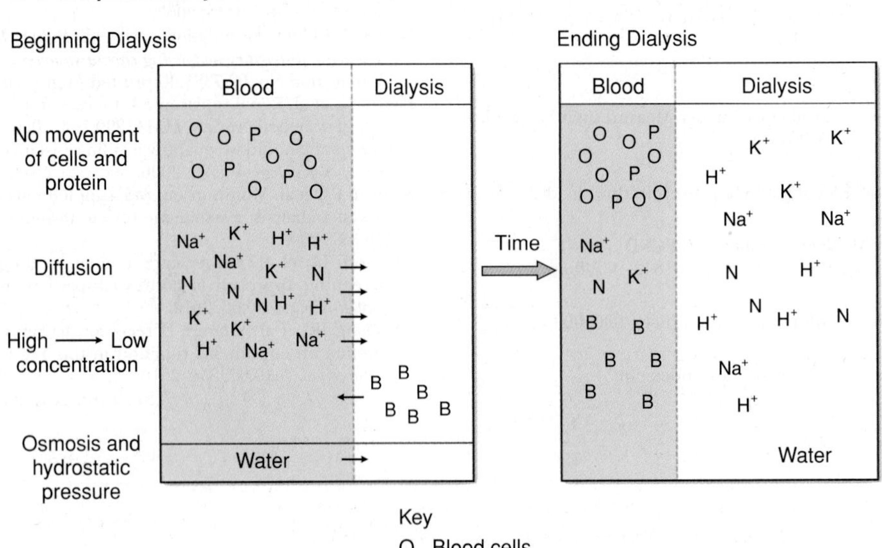

Adapted from: Premkumar K. *The Massage Connection Anatomy and Physiology*. Baltimore: Lippincott Williams & Wilkins 2004.

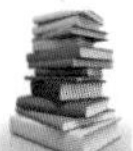

DEFINITIONS AND BACKGROUND

Dialysis specifically involves artificial filtering of blood by a machine. It is a catabolic process. Among patients on dialysis, 33% have diabetes, and 50% of deaths are related to cardiovascular disease. Morbidity is largely related to physical fitness at the start of therapy. Chronic long-term dialysis can aggravate bone disease, anemia, endocrine disorders and can lead to malnutrition if not monitored carefully.

Peritoneal dialysis (PD) involves artificial filtering of the blood by a hyperosmolar solution (with osmosis to remove water and diffusion for glucose exchange/waste removal). The patient and doctor select continuous ambulatory PD (CAPD) or intermittent PD. CAPD does not require a machine. Continuous cycler-assisted PD (CCPD) requires a machine called a *cycler* to fill and drain the abdomen, usually during sleep; this is called *automated PD (APD)*. PD removes metabolic wastes and excess fluid from the body but not so thoroughly that diet therapy is unnecessary. Between dialysis treatments, the patient must return to a strict renal diet. Sometimes alternative methods are required. Intradialytic parenteral nutrition (IDPN) is convenient since it is administered during dialysis treatment. Overweight is more prominent in this population than malnutrition, which occurs frequently in HD patients.

HD is the more common method used to treat advanced and permanent kidney failure. In HD, blood flows through a special filter that removes wastes and extra fluids and then is returned to the body. With HD, less protein is lost than with PD; nevertheless, amino acid losses still occur. Approximately 40% of patients undergoing **maintenance HD** suffer from varying degrees of PEM. Causes of PEM include the catabolic effects of HD treatments, acidemia associated with ESRD, comorbid conditions, and uremia-induced anorexia (Ohlrich et al, 2005). Toxins accumulate with renal failure that suppress appetite and contribute to nutritional decline. Pica (mostly ice but also starch, dirt, flour, and aspirin) has also been found in many dialysis patients.

Nutritional status in these patients should be assessed by a panel of measures rather than by any single measure. Criteria often used to diagnose malnutrition in dialysis patients include serum albumin <3.4 g/dL, average BW <90% of desired goal, or documented protein intake <0.8 g/kg. The NKF Kidney Disease Guidelines for Nutrition provide many clinical practice guidelines for adults and separate guidelines for children.

Higher dietary phosphorus intake and higher dietary phosphorus:protein ratios are each associated with increased death risk in HD patients, even after adjustments for serum phosphorus, phosphate binders and their types, and dietary protein, energy, and potassium intakes (Noori et al, 2010). Control of phosphorus levels must, therefore, be a priority. Nutritional intervention can decrease both malnutrition and mortality in HD. The first step is careful evaluation of protein–energy status, followed by intensive nutrition counseling and then by oral nutrition supplementation, appetite stimulation, or enteral tube feedings (Ohlrich et al, 2005). Prealbumin concentrations <20 mg/dL are a concern, and a fall in serum prealbumin level over 6 months is independently associated with increased death risk (Rambod et al, 2008). However, albumin is more of a marker of illness severity than nutritional status (Friedman and Fadem, 2010).

EN or PN support may be needed; PN should be limited to patients who do not respond to other medical, psychiatric, and nutritional interventions.

Anemia can lead to chronic fatigue and debility if not corrected. Recombinant human erythropoietin beta (rHuEPO) is often given to improve nutritional status. Patients who do not respond to erythropoietin replacement may suffer from malnutrition and inflammation (Locatelli et al, 2006). Higher serum hemoglobin levels are associated with fewer hospitalizations and fewer hospital days (O'Connor et al, 2005).

CKD disrupts calcium homeostasis and causes high PTH, low calcitriol, reduced intestinal calcium absorption, low serum calcium, and high serum phosphorus at low GFR. In this secondary HPT, not enough phosphate is cleared from the body; phosphate is released from bone. Vitamin D is not produced. Absorption of calcium in the gut is low, and blood levels of calcium are lowered. Fortunately, treatment of secondary HPT has improved in recent years, and skeletal pain, disabling fractures, tendon ruptures, and other symptoms can be avoided. Parenteral vitamin D is associated with improved survival among long-term HD patients (Shoben et al, 2008).

Dyslipidemia is common; dialysis patients have increased cardiovascular morbidity and mortality. Excessive cardiovascular mortality of dialysis patients is related to chronic inflammation and muscle wasting (Kuhlmann and Levin, 2005; Workeneh and Mitch, 2010). The ATP-dependent ubiquitin–proteasome system causes skeletal muscle wasting not only from inflammation but also from metabolic acidosis, angiotensin II, and defective insulin signaling (Workeneh and Mitch, 2010). Elevated CRP levels can predict cardiovascular mortality. Eventually, 14-kD actin levels can be a marker of excessive muscle wasting (Workeneh and Mitch, 2010).

Children need adequate protein to encourage growth, and an intensive program of dialysis and nutrition intervention can be used in children on maintenance RRT. Monitor potassium and phosphorus restrictions carefully; protein choices are often high in these nutrients. For all patients, monitor trends and not just single biochemical numbers to identify the need for more education and counseling.

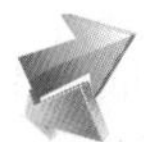

ASSESSMENT, MONITORING, AND EVALUATION

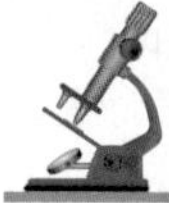

CLINICAL INDICATORS

Genetic Markers: Dialysis may be necessary for some of the genetic causes of renal failure.

Clinical/History

Height
Weight
aBWef
Edema
BMI
Diet history
Waist circumference
Waist:hip ratio
BP
I & O
Triceps skinfold (TSF)
Midarm circumference (MAC)
Midarm muscle circumference (nonaccess arm in HD)

- Temperature
- DEXA scan

Lab Work

- BUN
- Creat
- GFR
- CrCl (on HD, it will be <10)
- Urine urea nitrogen (UUN) or Kt/V
- Serum phosphorus (goal, <5.5 mg/dL)
- CRP (usually elevated)
- Serum PTH (goal, 100–200 pg/mL)
- Serum vitamin D
- Serum Ca^{++} (goal, 9.2–9.6 mg/dL)
- Mg^{++}
- Gluc, HgbA1c
- Transferrin
- Serum bicarbonate (low?)
- Na^{+}
- K^{+} (levels >6 mg/dL can trigger heart failure)
- Metabolic acidosis, hyperchloremia
- Uric acid
- Alb, transthyretin
- Urea
- Serum folacin
- Serum B_{12}
- Chol, Trig
- AST (decreased)
- Hemoglobin
- Hematocrit—target of 33–36%
- Serum Fe, ferritin
- N balance
- Serum zinc

INTERVENTION

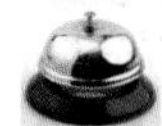

OBJECTIVES

- Normalize the volume and composition of the body fluids and remove uremic toxins.
- Compensate for lost amino acids without causing uremic symptoms.
- Spare protein adequately to allow for tissue repair and synthesis; ensure sufficient total energy intake. Inflammation may elevate resting energy expenditure levels (Utaka et al, 2005); monitor accordingly.
- In PD only: alter calorie intake according to glucose absorption from the solution (e.g., 20 kcal/L in 1.5% solution; 60 kcal/L in 2.5% solution; and 126 kcal/L in 4.5% solution).

SAMPLE NUTRITION CARE PROCESS STEPS

Excessive Mineral Intake

Assessment Data: HD patient returning to clinic; most labs within normal range, but phosphorus level at 7 mg/dL. Diet history indicates increased intake of dairy foods in the past week.

Nutrition Diagnosis (PES): NI-5.1.6 Excessive mineral (phosphorus) intake related to high intake of dairy foods in the past days as evidenced by serum phosphorus level of 7 mg/dL.

Interventions:

Food-Nutrient Delivery: Encourage return to renal dietary protocol.

Education: Review effects of hyperphosphatemia on quality of life.

Counseling: Discuss alternatives to dairy foods and provide recipes, menus, and other tips.

Coordination of Care: Review care plan with medical team and plan follow-up for the next clinic visit.

Monitoring and Evaluation: Improvement in serum phosphorus. No complaints with renal diet or dairy substitutes. Better able to plan menus and use recipes that are suitable and acceptable.

- Promote growth in children.
- Maintain fluid balance; modify electrolytes and fluid intake according to tolerance and lab values.
- Prevent or correct anorexia, constipation, growth delay, muscle weakness, cardiac arrhythmias, and hypertriglyceridemia.
- Correct metabolic acidosis to suppress muscle protein losses and improve bone metabolism (Workeneh and Mitch, 2010).
- Prevent the consequences of mineral dysregulation, including renal osteodystrophy, hyperphosphatemia, cardiovascular calcification, extraskeletal calcification, endocrine disturbances, neurobehavioral changes, compromised immune system and altered erythropoiesis. Severe dietary restrictions to control serum phosphorus reduce protein intake and can lead to protein–energy wasting and poor survival (Shinaberger et al, 2008). Dialysate concentrations should be prescribed with reference to plasma electrolyte levels. The KDOQI goals include the following:

Serum PTH	150–300 pg/mL
Serum Ca (albumin-corrected)	8.4–9.5 mg/dL
Serum P	3.5–5.5 mg/dL
Calcium-phosphorus (Ca-P) product	<55 mg/dL

- Improve patient survival, reduce morbidity, increase efficiency of care, and improve quality of life.
- Maintain follow-up contact for consistency of care in other settings or at home.

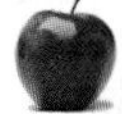

FOOD AND NUTRITION

- In many hospitals, a standard renal diet provides 60 g protein, 2 g sodium, and 2 g potassium, but this may not be appropriate for dialysis. Most dialysis patients are required to limit their intake of phosphorus to 800–1200 mg/d and total (dietary and medication) elemental calcium to ≤ 2000 mg/d.
- Keep open communication with the nephrologist to determine how to best manage the patient. See Table 16-9 for guidelines on managing dialysis nutrition.

Common Drugs Used and Potential Side Effects

- The drugs listed in Table 16-6 are used.
- Vitamin D deficiency is a common problem. In one study, 79% of the dialysis population was vitamin D deficient (25-hydroxyvitamin D < 30 ng/mL); black race, female sex, winter season, and serum albumin level <3.1 g/dL were the strongest predictors of vitamin D deficiency (Bhan et al, 2010). Vitamin D repletion guidelines are shown in Table 16-10.

Herbs, Botanicals, and Supplements

- Herbs and botanical supplements should not be used without discussing with the physician. These products

TABLE 16-9 Nutrition Therapy for Dialysis Patients

Nutrient	Hemodialysis (HD)	Peritoneal Dialysis (PD)
Protein for adults (50% from high biologic value sources)	1.2 g protein/kg/d. Urea kinetic modeling may also be used to devise a protein prescription.	1.2–1.3 g protein/kg/d. If there is peritonitis, 1.5 g/kg may be needed until infection subsides.
Protein for children	For children, base initial protein intake on recommended dietary allowance (RDA) for age plus an increment of 0.4 g/kg/d.	Children undergoing PD should be given RDA levels of protein, plus increments based on anticipated losses.
Energy	35 kcal/kg/d for patients who are <60 years of age and 30–35 kcal/kg for patients ≥60 years of age.	35 kcal/kg/d for patients who are <60 years of age and 30–35 kcal/kg for patients ≥60 years of age. Include dialysate calories in calculations. Extra calories may be needed in peritonitis.
Energy for children	For children, follow RDA levels by age for energy.	Same as HD
Carbohydrate (CHO) and fat	After protein is calculated, assess patient needs (e.g., less CHO in diabetes, fewer lipids with dyslipidemia), and calculate percentages accordingly. Try oral supplements before using other modes of feeding such as enteral or parenteral nutrition (PN).	Total energy intake increases from glucose in the dialysate in continuous ambulatory PD. This extra 300–450 kcal of glucose can increase weight and triglyceride levels. CHO absorption calculations must be individualized and altered as the diet prescription changes. Limit simple sugars and saturated fats.
Fluid	With ≥1 L fluid output = 2 L fluid needed. With <1 L fluid output = 1–1.5 L fluid needed. With anuria = 1 L fluid needed.	Fluid restriction is less common in PD; 1–3 L/d is suggested. Fluid intake should be determined by patient's state of hydration; encourage or restrict according to intake and output. No more than 1 kg should be gained in 1 day.
Potassium and phosphorus	Check levels of potassium and phosphorus; modify diet accordingly.	Same as HD
	Dialysis removes very little phosphorus; use 800–1000 mg or ≤17 mg/kg ideal body weight (BW). Calculate potassium as 40 mg/kg BW.	Adjust phosphorus intake according to serum levels; 800–1000 mg phosphorus or 10–15 mg phosphorus/g protein.
Sodium	Limit sodium intake unless there are large losses in dialysate, vomiting, or diarrhea. Restriction to 2–4 g of sodium is common.	Intake of sodium should be liberal, pending assessment of hydration, blood pressure, losses in dialysate, vomiting, and diarrhea.
Vitamins	Use water-soluble vitamin supplements to replace dialysate losses. Daily replacement may not be needed.	Supplement diet with water-soluble vitamins, especially vitamin B_6 and folic acid.
	Folic acid (often need 1 μg), vitamin B_6 (1.3–1.7 mg), vitamin C (75–90 mg), and vitamin B_{12} (2.4 μg)	Active vitamin D should be monitored and replaced at recommended levels. Avoid vitamin A excesses.
	For children use DRI levels for age.	Same as HD
Minerals	Monitor serum labs as available.	Same as HD
	Individualize calcium; dialysate concentrations should be prescribed according to plasma levels.	Same as HD
Enteral nutrition	Try oral supplements first. If tube feeding is necessary, use an appropriate product to meet protein, electrolyte, and volume needs. If low volume is needed, use a product with 1.5–2.0 kcal/mL with small free-water flushes. Monitor electrolytes.	Same as HD
Parenteral nutrition	Before considering PN as an intervention in a dialysis patient, all other methods should be used. Use caution with PN, especially for zinc, and vitamins A and D.	Same as HD
Omega-3 fatty acids	Fish oil supplementation may help reduce prostaglandin synthesis and may help improve hematocrit levels.	Same as HD
Mediterranean diet	A Mediterranean dietary pattern and regular soy intake may be considered.	Same as HD

TABLE 16-10 Vitamin D_3 Repletion

Serum 25(OH)D (ng/mL)	Vitamin D Status	Dose (IU)	Route	Duration (months)[a]
<5	Severe deficiency	50,000/wk × 12 weeks; then monthly	*po*	6
		500,000 once	*im*	
5–15	Mild deficiency	50,000/wk × 4 weeks, then monthly	*po*	6
16–30	Insufficiency	50,000/mo	*po*	6

[a]Duration for all methods is 6 months, after which assay is needed.

contain pharmacologically active compounds that may be hazardous to patients with kidney problems (Burrowes and Van Houten, 2005). For example, noni juice has a high potassium content and should be avoided.

- Approximately half of dialysis and transplant patients use CAM. Mineral supplements and vitamins rank first, followed by herbal teas and other products that contain ingredients that may accumulate in renal failure (Nowack et al, 2009).

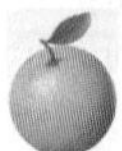

NUTRITION EDUCATION, COUNSELING, CARE MANAGEMENT

Dialysis: General

- Public Law 92-603 provides financial assistance via Medicaid to all persons covered by Social Security who have ESRD with dialysis. Table 16-11 discusses the role of dietitians in dialysis care.
- Discuss signs of uremia (nausea, vomiting, hiccups, fatigue, and weakness).

TABLE 16-11 Role of the Renal Dietitian in Dialysis Care

Patients with end-stage renal disease often experience malnutrition as a result of decreased dietary intake; inadequate dialysis; loss of nutrients into the dialysate; abnormal protein, carbohydrate, and lipid metabolism; and concomitant diseases, which may contribute to an increase in morbidity and mortality.

Close monitoring of nutritional status is completed by evaluating serum albumin and relevant biochemical data, appetite assessments, dietary energy and protein intakes, consumption of vitamins and minerals, and intake of oral supplemental foods, tube feeding, and parenteral nutrition.

Anthropometry is performed at baseline and on a yearly basis.

Specified changes in serum albumin level or body weight trigger action by the dietitian to prevent protein–energy malnutrition.

Multiple diet parameters are necessary to provide optimal nutritional health, including monitoring of calories, protein, sodium, fluid, potassium, calcium, and phosphorus, as well as other individualized nutrients. Consider all modes of nutritional intervention; use that which is best accepted by the patient and the least invasive.

- Discuss high-energy, low-protein, electrolyte-controlled food choices and supplements. Adequate care must be taken to ingest the designated protein and energy levels, according to current lab reports.
- When patients participate in an exercise program, appetites often improve. Exercise training is a potentially beneficial approach to correct muscle wasting, but more information is needed to optimize exercise regimens (Workeneh and Mitch, 2010).
- Counsel patient regarding managing a healthy diet to prevent or control heart disease or diabetes. A Mediterranean dietary pattern and regular soy intake both have been shown to attenuate chronic inflammation, and this may be useful in CKD patients (Kuhlmann and Levin, 2005).
- If avoiding potassium-rich foods is needed, salt substitutes should be monitored closely. Use of longer cooking times and extra water may help leach out excess potassium.
- Taste alterations are common, especially distaste for red meats, fish, poultry, eggs, sweets, and vegetables. Work individually with the patient to plan meals for adequacy of protein intake.
- Discuss sodium alternatives; see Table 16-5 for spices and condiments to use instead of salt.
- Provide information about dining away from home, home-delivered meals, and meals while traveling.
- Establishing trust, mutual respect, and emotional support are essential to promote a successful set of nutritional outcomes.

Hemodialysis

- Discuss maximum fluid gain (usually 3–5% of BW) between dialysis sessions. Noncompliance with fluid restriction is common and can lead to systemic and cardiac overload.
- Teach fluid management to motivate patients to comply with their regimens; patients report that they feel better when their weight gains are within acceptable limits.

Peritoneal Dialysis

- Fluid restrictions are not always needed with PD. Patient should learn how to recognize significant changes in dry weight (adjusted edema-free BW) or food intake. Discuss actions to be taken. Usually, 3–4 lb between intermittent PD is allowed.
- Teach the patient and family about managing diet to control phosphorus levels (goal is <5.5 mg/dL). Increasing patient knowledge may enhance dietary adherence to phosphorus restriction and use of phosphate binders. Avoid use of carbonated beverages that contain phosphates, such as colas.

Patient Education—Food Safety

Foodborne illness can occur when there is contamination of food at any point during the preparation process. Because renal patients are at high risk for foodborne illness, follow the four-step guidelines established by the U.S. Department of Agriculture: clean, separate, cook, and chill. More details are available at the Kidney Foundation Web site at http://www.kidney.org/atoz/content/foodsafety.cfm.

For More Information

- Dialysis
  http://www.nlm.nih.gov/medlineplus/dialysis.html
- HD
  http://kidney.niddk.nih.gov/kudiseases/pubs/hemodialysis/index.htm
- Merck Manual—HD
  http://www.merck.com/mmpe/sec17/ch234/ch234b.html
- Merck Manual—PD
  http://www.merck.com/mmpe/sec17/ch234/ch234d.html
- National Guidelines Clearinghouse
  http://www.guideline.gov/summary/summary.aspx?doc_id=10016&ss=15
- NKF Dialysis Cookbook
  http://www.kidney.org/atoz/pdf/dialysis_cookbook.pdf
- NKF—HD
  http://www.kidney.org/atoz/content/dietary_hemodialysis.cfm
- NKF—PD
  http://www.kidney.org/atoz/content/peritoneal.cfm
- PD
  http://kidney.niddk.nih.gov/kudiseases/pubs/peritoneal/index.htm

DIALYSIS—CITED REFERENCES

Bhan I, et al. Clinical measures identify vitamin D deficiency in dialysis. *Clin J Am Soc Nephrol.* 5:460, 2010.

Burrowes JD, Van Houten G. Use of alternative medicine by patients with stage 5 chronic kidney disease. *Adv Chronic Kidney Dis.* 12:312, 2005.

Friedman AN, Fadem SZ. Reassessment of albumin as a nutritional marker in kidney disease. *J Am Soc Nephrol.* 21:223, 2010.

Kuhlmann MK, Levin NW. Interaction between nutrition and inflammation in hemodialysis patients. *Contrib Nephrol.* 149:200, 2005.

Locatelli F, et al. Nutritional-inflammation status and resistance to erythropoietin therapy in haemodialysis patients. *Nephrol Dial Transplant.* 21:991, 2006.

Noori N, et al. Association of dietary phosphorus intake and phosphorus to protein ratio with mortality in hemodialysis patients [published online ahead of print February 25, 2010]. *Clin J Am Soc Nephrol.* 5:683, 2010.

Nowack R, et al. Complementary and alternative medications consumed by renal patients in southern Germany. *J Ren Nutr.* 19:211, 2009.

O'Connor AS, et al. The morbidity and cost implications of hemodialysis clinical performance measures. *Hemodial Int.* 9:349, 2005.

Ohlrich H, et al. The use of parenteral nutrition in a severely malnourished hemodialysis patient with hypercalcemia. *Nutr Clin Pract.* 20:559, 2005.

Rambod M, et al. Association of serum prealbumin and its changes over time with clinical outcomes and survival in patients receiving hemodialysis. *Am J Clin Nutr.* 88:1485, 2008.

Shinaberger CS, et al. Is controlling phosphorus by decreasing dietary protein intake beneficial or harmful in persons with chronic kidney disease? *Am J Clin Nutr.* 88:1511, 2008.

Shoben AB, et al. Association of oral calcitriol with improved survival in nondialyzed CKD. *J Am Soc Nephrol.* 19:1613, 2008.

Utaka S, et al. Inflammation is associated with increased energy expenditure in patients with chronic kidney disease. *Am J Clin Nutr.* 82:801, 2005.

Workeneh BT, Mitch WE. Review of muscle wasting associated with chronic kidney disease. *Am J Clin Nutr.* 91:1128S, 2010.

GLOMERULAR AND AUTOIMMUNE KIDNEY DISEASES

NUTRITIONAL ACUITY RANKING: LEVEL 2 ACUTE; LEVEL 3 CHRONIC

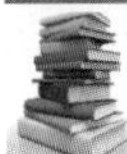

DEFINITIONS AND BACKGROUND

Glomerulonephritis is a collective term used for diseases with renal inflammation stemming from the glomeruli; immune mechanisms are involved in all of them (Segelmark and Hellman, 2010). Antigen–antibody complex reactions become trapped in the glomeruli with resulting edema, scarring, and inflamed glomeruli. Resolution can be promoted by anti-inflammatory clearance by macrophages and mesangial cells (Watson et al, 2006). Clinical trials have provided compelling evidence that omega-3 polyunsaturated fatty acid (eicosapentaenoic acid (EPA) and docosahexaenoic acid (DHA) supplementation is useful, although some other studies suggest such supplementation might be without benefit (Pestka, 2010).

Acute GN occurs with damage to the glomeruli from infection, lupus, or other forms of kidney disease. GN caused by lupus is classified on the basis of lesions, extent and severity of the involvement, immune complex deposition, activity, and chronicity (Seshan and Jennette, 2009). Postinfectious GN (PIGN) may be related to *Staphylococcus* (Wen and Chen, 2010) or to untreated *Streptococcal* infections. Anuria with <400 mL/24 hours of urinary output may require temporary dialysis. Most acute GN conditions resolve after 3–12 months.

In **chronic GN**, repeated episodes of nephritis lead to the loss of renal tissue and kidney function; glomeruli disappear, and normal filtering is lost. The kidneys can no longer concentrate urine, and more urine is voided in an effort to rid the body of wastes. Protein and blood are lost in the urine. Blood pressure rises, causing vascular changes and CKD. The level and type of proteinuria (only albumin or including other proteins) will determine the extent of damage and whether a patient is at risk for developing CKD. Decreasing proteinuria indicates an improved prognosis, whereas hypertension does not.

GN is the second most common cause of renal failure. Conservative treatment uses protein restriction (0.6 g protein/kg BW) to correct metabolic and hormonal derangements; restriction is contraindicated in cases of protein malnutrition, neoplasm, growth, or infection. Sufficient energy intake is essential. Four forms of primary GN include Goodpasture or anti-GBM disease, IgA nephritis (IgAN, Berger disease), membranous nephropathy, and membranoproliferative GN (MPGN), which occurs in adults of African descent and is a common cause of nephrotic syndrome. Much of the ESRD in African Americans is attributable to variants in the gene that encodes motor protein myosin 2 a (MYH9) in this haplotype (Freedman and Sedor, 2008).

Glomerulosclerosis involves hardening (scarring or sclerosis) of the glomeruli from lupus, HIV infection, or diabetes. Significant reduction of renal mass initiates a series of events that lead to proteinuria and glomerulosclerosis

(An et al, 2009). Albumin is lost in the urine, nitrogen waste products are retained, and retinal changes occur. **Focal segmental glomerulosclerosis (FSGS)** may cause nephrotic syndrome secondary to chronic pyelonephritis or diabetes; it is more common in Caucasian adults. Omega-3 fatty acid supplementation may reduce or reverse upregulation of prooxidant, proinflammatory, and profibrotic pathways in the remnant kidney (An et al, 2009).

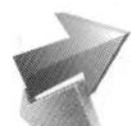

ASSESSMENT, MONITORING, AND EVALUATION

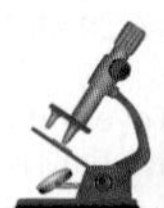

CLINICAL INDICATORS

Genetic Markers: Both genetics and infection seem to play a role. MYH9 is a gene that promotes MPGN in African Americans. Genes that cause the hereditary forms of FSGS that affect Caucasians include ACTN4, TRPC6, and CD2AP.

Clinical/History

- Height
- Weight
- aBWef
- BMI
- Diet history
- Waist:hip circumference
- BP
- Edema of face, ankles, feet, legs
- Fever?
- I & O
- Shortness of breath
- Decrease in urine volume (oliguria)
- Urine smell on breath and sweat
- Itching
- Abdominal pain, vomiting
- Dark or rust-colored urine
- Foamy urine
- Yellowish–brown skin discoloration
- Renal radiographs
- Kidney biopsy

Lab Work

- Alb, transthyretin (low?)
- CRP
- GFR
- CrCl level
- Complement levels
- Anti-glomerular basement membrane antibody test
- Uremia (accumulation in the blood of wastes)
- Transferrin
- BUN, Creat
- Proteinuria
- Gluc
- Urinary ketones
- Chol (increased from proteinuria?)
- Trig
- White blood cell (WBC) count
- H & H
- MCV
- Serum Fe, ferritin
- TIBC
- Specific gravity (decreased?)
- PTH
- Na^+, K^+
- Serum phosphorus
- AST
- Ca^{++}, Mg^{++}
- Serum copper (increased?)

INTERVENTION

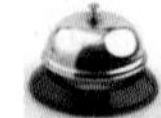

OBJECTIVES

- Improve renal functioning; prevent systemic complications where possible.
- Monitor abnormal protein status and serum nitrogen retention.
- Spare protein for tissue repair. Prevent further catabolism of protein to lessen production of urea and other protein waste products.
- Control hypertension and edema.
- Manage hyperglycemia or dyslipidemia.
- Correct metabolic abnormalities. Improve nutritional status and appetite.
- Prevent or correct growth failure in children.
- Reduce inflammation and attenuate oxidative damage.
- Reduce workload of circulatory system by decreasing excess weight, where needed.

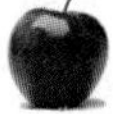

FOOD AND NUTRITION

- Modify patient's diet according to disease progression; maintain sufficient levels of protein as long as kidneys can eliminate waste products of protein metabolism.
- Use sufficient energy to spare protein (60% CHOs, 30% fat). For adults, 30–40 kcal/kg adjusted edema-free BW is needed to spare protein for tissue synthesis and wound healing.
- In **uremia**, diet should include 50% high–biologic value proteins (such as from cheese, meats, fish, eggs, and dairy foods), or essential amino acids at 2–3 times the normal should be included. Limit protein to 0.6–0.8 g/kg.
- In **oliguria**, restrict fluid intake to 500–700 mL. Limit protein to 0.6–0.8 g/kg. When urinary output is reduced greatly, restrict phosphorus intakes if needed. Potassium is often controlled by medications, but monitor and

SAMPLE NUTRITION CARE PROCESS STEPS

Inadequate Energy Intake

Assessment Data: I & O records. BMI of 21. Diet hx shows an average daily intake of 1300 kcal but requirements of 1750 kcal daily. Intake of protein (60 g) meets needs.

Nutrition Diagnosis (PES): Inadequate energy intake NI 1.4 related to poor renal status and sufficient protein intake without calories for sparing as evidenced by diet hx of 1300 kcal, 60 g protein but estimated needs of 1750 kcal/d.

Interventions:

Food-Nutrient Delivery: Increase the use of CHO and fats to spare protein.

Education: Provide instruction and education about the role of protein and the need for sufficient intake of calories from CHO and fat.

Counseling: Provide individualized tips for increasing calories to enhance total energy by using preferred foods.

Coordination of Care: Work with the medical team to assess the effectiveness of extra calories to keep lab values closer to normal and to gain a few pounds over time.

Monitoring and Evaluation: BMI improving; now 23 after 3 months of higher-energy intake. Protein intake remains approximately 60 g, calorie intake between 1700 and 1800 kcal/d. No undesirable side effects.

adjust as needed. Some patients will require dialysis to remove waste products.

- With **edema** or **high blood pressure**, restrict sodium intake to 2–3 g/d. In a child, a restriction of 500–1000 mg may be needed. Carefully monitor sodium levels because sodium depletion can occur during the diuretic phase of chronic GN.
- Vegetarian diets, soy products, and use of omega-3 fatty acids may be beneficial for dyslipidemia. Restrict fat and cholesterol if needed; monitor diet carefully.
- Control CHO intake with diabetes or hyperglycemia.
- If patient is obese, use an energy-controlled diet, but avoid fasting and very low–calorie diets.
- Determine vitamins and nutrients provided by therapeutic diet and supplement to meet daily requirements, especially for calcium, niacin, and other B vitamins, which are easily lost in urine. Children with uremia require vitamin D_3 replacement for growth and to improve appetite; adults will need it to maintain bone health.

Common Drugs Used and Potential Side Effects

- When diuretics such as furosemide are used to reduce edema, watch for potassium wasting or dehydration. Dehydration can elevate BUN; assess carefully.
- ACE inhibitors are useful for reducing hypertension.
- Immunosuppressants may be used.
- See Table 16-6 for more specific medications.

Herbs, Botanicals, and Supplements

- Herbs and botanical supplements should not be used without discussing with physician.
- Omega-3 fatty acid supplementation may be beneficial (An et al, 2009).

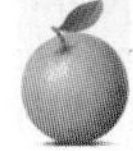

NUTRITION EDUCATION, COUNSELING, CARE MANAGEMENT

- A renal dietitian should provide nutrition therapy and counseling. A diet controlled in protein, fluid, phosphorus, sodium, and potassium may be needed; it must be individualized and is likely to change frequently.
- Commitment from the patient and family is needed; extra expense may be incurred for low-protein foods and amino acid analogs.
- Fluid intake should be distributed carefully throughout the patient's waking hours (see Table 16-7). Check for changes needed during diarrhea or related problems.
- Edema is better controlled by sodium restriction than by fluid restriction; monitor patient carefully. Patients with edema are often thirsty; edema water is trapped and unavailable for body's use.
- Encourage frequent doctor or clinic visits to monitor renal functioning.
- Patients with ascites may become anorexic in the upright position. Position patient carefully for food intake.

Patient Education—Food Safety

- Foodborne illness can occur when there is contamination of food at any point during the preparation process.
- Because renal patients are at high risk for foodborne illness, follow the four-step guidelines established by the U.S. Department of Agriculture: clean, separate, cook, and chill.
- Details are available at the Kidney Foundation Web site at http://www.kidney.org/atoz/content/foodsafety.cfm.

For More Information

- Acute GN
  http://www.nephrologychannel.com/agn/
- MEDLINE—GN
  http://www.nlm.nih.gov/medlineplus/ency/article/000484.htm

GLOMERULAR DISORDERS—CITED REFERENCES

An WS, et al. Omega-3 fatty acid supplementation attenuates oxidative stress, inflammation, and tubulointerstitial fibrosis in the remnant kidney. *Am J Physiol Renal Physiol.* 297:895, 2009.

Freedman BI, Sedor JR. Hypertension-associated kidney disease: perhaps no more. *J Am Soc Nephrol.* 19:2047, 2008.

Pestka JJ. n-3 Polyunsaturated fatty acids and autoimmune-mediated glomerulonephritis. *Prostaglandins Leukot Essent Fatty Acids.* 82:251, 2010.

Segelmark M, Hellman T. Autoimmune kidney diseases [published online ahead of print November 10, 2009]. *Autoimmun Rev.* 9:366, 2010.

Seshan SV, Jennette JC. Renal disease in systemic lupus erythematosus with emphasis on classification of lupus glomerulonephritis: advances and implications. *Arch Pathol Lab Med.* 133:233, 2009.

Watson S, et al. Apoptosis and glomerulonephritis. *Curr Dir Autoimmun.* 9:188, 2006.

Wen YK, Chen ML. The significance of atypical morphology in the changes of spectrum of postinfectious glomerulonephritis. *Clin Nephrol.* 73:173, 2010.

KIDNEY STONES

NUTRITIONAL ACUITY RANKING: LEVEL 1–2

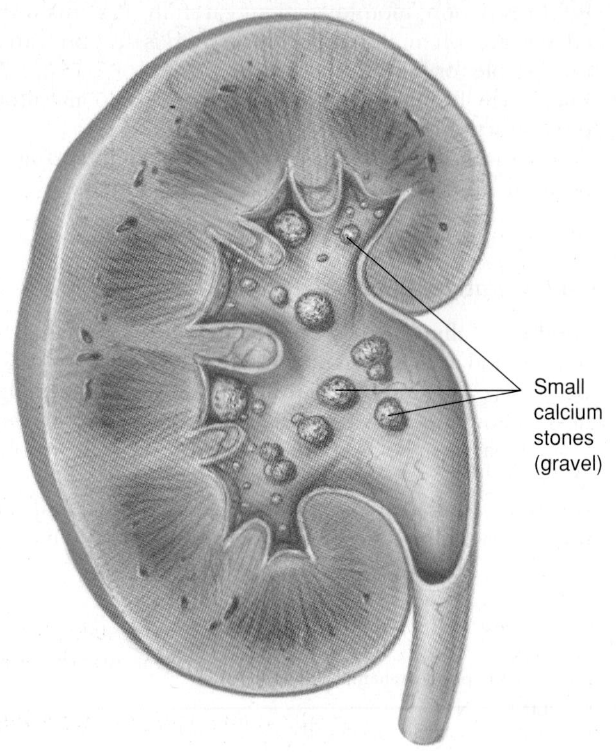

TABLE 16-12 Causes of and Predisposition to Kidney Stones

Climate	Hot climate and dehydration during summer months
Diet	Low intakes of dietary calcium and fluid, high intakes of sodium in susceptible individuals
Diminished water intake	During sleep, travel, or illness or from poor habits
Family	Family history of kidney stones
Genetic disorders	Gout, primary hyperoxaluria, hyperparathyroidism, renal tubular acidosis, cystinuria, and hypercalciuria
Gender	Three times more common in males
Intestinal changes	Inflammatory bowel disease, intestinal bypass surgery, ostomy surgery
Medications	Certain diuretics, use of the protease inhibitor indinavir, excessive intake of supplemental vitamin D
Urinary tract issues	Urinary tract infection or stagnation from blockage

REFERENCE

National Institute of Diabetes and Digestive and Kidney Diseases. Kidney stones in adults, http://kidney.niddk.nih.gov/kudiseases/pubs/stonesadults/, accessed February 22, 2010.

DEFINITIONS AND BACKGROUND

Kidney stones are masses made of crystals; when they move down through the ureters, they cause severe pain. Unfortunately, kidney stones are common due to modern lifestyles, dietary habits, and obesity (Straub and Hautmann, 2005). The process is officially known as *urolithiasis* or *nephrolithiasis.* While all humans form calcium oxalate crystals, most do not form stones. However, prevalence is rising in both sexes (Moe, 2006). Annually, approximately 400,000 people are treated for this problem. Stones affect 5% of adults but may even occur in premature infants.

Kidney stones develop when salt and minerals in urine form crystals that coalesce and grow in size. Stones are formed by progressive deposition of crystalline material around an organic nidus. Decreased fluid intake and consequent urine concentration are among the most important factors influencing stone formation. Other major causes of renal stones are urinary tract infections (UTIs), cystic kidney diseases, metabolic disorders such as HPT, and renal tubular acidosis (see Table 16-12). A person who has had kidney stones or has a family history of kidney stones is at high risk.

Fluid is a key factor. It is not the quantity of fluid consumed but that which is voided that is important. Extra fluid intake will be needed by those who live in hot, dry conditions and by those who exercise or perspire significantly. Many stones can be prevented through changes in diet (Grases et al, 2006). Apple or grapefruit juices may aggravate risk whereas wine, beer, and some diet sodas are protective against stones. Orange and lemon–lime flavors contain alkalis of citrate and malate, which inhibit calcium formation; good choices include Fresca, diet Sunkist orange, diet 7-Up, and diet Canada Dry.

Approximately 80% of stones are composed of calcium oxalate and calcium phosphate (Reynolds, 2005). Ten percent are composed of struvite (magnesium ammonium phosphate produced during infection with bacteria that possess the enzyme urease). The remaining 10% are composed of uric acid, cystine or ammonium acid urate, or melamine. Melamine contamination of infant formula has been noted by the FDA (Skinner et al, 2010).

Struvite stones are mostly found in women who have UTIs. **Cystine stones** may form in individuals who have cystinuria, a familial disorder.

Uric acid stones may result from purine metabolism, gout, leukemia, cancer, or colectomy; they are more common in men. An abnormally low urinary pH (UpH) contributes to the problem. Creating an alkaline urine is the goal; a UpH of 6.2–6.8 is desirable (Hess, 2006). A lower-purine food intake (such as sardines) is also beneficial.

Most studies show no increase in **calcium oxalate** stone risk with high calcium intake (from either diet or supplements) but a high rate of stone risk from a low calcium intake (Heany, 2008). In the Health Professionals Follow-up Study, the Nurses' Health Study I and II, spinach accounted for >40% of oxalate intake; risks were higher in men with low dietary calcium intake, but dietary oxalate was *not* a major risk factor (Taylor and Curhan, 2007). Therefore, diets need not be excessively low in oxalates (see list in Table 16-12).

Diets high in animal protein provide a high acid load; sufficient potassium and alkali are required to neutralize the effect (Straub and Hautmann, 2005). Vegetarians form stones at one third of the rate of those eating a mixed diet. Balanced diets containing moderate amounts of meat and plant proteins (legumes, seeds, nuts, and grains) may keep urinary composition within guidelines. Untreated **calcium oxalate stones** can lead to a greater chance of forming additional stones within later decades.

Citrate inhibits calcium oxalate stone formation by complexing with calcium in the urine, inhibiting spontaneous nucleation, and preventing growth and agglomeration of crystals; hypocitraturia is a metabolic abnormality found in 20–60% of stone formers (Zuckerman and Assimos, 2009). A normal calcium, low animal-protein diet with lemonade and citrus juices is effective for these individuals.

Extracorporeal shockwave lithotripsy remains the preferred method of treatment of urinary stones. Medical expulsive therapy is under review as a new treatment.

SAMPLE NUTRITION CARE PROCESS STEPS

Inadequate Fluid Intake

Assessment Data: I & O records showing low intake of fluids throughout the average day (<6 cups total). Recently hospitalized with uric acid stones; Hx of gout for 3 years.

Nutrition Diagnosis (PES): NI-3.1 Inadequate fluid intake related to poor daily habits as evidenced by uric acid stones and intake records showing <6 cups of fluid per average day.

Interventions:

Food-Nutrient Delivery: Increase fluid intake to 10–12 cups per day from water and other liquids.

Education: Discuss the importance of fluid intake and taking appropriate medicines as prescribed.

Counseling: Discuss purine-rich foods and that diet is seldom needed if the medicine is taken and works properly.

Coordination of Care: Work with pharmacist to ensure that medications will suffice.

Monitoring and Evaluation: Resolution of high urinary uric acid levels and no more renal stones. Intake of fluid averaging between 11 and 12 cups daily.

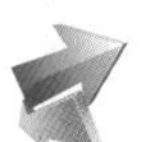

ASSESSMENT, MONITORING, AND EVALUATION

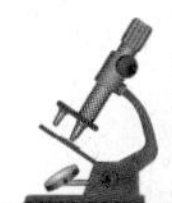

CLINICAL INDICATORS

Genetic Markers: Hypercalciuria is inherited, and it may be the cause of stones in more than half of the population who have calcium oxalate stones. Cystinuria runs in families and affects both men and women.

Clinical/History

- Height
- Weight
- BMI
- Diet history
- BP
- I & O
- Excruciating groin or flank pain
- Fever
- Hematuria or mild pyuria
- Abnormal urine color
- Excessive nocturia
- Nausea, vomiting
- Burning and urinary frequency
- Kidney ultrasound
- Intravenous pyelogram
- Abdominal radiographs or computed tomography scan

Lab Work

- Urinalysis (crystals, RBCs)
- 24-hour urine studies:
  - Total urine volume
  - Urinary calcium (normal, 300–400 mg)
  - Urinary sodium
  - Urinary citrate
- Uric acid
- UpH
- Serum oxalate levels
- Gluc
- Ca^{++}
- Mg^{++}
- Alb
- CRP
- Lactose intolerance
- Serum Na^+, K^+
- BUN
- Creat
- H & H
- Serum Fe

INTERVENTION

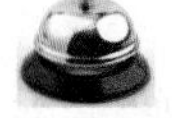

OBJECTIVES

- Determine predominant components and prevent recurrence by normalization of BMI, adequate physical activity, balanced nutrition, and sufficient daily fluid intake. Modify diet according to predominant components; there is seldom a single cause.
- To increase excretion of salts, dilute urine by increasing fluid volume to at least 2 L/24 h.
- Prevent scarring, recurrence of stones, obstruction, bone demineralization, or kidney damage.
- Promote use of a heart-healthy diet (Mitka, 2009).
- Repeat urinary studies approximately 6–8 weeks after initial metabolic testing to evaluate effectiveness of dietary changes. Once stable, where the patient's urine demonstrates decreased risk of stone formation, metabolic testing and radiographs should be performed at least annually.

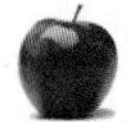

FOOD AND NUTRITION

- General guidelines: Fluid intake should be high, as tolerated (2 L/d). Colorless urine is sought. Individuals with cystinuria will need 3.5 L/d fluid intake (Reynolds, 2005). Limit the use of apple or grapefruit juices.
- Consume a diet that is balanced. Fruits and vegetables may reduce the low potassium/high sodium intake (Reynolds, 2005). The DASH diet is a good recommendation as it is associated with a marked decrease in kidney stone risk (Taylor et al, 2009).
- A heart-healthy weight loss and exercise plan may be needed if the patient is obese (Mitka, 2009; Taylor et al, 2005).
- Specific guidelines by stone content are provided in Table 16-13.
- Calcium should not be restricted, except in absorptive hypercalciuria where calcium restriction remains beneficial in combination with a drug (Straub and Hautmann, 2005). Hypocitraturia should be managed through a combination of oral alkali, dietary modifications, and

TABLE 16-13 Dietary Treatment of Specific Renal Stones

Type	Treatment
Calcium oxalate stones	Calcium intake should be increased to >1000 mg/d; good sources include skim milk, yogurt, low-fat dairy products, broccoli, fortified orange juice, and ricotta or other cheese. Fortified foods and almonds are several nondairy choices. Reducing urinary oxalates has a more powerful effect on stone formation than reduction of urinary calcium. However, diet has a limited role. Omit **very high sources** from rhubarb, spinach, strawberries, beets, All Bran, Swiss chard, almonds and mixed nuts, chocolate soy milk, miso, tahini, and soybeans. Limit **high sources**: okra, sweet potatoes, tomatoes, greens, fried potatoes, navy or black beans, apricots, figs, kiwifruit, some grains, soy milk, soy ice cream, chocolate candy bars, poppy seed, and turmeric. See Web site http://www.ohf.org/docs/Oxalate2008.pdf.
Citrate stones	Hypocitraturia is found in up to 20% of stone formers and may be idiopathic or secondary to intestinal, renal, dietary, or pharmacological causes.
Cystine stones	Individuals with cystinuria will need 3.5 L of fluid daily. Use a diet low in cystine, methionine, and cysteine. Protein intake should be mildly reduced. Cystine stones usually are the result of a rare hereditary defect. Alkalize urine with agents like D-penicillamine.
Struvite stones	Struvite stones contain magnesium ammonium phosphate and may form after an infection in the urinary system. They can grow very large and may obstruct the kidney, ureter, or bladder if not removed.
Uric acid stones	Urate stones can be dissolved by urine alkalinization with citrate or bicarbonate. There is no inhibitor of uric acid crystal formation; dietary measures focus on reducing uric acid and increasing urine volume. Nonfat milk, low-fat yogurt, and other dairy products are useful. High intake of fruits such as cherries and vegetable protein may reduce serum urate levels.

lemonade or other citrus juice–based therapy (Zuckerman and Assimos, 2009). Include legumes and dried beans for their health-promoting saponins, which are useful in the treatment of hypercalciuria.

Common Drugs Used and Potential Side Effects

- Certain medications, such as triamterene (Dyrenium), indinavir (Crixivan), and acetazolamide (Diamox), are associated with urolithiasis.
- Approximately 15% of patients forming stones require specific pharmacological prevention (Straub and Hautmann, 2005).
- For **calcium oxalate** or **uric acid stones**, allopurinol (Zyloprim) and probenecid are usually used; a purine-restricted diet is not always needed (Cameron and Sakhaee, 2007). Drink 10–12 glasses of fluid daily; avoid concomitant intake of vitamin C supplements. Maintain alkaline urine (may need to use sodium bicarbonate). Thiazide diuretics may reduce hypercalciuria (Reynolds, 2005).
- **Hypocitraturia** should be managed through diet and oral alkali (Zuckerman and Assimos, 2009). Potassium citrate and potassium bicarbonate help to alkalinize the urine. Sodium restriction may be inappropriate; sodium supplementation is beneficial in these patients because it results in voluntary increased fluid intake (Stoller et al, 2009).
- For **cystine stones:** D-penicillamine use requires vitamin B_6 and zinc supplementation. Increase fluid intake. Take the drug 1–2 hours before or after meals. Stomatitis, diarrhea, nausea, vomiting, and abdominal pain may occur.
- **Struvite** stones will require use of antibiotics.
- Uric acid stones are often dissolved by using potassium citrate/bicarbonate. Acetazolamide increases UpH in patients with uric acid and cystine stones who are already taking potassium citrate; however, it may be poorly tolerated and can induce calcium phosphate stone formation (Sterrett et al, 2008).
- Potassium citrate (Polycitra K) reduces kidney stone incidence in children treated for seizures with the ketogenic diet (McNally et al, 2009).

Herbs, Botanicals, and Supplements

- Herbs and botanical supplements should not be used without discussing with the physician.
- The use of probiotics such as *Oxalobacter formigenes* in the prevention of calcium oxalate stone disease needs further investigation.

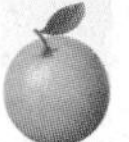

NUTRITION EDUCATION, COUNSELING, CARE MANAGEMENT

- The most important lifestyle change to prevent stones is to drink more liquids, especially water; try to produce at least 2 quarts of urine in every 24-hour period.
- Teach the principles of a heart-healthy DASH diet (Mitka, 2009; Taylor et al, 2009).
- A patient's 24-hour urine chemistry profile should guide the dietary adjustments. Use dietary measures that are appropriate for condition and content of the stone.
- Discuss occupational risks for stone formation, including working in hot, dry environments, or working with metals such as cadmium.

Patient Education—Food Safety

Foodborne illness can occur when there is contamination of food at any point during the preparation process. Follow standard practices in food safety and handling.

For More Information

- Kidney Stone Diet
  http://www.gicare.com/pated/edtgs29.htm.
- Kidney Stones in Adults
  http://www.niddk.nih.gov/health/kidney/pubs/stonadul/stonadul.htm
- National Library of Medicine
  http://www.nlm.nih.gov/medlineplus/ency/article/000458.htm
- Oxalosis and Hyperoxaluria Foundation
  http://www.ohf.org/
- Renal Stones in Adults
  http://kidney.niddk.nih.gov/Kudiseases/pubs/stonesadults/

KIDNEY STONES—CITED REFERENCES

Cameron MA, Sakhaee K. Uric acid nephrolithiasis. *Urol Clin North Am.* 34:335, 2007.
Grases F, et al. Renal lithiasis and nutrition. *Nutr J.* 5:23, 2006.
Heany RP. Calcium supplementation and incident kidney stone risk: a systematic review. *J Am Coll Nutr.* 27:519, 2008.
Hess B. Acid-base metabolism: implications for kidney stones formation. *Urol Res.* 34:134, 2006.
McNally MA, et al. Empiric use of potassium citrate reduces kidney-stone incidence with the ketogenic diet. *Pediatrics.* 124:e300, 2009.
Mitka M. Findings suggest heart-healthy diets may reduce risk of kidney stones. *JAMA.* 302:1048, 2009.
Moe OW. Kidney stones: pathophysiology and medical management. *Lancet.* 367:333, 2006.
Reynolds TM. ACP Best Practice No 181: chemical pathology clinical investigation and management of nephrolithiasis. *J Clin Pathol.* 58:134, 2005.
Skinner CG et al. Melamine Toxicity. *J Med Toxicol.* 6:50, 2010.
Sterrett SP, et al. Acetazolamide is an effective adjunct for urinary alkalization in patients with uric acid and cystine stone formation recalcitrant to potassium citrate. *Urology.* 72: 278, 2008.
Stoller ML, et al. Changes in urinary stone risk factors in hypocitraturic calcium oxalate stone formers treated with dietary sodium supplementation. *J Urol.* 181:1140, 2009.
Straub M, Hautmann RE. Developments in stone prevention. *Curr Opin Urol.* 15:119, 2005.
Taylor EN, Curhan GC. Oxalate intake and the risk for nephrolithiasis. *J Am Soc Nephrol.* 18:2198, 2007.
Taylor EN, et al. DASH-style diet associates with reduced risk for kidney stones. *J Am Soc Nephrol.* 20:2253, 2009.
Taylor EN, et al. Obesity, weight gain, and the risk of kidney stones. *JAMA.* 293:455, 2005.
Zuckerman JM, Assimos DG. Hypocitraturia: pathophysiology and medical management. *Rev Urol.* 11:134, 2009.

NEPHROTIC SYNDROME

NUTRITIONAL ACUITY RANKING: LEVEL 2–3

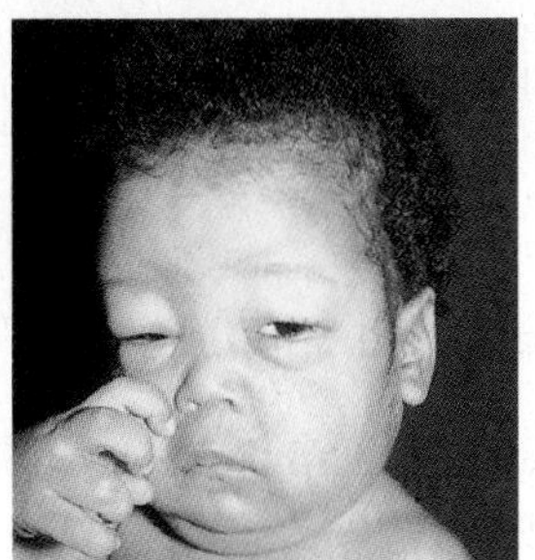

DEFINITIONS AND BACKGROUND

Nephrotic syndrome is not a disease but causes massive proteinuria, with 3.5 g or more of protein lost within 24 hours. As much as 30 g can be lost as a result. Serum albumin is especially affected. The common nephrotic syndrome in children is called "minimal change disease." In approximately 20% of children with nephrotic syndrome, kidney biopsy reveals scarring or deposits in the glomeruli.

Adults who have nephrotic syndrome usually have some form of GN, with renal failure not far behind. FSGS is the most common cause in Caucasians; MPGN is the common cause in African Americans. Other causes include DKD, lupus, amyloidosis, HIV infection, hepatitis B or C, malaria, and heart failure.

Elevated LDL cholesterol is common because of altered lipoprotein production. When the liver makes more albumin in an effort to replace that which is lost, more cholesterol and triglycerides are released.

MNT centers on the problem of salt and water retention, protein depletion, hyperlipidemia, and loss of carrier proteins for vitamins and minerals. Patients have normal anabolic responses to dietary protein restriction (decreased amino acid oxidation) and feeding (increased protein synthesis and decreased degradation). A very high–protein diet will alter GFR; limit protein to decrease hyperfiltration. A moderate-protein diet that provides adequate energy can maintain nitrogen balance in nephrotic syndrome. Immunosuppressive medication is not helpful in the genetic forms of congenital nephrotic syndrome (CNS); a high-energy diet is needed and kidney transplantation is the only curative therapy (Jalanko, 2009).

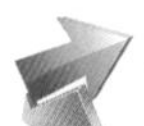

ASSESSMENT, MONITORING, AND EVALUATION

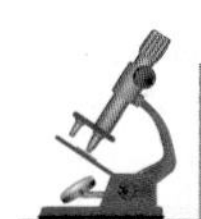

CLINICAL INDICATORS

Genetic Markers: CNS is a rare kidney disorder caused by genetic defects in the components of the glomerular filtration barrier, especially nephrin and podocin (Jalanko, 2009).

Clinical/History	Lab Work	
Height	Alb, transthyretin	Ceruloplasmin (decreased)
Weight	Proteinuria, uremia	AST (increased)
Weight gains?	CRP	Na^+
aBWef	LDL Chol and Trig (increased)	K^+ (hypokalemia?)
Edema	H & H	Serum phosphorus
BMI	Serum Fe	Hypovitaminosis D?
Diet history	TIBC, percent saturation	Ca^{++}, Mg^{++}
BP	Serum ferritin	BUN, Creat
I & O	Transferrin (increased)	GFR, CrCl
Foamy urine		
Chest pains		
Weakness		
Renal biopsy		
Renal radiographs		

INTERVENTION

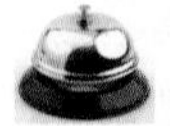

OBJECTIVES

- Treat the underlying condition and take appropriate medications.

SAMPLE NUTRITION CARE PROCESS STEPS

Inadequate Protein Intake

Assessment Data: Dietary recall and laboratory analysis.

Nutrition Diagnosis (PES): NI-5.7.1 Inadequate protein intake, of only 40 g/d, and worsening proteinuria as evidenced by urinary losses of more than 20% of the usual status.

Intervention: Education on protein requirements and sources. Counseling about ways to increase protein without exceeding the recommended level.

Monitoring and Evaluation: Lab values and dietary intake.

- Prevent thrombotic episodes and manage infectious complications (Jalanko, 2009).
- Ensure efficient utilization of fed proteins, spared by use of adequate calories. Prevent muscle catabolism. Rarely, if protein losses are severe, albumin infusion is used.
- Correct anorexia and prevent malnutrition.
- Reduce edema, control sodium intake, prevent or control renal failure.
- Manage hyperlipidemia and elevated triglycerides.
- Monitor for potassium deficits with certain diuretics.
- Replace any other nutrients, especially those at risk (e.g., calcium, vitamin D).

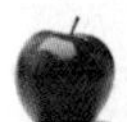

FOOD AND NUTRITION

- Use a diet of modest protein restriction (0.8 g/kg in adults, with 50% of high biological value). Children should be given the RDA for their age because high protein levels may worsen proteinuria and will not improve serum albumin levels.
- Diet should provide 35–40 kcal/kg/d. CHO intake should be high to spare protein for lean body mass; use high–complex CHO and high-fiber foods.
- With dyslipidemia, limit saturated fats and cholesterol; decrease intake of concentrated sugars and alcohol. Encourage use of linoleic acid and omega-3 fatty acids. A vegetarian, soy-based diet with amino acid replacements may be beneficial.
- If patient has edema, restrict sodium intake to 2–3 g. The DASH diet may be useful.
- Provide adequate sources of potassium, vitamin D, and calcium. Replace zinc, vitamin C, folacin, and other nutrients. Monitor the need for iron but do not use excesses, especially with infections.
- Fluid restrictions may be necessary if edema is refractory to diuretic therapy.
- Offer appetizing meals to increase intake. If required, use tube feedings (specialty renal products if needed). Nocturnal feedings can help children with growth.

Common Drugs Used and Potential Side Effects

- ACE inhibitors such as benazepril (Lotensin), captopril (Capoten), and enalapril (Vasotec) are used to lower blood pressure; they may help prevent protein from leaking into urine and damaging the kidneys. Angiotensin II receptor blockers losartan (Cozaar) and valsartan (Diovan) may also be prescribed.
- Antibiotics may be needed when infection is present. Evaluate effects of diet accordingly on drug effectiveness.
- Blood thinners such as warfarin (Coumadin) are prescribed if blood clots are a risk.
- Cholesterol-lowering drugs are often prescribed. If statins such as atorvastatin (Lipitor), fluvastatin (Lescol), lovastatin (Altoprev, Mevacor), pravastatin (Pravachol), rosuvastatin (Crestor), and simvastatin (Zocor) are used, CoQ10 may be depleted.
- Diuretics are used to excrete excess fluid. Thiazide diuretics such as furosemide (Lasix) will deplete potassium; others may spare or retain potassium (e.g., spironolactone). Monitor closely.
- Immune system–suppressing medications, such as corticosteroids, are used to decrease renal inflammation. With prednisone, sodium restrictions may be needed and losses of potassium, nitrogen, or calcium may result. Muscle wasting, weight gain, and other side effects are common. Cyclophosphamide has fewer side effects (du Boef-Vereijken et al, 2005).

Herbs, Botanicals, and Supplements

- Herbs and botanical supplements should not be used without discussing with the physician.
- With cyclosporine, avoid echinacea and St. John's wort because of their counterproductive effects on the drug.
- The use of soy to slow down the progression of diabetic nephropathy and proteinuria warrants further study.

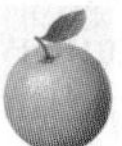

NUTRITION EDUCATION, COUNSELING, CARE MANAGEMENT

- Help patient plan appetizing meals. Sodium restriction is common.
- If patient has abdominal edema, careful positioning may increase comfort at mealtimes.
- Weight management plans will be needed if steroid use will be long-term.
- Nephrotic syndrome can increase the risk of infections and blood clots; medical follow-up is needed.
- In steroid-dependent nephrotic syndrome (SDNS), doses of prednisone lower than 0.75 mg/kg/d do not seem to stunt growth in children (Simmonds et al, 2010).

Patient Education—Food Safety

Foodborne illness can occur when there is contamination of food at any point during the preparation process. Because renal patients are at high risk for foodborne illness, follow the four-step guidelines established by the U.S. Department of Agriculture: clean, separate, cook, and chill. More details are available at the Kidney Foundation Web site at http://www.kidney.org/atoz/content/foodsafety.cfm.

For More Information

- Mayo Clinic
  http://www.mayoclinic.com/health/nephrotic-syndrome/DS01047
- NephCure Foundation
  http://www.nephcure.org/
- University of North Carolina Kidney Center
  http://www.unckidneycenter.org/kidneyhealthlibrary/nephroticsyndrome.html

NEPHROTIC SYNDROME—CITED REFERENCES

du Boef-Vereijken PW, et al. Idiopathic membranous nephropathy: outline and rationale of a treatment strategy. *Am J Kidney Dis.* 46:1012, 2005.

Jalanko H. Congenital nephrotic syndrome. *Pediatr Nephrol.* 24:2121, 2009.

Simmonds J, et al. Long-term steroid treatment and growth: a study in steroid-dependent nephrotic syndrome. *Arch Dis Child.* 95:146, 2010.

RENAL METABOLIC DISORDERS: HYPOPHOSPHATEMIC RICKETS AND HARTNUP DISORDER

NUTRITIONAL ACUITY RANKING: LEVEL 3–4

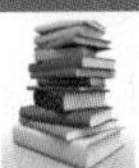

DEFINITIONS AND BACKGROUND

X-linked hypophosphatemic rickets (XLH) associated with decreased renal tubular reabsorption of phosphorous. A defect in the skeletal response to PTH contributes to HPT in XLH (Levine et al, 2009). Incidence is 1 in 20,000 births. XLH is characterized by low to normal serum levels of 1,25-dihydroxyvitamin D_3, normocalcemia, and hypophosphatemia. There is abnormal regulation of production and/or degradation of PTH. Because vitamin D is metabolized abnormally, skeletal and dental structures are affected. Hypophosphatemia is responsible for the clinical manifestations, which vary with the age of the patient and the severity of wasting (Laroche and Boyer, 2005). In poorly growing patients, growth hormone therapy improves final height, phosphate retention, and radial bone mineral density.

Hartnup disorder is an autosomal recessive abnormality of renal and GI neutral amino acids, especially tryptophan and histidine. It is a rare familial condition characterized by hyperaminoaciduria. A red, scaly, photosensitive pellagra-like skin rash is seen on the face, neck, hands, and legs. Cerebellar changes occur, including delirium. Without the absorption of tryptophan, conversions into serotonin, melatonin and niacin are inefficient. Because niacin is a precursor to nicotinamide, part of NAD+, those metabolic functions are also altered. The failure to resorb amino acids in this disorder is compensated by a protein-rich diet (Broer et al, 2005). Bone deformities, pain, and small stature can occur even in children with good compliance, requiring surgical correction and bone lengthening (Fucentese et al, 2008).

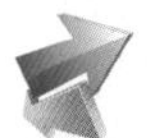

ASSESSMENT, MONITORING, AND EVALUATION

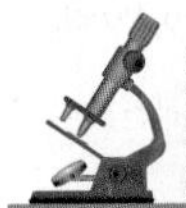

CLINICAL INDICATORS

Genetic Markers: XLH consists of a genetic alteration in the handling of phosphate in the proximal tubule. It is inherited as a sex-linked dominant trait with mutations of the metalloproteinase PHEX on chromosome Xp22.1; FGF23, DMP1, and ENPP1 may also be involved. Hartnup disorder is an autosomal recessive disorder with alterations in the neutral amino acid transporter B(0)AT1 (SLC6A19) on chromosome 5, the major luminal, sodium-dependent neutral amino acid transporter. Its expression in the kidney depends on collectrin (Tmem27), a protein related to ACE2, which maintains blood pressure and glomerular structure (Camargo et al, 2009).

Clinical/History

- Birth weight
- Present weight
- Length
- Growth percentile
- BMI
- Diet history
- BP
- For XLH:
  - Bowing of lower limbs
  - Bone pain
  - Seizures
  - Short stature, delayed growth
  - Skeletal radiograph
- For Hartnup disorder:
  - Red, scaly rash
  - Abnormal muscle tone
  - Cerebral ataxia

Lab Work

- Usual Chemistry panels plus those listed
- For XLH:
  - Serum phosphorus (low)
  - Serum vitamin D
  - Ca^{++} (normal)
  - Alk Phos (elevated with high bone turnover)
  - PTH
  - Hyper-phosphaturia (rickets)
  - BUN, Creat (normal)
- For Hartnup disorder:
  - Tryptophan-loading test

INTERVENTION

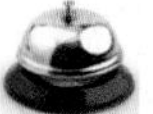

OBJECTIVES

- **XLH:** Correct malabsorption of phosphorus to establish homeostasis with adequate bone and skeletal mineralization. Avoid overly aggressive therapy to avoid hypercalcemia and secondary extraskeletal calcification.

SAMPLE NUTRITION CARE PROCESS STEPS

Abnormal Nutritional Labs

Assessment Data: Child with low rate of growth, percentile for height and weight at 15th percentile. Genetic testing is positive for XLH. Serum phosphate levels very low; calcium is normal, alk phos level elevated.

Nutrition Diagnosis (PES): Abnormal nutritional labs related to new diagnosis of genetic condition (vitamin D-resistant rickets, XLH) as evidenced by very low serum phosphate level with high alk phos and normal calcium levels and genetic test results.

Interventions:

Food-Nutrient Delivery: Maintain a balanced intake of calcium, phosphorus, and vitamin D-rich foods.

Education: Discuss the genetics of this disorder and how diet alone will not correct it.

Counseling: Counsel about the importance of taking all prescribed medications as ordered and not taking over-the-counter vitamins and minerals without first discussing with the doctor.

Coordination of Care: Discuss with the medical team any implications for diet. Support the importance of taking prescribed phosphate and vitamin D exactly as ordered.

Monitoring and Evaluation: Improved serum phosphate. Eventual improvement in growth, which may require growth hormone replacement.

- **Hartnup disorder:** Correct skin changes and behavioral side effects of this pellagra-like condition. Ensure adequacy of protein. Support measures such as psychiatric treatment as needed.

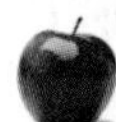

FOOD AND NUTRITION

- **XLH:** Diet should provide adequate amounts of calcium. Monitor to avoid mineral toxicities.
- **Hartnup disorder:** A high-protein diet with supplements will be needed.

Common Drugs Used and Potential Side Effects

- In **XLH,** ergocalciferol is a vitamin D analog that is used with phosphate supplements. Organic phosphate should be given every 4 hours along with supportive vitamin D therapy. After growth is completed, the drug is often reduced. If growth hormone therapy is used, monitor for undesirable side effects.
- **Hartnup disorder:** Patients are given oral nicotinamide therapy (40–200 mg/d) and oral neomycin. Psychiatric medications, such as antidepressants or mood stabilizers, may be needed.

Herbs, Botanicals, and Supplements

- Herbs and botanical supplements should not be used without discussing with the physician.

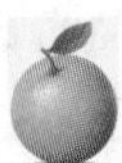

NUTRITION EDUCATION, COUNSELING, CARE MANAGEMENT

- Explain measures that are appropriate to the specific condition. Encourage regular medical visits and nutritionist follow-up.
- Patients with **XLH** will need counseling about desired intake of phosphorus and vitamin D to ensure adequate growth and development.
- Patients with **Hartnup disorder** should use sunscreen and avoid sun exposure as much as necessary. They will need counseling about high-protein diets.

Patient Education—Food Safety

Foodborne illness tips are available at the Kidney Foundation Web site at http://www.kidney.org/atoz/content/foodsafety.cfm.

For More Information

- Hartnup Disorder
  http://www.nlm.nih.gov/medlineplus/ency/article/001201.htm
- Merck Manual—Vitamin D-Resistant Rickets
  http://www.merck.com/mmhe/print/sec11/ch146/ch146g.html
- Office of Rare Diseases
  http://rarediseases.info.nih.gov/
- Vitamin D-Resistant Rickets
  http://www.xlhnetwork.org/site/Diagnosis.html

RENAL METABOLIC DISORDERS—CITED REFERENCES

Broer S, et al. Neutral amino acid transport in epithelial cells and its malfunction in Hartnup disorder. *Biochem Soc Trans.* 33:233, 2005.

Camargo SM, et al. Tissue-specific amino acid transporter partners ACE2 and collectrin differentially interact with hartnup mutations. *Gastroenterology.* 136:872, 2009.

Fucentese SF, et al. Metabolic and orthopedic management of X-linked vitamin D-resistant hypophosphatemic rickets. *J Child Orthop.* 2:285, 2008.

Laroche M, Boyer JF. Phosphate diabetes, tubular phosphate reabsorption and phosphatonins. *Joint Bone Spine.* 72:376, 2005.

Levine BS, et al. The journey from vitamin D-resistant rickets to the regulation of renal phosphate transport. *Clin J Am Soc Nephrol.* 4:1866, 2009.

POLYCYSTIC KIDNEY DISEASE

NUTRITIONAL ACUITY RANKING: LEVEL 2

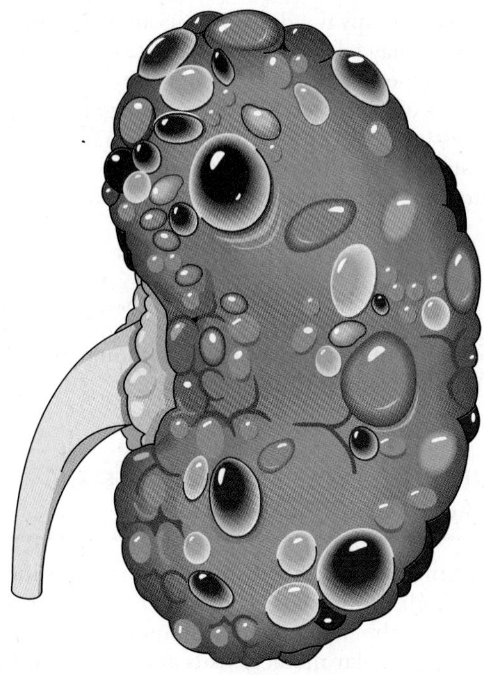

LifeART Super Anatomy Collection 9, CD-ROM. Baltimore: Lippincott Williams & Wilkins.

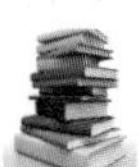

DEFINITIONS AND BACKGROUND

PKDs are disorders that cause multiple, fluid-filled, bilateral cysts in the kidneys and may also affect the liver, pancreas, colon, blood, and heart valves. Fluid-filled sacs or cysts of varying sizes that become larger as the disease progresses replace normal kidney tissue. Intracellular calcium signaling is important in kidney development, and defects in this signaling pathway cause the cyst formation. PKD results from loss of function of either of two proteins, polycystin-1 or polycystin-2. Increased understanding of genetic and pathophysiologic mechanisms has laid the foundation for development of more effective therapies.

PKD in its **autosomal dominant form (ADPKD)** affects 600,000 adults in the United States, at a rate of 1 in 400–1000 persons. ADPKD is one of the most common human genetic disorders. The antidiuretic hormone, arginine vasopressin (AVP), operates continuously in ADPKD patients to stimulate the formation of cyclic adenosine monophosphate (cAMP), thereby contributing to cyst and kidney enlargement and renal dysfunction (Torres et al, 2009). Patients with ADPKD remain clinically asymptomatic for decades while significant anatomic and physiologic systemic changes take place (Rizk and Chapman, 2008). Symptoms most often appear between 30 and 40 years of age. There is a close correlation between the extent of hypertension, left ventricular hypertrophy, deterioration of GFR, and progressive enlargement of the cystic kidneys in adult ADPKD (Schrier, 2009).

The rare **autosomal recessive form (ARPKD)** occurs in 1 per 44,000 births. ARPKD is the neonatal form of PKD and is associated with enlarged kidneys and biliary dysgenesis (Harris and Torres, 2009). Infants who are not treated may die before 1 month of age. Most infants with autosomal recessive PKD have unusual facial features (Potter face) and failure to thrive. Children with ARPKD experience high blood pressure, UTIs, and frequent urination. Their disease affects the liver, spleen, and pancreas, resulting in low blood cell counts, varicose veins, and hemorrhoids. Because kidney function is crucial for early physical development, children with autosomal recessive PKD are usually smaller than average size. Rare, syndromic forms of ARPKD cause defects of the eye, central nervous system, digits, or neural tube (Harris and Torres, 2009).

Treatment of PKD involves efforts to identify patients at greatest risk for disease progression, thus targeting therapy to retard disease progression and renal functional deterioration. The effect of renin–angiotensin–aldosterone system inhibition on renal volume and kidney function is being studied in the Halt Progression of Polycystic Kidney Disease (HALT PKD) trial (Schrier, 2009). Laparoscopic surgery to remove the cysts may be beneficial for some patients. Half of patients with PKD will require dialysis (Barash et al, 2010). For others, transplantation is needed.

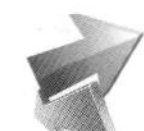

ASSESSMENT, MONITORING, AND EVALUATION

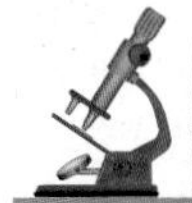

CLINICAL INDICATORS

Genetic Markers: ADPKD is the most common life-threatening hereditary disorder (Belibi and Edelstein, 2010); it is caused by mutations in the *PKD1* gene in 85% of cases and the *PKD2* gene in the rest of the cases.

ARPKD is caused by mutation in *PKHD1*; the ARPKD protein, fibrocystin, is localized to cilia/basal body and complexes with polycystin-2 (Harris and Torres, 2009).

Clinical/History

- Length or height
- Birth weight
- Present weight
- Growth percentile
- BMI
- Diet history
- BP (abnormally high)
- Vomiting
- Chronic headaches
- UTIs
- Hematuria
- Liver or pancreatic cysts
- Abnormal heart valves
- Kidney stones
- Brain aneurysms
- Diverticulosis, hemorrhoids
- Back or side pain
- Ultrasound

Lab Work

- Proteinuria, microalbuminuria
- Serum AVP
- BUN, Creat
- H & H
- Serum Fe, ferritin
- Na^+, K^+
- Chol, Trig
- Gluc
- Serum vitamin D
- Alb, transthyretin
- CRP
- Ca^{++}, Mg^{++}
- Serum phosphorus

SAMPLE NUTRITION CARE PROCESS STEPS

Excessive Mineral Intake

Assessment Data: I & O records, nursing flow sheets. Adult 50-year-old male with ADPKD. Blood pressure very high, 190/90 mm Hg on three separate measurements. Diet hx indicates use of bacon every breakfast, luncheon meats and cheese for midday meal, and canned soups for dinner at least four times weekly.

Nutrition Diagnosis (PES): NI-5.10.7 Excessive mineral (sodium) intake related to intake of high sodium foods as evidenced by BP 200/90 mm Hg and diet hx of high sodium food choices consumed every day.

Interventions:

Food-Nutrient Delivery: Suggest alternatives for meal planning that are lower in sodium. Discuss appropriate fluid intake as well.

Education: Educate the patient and his family members about the importance of lowering blood pressure by using medications and a lower sodium diet.

Counseling: Work with family members to plan menus that are easy to prepare for daily meals; discuss tips for restaurant and shopping choices.

Coordination of Care: If high fluid intake is recommended, work with the medical team accordingly.

Monitoring and Evaluation: Blood pressure gradually down to 120/80 mm Hg. Sodium intake within 2–3 g guideline on a daily basis.

INTERVENTION

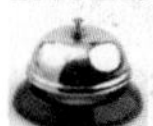

OBJECTIVES

- Prevent renal failure; manage CKD.
- Minimize or alleviate nausea, vomiting, and anorexia.
- Bring hypertension under control where present. The goal BP is 120/80 mm Hg.
- Control AVP secretion.
- Correct or alleviate proteinuria or microalbuminuria.
- Manage dialysis when and if needed. Prepare for transplantation if planned.

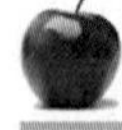

FOOD AND NUTRITION

- Modify diet according to symptoms; sodium restriction may be beneficial for lowering blood pressure. The DASH diet may be beneficial.
- Meet protein dietary allowance for age unless proteinuria is excessive, in which case lower levels are needed.
- Fluid intake should be tailored to the individual. Water loading, by suppressing AVP-stimulated cAMP production, is a proposed therapy for ADPKD; more trials are needed (Barash et al, 2010; Torres et al, 2009).
- Use more antioxidant-rich, anti-inflammatory foods, such as berries, apples, soy, flax oil, fish including salmon, and fish oils.

Common Drugs Used and Potential Side Effects

- ACE inhibitors are most frequently prescribed for hypertension (Jafar et al, 2005). Calcium channel blockers, diuretics, and beta-blockers may also be used. A common combined therapy is a diuretic plus an ACE inhibitor.
- Antibiotics may be used to treat infections; monitor specific medicines for nutritional side effects.
- Analgesics may be useful for pain management.
- Vasopressin V2 receptor antagonists, mTOR inhibitors, and statins that reduce cyst formation and improve renal function are being tested (Belibi and Edelstein, 2010).

Herbs, Botanicals, and Supplements

- Herbs and botanical supplements should not be used without discussing with the physician.

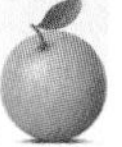

NUTRITION EDUCATION, COUNSELING, CARE MANAGEMENT

- Explain measures that are appropriate to specific condition. If high fluid intake is desirable, discuss goals and options with the patient and/or family.
- Encourage regular medical visits and nutritionist follow-up.

Patient Education—Food Safety

- Renal patients are at high risk for foodborne illness. Follow the four-step guidelines established by the U.S. Department of Agriculture: clean, separate, cook, and chill.
- Details are available at the Kidney Foundation Web site at http://www.kidney.org/atoz/content/foodsafety.cfm.

For More Information

- National Kidney and Urologic Diseases Information Clearinghouse http://kidney.niddk.nih.gov/kudiseases/pubs/polycystic/index.htm
- Polycystic Kidney Disease Foundation http://www.pkdcure.org

POLYCYSTIC KIDNEY DISEASE—CITED REFERENCES

Barash I, et al. A pilot clinical study to evaluate changes in urine osmolality and urine cAMP in response to acute and chronic water loading in autosomal dominant polycystic kidney disease. *Clin J Am Soc Nephrol.* 5:693, 2010.

Belibi FA, Edelstein CL. Novel targets for the treatment of autosomal dominant polycystic kidney disease. *Expert Opin Investig Drugs.* 19:315, 2010.

Harris PC, Torres VE. Polycystic kidney disease. *Annu Rev Med.* 60:321, 2009.

Jafar TH, et al. The effect of angiotensin-converting-enzyme inhibitors on progression of advanced polycystic kidney disease. *Kidney Int.* 67:265, 2005.

Rizk D, Chapman A. Treatment of autosomal dominant polycystic kidney disease (ADPKD): the new horizon for children with ADPKD. *Pediatr Nephrol.* 231029, 2008.

Schrier RW. Renal volume, renin-angiotensin-aldosterone system, hypertension, and left ventricular hypertrophy in patients with autosomal dominant polycystic kidney disease. *J Am Soc Nephrol.* 20:1888, 2009.

Torres VE, et al. A case for water in the treatment of polycystic kidney disease. *Clin J Am Soc Nephrol.* 4:1140, 2009.

RENAL TRANSPLANTATION

NUTRITIONAL ACUITY RANKING: LEVEL 4

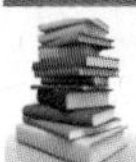

DEFINITIONS AND BACKGROUND

Renal transplantation may be completed in ESRD when GFR drops to 10 mL/min. Persons with poor health or history of cancer often cannot receive a transplantation. Patient and graft survival rates, as well as long-term quality of life, have improved dramatically, a result of advances in surgical techniques, immunosuppression, and perioperative care. Laparoscopic living-donor nephrectomy has improved the possibility of live renal donations. In addition, pediatric kidney transplants are an option for children with ESRD. A child must reach a certain body surface area or weight (such as 20 kg) to receive a parent's kidney; siblings younger than 18 years are generally not allowed to donate a kidney.

Malnutrition prior to transplantation is associated with an increased risk of infection, delayed wound healing, and muscle weakness. Delaying surgery for nutrition therapy (enteral and parenteral) is indicated only if severe malnutrition is present. Preoperative nutrition therapy should be conducted prior to hospital admission to lower the risk of nosocomial infections (Weimann et al, 2009).

An adequate nutritional status may improve outcomes after transplantation. In addition, a weight loss program may be needed prior to surgery if the patient is obese. Orlistat (alli® or Xenical®) and a structured low-fat, low-calorie diet and exercise program may be beneficial (MacLaughlin et al, 2010).

After a renal transplantation, the patient has a functioning donor kidney. High doses of glucocorticoid drugs are given to prevent rejection. Elimination of donor-specific anti–human leukocyte antigen antibodies during antibody-mediated rejection (AMR) is important; proteasome inhibitor–based therapy has been shown to effectively treat refractory AMR (Walsh et al, 2010).

The acute posttransplantation phase lasts up to 2 months; the chronic phase starts after 2 months. Complications of corticosteroid use include new-onset diabetes, osteoporosis, and hyperlipidemia. In the long term, cardiovascular morbidity remains the greatest risk (Roberts et al, 2006), followed by cancer and infections. Complications are listed in Table 16-14.

Early intensive dietary advice and follow-up helps control complications after renal transplantation. Prognosis is good for transplant patients who take care of themselves and attend to medical follow-up.

TABLE 16-14 Complications After Renal Transplantation

Complication	Description
Anemia	Posttransplantation anemia is a prevalent and undertreated condition.
Cancer	Lymphomas may occur. Malignancies are rapidly becoming a major cause of mortality.
Cardiovascular complications	Hyperlipidemia is one of the consequences of long-term use of corticosteroids. Elevated triglycerides and metabolic syndrome can also persist. Renal transplantation recipients are at high risk for ischemic heart disease or heart failure and will benefit from lifestyle modifications.
Diabetes	Patients are at risk for posttransplantation diabetes because of the use of corticosteroids. Higher BMI, elevated fasting blood glucose levels, and high blood pressure should be managed carefully.
Infection	Acute meningitis or Guillain–Barré syndrome triggered by *Campylobacter jejuni* infection are examples of infections in this population.
Neurological complications	Neurotoxic immunosuppressive medications may cause mild symptoms, such as tremors and paresthesia.
Osteoporosis	Bone density declines after long-term use of corticosteroids. Tertiary hyperparathyroidism may occur after kidney transplantation.
Pulmonary complications	Infectious pulmonary complications may occur. Noninfectious pulmonary complications arise because of the toxicity of posttransplantation medications.
Stroke	Stroke may occur in a small number of renal transplant recipients.
Weight gain or obesity	Obesity decreases effectiveness of insulin receptors, increasing the tendency for glucose intolerance. It may also delay wound healing.

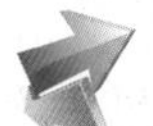

ASSESSMENT, MONITORING, AND EVALUATION

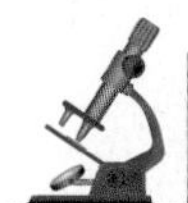

CLINICAL INDICATORS

Genetic Markers: Renal transplantation may be needed for some of the inherited disorders, such as PKD.

Clinical/History

Height
Present weight
aBWef
Edema
BMI
Weight changes
Diet history
I & O
BP
Temperature
DEXA scan

Lab Work

CRP
Alb
Ca^{++}, Mg^{++}
Phosphorus
Na^+, K^+
H & H
Serum Fe
BUN, Creat
GFR
WBC
Total lymphocyte count (TLC)
Gluc
tHcy levels
Lipid profile (LDL goal <100 mg/dL)
Trig
N balance
GFR, CrCl
Serum phosphorus
AST, ALT
Bilirubin
PTH

SAMPLE NUTRITION CARE PROCESS STEPS

Obesity

Assessment Data: Female patient 6 months posttransplant with weight gain of 30#; BMI now 32. Diet history indicates patient is eating small meals every 2–3 hours, consuming 300–400 kcal in excess of goal intake of 1700 kcal/d. Glucose and lipid levels slightly elevated over past reports.

Nutrition Diagnosis (PES): Obesity related to excess oral food and beverage intake as evidenced by weight gain of 30# since transplant 6 months ago and current BMI 32.

Interventions:

Education: Reduce overall energy intake to the goal range of 1700 kcal/d. Suggest lower calorie alternatives for food choices and preparation methods.

Counseling: Develop menu plans together to support goal achievement.

Coordination of Care: Discuss plans with medical team to support the patient goals during monthly clinic visits. Patient will see RD again in 3 months.

Monitoring and Evaluation: Improved weight status; loss of 10# in 3 months. Patient expresses satisfaction with meeting weight loss goal thus far. Lab values within normal limits for glucose and lipids.

INTERVENTION

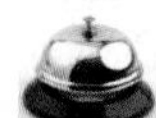

OBJECTIVES

- Promote healing and prevent infections, especially during acute phase.
- Prevent or control AMR.
- Support immunity and prevent new infections.
- Food intake is recommended within 24 hours postsurgery. Modify diet according to drug therapy to enhance outcome.
- Initiate immediate postoperative EN or PN in patients who did not receive oral intake for more than 7 days perioperatively or whose oral food intake is less than 60–80% for more than 14 days (Weimann et al, 2009).
- Prevent abnormalities in calcium or phosphorus metabolism with HPT.
- Monitor for abnormal electrolyte levels (sodium, potassium). Control blood pressure carefully to prevent cardiac problems.
- Maintain good blood pressure control and near-normal fasting blood glucose levels and HbA1c levels. Manage CHO intake, but provide enough energy to spare protein for healing.
- Manage fluid intake according to intake and output. Most patients can return to a normal or increased fluid intake after transplantation.
- Help patient adjust to a lifelong medical regimen during chronic phase. Improve survival rate by supporting immune response.
- Correct or manage complications that occur, such as posttransplantation anemia.
- Minimize long-term weight gain.

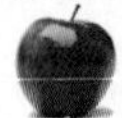

FOOD AND NUTRITION

- Progress to solids as quickly as possibly postoperatively. Monitor fluid status and adjust as needed.
- Energy should be calculated as 30–35 kcal/kg. Needs may increase with postoperative complications.
- Daily intake of protein should be 1.3–2.0 g/kg in the acute phase and 0.8–1.0 g/kg in the chronic phase. Soy proteins can be used in most cases and may help lower LDL cholesterol level.
- Control CHO intake; 50% of total calories is usual. Limit concentrated sweets and encourage the use of complex CHO.
- Encourage monounsaturated fats, omega-3 fatty acids, and the Mediterranean diet. Use more fish and fish oils and olive oil.
- Fluid is not restricted unless there are problems with graft functioning.
- Daily intake of sodium should be 2–4 g until drug regimen is reduced. Careful management of sodium efficiently controls blood pressure in patients who are hypertensive (Keven et al, 2006).
- Adjust potassium levels as needed (2–4 g if hyperkalemic).
- Daily intake of calcium should be 1200–1500 mg. Children especially will need adequate calcium for growth.
- Supplement diet with vitamin D, magnesium, phosphorus, and thiamine if needed. If homocysteine-lowering multivitamin therapy is needed; folic acid and vitamins B_6 and B_{12} are needed.
- Reduce gastric irritants as necessary, if GI distress or reflux occurs.
- Encourage exercise and a weight control plan for the long-term recovery phase.

Common Drugs Used and Potential Side Effects

- See Table 16-15 for a description of immunosuppressive drugs that are used.
- Calcium or vitamin D supplements may be needed to correct osteopenia.
- Most adult renal transplantation recipients develop dyslipidemia within 1 month of the initiation of immunosuppressive therapy. Statins and diet therapy are required.
- Chronic allograft nephropathy remains a cause of graft attrition over time (Afzali et al, 2005). Switching to tacrolimus due to cyclosporine-related side effects improves disease-specific quality-of-life indicators within a short time (Franke et al, 2006).

Herbs, Botanicals, and Supplements

- Herbs and botanical supplements should not be used without discussing with the physician.

TABLE 16-15 Immunosuppressant Drugs Used After Renal Transplantation

Drugs may be either *induction agents*, powerful drugs at the time of transplant, or *maintenance agents* used for long-term antirejection. Most patients are on a combination of the drugs listed below. Many transplant centers use tacrolimus, mycophenolate mofetil, and prednisone.

Medication	Comments
Antiproliferative agents: (mycophenolate mofetil, mycophenolate sodium, azathioprine)	These drugs lower the number of T cells and may cause leukopenia, thrombocytopenia, oral and esophageal sores, macrocytic anemia, pancreatitis, vomiting, diarrhea, and other complex side effects. Folate supplementation, liquid or soft diet, and use of oral supplements may be needed.
Belatacept	This is an investigational biologic agent, injected following renal transplantation to prevent rejection, maintain kidney function, and sustain lower blood pressure. "Posttransplant lymphoproliferative disorder"—a type of lymphoma associated with organ-transplant patients is one risk.
Corticosteroids (prednisone, Solu-Cortef)	Used for immunosuppression. Side effects include increased catabolism of proteins, negative nitrogen balance, hyperphagia, ulcers, decreased glucose tolerance, sodium retention, fluid retention, and bone thinning/osteoporosis. Cushing syndrome, obesity, muscle wasting, and increased gastric secretion may result. A higher protein intake and controlled carbohydrate intake are needed.
Calcineurin inhibitors: Cyclosporine (Sandimmune, Neoral, Gengraf)	Cyclosporine does not retain sodium as much as corticosteroids. Nausea, vomiting, and diarrhea are common side effects. Hyperlipidemia, hypertension, and hyperkalemia, hyperglycemia, hyperlipidemia, hair growth, gum enlargement, or tremors may occur. The drug is also nephrotoxic; a controlled renal diet may be beneficial.
Calcineurin inhibitor: Tacrolimus (Prograf, FK506)	Being 100 times more potent than cyclosporine, smaller doses are required to suppress T-cell immunity. Side effects include gastrointestinal distress, nausea, vomiting, hyperkalemia, headaches, hair loss, tremors, and hyperglycemia.
Monoclonal antibodies (mAbs) (basiliximab, daclizumab)	Less nephrotoxic than cyclosporine but can cause nausea, anorexia, diarrhea, fever, stomatitis, and vomiting. Monitor carefully. Anti-CD25 mAbs (basiliximab and daclizumab) are well tolerated. Anti-CD52 (Campath-1 H), anti-CD20 (rituximab), anti-LFA-1, anti-ICAM-1, and anti-tumor necrosis factor-α (infliximab) show potential.
Proteasome inhibitors (bortezomib, rituximab)	Proteasome inhibitor–based therapy may reduce early graft rejection (Walsh et al, 2010).
mTOR inhibitor (sirolimus)	Side effects may include rash, bone marrow problems (anemia, low white blood cell count and low platelet count), swelling of ankles, and frothy urine because of protein leakage from urine.

REFERENCE

Walsh RC, et al. Proteasome inhibitor-based primary therapy for antibody-mediated renal allograft rejection. *Transplantation*. 89:277, 2010.

- With cyclosporine, avoid use with echinacea and St. John's wort because of counterproductive effects on the drug.

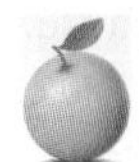

NUTRITION EDUCATION, COUNSELING, CARE MANAGEMENT

- Share, as appropriate, details of the DASH diet and Mediterranean diet. Discuss food sources of protein, calcium, magnesium, potassium, and sodium.
- Increase intakes of fiber-rich foods as a primary preventive approach against metabolic syndrome and cardiovascular disease, which are very prevalent after renal transplant (Noori et al, 2010).
- Avoid smoking and keep alcohol intake to a minimum.
- Rigorous efforts should be made to optimize weight before and after solid-organ transplantation by a judicious combination of diet, exercise, minimization of steroid therapy, surgery, and psychological therapies. Encourage moderation in diet; promote adequate exercise.
- Discuss the importance of bone health and how diet affects prevention of osteoporosis. If patient does not drink milk, describe other sources of calcium.
- Patients should learn how to apply self-management and when to seek medical attention. UTIs are the most common infection after renal transplantation.

Patient Education—Food Safety

- Foodborne illness can occur when there is contamination of food at any point during the preparation process. Follow the four-step guidelines established by the U.S. Department of Agriculture: clean, separate, cook, and chill.
- Details are available at the Kidney Foundation Web site at http://www.kidney.org/atoz/content/foodsafety.cfm.

For More Information

- MEDLINE—Renal Transplantation
  http://www.nlm.nih.gov/medlineplus/ency/article/003005.htm
- NKF—Transplantation
  http://www.kidney.org/atoz/atozTopic_Transplantation.cfm
- Nephrology Channel
  http://www.nephrologychannel.com/rrt/transplant.shtml
- Transplant Experience
  http://www.transplantexperience.com/kidney.php
- University of Maryland Transplant Center
  http://www.umm.edu/transplant/kidney/index.html

RENAL TRANSPLANTATION—CITED REFERENCES

Afzali B, et al. What we CAN do about chronic allograft nephropathy: role of immunosuppressive modulations. *Kidney Int.* 68:2429, 2005.

Franke GH, et al. Switching from cyclosporine to tacrolimus leads to improved disease-specific quality of life in patients after kidney transplantation. *Transplant Proc.* 38:1293, 2006.

Keven K, et al. The impact of daily sodium intake on posttransplant hypertension in kidney allograft recipients. *Transplant Proc.* 38:1323, 2006.

MacLaughlin HL, et al. Nonrandomized trial of weight loss with orlistat, nutrition education, diet, and exercise in obese patients with CKD: 2-year follow-up. *Am J Kidney Dis.* 55:69, 2010.

Noori N, et al. Dietary intakes of fiber and magnesium and incidence of metabolic syndrome in first year after renal transplantation. *J Ren Nutr.* 20:101, 2010.

Roberts MA, et al. Cardiovascular biomarkers in CKD: pathophysiology and implications for clinical management of cardiac disease. *Am J Kidney Dis.* 48:341, 2006.

Walsh RC, et al. Proteasome inhibitor-based primary therapy for antibody-mediated renal allograft rejection. *Transplantation.* 89:277, 2010.

Weimann A, et al. Surgery and transplantation—guidelines on parenteral nutrition, chapter 18. *Ger Med Sci.* 7:Doc10, 2009.

URINARY TRACT INFECTIONS

NUTRITIONAL ACUITY RANKING: LEVEL 1 (3 IF CHRONIC)

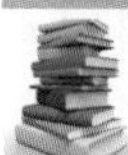

DEFINITIONS AND BACKGROUND

UTIs are associated with significant morbidity (Nanda and Juthani-Mehta, 2009). Single UTI episodes are very common, especially in adult women where there is a 50-fold predominance compared with adult men (Guay, 2009).

Acute pyelonephritis affects the renal parenchyma and is the most common cause of UTIs. *E. coli* most often cause upper UTIs; other organisms are found in complicated infections associated with diabetes mellitus (e.g., *Candida* spp), urinary stones, or immunosuppression. With effective antibacterial therapy, the immune response by both T and B lymphocytes supports antibodies that can eradicate the infectious agent.

There are approximately 250,000 cases of acute pyelonephritis each year. When the patient is septic, hospitalization and treatment with parenteral antibiotics may be needed. Indications for inpatient treatment include complicated infections, sepsis, persistent vomiting, failed outpatient treatment, or extremes of age (Ramakrishnan and Scheid, 2005). If patient does not improve rapidly, ultrasound and computed tomography are used to diagnose obstruction, abscess, or emphysematous pyelonephritis. Emphysematous pyelonephritis is a life-threatening infection especially seen in patients with poorly controlled diabetes mellitus. Mortality is high in that population, especially in the elderly. Most complications are treated percutaneously with broad-spectrum antibiotics and fluid resuscitation, followed by surgical therapy if needed.

In acute pyelonephritis in pregnancy, changes in innate immunity are present. Low maternal plasma concentrations of adiponectin are found in these cases; adiponectin has profound anti-inflammatory properties (Mazaki-Tovi et al, 2010). Further study is needed to identify measures that can be taken to enhance immunity during pregnancy.

Chronic pyelonephritis results from treatment failure and may be caused by resistant organisms, underlying anatomic/functional abnormalities, or immunosuppressed states (Ramakrishnan and Scheid, 2005). Fibrosis, scarring, and dilatation of the tubules impair renal function. Scarring from chronic pyelonephritis leads to loss of renal tissue and function, even progressing to ESRD. Hypertension is often present in this population.

Cystitis affects the lower urinary tract. **Interstitial cystitis (IC)** is a painful bladder syndrome with an inflamed bladder wall, pelvic discomfort, and urinary frequency and urgency. Omission of alcohol, caffeine, citrus beverages, and tomatoes gives relief to some individuals.

Cranberry inhibits the adhesion of uropathogens through anthocyanidin/proanthocyanidin as potent antiadhesion compounds (Guay, 2009). It may decrease the number of symptomatic UTIs over a 12-month period, particularly for women, but it is not clear whether juice, tablets, or capsules are the most effective source (Jepson and Craig, 208). GI intolerance, weight gain from excessive calorie load, and drug–cranberry interactions due to the inhibitory effect of flavonoids on cytochrome P450–mediated drug metabolism may occur (Guay, 2009).

Urinary incontinence requires attention, even if there are no UTIs. Check for vitamin B_{12} deficiency, decrease caffeine intake, and try bladder training (use of toilet every 2 hours). Maintain adequate fluid intake to prevent the onset of any UTIs. Women may need guidance on pelvic floor exercises to strengthen those muscles after childbirth or menopause.

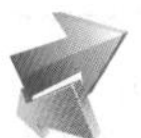

ASSESSMENT, MONITORING, AND EVALUATION

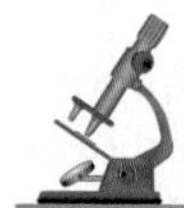

CLINICAL INDICATORS

Genetic Markers: UTIs are not genetic, but many inherited conditions can aggravate them. Elevated procalcitonin is a biomarker that differentiates lower UTI from pyelonephritis in the pediatric age group (Nanda and Juthani-Mehta, 2009).

Clinical/History		
Height	Edema	BP (increased?)
Weight	Diet history	Intravenous pyelogram
BMI	Temperature	
	I & O	

Lab Work		
Urine culture	Transferrin	Na^+, K^+
Procalcitonin (elevated?)	H & H	Urinary Na^+
Alb, transthyretin	Serum Fe, ferritin	Gluc
CRP	Ca^{++}, Mg^{++}	RBP
	Serum phosphorus	BUN, Creat

INTERVENTION

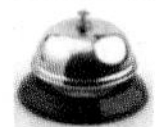

OBJECTIVES

- Preserve kidney function.
- Control blood pressure.
- Acidify urine to decrease additional bacterial growth. Prevent bacteremia.
- Force fluids unless contraindicated.

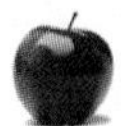

FOOD AND NUTRITION

- Restrict protein intake only if renal function is decreased. Otherwise, use sufficient amounts of high biological–value proteins, including foods such as meat, fish, poultry, eggs, and cheese.

SAMPLE NUTRITION CARE PROCESS STEPS

Inadequate Oral Food-Beverage Intake

Assessment Data: I & O records, nursing flow sheets for hospitalized elderly patient, coming from long-term care facility with UTI and temperature of 102°F. Diet Hx reveals poor intake for 3 days related to fever and anorexia. Signs of dehydration.

Nutrition Diagnosis (PES): NI-2.1 Inadequate oral food and beverage intake related to UTI with fever and resulting anorexia as evidenced by temperature of 102°F and I & O records showing very low intake for 3 days.

Interventions:

Food-Nutrient Delivery: Add extra fluids to trays and encourage 4 oz intake with all medications 3 times daily; goal is 30–35 mL/kg daily. Offer preferred foods; enhance with extra calories as needed (such as extra gravy with potatoes, extra margarine on bread). Include yogurt and cranberry juice if tolerated.

Education: Discuss the need to increase intake of fluids and nutrient-dense foods to support immunity, fight the infection, and reduce fever.

Counseling: Discuss food choices and ways to enhance total intake without being overwhelmed by large quantities of food.

Coordination of Care: Support the antibiotic therapy by providing high-quality food choices.

Monitoring and Evaluation: Temperature back to normal; resolution of UTI. Improved food and nutrient intake. Able to be discharged from hospital with guidance on how to prevent further dehydration and UTIs.

- Cranberries, plums, and prunes produce hippuric acid, which acidifies urine. Corn, lentils, breads/starches, peanuts, and walnuts also acidify the urine.
- Although vitamin C is not necessarily effective in lowering the UpH, sufficient levels of intake are needed to stimulate the anti-infective process.
- Avoid an excess of caffeine because of its diuretic effect. Stimulants such as caffeine rapidly leave the bladder, a vulnerable site where additional infections may begin.
- Vitamin A may be low; encourage improved intake, especially from beta-carotene–rich foods.
- Non-antimicrobial-based approaches undergoing investigation include probiotics, vaccines, oligosaccharide inhibitors of bacterial adherence and colonization, and bacterial interference with immunoreactive extracts of *E. coli* (Guay, 2009). Offer probiotic choices, such as yogurt or kefir, to replenish good intestinal bacteria.

Common Drugs Used and Potential Side Effects

- Outpatient oral antibiotic therapy with a fluoroquinolone is successful in most patients with mild uncomplicated pyelonephritis (Ramakrishnan and Scheid, 2005).
- Ceftriaxone and gentamicin are cost-effective because only once-daily dosing is needed. With urinary anti-infectives, sufficient water and fluids should be ingested. Be careful with forced water diuresis, which impairs antibiotic effectiveness. Monitor responses to glucose changes in people with diabetes. Avoid use with alcohol.
- Liposome treatments are under study for interstitial cystitis. The interstitial cystitis-related liposomes coat the bladder and may reduce inflammation there.
- Nitrofurantoin (Furadantin, Macrodantin) should be consumed with food, milk, and a diet adequate in protein. Nausea, vomiting, and anorexia are common; diarrhea is rare.
- Penicillin products such as amoxicillin (Amoxil, Trimox, Wymox) and ampicillin may be used. With penicillin allergy, vancomycin may be used.
- Quinolones include ofloxacin (Floxin), norfloxacin (Noroxin), ciprofloxacin (Cipro), and trovafloxacin (Trovan). If Cipro (ciprofloxacin) is used, avoid taking with calcium supplements, milk, and yogurt; limit use of caffeine and monitor for nausea. If a fluoroquinolone (Floxin, Maxaquin) is used, nausea is a side effect. Take separately from vitamin supplements.
- Sulfisoxazole (Gantrisin) can deplete folacin and vitamin K. Nausea and vomiting may also occur.
- Trimethoprim (Trimpex) and trimethoprim/sulfamethoxazole (Bactrim, Septra, Cotrim) may cause diarrhea, GI distress, and stomatitis. Use adequate fluid.

Herbs, Botanicals, and Supplements

- Herbs and botanical supplements should not be used without discussing with the physician.
- Probiotics may be useful to prevent and treat recurrent complicated and uncomplicated UTIs. Blueberry, parsley, bearberry, yogurt, birch, and couch grass have been suggested, but no clinical trials have proven efficacy.

- Cranberry juice may be useful for women but not necessarily for the elderly who require catheterization (Jepson and Craig, 2008). It may be useful also for pregnant women (Wing et al, 2008).

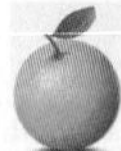

NUTRITION EDUCATION, COUNSELING, CARE MANAGEMENT

- Indicate which foods are palatable as sources of nutrients for dietary restrictions and for nutrients that tend to be low.
- Encourage appropriate fluid intake. Schedule voiding frequency and fluid intake if needed.
- Discuss the use of probiotics to support a healthy immune system, especially after antibiotic use.
- Limit caffeine and oral fluid intake at night, if needed.
- Showers, instead of baths, may be preventive.

Patient Education—Food Safety

Foodborne illness can occur when there is contamination of food at any point during the preparation process. Because renal patients are at high risk for foodborne illness, follow the four-step guidelines established by the U.S. Department of Agriculture: clean, separate, cook, and chill. More details are available at the Kidney Foundation Web site at http://www.kidney.org/atoz/content/foodsafety.cfm.

For More Information

- Interstitial Cystitis Association
  http://www.ichelp.org/
- Mayo Clinic—Pyelonephritis
  http://www.mayoclinic.com/health/kidney-infection/DS00593
- National Bladder Foundation
  http://www.bladder.org/

PYELONEPHRITIS AND URINARY TRACT INFECTIONS—CITED REFERENCES

Guay DR. Cranberry and urinary tract infections. *Drugs.* 69:775, 2009.

Jepson RG, Craig JC. Cranberries for preventing urinary tract infections. *Cochrane Database Syst Rev.* 1:CD001321, 2008.

Mazaki-Tovi S, et al. Low circulating maternal adiponectin in patients with pyelonephritis: adiponectin at the crossroads of pregnancy and infection. *J Perinat Med.* 38:9, 2010.

Nanda N, Juthani-Mehta M. Novel biomarkers for the diagnosis of urinary tract infection-a systematic review. *Biomark Insights.* 4:111, 2009.

Ramakrishnan K, Scheid DC. Diagnosis and management of acute pyelonephritis in adults. *Am Fam Physician.* 71:933, 2005.

Wing D, et al. Daily cranberry juice for the prevention of asymptomatic bacteriuria in pregnancy: a randomized, controlled pilot study. *J Urol.* 180:1367, 2008.

Enteral and Parenteral Nutrition Therapy

CHIEF ASSESSMENT FACTORS

- Availability of Appropriate Lab Work
- Benefits of Nutritional Intervention Outweigh Risks?
- Inadequate Oral Intake (Mechanical, Gastrointestinal, Psychological, or Surgical Reasons)
- Indirect Calorimetry (IC)[a]
- Nitrogen Balance[b]
- Other Planned Procedures and Impact of Delayed Nutrition Therapy
- Presence or Absence of Sepsis (in EN vs. PN)
- Risk for Refeeding Syndrome in Patients with Poor Intake, Maldigestion, and Malabsorption[c]
- Serial Anthropometric Measures
- Signs of Micronutrient Deficiency (selenium, copper, zinc)
- Systemic Inflammatory Response to Injury or Infection or Protein-Energy Undernutrition
- Surgery Affecting Oral Intake, Digestion, or Absorption
- Treatment, Timing, and Condition:
  - Cancer Having Intake or GI Consequences (Radiation, Chemotherapy, Surgery)
  - Cystic Fibrosis
  - Failure to Thrive, Chronic Malnutrition
  - GI Obstruction, Chronic Diarrhea, Crohn's Disease, Short Bowel Syndrome (SBS)
  - GI Disease from HIV Infection or AIDS
  - Organ Transplantation
  - Pancreatic Disease
  - Pulmonary Aspiration, Complications, or Ventilator Use
  - Sepsis, Trauma, Burns, or Other Causes of High Rates of Catabolism

[a]Indirect Calorimetry = measure of gas exchange based on oxygen used and carbon dioxide released, using the formula $RQ = VCO_2/VO_2$)

[b]Nitrogen Balance = net gain or loss of nitrogen per day; helps to determine if patient is in catabolic or anabolic state. 1 g Nitrogen = 6.25-g protein. N balance calculation = 24 hour protein intake (total g)/6.25 minus (24 hour UUN + 4)

Key: 0 balance implies equilibrium. 4–6 g (+) is anabolic/positive balance. Negative (−) implies catabolism. Goals: To maintain status, use 1-g N:200–300 kcal. For anabolism, use 1-g N:150 kcal. Interpretation: renal disease, liver disease, burns, or trauma may skew the results.

[c]Patients at risk for refeeding syndrome may have low serum levels of phosphorus (<3.0 mg/dL), magnesium (<1.3 mg/d/L), and potassium (<3.5 mEq/L) from poor intake. Feeding causes increased demand for these electrolytes so the macronutrients provided can be utilized. The increased metabolic demand causes further drops in these levels

unless they are repleted BEFORE feeding is initiated. Reintroduction of carbohydrate after a period of 24–72 hours of fasting, when blood glucose and insulin levels have both declined, sends out a surge of insulin. This insulin surge pulls glucose and the electrolytes into the cells, leading to hypophosphatemia (<1.0–1.5 mg/dL), hypomagnesemia (<1 mg/dL), and hypokalemia (<2.5 mEq/dL) and life-threatening results, as it has cardiac, pulmonary, hepatic, renal, neuromuscular, metabolic, and hematological consequences (Tresley and Sheean, 2008).

Note: Jensen et al (2009) indicate that the presence or absence of the systemic inflammatory response and whether the inflammation is severe or sustained distinguishes the forms of malnutrition described here. **Sarcopenia** is a smoldering inflammatory state partially driven by cytokines and oxidative stress, cachexia overlapping with failure to thrive. **Cachexia** as a systemic proinflammatory process with associated insulin resistance, increased lipolysis, increased lipid oxidation, increased protein turnover, and loss of body fat and muscle, as in pancreatic cancer or organ failure. **Marasmus** is pure starvation with reduced food intake or assimilation with loss of body cell mass and weight, but no underlying inflammatory condition; visceral proteins are generally preserved and edema is not present. If marasmic individuals subsequently develop inflammatory conditions and edema, the term **marasmic kwashiorkor** is used.

OVERVIEW OF ENTERAL AND PARENTERAL NUTRITION THERAPY

There are about 1000 kcal available as glucose or glycogen in the muscles, liver, and bloodstream, supplying energy for only 18–24 hours. Daily glucose replacement is crucial for brain and red blood cell survival. When oral feeding is not possible or safe, nutrients should be replaced by other means. Specialized nutrition therapy includes both tube (enteral) and IV (parenteral) feeding methods and must be carefully planned and administered.

Nutrition therapy has grown steadily over the past four decades. Table 17-1 lists definitions important in nutrition therapy. Initially, central parenteral nutrition (CPN, formerly total parenteral nutrition or TPN) was the ultimate standard of care. Later, tube feeding (enteral nutrition [EN]) was found to protect gut immunity and function more effectively. A critically ill patient who has been inadequately fed for 10–14 days will manifest characteristics of both the systemic inflammatory response and protein-energy undernutrition, even loss of up to 30% of body cell mass; nutrition modulation of the systemic inflammatory response can occur with early feeding (Jensen et al, 2009). Integrated approaches are required, including anti-inflammatory diets, glycemic control, physical activity and resistance training, appetite stimulants, anabolic agents, anti-inflammatory agents, anti-cytokines, and probiotics (Jensen, 2006). Because there are over 500 types of bacteria living in the human gut, the goal is to keep the healthy ones and reduce those that are detrimental. Temperature, osmolality, pH, and substrate availability can alter the host–bacteria relationship very quickly. Probiotics may help maintain the beneficial flora and reduce

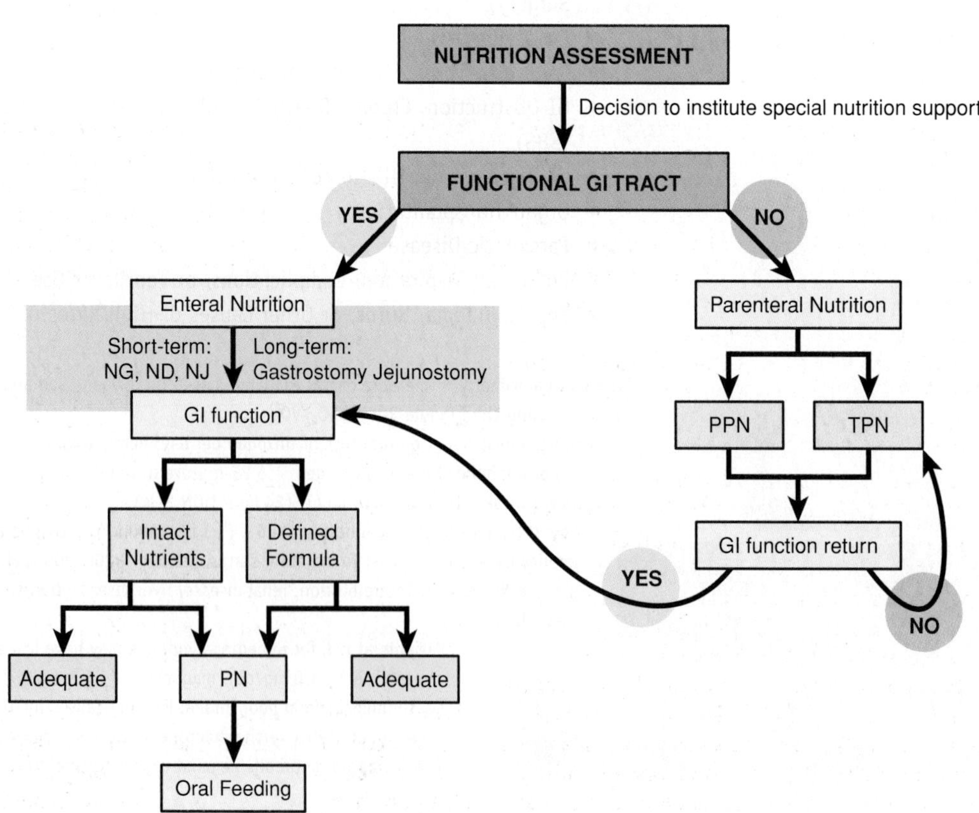

TABLE 17-1 ASPEN Definition of Terms Related to Nutrition Support

Admixture: The result of combining two or more fluids

Closed Enteral System: A closed enteral container prefilled with sterile, liquid formula by the manufacturer, which is considered ready to hang

Compatibility: The ability to combine two or more products such that the physical integrity and stability of each product is not altered when combined

Formulation: A mixture of nutrients suitable for administration to a patient

Hang Time: The length of time a formulation is considered safe for administration to the patient beginning with the time the formulation has been compounded, reconstituted, warmed, decanted, or has had the original package seal broken

Intravenous fat emulsion (IVFE): An IV oil-in-water emulsion of oils, egg phosphatides, and glycerin; the term is used in preference to lipids

Nutrition Support Process: The assessment, diagnosis, ordering, preparation, distribution, administration, and monitoring of nutrition support therapy

Nutrition Support Service (or Team): An interdisciplinary group that may include physicians, nurses, dietitians, pharmacists, and/or other healthcare professionals with expertise in nutrition who manage the provision of nutrition support therapy

Osmolality: The measured osmotic concentration of a liquid expressed in osmoles or milliosmoles per kilogram of solvent (Osmol per kg or mOsmol per kg, respectively). Osmolality indicates the osmotic pressure exerted by a liquid across a semipermeable membrane

Modular Enteral Feeding: Formulation created by combination of separate nutrient sources or by modification of existing formulations

Multichamber Bag: A container designed to promote extended stability of a parenteral nutrition formulation by separating some components (e.g., IV fat emulsion) from the rest of the formulation

Parenteral Nutrition: The IV administration of nutrients

- Central (CPN): Parenteral nutrition delivered into a large-diameter vein, usually the superior vena cava adjacent to the right atrium
- Peripheral (PPN): Parenteral nutrition delivered into a peripheral vein, usually of the hand or forearm

Preparation: A food, drug, or dietary supplement (or mixtures thereof) compounded in a licensed pharmacy or other healthcare-related facility pursuant to the order of a licensed prescriber

Product: A commercially manufactured food, drug, or dietary supplement. Drug products are accompanied by full prescribing information, which is commonly known as the Food Drug Administration-approved manufacturer's labeling or product package insert

Stability: The extent to which a product retains, within specified limits and throughout its period of storage and use (i.e., its shelf life), the same properties and characteristics that it possessed at the time of its manufacture

Standardized Parenteral Nutrition Formulation: A parenteral nutrition formulation intended to meet the daily maintenance requirements of a specific patient population (e.g., age-, stress-, or disease state specific) and differentiated by the route of administration (central vs. peripheral vein)

Total Nutrient Admixture: A parenteral nutrition formulation containing IV fat emulsion as well as the other components of parenteral nutrition (dextrose, amino acids, vitamins, minerals, water, and other additives) in a single container

Vascular Access Device: Catheter placed directly into the arterial or venous system for infusion therapy and/or phlebotomy

Adapted from: ASPEN, http://www.nutritioncare.org/, accessed March 15, 2010,

those that are pathogenic. This can be especially useful in patients with *Clostridium difficile* or vancomycin-resistant enterococci (VRE) colonization and may even prevent ventilator-associated pneumonia. Taking yogurt containing live *Lactobacillus* GG daily as 100 g for at least 1 month may help. More studies are warranted. The American Society for Parenteral and Enteral Nutrition (ASPEN) recently updated their Clinical Guidelines for various ages and facilities (ASPEN, 2009). ASPEN has published a series of related documents that may be referred to when using these guidelines, available at their web site at: http://www.nutritioncare.org/Library.aspx. For pediatrics, where nutrition therapy is needed for many acute or chronic conditions, various guidelines are also available from ASPEN. One of the more recent documents addresses management of the obese, hospitalized pediatric patient (ASPEN, 2010). There are ASPEN guidelines for managing critically ill patients who need nutrition therapy and will be in the ICU for 2–3 days or longer (McClave et al, 2009). Critically ill patients are at high risk for infections, organ dysfunction, and death. Feeding obese, critically ill adults is a bigger challenge; they are at high risk for infectious complications, slow healing postoperative wounds, nosocomial infections, and mortality. Protein stores are mobilized and less protein is synthesized during critical illness. The goal for feeding the critically ill obese patient is to attenuate hypermetabolism, lessen inflammation, and minimize catabolic losses. If the critically ill ICU patient is hemodynamically stable with a functional gastrointestinal (GI) tract, EN is recommended over parenteral nutrition (PN) because it has benefits such as less septic morbidity, fewer infectious complications, and significant cost savings (American Dietetic Association, 2010). Nutrition therapy is not always applied effectively or consistently, despite scientific evidence and protocols. PN must be carefully managed, especially since overfeeding may aggravate sepsis. Generally, if well managed, CPN is an effective alternative to EN in patients who cannot be fed via the GI tract. Payments for PN infusions, EN formulas, and prosthetic devices are managed under the U.S. federal guidelines. Therefore, prudent use of expensive products is expected. Generally, EN is preferred over PN where possible (American Dietetic Association, 2010; McClave et al, 2009). Advances in nutrition therapy and technology have contributed to improved quality of life for many patients in hospitals, long-term care, and home settings. Note that special guidelines should be used in home care, including an evaluation for sanitary preparation, administration, and storage of the products (Kovacevich et al, 2006). Home preparation tips for EN and parenteral (PN) therapies are available from a number

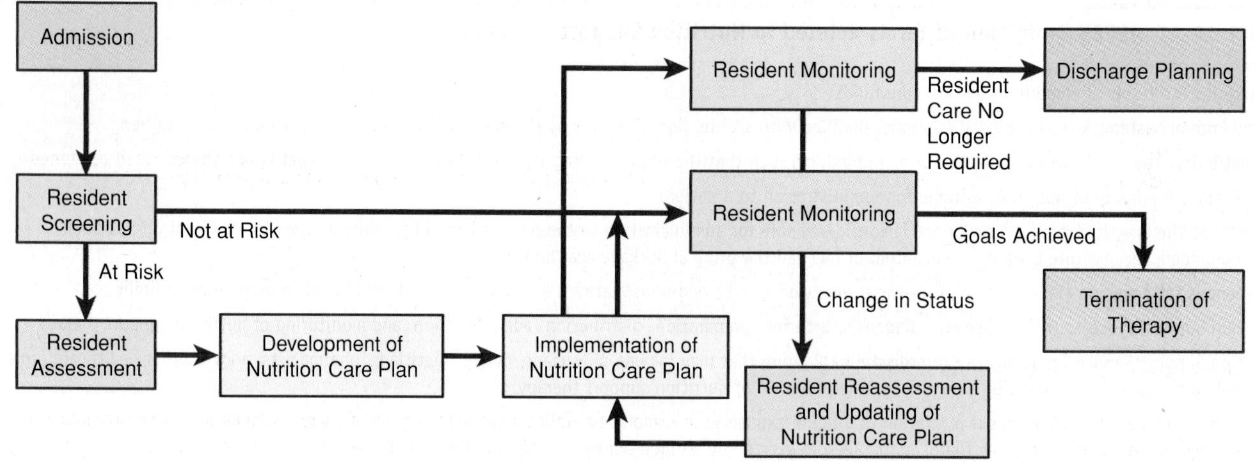

of hospitals, web sites, and formula companies. Selection of patients in long-term care who could receive tube feeding (TF) must include consideration of long-term goals and ethical issues. Because of the potential complications of permanent enteral access, percutaneous gastrostomy (PEG) or jejunostomy (PEJ) should be considered only when anticipated length of use is 1 month or longer (McMahon et al, 2005). When considering initiation of feedings, the treatment goal should be taken into account, whether palliative, curative, or rehabilitative. Additionally, the patient's wishes should be considered above all. In long-term care, the following flow chart is useful in designing protocols.

In a **coma (persistent vegetative state)**, the patient is completely unaware of self and the environment. This is accompanied by normal sleep–wake cycles and hypothalamic/brainstem autonomic functions. Coma may occur as a complication of an underlying illness or as a result of injury. Everyone who is in a coma has the nutrition diagnosis of "inadequate oral food and beverage intake" and requires some form of nutrition therapy to prevent malnutrition. While medically assisted nutrition can maintain life, it is considered futile if it cannot improve the prognosis, comfort, or general status of health of an individual (Andrews and Marian, 2006). Nutrition therapy has not necessarily improved outcomes in end-stage cancer, dementia, or other terminal illnesses. Many healthy elderly persons do not desire to be tube fed, especially with advanced disease or dementia. EN is of questionable benefit for nursing home residents with advanced dementia, yet two thirds of U.S. nursing home residents on EN had their feeding tube inserted during an acute care hospitalization; this practice should be discouraged (Teno et al, 2010). Quality of life must be considered. Some patients have "nutritional distress" if they cannot eat orally (Winkler, 2010). Other individuals receiving long-term EN or home PN have expressed anger, anxiety, or depression resulting from losses of independence and control of body functions and from the altered psychological and emotional aspects of eating (Winkler, 2007). Dietitians must help the patient, family, or guardian in deciding whether to initiate, withhold, or withdraw nutrition therapy (Table 17-2). The social, legal, emotional, and ethical needs and wants must be considered

TABLE 17-2 Ethics of Nutrition Support Therapy and End-of-Life Care

ASPEN Guidelines on Withholding or Withdrawing Nutrition Support
Withholding or withdrawing nutrition support therapy often involves different considerations than other life-sustaining therapies, in part because of emotional, religious, and symbolic meanings
Legally and ethically, nutrition support therapy should be considered a medical therapy
The decision to receive or refuse nutrition support therapy should reflect the autonomy and wishes of the patient. The benefits and burdens of nutrition support therapy, and the interventions required to deliver it, should be considered before offering this therapy
Care providers should be familiar with current evidence of the benefits and burdens of nutrition support therapy
Patients should be encouraged to have living wills and/or advance directives and to discuss with their loved ones their wishes in the event of a serious or terminal accident or disease. This directive should include nutrition support therapy
Competent patients or the legal surrogate of incompetent patients shall be involved in decisions regarding withholding or withdrawing of treatment
Incompetent patients' wishes (as documented in advance directives) shall be considered in making decisions to withhold/withdraw nutrition support therapy.
If there is no family and the patient is not competent, consider a conference with the physician, nursing director, social worker, dietitian to discuss the feeding options
Nutrition support therapy should be modified or discontinued when there are disproportionate burdens or when benefit can no longer be demonstrated
Institutions should develop clear policies regarding the withdrawal or withholding of nutrition support therapy and communicate these policies to patients in accordance with the Patient Self-Determination Act

(continued)

TABLE 17-2 Ethics of Nutrition Support Therapy and End-of-Life Care *(continued)*
Artificial Nutrition at the End of Life
Treat each case individually
When oral feeding is medically appropriate as per swallowing examination, do not artificially feed. Minimize suffering and discomfort; provide comfort foods without dietary restrictions
In dysphagia without complications, recommend as patient usually benefits
In dysphagia with complications, determine if patient will equivocally benefit. Will the benefits outweigh potential risks?
In persistent vegetative state, do not recommend as patients are unable to experience satisfying quality of life
The Dying Process, Palliative Care, Hospice
Dickinson Law School: Starvation is a long, drawn out, and painful process that can take anywhere from 30 to 60 days. Dying patients who stop taking in food and fluids *do not* starve to death. While the body can sustain itself for up to 2 months without food, it can sustain itself no more than about 2 weeks (at most) without fluid intake. Unlike starvation, dehydration is typically not a painful or even an uncomfortable process, especially when good comfort care measures are undertaken. Many patients report less discomfort, and there is less request for pain medication as dehydration runs its course
Patients who stop taking food and fluids drift into a state of unconsciousness. This phase of the process may take 5–8 days if the patient is fully hydrated when food and fluid intake is stopped. Patients will typically die peacefully several days after that. If the patient is already partly dehydrated when fluid intake is stopped, the dying process will be compressed and may only last a couple of days or less
American Academy of Hospice and Palliative Medicine: While most patients with complex medical conditions at the end of life do not experience hunger even with low energy intake, they do experience dry mouth
American Nurses Association: It is not common to hydrate in the presence of symptoms of edema or vomiting
Pediatrics: There is a need for more ethics education and more interdisciplinary discussion of inherently complex and stressful pediatric end of life cases. Appropriate goals of care and use of medically supplied nutrition and hydration are part of this educational process (Solomon et al, 2005).

REFERENCES

American Academy of Hospice and Palliative Medicine. Statement on the use of nutrition and hydration. Web site accessed March 6, 2010, at http://www.aahpm.org/positions/nutrition.html.

American Nurses Association. Position statement on foregoing nutrition and fluid. Web site accessed February 13, 2010, at http://www.nursingworld.org/readroom/position/ethics/etnutr.htm.

ASPEN. American Society for Parenteral and Enteral Nutrition, September 2008. Web site accessed March 5, 2010, at http://www.nutritioncare.org/wcontent.aspx?id=218.

Dickinson Law School. Tube feeding options at the end of life. Web site accessed March 6, 2010, at http://www.dickinson.edu/endoflife/.

Solomon MZ, et al. New and lingering controversies in pediatric end-of-life care. *Pediatrics* 116:872, 2005.

with each individual. Full authorization to write diet, EN, and CPN orders expedites patient-centered care and expands the dietitian's responsibilities beyond traditional dietetic practice (Braga et al, 2006). When dietitians are granted full authority to implement nutritional recommendations, they write orders on the physician's order sheets, change existing orders, and implement new orders immediately. While state licensure boards differ on their defined scopes of practice, several have approved order writing capacity by dietitians.

CITED REFERENCES

American Dietetic Association. Critical illness nutrition evidence analysis project. Evidence Analysis Library, accessed March 11, 2010 at http://www.adaevidencelibrary.com/topic.cfm?cat=1032.

Andrews M, Marian M. Ethical framework for the registered dietitian in decisions regarding withholding/withdrawing medically assisted nutrition and hydration. *J Am Diet Assoc.* 106:206, 2006.

ASPEN. Clinical guidelines for the use of parenteral and enteral nutrition in adult and pediatric patients. *JPEN J Parenter Enteral Nutr.* 33:255, 2009.

ASPEN. Clinical guidelines: nutrition support of hospitalized pediatric patients with obesity. *JPEN J Parenter Enteral Nutr.* 34:13, 2010.

Braga JM, et al. Implementation of dietitian recommendations for enteral nutrition results in improved outcomes. *J Am Diet Assoc.* 106:281, 2006.

Jensen GL. Inflammation as the key interface of the medical and nutrition universes: a provocative examination of the future of clinical nutrition and medicine. *JPEN J Parenter Enteral Nutr.* 30:453, 2006.

Jensen GL, et al. Malnutrition syndromes: a conundrum vs continuum. *JPEN J Parenter Enteral Nutr.* 33:710, 2009.

Kovacevich D, et al. Standards for specialized nutrition support: home care patients. *JPEN J Parenter Enteral Nutr.* 20:582, 2006.

McClave S, et al. Guidelines for the provision of nutrition support therapy in the critically ill patient. *JPEN J Parenter Enteral Nutr.* 33:277, 2009.

McMahon M, et al. Medical and ethical aspects of long-term enteral tube feeding. *Mayo Clin Proc.* 80:1461, 2005.

Teno JM, et al. Hospital characteristics associated with feeding tube placement in nursing home residents with advanced cognitive impairment. *JAMA.* 303:544, 2010.

Tresley J, Sheean P. Refeeding syndrome: recognition is the key to prevention and management. *J Am Diet Assoc.* 108:2105, 2008.

Winkler MF. American Society of Parenteral and Enteral Nutrition Presidential Address: food for thought: it's more than nutrition. *JPEN J Parenter Enteral Nutr.* 31:334, 2007.

Winkler MF. 2009 Lenna Frances Cooper Memorial Lecture: living with enteral and parenteral nutrition: how food and eating contribute to quality of life. *J Am Diet Assoc.* 110:169, 2010.

ENTERAL NUTRITION

NUTRITIONAL ACUITY RANKING: LEVEL 4 IF AT HOME

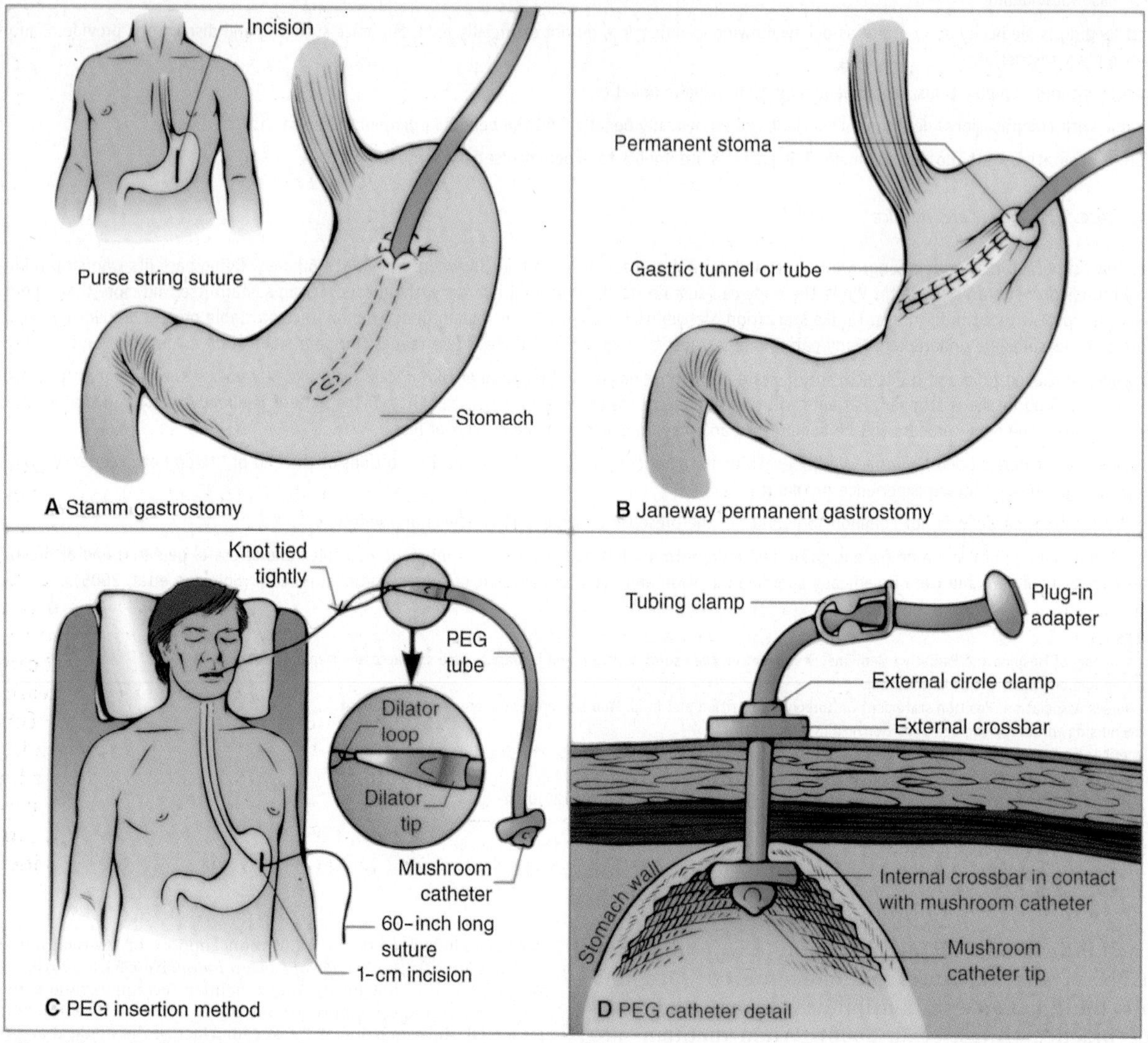

A Stamm gastrostomy

B Janeway permanent gastrostomy

C PEG insertion method

D PEG catheter detail

Adapted from: Smeltzer SC, Bare BG, *Brunner & Suddarth's Textbook of Medical-Surgical Nursing*, 9th ed. Philadelphia, Lippincott Williams & Wilkins, 2000.

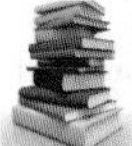

DEFINITIONS AND BACKGROUND

EN makes it possible to provide important substrates for those who cannot or will not meet daily requirements via oral intake but who have an intact digestive system (Chen and Peterson, 2009). EN involves nutrition therapy via nasogastric tube, orogastric tube, gastrostomy, nasoduodenal or nasoenteric feeding, or jejunostomy. PN is reserved for conditions in which EN is contraindicated, unsuccessful, or inadequate. EN is economical, yields effective nutrient utilization, and maintains gut mucosal integrity. Trophic stimulation of the gut occurs with EN but not with PN. Trophic feedings of 10–30 mL/hr may prevent some gut atrophy but will not yield as much benefit as using a more sufficient quantity for the individual. Prevention of intestinal permeability, faster return of cognitive function, and better outcomes have been noted with EN versus PN. EN has also been associated with a reduction in infection rates, hospital-associated infectious complications, ventilator dependency, and intensive care use. Immunoglobulin A (IgA) prevents absorption of enteric antigens; IgA levels increase with EN but not with PN. Immunoenhancement occurs when arginine, glutamine, long-chain polyunsaturated fatty acids (PUFAs), omega-3 fatty acids, vitamins A, C, E, and ribonucleic acids have pharmacological effects. Arginine is an intermediary in the urea cycle, making urea and ornithine via arginase. It is also useful for ammonia detoxification and the synthesis of glutamate and nitric oxide. With infection, the body catabolizes more protein to provide substrate (citrulline) for do novo arginine synthesis. Thus, in stress, trauma, or catabolic states, arginine becomes conditionally essential. Most people consume 5–6 g daily of arginine from dairy, beef, poultry, seafood, soybeans, nuts, seeds, or wheat germ. Enteral formulas vary in content, with an average of 1–2 g/L; enriched formulas may be 12 g/L or higher. Improved wound healing and net nitrogen retention have been noted with arginine supplementation. Glutamine is a primary substrate for the GI tract and lymphocytes; it helps to maintain acid–base balance. Because glutamine is a heat shock protein regulator, pneumonia, sepsis, and bacteremia are less frequent among patients who receive supplemented feedings. Glutamine is useful in attenuating the systemic inflammatory response syndrome (SIRS) response in highly stressed, critically ill patients (such as major elective surgery, trauma, burns, head and neck cancer, or ventilator patients). While its supplementation can decrease infectious complications, routine use is not warranted (American Dietetic Association, 2010).

There are some disadvantages of EN. Judicious use of EN should be considered in low birth weight or premature infants because feeding intolerance is common. Although EN is often started to prevent aspiration pneumonia from oral intake in stroke or demented patients, it may also increase the risk if positioning is poor or if tube placement is wrong. Tube dislodgement or occlusion, infection at the gastrostomy or jejunostomy site, hyperglycemia, azotemia, and fluid and electrolyte imbalances may also occur if not managed carefully. In some patients, maldigestion, malabsorption, abdominal distention, high residuals, nausea, vomiting, constipation, and other signs of GI intolerance are present. Home EN (HEN) for SBS, bowel obstruction, chronic pancreatitis, enterocutaneous fistula, cancer, or severe dysphagia requires careful and regular monitoring from the team.

The traditional assessments using albumin, transthyretin, and anthropometry are not useful in critical care settings. Weight loss prior to admission, disease severity, comorbidities or complications, and GI tract function are more useful. When possible, a nutritionally focused physical examination is needed, including state of hydration, abdominal examination for possible GI intolerance, state of consciousness, general overall appearance, body composition, presence of respiratory distress, nausea, vomiting, abdominal distention, diarrhea, abdominal cramping, constipation, weight changes, hydration status, and abnormal laboratory values. As appropriate, malnourished patients at risk can be fed early without observed negative clinical consequences.

Early EN is beneficial if the patient is hemodynamically stable, depending on where the tube must be placed. Improved clinical outcomes, lower rates of infection, and decreased hospital stays have been observed when EN was initiated within 24 hours and advanced to goal within 48–72 hours. A review of 13 trials with 1173 GI surgical patients found that early commencement of feeding (within 24 hours) reduces risk of postsurgical complications, length of hospital stay, and mortality (Lewis et al, 2009).

Either gastric or small bowel feedings work well; the latter used when aspiration or intolerance is noted. After mechanical ventilator extubation, oral intake is often low and nutrition therapy may be needed (Peterson et al, 2010). When patients are hemodynamically unstable, EN is usually held or combined with PN as needed. Use of an ICU nutrition protocol increases the likelihood of patients receiving the proper nutrition therapy.

Pediatric nutrition therapy protocols are not readily available for critically ill children (Joffe et al, 2009). After intestinal failure with SBS, children are often dependent on PN. However, this dependency can lead to intestinal failure-associated liver disease (IFALD) unless transition to trophic feeds and, eventually, full EN is attempted (Le et al, 2010). Use of omega-3 fatty acids is under study for this population, and more research is needed for pediatric critical care.

Because tube-fed patients in long-term acute-care facilities may be routinely over- or underfed, monitoring how much feeding is actually given to a patient should be done to determine if needs are being met. Both underfeeding and overfeeding affect ventilatory status. Therefore, it is ideal to measure a patient's energy requirements using indirect calorimetry (IC) at least once, especially for the critically ill,

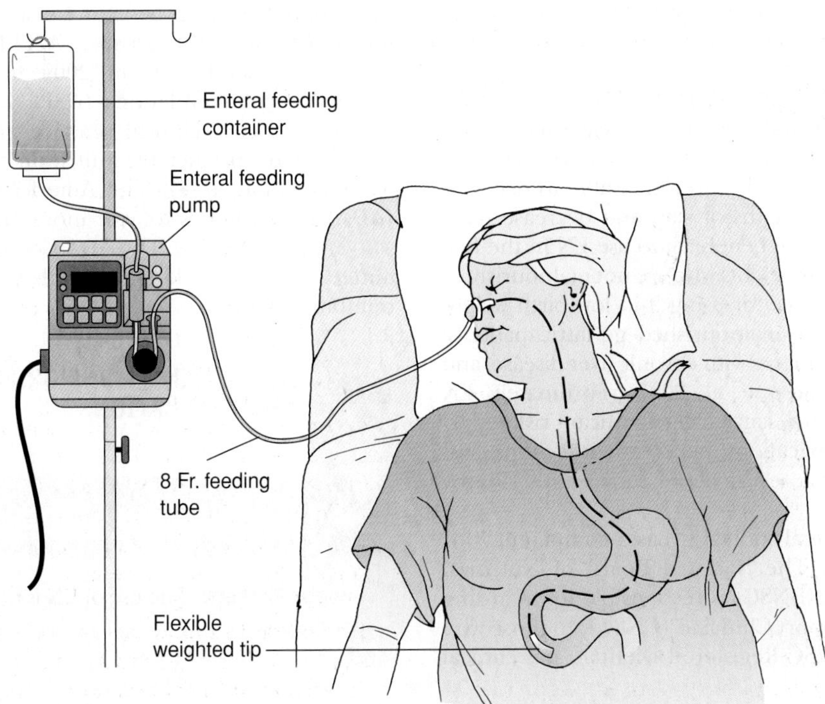

TABLE 17-3 Consequence Statement: Not Feeding a Resident/Patient When Oral Intake Is Inadequate

"The clinical manifestations of protein-energy undernutrition are related to length of time and extent of nutritional deprivation and the prior health status of the person. On the basis of both animal and human studies, there are serious detrimental effects on the function of every organ system, including the **heart, respiratory muscles, and the brain.** When maintained on a prolonged semi-starvation diet, otherwise healthy individuals experience a **loss of heart tissue** that parallels their loss of body mass. Respiratory rate, vital capacity, and minute volume of ventilation also decrease. These **changes in pulmonary function** are thought to result from reduced basal metabolic rate that accompanies starvation. In addition, **liver function declines, kidney filtration rates decline, and nearly every aspect of the immune system is compromised.** Defective ability to fight bacterial and viral infections occurs. Starvation therefore leads to **increased susceptibility to infection, delayed wound healing, reduced rate of drug metabolism, and impairment of both physical and cognitive function.** If starvation is prolonged, complications develop, **leading eventually to death.**"—*Sullivan, D. The role of nutrition in increased morbidity and mortality. Clin Geriatr Med. 11:663, 1995.*

Other documented consequences of not tube feeding a resident/patient who *will not* or *cannot* eat enough orally:

- **Dehydration** with increased risk of urinary tract infections, fever, swollen tongue, sunken eyeballs, decreased urine output, constipation, nausea and vomiting, decreased blood pressure, mental confusion, electrolyte disturbances
- **Decreased awareness** of environment from decreased glucose availability for the brain
- **Development of pressure ulcers** over bony prominences from lack of sufficient protein, calorie, vitamin, and mineral intakes and decreased body fat
- **Decreased ability to participate in activities of daily living** (self-feeding, dressing, bathing, toileting)
- **Low body weight and rapid, involuntary weight loss** that are highly predictive of illness and imminent death. (Note: seniors are especially unable to regain weight after a stress situation)

I, the undersigned, understand and acknowledge that these consequences have been reviewed with me. I am deciding not to tube feed __________________ (resident/patient) and accept the outcome of this decision.

Signed:__________________Date:_______ Witness:____________________________ Date_______

Power of Attorney, Guardian or Other Representative Witness:____________________________ Date_______

obese, or in whom estimation of requirements are difficult (American Dietetic Association, 2010).

For terminally ill individuals, consider the patient's advance directives. When a patient's wishes are not known, TF is viewed as humane by many internists. The ramifications of not feeding a patient should be discussed with all parties (see example form in Table 17-3).

The definition of what constitutes gastric residual volumes as indicators of EN tolerance will vary. Volume of gastric residuals, which prompts holding or cessation of feeding, varies from one facility to the next. One high volume should probably not prompt the clinician to stop TF but to monitor carefully and recheck frequently. Optimal patient positioning, use of prokinetic agents to improve gastric emptying, continuous infusion, and abdominal examinations to evaluate for distention are helpful.

Medical nutrition therapy (MNT) for patients who are tube fed saves thousands of dollars per case each year. Nutrition support teams (NSTs) are associated with improved quality and cost-effective care. Teams are often able to decrease complications, decrease lengths of stay, and decrease readmission rates. While it is not beneficial to use EN in the first week for dysphagic stroke patients who are not malnourished, there is reasonable evidence for using it in low birth weight infants (trophic feeding), malnourished geriatric patients, perioperative patients, patients with chronic liver disease, and critically ill patients (Koretz et al, 2007). Fortunately, EN results in clinically relevant, statistically significant risk reduction for infectious complications, pancreatic infections, and mortality in patients with severe acute pancreatitis (Petrov et al, 2008).

The "CNSC" credential indicates basic competency for managing EN therapy. The National Board of Nutrition Support Certification (NBNSC) is responsible for awarding Certified Nutrition Support Clinician (CNSC), to those who pass the exam. The CNSC Registered Dietitian has clinical expertise in nutrition therapy obtained through education, training, and experience. The CNSC assures optimal therapy for the nutrition diagnosis of "inadequate oral food and beverage intake" from a variety of etiologies. Interventions usually include alternative feeding methods for delivery of nutritional requirements. The CNSC practices in a variety of settings (acute facilities, subacute facilities, ambulatory/outpatient clinics, rehabilitation centers, long-term care facilities, home care, and hospice) and cares for patients of all age groups and types of illness.

Registered dietitians with special training and demonstrated competency in nutrition support therapy are able to evaluate, write, or recommend TF orders. A multidisciplinary approach works best for consideration of all medical, nutritional, and ethical issues. ASPEN published EN Practice Recommendations in 2009 that provide excellent, detailed recommendations (ASPEN, 2009). Standardized forms, protocols, clinical practice guidelines or pathways help provide predictable nutrition therapy outcomes for patients (Table 17-4). The American Dietetic Association (ADA) recommends four or more MNT services for adults who are receiving EN. The ADA Coding and Coverage Committee (CCC) is working diligently to expand coverage and reimbursement.

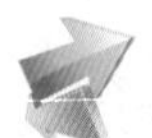

ASSESSMENT, MONITORING, AND EVALUATION

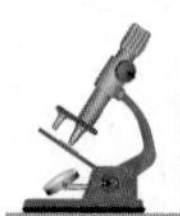

CLINICAL INDICATORS

Genetic Markers: The use of EN is not specific to genetic conditions.

Clinical/History	Lab Work	As Needed:			
Height	Initially and once weekly thereafter:	C-reactive protein (CRP)	Ca^{++}	Chloride	Prothrombin time (PT)
Weight	Glucose (Gluc)	Partial pressure of carbon dioxide (pCO_2)	Hemoglobin and hematocrit (H & H)	Respiratory quotient (RQ) (>1.0, energy delivery is excessive)	International normalized ratio (INR)
Body mass index (BMI)	Na^+ and K^+	Partial pressure of oxygen (pO_2)	Transferrin		
Intake and output (I & O)	Phosphorus	Cholesterol (Chol)			
Blood pressure (BP)	Magnesium	Triglycerides (Trig)			
Diarrhea	Blood urea nitrogen (BUN)				
Temperature	Creatinine (Creat)				
Nausea, vomiting	Albumin (Alb)				
Chest x-ray					
Residuals					

INTERVENTION

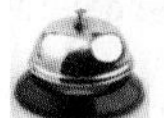

OBJECTIVES

- Prevent or reverse malnutrition, cachexia, impaired immunity, and loss of lean body mass related to inadequate oral food and beverage intake. If the gut works, use

TABLE 17-4 Clinical Practice Guidelines for Nutrition Support

Issue	Considerations or Evidence
EN vs. PN	When considering nutrition support in critically ill patients, strongly recommend that EN be used in preference to PN
Early vs. late EN	Recommend that standard, polymeric enteral formula be initiated within 24–48 hours after admission to an ICU
Formula composition of EN	Standard formula is acceptable for most patients
Positioning of patient for EN	When clinically feasible, patients should be placed in a 30–45° head of bed elevation during gastric feedings to decrease reflux of gastric contents into pharynx and esophagus and possibly to decrease pneumonia
Dose and actual delivery of EN	Actual delivery of threshold intake of approximately 14–18 kcal/kg/d or 60–70% of enteral feeding goal in the first week of ICU admission is associated with improved outcomes (e.g., length of hospital stay, time on ventilator, infectious complications), particularly when initiated within 48 hours of injury or admission
EN in combination with supplemental PN	When initiating EN, strongly recommend that PN not be used in combination with EN
Optimize delivery of EN	Start at the target rate, promotility agents (metoclopramide) or postpyloric feeding should be considered to reduce the gastric residual volume
Minimize risks in EN	Manage rate of advancement, check residuals, use bedside algorithms, consider motility agents, use small bowel vs. gastric feedings when needed, elevate head of the bed, use closed delivery systems, consider use of probiotics, and evaluate bolus administration
Dose of PN and composition of PN	Calculate needs for protein, carbohydrates, IV lipids, additives, vitamins, trace elements, and immune-enhancing substances
Insulin therapy	With elevated glucose levels (as in diabetes, infection, and sepsis), insulin therapy will help to achieve better control
Outcomes	Length of stay (ICU and hospital), quality of life, and specific complications should be considered: EN is associated with decreased infectious complications in comparison to PN
Tube placement	Placement of the tip of the feeding tube in the postpyloric position is associated with decreased gastric residual volume, a factor associated with reduced reflux of formula. Postpyloric feeding tube placement may not be necessary or feasible for all patients but may be useful in patients with large gastric residual volumes
Protocol	An enteral feeding protocol should address the following • When to use enteral vs. parenteral feeding • When to initiate enteral feeding • Positioning of patient • Energy goal per kilogram BW per day • Policy not to use blue dye • Indications for holding feedings • Tube placement • Prokinetic/promotility agents

Adapted from: American Dietetic Association. Critical Illness Nutrition Evidence Analysis Project. Evidence Analysis Library, http://www.adaevidencelibrary.com/topic.cfm?cat=1032, accessed March 11, 2010.

SAMPLE NUTRITION CARE PROCESS STEPS

Swallowing Difficulty

Assessment: 71-year-old male recently discharged from hospital for GI bleeding. Status post-cerebral infarction (CVA) resulting in left hemiparesis, moderate dementia, HTN. Admitted to long-term care unit with PEG tube placed secondary to new-onset dysphagia.

Medical HX: GI hemorrhage, dementia with behavioral disturbances, hx of aspiration, dysphagia.

Current Medications: Aricept, Lasix.

Height: 67 in. Current Weight: 138.1 lb (62 kg). IBW Range: 133–162 lb. IBW: 100%. BMI: 21.6.

Most laboratories are within normal limits (WNL) except for slightly elevated BUN (25) and low albumin (2.8).

Estimated Needs: Energy (25–30 kcal/kg): 1550–1860 kcal; protein (1.0–1.25 g/kg): 62–77 g; fluids (30 mL/kg): 1860 mL.

TF and Flush Order: Enteral formula with 1.5 kcal/mL; 1 can or 240 mL, 5 times a day (6 AM, 10 AM, 2 PM, 6 PM, 10 PM). Bolus feeding via syringe. Flush tube with 50-mL water before and after medications. Flush tube with 100-mL water every shift.

Nutrition Diagnoses: Swallowing difficulty (NC-1.1) related to recent stroke as evidenced by abnormal video swallow study done by speech language pathologist upon admission to long-term care facility.

Increased need for protein (NI-5.1) related to inflammation and depleted visceral protein status as evidenced by a low albumin level of 2.8.

Nutrition Interventions: Administer enteral feeding as ordered (ND-2). Implement nutrition-related medication management (ND-6) of protein additive three times daily (TID).

Goal 1: no significant weight changes; no signs of dehydration.

Goal 2: no episodes of nausea, vomiting, diarrhea, constipation, or aspiration.

Goal 3: albumin level of 3.0 and other laboratories WNL.

Monitoring and Evaluation: Tolerating TF well; currently meeting daily estimated nutrition and hydration needs. Monitor monthly weights. Monitor tolerance to TF order. Monitor albumin and significant laboratories as ordered.

it and check tube placement, laboratories, electrolytes, and fluid boluses to be sure the patient is tolerating the product well.

- Write or edit **nutrition prescription** to provide adequate protein, carbohydrate, fat, vitamins, minerals, and water. Nitrogen needs will increase for burn, pressure ulcer, or trauma patients; the percentage of total kilocalories from protein should be increased in these cases. Aim for 100% of dietary reference intakes (DRIs) for vitamins and minerals; provide explanation if order is excessive or insufficient. Additional liquid vitamins and minerals may be needed if formula volume does not meet micronutrient needs. Alter TF prescriptions as appropriate according to results of the nutritionally focused physical examinations.
- Choose **timing** wisely. If the critically ill patient is adequately fluid resuscitated, EN should be started within 24–48 hours following injury or admission to the ICU (American Dietetic Association, 2010).
- Recommend or select **feeding tube** and **site/location** on the basis of clinical condition, GI anatomy, and anticipated length of treatment. For patients at high risk for aspiration, who will be fed longer than 1 month, try a PEG tube with continuous feeding. If aspiration persists, try a transjejunal tube with lower placement in the GI tract. Gastrostomy buttons have minimal complications, acceptable longevity, and good tolerance in children and adults.
- **Formula selection** includes type of feeding needed by individual, the disorder, viscosity, and kcal/mL. Elemental formulas should be limited to specific conditions in which digestion or absorption is impaired or in which polymeric diets have failed. See Table 17-5 for types of formula selections.
- Monitor patient **positioning.** The head of the bed should be elevated 30–45° during feeding. To decrease the incidence of aspiration pneumonia and reflux of gastric contents into the esophagus and pharynx, patients should be placed in a 45-degree head of bed elevation, if not contraindicated (American Dietetic Association, 2010). For the unconscious patient, turn to the side to help with gastric emptying. For intermittent or bolus feedings, keep patient on his/her right side or keep head of bed elevated for 30 minutes after feeding to prevent aspiration.
- Ensure **adequate free water** is provided (usually 30 mL/kg in young adults with normal renal function). Determine percentage of free water in the formula (usually 70–85%), and subtract this amount from estimated needs; flushes should provide the difference.
- Monitor for **signs of intolerance;** adjust formula type, volume, or concentration as needed:
  - With diabetic gastroparesis, tube feeding may not be well tolerated; insulin adjustments may be required.

TABLE 17-5 Sample Types of Formulas

Formula Type	Macronutrient Content
Blenderized	Whole protein, carbohydrates, and fats from regular foods and liquids blended together
Polymeric—1 kcal/mL	Intact proteins, complex carbohydrates, and mainly LCTs
Added fiber	Varies but usually polymeric
Energy Dense—1.5–2.0 kcal/mL	Varies but usually polymeric
Disease specific	Varies by condition (liver, renal, diabetes, HIV-AIDS)
Peptide based (semi-elemental; oligomeric)	Peptides of varying chain length, simple sugars, glucose polymers or starch and fat, combination of LCT/MCT
Elemental (monomeric)	Individual amino acids, glucose polymers, typically low in fat. Some with only 2–3% of fat as LCT
Immune enhancing	Varies but usually polymeric. Usually has arginine, glutamine, or RNA added
High nitrogen	May be polymeric or monomeric
Critical care	May be polymeric or monomeric

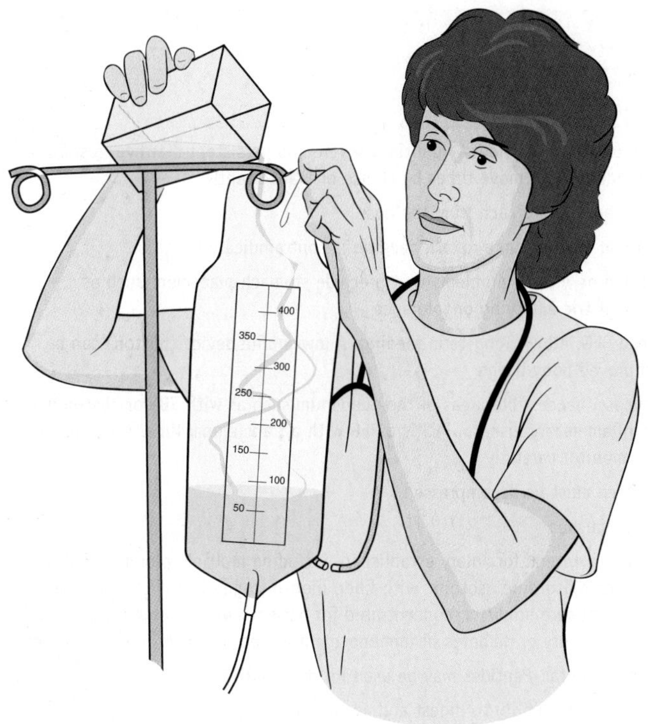

  - Monitor fluid carefully in organ failure where fluid restriction is needed; a more concentrated product can achieve energy and protein goals.
  - Evaluate medications or infection as potential causes of diarrhea or feeding intolerance.
  - Fiber-added formulas may be appropriate with diarrhea or constipation.
  - Optimal oral health, tight glycemic control, minimal use of narcotics, and continuous feedings are recommended for patients at high risk for aspiration.
- Evaluating **gastric residual volume (GRV)** is an optional part of a monitoring plan to assess tolerance; EN should be held when a GRV greater than or equal to 250 mL is documented on two or more consecutive occasions (American Dietetic Association, 2010). Replace aspirate for the electrolytes and gastric juice. Do NOT use blue dye added to the formula to test for aspiration (American Dietetic Association, 2010).
- **Weights** are also important. Patient should be weighed on same scale at regular intervals, wearing similar clothing. Check twice if weights differ significantly from previous weights.

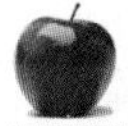

FOOD AND NUTRITION

- Calculate energy requirements and protein, fluid, and nutrient needs according to age, sex, and medical status. See Table 17-6 for considerations.
- For weight loss, 20 kcal/kg is recommended. Use 25 kcal/kg to maintain weight, 30 kcal/kg with mild stress factors, and 35–40 kcal/kg in moderately stressed patients.
- Protein is generally 0.8–1.0 g/kg to maintain status, 1.25 g/kg for mild stress, 1.5 g/kg for moderate stress, and 1.75–2.0 g/kg for severe stress, trauma, or burns. The critically ill may need more calories and protein than other patients.
- Estimate fluid needs at 30–35 mL free H_2O/kg body weight (BW) or 1 mL/kcal.
- Check patient's tolerance and side effects; alter formula content as appropriate. Sample new products to determine costs and convenience for home or institutional use. Numerous EN formulas are currently available, with a large portion of them targeting specific disease conditions (Chen and Peterson, 2009).
- Flush tubing with water (25–100 mL) every 3–6 hours for tube patency and before/after medications are given.
- With a gastrostomy tube, bolus or intermittent feeding is possible. For postpyloric or transpyloric placement, cyclic feedings may be better tolerated than continuous feedings.
- If the patient is in transition back to oral diet or works during the day, night feeding may be used. It may be more energy efficient than continuous feeding over 24 hours.
- Interdisciplinary teamwork is a crucial factor. The following guidelines are useful for managing tube feeding and transitioning from tube to oral feeding. (See figure on page 909)

Common Drugs Used and Potential Side Effects

Drug–nutrient interactions are complex and can cause malabsorption of either the drug or the nutrient in tube feedings. Depending on the physical properties of a drug, it may be absorbed in a limited area of the GI tract or along much of the entire length. Monitor carefully for toxicity. Flush with 5- to 10-mL water after each medication is administered to prevent clogging.

- Antibiotics, H_2-receptor antagonists, and sorbitol elixirs alter gut flora and can cause diarrhea because of their high osmolality.
- Antidiarrheal drugs can be used to slow GI motility. Their use should not preclude a carefully planned fiber intake. Dry mouth is one common side effect.
- Metoclopramide (Reglan) has been used to prevent reflux and aspiration in patients who are tube fed. Administration 10 minutes before tube insertion seems to increase success rate of tube passage. Gastric motility and relaxation of the pyloric sphincter are improved with this drug. However, chronic use may dislodge gastrostomy tubes; monitor closely.
- Phenytoin (Dilantin) administration should be separated from TF by 1–2 hours to prevent decreased medication absorption. TF rate may need to be recalculated, accounting for time TF is held before and after phenytoin administration, and adjusted accordingly.

Herbs, Botanicals, and Supplements

- Herbs and botanical supplements should not be mixed with enteral feedings without discussing with the physician and the pharmacist.
- Gastric feeding supplementation with ginger extract might reduce delayed gastric emptying, but more research is needed.

TABLE 17-6 **Key Enteral Issues**

Issue	Comments
Feeding site selection	Consider any GI impairments or inability to absorb nutrients, vomiting, severe and persistent diarrhea, respiratory disease or skull surgery/fracture, or tendency to remove tubes by choice or inadvertently
Nasogastric	Often used for temporary needs; tube placed into stomach from the nose
Nasoenteric	For patients with impaired gastric emptying or in whom a gastric feeding is contraindicated
Nasojejunal	For patients at risk of pulmonary aspiration or with GI problems that preclude stomach placement such as mechanical problems or problems with gastric emptying or tolerance
Gastrostomy	Surgical incision or endoscopically placed PEG. Allows long-term feeding. A low-profile device (button) can be used for long-term feedings or for improved body image
Jejunostomy	Surgical incision into the jejunum to bypass inaccessible areas of the duodenum such as with SBS or obstructions from cancer, adhesions, stricture, or inflammatory disease. PEJ is a PEG with a transjejunal limb. A jejunostomy tube may cause some bowel necrosis; monitor carefully
Gastrojejunostomy	Good for small bowel feeding when stomach must be decompressed
Contraindications for tube feeding	Severe malabsorption; severe, intractable diarrhea
Formula selection	It is generally more cost effective to have an enteral formulary established, including multiple products, but one main brand of each category (e.g., standard/isotonic, isotonic with fiber, high-nitrogen isotonic, elemental, high-protein/high calorie for stress, critical care products, concentrated for patients with volume intolerance, malabsorption, specialty products for pulmonary or diabetes or immunocompromised, renal, or hepatic patients)
Elemental vs. intact formulas	No superiority has been documented for elemental. Peptides may be used for most patients
Substrates	Carbohydrate, protein, and fat (consider patient's ability to digest and absorb nutrients)
Tolerance factors	Osmolality, calorie, and nutrient densities. In general, more free water is needed with a more concentrated formula
Fluid needs	Generally, 1 mL/kcal is recommended, unless patient needs fluid restriction; 30 mL/kg is most common for adults. Elderly individuals may require slight alterations, depending on organ function. Children must receive adequate fluid, calculated by body weight
Organ failure	Heart failure, renal failure, or liver failure with ascites; 20 mL/kg can also be used initially, progressing to 25 mL/kg as tolerated
Risk for dehydration	Risk of abnormal losses due to GI drainage, diarrhea, and dehydration, and for those with other needs for extra water, 35–40 mL/kg may be used
Delivery methods	Patient tolerance is a key. Goal: meet needs without complications such as nausea, vomiting, diarrhea, or glucosuria
Bolus	Set amount given every 3–4 hours as a rapid syringe feeding; this closely resembles an oral diet for patients who are ambulatory or with long-term and well-established feedings
Continuous	Controlled delivery of feeding over 24 hours. Less nausea and diarrhea are likely. Once stable, most patients may transfer to intermittent
Cycled	Controlled delivery over 8–16 hours, allowing some rest periods for patient during 24 hours. Cyclic is well tolerated by ambulatory patients
Intermittent	Prescribed amount given every 3–4 hours by drip over 20–30 minutes
Complications	Evaluate for metabolic complications. Electrolyte shifts and elevated glucose may occur; an insulin regimen may be needed until hyperglycemia is resolved
Aspiration	Proper positioning greatly reduces risks of pulmonary aspiration
GI side effects	For GI concerns, check for residuals and hold feedings for amounts greater than 150 mL; stop for 4 hours and recheck. For diarrhea, check osmolality of feeding, rate, albumin level, and medications (e.g., sorbitol, magnesium)
Mechanical ventilation	Use enteral nutrition with H_2 antagonists to facilitate gastric emptying
PEG tube problems	Possible complications include pain at the PEG site, leakage of stomach contents around the tube site, dislodgment or malfunction of the tube, aspiration, bleeding, and perforation
Tube clogging	Small-bore tubes are associated with clogging. To prevent or correct mechanical clogging in small-bore tubes, flush regularly with water before and after all medications

See also: ASPEN Guidelines for enteral nutrition at Web site http://www.nutritioncare.org/WorkArea/showcontent.aspx?id=3128.

INTERDISCIPLINARY NUTRITION CARE PLAN
Transitioning from Tube Feeding to Oral Diet

Client Name: ______________________ **#:** ________ **Initiated by:** ________ **Date:** ________

SCREENING
Nutrition Screen diagnosis: Transition From Enteral Tube Feeding to Oral Intake
Signed: ____________ Date: ________

GOALS (Check any/all):

❑ Maintain or improve nutritional status in ____ (goal time).

❑ Increase weight by ____ lb in ____ (goal time).

❑ Successful transition from enteral tube feeding in ____ (goal time).

❑ Maintain or improve hydration status in ____ (goal time).

❑ Increase oral intake to meet nutritional needs in ____ (goal time).

ASSESS *(Check any/all)*
❑ **Oral feeding readiness**
❑ **Dehydration**
❑ **Poor strength**
Weight/BMI
❑ Weight change >3 lb/wk, >5%/mo, or >10%/6mo
❑ BMI <20
❑ BMI <27
Poor Oral Intake Symptoms
❑ Lack of appetite
❑ Complex diet order
❑ Vomiting
❑ Decreased ability to chew/swallow
❑ Nausea
❑ Depression/anxiety

Signed: ____________ Date: ________

None →

MODERATE-RISK INTERVENTIONS
(Check any/all)
❑ **H4 Ways to Improve Nutrition** provided and explained
❑ **Food Record** provided and explained
❑ **Fluid intake discussed and encouraged**
Obtain Dr. orders as needed:
❑ RD chart consult
❑ SLP chart consult
❑ Monitor Weight q:_____
❑ BID/TID supplements
❑ **Other:**____________
(See notes for documention.)

Signed: ____________ Date: ________

↓ Next visit

ASSESS RESPONSE *(Check any/all)*
❑ Further weight loss
❑ Dehydration
❑ Poor strength
❑ Cannot tolerate oral feeding
❑ Exhibiting Poor Oral Intake Symptoms
❑ **Other:**____________
(See notes for documention.)

Signed: ____________ Date: ________

← 1 or more | None →

OUTCOMES ACHIEVED
❑ Oral diet tolerated
❑ Weight gained
❑ Hydration status maintained or improved
❑ Absence of Poor Oral Intake Symptoms
❑ Strength maintained or improved
❑ **Other:**____________
(See notes for documention.)
❑ Repeat Nutrition Risk Screen in ____ days
Signed: ____________ Date: ________

↓ 1 or more

HIGH-RISK INTERVENTIONS *(Check any/all)*
❑ **4 Ways to Improve Nutrition** provided and explained
❑ **Food Record** provided and explained
❑ **Fluid intake stressed**
Obtain Dr. orders as needed:
❑ RD referral for home visit/nutrient analysis
❑ Speech Language Pathologist (SLP) referral for oral feeding readiness/problems
❑ Tube feeding
❑ Monitor weight q:_____
❑ Monitor I & O q:_____
❑ BID/TID supplements
❑ **Other:**____________
(See notes for documention.)

Signed: ____________ Date: ________

↓ Next visit

ASSESS RESPONSE *(Check any/all)*
❑ Further weight loss
❑ Continued dehydration
❑ Continued loss of strength
❑ Cannot tolerate oral feeding
❑ Exhibiting Poor Oral Intake Symptoms
❑ **Other:**____________
(See notes for documention.)
Signed: ____________ Date: ________

None →

OUTCOMES ACHIEVED
❑ Oral diet tolerated
❑ Weight gained
❑ Hydration status maintained or improved
❑ Absence of Poor Oral Intake Symptoms
❑ Strength maintained or improved
❑ **Other:**____________
(See notes for documention.)
❑ Repeat Nutrition Screen in ____ days
Signed: ____________ Date: ________

↓ 1 or more

OUTCOMES NOT ACHIEVED
Reassess/evaluate need for further enteral feeding. Document on Nutrition Variance Tracking form.

Adapted with permission from www.RD411.com, Inc.

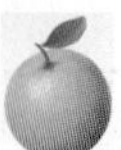

NUTRITION EDUCATION, COUNSELING, CARE MANAGEMENT

- Patient/caretaker should be taught to review signs and symptoms of intolerance, how to manage simple problems, when to call for registered dietitian (RD) guidance versus when to call the physician.
- At least one follow-up phone call or home visit should be made to patients on HEN.
- Patient should be allowed and encouraged to maintain social contacts at mealtime.
- When transitionally weaning young children to an oral diet, oral–motor, sensory, and developmental feeding problems may occur. Check for feeding readiness via oral stimulation and develop a feeding plan.

Patient Education—Formula Safety

- Safe preparation of TF is essential. Homemade feedings are not recommended in most cases.
- Table 17-7 describes a Hazard Analysis Critical Control Points (HACCP) procedure for maintaining a safe enteral feeding system in the hospital setting. Hang time for open-system containers (feeding bags) is 4 hours; hang time for closed-system containers is 24–48 hours.
- Always wash hands carefully and sanitize counter before handling the equipment or preparing the formula. Use a clean tube each time; wash in dishwashing liquid and rinse well between uses.
- Wash feeding bags with water. Do not use soap as it will stick to the inside of the bag and get into the formula and may lead to diarrhea and other unpleasant consequences.
- Temperature standards for refrigeration and storage of enteral feeding product must be met.
- Open cans of formula could be kept in the refrigerator and discarded if not used within 24 hours. Take out and allow to warm up to room temperature 15–20 minutes before a feeding. Feedings should be given at room temperature to minimize risk of cramping or diarrhea. Unopened commercially prepared formulas do not require refrigerated storage.
- Always flush the feeding tube with water after a feeding to prevent dehydration and prevent the food from getting clogged. The RD should always monitor that the feeding

TABLE 17-7 Critical Control Point Checklist for Tube Feedings

Purchasing, Receiving, and Storage

- Enteral feeding product(s) received according to specification
- Temperature standards for refrigeration and dry storage of enteral feedinq product(s) met
- Product usage according to FIFO (first in, first out); those exceeding expiration date returned/discarded
- Liquid protein module and frozen shakes (labeled with date) placed in refrigerator for thawing
- Open cartons discarded after 48 hours
- Unopened and unused thawed liquid protein module discarded after 5 days
- Unopened and unused thawed shakes discarded after 12 days
- Medium-chain triglyceride oil, dry carbohydrate powder, and protein powder stored at room temperature; labeled with date opened. Opened cases and unused bottles/cans discarded after 1 month
- Inventory of reconstituted, mixed enteral formulas and portioned protein, fat, and carbohydrate modules reveals none are past expiration date
- Prepared enteral feedings kept separate from raw or processed food items and cleaning compounds

Preparation and Delivery

- Employees wash hands prior to preparing enteral feedings or modular components
- Cleaned and sanitized surface and equipment used to prepare enteral feedings or modular components
- Enteral formula prepared according to recipe
- Tap water used to reconstitute pediatric powdered formulas and Ceralyte; distilled or sterile water used in the preparation of enteral formulas upon specific order
- Reconstituted mixed enteral formulas and portioned protein, fat, and carbohydrate modules sealed and labeled (formula, rate of administration, patient name and room number, date prepared)
- Temperature standards for refrigerated storage of reconstituted, mixed enteral formulas and portioned protein, fat, and carbohydrate modules met
- Nursing staff washes hands prior to handling feedings and administration systems
- Nursing staff avoids touching any part of the container or administration system that will come in contact with the feeding
- Nursing staff assembles feeding system on a disinfected surface and inspects seals/reservoirs for damage
- Medications are not added to feeding unless necessary. If added, tube is flushed with tap water (or as specified) after administration
- Date/time each component of feeding system; also feeding bag is labeled with patient name and formula
- Hang time of feeding limited to 4 hours
- Feeding bags completely emptied of product prior to pouring newly opened product into the bag
- Disconnected sets are capped
- Container is positioned to prevent reflux of feeding up set
- Feeding tube is irrigated with tap water (or as specified)
- Administration sets changed every 24 hours

Adapted with permission from New York-Presbyterian Hospital/New York Weill Cornell Medical Center.

and flushes provide sufficient water. If the tube clogs, try 100 mL of cola or a small amount of meat tenderizer to rinse.

For More Information

- American Society for Gastrointestinal Endoscopy http://www.askasge.org/pages/brochures/peg.cfm
- Enteral Formula Selection http://www.healthsystem.virginia.edu/internet/digestive-health/nutritionarticles/MaloneArticle.pdf
- Home Enteral Nutrition http://www.mayoclinic.org/gi-jax/enteral.html
- Home Enteral Nutrition Self-Help Guide http://www.copingwell.com/copingwell/HENCopingManual.pdf
- University of Washington TF Guidelines http://healthlinks.washington.edu/nutrition/section5.html

ENTERAL NUTRITION—CITED REFERENCES

American Dietetic Association. Critical Illness Nutrition Evidence Analysis Project. Evidence Analysis Library. Web site accessed March 11, 2010, at http://www.adaevidencelibrary.com/topic.cfm?cat=1032.

ASPEN. Enteral Nutrition Practice Recommendations, 2009. *J Parenteral Enter Nutr.* Web site accessed March 9, 2009, at http://jpen.sagepub.com.

Chen Y, Peterson S. Enteral nutrition formulas: which formula is right for your adult patient? *Nutr Clinical Practice.* 24:344, 2009.

Joffe A, et al. Nutritional support for critically ill children. *Cochrane Database Syst Rev.* 2:CD005144, 2009.

Koretz RL, et al. Does enteral nutrition affect clinical outcome? A systematic review of the randomized trials. *Am J Gastroenterol.* 102:412, 2007.

Le HD, et al. Innovative parenteral and enteral nutrition therapy for intestinal failure. *Semin Pediatr Surg.* 19:27, 2010.

Lewis SJ, et al. Early enteral nutrition within 24 h of intestinal surgery versus later commencement of feeding: a systematic review and meta-analysis. *J Gastro Surg.* 13:569, 2009.

Peterson S, et al. Adequacy of oral intake in critically ill patients 1 week after extubation. *J Am Diet Assoc.* 110:427, 2010.

Petrov MS, et al. Enteral nutrition and the risk of mortality and infectious complications in patients with severe acute pancreatitis: a meta-analysis of randomized trials. *Arch Surg.* 143:1111, 2008.

PARENTERAL NUTRITION

NUTRITIONAL ACUITY RANKING: LEVEL 4 (HOME)

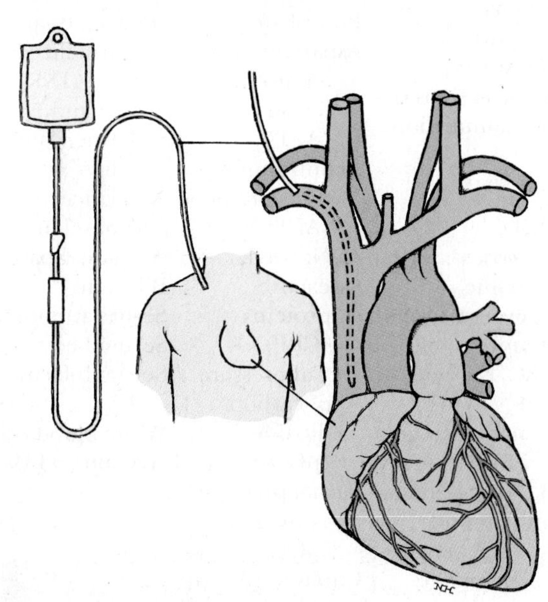

Adapted from: Neil O. Hardy, Westpoint, CT.

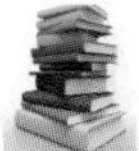

DEFINITIONS AND BACKGROUND

PN refers to IV nutrient admixture administered into the blood with a catheter placed in a vein. PN contains protein, carbohydrate, fat, vitamins, minerals, or other nutrients and is referred to as CPN if it meets the needs of the patient.

CPN can meet estimated nutritional needs, promote nitrogen balance, and improve anabolism. When there is a risk of malnutrition and EN is not tolerated or where there is gut failure, CPN is safe and encouraged. Start CPN only if EN attempts have failed; delay for at least a week unless malnourished before admission to a critical care unit. Short-term CPN is not recommended, especially for 1–2 days. Some medications can be infused into a parenteral solution, such as heparin, insulin, ranitidine; Y-site coinfusion saves time for the nursing staff.

Disadvantages of PN include pneumothorax, infection from the central line, metabolic complications, and the potential for overfeeding. Overfeeding may lead to sepsis. Finally, PN is more expensive than EN and oral diets and does not provide support for healthy gut immunity.

CPN and peripheral PN (PPN) are options for IV feeding. Indications for PPN include temporary losses of GI function (e.g., acute ileus) and occasions when short-term use is indicated such as after minor GI surgery. CPN may be most useful in patients undergoing surgery for esophageal or stomach cancers, in preoperative GI patients who are severely malnourished, and in patients with prolonged GI tract failure. Other indications for adults are listed in Table 17-8.

PN is used judiciously in metastatic cancer or chronic obstructive pulmonary disorder (COPD) because of complications, costs, and decreased quality of life (Ferreira et al, 2005; Joque and Jatoi, 2005). The limited nutritional response of cancer patients to PN reflects the metabolic derangements of cachexia; in nonsurgical, well-nourished oncologic patients, routine PN is not recommended because it offers no advantage and is associated with increased morbidity (Bozzetti et al, 2009). It may sometimes be used in long-term home care to manage radiation enteropathy.

Initiation of PN and metabolic complications are best managed by an expert in nutrition therapy. The skills that distinguish them from other practitioners include competency in fluid and electrolyte monitoring, acid–base monitoring, metabolic monitoring, management of refeeding syndrome, and related areas. Specially trained and certified registered

TABLE 17-8 Candidates for Central Parenteral Nutrition (CPN) in Adults

1. Someone with a nonfunctional or inaccessible gastrointestinal tract
   a. Massive bowel resection or SBS
   b. Radiation enteritis
   c. Ischemic bowel or bowel obstruction
   d. Chronic, severe malabsorption
   e. Inflammatory bowel disease, gastrointestinal obstruction, inflammatory adhesions
   f. Severe diarrhea as in AIDS when enteral feeding is not successful
   g. Enterocutaneous fistula—high-output, proximal fistula
2. Someone who cannot be adequately nourished with an oral diet or enteral nutrition (EN)
   a. After bone marrow transplantation, specifically in cases of graft vs. host disease accompanied by inadequate oral intake
   b. Intractable vomiting such as hyperemesis gravidarum
   c. In pregnancy when oral intake is compromised and when EN is not tolerated, as with SBS
   d. After major surgery when enteral access cannot be established
3. Someone with inadequate oral and enteral intake anticipated to persist for at least 7–14 days
   a. Severely catabolic patients whose gut cannot be used within 3–5 days (such as closed head trauma, fractures, burns)
   b. Cases with a high risk of aspiration
   c. Severe acute necrotizing pancreatitis when EN fails after a trial of 5–7 days
   d. Home parenteral nutrition (HPN) may be suggested for malnourished cancer patients who have a reasonable prognosis and cannot have EN

dietitians may write PN orders if granted clinical privileges by their institution or facility. To determine energy and nutrient requirements accurately, IC and use of programmed calculation software are recommended to prevent administration of excessive glucose and energy. The main consideration when administering fat and carbohydrates in PN is to prevent overfeeding the patient. (Braga et al, 2009).

Perioperative nutritional therapy can minimize negative protein balance by avoiding starvation; maintaining muscle, immune, and cognitive function; and enhancing postoperative recovery. Giving 7–10 days of preoperative PN improves postoperative outcome in patients with severe undernutrition who cannot be adequately orally or enterally fed (Braga et al, 2009).

Adequate nutrition therapy criteria include reaching a nutritional goal within 72 hours after initiation. PN may be given by continuous or cyclic infusion, altered according to patient tolerance. In most cases, gradual transition from PN to EN or oral nutrition is required to prevent periods of inadequate nutrition. The energy deficit accumulated by underfed ICU patients during the first days of stay may play an important role in outcomes for long-staying patients; how to reach calorie requirements by PN without harming the patient is a subject of debate (Singer et al, 2010).

With proper training and monitoring, CPN may be performed safely at home. CPN will drip through a needle or catheter placed into the central vein for 10–12 hours, once a day or five times a week. However, dependence on PN significantly impacts quality of life. Travel, sleep, exercise, and leisure activities are altered by home PN; quality of life issues must be addressed for each individual (Winkler, 2010).

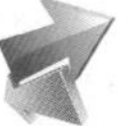

ASSESSMENT, MONITORING, AND EVALUATION

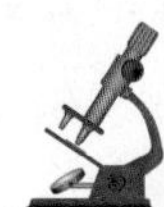

CLINICAL INDICATORS

Genetic Markers: PN is used for a variety of conditions; some of which have a genetic origin.

Clinical/History

Height
Weight (measure daily)
BMI
Resting energy expenditure (REE)
BP
I & O (monitor continuously)
Edema
Skin turgor
Chest x-ray
Physical signs of malnutrition

Lab Work

Daily:
Glucose (Gluc)—every 6 hours until stable
CBC, Na^+ and K^+, Blood urea nitrogen (BUN)—daily for in-patients
Initially and once weekly thereafter:
Creatinine (Creat)
Transthyretin
Triglycerides (if receiving IVFEs)
Urinary Gluc
Twice Weekly at First, Then As Needed:
Albumin (Alb)
Calcium (Ca^{++})
Magnesium (Mg^{++})
Phosphate
Aspartate aminotransferase (AST)
Alanine aminotransferase (ALT)
As Needed:
C-reactive protein (CRP)
Partial pressure of carbon dioxide (pCO_2)
Partial pressure of oxygen (pO_2)
Cholesterol (Chol)
Hemoglobin and hematocrit (H & H)
Transferrin
Chloride
Respiratory quotient (RQ) (>1.0, energy delivery is excessive)
Prothrombin time (PT)
International normalized ratio (INR)
Serum and Urine Osmolality
N balance
Serum selenium
Amylase, lipase
Bilirubin
Serum ammonia
Serum Fe
Serum folacin, B_{12}
White blood cell count, TLC

INTERVENTION

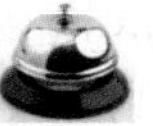

OBJECTIVES

- If early EN is not feasible in first 7 days of hospitalization for a malnourished patient, consider PN to replete lean body mass.
- Assess estimated needs using IC, where possible. Determine appropriate patient requirements for calories, protein, vitamins, minerals, and fluid.

SAMPLE NUTRITION CARE PROCESS STEPS

Inadequate Oral Food and Beverage Intake

Assessment: BMI: 23. Loss of 12# in past year from inflammatory bowel disease and recent intestinal surgery to remove a small segment of the colon. Status 1 week postoperation; not tolerating enteral feedings at this time. Central line placed for CPN feedings. Most laboratories are WNL.

Estimated Needs: Energy (30–35 kcal/kg): 1700–1920 kcal; Protein (1.25 g/kg): 75 g. Fluids (30 mL/kg): 1700 mL. PN Order: Start CPN as directed by RD consultation.

Nutrition Diagnoses: NI-2.1 Inadequate oral food and beverage intake related to inability to eat orally because of IBD, GI distress, intestinal surgery as evidenced by weight loss of 12# in past year and intolerance for enteral feeds.

Nutrition Interventions: Write and administer CPN infusion to meet energy, protein, and fluid requirements without overfeeding.

Goal 1: very gradual increase in weight; no signs of dehydration or refeeding syndrome

Goal 2: no sepsis, fever

Goal 3: laboratories WNL

Monitoring and Evaluation: Tolerating CPN well; currently meeting daily estimated nutrition and hydration needs. Monitor weekly weights, tolerance to CPN order, significant laboratories as ordered.

- Fat and carbohydrate (CHO) make the balance of non-protein calories after protein needs are estimated. When hypertonic dextrose is provided in substantial amounts without protein, mortality is high; CPN should provide balanced macronutrients and micronutrients (Jensen et al, 2009).
- Formulate solutions according to individual needs. For renal patients, review fluid and electrolytes and monitor essential amino acids (EAAs) in the solution. For hepatic patients, evaluate needs for fluid, electrolytes, and specialty amino acid solutions. For pulmonary conditions and diabetes, increased fat content and decreased dextrose may be needed.
- Maintain aseptic technique in all procedures for safe parenteral therapy. IVFEs support rapid growth of microorganisms, and PN solutions containing these fat emulsions should be changed every 12 hours. All PN solutions regardless of IVFE content should be used within 24 hours.
- Avoid substrate shifts. Because glucose abnormalities occur in >90% of patients, monitor plasma glucose often and adjust the insulin dose as needed.
- Avoid suddenly stopping constant concentrated dextrose infusions, which can cause hypoglycemia.
- Prevent refeeding syndrome. The hallmark sign is hypophosphatemia, along with neurologic, pulmonary, cardiac, neuromuscular, and hematologic complications. Dextrose infusion followed by increased insulin release causes shifts in phosphorus, potassium, and magnesium, often within 2–4 days of starting to feed. This sudden shift from fat to carbohydrate metabolism increases the basal metabolic rate and may lead to confusion, coma, convulsions, or death.
- Prevent or correct other complications associated with PN: weight gain over 2 lb or 1 kg daily, indicating syndrome of inappropriate antidiuretic hormone; mouth sores; skin changes; poor night vision; fluid overload; cardiac arrhythmias; metabolic bone disease. Catheter-related sepsis occurs in about 50% of patient cases. Manage liver complications that are common in young children.
- Select patients carefully. The incidence of inappropriate PN prescription is low when multidisciplinary NSTs are closely involved and when written guidelines are used (Kohli-Seth et al, 2009).
- Maintain fluid requirements. Avoid fluid overload that is more common than dehydration.
- Prevent essential fatty acid deficiency (EFAD); need 2–4% linoleic acid (LA) (as from soybean, corn, sunflower, or safflower). Avoid excesses.
- For home PN, support patient goals to continue usual activity, employment, and a pleasant daily life.
- Transition back to EN or oral intake, when and if feasible.

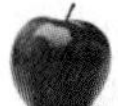

FOOD AND NUTRITION

- Calculate needs for PN related to requirements for energy, protein, fluid, vitamins, and minerals. The commonly used formula of 25 kcal/kg ideal body weight furnishes an approximate estimate of daily energy expenditure and requirements; in severe stress, requirements may approach 30 kcal/kg (Braga et al, 2009). CPN usually provides water (30–40 mL/kg/d), energy (30–60 kcal/kg/d, depending on estimated needs), amino acids (1–2.0 g/kg/d, depending on catabolism), essential fatty acids, vitamins, and minerals.
- Children need energy (up to 120 kcal/kg/d) and amino acids (up to 2.5 or 3.5 g/kg/d). They may also need a different fluid requirement. For neonates, use lower dextrose concentrations (17–18%).
- In older patients, lower glucose tolerance, electrolyte and micronutrient deficiencies, and lower fluid tolerance are common (Sobotka et al, 2009). In heart or renal failure, patients may need a fluid restriction.
- Dextrose monohydrate in CPN yields 3.4 kcal/g, not 4 kcal/g. For unstable blood glucose, use fat at 10–20% of energy intake; avoid overfeeding and consider use of insulin. Maximum rate of glucose infusion should not exceed 5–6 mg/kg/min, the rate of glucose oxidation or utilization.
- Amino acid infusions should not include enhanced arginine in sepsis, whereas it can be beneficial in postsurgical patients. Glutamine deficiency is common in critical illness, inflammatory bowel disease and stress; it is available for IV use but not in the United States. Glutamine infusion should not be used in hepatic encephalopathy. For liver failure or non-dialyzed renal insufficiency, reduce protein content and use a high percentage of EAAs.
- Fat should be given daily as an energy source. A 10% IVFE generally yields 1.1 kcal/mL. IVFE should not exceed 2.5 g/kg in adults or 1 g/kg in septic patients.

- Give 2–4% total kilocalories as LA to prevent EFAD. Avoid excessive use of LA, which is metabolized to the immunosuppressive and proarrhythmic arachidonic acid and to prostaglandins, thromboxanes, and leukotrienes. The omega-3 fatty acids (alpha-linolenic [ALA], docosapentanoic acid [DPA], DHA, EPA, gamma linolenic acid [GLA]) promote vasodilation, enhanced immunity, decreased inflammation and platelet aggregation, and antiarrhythmic effects.
- Medium-chain triglyceride (MCT) oil is made from coconut or palm oils but contains no EFA. In sepsis, transport of long-chain triglycerides (LCT) is impaired; MCT may be useful because no carnitine or lipases are needed.
- Structured lipids that contain a mixture of fish oil (Omegaven) and olive oil (Clinoleic) may provide better tolerance and fewer infections (Hardy and Puzovic, 2009). They are useful for decreasing the time needed for ventilator support in respiratory patients. Fish oil IV lipids are available in Europe and Asia but not necessarily in the United States or Canada. EPA and DHA help to stabilize NFκB in the cytoplasm, which decreases an excessive inflammatory response; they also increase vagal tone that improves GI motility.
- Sample nutrient requirements are listed in Table 17-9. Antioxidants are important; assure sufficient infusion of vitamins. IV vitamin A is only 25–33% available because it attaches to the plastic bags; vitamin E may also be less available. Vitamin E may be given as 1000 IU every 8 hours, sometimes orally. IV vitamin C is often given as 1000 mg every 8 hours; vitamin D is given as ergocalciferol. Vitamin K is part of the multivitamin infusate. Choline is important in metabolic pathways but is not generally given daily.
- Zinc, glutathine (from selenium), beta carotene, lipoic acid, melatonin, and *N*-acetylcysteine are other antioxidants that are important. However, avoid toxic IV mineral levels (e.g., >50 mg/d zinc; >1000 μg/d selenium for more than 10 days).
- Iodine deficiency has adverse effects on thyroid hormone production, and because most PN formulations do not contain iodine, monitoring is recommended (Zimmerman and Crill, 2009).
- Osmolality is important to monitor to prevent dehydration and other complications. For example, D5 W 5 has an osmolality of 252 mOsm/L, whereas D20 W 5 has an osmolality of 1008 mOsm/L.
- Special considerations will vary according to the patient's condition. Examples include:
  1. Short-chain fatty acids, soy, and fermentable fiber may be needed to reduce CPN-induced bowel atrophy.
  2. For respiratory failure, suggest a lipid emulsion that provides most of the nonprotein calories to lower the RQ.
- Follow practice guidelines, especially for children and home care patients (Kovacevich et al, 2005; Wessel et al, 2005). The increasing numbers of older (>65 years) Americans will increase the demand for home health services including support services (nursing, physical therapy, occupational therapy, durable medical equipment, respiratory therapy), infusion therapies, palliative care, and hospice; certification in gerontological care is encouraged and ASPEN Guidelines should be followed for optimal outcomes (Fuhrman, 2009).
- For management of complications of PN, see Table 17-10.

TABLE 17-9 Sample Basic Adult Daily Requirements for CPN

Nutrient	Amount
Water (/kg body wt/d)	30–40 mL
Energy[a] (/kg body wt/d)	
Medical patient	30 kcal
Postoperative patient	30–45 kcal
Hypercatabolic patient	45–60 kcal
Amino acids (/kg body wt/d)	
Medical patient	1.0 g
Postoperative patient	2.0 g
Hypercatabolic patient	3.0 g
Minerals	
Acetate/gluconate	90 mEq
Calcium	15 mEq
Chloride	130 mEq
Chromium	15 μg
Copper	1.5 mg
Iodine	120 μg
Magnesium	20 mEq
Manganese	2 mg
Phosphorus	300 mg
Potassium	100 mEq
Selenium	100 μg
Sodium	100 mEq
Zinc	5 mg
Vitamins	
Ascorbic acid	100 mg
Biotin	60 mcg
Cobalamin	5 μg
Folate (folic acid)	400 μg
Niacin	40 mg
Pantothenic acid	15 mg
Pyridoxine	4 mg
Riboflavin	3.6 mg
Thiamin	3 mg
Vitamin A	4000 IU
Vitamin D	400 IU
Vitamin E	15 mg
Vitamin K	200 μg

[a]Requirements for energy increase by 7% per 1°F or 12% per 1°C of fever.
Reference: Merck–Total Parenteral Nutrition, http://www.merck.com/mmpe/sec01/ch003/ch003c.html, accessed March 11, 2010.

- Do not overfeed; hyperglycemia, fatty liver, and excessive CO_2 production may occur. Monitor phosphate levels to assess levels of anabolism, risk for refeeding syndrome, and malnutrition.
- Provide weaning when patient is ready; use TF for interim nourishment if necessary. Progress to liquids and solids when patient is ready. Infusion of PN nutrients may suppress appetite, excessively prolonging PN use.

TABLE 17-10 **Complications in Parenteral Nutrition (PN)**

Complication	Comments
Catheter occlusion, venous thrombosis, phlebitis, sepsis	Contact physician or designated member of health care team for evaluation, diagnosis, and treatment of lines. For air embolism, place patient on his or her left side and lower head of the bed until resolved. Monitor for pneumothorax and ensure that trained staff handles catheters
Dehydration	Elevated BUN is noted. MD gives free water as 5% dextrose via peripheral vein Calculate needs as 30 mL/kg body weight or as 1 mL/kcal given. Alter as needed for diarrhea, medications used, ostomy, and losses from exudates such as burns or pressure ulcers
Electrolyte abnormalities	Monitor fluid status, organ system function, and serum sodium, potassium, phosphorus, calcium and magnesium regularly. Determine relevant cause or mechanism
Fluid overload	Greater than 1-kg gain per day is noted. Calculate needs and decrease volume to meet needs; diuretics or dialysis may be needed; a higher concentration of dextrose or lipids may be needed if fluid restriction is required
Gallbladder disorder	Cholelithiasis, gallbladder sludge, or cholecystitis can be caused or worsened by prolonged gallbladder stasis. Stimulate contraction by providing about 20–30% of calories as fat and stop glucose infusion several hours a day. Oral or enteral intake also helps. Treatment with metronidazole, ursodeoxycholic acid, phenobarbital, or cholecystokinin helps some patients with cholestasis
Hypocalcemia	Consider endocrine causes. Evaluate for hypoalbuminemia. Add additional calcium if needed
Hypercalcemia	Consider endocrine causes. Evaluate vitamin D, use isotonic saline, and add inorganic phosphate to solution until normal
Hypoglycemia	Administer more dextrose; reduce or discontinue insulin use; gradually taper infusion rate during weaning
Hyperglycemia	Reduce total grams of dextrose in the solution; add or increase insulin; consider use of lipids as partial substrate; advance feedings more slowly. Sometimes use of PN with a small amount of EN or oral intake can be helpful. Blood glucose >220 mg/dL can cause hyperinsulinemia, increased intracellular transport of potassium and phosphate with hypokalemia and hypophosphatemia. Impaired phagocytosis and neutrophil clearance may also occur
Hypokalemia	Increase potassium in solution and monitor potassium-depleting diuretic use such as furosemide. Add additional potassium if needed
Hyperkalemia	Evaluate renal function; decrease potassium in solution and evaluate medications used; reduce exogenous supplements
Hypomagnesemia	Increase magnesium in solution and monitor refeeding. Consider if magnesium-wasting medications are being used. Additional magnesium may be needed
Hypermagnesemia	Decrease magnesium in solution
Hyponatremia	Sometimes this occurs with fluid overload and total body water excess. Only occasionally is added sodium required
Hypernatremia	Replace fluids with a more dilute CPN solution; decrease sodium
Hyperphosphatemia	Evaluate renal function; decrease phosphate in solution and use phosphate binders if necessary
Hypophosphatemia	Increase phosphate in solution and monitor for refeeding syndrome
Lipid abnormalities	Decrease lipids if triglycerides are higher than 300 mg/dL; infuse over a longer time period; calculate that total kilocalories are not greater than 60% from lipids. Lipids over 2 g/kg/d can increase congestion of reticuloendothelial system and impair clearance of triglycerides. Some studies suggest use of omega-3 fatty acids to reverse cholestasis
Liver function changes	Altered liver function from excess energy may cause fatty infiltration and increased alkaline phosphatase. Liver dysfunction may be transient, evidenced by increased transaminases, bilirubin, and alkaline phosphatase; it commonly occurs when CPN is started. Delayed or persistent elevations may result from excess amino acids. Pathogenesis is unknown, but cholestasis and inflammation may contribute. Progressive fibrosis occasionally develops. Reducing protein delivery may help. For painful hepatomegaly, reducing CHO infusion may be needed
Metabolic Bone Disease	Bone demineralization develops in some patients given CPN for >3 months. Temporarily or permanently stopping CPN is the only known treatment
Pulmonary complications	Calculate needs and avoid overfeeding. Minimal kilocalories may be best, e.g., 20–25 kcal/kg. CHO provision should not exceed 4–5 mg/kg/min; avoid fluid excesses. Respiratory failure may occur in patients with limited pulmonary reserve. Prolonged mechanical ventilation can occur with carbon dioxide retention associated with overfeeding
Renal function changes	Protein excesses >2 g/kg daily can increase ureagenesis and decrease renal function or cause dehydration

Adapted from: Merck–Total Parenteral Nutrition, http://www.merck.com/mmpe/sec01/ch003/ch003c.html, accessed March 11, 2010.

Common Drugs Used and Potential Side Effects

- Basic CPN solutions are prepared using sterile techniques, usually in liter batches. Normally, 2 L/d of the standard solution is needed for adults. An effective, standardized PN process uses standardized formulations and products, ordering, labeling, screening, compounding, and administration (Kochevar et al, 2007).
- Contact the pharmacy for a list of drugs that are stable and compatible with PN solutions or nutrient additives. Often, H_2-blockers, steroids, and insulin are added to PN solutions.

- Intestinal tropic factors, such as recombinant human growth hormone (r-hGH), are used for SBS patients as part of intestinal rehabilitation regimens (Matarese et al, 2005).
- There are potential therapeutic roles for growth hormone, testosterone, oxandrolone, and megestrol acetate (Gullett et al, 2010).
- Loss of muscle mass occurs from increased protein degradation (cachexia), decreased rate of muscle protein synthesis (inactivity or bed rest), or both (sarcopenia). Nutrition therapy with an emphasis on high-quality protein plus use of an anabolic agent can slow or prevent muscle loss (Evans, 2010).
- Parenteral omega-3 fatty acids, such as Omegaven, may benefit patients with SBS who develop PN-associated liver disease (PNALD) with their CPN (Diamond et al, 2009).

Herbs, Botanicals, and Supplements

- Obesity creates a low-grade SIRS with lipotoxicity and cytokine dysregulation that may respond to arginine, fish oil, and carnitine at the molecular level (Cave et al, 2008).
- Herbs and botanical supplements should not be added to any IV feedings.
- Prescription and nonprescription medications are commonly used together; nearly 1 in 25 individuals may be at risk for a major drug–drug interaction (Qato et al, 2008).
- Prebiotics or probiotics may be useful for the prevention of infection.

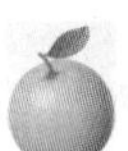

NUTRITION EDUCATION, COUNSELING, CARE MANAGEMENT

- Discuss with patient/caretakers the goals of the PN, especially if home CPN will be used. Discuss aseptic technique, input and output records, CPN pump use, medications, additives, and complications. Long-term consequences should be discussed, such as trace element deficiencies and metabolic problems.
- Teach transition processes when and if patient is ready. Nutrition therapy is challenging; the objective is to restore enteral autonomy to a patient with a complex medical and surgical history, and a coordinated team effort is needed to wean from PN eventually (Weseman and Gilroy, 2005). Assistance from a registered dietitian is recommended.
- Wean from CPN to TF if patient tolerates one third to one half of kilocalorie needs by that route.
- To wean from CPN to oral diet, start with sips of clear liquids and advance, if tolerated, to lactose-free full liquids by the second day. When intake is >500 kcal orally, reduce CPN by 50%. When patient is consuming two thirds to three fourths of estimated needs orally, discontinue CPN by tapering (first hour by 50%, second hour by 75%, and third hour 100%). Nausea and vomiting may occur; eating some type of concentrated CHO during transition to oral diet is helpful.
- Discuss potential problems and when to call the doctor, the dietitian, the pharmacist, or the nurse.
- Discuss psychosocial issues related to adaptation to PN, oral deprivation, sense of loss, grief, and lifestyle changes. Quality of life tends to decline with long-term CPN use (Winkler, 2010). Encourage the patient to participate in favorite activities and physical activity as much as possible (Oz et al, 2008).
- Promote positive communications and collaboration among members of the health care team. A safe PN system must minimize procedural incidents; clinicians with nutrition therapy expertise are essential team members (Kochevar et al, 2007).

Patient Education—Infusion Safety

- Solutions must always be prepared and handled under sterile conditions. A standardized process for PN must be explored to improve patient safety and clinical appropriateness and to maximize resource efficiency (Kochevar et al, 2007).
- Home CPN requires aseptic technique and meticulous catheter care. Discuss infection control measures because catheter-related bloodstream infections are serious, critical complications.
- Change bag, tubing, and cassette every 24 hours or as recommended by the facility or agency.

For More Information

- American Society for Nutrition
  http://www.nutrition.org/
- ASPEN
  http://www.nutritioncare.org/
- Certification in Nutrition Therapy
  http://www.nutritioncare.org/nbnsc/
- NIH
  http://www.nlm.nih.gov/medlineplus/druginfo/meds/a601166.html

PARENTERAL NUTRITION—CITED REFERENCES

Bozzetti F, et al. ESPEN Guidelines on parenteral nutrition: non-surgical oncology. *Clin Nutr.* 28:445, 2009.

Braga M, et al. ESPEN Guidelines on parenteral nutrition: surgery. *Clin Nutr.* 28:378, 2009.

Cave MC, et al. Obesity, inflammation, and the potential application of pharmaconutrition. *Nutr Clin Pract.* 23:16, 2008.

Diamond IR, et al. Changing the paradigm: omegaven for the treatment of liver failure in pediatric short bowel syndrome. *J Pediatr Gastroenterol Nutr.* 48:209, 2009.

Evans WJ. Skeletal muscle loss: cachexia, sarcopenia, and inactivity[published online ahead of print Feb 17, 2010]. *Am J Clin Nutr.*

Ferreira IM, et al. Nutritional supplementation for stable chronic obstructive pulmonary disease. *Cochrane Database Syst Rev.* 2:CD000998, 2005.

Fuhrman MP. Home care for the elderly. *Nutr Clin Pract.* 24:196, 2009.

Gullett NP, et al. Update on clinical trials of growth factors and anabolic steroids in cachexia and wasting. *Am J Clin Nutr.* 91:1143S, 2010.

Hardy G, Puzovic M. Formulation, stability and administration of parenteral nutrition with new lipid emulsions. *Nutr Clin Pract.* 24:616, 2009.

Jensen GL, et al. Malnutrition syndromes: a conundrum vs continuum. *JPEN J Parenter Enteral Nutr.* 33:710, 2009.

Joque L, Jatoi A. Total parenteral nutrition in cancer patients: why and when? *Nutr Clin Care.* 8:89, 2005.

Kohli-Seth R, et al. Adult parenteral nutrition utilization at a tertiary care hospital. *Nutr Clin Pract.* 24:728, 2009.

Kovacevich DS, et al. Standards for specialized nutrition support: home care patients. *Nutr Clin Pract.* 20:579, 2005.

Kochevar M, et al. A.S.P.E.N. Statement on parenteral nutrition standardization. JPEN *J Parenter Enteral Nutrition.* 31:441, 2007.

Matarese LR, et al. Short bowel syndrome: clinical guidelines for nutrition management. *Nutr Clin Pract.* 20:493, 2005.

Oz P, et al. Eating habits and quality of life of patients receiving home parenteral nutrition in Israel. *Clin Nutr.* 27:95, 2008.

Qato DM, et al. Use of prescription and over-the-counter medications and dietary supplements among older adults in the United States. *JAMA.* 300:2867, 2008.

Singer P, et al. Considering energy deficit in the intensive care unit. *Curr Opin Clin Nutr Metab Care.* 13:170, 2010.

Sobotka L, et al. ESPEN Guidelines on parenteral nutrition: geriatrics. *Clin Nutr.* 28:461, 2009.

Weseman RA, Gilroy R. Nutrition management of small bowel transplant patients. *Nutr Clin Pract.* 20:509, 2005.

Wessel J, et al. Standards for specialized nutrition support: hospitalized pediatric patients. *Nutr Clin Pract.* 20:103, 2005.

Winkler MF. 2009 Lenna Frances Cooper Memorial Lecture: living with enteral and parenteral nutrition: how food and eating contribute to quality of life. *J Am Diet Assoc.* 110:169, 2010.

Zimmerman MB, Crill CM. Iodine in enteral and parenteral nutrition. *Best Pract Res Clin Endocrinol Metab.* 24:143, 2010.

APPENDIX

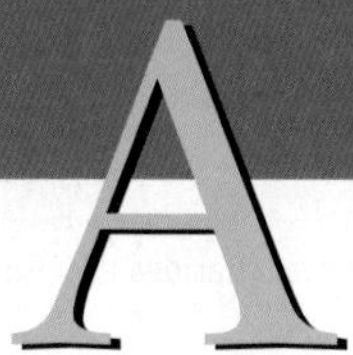

Nutritional Review

RECOMMENDED DIETARY ALLOWANCES AND DIETARY REFERENCE INTAKES

The Dietary Reference Intakes (DRIs) are nutrient-based reference values for use in planning and assessing diets and for other purposes (IOM, 2010). DRIs replaced older tools first published by the National Academy of Sciences in 1941. The DRI values comprise seven reports with more detailed guidance than the old system. The DRIs are composed of the following:

- **Estimated average requirements** (EAR), expected to satisfy the needs of 50% of the people in that age group.
- **Recommended dietary allowances** (RDA). After computing the EARs for each age/gender category, the Food and Nutrition Board (FNB) then established RDAs to meet the nutrient requirements of each category.
- **Adequate intake** (AI), where no RDA has been established
- **Tolerable upper intake levels** (UL), to caution against excessive intake of nutrients (like vitamin D) that can be harmful in large amounts.

REFERENCE

IOM. Institute of Medicine, National Academy of Sciences. Dietary Reference Intakes, 2001. Web site accessed 3/14/10. http://www.iom.edu/Object.File/Master/7/294/0.pdf

<u>**Reader Please Note:**</u> All tables in this Appendix A are derived from the ARS Nutrient Database for Standard Reference, Release 17.
Foods are from single nutrient reports, sorted either by food description or in descending order by nutrient content in terms of common household measures. Mixed dishes are not included here. The food items and weights in these reports are adapted from those in 2002 revision of USDA Home and Garden Bulletin No. 72, Nutritive Value of Foods.

MACRONUTRIENTS

Acceptable macronutrient distribution ranges for individuals have been set for carbohydrate, fat, *n*-6 and *n*-3 polyunsaturated fatty acids, and protein on the basis of evidence through the Institute of Medicine.

Carbohydrates and Fiber

Carbohydrates (CHO) are essential for life and to provide energy to the body. The brain and central nervous system (CNS) require a continuously available glucose supply. When it is necessary, lean body mass is metabolized to provide glucose for these tissues. Generally, 90% of carbohydrates are absorbed from a mixed diet. The RDA for carbohydrate is set at 130 g/d for adults and children, based on the average minimum amount of glucose used by the brain. The median intake of carbohydrates is approximately 220–330 g/d for men and 180–230 g/d for women. To plan a balanced intake between 45 and 65% of kcal/d, it would equal 135 to 195 g carbohydrate on a 1200 kcal diet; 202–292 g CHO on an 1800 kcal diet; or 270–390 g CHO for a 2400-kcal diet.

No recommendations based on glycemic index have been made. Intensely flavored artificial sweeteners that are approved for use in the United States include aspartame (NutraSweet), acesulfame-K (Sunette), neotame, saccharin (Sweet n Low), sucralose (Splenda), and stevia (Truvia). These are many times sweeter than natural sugars. Sugar replacers are natural sugar-free sugar alcohols such as mannitol, erythritol, isomalt, lactitol, maltitol, xylitol, and sorbitol. Unlike artificial sweeteners, these are used in the same amount as sugars and have the same bulk and volume. Labels indicate "sugar free" or "no sugar added. Sorbitol has a sweetness value of 60; mannitol has sweetness value of 50, or half that of table sugar.

Both soluble and insoluble fiber play an important role in maintenance of health. Except in a few therapeutic situations, fiber should be obtained from food sources (20 and 35 g/d for adults). Men up to age 50 need 38 g/d; over age 50, 30 g/d. Women up to age 50 need 25 g fiber per day, women over age 50, 21 g fiber per day. All dietary fibers, regardless of type, are readily fermented by microflora of the small intestines, producing short-chain fatty acids (acetate, propionate, and butyrate). An overview of carbohydrate and fiber classifications is provided in Table A-1. A food list of fiber sources can be found in Table A-2.

TABLE A-1 Carbohydrate and Fiber

Class	Type	Food Sources	Comments
Monosaccharides	Glucose (dextrose)	Corn syrup, honey, fruits, vegetables	Most important; most widely distributed. Sweetness value = 74.
	Fructose (levulose, fruit sugar)	High-fructose corn syrup, honey, fruits, vegetables	Sweetest, especially when fruit ripens. Most fruits contain 1–7%. Makes up 40% of the weight of honey. Sweetness value = 173.
	Galactose	Milk sugar	Part of the lactose molecule. Sweetness value = 32.
	Mannose	Found in poorly digested fruit structures	Of little nutritional value
Disaccharides	Sucrose (table sugar)	Cane or beet sugars, maple sugar, grape sugar, some natural fruits and vegetables	Formed when glucose and fructose are linked together. Honey is a form of sucrose known as an invert sugar. Sweetness value = 100.
	Lactose (milk sugar)	Milk, cream, whey	Glucose + galactose molecules in the mammary glands of lactating mammals. 7.5% of the composition of human milk, 4.5% of cow's milk. Sweetness value = 16.
	Maltose (malt sugar)	Malt, sprouting grains, partially digested starch	Made of two glucose molecules. Sweetness value = 32.
Polysaccharides—digestible	Starch (amylose and amylopectin)	Modified food starch, potatoes, beans, breads, rice, pasta, starchy products such as tapioca	Most starches require cooking for best digestion. When cooked and cooled, they are effective thickeners (such as modified food starch).
	Glycogen	No foods	Muscle and liver storage form of glucose; only 18 hours can be stored in one day.
Polysaccharides—indigestible (fiber)	**Insoluble fibers:** Cellulose	Soybean hulls, fruit membranes, legumes, carrots, celery, broccoli, and many other vegetables. The most abundant organic compound in the world.	Insoluble fibers increase fecal volume (bulk) and decrease colonic transit time by their ability to increase water-holding capacity; excess may deplete mineral status.
	Insoluble hemicelluloses (xylan, galactan, mannan, arabinose, galactose)	Corn hulls, wheat and corn brans, brown rice, cereal	The predominant sugar is used to name it.
	Algal polysaccharides (carrageenan)	Processed foods such as baby food, ice cream, sour cream	Extracted from seaweed and algae.
	Lignin (noncarbohydrate)	Wheat straw, alfalfa stems, tannins, cottonseed hulls	Polymer made of phenylpropyl alcohols and acids. Flaxseed lignin is an excellent antioxidant. Lignin may lower serum cholesterol levels.
	Cutin (noncarbohydrate)	Apple or tomato peels, seeds in berries, peanut or almond skins, onion skins	
	Soluble fibers: Pectin (polygalacturonic acid)	Citrus pulp, apple pulp, strawberries, sugar beet pulp, banana, cabbage and *Brassica* foods, legumes (such as kidney beans), sunflower heads	Soluble fibers decrease serum cholesterol by decreasing the enterohepatic recycling of bile acids and increasing use of cholesterol in bile synthesis. This stabilizes blood glucose levels and maintains mineral nutriture. Little effect on fecal bulk or transit time.
	Beta-glucans (glucopyranose)	Oat and barley bran; soy fiber concentrate.	Lowers serum cholesterol
	Gums (galactose and glucuronic acid)	Oats, guar gum, legumes, barley, xanthan from prickly ash trees	Useful for gel formation which slow digestion and slows down transit time; helpful in diarrhea.
	Psyllium	Extracted from psyllium seeds or plantains	High water binding capacity (choking hazard)
Oligosaccharides	Raffinose and stachyose	Beans and other legumes	Low-molecular-weight polymers containing 2–20 sugar molecules.
	Fructans [fructooligosaccharides (FOSs), inulin, oligofructose]	Wheat, onions, garlic, bananas, chicory, tomatoes, barley, rye, asparagus, and Jerusalem artichokes	They add flavor and sweetness to low-calorie foods and provide prebiotics to stimulate the growth of intestinal bacteria, especially *bifidobacteria*. May be used as a fat replacer.
Miscellaneous carbohydrates	Chitin (Glucopyranose)	Supplement made from crab or lobster shells	May reduce serum cholesterol
	Polydextrose, polyols (sorbitol, mannitol, etc.)	Synthesized	Bulking agent or sugar substitute.
	Algal polysaccharides (carrageenan)	Isolated from algae and seaweed	Forms a gel used as thickening agent. Can be toxic.

Sources: Byrd-Brenner C, et al. *Wardlaw's perspectives in nutrition*. 8th ed. New York: McGraw-Hill, 2008; Gallagher M. *Macronutrients in Krause's food and nutrition therapy*. Mahan LK, Escott-Stump S, editors. 12th ed. St Louis, MO: Elsevier, 2008.

TABLE A-2 **Food Sources of Dietary Fiber**[a]

Food, Standard Amount	Dietary Fiber (g)	Calories	Food, Standard Amount	Dietary Fiber (g)	Calories
Navy beans, cooked, 1/2 cup	9.5	128	Potato, baked, with skin, one medium	3.8	161
Bran ready-to-eat cereal (100%), 1/2 cup	8.8	78	Soybeans, green, cooked, 1/2 cup	3.8	127
Kidney beans, canned, 1/2 cup	8.2	109	Stewed prunes, 1/2 cup	3.8	133
Split peas, cooked, 1/2 cup	8.1	116	Figs, dried, 1/4 cup	3.7	93
Lentils, cooked, 1/2 cup	7.8	115	Dates, 1/4 cup	3.6	126
Black beans, cooked, 1/2 cup	7.5	114	Oat bran, raw, 1/4 cup	3.6	58
Pinto beans, cooked, 1/2 cup	7.7	122	Pumpkin, canned, 1/2 cup	3.6	42
Lima beans, cooked, 1/2 cup	6.6	108	Spinach, frozen, cooked, 1/2 cup	3.5	30
Artichoke, globe, cooked, one each	6.5	60	Shredded wheat ready-to-eat cereals, various, ~1 ounce	2.8–3.4	96
White beans, canned, 1/2 cup	6.3	154	Almonds, 1 ounce	3.3	164
Chickpeas, cooked, 1/2 cup	6.2	135	Apple with skin, raw, one medium	3.3	72
Great northern beans, cooked, 1/2 cup	6.2	105	Brussels sprouts, frozen, cooked, 1/2 cup	3.2	33
Cowpeas, cooked, 1/2 cup	5.6	100	Whole-wheat spaghetti, cooked, 1/2 cup	3.1	87
Soybeans, mature, cooked, 1/2 cup	5.2	149	Banana, one medium	3.1	105
Bran ready-to-eat cereals, various, ~1 ounce	2.6–5.0	90–108	Orange, raw, one medium	3.1	62
Crackers, rye wafers, plain, two wafers	5.0	74	Oat bran muffin, one small	3.0	178
Sweet potato, baked, with peel, one medium (146 g)	4.8	131	Guava, one medium	3.0	37
Asian pear, raw, one small	4.4	51	Pearled barley, cooked, 1/2 cup	3.0	97
Green peas, cooked, 1/2 cup	4.4	67	Sauerkraut, canned, solids, and liquids, 1/2 cup	3.0	23
Whole-wheat English muffin, one each	4.4	134	Tomato paste, 1/4 cup	2.9	54
Pear, raw, one small	4.3	81	Winter squash, cooked, 1/2 cup	2.9	38
Bulgur, cooked, 1/2 cup	4.1	76	Broccoli, cooked, 1/2 cup	2.8	26
Mixed vegetables, cooked, 1/2 cup	4.0	59	Parsnips, cooked, chopped, 1/2 cup	2.8	55
Raspberries, raw, 1/2 cup	4.0	32	Turnip greens, cooked, 1/2 cup	2.5	15
Sweet potato, boiled, no peel, one medium (156 g)	3.9	119	Collards, cooked, 1/2 cup	2.7	25
Blackberries, raw, 1/2 cup	3.8	31	Okra, frozen, cooked, 1/2 cup	2.6	26
			Peas, edible-pod, cooked, 1/2 cup	2.5	42

[a]Food sources of dietary fiber are ranked by grams of dietary fiber per standard amount; also calories in the standard amount. All are ≥10% of AI for adult women, which is 25 g/d.

Fatty Acids and Lipids

The usual American diet contains 35–40% fat kcal. Fats are carriers for fat-soluble vitamins and essential fatty acids (EFAs). Fat is essential for cell membranes (especially the brain) serves as an insulating agent for organs and is a rich energy source. Generally, 95% of fat from the diet is absorbed. One to two percent of calories should be available as linoleic acid to prevent EFA deficiency. People with low body fat stores, very malnourished persons, psychiatric patients, and premature low birth weight (LBW) infants are at risk for EFA deficiency.

Lipase is needed to metabolize long-chain triglycerides (LCT) into free fatty acids (FFAs). When parenteral fat emulsions contain LCT, large doses may compromise immune function, elevate serum lipids, impair alveolar diffusion capacity, or decrease reticular endothelial system function. Medium-chain fatty acids (MCFAs) are produced from medium-chain triglycerides (MCTs). MCTs are transported to the liver via the portal vein and, therefore, do not require micelle or chylomicron formation.

Omega-3 fatty acids reduce inflammation and help prevent certain chronic diseases. These essential fatty acids are highly concentrated in the brain. Two to three servings of fatty fish per week (about 1250 mg EPA and DHA per day) are beneficial for most people. If using fish oil supplements, 3000–4000 mg standardized fish oils would be needed per day. Safe and effective doses of omega-3 fatty acid supplements have not been established in children. EPA and arachidonic acids are transformed into eicosanoids for prostaglandin, leukotriene, thromboxane, and prostacyclin synthesis. Prostaglandins are used in many diverse hormone-like compounds. Omega-3 fatty acids should be used cautiously by people who have a bleeding disorder, take blood thinners, or are at an increased risk for hemorrhagic stroke.

It is very important to maintain a balance between omega-3 and omega-6 fatty acids in the diet. The Mediterranean diet consists of a healthier balance between omega-3 and omega-6 fatty acids than the typical American diet. Omega-6 fatty acids play a role as proinflammatory agents and are useful when initiating a stress response.

Sphingolipids are hydrolyzed throughout the GI tract to regulate growth, differentiation, apoptosis, and other cellular functions. They reduce low-density lipoprotein (LDL) levels and increase high-density lipoprotein (HDL) levels. Dietary constituents such as cholesterol, fatty acids, and mycotoxins alter their metabolism.

The recommended intakes of total fat per day equal 20–35% of kcal. Of this, consume 1–2% from omega-3 fatty acids and 5–8% from omega-6 fatty acids. Table A-3 describes more details.

Proteins and Amino Acids

Amino acids and proteins are the building blocks of life. All growth and repair functions of the body require utilization and availability of amino acids in the proper proportion and amounts. Average total essential amino acid needs are as follows: infants, 40% essential; children, 36% essential; and adults, 19% essential. This translates into 52 g protein for teenaged boys aged 14–18 years and 46 g for teenaged girls aged 14+, and women. Pregnant or nursing women need 71 g/d. Men aged 19+ need 56 g protein per day. Need increase with injury, trauma, and certain medical conditions.

TABLE A-3 Fats and Lipids

Class	Fatty Acid Component	Key Food Sources	Comments
Simple lipids *Neutral fats (acyl-glycerols)*	Mono- and diglycerides	Additive in low-fat foods	Glycerol with one or two esterified fatty acids
	Triglycerides (triacylglycerols)	Fats and oils	Glycerol with three esterified fatty acids
Fatty acids, polyunsaturated Omega-3 family	Alpha linolenic acid (ALA)	Vegetable oils (soybean, canola, or rapeseed), flaxseeds, flaxseed oil, soybeans, pumpkin seeds, pumpkin seed oil, purslane, perilla seed oil, walnuts, walnut oil. Flaxseed and flaxseed oil should be kept refrigerated; whole flaxseeds should be ground within 24 hours of use.	**An essential fatty acid.** Once eaten, the body converts ALA to EPA and DHA, the two types of omega-3 fatty acids more readily used by the body. The adequate daily intake of ALA should be 1.6 and 1.1 g for men and women, respectively.
	Eicosapentaenoic acid (EPA) and Docosahexanoic acid (DHA)	Cold-water fish such as salmon, mackerel, eel, tuna, herring, halibut, trout, sardines, and herring. Fish oil capsules should be refrigerated.	EPA and DHA (1 g/d) from fatty fish can reduce CHD and some types of cancer. Infants who do not receive sufficient DHA from their mothers during pregnancy are at risk for nerve or vision problems.
Omega-6 family	Linoleic acid	Safflower, sunflower, corn, soybean, peanut oils.	**An essential fatty acid**
	Conjugated linoleic acid (CLA)	Naturally rich in milk fat	Group of isomers produced by rumen bacteria. CLA may have a role in weight management and other functions.
	Arachidonic acid	Animal tissues (very low). There is no good dietary source.	
Monounsaturated Omega-9 family	Oleic acid	Olive oil, canola oil, peanut oil, sunflower oil, and sesame oil. Avocados, olives, nut butters, such as peanut butter, nuts and seeds, such as macadamia nuts, pecans, and almonds	
Compound lipids *Phospholipids*	Glycerophosphatides (lecithins, cephalins, plasmologens)	Egg yolks, liver, wheat germ, peanuts	Glycerol with two fatty acids and a nitrogen
	Glycosphingolipids (ceramides, sphingomyelins)	Low in the food supply, mainly in dairy products, eggs, soybeans. Fruit has a tiny bit.	Sphingosine with one esterified fatty acid (a ceramide). Found in myelin of nerve tissue.
Glycolipids	Cerebrosides, gangliosides	Low in the food supply.	Found in nerve and brain tissue. A ceramide linked to a monosaccharide or an oligosaccharide

(continued)

TABLE A-3 Fats and Lipids *(continued)*

Class	Fatty Acid Component	Key Food Sources	Comments
Lipoproteins	Protein–lipid combination	Made by the liver	VLDL, LDL, HDL have various roles in health maintenance.
Miscellaneous lipids *Sterols*	Cholesterol	Liver, heart, and other organ meats	Steroid nucleus (synthesized from acetyl-coenzyme A). Technically a wax.
Fat-soluble vitamins	A,D, E, and K	Various food sources	Lipid soluble; some are esterified with 1 fatty acid
Trans fatty acids		Margarines, some cookies and crackers. The new food label includes the amount of trans fat in a serving.	These are made by hydrogenation of vegetable oils to form more solid products (i.e., margarine).The process increases the amount of saturation and converts natural *cis* double bonds to *trans* double bonds. To decrease intake, use leaner cuts of meat, fewer cold cuts. Choose skim milk, fat-free products in food choices and in cooking.
Fat-related substances	Carnitine	Produced in the liver from essential amino acids lysine and methionine.	Carnitine transports fatty acids into mitochondria, where they undergo beta-oxidation. When in short supply, production of ATP slows down or halts altogether, affecting heart or skeletal muscle. In renal failure, it is a useful additive to improve fatty acid metabolism.
	Myo-inositol	Found as phospholipid in animals, phytic acid in plants.	Inositol phosphates liberated from glycerophosphatides acts as a secondary messenger in the release of intracellular of calcium, which in turn causes activation of certain cellular enzymes and produces hormonal responses. Possible role in diabetes mellitus or in renal failure.

The main protein source in the American diet is animal protein from beef and poultry.

To produce the nonessential amino acids from dietary intake of the essentials, it is recommended that the limited amino acids be consumed within a 24-hour period of each other. Protein synthesis requires all amino acids; an insufficient amount of any one may impede or slow formation of the polypeptide chain. For valine, leucine, and isoleucine, the requirement of each is increased by excess of the other branched-chain amino acids (BCAAs).

Protein requirement is inversely related to calories when the latter are deficient. Generally, more than 90% of protein is absorbed from the diet. Foods of high biological value (HBV) contain approximately 40% EAAs. Table A-4 indicates which amino acids are essential and which can be made by the body (nonessential). Eight amino acids are generally regarded as essential for humans: threonine, valine, tryptophan, isoleucine, leucine, lysine, phenylalanine, methionine (names of these amino acids are easy to remember by the phrase "**TV TILL PM**"). Foods that contain all of the essential amino acids are called complete proteins. Incomplete proteins tend to be deaminated for sources of energy rather than being available for new tissue, healing, and growth. For biological value of proteins see Table A-5 and see Table A-6 for sources of protein.

MICRONUTRIENTS

Minerals

Minerals are inorganic compounds containing no carbon structures. There are 22 essential minerals known to be needed from the diet. Macrominerals (needed in large amounts) include calcium, phosphorus, magnesium, potassium, sodium, chloride, and sulfur. Trace minerals include iron, copper, selenium, fluoride, iodine, chromium, zinc, manganese, molybdenum, cobalt, and others.

Major Minerals

Minerals that are needed at levels of 100 mg daily or more are known as macrominerals.

Calcium: Calcium absorption is dependent upon the calcium needs of the body, foods eaten, and the amount of calcium in foods eaten. Vitamin D, whether from diet or exposure to the ultraviolet light of the sun, increases calcium absorption. Calcium absorption tends to decrease with increased age for both men and women. *RDA for calcium is 1000 mg for most adults, 1300 mg for teenagers, and 1200 mg for those over 50 years.*

TABLE A-4 Amino Acids

Essential Amino Acids	Type	Food Sources	Comments: Must be Consumed
Histidine	Aromatic	Dairy, meat, poultry, fish.	Precursor of histamine. Important for red and white blood cells. An important source of carbon atoms in the synthesis of purines. Histidine is needed to help grow and repair body tissues, and to maintain the myelin sheaths that protect nerve cells. It also helps manufacture red and white blood cells, and helps to protect the body from heavy metal toxicity. Histamine stimulates the secretion of the digestive enzyme gastrin. Extra is needed by infants and renal failure patients.
Isoleucine	Neutral	Meats, fish, cheeses, nuts	Belongs to the branched-chain amino acid group (BCAAs), which help maintain and repair muscle tissue. Important for stabilizing and regulating blood sugar and energy levels. Needed for synthesis of hemoglobin and energy regulation. Need 20 mg/kg body weight
Leucine	Neutral	Soybeans, cowpeas, lentils, beef, peanuts, pork salami, salmon, shellfish, chicken, eggs	Belongs to the branched-chain amino acid group (BCAAs). Second most common amino acid found in proteins; necessary for the optimal growth of infants and for the nitrogen balance in adults. Needed for wound healing and healthy skin and bones. Need 39 mg/kg body weight
Lysine	Basic	Limited in corn, wheat, and rice.	It is an essential building block for all protein, and is needed for proper growth and bone development in children. Lysine helps the body absorb and conserve calcium, form collagen and muscle protein, and synthesize enzymes and hormones. Need 30 mg/kg body weight
Methionine	Sulfur	Limited in soy products.	Helps to initiate translation of messenger RNA by being the first amino acid incorporated into the N-terminal position of all proteins. Methionine supplies sulfur and other compounds required by the body for normal metabolism and growth. Reacts with ATP to form *S*-adenosyl methionine (SAM) which is the principal methyl donor in the body. It contributes to the synthesis of epinephrine and choline. Need 10.4 + 4.1 (15 total) mg/kg body weight
Phenylalanine	Aromatic	Soybeans, lentils, nuts, seeds, chicken, fish, eggs.	Exhibits ultraviolet radiation absorption properties with a large extinction coefficient. Phenylalanine is part of the composition of aspartame, a common sweetener found in prepared foods (particularly soft drinks, and gum). Key role in the biosynthesis of other amino acids and some neurotransmitters. Healthy nervous system, memory and learning. Useful against depression. Need, along with tyrosine, 25 (total) mg/kg body weight
Threonine	Neutral	Soybeans, pork, lentils, beef, fish.	Important component in the formation of protein, collagen, elastin and tooth enamel. It is also important for production of neurotransmitters and health of the nervous system and the immune system. Need 15 mg/kg body weight
Tryptophan	Aromatic	Rich in flaxseed, salami, lentils, turkey, nuts, eggs. Limited in corn.	Formed from proteins during digestion by the action of proteolytic enzymes. Tryptophan is also a precursor for serotonin (a neurotransmitter) and melatonin (a neurohormone). Precursor of niacin. Tryptophan may enhance relaxation and sleep, relieve minor premenstrual symptoms, sooth nerves and anxiety, and reduce carbohydrate cravings. Need 4 mg/kg body weight.
Valine	Neutral	Meat, eggs, milk, cereal proteins.	Belongs to the branched-chain amino acid group (BCAAs). Constituent of fibrous protein in the body. Useful in treatments involving muscle, mental, and emotional upsets, and for insomnia and nervousness. Valine may help treat malnutrition associated with drug addiction. Needed for muscle development. Need 26 mg/kg body weight

(continued)

TABLE A-4 **Amino Acids *(continued)***

Conditional Amino Acids	Type	Food Sources	Comments: Must be Consumed in the Diet During Stress or Illness
Arginine, citrulline, ornithine	Basic	Peanuts, almonds, seeds	These three amino acids are part of urea acid cycle. Arginine plays an important role in cell division, wound healing, removing ammonia from the body, immune function, and the release of hormones. Extra needed in growing children. Citrulline supports the body in optimizing blood flow through its conversion to L-arginine and then nitric oxide (NO). Ornithine is a precursor of citrulline, glutamic acid, and proline; it is an intermediate in arginine biosynthesis.
Cysteine	Sulfur	Can be made from homocysteine but cannot be synthesized on its own. Limited in soy products.	Spares methionine. Component of nails, skin and hair. Antioxidant when taken with vitamin E and selenium. Extra needed in infancy, liver failure. Naturally occurring hydrophobic amino acid with a sulfhydryl group; found in most proteins. *N*-acetyl cysteine (NAC) is the most frequently used form and it helps toxify harmful substances in the body. Both cysteine and NAC increase levels of the antioxidant glutathione.
Glutamine	Acidic	Beef, chicken, milk, eggs, what.	One of the 20 amino acids generally present in animal proteins; the most abundant amino acid in the body. Over 61% of skeletal muscle tissue is glutamine. It contains two ammonia groups, one from precursor glutamate, and the other from free ammonia in the bloodstream. Glutamine is converted to glucose when more glucose is required by the body as an energy source. Glutamine assists in maintaining the proper acid/alkaline balance in the body, and is the basis for the synthesis of RNA and DNA.
Glycine	Neutral	Abundant in fish, meat, dairy products, beans.	The simplest amino acid; it has no stereoisomers. The body uses it to help the liver in detoxification of compounds and for helping the synthesis of bile acids. Glycine is essential for the synthesis of nucleic acids, bile acids, proteins, peptides, purines, adenosine triphosphate (ATP), porphyrins, hemoglobin, glutathione, creatine, bile salts, one-carbon fragments, glucose, glycogen, and L-serine and other amino acids. Beneficial for skin and wound healing. It has a sweet taste.
Hydroxyproline			Derived from proline and used almost exclusively in structural proteins including collagen, connective tissue in mammals, and in plant cell walls. The nonhydroxylated collagen is commonly termed procollagen.
Proline	Cyclic	A diet low in ascorbic acid may lead to low levels of hydroxyproline. Derived from L-glutamate.	Needed for intracellular signaling. Involved in the production of collagen and in wound healing. Proline is the precursor for hydroxyproline, which the body incorporates into collagen, tendons, ligaments, and the heart muscle. Important component in certain medical wound dressings that use collagen fragments to stimulate wound healing.
Serine	Neutral; also an alcohol	Synthesized from glycine	Important for healthy brain and immunity. Variety of biosynthetic pathways including those involving pyrimidines, purines, creatine, and porphyrins. Serine has sugar-producing qualities, and is very reactive in the body. It is highly concentrated in all cell membranes, aiding in the production of immunoglobulins and antibodies. Need extra for hemodialysis patients.
Taurine		Found in seafood and meat.	Functions with glycine and gamma-aminobutyric acid as a neuroinhibitory transmitter. Also needed for brain function and metabolism of magnesium, calcium and potassium. Extra needed for infants and in trauma, infection, renal failure.
Tyrosine	Aromatic	Soy, poultry, dairy and other high protein foods.	Metabolically synthesized from phenylalanine to become the para-hydroxy derivative. Tyrosine is a precursor of the adrenal hormones epinephrine, norepinephrine, and the thyroid hormones L-tyrosine, through its effect on neurotransmitters, is used to treat conditions including mood enhancement, appetite suppression, and growth hormone (HGH) stimulation. Extra is needed for infants and in chronic renal failure.

(continued)

TABLE A-4 Amino Acids *(continued)*

Nonessential and Other Amino Acids/Proteins	Type	Food Sources	Comments: Made by the Body if Enough Nitrogen is Available
Alanine	Neutral		Removes toxic substances released from breakdown of muscle protein during intensive exercise. Part of glucose–alanine pathway. Alanine comes from the breakdown of DNA or the dipeptides, anserine and carnosine, and the conversion of pyruvate for carbohydrate metabolism.
Asparagine	Acidic	Seafood, meat, casein, dairy products, eggs, beans, seeds, nuts, corn.	Healthy CNS. Asparagine is synthesized from aspartic acid and ATP. One of the principal and frequently the most abundant amino acids involved in the transport of nitrogen and in amination/transamination. It serves as an amino donor in liver transamination.
Aspartic acid	Acidic		Used for immunity and removal of toxins and ammonia from the body. Aspartic acid is alanine with one of the β hydrogens replaced by a carboxylic acid group. It supports metabolism during construction of asparagine, arginine, lysine, methionine, threonine, isoleucine, and several nucleotides.
Carnitine			Produced in the liver, brain and the kidneys from methionine and lysine; responsible for the transport of long-chain fatty acids into the energy-producing mitochondria. Carnitine helps maintain a healthy blood lipid profile and promote fatty acid utilization within heart muscle.
Creatine			Synthesized in the liver, kidneys and pancreas out of arginine, methionine and glycine; increases the availability of cellular ATP. Donates a phosphate ion to increase the availability of ATP. Stored in muscle cells as phosphocreatine; helps generate cellular energy for muscle contractions.
Glutamic acid	Acidic		Gamma-aminobutyric acid (GABA) is formed from glutamic acid with the help of vitamin B_6, is found in almost every region of brain, and is formed through the activity of the enzyme glutamic acid decarboxylase (GAD). GABA serves as an inhibitory neurotransmitter to block the transmission of an impulse from one cell to another in the CNS. The crystalline salt of glutamic acid, monosodium glutamate, contributes to the flavor called umami.
Glutathione		Seaweed	Glutathione (GSH) is a tripeptide composed of three different amino acids, glutamate, cysteine and glycine, which has numerous important functions within cells. Glutathione plays a role in such diverse biological processes as protein synthesis, enzyme catalysis, transmembrane transport, receptor action, intermediary metabolism, and cell maturation. Glutathione acts as an antioxidant used to prevent oxidative stress in most cells and help to trap free radicals that can damage DNA and RNA.
Theanine			L-theanine is the predominant amino acid in green tea and makes up 50% of the total free amino acids in the plant; the main component responsible for the taste of green tea. L-theanine is involved in the formation of the inhibitory neurotransmitter, gamma amino butyric acid (GABA). GABA influences the levels of two other neurotransmitters, dopamine and serotonin, producing a relaxation effect.

Adapted from: Furst P, Steele P. What are the essential elements needed for the determination of amino acid requirements in humans? The American Society for Nutritional Sciences *J Nutr* 134:1558, 2004;
Shils M, et al. *Modern nutrition in health and disease*. 9th ed. Baltimore: Lippincott Williams & Wilkins, 1999.

TABLE A-5 Biological Value of Proteins

Food Source	Biological Value	Food Source	Biological Value
Whey protein	104	Casein	77
Egg	100	Soybean	74
Cow's milk	95	Rice, white	67
Cottonseed	81	Wheat, whole	53
Beef	80	Sesame	50
Fish	79	Corn	49

From the Joint FAO/WHO Ad Hoc Expert Committee. Energy and protein requirements. WHO technical report no. 522. Geneva: World Health Organization, 1973, p. 67.

TABLE A-6 Protein Sources

Food	Serving	Weight (g)	Protein (g)
Hamburger, extra lean	6 ounces	170	48.6
Chicken, roasted	6 ounces	170	42.5
Fish	6 ounces	170	41.2
Tuna, water packed	6 ounces	170	40.1
Beefsteak, broiled	6 ounces	170	38.6
Cottage cheese or ricotta cheese	1 cup	225	28.1
Beef, fish, pork, chicken or turkey	3 ounces	85	21
Cheese pizza	2 slices	128	15.4
Yogurt, low fat	8 ounces	227	11.9
Tofu or vegetarian burger patty	1/2 cup	126	10–15
Lentils, cooked	1/2 cup	99	9
Skim milk	1 cup	245	8.4
Split peas, cooked	1/2 cup	98	8.1
Whole or chocolate milk	1 cup	244	8
Peanut or other nut butters	2 tablespoons	Varies	8
Kidney beans, cooked	1/2 cup	87	7.6
Cheddar cheese	1 ounce (1 slice)	28	7.1
Macaroni, cooked	1 cup	140	6.8
Soy milk	1 cup	245	6–9
Egg	1 large	50	6.3
Whole wheat bread	2 slices	56	5.4
White bread	2 slices	60	4.9
Rice, cooked	1 cup	158	4.3
Broccoli, cooked	5-inch piece	140	4.2
Nuts or seeds	2 tablespoons	Varies	3–5
Baked potato	2 × 5 inches	156	3
Corn, cooked	1 ear	77	2.6
Bread, cooked cereal or rice or pasta	1 slice	Varies	2

From: U. S. Department of Agriculture. Nutrient database, http://www.ars.usda.gov/SP2UserFiles/Place/12354500/Data/SR22/nutrlist/sr22w203.pdf, accessed January 22, 2010.

Roles. For strong bones and teeth, nerve irritability, muscle contraction, heart rhythm, blood coagulation, enzymes, osmotic pressure, intercellular cement, maintenance of cell membranes, and protection against high blood pressure. About 60% is bound to protein, mostly albumin. About 30–60% absorption occurs with intakes of 400–1000 mg.

Sources. Milk and cheese products remain the primary source of calcium for Americans. Phytates and excessive protein or zinc decrease absorption. Calcium from soy milk is absorbed only 75% as efficiently as from cow's milk. Calcium is lost in cooking some foods, even under the best conditions. To retain calcium, cook foods in a minimal amount of water and for the shortest possible time. Table A-7 lists both dairy and nondairy sources of calcium.

Signs of Deficiency. In hypocalcemia, there may be tetany, paresthesia, hyperirritability, muscle cramps, convulsions, and stunting in growth. No consistent data suggests that a high-protein diet depletes calcium.

Signs of Excess. With hypercalcemia, milk alkali syndrome, kidney stones or renal insufficiency can occur. Recommending excessive calcium use among the general, unsupervised public is not advisable. For bone health, vitamin D is the priority and should be given along with calcium.

Chloride: Chloride constitutes about 3% of total mineral content in the body. It is the main extracellular ion, along with sodium. *No RDA levels have been established for chloride. The upper limit (UL) for adults is 3.6 g/d.*

Roles. Digestion (HCl in stomach), acid–base balance, O_2/CO_2 exchange in red blood cells (RBCs), and fluid balance.

Sources. Table salt, salt substitutes containing potassium chloride, processed foods made with table salt, sauerkraut, snack chips, and green olives.

Signs of Deficiency. Hypochlorhydria and disturbed acid–base balance.

TABLE A-7 **Dairy Sources of Calcium**[a]

Dairy Food, Standard Amount	Calcium (mg)	Calories
Plain yogurt, nonfat (13 g protein/ 8 ounces), 8-ounce container	452	127
Romano cheese, 1.5 ounces	452	165
Pasteurized process Swiss cheese, 2 ounces	438	190
Plain yogurt, low-fat (12 g protein/ 8 ounces), 8-ounce container	415	143
Fruit yogurt, low-fat (10 g protein/ 8 ounces), 8-ounce container	345	232
Swiss cheese, 1.5 ounces	336	162
Ricotta cheese, part skim, 1/2 cup	335	170
Pasteurized process American cheese food, 2 ounces	323	188
Provolone cheese, 1.5 ounces	321	150
Mozzarella cheese, part-skim, 1.5 ounces	311	129
Cheddar cheese, 1.5 ounces	307	171
Fat-free (skim) milk, one cup	306	83
Muenster cheese, 1.5 ounces	305	156
Pudding, ready to eat, one cup	300	Varies
Macaroni and cheese, one cup prepared	300	Varies
1% low-fat milk, one cup	290	102
Low-fat chocolate milk (1%), one cup	288	158
2% reduced fat milk, one cup	285	122
Reduced fat chocolate milk (2%), one cup	285	180
Buttermilk, low-fat, one cup	284	98
Chocolate milk, one cup	280	208
Whole milk, one cup	276	146
Yogurt, plain, whole milk (8 g protein/ 8 ounces), 8-ounce container	275	138
Ricotta cheese, whole milk, 1/2 cup	255	214
Blue cheese, 1.5 ounces	225	150
Mozzarella cheese, whole milk, 1.5 ounces	215	128
Feta cheese, 1.5 ounces	210	113
Cottage cheese, one cup	150	
Frozen yogurt or ice cream	100	Varies
Non-food, standard amount	Calcium (mg)	Calories
Fortified ready-to-eat cereals (various), 1 ounce	236–1043	88–106
Soy beverage, calcium fortified, one cup	368	98
Sardines, Atlantic, in oil, drained, 3 ounces	325	177
Fortified orange juice, one cup	300	120
Tofu, firm, prepared with calcium, 1/2 cup	253	88
Bread, calcium-fortified, one slice	200	70
Pink salmon, canned, or sardines, with bone, 3 ounces	181	118
Collards, cooked from frozen, 1/2 cup	178	31
Molasses, blackstrap, one tbsp	172	47
Spinach, cooked from frozen, 1/2 cup	146	30
Soybeans, green, cooked, 1/2 cup	130	127
Turnip greens, cooked from frozen, 1/2 cup	124	24
Ocean perch, Atlantic, cooked, 3 ounces	116	103
Oatmeal, plain and flavored, instant, fortified, one packet prepared	99–110	97–157
Cowpeas, cooked, 1/2 cup	106	80
Almonds, 1 ounce	100	164
White beans, canned, 1/2 cup	96	153
Broccoli or kale, cooked from frozen, 1/2 cup	90–100	20
Okra, cooked from frozen, 1/2 cup	88	26
Soybeans, mature, cooked, 1/2 cup	88	149
Blue crab, canned, 3 ounces	86	84
Beet greens, cooked from fresh, 1/2 cup	82	19

Source: Nutrient values from Agricultural Research Service (ARS) Nutrient Database for Standard Reference, Release 17. Foods are from ARS single nutrient reports, sorted in descending order by nutrient content in terms of common household measures. Food items and weights in the single nutrient reports are adapted from those in 2002 revision of USDA Home and Garden Bulletin No. 72, Nutritive Value of Foods. Mixed dishes and multiple preparations of the same food item have been omitted from this table.

[a]Food sources of calcium ranked by milligrams of calcium per standard amount; also calories in the standard amount. All are ≥20% of AI for adults 19–50, which is 1,000 mg/d. Those containing 300 mg or more are highlighted in salmon, those with 200–299 mg are shaded lighter, and those with the lightest shading have 80–199 mg.

Note: Both calcium content and bioavailability should be considered when selecting dietary sources of calcium. Some plant foods have calcium that is well absorbed, but the large quantity of plant foods that would be needed to provide as much calcium as in a glass of milk may be unachievable for many. Many other calcium-fortified foods are available, but the percentage of calcium that can be absorbed is unavailable for many of them.

Signs of Excess. Disturbed acid–base balance.

Magnesium: Magnesium is a mineral needed by every cell of the body; half of the stores are found inside cells of body tissues and organs, and half are combined with calcium and phosphorus in bone. Only 1% of magnesium in the body is found in blood. The body works hard to keep blood levels of magnesium constant. Results of two national surveys indicated that the diets of most adult men and women do not provide the recommended amounts of magnesium. Adults aged 70 years and over eat less magnesium than younger adults, and non-Hispanic black subjects consume less magnesium than either non-Hispanic white or Hispanic subjects. Despite poor intakes, magnesium deficiency is rarely seen in the United States in adults. *RDA varies by age but is typically 420 mg for men and 320 mg for women. UL for supplemental magnesium for adolescents and adults is 350 mg/d.*

Roles. Magnesium is needed for more than 300 biochemical reactions including normal muscle contraction, nerve transmission and function, heart rhythm, energy metabolism and protein synthesis, enzyme activation (ADP, ATP), glucose utilization, bone matrix and growth, and normal Na^+/K^+ pump. Maintaining an adequate magnesium intake is a

TABLE A-8 Food Sources of Magnesium[a]

Food, Standard Amount	Magnesium (mg)	Calories	Food, Standard Amount	Magnesium (mg)	Calories
Pumpkin and squash seed kernels, roasted, 1 ounce	151	148	Bulgur, dry, 1/4 cup	57	120
Brazil nuts, 1 ounce	107	186	Oat bran, raw, 1/4 cup	55	58
Bran ready-to-eat cereal (100%), ~1 ounce	103	74	Soybeans, green, cooked, 1/2 cup	54	127
Halibut, cooked, 3 ounces	91	119	Tuna, yellowfin, cooked, 3 ounces	54	118
Quinoa, dry, 1/4 cup	89	159	Artichokes (hearts), cooked, 1/2 cup	50	42
Spinach, canned, 1/2 cup	81	25	Peanuts, dry roasted, 1 ounce	50	166
Almonds, 1 ounce	78	164	Lima beans, baby, cooked from frozen, 1/2 cup	50	95
Spinach, cooked from fresh, 1/2 cup	78	20	Beet greens, cooked, 1/2 cup	49	19
Buckwheat flour, 1/4 cup	75	101	Navy beans, cooked, 1/2 cup	48	127
Cashews, dry roasted, 1 ounce	74	163	Tofu, firm, prepared with nigari,[b] 1/2 cup	47	88
Soybeans, mature, cooked, 1/2 cup	74	149	Okra, cooked from frozen, 1/2 cup	47	26
Pine nuts, dried, 1 ounce	71	191	Soy beverage, one cup	47	127
Mixed nuts, oil roasted, with peanuts, 1 ounce	67	175	Hazelnuts, 1 ounce	46	178
White beans, canned, 1/2 cup	67	154	Oat bran muffin, 1 ounce	45	77
Pollock, walleye, cooked, 3 ounces	62	96	Great northern beans, cooked, 1/2 cup	44	104
Black beans, cooked, 1/2 cup	60	114	Oat bran, cooked, 1/2 cup	44	44
			Brown rice, cooked, 1/2 cup	42	108
			Haddock, cooked, 3 ounces	42	95

Source: Nutrient values from Agricultural Research Service (ARS) Nutrient Database for Standard Reference, Release 17. Foods are from ARS single nutrient reports, sorted in descending order by nutrient content in terms of common household measures. Food items and weights in the single nutrient reports are adapted from those in 2002 revision of USDA Home and Garden Bulletin No. 72, Nutritive Value of Foods. Mixed dishes and multiple preparations of the same food item have been omitted from this table.

[a]Food Sources of Magnesium ranked by milligrams of magnesium per standard amount; also calories in the standard amount. (All are ≥ 10% of RDA for adult men, which is 420 mg/d).

[b]Calcium sulfate and magnesium chloride.

positive lifestyle modification for preventing and managing high blood pressure. Elevated blood glucose levels increase the loss of magnesium in the urine, which in turn lowers blood levels of magnesium; this explains why low blood levels of magnesium are seen in poorly controlled type 1 and type 2 diabetes.

Sources. Magnesium is present in many foods but usually in small amounts. Eating a wide variety of foods, including five servings of fruits and vegetables daily and plenty of whole grains, helps to ensure an AI. The center of the chlorophyll molecule in green vegetables contains magnesium. Intake from a meal may be 45–55% absorbed. Beware of excess phytates. Water can provide magnesium, but the amount varies according to the water supply. "Hard" water contains more magnesium than "soft" water. Dietary surveys do not estimate magnesium intake from water, which may lead to underestimating total magnesium intake and its variability (see Table A-8).

Signs of Deficiency. When magnesium deficiency occurs (hypomagnesemia), it is usually due to excessive loss of magnesium in urine from diabetes, antibiotics, diuretics, or excessive alcohol use; gastrointestinal (GI) system disorders; chronically low intake of magnesium; chronic or excessive vomiting, diarrhea, and fat malabsorption. Magnesium deficiency can cause metabolic changes that may contribute to heart attacks, strokes, and postmenopausal osteoporosis. Poor growth, confusion, disorientation, loss of appetite, depression, tetany with muscle contractions and cramps, tingling, numbness, abnormal heart rhythms, coronary spasm, abnormal nerve function with seizures or convulsions, hyperirritability, and even death can occur.

Signs of Excess. Magnesium toxicity (hypermagnesemia) is often associated with kidney failure, when the kidney loses the ability to remove excess magnesium. Mental status changes, nausea, osmotic diarrhea, appetite loss, muscle weakness, difficulty breathing, respiratory failure, extremely low blood pressure, and irregular heartbeat can occur. High doses of magnesium from laxatives can promote diarrhea, even with normal kidney function. The elderly are at risk of magnesium toxicity; kidney function declines with age and use of magnesium-containing laxatives and antacids is common.

Phosphorus: Phosphorus is second only to calcium in quantity in the human body. About 80% is in the skeleton and teeth as calcium phosphate; 20% is in extracellular fluid and cells. About 10% is bound to protein. *RDA for adult men and women is 700 mg/d. UL for adults varies from 3–4 g/d.*

Roles. Energy metabolism (ADP, ATP); fat, amino acid, and carbohydrate metabolism; calcium regulation; vitamin utilization; bones and teeth; osmotic pressure; DNA coding; buffer salts; fatty acid transport; oxygen transport and release; leukocyte phagocytosis; and microbial resistance.

Sources. Protein-rich foods such as meat, poultry, fish, egg yolks, dried beans and nuts, whole grains, enriched breads and cereals, milk, cheese, and dairy products. Also found in peas, corn, chocolate, and seeds. Excessive intake of soft drinks increases phosphorus intake, often causing an unbalanced intake of calcium. About 70% of oral intake is absorbed. In the United States, milk and cheese products contribute the main sources of phosphorus for infants, toddlers, and adolescents; meat, poultry, and fish products contribute more to the diets of adults.

Signs of Deficiency. Hypophosphatemia leads to neuromuscular, renal and hematological changes, as well as rickets or osteomalacia. Deficiency is rare but may occur in those persons who take phosphate binders, persons receiving total parenteral nutrition without phosphate, and prematurity.

Signs of Excess. Hyperphosphatemia is especially problematic in renal failure. Nutritional secondary hyperparathyroidism may occur, with fragile bones and fractures.

Potassium: Potassium constitutes about 5% of total mineral content in the body. It is the main intracellular ion. *No specific RDA exists.*

Roles. Nerve conduction, muscle contraction, glycolysis, glycogen formation, protein synthesis and utilization, acid–base balance, cellular enzyme functioning, and water balance.

Sources. Fruits and vegetables, dried beans and peas, whole grains, and whole and skim milk. In the United States, milk and cheese products, meat, poultry, and fish products contribute the most; vegetables follow. Table A-9 provides a list of foods that contain over 500 mg potassium per serving.

Signs of Deficiency. Hypokalemia includes muscle weakness, cardiac arrhythmia, paralysis, bone fragility, decreased growth, weight loss, and even death.

Signs of Excess. Hyperkalemia promotes paralysis, muscular weakness, arrhythmias, heart disturbances, and even death.

Sodium: Sodium constitutes about 2% of total mineral content in the body. It is the main extracellular ion, along with chloride. *No specific RDA is set; 2300 mg/d is the UL for adults.*

Roles. Nerve stimulation, muscle contraction, acid–base balance, regulation of blood pressure, and glucose transport into cells. Sodium is the major extracellular fluid cation.

Sources. Milk, cheese, eggs, meat, fish, poultry, beets, carrots, celery, spinach, chard, seasoned salts, baking powder and soda, table salt (NaCl), many drugs and preservatives, some drinking water. High-sodium processed foods include: salty snack foods; ketchup and mustard; cured and processed meats; processed cheese; canned soups, vegetables, beans, and meats; soup, rice, and pasta mixes; soy sauce or hoisin sauce; monosodium glutamate (MSG); garlic salt, onion salt, celery salt, and seasoned salts. More than 95% of sodium from a mixed diet is absorbed.

TABLE A-9 Food Sources of Potassium[a]

Food, Standard Amount	Potassium (mg)	Calories
Sweet potato, baked, one potato (146 g)	694	131
Tomato paste, 1/4 cup	664	54
Beet greens, cooked, 1/2 cup	655	19
Potato, baked, flesh, one potato (156 g)	610	145
White beans, canned, 1/2 cup	595	153
Yogurt, plain, nonfat, 8-ounce container	579	127
Tomato puree, 1/2 cup	549	48
Clams, canned, 3 ounces	534	126
Yogurt, plain, low-fat, 8-ounce container	531	143
Prune juice, 3/4 cup	530	136
Carrot juice, 3/4 cup	517	71
Blackstrap molasses, one tbsp	498	47
Halibut, cooked, 3 ounces	490	119
Soybeans, green, cooked, 1/2 cup	485	127
Tuna, yellowfin, cooked, 3 ounces	484	118
Lima beans, cooked, 1/2 cup	484	104
Winter squash, cooked, 1/2 cup	448	40
Soybeans, mature, cooked, 1/2 cup	443	149
Rockfish, Pacific, cooked, 3 ounces	442	103
Cod, Pacific, cooked, 3 ounces	439	89
Banana, one medium	422	105
Spinach, cooked, 1/2 cup	419	21
Tomato juice, 3/4 cup	417	31
Tomato sauce, 1/2 cup	405	39
Peaches, dried, uncooked, 1/4 cup	398	96
Prunes, stewed, 1/2 cup	398	133
Milk, nonfat, one cup	382	83
Pork chop, center loin, cooked, 3 ounces	382	197
Apricots, dried, uncooked, 1/4 cup	378	78
Rainbow trout, farmed, cooked, 3 ounces	375	144
Pork loin, center rib (roasts), lean, roasted, 3 ounces	371	190
Buttermilk, cultured, low-fat, one cup	370	98
Cantaloupe, 1/4 medium	368	47
1–2% milk, one cup	366	102–122
Honeydew melon, 1/8 medium	365	58
Lentils, cooked, 1/2 cup	365	115
Plantains, cooked, 1/2 cup slices	358	90
Kidney beans, cooked, 1/2 cup	358	112
Orange juice, 3/4 cup	355	85
Split peas, cooked, 1/2 cup	355	116
Yogurt, plain, whole milk, 8-ounce container	352	138

Source: Nutrient values from Agricultural Research Service (ARS) Nutrient Database for Standard Reference, Release 17. Foods are from ARS single nutrient reports, sorted in descending order by nutrient content in terms of common household measures. Food items and weights in the single nutrient reports are adapted from those in 2002 revision of USDA Home and Garden Bulletin No. 72, Nutritive Value of Foods.

[a]Food sources of potassium ranked by milligrams of potassium per standard amount, also showing calories in the standard amount. The AI for adults is 4700 mg/d potassium.

Signs of Deficiency. Hyponatremia occur from water intoxication with resulting anorexia, nausea, muscle atrophy, poor growth, weight loss, confusion, coma, and even death.

Signs of Excess. Hypernatremia may cause confusion, high blood pressure, calcium excretion from bones, heart failure, edema, and coma.

Sulfur: Sulfur exists as part of the amino acids methionine, cystine, and cysteine and as part of the antioxidant glutathione peroxidase and other organic molecules. *No specific RDA is set.*

Roles. Amino acids (methionine, cystine, cysteine), thiamin molecule, coenzyme A, biotin and pantothenic acid, connective tissue metabolism, penicillin, sulfa drugs, insulin molecule, heparin, and keratin of skin, hair, and nails.

Sources. Meat, poultry, fish, eggs, dried beans and legumes, *Brassica* family vegetables (broccoli, cabbage, cauliflower, Brussels sprouts), and wheat germ.

Signs of Deficiency. Not specific but likely to occur with hypoalbuminemia.

Signs of Excess. Uncommon because excess is excreted in the urine as sulfate, usually in combination with calcium. This may result in hypercalciuria (often after a high-protein meal).

Trace Minerals

Trace minerals are elements that are found in minute amounts in body tissues and are specific to the function of certain enzymes. They are typically not found in free ionic state but are bound to other proteins.

Copper: Copper is an antioxidant. Concentrations of copper are highest in the liver, brain, heart, and kidney; skeletal muscle also contains a large percentage because of total mass. About 90% of copper is bound as ceruloplasmin and is transported to other tissues mainly by albumin. Absorption occurs in the proximal jejunum. *RDA is 900 mg* daily for men and women. UL was set at 10 mg/d.

Roles: Skeletal development, immunity, formation of RBCs and leukopoiesis, phospholipid synthesis, electron transport, pigmentation, aortic elasticity, connective tissue formation, and CNS and myelin sheath structure. Part of metalloenzymes including cytochrome c-odixase.

Sources: Barley and whole grains, oysters and shellfish, nuts, dried beans and legumes, cocoa, eggs, prunes, and potatoes. Note: Milk is low in copper. Daily intake of copper in the United States is 2–5 mg; however, many persons have a lower intake than this because fresh foods are low in copper. Meat, poultry, and fish are primary sources in the United States. Approximately 30–60% of oral intake is absorbed, enhanced by acid and decreased by calcium. 94% of copper is tightly bound to ceruloplasmin.

Signs of Deficiency. Hypochromic anemia, cardiomyopathy, leukopenia, neutropenia, skeletal abnormalities and osteoporosis, decreased skin and hair pigmentation, Menke's steel hair (kinky-hair) syndrome, and reduced immune response. Deficiency is rare in adults, except with celiac disease, protein-losing enteropathies, and nephrotic syndrome. Requirement is increased by excessive zinc intake.

Signs of Excess. Excess is rare, but liver cirrhosis, biliary cirrhosis, and Wilson's disease may contribute to the retention of copper. Abnormalities in RBC formation, copper deposits in the brain, diarrhea, tremors, and liver damage occur. Eye rings are present in Wilson's disease. Excesses may decrease vitamin A absorption.

Fluoride: Fluoride is found in nearly all drinking waters and soils. The American Dietetic Association affirms that fluoride is an important element for all mineralized tissues and that appropriate consumption aids bone and tooth health (American Dietetic Association, 2005). Eighty to ninety percent of oral intake is absorbed. *RDA is 3–4 mg/d for men and women. UL is set at 10 mg/d.*

Roles.: Calcium uptake; some role in prevention of calcified aortas; resistance to dental caries, collapsed vertebrae, and osteoporosis; formation of hydroxyapatite; and enamel growth.

Sources. Fluoridated water, tea, mackerel, salmon with bones, infant foods to which bone meal has been added.

Signs of Deficiency. Dental caries, calcification of aorta, and anemia. Possibly bone thinning and osteoporosis.

Signs of Excess. Bony outgrowths at the spine. Tooth mottling, pitting, and discoloration (fluorosis) occur at doses of greater than 2–3 ppm in the drinking water. Excess can result in neurological problems; this feature is used in rat poison, for example.

Iron

Functional iron is found in hemoglobin (two-thirds), myoglobin (almost one-third), and enzymes. Storage iron is found in ferritin, hemosiderin, and transferrin. Iron is conserved and reused at a rate of 90% daily; the rest is excreted, mainly in bile. Dietary iron must be consumed to meet the 10% gap to prevent deficiency. To increase iron absorption, use sulfur amino acids and vitamin C (especially with nonheme foods); cook foods in an iron skillet; choose iron-enriched rice and do not rinse before cooking. Take iron separately from calcium supplements. Excessive calcium intake and oxalic, tannic, and phytic acids can reduce absorption. Avoid coffee and tea for 1 hour after eating; the tannic acid blocks iron absorption. Serum iron is largely bound to transferrin. About 5–15% is absorbed as ferrous iron; 15–25% of oral intake of heme iron is absorbed (meat, fish, and poultry); 2–20% of oral intake of nonheme iron is absorbed (legumes, grains, and fruit). *The RDA is 8 mg for men and postmenopausal women; 18 mg for premenopausal women. Pregnant women need 27 mg/d and breastfeeding women need 9 mg. Teenage girls (ages 14–18 years) need 15 mg iron per day (27 mg if pregnant; 10 mg if breastfeeding). Teenage boys (ages 14–18 years) need 11 mg iron per day The UL for iron is 45 mg/d.*

Roles. Responsible for carrying oxygen to cells through hemoglobin and myoglobin, skeletal muscle functioning, cognitive functioning, leukocyte functions and T-cell immunity, cellular enzymes, and cytochrome content for normal cellular respiration.

Sources: Beans, beef, dried fruit, enriched grains, fortified cereals, pork. In the United States, grain products provide the highest amount of dietary iron (see Table A-10).

Signs of Deficiency. Hypochromic and microcytic anemia, fatigue and weakness, pallor, pale conjunctiva, koilonychia (thin, spoon-shaped nails), impaired learning ability, cheilosis, glossitis, pica, tachycardia. Deficiency is defined as having an abnormal value for two of three laboratory tests of iron status (erythrocyte protoporphyrin, transferrin saturation, or serum ferritin). Iron deficiency anemia is defined as iron deficiency plus low hemoglobin. Iron deficiency anemia is the most common nutrient deficiency in the world, especially among toddlers, teenage girls, and women of childbearing age.

Signs of Excess. Iron deposits (hemosiderosis); vomiting or diarrheas with GI distress, hemochromatosis, drowsiness. Excess may occur from taking iron supplements daily or from consuming multiple sources, including transfusion overload with sickle cell anemia or thalassemia major.

Zinc: Zinc is distributed in the body with proteins such as albumin, transferrin, ceruloplasmin, and gamma-globulin.

TABLE A-10 Food Sources of Iron[a]

Food, Standard Amount	Heme (H) or Nonheme (N)	Iron (mg)	Calories
Clams, canned, drained, 3 ounces	H	23.8	126
Fortified ready-to-eat cereals (various), ~1 ounce	N	1.8–21.1	54-127
Oysters, eastern, wild, cooked, moist heat, 3 ounces	H	10.2	116
Organ meats (liver, giblets), various, cooked, 3 ounces[b]	N	5.2–9.9	134–235
Fortified instant cooked cereals (various), one packet	N	4.9–8.1	Varies
Soybeans, mature, cooked, 1/2 cup	N	4.4	149
Pumpkin and squash seed kernels, roasted, 1 ounce	N	4.2	148
White beans, canned, 1/2 cup	N	3.9	153
Blackstrap molasses, one tbsp	N	3.5	47
Lentils, cooked, 1/2 cup	N	3.3	115
Spinach, cooked from fresh, 1/2 cup	N	3.2	21
Beef, chuck, blade roast, lean, cooked, 3 ounces	H	3.1	215
Beef, bottom round, lean, 0 inch fat, all grades, cooked, 3 ounces	H	2.8	182
Kidney beans, cooked, 1/2 cup	N	2.6	112
Sardines, canned in oil, drained, 3 ounces	H	2.5	177
Beef, rib, lean, 1/4 inches fat, all grades, 3 ounces	H	2.4	195
Chickpeas, cooked, 1/2 cup	N	2.4	134
Duck, meat only, roasted, 3 ounces	H	2.3	171
Lamb, shoulder, arm, lean, 1/4 inches fat, choice, cooked, 3 ounces	H	2.3	237
Prune juice, 3/4 cup	N	2.3	136
Shrimp, canned, 3 ounces	H	2.3	102
Cowpeas, cooked, 1/2 cup	N	2.2	100
Ground beef, 15% fat, cooked, 3 ounces	H	2.2	212
Tomato puree, 1/2 cup	N	2.2	48
Lima beans, cooked, 1/2 cup	N	2.2	108
Soybeans, green, cooked, 1/2 cup	N	2.2	127
Navy beans, cooked, 1/2 cup	N	2.1	127
Refried beans, 1/2 cup	N	2.1	118
Beef, top sirloin, lean, 0 inch fat, all grades, cooked, 3 ounces	H	2.0	156
Tomato paste, 1/4 cup	N	2.0	54

Source: Nutrient values from Agricultural Research Service (ARS) Nutrient Database for Standard Reference, Release 17. Foods are from ARS single nutrient reports, sorted in descending order by nutrient content in terms of common household measures. Food items and weights in the single nutrient reports are adapted from those in 2002 revision of USDA Home and Garden Bulletin No. 72, Nutritive Value of Foods. Mixed dishes and multiple preparations of the same food item have been omitted from this table.

[a]Food Sources of iron ranked by milligrams of iron per standard amount; also calories in the standard amount. All are ≥ 10% of RDA for teen and adult females, which is 18 mg/d.

[b]High in cholesterol.

Animal sources are better utilized; vegetarian diets must be monitored for zinc deficiency. Ten to forty percent of zinc from meals is absorbed in the duodenum and the jejunum. Vitamin D can increase bioavailability. Phytates, excess copper, and fiber form complexes and reduce absorption, as do calcium and phosphate salts. Zinc absorption is affected by level of zinc in the diet and interfering substances, such as phytates, calcium, cadmium, folic acid, copper, or excessive fiber. Albumin is the major plasma carrier. *RDA is 11 mg for men and 8 mg for women. UL is 40 mg.*

Roles. ACTH-stimulated steroidogenesis in adrenals; sexual maturation; fatty acid, carbohydrate, protein, and nucleic acid metabolism; CO_2 transport; amino acid breakdown from peptides; oxidation of vitamin A; reproduction; growth; enzymes including alcohol dehydrogenase, alkaline phosphatase, and lactic acid dehydrogenase; wound healing; catalyst for hydrogenation; immunity; night vision; alcohol detoxification in the liver; heme synthesis; taste and smell acuity; synthesis of glutathione; and collagen precursors. Zinc supplementation has been shown to be effective in reducing morbidity and mortality from diarrhea, malaria, HIV infection, sickle cell anemia, renal disease, and GI disorders. Zinc gluconate lozenges do not always alleviate cold symptoms in children and adolescents but may be somewhat helpful.

Sources. Beans, seafood (e.g., lobster, shrimp, oysters), poultry, meat (red meat such as beef and liver especially), eggs, milk, peanuts, oatmeal, whole grains (e.g., whole wheat, rye bread, wheat germ), and yeast. The average American diet contains 10–15 mg/d. Meat, poultry, and fish are the primary sources of zinc.

Signs of Deficiency. Zinc is so prevalent in cellular metabolism that even minor impairment in supply is likely to have multiple biological and clinical effects. Deficiency reduces antibody responses and cell-mediated immunity and may cause dermatitis, skin lesions, growth failure (dwarfism), hypogonadism, decreased taste acuity (hypogeusia), alopecia, diarrhea, glossitis, stomatitis, and impaired wound healing. Zinc deficiency has a significant impact on development and on immune function; premature infants and children are at greatest risk. In children with zinc deficiency, severe growth depression is seen. Strict vegetarians, preschoolers who do not eat meat, adolescent females, and those on a chronically high-phytate diet may also be at risk, especially if other disease states are present.

Signs of Excess. Vomiting, diarrhea, low levels of serum copper, hyperamylasemia may result. Excessive zinc intake is probably self-limiting because of GI distress that occurs. Zinc toxicity can occur in renal dialysis if not carefully monitored.

Ultra-Trace Minerals

Boron: Boron can be found in the brain and the bone; it is also found in the spleen and thyroid. It is found in foods such as sodium borate; it is absorbed at a rate of 90%. *No RDA has been set, but a UL of 20 mg was established.*

Roles. Mineral metabolism in animals and humans, cell membrane functioning. It may function in a role similar to estrogen in bone metabolism and strengthening.

Sources. Drinking water, wine, cider and beer, noncitrus fruits, potatoes, peanuts, and legumes. Note: Protein foods and grains are low in boron. Infant foods, fruits and fruit juices, milk and cheese foods, and beverages provide the most.

Signs of Deficiency. None known at this time.

Signs of Excess. Reproductive and developmental effects are possible.

Chromium: Chromium is closely related to insulin action. Absorption ranges from 0.5 to 2%. Chromium needs transferrin for distribution. *RDA is 20 mg/d for women and 35 mg/d for men.* No UL has been set.

Roles. Insulin molecule (part of glucose tolerance factor known as chromodulin); fatty acid, triglyceride, and cholesterol metabolism; normal glucose metabolism; nucleic acid stability; regulation of gene expression; and peripheral nerve functioning.

Sources. Oysters, liver, potatoes, eggs, vegetable oil, brewer's yeast, whole grains and bran, shortening, nuts, and peanuts. Dairy products, fruits, and vegetables are low in chromium. Phytates and oxalates can decrease absorption.

Signs of Deficiency. Hyperglycemia refractory to insulin, weight loss, glucosuria, peripheral neuropathy, encephalopathy. Deficiency may be found in severe malnutrition, in diabetes, or in elderly patients with cardiovascular disease.

Signs of Excess. Dermatological allergy, nausea, vomiting, convulsions, irritation, gastrointestinal ulcers.

Cobalt: Most cobalt is in vitamin B_{12} stores in the liver. Cobalt may share intestinal transport with iron and is increased in patients with low iron intake and iron stores. *No specific RDA is set.*

Roles. Treatment of some anemias, part of structure of cobalamin in vitamin B_{12}, role in immunity, and healthy nerves and RBCs.

Sources. Seafood (such as oysters and clams), meats (such as liver), poultry, some grains, and cereals. Note: Cow's milk is very low. More than 50% of dietary cobalt is absorbed.

Signs of Deficiency. Weakness, anemia, and emaciation. Deficiency is usually in conjunction with vitamin B_{12} deficiency and low intake of protein foods. Lack of intrinsic factor, gastrectomy, or malabsorption syndromes may also cause deficiency.

Signs of Excess. Polycythemia, bone marrow hyperplasia, reticulocytosis, and increased blood volume may result.

Iodine: With the iodization of salt, iodine deficiency has been almost eliminated in the United States and Western nations. Fortification results in fewer goiters and less cretinism, stillbirths, spontaneous abortions, and mental or growth retardation. Millions of people are at risk in other nations. The thyroid gland maintains 75% of the body's iodine; the rest is in the gastric mucosa and bloodstream. Iodide content of vegetables varies by the content of the local soil. Absorption is 50–100% from the gut. *RDA is 150 mg*/d for both men and women. UL is 1.1 mg/d.

Roles. Energy metabolism, proper thyroid functioning, normal growth and reproduction, prevention of goiter, and regulation of cellular metabolism and temperature. Iodine is found with T3 and T4 distribution.

Sources. Iodized salt, seaweed, and seafood (clams, oysters, sardines, lobster, and saltwater fish). Other lesser sources may include cream (in milk), eggs, drinking water in various areas, plant leaves (broccoli, spinach, and turnip greens), cranberries, and legumes. Iodized salt should be encouraged for pregnant women. Goitrogens in cabbage, turnips, rapeseeds, peanuts, cassava, and soybeans may block uptake of iodine by body cells; heating and cooking inactivate them.

Signs of Deficiency. Enlarged thyroid gland or related goiter; hypercholesterolemia; weight gain; cold intolerance; thinning hair; cognitive impairment; deafness; decreased metabolic rate; neuromuscular impairments. In infants, abnormal fetal growth, brain development, and cretinism can result.

Signs of Excess. Excess may depress thyroid activity and elevate thyroid-stimulating hormone (TSH) levels. High levels of thyroid hormone with goiter or myxedema can occur.

Manganese: Manganese affects reproductive capacity, pancreatic function, and carbohydrate metabolism. Less than 5% is absorbed from diet. It is transported bound to a macroglobulin, transferrin, or transmanganin. Manganese, cobalt, and iron compete for pathways. Human milk tends to be low in manganese levels. *An AI level has been set at 2.3 mg for men and 1.8 mg for women. The UL has been established at 11 mg.*

Roles. Polysaccharide and fatty acid metabolism, enzyme activation, tendon and skeletal development, possible role in hypertension, fertility and reproduction (role in squalene as a precursor of cholesterol and sex hormones), melanin and dopamine production, energy and glucose production.

Sources. Tea, coffee, whole grains, wheat germ and bran, blueberries, peas, beans and dried legumes, nuts, spinach, and cocoa powder. Sources of manganese are plant foods, not animal foods. In the United States, grain products are primary sources.

Signs of Deficiency. Nausea, vomiting, transient dermatitis, weight loss, ataxia, skeletal and cartilage abnormalities occur. Beware of excess calcium, phosphorus, iron, or magnesium supplementation.

Signs of Excess. Excesses accumulate in the liver and CNS. Parkinsonian tremors, difficulty in walking, facial muscle spasms, ataxia, hyperirritability, or hallucinations can occur.

Molybdenum: Molybdenum is important mostly for its role in xanthine oxidase. About 40–100% of intake is absorbed from the duodenum in protein-bound form. It is readily absorbed from the stomach and small intestine and excreted in the urine. *RDA is 45 mcg for both men and women. The UL is 2 mg.*

Roles. Flavoproteins; copper antagonist; component of sulfite oxidase, aldehyde oxidase, and xanthine oxidase; iron storage; energy metabolism; and degradation of cysteine and methionine through sulfite oxidase.

Sources. Legumes, whole-grain breads and cereals, dark green leafy vegetables, milk and dairy products, and organ meats. Milk and cheese products and grains provide the most from diet.

Signs of Deficiency. Tachycardia, tachypnea, visual and mental changes, elevated plasma methionine, low-serum uric acid, headache, lethargy, nausea, and vomiting. Long-term parenteral nutrition that is deficient in molybdenum is a concern.

Signs of Excess. Hyperuricemia and gout-like syndrome can occur. Excesses are rare.

Selenium: Cellular and plasma glutathione are the functional parameters for measuring selenium status. Selenium intake in the United States is generally very good; deficiency is rare. More than 50% dietary intake is absorbed (average range, 35–85%). It is transported via albumin from the duodenum. *RDA level for selenium was set at 55 mg*/d; *UL was set at 400 mg.*

Roles. Selenium functions within mammals primarily as selenoproteins. Glutathione catalyzes the reduction of peroxides that can cause cellular damage. Protein biosynthesis (selenomethionine and selenocysteine), sparing of vitamin E, protection against mercury toxicity; some role in thyroid function and immunity.

Sources. Seafood and fish, chicken, egg yolks, meats (especially kidney and liver), whole-grain breads and cereals, wheat germ, foods grown in selenium-rich soil including garlic, dairy products, Brazil nuts, and onions. Dietary selenium is found with protein in animal tissue (muscle meats, organ meats, and seafood). Grains and seeds have variable amounts dependent on the soil.

Signs of Deficiency. Muscle weakness and pain, carcinogenesis, and cardiomyopathy. Keshan's disease with cardiomyopathy is a selenium deficiency in China where soil levels are quite low. Kashin-Beck's disease occurs in preadolescents and adolescents; it has effects similar to osteoarthritis with stiffness and swelling of the elbows, knees, and ankles.

Signs of Excess. Selenosis causes garlicky odor on the breath and decaying of teeth. Nausea, vomiting, hair and nail loss, fatigue, headache, and chronic dermatitis can also occur.

Less-Studied Ultra-Trace Minerals

Aluminum, Arsenic, Cadmium, Lead, Lithium, and Tin: Not much is known about the roles, functions, or purpose in the human body of these minerals. For all age groups, grain products (mainly cornbread, pancakes, biscuits, muffins, and yellow cake) provide the highest amount of aluminum in the diet. Organic arsenic is found in dairy products, meats, poultry, fish, grains and cereal. Inorganic arsenic is toxic.

Nickel: There may be roles in iron and zinc metabolism, hematopoiesis, DNA and RNA, and enzyme activation. Less than 10% of nickel is absorbed. It is transported by serum albumin. Nickel hypersensitivity can occur from prior dermal contact. *No RDA has been set, but UL was established at 1 mg/d.*

Sources. Nuts, legumes, cereals, sweeteners, chocolate candy, and chocolate milk powders.

Silicon: There may be roles in normal bone growth and calcification; collagen and connective tissue formation in the presence of calcium.

Natural food and water sources do not seem to cause adverse health effects. *No RDA or UL have been established.*

Sources. Most plant-based foods. Grains and beer are good sources.

Vanadium: Vanadium seems to have a role in thyroid metabolism. High doses may cause biochemical changes that precede cancer. *No RDA has been set. UL was established at 1.8 mg/d.*

Sources. Shellfish, whole grains, mushrooms, black pepper, parsley, and dill seed.

VITAMINS

Vitamins were first named "vital amines" in 1912 because they seemed to be important to life. Once it was known that they contain few amine groups, the "e" was dropped. There are 13 known vitamins (four fat-soluble and nine water-soluble vitamins). They are organic compounds, containing carbon structures. The best nutritional strategy for promoting optimal health and reducing the risk of chronic disease is to obtain adequate nutrients from a wide variety of foods. Eating more whole grains, fruits and vegetables is the recommendation, rather than taking supplements. Supplements are needed in special cases, such as in pregnancy and in some medical conditions. Supplements are most useful when taken as a multivitamin supplement that meets 100% of the daily recommended values. Although fat-soluble vitamins should not be consumed above UL doses, meeting 100% DRI levels is safe.

Fat-Soluble Vitamins

Vitamin A (Retinol, Retinal, Retinoic Acid): Vitamin A is best known for its role in vision and skin integrity. From 7–65% of vitamin A from the diet is absorbed in the mucosal cells of the small intestine. There, dietary retinyl esters are hydrolyzed by pancreatic triglyceride lipase (PTL), and the intestinal brush border phospholipase. Once in the cell, retinol is complexed with cellular retinol-binding protein type 2 (CRBP2), a substrate for reesterification of the retinol by the enzyme lecithin/retinol acyltransferase (LRAT). Retinol-binding protein (RBP) is used for transport. Retinyl esters are incorporated into chylomicrons. Stress can increase excretion; zinc or protein deficiency can decrease transport. Dietary vitamin A is transported via chylomicrons; 90% of vitamin A is stored in the liver. Its provitamins include beta-carotene and cryptoxanthin. *AI for infants is based on the amount of retinol found in human milk. RDA is 900 mg for men and 700 mg for women, adjusted for differences in average body size. UL is 3000 mg/d.*

Functions. Vision (especially night), gene regulation, growth, prevention of early miscarriage, immunity against infection (measles and many others), corticosterones, weight gain, proper bone, tooth, and nerve development, membrane functions, and epithelial tissue integrity in lungs and trachea especially. Vitamin A supplementation is used to treat some forms of cancer and degenerative retinitis pigmentosa.

Sources. See Table A-11 for sources.

TABLE A-11 Food Sources of Vitamin A[a]

Food, Standard Amount	Vitamin A (μg RAE)	Calories
Organ meats (liver, giblets), various, cooked, 3 ounces[b]	1490–9126	134–235
Carrot juice, 3/4 cup	1692	71
Sweet potato with peel, baked, one medium	1096	103
Pumpkin, canned, 1/2 cup	953	42
Carrots, cooked from fresh, 1/2 cup	671	27
Spinach, cooked from frozen, 1/2 cup	573	30
Collards, cooked from frozen, 1/2 cup	489	31
Kale, cooked from frozen, 1/2 cup	478	20
Mixed vegetables, canned, 1/2 cup	474	40
Turnip greens, cooked from frozen, 1/2 cup	441	24
Instant cooked cereals, fortified, prepared, one packet	285–376	75–97
Various ready-to-eat cereals, with added vitamin A, ~1 ounce	180–376	100–117
Carrot, raw, one small	301	20
Beet greens, cooked, 1/2 cup	276	19
Winter squash, cooked, 1/2 cup	268	38
Dandelion greens, cooked, 1/2 cup	260	18
Cantaloupe, raw, 1/4 medium melon	233	46
Mustard greens, cooked, 1/2 cup	221	11
Pickled herring, 3 ounces	219	222
Red sweet pepper, cooked, 1/2 cup	186	19
Chinese cabbage, cooked, 1/2 cup	180	10

Source: Nutrient values from Agricultural Research Service (ARS) Nutrient Database for Standard Reference, Release 17. Foods are from ARS single nutrient reports, sorted in descending order by nutrient content in terms of common household measures. Food items and weights in the single nutrient reports are adapted from those in 2002 revision of USDA Home and Garden Bulletin No. 72, Nutritive Value of Foods. Mixed dishes and multiple preparations of the same food item have been omitted from this table.

[a]Food Sources of vitamin A ranked by micrograms. Retinol Activity Equivalents (RAE) of vitamin A per standard amount; also calories in the standard amount. (All are ≥20% of RDA for adult men, which is 900 mg/d RAE).

[b]High in cholesterol.

Signs of Deficiency. Impaired vision is the first sign. Xerophthalmia, night blindness (nyctalopia), follicular hyperkeratosis or thickening of skin around hair follicles, drying of the whites of the eyes, eventual blindness, spots on the whites of the eyes, infections, and death.

Vulnerable Populations. Anorexia nervosa, burns, biliary obstruction, cancer, cirrhosis, celiac disease, cystic fibrosis, drug use (cholestyramine, mineral oil, and neomycin), hookworm, hepatitis of infectious origin, giardiasis, kwashiorkor, malaria, measles, pancreatic disease, pneumonia, pregnancy, prematurity, rheumatic fever, tropical sprue, and zinc deficiency.

Signs of Excess. Headache, anorexia, abdominal pain, blurred vision, muscle weakness, drowsiness, irritability, peeling of skin, peripheral neuritis, papilledema, serum vitamin A >100 μg/dL. Long-term supplementation with retinol (such as 25,000 IU/d) may have adverse effects on blood lipid levels and bone health. Vitamin A is known for its teratogenic affects; pregnant women should consider taking it in the form of beta-carotene. Caution should be given to supplement use in women of childbearing age because many women don't know they are pregnant in the earliest stages; supplements with retinol should be avoided during the first trimester.

Carotenoids: There are more than 500 natural carotenoids. Two beta-carotene molecules are equivalent to one molecule of vitamin A. The bioavailability of carotenoids from vegetables is low; fat is required for adequate absorption. Between 9 and 17% of dietary carotenes are absorbed. Dietary carotenoids may prevent some types of cancer through enhancement of immune response, inhibition of mutagenesis, and protection against oxidative damage to cells; alpha-carotenes, beta-cryptoxanthin, lutein, zeaxanthin, and lycopene contribute to these important functions. Persons at risk for developing lung cancer (i.e., current smokers and workers exposed to asbestos) should *not* take beta-carotene supplements. *No specific RDA recommendations were made for beta-carotene.*

Sources. Beta-carotene is found in deep yellow, orange, or dark green fruits and vegetables such as pumpkin, sweet potato, carrots, spinach, kale, turnip greens, cantaloupe, apricots, romaine lettuce, broccoli, papaya, mango, and tangerine.

Signs of Excess. Hypercarotenodermia involves yellowing of skin and the whites of eyes.

Vitamin D (Calcitriol, D_3): Vitamin D for humans is obtained from sun exposure, food and supplements. It is biologically inert and has to undergo two hydroxylation reactions to become active as Calcitriol (1,25-dihydroxycholecalciferol), or 1,25-dihydroxyvitamin D_3. Steps in metabolism include 7-dehydrocholesterol → previtamin D_3 → cholecalciferol (D_3) → 25-hydroxycholecalciferol → calcitriol (1,25-dihydroxycholecalciferol, the active form). Bile salts are required for absorption; 90% of dietary intake is absorbed. Dietary vitamin D is absorbed with lipid into the intestine by passive diffusion; it is synthesized in the skin from cholesterol that enters the capillary system.

Transport occurs via chylomicrons to the liver. Although five forms of vitamin D have been discovered, the two forms that matter are vitamins D_2 (ergocalciferol) and D_3 (cholecalciferol). There is decreased production from the skin with aging. *2.5 mcg of vitamin D is considered sufficient to prevent vitamin D-deficiency rickets, higher levels of 5* μg/d are recommended for infants and children throughout the period of skeletal development. The AI increases to 10 μg/d for adults aged 51 and older and to 15 μg/d for adults 71 years and older. The UL for infants is 25 μg/d and for children and adults, 50 μg/d.

Functions. The main functions of vitamin D are bone metabolism, calcium homeostasis, and expression of hundreds of genes. Calcitriol plays a key role in the maintenance of many organ systems; the volume and acidity of gastric secretions; growth of soft tissues including skin and pancreas; bone calcification, growth and repair; tooth formation; parathormone (PTH) management; and renal/intestinal phosphate absorption.

Sources. Brief and casual exposure (10–20 minutes daily) to natural sunlight can be encouraged. Check nutrition labels for vitamin D fortification when using soy or rice milks. Food sources of vitamin D are listed in Table A-12.

TABLE A-12 Food Sources of Vitamin D

Foods with Naturally Occurring Vitamin D	International Units
Herring, 3 ounces	1384
Cod liver oil, one tablespoon	1350
Halibut, 3 ounces	510
Catfish, 3 ounces	425
Salmon, canned, 3 ounces	390
Mackerel, 3 ounces	306
Sardines, canned in oil, 1.75 ounces	250
Tuna, canned in oil, 3 ounces	200
Egg yolk, one yolk	20
Beef liver, 3 ounces	15
Swiss cheese, 1 ounce	12
Vitamin D–Fortified Foods	
Soy milk, one cup	119
Milk, one cup	100
Fortified orange juice, one cup	100
Fortified breakfast cereal, one cup	20–100
Fortified yogurt, one cup	80
Fortified margarine, one tablespoon	60

Source: Nutrient values from Agricultural Research Service (ARS) Nutrient Database for Standard Reference, Release 17. Foods are from ARS single nutrient reports, sorted in descending order by nutrient content in terms of common household measures. Food items and weights in the single nutrient reports are adapted from those in 2002 revision of USDA Home and Garden Bulletin No. 72, Nutritive Value of Foods. Mixed dishes and multiple preparations of the same food item have been omitted from this table.

Signs of Deficiency. Hypocalcemic tetany is a low calcium condition in which the patient has overactive neurological reflexes, spasms of the hands and feet, cramps and spasms of the voice box (larynx). Vitamin D from sunlight exposure is low during the winter months. Hypovitaminosis D is related to lowered vitamin D intake, less exposure to ultraviolet light (UVB), anticonvulsant use, renal dialysis, nephrotic syndrome, hypertension, diabetes, winter season, and high PTH and alkaline phosphatase levels. Hypovitaminosis D is common in general medical in-patients. Bowed legs, rickets in children, and osteomalacia in adults may occur.

Vulnerable Populations. The prevalence of vitamin D deficiency is high. The National Health and Nutrition Examination Survey (NHANES) team found that 9% of U. S. children were vitamin D deficient (<15 ng/mL of blood) and another 61% were vitamin D insufficient (15–29 ng/mL). Those individuals with dark skin or who wear protective clothing may also not absorb sufficient vitamin D from sun exposure alone. Living near the North or South Pole in winter is a risk for deficiency. Biliary obstruction, celiac disease, cystic fibrosis, drug use (bile salt binders, glucocorticoids, phenobarbital, primidone, and mineral oil), end-organ failure, Fanconi's disease, hepatic disease, hypertension, primary hypophosphatemia, hypoparathyroidism, inflammatory bowel disease, intestinal malabsorption, lymphatic obstruction, multiple sclerosis, nephrotic syndrome, neurological and psychiatric conditions such as depression and bipolar disorders, pancreatitis, parathyroid surgery, postmenopausal status, prematurity, renal disease and dialysis, small bowel resection, and tropical sprue. Pregnant women should enjoy a few minutes in the sun each day, if possible. Low levels may increase the risk of breast, colon, and prostate cancers; depression, poor brain function, severe dementia in older adults; tuberculosis; pneumonia; bacterial infections and gum disease; autoimmune diseases, such as multiple sclerosis and type 1 diabetes.

Signs of Excess. Patients often complain of headache and nausea, and infants given excessive amounts of vitamin D may have GI upset, bone fragility, and retarded growth. Stupor, confusion, anorexia, nausea, vomiting, constipation, weakness, hypertension, renal stones, polyuria, polydipsia, cardiac arrhythmias, itchy skin, increased bone density on x-ray, calcium deposits throughout the body, increased serum calcium, increased calcium in the urine, elevated serum 25-hydroxycholecalciferol or elevated serum 1,25-dihydroxycholecalciferol levels. In the absence of sufficient vitamin K, excessive vitamin D can cause soft tissue calcification.

Vitamin E (Tocopherol, Tocotrienols): Tocotrienols plus other forms affect cholesterol metabolism, carotid arteries, and immunity against cancer. The natural form is D-alpha-tocopherol (need 22 IU). The DL-alpha-tocopherol form is synthetic and less effective. Vitamin E is absorbed in the upper small intestine by micelle-dependent diffusion. Overall, 20–40% is absorbed with meals; bile and pancreatic secretions are needed and VLDLs and LDLs carry it to tissues. An IU of vitamin E is equal to 0.67 mg of RRR-alpha-tocopherol and 1 mg of all-rac-alpha-tocopherol. *RDA is 15 mg for adults. UL is 1000 mg.*

Functions: The main function of vitamin E is as a lipid-soluble membrane antioxidant, along with vitamin C and selenium. It protects unsaturated phospholipids of the membrane from oxidative degradation through free-radical scavenging. Other roles include anticoagulant and vitamin K antagonist; intracellular respiration; hemopoietic agent; roles in muscular, vascular, reproductive, and CNS systems; some role in reproduction; neutralizes free radicals; protects against cataracts; may relieve discomforts of rheumatoid arthritis; protects against effects of the sun, smog, and lung disease; protects brain cell membranes.

Sources. Tocopherols and tocotrienols are synthesized only by plants so plant products, especially oils, are the best sources of Vitamin E.

Requirements increase with use of PUFAs; if normal needs are 15 mg/d, normal requirements double daily with high PUFA intakes. Gamma-tocopherol is more common in the U. S. food supply (as from soybean oil); it is less useful to the body (see Table A-13).

Signs of Deficiency. Symptoms of deficiency in humans are rare, but can manifest clinically as loss of deep tendon reflexes, impaired vibratory and position sensation, changes in balance and coordination, muscle weakness and visual disturbances. Other targets of deficiency include the vascular and reproductive systems. Rupture of RBCs, impaired vitamin A storage, and prolonged blood coagulation may also occur. For supplementation, pharmacists evaluate equivalent vitamin E dosing as follows:

DL-alpha-tocopheryl acetate	1 mg	1 IU
DL-alpha-tocopherol	0.91 mg	1.1 IU
DL-alpha-tocopheryl acid succinate	1.12 mg	0.89 IU
D-alpha-tocopheryl acid succinate	0.826 mg	1.21 IU

Vulnerable Populations. Alzheimer's disease, arthritis, biliary cirrhosis, bronchopulmonary dysplasia, cardiovascular diseases, cystic fibrosis, drug use (cholestyramine, clofibrate, oral contraceptives, and triiodothyronine), high intake of PUFA in diet, malabsorption syndromes, malnutrition, musculoskeletal disorders, pancreatic diseases, pregnancy, prematurity, pulmonary diseases, and steatorrhea.

Signs of Excess. Vitamin E is one of the least toxic vitamins, but at high doses, it can antagonize the utilization of other fat-soluble vitamins. Excessive intake has caused isolated cases of dermatitis, fatigue, pruritus ani, acne, vasodilation, hypoglycemia, GI symptoms, increased requirement for vitamin K, impaired coagulation, and muscle damage.

Vitamin K: First isolated from alfalfa, the forms of vitamin K are **phylloquinone (K_1)** in green plants; **menaquinone (K_2)** from human bacterial synthesis and **menadione (K_3)** in pharmaceutical form. Vitamin K absorption is optimal with bile and pancreatic juice; 10–70% of dietary intake is usually absorbed. The phylloquinones are absorbed by and energy-dependant process in the small intestine; the menaquinones and menadione are absorbed in the small intestine and colon by passive diffusion. Because intestinal bacteria make about 50% of the bodily requirement, a sterile gut or malabsorption can create deficiency. Vitamin E excesses can reduce absorption of vitamin K. Warfarin (Coumadin) blocks regeneration of active, reduced vitamin K, thus prolonging clotting time,

TABLE A-13 Food Sources of Vitamin E[a]

Food, Standard Amount	AT (mg)	Calories
Fortified ready-to-eat cereals, ~1 ounce	1.6–12.8	90–107
Sunflower seeds, dry roasted, 1 ounce	7.4	165
Almonds, 1 ounce	7.3	164
Sunflower oil, high linoleic, one tbsp	5.6	120
Cottonseed oil, one tbsp	4.8	120
Safflower oil, high oleic, one tbsp	4.6	120
Hazelnuts (filberts), 1 ounce	4.3	178
Mixed nuts, dry roasted, 1 ounce	3.1	168
Turnip greens, frozen, cooked, 1/2 cup	2.9	24
Tomato paste, 1/4 cup	2.8	54
Pine nuts, 1 ounce	2.6	191
Peanut butter, two tbsp	2.5	192
Tomato puree, 1/2 cup	2.5	48
Tomato sauce, 1/2 cup	2.5	39
Canola oil, one tbsp	2.4	124
Wheat germ, toasted, plain, two tbsp	2.3	54
Peanuts, 1 ounce	2.2	166
Avocado, raw, 1/2 avocado	2.1	161
Carrot juice, canned, 3/4 cup	2.1	71
Peanut oil, one tbsp	2.1	119
Corn oil, one tbsp	1.9	120
Olive oil, one tbsp	1.9	119
Spinach, cooked, 1/2 cup	1.9	21
Dandelion greens, cooked, 1/2 cup	1.8	18
Sardine, Atlantic, in oil, drained, 3 ounces	1.7	177
Blue crab, cooked/canned, 3 ounces	1.6	84
Brazil nuts, 1 ounce	1.6	186
Herring, Atlantic, pickled, 3 ounces	1.5	222

Source: Nutrient values from Agricultural Research Service (ARS) Nutrient Database for Standard Reference, Release 17. Foods are from ARS single nutrient reports, sorted in descending order by nutrient content in terms of common household measures. Food items and weights in the single nutrient reports are adapted from those in 2002 revision of USDA Home and Garden Bulletin No. 72, Nutritive Value of Foods. Mixed dishes and multiple preparations of the same food item have been omitted from this table.
[a]Food sources of vitamin E ranked by milligrams of vitamin E per standard amount; also calories in the standard amount. (All provide ≥10% of RDA for vitamin E for adults, which is 15 mg a-tocopherol [AT]/d).

which is best monitored through international normalized ratio (INR) where the timing level of 2–3 is desired. *AI is 120 mg for men and 90 mg for women. No UL has been established, but data are limited and one should not assume that high vitamin K consumption is harmless.*

Functions. Vitamin K is important for normal blood clotting, calcium metabolism, and bone mineralization. Low vitamin K intakes are associated with an increased incidence of hip fractures. Genetic loss of less critical vitamin K–dependent proteins, dietary vitamin K inadequacy, human polymorphisms or mutations, and vitamin K deficiency induced by chronic anticoagulant (warfarin/Coumadin) therapy are all linked to age-associated conditions: bone fragility after estrogen loss (osteocalcin) and arterial calcification linked to cardiovascular disease (McCann and Ames, 2009). Vitamin K is also linked with sphingolipid metabolism in the brain.

Sources. Plant foods such as green leafy vegetables are better sources of vitamin K than animal foods. Fish, liver, meat, eggs, cereal, and some fruits contain smaller amounts (see Table A-14).

Signs of Deficiency. Hemorrhage with prolonged clotting time is the key sign of deficiency, which might even lead to a fatal anemia. Vitamin K deficiency can be found in lipid malabsorption, chronic antibiotic therapy, and liver disease where

TABLE A-14 Food Sources of Vitamin K

Food and Serving Size	Vitamin K (μg)
Kale, cooked 1/2 cup	531
Spinach, cooked 1/2 cup	444
Collard greens, cooked 1/2 cup	418
Beet greens, cooked 1/2 cup	348
Swiss chard, cooked 1/2 cup	286
Turnip greens, cooked, 1/2 cup	265
Mustard greens, cooked 1/2 cup	210
Spinach, raw one cup	145
Broccoli 1/2 cup	110 cooked, 45 raw
Brussels sprouts, cooked 1/2 cup	109
Scallions (including bulb and green tops), raw 1/2 cup	104
Cabbage, cooked 1/2 cup	81
Lettuce (green leaf), raw one cup	97
Prunes, stewed one cup	65
Okra, cooked one cup	64
Parsley one tablespoon	62
Cucumber, raw one large	49
Asparagus, cooked four spears	48
Tuna, canned 3 ounces	37
Celery, raw one cup	35
Black-eyed peas, cooked 1/2 cup	31
Kiwi one medium	30
Blackberries or blueberries, raw one cup	29
Artichoke, cooked one cup	25
Peas 1/2 cup	24
Grapes (red or green) one cup	23
Strawberries, sliced one cup	23
Green beans, cooked 1/2 cup	20
Soy beans or mung beans, cooked 1/2 cup	16–17
Oil, canola, or olive one tablespoon	8–10

Source: Nutrient values from Agricultural Research Service (ARS) Nutrient Database for Standard Reference, Release 17. Foods are from ARS single nutrient reports, sorted in descending order by nutrient content in terms of common household measures. Food items and weights in the single nutrient reports are adapted from those in 2002 revision of USDA Home and Garden Bulletin No. 72, Nutritive Value of Foods. Mixed dishes and multiple preparations of the same food item have been omitted from this table.

bleeding and hypoprothrombinemia can result. Giving an injection of vitamin K upon birth prevents hemorrhagic disease of newborns. In addition, there are 16 known vitamin K–dependent (VKD) proteins; five of them have critical functions with preferential distribution of dietary vitamin K1 to the liver to preserve coagulation function when vitamin K1 is limiting (McCann and Ames, 2009).

Vulnerable Populations. Individuals who practice pica or have calcium disorders, use certain medications (anticoagulants, cholestyramine, mineral oil, phenytoin, neomycin or other antibiotics, or large doses of aspirin), hepatic biliary obstruction, hepatocellular disease, malabsorption syndromes, postmenopausal women at risk for hip fractures, prematurity, and small bowel disorders. Individuals who take large doses of vitamin A or E may also acquire a vitamin K deficiency.

Signs of Excess. Prolonged bleeding time. Menadione can be toxic if given in excessive dose; severe jaundice in infants or hemolytic anemia may result. Seek consistency in vitamin K intake while using warfarin; aim for 120 μg/d for men and 90 μg/d for women. Although dietary sources do not appear to be dangerous, excessive menadione can be toxic and may cause hemolytic anemia.

REFERENCE

McCann JC, Ames B. Vitamin K, an example of triage theory: is micronutrient inadequacy linked to diseases of aging? *Am J Clin Nutr.* 90:889, 2009.

Water-Soluble Vitamins

Thiamin (Vitamin B_1): Known as the "morale" vitamin, thiamin is beneficial for nerve and heart function. Thiamin is absorbed by the proximal small intestine by active transport in low doses and passive diffusion in high doses. High-CHO intakes, pregnancy, lactation, increased basal metabolic rate, and antibiotic use will all increase needs. As energy intake from protein and fat increases, thiamin requirement decreases. The extent of absorption varies widely. Thiamin hydrochloride is the common supplemental form. The DRIs for thiamin include AIs for infants as found in human milk; RDAs are based on levels of energy intake. *RDA is 1.2 mg/d for men and 1.1 mg/d for women. No UL was established.*

Functions. Thiamin is mainly a coenzyme for decarboxylations of 2-keto acids and transketolations. It prevents beriberi and has a role in cell respiration, RNA and DNA formation, protein catabolism, growth, appetite, normal muscle tone in cardiac and digestive tissues, neurologic functioning. It is a coenzyme in the energy-producing Krebs' cycle, with thiamin pyrophosphate (TPP) at the pyruvic acid step. Magnesium, manganese, riboflavin, and vitamin B_6 are synergists. Thiamin is essential for conversions derived from the amino acids methionine, threonine, leucine, isoleucine, and valine. Acetylcholine synthesis also requires thiamin.

Sources. Liver, fortified cereals, dried legumes such a split peas, brown rice, organ and lean meats, whole grains such as oats and whole wheat, nuts, cornmeal, enriched flour or bread, dried milk, wheat germ, dried egg yolk or whole egg, green peas, and seeds. Note: Two slices of bread or one slice of bread and one serving of cereal will provide 15% of the daily RDA. Some nutrients are thiamin sparing; others destroy the nutrient. Thiamin is spared by fat, protein, sorbitol, and vitamin C; antagonists include raw fish, tea, coffee, blueberries, and red cabbage. Avoid cooking with excessive water and alkaline products such as baking soda; thiamin is lost readily.

Signs of Deficiency. Anorexia, calf muscle weakness, weight loss, cardiac and neurologic signs. Eventually, beriberi occurs with mental confusion, muscular wasting, edema, peripheral neuropathy, and tachycardia. Energy deprivation and inactivity are causes of dry (nonedematous) beriberi. Wernicke's encephalopathy is due to thiamin deficiency and often associated with malnutrition and alcoholism. TPN without multivitamin use can lead to symptoms of Wernicke's encephalopathy.

Vulnerable Populations. Individuals who have alcoholism, cancers, cardiomyopathies, CHO (high intakes), celiac disease, children with congenital heart disease before and after surgery, congestive heart failure, fever, high parenteral glucose loading, lactation and pregnancy, tropical sprue, and thyrotoxicosis are at risk.

Signs of Excess. Respiratory failure and death with large doses (1000 times nutritional needs). With 100 times the normal dose, headache, convulsions, muscular weakness, cardiac arrhythmia, and allergic reactions have been noted. Massive doses greater than 1000 times the estimated needs suppress the respiratory center and lead to death.

Riboflavin (Vitamin B_2): Riboflavin is important in CHO metabolism and maintenance of healthy mucous membranes.

Riboflavin is absorbed in the free form by a carrier-mediated process in the proximal small intestine. The DRIs for riboflavin include AIs for infants and RDAs based on the amount required to maintain normal tissue reserves based on urinary excretion, RBC riboflavin contents, and erythrocyte glutathione reductase activity. *RDA is 1.3 mg/d for men and 1.1 mg/d for women.* Requirements are higher during pregnancy and lactation. *No UL was established.*

Functions. It is the main coenzyme in redox reactions of fatty acids and the tricarboxylic acid (TCA) cycle. Cell respiration, oxidation reduction, conversion of tryptophan to niacin, component of retinal pigment, involvement in all metabolisms (especially fat), purine degradation, adrenocortical function, coenzyme in electron transport as flavin adenine dinucleotide (FAD) and flavin mononucleotide (FMN), healthy mucous membranes, skin and eyes, growth, and proper functioning of niacin and pyridoxine.

Sources. Milk, yogurt, cheese, egg whites, liver, beef, chicken, fish, legumes, peanuts, enriched grains and fortified cereals. Body size, growth, activity excesses, and fat metabolism affect daily requirements. Avoid excesses of niacin and methylxanthines. Light destroys riboflavin; buy milk in opaque cartons. As protein intake increases, the need for riboflavin decreases. Riboflavin is spared by dextrins and starch and is found in greater amounts in protein foods. Cheilosis causes a magenta-colored tongue.

Signs of Deficiency. Deficiencies are first evident in the tissues that have rapid cellular turnover such as the skin and epithelia. Seborrheic dermatitis of the nasolabial folds, ears, and/or eyelids; itchy and burning eyes or lips, mouth, and tongue; cheilosis (fissures and scaling of lips); angular stomatitis; glossitis with purplish-red, swollen tongue; peripheral neuropathy; dyssebacea (sharkskin); corneal vascularization; photophobia; lacrimation; normochromic normocytic anemia with erythroid hypoplasia; pancytopenia due to generalized marrow hypoplasia. Riboflavin deficiency is most commonly found in developing countries like India and can lead to deficiency of vitamins B_6 and B_2 and impairment of psychomotor function. Riboflavin metabolism is affected by infections, drugs, and hormones.

Vulnerable Populations. Alcoholism, cancers, chronic infections, drug use (broad-spectrum antibiotics and chloramphenicol), gastrectomy, and low oral intake during childhood, pregnancy, or lactation.

Signs of Excess. There is no known toxicity.

Niacin (Nicotinic Acid, Nicotinamide): Niacin is absorbed in the stomach and small intestine by carrier-mediated facilitated diffusion. Niacin requirements are related to protein and calorie intake. Intake for infants is established as AIs. *RDA is 16 mg/d for men and 14 mg/d for women. UL was established at 35 mg for men and women.*

Functions. Niacin serves as coenzyme for several dehydrogenases. It is part of nicotinamide adenine dinucleotide (NAD) and NADH in over 200 enzymes involved with metabolism of CHO, protein, and fat. It is involved with intracellular reactions and biosynthetic pathways; energy metabolism; growth; conversion of vitamin A to retinol; metabolism of fatty acids, serum cholesterol, and triglycerides. It has a role in DNA repair and gene stability, thus affecting cancer risk. It prevents pellagra (along with other B-complex vitamins). It is needed to treat tuberculosis as Isoniazid. Nicotinic acid is used as a vasodilator; nicotinamide is less vasodilating.

Sources. Beef and lean meats, organ meats, poultry, tuna and salt water fish, peanut butter, peanuts and legumes, enriched breads and fortified cereals. Diet supplies 31% of niacin intake as tryptophan. Milk and eggs are good sources of tryptophan but not niacin. Sixty milligrams of tryptophan are needed to equal 1 mg of niacin.

Signs of Deficiency. Signs start with beefy tongue, stomatitis with swelling and soreness of the oral mucosa; esophagitis with gastritis; diarrhea with proctitis; inflammation and erythema of the mucosal surfaces of the genitourinary tract; symmetric pigmented rash with scaling and hyperkeratosis; worsening of the skin rash in areas of sun exposure or trauma; headaches, insomnia, depression, anxiety; tremors or rigidity of limbs; loss of tendon reflexes; numbness and paresthesias in limbs. Severe deficiency leads to **pellagra** with Casal's collar, a rough, red **d**ermatitis, **d**iarrhea, **d**ementia (the three Ds of pellagra).

Vulnerable Populations. Alcoholism, cancers, chronic diarrhea, cirrhosis, diabetes, and tuberculosis. Undernourished people in Africa.

Signs of Excess. Toxicity is generally low but may cause histamine release, flushing of skin (when using 1–2 g of nicotinic acid daily in an effort to lower cholesterol levels), or even liver toxicity. Megadoses should be avoided.

Pantothenic Acid (Vitamin B-5): Pantothenic acid is a coenzyme in fatty acid metabolism. Pantothenic acid is available "from everywhere." It is absorbed by passive diffusion and active transport in the jejunum. Fifty percent is bioavailable from diet. Needs increase by one-third in pregnancy and lactation. *AI for adult men and women is 5 mg/d. UL is not established.*

Functions. Coenzyme A is essential in the formation of acetyl CoA and energy production from the macronutrients. It also affects synthesis of cholesterol and fatty acids, adrenal gland activity, acetyl transfer, antibodies, normal serum glucose, electrolyte control and hydration, heme synthesis, and healthy RBCs. It changes choline to acetylcholine and prevents premature graying in some animals.

Sources. Pantothenic acid is present in all plant and animal tissues. The most important sources are meats, particularly heart and liver, but mushrooms, avocados, broccoli, egg yolks, yeast, skim milk, and sweet potatoes are also good sources.

Signs of Deficiency. Deficiency is rare but can impair lipid synthesis and energy production. Symptoms include paresthesia in the toes and soles of the feet, burning sensations in the feet, depression, fatigue, insomnia, and weakness.

Vulnerable Populations. Alcoholism, elderly women, liver disease, chronic ulcerative colitis, and pregnancy.

Signs of Excess. Rarely, excess causes mild intestinal distress or diarrhea.

Vitamin B_6 (Pyridoxine): This group includes numerous 2-methyl-3,5-dihydroxymethylpyridine derivatives exhibiting the biologic activity of PN, including pyridoxol, pyridoxal, and pyridoxamine. Vitamin B_6 is absorbed by passive diffusion of the dephosphorylated forms PN, PL, or PM, primarily in the jejunum and ileum. Pyridoxal phosphate (PLP) is the active form. Some studies suggest that a higher RDA is desirable for some individuals. About 96% of dietary vitamin B_6 is absorbed. High-protein intakes may deplete vitamin B_6 levels, thus needs increase with increased protein intake. Needs decrease with fatty acids or with other B-complex vitamins. The DRIs for vitamin B_6 include AIs for infants. Infants need three times as much vitamin B_6 as adults. *RDA is 1.3–1.7 mg/d for men and 1.3–1.5 mg/d for women. The UL was established at 100 mg/d for adult men and women.*

Functions. Vitamin B_6 is primarily known for its role in amino acid metabolism, histamine synthesis, gene expression, and hemoglobin synthesis. PLP is involved in practically all reactions in the metabolism of amino acids and in several aspects of the metabolism of neurotransmitters, glycogen, sphingolipids, heme, steroids, coenzymes (-ases), conversion of tryptophan to niacin, fat metabolism (changing linoleic to arachidonic acid), synthesis of folic acid, homocysteine metabolism, glandular and endocrine functions, antibodies, dopamine and serotonin metabolism, glycogen phosphorylase, and immunity.

Sources. Wheat and whole-grain cereals (such as oatmeal), legumes and nuts (garbanzo beans, soybeans, and peanuts) are the highest sources.

Signs of Deficiency. The vitamin is widely distributed throughout the diet; deficiency is rare but may present as convulsions in infants; depression, confusion, irritability; hypochromic, microcytic anemia. Peripheral neuropathies; glossitis, cheilosis, angular stomatitis; impaired immunity; seborrheic dermatitis involving the face and neck; blepharitis may also occur.

Vulnerable Populations. Alcoholism, use of certain medications (cycloserine, Dilantin, hydralazine, isoniazid, oral contraceptives, and penicillamine), elderly status, pregnancy, schizophrenia, isoniazid treatment and no vitamin replacement for tuberculosis.

Signs of Excess. Toxicity is relatively low. Sensory neuropathy with gait changes, peripheral sensations, and muscle incoordination.

Biotin (Vitamin B-7): Biotin is a coenzyme for carboxylations. *RDA is 30 mg/d for adult men and women. UL is not established.*

Functions. Coenzyme in CO_2 fixation, deamination, decarboxylation, synthesis of fatty acids, CHO metabolism, oxidative phosphorylation, leucine catabolism, and carboxylation of pyruvic acid to oxaloacetate.

Sources. Liver, kidney, pork, milk, egg yolk, yeast, cereal, nuts, legumes, and chocolate. Note: Biotin can be synthesized by intestinal bacteria. Be wary of extended antibiotic use or prolonged unsupplemented TPN use. Probably, 50% of dietary biotin is absorbed from the small intestine. Biotin is called the "anti–raw egg white" factor; avidin in raw egg white decreases biotin availability.

Signs of Deficiency. Inflammation of the skin and lips. Other symptoms include dermatitis, alopecia, paralysis, depression, nausea, hepatic steatosis, hypercholesterolemia, and glossitis.

Vulnerable Populations. Individuals who consume excessive intake of avidin from raw egg whites. People with genetic conditions (beta-methylcrotonylglycinuria and propionic acidemia), or inadequate provision with long-term parenteral nutrition.

Signs of Excess. There are no known toxic effects.

Folic Acid (Vitamin B-9): Folate generally refers to pteroylmonoglutamin acid and its derived compounds. Folate is found naturally in food; folic acid is the supplemental form. Pteroylglutamic acid is the pharmacological form. Folic acid works primarily as a coenzyme in single-carbon metabolism. Some folic acid can be made in the intestines with help from biotin, protein, and vitamin C. Synthetic folic acid increases serum levels more effectively than food sources of folate. Only 25–50% of dietary sources are bioavailable. Absorption occurs by active transport mainly in the jejunum, but can also be absorbed by passive diffusion when ingested in large amounts.

The DRIs express folate in "dietary folate equivalents or DFEs," which account for the difference between food sources and the more bioavailable supplemental sources. DFEs from fortified foods provide 1.7 times the micrograms of natural folic acid. Fortification of more commonly eaten foods has been implemented to provide adequate folic acid for vulnerable populations. About 90% of circulating folacin is bound to albumin. Drugs that interfere with utilization include aspirin, sulfasalazine (Azulfidine), methotrexate, antacids, anticonvulsants such as phenytoin (Dilantin), oral contraceptives, pyrimethamine, trimethoprim. *The DRI is described as AIs for infants. RDA is 400 mcg for adults. Pregnant women need 600 mcg and lactating women need 500 mcg. UL is 1000 mcg/d.*

Functions. Needed for growth; hemoglobin; amino acid metabolism. Prevents excessive buildup of homocysteine to protect against heart disease and some forms of cancer. Prevents megaloblastic and macrocytic anemias. Reduces the incidence of neural tube defects. Folate is required for synthesis of phospholipids, DNA, proteins, new cells, and neurotransmitters. Choline is used as a methyl donor (to convert homocysteine to methionine) when folate intake is low. Folic acid is needed during pregnancy to prevent spina bifida, cleft palate, some heart or other birth defects.

Sources. Foods with highest folate content include fortified cereals, pinto and navy beans (cooked), lentils, beets, asparagus, spinach, romaine lettuce, broccoli, and oranges. Analysis of foods for their folate content is complex and difficult. Folate exists in 150 different forms, and losses of 50–90% typically occur during storage, cooking, or processing at high temperatures (see Table A-15).

Signs of Deficiency. Decrease in total number of cells (pancytopenia) and large RBCs with a macrocytic or megaloblastic anemia. Deficiency is common, especially during pregnancy, with oral contraceptive use, in malabsorption syndromes, in alcoholics, in teens, and in elderly individuals. Neural tube defects such as spina bifida or anencephaly may result from impaired biosynthesis of DNA and RNA.

Vulnerable Populations. Alcoholics, cancer, medication use (aspirin, cycloserine, Dilantin, methotrexate, oral contraceptives, primidone, and pyrimethamine), hematological diseases (pernicious anemia, sickle cell anemia, and thalassemia), vitamin B_{12} deficiency, malabsorption syndromes, and pregnancy.

Signs of Excess. No adverse effects of high oral doses of folate have been reported. Although parenteral administration of amounts some 1000 times the dietary requirement produce epileptiform seizures in the rat.

Vitamin B_{12} (Cobalamin, Cyanocobalamin): Vitamin B_{12} is known for its role as a coenzyme in metabolism of propionate, amino acids, and single-carbon fragments. It is known as a blood cell and nerve cell growth stimulator, along with folic acid. It is the "extrinsic factor" needed from diet to complement the "intrinsic factor" found in the stomach. Many people with achlorhydria or over age 50 lose the ability to absorb vitamin B_{12} from foods and should consider using more fortified foods. *RDA is 2.4 mcg for adults. Pregnant women need 2.6* μg and lactating women need 2.8 μg. No UL was established.

TABLE A-15 Food Sources of Folic Acid

Food	Folic Acid or Folate (μg)
Cereal, ready to eat, one cup	100–400
Cereal, cooked (oatmeal, farina, grits), one cup	75–300
Turkey giblets, cooked, one cup	486
Lentils or black-eyed peas, cooked, one cup	358
Pinto beans, cooked, one cup	294
Chickpeas (garbanzo beans), one cup	282
Okra, frozen, cooked, one cup	269
Spinach, cooked, one cup	263
Black beans, cooked, one cup	256
Enriched long-grain white rice, cooked, one cup	238
Beef liver, cooked, 3 ounces	221
Enriched egg noodles, cooked, one cup	221
Spinach, canned, one cup	210
Collards, cooked, one cup	177
Turnip greens, cooked, one cup	170
Broccoli, cooked, one cup	168
Enriched spaghetti, cooked, one cup	167
Brussels sprouts, cooked, one cup	157
Artichokes, cooked, one cup	150
Beets, cooked, one cup	136
Peas, cooked, one cup	127
Papaya, one whole	116
Cream-style corn, canned, one cup	115
Orange juice, one cup	110

Source: Nutrient values from Agricultural Research Service (ARS) Nutrient Database for Standard Reference, Release 17. Foods are from ARS single nutrient reports, sorted in descending order by nutrient content in terms of common household measures. Food items and weights in the single nutrient reports are adapted from those in 2002 revision of USDA Home and Garden Bulletin No. 72, Nutritive Value of Foods. Mixed dishes and multiple preparations of the same food item have been omitted from this table.

Functions. Coenzymes, blood cell formation, nucleoproteins and genetic material, nutrient metabolism, growth, nerve tissue, thyroid functions, metabolism, transmethylation, myelin formation, homocysteine metabolism and prevention of heart disease.

Sources. Vitamin B_{12} is not found in plant foods; monitor vegetarian diets. For best absorption, riboflavin, niacin, magnesium, and vitamin B_6 are also needed (see Table A-16).

Signs of Deficiency. Constipation, poor balance, loss of appetite, numbness and tingling in hands and feet, megaloblastic anemia. Some psychiatric disturbances such as depression, poor memory, dementia, or confusion. Biochemical deficiency such as serum cobalamin level $<$150–170 pg/mL or serum methylmalonic acid (MMA) $<$0.35 μg/dL; a return in MMA to normal after cobalamin therapy indicates prior deficiency.

Vulnerable Populations. Adolescents with poor diet with low intake of meat/fish/dairy products or strict vegetarian (vegan) diets are at risk. Senior citizens and those with severe, chronic malnutrition are also at risk. Others at risk include those with pernicious anemia (autoimmune atrophic gastritis), disorders of the gastric mucosa, genetic defects (apoenzymes, absence of transcobalamin II, absence of ileal receptors), extensive disease affecting the stomach, intestinal infections, malabsorption (tropical sprue, celiac sprue, pancreatic insufficiency, Crohn's disease, fish tapeworm, HIV infection, or ileal resection), prolonged exposure to nitrous oxide or megadoses of folic acid. Monitor persons after total gastrectomy for megaloblastic anemia because intrinsic factor is not available. Some gastric bypass patients may also become deficient. Individuals who take zantac, pepcid, tagamet, metformin, omeprazole (Prilosec), lansoprazole (Prevacid) may also be at risk.

Signs of Excess. No toxicity is known.

Choline: Choline is a methyl-rich nutrient that is required for phospholipid synthesis and neurotransmitter function. Internal synthesis of phosphatidylcholine is insufficient to maintain choline status when intakes of folate and choline are low. *AI is set at 550 mg/d for adult men and 425 mg/d for adult women. UL level has been set at 3.5 g/d.*

Functions. Lipotropic agent, some role in muscle control and in short-term memory with the neurotransmitter acetylcholine, component of sphingomyelin, emulsifier in bile, and component of pulmonary surfactant (CO_2/O_2 exchange). It helps the body absorb and use fats, especially for cell membranes. Choline is used as a methyl donor to convert homocysteine to

TABLE A-16 Food Sources of Vitamin B_{12}

Food	Vitamin B_{12} (μg)
Boneless lamb chop, cooked, 3 ounces	2.7
Fortified cereals, one cup	1–6 (varies)
Light tuna canned in water, drained, 3 ounces	2.5
Salmon, cooked, 3 ounces	2.4
Ground beef, 90% lean, cooked, 3 ounces	2.3
Eye round roast and steak, cooked, 3 ounces	1.4
Plain yogurt, low fat, one cup	1.4
Roast turkey, 3 ounces	1.3
Milk, skim, one cup	1.3
Beef hot dog, cooked	0.9
Cottage cheese, low-fat, 4 ounces	0.7
Boneless top loin pork roast, cooked, 3 ounces	0.6
Fortified soy milk or rice milk, one cup	0.6
Chicken breast, cooked, one cup	0.5
Dark meat chicken, cooked, one cup	0.4
Cheddar cheese, one slice	0.2
American cheese, one ounce	0.2

Source: Nutrient values from Agricultural Research Service (ARS) Nutrient Database for Standard Reference, Release 17. Foods are from ARS single nutrient reports, sorted in descending order by nutrient content in terms of common household measures. Food items and weights in the single nutrient reports are adapted from those in 2002 revision of USDA Home and Garden Bulletin No. 72, Nutritive Value of Foods. Mixed dishes and multiple preparations of the same food item have been omitted from this table.

methionine when folate intake is low. Choline magnesium trisalicylate is used to relieve pain, inflammation and tenderness caused by arthritis as a form of nonsteroidal anti-inflammatory medications

Sources. Eggs, high-protein animal products such as liver, dairy foods, soybeans, peanuts, cauliflower, lettuce, and chocolate. Lecithin is a choline precursor, as is phosphatidylcholine. Liver can synthesize or resynthesize. Average daily intake is 400–900 mg. High-fat intake accelerates deficiency.

Signs of Deficiency. Insufficient phospholipid synthesis occurs; neurotransmitter function and liver damage might occur.

Signs of Excess. Anorexia, fishy body odor, upset stomach.

Vitamin C (Ascorbic Acid, Dehydroascorbic Acid): Vitamin C is needed via an exogenous source by all humans and is found in fruits and vegetables. About 90% of dietary intake is absorbed. Concentration of vitamin C in plasma and other body fluids does not increase in proportion to increasing daily doses of vitamin C. Saturation is complete at 200 mg. *RDA for vitamin C is 75 mg for women and teen boys. Pregnant women need 85 mg and lactating women need 120 mg. Teen girls need 65 mg; 80 if pregnant or 115 if lactating.*

Men need 90 mg. Smokers need an extra 35 mg daily. The UL for vitamin C is 2000 mg/d.

Functions. Hydroxylation (lysine and proline) in collagen formation and wound healing, norepinephrine metabolism, tryptophan to serotonin transformation, folic acid metabolism, antioxidant as a scavenger of superoxide radicals and to protect vitamins A and E, changing ferric iron to ferrous iron, healthy immunity and prevention of infection, intracellular respiration, tyrosine metabolism, intercellular structures of bone, teeth, and cartilage, prevention of scurvy. It may defer aging through the collagen turnover process. Vitamin C also serves as a reducing agent, elevates HDL cholesterol in the elderly, and lowers total serum cholesterol. It is also needed for biosynthesis of carnitine and for metabolism of drugs and steroids. Dietary antioxidants, including vitamins C and E, may protect against atherosclerotic disease and cognitive impairment.

Sources. For details see Table A-17. No more than 1 g/d is stored in liver tissue. An excretion of 50% of intake is normal. Men are found to have lower serum levels than women. Smoking decreases serum levels; increased intake removes greater amounts of nicotine. Avoid high levels of pectin, iron, copper, or zinc from the diet and do not cook fruits or vegetables in copper pans.

Signs of Deficiency. The first symptom of deficiency is fatigue; treatment with vitamin C results in quick recovery and alleviation of symptoms. Insufficient (depletion) is 11–28 μmol/L, considered latent scurvy with mood changes; mild but distinct fatigue and irritability; vague, dull, aching pains. Deficient is <11 μmol/L with failure of wounds to heal, petechial hemorrhage, follicular hyperkeratosis, bleeding gums, eventual tooth loss, weak bones or cartilage and connective tissues, rheumatic pains in the legs, muscular atrophy, skin lesions, and psychological changes including depression and hypochondria. High blood lead levels will also deplete serum vitamin C.

TABLE A-17 Food Sources of Vitamin C[a]

Food, Standard Amount	Vitamin C (mg)
Guava, raw, 1/2 cup	188
Red sweet pepper, raw, 1/2 cup	142
Red sweet pepper, cooked, 1/2 cup	116
Kiwi fruit, one medium	70
Orange, raw, one medium	70
Orange juice, 3/4 cup	61–93
Green pepper, sweet, raw, 1/2 cup	60
Green pepper, sweet, cooked, 1/2 cup	51
Grapefruit juice, 3/4 cup	50–70
Vegetable juice cocktail, 3/4 cup	50
Strawberries, raw, 1/2 cup	49
Brussels sprouts, cooked, 1/2 cup	48
Cantaloupe, 1/4 medium	47
Papaya, raw, 1/4 medium	47
Kohlrabi, cooked, 1/2 cup	45
Broccoli, raw, 1/2 cup	39
Edible pod peas, cooked, 1/2 cup	38
Broccoli, cooked, 1/2 cup	37
Sweet potato, canned, 1/2 cup	34
Tomato juice, 3/4 cup	33
Cauliflower, cooked, 1/2 cup	28
Pineapple, raw, 1/2 cup	28
Kale, cooked, 1/2 cup	27
Mango, 1/2 cup	23

Source: Nutrient values from Agricultural Research Service (ARS) Nutrient Database for Standard Reference, Release 17. Foods are from ARS single nutrient reports, sorted in descending order by nutrient content in terms of common household measures. Food items and weights in the single nutrient reports are adapted from those in 2002 revision of USDA Home and Garden Bulletin No. 72, Nutritive Value of Foods.

[a]Food sources of vitamin C ranked by milligrams of vitamin C per standard amount; also calories in the standard amount. (All provide ≥ 20% of RDA for adult men, which is 90 mg/d).

Vulnerable Populations. Those with achlorhydria, Alzheimer's disease, burns, cancers, chronic diarrhea, nephrosis, pregnancy, severe trauma, surgical wounds, and tuberculosis. Older and very young are more likely to have weaker immune systems and need more vitamin C. Moderate-to-high alcohol intake reduces immune effectiveness; alcoholics are at risk of scurvy. High blood pressure and cholesterol can lead to immune problems and heart disease. Disease agents originating in the mouth may travel in addition to causing dental problems. Diabetes, high glucose, other abnormal labs can stress the immune system; pollutant exposure, steroid use, and radiation can deplete vitamin C levels. Individuals with gout, arthritis, bladder cancer, reflex pain after hip fracture, pneumonia, risk for stroke or macular degeneration or hip fracture, renal oxalate stones, pregnancy, *Helicobacter pylori* infection, or prolonged proton pump use should be evaluated closely.

Signs of Excess. GI distress and diarrhea are most common.

A P P E N D I X 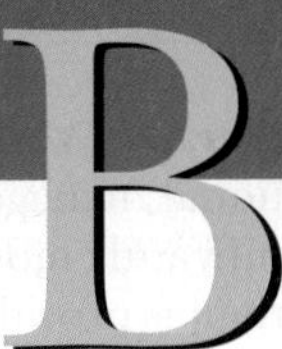

Dietetic Process, Forms, and Counseling Tips

INTRODUCTION TO THE PRACTICE OF DIETETICS

The American Dietetic Association (ADA) is responsible for establishing the expectations for required education, practice guidelines, and standards of professional performance for dietetic professionals. The Commission on Dietetic Registration maintains credentialing authority for the roles of Registered Dietitian (RD) and Dietetic Technician Registered (DTR). A scope of practice framework can be used to assist dietetic professionals in defining their responsibilities and refining practice according to professional job analyses that are conducted every few years.

Dietitians and dietetic technicians work in a variety of settings but tend to be **concentrated in healthcare settings:** acute care, long-term care, dialysis units, psychiatric facilities, community sites, and home health. They perform a variety of tasks including clinical services, food systems management, nutrition education, and public health functions. See Figure B-1.

There are over 59 core dietetics position descriptions including not only the roles of traditional clinical dietitian; outpatient dietitian; or Special Supplemental Nutrition Program for Women, Infants, and Children (WIC) nutritionist but also covering areas such as consulting, sales, and communications. Generally, dietetics professionals aim to improve the health of their clientele by influencing their food and nutrition decisions. Many dietetics practice groups have now established standards of practice that are specific to their area of expertise. The following guidelines are useful in consideration of an effective practice in dietetics.

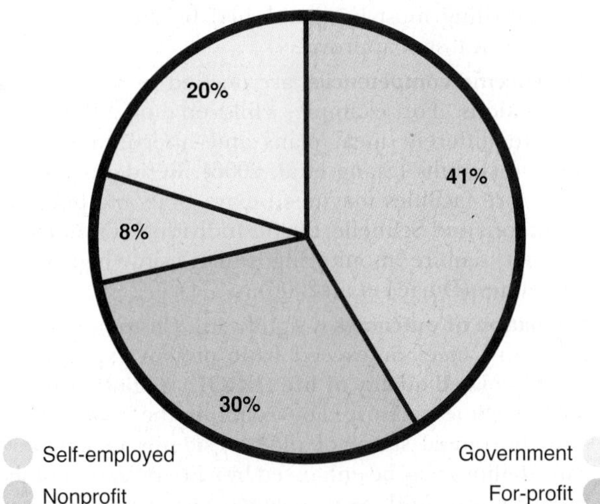

Figure B-1 Employment sector of dietetics practitioners ($n = 8115$) (Image courtesy of Compensation & Benefits Survey of the Dietetics Profession 2009.)

1. **Standards** from The Joint Commission and other organizations set the expectation that quality care will lead to positive outcomes. Effective leadership and continuous performance improvement are critical for maintaining quality.
2. **Regulations,** such as those from the Centers for Medicare and Medicaid Services (CMS), have been written to protect vulnerable patients/residents from inadequate care. For example, in long-term care, the F325 tag related to **§483.25 Nutrition** states that, based on a resident's comprehensive assessment, the facility must ensure that a resident (1) maintains acceptable parameters of nutritional status, such as body weight and protein levels, unless the resident's clinical condition demonstrates that this is not possible; and (2) receives a therapeutic diet when there is a nutritional problem. All of the guidelines and directives are to be followed by dietitians and their supporting staff members accordingly.
3. Most dietitians work in settings that are supportive of **interdisciplinary teamwork.** Dietitians must be proactive, take on new skills, and overcome traditional stereotypes. The roles are expanding, for example, in bariatric surgery, in functional medicine, and in home care.
4. Many dietetics positions now include **enhanced responsibilities** in nutritionally focused physical assessment, certification in cardiopulmonary resuscitation, assessment for the use of adaptive feeding equipment, worksite wellness, swallowing evaluations, exercise prescription and education, functional nutrition assessments, and home care services.
5. For **basic nutrition education,** advice can be provided by many healthcare professionals. However, **medical nutrition**

therapy (MNT) is an intensive approach to the nutritional management of chronic disease and requires significantly more education in food and nutrition science than is provided by other professional curricula. The RD is the single identifiable healthcare professional to have the most standardized education, supervised clinical training, and national credentialing, who meets the continuing education requirements for reimbursement as a direct provider of MNT.

6. **State licensure laws** protect the public from unscrupulous practices. Each licensure board establishes a relevant scope of practice for dietitians and nutritionists who practice in that state. Scopes of practice detail what can or cannot be performed by a person using the title of dietitian or nutritionist.
7. Application of the American Dietetic Association's **Nutrition Care Process** with **standardized terminology** enables dietitians to perform at a higher level of comprehensive care than in the past. See Figure B-2.
8. The best patient care emphasizes **coordinated, comprehensive care along the continuum of the healthcare delivery system**. Multidisciplinary teams are best suited to develop, lead, and implement evidence-based disease management programs. Evidence-based care integrates research into practice, regardless of the setting. Indeed, research is the basis of the profession (Pavlinac, 2010).
9. Dietitians must take an **evidence-based approach to care** based on their education, training, skill level, and work experiences. Science and evidence-based education can help to overcome dangerous perceptions of consumers or misunderstandings by members of the medical community (Krebs and Primak, 2006).
10. **Unique nutritional care guidelines** should be used in specialty areas such as cancer, diabetes, cardiology and pulmonary, gastroenterology, geriatrics, HIV-AIDS, liver disease, nutrition support, pancreatic disease, renal failure, surgical or transplantation units, intensive care, and functional nutrition therapy. See Figure B-3 for the Functional Medicine Matrix Model™ that was used as part of a holistic assessment format.
11. **Medical classification systems** are used for a variety of purposes including statistical analyses, reimbursement, decision-support systems, and procedures.
12. **Diagnostic-related groups (DRGs)** classify hospital cases into similar categories for reimbursement, assuming a similar use of resources. In 2007, Medical Severity DRG (MS-DRG) codes were added to enhance payment for conditions that involve greater morbidity or risk for mortality. In 2008, Hospital Acquired Condition (HAC) was described, and some conditions were no longer considered to be complications if they were not present upon admission (POA).
13. Use correct **nutrition diagnosis nomenclature** for malnourished adults in clinical practice settings: *"starvation-related malnutrition"* when there is chronic starvation without inflammation; *"chronic disease–related malnutrition"* when a mild to moderate inflammation is chronic; and *"acute disease or injury–related malnutrition"* for acute, severe inflammation (Jensen et al, 2009).
14. For the **coding of malnutrition** in the medical record, use ICD-9 code 262.
15. **Sentinel events** are defined by The Joint Commission as unexpected occurrences leading to serious physical or psychological injury or death. The risk for a sentinel event requires an immediate investigation and response. Issues such as changes in functional status, the severity of a nutrition diagnosis, unintended weight changes (>10% in 6 months), and changes in body composition such as the loss of subcutaneous fat are risks that should be examined.
16. **Order-writing privileges** by dietitians allow orders for nutritional prescriptions for enteral and parenteral nutrition to be implemented quickly and effectively. Order-writing must be established by the local facility with medical staff approval.
17. **Age-specific competencies** are needed to serve various populations. For example, children and adolescents require different meal plans and interventions from those for adults (Stang et al, 2006). Residents in long-term care facilities may need extra time and attention (Simmons and Schnelle, 2006). Individuals on nutrition support require monitoring while using age-specific guidelines (Durfee et al, 2006).
18. **Evaluation of outcomes** is significant. Customer satisfaction must meet or exceed basic patient expectations. **Health-related quality of life (HRQL)** is another important outcome measure. For example, the quality of life and nutritional status of older residents in long-term care facilities may be enhanced by a liberalization of diet prescriptions and person-centered care. This care involves residents in decisions about schedules, menus, and dining locations; weight loss, undernutrition, and other effects of poor nutrition and hydration are then decreased (Neidert, 2005).

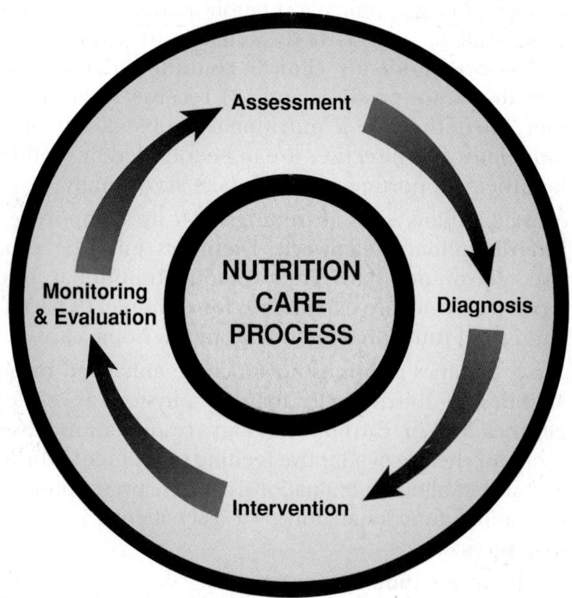

Figure B-2

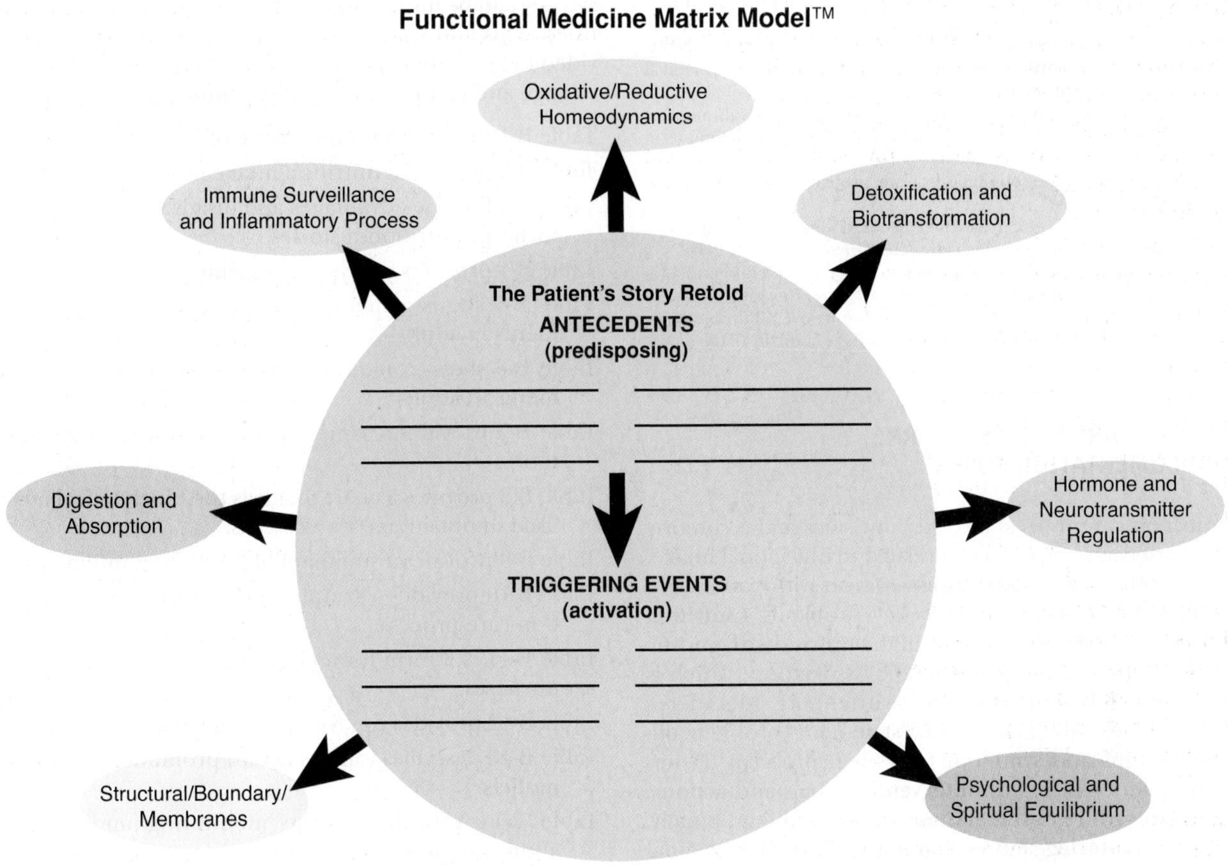

Functional Medicine Matrix Model™

Oxidative/Reductive Homeodynamics

Immune Surveillance and Inflammatory Process

Detoxification and Biotransformation

The Patient's Story Retold

ANTECEDENTS (predisposing)

______________ ______________

______________ ______________

______________ ______________

TRIGGERING EVENTS (activation)

______________ ______________

______________ ______________

______________ ______________

Digestion and Absorption

Hormone and Neurotransmitter Regulation

Structural/Boundary/ Membranes

Psychological and Spirtual Equilibrium

Nutrition Status	Exercise	Sleep	Beliefs & Self-Care	Relationships

Date:_______ Name: ________________ Age:____ Sex:____ Chief Complaints:______________

Figure B-3 Used with permission from The Institute for Functional Medicine.

19. **Ongoing review** is needed to monitor progress. Difficulty in obtaining current laboratory values makes it hard to follow patient outcomes after discharge. With electronic medical records and careful maintenance of confidentiality, monitoring can be more effective.
20. Dietetics professionals are likely to advance to **management positions**, such as food service director, consultant, or patient case manager, because they possess strong nutrition knowledge and management skills. Nearly half of all RDs and DTRs supervise other employees (Ward, 2010).
21. Having supervisory responsibility is strongly associated with higher wages (Ward, 2010). In addition, having a masters degree or PhD and one or more specialty certifications (e.g., CDE, CNSD, and the various Certified Specialist credentials offered by the Commission on Dietetic Registration) leads to an increased median wage (Ward, 2010).
22. **Food and nutrition managers** are in opportune positions to influence other managers, acquire resources, identify opportunities, and achieve desirable outcomes.
23. **Levels of responsibility** tend to increase with years of experience and with business skills such as leadership, marketing, and negotiation. Dietitians are encouraged to include management and leadership development as part of their continuing education portfolio.

REFERENCES

Durfee SM, et al. Standards for specialized nutrition support for adult residents of long-term care facilities. *Nutr Clin Pract.* 21:96, 2006.

Jensen GL, et al. Adult starvation and disease-related malnutrition: a proposal for etiology-based diagnosis in the clinical practice setting from the International Consensus Guideline Committee. *Clin Nutr.* 29:151, 2009.

Krebs NF, Primak LE. Comprehensive integration of nutrition into medical training. *Am J Clin Nutr.* 83:945S, 2006.

Neidert K. Position of the American Dietetic Association: liberalization of the diet prescription improves quality of life for older adults in long-term care. *J Am Diet Assoc.* 105:1955, 2005.

Pavlinac JM. Research is the foundation of our profession. *J Am Diet Assoc.* 110:499, 2010.

Simmons SF, Schnelle JF. Feeding assistance needs of long-stay nursing home residents and staff time to provide care. *J Am Geriatr Soc.* 54:919, 2006.

Stang J, et al. Position of the American Dietetic Association: child and adolescent food and nutrition programs. *J Am Diet Assoc.* 106:1467, 2006.

Ward B. Compensation & benefits Survey 2009: despite overall downturn in economy, RD and DTR salaries rise. *J Am Diet Assoc.* 110:25, 2010.

NUTRITION CARE PROCESS, FORMS, AND DOCUMENTATION TOOLS

The nutrition care process involves four steps and a comprehensive understanding of factors related to nutritional intake. Following a thorough **nutrition assessment** with patient history and current status, identify key problems (**nutrition diagnoses**). Use the latest edition of the nutrition diagnostic language from the American Dietetic Association, which is available to members at http://www.eatright.org/Members/content.aspx?id=5477. Write a PES statement (problem, etiology, and signs and symptoms) for each problem. Determine the plan of care, with **intervention** goals and actions, designed according to the etiology of the problem. Finally, plan how **monitoring and evaluation** will occur. The final step should be measurable and should be related to the identified signs and symptoms. **Sample tools and forms** are provided here; all tools should be adapted for the facility and for the age and complexity of patients in the population.

Table B-1 provides a sample scope of practice policy.

Table B-2 provides a nutrition intake history form for adults.

Table B-3 lists the advantages and disadvantages of different forms of nutrition histories.

Table B-4 provides a physical assessment checklist.

Table B-5 shows a method for estimating energy requirements in adults.

Table B-6 shows a method for estimating protein requirements in adults.

Table B-7 provides a sample pediatric nutrition assessment tool.

Table B-8 provides a chart that lists the biochemical analyses used in nutritional assessments.

Table B-9 provides a summary of food–drug interactions.

Table B-10 provides a sample worksheet for using the nutrition care process.

Table B-11 is a form for a clinical case review and for audit purposes.

Table B-12 provides tips for adult education and counseling.

Table B-13 describes various health promotion intervention models.

Table B-14 provides sample monitoring and evaluation audits for patient education.

TABLE B-1 Sample Hospital Nutrition Department Scope of Services

PURPOSE

In order to provide care consistent with the mission of the hospital system, the nutrition department has defined its scope of services and goals.

POLICY

It is the policy of the hospital system for each department to provide care and/or services based on the defined scope of services and goals and to implement policies and procedures based on the scope of services and goals.

DEPARTMENT MISSION

The nutrition department commits itself to enhancing the quality of life throughout the patient's life cycle and promoting and restoring health through the provision of quality nutritional care services in an environment that ensures dignity and respect for each person. The nutrition department has an obligation to ensure continuous quality improvement in the care and services it provides.

PROCEDURE

Care/Services Provided

The department provides timely nutrition assessment, monitoring, counseling, education, discharge planning, and diet instruction, as defined in department policies, to meet the needs of patients' various backgrounds, which affect nutritional preferences and habits. Administration evaluates the activities of the department with regard to the provision of quality dietary intervention, patient treatment and outcomes, and the quality of meal service.

Types of Patients/Customers Served

Nutrition services are available for all segments of the hospital population—newborn, infant, child, adolescent, adult, and geriatric—including outpatient services, cardiopulmonary rehabilitation, emergency department, corporate wellness, and community events.

Timeliness

Clinical dietitians are scheduled for Monday through Saturday, with shift availability at all meal periods. One dietitian is scheduled for weekend coverage; Sunday coverage is an on-call assignment. When appropriate, formula calculations, calorie counts or nutrient analyses, and basic nutrition assessments can be completed via the computer system and any telephone within the system to facilitate timely treatments.

STAFFING

The clinical nutrition manager sets a staffing plan to meet the needs of the patient population. A staffing assessment is completed every 2 years or when deemed necessary. Dietitian schedules are prepared in advance, including hours of duty and on-call schedules.

(continued)

TABLE B-1 Sample Hospital Nutrition Department Scope of Services *(continued)*

STAFF CREDENTIALS AND REQUIREMENTS

Dietitians are registered through the Commission on Dietetic Registration; each must maintain their registration through continuing education. The education requirement is 75 hours during each 5-year period. Competency standards are developed, updated, and reviewed regularly by the clinical nutrition manager to meet the specific, changing needs of the facility.

ASSIGNMENTS

Full-time equivalents of clinical dietitians are assigned to patient care and ambulatory clinics. One full-time equivalent of a clinical nutrition manager leads the clinical/outpatient staff. Staff are assigned to community education programs upon request and scheduling allows. Based on the daily census and acuity, clinical and outpatient dietitians may adjust the daily staffing pattern to meet needs according to changes in patient acuity.

STANDARDS OF CARE

Clinical dietitians apply the hospital-approved standards of nutrition care and the evidence-based guidelines of the American Dietetic Association.

SCREENING

All inpatients are screened by the nursing department within 24 hours of admission to determine the need for further nutrition assessment. Clinical dietitians develop the screening triggers, which are approved by the medical staff. Patients receive nutrition intervention based on the priority/acuity levels assigned by the dietitians. The clinical dietitians perform subsequent re-screening according to policy and regulatory guidelines.

Priority for Nutrition Services	High Priority	Moderate Priority	Low Priority
Definitions/Indications	Nutrition interventions that warrant frequent comprehensive patient reassessment to document the impact of the intervention on critical nutrition outcomes, medical status (i.e., labs, GI tolerance, etc.), and/or clinical progress. Examples: New or modified EN/PN or use of medical food supplements. Comprehensive nutrition education or counseling.	Nutrition interventions that warrant early evaluation, which can be sufficiently tracked via brief f/u notes. Less frequent comprehensive patient reassessment is needed. Examples: Stable EN or PN. Brief nutrition education for survival skills. Coordination of care.	Nutrition interventions that bring closure and/or immediately resolve a patient's nutrition diagnosis/problem OR when no nutrition intervention is needed. F/U is expected in the form of rescreening with reassessment as indicated by a change in status. Examples: Brief nutrition education. No nutrition diagnosis. Palliative care only.
Plan of care review standard	Update POC when reassessing patient.	Within 5 days, based on a brief chart review, communication w/ other patient care providers as appropriate and patient contact. State the nutrition diagnosis, response to intervention, and the new or modified plan.	Per rescreening standards
Reassessment standard	Within 3 days	Within 7 days	Per rescreening standards

ASSESSMENT AND NUTRITION DIAGNOSES

The clinical dietitians assess patients using the guidelines in the standards of care approved by the medical staff. Following the profession's nutrition care process, a nutrition diagnosis is established as needed. The etiology of the diagnosis selected determines the type and extent of intervention that will be provided. The most common nutrition diagnoses in this facility are as follows:

Inadequate oral food/beverage intake (NI-2.1)
Inadequate protein-energy intake (NI-5.3)
Increased nutrient needs (NI-5.1)
Evident malnutrition (NI-5.2)
Inadequate energy intake (NI-1.4)
Swallowing difficulty (NC-1.1)
Involuntary weight loss (NC-3.2)
Inadequate intake from enteral/parenteral nutrition (NI-2.3)
Food and nutrition-related knowledge deficit (NB-1.1)
Underweight (NC-3.1)
Overweight/obesity (NC-3.3)
Excessive energy intake (NI-1.5)

INTERVENTIONS: FOOD AND NUTRIENT DELIVERY

According to the patient's ability to take in sufficient energy, protein, carbohydrate, fat, vitamins, minerals and water, the clinical dietitian will approve or recommend alterations in the nutrition prescription, the addition or discontinuation of enteral/parenteral nutrition, and the use of specific supplements or bioactive substances (e.g., fish oil, lycopene, lutein, ginger, and multivitamin–mineral supplements).

Most common food–nutrient delivery interventions in this facility are as follows:

General/healthful diet (ND- 1.1)
Commercial beverages (ND-3.1.1)
Initiate EN or PN (ND-2.1)
Modify rate, concentration, composition or schedule (ND-2.2)
Modify distribution, type, or amount of food and nutrients within meals or at specified times (ND-1.2)
Modified beverages (ND-3.1.3)
Modified food (ND-3.1.4)
Multivitamins/minerals (ND-3.2.1)
Nutrition-related medication management (ND-6.1)

(continued)

TABLE B-1 Sample Hospital Nutrition Department Scope of Services *(continued)*

INTERVENTIONS: EDUCATION

The clinical dietitian performs a nutrition education needs assessment to determine patient/family knowledge and skill level. The patient's age, barriers to learning, assessed needs, abilities, readiness, and length of stay will determine the level of education to provide. Because lifestyle factors, financial concerns, patient/family expectations, and food preferences affect the individualized education plan, most patients will be referred to ambulatory clinics if extensive education is required to resolve a nutrition diagnosis. The most common education intervention in this facility is Nutrition Education—Survival Information (E-1.3).

INTERVENTIONS: COUNSELING

The clinical dietitian provides individualized guidance and nutritional advice to the patient and/or family members. Techniques to promote behavioral change are used, as appropriate, and documented accordingly. Readiness to change is noted. Follow-up counseling includes an evaluation of the effectiveness of counseling given and recommendations for additional follow-up. There are no specific counseling interventions most often noted for the in-patient setting; this type of intervention is handled in the ambulatory clinics.

INTERVENTIONS: COORDINATION OF CARE

The clinical dietitians participate in both weekly and patient care meetings on assigned units. Discharge planning needs are identified throughout the assessment, re-assessment, and education processes. These needs are referred to the social worker or case manager and communicated to the team during meetings. The dietitian communicates with the referring agency, facility, or next dietitian provider when a specialized care plan is needed. The most common coordination of care interventions in this facility are as follows:

Team meeting (RC-1.1)

Referral to an RD with different expertise (RC-1.2)

Collaboration/referral to other providers (RC-1.3)

MONITORING AND EVALUATION

The clinical dietitian selects the appropriate measures to monitor and evaluate the effectiveness of interventions. The top nutrition monitors used in this facility are as follows:

Total energy intake (FI-1.1)

Enteral/Parenteral nutrition intake formula/solution (FI-3.1.2), initiation (FI-3.1.4), rate/schedule (FI-3.1.5)

Nutrition physical exam findings: skin (S-3.1.6), gastrointestinal (S-3.1.3)

Weight/weight change (S-1.1.4)

DEPARTMENT GOALS

In support of the hospital mission to provide high-quality healthcare through continuous improvement and to exceed the expectations of patients and customers, the clinical nutrition staff of the food and nutrition department have the following goals:

1. Staff qualified, progressive Registered Dietitians who exceed baseline knowledge proficiency standards set by the American Dietetic Association. To accomplish this, all Registered Dietitians must set annual professional development goals on their performance evaluations. These goals are supported by the clinical nutrition manager, funded by Food and Nutrition Services, and tracked through the professional development portfolio of the Commission on Dietetic Registration (CDR).
2. Provide timely nutrition therapy, which results in measurable improvements to patient health from the time of admission to the time of discharge from therapy. Dietitians will follow outcomes of therapy via objective measures (e.g., weight, verbalization of learning, and blood glucose improvements) and chart them in their documentation.
3. Ensure that outpatient medical nutrition therapy and diabetes education programs, combined, will break-even financially. Billing and accounts receivable will be monitored by the program coordinator. Two or three free community education nutrition programs will be offered yearly to local county residents.
4. Ensure that patients will indicate >90% satisfaction rating with their inpatient nutrition care and ambulatory services.
5. Review and administer the expanded dietitian scope of practice for those staff members who have demonstrated competency and have certification (where available) in their specialty area.

EXPANDED SCOPE OF PRACTICE

Because malnutrition is a key factor in determining the prognosis of a patient, protein, energy, vitamin and mineral deficiencies can be detected and corrected earlier through a better utilization of RD skills by assigning order-writing and prescribing privileges to the qualified dietitian specialists on staff. Prescribing authority boosts patient satisfaction by offering quicker interventions, reduces costs with shorter lengths of stays, improves nutrition outcomes, and promotes greater professional satisfaction by those qualified dietitians. Currently, there are three levels of prescriptive authority for dieticians, which are implemented in healthcare facilities and defined as follows:

- **No prescriptive authority:** RDs recommend supplements, diets or diet changes, nutrition-related tests, or procedures to the physician. Recommendations may be written in the medical record or discussed with the physician, but a physician must write an order before recommendations are implemented.
- **Dependent prescriptive authority:** RDs have the authority to order diets, nutritional supplements, nutrition-related tests, or procedures according to protocols, algorithms, policies, or preapproved criteria that specify the type and magnitude of change. Physician approval of the nutritional treatment is not required as long as the orders and treatments provided fall within the guidelines of the protocol, algorithm, policy, or criteria approved in advance by the appropriate institutional authority (e.g., patient-care committee, medical executive committee). However, the RD can discuss the nutritional care provided with the physician and document the order appropriately in the medical record.
- **Independent prescriptive authority:** The RD may act autonomously to provide nutritional services that include ordering diets, nutrition-related tests, or procedures authorized by the clinical privileges granted to the practitioner by the appropriate institutional authority. Physician approval is not required; however, the RD can discuss the nutritional care provided with the physician and document the order appropriately in the medical record.

Steps for Expanded Nutrition Scope of Practice with Dietitian Order-Writing Privileges:

- Evaluate state licensure laws.
- Investigate the level of prescriptive authority permitted at the facility.
- Assure that current licensure and board certifications are accurate in the staff database.
- Discuss plans with each RD staff member with regard to credentialing, graduate study, fellowships, and other measures of basic and continuing competency.

(continued)

TABLE B-1 Sample Hospital Nutrition Department Scope of Services *(continued)*

- When RDs are allowed to have complete order-writing privileges, patient care and outcome are better than they would be if a physician must first sign off on orders.
  - A literature review conducted on the clinical nutrition management list-serv noted that 42–57% of nutrition recommendations were actually put into action by the physician.
  - An average of 17 hours was required before orders were implemented by the MD.
  - Length of stay decreased by up to 5 days for patients who were given nutrition interventions earlier.
- Document success stories, cost savings, improved timeliness of care, shorter LOS than average related to early detection and intervention by the RD.
- Detail the desired scope of dietetics practice using the ADA evidence analysis library, the appropriate standards of professional practice, and other evidence-based guidelines.
- Draft new nutrition policies and procedures. Define the desirable steps for expanded scope of practice (e.g., ordering nutrition-related lab tests; prescribing basic diet orders; changing therapeutic diet orders according to measures such as weight loss or gain, decreased functional ability, significant appetite change; developing standing orders for common nutrition problems and interventions; and writing or updating enteral/parenteral infusion orders).
- Construct an **approval packet with letters of support** for the nutrition committee to establish medical review/consent. When approved by the nutrition committee, obtain signatures from the executive board, chief of medical staff, director of nursing, and hospital director. Include the time period for the scope and a date of review.

TABLE B-2 Dietary Intake Assessment and Nutrition History

Methods for Assessing Dietary Intake	Advantages	Disadvantages
24-Hour Recall: An informal, qualitative method in which the patient recalls all of the foods and beverages that were consumed in the last 24 hours, including the quantities and methods of preparation.	Dietary information is easily obtained. It is also good during a first encounter with a new patient in which there are no other nutritional data. Patients should be able to recall all that they have consumed in the last 24 hours.	It is very limited and may not represent an adequate food intake for the patient. Data achieved using this method may not represent the long-term dietary habits of the patient. Estimating food quantities and food ingredients may be difficult, especially if the patient ate in restaurants.
Usual Intake/Diet History: This method asks the patient to recall a typical daily intake pattern, including amount, frequencies, and methods of preparation. This intake history should include all meals, beverages, and snacks. Include discussion of usual intake and lifestyle recall. This consists of asking the patient to run through a typical day in chronological order, describing all food consumption as well as activities. This method is very helpful because it may reveal other factors that affect patient's nutritional and overall health.	This method evaluates long-term dietary habits and is quick and easy to do. Components usually include the following: Ability to secure and prepare food Activity pattern Alcohol or illicit drug use Appetite Bowel habits—diarrhea, constipation, steatorrhea Chewing/swallowing ability Diet history—usual meal pattern Disease(s) affecting use of nutrients Food allergies/intolerances Medications Nausea or vomiting NPO status or dietary restrictions Pain when eating Satiety level Surgical resection or disease of the GI tract Taste changes or aversions Vitamin/mineral or other nutritional supplements Weight changes	A limited amount of information on the actual quantities of food and beverages is obtained. Also, this method only works if a patient can actually describe a "typical" daily intake, which is difficult for those who vary their food intake greatly. In these patients, it is advisable to use the 24-hour recall method. Another disadvantage is that patients may not include foods that they know are unhealthy.

(continued)

TABLE B-2 Dietary Intake Assessment and Nutrition History *(continued)*

Methods for Assessing Dietary Intake	Advantages	Disadvantages
Food Frequency Questionnaire: This method makes use of a standardized written checklist where patients check off the particular foods or type of foods they consume. It is used to determine trends in patients' consumption of certain foods. The checklist puts together foods with similar nutrient content, and frequencies are listed to identify daily, weekly, or monthly consumption.	It is possible to identify inadequate intake of any food group so that dietary and nutrient deficiencies may be identified. The questionnaire can be geared to a patient's pre-existing medical conditions.	Patient error may occur in filling out how foods are prepared. Patients may over- or underestimate food quantities.
Dietary Food Log: Patient records all food, beverage, and snack consumption for a 1-week period. Specific foods and quantities should be recorded. The data from the food log may later be entered into a computer program, which will analyze the nutrient components of the foods eaten according to specific name brands or food types. Patients are asked to enter data into the food log immediately after food is consumed.	A computer can objectively analyze data obtained. Data on calorie, fat, protein, and carbohydrate consumption can be obtained. Also, since patients are asked to enter data immediately after eating, the data are more accurate than other methods.	Patients may err in entering accurate food quantities. In addition, it is possible that the week-long food log does not accurately represent a patient's normal eating habits since he or she knows that the foods eaten will be analyzed, and thus, he or she may eat healthier for that week.

TABLE B-3 Adult Nutrition History Questionnaire

Patient Name ______________________________ Date__________

1. Height ______feet ______inches
2. How much weight have you gained or lost in the past month? ____ 3 months? ____ 1 year? ________ Present weight ________ BMI ________ Usual weight ________ Desirable weight for height _____
3. Have you ever had problems with your weight? Overweight Underweight Comment:_________________
4. Describe your eating habits: Good Fair Poor
5. How often do you skip meals? Daily Seldom Never
6. Describe your appetite recently: Hearty Moderate Poor
7. If you snack between meals, describe your typical snack _______________ How often? ______
8. When you chew your food, do you have problems or take a long time? Yes No
9. Do you wear dentures at mealtime? Yes No. If yes, do they fit comfortably? Yes No
10. List the vitamin/mineral supplements/herbs and botanicals you take:_________________
11. How many alcoholic drinks do you consume in a day? None 1–2 drinks More than 2 drinks
12. Describe foods you **DO NOT** tolerate: ______________________ Why? ____________________
13. List foods that you especially dislike:_______________________________________
14. List your favorite foods:____
15. List foods that you are **ALLERGIC** to: _____________What symptoms do you experience? ______
16. What type of modified diet do you follow? __________ What types in the past? ______________ Who prescribed or suggested this diet for you? Doctor Friend Self-selected
17. How many meals do you eat at home each week? _____ at school(s)? ____ in restaurants? ____
18. What is your current occupation? ____________________________
19. How active are you on a daily basis? Sedentary ___ Moderate ___ Active ____

TABLE B-3 Adult Nutrition History Questionnaire *(continued)*

Usual Daily Intake

Time	Meal	Food/Method of Preparation	Amount Eaten	RD Calculations
	Morning			
	Snack			
	Noon			
	Snack			
	Dinner			
	Snack			
	During the night			

24-Hour Diet Recall Form

Please be as specific as possible. Include all beverages, condiments, and portion sizes.

Time	Food Item and Method of Preparation	Amount Eaten	Where

Dietitian Comments:

Calculations: Estimated energy needs: ___kcal/kg Est protein needs: ___g/kg Est fluid needs: __ml/kg

Signed: ______________________________RD Date:____________

TABLE B-4 Physical Assessment for Clinical Signs of Malnutrition

Certain risk factors and signs of nutrient deficiency or excess can be identified during the physical examination. One sign is rarely diagnostic; the more signs present, the more likely it is that they reflect a malnourished individual.

Nutrient	Physical Signs of Deficiency
Energy	Severe undernutrition, emaciation
Protein	Dull, dry depigmented hair; easily pluckable
	Edematous extremities
	Poor wound healing; pressure ulcers
	Pneumonia
Carbohydrate	Irritability, fatigue
	Respiratory or neurological changes
Fat	Skin rashes
	Dry, flaky skin
	Loss of subcutaneous fat
Vitamin A	Hair follicle blockage with a permanent "goose-bump" appearance
	Dry, rough skin
	Small, grayish, foamy deposits on the conjunctiva adjacent to the cornea
	Drying of the eyes and mucous membranes
Vitamin K	Small hemorrhages in the skin or mucous membranes
	Prolonged bleeding time
Thiamin	Weight loss
	Muscular wasting
	Occasional edema (wet beriberi)
	Malaise
	Tense calf muscles
	Distended neck veins
	Jerky eye movement
	Staggering gait and difficulty walking
	Infants may develop cyanosis
	Round, swollen (moon) face
	Foot and wrist drop
Riboflavin	Tearing, burning, and itching of the eyes with fissuring in the corners of the eyes
	Soreness and burning of the lips, mouth, and tongue
	Cheilosis (fissuring and/or cracking of the lips and corners of the mouth)
	Purple swollen tongue
	Seborrhea of the skin in the nasolabial folds, scrotum, or vulva
	Capillary overgrowth around the corneas
Niacin	Dermatitis or skin eruptions
	Tremors
	Sore tongue
	Skin that is exposed to sunlight develops cracks and a scaly form of pigmented dermatitis
	May also show signs of riboflavin deficiency
Vitamin B_6	Tongue inflammation
	Inflammation of the lining of the mouth
	Fissures in the corners of the mouth
Folate	Weakness, fatigue, and depression
	Pallor
	Dermatologic lesions
Vitamin B_{12}	Lemon-yellow tint to the skin and eyes
	Smooth, red, thickened tongue
Vitamin C	Impaired wound healing
	Edema
	Swollen, bleeding, and/or retracted gums or tooth loss; mottled teeth; enamel erosion
	Lethargy and fatigue
	Skin lesions
	Small red or purplish pinpoint discolorations on the skin or mucous membranes (petechiae)
	Darkened skin around the hair follicles
	Corkscrew hair
Chromium	Corneal lesions
Copper	Hair and skin depigmentation
	Pallor
Iodine	Goiter
Iron	Skin pallor
	Pale conjunctiva
	Fatigue
	Thin, concave nails with raised edges
Magnesium	Tremors, muscle spasms, tetany
	Personality changes
Potassium	Severe hypertension
	Arrhythmias
Zinc	Delayed wound healing
	Hair loss
	Skin lesions
	Eye lesions
	Nasolabial seborrhea
	Pressure ulcers

Adapted from: Halsted C, et al. Preoperative nutritional assessment. In Quigley E, Sorrell M, eds. *The gastrointestinal surgical patient: preoperative and postoperative care.* Baltimore: Williams & Wilkins, 1994; pp. 27–49.

TABLE B-5 Calculation of Adult Energy Requirements

For adults, body mass index is a useful guide. BMI = Weight (kg)/Height ^{2} (m) [Where 1 kg = 2.2 lb; 1 in = 2.54 cm] or [Weight (lb) × 705/Height (in)]. Basal metabolic rate (BMR) or basal energy expenditure (BEE) is energy expenditure at rest. It involves energy required to maintain minimal physiological functioning (i.e., heart beating, breathing). Various methods are used to determine BEE and energy needs. Resting energy expenditure (REE) includes specific dynamic action for digestion and absorption (slightly above basal) and is considered relatively equivalent to BEE in a clinical context. Factors affecting energy requirements and BMR include the following:

1. Age. Infants need more energy per square meter of body surface than any other age group. BMR declines after maturity.
2. Body Size. Total BMR relates to body size; large persons require more energy for basal needs and for activity.
3. Body Composition. Lean tissue is more active than adipose tissue.
4. Climate. A damp or hot climate often decreases BMR, and a cold climate increases BMR slightly.
5. Hormones. Thyroxine increases BMR; sex hormones and adrenaline alter BMR mildly; low zinc intake may lower BMR.
6. Fever. BMR increases by 7% for each degree above normal in Fahrenheit; 10% for each degree Centigrade.
7. Growth. BMR increases during anabolism in pregnancy, childhood, teen years, and the anabolic phase of wound healing.

REE can be from normal to below normal in mild starvation, such as that which occurs in the hospital setting. **Unplanned weight loss** can affect morbidity and mortality. Problematic % weight change in adults is considered to be: >2% in 1 week, >5% in 1 month, >7.5% in 3 months, > 20% in any period of time. >40% is incompatible with life.

Indirect calorimetry is useful for the critically ill where the calculation of energy expenditure is measured by gas exchange (VO_2 and VCO_2 represent intracellular metabolism). However, note that the energy needs of critically ill or injured adults are lower than previously thought; estimates are based on body mass index (BMI) if indirect calorimetry is not available. Overfeeding can cause fluid overload, increased CO_2 production, and hepatic aberrations. Defer weight repletion until a patient's critical episode subsides; needs generally normalize again in 3–6 weeks. Feeding programs should support a patient being within 10–15 pounds of desirable BMI range. Use these guidelines:

For Adults	Sedentary (kcal/kg)	Moderate	Active (kcal/kg)	Critically Ill (kcal/kg)
Overweight BMI >30	20–25	30	35	15–20
Normal weight BMI 20–29	30	35	40	20–25
Underweight BMI 15–19	30	40	45–50	30–35

(continued)

TABLE B-5 Calculation of Adult Energy Requirements *(continued)*

Mifflin – St. Jeor Equation Sheet

Weight^			Height				Age	
Pounds	**Kilograms**	**MSJ***	**Feet and Inches**	**Inches**	**Centimeters**	**MSJ***	**Years**	**MSJ***
85	38.64	**386.36**	4′ 9″	57	144.78	**904.88**	70	**350**
90	40.91	**409.09**	4′ 10″	58	147.32	**920.75**	72	**360**
95	43.18	**431.82**	4′ 11″	59	149.86	**936.63**	74	**370**
100	45.45	**454.55**	5′	60	152.4	**952.50**	76	**380**
105	47.73	**477.27**	5′ 1″	61	154.94	**968.38**	78	**390**
110	50.00	**500.00**	5′ 2″	62	157.48	**984.25**	80	**400**
115	52.27	**522.73**	5′ 3″	63	160.02	**1000.13**	81	**405**
120	54.55	**545.45**	5′ 4″	64	162.56	**1016.00**	82	**410**
125	56.82	**568.18**	5′ 5″	65	165.1	**1031.88**	83	**415**
130	59.09	**590.91**	5′ 6″	66	167.64	**1047.75**	84	**420**
135	61.36	**613.64**	5′ 7″	67	170.18	**1063.63**	85	**425**
140	63.64	**636.36**	5′ 8″	68	172.72	**1079.50**	86	**430**
145	65.91	**659.09**	5′ 9″	69	175.26	**1095.38**	87	**435**
150	68.18	**681.82**	5′ 10″	70	177.8	**1111.25**	88	**440**
155	70.45	**704.55**	5′ 11″	71	180.34	**1127.13**	89	**445**
160	72.73	**727.27**	6′	72	182.88	**1143.00**	90	**450**
165	75.00	**750.00**	6′ 1″	73	185.42	**1158.88**	91	**455**
170	77.27	**772.73**	6′ 2″	74	187.96	**1174.75**	92	**460**
175	79.55	**795.45**	6′ 3″	75	190.5	**1190.63**	93	**465**
180	81.82	**818.18**					94	**470**
185	84.09	**840.91**					95	**475**
190	86.36	**863.64**					96	**480**
195	88.64	**886.36**					97	**485**
200	90.91	**909.09**					98	**490**
205	93.18	**931.82**					99	**495**
210	95.45	**954.55**					100	**500**
215	97.73	**977.27**					101	**505**
220	100.00	**1000.00**					102	**510**
225	102.27	**1022.73**					103	**515**

*REE for males = (MSJ weight + MSJ Height − MSJ age) + 5
*REE for females = (MSJ weight + MSJ Height − MSJ age) − 161
^Always use actual body weight. Activity factor is 1.2 if confined to bed; 1.3 if ambulatory.

Body Mass Index (BMI)
Weight (lb)

Height	**100**	**105**	**110**	**115**	**120**	**125**	**130**	**135**	**140**	**145**	**150**	**155**	**160**	**165**	**170**	**175**	**180**	**185**	**190**	**195**	**200**	**205**
5′0″	20	21	21	22	23	24	25	26	27	28	29	30	31	32	33	34	35	36	37	38	39	40
5′1″	19	20	21	22	23	24	25	26	26	27	28	29	30	31	32	33	34	35	36	37	38	39
5′2″	18	19	20	21	22	23	24	25	26	27	27	28	29	30	31	32	33	34	35	36	37	37
5′3″	18	19	19	20	21	22	23	24	25	26	27	27	28	29	30	31	32	33	34	35	35	36
5′4″	17	18	19	20	21	21	22	23	24	25	26	27	27	28	29	30	31	32	33	33	34	35
5′5″	17	17	18	19	20	21	22	22	23	24	25	26	27	27	28	29	30	31	32	32	33	34
5′6″	16	17	18	19	19	20	21	22	23	23	24	25	26	27	27	28	29	30	31	31	32	33
5′7″	16	16	17	18	19	20	20	21	22	23	23	24	25	26	27	27	28	29	30	31	31	32
5′8″	15	16	17	17	18	19	20	21	21	22	23	24	24	25	26	27	27	28	29	30	30	31
5′9″	15	16	16	17	18	18	19	20	21	21	22	23	24	24	25	26	27	27	28	29	30	30
5′10″	14	15	16	17	17	18	19	19	20	21	22	22	23	24	24	25	26	27	27	28	29	29
5′11″	14	15	15	16	17	17	18	19	20	20	21	22	22	23	24	24	25	26	26	27	28	29
6′0″	14	14	15	16	16	17	18	18	19	20	20	21	22	22	23	24	24	25	26	26	27	28
6′1″	13	14	15	15	16	16	17	18	18	19	20	20	21	22	22	23	24	24	25	26	26	27
6′2″	13	13	14	15	15	16	17	17	18	19	19	20	21	21	22	22	23	24	24	25	26	26
6′3″	12	13	14	14	15	16	16	17	17	18	19	19	20	21	21	22	22	23	24	24	25	26
6′4″	12	13	13	14	15	15	16	16	17	18	18	19	19	20	21	21	22	23	23	24	24	25

TABLE B-6 Calculations of Adult Protein Requirements

It requires 6.25 g of dietary protein to equal 1 g of nitrogen. Therefore, estimated nitrogen requirements × 6.25 = estimated protein needs in grams. If energy is not provided in adequate amounts, protein tissues become a substrate. Extra protein intake may be needed to compensate for excess protein loss in specific patient populations such as those with burn injuries, open wounds, and protein-losing enteropathy or nephropathy. Lower protein intake may be necessary in patients with chronic renal insufficiency who are not treated by dialysis and certain patients with hepatic encephalopathy. The following table provides an estimate for protein needs in adults.

Clinical Condition	Daily Protein Requirement (g/kg body weight)
Normal	0.8
Metabolic stress (illness/injury)	1.0–1.5
Acute renal failure (undialyzed)	0.8–1.0
Hemodialysis	1.2–1.4
Peritoneal dialysis	1.3–1.5

Adapted from the American Gastroenterological Association. Medical position statement: parenteral nutrition. *Gastroenterol.* 121:966, 2001.

TABLE B-7 Pediatric Nutrition Assessment

Date of Birth _______________ Hx of LBW or other birth problems __________ Present Illness: ____________________
Medical History: _______________ Social History: _______________ Family Medical Hx: ____________________
Height (Length): ______(cm) Height for Age: _______(%ile) % Height for Age: _______ Interpretation: _______
Current weight: _______(kg) Weight for Age: _______(%ile) % Weight for Height: ______ Interpretation: _________
Ideal Weight for Height: _______(kg) Ideal Height for Age: ____(cm) Weight change? (days, weeks, or months) __________
Head circumference: ______(cm) ______(%ile) ______ (For children <3 years old, use the growth chart.)
Review of Systems for Nutritional Deficiencies:
General: ____
Skin: ___________________ Hair: _________ Nails: ____________ Head: _______________
Eyes: _____________ Mouth: ___________ GI/Abdomen: ___________ Cardiac: ____________
Extremities: ____________ Neurological: __________ Musculoskeletal: ___________________
Laboratory Test Results: ____
Child allergic to any food or drinks? Yes / No If yes, allergic to what? ____________ Rash or eczema? Yes / No
Does the child avoid any specific foods such as milk or meats? Yes / No If yes, which ones? __________________
Does the child take any vitamins, minerals, or food supplements? Yes / No If yes, which? ___________ With fluoride Yes / No
If not taking a vitamin, does the water supply contain fluoride? Yes / No
Using formula? ________ How much given and how much water is added? ________ Put to bed with a bottle? Yes / No
What type of milk? ____________ # ounces/day? ______ Other beverages during the day? Iced tea Soda

Diet soda Kool-aid Juice Water Other _______

If eating foods, at what age were solids introduced into the diet? __________ How many meals are eaten during the day? ___
How many snacks are eaten during the day? _______________ What types? _______________
Does the child usually eat the food that is prepared for the family? Yes / No
Does the child chew on any of the following: Dirt Clay Paint chips Woodwork Ice Plaster Newspaper
How old is the house? Are there lead pipes? Yes / No Has the water been tested for lead? Yes / No
Estimated energy needs: ____________ Protein needs: ___________ Fluid needs: _______________

Patient Age	Energy Requirements	Fluid
Infants, up to 6 months	108 kcal/kg	1–10 kg = 100 cc/kg body weight
Infants, 6 months to 1 year	98 kcal/kg	11–20 kg = 1000 cc plus 50 cc/kg body weight >10 kg
Children	Requirements increase to 102 kcal/kg from 1–3 years of age.	≥21 kg = 1500 cc plus 20 cc/kg body weight >20 kg
	Requirements gradually decrease with age to 70 kcal/kg at age 10.	—
Adolescents	45–55 kcal/kg male; 40–47 kcal/kg female	Can use 30 cc/kg body weight; increase with fever, illness, diseases

Dietitian Comments:
Calculations: Estimated energy needs: ___kcal/kg Estimated protein needs: ___g/kg Estimated fluid needs: __ml/kg
Signed: ______________________________ RD Date: ______________

Adapted from: University of California, Los Angeles Nutrition Department. Pediatric Nutrition Assessment Checklist. Accessed April 8, 2010 at http://apps.medsch.ucla.edu/nutrition/chklst2.htm.

TABLE B-8 Interpretation of Lab Values

Many lab tests can provide useful information on patients' nutritional status along with information on their medical status. Age-specific criteria should be used to evaluate data. Common tests include the following.

Allergy Antibody Assessment

Allergy blood and skin testing
C-reactive protein
Helicobacter pylori Antibodies Test
Immunoglobulins: IgG, IgM, IgA, IgD, and IgE; specific IgE for molds, IgG for spices and herbs
Rheumatoid factor (RF)

Blood Chemistry and Renal Tests

Albumin
Blood urea nitrogen (BUN)
Creatinine clearance
Glomerular filtration rate (GFR)
Nitrogen balance
Serum creatinine
Serum proteins, total protein

Cardiopulmonary System

Arterial blood gases
Cardiac enzymes
Creatine kinase
Homocysteine
Lactate dehydrogenase, aspartate transaminase (AST)
Lipid profile: Cholesterol, lipoproteins, triglycerides

Celiac Assessment

IgA-antitissue transglutaminase (tTG)
IgA-antiendomysial antibodies (IgA-EMA)
IgA-antigliadin antibodies (IgA-AGA)

Coagulation Tests

Bleeding or coagulation time
International normalized ratio (INR)
Prothrombin time (PT)

Endocrine System

Aldosterone
Antidiuretic hormone
Blood glucose
C-peptide
Calcium
Calcitonin
Glucose tolerance test (GTT)
Insulin
Parathormone (PTH)
Phosphorus
Thyroxine (T4)
Thyroid-stimulating hormone (TSH)
Triiodothyronine (T3)

Gastrointestinal System and Stool Tests

Bacterial overgrowth of small intestine breath test
Comprehensive digestive stool analysis
Gastric analysis
Lactose intolerance breath test
Parasitology assessment
Serum gastrin

Hepatic System

Albumin, gamma-globulin, A-G ratio
Alanine aminotransferase (ALT)
Aspartate aminotransferase (AST)
Alkaline phosphatase (ALP)
Ammonia
Bilirubin
Gamma-glutamyl transpeptidase (GGT)
Hepatitis virus
Prothrombin time (PT)
Partial thromboplastin time (PTT)
Total protein
Urobilinogen

Musculoskeletal System

Alkaline phosphatase (ALP)
Acid phosphatase
Creatine phosphokinase (CPK)
Enzymes, isoenzymes
Lactate dehydrogenase (LDH)

Pancreatic Tests

Serum amylase
Serum lipase

Red Cell Indices

Carbon dioxide
Mean cell volume (MCV)
Mean cell hemoglobin (MCH)
MCH concentration
Reticulocyte cell count
Serum ferritin
Serum iron and total iron-binding capacity
Sodium, potassium, chlorine

(continued)

TABLE B-8 Interpretation of Lab Values *(continued)*

Vitamin and Mineral Assessment

Calcium
Zinc
Vitamin A
Vitamin C
Vitamin B_6
Vitamin B_{12}
Folate

Urinary System

Physical observation: Color, clarity, odor
Microscopic examination: Cells, casts, crystals, bacteria, yeast
Urine volume
Chemical tests: Specific gravity, pH, protein, glucose, ketones, blood, bilirubin, urobilinogen, nitrite, leukocyte esterase

Value	Normal Range	Purpose or Comment	Increased In	Decreased In
Hematology: Coagulation Tests and Bleeding Time				
Prothrombin time (PT), international normalized ratio (INR)	11–16 seconds control; 70–110% of control value Patients on anticoagulant drugs should have an INR of 2.0–3.0 for basic "blood thinning" needs. For some patients who have a high risk of clot formation, the INR needs to be higher—about 2.5–3.5.	Since PT and INR evaluate the ability of blood to clot properly, they can be used to assess both bleeding and clotting tendencies. One common use is to monitor the effectiveness of blood thinning drugs such as warfarin (Coumadin). Anticoagulant drugs must be carefully monitored to maintain a balance between preventing clots and causing excessive bleeding.	A prolonged or increased prothrombin time means that blood is taking too long to form a clot. Antibiotics, aspirin, and cimetidine can increase the PT/INR.	Too much anticoagulation (warfarin, for example). Barbiturates, oral contraceptives, hormone-replacement therapy (HRT), and vitamin K (either in a multivitamin or liquid nutrition supplement) can decrease PT. Beef and pork liver, green tea, broccoli, chickpeas, kale, turnip greens, and soybean products contain large amounts of vitamin K and can alter PT results if consumed in large amounts.
Hematology: Blood Cell Values				
Erythrocyte count (red blood cells [RBC])	4.5–6.2 million/mm^3 in males; 4.2–5.4 million/mm^3 in females	Made in bone marrow; production controlled by erythropoietin.	Polycythemia, dehydration, severe diarrhea	Anemias such as vitamin B_{12}, iron, folic acid, and protein; chronic infections; hemorrhage
Erythrocyte sedimentation rate	0–15 mm/hour in males; 0–25 mm/hour in females	Sedimentation rate measures how quickly RBCs (erythrocytes) settle in a test tube in 1 hour. Often used with C-reactive protein (CRP) for testing of inflammation.	Inflammation, pneumonia, appendicitis, pelvic inflammatory disease, lymphoma, multiple myeloma, lupus, rheumatoid arthritis (RA), osteomyelitis, temporal arteritis	
Ferritin	20–300 mg/mL in males; 20–120 mg/mL in females	Chief iron storage protein in the body. Reflects reticuloendothelial iron storage. Usually 23% of total iron stores.	Hemochromatosis, leukemias, anemias other than iron deficiency, Hodgkin's disease, liver diseases	Iron deficiency anemia
Folate, serum	0.3 μg/dL (7 nmol/L)	Important for DNA functioning	Blind loop syndrome	Pregnancy, lactation, macrocytic anemia, intestinal malabsorption syndrome, alcoholism, use of goat's milk in childhood, use of anticonvulsants, cycloserine, methotrexate, and oral contraceptives

(continued)

TABLE B-8 Interpretation of Lab Values *(continued)*

Value	Normal Range	Purpose or Comment	Increased In	Decreased In
Iron, serum	75–175 mg/dL in males; 65–165 mg/dL in females; 40–100+ mg/dL in children up to 2 years old; 50–120 mg/dL in children >2 years.	Iron found in blood, largely in hemoglobin	Hemochromatosis, acute or chronic liver disease, hemolytic anemia, leukemia, lead poisoning, thalassemia, vitamin B_{12} or folate deficiency, dehydration, small bowel surgery	50 µg/dL (9 mmol/L) may indicate iron deficiency anemia or blood loss. Chronic diseases, pregnancy, cancer, end-stage renal disease (ESRD) or chronic renal disease, malnutrition or poor dietary intake, sickle cell disease, viral hepatitis, thalassemia
Iron-binding capacity, total (TIBC)	240–450 mg/dL	Measure of the capacity of serum transferrin. 18–59% transferrin saturation is normal. As serum iron decreases, TIBC goes up, at least initially.	Iron deficiency, blood loss, later in pregnancy, oral contraceptive use, hepatitis, low serum iron, gastrectomy	High serum iron, renal disease, hemochromatosis, pernicious anemia, cancer, thalassemia, hemolytic diseases, small bowel surgery, sepsis, liver disease; may be low in malnutrition
Hematocrit (% packed cell volume)	40–54% in males; 37–47% in females; 33–35% in children; 37–49% in 12- to 18-year-old males; 36–46% in 12- to 18-year-old females	Cell volume % of RBCs in whole blood. Elevated when iron level is low.	Polycythemia	Anemias, prolonged dietary deficiency of protein and iron, sepsis, small bowel surgery, gastrectomy, renal or liver disease, blood loss
Hemoglobin, whole blood	14–17 g/dL in males; 12–15 g/dL in females; ≥10 g/dL in babies 6–23 months old; ≥11 in children 2–5 years old; 11.5–15.5 g/dL in children 6–12 years old; 13.0–16.0 g/dL in 12- to 18-year-old males; 12.0–16.0 g/dL in 12- to 18-year-old females	Oxygen carrier from lung to tissues. Binds CO_2 on return to the lung.	Polycythemia, dehydration, hemolysis, sickle cell anemia, recent blood transfusions, chronic obstructive pulmonary disease (COPD), heart failure, high altitude, burns, dehydration	Anemias, prolonged dietary deficiency of iron, excessive bleeding, cancer, lupus, overhydration, Hodgkin's disease, malnutrition, renal or liver disease, pregnancy, lead poisoning, sepsis, small bowel surgery, gastrectomy
Mean corpuscular hemoglobin (MCH)	26–32 pg; concentration is 32–36%	High concentration of individual RBCs (Hgb/RBC)	Macrocytic anemia	Hemoglobin deficiency, hypochromic anemia
Mean corpuscular volume (MCV)	80–94 cu/µm	Individual RBC size	High MCV or macrocytosis: folate, vitamin B_{12} deficiency. Alcoholic or liver disease, blood loss, hypothyroidism, small bowel surgery	Low MCV or microcytosis: iron, copper, pyridoxine deficiency. Thalassemia, anemia of chronic disease, cancer, blood loss
Transferrin (siderophilin)	170–370 mg/dL (1.7–3.7 g/L)	Glycoprotein in blood plasma that transports iron to liver and spleen for storage and to bone marrow for hemoglobin synthesis	Iron deficiency, acute hepatitis, oral contraceptive use, pregnancy, chronic blood loss, dehydration, gastrectomy	Acute or chronic inflammation, chronic liver disease, lupus, zinc deficiency, sickle cell anemia, pernicious anemia with vitamin B_{12} or folate deficiency, chronic infection and inflammatory diseases, malnutrition, burns, iron overload, nephrotic syndrome, sepsis, small bowel surgery

(continued)

TABLE B-8 Interpretation of Lab Values *(continued)*

Value	Normal Range	Purpose or Comment	Increased In	Decreased In
White blood cells (WBC), leukocytes	4.8–11.8 thousand/mm^3	Highly variable lab value; protect against disease or infection	Metabolic acidosis, acute hemorrhage, acute bacterial infections, leukemias, burns, gangrene, exercise, stress, eclampsia	Chemotherapy, ABT. Neutropenia is often seen in deficiency states. Some viral conditions, cachexia, anaphylactic shock, bone marrow suppression, pernicious or aplastic anemia, diuretic use
Hematology and Lymphatic System: Differential				
Lymphocytes	Total lymphocyte count (TLC) = normal, 12,000/mm^3; deficient, <900/mm^3; 24–44% total WBC count	Made in thymus and lymph nodes; produce antibodies	Infectious mononucleosis, mumps, German measles, convalescence from acute infections	Infections, malnutrition
Leukocytes: basophils	0–1.5% total WBC count	They release substances that cause smooth muscle contraction, vasoconstriction, and an increased permeability of small blood vessels. Basophils are stimulated by allergens.	Postsplenectomy, chronic myelogenous leukemia, polycythemia, Hodgkin's disease, chicken pox	Hyperthyroidism, acute infections,pregnancy, anaphylaxis
Leukocytes: eosinophils	0.5–4% total WBC count	Eosinophils are stimulated by parasites and some bacteria. They release substances that cause vasoconstriction, smooth muscle contraction, and an increased permeability of small blood vessels. Related to allergies.	Allergies, parasitic infections, pernicious anemia, ulcerative colitis, Hodgkin's disease	Use of β-blockers, corticosteroids; stress, and bacterial and viral infections including trichinosis
Leukocytes: monocytes	4–8% total WBC count	Phagocytosis. Produced in bone marrow.	Monocytic leukemia, lipid storage disease, protozoan infection, chronic ulcerative colitis	
Leukocytes: neutrophils	60–65% total WBC count	Phagocytosis	Wound sepsis in burns, bacterial infections, inflammation, cancer, traumas, stress, diabetes, acute gout	Folate or vitamin B_{12} deficiency, sickle cell anemia, steroid therapy, postsurgical status
Platelets (thrombocytes)	125,000–300,000 mm^3	Largely polysaccharides and phospholipids. Role in coagulation.	Malignancy, polycythemia vera, splenectomy, iron deficiency anemia, cirrhosis, chronic pancreatitis	Thrombocytopenic purpura
General Serum Values and Enzymes				
Amylase	60–180 Somogyi units/dL	Pancreatic enzyme for hydrolysis of starch and glycogen	Increased in perforated peptic ulcer, acute pancreatitis, mumps, cholecystitis, renal insufficiency, alcohol poisoning, partial gastrectomy	Decreased in hepatitis, severe burns, pancreatic disease, advanced cystic fibrosis, toxemia of pregnancy, hepatitis
Bicarbonate	22–28 mEq/L	Acid–base balance	Metabolic alkalosis, large intake of sodium bicarbonate, excessive vomiting, potassium deficiency, respiratory acidosis, emphysema	Diabetic acidosis, starvation, chronic diarrhea, renal insufficiency, respiratory alkalosis (hyperventilation), fistula drainage

(continued)

TABLE B-8 Interpretation of Lab Values *(continued)*

Value	Normal Range	Purpose or Comment	Increased In	Decreased In
Bilirubin	Direct: ≤0.3 mg/dL; total: ≤1 mg/dL	Hemoglobin is converted to bilirubin when RBCs are destroyed.	Hepatitis, jaundice, biliary obstruction, drug toxicity, hemolytic disease, prolonged fasting	Seasonal affective disorder
Calcium	9–11 mg/dL (2.3–2.8 mmol/L); 3.9–5.4 mg/dL serum ionized	50% is protein bound, so protein intake affects serum calcium level more than dietary calcium. Regulated by parathormone (PTH) and thyrocalcitonin. Coma above 13 mg/dL; death below 7 mg/dL.	Hyperparathyroidism, renal calculi, vitamin D excess, osteolytic disease, milk-alkali syndrome, immobilization, tuberculosis, Addison's disease, antibiotic therapy, cancer	Steatorrhea, renal failure, malabsorption, vitamin D deficiency, hypoparathyroidism, sprue, celiac disease, overhydration, hypoalbumenia, hyperphosphatemia
Ceruloplasmin	27–37 mg/dL	Form of copper found in the bloodstream	Leukemias, anemias, cirrhosis of the liver, hypo/hyperthyroidism, collagen diseases, pregnancy	Wilson's disease, severe copper deficiency, nephrosis, leukemia remission, prolonged total parenteral nutrition (TPN) without copper, cystic fibrosis
Copper	70–140 μg/dL in males; 80–155 μg/dL in females	Found bound to albumin or as ceruloplasmin	Leukemias, anemias, cirrhosis of the liver, hypo/hyperthyroidism, collagen diseases, pregnancy	Wilson's disease, severe copper deficiency, nephrosis, leukemia remission, prolonged TPN without copper, cystic fibrosis
Creatine phosphokinase (CPK)	0–145 IU/L	Catalyst for phosphorylation of creatine by adenosine triphosphate (ATP). Mostly found in skeletal and cardiac muscle. Increases 2–4 hours after myocardial infarction (MI), returning to normal after 3 days.	Hepatic or uremic coma, striated muscle disease, muscular dystrophy, MI, cerebrovascular accident (CVA), trauma, alcoholic liver disease, encephalitis	
D-xylose, 25-g dose	30–40 mg/dL	This test measures the intestines' ability to absorb D-xylose—a simple sugar—as an indicator of whether nutrients are being properly absorbed.		Xylose malabsorption
Gamma-glutamyl transpeptidase (GGT)	5–40 IU/L	GGT participates in the transfer of amino acids across the cellular membrane and in glutathione metabolism. Used to detect diseases of the liver, bile ducts, and kidney and to differentiate liver or bile duct (hepatobiliary) disorders from bone disease.	Coronary heart failure (CHF), MI, cholecystitis, liver disease, alcoholism, hepatic biliary disease, pancreatitis, nephritic syndrome	
Lactic acid dehydrogenase (LDH)	200–680 IU/mL	Catalyzes conversion between pyruvate and lactic acid in glycolytic cycle. Has 5 isoenzymes. Increases 8–10 hours after MI, returning to normal after 7–14 days.	Untreated pernicious anemia, acute MI, heart failure, malignancy, alcoholic liver damage, cardiovascular surgery, hepatitis, pulmonary embolus, leukemia, cancer, renal failure, hemolytic or megaloblastic anemia, muscular dystrophy, nephrotic syndrome	Radiation therapy
Lipase	0.2–1.5 IU/mL	Synthesized by the pancreas	Pancreatic disease, acute pancreatitis, perforated ulcer, pancreatic duct obstruction, biliary tract infection, renal insufficiency	

(continued)

TABLE B-8 Interpretation of Lab Values *(continued)*

Value	Normal Range	Purpose or Comment	Increased In	Decreased In
Phenylalanine, serum	<3 mg/dL	An amino acid of importance in phenylketonuria (PKU) patients	Levels might be high in PKU	Severe protein deficiency and malnutrition
Phosphatase, acid	0.5–2 Bodansky units	A blood test that measures prostatic acid phosphatase (an enzyme found primarily in men in the prostate gland and semen) to determine the health of the prostate gland	Prostate dysfunction results in the release of prostatic acid phosphatase into the blood.	
Phosphatase, alkaline (ALP)	2–4.5 Bodansky units (30–135 IU/L); children = 3× that of adults	ALP is an enzyme found in all tissues. Tissues with particularly high concentrations of ALP include the liver, bile ducts, placenta, and bone. Indirect test for calcium, phosphorus, vitamin D nutriture. Used to determine the presence of liver or bone cell disorders.	Anemia, Paget's disease, biliary obstruction, leukemia, hyperparathyroidism, rickets, bone disease, healing fracture	Malnutrition, protein deficiency
Sulfate, inorganic	0.5–1.5 mg/dL	Usual sulfur intake is 0.6–1.6 grams on a mixed diet containing 100 grams of protein.	Supplemental overdose; high sulfate intake from water supply	Protein deficiency; injury to the bones, cartilage, or tendons
Transaminase: aspartate aminotransferase (AST)	5–40 IU/mL	Found in the liver, muscle, and the brain. Functional measure of vitamin B_6 nutriture. Released in tissue injury. Formerly SGOT (serum glutamic oxaloacetic transaminase).	Hepatic cancer, shock/trauma, cirrhosis, neoplastic disease, MI	Uncontrolled diabetes mellitus; Beriberi
Transaminase: alanine aminotransferase (ALT)	4–36 IU/L	Found in the liver. Generally parallels AST levels. Functional measure of vitamin B_6 nutriture. Formerly SGPT (serum glutamic pyruvic transaminase).	Hepatitis, cirrhosis, trauma, hepatic cancer, shock, mononucleosis	Wilson's disease
Glucose Control				
Glucose, fasting serum	70–110 mg/dL (3.9–6.1 mmol/L)	Principle fuel for cellular function, particularly for the brain and RBCs.	DM, hyperthyroidism pancreatitis, MI, hyperfunction of endocrine, stress, CHF infection, surgery, CVA, hepatic dysfunction, cancer, Cushing's syndrome, burns, steroids, chromium deficiency	Postprandial hypoglycemia, sepsis, cancer, malnutrition, hypothyroid, gastrectomy, liver damage or disease, Addison's disease
Glucose tolerance test (GTT)	2-hour post load glucose <200 mg/dL	Test done when blood glucose levels are >120 mg/dL.	Diabetes, hyperthyroidism, pancreatic cancer, Cushing's syndrome, acromegaly, pheochromocytoma.	Hypoglycemia, hypothyroidism, malabsorption, malnutrition, insulinoma, hypopituitarism
Glycosylated hemoglobin–HbA1 C	4–7% (nondiabetic); good, <9%; fair, 9–12%; poor, >12%	May reflect poor glucose control over the past 2–4 months	Poor blood sugar control, newly diagnosed diabetes, pregnancy	Low RBC (chronic blood loss, hemolytic anemia), chronic renal failure (CRF), sickle cell anemia
Protein Factors				
Albumin	3.5–5 g/dL (35–50 g/L); 3.2–5.1 g/dL in infants up to 1 year old; 3.2–5.7 in children aged 1–2 years; 3.5–5.8 for ages 2 years to adult. Albumin is usually 40% of proteins.	Nonspecific protein nutriture measure. Mostly synthesized in the liver. Transports fatty acids, thyroxin, bilirubin, and many drugs. Albumin–globulin ratio (A:G) is 1.2–1.9; low in renal or liver diseases.	Dehydration, multiple myeloma	Decreased with inflammation and severity of illness, acute stress, starvation, malabsorption of protein, cirrhosis, nephritis with edema, liver disease, malnutrition

(continued)

TABLE B-8 Interpretation of Lab Values *(continued)*

Value	Normal Range	Purpose or Comment	Increased In	Decreased In
C-reactive protein (CRP)	0	Elevated in inflammation	Systemic inflammation, obesity, diabetes, heart disease, arthritis, smoking	Vitamin C supplements may lower an elevated CRP. Marathon runners may have very low levels.
Creatinine	0.6–1.2 mg/dL	A basic creatine anhydride, nitrogenous end product of skeletal muscle metabolism. Indirect measure of renal filtration rate.	Hyperthyroidism, CHF, diabetic acidosis, dehydration, muscle disease, some cancers, nephritis, urinary obstruction	Overhydration, multiple sclerosis (MS), pregnancy, eclampsia, increased age, severe wasting
Creatinine–height index (CHI)	CHI = (measured 24-hour creatine excretion × 100)/predicted 24-hour creatine excretion	Estimates skeletal muscle mass. CHI values of 60–80% represent mild marasmus. CHIs of 40–59% represent moderate marasmus. CHIs of <40% represent severe marasmus.	High doses of creatine supplementation	Marasmus, malnutrition
Globulin	2.3–3.5 g/dL	5 fractions; transport antibodies	Infections, leukemia, dehydration, shock, tuberculosis (TB), chronic alcoholism, Hodgkin's disease	Malnutrition, immunological deficiency
Nitrogen balance	Goal of 1–4 g/24 hours urinary urea nitrogen (UUN)	Nitrogen balance is the result of nitrogen intake (from the diet) and nitrogen losses, which consist of nitrogen recovered in urine and feces and miscellaneous losses.	Severe liver disease	Nephrosis
Prealbumin (transthyretin)	16–35 mg/dL	Reflects the past 3 days of protein intake but is affected by inflammation	Renal failure, Hodgkin's disease, pregnancy, dehydration	Acute catabolic states, hepatic disease, stress infection, surgery, low protein intake, malnutrition, hyperthyroidism, nephritic syndrome, overhydration, inflammation
Proteins, total serum	6–8 g/dL; 5.6–7.2 in infants to 1 year; 5.4–7.5 in children 1–2 years old; 5.3–8.0 in ages 2 years to adult	Amount of protein in the bloodstream. Reflects depletion of tissue proteins. Act as buffers in acid–base balance. Plasma proteins equal approximately 7% of total plasma volume.	Dehydration, shock	Hepatic disease, leukemia, malnutrition, infection, pregnancy, malabsorption, severe burns
Nutrient Values				
Ascorbic acid (vitamin C)	0.2–2.0 mg/dL	Serum levels of vitamin C	Oxalate stones, diarrhea, high uric acid	Large doses of aspirin, barbiturates, stress, anemia, tetracycline, oral contraceptives, cigarette smoking, alcoholism, dialysis
Essential fatty acids (EFA) (triene to tetraene [T/T] ratio)	0.2 is normal; a ratio >0.4 in serum phospholipids indicates EFA deficiency in healthy people	Ratio 20:39/20:46 (T/T ratio) is measured. T/T ratios are assessed in RBCs, RBC phospholipids, and serum phospholipids.		EFA deficiency occurs in starvation, marasmus, and strict low-fat diets.
Niacin: *N*-methylnicotinamide	5.8 μmol/d	For niacin assessment. Usual dietary intake is 16–33 mg/d.	Large doses of nicotinic acid	Pregnancy, lactation, Hartnup disease, pellagra, schizophrenia
Riboflavin: glutathione reductase, erythrocyte	1.2 IU/g hemoglobin	Dietary intake is related to CHO and total energy intake.		Tetracycline or thiazide diuretic use, probenecid, oral contraceptives, sulfa drugs, pellagra, cheilosis, some forms of glossitis, vegetarians using no dairy products or supplements

(continued)

TABLE B-8 Interpretation of Lab Values *(continued)*

Value	Normal Range	Purpose or Comment	Increased In	Decreased In
Selenium: glutathione peroxidase	Serum enzyme levels	Works with vitamin E to protect RBCs as part of the enzyme.	Excessive lipid peroxidation	PCM, hypoproteinemia
Thiamin: transketolase activity, erythrocyte	1.20 μg/mL/hr	Dietary requirements increase when CHO intake is high.		Use of baking soda in cooking, high CHO intake, infantile beriberi, dry or edematous (cardiac) beriberi, excessive intake of caffeic or tannic acids, pellagra, chronic alcoholism, lactic acidosis in metabolic disorders such as maple syrup urine disease (MSUD)
Vitamin B_6: pyridoxal 5′−phosphate, plasma	5 ng/mL (20 nmol/L)	Usual dietary intake is 2 milligrams, assuming 100 grams of protein is consumed.		Acute celiac disease, chronic alcoholism, pellagra, high protein intake, pregnancy, oral contraceptive use, isoniazid (INH) and other TB drug use, use of anticonvulsants, malarial drugs
Vitamin A: carotene; retinol, serum	48–200 mg/dL; 10–60 μg/dL	Serum levels of carotenoids	Excessive intake, such as from carrots; postprandial hyperlipidemia; diabetes; hypothyroidism	High fever, liver disease, malabsorption syndrome
Retinol-binding protein	2.6–7.6 mg/dL	Used less often to determine status of retinol	May be high in renal failure	Protein deficiency
Serum vitamin A	125–150 IU/dL or 20–80 mg/dL		Hypervitaminosis A	Cirrhosis, infectious hepatitis, myxedema, night blindness, malabsorption, starvation, infections such as measles
Vitamin B_{12}: serum B_{12}	24.4–100 ng/dL (180 pmol/L)	Vitamin B_{12} is less well absorbed in the elderly and in persons who have less intrinsic factor or the ability to reabsorb in the intestines.	Leukemia such as acute myelogenous leukemia (AML) or CML, leukocytosis, polycythemia vera, liver metastasis, hepatitis, cirrhosis	Macrocytic anemia, iron or vitamin B_6 deficiency, gastritis, dialysis, congenital intrinsic factor deficiency, pernicious anemia, tapeworm, ileal resection, strict vegetarian diets, pregnancy
Vitamin D: 1,25-HCC, blood	0.7–3.3 IU/dL	Indirect measures are available from serum alkaline phosphatase, calcium levels, and serum phosphorus.	Hypervitaminosis D	Rickets; osteomalacia; steroid therapy; fracture; poorly calcified teeth; drug therapy such as anticonvulsants, cholestyramine, and barbiturates
Vitamin E: alpha-tocopherol; plasma vitamin E	<18 μmol/g (41.8 μmol/L); 0.5–2.0 mg/dL	Usual dietary intake is 14 milligrams of d-alpha-tocopherol	High vitamin E intake (this affects coagulation because it works against vitamin K)	High polyunsaturated fatty acid (PUFA) intake, premature infants, cystic fibrosis, hemolytic anemia
Vitamin K: INR or PT	PT, 10–15 seconds	Combined low levels of prothrombin activity, serum calcium, and serum carotene may indicate abnormal fat and fat-soluble vitamin absorption.	Menadione use, intravenous (IV) administration of vitamin K, parenchymal liver disease	PT is prolonged in salicylates, sulfa, and tetracycline use. Liver disease, fat malabsorption, prematurity, small bowel disorders.
Zinc: serum zinc	0.75–1.4 mg/mL or up to 79 μg/dL in plasma; 100–140 μg/dL in serum	Large amounts are found in liver, skeletal muscle, and bone. Part of the insulin molecule. Usual intake is 10–15 mg/d.	Eating foods stored in galvanized containers. Excesses from supplements.	Wounds, geophagia, high-calcium or high-phytate diets, growth, stress, skin lesions, poor taste or olfactory acuity, upper respiratory infections, MI, oral contraceptive use, cancer, pregnancy, cirrhosis, sickle cell or pernicious anemias

(continued)

TABLE B-8 Interpretation of Lab Values *(continued)*

Value	Normal Range	Purpose or Comment	Increased In	Decreased In
Electrolytes				
Chloride	95–105 mEq/L	Acid–base balance. Major anion. Follows sodium passively in its transport.	Eclampsia, metabolic acidosis, dehydration, pancreatitis, anemia, renal insufficiency, Cushing's syndrome, head injury, hyperventilation, hyperlipidemia, hypoproteinemia	Diabetic acidosis, metabolic alkalosis, gastroenteritis, fever, potassium deficiency, excessive sweating, heart failure, hyponatremia, infection, diuretics, overhydration
Magnesium	1.8–3 mg/dL	Influences muscular activity. Coenzyme in CHO and protein metabolism.	Renal insufficiency, uncontrolled diabetes, Addison's disease, hypothyroidism, ingestion of magnesium-containing antacids or salts	Malnutrition, potassium-depleting diuretics, malabsorption, alcohol abuse, starvation, renal disease, acute pancreatitis, severe diarrhea, ulcerative colitis
Phosphorous phosphate (PO_4)	2.3–4.7 mg/dL	Influenced by diet and absorption; regulated by kidneys.	Liver disease, bone tumors, hypervitaminosis D, end-stage renal disease, renal insufficiency, hypoparathyroidism, diabetic ketoacidosis (DKA), Addison's disease, childhood	Malnutrition, gout, hyperparathyroidism, osteomalacia, hyperinsulinism, hypovitaminosis D, alcoholism, overuse of phosphate-binding antacids, rapid refeeding after prolonged starvation
Potassium, serum	3.5–5.5 mEq/L (16–20 mg/dL)	Intracellular. Cellular metabolism; muscle protein synthesis. Enzymes.	Renal insufficiency or failure, overuse of potassium supplements, Addison's disease, dehydration, acidosis, cell damage, poorly controlled diabetes	Decreased potassium intake, renal disease, burns, trauma, diuretics, steroids, vomiting, stress, diarrhea, crash diet, overhydration, malnutrition, estrogen, steroid therapy, cirrhosis, hemolysis, fistula drainage
Sodium, serum	136–145 mEq/L	Absorbed almost 100% from gastrointestinal (GI) tract. Major cation; extracellular ion. Controls osmotic pressure. Acid-base balance.	Vitamin K deficiency, vomiting, heart failure, hypervitaminosis, dehydration, diabetes insipidus, Cushing's disease, primary aldosteronism, diarrhea, steroids	Decreased sodium intake, diuretic use, burns, diarrhea, vomiting, nephritis, diabetic acidosis, hyperglycemia, overhydration
Lipids				
Total serum cholesterol (TC)	Adults: Desirable: 120–199 mg/dL; borderline high: 200–239 mg/dL; high: ≥240 mg/dL Child: Desirable: 70–175 mg/dL; borderline: 170–199 mg/dL; high: ≥200 mg/dL	Fat-related compound; component of plaque. Need fasting sample. Usually 30% high-density lipoprotein (HDL) and 70% low-density lipoprotein (LDL).	High: >200 mg/dL. Hyperlipidemia, diabetes, MI, hypertension (HTN), high-cholesterol diet, nephrotic syndrome, hypothyroidism, pregnancy, cardiovascular disease (CVD)	Low: <160 mg/dL. Low dietary fat ingestion, malnutrition, malabsorption or starvation, fever, acute infections, liver damage, steatorrhea, hyperthyroidism, cancer, pernicious anemia
High-density lipoprotein (HDL)	Males: >45 mg/dL; females: >55 mg/dL	Usually higher in females. Low levels may indicate risk for heart disease.	Vigorous exercise, weight reduction, liver disease, alcoholism	Starvation, obesity, liver disease, DM, smoking, hyperthyroidism
Low-density lipoprotein (LDL)	Desirable: <130 mg/dL; borderline high: 130–159 mg/dL; high: ≥160 mg/dL	May indicate cardiac risk when elevated.	Familial hyperlipidemia, diet high in saturated fat and cholesterol, hypothyroidism, MI, DM, nephrotic syndrome, pregnancy, hepatic disease	Nephritic syndrome

(continued)

TABLE B-8 Interpretation of Lab Values *(continued)*

Value	Normal Range	Purpose or Comment	Increased In	Decreased In
Phospholipids	60–350 mg/dL	Measure of EFAs, indirect. Includes lecithin, sphingomyelins, cephalins, and plasmogens.		EFA deficiency
Triglycerides (TG)	Desirable: 10–190 mg/dL; borderline high: 200–400 mg/dL; high: 400–1000 mg/dL; very high: >1000 mg/dL	Neutral fats are the main transport form of fatty acids. Need fasting sample.	High-carbohydrate diet, alcohol abuse (secondary), hyperlipoproteinemias, nephrotic syndrome, CRF, MI, HTN, DM, respiratory distress, pancreatitis, hypothyroidism	Malnutrition, COPD, malabsorption, hyperthyroidism, hyperparathyroidism, brain infarct
Osmolality and pH				
pH, arterial, plasma	7.36–7.44	Hydrogen ion concentration. Enzymes work within narrow pH ranges.	Alkalosis (uncompensated), hyperventilation, pyloric obstruction, HCl losses, diuretic use	Acidosis (uncompensated), emphysema, diabetic acidosis, renal failure, vomiting, diarrhea, intestinal fistula
Osmolality, serum	270–280 mOsm/L	Maintaining normal serum level is desirable.	Elevated in dehydration	Low in overhydration
Respiratory Factors				
Respiratory quotient (RQ)	0.85 from mixed diet	1.0 from CHO; 0.80 from protein; 0.70 from fat	High-CHO diet	High-fat diet
Oxygen: partial pressure of oxygen (pO_2)	80–100 mm Hg	Reflects hemoglobin concentration. Arterial blood is used.	Hyperoxia	Hypoxia (anemic, stagnant, chronic, anoxic)
Carbon dioxide: partial pressure of carbon dioxide (pCO_2)	35–45 mm Hg; 24–30 mEq/L		Pulmonary problems, metabolic alkalosis due to ingestion of excess sodium bicarbonate, protracted vomiting with potassium deficiency, Cushing's syndrome, heart failure with edema	Diabetic ketosis or ketoacidosis, starvation, renal insufficiency, persistent diarrhea, lactic acidosis, respiratory alkalosis, diarrhea
Renal Values				
Glomerular filtration rate (GFR)	110–150 mL/min in males; 105–132 mL/min in females	GFR reflects kidney function		Renal failure: <90 mL/min/1.73 m^2 indicates renal decline
Urea clearance	40–65 mL/min standard; 60–100 mL/min maximum	Part of the assessment of renal status		Uremia
Blood urea nitrogen (BUN) to creatinine ratio	>10:1	Measure of impaired renal function.	Renal disease, excess protein intake, bleeding in small intestine, burns, high fever, steroid therapy, decreased renal blood flow, urinary tract obstruction	Low-protein intake, repeated dialysis without repletion, severe vomiting and diarrhea, hepatic insufficiency
BUN	8–18 mg/dL (3–6.5 mmol/L); slightly higher in males	Urea is the end product of protein metabolism. Varies directly with dietary intake. Formed in the liver from amino acids and other ammonia-containing compounds.	Renal failure, azotemia, DM, burns, dehydration, shock, heart failure, infection, chronic gout, excessive protein intake, catabolism, GI bleed, MI, urinary obstruction, starvation, steroid therapy, trauma	Hepatic failure, malnutrition, malabsorption, overhydration, pregnancy, acromegaly, low-protein diet

(continued)

TABLE B-8 Interpretation of Lab Values *(continued)*

Value	Normal Range	Purpose or Comment	Increased In	Decreased In
Uric acid	4.0–9.0 mg/dL in men; 2.8–8.8 mg/dL in women	Metabolite from purine metabolism. Excreted by kidney. Serum level reflects balance between production and excretion.	Higher in winter, stress, gout, leukemia, hypoparathyroidism, total fasting, toxemia of pregnancy, elevated triglycerides, DKA, hypertension, hemolytic or sickle cell anemia, renal disease, alcoholism, multiple myeloma, polycythemia, use of vincristine or mercaptopurine	Acute hepatitis, Wilson's disease, celiac disease, Fanconi's syndrome, Hodgkin's disease, use of allopurinol or large doses of Coumadin, folic acid anemia, burns, pregnancy, malabsorption, lead poisoning
Hormones				
Adrenocorticotropic hormone (ACTH)	5–95 pg/mL at 9 AM; 0–35 pg/mL at midnight		Cushing's syndrome, secondary hypoadrenalism	Pituitary, Cushing's syndrome, primary adrenal insufficiency
Cortisol	5–25 μg/dL at 8 AM; 10 μg/dL at 8 PM	Lower in women	Extreme stress, elevated in patients with night-eating syndrome	
Gastrin	0–200 pg/mL		Zollinger–Ellison syndrome, pyloric obstruction, short bowel syndrome, pernicious anemia, atrophic gastritis	
Growth hormone (GH)	<6 ng/mL in men; <10 ng/mL in women	Being administered in some medical conditions		
Insulin	6–26 IU/mL, fasting	Serum levels are useful.	Untreated obese patients who have diabetes, metabolic syndrome, insulinoma	Severe diabetic acidosis with ketosis and weight loss
Iodine, total	8–15 mEq/L	Affects the activity of the thyroid gland; usual intake with 10 grams of NaCl is 1000 micrograms of iodine.	Hyperthyroidism	Cretinism, simple goiter, low-iodine diet or high-goitrogenic dietary intake
Protein-bound iodine (PBI)	3.6–8.8 mg/dL	Most iodine is protein-bound in the thyroid hormones.	Hyperthyroidism, thyroiditis, pregnancy, oral contraceptive use, hepatitis	Cretinism, simple goiter, low-iodine diet or high-goitrogenic dietary intake
Serotonin (5-HIAA)	0.05–0.20 μg/mL	Neurotransmitter		Depression
Thyroxine (T4); triiodothyronine (T3)	T4: 4–12 μg/100 mL; T3: 75–95 μg/100 mL	Tests of thyroid function	Myasthenia gravis, nephrosis, pregnancy, preeclampsia, Graves' disease, hyperthyroidism	Increased thyroid-stimulating hormone (TSH), decreased T4, T3 (hypothyroidism); malnutrition; hypothyroidism; nephrosis; cirrhosis; Simmonds' disease
Thyroid-stimulating hormone (TSH)	≤0.2 μU/L	Thyroid function tests (TSH, T4, T3)	Primary untreated hypothyroidism, post subtotal thyroidectomy	Hyperthyroidism
Stool Values				
Fat, fecal	<7 g/24 hr		Fat malabsorption	
Nitrogen	<2.5 g/d			
Urinalysis	Normal is pale golden yellow	Abnormal color changes: orange = high level of bile; red = blood, porphyria, urates, or bile or ingestion of beets, blackberries, or food dyes; brown = blood; melanin may turn black on standing.	Dehydration: dark golden color	Overhydration: clear color (diluted)

(continued)

TABLE B-8 Interpretation of Lab Values *(continued)*

Value	Normal Range	Purpose or Comment	Increased In	Decreased In
Acetone, ketones	0	Elevation indicates ketosis.	Diabetic ketoacidosis; starvation; fever; prolonged vomiting; high-protein, high-fat, or low-CHO diet; diarrhea; anorexia	
Aldosterone	6–16 mg/24 h			
Ammonia	20–70 mEq/L		Hepatic disease or coma, renal failure, severe heart failure, high-protein diet	Essential hypertension
Amylase	260–950 Somogyi units/24 h		Perforated peptic ulcer, acute pancreatitis, mumps, cholecystitis, renal insufficiency, alcohol poisoning	Hepatitis, pancreatic insufficiency, severe burns
Calcium, normal diet	<250 mg/24 h		Hyperparathyroidism, high calcium or vitamin D in diet, immobilization, metastatic bone disease, multiple myeloma, renal tubular acidosis	Decreased levels may reflect poor intake. Hypoparathyroidism, rickets, renal failure, steatorrhea, osteomalacia
Cortisol, urinary free	10–100 μg/dL		Elevated in stress	Adrenal insufficiency
Creatinine clearance	Males (20 years old): 90 mL/min/SA; females (20 years old): 84 mL/min/SA; decreases by 6 mL/min/SA per decade		Pregnancy, childhood, exercise.	Ascites, dehydration, renal failure, heart failure, shock, cirrhosis
Epinephrine, norepinephrine	Epinephrine: <10 μg/24 h; Norepinephrine <100 μg/24 h		Stress	
Estrogens	4–25 mg/24 h in males; 4–60 mg/24 h in females, higher in pregnancy			
Hemoglobin, myoglobin	0	Any amount	Blood loss, urinary tract injury	
5-Hydroxyindoleacetic acid	0	Serotonin excretion		
(5-HIAA)	20–60 mg/24 h		Calcium oxalate stones	
Oxalate pH	4.6–8; average of 6 (dependent on diet)	Depends on time of sampling and food ingested	Alkaline: metabolic alkalemia, proteus infection, aged specimen, large amount of fruits and vegetables eaten	Acidic: high-protein intake
Protein (albumin)	<30 mg/24 h (0 qualitative)	Amino acids in urine should be 0.4–1 g/L.	Nephrotic syndrome	
Specific gravity	1.003–1.030	Ability to concentrate urine	High in antidiuretic hormone deficiency	Low in renal tubular dysfunction
Sugar	0		Hyperglycemia, ketosis, DKA	
3-Methyl histidine, urine		Indicator of lean body mass turnover	Increased levels may reflect loss of lean body mass.	
Urea	20–35 g/L			
Uric acid	0.2–2.0 g/L			
Vanillylmandelic acid (VMA)	<6.8 mg/24 h	Metabolite of both epinephrine and norepinephrine		
Volume	1000–1500 mL	Varies slightly between individuals	Diabetes insipidus	Dehydration

The table provides estimated and sample normal values; normal ranges will vary by the techniques used by the laboratory completing the tests.
Developed from: Pagana KD, Pagana TJ. *Mosby's manual of diagnostic and laboratory tests*. 4th ed. Philadelphia: Mosby, 2009.

TABLE B-9 Quick Reference: Food–Drug Interactions

Drugs	Effects and Precautions
Antibiotics	
Cephalosporins, penicillin	Take on an empty stomach to speed absorption of the drugs.
Erythromycin	Do not take with fruit juice or wine, which decrease the drug's effectiveness.
Sulfa drugs	Increase the risk of vitamin B_{12} deficiency.
Tetracycline	Dairy products reduce the drug's effectiveness. Lowers vitamin C absorption.
Anticonvulsants	
Dilantin, phenobarbital	Increases the risk of anemia and nerve problems due to a deficiency in folate and other B vitamins.
Antidepressants	
Fluoxetine	Reduces appetite and can lead to excessive weight loss.
Lithium	A low-salt diet increases the risk of lithium toxicity; excessive salt reduces the drug's efficacy.
Monoamine oxidase (MAO) inhibitors	Foods high in tyramine (e.g., aged cheeses, processed meats, legumes, wine, and beer) can bring on a hypertensive crisis.
Tricyclics	Many foods, particularly legumes, meat, fish, and foods high in vitamin C, reduce absorption of the drugs.
Antihypertensives, Heart Medications	
Angiotensin-converting enzyme (ACE) inhibitors	Take on an empty stomach to improve the absorption of the drugs.
Alpha-blockers	Take with liquid or food to avoid excessive drop in blood pressure.
Antiarrhythmic drugs	Avoid caffeine, which increases the risk of an irregular heartbeat.
Beta-blockers	Take on an empty stomach; food, especially meat, increases the drug's effects and can cause dizziness and low blood pressure.
Digitalis	Avoid taking with milk and high-fiber foods, which reduce absorption; increases potassium loss.
Diuretics	Increases the risk of potassium deficiency.
Potassium-sparing diuretics	Unless a doctor advises otherwise, do not take diuretics with potassium supplements or salt substitutes, which can cause potassium overload.
Thiazide diuretics	Increases the reaction to MSG.
Asthma Drugs	
Pseudoephedrine	Avoid caffeine, which increases feelings of anxiety and nervousness.
Theophylline	Charbroiled foods and a high-protein diet reduce absorption. Caffeine increases the risk of drug toxicity.
Cholesterol-Lowering Drugs	
Cholestyramine	Increases the excretion of folate and vitamins A, D, E, and K.
Gemfibrozil	Avoid fatty foods, which decrease the drug's efficacy in lowering cholesterol.
Heartburn and Ulcer Medications	
Antacids	Interfere with the absorption of many minerals; for maximum benefit, take medication 1 hour after eating.
Cimetidine, famotidine, sucralfate	Avoid high-protein foods, caffeine, and other items that increase stomach acidity.
Hormone Preparations	
Oral contraceptives	Salty foods increase fluid retention. Drugs reduce the absorption of folate, vitamin B_6, and other nutrients; increase intake of foods high in these nutrients to avoid deficiencies.
Steroids	Salty foods increase fluid retention. Increase intake of foods high in calcium, vitamin K, potassium, and protein to avoid deficiencies.
Thyroid drugs	Iodine-rich foods may lower the drug's efficacy.
Laxatives	
Mineral oils	Overuse can cause a deficiency of vitamins A, D, E, and K.
Painkillers	
Aspirin and stronger nonsteroidal anti-inflammatory drugs	Always take with food to lower the risk of gastrointestinal irritation; avoid taking with alcohol, which increases the risk of bleeding. Frequent use of these drugs lowers the absorption of folate and vitamin C.
Codeine	Increase fiber and water intake to avoid constipation.
Sleeping Pills, Tranquilizers	
Benzodiazepines	Never take with alcohol. Caffeine increases anxiety and reduce drug's effectiveness.
Weight Loss–Inducing Drugs	
Many drugs cause weight loss because of changes in appetite or other side effects.	

TABLE B-10 Sample Worksheet for Using Standardized Nutrition Terminology

***Nutrition Care Process*—**Critical thinking worksheet to help determine the appropriate standardized language to document and support the NCP

STEP ONE: NUTRITION ASSESSMENT

Complete a comprehensive assessment of a patient using the established assessment standards/guidelines set by your facility or practice setting. Be sure to include "comparative standards:" anthropometrics, estimated needs, and nutrient intake as well as identify the reference standards used to analyze the calculated/numerical data such as the DRIs, BMI, and NCHS charts.

STEP TWO: NUTRITION DIAGNOSIS

(1) List all of the patient's problems/issues:

(2) Cross off medical problems/medical diagnoses.

(3) Cross off issues that do not have supporting evidence (of signs/symptoms).

(4) Cross off issues where the root etiology (cause of) cannot be determined.

(5) Place a "✓" by the issues you will be able to re-evaluate upon follow-up; be sure to have updated signs/symptoms data on the reassessment date.

(6) Of the checked issues, circle those that are the most urgent nutrition problem(s) to resolve and the priority issue to start addressing.

(7) Based on the problem(s) circled, choose the diagnosis that best suits the nutrition issue in its most detailed form.

(8) Write P.E.S statement(s) with the appropriate "root" etiology and signs/symptoms:

P: ______________________ related to **E:** ______________________ as evidenced by
S/S: ______________________ ***See examples

STEP THREE: NUTRITION INTERVENTION (Direct interventions at the **etiology.** If a dietitian cannot change the etiology, then direct the interventions at reducing the signs/symptoms of the nutrition diagnosis).

Nutrition Prescription: (Proper diet and regimen to meet the nutrient needs of what?) ______________________

Based upon scope of practice and clinical privilege established by your facility or practice setting, choose:

1) Recommended Interventions (other practitioner must do)

- intervention term: ______________________

  goal of intervention: ______________________
- intervention term: ______________________

  goal of intervention: ______________________
- intervention term: ______________________

  goal of intervention: ______________________

2) Interventions you can/will do on your own (actions)

- intervention term: ______________________

  goal of intervention: ______________________
- intervention term: ______________________

  goal of intervention: ______________________
- intervention term: ______________________

  goal of intervention: ______________________

Goal of intervention = why you chose that intervention/strategy — what the intervention is intended to do/accomplish

STEP FOUR: MONITORING & EVALUATION (Directed at the **signs/symptoms to** monitor the success of intervention(s) and progress toward goal(s)

1) Indicate when/timeframe during which you plan to reassess: within __________ days/weeks/months

2) List signs/symptoms from PES above and match to M&E Terms (unshaded) from Assess/M&E list (indicators)

3) Establish criteria for each M&E indicator (pt goals)

- Signs/Symptoms: ______________________

  M&E term: ______________________

  Criteria-Pt will: ______________________
- Signs/Symptoms: ______________________

  M&E term: ______________________

  Criteria-Pt will: ______________________
- Signs/Symptoms: ______________________

  M&E term: ______________________

  Criteria-Pt will: ______________________

Criteria = measurable patient-centered goals

Reassessment or follow-up encounter

1) Do you have the info/data needed to compare previous signs/symptoms to the current time? If no, you need to address this as an intervention recommendation, and check it at the next encounter. If yes, evaluate progress toward the M&E criteria on the left (pt goals).

   ☐ Pt met goal/criteria ☐ Pt did not meet goal/criteria

2) Based upon progress toward pt goals, evaluate progress toward the resolution of the nutrition problem from the PES:

   ☐ Resolved (nutrition problem no longer exists)

   ☐ Improvement shown (nutrition problem still exists)

   ☐ Unresolved no improvement shown

   ☐ No longer appropriate (change in condition)

3) If no improvement is shown, you may need to change intervention(s).

(continued)

TABLE B-10 Sample Worksheet for Using Standardized Nutrition Terminology *(continued)*

***SAMPLE COMMON PES STATEMENTS			
Diagnostic Label	**Domain Code**	• **Common Etiology** • **"as related to . . ."**	**Common Signs/Symptoms "as evidenced by . . ." [with M/E codes]**
Inadequate oral food/ beverage intake	NI-2.1	• Decreased appetite • Nausea • Emesis • Altered mental status	• Poor po intake of ≤25% of meals [M&E – FH-1.3.2]
		• Increased needs with advanced Ca • Increased needs due to wound healing, infection, multiple frax • Increased needs secondary to catabolic state	• Wt loss of >5% in 1–2 months [M&E - AD-1.1.4] • Poor po intake of ≤25% of meals [M&E - FH-1.3.2]
		• Comfort measures only (Hospice)	• Consumption of minimal comfort foods <10% needs [M&E - FH-1.2.1]
Inadequate intake from enteral/ parenteral nutrition	NI-2.3	• Current TF formula/rate • Increased needs sec to surgery • Infusion goal not reached due to intolerance of feeding	• Current nutrition regimen only meeting __% of est. needs [M&E - FH-1.2.1] • TF/TPN only meeting __% of est. needs [M&E - FH-1.4.1] • Wt loss of ___% in ___ weeks/months [M&E - AD-1.1.4] • Delayed wound healing [M&E - PD-1.1.8]
Excessive intake from enteral/parenteral nutrition	NI-2.4	Decreased needs due to ventilator	• Current nutrition regimen meeting ≥100% of est. needs [M&E - FH-1.2.1] • TF/TPN meeting ≥100% of est. needs [M&E - FH-1.4.1]
Increased nutrient needs (protein)	NI-5.1	• Increased nutrient demands (PRO) for: • Wound healing • Surgical wounds	• Prealb or alb of __g/L (decreased) [M&E - BD-1.11.1] • Loss of skin integrity (surgical wounds) [M&E - PD-1.1.8] • Loss of muscle mass [M&E - PD-1.1.4] • Stage __ pressure ulcer [M&E - PD-1.1.8] • Inadequate protein intake– consuming only __% pro needs [M&E - FH-1.6.2]
Malnutrition	NI-5.2	• End-stage liver disease • Short gut • Small bowel transplant • Mental illness • Ascites • ETOH dependency	• Decreased albumin of ____g/L [M&E - BD-1.11.1] • Decreased food intake, consuming only ___% meals [M&E - FH-1.3.2] • Pt refusing to eat [M&E - FH-1.3.2] • Wt loss of ___% in ___weeks/months [M&E - AD-1.1.4] • Evident temporal wasting [M/E - PD-1.1.6] • Evident minimal body fat / fat stores [M/E - PD-1.1.4] • Evident cachexia [M/E - PD-1.1.4] • Delayed wound healing [M/E - PD-1.1.8]

Provided courtesy of Sherri Jones, MS, MBA, RD, LDN. UPMC Presbyterian Shadyside, Pittsburgh PA.

TABLE B-11 Clinical Case Review and Audit

Assessment	3 Exceeds Very detailed	2-Met Goals Competent	1-Unsat. Large amt missing	Comments
Pathophysiology of disease/disorder				
Stage/phase (if applicable)				
Relevance of nutrition status in this disorder/disease				
Prognosis for this disease				
Up-to-date interpretation of evidence-based research				
General information noted- Ht, Wt				
Social background reviewed				
Past medical status/socioeconomic status				
Family history; genetics, if relevant				
Pertinent medical/surgical status reviewed/documented				
Medications and potential drug/nutrient interactions assessed/noted				
Laboratory values: skewed values and relevance noted				
Typical diet recall or diet Hx analyzed				
Correct calculations/anthropometrics used to estimate nutrition needs				
Nutrition Diagnoses	**3 Exceeds** Very detailed	**2-Met Goals** Competent	**1-Unsat.** Large amt missing	**Comments**
1–2 Nutrition diagnosis(es) identified & appropriate				
P.E.S statements: logical, able to be managed by an RD in this setting				
Nutrition Interventions	**3 Exceeds** Very detailed	**2-Met Goals** Competent	**1-Unsat.** Large amt missing	**Comments**
Short- and long-term goals set with pt/significant other				
Recommendations based on etiologies of problems				
Food–nutrient delivery:				
Education:				
Counseling:				
Coordination of care:				
Monitoring and Evaluation	**3 Exceeds** Very detailed	**2-Met Goals** Competent	**1-Unsat.** Large amt missing	**Comments**
Progress: day to day analysis – Intake				
Progress: day to day analysis – Clinical				
Progress: day to day analysis – Behavioral/Environmental				
Documented need for f/up; timeframe noted				
If education provided, pt/family understanding is documented				
Nutrition support – kilocalories, protein, fluid, recommendations proper				
Nutrition care plans updated in a timely manner				
Meal plan established if warranted				
Age-appropriate standards and assessment tools used if needed				
Discharge plan or needs discussed				
Communication and Documentation	**3 Exceeds** Very detailed	**2-Met Goals** Competent	**1-Unsat.** Large amt missing	**Comments**
Organized; follows a comprehensible sequence				
Educational flow sheets documented accurately				
Uses correct grammar and terms				
Follow-up notes re-evaluate nutrition diagnoses, status, plans				

Evaluator:________________________ Date:____________ Medical Record #______________

TOTAL POINTS:____________

TABLE B-12 Tips for Adult Education and Counseling

The adult as a learner	During the process of maturation, a person moves from dependency toward increasing self-directedness but at different rates for different people and in different dimensions of life. Teachers have a responsibility to encourage and nurture this movement. Adults have a deep psychological need to be generally self-directing, but they may be dependent in certain temporary situations.
The learner's experience	As people grow and develop, they accumulate an increasing reservoir of experience that becomes an increasingly rich resource for learning—for themselves and for others. Furthermore, people attach more meaning to lessons they gain from experience than those they acquire passively. Accordingly, the primary techniques in education are experiential ones—laboratory experiments, discussion, problem-solving cases, field experiences, case reports.
Readiness to learn	People become ready to learn something when they experience a need to learn it in order to cope more satisfyingly with real-life tasks and problems. The educator has a responsibility to create conditions and provide tools and procedures for helping learners discover their "need to know." Learning programs should be organized around life-application categories and sequenced according to the learners' readiness to learn. Key: Attend to learners' developmental readiness.
Orientation to learning	Adult learners see education as a process of developing increased competence to achieve their full potential in life. They want to be able to apply whatever knowledge and skill they gain today to living more effectively tomorrow. Accordingly, learning experiences should be organized around competency-development categories. People are performance-centered in their orientation to learning.
Assumptions	1. All learners can think; critical and creative thinking are goals. 2. There needs to be a safe, risk-taking environment and sufficient time to learn. 3. The environment for learning should be rich and responsive. 4. Offer challenging problem-solving opportunities.
Chief assessment factors for learning	1. Socioeconomic factors 2. Cultural/religious beliefs and background 3. Age and sex of patient and significant others (SOs) 4. Birth order of patient and family involvement 5. Occupation 6. Medical status and medical history 7. Marital status; number and ages of children 8. Cognitive status; educational level 9. Readiness to learn and staging: precontemplation, contemplation, preparation, action, or maintenance 10. Emotional status (stress, acceptance of illness, chronic disease, or condition)
Health literacy and teaching tools	Low health literacy (the ability to read, understand, and act on health information) is a public health issue. One out of five American adults reads at the fifth-grade level or below, and the average American reads at the eighth to ninth grade level. Most consumers need help understanding healthcare information. Patients prefer medical information that is easy to read and understand. Easy-to-read healthcare materials are *essential*. Provide important information first.
Written materials	Print very clearly and avoid handwritten messages. Use large print; font size should be a minimum of 12 points. Double space text to avoid crowding. Avoid using all capital letters. Use headings to introduce the upcoming topic. Avoid abbreviations, and use black ink on light-colored paper. Information must be current and accurate. Provide important information first. Highlight the "need to know" versus the "nice to know." Present information in a "how to" manner. Use a conversational style. Spell out numbers below 10. Limit syllables to —one or two per word. Keep sentences short, and use bullets when possible.
Educational tools	Newsletters and bulletin boards Demonstrations or role-playing Laboratory reports, flip charts Food recall or intake records with feedback Educational games and fun quizzes Group classes or supermarket tours Educational video and audio tapes

(continued)

TABLE B-12 Tips for Adult Education and Counseling *(continued)*

Visual aids	Visuals should be able to stand alone, without words. Use photographs and realistic images. Use culturally appropriate food models, empty packages of real foods, and measuring cups and spoons. Work with restaurant menus where needed. Share simple recipes.
Principles of learning	The recipient must value the information. Pace should be adequate for learner; take small steps. Environment should be conducive to learning (free of distractions and stress), and patient should be ready to learn (free from pain). Information must be meaningful, relevant, and organized. Material should be logical in sequence. Counselor must be truly interested in sharing the information. Adequate follow-up should be available for the reinforcement of facts and principles. For adult learners, information that is useful in the present is more meaningful than facts learned for the "future." Adults tend to prefer problem-solving information (survival skills) over learning facts.
Principles of teaching	The counselor must first listen to the patient. Involve the patient in setting mutual objectives. Small segments of information should be presented in understandable language in small, manageable "sound bytes." An organized plan should be used to teach. Clear objectives should be established, with timelines and short- and long-term outcomes. Feedback should be used with each step. Be prepared to receive evaluation (peer review) from the patient; improve as needed. Good eye contact should be maintained with the patient. Be aware, however, that direct or prolonged eye contact can be seen as rude or threatening by some cultures; know your client. Appropriate teaching tools or audiovisual aids should be used as appropriate. Using a sixth- to eighth-grade reading level is suggested, preferably with an easy layout, visual appeal, and illustrations. Questions must be allowed for clarification. Praise and positive reinforcement should be offered to the learner. Carl Rogers emphasizes the use of "unconditional positive regard" for all persons.
Counseling tips	Knowledge does not automatically ensure compliance. Behavioral change takes time and encouragement. Trial and error will be common for the patient in learning new behaviors. An increase in self-esteem comes with an improvement in behavior. The counselor should appropriately foster independence. Empathy is an important part of humanistic care. The counselor serves as an intervention specialist. The "patient-centered" approach to counseling is effective. Assess the stage of change and motivation level of client. Evaluate past experiences with dietary changes and anticipated challenges. Goal-setting requires the patient to recognize the need for change, establish a goal, monitor goal-related activity, and use self-reward for goal attainment. Identify challenges, obstacles, coping strategies, and skills. Help the client to anticipate lapses and relapses.
Patient assessment of chronic illness care (PACIC tool)	Patient-centered model of behavioral counseling using the **5 As**: **Assess:** Beliefs, behavior, and knowledge. **Advise:** Provide specific information about health risks and benefits of change. **Agree:** Collaboratively set goals based on the patient's interest and confidence in their ability to change behavior. **Assist:** Identify personal barriers, strategies, problem-solving techniques, and social/environmental support. **Arrange:** Specify a plan for follow-up (e.g., visits, phone calls, mailed reminders).
Counseling in hospice care	Attempt to reduce fears related to eating. Recognize stages of terminal illness: fear of abandonment, finding a natural and realistic approach, building bridges, and ownership of the experience. Pain management is most important for quality of life. Respect the individual's cultural beliefs and needs. Identify a patient advocate who will address concerns as care progresses. Help maintain self-esteem and dignity. Comfort foods can be important to patient satisfaction; address these needs on a meal-to-meal basis. Listen for hidden messages from the patient; communicate with other healthcare team members.

TABLE B-13 Health-Promotion Intervention Models

Because increasing evidence suggests that health-promotion interventions that are based on social and behavioral science theories are more effective than those lacking a theoretical base, five models are described here (Glanz and Bishop, 2010.)

Behavioral Ecological Model (BEM)

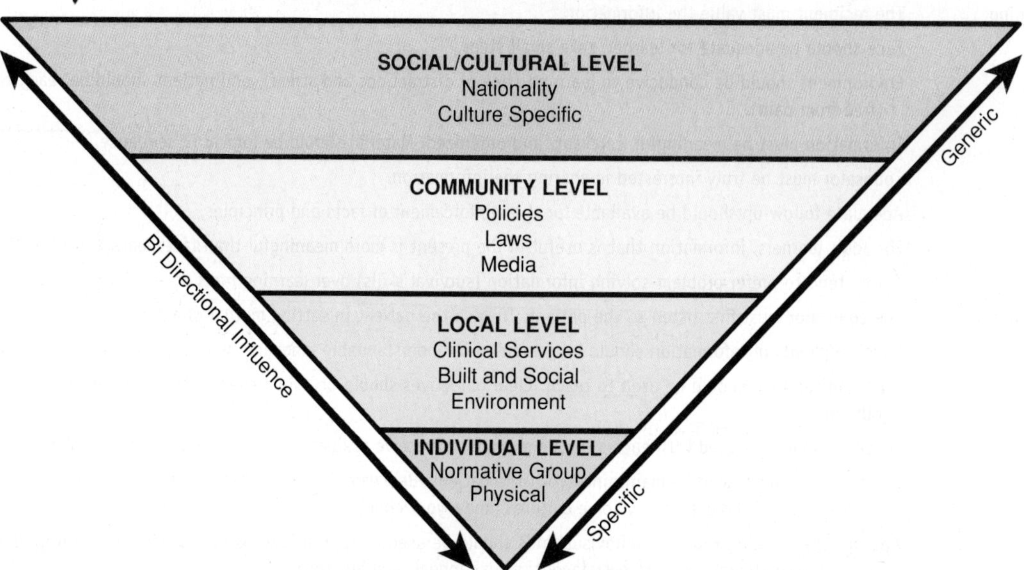

Figure B-4 Behavioral Ecological Model (BEM). (Image courtesy of Hovell et al [2002].)

Behavioral Ecological Model (BEM) Principle	Processes	Application
Environment influences behavior	Consequences are produced by the behavior	Control or change risky environment
Hierarchy of interacting reinforcement contingencies	Interaction is key	Interaction among both physical and social contingencies explain and ultimately control health behavior.

Hovell MF, Wahlgren DR, Gehrman C. The Behavioral Ecological Model: Integrating public health and behavioral science. In DiClemente RJ, Crosby R, Kegler M, (eds.). *New and Emerging Theories in Health Promotion Practice & Research.* Jossey-Bass Inc., San Francisco, California, 2002.

(continued)

TABLE B-13 **Health-Promotion Intervention Models *(continued)***

Health Belief Model

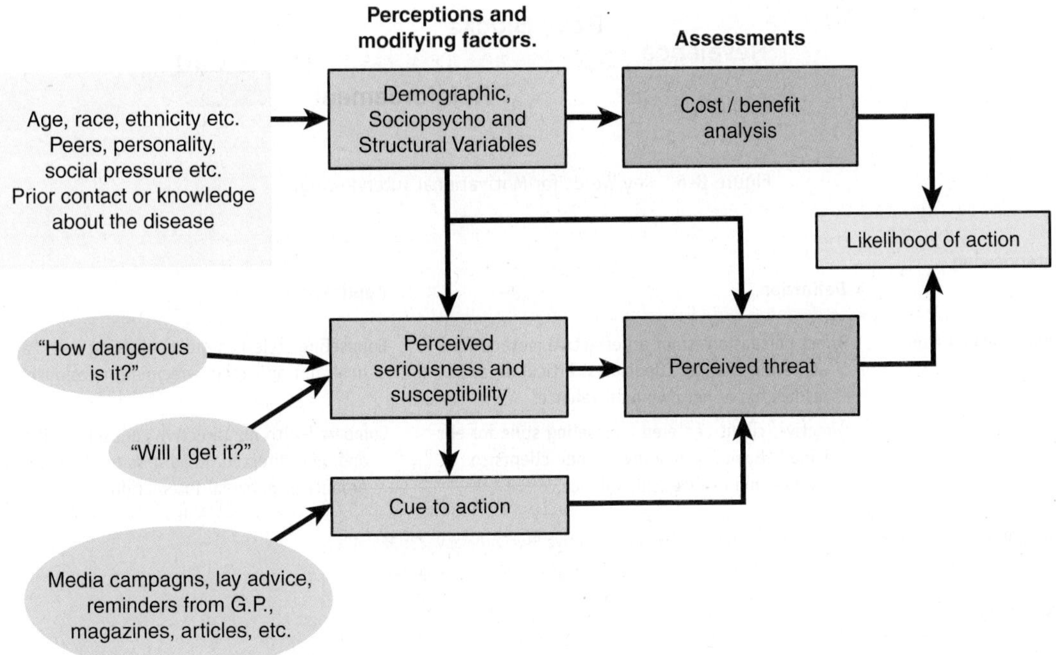

Figure B-5 Health Belief Model (HBM). (Image courtesy of Glanz et al (2002).)

Health Belief Model Concept	Definition	Application
Perceived susceptibility	One's opinion of chances of getting a condition.	Define population(s) at risk, risk levels. Personalize risk based on a person's features or behavior. Heighten perceived susceptibility if too low.
Perceived severity	One's opinion of how serious a condition and its sequelae are.	Specify consequences of the risk and the condition.
Perceived benefits	One's opinion of the efficacy of the advised action to reduce risk or the seriousness of impact.	Define action to take: how, where, when; clarify the positive effects to be expected.
Perceived barriers	One's opinion of the tangible and psychological costs of the advised action.	Identify and reduce barriers through reassurance, incentives, and assistance.
Cues to action	Strategies to activate readiness.	Provide how-to information; promote awareness, reminders.
Self-efficacy	Confidence in one's ability to take action.	Provide training, guidance in performing action.

Glanz K, Bishop DB. The role of behavioral science theory in development and implementation of public health interventions. *Annu Rev Public Health.* 31:399, 2010.
Glanz, K., Rimer, BK, Lewis, FM. *Health Behavior and Health Education. Theory, Research and Practice.* San Francisco: Wiley & Sons., 2002.

(continued)

TABLE B-13 Health-Promotion Intervention Models *(continued)*

Motivational Interviewing

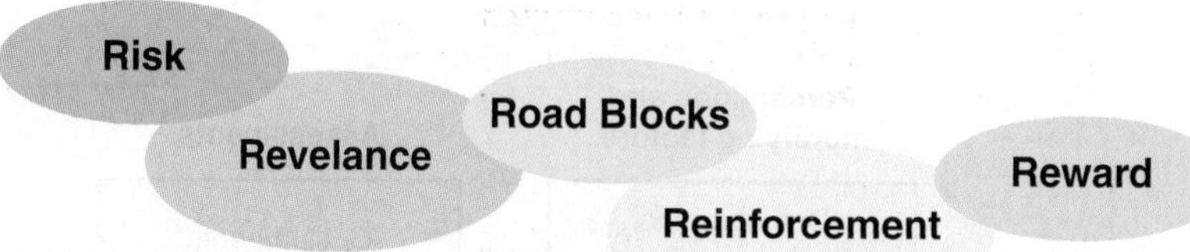

Figure B-6 Key Words for Motivational Interviewing.

Motivational Interviewing (MI) Concept	Definition	Application
Motivation to change comes from the client, not the counselor	Direct persuasion is not an effective method for achieving change. Client must articulate and resolve his or her own ambivalence.	Counseling style is a quiet, eliciting one. Partnership is the goal, not an expert—recipient relationship.
Resolution of ambivalence	Directive, client-centered counseling style for eliciting behavior change by helping clients to explore and resolve ambivalence.	Compared with nondirective counseling, it is more focused and goal-directed. Readiness to change is a fluctuating product of personal interaction.

Rollnick S., & Miller, W.R. What is motivational interviewing? Behavioural and Cognitive Psychotherapy, 23: 325, 1995.

Social Cognitive Theory

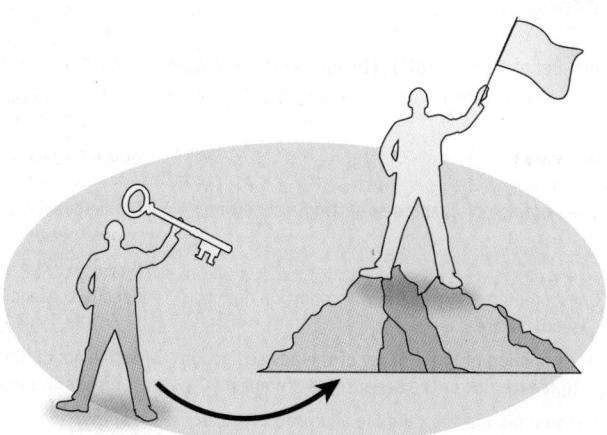

Figure B-7 Self-Efficacy as part of Social Cognitive Theory.

Social Cognitive Theory Principle	Processes	Application
Human functioning is self-regulated	Cognitive, vicarious, and self-reflective processes	Human adaptation to change
Dynamic interplay of personal, behavioral, and environmental influences	Self as organizing, proactive, self-reflective	People are not reactive organisms shepherded by environmental forces or concealed inner impulses
People watch and learn from others	Interactive learning	Confidence comes from practice
Self-efficacy is the belief in the ability to succeed in specific situations	Positive approaches to goals, tasks, and challenges.	Those who believe they can perform well are more likely to view difficult tasks as something to be mastered rather than something to be avoided.

Bandura, A. *Social foundations of thought and action: A social cognitive theory.* Englewood Cliffs, NJ: Prentice Hall, 1986.

(continued)

TABLE B-13 Health-Promotion Intervention Models *(continued)*

Transtheoretical Model (TTM)

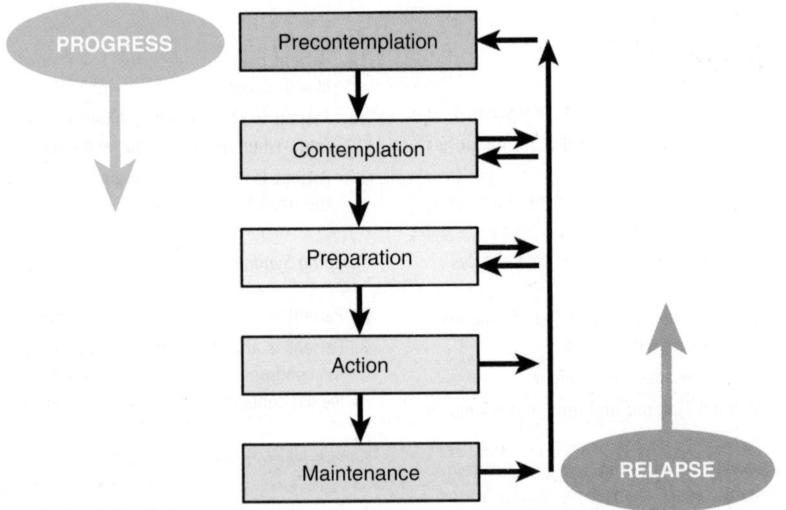

Figure B-8 Transtheoretical Model (TTM). (Image courtesy of Prochaska and DiClemente (1982).)

TTM Stage	Definition	Helping Processes
Precontemplation	Individual has the problem (whether he/she recognizes it or not) and has no intention of changing.	Consciousness raising (information and knowledge) Dramatic relief (role-playing) Environmental reevaluation (how problem affects physical environment)
Contemplation	Individual recognizes the problem and is seriously thinking about changing.	Self-reevaluation (assessing one's feelings regarding behavior)
Preparation for action	Individual recognizes the problem and intends to change the behavior within the next month. Some behavior change efforts may be reported but the defined behavior change criterion has not been reached consistently.	Self-liberation (commitment or belief in the ability to change)
Action	Individual has enacted consistent behavior change for less than six months.	Reinforcement management (overt and covert rewards) Helping relationships (social support, self-help groups) Counterconditioning (alternatives for behavior) Stimulus control (avoid high-risk cues)
Maintenance	Individual maintains new behavior for six months or more.	Support and encouragement

Prochaska JO, DiClemente CC. Trans-theoretical therapy – toward a more integrative model of change. *Psychotherapy: Theory, Research & Practice.* 19(3):276, 1982.

TABLE B-14 Sample Monitoring and Evaluation Audits for Patient Education

This patient education audit identifies the ability of the patient to demonstrate or verbalize how he or she will or has changed behaviors after nutritional instructions.

Any Patient

1. Patient is able to personalize the MyPyramid food guidance system.
2. Patient is able to explain the importance of his or her diet for his or her health.
3. Patient is able to plan ____ day's menus and snacks from his/her dietary pattern.
4. Patient is able to incorporate desirable economic/ethnic food choices into his/her prescribed diet.
5. Patient has been following _____ diet at home for a period of time and is able to describe the elements of this diet with accuracy.
6. Patient expresses recognition of a need to lose/gain weight.
7. Patient is able to describe specific food allergies and food ingredients to avoid.
8. Patient is able to describe the reasons for following _______ diet (e.g., improve appearance, increase energy, reduce chances for complications, improve quality of life).
9. Patient is able to describe the impact of appropriate activity or exercise on health and nutritional well-being.

Cardiac Diet

1. Patient is able to name three beverages that are high in caffeine.
2. Patient is able to describe modifications in his or her diet that will be needed to prevent further coronary complications: saturated versus poly- and monounsaturated fats, sodium and potassium, fiber, and use of the DASH diet.
3. Patient is able to categorize correctly into the proper food pyramid lists.
4. Patient is able to plan menus for home use that include appropriate modifications.
5. Patient is able to name snack foods that can be included in dietary plan.

Diabetes Diet

1. Patient is able to explain the relationship of diet with complications of diabetes.
2. Patient is able to name foods that contain CHO.
3. Patient is able to preplan meals for _____ weeks.
4. Patient is able to verbalize a simple definition of diabetes.
5. Patient is able to describe the role of medications related to food intake.
6. Patient is able to explain the rationale for following a prudent diet to prevent complications such as heart disease.
7. Patient is able to explain how proper spacing of meals affects his/her disorder.
8. Patient is able to describe symptoms of ketoacidosis and insulin shock and can name foods to take or avoid for each condition.
9. After looking at several food labels, patient is able to point out ingredients that mean carbohydrate.
10. Patient is able to describe techniques for managing special events (travel, parties, restaurants, holiday meals, weekends).
11. Patient is able to describe his or her personal exercise prescription as ___ minutes of activity ___ times per week.
12. Patient is able to describe 1–2 items to carry in case of episodes of low blood glucose.
13. Patient is able to define when to call his or her health provider (e.g., when glucose is above/below normal ___ times).
14. Patient is able to discuss proper foot care, the need for eye exams, and the need for foot exams.

Dumping Syndrome Diet

1. Patient is able to verbalize the effects of diet on dumping syndrome.
2. Patient is able to explain the guidelines to be followed to prevent dumping syndrome (e.g., beverages are served 30 minutes before or after meals; concentrated sweets are omitted or severely limited).

Gliadin-Free/Gluten-Restricted Diet

1. Patient is able to examine food labels and to name ingredients that must be avoided.
2. Patient is able to list products that must be avoided in diet.
3. Patient is able to plan menus that can be used at home.
4. Patient is able to adapt recipes for use at home.

High-Fiber Diet

1. Patient is able to verbalize foods that can be used to increase fiber in his or her diet, to desired level of ___ grams daily.
2. Patient is able to explain the role of fiber in his or her particular disorder.
3. Patient is able to describe the purpose of adequate fluids in the dietary regimen and is able to consume ___ milliliters daily.

Lactose Intolerance Diet

1. Patient is able to name foods or beverages that must be avoided.
2. Patient is able to plan menus that are nutritionally complete for calcium but are lactose restricted.
3. Patient demonstrates awareness that he or she can tolerate up to ___ milliliters of lactose per day at this time.
4. Patient is able to discuss the difference between lactose intolerance and milk allergy.

Low-Cholesterol and Dyslipidemia Diets

1. Patient is able to describe simple definitions for cholesterol and saturated, polyunsaturated, and monounsaturated fats.
2. Patient is able to identify foods that have high cholesterol content.
3. Patient is able to name vegetable oils that may be used in the diet.
4. Patient is able to describe three cooking methods that are acceptable for the dietary regimen.
5. Patient is able to name foods that are good sources of monounsaturated fats.

(continued)

TABLE B-14 Sample Monitoring and Evaluation Audits for Patient Education *(continued)*

Low-Fat Diet

1. Patient is able to name foods that he or she must omit for the low-fat diet.
2. Patient is able to explain the role of fat in his or her condition.
3. Patient is able to note grams of fat from a given food label.

Mineral-Altered Diets (Iron, Potassium, Calcium, Sodium)

1. Patient is able to name foods that are high/low in minerals.
2. Patient is able to accurately select menu choices for days that include/exclude foods that are high in mineral.
3. Patient is able to plan menus for home that are high/low in minerals.

Pregnancy Diet

1. Patient is able to describe nutritional changes to her diet in order to have a healthy baby.
2. Patient is able to describe why breastfeeding is an important consideration.

Protein-Altered Diets

1. Patient can identify foods that contain protein of high biological value.
2. Patient can name foods to include/omit in diet to increase/decrease the protein content of meals and snacks.

Renal Diets

1. Patient is able to describe restrictions that are needed in regard to protein, sodium, potassium, fluid, calories, and phosphorus.
2. Patient is able to plan menus that are balanced for the restricted nutrients.
3. Patient is able to name "free" foods that he or she can eat as desired.
4. Patient is able to discuss how foods, nutrients, and prescribed medications may interact.

Sodium Restrictions

1. Patient is able to name foods that are naturally high in sodium.
2. Patient is able to name foods that have been processed or prepared with an excess of sodium.
3. Patient is able to explain the difference between "salt" and "sodium" in foods.
4. Patient is able to list seasonings that can be used at home in place of salt and salt-containing seasonings.
5. Patient is able to plan menus for home that will be low in sodium.
6. Patient is able to identify salt substitutes that he or she can use for his or her condition.
7. Patient is able to discuss how other minerals (potassium, calcium, magnesium) play a role in the specific condition.

Vegetarian Diet

1. Patient is able to identify correctly two or more complementary protein foods.
2. Patient is able to plan menus that provide adequate protein and vitamin B_{12}, zinc, and so on for age and gender.

Weight Management Diet

1. Patient is able to verbalize his or her primary motivation for losing weight and current readiness for a change in behaviors.
2. Patient is able to describe his or her realistic goal for weight loss—either short term or long term, including a timetable.
3. Patient is able to list foods that are low in energy and may be eaten as snacks.
4. Patient is able to categorize foods into the proper pyramid food categories.
5. Patient is able to demonstrate a proper technique for recording food intake at home.
6. Patient has demonstrated weight loss over a certain timeframe.

APPENDIX

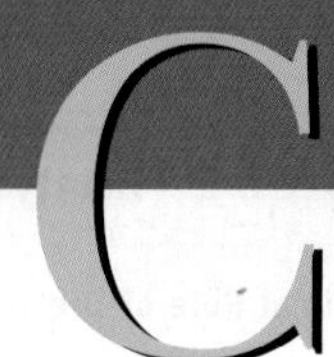

Acuity Ranking for Dietitian Services and Concept Map

Over 100 dietitians, clinical nutrition managers, and specialists were surveyed for this acuity ranking for dietitian services, and a summary is given below. Levels of consensus on acuity are indicated for the medical diagnoses and conditions in this text. Where strong consensus was available, this table provides the acuity ranking for the nutritional involvement needed from a registered dietitian (RD). The survey asked the questions listed in Table C-1. Table C-2 summarizes the rankings given by participants to the nutrition acuity by condition or disease. Concept maps are useful for organizing data to prepare assessments or case reviews. Figure C-1 can be used or adapted as a teaching tool for skill development. Figure C-2 provides an example of a process chart for considering all aspects of data for a comprehensive functional nutrition plan.

TABLE C-1 Nutrition Acuity and Medical Diagnosis–Related Survey Questions

Rate your opinion about the level of dietitian involvement (over time, not just per visit) for the following diagnoses on a 1 to 5 rating scale where

1 = Little involvement; minimal, can be delegated to others
2 = Some roles in oversight of nutrition care
3 = Moderate involvement needed over time
4 = Extensive involvement needed over time
5 = Unable to determine; no opinion or experience

TABLE C-2 Acuity for Dietitian Roles in Medical Diagnoses

Minimal Role of Dietitian–1	Some Roles of Dietitian–2	Moderate Role of Dietitian–3	Extended Role of Dietitian–4
NORMAL LIFE-CYCLE CONDITIONS			
Pregnancy, normal	Child, normal (1–2)	Pregnancy, high risk	
Lactation	Teenager, normal		
Infant, normal (birth up to 6 months)	Adult male, normal		
Infant, normal (6–12 months) (1–2)	Adult female, normal		
	Elderly male, normal		
	Elderly female, normal		
DIETARY PRACTICES AND MISCELLANEOUS CONDITIONS			
Periodontal disease (1–2)	Complementary medicine and herbal/ botanical counseling	Pressure ulcer, stages 1 or 2 (2–3)	Pressure ulcer, stages 3 or 4 or multiple
Temporomandibular joint (TMJ) dysfunction	Cultural food pattern, advisement and planning	Vitamin deficiency prevention or counseling	
Skin disorders (acne, rosacea, eczema, psoriasis)	Vegetarian diet advisement or planning	Food allergy, multiple or complex (3–4)	
Ménière's syndrome	Religious dietary patterns, advisement/ planning		
	Dental difficulties (caries, wired jaw, mouth pain, xerostomia) (2–3)		
	Vision and self-feeding problems (low vision or chewing problems) (1–2) blindness, coordination		
	Food allergy, simple (2–3)		
	Foodborne illness, prevention or counseling		

(continued)

TABLE C-2 Acuity for Dietitian Roles in Medical Diagnoses *(continued)*

Minimal Role of Dietitian–1	Some Roles of Dietitian–2	Moderate Role of Dietitian–3	Extended Role of Dietitian–4
PEDIATRICS: BIRTH DEFECTS, GENETIC, ACQUIRED DISORDERS			
Attention deficit disorders	Abetalipoproteinemia (variable)	Bronchopulmonary dysplasia (3–4)	Failure to thrive, pediatric
Autism spectrum disorders (1–2)	Biliary atresia (2–3)	Cerebral palsy	Inborn errors of carbohydrate metabolism
Adrenoleukodystrophy (variable)	Congenital heart disease	Cleft palate	Hirschsprung's disease (congenital megacolon)
Leukodystrophies (variable)	Cystinosis and Fanconi's syndrome (variable)	Homocystinuria (3–4)	HIV infection and AIDS, pediatric
Otitis media	Down syndrome	Maple syrup urine disease (MSUD) (3–4)	Low birth weight or premature infant (3–4)
	Fetal alcohol syndrome (1–2)	Medium-chain acyl-CoA dehydrogenase deficiency (MCADD)	Necrotizing enterocolitis
	Large for gestational age infant (variable)	Myelomeningocele (variable)	Phenylketonuria (PKU)
		Obesity, childhood (prevention, treatment) (3–4)	Tyrosinemia (variable)
		Prader–Willi syndrome (3–4)	Urea cycle disorders (variable)
		Rickets, nutritional	
		Spina bifida and neural tube defects	
		Wilson's disease (hepatolenticular degeneration)	
NEUROLOGICAL AND PSYCHIATRIC CONDITIONS			
Neurological Disorders			
Migraine headache, prevention or counseling	Epilepsy or seizure disorders	Amyotrophic lateral sclerosis	Brain trauma
Trigeminal neuralgia (1–2)	Multiple sclerosis	Cerebral aneurysm	Coma
	Myasthenia gravis and neuromuscular junction disorders	Guillain-Barré syndrome	
	Parkinson's disease	Huntington's chorea (variable)	
	Tardive dyskinesia	Spinal cord injury	
		Stroke (cerebrovascular accident)	
Eating Disorders		Anorexia nervosa	
		Binge eating disorder (3–4)	
		Bulimia (3–4)	
		Other disordered eating patterns (3–4)	
Psychiatric Disorders			
Bipolar disorder (1–2)		Alzheimer's disease or other dementias	
Depression with numerous medications (1–2)			
Schizophrenia and psychoses (1–2)			
Substance use disorders			

(continued)

TABLE C-2 Acuity for Dietitian Roles in Medical Diagnoses *(continued)*

Minimal Role of Dietitian–1	Some Roles of Dietitian–2	Moderate Role of Dietitian–3	Extended Role of Dietitian–4
PULMONARY DISORDERS			
Asthma	Cor pulmonale (variable)	Chronic obstructive pulmonary diseases (emphysema or chronic bronchitis)	Chylothorax
Bronchiectasis	Interstitial lung disease (1–2)	Cystic fibrosis	
Bronchitis, acute	Sarcoidosis	Respiratory distress syndrome (3–4)	Respiratory failure and ventilator dependency
Pneumonia (1–2)	Sleep apnea	Transplantation, lung (3–4)	
Pulmonary embolism (1–2)	Thoracic empyema		
	Tuberculosis		
CARDIOVASCULAR DISORDERS			
Angina pectoris	Peripheral artery disease	Atherosclerosis, coronary heart disease, and dyslipidemias	Cardiac cachexia
Arteritis		Cardiomyopathies	Heart transplantation or heart-lung transplantation
Pericarditis and cardiac tamponade		Heart failure	
Thrombophlebitis		Hypertension	
		Myocardial infarction	
GASTROINTESTINAL DISORDERS			
Upper GI			
Dyspepsia or indigestion (1–2)	Esophageal varices (2–3)	Dysphagia (3–4)	
	Hiatal hernia, esophagitis, and gastroesophageal reflux (GERD) (2–3)	Esophageal stricture or spasm, achalasia, or Zenker's diverticulum	
	Gastric retention or gastroparesis (2–3)	Esophageal trauma (3–4)	
	Peptic ulcer	Gastritis and gastroenteritis	
		Giant hypertrophic gastritis (Ménétrier's disease)	
		Gastrectomy and/or vagotomy (3–4)	
		Vomiting, pernicious	
Lower GI			
Lactose malabsorption (lactase deficiency) (variable)	Diarrhea, dysentery, and traveler's diarrhea	Fat malabsorption syndrome	Tropical sprue
Constipation (1–2)	Diverticular diseases (2–3)	Megacolon, acquired	Celiac disease
Fecal incontinence	Peritonitis	Irritable bowel disease	Crohn's disease (3–4)
Hemorrhoids, hemorrhoidectomy	Colostomy (2–3)	Carcinoid syndrome	Ulcerative colitis
Proctitis		Ileostomy	Short bowel syndrome
		Intestinal lymphangiectasia (variable)	Intestinal fistula
		Whipple's disease (intestinal lipodystrophy) (3–4)	Intestinal transplantation

(continued)

TABLE C-2 Acuity for Dietitian Roles in Medical Diagnoses *(continued)*

Minimal Role of Dietitian–1	Some Roles of Dietitian–2	Moderate Role of Dietitian–3	Extended Role of Dietitian–4
HEPATIC, PANCREATIC, AND BILIARY DISORDERS			
Jaundice	Ascites and chylous ascites	Alcoholic liver disease	Liver transplantation
	Hepatitis	Hepatic cirrhosis	
	Pancreatic insufficiency (2–3)	Hepatic encephalopathy, failure or coma (3–4)	
	Gallbladder disease, surgical or nonsurgical	Pancreatitis, acute (3–4)	
	Biliary cirrhosis	Pancreatitis, chronic	
	Cholestatic liver disease (2–3)	Zollinger–Ellison syndrome (variable)	
ENDOCRINE DISORDERS			
Adrenocortical insufficiency, chronic	Pregnancy-induced	Metabolic syndrome (3–4)	Type 1 diabetes
	Hypertension and preeclampsia	Prediabetes (3–4)	Pancreatic transplantation
Addison's disease (variable)	Syndrome of inappropriate antidiuretic hormone (SIADH)	Diabetic gastroparesis (3–4)	Type 2 diabetes mellitus, adults
Cushing's syndrome (variable)		Diabetic ketoacidosis (3–4)	Type 2 diabetes mellitus, children and teens
Acromegaly (variable)	Parathyroid disorders	Hyperosmolar hyperglycemic state (3–4)	Gestational diabetes
Hyperaldosteronism (variable)	(altered calcium)	Hypoglycemia, iatrogenic	
Hypopituitarism (variable)		Hyperinsulinism and spontaneous hypoglycemia (3–4)	
Pheochromocytoma (variable)		Diabetes insipidus	
Hyperthyroidism			
Hypothyroidism			
WEIGHT MANAGEMENT, UNDERNUTRITION, AND MALNUTRITION		Underweight or unintentional weight loss (3–4)	Overweight or uncomplicated obesity
		Protein-calorie malnutrition, mild (3–4)	Obesity, medical (with comorbidities)
			Protein–calorie malnutrition, moderate or severe
			Energy malnutrition
			Refeeding syndrome
MUSCULOSKELETAL AND COLLAGEN DISORDERS			
Ankylosing spondylitis (variable)	Immobilization, extended	Rhabdomyolysis (variable)	
Myofascial pain syndromes: fibromyalgia or polymyalgia rheumatica	Muscular dystrophy		
Osteomyelitis, acute (1–2)	Osteoarthritis and degenerative joint disease		
Paget's disease (osteitis deformans) (variable)	Osteopenia and osteomalacia		
Polyarteritis nodosa (variable)	Osteoporosis		
Rheumatoid arthritis	Systemic lupus erythematosus		
Ruptured intervertebral disc			
Scleroderma (systemic sclerosis) (1–2)			

(continued)

TABLE C-2 Acuity for Dietitian Roles in Medical Diagnoses *(continued)*

Minimal Role of Dietitian–1	Some Roles of Dietitian–2	Moderate Role of Dietitian–3	Extended Role of Dietitian–4
HEMATOLOGY: ANEMIAS AND BLOOD DISORDERS			
Aplastic anemia	Anemia, hemolytic from vitamin E deficiency (2–3)		
Anemia from parasitic infestation	Anemia, iron deficiency		
Anemia, sickle cell	Anemia, nutritional (folic acid, copper, etc.)		
Anemia, sideroblastic	Anemia, pernicious or vitamin B_{12} deficiency		
Polycythemia vera (Osler's disease)	Hemochromatosis (iron overloading)		
Thalassemia (Cooley's anemia)	Hemorrhage, acute or chronic		
Thrombocytic purpura			
CANCER	Breast cancer	Brain tumor	Bone marrow transplantation
	Choriocarcinoma	Esophageal cancer (3–4)	
	Leukemia, chronic	Gastric carcinoma (3–4)	
	Lung cancer	Hepatic carcinoma	
	Myeloma (simple or multiple) (2–3)	Intestinal carcinoma (3–4)	
	Prostate cancer	Leukemia, acute	
		Lymphoma, Hodgkin's disease	
		Lymphoma, non-Hodgkin's	
		Oral cancer (3–4)	
		Osteosarcoma (2–3)	
		Pancreatic carcinoma	
		Radiation colitis or enteritis (3–4)	
		Wilms' tumor (embryoma of kidney)	
SURGICAL DISORDERS			
Appendectomy	Surgery, general	Bowel surgery	Gastric bypass surgery
Cesarean delivery	Sodium imbalances: hyponatremia or hypernatremia	Open heart surgery	
Hysterectomy, abdominal	Potassium imbalances: hypokalemia or hyperkalemia	Pancreatic surgery (3–4)	
Pelvic exenteration	Calcium imbalances: hypocalcemia or hypercalcemia		
Spinal surgery (1–2)	Magnesium imbalances: hypomagnesemia or hypermagnesemia		
Total hip arthroplasty	Phosphate imbalances: hypophosphatemia or hyperphosphatemia		
Tonsillectomy and adenoidectomy	Amputation, one or more limbs		
	Parathyroidectomy		

(continued)

TABLE C-2 Acuity for Dietitian Roles in Medical Diagnoses *(continued)*

Minimal Role of Dietitian–1	Some Roles of Dietitian–2	Moderate Role of Dietitian–3	Extended Role of Dietitian–4
AIDS, INFECTIONS, BURNS, IMMUNOLOGY, AND TRAUMA			
Candidiasis	Bacterial endocarditis	AIDS and HIV infection, adult (3–4)	Burns, major thermal injury
Chronic fatigue syndrome (1–2)	Burns, minor thermal injury	Sepsis or septicemia	Multiple organ dysfunction
Fever >102°F	Encephalitis or Reye's syndrome	Trauma, major	
Herpes simplex 1 or 2	Fracture, hip or long bone		
Herpes zoster (shingles)	Trauma, minor		
Infection, general			
Influenza (flu, respiratory)			
Intestinal parasites			
Meningitis			
Mononucleosis			
Pelvic inflammatory disease			
Poliomyelitis			
Rheumatic fever			
Toxic shock syndrome			
Trichinosis			
Typhoid fever			
RENAL DISORDERS			
Pyelonephritis	Inborn errors: polycystic kidney disease	Inborn errors: vitamin D–resistant rickets (3–4)	Chronic kidney disease
Urolithiasis (renal stones) (1–2)	Glomerulonephritis, acute	Inborn errors: Hartnup disease (variable)	Hemodialysis
	Glomerulonephritis, chronic	Nephrosclerosis (2–3)	Peritoneal renal dialysis
	Nephritis (Bright's disease) (2–3)	Renal failure, acute	Renal transplantation
	Nephrotic syndrome (2–3)		
ENTERAL–PARENTERAL NUTRITION			Tube feeding, initiation, monitoring, or home
			Parenteral nutrition, initiation, monitoring, or home

Thanks to Matthew Dallas, MS, RD, for summarizing this table.

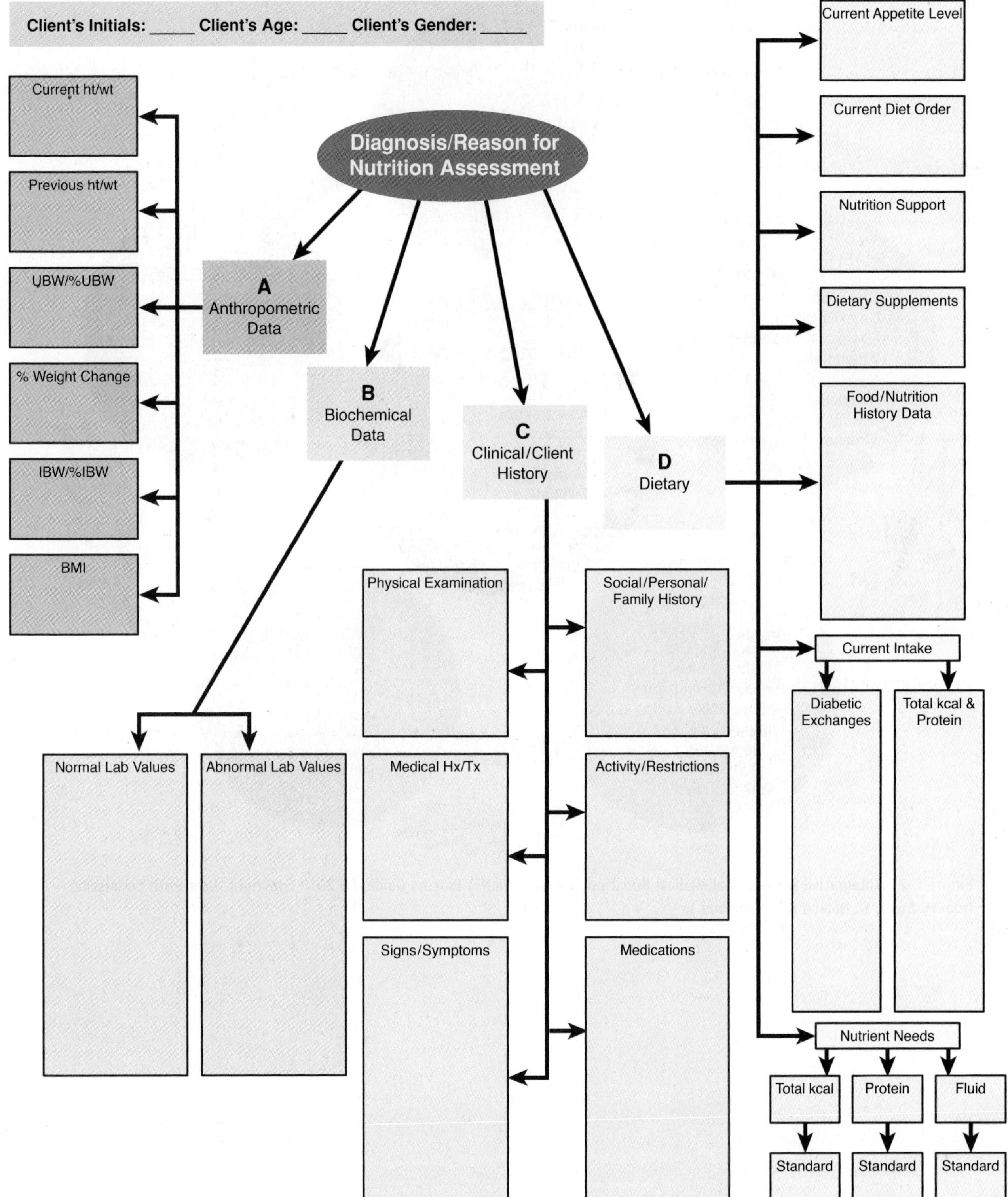

Figure C-1 Concept Map. Used with permission from Molaison, E.F., Taylor, K., Erickson, D., and Connell, C.L. (2009). Perception of concept mapping as a learning tool by dietetic internship students and preceptors. *Journal of Allied Health*, 38, e-97–e-103.

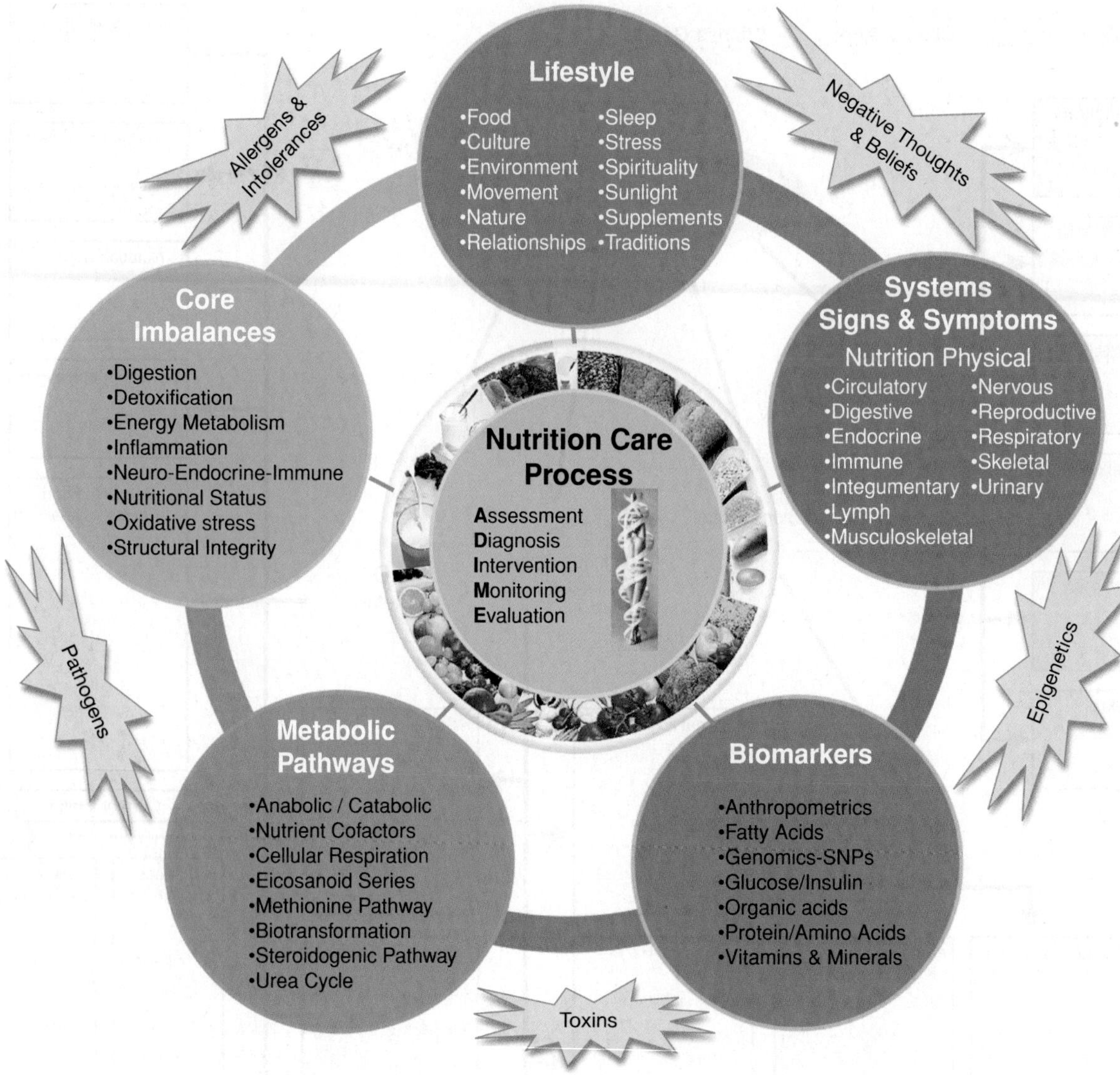

Figure C-2 Integrative & Functional Medical Nutrition Therapy (IFMNT) Process Guide. (© 2010 Copyright. Used with permission from M. Swift, D. Noland & E. Redmond.)

APPENDIX

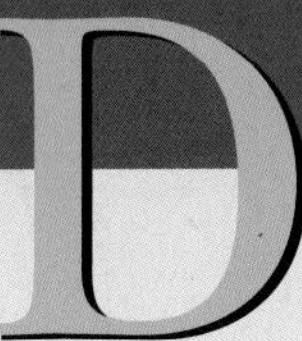

Dietary Reference Intakes

Dietary Reference Intakes (DRIs): Recommended Intakes for Individuals, Vitamins

Food and Nutrition Board, Institute of Medicine, National Academies

Life Stage Group	Vit A (µg/d)[a]	Vit C (mg/d)	Vit D (µg/d)[b,c]	Vit E (mg/d)[d]	Vit K (µg/d)	Thiamin (mg/d)	Riboflavin (mg/d)	Niacin (mg/d)[e]	Vit B_6 (mg/d)	Folate (µg/d)[f]	Vit B_{12} (µg/d)	Pantothenic Acid (mg/d)	Biotin (µg/d)	Choline[g] (mg/d)
Infants														
0–6 mo	400*	40*	5*	4*	2.0*	0.2*	0.3*	2*	0.1*	65*	0.4*	1.7*	5*	125*
7–12 mo	500*	50*	5*	5*	2.5*	0.3*	0.4*	4*	0.3*	80*	0.5*	1.8*	6*	150*
Children														
1–3 y	**300**	**15**	5*	**6**	30*	**0.5**	**0.5**	**6**	**0.5**	**150**	**0.9**	2*	8*	200*
4–8 y	**400**	**25**	5*	**7**	55*	**0.6**	**0.6**	**8**	**0.6**	**200**	**1.2**	3*	12*	250*
Males														
9–13 y	**600**	**45**	5*	**11**	60*	**0.9**	**0.9**	**12**	**1.0**	**300**	**1.8**	4*	20*	375*
14–18 y	**900**	**75**	5*	**15**	75*	**1.2**	**1.3**	**16**	**1.3**	**400**	**2.4**	5*	25*	550*
19–30 y	**900**	**90**	5*	**15**	120*	**1.2**	**1.3**	**16**	**1.3**	**400**	**2.4**	5*	30*	550*
31–50 y	**900**	**90**	5*	**15**	120*	**1.2**	**1.3**	**16**	**1.3**	**400**	**2.4**	5*	30*	550*
51–70 y	**900**	**90**	10*	**15**	120*	**1.2**	**1.3**	**16**	**1.7**	**400**	**2.4**[i]	5*	30*	550*
> 70 y	**900**	**90**	15*	**15**	120*	**1.2**	**1.3**	**16**	**1.7**	**400**	**2.4**[i]	5*	30*	550*
Females														
9–13 y	**600**	**45**	5*	**11**	60*	**0.9**	**0.9**	**12**	**1.0**	**300**	**1.8**	4*	20*	375*
14–18 y	**700**	**65**	5*	**15**	75*	**1.0**	**1.0**	**14**	**1.2**	**400**[i]	**2.4**	5*	25*	400*
19–30 y	**700**	**75**	5*	**15**	90*	**1.1**	**1.1**	**14**	**1.3**	**400**[i]	**2.4**	5*	30*	425*
31–50 y	**700**	**75**		**15**	90*	**1.1**	**1.1**	**14**	**1.3**	**400**[i]	**2.4**	5*	30*	425*
51–70 y	**700**	**75**	10*	**15**	90*	**1.1**	**1.1**	**14**	**1.5**	**400**	**2.4**[h]	5*	30*	425*
> 70 y	**700**	**75**	15*	**15**	90*	**1.1**	**1.1**	**14**	**1.5**	**400**	**2.4**[h]	5*	30*	425*
Pregnancy														
14–18 y	**750**	**80**	5*	**15**	75*	**1.4**	**1.4**	**18**	**1.9**	**600**[j]	**2.6**	6*	30*	450*
19–30 y	**770**	**85**	5*	**15**	90*	**1.4**	**1.4**	**18**	**1.9**	**600**[j]	**2.6**	6*	30*	450*
31–50 y	**770**	**85**	5*	**15**	90*	**1.4**	**1.4**	**18**	**1.9**	**600**[j]	**2.6**	6*	30*	450*
Lactation														
14–18 y	**1,200**	**115**	5*	**19**	75*	**1.4**	**1.6**	**17**	**2.0**	**500**	**2.8**	7*	35*	550*
19–30 y	**1,300**	**120**	5*	**19**	90*	**1.4**	**1.6**	**17**	**2.0**	**500**	**2.8**	7*	35*	550*
31–50 y	**1,300**	**120**	5*	**19**	90*	**1.4**	**1.6**	**17**	**2.0**	**500**	**2.8**	7*	35*	550*

NOTE: This table (taken from the DRI reports, see www.na p.edu) presents Recommended Dietary Allowances (RDA s) in **bold type** and Adequate Intakes (AIs) in ordinary type followed by an asterisk (*). RDAs and AIs may both be used as goals for individual intake. RDAs are set to meet the needs of almost all (97 to 98 percent) individuals in a group. For healthy breastfed infants, the AI is the mean intake. The AI for other life stage and gender groups is believed to cover needs of all individuals in the group, but lack of data or uncertainty in the data prevent being able to specify with confidence the percentage of individuals covered by this intake.

[a] As retinol activity equivalents (RAEs). 1 RAE = 1 µg retinol, 12 µg β-carotene, 24 µg α-carotene, or 24 µg β-cryptoxanthin. The RAE for dietary provitamin A carotenoids is twofold greater than retinol equivalents (RE), whereas the RAE for preformed vitamin A is the same as RE.

[b] As cholecalciferol. 1 µg cholecalciferol = 40 IU vitamin D.

[c] In the absence of adequate exposure to sunlight.

[d] As α-tocopherol. α-Tocopherol includes *RRR*-α-tocopherol, the only form of α-tocopherol that occurs naturally in foods, and the *2R*-stereoisomeric forms of α-tocopherol (*RRR*-, *RSR*-, *RRS*-, and *RSS*-α-tocopherol) that occur in fortified foods and supplements. It does not include the *2S*-stereoisomeric forms of α-tocopherol (*SRR*-, *SSR*-, *SRS*-, and *SSS*-α-tocopherol), also found in fortified foods and supplements.

[e] As niacin equivalents (NE). 1 mg of niacin = 60 mg of tryptophan; 0–6 months = preformed niacin (not NE).

[f] As dietary folate equivalents (DFE). 1 DFE = 1 µg food folate = 0.6 µg of folic acid from fortified food or as a supplement consumed with food = 0.5 µg of a supplement taken on an empty stomach.

[g] Although AIs have been set for choline, there are few data to assess whether a dietary supply of choline is needed at all stages of the life cycle, and it may be that the choline requirement can be met by endogenous synthesis at some of these stages.

[h] Because 10 to 30 percent of older people may malabsorb food-bound B_{12}, it is advisable for those older than 50 years to meet their RDA mainly by consuming foods fortified with B_{12} or a supplement containing B_{12}.

[i] In view of evidence linking folate intake with neural tube defects in the fetus, it is recommended that all women capable of becoming pregnant consume 400 µg from supplements or fortified foods in addition to intake of food folate from a varied diet.

[jk] It is assumed that women will continue consuming 400 µg from supplements or fortified food until their pregnancy is confirmed and they enter prenatal care, which ordinarily occurs after the end of the periconceptional period—the critical time for formation of the neural tube.

Dietary Reference Intakes (DRIs): Recommended Intakes for Individuals, Elements

Food and Nutrition Board, Institute of Medicine, National Academies

Life Stage Group	Calcium (mg/d)	Chromium (μg/d)	Copper (μg/d)	Fluoride (mg/d)	Iodine (μg/d)	Iron (mg/d)	Magnesium (mg/d)	Manganese (mg/d)	Molybdenum (μg/d)	Phosphorus (mg/d)	Selenium (μg/d)	Zinc (mg/d)	Potassium (g/d)	Sodium (g/d)	Chloride (g/d)
Infants															
0–6 mo	210*	0.2*	200*	0.01*	110*	0.27*	30*	0.003*	2*	100*	15*	2*	0.4*	0.12*	0.18*
7–12 mo	270*	5.5*	220*	0.5*	130*	**11**	75*	0.6*	3*	275*	20*	**3**	0.7*	0.37*	0.57*
Children															
1–3 y	500*	11*	**340**	0.7*	**90**	**7**	**80**	1.2*	**17**	**460**	**20**	**3**	3.0*	1.0*	1.5*
4–8 y	800*	15*	**440**	1*	**90**	**10**	**130**	1.5*	**22**	**500**	**30**	**5**	3.8*	1.2*	1.9*
Males															
9–13 y	1,300*	25*	**700**	2*	**120**	**8**	**240**	1.9*	**34**	**1,250**	**40**	**8**	4.5*	1.5*	2.3*
14–18 y	1,300*	35*	**890**	3*	**150**	**11**	**410**	2.2*	**43**	**1,250**	**55**	**11**	4.7*	1.5*	2.3*
19–30 y	1,000*	35*	**900**	4*	**150**	**8**	**400**	2.3*	**45**	**700**	**55**	**11**	4.7*	1.5*	2.3*
31–50 y	1,000*	35*	**900**	4*	**150**	**8**	**420**	2.3*	**45**	**700**	**55**	**11**	4.7*	1.5*	2.3*
51–70 y	1,200*	30*	**900**	4*	**150**	**8**	**420**	2.3*	**45**	**700**	**55**	**11**	4.7*	1.3*	2.0*
> 70 y	1,200*	30*	**900**	4*	**150**	**8**	**420**	2.3*	**45**	**700**	**55**	**11**	4.7*	1.2*	1.8*
Females															
9–13 y	1,300*	21*	**700**	2*	**120**	**8**	**240**	1.6*	**34**	**1,250**	**40**	**8**	4.5*	1.5*	2.3*
14–18 y	1,300*	24*	**890**	3*	**150**	**15**	**360**	1.6*	**43**	**1,250**	**55**	**9**	4.7*	1.5*	2.3*
19–30 y	1,000*	25*	**900**	3*	**150**	**18**	**310**	1.8*	**45**	**700**	**55**	**8**	4.7*	1.5*	2.3*
31–50 y	1,000*	25*	**900**	3*	**150**	**18**	**320**	1.8*	**45**	**700**	**55**	**8**	4.7*	1.5*	2.3*
51–70 y	1,200*	20*	**900**	3*	**150**	**8**	**320**	1.8*	**45**	**700**	**55**	**8**	4.7*	1.3*	2.0*
> 70 y	1,200*	20*	**900**	3*	**150**	**8**	**320**	1.8*	**45**	**700**	**55**	**8**	4.7*	1.2*	1.8*
Pregnancy															
14–18 y	1,300*	29*	**1,000**	3*	**220**	**27**	**400**	2.0*	**50**	**1,250**	**60**	**13**	4.7*	1.5*	2.3*
19–30 y	1,000*	30*	**1,000**	3*	**220**	**27**	**350**	2.0*	**50**	**700**	**60**	**11**	4.7*	1.5*	2.3*
31–50 y	1,000*	30*	**1,000**	3*	**220**	**27**	**360**	2.0*	**50**	**700**	**60**	**11**	4.7*	1.5*	2.3*
Lactation															
14–18 y	1,300*	44*	**1,300**	3*	**290**	**10**	**360**	2.6*	**50**	**1,250**	**70**	**14**	5.1*	1.5*	2.3*
19–30 y	1,000*	45*	**1,300**	3*	**290**	**9**	**310**	2.6*	**50**	**700**	**70**	**12**	5.1*	1.5*	2.3*
31–50 y	1,000*	45*	**1,300**	3*	**290**	**9**	**320**	2.6*	**50**	**700**	**70**	**12**	5.1*	1.5*	2.3*

NOTE: This table presents Recommended Dietary Allowances (RDAs) in **bold type** and Adequate Intakes (AIs) in ordinary type followed by an asterisk (*). RDAs and AIs may both be used as goals for individual intake. RDAs are set to meet the needs of almost all (97 to 98 percent) individuals in a group. For healthy breastfed infants, the AI is the mean intake. The AI for other life stage and gender groups is believed to cover needs of all individuals in the group, but lack of data or uncertainty in the data prevent being able to specify with confidence the percentage of individuals covered by this intake.

SOURCES: *Dietary Reference Intakes for Calcium, Phosphorous, Magnesium, Vitamin D, and Fluoride* (1997); *Dietary Reference Intakes for Thiamin, Riboflavin, Niacin, Vitamin B_6, Folate, Vitamin B_{12}, Pantothenic Acid, Biotin, and Choline* (1998); *Dietary Reference Intakes for Vitamin C, Vitamin E, Selenium, and Carotenoids* (2000); *Dietary Reference Intakes for Vitamin A, Vitamin K, Arsenic, Boron, Chromium, Copper, Iodine, Iron, Manganese, Molybdenum, Nickel, Silicon, Vanadium, and Zinc* (2001); and *Dietary Reference Intakes for Water, Potassium, Sodium, Chloride, and Sulfate* (2004). These reports may be accessed via http://www.nap.edu.

Dietary Reference Intakes (DRIs): Tolerable Upper Intake Levels (UL[a]), Vitamins

Food and Nutrition Board, Institute of Medicine, National Academies

Life Stage Group	Vitamin A (μg/d)[b]	Vitamin C (mg/d)	Vitamin D (μg/d)	Vitamin E (mg/d)[c,d]	Vitamin K	Thiamin	Ribo-flavin	Niacin (mg/d)[d]	Vitamin B_6 (mg/d)	Folate (μg/d)[d]	Vitamin B_{12}	Pantothenic Acid	Biotin	Choline (g/d)	Carote-noids[e]
Infants															
0–6 mo	600	ND[f]	25	ND	ND	ND	ND	ND	ND	ND	ND	ND	ND	ND	ND
7–12 mo	600	ND	25	ND	ND	ND	ND	ND	ND	ND	ND	ND	ND	ND	ND
Children															
1–3 y	600	400	50	200	ND	ND	ND	10	30	300	ND	ND	ND	1.0	ND
4–8 y	900	650	50	300	ND	ND	ND	15	40	400	ND	ND	ND	1.0	ND
Males, Females															
9–13 y	1,700	1,200	50	600	ND	ND	ND	20	60	600	ND	ND	ND	2.0	ND
14–18 y	2,800	1,800	50	800	ND	ND	ND	30	80	800	ND	ND	ND	3.0	ND
19–70 y	3,000	2,000	50	1,000	ND	ND	ND	35	100	1,000	ND	ND	ND	3.5	ND
> 70 y	3,000	2,000	50	1,000	ND	ND	ND	35	100	1,000	ND	ND	ND	3.5	ND
Pregnancy															
14–18 y	2,800	1,800	50	800	ND	ND	ND	30	80	800	ND	ND	ND	3.0	ND
19–50 y	3,000	2,000	50	1,000	ND	ND	ND	35	100	1,000	ND	ND	ND	3.5	ND
Lactation															
14–18 y	2,800	1,800	50	800	ND	ND	ND	30	80	800	ND	ND	ND	3.0	ND
19–50 y	3,000	2,000	50	1,000	ND	ND	ND	35	100	1,000	ND	ND	ND	3.5	ND

[a] UL = The maximum level of daily nutrient intake that is likely to pose no risk of adverse effects. Unless otherwise specified, the UL represents total intake from food, water, and supplements. Due to lack of suitable data, ULs could not be established for vitamin K, thiamin, riboflavin, vitamin B_{12}, pantothenic acid, biotin, carotenoids. In the absence of ULs, extra caution may be warranted in consuming levels above recommended intakes.

[b] As preformed vitamin A only.

[c] As α-tocopherol; applies to any form of supplemental α-tocopherol.

[d] The ULs for vitamin E, niacin, and folate apply to synthetic forms obtained from supplements, fortified foods, or a combination of the two.

[e] β-Carotene supplements are advised only to serve as a provitamin A source for individuals at risk of vitamin A deficiency.

[f] ND = Not determinable due to lack of data of adverse effects in this age group and concern with regard to lack of ability to handle excess amounts. Source of intake should be from food only to prevent high levels of intake.

SOURCES: *Dietary Reference Intakes for Calcium, Phosphorous, Magnesium, Vitamin D, and Fluoride* (1997); *Dietary Reference Intakes for Thiamin, Riboflavin, Niacin, Vitamin B_6, Folate, Vitamin B_{12}, Pantothenic Acid, Biotin, and Choline* (1998); *Dietary Reference Intakes for Vitamin C, Vitamin E, Selenium, and Carotenoids* (2000); and *Dietary Reference Intakes for Vitamin A, Vitamin K, Arsenic, Boron, Chromium, Copper, Iodine, Iron, Manganese, Molybdenum, Nickel, Silicon, Vanadium, and Zinc* (2001). These reports may be accessed via http://www.nap.edu.

Dietary Reference Intakes (DRIs): Tolerable Upper Intake Levels (UL[a]), Elements

Food and Nutrition Board, Institute of Medicine, National Academies

Life Stage Group	Arsenic[b]	Boron (mg/d)	Calcium (g/d)	Chromium	Copper (μg/d)	Fluoride (mg/d)	Iodine (μg/d)	Iron (mg/d)	Magnesium (mg/d)[c]	Manganese (mg/d)	Molybdenum (μg/d)	Nickel (mg/d)	Phosphorus (g/d)	Potassium	Selenium (μg/d)	Silicon[d]	Sulfate	Vanadium (mg/d)[e]	Zinc (mg/d)	Sodium (g/d)	Chloride (g/d)
Infants																					
0–6 mo	ND[f]	ND	ND	ND	ND	0.7	ND	40	ND	ND	ND	ND	ND	ND	45	ND	ND	ND	4	ND	ND
7–12 mo	ND	ND	ND	ND	ND	0.9	ND	40	ND	ND	ND	ND	ND	ND	60	ND	ND	ND	5	ND	ND
Children																					
1–3 y	ND	3	2.5	ND	1,000	1.3	200	40	65	2	300	0.2	3	ND	90	ND	ND	ND	7	1.5	2.3
4–8 y	ND	6	2.5	ND	3,000	2.2	300	40	110	3	600	0.3	3	ND	150	ND	ND	ND	12	1.9	2.9
Males, Females																					
9–13 y	ND	11	2.5	ND	5,000	10	600	40	350	6	1,100	0.6	4	ND	280	ND	ND	ND	23	2.2	3.4
14–18 y	ND	17	2.5	ND	8,000	10	900	45	350	9	1,700	1.0	4	ND	400	ND	ND	ND	34	2.3	3.6
19–70 y	ND	20	2.5	ND	10,000	10	1,100	45	350	11	2,000	1.0	4	ND	400	ND	ND	1.8	40	2.3	3.6
>70 y	ND	20	2.5	ND	10,000	10	1,100	45	350	11	2,000	1.0	3	ND	400	ND	ND	1.8	40	2.3	3.6
Pregnancy																					
14–18 y	ND	17	2.5	ND	8,000	10	900	45	350	9	1,700	1.0	3.5	ND	400	ND	ND	ND	34	2.3	3.6
19–50 y	ND	20	2.5	ND	10,000	10	1,100	45	350	11	2,000	1.0	3.5	ND	400	ND	ND	ND	40	2.3	3.6
Lactation																					
14–18 y	ND	17	2.5	ND	8,000	10	900	45	350	9	1,700	1.0	4	ND	400	ND	ND	ND	34	2.3	3.6
19–50 y	ND	20	2.5	ND	10,000	10	1,100	45	350	11	2,000	1.0	4	ND	400	ND	ND	ND	40	2.3	3.6

[a] UL = The maximum level of daily nutrient intake that is likely to pose no risk of adverse effects. Unless otherwise specified, the UL represents total intake from food, water, and supplements. Due to lack of suitable data, ULs could not be established for arsenic, chromium, silicon, potassium, and sulfate. In the absence of ULs, extra caution may be warranted in consuming levels above recommended intakes.

[b] Although the UL was not determined for arsenic, there is no justification for adding arsenic to food or supplements.

[c] The ULs for magnesium represent intake from a pharmacological agent only and do not include intake from food and water.

[d] Although silicon has not been shown to cause adverse effects in humans, there is no justification for adding silicon to supplements.

[e] Although vanadium in food has not been shown to cause adverse effects in humans, there is no justification for adding vanadium to food and vanadium supplements should be used with caution. The UL is based on adverse effects in laboratory animals and this data could be used to set a UL for adults but not children and adolescents.

[f] ND = Not determinable due to lack of data of adverse effects in this age group and concern with regard to lack of ability to handle excess amounts. Source of intake should be from food only to prevent high levels of intake.

SOURCES: *Dietary Reference Intakes for Calcium, Phosphorous, Magnesium, Vitamin D, and Fluoride* (1997); *Dietary Reference Intakes for Thiamin, Riboflavin, Niacin, Vitamin B_6, Folate, Vitamin B_{12}, Pantothenic Acid, Biotin, and Choline* (1998); *Dietary Reference Intakes for Vitamin C, Vitamin E, Selenium, and Carotenoids* (2000); *Dietary Reference Intakes for Vitamin A, Vitamin K, Arsenic, Boron, Chromium, Copper, Iodine, Iron, Manganese, Molybdenum, Nickel, Silicon, Vanadium, and Zinc* (2001); and *Dietary Reference Intakes for Water, Potassium, Sodium, Chloride, and Sulfate* (2004). These reports may be accessed via http://www.nap.edu.

Dietary Reference Intakes (DRIs): Estimated Energy Requirements (EER) for Men and Women 30 Years of Age[a]

Food and Nutrition Board, Institute of Medicine, National Academies

Height (m [in])	PAL[b]	Weight for BMI[c] of 18.5 kg/m^2 (kg [lb])	Weight for BMI of 24.99 kg/m^2 (kg [lb])	EER, Men[d] (kcal/day)		EER, Women[d] (kcal/day)	
				BMI of 18.5 kg/m^2	BMI of 24.99 kg/m^2	BMI of 18.5 kg/m^2	BMI of 24.99 kg/m^2
1.50 (59)	Sedentary	41.6 (92)	56.2 (124)	1,848	2,080	1,625	1,762
	Low active			2,009	2,267	1,803	1,956
	Active			2,215	2,506	2,025	2,198
	Very active			2,554	2,898	2,291	2,489
1.65 (65)	Sedentary	50.4 (111)	68.0 (150)	2,068	2,349	1,816	1,982
	Low active			2,254	2,566	2,016	2,202
	Active			2,490	2,842	2,267	2,477
	Very active			2,880	3,296	2,567	2,807
1.80 (71)	Sedentary	59.9 (132)	81.0 (178)	2,301	2,635	2,015	2,211
	Low active			2,513	2,884	2,239	2,459
	Active			2,782	3,200	2,519	2,769
	Very active			3,225	3,720	2,855	3,141

[a] For each year below 30, add 7 kcal/day for women and 10 kcal /day for men. For each year above 30, subtract 7 kcal/day for women and 10 kcal/day for men.

[b] PAL = physical activity level.

[c] BMI = body mass index.

[d] Derived from the following regression equations based on doubly labeled water data:

Adult man: EER = 662 – 9.53 × age (y) + PA × (15.91 × wt [kg] + 539.6 × ht [m])

Adult woman: EER = 354 – 6.91 × age (y) + PA × (9.36 × wt [kg] + 726 × ht [m])

Where PA refers to coefficient for PAL

PAL = total energy expenditure ÷ basal energy expenditure

PA = 1.0 if PAL ≥ 1.0 < 1.4 (sedentary)

PA = 1.12 if PAL ≥ 1.4 < 1.6 (low active)

PA = 1.27 if PAL ≥ 1.6 < 1.9 (active)

PA = 1.45 if PAL ≥ 1.9 < 2.5 (very active)

Dietary Reference Intakes (DRIs): Acceptable Macronutrient Distribution Ranges

Food and Nutrition Board, Institute of Medicine, National Academies

Macronutrient	Range (percent of energy)		
	Children, 1–3 y	Children, 4–18 y	Adults
Fat	30–40	25–35	20–35
n-6 polyunsaturated fatty acids[a] (linoleic acid)	5–10	5–10	5–10
n-3 polyunsaturated fatty acids[a] (α-linolenic acid)	0.6–1.2	0.6–1.2	0.6–1.2
Carbohydrate	45–65	45–65	45–65
Protein	5–20	10–30	10–35

[a] Approximately 10% of the total can come from longer-chain *n*-3 or *n*-6 fatty acids.

SOURCE: *Dietary Reference Intakes for Energy, Carbohydrate, Fiber, Fat, Fatty Acids, Cholesterol, Protein, and Amino Acids* (2002).

Dietary Reference Intakes (DRIs): Recommended Intakes for Individuals, Macronutrients
Food and Nutrition Board, Institute of Medicine, National Academies

Life Stage Group	Total Water[a] (L/d)	Carbohydrate (g/d)	Total Fiber (g/d)	Fat (g/d)	Linoleic Acid (g/d)	α-Linolenic Acid (g/d)	Protein[b] (g/d)
Infants							
0–6 mo	0.7*	60*	ND	31*	4.4*	0.5*	9.1*
7–12 mo	0.8*	95*	ND	30*	4.6*	0.5*	**13.5**
Children							
1–3 y	1.3*	**130**	19*	ND	7*	0.7*	**13**
4–8 y	1.7*	**130**	25*	ND	10*	0.9*	**19**
Males							
9–13 y	2.4*	**130**	31*	ND	12*	1.2*	**34**
14–18 y	3.3*	**130**	38*	ND	16*	1.6*	**52**
19–30 y	3.7*	**130**	38*	ND	17*	1.6*	**56**
31–50 y	3.7*	**130**	38*	ND	17*	1.6*	**56**
51–70 y	3.7*	**130**	30*	ND	14*	1.6*	**56**
> 70 y	3.7*	**130**	30*	ND	14*	1.6*	**56**
Females							
9–13 y	2.1*	**130**	26*	ND	10*	1.0*	**34**
14–18 y	2.3*	**130**	26*	ND	11*	1.1*	**46**
19–30 y	2.7*	**130**	25*	ND	12*	1.1*	**46**
31–50 y	2.7*	**130**	25*	ND	12*	1.1*	**46**
51–70 y	2.7*	**130**	21*	ND	11*	1.1*	**46**
> 70 y	2.7*	**130**	21*	ND	11*	1.1*	**46**
Pregnancy							
14–18 y	3.0*	**175**	28*	ND	13*	1.4*	**71**
19–30 y	3.0*	**175**	28*	ND	13*	1.4*	**71**
31–50 y	3.0*	**175**	28*	ND	13*	1.4*	**71**
Lactation							
14–18 y	3.8*	**210**	29*	ND	13*	1.3*	**71**
19–30 y	3.8*	**210**	29*	ND	13*	1.3*	**71**
31–50 y	3.8*	**210**	29*	ND	13*	1.3*	**71**

NOTE: This table presents Recommended Dietary Allowances (RDAs) in **bold** type and Adequate Intakes (AIs) in ordinary type followed by an asterisk (*). RDAs and AIs may both be used as goals for individual intake. RDAs are set to meet the needs of almost all (97 to 98 percent) individuals in a group. For healthy infants fed human milk, the AI is the mean intake. The AI for other life stage and gender groups is believed to cover the needs of all individuals in the group, but lack of data or uncertainty in the data prevent being able to specify with confidence the percentage of individuals covered by this intake.

[a] *Total* water includes all water contained in food, beverages, and drinking water.

[b] Based on 0.8 g/kg body weight for the reference body weight.

Dietary Reference Intakes (DRIs): Additional Macronutrient Recommendations
Food and Nutrition Board, Institute of Medicine, National Academies

Macronutrient	Recommendation
Dietary cholesterol	As low as possible while consuming a nutritionally adequate diet
Trans fatty acids	As low as possible while consuming a nutritionally adequate diet
Saturated fatty acids	As low as possible while consuming a nutritionally adequate diet
Added sugars	Limit to no more than 25% of total energy

SOURCE: *Dietary Reference Intakes for Energy, Carbohydrate, Fiber, Fat, Fatty Acids, Cholesterol, Protein, and Amino Acids* (2002).

Dietary Reference Intakes (DRIs): Estimated Average Requirements for Groups

Food and Nutrition Board, Institute of Medicine, National Academies

Life Stage Group	CHO (g/d)	Protein (g/d)	Vit A (µg/d)[a]	Vit C (mg/d)	Vit E (mg/d)[b]	Thiamin (mg/d)	Riboflavin (mg/d)	Niacin (mg/d)[c]	Vit B_6 (mg/d)	Folate (µg/d)[a]	Vit B_{12} (µg/d)	Copper (µg/d)	Iodine (µg/d)	Iron (mg/d)	Magnesium (mg/d)	Molybdenum (µg/d)	Phosphorus (mg/d)	Selenium (µg/d)	Zinc (mg/d)
Infants																			
7–12 mo		10												6.9					2.5
Children																			
1–3 y	100	11	210	13	5	0.4	0.4	5	0.4	120	0.7	260	65	3.0	65	13	380	17	2.5
4–8 y	100	15	275	22	6	0.5	0.5	6	0.5	160	1.0	340	65	4.1	110	17	405	23	4.0
Males																			
9–13 y	100	27	445	39	9	0.7	0.8	9	0.8	250	1.5	540	73	5.9	200	26	1,055	35	7.0
14–18 y	100	44	630	63	12	1.0	1.1	12	1.1	330	2.0	685	95	7.7	340	33	1,055	45	8.5
19–30 y	100	46	625	75	12	1.0	1.1	12	1.1	320	2.0	700	95	6	330	34	580	45	9.4
31–50 y	100	46	625	75	12	1.0	1.1	12	1.1	320	2.0	700	95	6	350	34	580	45	9.4
51–70 y	100	46	625	75	12	1.0	1.1	12	1.4	320	2.0	700	95	6	350	34	580	45	9.4
> 70 y	100	46	625	75	12	1.0	1.1	12	1.4	320	2.0	700	95	6	350	34	580	45	9.4
Females																			
9–13 y	100	28	420	39	9	0.7	0.8	9	0.8	250	1.5	540	73	5.7	200	26	1,055	35	7.0
14–18 y	100	38	485	56	12	0.9	0.9	11	1.0	330	2.0	685	95	7.9	300	33	1,055	45	7.3
19–30 y	100	38	500	60	12	0.9	0.9	11	1.1	320	2.0	700	95	8.1	255	34	580	45	6.8
31–50 y	100	38	500	60	12	0.9	0.9	11	1.1	320	2.0	700	95	8.1	265	34	580	45	6.8
51–70 y	100	38	500	60	12	0.9	0.9	11	1.3	320	2.0	700	95	5	265	34	580	45	6.8
> 70 y	100	38	500	60	12	0.9	0.9	11	1.3	320	2.0	700	95	5	265	34	580	45	6.8
Pregnancy																			
14–18 y	135	50	530	66	12	1.2	1.2	14	1.6	520	2.2	785	160	23	335	40	1,055	49	10.5
19–30 y	135	50	550	70	12	1.2	1.2	14	1.6	520	2.2	800	160	22	290	40	580	49	9.5
31–50 y	135	50	550	70	12	1.2	1.2	14	1.6	520	2.2	800	160	22	300	40	580	49	9.5
Lactation																			
14–18 y	160	60	880	96	16	1.2	1.3	13	1.7	450	2.4	985	209	7	300	35	1,055	59	10.9
19–30 y	160	60	900	100	16	1.2	1.3	13	1.7	450	2.4	1,000	209	6.5	255	36	580	59	10.4
31–50 y	160	60	900	100	16	1.2	1.3	13	1.7	450	2.4	1,000	209	6.5	265	36	580	59	10.4

NOTE: This table presents Estimated Average Requirements (EARs), which serve two purposes: for assessing a dequacy of population intakes, and as the basis for calculating Recommended Dietary Allowances (RDAs) for individuals for those nutrients. EARs have not been established for vitamin D, vitamin K, pantothenic acid, biotin, choline, calcium, chromium, fluoride, manganese, or other nutrients not yet evaluated via the DRI process.

[a] As retinol activity equivalents (RAEs). 1 RAE = 1 µg retinol, 12 µg β-carotene, 24 µg α-carotene, or 24 µg β-cryptoxanthin. The RAE for dietary provitamin A carotenoids is two-fold greater than retinol equivalents (RE), whereas the RAE for preformed vitamin A is the same as RE.

[b] As α-tocopherol. α-Tocopherol includes *RRR*-α-tocopherol, the only form of α-tocopherol that occurs naturally in foods, and the *2R*-stereoisomeric forms of α-tocopherol (*RRR*-, *RSR*-, *RRS*-, and *RSS*-α-tocopherol) that occur in fortified foods and supplements. It does not include the *2S*-stereoisomeric forms of α-tocopherol (*SRR*-, *SSR*-, *SRS*-, and *SSS*-α-tocopherol), also found in fortified foods and supplements.

[c] As niacin equivalents (NE). 1 mg of niacin = 60 mg of tryptophan.

[d] As dietary folate equivalents (DFE). 1 DFE = 1 µg food folate = 0.6 µg of folic acid from fortified food or as a supplement consumed with food = 0.5 µg of a supplement taken on an empty stomach.

SOURCES: *Dietary Reference Intakes for Calcium, Phosphorous, Magnesium, Vitamin D, and Fluoride* (1997); *Dietary Reference Intakes for Thiamin, Riboflavin, Niacin, Vitamin B_6, Folate, Vitamin B_{12}, Pantothenic Acid, Biotin, and Choline* (1998); *Dietary Reference Intakes for Vitamin C, Vitamin E, Selenium, and Carotenoids* (2000); *Dietary Reference Intakes for Vitamin A, Vitamin K, Arsenic, Boron, Chromium, Copper, Iodine, Iron, Manganese, Molybdenum, Nickel, Silicon, Vanadium, and Zinc* (2001), and *Dietary Reference Intakes for Energy, Carbohydrate, Fiber, Fat, Fatty Acids, Cholesterol, Protein, and Amino Acids* (2002). These reports may be accessed via www.nap.edu.

INDEX

Note: Italicized *f*'s and *t*'s refer to figures and tables

EVERYTHING YOU NEED TO DEVELOP AN EFFECTIVE MEDICAL NUTRITION PLAN—ALL IN ONE PLACE!

Nutrition and Diagnosis-Related Care

SEVENTH EDITION

SYLVIA ESCOTT-STUMP, MA, RD, LDN

Developed by well-known author and leader in dietetics, Sylvia Escott-Stump, the Seventh Edition of **Nutrition and Diagnosis-Related Care** remains the premiere publication for creating and implementing sound medical nutrition therapy plans. Meeting the needs of busy students and practitioners, it offers quick access to the available research evidence and best clinical practices.

Inside the book, you'll find resources to manage the nutritional needs of patients dealing with more than 360 diseases and disorders. Each entry, covering a distinct disease or disorder, offers vital background information, objectives for care, patient education information, and dietary and nutritional recommendations. Each entry also includes commonly used medications as well as herbal and botanical remedies and their potential side effects.

Reflects the Latest Findings and Practices!

Thoroughly updated, this edition features the most recent information on nutritional genetics. In addition, it includes more nutrition care process examples throughout the text, supporting the American Dietetic Association's guidelines.

Features to Help You Quickly Develop Effective Nutrition Plans—

- **New full-color illustrations and photographs** help you better understand the nature of various diseases and the therapeutic role of nutrition.
- **Nutritional acuity level rankings**, based on surveys of clinical practitioners, help you categorize patients by complexity of nutritional risk.
- **Clinical indicators** for each disease and disorder set forth the associated tests, disease markers, and common biochemical evaluations needed to support assessment, monitoring, and evaluation.
- **Nutrition care process language** stimulates your critical thinking skills to manage a range of actual clinical practice issues.

Refer to this Seventh Edition any time you need to write protocols, establish priorities in nutrition care, evaluate costs, or determine the effectiveness of nutrition interventions in improving patient outcomes.

LWW.com

ISBN-13: 978-1-60831-017-3
ISBN-10: 1-60831-017-5

90000

9 781608 310173

Wolters Kluwer Health | Lippincott Williams & Wilkins